JOSLIN'S
DIABETES MELLITUS

13th Edition

JOSLIN'S DIABETES MELLITUS

13th Edition

Edited by

C. RONALD KAHN, M.D.

Director, Elliott P. Joslin Research Laboratory
Joslin Diabetes Center;
Mary K. Iacocca Professor of Medicine
Harvard Medical School
Boston, Massachusetts

GORDON C. WEIR, M.D.

Medical Director, Joslin Diabetes Center;
Professor of Medicine
Harvard Medical School
Boston, Massachusetts

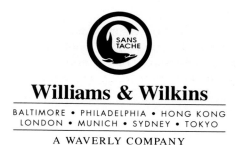

Williams & Wilkins

BALTIMORE • PHILADELPHIA • HONG KONG
LONDON • MUNICH • SYDNEY • TOKYO

A WAVERLY COMPANY

Williams & Wilkins
Rose Tree Corporate Center, Building II
1400 North Providence Road, Suite 5025
Media, PA 19063-2043 USA

Executive Editor—R. Kenneth Bussy
Development Editor—Tanya Lazar
Project Editor—Dorothy DiRienzi
Production Manager—Michael DeNardo

First Edition, 1916
Second Edition, 1917
Third Edition, 1923
Fourth Edition, 1928
Fifth Edition, 1935
Sixth Edition, 1937
Seventh Edition, 1940
Eighth Edition, 1946
Ninth Edition, 1952
Tenth Edition, 1959
Eleventh Edition, 1971
Twelfth Edition, 1985
Thirteenth Edition, 1994

Library of Congress Cataloging-in-Publication Data

Joslin, Elliott P. (Elliott Proctor), 1869–1962.
    Joslin's diabetes mellitus. — 13th. / edited by C. Ronald Kahn,
Gordon C. Weir.
      p.   cm.
    Includes bibliographical references and index.
    ISBN 0-8121-1531-7
    1. Diabetes.   I. Kahn, C. Ronald.   II. Weir, Gordon C.
III. Title.   IV. Title: Diabetes mellitus.
    [DNLM: 1. Diabetes Mellitus.   WK 810 J83t 1994]
RC660.J6   1994
616.4'62—dc20
DNLM/DLC   93–4766
for Library of Congress   CIP

NOTE: Although the author(s) and the publisher have taken reasonable steps to ensure the accuracy of the drug information included in this text before publication, drug information may change without notice and readers are advised to consult the manufacturer's packaging inserts before prescribing medication.

PRINTED IN THE UNITED STATES OF AMERICA

Print number: 5 4 3

Dedicated to Alexander Marble, M.D.

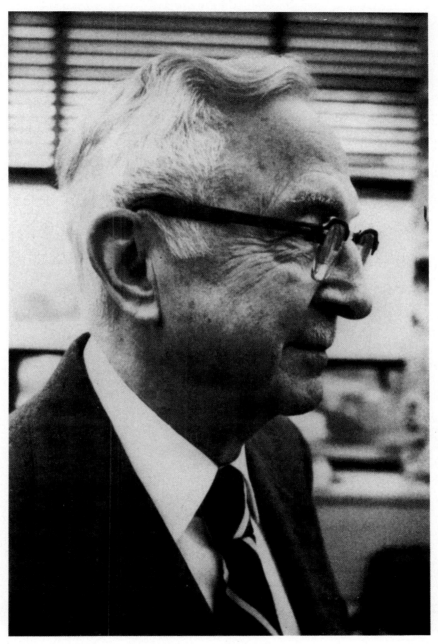

1902–1992

PREFACE

The 13th edition of *Joslin's Diabetes Mellitus* represents a fascinating point in the evolution of a book devoted to a single disease. The first edition was published in 1916, a single-handed contribution by a man of extraordinary dedication, vision, and energy—Dr. Elliott P. Joslin. Dr. Joslin began his practice in 1898 in the pre-insulin era, and in this setting developed a unique understanding of the natural history of diabetes, as is evident in the first edition. The editions published shortly after the discovery of insulin show how quickly and clearly he grasped the principles of insulin therapy, adopting approaches that would be considered modern even by today's standards. He was unwavering in his conviction that blood glucose levels should be kept as close to normal as possible, even though the importance and even the existence of chronic complications of diabetes were not appreciated at that point. He clearly understood the critical role of education for people with diabetes and made it the cornerstone of all treatment programs. He quickly found that diet and exercise were a fundamental part of any regimen. His descriptions of the symptoms of hypoglycemia are as well defined as can be found anywhere today, and he rapidly determined the small quantity of carbohydrate required to treat insulin reactions. Any serious student of diabetes should spend time with these early editions.

The evolution of the book mirrors the development of the field of diabetes and of the Joslin Diabetes Center. Although the book was originally written entirely by one man, in subsequent editions Dr. Joslin included some of his colleagues in the task. Eventually, substantial contributions to the book were provided not only by the staff of the Joslin Diabetes Center, but also by clinicians from the adjacent New England Deaconess Hospital, where most Joslin patients were hospitalized. Research has always been a fundamental activity at Joslin and as such has been reflected in all of the editions. Dr. Joslin himself was a fine clinical investigator who made astute observations about his patients and recorded the information in a meticulous fashion, as can be appreciated in his numerous publications. He also recognized the need for a more organized approach to research and appointed Dr. Alexander Marble as the first head of research in 1934. The research programs were greatly expanded when Dr. Albert Renold took over the leadership in 1957, with the ties to Harvard Medical School and Peter Bent Brigham Hospital (now Brigham and Women's Hospital) being greatly strengthened.

The most recent editions of *Joslin's Diabetes Mellitus* have reflected both the practice and experiences of the physicians of the Joslin Diabetes Center and the new science that had such an impact on the field of diabetes. The chapters were written almost exclusively by individuals working at Joslin or Deaconess. Patients came to the Joslin from all over the world, knowing that whatever problems they had could be dealt with by someone who understood diabetes. The Joslin staff has consisted of adult and pediatric diabetologists, nephrologists, ophthalmologists and optometrists, podiatrists, and mental health professionals, as well as nurse educators and nutrition specialists. Problems in vascular disease, cardiology, and neurology, and in virtually all other areas of medicine, are managed in collaboration with colleagues at the Deaconess. Women with diabetes traditionally have delivered their babies at Brigham and Women's Hospital, and sick children often are hospitalized at Children's Hospital Medical Center. Because there were experts at these institutions who had extensive experience in virtually every aspect of diabetes care, they joined with the Joslin staff to write the clinical chapters, describing the characteristics and outcomes of their patients within the context of the larger literature. Advances in basic and clinical research usually were described by present or former members of the research division at the Joslin. Because diabetes care and research have become so complicated and international in scope it was decided to extend the authorship of the present edition to include a number of authorities not directly connected with Joslin.

The broadening of the scope of the book is consistent with Joslin's current efforts to expand its size and influence. For example, in 1985 Joslin embarked on a plan to establish affiliated centers in different parts of the country. As of 1992, eight Joslin clinical centers had been started: three in Florida (Clearwater, Jacksonville, and Miami) and the others in Chicago, Illinois; Charlotte, North Carolina; Indianapolis, Indiana; Livingston, New Jersey; and Pittsburgh, Pennsylvania. This development has been associated with an expansion of Joslin's publication program to provide more information about diabetes to patients, health-care providers, and other interested parties. In addition, construction was begun in 1992 to add three more floors to the Boston building, with two floors designed for research activities and the other for expanded clinical services. The project should be completed in 1994.

The 13th edition is very different from the 12th, which was published in 1985. Some differences reflect the dramatic advances in knowledge and research. In addition, less emphasis is given to the local Joslin and Deaconess experience with various aspects of diabetes care and more to other experiences described in the literature. Nonetheless, an effort has been made to retain the flavor of Joslin's clinical strategies and the emphasis on the importance of the team approach. Progress in the basic sciences has been explosive in recent years, particularly in the area of molecular biology, with a resultant major impact on diabetes research. This progress is reflected particularly in the more basic aspects of diabetes research. Because of the rapid rate of appearance of new knowledge, many authors were concerned that their chapters would not be fully up to date when the book was published. This problem is a reality faced by authors dealing with books in medical research, but every reasonable effort has been made to have the 13th edition closely reflect our understanding of diabetes in 1993.

In this preface, special mention must be made of Albert Y. Samuelian, an important friend of the Joslin. Mr. Samuelian, who died in 1980, had built a successful business specializing in textbooks. His family has continued to be involved in activities at Joslin and has shown particular interest in this book, which contains so much of the essence of the mission of the Joslin. The Joslin Diabetes Center is a private nonprofit institution that has been a symbol of excellence in the care of people with diabetes and a center of scientific excellence devoted to finding ways of preventing, curing, and reducing the complications of this terrible disease. Support from Joslin patients and their families and friends is critical to Joslin's ability to pursue its mission. We thank the Samuelian family for its generous support and interest in this textbook on diabetes.

This 13th edition of *Joslin's Diabetes Mellitus* is dedicated to Dr. Alexander Marble, who died at the age of 90 in September of 1992. Dr. Marble is an important part of the history of Joslin. Born and raised in Kansas, he graduated from Harvard Medical School in 1927 and received training in medicine at Johns Hopkins Hospital and Massachusetts General Hospital. In 1932 he began practicing medicine with Dr. Elliott P. Joslin. He founded the Baker Research Laboratory in 1933, served as president of the Joslin from 1967 to 1976, and was Clinical Professor of Medicine at Harvard Medical School. Although superb as a clinician, teacher, and administrator, he will be remembered most for his research and scholarship, as evidenced by his authorship of over 350 articles in medical and scientific books and journals. One of his particular interests was the relationship between control of blood glucose levels and the complications of diabetes. Dr. Marble was deeply involved in many editions of the Joslin textbook, serving as the principal editor of the 11th and 12th editions, and is still revered for the extraordinary attention to excellence and detail he devoted to these projects. It is somewhat intimidating for the current editors to follow on Dr. Marble's heels; the mistakes and omissions that will be found in this 13th edition would not have passed by Dr. Marble had he still been involved. Because of his devotion to scholarship and the subject of diabetes, it is fitting that the new library at the Joslin Diabetes Center will bear his name. It is equally fitting that we dedicate this 13th edition of *Joslin's Diabetes Mellitus* to Alexander Marble, M.D.

Finally, a large group of individuals must work together to bring such a project to fruition. The authors of the various chapters spent untold hours of thinking, researching, and writing to reach the level of excellence expected of a book of this stature. It is remarkable that every author who originally agreed to contribute a chapter was able to make a final delivery. Two individuals, with whom it has been a pleasure to work, have made great contributions to the project. Terri-Lyn Bellman, the coordinator of the book at Joslin, was remarkably efficient at keeping track of all the manuscripts, disks, correspondence, and telephone calls. Nancy K. Voynow, the editorial assistant in Boston, was thoroughly professional, skilled, and efficient throughout, doing a wonderful job editing this enormous amount of complicated material. All of the editions of this book—from the first in 1916 to the current 13th edition—have been published by Lea & Febiger in Philadelphia. We continue to appreciate our long-standing relationship with this fine company. And, of course, we most of all thank our wives and children for their support and tolerance of the never-ending intrusion of this book into evenings, weekends, and at times even vacations.

Boston, Massachusetts   GORDON C. WEIR
                                                          C. RONALD KAHN

CONTRIBUTORS

Lloyd M. Aiello, M.D.,
Director, Beetham Eye Institute,
Joslin Diabetes Center;
Chief, Section of Ophthalmology,
New England Deaconess Hospital;
Associate Clinical Professor of Ophthalmology,
Harvard Medical School,
Boston, Massachusetts.

Barbara J. Anderson, Ph.D.,
Psychologist,
Mental Health Unit,
Joslin Diabetes Center;
Associate Professor in Psychology and Psychiatry,
Harvard Medical School,
Boston, Massachusetts.

Lloyd Axelrod, M.D.,
Physician and Chief,
James Howard Means Firm,
Massachusetts General Hospital;
Associate Professor of Medicine,
Harvard Medical School,
Boston, Massachusetts.

Nirmal K. Banskota, M.D.,
Consultant Endocrinologist,
Department of Diabetes, Endocrinology and
    Metabolism,
City of Hope National Medical Center,
Duarte, California.

Donald M. Barnett, M.D.
Senior Physician,
Joslin Diabetes Center and New England Deaconess
    Hospital;
Assistant Clinical Professor of Medicine,
Harvard Medical School,
Boston, Massachusetts.

Richard S. Beaser, M.D.,
Chief, Patient Education and Senior Physician,
Joslin Diabetes Center;
Medical Director of Diabetes Treatment Unit,
Joslin Diabetes Center, and the
New England Deaconess Hospital
Assistant Clinical Professor of Medicine,
Harvard Medical School,
Boston, Massachusetts.

Peter H. Bennett, M.B., F.R.C.P., F.F.C.M.,
Chief, Phoenix Epidemiology and Clinical Research
    Branch,
National Institute of Diabetes and Digestive and Kidney
    Diseases,
Phoenix, Arizona.

Edwin L. Bierman, M.D.,
Professor of Medicine and Head,
Division of Metabolism, Endocrinology and Nutrition,
University of Washington School of Medicine,
Seattle, Washington.

Bruce R. Bistrian, M.D., Ph.D.,
Chief, Division of Clinical Nutrition,
New England Deaconess Hospital;
Professor of Medicine,
Harvard Medical School,
Boston, Massachusetts.

Stephen R. Bloom, M.A., M.D., D.Sc., F.R.C.P.,
Professor of Endocrinology,
Hammersmith Hospital,
London, United Kingdom.

Susan Bonner-Weir, Ph.D.
Investigator, Section on Islet Transplantation and Cell
    Biology,
Joslin Diabetes Center;
Assistant Professor,
Harvard Medical School;
Boston, Massachusetts.

Jerry D. Cavallerano, O.D., Ph.D.,
Staff Optometrist,
Beetham Eye Institute,
Joslin Diabetes Center,
Boston, Massachusetts.

Alan Chait, M.D.,
Professor of Medicine,
University of Washington,
Seattle, Washington.

Stuart R. Chipkin, M.D.
Director, Clinical Endocrinology, Diabetes and
  Metabolism
Assistant Professor of Medicine and Physiology,
Boston University School of Medicine,
Boston, Massachusetts.

A. Richard Christlieb, M.D.,
Senior Physician,
Joslin Diabetes Center;
Associate Professor of Medicine,
Harvard Medical School,
Boston, Massachusetts

Anne Clark, Ph.D.,
Research Fellow,
Diabetes Research Laboratories and Laboratory of
  Cellular Endocrinology,
Department of Human Anatomy, Oxford University,
Oxford, United Kingdom.

David R. Clemmons, M.D.,
Chief, Division of Endocrinology and Professor of
  Medicine,
Department of Medicine,
University of North Carolina,
Chapel Hill, North Carolina.

Peter A. Colman, M.B.B.S., M.D., F.R.A.C.P.,
Director, Endocrine Laboratory and Department of
  Diabetes and Endocrinology,
Royal Melbourne Hospital,
Victoria, Australia.

Ramachandiran Cooppan, M.D.,
Senior Physician,
Joslin Diabetes Center and New England Deaconess
  Hospital;
Instructor in Medicine,
Harvard Medical School,
Boston, Massachusetts.

Phyllis A. Crapo, R.D.,
Associate Adjunct Professor,
Department of Medicine,
University of California, San Diego,
La Jolla, California.

Jeffrey S. Dover, M.D., F.R.C.P.C.,
Chief, Division of Dermatology,
New England Deaconess Hospital;
Assistant Professor of Dermatology,
Harvard Medical School,
Boston, Massachusetts.

George S. Eisenbarth, M.D.,
Executive Director and Chief, Section of Clinical
  Immunology,
Barbara Davis Center for Childhood Diabetes;
Professor of Pediatrics/Medicine,
University of Colorado Health Sciences Center,
Denver, Colorado.

George M. Eliopoulos, M.D.,
Assistant Chairman, Department of Medicine,
New England Deaconess Hospital;
Associate Professor of Medicine,
Harvard Medical School,
Boston, Massachusetts.

Joseph N. Fisher, M.D.,
Professor of Medicine and Pediatrics;
Chief of Medicine,
William F. Bowld Hospital;
Co-Associate Program Director,
Clinical Research Center,
University of Tennessee,
Memphis, Tennessee.

Jeffrey S. Flier, M.D.,
Chief, Endocrine Division,
Beth Israel Hospital;
Professor of Medicine,
Harvard Medical School,
Boston, Massachusetts.

Alan K. Foulis, M.D.,
Consultant Pathologist and Honorary Clinical Senior
  Lecturer,
Royal Infirmary,
University of Glasgow,
Glasgow, United Kingdom.

Roy Freeman, M.D.,
Staff Neurologist, Division of Neurology,
New England Deaconess Hospital;
Assistant Professor of Neurology,
Harvard Medical School,
Boston, Massachusetts.

Om P. Ganda, M.D.,
Senior Physician,
Joslin Diabetes Center;
New England Deaconess Hospital;
Associate Clinical Professor of Medicine,
Harvard Medical School;
Boston, Massachusetts.

Gary W. Gibbons, M.D.,
Clinical Chief,
Division of Vascular Surgery,
New England Deaconess Hospital;
Associate Clinical Professor of Surgery,
Harvard Medical School,
Bostin, Massachusetts.

Stephen G. Gilbey, B.A., M.D., M.R.C.P.,
Consultant Physician,
St. James University Hospital,
Leeds, United Kingdom.

Barry J. Goldstein, M.D., Ph.D.,
Associate Professor of Medicine and Pharmacology, and
Director, Division of Endocrinology and Metabolic
 Diseases,
Jefferson Medical College of Thomas Jefferson
 University
Philadelphia, Pennsylvania.

Irwin Goldstein, M.D.,
Professor of Urology,
Boston University School of Medicine,
Boston, Massachusetts.

Laurie J. Goodyear, Ph.D.,
Research Associate,
Joslin Diabetes Center;
Instructor in Medicine,
Harvard Medical School,
Boston, Massachusetts.

David Gough, Ph.D.,
Professor of Bioengineering, and Vice Chair,
Department of Applied Mechanics and Engineering
 Sciences,
University of California, San Diego,
La Jolla, California.

Raj K. Goyal, M.D.,
Chief, Gastroenterology Division,
Beth Israel Hospital,
Charlotte F. and Irving W. Rabb Professor of Medicine,
Harvard Medical School,
Boston, Massachusetts.

Geoffrey Habershaw, D.P.M.,
Chief, Division of Podiatry,
New England Deaconess Hospital;
Chief, Podiatry,
Joslin Diabetes Center;
Chief, Podiatry,
Quincy Hospital;
Clinical Instructor in Surgery,
Harvard Medical School,
Boston, Massachusetts.

Philippe A. Halban, Ph.D.,
Professor of Medicine,
Director, Louis Jeantet Research Laboratories,
University of Geneva Medical Center,
Geneva, Switzerland.

Jeffrey B. Halter, M.D.,
Professor of Internal Medicine,
Chief, Division of Geriatric Medicine,
Research Scientist and Medical Director of Institute of
 Gerontology, and
Director of Geriatrics Center,
University of Michigan;
Director, Geriatric Research, Education, and Clinical
 Center, Department of Veterans Affairs Medical
 Center,
Ann Arbor, Michigan.

John W. Hare, M.D.,
Senior Physician,
Joslin Diabetes Center;
Consultant (Obstetrics),
Brigham and Women's Hospital;
Associate Clinical Professor of Medicine,
Harvard Medical School,
Boston, Massachusetts.

Masakazu Hattori, M.D., Ph.D.,
Investigator, Section on Immunology and
 Immunogenetics,
Joslin Diabetes Center;
Assistant Professor of Medicine,
Harvard Medical School,
Boston, Massachusetts.

Stuart T. Hauser, M.D., Ph.D.,
Professor of Psychiatry,
Harvard Medical School;
Massachusetts Mental Health Center,
Boston, Massachusetts.

Jean-Claude Henquin, M.D., Ph.D.,
Professor of Physiology and Research Director,
Endocrinology and Metabolism Unit,
University of Louvain Faculty of Medicine,
Brussels, Belgium.

Hugo J. Hollerorth, Ed.D.,
Formerly, Health Curriculum Specialist,
Joslin Diabetes Center,
Boston, Massachusetts.

Barbara V. Howard, Ph.D.,
President, Medlantic Research Institute,
Washington, D.C.

Wm. James Howard, M.D.,
Senior Vice President and Medical Director,
Washington Hospital Center;
Professor of Medicine,
George Washington University,
Washington, D.C.

Alan M. Jacobson, M.D.,
Chief, Mental Health Unit,
Joslin Diabetes Center;
Associate Professor in Psychiatry,
Harvard Medical School,
Boston, Massachusetts.

Richard M. Jacoby, M.D.,
Staff Cardiologist at Fairfax Hospital,
Falls Church, Virginia;
Former Fellow in Cardiology,
New England Deaconess Hospital,
Boston, Massachusetts.

Leonard S. Jefferson, Jr., Ph.D.,
Professor and Chairman of Cellular and Molecular
    Physiology, The Milton S. Hershey Medical Center,
The Pennsylvania State University,
Hershey, Pennsylvania.

C. Ronald Kahn, M.D.,
Director, Elliott P. Joslin Research Laboratory,
Joslin Diabetes Center;
Mary K. Iacocca Professor of Medicine,
Harvard Medical School,
Boston, Massachusetts.

Masoor Kamalesh, M.D.,
Cardiology Fellow,
New England Deaconess Hospital;
Research Fellow,
Institute for Prevention of Cardiovascular Disease;
Fellow in Medicine,
Harvard Medical School,
Boston, Massachusetts.

Avraham Karasik, M.D.
Director, Institute of Endocrinology,
Sheba Medical Center,
Tel Hashomer;
Senior Lecturer,
Sackler Medical School,
Tel Aviv University,
Tel Aviv, Israel.

Anne M. Karinch, Ph.D.
Postdoctoral Fellow,
Department of Cellular and Molecular Physiology,
The Milton S. Hershey Medical Center,
The Pennsylvania State University,
Hershey, Pennsylvania.

Kathleen L. Kelly, Ph.D.,
Research Associate,
Department of Medicine,
Boston University School of Medicine,
Boston, Massachusetts.

Scot R. Kimball, Ph.D.
Assistant Professor of Cellular and Molecular
    Physiology, The Milton S. Hershey Medical Center,
The Pennsylvania State University,
Hershey, Pennsylvania.

George L. King, M.D.,
Senior Investigator,
Joslin Diabetes Center;
Associate Professor,
Harvard Medical School,
Boston, Massachusetts.

Abbas E. Kitabchi, Ph.D., M.D.,
Professor of Medicine and Biochemistry,
Director, Division of Endocrinology and Metabolism,
and Chief, Endocrinology and Diabetes Program,
William F. Bowld Hospital and Memphis Regional
    Medical Center,
University of Tennessee,
Memphis, Tennessee.

Leo P. Krall, M.D.,
Consultant,
Joslin Diabetes Center;
Consultant,
New England Deaconess Hospital;
Lecturer on Medicine,
Harvard Medical School;
Past and Honorary President,
International Diabetes Federation;
Chairman of the Board,
Diabetes Research and Educational Foundation,
Boston, Massachusetts.

Susan F. Kroop, M.D.,
Staff Physician,
New England Deaconess Hospital;
Instructor in Medicine,
Harvard Medical School,
Boston, Massachusetts.

Andrzej S. Krolewski, M.D., Ph.D.,
Chief, Section on Epidemiology and Genetics,
Joslin Diabetes Center;
Assistant Professor of Medicine,
Harvard Medical School,
Boston, Massachusetts.

Jack L. Leahy, M.D.,
Assistant Professor in Medicine,
New England Medical Center and Tufts University
    School of Medicine,
Boston, Massachusetts.

Harold E. Lebovitz, M.D.,
Professor of Medicine, and Chief, Section of
    Endocrinology and Diabetes,
State University of New York Health Science Center at
    Brooklyn,
Brooklyn, New York.

Rachmiel Levine, M.D.,
Medical Director Emeritus,
City of Hope National Medical Center,
Duarte, California.

Lynne L. Levitsky, M.D.,
Chief, Pediatric Endocrine Unit,
Massachusetts General Hospital;
Associate Professor of Pediatrics,
Harvard Medical School,
Boston, Massachusetts.

Frank W. LoGerfo, M.D.,
Chief, Division of Vascular Surgery,
New England Deaconess Hospital;
Professor of Surgery,
Harvard Medical School,
Boston, Massachusetts.

Mark H. Lowitt, M.D.,
Assistant Professor of Dermatology,
University of Maryland School of Medicine,
Baltimore, Maryland.

Bonnie T. Mackool, M.D., M.S.P.H.,
Director, Consultation Service,
Department of Dermatology,
Massachusetts General Hospital;
Instructor, Harvard Medical School,
Boston, Massachusetts.

Edward A. Mascioli, M.D.,
Attending Physician,
New England Deaconess Hospital;
Assistant Professor of Medicine,
Harvard Medical School,
Boston, Massachusetts.

Roger J. May, M.D.,
Physician,
Marshfield Clinic,
Marshfield, Wisconsin.

Jeannie Messent, M.B., M.R.C.P.,
Research Registrar,
Unit for Metabolic Medicine,
United Medical and Dental Schools,
Guy's Hospital,
London, United Kingdom.

Anthony P. Monaco, M.D.,
Director, Division of Organ Transplantation,
New England Deaconess Hospital;
Professor of Surgery,
Harvard Medical School,
Boston, Massachusetts.

Linda A. Morrow, M.D.,
Physician/Scientist,
Brockton/West Roxbury Veterans Affairs Medical
 Center, Division of the Boston Geriatric Research,
 Education, and Clinical Center;
Instructor in Medicine,
Division of Aging,
Harvard Medical School,
Boston, Massachusetts.

Alan C. Moses, M.D.,
Program Director,
Harvard-Thorndike General Clinical Research Center;
Associate Director, Division of Endocrinology,
Beth Israel Hospital;
Associate Professor of Medicine,
Harvard Medical School,
Boston, Massachusetts.

Mary Beth Murphy, M.S.N., M.B.A.,
Consultant/Special Projects,
Memphis Regional Medical Center,
Memphis, Tennessee.

David M. Nathan, M.D.,
Director, Mallinckrodt General Clinical Research
 Center;
Associate Physician, Diabetes Unit,
Massachusetts General Hospital;
Associate Professor of Medicine,
Harvard Medical School,
Boston, Massachusetts.

Richard W. Nesto, M.D.,
Co-Director of Institute for Prevention of
 Cardiovascular Disease,
New England Deaconess Hospital;
Assistant Professor of Medicine,
Harvard Medical School,
Boston, Massachusetts.

Niall M. O'Meara, M.D.,
Consultant Endocrinologist,
Department of Diabetes/Endocrinology,
Mater Misericordiae Hospital,
Dublin, Ireland.

Joanne J. Palmisano, M.D.,
Senior Physician,
Joslin Diabetes Center and New England Deaconess
 Hospital;
Associate Physician,
Brigham and Women's Hospital;
Instructor in Medicine,
Harvard Medical School,
Boston, Massachusetts.

Cynthia Pasquarello, R.N., B.S., C.D.E.,
Pediatric and Adolescent Diabetes Nurse Specialist,
Joslin Diabetes Center,
Boston, Massachusetts.

José R. Pinto, M.D.,
Consultant in Nephrology,
Guest Lecturer in Nephrology,
Lisbon University,
Lisbon, Portugal.

Kenneth S. Polonsky, M.D.,
Professor of Medicine and Chief, Section of
 Endocrinology,
Pritzker School of Medicine,
University of Chicago,
Chicago, Illinois.

William Polonsky, Ph.D.,
Psychologist,
Mental Health Unit,
Joslin Diabetes Center;
Instructor in Psychology/Psychiatry,
Harvard Medical School,
Boston, Massachusetts.

Kenneth E. Quickel, Jr., M.D.,
President, Joslin Diabetes Center;
Lecturer on Medicine,
Harvard Medical School,
Boston, Massachusetts.

Stephen S. Rich, Ph.D.,
Professor of Laboratory Medicine and Pathology, and
Director, Genetic Epidemiology,
Institute of Human Genetics,
University of Minnesota,
Minneapolis, Minnesota.

Donna L. Richardson, R.N., M.S., C.D.E.,
Director of Patient Education,
Joslin Diabetes Center,
Boston, Massachusetts.

James. L. Rosenzweig, M.D.,
Senior Physician,
Joslin Diabetes Center;
Physician,
New England Deaconess Hospital;
Assistant Professor of Medicine,
Harvard Medical School,
Boston, Massachusetts.

Neil B. Ruderman, M.D., D. Phil.,
Professor of Medicine and Physiology, Chief, Division
    of Diabetes and Metabolism,
Boston University School of Medicine;
Boston, Massachusetts.

Mark J. Rumbak, M.D.,
Assistant Professor of Medicine,
Pulmonary, Critical Care and Occupational Medicine,
College of Medicine,
University of South Florida,
Tampa, Florida.

Iñigo Saenz de Tejada, M.D.,
Associate Professor of Urology,
Director, Urology Research Laboratories,
Boston University School of Medicine,
Boston, Massachusetts.

Deborah E. Sentochnik, M.D.,
Attending Staff,
Infectious Diseases,
Lahey Clinic,
Burlington, Massachusetts.

David Shaffer, M.D.,
Staff Surgeon,
Division of Organ Transplantation,
New England Deaconess Hospital;
Assistant Professor of Surgery,
Harvard Medical School,
Boston, Massachusetts.

Steven E. Shoelson, M.D., Ph.D.,
Investigator, Joslin Diabetes Center;
Associate Physician,
Brigham and Women's Hospital;
Assistant Professor,
Harvard Medical School,
Boston, Massachusetts.

David A. Simmons, M.D.,
Associate Professor of Medicine,
Division of Endocrinology, Diabetes and Metabolism,
Department of Medicine,
University of Pennsylvania School of Medicine,
Philadelphia, Pennsylvania.

Lee S. Simon, M.D.,
Assistant to the President,
Medical Education Staff,
New England Deaconess Hospital;
Clinical Associate,
Massachusetts General Hospital;
Clinical Associate,
Dana Farber Cancer Center;
Assistant Professor of Medicine,
Harvard Medical School,
Boston, Massachusetts.

Donald C. Simonson, M.D.,
Head, Section of Clinical Physiology,
Joslin Diabetes Center;
Chief, Section of Diabetes and Metabolism,
Brigham and Women's Hospital;
Assistant Professor of Medicine,
Harvard Medical School,
Boston, Massachusetts.

Fannie E. Smith, M.D., Ph.D.,
Research Associate, Section of Islet Transplantation and
    Cell Biology,
Joslin Diabetes Center;
Instructor in Medicine,
Harvard Medical School,
Boston, Massachusets.

Robert J. Smith, M.D.,
Assistant Director of Research, and
Head of Section on Metabolism,
Joslin Diabetes Center;
Associate Professor of Medicine,
Harvard Medical School,
Boston, Massachusetts.

Daniel Tarsy, M.D.,
Chief, Division of Neurology,
New England Deaconess Hospital;
Assistant Professor of Neurology,
Harvard Medical School,
Associate Professor of Neurology,
Boston University School of Medicine,
Boston, Massachusetts.

Robert C. Turner, M.D., F.R.C.P.,
Clinical Reader,
Oxford University,
Oxford, United Kingdom.

Roger H. Unger, M.D.,
Director, Center for Diabetes Research;
Professor of Internal Medicine,
Touchstone/West Distinguished Chair in Diabetes
    Research,
University of Texas Southwestern Medical Center;
Senior Medical Investigator,
Department of Veterans Medical Center,
Dallas, Texas.

GianCarlo Viberti, M.D., F.R.C.P.,
Professor of Diabetes and Metabolic Medicine, and
Head, Department of Metabolic Medicine,
United Medical and Dental Schools;
Consultant Physician,
Guy's Hospital,
London, United Kingdom.

James H. Warram, M.D., Sc.D.,
Investigator, Epidemiology and Genetics Section,
Research Division,
Joslin Diabetes Center;
Lecturer in Epidemiology,
Harvard School of Public Health,
Boston, Massachusetts.

Gordon C. Weir, M.D.,
Medical Director, and Chief,
Section on Islet Transplantation and Cell Biology,
Joslin Diabetes Center;
Professor of Medicine,
Harvard Medical School,
Boston, Massachusetts.

Morris F. White, Ph.D.,
Investigator,
Section on Cellular and Mollecular Physiology,
Joslin Diabetes Center;
Associate Professor of Biological Chemistry in the
    Department of Medicine,
Harvard Medical School,
Boston, Massachusetts.

Barbara Widom, M.D.,
Physician,
Aspen Medical Center,
Loveland, Colorado.

Martin J. Wiseman, M.D.,
Head, Nutrition Unit,
Department of Health,
London, United Kingdom.

Joseph I. Wolfsdorf, M.B., B.Ch.,
Chief of Pediatrics,
Joslin Diabetes Center;
Associate in Endocrinology and Director of Diabetes
    Program,
The Children's Hospital;
Associate Physician,
New England Deaconess Hospital;
Assistant Professor of Pediatrics,
Harvard Medical School,
Boston, Massachusetts.

David Wynick, B.Sc., M.R.C.P., M.D.,
Medical Registrar,
Division of Endocrinology and Metabolism,
Royal Postgraduate Medical School,
Hammersmith Hospital,
London, United Kingdom.

Stuart W. Zarich, M.D.,
Director, CCU,
New England Deaconess Hospital;
Instructor in Medicine,
Harvard Medical School,
Boston, Massachusetts.

Priv. Doz. Dr. med. Anette G. Ziegler,
Diabetes Research Institute and Schwabing City
    Hospital,
Munich, Germany.

CONTENTS

Obesity and Lipoprotein Disorders

Treatment of Diabetes Mellitus

Onset of the Complications of Diabetes

COMPLICATIONS: CLINICAL ASPECTS

HYPOGLYCEMIA AND ISLET-CELL TUMORS

Chapter 1

THE HISTORY OF DIABETES

LEO P. KRALL
RACHMIEL LEVINE
DONALD BARNETT

Diabetes was described more than 2000 years ago. For the past 200 years, it has featured in the history of modern medicine. Since the discovery of insulin, work on diabetes at both cellular and clinical levels has expanded as fast as new laboratory and diagnostic techniques allow. To chart even the recent history of diabetes is a formidable task requiring substantial knowledge of internal medicine and the basic sciences underlying the pathology of the disease complex. This chapter attempts an overview by citing key topics of historical significance and quotes from principal figures in this important story.

It is fitting for a chapter on the history of diabetes to be included in the 13th edition of *Joslin's Diabetes Mellitus*, as Dr. Elliott P. Joslin, the founder of the Joslin Clinic and the editor of the book through the first 10 editions, was himself a historian. Early editions of this text show Dr. Joslin diligently searching in both the remote and more-recent literature for clues on how to better "study and care" for patients with diabetes.

In 1956, when Dr. Joslin was planning the first phase of the present modern facility that houses the Joslin Clinic, now known as the Joslin Diabetes Center, he turned to a history of medicine. He invited a sculptor to compose a bas relief portraying the history of medicine from ancient times to the present day, with an emphasis on the history of diabetes. Two examples depicted on these panels are noteworthy: references to John Hunter (1728–1793), the first modern physiologist, and to George Minot (1885–1950), a patient of Dr. Joslin who was "saved" by insulin in 1922 while still a young physician and who subsequently received the Nobel Prize in 1934 for the codiscovery of treatment of pernicious anemia (Fig. 1–1). Sir John Hunter's portrait hung prominently in Dr.

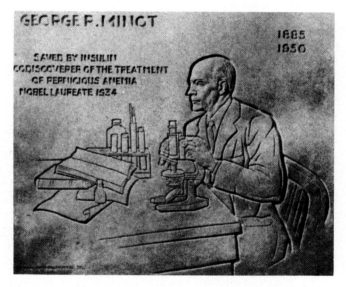

Fig. 1–1. Panel on outside wall of Joslin Diabetes Center.

Joslin's home office at 81 Bay State Road in the Back Bay section of Boston for 50 years. From his love of comparative anatomy, to his skills as a surgeon (a practical specialty that Dr. Joslin greatly admired), and to his courage as a clinical researcher, Dr. Hunter's life reflected an unending sense of wonder at the glories of nature "in health and disease."[1] In a sense, these examples prophetically mark Dr. Joslin's own life as a complete student of diabetes. The quotation on the lead panel on the Joslin Diabetes Center serves as a fitting introduction to this chapter and the events of the pre-insulin era.

The evolution of medicine is in reality the history of man and his religion. Those who have contributed to its advancement are legion. Progressive steps in the art of healing, especially as related to diabetes are here recorded.

THE ROAD TO INSULIN

The struggle for recognition of the role of the pancreas in diabetes was long and arduous. The fascinating, tortuous road to discovery involved a host of clinicians, chemists, physiologists, and pathologists. The tale is filled with marvelous insights as well as egregious errors, serendipity and futile labors, triumphs, and defeats.

The following masterly description of severe clinical diabetes by Aretaeus of Cappadocia (about 150 A.D.) represents the sum of our knowledge up until the second half of the seventeenth century.

> Diabetes is a remarkable disorder, and not one very common to man. It consists of a moist and cold wasting of the flesh and limbs into urine, from a cause similar to that of dropsy; the secretion passes in the usual way, by the kidneys and the bladder. The patients never cease making water, but the discharge is as incessant as a sluice let off. This disease is chronic in character, and is slowly engendered, though the patient does not survive long when it is completely established for the marasmus produced is rapid and death is speedy.[2]

In 1674, Thomas Willis, a physician, anatomist, and a professor of natural philosophy at Oxford, discovered (by tasting) that the urine of diabetic persons was sweet. This was actually a rediscovery, for unbeknownst to him, an ancient Hindu document by Susruta in India in about 400 B.C. had described the diabetic syndrome as characterized by a "honeyed urine."[2,3] Willis could not pinpoint the chemical nature of the "sweet" substance since a variety of different chemical substances could be equally sweet to the sense of taste.[4]

It was Matthew Dobson of Manchester, England, who in 1776 demonstrated that diabetics actually excrete sugar in the urine. He evaporated urine to dryness by boiling and noted that the residue, a crystalline material, had the appearance and taste of "brown sugar."[5]

Dobson's definitive finding soon began influencing clinicians as to the possible causes of the disease and the bodily organs primarily involved. The prevalent view up to that time was that the kidneys were the central organ affected by the disease, since its most striking signs and symptoms related to the frequency and degree of urination. Some clinical observers also noted a tendency towards enlargement of the liver, which we now know to be due to intense infiltration of the organ with fat in diabetic persons with uncontrolled diabetes. In a case report, which also gave a detailed description of postmortem findings, Cawley reported in 1788 (without particular comment) that he observed a shriveled pancreas with stones in a diabetic patient at autopsy. This may have been the first published reference to the pancreas in relation to human diabetes, but no deductions were drawn as to etiology.[6]

It was John Rollo, Surgeon General of the Royal Artillery, who first applied the discovery of glycosuria by Dobson to the quantitative metabolic study of diabetes. Aided by Cruickshank, "apothecary and chemist to the ordinance," Rollo devised the first rational approach to the dietary treatment of the disease and shifted the view then current that the primary seat of the disorder was the kidneys to its being the gastrointestinal tract.[7]

Rollo studied Captain Meredith, a corpulent man with adult-onset diabetes with severe glycosuria. Rollo made daily recordings of the amounts and kinds of food Meredith ate and weighed the sugar cake obtained by boiling and evaporating the urine excreted every day. He noted that the amount of sugar excreted varied from day to day, depending primarily on the type of food ingested. "Vegetable" matter (i.e., breads, grains, fruits) increased glycosuria, whereas "animal" matter (i.e., meat) resulted in a comparatively lower excretion of sugar. Rollo and Cruickshank concluded, therefore, that the glycosuria was secondary to the "saccharification" of "vegetable" matter (i.e., carbohydrate foods in the stomach and the influx of sugar into the body) and considered that the "morbid" organ in diabetes was not the kidney but the "stomach," which overproduced sugar from "vegetable" matter. Excretion of sugar by the kidney was thus a secondary event caused by hyperglycemia. The indicated treatment was thus a diet low in carbohydrates and high in fat and protein.[7] It was not until the advent of insulin that this dietary prescription was altered significantly.

Although Rollo assumed the presence of hyperglycemia in diabetes, at that time there was no convincing proof that hyperglycemia existed. Wollaston (the renowned chemist and physician) tried to measure "sugar" in the blood but failed to detect it, primarily because he based his technique, a primitive kind of paper chromatography, on the assumption that the sugar in the blood was identical to the table sugar that he used as a standard.[2] In 1815, Chevreuil showed that blood sugar behaved chemically as if it were "grape" sugar (i.e., dextrose or glucose).[8] Later, specific methods of analysis were devised and used to measure glucose as the major "reducing substance" in the serum and urine.[9-11] Rollo's predictions were confirmed—that in diabetes a rise in blood sugar level causes the excretion of sugar and that the "seat" of diabetes was outside the kidneys.

Over the next 40 to 50 years (1830–1880), clinicians in England, France, and Germany described cases of diabetes with postmortem findings of diseased, atrophic, or stone-filled pancreases. Speculations as to the role of this organ in diabetes abounded. However, the evidence was not at all convincing, since in the vast majority of diabetic patients, the pancreas was of normal size and appearance at autopsy. With the functions of the pancreas regarding digestion of foodstuffs being only barely surmised at that time and the organ itself known only as a purely exocrine gland, the finding of pathologic lesions in the pancreas in a small group of diabetic individuals was interpreted as a chance phenomenon rather than a possible guide to the etiology of the disease.

In France, Claude Bernard was, of course, aware of the findings and speculations regarding the possible role of the pancreas in diabetes. To test such a hypothesis, he devised a "crucial" experiment in dogs. He ligated pancreatic ducts and/or injected them with oil or paraffin to block all secretion. This led to profound atrophy of the gland. Since only a few strands of what appeared to him to be lifeless scar tissue remained, Bernard assumed that the atrophy was indeed complete. Despite this, the animals showed neither glycosuria nor any other indication of diabetes.[12] Such experiments also were performed by Schiff, with equally negative results. The "anti-pancreatic" viewpoint was thus immeasurably strengthened by the authoritative voices of the foremost physiologists of the age. Bernard's celebrated findings of glycosuria after "piqûre" of the IVth ventricle also drew attention to the possibility that alterations in the central nervous system could be etiologically related to diabetes. A lesion in the brain would cause hyperglycemia by way of the "visceral" nerves acting on the liver. And yet, thoughtful clinical observers could not overlook the admittedly inconsistent, yet very real, pathologic findings of pancreatic lesions in some diabetic individuals.

The two strongest forces arguing for a "pancreatic" factor in the etiology of diabetes were Bouchardet and Lancereaux. Bouchardet, trained by Chevreuil in organic chemistry and an early pioneer in the study of fermentation and a professor of public health, did meticulous long-term studies on human diabetes. These began in 1835 and were gathered into his 1875 book, *De la Glycosuria ou Diabète Sucré*.[13] He followed the essentials of Rollo's dietary regimen in treating diabetes. He added a very important therapeutic arm, encouraging hard physical labor, having observed ameliorative effects of muscular work on glycosuria and hyperglycemia. But above all, his clinical experience taught him to distinguish at least two different types of diabetes: the severe type in younger persons that responded poorly to his regimen, and the type in older, obese persons for which the prescribed therapy of diet and physical exertion worked admirably. The clinical behavior of the two types of diabetes and the postmortem findings led Bouchardet and Lancereaux to suggest that the severe form resistant to dietary treatment was pancreatic in origin. Lancereaux and his students came to identical conclusions about etiology and introduced the terms *diabète maigre* (diabetes of the thin) and *diabète gras* (diabetes of the fat) for the two common clinical forms of the disease.[14] Since *diabète gras* was the more frequently occurring type, it now became understandable why severe pancreatic damage was found less frequently than expected. A pancreatic etiology for *diabète maigre* thus became an acceptable postulate, even though one could not yet form a sound notion as to the mechanisms involved.

The concept that the body possesses glands that deliver their products directly to the blood (ductless or "blood" glands) gained substantial ground through Berthold's study of castration (1849), the clinical description of Addison's disease (1849), and the experimental ablation of the adrenal gland by Brown-Sequard (1855). In 1869, Paul Langerhans, a senior medical student in Berlin, published a short paper, his medical dissertation, on pancreatic histology in which he described a previously

CONTRIBUTIONS

TO THE MICROSCOPIC ANATOMY OF THE PANCREAS.

INAUGURAL-DISSERTATION

FOR THE DOCTOR'S DEGREE IN

MEDICINE AND SURGERY

PRESENTED TO THE MEDICAL FACULTY

FRIEDRICH–WILHELMS–UNIVERSITY

BERLIN

AND TO DEFEND PUBLICLY ON

FEBRUARY 18, 1869

BY PAUL LANGERHANS

BERLIN.

Fig. 1–2. Introduction to the thesis of Paul Langerhans, who, while a medical student, discovered what were later called the islets of Langerhans.

unknown cell type in the gland (Fig. 1–2).[15] These cells were situated between the acini and did not communicate directly with the excretory ducts. He described them as occurring in small heaps or islands. The key paragraph giving microscopic details includes the following: "Under high power these specks are seen to consist of masses 0.12–0.24 millimeters in diameter distributed at regular intervals in the parenchyma and can be easily seen in fragment preparations of the fresh gland or in that treated for a short time in iodized serum."[16]

Langerhans could assign no particular function to these cells. The paper disappeared, without much ado, into the literature until the 1890s.

Lavoisier's Legacy

A set of developments in the early 1800s that deepened understanding of the basic metabolic principles of human physiology had far-reaching consequences for all medicine and for diabetes in particular. Lavoisier (1743–1794) established the concept of the respiratory quotient and with the aid of calorimetric studies measured oxygen consumption at rest and under different conditions, such as during food ingestion and work. His intended studies on digestion were interrupted by his death under the guillotine during the French Revolution. A generation later, Liebig (1803–1873) advanced the field of physiologic chemistry by determining that there were three categories of food: protein, carbohydrate, and fat. In his study of the development of physiology, Rosen wrote of the crucial link between this information and the understanding of metabolism and endocrinology of today.

Liebig showed how protein was used to build up or repair the organism while the last two (carbohydrate and fat) were used for fuel. He determined how much oxygen was needed to burn the different classes of food and how much energy was released as measured by heat. Carl Voit, writing in 1865, described his teacher's work with these terms: "Liebig was the first to establish the importance of chemical transformations in the body. He stated that the phenomena of motion and activity which we call life arise from the interaction of oxygen, food and the components of the body. He clearly saw the relation between metabolism and activity and that not only heat but all motion was derived from metabolism. . . ." Voit's work as carried on by his student Max Rubner in Germany, and by his American students, Graham Lusk and W. O. Atwater, made it possible to study metabolic activities more precisely and to apply the results to clinical and theoretical problems. It was Rubner who in 1888–90 finally produced incontrovertible experimental proof that the principle of the conservation of energy held for living systems. This was confirmed for man by Atwater and Benedict in 1903. Rubner introduced a new point of view. He endeavored to see metabolism as a totality in energetic terms.[17]

Between 1840 and 1860 physiologic studies in metabolism as they relate to diabetes began their advance, especially in France under the leadership of Claude Bernard. His epoch-making discovery that blood glucose was derived in part from glycogen as a "secretion" of the liver thus identified the liver as a central organ in diabetes and explained how a diabetic patient whose liver was scarred by the end stages of cirrhosis might be "cured" of his hyperglycemia and glycosuria.

Pancreatic Diabetes

The decisive turning point in the history of diabetes was marked by the experimental work of von Mering and Minkowski[18] in 1889. Von Mering was interested in the possible role of the pancreas in the digestion and absorption of fats. From the literature then available, primarily the writings of Claude Bernard, von Mering understood that it was virtually impossible for an animal to survive total removal of the pancreas. He counseled with Minkowski, the assistant to Albert Naunyn, the foremost European clinician in diabetes at that time. Not daunted by the previous experiments, von Mering and Minkowski operated on two dogs, and both animals survived the complete pancreatectomy. Within less than a day, these animals exhibited unexpected behavior— in particular, frequent and voluminous urination. Minkowski's experience with severe human diabetes led him to examine the urine for sugar. With the next 2 years, Minkowski extended this serendipitous finding into an in-depth, now classic, study of experimental diabetes and its metabolic deviations. The study remains a model of scientific, physiologic inquiry. He demonstrated clearly that the pancreas was a gland of internal secretion and that a small portion of the gland, when implanted under the skin of a freshly depancreatized dog, prevented the appearance of hyperglycemia until the implanted tissue was removed or had degenerated spontaneously.

Confirmation of this finding came very quickly from Hedon and co-workers in France. Between 1891 and 1894 Laguesse drew proper attention to the almost forgotten original observations of Langerhans and suggested the collections of interacinar cells (which he designated the "islets of Langerhans") as a gland of secretion within the pancreas.[19,20]

Modern experimental and clinical endocrinology was conceived during the last decade of the nineteenth century. The date of birth was marked by the introduction of the term "hormone" by Starling in 1902, a term that he used to designate the specific chemical material elaborated into the blood by a ductless gland that is conveyed to other parts of the body and exerts a specific set of functional changes on its "target" tissues. In 1910, Jean de Meyer suggested that the pancreatic secretion that was lacking in the diabetic state should, when found, be called "insulin" to denote its origin from the "insulae" of Langerhans.[2]

Between 1895 and 1921 experimental work developed in two directions. One was the careful histologic study of the islets, which led to the finding of several distinct cell types, thus foreshadowing our present knowledge that the islets of Langerhans are the site of production and secretion of several hormones in addition to insulin.[21] The other was a search for insulin itself. The requirements for insulin as a potential therapeutic agent were stringent: 1) the preparation had to be of consistent potency; 2) it should reverse the metabolic abnormalities of the depancreatized animal; 3) it should reverse the signs, symptoms, and chemical abnormalities of human diabetes; and 4) it should produce no harmful side effects.

The difficulties in the early attempts to isolate insulin were legion. There was total ignorance of the chemical nature of the postulated antidiabetic substance, making the extraction procedure a hit-or-miss proposition. At that time, quantitative estimates of the blood sugar required inordinate amounts of blood and the procedure was not generally available. Because of ignorance about the profound effects of low blood sugar levels on the nervous system (hypoglycemic convulsions), they were also not recognized as such and were initially attributed to a "toxic" action of the extract. In addition, fever and infections were frequent sequelae of the injections of extracts. In view of the protein nature of the hormone (which, of course, was not yet known), it is obvious that those workers who used oral administration of the extract were bound to fail. Of the many forerunners of Banting and Best, those who came closest to the mark were E. L. Scott, Israel Kleiner, Ludwig Zuelzer, and Nicolas Paulesco. Indeed, Paulesco, a distinguished Romanian physiologist, produced a pancreatic extract that fulfilled all the criteria on animal experimentation for an "insulin," but he did not succeed in showing its application in human diabetes.[21] Thus, the significance of his contribution was appreciated only much later.

Frederick Banting, a young surgeon, and Charles Best, a medical student, with the help of the skilled chemist J. B. Collip, succeeded in fulfilling all of the criteria for a therapeutically active insulin and produced the first useful and consistently successful insulin preparation for the treatment of human diabetes. This discovery also became a powerful stimulus to the exploration of intermediary metabolism, the nature of hormone action, details of protein structure, and a host of other biologic questions. Thus, the pancreatic etiology of diabetes was finally established.[22–24]

As such things commonly proceed, there was a tendency to overdo the interpretation. First, all diabetes was ascribed to insulin deficiency. The role of other hormones in metabolic control and an awareness of the bewildering heterogeneity of the diabetic syndrome belong to the half century and more that has elapsed since that momentous summer in Toronto in 1921. In 1922 Banting and Macleod received a Nobel Prize for this historic discovery. There was immediate controversy over the omission of Best and Collip from the prize, a controversy that has continued to the present day. Recent historical research into the details of the Banting and Best collaboration confirm that J. J. R. Macleod, Professor of Physiology at the University of Toronto, facilitated as much as he could the research suggested by Banting and was probably an appropriate corecipient of the Nobel Prize.[25] It has always been clear that of the participants, Macleod was certainly the most knowledgeable in the fields of carbohydrate metabolism and diabetes mellitus. The success of the work by Banting and Best was due to Macleod's basic knowledge, Banting's stubborn persistence, and the important specific skills of Best and Collip.

THE INSULIN ERA

The Discovery of Insulin

The discovery of insulin was a seminal event in both the study of diabetes and the care of diabetic patients. The development of procedures for purifying and modifying insulin took an additional 30 years. Table 1–1 charts these and other developments from the initial discovery of insulin to the early 1980s.

In his masterful rendition of these developments, Michael Bliss recounts the remarkable story surrounding the discovery of insulin and notes that "the discovery of insulin at the University of Toronto in 1921–22 was one of the most dramatic events in the history of the treatment of disease."[25]

Insulin was to become the first major "replacement" therapy and elevated medical therapeutics to a stature equal to that conferred on surgery by the advances of the previous 50 years. Although liver, adrenal, and thyroid extracts became available in the 30 or more years following the discovery of insulin, even today they are less used than insulin. By 1952, the basic array of insulin options that are available today had been developed (Table 1–1).[26] With the advent of recombinant technology, insulin also became the first hormone produced by genetic engineering to be used for treatment of a human disease.

Several years after the discovery of insulin, Minkowski himself commented on the success of Banting and Best. He felt their success was due primarily to the advent of microanalytic techniques that enabled these researchers to measure glucose in small amounts of blood (rather than urine) and to repeat the determinations at will. In a sense, his comment was prophetic for the future treatment of diabetes. Today, with the advance and use of self-monitoring of blood glucose rather than urinary glucose determinations, treatment of diabetes has improved considerably. Minkowski also felt that the additional benefits that Banting, Best, and Macleod had at their disposal were an unlimited supply of pancreatic extract and their failure to be deterred by the toxic properties of their extracts.[27] However, their greatest attribute was their persistence in the investigation to the point of success.

Even though insulin had been discovered, during the early period following the observation of Banting and Best, a death sentence still hung over many patients with insulin-dependent diabetes (IDDM) because of the insufficiency of insulin supply. Many experiences of patients who needed this hormone are part of the memories of physicians working during the 1920s. There is no better recounting of the way in which insulin reclaimed lives

Table 1–1. Insulin Timetable: 1921 through the Present

1921	Pancreatic extracts demonstrated to lower blood sugar levels in experimental diabetic dogs (Banting and Best, Toronto)
1922	Insulin first used in human (Leonard Thompson, Toronto)
1923	"Isoelectric point" produced larger quantities of higher-potency insulin from animal sources—enough to satisfy commercial supply (Lilly Company)
1925	First international insulin unit defined (1 unit = 0.125 mg of standard material). U40/80 insulins become available
1926	Crystallized amorphous insulin adds to insulin stability (Abel)
1936	Addition of zinc to protamine insulin (PZI) to create a prolonged duration of action of the hormone (Scott, Fisher, Hagedorn)
1939	Globin insulin with a shorter duration of action than PZI developed
1950	NPH (neutral protamine Hagedorn) insulin developed with controlled amounts of protamine (Nordisk Company)
1951	Lente insulins developed by acetate buffering of zinc insulin (Novo Company, Hallas-Moller)
1955	Structure of insulin delineated (Sanger and co-workers)
1960	Radioimmunoassay of insulin becomes available (Berson and Yalow)
1967	Proinsulin discovered (Steiner and Oyer)
1971	Insulin receptor defined (Roth, Cuatrecasas, and co-workers)
1972	U-100 insulin introduced to promote better accuracy in administration
1973 ±	Small-dose intravenous insulin treatment for acidosis emerges as alternative to large-dose subcutaneous treatment
1976	C-peptide becomes clinical tool (Rubenstein et al.)
1977	Insulin gene cloned (Ullrich, Rutter, Goodman, and co-workers)
1978	Purified "single-peak" pork insulins introduced (Lilly Company)
1979	Open-loop insulin delivery system clinically available (Tamborlane)
1981	Insulin-receptor kinase activity described (Kasaga, Kahn, and co-workers)
1982	Recombinant DNA insulin becomes available (Lilly Company), and enzymatic conversion of pork insulin sequence to human insulin sequence developed (Novo Company)

This chart is modified from Haycock.[26]

than that of R. D. Lawrence, a British physician with diabetes who was to become a leader in the field. On the 25th anniversary of insulin, he wrote the following in a seminar sponsored by the Eli Lilly Company.

> When I started insulin early in 1923, nearly twenty-four years ago, it had only begun to come into commercial production in England. . . . About April, 1923, wasted, thin, fit for nothing, in a cautious way I began to use insulin. . . . I understood that there was enough for me in my hospital to carry me on for about a month, then the grace of God would have to supply me with a new set-up. But something developed. A girl (a doctor's daughter) in diabetic coma was admitted. To bring her out, she got the insulin on which I had hoped to live the next fortnight. Well, I was in a jam. . . . Somebody somehow brought me a bottle of Lilly insulin the next day. I looked at it with suspicion, but I was glad to have that, really—anything with an insulin label on the bottle. By the end of the fortnight I had complete confidence [in the new insulin] which I have never had any reason to change in supervening years.[28]

Figure 1–3 is a photograph of a core group of the first generation of physician-investigators at the 25th anniversary of the discovery of insulin in Toronto.

The Early Years (before 1960)

Over the 35-year period from the discovery of insulin through the 1950s, the effects of the availability of insulin were felt in three ways: an improved life expectancy for patients with IDDM, a surge of interest in understanding the mechanism of action of insulin upon intermediary metabolism, and an increasing recognition of the syndromes we have come to appreciate as the chronic complications of diabetes. Certainly, the major emphasis during that time was on IDDM and the elimination of death from diabetic coma. As enzymatic and hormonal regulation of glucose metabolism was clarified, the study focus on intermediary metabolism included the pituitary-adrenal axis, as well as carbohydrate metabolism in hepatic, adipose, and muscle tissues in the uncontrolled diabetic state.

Modern Endocrinology Comes of Age

The centerpiece of the new age in the study of metabolism came with the Nobel-laureate work of Bernardo Houssay of Argentina. A 30-year perspective of the field of metabolism following the discovery of insulin was summarized in Houssay's address at the dedication of the new Banting and Best Institute in Toronto in 1952.[29]

> Working with Biasotti; I found the hypophysectomies diminished the severity of diabetes by pancreatectomy in the dog. Implantation of the pars distalis (anterior lobe of mammals) again increases the severity of diabetes. The diabetogenic effect of the hypophysis was thus demonstrated. The severe symptoms of pancreatic diabetes were due to two factors: (a) presence of a hypophyseal hormone, and (b) a lack of secretion of insulin. The diabetogenic effect of hy-

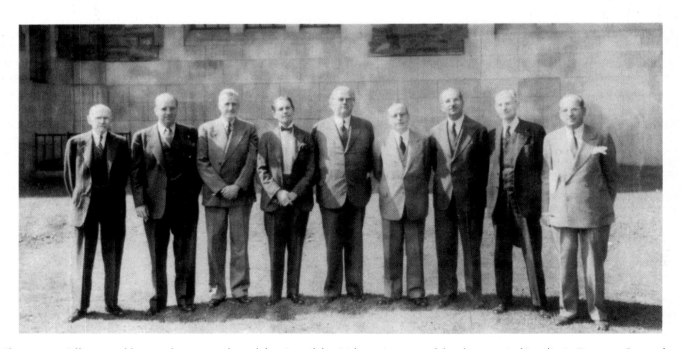

Fig. 1–3. Officers and honored guests at the celebration of the 25th anniversary of the discovery of insulin in Toronto, September 16–18, 1946. Left to right: Elliot P. Joslin, Boston, honorary president, American Diabetes Association; Charles H. Best, Toronto, codiscoverer of insulin; Russell M. Wilder, Rochester, Minnesota; president-elect, American Diabetes Association; Robert D. Lawrence, London, founder, The Diabetic Association; H. C. Hagedorn, Denmark, discoverer of protamine insulin; B. A. Houssay, Buenos Aires, researcher, "Houssay phenomenon"; Joseph H. Barach, Pittsburgh, president, American Diabetes Association. Eugene L. Opie, New York, discoverer, islets of Langerhans pathology; Cecil Striker, Cincinnati, first president, American Diabetes Association.

pophyseal extract in mammals was demonstrated in 1932 simultaneously in three laboratories: in Evan's, in Marine's, and in mine. In 1932, I was able to provoke a permanent diabetes by hypophyseal treatment in dogs previously submitted to partial pancreatectomy. Young obtained this effect in dogs with intact pancreas in 1937.

Dr. Houssay's work became the needed fulcrum for the advancements in understanding of the whole endocrine network that we appreciate today. In the 10 years following the availability of insulin, he was able to study the action of insulin by applying his earlier investigations on the effects of thyroid, adrenal, and pituitary ablation upon glucose regulation. Diabetes became a convenient and measurable parameter in the study of metabolism for him and his contemporaries.

During the 1930s there was an eruption in information about hormonal regulation of intermediary metabolism. C. F. Cori[30] and H. A. Krebs[31] were defining steps in glucose regulation. The adrenal gland became a continued focus of investigation, aided by Cushing's inclusion of human adrenal pathology earlier in the decade.[32] Also, as Harvey points out in his *Classics in Clinical Science*, Atchley and Loeb made major contributions to the understanding of the treatment of diabetic acidosis.[34]

In the early 1930's Atchley and Loeb conducted their studies on the electrolyte changes in diabetic acidosis. Their clinical experience with critically ill patients in diabetic acidosis led to realization of the state of ignorance as to how this syndrome evolved. Atchley suggested that they bring well regulated diabetic patients into the hospital and follow the sequential metabolic changes after discontinuing their insulin. They selected three patients: in the first, when insulin was taken away, the diabetes was so mild that little change occurred. The second had more severe diabetes, and the third had very severe diabetes and became seriously ill within a few hours after his insulin was discontinued. Their quantitative observations demonstrated the progressive loss of body water, sodium and potassium. These elegant balance studies represent one of the classic contributions in the evolution of our knowledge of the electrolyte changes in diabetes mellitus.

It took another decade and a half for the practical implementation of correct replacement of electrolytes in diabetic acidosis to be completed. The better availability of infection-free intravenous solutions was crucial to the achievement of optimal care for the acutely ill diabetic patient. The arrival in 1948 of the flame photometer for more-rapid determination of potassium levels also brought into perspective a requirement for this electrolyte in almost all cases of diabetic acidosis.

From today's perspective the final "conquest" of diabetic coma came with the use of intravenous insulin infusions. Since 1980, the formula for correcting the insulin deficit in patients with ketoacidosis has been contained in a mere half page of the guidelines of the American Diabetes Association.[34] This abbreviation of the treatment of diabetic acidosis parallels the marked decrease in mortality that has been observed over the past several decades.

The Study of Clinical Diabetes and Its Impact on Care

The original physicians on the first Insulin Committee of the University of Toronto in 1922 were Dr. Elliott P. Joslin of Boston; Dr. Robert Williams of Rochester, New York; Dr. Frederick Allen of Morristown, New Jersey; Dr. Woodyatt of Chicago, Illinois; Dr. Russell Wilder of the Mayo Clinic, Rochester, Minnesota; and Dr. Richard Geyelin, of New York City.[35] These men, each in his own way, were leaders in the new treatment of diabetes in the first decade after the discovery of insulin. New descriptions of problems in diabetes, as well as the need to help the patient with practical suggestions on daily planning required by the use of insulin, dominated that era. Patient manuals with practical pointers in daily care by Drs. Joslin, Wilder, and Lawrence were prime examples among many on the subject. These instructional renditions went through many editions. In the 1920s such monographs, rather than the all-purpose textbooks of the later years or the rapidly published journal articles of today, were the major sources of medical information.

Some of the best examples of this type of medical communication were the 10 monographs by Dr. Elliott P. Joslin and his original group of collaborators published from 1912 through 1946 (Table 1–2).[36–45] Their very titles illustrate the concerns of the clinician in the early insulin era and are a tribute to Dr. Joslin's guidance. In 1936 Kimmelstiel and Wilson's article on a kidney lesion that seemed pathognomonic for diabetes rounded out the early description of diabetic complications.[46]

Implicit in many of the discussions in the listed monographs, particularly those on pathology, diabetic coma, and retinopathy, was the feature of severe macrovascular disease. The suggestions of a much higher incidence of coronary artery disease emphasized in these publications was clearly substantiated in several surveys of diabetic patients in the 1940s and 1950s. Bell's monumental study on atherosclerosis documents the problem.[47]

Table 1–2. Joslin Monographs: 1912–1946

1912	*A Study of Metabolism in Severe Diabetes*, F. G. Benedict and E. P. Joslin[36]
1916	*The Treatment of Diabetes*, E. P. Joslin[37]
1918	*Diabetic Manual for the Mutual Use of Doctor and Patient*, E. P. Joslin[38]
1907–1946	*Diabetic Coma*, E. P. Joslin and staff of Baker Clinic (forerunner of Joslin Clinic-Center)[39]
1928	*Diabetic Surgery*, L. S. McKittrick and H. F. Root[40]
1930	*The Pathology of Diabetes*, S. Warren[41]
1932	*Diabetes in Childhood and Adolescence*, P. White[42]
1934	*The Association of Diabetes and Tuberculosis*, H. F. Root[43]
1935	*Neuritic Manifestations in Diabetes Mellitus*, W. R. Jordan[44]
1935	*The Visual Mechanism in Diabetes Mellitus*, J. H. Waite and W. P. Beetham[45]

Classification of neuropathy was to be continuously readdressed in the 30 years following the publication of the Jordan monograph[44] (Table 1–2). However, this attempt to describe the forms of diabetic neuropathy represented one of the earliest notations of severe joint neuropathy now called the "Charcot" phenomenon. It was thought to resemble the syphilitic involvement of lower extremity joints described by the French neurologist in the nineteenth century.

A monograph on the visual problems in diabetes in 1935 by Waite and Beetham[45] was to be a basis for Beetham's later studies on the natural history of retinopathy.[48] It formed a foundation for some of the initial assumptions used in treating retinopathy with laser photocoagulation.[49]

It is difficult for those involved with diabetes in the post-insulin period to comprehend fully the changes that have taken place since the introduction of insulin. The first Joslin patient to receive insulin was Elizabeth Mudge, R.N., who received insulin on August 7, 1922, at the Broadbeck Cottage of the New England Deaconess Hospital in Boston. She had not been able to leave her apartment for 9 months. After 6 weeks of insulin therapy she could walk 4 miles daily, and she lived for 25 more years. Regarding the pre-insulin days, Dr. Joslin noted, "I used to count the days my diabetic children lived."[42] This is emphasized by an episode that took place in the crowded original offices of the clinic on Bay State Road in the 1940s when a child patient was more than a bit noisy, much to the annoyance of younger physicians. Dr. Joslin came by and said, "Make all the noise you want. We love noisy children around here. For many years there were no normal children. They were very quiet and after a visit or two they did not return" (L. P. Krall, personal communication). Somehow the noise did not seem so annoying.

Prior to the use of insulin, most young diabetic patients died shortly after diagnosis. The Joslin Clinic experience[50] showed the commonest cause of death to be ketoacidosis (63.8% until 1914 and 41.5% until August 1921). The improvement from 1914 to 1921 was probably due to the introduction of Frederick Allen's "semistarvation" therapy in about 1915. Even though patients with IDDM could sometimes survive for years using this form of starvation therapy, most died sooner. By comparison, in the best of circumstances, the rate of death due to coma is now less than 1%, although in some developing countries, death rates still approach pre-insulin levels.

Joslin noted these improvements in the preface of the first edition of *The Treatment of Diabetes Mellitus* in 1916.[37] "I have honestly tried in these pages to let the 400 fatal cases tell their lessons to the 600 living. I would not have wished to write a book on diabetes three years ago." One must contrast this with the preface to his third edition of the book in 1923 based on 3,000 cases[51]: "Compared to the last decade, the doctor now has twice as many diabetics to treat. . . . Whereas formerly 10% of all diabetics seen in a year died the same year, the mortality has now fallen to 6.7% of my 293 patients treated with insulin. . . . Of the 48 children cared for in this period, 46 remain alive . . . and as for Bouchardat,

Cantani, Kulz, Lepine and all the other diabetic saints, how they would have enjoyed this year!"

The Birth of Diabetes Epidemiology

Dr. Elliott P. Joslin was the first diabetes epidemiologist. Born in 1869 in Oxford, Massachusetts, a small town of about 5,000 inhabitants some 50 miles west of Boston,[52] Joslin was a true "Yankee," although his ancestors came from France. The story has often been told, and is narrated in Arthur Miller's play *The Crucible*, that his great-great-great-great-great-grandmother was accused of being a witch in the frenetic Salem witch trial days and was sentenced to death; she was spared by the English governor, however, because she was pregnant. Her name was Proctor (Dr. Joslin's middle name), and in later years when he was awarded an honor in England, he told the story and thanked the British Crown for saving his life. A little known fact is that Dr. Joslin's mother had diabetes. In his *Diabetes Manual* (1959) he described her diabetes (case #8), found in 1900, adding, "Naturally I went to Strassburg to learn from Naunyn how to treat her."[53] She remained healthy for an additional 13 years.

From the very start of his practice, Dr. Joslin kept meticulous records and careful statistics. Salient points were noted and carefully recorded not only on the first visit but throughout the patient's life. Most of these were entered in large registers known as the "black books." For many years these data were transferred to cards and analyzed by the Statistical Bureau of the Metropolitan Life Insurance Company. In fact, each of his publications was replete with patient case numbers. In 1928 he stated: "Private statistics foreshadow future public statistics."[54]

Just after World War II, while a guest at a banquet, Joslin sat next to the Surgeon General of the U.S. Public Health Service and lamented that no one knew the prevalence of diabetes. He suggested that a study be done encompassing an entire town. Indeed, he had just such a town in mind: Oxford, Massachusetts, the site of his birth as well as that of Clara Barton, founder of the American Red Cross. Many years earlier he had made what was probably the first reference[55] to diabetes as a public health problem.

> In a country town in New England . . . on its peaceful, elm-lined Main Street, there once stood three houses, side by side, as commodious and attractive as any in the village. In these three houses lived in succession four women and three men—heads of families—and of this number, all but one has subsequently succumbed to diabetes. . . . Although six of the seven persons dwelling in these adjoining houses died from a single complaint, no one spoke of an epidemic. Contrast the activities of the local and state boards of health if these deaths had occurred from scarlet fever, typhoid fever or tuberculosis. Consider the measure which would have been adopted to discover the source of the outbreak and to prevent a recurrence. Because the disease was diabetes, and because the deaths occurred over a considerable interval of time, the fatalities passed unnoticed.

As a result of this interest, Dr. H. L. C. Wilkerson, a career health officer and a young physician, was sent by the U.S. Public Health Service to Joslin to learn about diabetes. He organized a study in Oxford, Massachusetts, a town of 4,983, and completed blood and urine glucose tests for 3,516 of the inhabitants (70.6%). He found that the prevalence of diabetes was about 4%, with almost one previously unknown case of diabetes for every known case.[56] This 4% prevalence has essentially been reaffirmed.[57] The study continued for almost 20 years and was the forerunner of the Framingham Heart Study.

New Approaches to the Treatment of Diabetes

Joslin was a highly organized person who not only was interested in his patients' health but found time to inquire into the details of their lives. He recognized the value of hospitalization in a hospital cottage dedicated to patient treatment and education. These cottages later evolved into the present-day Diabetes Treatment Unit, a sort of medical motel.

A very early and unique approach introduced by Joslin in management of the diabetic patient was the use of the "wandering" or "visiting nurse."[58] When younger patients were discharged to their homes, a nurse followed to aid families in using the new insulin.

Always a pioneer, Joslin appointed Priscilla White to his practice team "to study and care for children with diabetes."[59] This, in turn, prompted the initiation of camps for diabetic children in 1925. Later she gained experience with pregnancy and diabetes, for which she favored the emphasis as "pregnancy complicated by diabetes,"[60] not vice versa.

Education of persons with diabetes is considered one of the cornerstones of treatment. Here, Joslin led the way and so successfully that the concept is now accepted and educational programs are used throughout the world. He was so devoted to the idea of education that hospitalized patients were exposed to about 16 hours of teaching weekly.

The patient histories in the record room of the Joslin Diabetes Center have climbed towards 200,000, and Elliott P. Joslin's heritage passes the century mark. His influence is memorialized by a simple plaque on the wall of the Joslin auditorium presented by patients and staff of the New England Deaconess Hospital. The statement under his picture reads, "Gladly would he learn and gladly teach," and the last panel in the teaching unit tells it all: "This building given by thousands of patients and their friends provides an opportunity for many to control their diabetes by methods of teaching hitherto available to a privileged few."

ORAL HYPOGLYCEMIC AGENTS AND THE CONTROVERSY OVER DIABETIC CONTROL

Oral Hypoglycemic Agents

The sulfonylurea agents presented at least three new opportunities to the field of diabetes. These included greater access of insulin-fearing patients to physician care, particularly in the first 10 years following the availability of these agents; the addition of a new tool for the study of the action of insulin on non-insulin-dependent diabetes (NIDDM); and a new treatment option with first- and second-generation agents in use and a third generation of agents in preparation. The pharmacology of these agents is dealt with elsewhere (Chapter 29). In 1957, two years after the oral agents became available, a symposium on these agents was held at the New York Academy of Sciences. Dr. Rachmiel Levine encapsulated the past and predicted the future in the following excerpt from his concluding remarks.[61] "To me the most important aspect of the research in this field has been the stimulus it has provided to renewed work on the etiology of diabetes mellitus and on the synthesis of insulin, its storage, and the control of its release. We may say that, in addition to stimulating the B cells, the sulfonylureas have stimulated the investigators."

The Diabetic Control Controversy

Any history of diabetes since the discovery of insulin would be incomplete without a definition and explanation of the control and complications controversy (see Chapter 36). The first generation of physicians after the discovery of insulin, many of whom had nursed along dying patients during the decade before 1923, felt that tight control of diabetes by blood glucose and urine determinations was of paramount importance. In the 1920s, Dr. Joslin, having been interested in diabetes as long as any physician at that time, felt that the careful treatment of diabetes would lead to partial remission of the condition. He felt that restricted nutrition had been helpful in prolonging the life of some patients between 1915 and 1923 and that these dietary measures should be extended with modification to the insulin era. Many practitioners, however, felt that with the advent of insulin treatment, the diet could be greatly liberalized. Therefore, the diabetic "diet" became the target of debate in the earliest years of insulin use.

The founding members of the American Diabetes Association quickly became polarized on this issue. For instance, Dr. Joslin along with Dr. Ricketts of Chicago often faced off with Dr. Mosenthal and Dr. Tolstoi of New York City.[62] Indeed, about the time of the 25th anniversary of insulin, Dr. Tolstoi wrote a monograph that was a rallying cry for "purely symptomatic" care of diabetes.[63]

Some of the best summaries of this matter can be found in debates published in 1966[64] and 1974[65] entitled *Controversy in Internal Medicine*. The earlier dialogue on diabetes was titled "Are the Complications of Diabetes Preventable?" Dr. Alexander Marble of the Joslin Clinic and Harvard Medical School paired off with Dr. Philip Bondy of Yale Medical School. As usual, these discussions were energetic but inconclusive. All agreed this area would be aided by future prospective studies.

The considerations regarding the value of "loose" or "tight" control led to the development of a well-intended, but flawed, long-term prospective clinical trial with insulin, oral agents, and diet that was termed the University Group Diabetes Program (UGDP). The UGDP failed to show that improved control prevented or slowed the development of complications. In addition, it concluded that tolbutamide was associated with an increase in cardiovascular-related mortality. These findings caught the attention of the entire medical community in 1970 and were subsequently debated and discussed almost ad infinitum in the literature.[66,67] Although the UGDP study was a laudable attempt, if it were designed today, there is no doubt that the protocol would be quite different. However, since no effort has been made to repeat the study, the conclusions are largely ignored today, although the package inserts for the sulfonylureas state that they are to be used with some caution. Furthermore, despite this study, the Food and Drug Administration has made no attempt to ban or seriously restrict the use of the second generation of oral agents that emerged in the 1980s, consistent with the general feeling that sulfonylureas are of more benefit than potential harm.

A decade after the UGDP, the National Institute of Diabetes and Digestive and Kidney Diseases developed a plan for a study called the Diabetes Control and Complications Trial (DCCT).[68] In a sense, this is the third phase of the 40-year debate on the control of diabetes and its relationship to complications, but this trial has focused on insulin therapy only. The first analysis of this well-designed study on patients with Type I diabetes is scheduled for release in early 1994. It is hoped that the findings can help settle the issue on the importance of control of blood glucose levels.

THE CURRENT ERA

In an address published in 1960,[69] Dr. Charles Best considered diabetes since 1920 and tried to look ahead to possible future developments. When he gave the address, he was five years from retirement and had a distinguished career apart from his work on insulin.[70] He played a major role in the development of heparin and in extending the understanding of the function of choline in nutrition and was interested in the action of histamine. He had co-authored a physiology text used by several generations of medical students.

In this address, Best acknowledged the surge of work that the younger generation had produced in the post-insulin period. He praised by name those who had defined various metabolic and enzymatic pathways, and particularly admired work on the enzyme phosphorylase and the effects of glucagon and adrenalin. He also noted that in insulin deficiency the rate-limiting step in the uptake of glucose by muscle appears to be at the level of the "transporter" required to bring glucose into the cell, a transporter that would be defined at the molecular level more than 25 years later.

Advances in Diabetes Research (1960 to the Present)

Dr. Best would have been amazed and impressed by the remarkable amount of new information about the pathogenesis of diabetes and its complications that have been generated in the past 30 years. The following overview is provided to give readers a general sense of how knowledge has moved forward during this time. All of these subjects are covered in detail in various chapters of this textbook.

The development of the radioimmunoassay for insulin in 1960 led to important insights about insulin secretion and helped clarify some of the differences between IDDM and NIDDM.[71] The discovery that proinsulin was a biosynthetic precursor for insulin provided a fundamental insight into how cells process proteins and led the way to the useful radioimmunoassay for C-peptide. The insulin gene was cloned in 1977, which made human insulin available for clinical use and introduced diabetes research to the important new tools of molecular biology.

Important progress has also been made in understanding NIDDM. Although there has been interesting debate about the relative roles of insulin resistance and insulin deficiency, there is now general agreement that both are important. Insulin resistance is essential to the pathogenesis in most cases, and frank hyperglycemia does not develop unless β-cells fail to compensate. Furthermore, the contributions of a Western lifestyle (obesity and lack of exercise) to the development of NIDDM have been greatly clarified by epidemiologic and physiologic studies. The strong genetic contribution to its pathogenesis was clarified with the finding of a concordance rate of about 90% in identical twins. The specific genetic basis for most cases of NIDDM is not yet known, but the search for contributing genes has become very intense. Multiple mutations of the insulin receptor have been described, but these appear to account for only a small fraction of the cases of NIDDM. Likewise, a small number of individuals with NIDDM have been found to have mutations in one allele of the insulin gene. Recently, a substantial proportion of subjects with maturity-onset diabetes of the young (MODY) and a few with NIDDM have been found to have mutations of glucokinase, an enzyme that plays a key role in glucose recognition by β-cells.

Research in the biochemistry of intermediary metabolism has moved forward with great strides. Much has been learned about the insulin receptor: how it is phosphorylated and in turn promotes the phosphorylation of other substrates such as the insulin-receptor substrate 1. Glucose transport is much better understood now that the GLUT family of glucose transporters has been discovered. In particular, GLUT-2 has been found to be the major glucose transporter in liver and β-cells, and GLUT-4 is the key insulin-regulated transporter in muscle and adipose tissue.

Insulin sensitivity in vivo can now be measured using the insulin-glucose clamp technique or a modified intravenous glucose tolerance test. Furthermore, the flow of fuels in the states of fasting, feeding, diabetes, and exercise has been greatly clarified through the use of new techniques and a variety of isotopes. It has been possible to define precisely the relative roles of liver, brain, muscle, and adipose tissue. The important role of glucagon in carbohydrate and ketone metabolism was elucidated beautifully between 1970 and 1985. In addition, the counterregulatory responses to insulin-induced hypoglycemia in normal subjects and persons with diabetes have received intensive study. In particular, the important roles of glucagon and epinephrine in the defense against hypoglycemia in various types and stages of diabetes are now appreciated.

Much work has been carried out on the pathogenesis of the complications of diabetes. The contributions of glomerular hyperfiltration to the development of diabetic nephropathy are now partially understood. An understanding of the biochemical basis of neuropathy has also moved forward, with delineation of the contributions of the sorbitol pathway and myoinositol. Much work has also been done on the glycosylation of proteins, with particular recent attention to advanced glycosylation intermediates. A potential involvement of protein kinase C in the pathogenesis of diabetic retinopathy is also being explored. It is hoped that these biochemical studies will lead to new drugs that can prevent these damaging complications.

There have been great advances in the understanding of the pathogenesis of IDDM. The finding of a strong genetic linkage to the major histocompatibility antigens has provided important insight into the genetic basis of IDDM. Also, it is now well accepted that the autoimmune destruction of islets in IDDM is a chronic process that can smolder for many years before the development of frank hyperglycemia. Indeed, it is now possible to use markers such as antibodies to islet cells, antibodies to insulin, and impaired first-phase insulin secretion for predicting the development of diabetes. The finding that the progression of IDDM can be slowed with the immunosuppressive agent cyclosporine raises the hope that in the future IDDM may be prevented. There are excellent animal models of IDDM, the NOD mouse and the BB rat, which may help in the development of future therapeutic strategies.

Major insights into the cell biology of the islets of Langerhans have emerged. The molecular events that link glucose metabolism in β-cells to insulin secretion are now partially worked out. Evidence has been provided to support the concept that the loss of early glucose-induced insulin secretion in diabetes is secondary to the effects of chronic hyperglycemia on the β-cell. In addition, the interactions among the different cell types of the islet have been partially unraveled, with it now being accepted that glucose suppression of glucagon secretion is at least partially dependent upon intra-islet insulin release. Furthermore, many new insights into the growth and development of islets has emerged.

There have been important advances in the area of pancreas and islet transplantation. Pancreas transplantation went through a long experimental period but by 1990 had become a recognized therapeutic option. A pancreatic transplant is usually provided to individuals who also need a kidney transplant, with its required immunosuppression, and in about 75% of cases, recipients will be normoglycemic and off insulin one year later. Islet transplantation is still in an experimental stage, but there are now a few immunosuppressed recipients of isolated human islets who have not required insulin for over a year.

The New Classification of Diabetes

A major step in world recognition and confirmation of diabetes as a major health problem was the development of improved criteria for diagnosis or classification of the types of diabetes, particularly IDDM (Type I) and NIDDM (Type II), and various subtypes. The classification of diabetes started a decade before von Mering and Minkowski's work defining the role of the pancreas in the disease.[18] In 1877 Lancereaux, a student of Bouchardet, divided diabetes into a "lean" and a "fat" category.

During the pre- and post-insulin eras, various adjectives were used to classify and describe diabetes (Table 1–3), but by the mid-1970s these descriptions and the half dozen criteria used in diagnosing diabetes had become unworkable. The 1979 National Data Group Committee, with a wide assembly of epidemiologists and students of the disease, agreed upon our present system.[73,74] Although it was a compromise, it was accepted by the National Institutes of Health, the American Diabetes Association, the European Association for the Study of Diabetes, the International Diabetes Federation, and the World Health Organization (see Chapter 11 for up-to-date classification).

From a historical perspective, the 1979 classification "institutionalized" the concept that diabetes is fundamentally a disease governed by degrees of insulin sensitivity. Reaven noted in his 1988 Banting lecture, "The Role of Insulin Resistance in Human Disease," that the British investigator Himsworth should be credited with the initial formulation on the subject 50 years ago.[75] Prophetically, Himsworth stated: "Diabetes mellitus is a disease in which the essential lesion is a diminished ability of the tissues to utilize glucose . . . [this disease] is referable either to deficiency of insulin or to insensitivity to insulin, although it is possible that both factors may operate simultaneously."[76]

Table 1–3 Understanding Diabetes: A Century of Effort in Classifying the Disease (1880–1979)

Type I (insulin-dependent diabetes mellitus; IDDM)	
Pre-insulin era	Diabète maigre (lean)
	True diabetes (Naunyn) Asthenic/Unterdruk type
Insulin era	Juvenile-onset type
	(JODY = juvenile-onset diabetes of youth) Ketosis prone Brittle diabetes
Type II (non-insulin-dependent diabetes mellitus; NIDDM)	
Pre-insulin era	Diabète gras (big)
	Sthenic, Überdruk type
Insulin era	Adult-onset diabetes
	Maturity-onset type diabetes Ketosis-resistant diabetes Stable diabetes (MODY = maturity-onset diabetes of youth)
Other types	Secondary diabetes
(associated with conditions and pancreatic diseases, removal endocrinopathies, genetic syndromes)	Naunyn—"organic diabetes" . . . disease of the "diabetic organs" . . . liver, nervous system, thyroid
Gestational diabetes	Established firmly in 1964 (O'Sullivan and Mahan[72])

From Joslin et al.,[20] the National Diabetes Data Group,[73] and Fajans et al.[74]

The terms Type I and Type II diabetes quickly became accepted and used easily in the decade or more since their publication. Although communication with laymen and professional was enhanced, this simplistic terminology can overlook the complexity of the diabetic syndromes. The classic review by Fajan et al. in 1978 is a reminder of the marked syndrome variability that this disease can present to physician and researcher alike.[74]

New Milestones in Diabetes Management

The layman's role in developing concepts of diabetes management paralleled the evolution from a patient to a "consumer" role. Self-monitoring of blood glucose is both a significant advance in management and an important symbol of the role of the patient in treatment in the present decade. To be able to monitor blood glucose at will is a powerful tool that allows mastery by both patient and physician over the vagaries of diabetes management. It allows the patient to be in the pilot seat throughout a life with diabetes. No less important than the various intervention techniques such as laser treatment, arterial bypass operations, and advances in dialysis techniques, during 1972 a "rider" on another item of legislation passed by Congress stipulated that chronic renal failure was to be covered as a disability by Medicare.[77] This development removed treatment of diabetic kidney disease by dialysis or transplantation from a rationing system that was prevalent in most other countries. As a result, thousands of patients, a majority of them with IDDM and under the age of 40, have avoided almost certain death from chronic renal failure.

Another milestone was the development of the laser treatment for diabetic retinopathy, which followed earlier, much less successful, treatments such as pituitary ablation and the use of various drugs. Laser therapy moved rapidly from the research phase to acceptance and use. A long-term multicenter Diabetes Retinopathy Study (DRS) started in 1971 reached conclusions by 1975 that confirmed the value of laser therapy in preventing blindness.[78] Furthermore, the Early Treatment of Diabetic Retinopathy Study (ETDRS) was completed in 1990 and clearly showed that laser treatment could preserve vision in patients with macular edema (see Chapter 42).

Organizational Growth

The organization and mobilization of worldwide resources in the fight against diabetes by researchers, clinicians, and diabetic individuals themselves has been one of the most remarkable advances of the last several decades. In 1935 the British Diabetes Association was established. In 1937 a group of American physicians interested in diabetes met during a meeting of the American College of Physicians in New Orleans,[79] and after many discussions, started the American Diabetes Association (ADA) in 1941. The first meeting, held in Cleveland, Ohio, on June 1, 1941, was attended by about 300 physicians, who discussed the scientific aspects of diabetes. Dr. Cecil Striker of Cincinnati was the founder and first president. The ADA grew rapidly and suffered many growing pains; however, by 1960, there were over 25,000 members. The organization, which had started as a physicians-only group, recognized that its many goals could only be fulfilled by including lay persons, particularly those with diabetes and their families and friends, in the organization. In July 1964 the Board of Directors recommended this change, although it was years before the ADA became a truly voluntary health association.[62]

Vigorous growth has continued in many directions, and the ADA is now at the forefront of all issues relating to diabetes, with more than 9,000 professional members, 250,000 general members, and numerous affiliates throughout the United States. The ADA raises money for research, hosts meetings, publishes four journals, and is concerned with the well-being of those with diabetes. One of its major publications for the lay public is the journal *Diabetes Forecast*, which started with a circulation of 50,000 in 1948 and now has a worldwide circulation of 275,000.

The need for more emphasis on funding for research also spawned the Juvenile Diabetes Foundation, whose primary goal is the prevention and cure of juvenile diabetes through increased research. Indeed, since its founding, the Juvenile Diabetes Foundation has provided more than $100 million for diabetes-related research.

This same movement toward research and education was taking place in Europe, where the European Association for the Study of Diabetes was formed for that purpose. Its influence has grown remarkably, and its publication, *Diabetologia*, is respected throughout the world. Parallelling these developments is the organization by diabetes educators of the American Association of Diabetes Educators for training and certification in their field.

Since diabetes is a world problem, all nations—both developed and developing—now recognize the need for attention to the problem. In June 1949, at a meeting in an area much affected by World War II, the president of the Belgian Diabetic Association, Prof. J. P. Hoet, and his counterpart from England, Prof. R. D. Lawrence, and 75 other physicians and patients from 11 countries discussed their mutual problems. Meeting again in Amsterdam in 1950, they started the International Diabetes Federation (IDF)[80] with one lay delegate and one medical delegate from each country. The first congress of the new organization was held in Leiden, The Netherlands, in 1952. This initial meeting attracted 241 representatives from 20 countries, and the IDF has since held congresses triennially in Cambridge, U.K. (1955), Dusseldorf (1958), Geneva (1961), Toronto (1964), Stockholm (1967), Buenos Aires (1970), Brussels (1973), New Delhi (1976), Vienna (1979), Nairobi (1982), Madrid (1985), Sydney (1988), and Washington, D.C., under the auspices of the ADA (1991), and future congresses are planned for Kobe (1994) and Helsinki (1997).

The IDF is a confederation of some 85 world diabetes associations, the largest of which is the ADA. The international organization has developed many education and service programs worldwide, and its direction is moving increasingly toward the regions that need the most help. The coordination of activities with the World Health Organization (WHO), the health arm of the United Nations, is also vital. WHO can speak to governments while the IDF can muster the energies of academic and voluntary organizations. Together they are placing diabetes on the world agenda for action.

CONCLUSION

A few years ago, the president of the American Diabetes Association postulated in his valedictory address that the ADA might be better served by changing the name of the specialty to Endocrinology, Diabetes, and Metabolism.[81] The proposal marked, symbolically, the completion of the circle of thinking about diabetes in the past century. The study of diabetes emerged from questions about the metabolic basis of organ functions in digestion. Later, with the discovery of insulin, diabetes became the prime example of abnormal carbohydrate chemistry in humans and a major force in the rapid development of understanding of hormone interactions, i.e., endocrinology.

To understand metabolism and better treat diabetes and its related disorders today requires a demanding spectrum of knowledge about chemical, immunologic, vascular, and endocrinologic factors in humans, as well as a basic understanding of energy metabolism. Now, over 100 years since the work of Minkowski and von Mering, the knowledge required to understand this condition demands a comprehensive view of all that is known of the human normal and morbid state. Today, more than ever, "to know diabetes is to know medicine."

REFERENCES

1. Nuland SH. Why the leaves changed color in the autumn, surgery, science and John Hunter. In: Nuland SH. Doctors: the biography of medicine. New York: A Knopf, 1988:177–237.
2. Schadewaldt H. The history of diabetes mellitus. In: van Engelhardt D, ed. Diabetes: its medical and cultural history. Berlin: Springer Verlag, 1987:43–100.
3. Susruta Samhita (500 n. Chr.): BD.1–3, Calcutta 1907–16 (in reference 2).
4. Willis T. Pharmaceutica rationalis sive diatriba de medicamentorum operationibus in humano corpore. 2 vols. London 1674–5.
5. Dobson M. Experiments and observations on the urine in diabetes. In: Medical observations and inquiries by a society of physicians in London, Bd. 5, London 1776, S.298–316.
6. Cawley T. A singular case of diabetes, consisting entirely in the quality of the urine; with an inquiry into the different theories of that disease. London Med J 1788;9:286–308.
7. Rollo J. An account of two cases of the diabetes mellitus, with remarks as they arose during the progress of the cure. London: Dilly, 1797.
8. Chevreuil ME. Note sur le sucre de diabète. Ann Chim (Paris) 1815;95:319.
9. Benedict SR. A modification of the Lew-Benedict method for the determination of sugar in the blood. J Biol Chem 1918;34:203–7.
10. Folin O, Wu H. A system of blood analysis. J Biol Chem 1919;38:81–110.
11. Epstein AA. An accurate microchemical method of estimating sugar in the blood. JAMA 1914;63:1667–8.
12. Bernard C. Du suc pancréatique et de son rôle dans les phénomènes de la digestion. CR Soc Acad Sci (Paris 1850;1849:99–119.)
13. Bouchardat A. De la glycosurie ou diabète sucré. Paris, 1875.
14. Lancereaux E. Le diabète maigre: ses symptômes, son évolution, son pronostic et son traitement; ses rapports avec les altérations du pancréas. Union Med (Paris) 1880;29:161–8.
15. Langerhans P. Beitrage zur mikroskopischen Anatomie der Bauchspeicheldruse. Med Diss (Berlin), 1869.
16. Morrison H. Translation and introductory essay. Langerhans P. Contributions to the microscopic anatomy of the pancreas. Bull Inst Hist Med 1937;5:259–69.
17. Rosen G. The conservation of energy and the study of metabolism. In: Chandler McC, Brooks C, Cranefield PF, eds. The historical development of physiological thought. New York: Hafner Publishing Company, 1959:243–63.
18. Von Mering J, Minkowski O. Diabetes Mellitus nach Pankreasexstirpation. Zentralbl Klin Med 1889;10:393–4.
19. Laguesse E. Structure et développement du pancréas d'après les travaux récents. J Anat (Paris) 1894;30:591–608.
20. Joslin EP, Root H, White P, et al. The treatment of diabetes mellitus. 8th ed. Philadelphia: Lea & Febiger, 1946:312.
21. Paulesco NC. Action de l'extrait pancréatique injecté dans le sang, chez un animal diabétique. CR Soc Biol 1921;85:555–9.
22. Banting FG, Best CH. The internal secretion of the pancreas. Lab Clin Med 1922;7:251–66.
23. Banting FG, Best CH. Pancreatic extracts. J Lab Clin Med 1922;7:464–72.
24. Banting FG, Best CH, Collip JB, et al. Pancreatic extracts in the treatment of diabetes mellitus. Can Med Assoc J 1922;12:141–6.
25. Bliss M. The discovery of insulin. Chicago: University of Chicago Press, 1982.
26. Haycock P. History of insulin therapy. In: Schade DS, Santiago JV, Skyler JS, Rizza RA. Intensive insulin therapy. Princeton: Excerpta Medica, 1983:1–19.
27. Minkowski O. Historical development of the theory of pancreatic diabetes (introduction and translation by R. Levine). Diabetes 1989;38:1–6.
28. Lawrence RD. Hemochromatosis and complications of diabetes. In: 25th anniversary of the discovery of insulin. Physicians Bull 1947;7:34–35.
29. Houssay B. Memorable experiences in research. In: Banting and Best Research Institute inaugural dedication program, Toronto, 1952:31–32.
30. Cori CF. Enzymatic reactions in carbohydrate metabolism. Harvey Lectures 1945–46;41:253–72.
31. Krebs HA. The intermediate metabolism of carbohydrates. Lancet 1937;2:736–8.
32. Cushing H. The basophil adenomas of the pituitary body and their clinical manifestations (pituitary basophilism). Bull Johns Hopkins Hosp 1932;50–137.
33. Harvey AM. Classics in clinical science: the electrolytes in diabetic acidosis and Addison's disease. Am J Med 1980;68:322–24.
34. The American Diabetes Association. The physician's guide to type I diabetes (IDDM): diagnosis and treatment. Alexandria, VA: American Diabetes Association, 1988.
35. Colwell AR. The Banting memorial lecture 1968: fifty years of diabetes in perspective. Diabetes 1968;17;599–610.
36. Benedict FG, Joslin EP. The study of metabolism in severe diabetes. Washington, DC: Carnegie Institution of Washington, 1912:176.

37. Joslin EP. The treatment of diabetes, with observations upon the disease based upon one thousand cases. Philadelphia: Lea & Febiger, 1916.

38. Joslin E. A diabetic manual for mutual use of doctor and patient. Philadelphia: Lea & Febiger, 1918.

39. Joslin EP, Root HF, White P, Marble A. Diabetic coma. JAMA 1942;119:1160–5.

40. McKittrick LS, Root HF. Diabetic surgery. Philadelphia: Lea & Febiger, 1928.

41. Warren S. The pathology of diabetes mellitus. Philadelphia: Lea & Febiger, 1930.

42. White P. Diabetes in childhood and adolescence. Philadelphia: Lea & Febiger, 1932.

43. Root HF. The association of diabetes and tuberculosis: epidemiology, pathology, treatment and prognosis. N Engl J Med 1934;210:1–13.

44. Jordan WR. Neuritic manifestations in diabetes mellitus. Arch Intern Med 1936;57:307–66.

45. Waite JH, Beetham WP. The visual mechanism in diabetes mellitus: a comparative study of 2002 diabetics, and 457 non-diabetics for control. N Engl J Med 1935;212:429–43.

46. Kimmelstiel P, Wilson C. Intercapillary lesions in the glomeruli of the kidney. Am J Pathol 1936;12:83–97.

47. Bell ET. A postmortem study of vascular disease in diabetics. Arch Pathol 1952;53:444–55.

48. Beetham WP. Visual prognosis of proliferating diabetic retinopathy. Br J Ophthalmol 1963;611–9.

49. Aiello L, Beetham W, Balodimos, et al. Ruby laser photocoagulation in treatment of diabetic proliferating retinopathy: preliminary report. In: Symposium on the treatment of diabetic retinopathy. Airlie House Conference. Public Health Service publication no. 1890. Washington, DC: US Department of Health, Education and Welfare, 1968:437–63.

50. Marble A, Krall LP, Bradley RF, et al, eds. Joslin's diabetes mellitus. 12th ed. Philadelphia, Lea & Febiger, 1985:296.

51. Joslin EP. The treatment of diabetes mellitus, with observations based upon three thousand cases. 3rd ed. Philadelphia: Lea & Febiger, 1923.

52. Holt AC. Elliott Proctor Joslin: a memoir, 1869–1962. Worcester, MA: ASA Bartlett Press, 1969:1.

53. Joslin EP, Root HF, White P, Marble A. The treatment of diabetes mellitus. 10th ed. Philadelphia: Lea & Febiger, 1959.

54. Joslin EP. Preface. In: Treatment of diabetes mellitus. 4th ed. Philadelphia: Lea & Febiger, 1928.

55. Joslin EP. The prevention of diabetes mellitus. JAMA 1921;76:79–84.

56. Wilkerson HLC, Krall LP. Diabetes in a New England town: a study of 3,516 persons in Oxford, Mass. JAMA 1947;135:209–16.

57. Zimmet P, Dowse GK, Finch C. The epidemiology of NIDDM. IDF Bull 1990;35:3.

58. Joslin EP. The nurse and the diabetic. Boston, New England Deaconess Hospital, Annual Report, 1924.

59. Joslin EP. Annual report for Diabetes Foundation. In: Joslin archives, 1960:10.

60. White P. Pregnancy and diabetes. In: Marble A, White P, Bradley, RF, Krall LP, eds. Joslin's diabetes mellitus. 11th ed. Philadelphia: Lea & Febiger, 1971:584–93.

61. Levine R. Concluding remarks: the effects of the sulfonylureas and related compounds in experimental and clinical diabetes. Ann NY Acad Sci 1957;71:291.

62. The journey and the dream (a history of American Diabetes Association). Alexandria, VA: American Diabetes Association, 1990:16,57.

63. Tolstoi E. The practical management of diabetes. Springfield, IL: Thomas Publications, 1953.

64. Are the complications of diabetes preventable? In: Ingelfinger FJ, Relman AS, Finland M, eds. Controversy in internal medicine. Vol 1. Philadelphia: WB Saunders, 1966:489–514.

65. Management of adult-onset diabetes. In: Ingelfinger FJ, Ebert RV, Finland M, Relman AS, eds. Controversy in internal medicine II. Philadelphia: WB Saunders, 1974:387–417.

66. Prout TE. A Prospective view of the treatment of adult-onset diabetes: with special reference to the University Group diabetes program and oral hypoglycemic agents. Med Clin N Am 1971;55(4):1065–76.

67. Bradley RF. Oral hypoglycemic agents are worthwhile. In: Ingelfinger FJ, Ebert RV, Finland M, Relman AS, eds. Controversy in internal medicine II. Philadelphia: WB Saunders, 1974:408–15.

68. DCCT Research Group. Diabetes control and complications trial (DCCT) update. Diabetes Care 1990;13:427–33.

69. Best CH. Diabetes since nineteen hundred and twenty. Can Med Assoc J 1960;82:1061–6.

70. Marble A. Obituary: Charles Herbert Best 1899–1978. Diabetologia 1978;15:141–2.

71. Yalow RS. Remembrance project: origins of RIA. Endocrinology 1991;129:1694–5.

72. O'Sullivan JB, Mahan CM. Criteria for oral glucose tolerance test in pregnancy Diabetes 1964;13:278.

73. National Diabetes Data Group. Classification and diagnosis of diabetes mellitus and other categories of glucose intolerance. Diabetes 1979;28:1039–57.

74. Fajans SS, Cloutier MC, Crowther RL. Banting Memorial Lecture. Clinical and etiologic heterogeneity of idiopathic diabetes mellitus. Diabetes 1978;27:1112–25.

75. Reaven GM. Banting Memorial Lecture. Role of insulin resistance in human disease. Diabetes 1988;37:1595–607.

76. Himsworth HP. The Goulstonian lectures on the mechanism of diabetes mellitus. Lancet 1939;2:1,65,118,171.

77. U.S. Public Law 92–603 (1972). In: Evans RW, Blagg CR, Bryan FA. Implications for health care policy: a social and demographic profile of hemodialysis patients in the United States. JAMA 1981;245:487–91.

78. The Diabetic Retinopathy Study Research Group. Preliminary report on effects of photocoagulation therapy. The diabetic retinopathy study. Am J Ophthalmol 1976;81:383–96.

79. Striker C. The American Diabetes Association. Med Clin North Am 1947;31:483–7.

80. Krall LP. A prescription for world diabetes. In: Serrano-Rios M, Lefèbvre PJ, eds. Diabetes 1985. Amsterdam: Elsevier, 1986:3–24.

81. Colwell AR. President's address. Diabetes 1988;37:1449–52.

Chapter 2

ISLETS OF LANGERHANS: MORPHOLOGY AND ITS IMPLICATIONS

SUSAN BONNER-WEIR
FANNIE E. SMITH

The islets of Langerhans are clusters of endocrine tissue scattered throughout the exocrine pancreas in all vertebrates higher in evolutionary development than the bony fish (teleosts). In the adult mammal, the islets are 1 to 2% of the pancreatic mass and thus comprise around 1 g of tissue in the adult human. Islets are a complex mixture of cells and function both separately as micro-organs and in concert as the endocrine pancreas. Although the direct secretion of insulin and glucagon from islets into the portal vein has obvious advantages with respect to influence on hepatic function, it is not clear why the endocrine pancreas is dispersed throughout the exocrine pancreas. One suggestion is that the local insular-acinar portal system helps regulate the exocrine function of the pancreas, with this function providing some evolutionary advantage.[1]

The islet mass is dynamic, adjusting to meet the changing needs of the individual, whose size and level of activity vary at different stages of life. When the islet mass cannot adjust to meet the demand, diabetes results.

The pancreas of the adult human contains about 200 units, or 8 mg, of insulin[2] and that of the adult rat contains about 10 μg of insulin. The size of an islet can range from only a few cells and less than 40 μm in diameter to about 5000 cells and 400 μm in diameter. The average rat islet is 150 μm in diameter and contains about 45 ng of insulin. In the rat, and probably in other mammals, islets smaller than 160 μm in diameter represent 75% of the islets in number but only 15% of the islet volume, whereas islets larger than 250 μm in diameter represent only 15% of the islets in number but 60% of the islet volume.[3]

Although studies of the islets of nonmammalian vertebrates have been useful in extending our knowledge, we have a far more detailed understanding of the structure and function of mammalian islets. In a text on diabetes, the emphasis should be on the human islet, but our present understanding of islets is based mainly on rodent studies. Thus, the rodent islet will be used as the paradigm.

This chapter will first address the issues of islet development and growth and then define the cellular components of the islet and their organization. We now know that islets are not all the same, and this heterogeneity will be discussed. Finally, the manner in which the structural organization of an islet defines its function will be addressed.

PANCREATIC DEVELOPMENT

The pancreas is derived from outpocketings of endoderm from the primitive gut. There are two (sometimes three) pancreatic anlagen or primordia: a dorsal outpocketing of the gut opposite the developing liver and—after a short temporal lag—one or two (which quickly fuse into one) ventral buds from the base of the biliary floor of the gut.[4,5] The dorsal anlage, which gives rise to the splenic portion (tail and body) of the pancreas, fuses to various degrees with the ventral anlage(n), which give rise to the inferior aspect of the head or duodenal portion of the pancreas.

In mammals, 70 to 80% of the islet is insulin-producing β-cells; 5% is somatostatin-producing δ-cells, and 15 to 20% is either glucagon-producing α-cells or pancreatic polypeptide-producing PP cells. The origin of the pancreas as separate primordia is thought to be the basis of the regional distribution of glucagon-producing and pancreatic polypeptide-producing cells.[6] The dorsal pancreas, supplied with blood by the celiac trunk via the gastroduodenal and splenic arteries and drained by one main pancreatic duct, contains the glucagon-rich islets with few pancreatic polypeptide-containing cells. The opposite distribution is found in the ventral pancreas, which is supplied with blood from the superior mesenteric artery via the inferior pancreaticoduodenal artery and is drained by a separate exocrine duct. Here the islets contain pancreatic polypeptide-producing cells and few, if any, glucagon-producing cells. The degree of fusion of these ducts differs among species.

The question of whether pancreatic endocrine and exocrine cells have the same origin has been debated for many years. The APUD (amine precursor uptake and decarboxylation) concept of Pearse and Polak, which unifies the neuroendocrine system, led to the proposal that whereas the exocrine pancreas is endodermal in origin the islet cells are of neural crest origin.[7] However, in the late 1970s, elegant experiments in which the neuroectoderm was extirpated (rat)[8] or transplanted (using the quail-chick chimera marking system)[9,10] excluded a neuroectodermal origin for any of the four types of islet cells. The strongest evidence was from experiments in which the chimeric embryos were constructed before the neural crest had migrated, i.e., at the early neurula stage, by associating neuroectoderm of quail with endomesoderm of chick. The enteric ganglia of these embryos were of quail origin, but all the endocrine cells of the gut and pancreas were of chick origin.[9,11]

More recently, three lines of evidence again were used to suggest a neural origin of islet cells. The first was evidence of the presence of tyrosine hydroxylase, the first enzyme in the biogenic amine synthetic pathway, in 10 to 40% of the glucagon-staining cells at days 12 to 14 of fetal development.[12] The second was the finding that transgenic mice with the SV40 large T antigen linked to the insulin gene promoter transiently expressed the T antigen in the neural crest, the neural tube, and in pancreatic cells before they expressed insulin.[13] Teitelman and her co-workers suggested that these two lines of evidence implied a common ontogenic origin of nerves and islets.

However, another plausible explanation, as the authors acknowledged, is that the transgene may have been inappropriately expressed because of the absence of a negative regulatory element, a "silencer," identified further upstream than any of the constructs used. The third line of evidence is the localization by immunochemical means of a transcription factor, isl-1, which binds to the enhancer region of the insulin gene, in all polypeptide-secreting endocrine cells, the autonomic nervous system, and two primitive nuclei of the brain,[14,15] a finding that reveals yet another similarity between the developmental patterns of islets and nerves. All three of these lines of evidence are based on the commonality of gene expression in islets and nerves. However, such a commonality does not give definitive evidence of a common cell lineage.[16] Instead, the modular nature of transcription factor complexes[17] is conducive to a recurrence of certain patterns of gene expression such as that seen in islets and nerves and could have little to do with embryonic origin.

Islets differentiate from the pancreatic ductal epithelium as do exocrine cells, but the question of whether they are derived from the same or different precursor/stem cell populations remains unanswered. Embryonic development of the pancreas as ductules that proliferate, branch, and then differentiate was described by Pictet and Rutter.[4] Islet hormone-containing cells are first seen as single cells among the exocrine cells of the terminal pancreatic tubules and then as clusters of cells within the exocrine basement membrane. These clusters then become separated from the exocrine tissue to form distinct islets.[4] In the adult pancreas, sometimes the only separation between exocrine and islet cells are their respective basement membranes (Fig. 2–1). However, islets are usually surrounded by at least a partial capsule of fibroblasts and collagen fibers.

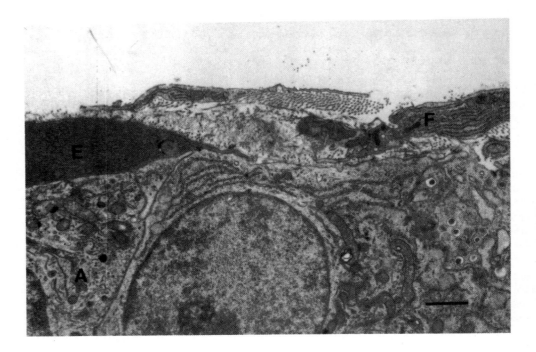

Fig. 2–1. The periphery of a rat islet showing the capsule of a single layer of fibroblasts (F) and collagen fibers laid down by these cells. No capsule is seen between the exocrine cell (E) and the endocrine α-cell (A); the capsule often incompletely surrounds the islet. Scale bar = 1 μm.

Pancreatic development can occur in culture if either mesenchymal tissue or extract is included with rat pancreas explant or if older fetal (day 17 or later) tissue is used.[18] The factors involved in this differentiation are still unknown. In the pancreas of adults of many species, islet cells of all types can be immunolocalized in the pancreatic ducts as occasional single cells or small budding islets. An increased occurrence of these cells has been observed under numerous experimental conditions, including dietary treatment with soybean trypsin inhibitor,[19] overexpression of interferon-γ in the β-cells of transgenic mice,[20] after partial pancreatectomy[21] and after cellophane wrapping of the head of the pancreas[22] and with some human diseases, including recent-onset Type I diabetes (insulin-dependent)[23] and severe liver disease. Adult ductal epithelium can be stimulated to undergo morphogenic changes that result in a substantial formation of new islets. When adult ductal epithelium was wrapped in fetal mesenchyme and implanted in nude mice, about 20% of the grafts resulted in the budding of "islet-like cell clusters" from the ducts, and islet hormone immunostaining was recently shown in these cells.[24,25] In the young adult rat, 3 days after a 90% pancreatectomy 10 to 15% of the pancreatic remnant volume is composed of proliferating ductules, which differentiate into new islets and exocrine tissue within another 3 to 4 days.[21]

Molecular biology may provide clues to the factors involved in the tissue-specific gene expression of these differentiated cells. A number of transcription factors that bind to the insulin gene have been identified,[14,26,27] but it is still unclear what factors determine the differences between β-cells and other neighboring cells of endodermal origin, such as α-cells, exocrine cells, or even liver cells. Intriguing data regarding differentiation come from the finding that adult rats depleted of copper show a resultant destruction of acinar tissue but retain "normal islets and ducts" and that after copper repletion the animals show a transdifferentiation, i.e., the regenerating cells in the pancreas are hepatocytes rather than exocrine cells.[28] These data show that the differentiation process can be reprogrammed.

The different islet cells do not have the same pattern of growth. Embryologically, the α-cells develop before the others, appearing in the dorsal pancreatic bud as it forms. Shortly thereafter, β- and PP-cells are seen budding from the exocrine tubules; these are followed by the δ-cells and gastrin immunoreactive cells.[29] The normal organization of the islet, with its central core of β-cells and its peripheral non-β-cells, is observed only after fetal day 18.5.[30] The proportions of the different cell types differ with age; the functional significance of these changes is unclear. For example, in the rat and human, the percentage of islet cells that are δ-cells is considerably greater in perinatal than in adult individuals.[31]

This schema may need to be reexamined because of recent evidence that developing islet cells coexpress more than one islet hormone. Such coexpression was first reported for single cell clones of a transplantable tumor cell line (MSL). These clones simultaneously expressed insulin, glucagon, somatostatin, and cholecystokinin (CCK).[32] When insulin was first detectable in fetal rat[30] and fetal mouse,[13] all insulin-immunoreactive cells also contained glucagon immunoreactivity. Four days later only 15 to 20% of the insulin-immunoreactive cells also had glucagon immunoreactivity. A similar overlap of insulin with either somatostatin or pancreatic polypeptide was observed at later times.[13] Teitelman and co-workers suggested a multistage maturation of islet cell: the progenitor cells first show tyrosine hydroxylase activity; then glucagon expression, which is followed in some cases by the additional expression of insulin; in turn the eventual segregation of populations of cells producing either glucagon or insulin; a repeat of the overlap of hormone expression of insulin first with somatostatin and then pancreatic polypeptide; and eventually four separate islet cell types. The appearance of tyrosine hydroxylase in these developing islet cells, which was reported in the fetal mouse,[13] was not seen in fetal rats.[30] Another interesting facet of the sequential differentiation of the mature islet cells is the ability of the MSL cell line to produce glucagon in vitro but insulin in vivo.[33] Our understanding of this complex process of differentiation of the islet cells is still at a primitive stage.

PHYLOGENETIC CONSIDERATIONS

The comparative aspects of the endocrine pancreas was the focus of much study in the 1970s.[34-37] The first step in the development of a separate islet organ is found in the vertebrate class Agnatha, the primitive jawless fish (represented today by hagfish and lampreys). In the hagfish all of the β-cells and most of the δ-cells are no longer in the gut mucosa and are restricted to the bile duct and adjacent islet organ whereas the glucagon/gastrin-producing cells remain in the gut mucosa.[34] The first appearance of a pancreas with all β-, α-, δ-, and PP-cells is in the cartilaginous fish (class Chrondrichthyes), in which the islet cells are found in the parenchyma, in the pancreatic ducts, or disseminated in the exocrine pancreas.[34,38] The bony fish (class Osteichthyes) have large accumulations of endocrine tissue, sometimes called the Brockmann bodies, near the spleen and pylorus and in addition have small islets scattered throughout the exocrine tissue, often in association with small ducts. The descriptions of islets in amphibians and reptiles are widely variant, but there seems to be a pattern of three types of islets: large splenic islets with the α-cell population greater than the β-cell population, islets of intermediate size with more β-cells but still a majority of α-cells, and small islets with mostly β-cells. This heterogeneity of islets has been better defined for the birds (class Aves): dark or α islets are composed of α- and δ-cells, and light or β islets are composed of β- and δ-cells. (PP-cells are often extrainsular.) In this class, as in mammals, there is a regional distribution of islet types with an embryologic derivation.

ISLET GROWTH

Islet mass increases considerably from the embryo to the adult, but the volume of islet tissue relative to that of the pancreas decreases from birth to adulthood. In newborn humans, islets comprise 20% of the pancreatic tissue; in children (1.5 to 11 years), 7.5%; and in adults, 1%.[39] Similar data have been reported for cattle[40] and rats.[41] These relative values can be misleading, for by adulthood the islet mass has grown and increased about fivefold from that at birth; only its relative amount decreases, as the exocrine tissue increases about 15-fold in the same time period. Thus, the growth of islet tissue is diluted by the more exuberant postnatal growth of the exocrine tissue.

The increase in islet mass is achieved by 1) neogenesis or neoformation of islet cells budding from ductules; 2) enlargement of individual cells; and 3) replication of existing islet cells. Neogenesis is responsible for most of the islet growth during the fetal and perinatal stages. In the adult, neogenesis is seen (discussed above), but the extent of its contribution to growth of the islet mass is unclear. Enlargement of individual cells with increased age or activity has been reported,[42] but there has been no estimate of the contribution of this growth to the islet mass. Replication of existing islet cells occurs late in fetal development and has been thought to be the principal means by which islet mass increases mass after birth.[42]

Studies of the growth of islet cells have utilized intact animals as well as cultured islet cells. Isolated rat islets synchronized in culture by temporary exposure to hydroxyurea were found to have a cell cycle of 14.9 hours. This cell cycle has been assumed to reflect that of the β-cell, the predominant cell of the islet.[43] The length of the cell cycle does not change with glucose stimulation or with the age of the animals whose islets are used.[43,44] Instead the growth rate is regulated by the number of β-cells that can enter the division phase (G1) from the resting (Go) phase. The size of this proliferative pool varies with age and stimulus, being 10% per 24 hours perinatally and only 3% per 24 hours in the adult. The accuracy of determinations of β-cell replication made by measuring the incorporation of thymidine in whole islets has been questioned, since nonendocrine cells found in islets incorporate thymidine at a far greater rate than do islet endocrine cells.[45] Only with nuclear labeling of insulin-immunostained cells can β-cell replication be measured accurately.

The growth capacity of the β-cell depends on the stimulus and the ability of the cell to recognize the stimulus as well as on the number of β-cells that can enter the cell cycle and undergo mitosis. There is an increased incidence of polyploid β-cells in the diabetic human, mouse, and rat, an increase that may reflect the inability of some cells to complete mitosis after entering the proliferative pool.[46,47]

Although there may be numerous stimuli for β-cell growth, three major stimuli are known. Glucose is a stimulus both in vivo and in vitro. As early as 1938, Woerner reported an increase in islet tissue in guinea pigs after continuous glucose infusions.[48] Such an increase has since been confirmed by several other studies.[49-53] Glucose has been shown to stimulate modest growth of either neonatal or adult pancreatic β-cells in culture.[54-56] Pregnancy has been shown to cause both increased replication and mass of β-cells.[57-61] As a parallel finding, in vitro studies have shown that prolactin, placental lactogen, and growth hormone can stimulate replication of β-cells.[56,62,63] A neural stimulus or perhaps a neural inhibitor has been suggested by the increase in islet mass after a ventromedial hypothalamic (VMH) lesion.[64] In addition to these stimuli, there may be a complex orchestration of as yet unidentified factors. As a means of identifying some of these, peptide growth factors have been studied in islet cultures. The most commonly tested factor has been insulin-like growth factor I (IGF-I), but results have varied.[56,63,65] None of the factors studied so far have produced marked stimulation of replication in vitro, but the importance of their contribution to growth and development should not be discounted. Small increases that continue over time may have a significant impact.

Because normally few mitotic figures are seen in adult islets and the rate of DNA replication is low, it has been thought that their capacity for β-cell growth or regeneration is limited. However, even at the low replicative level of 3% per day, the number of β-cells could double in 30 days if cell death is not appreciable.[42] In fact, the β-cell mass in the adult rat does double between the ages of 6 and 10 weeks. In addition, substantial β-cell growth has been shown in vivo in several animal models.[50,66,67] For example, after only 96 hours of glucose infusion, the β-cell mass in adult rats was selectively increased 50%; both hypertrophy of individual β-cells and hyperplasia contributed to this rapid and extensive increase of mass.[50] We must assume that the apparently low level of normal β-cell growth in the adult is all that is needed to counterbalance cell loss and to accommodate functional challenges. Diabetes results only if increased cell loss or functional demands cannot be met. This concept also points out our ignorance concerning the life span of the β-cell and what influences it. Does the turnover rate of the β-cell change? Does a differentiated β-cell have a finite ability to enter the cell cycle? If this ability is limited, a pancreas "under stress" ultimately may need to rely on its neogenic (e.g., new cells from ducts) rather than on its replicative (e.g., division of pre-existing β-cells) capabilities.

COMPONENTS OF THE ISLETS OF LANGERHANS

Endocrine Cells

There are four major endocrine cell types in mammalian islets: the insulin-producing β-cell, the glucagon-producing α-cell, the somatostatin-producing δ-cell, and the pancreatic polypeptide-producing PP-cell. (The latter three will be referred to collectively as the non-β-cells) (Fig. 2–2). Ultrastructural and immunocytochemical techniques are used to distinguish these cell types and have identified other minor cell types (Table 2–1). Numerous other peptides and hormones have been localized to the islet cells with the use of sensitive immunostaining techniques (Table 2–1). Localization of several of these peptides is confusing because the type of cells immunostained varies with species. For example, calcitonin gene-related peptide (CGRP) colocalizes with somatostatin in the rat δ-cell but with insulin in mouse β-cells.[68] Similarly, an antibody to pancreastatin stains

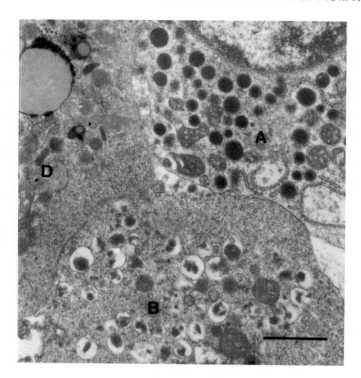

Fig. 2–2. The secretory granules of the islet endocrine cells have a characteristic morphology. Represented here are those of the β-cell (B), the α-cell (A), and the δ-cell (D) of a human islet. Scale bar = 1 μm.

α- and δ-cells in humans but β- and δ-cells in pigs.[69,70] An additional level of complexity is introduced by evidence that the hormones thyrotropin-releasing hormone (TRH) and gastrin are expressed in the islets but only during the perinatal period.[71,72] It is presently unclear how any of these other hormones/peptides function in the islet. The sensitivity of the techniques and the overlap of antibody recognition may be responsible for some of the confusing data. Another explanation for the overlap may be the sequential differentiation of the islet cell types, as discussed above. Another interesting example is islet

amyloid polypeptide (IAPP/amylin), which has been colocalized in the insulin granules.[73] Recent data showed that the occasional strongly stained cells in neonatal islet cultures stimulated with growth hormone were not immunoreactive for insulin but rather for glucagon or somatostatin (but the insulin-stained cells were weakly stained for IAPP/amylin).[74] Perhaps this confusion will be clarified as our knowledge of the regulation of differential gene expression is expanded.

The β-cells are polyhedral, being truncated pyramids, and are usually well granulated with secretory granules 250 to 300 nm in diameter (Fig. 2–3). It has been estimated that each rat β-cell contains about 10,000 granules.[75] There are two forms of insulin granules: mature granules that have an electron-dense core and a loosely fitting granule-limiting membrane with the appearance of a spacious halo; and immature granules with little or no halo, moderately electron-dense contents, and a clathrin coat. Immature granules have been shown to be the major, if not the only, site of conversion from proinsulin to insulin.[76] Other changes, such as the shedding of the clathrin coat, acidification of the granule contents, and crystallization of insulin, occur as the granule matures from a proinsulin-rich granule to an insulin-rich granule.[76] In some species the electron-dense core of the mature granule is visibly crystalline. Insulin is not the only peptide in the granules; in addition to the IAPP/amylin mentioned above, there are at least 100 other peptides.[77]

The α-cells are usually smaller and more columnar than the β-cells and well granulated with granules 200 to 250 nm in diameter (Fig. 2–2). The granules are electron dense with a narrow halo of less-dense material and a tightly fitting granule-limiting membrane; there is little species variation.

The δ-cells are usually smaller than either α- or β-cells, are well granulated, and are often dendritic in shape. Within a δ-cell the electron density of granules varies greatly (Fig. 2–2). Each granule, 200 to 250 nm in diameter, contains material of homogenous moderate density that fills the granule-limiting membrane.

PP-cells are the most variable among species. In humans the granules are elongated, very electron dense, and 120 to 160 nm in diameter. In dogs and cats the

Table 2–1.   Characteristcs of the Endocrine Cells of the Islets of Langerhans*

Cell type	Size of secretory granule (nm)	Percentage of islet cells	Hormonal content
β	250–350	60–80	Insulin (thyrotropin-releasing hormone, calcitonin gene-related peptide, IAPP/amylin, pancreastatin, 7B2 [novel protein], prolactin)
α	200–250	15–20	Glucagon (glicentin, TRH, CCK, endorphin, glucagon-like polypeptide-1, peptide YY, DKP histidyl-proline diketopiperazine, 7B2, pancreastatin)
δ	300–350 200–300	5–10	Somatostatin (met-enkephalin, CGRP, pancreastatin)
PP	120–160	15–20	Pancreatic polypeptide (met-enkephalin, PYY, 7B2)
δ₁	100–130	<1	Vasoactive intestinal polypeptide
EC	300–350	<1	Substance P, serotonin
G₁	300	<1	Gastrin (adrenocorticotropic hormone-related peptides)

*The secretory granules of each cell type have a characteristic size and morphology. The size of δ-cell secretory granules varies with species; hormonal content identified by immunostaining techniques; Peptides in parentheses found in at least one species. Some of these peptides, e.g., TRH and gastrin, are usually found only in perinatal islets. The physiologic significance of the islet location is unclear.

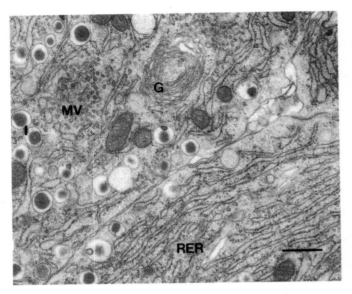

Fig. 2-3. The protein machinery of the insulin producing β-cell of a rat islet shown in three adjacent cells. RER = rough endoplasmic reticulum; MV = microvesicles; G = Golgi apparatus; I = insulin secretory granules. Scale bar = 0.5 μm.

granules are spherical, variable in electron density, and about 300 nm in diameter.[78]

Capsule

The existence of an islet capsule has been a controversial issue, perhaps because the capsule is a single layer of fibroblasts and the collagen fibers laid down by these fibroblasts (Fig. 2-1). Furthermore, frequently the capsule is absent between islet and exocrine cells. The extant capsule does overlay the efferent blood vessels of the islet and seems to define a subcapsular interstitial space.

Microvasculature

The islet is highly vascularized and has a direct arteriolar blood supply.[79] Islet capillaries are fenestrated, whereas fenestration is decreased or absent in capillaries in the surrounding exocrine tissue.[80] The fenestrae render these capillaries highly permeable. The passage of horseradish peroxidase into the pericapillary interstitial space of the islet takes only 45 seconds, whereas it takes 5 minutes in cardiac muscle.[81] The blood flow to the islets has been found to be disproportionately large (10 to 20% of the pancreatic blood flow) for the 1 to 2% of pancreatic volume.[82-85] Factors regulating islet blood flow may affect islet hormone secretion. High concentrations of glucose have been shown to enhance pancreatic blood flow and to preferentially increase islet blood flow.[86] In addition, several of the peptides immunochemically localized in islet nerves and/or endocrine cells, e.g., CGRP, are vasoactive.[87] The relation of the microvasculature to islet endocrine cells is discussed below. Lymphatic vessels, while common in the pancreas, have not been found within the islets.[88]

Nerves

The pancreas is innervated by sympathetic fibers from the celiac ganglion and by parasympathetic fibers from the vagus nerve.[89-91] These parasympathetic fibers synapse in small ganglia dispersed in the pancreas. They may act as pacemakers for the oscillations in hormone levels[92] that occur without extrinsic nervous connections, as in the isolated perfused canine pancreas.[93]

Within the pancreas, nerve fibers terminate in perivascular, periacinar, and perinsular areas. Within the islets, the nerves follow the blood vessels and terminate within the pericapillary space, within the capillary basement membrane, or closely apposed to the endocrine cells. Because no specialized synapses are found, it has been suggested that neurotransmitters released into the interstitial space may affect a number of neighboring islet cells. In some species, nerve cell bodies are close to or even within the islets.[91]

The distribution and number of the different types of nerve fibers differs among species.[89-91] Cholinergic nerves, as identified histochemically by cholinesterase activity or ultrastructurally by the presence of electron-lucent vesicles, are common in rat, cat, and rabbit islets. Adrenergic nerves, as identified immunochemically by antibodies to catecholamine-forming enzymes (including tyrosine hydroxylase)[91] and ultrastructurally by the presence of dense cored vesicles, are common in the hamster, dog, and cat. Peptidergic nerves are less well defined, being identified either immunochemically as containing substance P, enkephalin, vasoactive intestinal polypeptide (VIP), galanin, gastrin-releasing peptide, CGRP, or CCK or ultrastructurally by the presence of large granules. A further complication is introduced by the finding of neuropeptide Y and galanin in adrenergic nerves and the identification of VIP in cholinergic nerves.[94] Both substance P and CGRP seem to be localized in the sensory fibers. The presence of peptide-containing cell bodies in the pancreatic ganglia suggests that some of these peptidergic nerves are intrinsic to the pancreas and thus may be involved in the synchronization of islet secretion.[91]

The autonomic nervous system modulates islet hormone secretion.[89,91,95] Cholinergic stimulation elicits increased insulin, glucagon, and pancreatic polypeptide secretion. Its effects on somatostatin are less clear but appear to be inhibitory. β-Adrenergic stimulation similarly elicits increased secretion of insulin, glucagon, pancreatic polypeptide, and somatostatin.[96] α-Adrenergic stimulation decreases secretion of insulin and somatostatin, but its effects on glucagon secretion varies with species. The effects of α-adrenergic stimulation on secretion of pancreatic polypeptide are unknown.[96] The effects of stimulation of peptidergic nerves have not been studied as closely, but VIP, CCK, and galanin can affect islet cell secretion.

In the human and the rat, VIP neurons form a peri-insular network.[97] However, the relation of this network to the islet vasculature is uncertain. Therefore, it remains unknown whether these nerves influence islet secretions directly or indirectly via changes in the islet blood flow. To date the relationships among the various types of nerves and the other islet components have not been well defined.

ORGANIZATION OF THE COMPONENTS OF THE ISLETS OF LANGERHANS

The distribution of the endocrine cells is nonrandom, with a core of β-cells surrounded by a discontinuous mantle of non-β-cells 1 to 3 cells thick.[98,99] The islets of most mammalian species have this pattern, but those of human and other primates have a somewhat more complex pattern (Fig. 2−4). Sections of human pancreas show many different islet profiles, including oval and cloverleaf patterns, differences that have resulted in controversy about whether they actually have a mantle-core arrangement.[99−101] Nonetheless, in three dimensions, human islets can be considered as composites of several mantle-core subunits or as lobulated with mantle-core lobules.[99,101] In sectioned tissue, incomplete fusion of such subunits and penetrations of islet vasculature can appear as invaginations of the islet periphery. Most of the non-β-cells are found along these invaginations and the periphery,[99,100] thus maintaining a mantle-core arrangement. A new technique, confocal microscopy, allows a better appreciation of the three-dimensional organization of islet cells.[102] With confocal microscopy, α-cells are seen as a sheet or a peel at the islet periphery and δ-cells are seen as more peripheral to the α-cells in the human but less peripheral in the rat. This pattern of organization is based on intrinsic qualities of the cell surfaces of the different cell types, as shown by recent reaggregation studies. When single dispersed rat islet cells were allowed to reaggregate, the aggregates showed the same nonrandom organization as native islets, even when the proportions of β-cells and non-β-cells were reversed.[103] Both β-cells and non-β-cells have high levels of calcium-dependent cell-adhesion molecules (cadherins), but non-β-cells also contain calcium-independent cell-adhesion molecules.[104] It is thought that this differential expression of cell-adhesion molecules may be responsible for the segregation of β-cells and non-β-cells.

The microvasculature forms the infrastructure of an islet. The rat islet has been studied most extensively and will serve as the prototype in this discussion, but this generalization needs to be verified. Afferent vessels to an islet are 1 to 3 arterioles, depending on islet size. Each arteriole penetrates the islet though discontinuities of the non-β-cell mantle and enters directly into the β-cell core, where it branches into a number of fenestrated capillaries.[3] These capillaries follow a tortuous path, passing first through the β-cell core and then through the non-β-cell mantle. Often the vessels pass along the inside of the mantle before penetrating it. The efferent vessels are collecting or postcapillary venules. It is unclear where the transition from capillary to collecting venule occurs, but collecting venules can often be seen in indentations of the islet. The evidence is for a single continuous circulation through the islet. Although each capillary should have functionally different arterial and venous portions, no morphologic differences have yet been found.

The pattern of microvasculature varies, depending on islet size (Fig. 2−5). In large islets the efferent vessels coalesce into collecting venules within the subcapsular space. In small islets the efferent capillaries extend into the exocrine tissue for 50 to 100 μm before coalescing into collecting venules. Within the islet, endocrine cells are organized around the microvasculature (Fig. 2−6). In the rat the β-cells have been found to have two faces on capillaries.[105] In cross-section 8 to 10 β-cells are seen to form a rosette around one of the capillaries. In three dimensions this pattern would be tubelike. The outer face of each β-cell would be against a capillary, which is probably arterial and is usually not in cross-section. In β-cells experimentally degranulated with glyburide, the remaining granules are polarized toward the central "venous" capillary, suggesting an in situ polarity of the β-cells. Along the interface of three or more β-cells and extending from capillary face to capillary face are elaborate canaliculi.[106] Desmosomes that act as mechanical attachments are preferentially found near these canaliculi. These canaliculi contain large numbers of

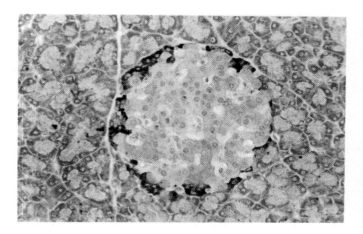
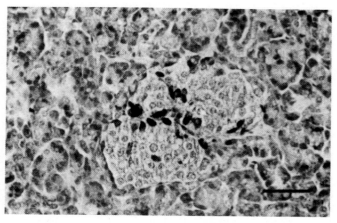

Fig. 2−4. The pattern of a mantle of non-β-cells (the glucagon-, somatostatin-, and pancreatic polypeptide-producing cells) around a core of insulin-producing β-cells is seen in the rat (left panel) and in the human (right panel) with immunostaining of the non-β-cells. Human islets can be considered composites of several subunits and those of the rat, only one subunit. Scale bar = 50 μm.

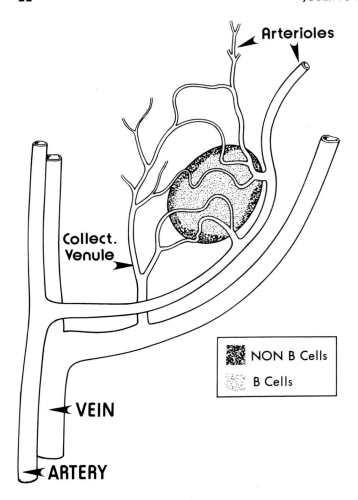

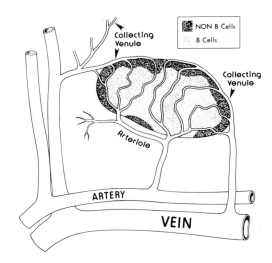

Fig. 2–5. Diagrams of the microvasculature of the rat islet based on corrosion casts and serial reconstructions of immuno-stained paraffin sections. In both small (left) and large (right) islets the efferent arteriole enters the islet in a gap or discontinuity of the non-β-cell mantle, such that it enters the β-cell core directly, where it breaks into a number of capillaries. These capillaries (fewer are drawn for diagrammatic purposes) traverse the β-cell core before passing along and through the non-β-cell mantle. In the small islets, the efferent capillaries pass 50 to 100 μm before coalescing into collecting venules, thus providing an insuloacinar portal system. However, in the large islets the efferent capillaries coalesce into collecting venules at the edge of the islet, even within the capsule. Thus, the drainage of large islets is directly into the venous system without passage through the exocrine tissue. Reprinted with permission from the American Diabetes Association from reference 3 (Bonner-Weir S, Orci L. New perspectives on the microvasculature of the Islets of Langerhans in the rat. Diabetes 1982;31:883–9).

microvilli,[106,107] which have been found to be enriched in the recently described β-cell glucose transporter (GLUT-2).[108] The presence of these elaborate structures suggests a bulk flow of interstitial fluid through these canaliculi in an arterial to venous direction and an uptake of glucose by the β-cells that is carried out mainly by the transporters on these microvilli. Thus, these canaliculi may serve as the initial interface for glucose sensing by the β-cell. Insulin secretory granules appear to be released from the lateral and apical surfaces to enter the venous (central) capillaries.

HETEROGENEITY WITHIN THE ISLETS

We now realize that the islets within one pancreas are not all alike. Islets differ in cellular composition. There is a regional distribution of the glucagon-producing α-cell and the pancreatic polypeptide-producing PP-cell that is based on the embryologic derivation of the pancreas from distinct anlage.[6] Thus, the splenic or dorsal portion (the tail, body, and superior part of the head) is glucagon-poor and pancreatic polypeptide-rich, while the duodenal or ventral portion (most of the head—sometimes designated as the uncinate process) of the pancreas is

glucagon-poor and pancreatic polypeptide-rich. Physiologic data from either islets or perfusion of regions of the pancreas suggest that islets from different regions function differently, with the splenic islets releasing more insulin than the duodenal islets in response to glucose.[109,110]

The different vascular relation to the exocrine tissue of islets of difference size was mentioned above.[3] Large islets (those >250 μm in diameter) are selectively located near the larger ducts and blood vessels. Their efferent vessels coalesce within the islet capsule; thus, they probably have little effect on surrounding exocrine tissue. However, the vascular pattern of the small islets and their abundance would lead to an effective insuloacinar portal system.

Another level of heterogeneity is indicated by the increasing evidence that not all β-cells within an islet are identical. Older physiologic data from studies of isolated islets suggested different sensitivities for insulin response.[111,112] More recently, work on single islet cells has shown that individual β-cells have different thresholds for glucose-induced insulin release. Thus, with increasing concentrations of glucose, more β-cells are recruited in the response.[113,114] This cellular heterogeneity has been

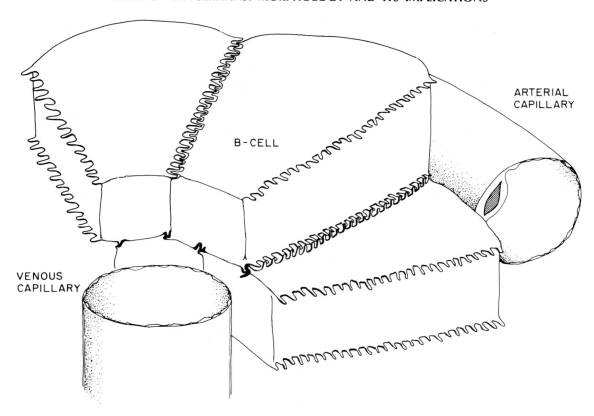

Fig. 2–6. Diagram of the intraislet arrangement of pancreatic β-cells. β-Cells have two capillary faces, one essentially arterial and one venous. The lateral interfaces of β-cells are smooth surfaces; however; where three or more β-cells meet, a canalicular system is found that extends from one capillary to the other. The canaliculi contain microvilli that are enriched in glucose transporters. This specialized arrangement suggests that there is a preferential bulk flow of interstitial fluid through these canaliculi in an arterial to venous direction. Reprinted with permission from the American Society of Clinical Investigation from reference 107 (Weir GC, Bonner-Weir S. Islets of Langerhans: the puzzle of intraislet interactions and their relevance to diabetes. J Clin Invest 1990;85:983–7).

extended to include the metabolic redox state and the threshold for glucose-induced biosynthesis of proinsulin.[115] It is unclear if these differences are constant for a particular cell through its lifetime or are related to the age of the cell. Furthermore, these differences may be intrinsic or may be imprinted by a factor from the environment. Even the β-cells from the same islet are heterogenous; in addition, the average insulin secretion per β-cell shows interislet variation.[116] On the basis of the anatomy of an islet, one can speculate that the environment of a central β-cell is quite different from that of a peripheral one (see below for further discussion). Important questions are raised by this heterogeneity. Are certain populations of β-cells more susceptible than others to autoimmune destruction? Is one population preferentially or selectively lost during the development of non-insulin-dependent diabetes?

The intercellular contacts between the endocrine cells influence their function. Stimulated secretion is enhanced when β-cells have contact with at least one other β-cell.[117,118] In addition β-cells in contact with another β-cell (but not with a non-β-cell) secrete more insulin per cell. Contact via gap junctions is thought to be involved, since heptanol, an alcohol that functionally uncouples gap-junction communication, causes paired β-cells to function as if they were single cells.

STRUCTURAL DEFINITIONS OF ISLET FUNCTION

Although this analysis of the anatomy of the islet essentially has ignored the islet nerves, the overall complexity of the three-dimensional organization of the islet is apparent. This knowledge is useful in interpreting the physiologic data on islet function. Experiments that administered islet hormones exogenously to isolated islets or to perfused pancreas preparations have provided data indicating that islet hormones are capable of influencing the other islet cells in feedback loops.[119,120] Thus, insulin can inhibit both α- and δ-cells, somatostatin can inhibit both α- and β-cells, and glucagon can stimulate both β- and δ-cells. (The role of pancreatic polypeptide or the PP-cell in these potential interactions has not been delineated.) These data have led to the concept that islet hormone secretion is regulated by specific intraislet interactions.[107] Three levels of interactions are possible: 1) cell to cell via junctional communication; 2) blood-borne via the vasculature; and 3) paracrine via the interstitium. What constraints on each of these levels does the anatomy of the islet provide?

Junctional Interactions

Gap junctions are the entities that allow cell-to-cell communication and coupling.[121,122] Such junctions have been seen between all types of islet endocrine cells in both heterologous and homologous links. They have been linked to metabolically coupled islet cells, but their effect on actual islet secretion is still being elucidated (see above). Islet hormones would not be expected to pass through these junctions because of molecular-size limitations and, more importantly, because the hormones within a cell would be enclosed within granule membranes.

Blood-borne Interactions

The microvascular pattern of the islet confers a directionality to the blood flow—from the point of arteriolar entry outward through the β-cell core to the peripheral non-β-cell mantle. This directionality has been demonstrated visually by passing a bolus of dye through the islet of a living rabbit[79] and by a video study of blood flow in the living mouse pancreas.[123] This pattern of flow would favor insulin's affecting the α- and δ-cells by its being transported in high concentrations from the core to the mantle. The reverse, that of the β-cells being influenced by local blood-borne somatostatin or glucagon, is not supported by the vascular pattern. Physiologic data from the approach of passive neutralization, using alternating anterograde and retrograde perfusions of dog, rat, monkey, and, recently, human pancreas, provide support for a β to α to δ (B-A-D) directional pattern of blood flow.[124] The local secretion of insulin is surely important for glucose control over α-cell function.[107] This pattern does not preclude the effects of the islet hormones via the systemic circulation. Somatostatin 28, which comes mainly from the gut and reaches the islets via systemic arterial circulation, may have more potent effects than somatostatin 14 on the islet cells of rats but not those of dogs.[126] However, it is not known if somatostatin is physiologically important to islets.

Paracrine Interactions

The paracrine effects are defined here as those local events that occur by simple diffusion through the interstitium. Such effects are difficult to evaluate because of the lack of good methods for studying the diffusion of peptides throughout this islet compartment. The pericapillary and subcapsular interstitial space is 6 ± 2% of the islet volume. In contrast, the vascular component (the endothelium and the luminal space) comprise approximately 14 ± 3% of the islet volume (S. Bonner-Weir, unpublished observations). Without having actual measurements, one can guess that the interstitial flow probably would be in the same direction as the blood flow. In such a case, diffusion inward to the core would be

severely limited. Thus, in large islets there would be a central core of β-cells that would be isolated by their distance from the non-β-cells and thus from all but systemically circulating levels of the other islet hormones. On the other hand, the peripheral β-cells could be under the local or paracrine influence of hormones secreted by adjacent or nearby non-β-cells. In small islets, essentially all β-cells might be close enough to the non-β-cells to be influenced by their hormones diffusing into the interstitial fluid. Thus, all β-cells could be regarded as peripheral. In fact, differences have been reported. Central β-cells of large islets have been reported to have smaller nuclei than either the peripheral β-cells of large islets or any β-cells in small islets.[125] Furthermore, in rats stimulated in vivo with either glucose or glibenclamide, central β-cells degranulate before peripheral β-cells.[127] These patterns may reflect the paracrine protection of the central β-cells or, conversely, the paracrine influence on peripheral β-cells. Presently, we do not know if these differences seen in the whole islets in vivo account for the heterogeneity found in single cells in vitro.

Somatostatin and glucagon, perfused in the isolated canine pancreas at concentrations only a small fraction of their estimated interislet concentration, have been shown to have profound effects on the other islet cells.[128] The implication of this finding was that at least some cells were protected from the secretory products of their neighbors, and a hypothesis of functional compartmentalization was suggested.[128] This hypothesis stated that the interstitial space within the islet was separated functionally into an "exocytotic-venous pathway" and an "arterial-receptor pathway."[128] Tight junctions were suggested as limiting domains of the plasma membrane of islet cells so as to segregate their sensing and secretory functions. However, tight junctions, which have been well documented in collagenase-isolated islets,[92] are not common in rodent islets fixed in situ[129,130] and therefore probably do not have important effect on compartments. A better anatomic basis for compartmentalization probably lies in the polarity of islet cells and the directionality of blood flow.[105]

SUMMARY

The islets of Langerhans are composed of various components that are organized to form microorgans. The architecture or three-dimensional structure imposes certain constraints on interactions between islet cells.

The mass of islets within a pancreas is dynamic and changes both with growth and development and with functional challenges. As we learn more about the regulation of differentiation of islet cell types, we also may learn how to enhance the growth of islet cells, particularly the β-cells.

Islets function both singly and in concert. Yet recent work has revealed greater diversity in islets than that previously recognized. There is functional heterogeneity between islets and between β-cells within the same islet. Numerous peptides other than the four main islet hormones (insulin, glucagon, somatostatin, and pancreatic polypeptide) have been immunolocalized in islets, but the roles of most are still unknown.

As our knowledge increases about the complex organization of the islet of Langerhans and the changes islets undergo throughout life, we will be able to develop more meaningful interpretations of the physiologic and pathophysiologic characteristics of islet function.

REFERENCES

1. Henderson JR. Why are the islets of Langerhans? Lancet 1969;2:469–70.

2. Wrenshall GA, Bogoch A, Ritchie RC. Extractable insulin of pancreas: correlation with pathological and clinical findings in diabetic and nondiabetic cases. Diabetes 1952;1:87–107.

3. Bonner-Weir S, Orci L. New perspectives on the microvasculature of the islets of Langerhans in the rat. Diabetes 1982;31:883–9.

4. Pictet R, Rutter WJ. Development of the embryonic endocrine pancreas. In: Greep RO, Astwood EB, Steiner DF, Freinkel N, eds. Endocrinology. Vol 1. Baltimore: Williams & Wilkins, 1972:25–66. (Geiger SR, ed. Handbook of physiology: a critical comprehensive presentation of physiologic knowledge and concepts. Section 7).

5. Frye BE. Extirpation and transplantation of the pancreatic rudiments of the salamanders *Amblystoma punctatum* and *Eurycea bislineata*. Anat Rec 1962;144:97–107.

6. Orci L, Baetens D, Ravazzola M, et al. Pancreatic polypeptide and glucagon: non-random distribution in pancreatic islets. Life Sci 1976;19:1811–6.

7. Pearse AGE, Polak JM. Neural crest origin of the endocrine polypeptide (APUD) cells of the gastrointestinal tract and pancreas. Gut 1971;12:783–8.

8. Pictet RL, Rall LB, Phelps P, Rutter WJ. The neural crest and the origin of the insulin-producing and other gastrointestinal hormone-producing cells. Science 1976; 191:191–2.

9. Fontaine J, Le Douarin NM. Analysis of endoderm formation in the avian blastoderm by the use of quail-chick chimaeras: the problem of the neurectodermal origin of the cells of the APUD series. J Embryol Exp Morphol 1977;41:209–22.

10. Fontaine J, LeLièvre C, Le Douarin NM. What is the developmental fate of the neural crest cells which migrate into the pancreas in the avian embryo? Gen Comp Endocrinol 1977;33:394–404.

11. Le Douarin NM. On the origin of pancreatic endocrine cells. Cell 1988;53:169–77.

12. Teitelman G, Joh TH, Reis DJ. Transformation of catecholaminergic precursors into glucagon (A) cells in mouse embryonic pancreas. Proc Natl Acad Sci USA 1981;78:5225–9.

13. Alpert S, Hanahan D, Teitelman G. Hybrid insulin genes reveal a developmental lineage for pancreatic endocrine cells and imply a relationship with neurons. Cell 1988;53:295–308.

14. Ohlsson H, Karlsson O, Edlund T. A beta-cell-specific protein binds to the two major regulatory sequences of the insulin gene enhancer. Proc Natl Acad Sci USA 1988;85:4228–31.

15. Karlsson O, Thor S, Norberg T, et al. Insulin gene enhancer binding protein isl-1 is a member of a novel class of proteins containing both a homeo- and a cys-his domain [Letter]. Nature 1990;344:879–82.

16. Baylin SB. APUD cells: fact and fiction. Trends Endocrinol Metab 1990;1:198–204.

17. Frankel AD, Kim PS. Modular structure of transcription factors: implications for gene regulation. Cell 1991; 65:717–9.

18. Pictet RL, Rall L, deGasparo M, Rutter WJ. Regulation of differentiation of endocrine cells during pancreatic development in vitro. In: Camerini-Davalos RA, Cole HS, eds. Early diabetes in early life. New York: Academic Press, 1991:25–39.

19. Weaver CV, Sorenson RL, Kaung HC. Immunocytochemical localization of insulin-immunoreactive cells in the ducts of rats treated with trypsin inhibitor. Diabetologia 1985;28:781–5.

20. Sarvetnick N, Shizuru J, Liggett D, et al. Loss of pancreatic islet tolerance induced by β-cell expression of interferon-γ [Letter]. Nature 1990;346:844–7.

21. Bonner-Weir S, Baxter LA, Schuppin GT, Smith FE. Two pathways for beta cell regeneration after 90% pancreatectomy [Abstract no. 650]. Diabetes 1991;40(Suppl 1):163A.

22. Rosenberg L, Duguid WP, Vinik AI. The effect of cellophane wrapping of the pancreas in the Syrian golden hamster: autoradiographic observations. Pancreas 1989; 4:31–7.

23. Gepts W. Pathologic anatomy of the pancreas in juvenile diabetes mellitus. Diabetes 1965;14:619–33.

24. Dudek RW, Lawrence IE Jr. Morphologic evidence of interactions between adult ductal epithelium of pancreas and fetal foregut mesenchyme. Diabetes 1988;37:891–900.

25. Dudek RW, Lawrence IE Jr, Hill RS, Johnson RC. Induction of islet cytodifferentiation by fetal mesenchyme in adult pancreatic ductal epithelium. Diabetes 1991;40:1041–8.

26. Karlsson O, Edlund T, Moss BJ, et al. A mutational analysis of the insulin gene transcription control region: expression in beta cells is dependent on two related sequences within the enhancer. Proc Natl Acad Sci 1987;84:8819–23.

27. Ohlsson H, Thor S, Edlund T. Novel insulin promoter- and enhancer-binding proteins that discriminate between pancreatic α- and β-cells. Mol Endocrinol 1991;5:897–904.

28. Reddy JK, Rao MS, Yeldandi AV, et al. Pancreatic hepatocytes: an in vivo model for cell lineage in pancreas of adult rat. Digest Dis Sci 1991;36:502–9.

29. Fujii S. Development of pancreatic endocrine cells in the rat fetus. Arch Histol Jpn 1979;42:467–79.

30. Hashimoto T, Kawano H, Daikoku S, et al. Transient coappearance of glucagon and insulin in the progenitor cells of the rat pancreatic islets. Anat Embryol 1988;178:489–97.

31. Rahier J, Wallon J, Henquin JC. Abundance of somatostatin cells in the human neonatal pancreas. Diabetologia 1980;18:251–4.

32. Madsen OD, Larsson LI, Rehfeld JF, et al. Cloned cell lines from a transplantable islet cell tumor are heterogeneous and express cholecystokinin in addition to islet hormones. J Cell Biol 1986;103:2025–34.

33. Madsen OD, Andersen LC, Michelsen B, et al. Tissue-specific expression of transfected human insulin genes in pluripotent clonal rat insulinoma lines induced during passage in vivo. Proc Natl Acad Sci USA 1988;85:6652–6.

34. Falkmer S, Ostberg Y. Comparative morphology of pancreatic islets in animals. In: Volk BW, Wellmann KF, eds. The diabetic pancreas. New York: Plenum Press, 1977:15–60.

35. Bonner-Weir S, Weir GC. The organization of the endocrine pancreas: a hypothetical unifying view of the phylogenetic differences. Gen Comp Endocrinol 1979; 38:28–37.

36. Epple A. The endocrine pancreas. In: Hoar WS, Randall DJ, eds. Fish physiology. Vol 2. New York: Academic Press, 1969:275–319.

37. Epple A, Brinn JE Jr. Islet histophysiology: evolutionary correlations. Gen Comp Endocrinol 1975;27:320–49.

38. Stefan Y, Falkmer S. Islet hormone cells in cartilaginous fish—the original pancreas? [Abstract no. 329] Diabetologia 1978;15:272.

39. Witte DP, Greider MH, DeSchryver-Kecshemeti K, et al. The juvenile human endocrine pancreas: normal vs idiopathic hypoinsulinemic hypoglycemia. Semin Diagn Pathol 1984;1:30.

40. Bonner-Weir S, Like AA. A dual population of islets of Langerhans in bovine pancreas. Cell Tissue Res 1980; 206:157–70.

41. McEvoy RC, Madson KL. Pancreatic insulin-, glucagon-, and somatostatin-positive islet cell populations during the perinatal development of the rat. I. Morphometric quantitation. Biol Neonate 1980;38:248–54.

42. Hellerstrom C, Swenne I, Andersson A. Islet cell replication and diabetes. In: Lefebvre PJ, Pipeleers DG, eds. The pathology of the endocrine pancreas in diabetes. Heidelberg: Springer-Verlag, 1988:141–70.

43. Swenne I. The role of glucose in the in vitro regulation of cell cycle kinetics and proliferation of fetal pancreatic B-cells. Diabetes 1982;31:754–60.

44. Swenne I, Andersson A. Effect of genetic background on the capacity for islet cell replication in mice. Diabetologia 1984;27:464–7.

45. De Vroede MA, In't Veld PA, Pipeleers DG. Deoxyribonucleic acid synthesis in cultured adult rat pancreatic B cells. Endocrinology 1990;127:1510–6.

46. Ehrie MG, Swartz FJ. Polyploidy in the pancreas of the normal and diabetic mutant mouse. Diabetologia 1976; 12:167–70.

47. Pohl MN, Swartz FJ. Development of polyploidy in B-cells of normal and diabetic mice. Acta Endocrinol 1979; 90:295–306.

48. Woerner, C.A Studies of the islands of Langerhans after continuous intravenous injection of dextrose. Anat Rec 1938;71:33–57.

49. Brosky GM, Heuck CC. Der Einfluss von Glukoseinfusionen auf die Proinsulin-und Insulinsynthese in den Langerhansschen Inseln bei der Ratte. Endokrinologie 1975;66:46–55.

50. Bonner-Weir S, Deery D, Leahy JL, Weir GC. Compensatory growth of pancreatic β-cells in adult rats after short-term glucose infusion. Diabetes 1989;38:49–53.

51. Kinash B, Haist RE. Continuous intravenous infusion in the rat and the effect on the islets of Langerhans of the continuous infusion of glucose. Can J Biochem Physiol 1954;32:428–33.

52. Brosky GM, Kern HF, Logothetopoulos J. Ultrastructure, mitotic activity and insulin biosynthesis of pancreatic beta cells stimulated by glucose infusions [Abstract no. 250]. Fed Proc 1972;31:256.

53. Logothetopoulos J, Valiquette N. Hormonal and nonhormonal protein biosynthesis in the pancreatic beta cell of the intact rat after prolonged hyperglycaemia. Acta Endocrinol 1984;107:382–9.

54. Chick WL. Beta cell replication in rat pancreatic monolayer cultures: effects of glucose, tolbutamide, glucocorti-coid, growth hormone and glucagon. Diabetes 1973; 22:687–93.

55. Chick WL, Lauris V, Flewelling JH, et al. Effects of glucose on beta cells in pancreatic monolayer cultures. Endocrinology 1973;92:212–8.

56. Nielsen JH. Growth and function of the pancreatic β cell in vitro: effects of glucose, hormones and serum factors on mouse, rat and human pancreatic islets in organ culture. Acta Endocrinol 1985;108(Suppl 266):1–39.

57. Hellerström C. The influence of pregnancy and lactation on the endocrine pancreas of mice. Acta Soc Med Uppsala 1963;68:17–28.

58. Green IC, Taylor KW. Effects of pregnancy in the rat on the size and insulin secretory response of the islets of Langerhans. J Endocrinol 1972;54:317–25.

59. Green IC, El Seifi S, Perrin D, Howell SL. Cell replication in the islets of Langerhans of adult rats: effects of pregnancy, ovariectomy and treatment with steroid hormones. J Endocrinol 1981;88:219–24.

60. Marynissen G, Aerts L, Van Assche FA. The endocrine pancreas during pregnancy and lactation in the rat. J Devel Physiol 1983;5:373–81.

61. Sorenson RL, Parsons JA. Insulin secretion in mammo-somatotropic tumor-bearing and pregnant rats: a role for lactogens. Diabetes 1985;34:337–41.

62. Nielsen JH, Linde S, Welinder BS, et al. Growth hormone is a growth factor for the differentiated pancreatic β-cell. Mol Endocrinol 1989;3:165–73.

63. Brelje TC, Sorenson RL. Role of prolactin versus growth hormone on islet B-cell proliferation in vitro: implications for pregnancy. Endocrinology 1991;128:45–57.

64. Jeanrenaud, B. An hypothesis on the aetiology of obesity: dysfunction of the central nervous system as a primary cause. Diabetologia 1955;28:502–13.

65. Rabinovitch A, Quigley C, Russell T, et al. Insulin and multiplication stimulating activity (an insulin-like growth factor) stimulate islet β-cell replication in neonatal rat pancreatic monolayer cultures. Diabetes 1982;31:160–4.

66. Brockenbrough JS, Weir GC, Bonner-Weir S. Discordance of exocrine and endocrine growth after 90% pancreatectomy in rats. Diabetes 1988;37:232–4.

67. Bonner-Weir S, Trent DF, Weir GC. Partial pancreatectomy in the rat and subsequent defect in glucose-induced insulin release. J Clin Invest 1983;71:1544–53.

68. Petersson M, Ahrén B, Böttcher C, Sundler F. Calcitonin gene related peptide: occurrence in pancreatic islets in the mouse and the rat and inhibition of insulin secretion in the mouse. Endocrinology 1986;119:865–9.

69. Schmidt WE, Siegel EG, et al. Pancreastatin: molecular and immunocytochemical characterization of a novel peptide in porcine and human tissues. Endocrinology 1986;123:1395–404.

70. Ravazzola M, Efendic S, Ostenson C-G, et al. Localization of pancreastatin immunoreactivity in porcine endocrine cells. Endocrinology 1988;123:227–9.

71. Aratan-Spire S, Wolf B, Czernichow P. Developmental pattern of TRH-degrading activity and TRH content in rat pancreas. Acta Endocrinol (Copenh) 1984;106:102–8.

72. Larsson L-I, Rehfeld JF, Sundler F, Håkanson R. Pancreatic gastrin in foetal and neonatal rats. Nature 1976;262:609–10.

73. Lukinius A, Wilander E, Westermark GT, et al. Co-localization of islet amyloid polypeptide and insulin in the B cell secretory granules of the human pancreatic islets. Diabetologia 1989;32:240–4.

74. Madsen OD, Nielsen JH, Michelsen B, et al. Islet amyloid

polypeptide and insulin expression are controlled differently in primary and transformed islet cells. Mol Endocrinol 1991;5:143–8.

75. Dean PM. Ultrastructural morphometry of the pancreatic β-cell. Diabetologia 1973;9:115–9.

76. Orci L. The insulin factory: a tour of the plant surroundings and a visit to the assembly line. Diabetologia 1985;28:528–46.

77. Guest PC, Bailyes EM, Rutherford NG, Hutton JC. Insulin secretory granule biogenesis: co-ordinate regulation of the biosynthesis of the majority of constituent proteins. Biochem J 1991;274:73–8.

78. Larsson L-I, Sundler F, Håkanson R. Pancreatic polypeptide—A postulated new hormone: identification of its cellular storage site by light and electron microscopic immunocytochemistry. Diabetologia 1976;12:211–26.

79. Henderson JR, Daniel PM. A comparative study of the portal vessels connecting the endocrine and exocrine pancreas, with a discussion of some functional implications. Q J Exp Physiol 1979;64:267–75.

80. Henderson JR, Moss MC. A morphometric study of the endocrine and exocrine capillaries of the pancreas. Q J Exp Physiol 1985;70:347–56.

81. Like AA. The uptake of exogenous peroxidase by the beta cells of the islets of Langerhans. Am J Pathol 1970;59:225–46.

82. Lifson N, Kramlinger KG, Mayrand RR, Lender EJ. Blood flow to the rabbit pancreas with special reference to the islets of Langerhans. Gastroenterology 1980;79:466–73.

83. Jansson L, Hellerström C. A rapid method of visualizing the pancreatic islets for studies of islet capillary blood flow using non-radioactive microspheres. Acta Physiol Scand 1981;113:371–4.

84. Lifson N, Lassa CV, Dixit PK. Relation between blood flow and morphology in islet organ of rat pancreas. Am J Physiol 1985;249:E43–8.

85. Meyer HH, Vetterlein F, Schmidt G, Hasselblatt A. Measurement of blood flow in pancreatic islets of the rat: effect of isoproterenol and norepinephrine. Am J Physiol 1982;242:E298–304.

86. Jansson L, Hellerström C. Stimulation by glucose of the blood flow to the pancreatic islets of the rat. Diabetologia 1983;25:45–50.

87. Brain SD, Williams TJ, Tippins JR, et al. Calcitonin gene-related peptide is a potent vasodilator [Letter]. Nature 1985;313:54–6.

88. Brunfeldt K, Hunhammar K, Skouby AP. Studies on the vascular system of the islets of Langerhans in mice. Acta Endocrinol 1958;29:473–80.

89. Smith PH, Porte D Jr. Neuropharmacology of the pancreatic islets. Annu Rev Pharmacol Toxicol 1976;16:269–85.

90. Polonsky KS, Given BD, Van Cauter E. Twenty-four-hour profiles and pulsatile patterns of insulin secretion in normal and obese subjects. J Clin Invest 1988;81:442–8.

91. Sundler F, Böttcher G. Islet innervation, with special reference to neuropeptides. In: Samols E, ed. The endocrine pancreas. New York: Raven Press, 1991:29–52.

92. Lang DA, Matthews DR, Peto J, Turner RC. Cyclic oscillations of basal plasma glucose and insulin concentrations in human beings. N Engl J Med 1979;301:1023–7.

93. Stagner JI, Samols E, Weir GC. Sustained oscillations of insulin, glucagon and somatostatin from the isolated canine pancreas during exposure to a constant glucose concentration. J Clin Invest 1980;65:939–42.

94. Ahrén B, Böttcher G, Kowalyk S, et al. Galanin is co-localized with noradrenaline and neuropeptide Y in dog pancreas and celiac ganglion. Cell Tissue Res 1990;261:49–58.

95. Ahrén B, Taborsky GJ Jr, Porte D Jr. Neuropeptidergic versus cholinergic and adrenergic regulation of islet hormone secretion. Diabetologia 1986;29:827–36.

96. Samols E, Weir GC. Adrenergic modulation of pancreatic A, B, and D cells. J Clin Invest 1979;63:230–36.

97. Larsson L-I, Fahrenkrug J, Holst JJ, Schaffalitzky de Muckadell OB. Innervation of the pancreas by vasoactive intestinal polypeptide (VIP) immunoreactive nerves. Life Sci 1978;22:773–80.

98. Orci L, Unger RH. Functional subdivision of islets of Langerhans and possible role of D cells. Lancet 1975;2:1243–4.

99. Erlandsen SL, Hegre OD, Parsons JA, et al. Pancreatic islet cell hormones distribution of cell types in the islet and evidence for the presence of somatostatin and gastrin within the D cell. J Histochem Cytochem 1976;24:883–97.

100. Grube D, Eckert I, Speck PT, Wagner H-J. Immunohistochemistry and microanatomy of the islets of Langerhans. Biomed Res 1983;4(Suppl):25.

101. Orci L. The microanatomy of the islets of Langerhans. Metabolism 1976;25(Suppl 1):1303–13.

102. Brelje TC, Scharp DW, Sorenson RL. Three-dimensional imaging of intact isolated islets of Langerhans with confocal microscopy. Diabetes 1989;38:808–14.

103. Halban PA, Powers SL, George KL, Bonner-Weir S. Spontaneous reassociation of dispersed adult rat pancreatic islet cells into aggregates with three-dimensional architecture typical of native islets. Diabetes 1987;36:783–90.

104. Rouiller GD, Cirulli V, Halban PA. Uvomorulin mediates calcium dependent aggregation of islet cells, whereas calcium independent cell adhesion molecules distinguish between islet cell types. Dev Biol 1991;148:233–42.

105. Bonner-Weir S. Morphological evidence for pancreatic polarity of β-cell within islets of Langerhans. Diabetes 1988;37:616–21.

106. Bonner-Weir S. Potential "sensing" and "secreting" domains of the pancreatic B-cell [Abstract no. 389]. Diabetes 1989;38(Suppl 2):98a.

107. Weir GC, Bonner-Weir S. Islets of Langerhans: the puzzle of intraislet interactions and their relevance to diabetes. J Clin Invest 1990;85:983–7.

108. Orci L, Thorens B, Ravazzola M, Lodish HF. Localization of the pancreatic beta cell glucose transporter to specific plasma membrane domains. Science 1989;245:295–7.

109. Stagner J, Samols E. Differential glucagon and insulin release from the isolated lobes of the in vitro canine pancreas [Abstract no. 156]. Diabetes 1982;31(Suppl 2):39A.

110. Trimble ER, Halban PA, Wolheim CB, Renold AE. Functional differences between rat islets of ventral and dorsal pancreatic origin. J Clin Invest 1982;69:405–13.

111. Grodsky GM. A threshold distribution hypothesis for packet storage of insulin. II. Effect of calcium. Diabetes 1972;21(Suppl 2):584–93.

112. Matthews EK, Dean PM. Electrical activity in islet cells. In: Falkmer S, Hellman B, Taljedal I.-B, eds. Structure and metabolism of pancreatic islets. Oxford: Pergamon Press, 1970:305.

113. Pipeleers D. The biosociology of pancreatic B-cells. Diabetologia 1987;30:277–91.

114. Salomon D, Meda P. Heterogeneity and contact-dependent

regulation of hormone secretion by individual B cells. Exp Cell Res 1986;162:507–20.

115. Schuit FC, In't Veld PA, Pipeleers DG. Glucose stimulates proinsulin biosynthesis by a dose-dependent recruitment of pancreatic beta cells. Proc Natl Acad Sci USA 1988;85:3865–9.

116. Hiriart M, Ramirez-Medeles MC. Functional subpopulations of individual pancreatic B-cells in culture. Endocrinology 1991;128:3193–8.

117. Bosco D, Orci L, Meda P. Homologous but not heterologous contact increases the insulin secretion of individual pancreatic B-cells. Exp Cell Res 1989;184:72–80.

118. Soria B, Chanson M, Giordano E, et al. Ion channels of glucose-responsive and -unresponsive β-cells. Diabetes 1991;40:1069–78.

119. Maruyama H, Hisatomi A, Orci L, et al. Insulin within islets is a physiologic glucagon release inhibitor. J Clin Invest 1984;74:2296–9.

120. Samols E, Marri G, Marks V. Promotion of insulin secretion by glucagon. Lancet 1965;2:415–6.

121. Meda P, Michaels RL, Halban PA, et al. In vivo modulation of gap junctions and dye coupling between B-cells of the intact pancreatic islet. Diabetes 1983;32:858–68.

122. Meda P, Perrelet A, Orci L. Gap junctions and cell-to-cell coupling in endocrine glands. Mod Cell Biol 1984;3:131–96.

123. Rooth P, Grankvist K, Täljedal I-B. In vivo fluorescence microscopy of blood flow in mouse pancreatic islets: adrenergic effects in lean and obese-hyperglycemic mice. Microvasc Res 1985;30:176–84.

124. Stagner JI, Samols E, Bonner-Weir S. β→α→δ pancreatic islet cellular perfusion in dogs. Diabetes 1988;37:1715–21.

125. Hellerström C, Petersson B, Hellman B. Some properties of the B-cells in the islets of Langerhans studied with regard to the position of the cells. Acta Endocrinol 1960;34:449–56.

126. Klaff LJ, Dunning BE, Taborsky GJ Jr. Somatostatin-28 does not regulate islet function in the dog. Endocrinology 1988;123:2668–74.

127. Stefan Y, Meda P, Neufeld M, Orci L. Stimulation of insulin secretion reveals heterogeneity of pancreatic B cells in vivo. J Clin Invest 1987;80:175–83.

128. Kawai K, Orci L, Ipp E, et al. Circulating somatostatin acts on the islets of Langerhans by way of a somatostatin-poor compartment. Science 1982;218:477–8.

129. In't Veld PA, Pipeleers DG, Gepts W. Evidence against the presence of tight junctions in normal endocrine pancreas. Diabetes 1984;33:101–4.

130. Yamamoto M, Kataoka K. A comparative study on the intercellular canalicular system and intercellular junctions in the pancreatic islets of some rodents. Arch Histol Jpn 1984;47:485–93.

Chapter 3

INSULIN BIOSYNTHESIS AND CHEMISTRY

STEVEN E. SHOELSON
PHILIPPE A. HALBAN

Insulin, the major hormonal regulator of glucose metabolism, was first isolated from pancreatic tissue in 1921 by Banting and Best.[1] Shortly after its discovery, the impure extract was used experimentally to treat pancreatectomized dogs[2] and patients with diabetes.[3] As soon as it became clear that the hormone was effective, both the amount of extract isolated and the degree of its purity were increased. Insulin was thus made available to patients with diabetes mellitus. The treatment of such patients underwent a remarkable revolution within one to two years of the initial discovery of insulin. However, many aspects of insulin biochemistry and chemistry were not understood until years later, and some of these topics remain as areas of intense investigation. This chapter will focus on the biosynthesis of insulin, from insulin gene to secretory granule; the chemistry and structure of insulin; and abnormalities in insulin structure that affect its action or biosynthetic processing.

THE INSULIN GENE AND REGULATION OF EXPRESSION

Structure of the Insulin Gene

The human insulin gene is located in region p13 of the short arm of chromosome 11, adjacent to the genes for insulin-like growth factor II (IGF-II) and tyrosine hydroxylase.[4-6] The insulin gene has been sequenced[6] and found to be polymorphic, mostly within a hypervariable region at the 5′ extremity.[7,8] While early analyses of restriction fragment length polymorphisms (RFLPs) suggested a correlation between non-insulin-dependent diabetes mellitus (NIDDM) and a repeating segment of DNA upstream from the insulin gene,[9-14] it is now thought that the observed heterogeneity of the insulin gene does not affect insulin gene expression directly and is not involved in the pathogenesis of diabetes.[15,16] The structure (Fig. 3–1) and evolution of the insulin gene have been reviewed comprehensively[17,18]; only essential details will be recalled here.

The insulin gene consists of three exons (protein-coding regions) separated by two introns (noncoding regions). A regulatory region, which is located 30 base-pairs from the transcription initiation site, precedes the "TATA" box (a DNA sequence necessary for transcription initiation). The first intron occurs in all insulin genes sequenced to date and presents a fairly constant length of some 100 to 200 base-pairs. The second intron is found in all sequenced insulin genes except the mouse and rat insulin I genes (these rodents have two nonallelic insulin genes) and shows considerable variability in length among species. The primary RNA transcript is close to 1500 nucleotides in length. There is no evidence for alternative splicing of the insulin gene.

Tissue Specificity

In mammals, insulin gene expression and insulin biosynthesis are restricted to the β-cells of the endocrine pancreas, with the possible exception of the yolk sac and

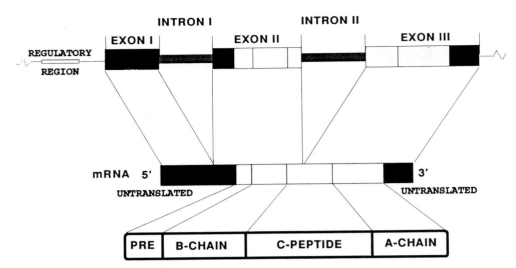

Fig. 3–1. The preproinsulin gene and mRNA. Most preproinsulin genes (including the human gene) consist of three exons interrupted by two introns. The first intron is a 5′ untranslated region and the second in the region of the C-peptide. The gene is shown above with the fully spliced transcript (mRNA) below. Regions of the mRNA encoding the different parts of the preproinsulin molecule are as indicated beneath the mRNA.

fetal liver.[19,20] This exquisite tissue selectivity is conferred upon the insulin gene by a complex interplay between upstream *cis*-elements (short DNA sequences) and cellular *trans*-acting factors (proteins) that bind to the DNA and regulate expression.[21–38] Both positive- and negative-acting regulatory elements of the human, rat, and mouse insulin genes have been mapped to a region within the 5′ flanking region of the insulin gene, 300 or so nucleotides upstream from the transcription start site.[21–26] The β-cell-specific enhancer and promoter activate transcription of the insulin gene in β-cells and have no apparent physiologic function in non-β-cells. Additional negative regulatory elements appear to prevent transcription of the insulin gene in cell types other than pancreatic β-cells.[29]

Two *cis*-elements 5′ to the insulin gene regulate (enhance) transcription of the insulin gene. These are 1) the related 9 base-pair DNA sequences IEB1 and IEB2 located at -108 and -233 of the rat insulin I gene and 2) the repeating TAAT/ATTA sequence located between -208 and -222. *Trans*-acting proteins that bind to the IEB1 and IEB2 regions have been identified,[31–36] and the interactions of these and other *cis*-elements and *trans*-acting factors provide the beginnings of an understanding of the mechanisms underlying tissue-specific aspects of gene regulation. Notably, the IEB1 and IEB2 sequences of the insulin gene are remarkably similar to and in some cases identical to immunoglobulin "E box" gene enhancer elements.[23,32,39] Proteins E12 and E47, which bind the immunoglobulin enhancer[40,41]; Pan-1 and Pan-2, which bind pancreatic exocrine gene enhancers[42]; and A1, which binds the insulin gene IEB1 and IEB2 sequences,[36] show extensive sequence and functional homology with one another. Thus, similar *cis*-elements and *trans*-acting factors regulate tissue specificity of diverse cellular products, including production of insulin in β-cells, of immunoglobulin in lymphocytes, and of digestive enzymes by the exocrine pancreas. While it is not yet understood how similar protein-DNA interactions turn on or off transcription of different genes, it is now thought that complexes of proteins (rather than a single *trans*-acting factor) must be involved.

A different binding protein interacts with the repeating TAAT/ATTA sequence at -222 to -208, which is part of the homeodomain-containing protein-binding motif.[43,44] A complementary DNA sequence encoding this protein, called Isl-1,[38] has been cloned and sequenced and shows extensive sequence homology with other homeodomain proteins from such diverse sources as *Drosophila* and *Caenorhabditis elegans*. In addition, a classical cyclic adenosine monophosphate (cAMP)-responsive element has been identified within the insulin gene regulatory region,[45] although the role of cAMP on insulin gene expression is not understood.

The identification of regulatory regions of the insulin gene and their cognate *trans*-acting factors represents a major advance in our understanding of the regulation of insulin gene expression in β-cells and non-β-cells alike. These factors are remarkably well conserved among animal species, which facilitates transfection of foreign insulin genes into cultured animal cells[46,47] and transgenic mice,[48,49] and ultimately may allow insulin gene transplantation into patients with Type I diabetes. In another sense, however, identification of β-cell-specific *trans*-factors raises a supplementary question concerning the mechanism underlying the tissue-specific expression of the factors themselves. We still have a long way to go in understanding the molecular programing responsible for tissue-selective insulin gene expression.

Regulation of Insulin Biosynthesis in the β-Cell

In addition to tissue-selective expression, the insulin gene is subject to environmental regulation within the β-cell (see references 17 and 50–52 for reviews). For secretion, glucose (and cAMP) is a major stimulus of insulin biosynthesis. The initial studies on the regulation of biosynthesis were limited to measuring the rate of incorporation of labeled amino acid into insulin or its precursors. The earliest of these studies, dating from the 1960s,[53–57] showed that glucose stimulated insulin biosynthesis in vitro. Subsequent studies on the rate of incorporation of labeled amino acid into proinsulin or insulin showed stimulation not only by glucose[58–62] but also by other sugars[62,63] and potential nutrients, including leucine,[64] inosine, guanosine, and ribose.[65] Unlike leucine, arginine has been found to inhibit insulin biosynthesis[66,67] despite its pronounced stimulatory impact on insulin release. Amino acid incorporation into proinsulin was also found to display stringent cationic requirements,[68] with a dependence on K^+ but not on Ca^{++} or Mg^{++}.[68,69] Cyclic AMP was found to stimulate proinsulin biosynthesis,[60,70-73] and, as discussed below, it now seems probable that cAMP participates in the glucose stimulation of proinsulin biosynthesis.[74]

The effects of a number of other agents on insulin synthesis have also been documented. Hypoglycemic agents, including sulfonylureas and diazoxide, have been shown to inhibit proinsulin biosynthesis.[75-77] Current interest in the potential role of cytokines in β-cell destruction in Type I diabetes has stimulated studies of their effect on proinsulin biosynthesis. Although one study reported an inhibition of proinsulin biosynthesis by human lymphoblastoid interferon,[78] the effect was not found with a purer preparation of interferon.[79] Depending upon the concentration used, interleukin-1 can either stimulate or inhibit proinsulin biosynthesis.[79-81] The inhibitory effect seems to be more selective for the synthesis of proinsulin than for other islet-cell proteins[80] and reflects both pre- and post-transcriptional levels of regulation.[80] The rate of conversion of proinsulin to insulin may also be inhibited by interleukin-1.[81] Finally, the phospho-oligosaccharide suggested to act as one of the second messengers mediating insulin action in insulin-sensitive cells has been shown to inhibit proinsulin biosynthesis,[82] but the physiologic relevance is unclear.

Measurements of the rates of incorporation of labeled amino acid into newly synthesized proteins reflects both pre- and post-transcriptional events. Even before it was possible to produce cDNA to quantify mRNA levels, attempts had been made to differentiate these levels of control. In the early 1970s Permutt and Kipnis convincingly demonstrated that glucose regulation occurred at both the pre- and post-transcriptional levels[83-85] and that translation was affected by modulating initiation and the rate of elongation.[85] Such translational regulation by glucose was confirmed in subsequent experiments using cell-free systems.[86,87]

When cDNA for measuring preproinsulin mRNA levels in insulin-producing cells became available, regulatory mechanisms for insulin biosynthesis were studied directly (see reference 52 for review). Most agents that stimulate proinsulin synthesis raise levels of preproinsulin mRNA in isolated islets following prolonged exposure.[74,88-94] This could be due either to stabilization of the mRNA (decreased degradation in the face of maintained transcription) or to stimulated transcription per se. Glucose, cAMP, and dexamethasone stimulate transcription of the insulin gene.[74,93] Glucose has also been shown to stabilize preproinsulin mRNA by inhibiting its degradation, possibly by inhibiting the synthesis or activity of protein(s) involved in degradation.[95] To date, the only specific responsive element identified in the insulin gene has been that for cAMP (cAMP-responsive element or CRE).[45] It remains to be seen whether discrete elements exist for other agents (or their metabolites in the case of glucose) able to stimulate insulin gene transcription or whether such agents alter binding of the *trans*-factors described above to their cognate regulatory regions on the insulin gene.

Stimulation of proinsulin biosynthesis over relatively short times (less than 1 hour) occurs without a change in levels of preproinsulin mRNA.[96,97] Glucose can stimulate translation of insulin mRNA directly by affecting initiation, elongation, and signal-recognition particle (SRP)-mediated elongation arrest.[98,99] Translational regulation of insulin biosynthesis is most probably the dominant mechanism under physiologic circumstances.

In addition to the in vitro studies described above, a number of studies have been performed in rats. Glucose infusion for 24 hours produces a lasting increase in insulin biosynthetic activity in islets isolated from the treated rats.[100] Pancreatic levels of preproinsulin mRNA are decreased by starvation and raised by a subsequent infusion of glucose or by refeeding.[101,102] Intensive exogenous insulin therapy in rats has also been shown to lead to a profound, but reversible, decrease in pancreatic mRNA levels.[103] Studies on two rat models of NIDDM (neonatal injection of streptozotocin and partial pancreatectomy) suggest that even though an initial insult to the endocrine pancreas leads to an adaptive increase in preproinsulin mRNA levels such adaptation is not sufficient to prevent the onset of a diabetic condition.[104,105] Finally, an age-related impairment in post-transcriptional regulation of insulin biosynthesis has been demonstrated in old rats.[106,107]

Unlike glucose-stimulation of insulin secretion (see Chapter 4), the stimulation of insulin biosynthesis by glucose is not dependent upon extracellular Ca^{++},[68,69] indicating the involvement of a different array of second messengers. As for stimulus-secretion coupling, however, it is almost certain that glucose metabolism is required for generation of the signals necessary for stimulating biosynthesis, but the dose response curve for the two stimulatory events is somewhat different,[62,73] suggesting again that different signals may be involved. The time-course of the cessation of stimulation of insulin biosynthesis upon glucose withdrawal is slower than that for secretion. It has been suggested that this lag in the decrease of insulin biosynthesis relative to the release that occurs with glucose withdrawal may be advantageous to the β-cell, ensuring that intra-β-cell insulin levels always are restored to the appropriate level even after an extended period of stimulated release.[108]

POST-TRANSCRIPTIONAL EVENTS

Translation of Preproinsulin and Conversion to Proinsulin

Although the two-chain structure of insulin had been known since 1955,[109] it was not until 1967 that Steiner et al. first presented evidence for a single-chain biosynthetic precursor, proinsulin.[110,111] The identification of a hormone precursor was to prove of profound importance for our understanding not only of insulin synthesis but of protein synthesis in general. It is now evident that there is also a protein precursor for proinsulin, called prepro-insulin[112-118] (Fig. 3–2). It is synthesized on the rough endoplasmic reticulum (RER), with the first 25 or so amino acids forming a signal peptide. As preproinsulin is synthesized, the signal peptide is bound by the signal-recognition particle (SRP), which in turn homes to the SRP receptor on the membrane of the RER. These events occur after the addition of the first 60 or so amino acids to the growing preproinsulin chain.[119] The signal peptide is rich in hydrophobic residues, facilitating the penetration of the RER membrane. Penetration occurs rapidly, and the rest of the nascent preproinsulin molecule then crosses into the lumen of the RER, perhaps with the assistance of additional biosynthetic machinery. A signal peptidase within the RER effects cleavage of the signal peptide from preproinsulin to yield intact proinsulin. Conversion arises for the most part cotranslationally, such that preproinsulin itself is a very minor constituent of the β-cell.[117] These events provide a paradigm for the synthesis and translocation to the lumen of the RER of secretory proteins, as well as a model for membrane and lysosomal proteins.[120] The preproinsulin signal sequence can direct the translocation of a non-insulin-related peptide across the membrane of the RER[121] and has even been shown to be functional if transposed to an internal (i.e., not N-terminal) location.[122] The universal nature of these functional features, including the signal peptide, translocation, and proteolytic conversion, is underscored by the fact that preproinsulin, when expressed in bacteria, is converted to proinsulin, which segregates to the periplasmic space.[123,124]

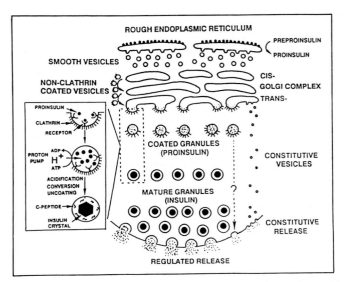

Fig. 3–3. Trafficking and processing events in the pathway of insulin production by the pancreatic β-cell. For clarity, some steps have been intentionally oversimplified and some critical processes have been omitted (e.g., transcription, translation, and degradation). The inset shows the major events involved in targeting proinsulin to nascent granules and in the transition between proinsulin-containing coated granules and insulin-containing mature granules. The *trans*-Golgi receptor presumed to be involved in the targeting process has yet to be identified in the β-cell. Proinsulin release by exocytosis of coated granule contents has never been directly documented. Little if any proinsulin is released via the constitutive pathway under normal circumstances. Reprinted with permission from reference 125 (Halban PA. Proinsulin trafficking and processing in the pancreatic B-cell. Trends Endocrinol Metab 1990;1:261–5).

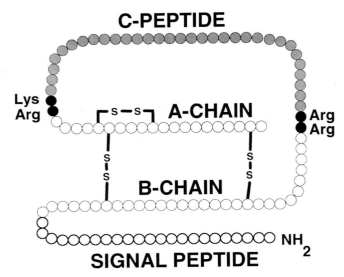

Fig. 3–2. Preproinsulin. The initial, high-molecular-weight precursor of insulin consists of four distinct domains. The signal (or pre-) peptide occupies the first (N-terminal) 23 residues and is cleaved off within the lumen of the rough endoplasmic reticulum to produce proinsulin. Conversion of proinsulin to insulin arises at the pairs of basic residues linking the two insulin (A- and B-) chains to the C- (connecting) peptide, as depicted in Figure 3–3. The two insulin chains are joined together by two disulfide bridges. The molecular mass of insulin is approximately 5,800 daltons.

Like all secretory proteins, from the moment of synthesis insulin and its precursors are enveloped in a limiting membrane and as such protected from the cytosol. The passage from one subcellular compartment to the next occurs by the successive budding and fusion of carrier vesicles, culminating in formation of the mature secretory granule and the ultimate fusion event, exocytosis (Fig. 3–3). These events, initially outlined in pioneering studies by Palade,[126] provided the point of departure for Orci's seminal studies on the cell biology of the insulin-producing β-cell (for reviews see references 127–130). Although our understanding of these events has increased dramatically in recent years, elucidation of the secretory pathway in molecular detail remains one of the great challenges of modern cell biology. This chapter simply outlines the major steps, many of which have been discussed in greater detail in review articles[125,127–136] dealing with secretory protein production in general[131–136] or the β-cell in particular.[125,127–130] Since the major elements of the secretory pathway in most secretory cells resemble one another, non-insulin-producing cells have provided information pertinent to the β-cell.

Intracellular Trafficking of Proinsulin

Unlike the majority of secretory proteins found within the lumen of the RER, proinsulin is never glycosylated.

Like its companions, however, proinsulin is transported from the transitional elements of the RER to the *cis*-cisternae of the Golgi complex in smooth vesicles. This transfer is energy (ATP) dependent,[137] depends upon the microfilamentous-microtubular network[138–140] and (by analogy with other cell types) most probably upon the participation of cytosolic proteins, including the N-ethylmaleimide (NEM)-sensitive fusion protein (NSF),[141,142] G proteins,[143] and members of the heat-shock protein family.[144] It is likely that members of this family of proteins also are involved in the folding of proinsulin within the lumen of the RER.[145,146] The identification of proteins and cofactors associated with vesicle budding, transport, and fusion has been made possible by the development of cell-free model systems,[147] and this list will likely continue to grow.

The next organelle to be involved in proinsulin trafficking and processing is the Golgi complex (reviewed in references 148–152), where proinsulin is sorted from proteins not destined for secretory granules. Once the proinsulin molecules have been delivered to the *cis*-Golgi, they are transferred from one Golgi stack to the next. This transport is assured by small vesicles typified by the presence of a coat protein (β-COP) (not clathrin) on their cytosolic face.[153–155] The coat is lost before fusion with the target stack.[156] The complete cycle of events involved in vesicular transport between Golgi stacks has been reviewed.[157] As for transfer from RER to Golgi, intercisternal transfer between Golgi stacks is mediated in part by the so-called NEM-sensitive fusion protein,[158] by G-proteins,[159,160] by a series of other proteins[161,162] that include "SNAPs" (NSF attachment proteins),[161] and by fatty acyl coenzyme A.[163] Once delivered to the *trans*-cisternae of the Golgi complex, proinsulin is separated from other secretory and integral membrane proteins destined for the constitutive pathway and from enzymes destined for lysosomes.

Sorting of Proinsulin to the Regulated Secretory Pathway

Secretion of insulin or other proteins can proceed through either constitutive or regulated pathways. All cells utilize the constitutive secretory pathway, both for secretion and to dispatch integral membrane proteins to their appropriate destinations.[131,133] Only a few, highly differentiated, secretory cell types can store products in secretory granules and release them in response to a secretagogue, however. The β-cell is equipped with both these pathways[164] but under normal circumstances directs proinsulin almost exclusively to the regulated pathway.[165] The pattern of release using these two pathways is quite different.[131,133] As its name implies, the constitutive pathway is not subject to control by secretagogues. It arises by the rapid transport of proteins from the *trans*-Golgi to the plasma membrane in small vesicles (transit time ~10 minutes). For proteins inserted in the vesicle membrane (i.e., cell-surface receptors), fusion of the vesicle with the plasma membrane results in presentation to the extracellular environment, whereas proteins in solution in the transport vesicles are secreted.

The internal milieu of transport vesicles is probably not inert. The conversion of proalbumin to albumin[166] or of the insulin proreceptor to receptor[167] may arise in this compartment, for example. The enzyme catalyzing such conversion is thought to be the mammalian equivalent of the yeast KEX2 enzyme[168,169] known as furin or PACE,[170] which cleaves at sequences of two or more basic residues. The substrate specificity of conversion is exemplified by the dramatic consequences of point mutations at the cleavage sites of proalbumin or the insulin proreceptor, which arise naturally in rare instances and lead to hyperproalbuminemia,[171] or insulin resistance due to inefficient conversion of the insulin proreceptor to receptor,[172] respectively. Proalbumin conversion can also be inhibited by replacing a native arginine within the cleavage site with canavanine.[173] The yeast KEX2 endoprotease also can cleave neuroendocrine prohormones if the enzyme is artificially overexpressed in mammalian cells.[174] Furthermore, if the insulin gene is expressed in yeast, proinsulin is converted to insulin[175] (presumably by the combined activity of KEX2 and the carboxypeptidase-like activity of the KEX1 gene product[176]). Finally, it has been shown that the neuropeptide Y precursor[177] and certain mutant forms of prosomatostatin,[178] although normally converted following their introduction into secretory granules, can be converted in cells that do not have a regulated secretory pathway. Taken together, these data suggest considerable overlap between the conversion enzymes used in widely differing cellular environments.

The regulated pathway involves the selective packaging of prohormones into secretory granules, followed by secretion (exocytosis) in response to a stimulus. As will be discussed later, conversion of prohormone to hormone occurs in the secretory granule itself, which also serves as the hormone storage compartment. Active selection of products destined for granules is known to take place in the *trans*-most cisternae of the Golgi complex.[128,131–134,179] The constitutive pathway is considered to be a default pathway, accepting any material in the *trans*-Golgi not previously singled out for shipment to a specific destination. The selection process for directing prohormones to granules is not well understood. By contrast, the targeting of enzymes to lysosomes, for example, is known to depend upon recognition by the mannose-6-phosphate receptor.[180–182] It is important to note, however, that there is morphologic evidence for an intimate association of proinsulin with the cisternal face of Golgi membranes, suggestive of the presence of receptors.[183] Although it remains possible that these receptors are members of a family of 25,000-dalton proteins found in crude Golgi preparations of dog pancreas,[184] further studies are required for confirmation. The recent demonstration of a cell-free model system for studying targeting to the regulated pathway[185] will facilitate the search for putative receptors.

Current dogma indicates that the sorting machinery is the same in all cells equipped with the regulated pathway.[184] This conclusion is based in part upon the results of experiments in which cells are transfected with genes for foreign proteins. For example, AtT20 (pituitary corticotroph) cells can target foreign secretory peptides such as proinsulin[186] or growth hormone,[187] as well as exocrine enzymes such as trypsinogen,[188] to secretory granules. Furthermore, a protein normally destined for the constitutive pathway can be rerouted to secretory granules and regulated release if fused to the appropriate sequences of the growth hormone molecule.[189] The last experiment indicates that functional domains on the secretory protein must be recognized by the targeting machinery. By analogy, there must be functional domains on the proinsulin molecule allowing for its recognition and targeting to the regulated pathway.[190]

The ability to selectively alter protein sequences by site directed mutagenesis, and to then express the mutant protein in the cell of choice by transfection, has led to numerous experiments designed to elucidate which structural domains are involved in protein targeting (for review see reference 191). Proinsulin has also been studied in this way. If native proinsulin is expressed in AtT20 cells, it is normally targeted to the regulated pathway.[186] The removal of some[192] or all[193] of the C-peptide sequence does not affect such targeting (although conversion is affected). Therefore, C-peptide does not seem to be implicated in the recognition of proinsulin by the targeting machinery. However, major truncation of the C-peptide can lead to inefficient secretion via the constitutive pathway in cells lacking the regulated pathway, perhaps due to abnormal retention in a compartment proximal to the constitutive secretory vesicle.[194]

To date, only one mutation has been shown to affect targeting of proinsulin to the regulated pathway. This mutation was first identified in a case of familial hyperproinsulinemia (see Mutations of the Insulin Gene below). It involved replacement of the histidine found in most insulin sequences at position 10 of the B-chain with aspartic acid. Diversion of the mutant proinsulin from the regulated to the constitutive pathway results following transfection into AtT20 cells[195] or expressed in transgenic mouse islets,[196] which might result from diminished recognition by regulated pathway receptors.

The earliest detectable form of the secretory granule in both β-cells[197] and non-β-cells[197,198] is formed from regions of the *trans*-Golgi characterized by the presence of clathrin on their cytosolic face. The immature granule carries a partial coating of clathrin. Clathrin consists of two chains, which can associate to form a network of triskelions and cover membranes with a basket-like coat.[199,200] The assembly of a clathrin coat depends upon associated proteins, including a specific binding domain on the cytosolic face of membrane-spanning receptors.[199,200] In the β-cell, the clathrin coat on the *trans*-Golgi membranes may be anchored to receptors proposed to be part of the prohormone targeting mechanism. If true, introduction of prohormones into granules would be similar to the process of hormone entry into endosomes that occurs during receptor-mediated endocytosis via clathrin-coated pits.[127–130,201] Although it is still not clear what role clathrin plays in either endosome or granule formation, it may be involved in retaining selected proteins within discrete subcellular compartments.[202]

The Clathrin-Coated, Immature Secretory Granule and Conversion of Proinsulin to Insulin

The conversion of proinsulin to insulin and C-peptide occurs in the immature, clathrin-coated secretory granule.[128,203–205] and is outlined in Figure 3–4. As mentioned earlier, Steiner et al. first demonstrated that proinsulin is the immediate single-chain precursor of insulin.[110,111] Shortly thereafter, Kemmler and Steiner[206] and Yip[207] started their search for the converting enzymes. It was immediately suggested that conversion could involve a two-step mechanism, with an initial tryptic cleavage on the C-terminal side of a basic residue followed by trimming, by a carboxypeptidase-like enzyme, of the newly generated C-terminal basic residue.[208,209] It has since become apparent that a similar, if not identical, two-step attack is also responsible for the conversion of most other proproteins.[210–213] For proinsulin, there are two pairs of basic residues at which the endoproteolytic conversion event occurs: Arg-Arg linking the insulin B-chain to the C-peptide and Lys-Arg linking the C-peptide to the insulin A-chain. Two enzymes thought to be involved in this initial cleavage event have been partially characterized. They display different cationic requirements and different affinities for the two cleavage sites.[214,215] Both enzymes display an acidic pH optimum. Only one of the two, however, shows significant activity at neutral pH, which has led to the suggestion that it may be active in a pregranular (presumably Golgi) compartment.[215] There is, however, no direct evidence for this, and morphologic data would seem to discount proinsulin conversion within the Golgi complex of the β-cell.[203–205] Experiments in vitro with the semipurified enzymes indicate that the initial cleavage arises preferentially at the B-chain/C-peptide junction. Cleavage at this site may facilitate subsequent cleavage at the C-peptide/A-chain junction. This order of cleavage events may explain why proinsulin that is cleaved and trimmed only at the B-chain/C-peptide junction is the major conversion intermediate encountered in human serum.[216]

Recently, two human cDNAs were identified that encode mammalian equivalents of the yeast KEX2 enzyme.[217,218] The gene products have been named PC1 (or PC3) and PC2.[170,217,218] It is presumed that the two semipurified enzymes just described correspond to these two gene products. Whereas the presence of both pairs of basic residues is mandatory in the occurrence of proinsulin conversion,[219–221] it has also been shown that removal of segments of the C-peptide, while retaining both pairs of basic residues, can inhibit conversion in secretory cells transfected with the mutant proinsulin gene.[192] This suggests that the cleavage sites must be presented to the conversion enzymes in a rather specific fashion, and this has indeed been shown for other prohormones.[221,222] The enzyme responsible for trimming off the residual C-terminal basic residues left at the ends of the insulin B-chain and C-peptide after the endoproteolytic attack of proinsulin is thought to be carboxypeptidase H.[223,224] This enzyme is not unique to the β-cell or to cells displaying the regulated

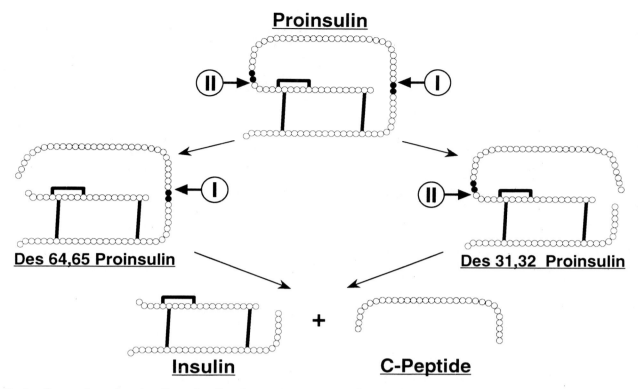

Fig. 3–4. Conversion of proinsulin to insulin. Conversion occurs within acidifying secretory granules. The initial event is an endoproteolytic cut on the C-terminal side of one of the basic residues linking the insulin chains to the C-peptide. According to Davidson et al.[215] two endopeptidases (I and II) are involved; each is postulated to display a preference for just one site. The residual basic amino acids left at the C-terminus of the cleaved proinsulin intermediate are trimmed off by carboxypeptidase H. These two sequential events lead to one of two proinsulin conversion intermediates: des 64,65 split proinsulin or des 31,32 split proinsulin. A further round of endoproteolytic cleavage and carboxypeptidase trimming of either intermediate generates insulin and C-peptide (as well as the four basic amino acids that originally linked C-peptide to the insulin chains).

secretory pathway, as it is secreted even by hepatoma cells.[225]

After an initial lag phase of approximately 15 minutes (presumably the time required for proinsulin to enter granules and for conversion to be initiated), the half-time for conversion is 30 to 45 minutes.[17,165] If β-cells are exposed to high glucose concentrations in vitro, there is a subsequent acceleration of conversion, which may be due to increased rates of granule formation and/or synthesis or turnover of conversion enzymes.[226] By contrast, it has been suggested that interleukin-1,[81] an insulin-sensitive phospho-oligosaccharide,[82] and diazoxide[227] can each decrease the rate of proinsulin conversion (with this effect being selective for rat proinsulin II in the case of interleukin-1[81]). It is unclear whether these agents can affect conversion directly or whether the postulated effects are secondary to some other action on the β-cell. Not all proinsulins are converted at the same rate. Thus, in rat or mouse β-cells, where two nonallelic proinsulins are synthesized in parallel, the rate of conversion of proinsulin I is more rapid than that for proinsulin II.[228] Although no explanation for this phenomenon exists at present, it seems likely that it reflects the relative affinity of the conversion enzymes for the two different proinsulin molecules, and a recent study indicates that

the B-chain/C-peptide junction of rat proinsulin II is more resistant to cleavage than is its counterpart on proinsulin I.[229]

Morphologic studies have shown that in the β-cell there is progressive acidification leading from the *trans*-most Golgi to the mature secretory granule.[230] The conversion of proinsulin to insulin occurs within the immature granule, which already displays a modest acidity.[128,230] Such an acidic environment would ensure maximal activity of the conversion enzymes, which, as mentioned earlier, display an acidic pH optimum.[215] The acidification of granules is assured by an ATP-dependent proton pump.[231,232] In studies on isolated secretory granules,[233] a direct correlation between the activity of this proton pump and proinsulin conversion was observed, again supporting the importance of acidification for conversion. The removal of clathrin from the immature granule would seem to occur in parallel with intragranular acidification and proinsulin conversion. Indeed, there is indirect evidence that preventing proinsulin conversion (by replacing the basic amino acids recognized by the conversion endoproteases with amino acid analogues) also prevents clathrin uncoating.[234] The mechanism of clathrin uncoating of immature secretory granules is not yet understood. By analogy with the uncoating of clathrin-coated vesicles in the brain,[235-238] an ATP-dependent enzyme may be involved; this enzyme has been shown to be a member of the 70-kilodalton heat-shock family of proteins.[235,239]

The Efficiency of Proinsulin Conversion

In a β-cell from a healthy rat,[165] and most likely a healthy human being as well, almost all (>99%) newly synthesized proinsulin appears to be destined for secretory granules. Despite this remarkably efficient targeting, there is always a detectable level of proinsulin-like material in the circulation, as became apparent almost as soon as proinsulin had been identified as the immediate precursor of insulin.[240-244] With the use of specific antibodies, it has been shown that this material consists not only of intact proinsulin but also of conversion intermediates.[245] The major intermediate encountered in the circulation results from cleavage at the B-chain/C-peptide junction,[216,245] leaving the C-peptide joined by its C-terminal extremity to the insulin A-chain. In the fasting state in healthy individuals, proinsulin and this intermediate have each been estimated to each account for some 10% of the total insulin-related material in the circulation.[245] The other major conversion intermediate (cleaved only at the C-peptide/A-chain junction) is present in much smaller amounts. The relative amounts of proinsulin, intermediates, and insulin in the peripheral circulation reflects not only rates of production by the pancreas but also rates of clearance. Proinsulin is cleared from the circulation less rapidly than insulin (primarily because the insulin receptor displays a lower affinity for proinsulin than for insulin), which explains why its relative concentration in the periphery is higher than that encountered in the portal vein.[242] Although the intermediate cleaved between the A-chain and C-peptide may be released in smaller amounts than the other intermediate,[216] it is also cleared more rapidly,[246] which will further reduce its relative concentration in the periphery.

It is not clear why such relatively large amounts of proinsulin and/or conversion intermediates are released. One must assume that all granules contain an adequate supply of conversion enzymes and that, since almost all proinsulin molecules are introduced into granules, the proinsulin should, in turn, be converted to insulin. One possible explanation is that some granules release their contents before conversion is complete. Since proinsulin conversion does not occur to any significant extent outside of the β-cell, any unconverted, or partially converted, proinsulin released in this way would be detected in the circulation. This concept will be discussed below (see Proinsulin Processing and Trafficking in Disease States).

Other Constituents of the β-Granule

Proinsulin is not the only protein introduced into the β-cell secretory granule (for a review see reference 247). As just discussed, proinsulin conversion occurs in the granule itself, which means that the conversion enzymes also must reside within this organelle. Among other granule constituents already characterized, two deserve special mention. The first is chromogranin A, which is found in many different secretory cell types, including β-cells.[248-250] Proteolytic conversion results in the generation of β-granin[250] as well as pancreastatin, which are co-released with insulin from the β-cell. β-granin is most probably liberated from its precursor by the proinsulin-processing enzymes,[250] whereas generation of pancreastatin most likely involves another set of enzymes.[247] Pancreastatin inhibits insulin release from the β-cell.[251,252] It is amidated within β-cells, presumably as a result of the action of peptidylglycine-amidating monooxygenase (PAM) believed to reside in β-cell granules.[247,253]

The other protein of interest is islet amyloid polypeptide (IAPP) (also known as amylin or diabetes-associated peptide), which displays considerable structural homology with calcitonin gene-related peptide (CGRP) (for reviews see references 254 and 255). IAPP is generated by proteolytic processing of a higher-molecular-weight precursor (pro-IAPP).[256] Again, the proinsulin conversion enzymes could be responsible for this conversion event. The active form of IAPP is amidated.[255] IAPP is the major constituent of islet amyloid deposits.[257] These deposits, first reported at the turn of the century, have been found in the pancreases of nearly all individuals with NIDDM[257,258] and often in insulinoma tissue.[257] Amyloid deposits also are found surrounding islets in diabetic cats, but, curiously, not in rodents. This difference between species is now ascribed to differences in IAPP primary structure, with formation of amyloid deposits being dependent upon specific structural domains.[259-261] Sequences unique to pro-IAPP have also been found in amyloid deposits,[262] and it has been suggested that inadequate pro-IAPP conversion in individuals with diabetes may in part be responsible for islet amyloidosis.[247,262,263] Since NIDDM also is associated with hyperproinsulinemia (see below), it has further been proposed that there may be a basic defect in precursor processing associated with this disease state.[247,263]

IAPP has attracted considerable attention in the last few years since it has been reported to display properties of a diabetogenic agent. IAPP has been reported to inhibit insulin release in vitro[264] and to cause insulin resistance,[265-267] although both of these effects are controversial.[268,269] IAPP also exerts calcitonin-like effects.[270] The relative physiologic impact of calcitonin itself and of these mimetic properties of IAPP remains to be established. Studies on the biologic role of IAPP (even if such studies are in their infancy), taken together with the presence of IAPP in islet amyloid deposits in individuals with NIDDM, have led to a host of reviews proposing a possible link between IAPP and diabetes.[254,258,263,270-274] Time will tell whether IAPP is involved in the pathogenesis of NIDDM and/or amyloid deposits reflect a lesion in β-cell function.

In common with other soluble granule constituents, IAPP is co-secreted with insulin.[275-277] Although the synthesis of some β-cell-granule proteins is regulated in concert with that of proinsulin,[278] this is not true for all of them.[278] It remains to be seen whether IAPP synthesis is subject to tight regulation, and as for all granule matrix proteins, including proinsulin itself, it will be fascinating to learn how its precursor finds its way to the secretory granule.

The Mature Granule and the Insulin Crystal

The combination of granule acidification and conversion of proinsulin to insulin provides the scenario for insulin crystallization within the mature granule. Insulin is known to be able to associate into dimers and, in the presence of Zn^{++}, the dimers can associate to form hexamers.[279,280] The Zn^{++} is coordinated by the histidine residue at position 10 of the insulin B-chain. The Zn-hexamers can then pack together to form a crystal lattice. Crystallization depends upon a very high local concentration of insulin and Zn^{++}, as well as an acidic milieu, with these conditions being satisfied within the granule.[247,281,282] The dense core of the secretory granule observed by electron microscopy is thus taken to be an insulin crystal.[279,283–285] C-peptide does not co-crystallize to any significant extent with insulin and is therefore excluded from the crystal, to be found in the clear halo surrounding the dense core of granules.[127,286] Proinsulin can also coordinate Zn^{++} and form hexamers.[279–281] The six C-peptides, however, are thought to lie on the surface of the proinsulin hexamer. This has two consequences: 1) the proinsulin hexamer is much more soluble than the insulin hexamer, and 2) the outlying C-peptides mask the faces involved in the assembly of insulin hexamers into the crystal form. It is thus possible that proinsulin hexamers form in immature granules (or possibly even in the Golgi complex), with crystallization arising only after conversion.[281] It is perhaps not coincidental that the presumed localization and orientation of the C-peptides in the proinsulin hexamer would expose the pairs of basic residues, linking the C-peptide with the two insulin chains, to the conversion enzymes. The preferred substrate for conversion may be the proinsulin hexamer.

THE FATE OF THE MATURE SECRETORY GRANULE

Insulin is stored in the mature secretory granule until it is either released, by exocytosis, or degraded, by crinophagy.

Insulin Release (Exocytosis)

Exocytosis arises by fusion of the granule membrane with the plasma membrane, with subsequent discharge of granule contents to the extracellular space, and is followed by pinocytosis of limited regions of the plasma membrane[287] (see references 126 and 288 for reviews). In this way, the total surface area of the cell is maintained even in the face of extensive exocytosis. Although insulin release and its regulation is discussed in detail in Chapter 4, it is appropriate to mention those features of this process related to intracellular trafficking and targeting of organelles.

There is good evidence, from both morphologic and biochemical studies, that transport within the regulated secretory pathway is dependent upon the cytoskeletal network of microtubules and microfilaments. Granules move along microtubules on their way from the Golgi complex to the plasma membrane.[138–140,289] By analogy with other cell types in which directional movement of organelles is rather better understood, accessory proteins, including microtubule-associated proteins (MAPs) and force-generating enzymes, are likely involved in granule movement in β-cells as in other secretory cells.[290–292] The stimulation of insulin release must involve not only facilitated fusion of granule and plasma membrane but also recruitment of granules to the plasma membrane. The margination of granules in proximity to the plasma membrane has been shown under certain situations for non-β-cells,[293–295] leading to the hypothesis that, under basal conditions, granule fusion with the plasma membrane is inhibited by factors in the immediate vicinity of the inner face of the plasma membrane. Stimulus-secretion coupling would then involve the generation of second messengers to override these inhibitory signals, thereby allowing for granule fusion.[130] This model also demands the existence of both granule and plasma membrane proteins that would be involved in the targeting, recognition, and fusion events of exocytosis.[131,296]

There have been reports in the literature that newly synthesized insulin is released in preference to older, stored material.[297–303] If this were true, it would imply heterogeneity among secretory granules, with new granules being recognized as such and tagged for preferential exocytosis. Clearly, the immature, clathrin-coated granule could be a candidate for preferential release of newly synthesized products. These granules, however, contain essentially only proinsulin, whereas the experimental data show preferential release of newly synthesized insulin. Another explanation for this phenomenon could be that it reflects the combination of the protocol employed for these studies and β-cell heterogeneity. In all cases, isolated islets were pulse-labeled with a radioactive amino acid and the release of labeled (newly synthesized) and unlabeled (stored) insulin then compared during a post-label, or chase, period. Since it is known that β-cells in the islet are composed of a mixed population,[304–306] with some cells being more active than others both in terms of biosynthesis[306] and secretion,[304] the so-called preferential release of new, labeled insulin could reflect different rates of turnover. Whether granule or cell heterogeneity accounts for this phenomenon remains open, but cell heterogeneity will probably be shown to play a major part.

Degradation of Insulin Stores in the β-Cell (Crinophagy)

If not released, insulin can be degraded within the β-cell.[307,308] Degradation arises by the fusion of granules with lysosomes,[309] an event referred to as crinophagy and first shown to occur in pituitary mammatroph cells[310] and pancreatic α-cells.[311] Degradation seems to act in concert with biosynthesis and release to regulate the amount of insulin housed in the β-cell at a given time.[307,308] Although the factors regulating crinophagy are not understood, it has been found that when insulin release is inhibited degradation increases, and vice versa.[307,308,312,313] Insulin is degraded only slowly, even after its introduction into lysosomes.[309,314,315] This is thought to be due to the stability of the insulin crystal in lysosomes, which display an acidic milieu similar to that of the secretory granule. By contrast, both proinsulin and C-peptide (neither of which exists in the crystal state within granules) are degraded rapidly within β-cells.[309,314-316]

PROINSULIN PROCESSING AND TRAFFICKING IN DISEASE STATES

There are situations in which the proportion of proinsulin, relative to insulin, in the circulation is unusually elevated. The possible reasons for such hyperproinsulinemia will be discussed in relation to proinsulin processing and trafficking in the β-cell.

Diabetes Mellitus

For the following discussion it will be important to distinguish between conditions leading to an increase in both serum proinsulin and insulin, with a normal ratio of proinsulin to insulin, and those leading to an elevated ratio of proinsulin to insulin regardless of the total amounts of immunoreactive products encountered. This second situation is of concern here. Such an increased ratio of proinsulin to insulin is found frequently in individuals with NIDDM[317-322] and in some with recent-onset insulin-dependent diabetes (IDDM)[323-325] or their nondiabetic twins[326] or siblings.[327] This ratio has also been found to be increased in patients with thyrotoxicosis[328] or hypokalemia,[329] in hyperinsulinemic/hypoglycemic subjects without known insulinoma,[330] and in patients with cystic fibrosis and impaired glucose tolerance.[331] It is of interest that elevated proinsulin-to-insulin ratios in persons with diabetes can be restored, or partially restored, to normal by improving their metabolic status.[332-334]

In most early studies, no attempt was made to distinguish between intact proinsulin and conversion intermediates. When this was achieved (e.g., reference 335) des 32,33 split proinsulin (proinsulin cleaved between the B-chain and C-peptide) was found to contribute significantly towards total "proinsulin-related" immunoreactivity in persons with Type II diabetes, just as in control subjects.[216]

The reasons for elevated ratios of proinsulin to insulin in persons with diabetes are not known. Available information would suggest, however, that there is no problem with targeting to secretory granules. Although there are studies showing that this ratio is increased because of decreased insulin levels in the face of preserved or elevated proinsulin levels,[336,337] there is no suggestion of constitutive release of proinsulin. Therefore, the problem must lie at the level of the conversion of proinsulin to insulin. There are two alternative explanations currently under evaluation: 1) proinsulin conversion per se is impaired; 2) granule turnover is so rapid that a significant amount of proinsulin is released before it can be converted.

According to the first explanation, the conversion system (enzymes) itself is at fault. This should lead to an increase not only in the amount of unprocessed proinsulin that leaves the β-cell but also in the amount any other pro-protein normally cleaved within β-cells by the same processing machinery. The precursor to IAPP (amylin), pro-IAPP, is one such protein. As mentioned earlier, islet amyloidosis and elevated proinsulin in persons with diabetes have indeed been ascribed to the same fundamental defect in β-cell precursor processing.[247,263,338] This hypothesis is certainly strengthened by the detection of pro-IAPP in islet amyloid deposits.[262]

The second explanation, that hyperproinsulinemia is caused by increased turnover, is based on the suggestion that the rate of turnover of secretory granules might be such that the residence time of some proinsulin molecules within the granules (before release) would be too short to permit conversion.[318] Such might be the case in Type II diabetes, under conditions of increased insulin demand caused by insulin resistance, in the face of a partially depleted population of β-cells.

Insulinoma

Aside from the unregulated overproduction of immunoreactive insulin by insulinoma cells, they also are characterized by the disproportionate amount of proinsulin they secrete.[339-344] There is considerable heterogeneity among insulinomas, and the relative amount of proinsulin produced has been correlated with the sensitivity of immunoreactive insulin output towards inhibitors such as somatostatin or diazoxide.[344] In addition to proinsulin itself, there have been several reports of the presence of insulin immunoreactive products of even higher molecular weight in the circulation of patients with insulinoma.[345-350] Although it is unclear whether such material is generated within insulinoma cells or in the circulation, it possibly consists of aggregated proinsulin or insulin,[348] similar to that encountered following exogenous insulin injection.[351]

Based upon the results of studies on human insulinoma tissue[352] or on cell lines derived from animal insulinomas,[353-356] it is possible that their unusually elevated production of proinsulin reflects a partial diversion of proinsulin from the regulated to the constitutive pathway. Why such a diversion should be provoked by cellular transformation is unclear. Certainly, tumor cells typically fail to express some of the differentiated features of the native parent cell. The failure to use the regulated pathway to full effect would be an example of such a lesion. Perhaps the need to synthesize unusual quantities of membrane and associated proteins to satisfy accelerated cell division leads to an impaired ability to satisfy luxury pathways such as granule formation. Amyloid deposits often are found in insulinoma tissue.[257] As for amyloidosis in islets of individuals with NIDDM, insulinoma amyloidosis also may reflect increased production of pro-IAPP in association with the observed hyperproinsulinemia.

INSULIN STRUCTURE

Amino Acid Sequence

Although insulin was recognized to be a protein shortly after its discovery,[357] the elucidation of its primary structure came many years later with the development by Sanger and co-workers of methods to determine primary sequences of proteins.[109,358] In fact, insulin was the first protein to have its entire primary sequence determined (a scientific feat for which Sir Frederic Sanger received the 1959 Nobel Prize in Chemistry). Figure 3—5 compares the primary sequences of insulins from different animal species. All known insulins are composed of two polypeptide chains that are linked to one another by disulfide bonds. The A- and B-chains of human, porcine, and bovine insulins, like most other vertebrate insulins, are composed of 21 and 30 amino acids, respectively. These two peptide chains are covalently linked to one another by two cystine disulfides, one between CysA7 and CysB7 and the other between CysA20 and CysB19. An additional intrachain disulfide connects cysteines A6 and A11.

For many years patients with diabetes were treated with insulins that had been isolated from porcine and bovine pancreases. The primary sequences of these insulins are closely related to the sequence of human insulin. There is only a single difference between the sequences of human and porcine insulins, at position B30, where human insulin has a threonine and porcine insulin has an alanine (Fig. 3—5). Bovine insulin differs from human insulin at three positions. Like porcine insulin, bovine insulin has an alanine at the B30 position. In addition, threonine and isoleucine at positions A8 and A10 of human insulin are replaced by alanine and valine in the bovine sequence. All of these are considered to be conservative changes in primary sequence that have no apparent effect on biologic activity, although they do affect solubility.[359]

In efforts to elucidate relationships between insulin structure and function, the sequences of insulins from nearly 50 additional species, including many mammalian species as well as other vertebrates (birds, fish, and reptiles), have been determined.[17,360] Thirty-three percent of insulin residues are strictly invariant (boxes, Fig. 3—5), suggesting unique structural requirements at these positions either for receptor recognition or maintenance of core structure directly or for the direction of proper protein folding, targeting to granules, or proteolytic processing during insulin biosynthesis. All six cysteines and their patterns of disulfide cross-linking are conserved throughout vertebrate evolution. In addition, residues of the amino (A1—A5) and carboxyl (A16, A19, A20, A21) termini of the A-chain and throughout the middle of the B-chain (B5—B8, B11—B16, B23—B26) are invariant or highly conserved, suggesting an important biologic role for all of these residues (solid and hatched boxes). Mutations and chemical modifications at invariant or highly conserved positions generally diminish or abolish receptor binding potency and biologic activity, emphasizing the importance of these positions in either creating

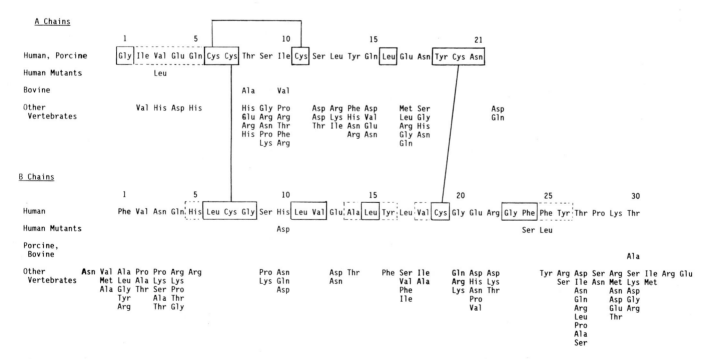

Fig. 3—5. Amino acid sequences of therapeutic and mutant human insulins and substitutions occurring in 46 additional vertebrate insulins. Solid lines denote disulfide bonds; solid and hatched boxes surround invariant and highly homologous residues, respectively.

or maintaining a three-dimensional surface suitable for receptor recognition.[361–363]

Three-Dimensional Structure

The pioneering studies of the x-ray diffraction patterns of insulin crystals, conducted simultaneously by Dorothy Hodgkin and co-workers at Oxford[364,365] and the Peking Insulin Structure Group,[366] have been the cornerstone for relating insulin's structure and function. These three-dimensional structural determinations were first obtained at resolutions of 2.8 Å and 2.5 Å, respectively, and have now been refined to a resolution of 1.5 Å.[367] Within each unit cell of 2-zinc insulin crystals, six insulin molecules compose a hexamer around two zinc atoms; each zinc atom is chelated by three HisB10 residues (Fig. 3–6). 2-Zinc insulin hexamers can be subdivided into three equivalent dimers, with each dimer being composed of two insulin molecules of similar but not identical structure.

The hydrophobic core of the 2-zinc insulin monomer is composed of all invariant or highly conserved residues, including leucine residues A16, B6, B11, and B15; the A6–A11 cystine; the TyrA19 ring; IleA2; and AlaB14, supporting the notion that core structure must be maintained for insulin action. These core residues with hydrophobic side chains contact additional more peripheral nonpolar residues, including ValA3, LeuA13, ValB12, ValB18, CysB19, and PheB24, which in turn contact the remaining nonpolar residues (PheB1, ValB3, LeuB17, and PheB25). The more peripheral nonpolar residues that are exposed partially on the monomer surface contribute to the surfaces of insulin involved in protein-protein interactions, including the dimer and hexamer interfaces and possibly the receptor-binding surface as well (discussed below).

Residues from both A- and B-chains comprise the hydrophobic core of insulin and the various binding surfaces. The A-chain forms two helical segments (A1–A8 and A13–A19), which are connected by a turn; the B-chain contains two regions of extended chain (B1–B8, B21–B30) connected by a region of α-helix (B9–B19). The two chains are connected to one another covalently by cystine disulfides (A7–B7, A20–B19) and the overall structure is stabilized by interchain hydrogen bonds (A11...B4, A6...B6, A21...B23, and A19...B25) and ionic interactions between the amino terminus of the A-chain and the carboxyl terminus of the B-chain.

Structural studies have also been conducted with hexameric 4-zinc[368,369] and phenol-induced porcine insulin crystals,[370] dimeric hagfish and zinc-free porcine insulins,[371,372] and monomeric despentapeptide (B26–B30) insulin.[373] The hydrophobic core structure is maintained in all crystallographic forms of insulin. However, comparisons of different subunit structures also reveal areas of the molecule that adopt dissimilar structures. For example, the two subunit structures of 4-zinc insulin are grossly different.[368,369] One monomer of 4-zinc insulin resembles the 2-zinc insulin structure in which the B-chain helix extends from B9 to B19, which is referred to as the T state.[370,374] In the apposing monomer

(termed the R state), the B-chain helix extends all the way to PheB1 such that the B1 positions of the 2 monomers are displaced 20 to 25 Å. Thus 2-zinc insulin has a T_6 structure, 4-zinc insulin is designated T_3R_3, and the phenol-induced structure is designated R_6 (the TR nomenclature for structural subunits follows the conventions adopted for allosteric changes in hemoglobin structure; R is liganded and T is unliganded, e.g., see reference 375). Differences in subunit structure appear to be propagated nonlocally through the helical bundles.[376]

In crystals, protein structures can be perturbed as a result of crystal packing forces. This is exemplified by the structural differences observed in various crystal forms of insulin[364–373,376] Therefore, efforts have been made to relate crystallographic structures of insulin to its structure in solution. Spectroscopic studies were designed to determine which of the crystallographic conformations reflect the structure of insulin monomer in solution. Circular dichroism,[377,378] rapid kinetic analyses,[379] and visible spectroscopy[379–381] all demonstrate that phenol or lyotropic anions (e.g., SCN^-, I^-, Br^-) induce the transition from T to R in solution. However, these are measures of global structure that do not provide details necessary for determining three-dimensional structures of proteins in solution.

Advances in nuclear magnetic resonance (NMR) technology now make it possible to assess the structures of small proteins (<10,000 daltons) in solution. Several groups have applied these methods to the study of insulin and related related analogues,[382–387] although initial studies were limited by the tendency of insulin to self-associate. Spectra have been obtained under highly basic conditions,[382] although disulfide interchange precluded accumulation of high-resolution spectra. In acidic, aqueous-organic co-solvent mixtures, formation of insulin dimers and hexamers is similarly suppressed, and under these conditions highly refined spectra have been obtained.[383–389] Most recently, methods for protein engineering have been used to prevent insulin self-association[390–393] (see below), and with such analogues, high-resolution spectra can now be obtained under more physiologic pH and solvent conditions.[386,393,394] Of note, the basic structure of insulin is similar in insulin crystals and in solution under both acidic conditions and at neutral pH. Molecule 2 of 2-zinc insulin crystals (Chinese nomenclature) best approximates the structure of insulin in solution, although insulin structure is remarkably flexible in solution, consistent with the notion that changes in insulin structure might accompany binding.

Receptor-Binding Surface

Comparisons among crystallographic structures of insulin and biologic potencies of different species and analogues of insulin have been used to deduce a putative surface of insulin that interacts with the insulin receptor.[361,363,367] It is thought that residues from both ends of the A-chain (GlyA1, GlnA5, TyrA19, AsnA21) and from several regions of the B-chain (ValB12, TyrB16, GlyB23,

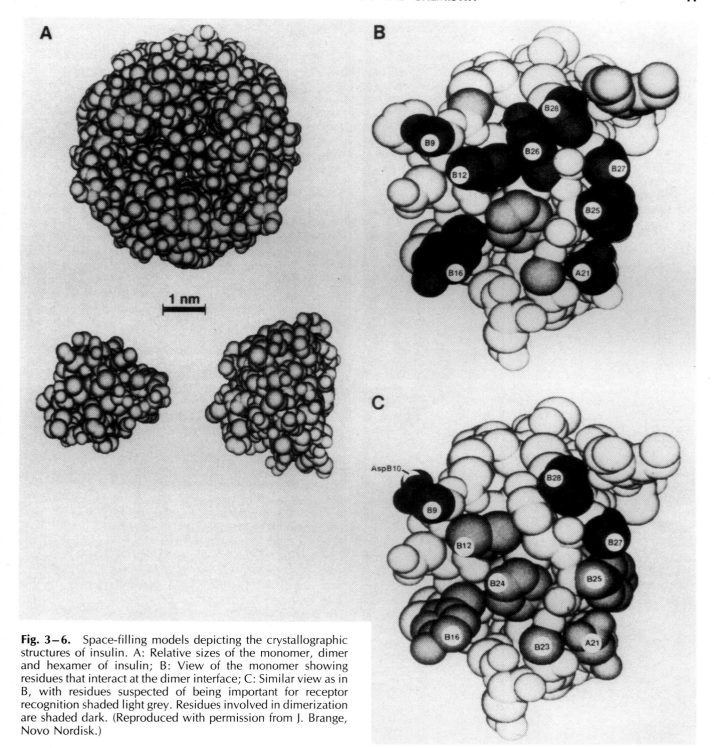

Fig. 3–6. Space-filling models depicting the crystallographic structures of insulin. A: Relative sizes of the monomer, dimer and hexamer of insulin; B: View of the monomer showing residues that interact at the dimer interface; C: Similar view as in B, with residues suspected of being important for receptor recognition shaded light grey. Residues involved in dimerization are shaded dark. (Reproduced with permission from J. Brange, Novo Nordisk.)

PheB24, PheB25) come together to form this binding surface (Fig. 3–6). It is worth noting that this is a static representation of the deduced binding surface of insulin and, as insulin is flexible in solution and may change structure upon binding to receptor (see below), this model may be an oversimplification.

Two recent studies with "anomalous" analogues—those whose binding and biologic activities cannot be

accounted for by crystallographic representations of native insulin structure—underscore the likelihood of a structural change associated with insulin binding. Crystal structures of insulin analogues that are either chemically cross-linked between the α-amino group of GlyA1 and the ε-amino group of LysB29 (diaminosuberic acid[395]) or directly connected between these residues by a peptide bond (single-chain insulin[396]) are essentially identical to the structures of native insulin, despite the markedly reduced[395,399] or undetectable[396] receptor-binding potencies of these analogues. Single-chain insulin retains the capacity to form both R and T structures, suggesting that this transition has little to do with the insulin binding process.[396] In fact, these results led Derewenda et al. to conclude that known crystal structures of insulin likely depict inactive conformers.[396] The solution structure of PheB24→AGly insulin, an insulin analogue with near-normal binding potency,[397] was examined in a separate study with NMR.[380] Whereas the core structure of the analogue, as defined by the α-helices, is intact, the B20−B23 β-turn and interactions between the carboxyl-terminus of the B-chain and the helical core are absent. That this analogue partially unfolds yet retains biologic potency suggests that separation of the C-terminal B-chain from the helical core does not interfere with receptor binding. Taken together with the aforementioned crystallographic studies conducted with cross-linked[395] or single-chain[396] insulin analogues, these studies suggest that separation of the carboxyl-terminus of the B-chain from insulin's helical core might be necessary during the receptor binding process.[378−398]

Modified Insulins

Much of what is known about insulin structure-function relationships comes from studies with modified insulins and comparisons of insulins from different animal species. Some of these studies have been the subjects of previous reviews.[17,362,363] An interesting recent application is the engineering of insulin analogues with altered pharmacokinetic characteristics. As discussed, insulin aggregates in solution to form dimers, which in turn form tetramers, hexamers, and additional higher-order aggregates (see Fig. 3−6). By selective substitution of amino acids within the dimer- and hexamer-forming surfaces of insulin, aggregation is dramatically altered.[390−393] For example, substitutions of SerB9 or HisB10 within the hexamer-forming surface or ThrB27 or ProB28 within the dimer-forming surface with charged residues substantially diminishes hexamer and dimer formation, respectively. Substitutions at both surfaces within the same analogue prevent aggregations altogether, resulting in monomeric insulin analogues with altered absorption characteristics following subcutaneous injection.[391] These and similar approaches are being used in attempts to provide diabetic patients with therapeutic insulins better matched to their metabolic requirements.

PROINSULIN STRUCTURE

Proinsulin is the biosynthetic precursor of insulin,[110,111] as discussed earlier in this chapter. The crystallographic structure of proinsulin has not yet been reported, although appropriate crystals have been obtained and diffraction studies have been undertaken. Structural studies by two-dimensional NMR indicate that overall the insulin moiety of proinsulin is similar to that of insulin, while the C-peptide portion of proinsulin appears to be unstructured.[400] Thus, the model of proinsulin structure proposed by Blundell et al.[401] appears to be

correct. There are, however, perturbations in the insulin moiety of proinsulin that are reverted by cleavage between the A-chain but not the B-chain and C-peptide, suggesting a structural recognition element for the type II endopeptidase.[400] To account for the reduced biologic potency of proinsulin (reviewed in reference 243), it has been suggested that the C-peptide obscures a portion of the receptor-binding surface of insulin[401] or, alternatively, prevents movement of the C-terminus of the B-chain during binding.[378]

For proinsulin the amino terminus of the insulin A-chain is connected to the carboxyl-terminus of the B-chain by a peptide sequence called the connecting peptide (or C-peptide). Unlike insulin, whose sequence is highly conserved, the sequence of the C-peptide portions of different proinsulins show little homology. These C-peptides differ markedly both in length and amino acid composition, suggesting that the C-peptide composition itself is not very important. Rather, it is likely that the C-peptide moiety of proinsulin acts as a tether between the A- and B-chains of insulin to guarantee appropriate folding and disulfide pairing during the biosynthetic process.

PREPARATION OF THERAPEUTIC INSULIN

Until recently insulin for therapeutic purposes was produced almost exclusively by extraction from bovine and porcine pancreases. Between 100 and 400 mg of insulin can be obtained from each kilogram of pancreatic tissue, and it has been estimated that there would be sufficient supplies of animal insulin to meet the requirements of diabetic patients into the next century.[402] Through modern purification procedures, animal insulins can be prepared in essentially pure form, which eliminates the possibility of the development of antibodies to impurities in the insulin preparations. However, patients treated with so-called pure insulins still develop antibodies to insulin, which suggested that differences in the primary structures of these insulins might be what stimulates antibody production. Therefore, enzymatic and biosynthetic methods have been developed for the preparation of therapeutic insulin identical to human insulin (for additional discussions see Chapters 27 and 33).

Isolation from Animal Sources

The underlying procedure for isolating insulin from pancreatic tissue has remained nearly unchanged for over 50 years.[403,404] Frozen pancreases are extracted in acidified aqueous ethanol to solubilize the insulin and inactivate exocrine proteases. After a neutralization step, the pH is readjusted to between 3 and 4 (near the isoelectric point of insulin), 2 to 3 M NaCl is added, and insulin precipitates. "Salt cake" insulin is then redissolved in acid and crystallized in the presence of zinc. After two crystallization steps, insulin is 80 to 90% pure,[359,403,404] although it still contains substantial amounts of proinsulin and related conversion intermediates, arginyl- and ethyl-insulins, covalent insulin dimers, and monodesamido insulin. Because these impurities have potentially harmful side effects, most insulin preparations used to treat diabetic patients are further purified by gel-filtration, ion-exchange chromatography, and/or reversed-phase liquid chromatography. Highly purified insulin preparations for treating diabetic patients, including single-component (SC) insulin (Lilly), monocomponent (MC) insulin (Novo), and porcine regular insulin (RI) (Nordisk), all contain less than 1 ppm of impurities.

Semisynthesis and Biosynthesis of Human Insulin

Porcine insulin can be converted to the human insulin sequence by an enzyme-catalyzed transpeptidation reaction.[405,406] Under the appropriate conditions, trypsin acts preferentially at LysB29 rather than ArgB22 to yield a covalent des[B30]insulin/trypsin complex (acyl-enzyme intermediate). In the presence of high concentrations of organic co-solvents and the *tert*-butyl ester of threonine, transpeptidation predominates over hydrolysis to yield the *tert*-butyl ester of human insulin. Following appropriate purification steps and acidolytic removal of the ester, human insulin suitable for treating patients is obtained.

Recent advances in recombinant DNA technology now make possible production of human insulin from protein products produced either in bacteria or yeast. Three different basic strategies have been used.[407-409] DNA sequences encoding individual A- and B-chains were synthesized with a codon for methionine at the position corresponding to the N-terminus of each chain, and inserted into the Trp synthetase gene.[407] The fusion proteins thus produced account for up to 20% of total protein in the *Escherichia coli*. The chimeric proteins precipitate as inclusion bodies, providing protection from bacterial proteases, and are harvested and treated with cyanogen bromide to release the desired A- and B-chains. All cysteine residues are converted to the respective S-sulfonates to ease handling and purification, after which mild reduction and air oxidation steps yield intact human insulin. Alternatively, full-length proinsulin is produced in *E. coli* following a similar strategy, but the postfermentation chemistry is simplified because proper chain combination is directed by the C-peptide.[408] The proinsulin product is cleaved enzymatically to yield intact human insulin. "Miniproinsulin" is a shortened form of proinsulin with intact A- and B-chains and an Ala-Ala-Lys connecting peptide segment. Following transfection, yeast (*Saccharomyces cerevisiae*) express the protein and export it into the media as a properly processed and folded product.[409] After purification steps and trypsin-catalyzed transpeptidation and acidolysis (see previous paragraph), intact human insulin is obtained.

MUTANT INSULINS AND PROINSULINS

Mutations in the insulin gene can occur in upstream or downstream flanking sequences, within one of the two introns or within the protein-encoding exons. Naturally, these different kinds of insulin gene mutations would present different biochemical profiles and possibly different phenotypic expressions. For example, mutations in the enhancer/promoter region might result in decreased transcription and in insulin deficiency, whereas mutations

in the gene sequence encoding the signal peptide of preproinsulin might affect transport into the RER and packaging into secretory vesicles. While considerable heterogeneity is observed distal to the 5' end of the insulin gene (cf. 7,8), the most notable mutations thus far reported occur in the coding regions for insulin and proinsulin.[410-429]

Insulinopathies

Tager and Rubenstein and co-workers were the first to recognize the relationship between diabetes and a structurally abnormal insulin molecule.[410,411] Subsequent advances in high-performance liquid chromatography (HPLC) separation and detection allowed characterization of additional abnormal forms of insulin,[412,414] and through advances in DNA sequencing methods, investigators in Steiner's laboratory found mutations in the insulin genes of these patients.[413,415,417] Three different altered forms of insulin with low biologic potency have now been associated with diabetes: "Insulin Chicago" results from a PheB25→Leu substitution,[412,413] "Insulin Los Angeles" involves a PheB24→Ser switch,[414,415] and "Insulin Wakayama" results from a ValA3→Leu substitution.[417] While additional, apparently unrelated, probands have been found who produce the same abnormal insulins from identical insulin gene mutations,[418-420] no additional abnormal insulins have yet been identified, although they surely exist.

These patients and their families define a new clinical syndrome, the insulinopathies, which are characterized by high circulating levels of insulin and a frequent association with mild carbohydrate intolerance.[411,416,420,421] What makes these subjects different from others with Type II diabetes, however, is a normal or slightly impaired sensitivity to exogenous insulin despite unusually high levels of their own circulating insulin.[416] Hyperinsulinemia in these patients is not explained by the presence of circulating antibodies or elevated levels of counterregulatory hormones (Table 3–1). In fact each of these patients produces normal and abnormal forms of insulin in equivalent amounts.[412] The more potent normal insulin is cleared more rapidly, resulting in accumulation of the abnormal insulin and in

Table 3–1. Characteristics of Patients with Mutant Insulins

1. Hyperinsulinemia
2. No evidence for insulin resistance
   Normal levels of contrainsulin hormones
   No antibodies to insulin
   No antibodies to insulin receptor
   No detectable defect in insulin receptor
3. Normal response to exogenous insulin
   Normal insulin tolerance test
   Normal euglycemic insulin-clamp study
4. Reduced biologic activity of endogenous insulin
   Abnormal glucose clamp study with hyperglycemia
   Reduced potency of isolated serum insulin
5. Reduced C-peptide:insulin molar ratio
6. Hyperglycemia/diabetes may or may not be present

a dramatic degree of hyperinsulinemia. The amounts of normal bioactive insulin in the circulations of these patients are actually inappropriately low, resulting in the observed impaired glucose tolerance and diabetes.[417,421]

Familial Hyperproinsulinemia

Mutations in the insulin gene can also result in impaired processing of proinsulin to insulin. As seen with abnormal insulins, individuals with hyperproinsulimemia caused by impaired processing may exhibit carbohydrate intolerance, but not necessarily.[422,423] For two of the three cases studied, large amounts of an insulin molecule with C-peptide still attached at the A-chain/C-peptide junction were found in the circulation.[422-426] In both cases, impaired processing appears to result directly from a mutation of arginine within the Lys64-Arg65 endopeptidase recognition sequence.[424,425] DNA sequencing studies reveal an Arg65→His mutation in one the patients.[426]

A third case of familial hyperproinsulinemia results from a HisB10→Asp mutation.[427,428] It is surprising that a defect in proinsulin structure distant from the paired basic cleavage sites prevents processing. However, transfection of the mutated gene into cells and expression in transgenic mice[196,429] both show that significant proportions of the mutated hormone are secreted from cells via the constitutive pathway. As proinsulins have substantially less biologic potency than the corresponding insulin molecules, and as much of insulin and proinsulin clearance occurs by receptor-mediated pathways, the proinsulin molecules are cleared more slowly and accumulate in the circulation of afflicted patients. The proteolytic product of HisB10→Asp proinsulin is HisB10→Asp insulin, which unlike other abnormal insulins exhibits enhanced potency.[393,429]

SUMMARY

From the initial seconds of the biosynthesis of its early precursor, preproinsulin, to its release or degradation, insulin is always protected from the cytosol by a limiting membrane. Insulin release reflects a well-orchestrated series of events involving the successive budding, directed movement, and fusion of transport vesicles or granules and intravesicular proteolytic conversion events. The three-dimensional structure and physicochemical properties of insulin and its precursors play an intimate role in this series of events, just as they do for the biologic activity of these molecules.

REFERENCES

1. Banting FG, Best CH. The internal secretion of the pancreas. J Lab Clin Med 1922;7:251–66.
2. Banting FG, Best CH. Pancreatic extracts. J Lab Clin Med 1922;7:464–72.
3. Banting FG, Best CH, Collip JB, et al. Pancreatic extracts in the treatment of diabetes mellitus. Can Med Assoc J 1922;12:141–6.
4. Bell GI, Pictet RL, Rutter WJ, et al. Sequence of the human insulin gene. Nature 1980;284:26–32.
5. Owerbach D, Bell GI, Rutter WJ, et al. The insulin gene is located on the short arm of chromosome 11 in humans. Diabetes 1981;30:267–70.
6. Dull TJ, Gray A, Hayflick JS, Ullrich A. Insulin-like growth factor II precursor gene organization in relation to insulin gene family. Nature 1984;310:777–81.
7. Bell GI, Karam JH, Rutter WJ. Polymorphic DNA region adjacent to the 5′ end of the human insulin gene. Proc Natl Acad Sci USA 1981;78:5759–63.
8. Bell GI, Selby MJ, Rutter WJ. The highly polymorphic region near the human insulin gene is composed of simple tandemly repeating sequences. Nature 1982;295:31–5.
9. Owerbach D, Poulsen S, Billesbølle P, Nerup J. DNA insertion sequences near the insulin gene affect glucose regulation. Lancet 1982;1:880–3.
10. Owerbach D, Nerup J. Restriction fragment length polymorphism of the insulin gene in diabetes mellitus. Diabetes 1982;31:275–7.
11. Rotwein PS, Chirgwin J, Province M, et al. Polymorphism in the 5′ flanking region of the human insulin gene: a genetic marker for non-insulin-dependent diabetes. N Engl J Med 1983;308:65–71.
12. Bell GI, Horita S, Karam JH. A polymorphic locus near the human insulin gene is associated with insulin-dependent diabetes mellitus. Diabetes 1984;33:176–83.
13. Permutt MA, Chirgwin J, Rotwein P, Giddings S. Insulin gene structure and function: a review of studies using recombinant DNA methodology. Diabetes Care 1984;7:386–94.
14. Cocozza S, Riccardi G, Monticelli A, et al. Polymorphism at the 5′ end flanking region of the insulin gene is associated with reduced insulin secretion in healthy individuals. Eur J Clin Invest 1988;18:582–6.
15. Elbein S, Rotwein P, Permutt MA, et al. Lack of association of the polymorphic locus in the 5′-flanking region of the human insulin gene and diabetes in American blacks. Diabetes 1985;34:433–9.
16. Permutt MA, Elbein SC. Insulin gene in diabetes: analysis through RFLP. Diabetes Care 1990;13:364–74.
17. Steiner DF, Bell GI, Tager HS. Chemistry and biosynthesis of pancreatic protein hormones. In: DeGroot LJ, Besser GM, Cahill GF Jr, et al, eds. Endocrinology. 2nd ed. Vol 2. Philadelphia: WB Saunders, 1989:1263–89.
18. Steiner DF, Chan SJ, Welsh JM, Kwok SCM. Structure and evolution of the insulin gene. Annu Rev Genet 1985;19:463–84.
19. Muglia L, Locker J. Extrapancreatic insulin gene expression in the fetal rat. Proc Natl Acad Sci USA 1984;81:3635–9.
20. Giddings SJ, Carnaghi LR. Selective expression and developmental regulation of the ancestral rat insulin II gene in fetal liver. Mol Endocrinol 1990;4:1363–9.
21. Selden RF, Skoskiewicz MJ, Russell PS, Goodman HM. Regulation of insulin-gene expression: implications for gene therapy. N Engl J Med 1987;317:1067–76.
22. Walker MD, Edlund T, Boulet AM, Rutter WJ. Cell-specific expression controlled by the 5′-flanking region of insulin and chymotrypsin genes. Nature 1983;306:557–61.
23. Edlund T, Walker MD, Barr PJ, Rutter WJ. Cell-specific expression of the rat insulin gene: evidence for role of two distinct 5′ flanking elements. Science 1985;230:912–6.
24. Karlsson O, Edlund T, Moss JB, et al. A mutational analysis of the insulin gene transcription control region: expression in beta cells is dependent on two related sequences within the enhancer. Proc Natl Acad Sci USA 1987;84:8819–23.

25. Takeda J, Ishii S, Seino Y, et al. Negative regulation of human insulin gene expression by the 5'-flanking region in non-pancreatic cells. FEBS Lett 1989;247:41–5.

26. Whelan J, Poon D, Weil PA, Stein R. Pancreatic β-cell-type-specific expression of the rat insulin II gene is controlled by positive and negative cellular transcriptional elements. Mol Cell Biol 1989;9:3253–9.

27. Hwung Y-P, Gu Y-Z, Tsai M-J. Cooperativity of sequence elements mediates tissue specificity of the rat insulin II gene. Mol Cell Biol 1990;10:1784–8.

28. Ohlsson H, Edlund T. Sequence-specific interactions of nuclear factors with the insulin gene enhancer. Cell 1986;45:35–44.

29. Nir U, Walker MD, Rutter WJ. Regulation of rat insulin I gene expression: evidence for negative regulation in nonpancreatic cells. Proc Natl Acad Sci USA 1986; 83:3180–4.

30. Sample CE, Steiner DF. Tissue-specific binding of a nuclear factor to the insulin gene promoter. FEBS Lett 1987; 222:332–6.

31. Ohlsson H, Karlsson O, Edlund T. A beta-cell-specific protein binds to the two major regulatory sequences of the insulin gene enhancer. Proc Natl Acad Sci USA 1988;85:4228–31.

32. Moss LG, Moss JB, Rutter WJ. Systematic binding analysis of the insulin gene transcription control region: insulin and immunoglobulin enhancers utilize similar transactivators. Mol Cell Biol 1988;8:2620–7.

33. Boam DSW, Docherty K. A tissue-specific nuclear factor binds to multiple sites in the human insulin-gene enhancer. Biochem J 1989;264:233–9.

34. Boam DSW, Clark AR, Docherty K. Positive and negative regulation of the human insulin gene by multiple trans-acting factors. J Biol Chem 1990;265:8285–96.

35. Whelan J, Cordle SR, Henderson E, et al. Identification of a pancreatic β-cell insulin gene transcription factor that binds to and appears to activate cell-type-specific expression: its possible relationship to other cellular factors that bind to a common insulin gene sequence. Mol Cell Biol 1990;10:1564–72.

36. Walker MD, Park CW, Rosen A, Aronheim A. A cDNA from a mouse pancreatic β cell encoding a putative transcription factor of the insulin gene. Nucleic Acids Res 1990;18:1159–66.

37. Karlsson O, Walker MD, Rutter WJ, Edlund T. Individual protein-binding domains of the insulin gene enhancer positively activate β-cell-specific transcription. Mol Cell Biol 1989;9:823–7.

38. Karlsson O, Thor S, Norberg T, et al. Insulin gene enhancer binding protein IsI-1 is a member of a novel class of proteins containing both a homeo- and a Cys-His domain. Nature 1990;344:879–82.

39. Lenardo M, Pierce JW, Baltimore D. Protein-binding sites in Ig gene enhancers determine transcriptional activity and inducibility. Science 1987;236:1573–7.

40. Murre C, McCaw PS, Baltimore D. A new DNA binding and dimerization motif in immunoglobulin enhancer binding, daughterless, myoD and myc proteins. Cell 1989;56:777–83.

41. Murre C, McCaw PS, Vaessin H, et al. Interactions between heterologous helix-loop-helix proteins generate complexes that bind specifically to a common DNA sequence. Cell 1989;58:537–44.

42. Nelson C, Shen L-P, Meister A, et al. Pan: a transcriptional regulator that binds chymotrypsin, insulin, and AP-4 enhancer motifs. Genes Dev 1990;4:1035–43.

43. Desplan C, Theis J, O'Farrell PH. The sequence specificity of homeodomain-DNA interaction. Cell 1988;54:1081–90.

44. Scott MP, Tamkun JW, Hartzell GW III. The structure and function of the homeodomain. Biochim Biophys Acta 1989;989:25–48.

45. Philippe J, Missotten M. Functional characterization of a cAMP-responsive element of the rat insulin I gene. J Biol Chem 1990;265:1465–9.

46. Madsen OD, Andersen LC, Michelsen B, et al. Tissue-specific expression of transfected human insulin genes in pluripotent clonal rat insulinoma lines induced during passage in vivo. Proc Natl Acad Sci USA 1988;85:6652–6.

47. Gold G, Walker MD, Edwards DL, Grodsky GM. Biosynthetic regulation of endogenous hamster insulin and exogenous rat insulin II in transfected HIT cells. Diabetes 1988;37:1509–14.

48. Selden RF, Skoskiewicz MJ, Howie KB, et al. Regulation of human insulin gene expression in transgenic mice. Nature 1986;321:525–8.

49. Bucchini D, Ripoche M-A, Stinnakre M-G, et al. Pancreatic expression of human insulin gene in transgenic mice. Proc Natl Acad Sci USA 1986;83:2511–5.

50. Ashcroft SJH. Glucoreceptor mechanisms and the control of insulin release and biosynthesis. Diabetologia 1980; 18:5–15.

51. Campbell IL, Hellquist LNB, Taylor KW. Insulin biosynthesis and its regulation. Clin Sci 1982:62:449–55.

52. Welsh M. Glucose regulation of insulin gene expression. Diabete Metab 1989;15:367–71.

53. Taylor KW, Parry DG, Smith GH. Biosynthetic labelling of mammalian insulins in vitro. Nature 1964;203:1144–5.

54. Parry DG, Taylor KW. The effects of sugars on incorporation of [³H] leucine into insulins. Biochem J 1966;100:2c–4c.

55. Howell SL, Taylor KW. Effects of glucose concentration on incorporation of [³H] leucine into insulin using isolated mammalian islets of Langerhans. Biochim Biophys Acta 1966;130:519–21.

56. Morris GE, Korner A. The effect of glucose on insulin biosynthesis by isolated islets of Langerhans of the rat. Biochim Biophys Acta 1970;208:404–13.

57. Lin BJ, Haist RE. Insulin biosynthesis: effects of carbohydrates and related compounds. Can J Physiol Pharmacol 1969;47:791–801.

58. Tanese T, Lazarus NR, Devrim S, Recant L. Synthesis and release of proinsulin and insulin by isolated rat islets of Langerhans. J Clin Invest 1970;49:1394–404.

59. Lin BJ, Nagy BR, Haist RE. Effect of various concentrations of glucose on insulin biosynthesis. Endocrinology 1972; 91:309–11.

60. Pipeleers DG, Marichal M, Malaisse WJ. The stimulus-secretion coupling of glucose-induced insulin release. XIV. Glucose regulation of insular biosynthetic activity. Endocrinology 1973;93:1001–11.

61. Zucker PF, Lin BJ. Differential effect of D-glucose anomers on proinsulin biosynthesis by the pancreatic islets. Can J Physiol Pharmacol 1977;55:1397–400.

62. Ashcroft SJH, Bunce J, Lowry M, Hansen SE, Hedeskov CJ. The effect of sugars on (pro)insulin biosynthesis. Biochem J 1978;174:517–26.

63. Jain K, Logothetopoulos J, Zucker P. The effects of D- and L-glyceraldehyde on glucose oxidation, insulin secretion and insulin biosynthesis by pancreatic islets of the rat. Biochim Biophys Acta 1975;399:384–94.

64. Anderson A. Stimulation of insulin biosynthesis in isolated

mouse islets by L-eucine, 2-aminonorbornane-2-carboxylic acid and α-ketoisocaproic acid. Biochim Biophys Acta 1976;437:345–53.

65. Jain K, Logothetolpoulos J. Stimulation of proinsulin biosynthesis by purine-ribonucleosides and D-ribose. Endocrinology 1977;100:923–7.

66. Bauer GE, Noe BD. Regulation of hormone biosynthesis in cultured islet cells from anglerfish. In Vitro Cell Dev Biol 1985;21:15–21.

67. Patzelt C. Differential inhibitory action of cationic amino acids on protein synthesis in pancreatic rat islets. Diabetologia 1988;31:241–6.

68. Pipeleers DG, Marichal M, Malaisse WJ. The stimulus-secretion coupling of glucose-induced insulin release. XV. Participation of cations in the recognition of glucose by the β-cell. Endocrinology 1973;93:1012–8.

69. Sener A, Malaisse WJ. The stimulus-secretion coupling of glucose-induced insulin release. XXXIX. Long term effects of K⁺ deprivation upon insulin biosynthesis and release. Endocrinology 1980;106:778–85.

70. Schatz H, Maier V, Hinz M, et al. Stimulation of H-3-leucine incorporation into the proinsulin and insulin fraction of isolated pancreatic mouse islets in the presence of glucagon, theophylline and cyclic AMP. Diabetes 1973;22:433–41.

71. Lin BJ, Haist RE. Effects of some modifiers of insulin secretion on insulin biosynthesis. Endocrinology 1973; 92:735–42.

72. Malaisse WJ, Pipeleers DG, Levy J. The stimulus-secretion coupling of glucose-induced insulin release. XVI. A glucose-like and calcium-independent effect of cyclic AMP. Biochim Biophys Acta 1974;362:121–8.

73. Maldonato A, Renold AE, Sharp GWG, Cerasi E. Glucose-induced proinsulin biosynthesis: role of islet cyclic AMP. Diabetes 1977;26:538–45.

74. Nielsen DA, Welsh M, Casadaban MJ, Steiner DF. Control of insulin gene expression in pancreatic β-cells and in an insulin-producing cell line, RIN-5F cells. I. Effects of glucose and cyclic AMP on the transcription of insulin mRNA. J Biol Chem 1985;260:13585–9.

75. Levy J, Malaisse WJ. The stimulus-secretion coupling of glucose-induced insulin release. XVII. Effects of sulfonylureas and diazoxide on insular biosynthetic activity. Biochem Pharmacol 1975;24:235–9.

76. Schatz H, Steinle D, Pfeiffer EF. Long-term actions of sulfonylureas on (pro-)insulin biosynthesis and secretion. I. Lack of evidence for a compensatory increase in (pro-)-insulin biosynthesis after exposure of isolated pancreatic rat islets to tolbutamide and glibenclamide in vitro. Horm Metab Res 1977;9:457–65.

77. Glatt M, Schatz H. The influence of an acyl-amino-alcyl-benzoic acid (HB 699) on biosynthesis and secretion of insulin in isolated rat islets of Langerhans. Diabete Metab 1981;7:105–8.

78. Rhodes CJ, Taylor KW. Effect of human lymphoblastoid interferon on insulin synthesis and secretion in isolated human pancreatic islets. Diabetologia 1984;27:601–3.

79. Sandler S, Andersson A, Hellerström C. Inhibitory effects of interleukin 1 on insulin secretion, insulin biosynthesis, and oxidative metabolism of isolated rat pancreatic islets. Endocrinology 1987;121:1424–31.

80. Spinas GA, Hansen BS, Linde S, et al. Interleukin 1 dose-dependently affects the biosynthesis of (pro)insulin in isolated rat islets of Langerhans. Diabetologia 1987; 30:474–80.

81. Hansen BS, Nielsen JH, Linde S, et al. Effect of interleukin-1 on the biosynthesis of proinsulin and insulin in isolated rat pancreatic islets. Biomed Biochim Acta 1988; 47:305–9.

82. Camara J, Albor A, Mato JM, et al. Inhibition of proinsulin biosynthesis and conversion by a putative insulin mediator. Biochem Int 1989;18:865–9.

83. Permutt MA, Kipnis DM. Insulin biosynthesis. I. On the mechanism of glucose stimulation. J Biol Chem 1972; 247:1194–9.

84. Permutt MA, Kipnis DM. Insulin biosynthesis: studies of islets polyribosomes. Proc Natl Acad Sci USA 1972; 69:505–9.

85. Permutt MA. Effect of glucose on initiation and elongation rates in isolated rat pancreatic islets. J Biol Chem 1974; 249:2738–42.

86. Lomedico PT, Saunders GF. Cell-free modulation of proinsulin synthesis. Science 1977;198:620–2.

87. Itoh N, Sei T, Nose K, Okamoto H. Glucose stimulation of the proinsulin synthesis in isolated pancreatic islets without increasing amount of proinsulin mRNA. FEBS Lett 1978;93:343–7.

88. Brunstedt J, Chan SJ. Direct effect of glucose on the preproinsulin mRNA level in isolated pancreatic islets. Biochem Biophys Res Commun 1982;106:1383–9.

89. Brunstedt J. Expression of the insulin gene: regulation by glucose, hydrocortisone and growth hormone in mouse pancreatic islets in organ culture. Acta Biol Med Germ 1982;41:1151–5.

90. Giddings SJ, Chirgwin JM, Permutt MA. Glucose regulated insulin biosynthesis in isolated rat pancreatic islets is accompanied by changes in proinsulin mRNA. Diabetes Res 1985;2:71–5.

91. Welsh M, Brunstedt J, Hellerström C. Effects of D-glucose, L-leucine and 2-ketoisocaproate on insulin mRNA levels in mouse pancreatic islets. Diabetes 1986;35:228–31.

92. Hammonds P, Schofield PN, Ashcroft SJH, et al. Regulation and specificity of glucose-stimulated insulin gene expression in human islets of Langerhans. FEBS Lett 1987; 223:131–7.

93. Welsh M, Weber T, Wrange O, et al. Regulation of insulin gene expression by dexamethasone, Ca²⁺ and a phorbol ester. Biomed Biochim Acta 1988;47:299–303.

94. Formby B, Ullrich A, Coussens L, et al. Growth hormone stimulates insulin gene expression in cultured human fetal pancreatic islets. J Clin Endocrinol Metab 1988; 66:1075–9.

95. Welsh M, Nielsen DA, MacKrell AJ, Steiner DF. Control of insulin gene expression in pancreatic β-cells and in an insulin-producing cell line, RIN-5F cells. II. Regulation of insulin mRNA stability. J Biol Chem 1985;260:13590–4.

96. Itoh N, Okamoto H. Translational control of proinsulin synthesis by glucose. Nature 1980;283:100–2.

97. Itoh N, Ohshima Y, Nose K, Okamoto H. Glucose stimulates proinsulin synthesis in pancreatic islets without a concomitant increase in proinsulin mRNA synthesis. Biochem Int 1982;4:315–21.

98. Welsh M, Scherberg N, Gilmore R, Steiner DF. Translational control of insulin biosynthesis: evidence for regulation of elongation, initiation and signal-recognition-particle-mediated translational arrest by glucose. Biochem J 1986;235:459–67.

99. Welsh N, Welsh M, Steiner DF, Hellerstöm C. Mechanism of leucine- and theophylline-stimulated insulin biosynthesis in isolated rat pancreatic islets. Biochem J 1987; 246:245–8.

100. Zucker P, Logothetopoulos J. Persisting enhanced proinsulin-insulin and protein biosynthesis (³H-leucine incorpo-

ration) by pancreatic islets of the rat after glucose exposure. Diabetes 1975;24:194–200.

101. Giddings SJ, Chirgwin J, Permutt MA. Effects of glucose on proinsulin messenger RNA in rats in vivo. Diabetes 1982;31:624–9.

102. Giddings SJ, Chirgwin J, Permutt MA. The effects of fasting and feeding on preproinsulin messenger RNA in rats. J Clin Invest 1981;67:952–60.

103. Kruszynska YT, Villa-Komaroff L, Halban PA. Islet B-cell dysfunction and the time course of recovery following chronic overinsulinisation of normal rats. Diabetologia 1988;31:621–6.

104. Orland MJ, Chyn R, Permutt MA. Modulation of proinsulin messenger RNA after partial pancreatectomy in rats: relationship to glucose homeostasis. J Clin Invest 1985;75:2047–2055.

105. Giddings SJ, Orland MJ, Weir GC, et al. Impaired insulin biosynthetic capacity in a rat model for non-insulin-dependent diabetes: studies with dexamthasone. Diabetes 1985;34:235–40.

106. Wang SY, Halban PA, Rowe JW. Effects of aging on insulin synthesis and secretion: differential effects on preproinsulin messenger RNA levels, proinsulin biosynthesis, and secretion of newly made and preformed insulin in the rat. J Clin Invest 1988;81:176–84.

107. Wang SY, Rowe JW. Age-related impairment in the short term regulation of insulin biosynthesis by glucose in rat pancreatic islets. Endocrinology 1988;123:1008–13.

108. Kaelin D, Renold AE, Sharp GWG. Glucose stimulated proinsulin biosynthesis: rates of turn off after cessation of the stimulus. Diabetologia 1978;14:329–35.

109. Ryle AP, Sanger F, Smith LF, Kitai R. The disulphide bonds of insulin. Biochem J 1955;60:541–56.

110. Steiner DF, Oyer PE. The biosynthesis of insulin and a probable precursor of insulin by a human islet cell adenoma. Proc Natl Acad Sci USA 1967;57:473–80.

111. Steiner DF, Cunningham D, Spigelman L, Aten B. Insulin biosynthesis: evidence for a precursor. Science 1967;157:697–700.

112. Yip CC, Hew C-L, Hsu H. Translation of messenger ribonucleic acid from isolated pancreatic islets and human insulinomas. Proc Natl Acad Sci USA 1975;72:4777–9.

113. Lomedico PT, Saunders GF. Preparation of pancreatic mRNA: cell-free translation of an insulin-immunoreactive polypeptide. Nucleic Acids Res 1976;3:381–91.

114. Chan SJ, Keim P, Steiner DF. Cell-free synthesis of rat preproinsulins: characterization and partial amino acid sequence determination. Proc Natl Acad Sci USA 1976;73:1964–8.

115. Shields D, Blobel G. Cell-free synthesis of fish preproinsulin, processing by heterologous mammalian microsomal membranes. Proc Natl Acad Sci USA 1977;74:2059–63.

116. Permutt MA, Routman A. Proinsulin precursors in isolated rat pancreatic islets. Biochem Biophys Res Commun 1977;78:855–62.

117. Patzelt C, Labrecque AD, Duguid JR, et al. Detection and kinetic behavior of preproinsulin in pancreatic islets. Proc Natl Acad Sci USA 1978;75:1260–4.

118. Albert SG, Permutt MA. Proinsulin precursors in catfish pancreatic islets. J Biol Chem 1979;254:3483–92.

119. Eskridge EM, Shields D. Cell-free processing and segregation of insulin precursors. J Biol Chem 1983;258:11487–91.

120. Walter P, Lingappa VR. Mechanism of protein translocation across the endoplasmic reticulum membrane. Annu Rev Cell Biol 1986;2:499–516.

121. Eskridge EM, Shields D. The NH_2 terminus of preproinsulin directs the translocation and glycosylation of a bacterial cytoplasmic protein by mammalian microsomal membranes. J Cell Biol 1986;103:2263–72.

122. Wiedmann M, Huth A, Rapoport TA. Internally transposed signal sequence of carp preproinsulin retains its functions with the signal recognition particle. FEBS Lett 1986;194:139–45.

123. Talmadge K, Kaufman J, Gilbert W. Bacteria mature preproinsulin to proinsulin. Proc Natl Acad Sci USA 1980;77:3988–92.

124. Chan SJ, Weiss J, Konrad M, et al. Biosynthesis and periplasmic segregation of human proinsulin in Escherichia coli. Proc Natl Acad Sci USA 1981;78:5401–5.

125. Halban PA. Proinsulin trafficking and processing in the pancreatic B-cell. Trends Endocrinol Metab 1990;1:261–5.

126. Palade G. Intracellular aspects of the process of protein synthesis. Science 1975;189:347–58.

127. Orci L. Macro- and micro-domains in the endocrine pancreas. Diabetes 1982;31:538–65.

128. Orci L. The insulin factory: a tour of the plant surroundings and a visit to the assembly line. Diabetologia 1985;28:528–46.

129. Orci L. The insulin cell: its cellular environment and how it processes (pro)insulin. Diabetes Metab Rev 1986;2:71–106.

130. Orci L, Vassalli JD, Perrelet A. The insulin factory. Sci Am 1988;259:85–94.

131. Kelly RB. Pathways of protein secretion in eukaryotes. Science 1985;230:25–32.

132. Pfeffer SR, Rothman JE. Biosynthetic protein transport and sorting by the endoplasmic reticulum and Golgi. Annu Rev Biochem 1987;56:829–52.

133. Burgess TL, Kelly RB. Constitutive and regulated secretion of proteins. Annu Rev Cell Biol 1987;3:243–93.

134. Moore H-PH. Factors controlling packaging of peptide hormones into secretory granules. Ann NY Acad Sci 1987;493:50–61.

135. Lingappa VR. Intracellular traffic of newly synthesized proteins: current understanding and future prospects. J Clin Invest 1989;83:739–51.

136. Huttner WB, Tooze SA. Biosynthetic protein transport in the secretory pathway. Curr Opinion Cell Biol 1989;1:648–54.

137. Howell SL. Role of ATP in the intracellular translocation of proinsulin and insulin in the rat pancreatic B-cell [Letter]. Nature New Biol 1972;235:85–6.

138. Lacy PE, Howell SL, Young DA, Fink CJ. New hypothesis of insulin secretion [Letter]. Nature 1968;219:1177–9.

139. Malaisse-Lagae F, Amherdt M, Ravazzola M, et al. Role of microtubules in the synthesis, conversion, and release of (pro)insulin. J Clin Invest 1979;63:1284–96.

140. Howell SL. The mechanism of insulin secretion. Diabetologia 1984;26:319–27.

141. Beckers CJM, Block MR, Glick BS, et al. Vesicular transport between the endoplasmic reticulum and the Golgi stack requires the NEM-sensitive fusion protein. Nature 1989;339:397–8.

142. Wilson DW, Wilcox CA, Flynn GC, et al. A fusion protein required for vesicle-mediated transport in both mammalian cells and yeast. Nature 1989;339:355–9.

143. Bourne HR. Do GTPases direct membrane traffic in secretion? Cell 1988;53:669–71.

144. Pelham HRB. Speculations on the functions of the major heat shock and glucose-regulated proteins. Cell 1986;46:959–61.

145. Flynn GC, Chappell TG, Rothman JE. Peptide binding and

release by proteins implicated as catalysts of protein assembly. Science 1989;245:385–90.

146. Rothman JE. Polypeptide chain binding proteins: catalysts of protein folding and related processes in cells. Cell 1989;59:591–601.

147. Balch WE. Biochemistry of interorganelle transport: a new frontier in enzymology emerges from versatile in vitro model systems. J Biol Chem 1989;264:16965–8.

148. Farquhar MG, Palade GE. The Golgi apparatus (complex)—(1954–1981)—from artifact to center stage. J Cell Biol 1981;91(Suppl):77s–103s.

149. Rothman JE. The Golgi apparatus: two organelles in tandem. Science 1981;213:1212–9.

150. Dunphy WG, Rothman JE. Compartmental organization of the Golgi stack. Cell 1985;42:13–21.

151. Farquhar MG. Progress in unraveling pathways of Golgi traffic. Annu Rev Cell Biol 1985;1:447–88.

152. Oster GF, Cheng LY, Moore H-PH, Perelson AS. Vesicle formation in the Golgi apparatus. J Theor Biol 1989; 141:463–504.

153. Serafini T, Stenbeck G, Brecht A, et al. A coat subunit of Golgi-derived non-clathrin-coated vesicles with homology to the clathrin-coated vesicle coat protein β-adaptin. Nature 1991;349:215–20.

154. Duden R, Griffiths G, Frank et al. β-COP, a 110 kd protein associated with non-clathrin-coated vesicles and the Golgi complex, shows homology to β-daptin. Cell 1991;64: 649–65.

155. Orci L, Glick BS, Rothman JE. A new type of coated vesicular carrier that appears not to contain clathrin: its possible role in protein transport within the Golgi stack. Cell 1986;46:171–84.

156. Orci L, Malhotra V, Amherdt M, et al. Dissection of a single round of vesicular transport: sequential intermediates for intercisternal movement in the Golgi stack. Cell 1989; 56:357–68.

157. Rothman JE, Orci L. Movement of proteins through the Golgi stack: a molecular dissection of vesicular transport. FASEB J 1990;4:1460–8.

158. Malhotra V, Orci L, Glick BS, et al. Role of an N-ethylmaleimide-sensitive transport component in promoting fusion of transport vesicles with cisternae of the Golgi stack. Cell 1988;54:221–7.

159. Melançon P, Glick BS, Malhotra V, et al. Involvement of the GTP-binding "G" proteins in transport through the Golgi stack. Cell 1987;51:1053–62.

160. Segev N, Mulholland J, Botstein D. The yeast GTP-binding YPT1 protein and a mammalian counterpart are associated with the secretion machinery. Cell 1988;52:915–24.

161. Clary DO, Griff IC, Rothman JE. SNAPs, a family of NSF attachment proteins involved in intracellular membrane fusion in animals and yeast. Cell 1990;61:709–21.

162. Clary DO, Rothman JE. Purification of three related peripheral membrane proteins needed for vesicular transport. J Biol Chem 1990;265:10109–117.

163. Pfanner N, Orci L, Glick BS, et al. Fatty acyl-coenzyme A is required for budding of transport vesicles from Golgi cisternae. Cell 1989;59:95–102.

164. Gold G, Wieland FT, Grodsky GM. Unregulated secretion of an exogenous glycotripeptide by rat islets and hit cells. Biochem Biophys Res Commun 1988;156:457–62.

165. Rhodes CJ, Halban PA. Newly synthesized proinsulin/insulin and stored insulin are released from pancreatic B cells predominantly via a regulated, rather than a constitutive, pathway. J Cell Biol 1987;105:145–53.

166. Judah JD, Quinn PS. Calcium ion-dependent vesicle fusion

in the conversion of proalbumin to albumin [Letter]. Nature 1978;271:384–5.

167. Hedo JA, Simpson IA. Biosynthesis of the insulin receptor in rat adipose cells: intracellular processing of the M_r-190000 pro-receptor. Biochem J 1985;232:71–8.

168. Bathurst IC, Brennan SO, Carrell RW, et al. Yeast KEX2 protease has the properties of a human proalbumin converting enzyme. Science 1987;235:348–50.

169. Brennan SO, Peach RJ. Calcium-dependent KEX2-like protease found in hepatic secretory vesicles converts proalbumin to albumin. FEBS Lett 1988;229:167–70.

170. Barr PJ. Mammalian subtilisins: the long-sought dibasic processing endoproteases. Cell 1991;66:1–3.

171. Brennan SO, Carrell RW. A circulating variant of human proalbumin [Letter]. Nature 1978;274:908–9.

172. Yoshimasa Y, Seino S, Whittaker J, et al. Insulin-resistant diabetes due to a point mutation that prevents insulin proreceptor processing. Science 1988;240:784–7.

173. Redman CM, Avellino G, Yu S. Secretion of proalbumin by canavanine-treated Hep-G2 cells. J Biol Chem 1983; 258:344–52.

174. Thomas G, Thorne BA, Thomas L, et al. Yeast KEX2 endopeptidase correctly cleaves a neuroendocrine prohormone in mammalian cells. Science 1988; 241:226–30.

175. Thim L, Hansen MT, Norris K, et al. Secretion and processing of insulin precursors in yeast. Proc Natl Acad Sci USA 1986;83:6766–70.

176. Cooper A, Bussey H. Characterization of the yeast KEX1 gene product: a carboxypeptidase involved in processing secreted precursor proteins. Mol Cell Biol 1989;9: 2706–14.

177. Wulff BS, O'Hare MT, Boel E, et al. Partial processing of the neuropeptide Y precursor in transfected CHO cells. FEBS Lett 1990;261:101–5.

178. Stoller TJ, Shields D. The role of paired basic amino acids in mediating proteolytic cleavage of prosomatostatin: analysis using site-directed mutagenesis. J Biol Chem 1989;264:6922–4.

179. Orci L, Ravazzola M, Amherdt M, et al. The trans-most cisternae of the Golgi complex: a compartment for sorting of secretory and plasma membrane proteins. Cell 1987;51:1039–51.

180. Pfeffer SR. Mannose 6-Phosphate receptors and their role in targeting proteins to lysosomes. J Membrane Biol 1988;103:7–16.

181. Dahms NM, Lobel P, Kornfeld S. Mannose 6-phosphate receptors and lysosomal enzyme targeting. J Biol Chem 1989;264:12115–8.

182. Kornfeld S, Mellman I. The biogenesis of lysosomes. Annu Rev Cell Biol 1989;5:483–525.

183. Orci L, Ravazzola M, Perrelet A. (Pro)insulin associates with Golgi membranes of pancreatic B cells. Proc Natl Acad Sci USA 1984;81:6743–6.

184. Chung K-N, Walter P, Aponte GW, Moore H-PH. Molecular sorting in the secretory pathway. Science 1989; 243:192–7.

185. Tooze SA, Huttner WB. Cell-free protein sorting to the regulated and constitutive secretory pathways. Cell 1990;60:837–47.

186. Moore H-PH, Walker MD, Lee F, Kelly RB. Expressing a human proinsulin cDNA in a mouse ACTH-secreting cell. Intracellular storage, proteolytic processing and secretion on stimulation. Cell 1983;35:531–8.

187. Moore H-PH, Kelly RB. Secretory protein targeting in a pituitary cell line: differential transport of foreign secre-

tory proteins to distinct secretory pathways. J Cell Biol 1985;101:1773–81.

188. Burgess TL, Craik CS, Kelly RB. The exocrine protein trypsinogen is targeted into the secretory granules of an endocrine cell line: studies by gene transfer. J Cell Biol 1985;101:639–45.

189. Moore H-PH, Kelly RB. Re-routing of a secretory protein by fusion with human growth hormone sequences. Nature 1986;321:443–6.

190. Halban PA. Structural domains and molecular lifestyles of insulin and its precursors in the pancreatic beta cell. Diabetologia 1991;34:767–78.

191. Garoff H. Using recombinant DNA techniques to study protein targeting in the eucaryotic cell. Annu Rev Cell Biol 1985;1:403–45.

192. Gross DJ, Villa-Komaroff L, Kahn CR, et al. Deletion of a highly conserved tetrapeptide sequence of the proinsulin connecting peptide (C-peptide) inhibits proinsulin to insulin conversion by transfected pituitary corticotroph (AtT20) cells. J Biol Chem 1989;264:21486–90.

193. Powell SK, Orci L, Craik CS, Moore H-PH. Efficient targeting to storage granules of human proinsulins with altered propeptide domain. J Cell Biol 1988;106:1843–51.

194. Shakur Y, Shennan KIJ, Taylor NA, Docherty K. A major C-peptide deletion prevents secretion of a mutant human proinsulin from transfected monkey kidney cells. J Mol Endocrinol 1989;3:155–62.

195. Gross DJ, Halban PA, Kahn CR, et al. Partial diversion of a mutant proinsulin (B10 aspartic acid) from the regulated to the constitutive secretory pathway in transfected AtT-20 cells. Proc Natl Acad Sci USA 1989;86:4107–11.

196. Carroll RJ, Hammer RE, Chan SJ, et al. A mutant human proinsulin is secreted from islets of Langerhans in increased amounts via an unregulated pathway. Proc Natl Acad Sci USA 1988;85:8943–7.

197. Orci L, Ravazzola M, Amherdt M, et al. Clathrin-immunoreactive sites in the Golgi apparatus are concentrated at the *trans* pole in polypeptide hormone-secreting cells. Proc Natl Acad Sci USA 1985;82:5385–9.

198. Tooze J, Tooze SA. Clathrin-coated vesicular transport of secretory proteins during the formation of ACTH-containing secretory granules in AtT20 cells. J Cell Biol 1986;103:839–50.

199. Pearse BMF. Clathrin and coated vesicles. EMBO J 1987;6:2507–12.

200. Brodsky FM. Living with clathrin: its role in intracellular membrane traffic. Science 1988;242:1396–402.

201. Hubbard AL. Endocytosis. Curr Opin Cell Biol 1989;1:675–83.

202. Payne GS, Schekman R. Clathrin: a role in the intracellular retention of a Golgi membrane protein. Science 1989; 245:1358–65.

203. Orci L, Ravazzola M, Amherdt M, et al. Direct identification of prohormone conversion site in insulin-secreting cells. Cell 1985;42:671–81.

204. Orci L, Ravazzola M, Storch M-J, et al. Proteolytic maturation of insulin is a post-Golgi event which occurs in acidifying clathrin-coated secretory vesicles. Cell 1987; 49:865–8.

205. Steiner DF, Michael J, Houghten R, et al. Use of a synthetic peptide antigen to generate antisera reactive with a proteolytic processing site in native human proinsulin: demonstration of cleavage within clathrin-coated (pro)secretory vesicles. Proc Natl Acad Sci USA 1987;84:6184–8.

206. Kemmler W, Steiner DF. Conversion of proinsulin to insulin in a subcellular fraction from rat islets. Biochem Biophys Res Commun 1970;41:1223–30.

207. Yip CC. A bovine pancreatic enzyme catalyzing the conversion of proinsulin to insulin. Proc Natl Acad Sci USA 1971;68:1312–5.

208. Kemmler W, Peterson JD, Rubenstein AH, Steiner DF. On the biosynthesis, intracellular transport and mechanism of conversion of proinsulin to insulin and C-peptide. Diabetes 1972;21(Suppl 2):572–81.

209. Steiner DF, Kemmler W, Tager HS, Peterson JD. Proteolytic processing in the biosynthesis of insulin and other proteins. Fed Proc 1974;33:2105–15.

210. Docherty K, Steiner DF. Post-translational proteolysis in polypeptide hormone biosynthesis. Annu Rev Physiol 1982;44:625–38.

211. Fisher JM, Scheller RH. Prohormone processing and the secretory pathway. J Biol Chem 1988;263:16515–8.

212. Harris RB. Processing of pro-hormone precursor proteins. Arch Biochem Biophys 1989;275:315–33.

213. Kreil G. Processing of precursors by dipeptidylaminopeptidases: a case of molecular ticketing. Trends Biochem Sci 1990;15:23–6.

214. Davidson HW, Peshavaria M, Hutton JC. Proteolytic conversion of proinsulin into insulin: identification of a Ca^{2+}-dependent acidic endopeptidase in isolated insulin-secretory granules. Biochem J 1987;246:279–86.

215. Davidson HW, Rhodes CJ, Hutton JC. Intraorganellar calcium and pH control proinsulin cleavage in the pancreatic β cell via two distinct site-specific endopeptidases. Nature 1988;333:93–6.

216. Given BD, Cohen RM, Shoelson SE, et al. Biochemical and clinical implications of proinsulin conversion intermediates. J Clin Invest 1985;76:1398–405.

217. Smeekens SP, Steiner DF. Identification of a human insulinoma cDNA encoding a novel mammalian protein structurally related to the yeast dibasic processing protease Kex2. J Biol Chem 1990;265:2997–3000.

218. Smeekens SP, Avruch AS, LaMendola J, et al. Identification of a cDNA encoding a second putative prohormone convertase related to PC2 in AtT20 cells and islets of Langerhans. Proc Natl Acad Sci USA 1991;88:340–4.

219. Noe BD. Inhibition of islet prohormone to hormone conversion by incorporation of arginine and lysine analogs. J Biol Chem 1981;256:4940–6.

220. Halban PA. Inhibition of proinsulin to insulin conversion in rat islets using arginine and lysine analogs: lack of effect on rate of release of modified products. J Biol Chem 1982;257:13177–80.

221. Docherty K, Rhodes CJ, Taylor NA, et al. Proinsulin endopeptidase substrate specificities defined by site-directed mutagenesis of proinsulin. J Biol Chem 1989; 264:18335–9.

222. Rholam M, Nicolas P, Cohen P. Precursors for peptide hormones share common secondary structures forming features at the proteolytic processing sites. FEBS Lett 1986;207:1–6.

223. Docherty K, Hutton JC. Carboxypeptidase activity in the insulin secretory granule. FEBS Lett 1983;162:137–41.

224. Davidson HW, Hutton JC. The insulin-secretory-granule carboxypeptidase H: purification and demonstration of involvement in proinsulin processing. Biochem J 1987;245:575–82.

225. Grimwood BG, Plummer TH Jr, Tarentino AL. Carboxypeptidase H: a regulatory peptide-processing enzyme produced by human hepatoma Hep G2 cells. J Biol Chem 1989;264:15662–7.

226. Nagamatsu S, Bolaffi JL, Grodsky GM. Direct effects of glucose on proinsulin synthesis and processing during desensitization. Endocrinology 1987;120:1225–31.

227. Valverde I, Alarcon C, Rovira A, et al. Diazoxide-induced long-term hyperglycemia. II. Slackening of proinsulin conversion. Diabetes Res 1989;10:59–62.

228. Gishizky ML, Grodsky GM. Differential kinetics of rat insulin I and II processing in rat islets of Langerhans. FEBS Lett 1987;223:227–31.

229. Sizonenko SV, Halban PA. Differential rates of conversion of rat proinsulin I and II. Biochem J 1991;278:621–5.

230. Orci L, Ravazzola M, Amherdt M, et al. Conversion of proinsulin to insulin occurs coordinately with acidification of maturing secretory vesicles. J Cell Biol 1986;103:2273–81.

231. Hutton JC, Peshavaria M. Proton-translocating Mg^{2+}-dependent ATPase activity in insulin-secretory granules. Biochem J 1982;204:161–70.

232. Hutton JC. The internal pH and membrane potential of the insulin-secretory granule. Biochem J 1982;204:171–8.

233. Rhodes CJ, Lucas CA, Mutkoski RL, et al. Stimulation by ATP of proinsulin to insulin conversion in isolated rat pancreatic islet secretory granules: association with the ATP-dependent proton pump. J Biol Chem 1987; 262:10712–7.

234. Orci L, Halban PA, Amherdt M, et al. Nonconverted, amino acid analog-modified proinsulin stays in a Golgi-derived clathrin-coated membrane compartment. J Cell Biol 1984;99:2187–92.

235. Schlossman DM, Schmid SL, Braell WA, Rothman JE. An enzyme that removes clathrin coats: purification of an uncoating ATPase. J Cell Biol 1984;99:723–33.

236. Schmid SL, Rothman JE. Enzymatic dissociation of clathrin cages in a two-stage process. J Biol Chem 1985; 260:10044–9.

237. Schmid SL, Rothman JE. Two classes of binding sites for uncoating protein in clathrin triskelions. J Biol Chem 1985;260:10050–6.

238. Schmid SL, Braell WA, Rothman JE. ATP catalyzes the sequestration of clathrin during enzymatic uncoating. J Biol Chem 1985;260:10057–62.

239. Chappell TG, Konforti BB, Schmid SL, Rothman JE. The ATPase core of a clathrin uncoating protein. J Biol Chem 1987;262:746–51.

240. Rubenstein AH, Cho S, Steiner DF. Evidence for proinsulin in human urine and serum. Lancet 1968;1:1353–5.

241. Roth J, Gorden P, Pastan I. "Big insulin": a new component of plasma insulin detected by immunoassay. Proc Natl Acad Sci USA 1968;61:138–45.

242. Horwitz DL, Starr JI, Mako ME, et al. Proinsulin, insulin, and C-peptide concentrations in human portal and peripheral blood. J Clin Invest 1975;55:1278–83.

243. Robbins DC, Tager HS, Rubenstein AH. Biologic and clinical importance of proinsulin. N Engl J Med 1984;310:1165–75.

244. Polonsky KS, Rubenstein AH. The kinetics and metabolism of insulin, proinsulin, C-peptide. In: DeGroot LJ, Besser GM, Cahill GR Jr, et al, eds. Endocrinology. 2nd ed. Vol 2. Philadelphia: WB Saunders, 1989:1304–17.

245. Sobey WJ, Beer SF, Carrington CA, et al. Sensitive and specific two-site immunoradiometric assays for human insulin, proinsulin, 65–66 split and 32–33 split proinsulins. Biochem J 1989;260:535–41.

246. Peavy DE, Brunner MR, Duckworth WC, et al. Receptor binding and biological potency of several split forms (conversion intermediates) of human proinsulin: studies

247. Hutton JC. The insulin secretory granule. Diabetologia 1989;32:271–81.

248. Hutton JC, Hansen F, Peshavaria M. β-Granins: 21 kDa co-secreted peptides of the insulin granule closely related to adrenal medullary chromogranin A. FEBS Lett 1985;188:336–40.

249. Hutton JC, Davidson HW, Grimaldi KA, Peshavaria M. Biosynthesis of betagranin in pancreatic β-cells: identification of a chromogranin A-like precursor and its parallel processing with proinsulin. Biochem J 1987;244:449–56.

250. Hutton JC, Davidson HW, Peshavaria M. Proteolytic processing of chromogranin A in purified insulin granules: formation of a 20 kDa N-terminal fragment (betagranin) by the concerted action of a Ca^{2+}-dependent endopeptidase and carboxypeptidase H (EC 3.4.17.10). Biochem J 1987;244:457–64.

251. Tatemoto K, Efendic S, Mutt V, et al. Pancreastatin, a novel pancreatic peptide that inhibits insulin secretion. Nature 1986;324:476–8.

252. Ahren B, Lindskog S, Tatemoto K, Efendic S. Pancreastatin inhibits insulin secretion and stimulates glucagon secretion in mice. Diabetes 1988;37:281–5.

253. Zhou A, Thorn NA. Evidence for presence of peptide-amidating activity in pancreatic islets from newborn rats. Biochem J 1990;267:253–6.

254. Cooper GJS, Day AJ, Willis AC, et al. Amylin and the amylin gene: structure, function and relationship to islet amyloid and to diabetes mellitus. Biochim Biophys Acta 1989;1014:247–58.

255. Nishi M, Sanke T, Nagamatsu S, et al. Islet amyloid polypeptide: a new β cell secretory product related to islet amyloid deposits. J Biol Chem 1990;265:4173–6.

256. Sanke T, Bell GI, Sample C, et al. An islet amyloid peptide is derived from an 89-amino acid precursor by proteolytic processing. J Biol Chem 1988;263:17243–6.

257. Westermark P, Wernstedt C, Wilander E, et al. Amyloid fibrils in human insulinoma and islets of Langerhans of the diabetic cat are derived from a neuropeptide-like protein also present in normal islet cells. Proc Natl Acad Sci USA 1987;84:3881–5.

258. Clark A. Islet amyloid and type 2 diabetes. Diabetic Med 1989;6:561–7.

259. Betsholtz C, Svensson V, Rorsman F, et al. Islet amyloid polypeptide (IAPP): cDNA cloning and identification of an amyloidogenic region associated with the species-specific occurence of age-related diabetes mellitus. Exp Cell Res 1989;183:484–93.

260. Betsholtz C, Christmansson L, Engstrom U, et al. Sequence divergence in a specific region of islet amyloid polypeptide (IAPP) explains differences in islet amyloid formation between species. FEBS Lett 1989;251:261–4.

261. Betsholtz C, Christmansson L, Engström U, et al. Structure of cat islet amyloid polypeptide and identification of amino acid residues of potential significance for islet amyloid formation. Diabetes 1990;39:118–22.

262. Westermark P, Engström U, Westermark GT, et al. Islet amyloid polypeptide (IAPP) and pro-IAPP immunoreactivity in human islets of Langerhans. Diabetes Res Clin Pract 1989;7:219–6.

263. Porte D Jr, Kahn SE. Hyperproinsulinemia and amyloid in NIDDM: clues to etiology of islet β-cell dysfunction? Diabetes 1989;38:1333–6.

264. Ohsawa H, Kanatsuka A, Yamaguchi T, et al. Islet amyloid polypeptide inhibits glucose-stimulated insulin secretion in cultured IM-9 lymphocytes and in vivo and in vitro in rats. J Biol Chem 1985;260:13989–94.

from isolated rat pancreatic islets. Biochem Biophys Res Commun 1989;160:961–7.

265. Sowa R, Sanke T, Hirayama J, et al. Islet amyloid polypeptide amide causes peripheral insulin resistance in vivo in dogs. Diabetologia 1990;33:118–20.

266. Yamaguchi A, Chiba T, Morishita T, et al. Calcitonin gene-related peptide and induction of hyperglycemia in conscious rats in vivo. Diabetes 1990;39:168–74.

267. Molina JM, Cooper GJS, Leighton B, Olefsky JM. Induction of insulin resistance in vivo by amylin and calcitonin gene-related peptide. Diabetes 1990;39:260–5.

268. Bretherton-Watt D, Gilbey SG, Ghatei MA, et al. Failure to establish islet amyloid polypeptide (amylin) as a circulating beta cell inhibiting hormone in man. Diabetologia 1990;33:115–7.

269. Nagamatsu S, Carroll RJ, Grodsky GM, Steiner DF. Lack of islet amyloid polypeptide regulation of insulin biosynthesis or secretion in normal rat islets. Diabetes 1990;39:871–4.

270. MacIntyre I. Amylinamide, bone conservation, and pancreatic β cells. Lancet 1989;2:1026–7.

271. Johnson KH, O'Brien TD, Betsholtz C, Westermark P. Islet amyloid, islet-myloid polypeptide, and diabetes mellitus. N Engl J Med 1989;321:513–8.

272. Leighton B, Cooper GJS. The role of amylin in the insulin resistance of non-insulin-dependent diabetes mellitus. Trends Biochem Sci 1990;15:295–9.

273. Johnson KH, O'Brien TD, Westermark P. Newly identified pancreatic protein islet amyloid polypeptide: what is its relationship to diabetes? Diabetes 1991;40:310–4.

274. Steiner DF, Ohagi S, Nagamatsu S, et al. Is islet amyloid polypeptide a significant factor in pathogenesis or pathophysiology of diabetes? Diabetes 1991;40:305–9.

275. Kanatsuka A, Makino H, Ohsawa H, et al. Secretion of islet amyloid polypeptide in response to glucose. FEBS Lett 1989;259:199–201.

276. Kahn SE, D'Alessio DA, Schwartz MW, et al. Evidence of cosecretion of islet amyloid polypeptide and insulin by β-cells. Diabetes 1990;39:634–8.

277. Mitsukawa T, Takemura J, Asai J, et al. Islet amyloid polypeptide response to glucose, insulin, and somatostatin analogue administration. Diabetes 1990;39:639–42.

278. Guest PC, Rhodes CJ, Hutton JC. Regulation of the biosynthesis of insulin-secretory-granule proteins: coordinate translational control is exerted on some, but not all, granule matrix constituents. Biochem J 1989;257:431–7.

279. Blundell T, Dodson G, Hodgkin D, Mercola D. Insulin: the structure in the crystal and its reflection in chemistry and biology. Adv Protein Chem 1972;26:279–402.

280. Grant PT, Coombs TL, Frank BH. Differences in the nature of the interaction of insulin and proinsulin with zinc. Biochem J 1972;126:433–40.

281. Emdin SO, Dodson GG, Cutfield JM, Cutfield SM. Role of zinc in insulin biosynthesis: some possible zinc-insulin interactions in the pancreatic B-cell. Diabetologia 1980;19:174–82.

282. Hutton JC, Penn EJ, Peshavaria M. Low-molecular-weight constituents of isolated insulin-secretory granules: bivalent cations, adenine nucleotides and inorganic phosphate. Biochem J 1983;210:297–305.

283. Greider MH, Howell SL, Lacy PE. Isolation and properties of secretory granules from rat islets of Langerhans: II. Ultrastructure of the beta granule. J Cell Biol 1969;41:162–6.

284. Coore HG, Hellman B, Pihl E, Täljedal I-B. Physicochemi-

cal characteristics of insulin secretion granules. Biochem J 1969;111:107–13.

285. Howell SL, Tyhurst M, Duvefelt H, et al. Role of zinc and calcium in the formation and storage of insulin in the pancreatic β-cell. Cell Tiss Res 1978;188:107–18.

286. Michael J, Carroll R, Swift HH, Steiner DF. Studies on the molecular organization of rat insulin secretory granules. J Biol Chem 1987;262:16531–5.

287. Orci L, Malaisse-Lagae F, Ravazzola M, et al. Exocytosis-endocytosis coupling in the pancreatic beta cell. Science 1973;181:561–2.

288. Orci L. A portrait of the pancreatic B-cell. Diabetologia 1974;10:163–87.

289. Kelly RB. Microtubules, membrane traffic, and cell organization. Cell 1990;61:5–7.

290. Sheetz MP, Vale R, Schnapp B, et al. Movements of vesicles on microtubules. Ann NY Acad Sci 1987;493:409–16.

291. Vale RD, Goldstein LSB. One motor, many tails: an expanding repertoire of force-generating enzymes. Cell 1990;60:883–5.

292. Cleveland DW. Microtubule MAPping. Cell 1990;60:701–2.

293. Tooze J, Burke B. Accumulation of adrenocorticotropin secretory granules in the midbody of telophase AtT20 cells: evidence that secretory granules move anterogradely along microtubules. J Cell Biol 1987;104:1047–57.

294. Matsuuchi L, Buckley KM, Lowe AW, Kelly RB. Targeting of secretory vesicles to cytoplasmic domains in AtT-20 and PC-12 cells. J Cell Biol 1988;106:239–51.

295. Rivas RJ, Moore H-PH. Spatial segregation of the regulated and constitutive secretory pathways. J Cell Biol 1989;109:51–60.

296. Schweizer FE, Schafer T, Tapparelli C, et al. Inhibition of exocytosis by intracellularly applied antibodies against a chromaffin granule-binding protein. Nature 1989;339:709–12.

297. Howell SL, Parry DG, Taylor KW. Secretion of newly synthesized insulin in vitro [Letter]. Nature 1965;208:487.

298. Sando H, Borg J, Steiner DF. Studies on the secretion of newly synthesized proinsulin and insulin from isolated rat islets of Langerhans. J Clin Invest 1972; 51:1476–85.

299. Sando H, Grodsky GM. Dynamic synthesis and release of insulin and proinsulin from perifused islets. Diabetes 1973;22:354–60.

300. Schatz H, Nierle C, Pfeiffer EF. (Pro-)insulin biosynthesis and release of newly synthesized (pro-)insulin from isolated islets of rat pancreas in the presence of amino acids and sulphonylureas. Eur J Clin Invest 1975;5:477–85.

301. Halban PA. Differential rates of release of newly synthesized and of stored insulin from pancreatic islets. Endocrinology 1982;110:1183–8.

302. Gold G, Landahl HD, Gishizky ML, Grodsky GM. Heterogeneity and compartmental properties of insulin storage and secretion in rat islets. J Clin Invest 1982;69:554–63.

303. Gold G, Gishizky ML, Grodsky GM. Evidence that glucose "marks" β cells resulting in preferential release of newly synthesized insulin. Science 1982;218:56–8.

304. Salomon D, Meda P. Heterogeneity and contact-dependent regulation of hormone secretion by individual B cells. Exp Cell Res 1986;162:507–20.

305. Stefan Y, Meda P, Neufeld M, Orci L. Stimulation of insulin secretion reveals heterogeneity of pancreatic B cells in vivo. J Clin Invest 1987;80:175–83.

306. Schuit FC, In't Veld PA, Pipeleers DG. Glucose stimulates

proinsulin biosynthesis by a dose-dependent recruitment of pancreatic beta cells. Proc Natl Acad Sci USA 1988;85:3865–9.

307. Halban PA, Wollheim CB. Intracellular degradation of insulin stores by rat pancreatic islets in vitro: an alternative pathway for homeostasis of pancreatic insulin content. J Biol Chem 1980;255:6003–6.

308. Halban PA, Renold AE. Influence of glucose on insulin handling by rat islets in culture: a reflection of integrated changes in insulin biosynthesis, release, and intracellular degradation. Diabetes 1983;32:254–61.

309. Orci L, Ravazzola M, Amherdt M, et al. Insulin, not C-peptide (proinsulin), is present in crinophagic bodies of the pancreatic B-cell. J Cell Biol 1984;98:222–8.

310. Smith RE, Farquhar MG. Lysosome function in the regulation of the secretory process in cells of the anterior pituitary gland. J Cell Biol 1966;31:319–47.

311. Orci L, Junod A, Pictet R, et al. Granulolysis in A-cells of endocrine pancreas in spontaneous and experimental diabetes in animals. J Cell Biol 1968;38:462–6.

312. Schäfer G, Daum H, Schatz H. Studies on insulin degradation inside the pancreatic B-cell: evidence for a regulating role of glucose. Mol Cell Endocrinol 1983;31:141–9.

313. Schnell AH, Swenne I, Borg LAH. Lysosomes and pancreatic islet function: a quantitative estimation of crinophagy in the mouse pancreatic B-cell. Cell Tissue Res 1988;252:9–15.

314. Halban PA, Mutkoski R, Dodson G, Orci L. Resistance of the insulin crystal to lysosomal proteases: implications for pancreatic B-cell crinophagy. Diabetologia 1987;30:348–53.

315. Halban PA, Amherdt M, Orci L, Renold AE. Proinsulin modified by analogues of arginine and lysine is degraded rapidly in pancreatic B-cells. Biochem J 1984;219:91–7.

316. Rhodes CJ, Halban PA. The intracellular handling of insulin-related peptides in isolated pancreatic islets: evidence for differential rates of degradation of insulin and C-peptide. Biochem J 1988;251:23–30.

317. Duckworth WC, Kitabchi AE, Heinemann M. Direct measurement of plasma proinsulin in normal and diabetic subjects. Am J Med 1972;53:418–27.

318. Gorden P, Hendricks CM, Roth J. Circulating proinsulin-like component in man: increased proportion in hypoinsulinemic states. Diabetologia 1974;10:469–74.

319. Mako ME, Starr JI, Rubenstein AH. Circulating proinsulin in patients with maturity onset diabetes. Am J Med 1977;63:865–9.

320. Ward WK, LaCava EC, Paquette TL, et al. Disproportionate elevation of immunoreactive proinsulin in type 2 (non-insulin-dependent) diabetes mellitus and in experimental insulin resistance. Diabetologia 1987;30:698–702.

321. Yoshioka N, Kuzuya T, Matsuda A, et al. Serum proinsulin levels at fasting and after oral glucose load in patients with type 2 (non-insulin-dependent) diabetes mellitus. Diabetologia 1988;31:355–60.

322. Hampton SM, Beyzavi K, Teale D, Marks V. A Direct assay for proinsulin in plasma and its applications in hypoglycaemia. Clin Endocrinol 1988;29:9–16.

323. Ludvigsson J, Heding L. Abnormal proinsulin/C-peptide ratio in juvenile diabetes. Acta Diabet Lat 1982;19:351–8.

324. Heding LG, Ludvigsson J, Kasperska-Czyzykowa T. B-cell secretion in non-diabetics and insulin-dependent diabetics. Acta Med Scand Suppl 1981;656:5–9.

325. Snorgaard O, Hartling SG, Binder C. Proinsulin and C-peptide at onset and during 12 months cyclosporin treatment of type 1 (insulin-dependent) diabetes mellitus. Diabetologia 1990;33:36–42.

326. Heaton DA, Millward BA, Gray IP, et al. Increased proinsulin levels as an early indicator of B-cell dysfunction in non-diabetic twins of type 1 (insulin-dependent) diabetic patients. Diabetologia 1988;31:182–4.

327. Hartling SG, Lindgren F, Dahlqvist G, et al. Elevated proinsulin in healthy siblings of IDDM patients independent of HLA identity. Diabetes 1989;38:1271–4.

328. Sestoft L, Heding LG. Hypersecretion of proinsulin in thyrotoxicosis. Diabetologia 1981;21:103–7.

329. Gorden P, Sherman BM, Simopoulos AP. Glucose intolerance with hypokalemia: an increased proportion of circulating proinsulin-like component. J Clin Endocrinol Metab 1972;34:235–40.

330. Duckworth WC, Kitabchi AE. Hyperproinsulinemia in hypoglycemic subjects. Horm Metab Res 1972;4:133–5.

331. Hartling SG, Garne S, Binder C, et al. Proinsulin, insulin, and C-peptide in cystic fibrosis after an oral glucose tolerance test. Diabetes Res 1988;7:165–9.

332. Kanazawa Y, Awata T, Shibasaki Y, et al. Alteration of beta-cell function in different diabetic states. Exp Clin Endocrinol 1984;84:346–51.

333. Glaser B, Leibovich G, Nesher R, et al. Improved beta-cell function after intensive insulin treatment in severe non-insulin-dependent diabetes. Acta Endocrinol 1988;118:365–73.

334. Yoshioka N, Kuzuya T, Matsuda A, Iwamoto Y. Effects of dietary treatment on serum insulin and proinsulin response in newly diagnosed NIDDM. Diabetes 1989;38:262–6.

335. Nagi DK, Hendra TJ, Ryle AJ, Cooper TM, et al. The relationships of concentrations of insulin intact proinsulin and 32–33 split proinsulin with cardiovascular risk factors in type 2 (non-insulin-dependent) diabetic subjects. Diabetologia 1990;33:532–7.

336. Deacon CF, Schleser-Mohr S, Ballmann M, et al. Preferential release of proinsulin relative to insulin in non-insulin-dependent diabetes mellitus. Acta Endocrinol 1988;119:549–54.

337. Temple RC, Carrington CA, Luzio SD, et al. Insulin deficiency in non-insulin-dependent diabetes. Lancet 1989;1:293–5.

338. Clark A, Matthews DR, Naylor BA, et al. Pancreatic islet amyloid and elevated proinsulin secretion in familial maturity-onset diabetes. Diabetes Res 1987;4:51–5.

339. Melani F, Ryan WG, Rubenstein AH, Steiner DF. Proinsulin secretion by a pancreatic beta-cell adenoma: proinsulin and C-peptide secretion. N Engl J Med 1970;283:713–9.

340. Gorden P, Sherman B, Roth J. Proinsulin-like component of circulating insulin in the basal state and in patients and hamsters with islet cell tumors. J Clin Invest 1971;50:2113–22.

341. Gutman RA, Lazarus NR, Penhos JC, et al. Circulating proinsulin-like material in patients with functioning insulinomas. N Engl J Med 1971;284:1003–8.

342. Cohen RM, Given BD, Licinio-Paixao J, et al. Proinsulin radioimmunoassay in the evaluation of insulinomas and familial hyperproinsulinemia. Metabolism 1986;35:1137–46.

343. Cohen RM, Camus F. Update on insulinomas or the case of the missing (pro)insulinoma [Editorial]. Diabetes Care 1988;11:506–8.

344. Berger M, Bordi C, Cuppers H-J, et al. Functional and morphologic characterization of human insulinomas. Diabetes 1983;32:921–31.

345. Yalow RS, Berson SA. "Big, big insulin". Metabolism 1973;22:703–13.

346. Nunes-Correa J, Lowy C, Sönksen PH. Presumed insulin-

oma secreting a high-molecular-weight insulin analogue. Lancet 1974;1:837–41.

347. Pipeleers DG, Levy J, Malaisse-Lagae F, Malaisse WJ. In vitro biosynthesis and release of three immuno-reactive insulin-like components by a human insulinoma. Diabete Metab 1975;1:7–11.

348. Beischer W, Melani F, Keller L, Pfeiffer EF. Chromatographic heterogeneity of insulin extracted from insulinomas. J Clin Endocrinol Metab 1975;40:393–400.

349. Villaume C, Beck B, Debry G. High molecular weight substances with insulin immunoreactivity. Diabete Metab 1979;5:159–65.

350. Villaume C, Beck B, Pointel JP, et al. Portal, hepatic and peripheral insulin immunoreactive substances before and after removal of an insulinoma. J Endocrinol Invest 1982;5:315–21.

351. Robbins DC, Shoelson SE, Tager HS, et al. Products of therapeutic insulins in the blood of insulin-dependent (type I) diabetic patients. Diabetes 1985;34:510–9.

352. Creutzfeld C, Track NS, Creutzfeld W. In vitro studies of the rate of proinsulin and insulin turnover in seven human insulinomas. Eur J Clin Invest 1973;3:371–84.

353. Gutman RA, Fink G, Shapiro JR, et al. Proinsulin and insulin release with a human insulinoma and adjacent nonadenomatous pancreas. J Clin Endocrinol Metab 1973; 36:978–87.

354. Gold G, Gishizky ML, Chick WL, Grodsky GM. Contrasting patterns of insulin biosynthesis, compartmental storage, and secretion: rat tumor versus islet cells. Diabetes 1984;33:556–61.

355. Valverde I, Barreto M, Malaisse WJ. Stimulation by D-glucose of protein biosynthesis in tumoral insulin-producing cells (RINm5F line). Endocrinology 1988;122:1443–8.

356. Wang SY: The acute effects of glucose on the insulin. biosynthetic-secretory pathway in a simian virus 40-transformed hamster pancreatic islet β-cell line. Endocrinology 1989;124:1980–7.

357. Wintersteiner O, du Vigeaud V, Jensen H. Studies on crystalline insulin. V. The distribution of nitrogen in crystalline insulin. J Pharmacol Exp Ther 1928;32:397–411.

358. Sanger F. Chemistry of insulin: determination of the structure of insulin opens the way to greater understanding of life processes. Science 1959;129:1340–4.

359. Brange J. Galenics of insulin. New York: Springer-Verlag, 1987.

360. Dayhoff ML. Atlas of protein sequences and structure. Vol 5, Suppl 3. Washington, DC: National Biomedical Research Foundation, 1978.

361. Pullen RA, Lindsay DG, Wood SP, et al. Receptor-binding region of insulin. Nature 1976;259:369–73.

362. Brandenburg D, Wollmer A, eds. Insulin: chemistry, structure and function of insulin and related hormones. Proceedings of the 2nd International Insulin Symposium. Aachen, 1979. Berlin: W de Gruyter, 1980.

363. Gammeltoft S. Insulin receptors: binding kinetics and structure-function relationship of insulin. Physiol Rev 1984;64:1321–78.

364. Adams MJ, Blundell TL, Dodson EJ, et al. Structure of rhombohedral 2 zinc insulin crystals. Nature 1969; 224:491–5.

365. Blundell TL, Cutfield JF, Cutfield SM, et al. Atomic positions in rhombohedral 2-zinc insulin crystals. Nature 1971;231:506–11.

366. Peking Insulin Structure Group. Insulin's crystal structure at 2.5 Å resolution. Peking Rev 1971;40:11–6.

367. Baker EN, Blundell TL, Cutfield JF, et al. The structure of 2Zn pig insulin crystals at 1.5 Å resolution. Philos Trans R Soc Lond [Biol] 1988;B319:389–456.

368. Cutfield JF, Cutfield SM, Dodson EJ, et al. Similarities and differences in the crystal structures of insulin. In: Dodson GG, Glusker J, Sayre D, eds. Structural studies on molecules of biological interest. Oxford: Oxford University Press, 1981:527–46.

369. Smith GD, Swenson DC, Dodson EJ, et al. Structural stability in the 4-zinc human insulin hexamer. Proc Natl Acad Sci USA 1984;81:7093–7.

370. Derewenda U, Derewenda Z, Dodson EJ, et al. Phenol stabilizes more helix in a new symmetrical zinc insulin hexamer. Nature 1989;338:594–6.

371. Dodson EJ, Dodson GG, Lewitova A, Sabesan M. Zinc-free cubic pig insulin: crystallization and structure determination. J Mol Biol 1978;125:387–96.

372. Dodson EJ, Dodson GG, Hodgkin DC. The conformations observed in the N terminal A chain residues of insulin. In: Ananchenko SN, ed. Frontiers of bioinorganic chemistry and molecular biology. Oxford: Pergamon Press, 1980:145–50.

373. Bi RC, Dauter Z, Dodson EJ, et al. Insulin's structure as a modified and monomeric molecule. Biopolymers 1984;23:391–5.

374. Roy M, Brader ML, Lee RW-K, et al. Spectroscopic signatures of the T to R conformational transition in the insulin hexamer. J Biol Chem 1989;264:19081–5.

375. Perutz MF. Regulation of oxygen affinity of hemoglobin: influence of structure of the globin on the heme iron. Annu Rev Biochem 1979;48:327–86.

376. Chothia C, Lesk AM, Dodson GG, Hodgkin DC. Transmission of conformational change in insulin. Nature 1983;302:500–5.

377. Wollmer A, Rannefeld B, Johansen BR, et al. Phenol-promoted structural transformation of insulin in solution. Biol Chem Hoppe-Seyler 1987;368:903–11.

378. Renscheidt H, Strassburger W, Glatter U, et al. A solution equivalent of the 2Zn→4Zn transformation of insulin in the crystal. Eur J Biochem 1984;142:7–14.

379. Kaarsholm NC, Ko H-C, Dunn MF. Comparison of solution structural flexibility and zinc binding domains for insulin, proinsulin, and miniproinsulin. Biochemistry 1989; 28:4427–35.

380. Wollmer A, Rannefeld B, Stahl J, Melberg SG. Structural transition in the metal-free hexamer of protein-engineered [B13 Gln] insulin. Biol Chem Hoppe-Seyler 1989; 370:1045–53.

381. Brader ML, Kaarsholm NC, Lee RW-K, Dunn MF. Characterization of the R-State insulin hexamer and its derivatives. The hexamer is stabilized by heterotropic ligand binding interactions. Biochemistry 1991;30:6636–45.

382. Bradbury JH, Ramesh V. [1]H n.m.r. studies of insulin: assignment of resonances and properties of tyrosine residues. Biochem J 1985;229:731–7.

383. Hua Q-X, Chen Y-J, Wang C-C, et al. High resolution ^{1}H-NMR studies of des-(B26-B30)-insulin; assignment of resonances and properties of aromatic residues. Biochim Biophys Acta 1989;994:114–20.

384. Weiss MA, Nguyen DT, Khait I, et al. Two-dimensional-NMR and photo-CIDNP studies of the insulin monomer: assignment of aromatic resonances with application to protein folding, structure and dynamics. Biochemistry 1989;28:9855–73.

385. Kline AD, Justice RM Jr. Complete sequence-specific ^{1}H NMR assignments for human insulin. Biochemistry 1990;29:2906–13.

386. Roy M, Lee RWK, Brange J, Dunn MF. ^{1}H NMR spectrum of

the native human insulin monomer: evidence for conformational differences between the monomer and aggregated forms. J Biol Chem 1990;265:5448–52.

387. Hua Q, Weiss MA. Comparative 2D NMR studies of human insulin and des-pentapeptide insulin: sequential resonance assignment and implications for protein dynamics and receptor recognition. Biochemistry 1991;30:5505–15.

388. Hua Q, Weiss MA. Toward the solution of human insulin: sequential 2D 1H NMR assignment of a des-pentapeptide analogue and comparison with crystal structure. Biochemistry 1990;29:10545–55.

389. Boelens R, Ganadu ML, Verheyden P, Kaptein R. Two-dimensional NMR studies on des-pentapeptide-insulin: proton resonance assignments and secondary structure analysis. Eur J Biochem 1990;191:147–53.

390. Brange J, Ribel U, Hansen JF, et al. Monomeric insulins obtained by protein engineering and their medical implications. Nature 1988;333:679–82.

391. Brange J, Owens DR, Kang S, Vølund A. Monomeric insulins and their experimental and clinical implications. Diabetes Care 1990;13:923–54.

392. Shoelson SE, Lu Z-X, Parlautan L, et al. Mutations at the dimer, hexamer and receptor-binding surfaces of insulin independently affect insulin-insulin and insulin-receptor interactions. Biochemistry 1992;31:1757–67.

393. Weiss MA, Hua Q-X, Lynch CS, et al. Heteronuclear 2D NMR studies of an engineered insulin monomer: assignment and characterization of the receptor-binding surface by selective ^{2}H and ^{13}C labeling with application to protein design. Biochemistry 1991;30:7373–89.

394. Kristensen SM, Jørgensen AMM, Led JJ, et al. Proton nuclear magnetic resonance study of the B9(Asp) mutant of human insulin: sequential assignment of secondary structure. J Mol Biol 1991;218:221–31.

395. Cutfield J, Cutfield S, Dodson E, et al. Evidence concerning insulin activity from the structure of a cross-linked derivative. Hoppe-Seyler's Z Physiol Chem 1981; 362:755–61.

396. Derewenda U, Derewenda Z, Dodson EJ, et al. X-ray analysis of the single chain B29-A1 peptide-linked insulin molecule: a completely inactive analogue. J Mol Biol 1991;220:425–33.

397. Mirmira RG, Tager HS. Role of the phenylalanine B24 side chain in directing insulin interaction with its receptor. J Biol Chem 1989;264:6349–54.

398. Hua Q-X, Shoelson SE, Kochoyan M, Weiss MA. Receptor binding redefined by a structural switch in a mutant human insulin. Nature 1991;354:238–41.

397. Nakagawa SH, Tager HS. Role of the phenylalanine B25 side chain in directing insulin interaction with its receptor: steric and conformational effects. J Biol Chem 1986;261:7332–41.

398. Nakagawa SH, Tager HS. Role of the COOH-terminal B-chain domain in insulin-receptor interactions: identification of perturbations involving the insulin mainchain. J Biol Chem 1987;262:12054–8.

399. Nakagawa SH, Tager HS. Perturbation of insulin-receptor interactions by intramolecular hormone cross-linking. J Biol Chem 1989;264:272–9.

400. Weiss MA, Frank BH, Khait I, et al. NMR and photo-CIDNP studies of human proinsulin and prohormone processing intermediates with application to endopeptidase recognition. Biochemistry 1990;29:8389–401.

401. Blundell TL, Bedarkar S, Rinderknecht E, Humbel RE. Insulin-like growth factor: a model for tertiary structure accounting for immunoreactivity and receptor binding. Proc Natl Acad Sci USA 1978;75:180–4.

402. WHO Expert Committee on Diabetes Mellitus. Second report. WHO Tech Rep Ser 1980;646;7–80.

403. Rolando RL, Torroba D. Heterogeneity of the fourth international standard for insulin by gel-chromatography on sephadex. Experientia 1972;28:1169.

404. Schlichtkrull J, Ege H, Jorgensen KH, et al. Die Chemie des Insulins. In: Oberdisse K, ed. Diabetes mellitus A (Handbuch der inneren Medizin, Bd 7/24). Berlin: Springer, 1975:77–127.

405. Morihara K, Oka T, Tsuzuki H. Semi-synthesis of human insulin by trypsin-catalyzed replacement of Ala-B30 by Thr in porcine insulin [Letter]. Nature 1979;280:412–3.

406. Markussen J. Human Insulin by tryptic transpeptidation of porcine insulin and biosynthetic precursors. Lancaster, UK: MTP Press, 1987.

407. Chance RE, Hoffmann JA, Kroeff EP, et al. Production of human insulin using recombinant DNA technology and a new chain combination procedure. In: Rich DH, Gross E, eds. Peptides: synthesis-structure-function. Rockford IL: Pierce Chemical Co, 1981:721–8.

408. Frank BH, Pettee JM, Zimmerman RE, Burck PJ. The production of human proinsulin and its transformation to human insulin and C-peptide. In: Rich DH, Gross E, eds. Peptides: synthesis-structure-function. Rockford, IL: Pierce Chemical Co, 1981:729–38.

409. Markussen J, Damgaard U, Jorgensen KH, et al. Biosynthesis of human insulin in yeast via single-chain precursors. In: Theodoropoulos D, ed. Peptides 1986: Proceedings of the 19th European Peptide Symposium. Berlin: Walter de Gruyter, 1986:189–94.

410. Tager H, Given B, Baldwin D, et al. A structurally abnormal insulin causing human diabetes. Nature 1979;281:122–5.

411. Given BD, Mako ME, Tager HS, et al. Diabetes due to secretion of an abnormal insulin. N Engl J Med 1980;302:129–35.

412. Shoelson S, Haneda M, Blix P, et al. Three mutant insulins in man. Nature 1983;302:540–3.

413. Kwok SCM, Steiner DF, Rubenstein AH, Tager HS. Identification of a point mutation in the human insulin gene giving rise to a structurally abnormal insulin (insulin Chicago). Diabetes 1983;32:872–5.

414. Shoelson SE, Fickova M, Haneda M, et al. Identification of a mutant human insulin predicted to contain a serine-for-phenylalanine substitution. Proc Natl Acad Sci USA 1983;80:7390–4.

415. Haneda M, Chan SJ, Kwok SCM, et al. Studies on mutant human insulin genes: identification and sequence analysis of a gene encoding [Ser^{B24}] insulin. Proc Natl Acad Sci USA 1983;80:6366–70.

416. Haneda M, Polonsky KS, Bergenstal RM, et al. Familial hyperinsulinemia due to a structurally abnormal insulin: definition of an emerging new clinical syndrome. N Engl J Med 1984;310:1288–9.

417. Nanjo K, Sanke T, Miyano M, et al. Diabetes due to secretion of a structurally abnormal insulin (insulin Wakayama): clinical and functional characteristics of [Leu^{A3}] insulin. J Clin Invest 1986;77:514–9.

418. Nanjo K, Miyano M, Kondo M, et al. Insulin Wakayama: familial mutant insulin syndrome in Japan. Diabetologia 1987;30:87–92.

419. Iwamoto Y, Sakura H, Ishii Y, et al. A new case of abnormal insulinemia with diabetes: reduced insulin values determined by radioreceptor assay. Diabetes 1986;35:1237–42.

420. Steiner DF, Tager HS, Chan SJ, et al. Lessons learned from molecular biology of insulin-gene mutations. Diabetes Care 1990;13:600–9.

421. Shoelson SE, Polonsky KS, Zeidler A, et al. Human insulin B24 (Phe→Ser): secretion and metabolic clearance of the abnormal insulin in man and in a dog model. J Clin Invest 1984;73:1351–8.

422. Gabbay KH, Bergenstal RM, Wolff J, et al. Familial hyperproinsulinemia: partial characterization of circulating proinsulin-like material. Proc Natl Acad Sci USA 1979;76:2881–5.

423. Kanazawa Y, Hayashi M, Ikeuchi M, et al. Familial proinsulinemia: a rare disorder of insulin biosynthesis. In: Baba S, Kaneko T, Yanaihara N, eds. Proinsulin, insulin, C-peptide. Amsterdam: Excerpta Medica, 1979:262–9.

424. Robbins DC, Blix PM, Rubenstein AH, et al. A human proinsulin variant at arginine 65. Nature 1981;291:679–81.

425. Robbins DC, Shoelson SE, Rubenstein AH, Tager HS. Familial hyperproinsulinemia: two cohorts secreting indistinguishable type II intermediates of proinsulin conversion. J Clin Invest 1984;73:714–9.

426. Shibasaki Y, Kawakami T, Kanazawa Y, et al. Posttranslational cleavage of proinsulin is blocked by a point mutation in familial hyperproinsulinemia. J Clin Invest 1985;76:378–80.

427. Gruppuso PA, Gorden P, Kahn CR, et al. Familial hyperproinsulinemia due to a proposed defect in conversion of proinsulin to insulin. N Engl J Med 1984;311:629–34.

428. Chan SJ, Seino S, Gruppuso PA, et al. A mutation in the B chain coding region is associated with impaired proinsulin conversion in a family with hyperproinsulinemia. Proc Natl Acad Sci USA 1987;84:2194–7.

429. Schwartz GP, Burke GT, Katsoyannis PG. A superactive insulin: [B10-aspartic acid] insulin (human). Proc Natl Acad Sci USA 1987;84:6408–11.

Chapter 4

CELL BIOLOGY OF INSULIN SECRETION

JEAN-CLAUDE HENQUIN

Under physiologic conditions, the concentration of blood glucose fluctuates only in a narrow range despite alternations in periods of food intake and fasting. This stability is due to a remarkably efficient hormonal system that exerts opposite effects on the organs of glucose storage and production. Whereas several hormones can prevent the blood glucose level from falling dangerously low by stimulating glycogenolysis and gluconeogenesis, insulin is the only efficient means by which the organism can prevent exaggerated elevations in blood glucose level. It is therefore not surprising that insulin secretion by β-cells of the islets of Langerhans is subject to tight control.

The principal characteristic of β-cells is that they function as "fuel-sensors" capable of adapting the rate of insulin secretion to the variations in plasma levels of glucose and other energetic substrates (amino acids, fatty acids, and ketone bodies). However, several hormones and neurotransmitters also exert a critical control on β-cell function, which can also be influenced by various pharmacologic agents. This multifactorial control necessitates rapid integration by β-cells of a host of signals generating distinct intracellular messengers.

Our understanding of stimulus-secretion coupling in β-cells has progressed considerably. Yet because of the great complexity of the phenomenon and of space constraints, I summarize here only the basic mechanisms of β-cell function and privilege references to studies made with normal β-cell models. Tumoral insulin-secreting cell lines are instrumental when large amounts of tissue are necessary to solve a problem, but some of their properties clearly differ from those of normal β-cells.

THE PREEMINENT ROLE OF GLUCOSE IN THE CONTROL OF INSULIN SECRETION

On the basis of in vitro experiments,[1,2] the numerous agents that increase insulin secretion can be subdivided into two broad categories: the initiators and the potentiators.

The initiators or primary stimuli are able to increase insulin secretion in the absence of any other stimulatory agent. These include D-glucose, D-glyceraldehyde, D-mannose, L-leucine and its derivative α-ketoisocaproic acid, inosine, and certain pharmacologic substances.

The potentiators or secondary stimuli are ineffective alone but increase insulin secretion in the presence of an initiator, particularly glucose. These include D-fructose, certain amino acids, fatty acids, ketone bodies, acetylcholine, glucagon, certain gastrointestinal hormones, and several drugs.

It is, however, essential to emphasize that glucose is by far the most important controller of insulin secretion. One may even consider glucose as the only physiologic initiator of insulin secretion in adult mammals. This concept is schematically illustrated in Figure 4–1.

When insulin secretion is studied in vitro, with isolated islets or the perfused pancreas and an artificial balanced-salt solution, a stimulatory effect of glucose can already be measured at concentrations within the physiologic range (depicted in hatched area in Fig. 4–1). In contrast, amino acids (alone or in combination) or drugs (e.g., sulfonylureas) must be used at concentrations well above the physiologic or therapeutic range to induce insulin release. Hormones have no effect when used alone. However, if the incubation or perfusion medium contains a physiologic concentration of glucose, insulin secretion can be increased by amino acids, hormones, or drugs at physiologic or therapeutic concentrations[3-7] (broken line in Fig. 4–1C,D). Glucose thus confers to otherwise ineffective or weakly effective agents the ability to increase insulin secretion, even at low concentrations. The mechanisms of this permissive action of glucose will be discussed in the section "Potentiation, Priming, and Desensitization of Insulin Secretion." If, on the other hand, the medium contains amino acids, hormones, or a drug at physiologic or therapeutic concentrations (substance X in Fig. 4–1A), the dose-response curve of glucose-induced insulin secretion is shifted to the left. Not only is the effect of glucose potentiated but β-cells apparently become more sensitive to the sugar. The difference between the two curves in Figure 4–1A is shown in Figure 4–1B. It shows that the change in insulin secretion brought about by the non-glucose stimulus increases as the concentration of glucose is raised. From this perspective one could describe the effect of glucose as a potentiation of the β-cell response to substance X. The terminology is unusual for in vitro studies in which "potentiators" are those agents that are ineffective alone, but it has been used in some in vivo studies.[8]

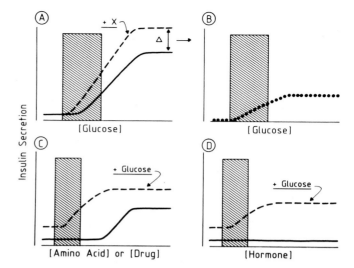

Fig. 4–1. Schematic representation of the effect of various concentrations of glucose, amino acids, drugs, and hormones on insulin secretion in vitro. Hatched areas correspond to the range of physiologic or therapeutic concentrations of the test substance. Solid lines show the effect of the substance alone. Broken lines show the effect of an amino acid or a drug (C) or a hormone (D) in the presence of a physiologic concentration of glucose. The broken line in A shows the effect of glucose in the presence of a physiologic or therapeutic concentration of another agent (X). The stippled line in B shows the difference between the effects of glucose alone and with agent X, i.e., the increase in insulin secretion produced by agent X at various concentrations of glucose.

With this background in mind, it is easy to understand how changes in the glucose concentration below the threshold value measured in vitro can control β-cell function in vivo. A small drop in plasma glucose level (e.g., during fasting) prevents inappropriate insulin secretion in response to non-glucose stimuli. On the other hand, relatively small increases in plasma glucose level (e.g., after meals) lead to larger insulin responses than those expected from dose-response curves defined in vitro because of the greater effect of non-glucose stimuli. The marked glucose dependency of the action of various stimuli on β-cells is thus an essential safeguard against both hypoglycemia and hyperglycemia.

GENERAL CHARACTERISTICS OF GLUCOSE-INDUCED INSULIN SECRETION

Kinetics

Insulin secretion depends not only on the ambient concentration of glucose but also on the rate of change of this concentration. When the glucose level increases slowly, the rate of insulin secretion increases in parallel. However, when the concentration of glucose is abruptly increased and then maintained at a high level, insulin secretion follows a biphasic time-course (Fig. 4–2A). A rapid peak (first phase) is followed by a nadir and a slowly rising second phase. This pattern, first described in the

<u>Insulin Secretion</u>   <u>Cytoplasmic Ca^{2+}</u>

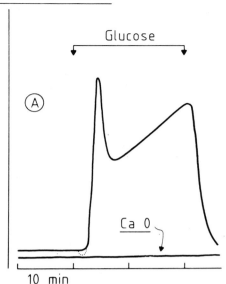

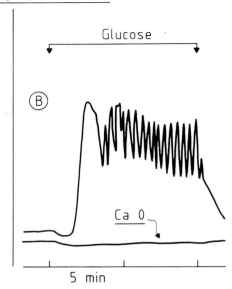

Fig. 4—2. A: Schematic representation of the biphasic pattern of insulin secretion observed in vitro in response to a sudden stimulation with glucose. No increase in secretion occurs in the absence of extracellular Ca^{++} (Ca 0). B: Schematic representation of the increase in cytoplasmic free Ca^{++} produced in β-cells within an intact mouse islet by a sudden stimulation with glucose (P. Gilon and J. C. Henquin, reference 17 and unpublished results). Glucose causes a slight decrease in cytoplasmic free Ca^{++} in the absence of extracellular Ca^{++}.

perfused rat pancreas,[9] is commonly observed in vitro. It is not seen in vivo after a meal or even after an oral glucose load but can be produced by a rapid increase in plasma glucose levels during intravenous glucose infusion.[10] This ability of β-cells to respond rapidly to glucose is thought to be essential for optimal glucose homeostasis. The loss of this ability has long been considered an early sign of β-cell dysfunction.[10,11]

Numerous hypotheses have been put forward to explain the biphasic time-course of glucose-induced insulin secretion. Since the glucose dependency of the two phases is similar in vitro[12] and in vivo,[10] there is no evidence that distinct mechanisms are involved. Early suggestions that the nadir between the two phases is due to a negative feedback exerted by insulin secreted during the first phase or to partial inhibition by somatostatin have been abandoned.[12,13] The concept that the first phase reflects release of preformed insulin and that the second phase reflects release of newly synthesized insulin is also not correct.[12]

According to a "storage-limited" model,[12,13] there could exist two compartments of insulin granules, the smaller one being readily released and responsible for the first phase. This functional segregation could reflect association of certain granules with different structures of the microtubular-microfilamentous system.[14,15]

According to a "signal-limited" model,[13,16] changes in the magnitude or effectiveness of the triggering signal produced by glucose could underlie the biphasic response. Evidence supporting this hypothesis is accumulating. The rise in cytoplasmic Ca^{++} concentration produced by glucose is biphasic in intact mouse islets[17] and often so in single β-cells from rats or mice.[18–20] However, no gradual increase occurs during the second phase. Therefore, the slowly rising second phase of secretion (which is more pronounced in the rat than in

the mouse) does not depend simply on the concentration of cytoplasmic Ca^{++} but probably also involves an increase in the efficacy of the Ca^{++} signal[21,22]

Under certain conditions, a small decrease in β-cell cytoplasmic Ca^{++} content[17–20,23] and insulin secretion[23] precedes the first-phase increase triggered by glucose (Fig. 4–2). There is no consensus about the mechanism of these transient inhibitory effects of glucose or about their possible links with the paradoxical decrease in plasma insulin levels that glucose sometimes produces in patients with non-insulin-dependent diabetes mellitus (NIDDM).[24,25]

It should also be mentioned that biphasic insulin secretion can be triggered by stimuli other than glucose and that the kinetics of the secretory response may be influenced by the concentration of the applied stimulus and by the prevailing concentration of glucose.[1,4,6] For instance, the common idea that sulfonylureas simply trigger a first phase of insulin secretion[9] holds true only for stimulation by high concentrations of the drugs in low-glucose environments. When used at a low concentration and in the presence of glucose, sulfonylureas induce a sustained secretion of insulin.[6,26,27] These are further arguments supporting the conclusion that the kinetics of insulin secretion does not depend simply on the existence of different pools of insulin granules.

A third phase of insulin secretion has also been described in vitro. It is characterized by a progressive fall of the secretory rate when glucose stimulation is prolonged over 3 to 4 hours.[28,29] It is not due to exhaustion of insulin reserves but reflects β-cell desensitization[30] (see section "Potentiation, Priming, and Desensitization of Insulin Secretion"). Its possible links with NIDDM are discussed in Chapter 14 on the pathogenesis of NIDDM.

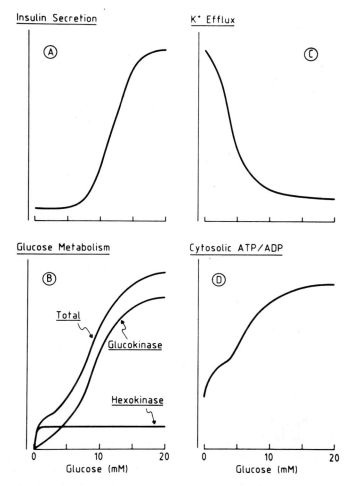

Fig. 4–3. Glucose dependency of insulin secretion (A), glucose metabolism (B), K⁺ efflux (C), and cytosolic ATP/ADP ratio (D) in rodent islets. A: This schematic curve is representative of results of insulin secretion that can be obtained with various preparations (perfused pancreas, isolated islets). B: Total glucose usage by islet cells is the sum of glucose phosphorylation by the hexokinase and the glucokinase. Redrawn with permission from reference 32 (Meglasson MD, Matschinsky FM. New perspectives on pancreatic islet glucokinase. Am J Physiol 1984;246:E1–13). C: K⁺ efflux was measured by monitoring the loss of ⁴²K⁺ from islets preloaded with the radioactive tracer. Redrawn with permission from reference 33 (Henquin JC. D-glucose inhibits potassium efflux from pancreatic islet cells. Nature 1978;271:271–3; copyright © 1978, Macmillan Magazines, Ltd.). D: The cytosolic ATP/ADP ratio was measured after brief permeabilization of islet cells by digitonin. Redrawn with permission from the reference 34 (Malaisse WJ, Sener A. Glucose-induced changes in cytosolic ATP content in pancreatic islets. Biochim Biophys Acta 1987;927:190–5).

Dose-Response Relationship

The relationship between the extracellular glucose concentration and the rate of insulin secretion in vitro is sigmoidal[31] (Fig. 4–3A). In isolated rat islets or in the perfused rat pancreas, the threshold concentration is around 5 to 6 mM, half-maximal and maximal responses are observed at 9 to 11 mM and 15 to 20 mM, respectively. This relationship is slightly shifted to the left in human islets and to the right in mouse islets. In vivo, circulating nutrients other than glucose, hormones, and neurotransmitters shift the dose-response relationship to glucose to the left (see first section).

The sigmoidal shape of this curve could be due to a Gaussian distribution of the thresholds for stimulation between β-cells. Raising the concentration of glucose would thus recruit more and more β-cells to secrete insulin. Functional heterogeneity between β-cells has been suggested by microscopic examination of islets in situ.[35] It has been directly demonstrated in vitro by measuring (with the reverse hemolytic plaque assay) insulin secretion from single β-cells obtained by dispersion of rat islets.[36] The number of secreting cells increases as the concentration of glucose is raised[37,38] The alternative possibility is that the response of each individual cell increases with the concentration of glucose. It has indeed been demonstrated that glucose causes a dose-dependent increase in the free cytoplasmic Ca⁺⁺ concentration[20] and in insulin release[37,38] in single isolated β-cells. In conclusion, it is likely that both the recruitment of β-cells and the increase in individual β-cell function participate in the response to glucose. The respective contribution of the two mechanisms when β-cells are coupled within the intact islets[39,40] is difficult to establish.

ISLET CELL INTERACTIONS

Dispersed islet cells or single purified β-cells secrete much less insulin in response to glucose than do intact islets.[41–43] This impaired secretion, which is not accounted for by alterations in glucose transport and oxidation or in cyclic adenosine monophosphate (cAMP) formation,[44] is partially corrected by reaggregation of the cells. It appears that the contact must be between β-cells (not with non-β-cells) for this increase in secretory function to occur.[45] Electrical[39] and functional[40] coupling of β-cells within subterritories of the islet may be essential for optimal insulin secretion.

It has been speculated that glucagon and somatostatin released by α-cells and δ-cells at the periphery of the islets could have a local influence on their neighboring β-cells. Both anatomic and functional evidence excludes that such an influence follows a vascular route.[46,47] Direct support for a paracrine mechanism is also lacking. More complete discussion of this question can be found in Chapter 2 on the morphology of the islets of Langerhans.

INSULIN BIOSYNTHESIS

Since the mechanisms of insulin biosynthesis are dealt with in detail in Chapter 3, the present section summarizes only the major aspects of this essential function of β-cells.

Proinsulin Synthesis and Insulin-Granules Formation

Translation of the insulin mRNA leads to the production of a precursor molecule, preproinsulin, with the following primary structure: signal peptide-B chain-Arg-

Arg-connecting peptide-Lys-Arg-A chain.[48] The hydrophobic signal peptide (24 amino acid residues) serves to direct the nascent molecule into the lumen of the endoplasmic reticulum. It is rapidly cleaved off and degraded, while the molecule of proinsulin (86 amino acid residues) folds and undergoes formation of disulfide bridges between A and B chains. Proinsulin is then transported in smooth microvesicles from the endoplasmic reticulum to the *cis* pole of the Golgi complex by an energy-requiring mechanism.[49,50] In the *trans* elements of the Golgi complex, proinsulin is packed in immature, clathrin-coated granules, where the conversion into insulin starts.[49] This conversion results from endoproteolytic cleavage at the pairs of dibasic amino acids linking the connecting peptide (C-peptide) to the two chains of insulin. Two endopeptidases appear to be involved in this cleavage,[51] and their sequential activation could be regulated by the progressive decrease in granular pH brought about by an adenosine triphosphate (ATP)-dependent proton pump.[52]

Removal of the C-peptide from proinsulin decreases the solubility of the molecule in an acidic milieu. Insulin precipitates with zinc contained in the granules and forms crystals that occupy the center of the granular sac, whereas C-peptide remains in soluble form at the periphery.[53] Mature granules contain insulin and C-peptide in equimolar concentrations and small amounts of proinsulin and incompletely processed proinsulin. All these molecules, and several others also present in the granules,[54] are released with insulin when the granules undergo exocytosis. There is no evidence that proinsulin can be released by a constitutive (unregulated) pathway involving small smooth vesicles coming from the Golgi.[55]

Regulation of Proinsulin Synthesis

Glucose stimulates the synthesis of proinsulin much more markedly than that of other islet proteins. Its rapid effects (within minutes) involve an increase in the translation of insulin mRNA.[56] Long-term stimulation by glucose (several hours) also leads to an increase in levels of proinsulin mRNA[57] by stimulating transcription of the insulin gene and stabilizing preexisting preproinsulin mRNA.[50]

Glucose stimulation of proinsulin biosynthesis requires metabolism of the sugar by β-cells. It is mimicked by other nutrients and appears to depend on increased metabolic fluxes in β-cells, rather than on the presence of a specific agent.[58] The second messengers involved are still unknown, although there is evidence for some role of cAMP.[50] The dose-response curve for the stimulation of insulin biosynthesis by glucose is sigmoidal, with a threshold around 2 mM and a half-maximal response around 5 mM.[59] Stimulation of insulin synthesis thus occurs at lower glucose concentrations than does stimulation of insulin secretion. It may involve recruitment of β-cells[59] in addition to an increase in the synthetic activity of individual cells.

Links between Insulin Synthesis and Secretion

Short-term control of insulin secretion does not depend on insulin synthesis. Pancreatic insulin stores largely exceed the maximal secretory rates (<10% of insulin content per hour). Moreover, synthesis and secretion are dissociated under several conditions. In contrast to glucose and other fuel secretagogues that stimulate both synthesis and secretion, several agents (e.g., arginine, acetylcholine, hypoglycemic sulfonylureas) increase insulin secretion without increasing its synthesis.[60,61] It also is possible to abolish the effects of glucose on secretion without affecting those on synthesis (e.g., by omitting extracellular Ca^{++}).[60,61]

Synthesis and secretion are, however, not completely independent events. Under certain circumstances, isolated islets release newly synthesized insulin in preference to older stored hormone.[62] This may indicate that insulin granules do not undergo exocytosis at random but that a subpopulation of newly formed granules is "marked" to be released rather than to be stored.[63] The mechanisms of this "marking" are not known. Alternatively, the phenomenon of preferential release of newly formed insulin could be due to β-cell heterogeneity within the islets.[64] If the rise in glucose concentration recruits the same β-cells to synthesize[59] and to release insulin, and if these cells have low stores of preformed insulin, an apparent preferential secretion of newly formed insulin may be measured.

IDENTIFICATION OF GLUCOSE BY β-CELLS

In many cells, an extracellular stimulus binds to a membrane receptor to produce intracellular second messengers that eventually trigger the specific response. The existence, in the plasma membrane of β-cells, of a glucoreceptor that would trigger insulin secretion upon binding of glucose itself has been considered but could never be proved. On the other hand, compelling evidence indicates that glucose must be metabolized by β-cells in order to induce insulin secretion. Small interferences with glucose metabolism have repercussions on insulin secretion, whereas marked interferences with insulin secretion may be without effect on glucose metabolism in β-cells. The experimental work on which this "fuel-concept" of insulin secretion is based has been discussed in detail in several review articles.[2,60,65–68] Even the observation that the α-anomer of D-glucose is a better stimulus of release than is the β-anomer (at first sight a "strong argument" for the glucoreceptor theory)[69] can be explained by differences in the rate of metabolism.[70]

Glucose enters β-cells by facilitated diffusion, through a high K_m (~17 mM) transporter that is structurally and functionally similar to the low-affinity glucose transporter (GLUT-2) present in liver cells.[71,72] The properties of this transporter are such that the intracellular glucose concentration rapidly equalizes with the extracellular glucose concentration.[73,74] Since the glucose-transport capacity far exceeds the glucose-phosphorylation capacity, glucose transport is not rate-limiting for insulin secretion (at least in normal β-cells).

Under physiologic conditions, glucose storage as glycogen and glucose transformation to sorbitol are quantitatively small. They seem to play no major role in the control of β-cell function. Glucose metabolism through the pentose phosphate pathway does not exceed 5%, and its relative contribution decreases as the glucose concentration is raised. This pathway is generally thought to be unimportant for the control of insulin secretion. Glycolysis is the major pathway of glucose metabolism in β-cells.[65,66]

Glucose is phosphorylated by two enzymes: a high-affinity ($K_m \sim 0.1$ mM) hexokinase and a low-affinity ($K_m \sim 10$ to 12 mM) glucokinase. This glucokinase is similar to that found in hepatocytes.[75,76] In islet extracts, more than 75% of glucose phosphorylation can be attributed to the hexokinase. However, in intact cells hexokinase is severely inhibited by glucose-6-phosphate, and glucokinase plays the predominant role. The relative contribution of the two phosphorylating enzymes to total glucose usage by islets incubated in the presence of various concentrations of glucose is shown in Figure 4–3B. It is evident that the low affinity of glucokinase for glucose allows changes in glucose metabolism to occur at physiologic concentrations of glucose. This and other properties of glucokinase have led to the suggestion that this enzyme is the glucose sensor and pacemaker of glycolysis in β-cells.[32,66,67] This view is not unanimously accepted, and the importance of control sites of glycolysis downstream from glucokinase has been emphasized.[77]

Approximately 25 to 30% of the pyruvate molecules formed by glycolysis are oxidized in mitochondria,[65,66] while the remainder of pyruvate leaves β-cells, largely after transformation to lactate. The fact that only a fraction of glucose is eventually oxidized does not mean that the triggering signal produced by the sugar is an intermediate of glycolysis and that oxidative metabolism has a secondary role. Actually, the relative acceleration of mitochondrial metabolism is larger than that of glycolysis when the concentration of glucose is raised.[68] This is, at least partly, attributable to an activation by Ca^{++} of the α-glycerophosphate shuttle that transfers reducing equivalents from the cytosol into mitochondria.[68,78] Moreover, some agents that are metabolized exclusively in mitochondria largely mimic the effects of glucose. There is now general agreement that an acceleration of mitochondrial oxidative metabolism plays a key function in the secretory response to glucose and other nutrients.[68,79]

Identification of the factor(s) coupling the changes in β-cell metabolism and the changes in insulin secretion is a fundamental but very complex question. Numerous hypotheses have been put forward, all of which have raised controversies. It is, however, now unanimously agreed that the signal triggering secretion is a rise in the concentration of free Ca^{++} in the cytoplasm of β-cells.

CALCIUM HOMEOSTASIS IN β-CELLS AND INFLUENCE OF GLUCOSE

The concentration of cytoplasmic Ca^{++} in β-cells is controlled by mechanisms essentially similar to those present in other excitable cells.[25,80–82] In unstimulated β-cells, the permeability of the plasma membrane to Ca^{++} is low but the large electrochemical gradient for Ca^{++} causes a small influx of the ion. This is counterbal-anced by two extrusion systems whose relative contributions are still unclear: a Ca^{++} ATPase (or calcium pump) and a Na^+/Ca^{++} countertransport driven by the electrochemical gradient for Na^+. An important role also is played by the endoplasmic reticulum, into which Ca^{++} is sequestered after pumping by a high-affinity Ca^{++} ATPase.[81,82] On the other hand, the Ca^{++} sequestration system of mitochondria (high-capacity but low-affinity) becomes involved only when the concentration of cytoplasmic Ca^{++} is markedly increased. Insulin granules are rich in Ca^{++} (largely bound to nucleotides and proteins) but do not appear to play any role in the short-term control of cytoplasmic Ca^{++}.[25,81]

Several mechanisms could underlie the increase in cytoplasmic Ca^{++} brought about by glucose: an inhibition of Ca^{++} extrusion; a mobilization of Ca^{++} sequestered in cellular organelles; and a stimulation of Ca^{++} influx through Ca^{++} channels. Measurements by microspectrofluorimetric techniques have shown conclusively that glucose does not increase cytoplasmic Ca^{++} in β-cells when Ca^{++} influx is impossible either because the medium does not contain Ca^{++} or because Ca^{++} channels are blocked.[17,20,83] Glucose may even lower cytosolic Ca^{++} under these conditions, an effect ascribed to sequestration of Ca^{++} by cellular organelles (Fig. 4–2B). The long-standing conflict between two theories suggesting that the first phase of insulin secretion induced by glucose requires Ca^{++} influx in β-cells[84] or depends on mobilization of intracellular Ca^{++}[80] is thus solved. The available evidence indicates that glucose neither mobilizes intracellular Ca^{++} nor reduces its efflux as previously proposed.[80,85] The mechanisms whereby glucose controls Ca^{++} influx in β-cells are discussed in the next section.

BIOPHYSICAL EFFECTS OF GLUCOSE IN β-CELLS

The following description is based on experiments with mouse β-cells, the experimental model that best lends itself to electrophysiologic studies of the control of insulin release.[86–92] However, the available evidence suggests that the general conclusions may be extended to other species.

In the absence of glucose, or in the presence of a nonstimulatory concentration of glucose (3mM), the membrane potential of β-cells is stable, between −60 and −70 mV (Fig. 4–4). This resting potential is determined mainly by a much higher membrane conductance for K^+ than for other ions.[90] When the concentration of glucose is raised from 3 to 10 mM, an initial, progressive depolarization by 10 to 15 mV occurs, to a threshold potential at which an oscillatory electrical activity appears. Each oscillation (slow wave) begins by a rapid depolarization from the threshold potential to a plateau potential on which action potentials (spikes) are superimposed and ends by a rapid repolarization to a potential slightly more negative than the threshold potential. During the intervals between the slow waves, the membrane progressively depolarizes to the threshold potential at which the cycle repeats.

The initial depolarization can be observed when the concentration of glucose exceeds 4 mM, and the thresh-

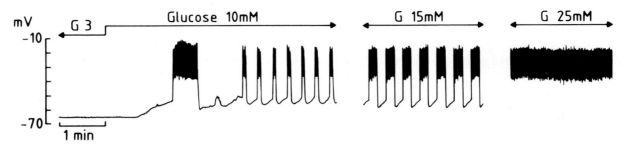

Fig. 4–4. Changes in the membrane potential of a mouse β-cell induced by successive increases in the concentration of glucose in the perifusion medium. The three recordings were obtained in the same cell, with an intracellular electrode. Adapted with permission from reference 93 (Henquin JC. Les mécanismes de contrôle de la sécrétion d'insuline. Arch Int Physiol Biochim 1990;98:A61–80).

old potential is reached at about 7 mM glucose. As the concentration of glucose increases from 7 mM to 25 mM, slow waves become longer and intervals shorter. The membrane eventually remains persistently depolarized at the plateau potential and exhibits continuous spike activity[88,90] (Fig. 4–4). The intensity of the electrical activity as a function of the concentration of glucose is thus characterized by a sigmoidal relationship similar to that of insulin secretion.[87]

Glucose-induced electrical activity corresponds to an influx of Ca^{++} through voltage-dependent Ca^{++} channels (during both slow waves and spikes).[90] It is therefore not surprising that the uptake of Ca^{++} by islet cells[25,85] and the rise in cytoplasmic Ca^{++} in β-cells[94] display the same glucose dependency as the electrical activity and insulin secretion (see Fig. 4–3A). It is also striking that a biphasic time-course characterizes the electrical activity (Fig. 4–4), the rise in cytoplasmic Ca^{++} (Fig. 4–2B), and insulin secretion (Fig. 4–2A) induced by a sudden increase in the concentration of glucose.

LINKS BETWEEN GLUCOSE METABOLISM AND CHANGES IN MEMBRANE POTENTIAL

Many effects of glucose in β-cells are thus characterized by nonlinear dose-response relationships. The threshold for stimulation of secretion appears to be linked to the existence of a threshold potential that must be reached for Ca^{++} influx to increase. Two key questions are thus: how does glucose depolarize the membrane to the threshold potential, and how does it control insulin secretion beyond the threshold?

Measurements of K^+ fluxes[33,95] and of electrical membrane resistance[96] first established that a decrease in K^+ permeability underlies the β-cell membrane depolarization between the resting and the threshold potential. As shown in Figure 4–3C, glucose-induced inhibition of K^+ efflux from islet cells is most marked when the concentration of the sugar is increased to about 7 mM. This inhibition totally depends on glucose metabolism.[33] An important further step was the demonstration, using the patch-clamp technique, that the decrease in K^+ conductance of the β-cell membrane is due to closure of one particular type of K^+ channel. These channels are voltage-independent and can be blocked by intracellular ATP.[97–100] Closure of these ATP-sensitive K^+ channels

requires glucose metabolism in β-cells[98,100] and shows a glucose dependency[100,101] similar to that of the inhibition of K^+ efflux shown in Figure 4–3C. The mechanisms by which glucose metabolism controls the activity of ATP-sensitive K^+ channels are complex and still incompletely elucidated.[101–104] It appears, however, that a major determinant could be the ratio of the concentrations ATP/ADP in the cytoplasm of β-cells. This ratio increases as the concentration of glucose is raised between 0 and 7 mM[34] (Fig. 4–3D). When enough ATP-sensitive K^+ channels have been closed (>95%) and, hence, when the decrease in K^+ conductance is sufficient,[92,102,105] the β-cell membrane depolarizes to the threshold potential at which voltage-dependent Ca^{++} channels open,[102–104,106,107] permitting Ca^{++} influx to occur (Fig. 4–5).

The second and probably most important question is how stimulatory concentrations of glucose (7 to 25 mM) control the duration of the phases of electrical activity during which Ca^{++} enters β-cells to trigger insulin secretion. Partial answers have recently been obtained. Although most ATP-sensitive K^+ channels are closed by subthreshold concentrations of the sugar,[100–102,105] the few that remain open can subserve the subtle control of membrane potential exerted by small variations in the glucose concentration within the physiologic range.[108,109] Changes in cytoplasmic ATP/ADP still occur under these conditions[34] (Fig. 4–3D). The voltage-dependent and voltage- and Ca^{++}-dependent K^+ channels also present in the β-cell membrane[101–104] (Fig. 4–5) are responsible for the repolarization of the spikes but play no role in the control of the slow waves by glucose.[92] It is possible that the metabolism of glucose also influences Ca^{++} influx by modulating the properties of Ca^{++} channels[102,314] (Fig. 4–5).

PUTATIVE MESSENGERS IN β-CELL RESPONSE TO GLUCOSE

It is currently thought that changes in the cytoplasmic ATP/ADP ratio in β-cells play a major role in coupling glucose metabolism to the biophysical events eventually leading to insulin release (see previous section). However, the possible intervention of other messengers should certainly not be formally excluded. Even though ATP-sensitive K^+ channels are the major target for

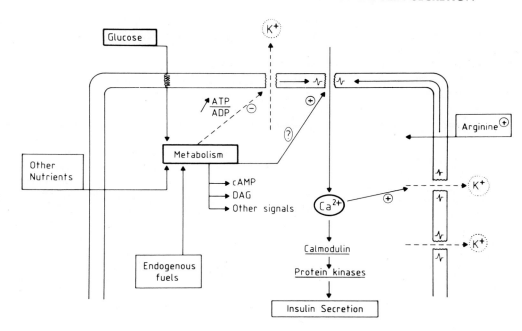

Fig. 4–5. Schematic representation of the major mechanisms by which glucose and other nutrients stimulate insulin secretion: + = stimulation; − = inhibition; DAG = diacylglycerol.

glucose, there exist still ill-defined mechanisms by which the sugar can amplify its own triggering action on insulin release independently from changes in membrane potential and cytosolic Ca^{++}.[22,315]

Metabolic Intermediates

The hypothesis that an intermediate of glucose metabolism (e.g., of glycolysis) is directly involved in triggering secretion has never received convincing support. It is even difficult to reconcile with the observation that fuel secretagogues metabolized through distinct pathways have largely similar effects.

Reduced Pyridine Nucleotides

It has often been proposed that a more-reduced state of the cytosol of β-cells could link glucose metabolism and insulin secretion by changing the thiol-disulfide equilibrium in various proteins.[79,110,111] Although reduced pyridine nucleotides are unlikely to be an essential triggering signal,[20,112,113] they may play a modulatory role (e.g. by favoring lipid synthesis).

Protons

Glucose metabolism increases H^+ production. However, contrary to expectations and early measurements,[110] recent studies have shown that stimulation of β-cells by glucose does not lower intracellular pH.[114,115] This is due to the presence of efficient buffers in the cytoplasm and of proton extruders in the plasma membrane. It remains possible that small variations in cytoplasmic pH play a modulatory role in stimulus-secretion coupling.[116]

cAMP

Glucose slightly increases the concentration of cAMP in β-cells,[117] probably through an activation of adenylate cyclase by protein kinase C[118] or by a Ca^{++}-calmodulin protein kinase.[119] There is no doubt that a rise in cAMP concentration in β-cells is not a sufficient signal to trigger insulin secretion but that it can amplify the response to various secretagogues.[80,81,117,119,120] The role of this amplification during hormonal stimulation of β-cells is well established (see "Neurohormonal Amplification of Insulin Secretion"). It is much less clear during stimulation by glucose alone.[121] Experiments with isolated β-cells suggest, however, that a minimal concentration of cAMP is necessary for glucose to stimulate insulin secretion normally.[44]

Coenzyme A Esters

Glucose inhibits the oxidation of endogenous fatty acids in pancreatic β-cells,[122,123] probably by increasing the levels of malonyl-CoA.[124,125] This might result in an increased availability of fatty acyl CoA that could serve as precursors of second messengers or as second messengers themselves.[81] This attractive hypothesis is in keeping with the observation that inhibition of palmitate oxidation by 2-bromostearate augments insulin release[123] but at odds with the observation that insulin secretion in response to various secretagogues is decreased when oxidation of endogenous fatty acids is inhibited by methylpalmoxirate.[126] The reasons for these discrepancies are unclear.

Inositol Phosphates

Glucose stimulates both the synthesis and hydrolysis of phospholipids in β-cells.[81,127–129] The significance of this acceleration of phospholipid turnover for glucose-induced insulin secretion is still unclear. However, the breakdown of phosphatidylinositol 4,5-biphosphate and accumulation of inositol 1,4,5-triphosphate are no longer considered to be primary signals (even for triggering of first-phase secretion), but rather to be consequences of the rise in cytoplasmic Ca^{++}.[128-130]

Diacylglycerol

Glucose stimulates de novo synthesis of diacylglycerol in β-cells.[131-133] However, this diacylglycerol is richer in palmitate and poorer in arachidonate than is the diacylglycerol generated by hydrolysis of preexisting glycerolipids and does not significantly increase the total mass of diacylglycerol in islet cells.[133] This may explain why glucose is usually found not to activate protein kinase C in β-cells.[134,135] Except in one study,[136] no insertion of the enzyme in the plasma membrane of β-cells has been observed upon stimulation by glucose.[134,135] The exact role of protein kinase C in glucose-induced insulin secretion remains disputed,[134-138] but there is much evidence that it is not a major one.[134,135,137]

Arachidonic Acid and Derivatives

Glucose stimulation of islet cells increases the release of arachidonic acid from phospholipids. However, decisive arguments that arachidonic acid itself plays a role in stimulus-secretion coupling are still missing.[127,139] On the other hand, metabolites of arachidonic acid could modulate glucose-induced insulin secretion. The latter is decreased by prostaglandins and increased by certain products formed by lipoxygenation.[127,139,140]

Other Lipid Derivatives

It has been suggested that phosphatidic acid, formed by activation of phospholipases or by de novo synthesis from glucose, and lysophospholipids formed by activation of phospholipase A_2 might be involved in glucose-induced insulin secretion.[139] However, definition of their exact role awaits further investigations.

OSCILLATIONS OF β-CELL RESPONSE TO GLUCOSE

Oscillations of the Triggering Signal

Measurements of electrical activity in β-cells show that Ca^{++} influx occurs intermittently during stimulation by physiologic concentrations of glucose (Fig. 4–4). One might thus expect that the concentration of cytoplasmic Ca^{++} oscillates with a similar period. Large oscillations in cytoplasmic Ca^{++} levels are often observed in single β-cells stimulated by glucose,[18,19,83] but their period (2 to 6 minutes) is much longer than that of the slow waves (10 to 30 seconds) during which Ca^{++} enters β-cells. However, in two studies using intact mouse islets, faster oscillations of intracellular Ca^{++} have been detected.[17,141] These oscillations were synchronous in all β-cells of the islets and were found to correlate with the

electrical activity, but their amplitude was sometimes variable between regions of the islets.

Oscillations of Insulin Secretion

Combined measurements of insulin secretion and cytoplasmic Ca^{++} concentration in single mouse islets have shown that both phenomena oscillate in phase during stimulation with glucose.[142] In isolated islets, synchronized by a sudden increase in the glucose concentration of the perifusion medium, insulin secretion has been found to oscillate with a period of about 5.5 minutes[143] or of 16 to 22 minutes.[144,145] Insulin secretion by the isolated canine pancreas displays sustained oscillations (7 to 10 minutes) even during perfusion at a constant concentration of glucose.[146] Neither the underlying mechanisms nor the links between these oscillations and those of plasma insulin levels recorded in humans or other species have been clearly identified.[147,148]

THE β-CELL RESPONSE TO NUTRIENTS OTHER THAN GLUCOSE

Sugars and Derivatives

Besides glucose, mannose is the only hexose that stimulates insulin secretion in the absence of any other secretagogue. The lower potency of mannose than that of glucose is ascribed to a lower rate of metabolism in β-cells.[60,70,149] Fructose is metabolized slowly by islet cells and causes a modest increase in insulin secretion only in the presence of glucose. Hexosamines (e.g., N-acetylglucosamine), glyceraldehyde, and dihydroxyacetone are well metabolized and stimulate insulin secretion. The coherent picture that has emerged from a number of studies is that the insulin-releasing capacity of these sugars and derivatives correlates well with their rate of metabolism in β-cells.[60,65,70,149] The links between the recognition of these "other substrates" and the exocytosis of insulin granules are similar to those implicated in the response to glucose (Fig. 4–5).

Amino Acids

The ability of amino acids to increase insulin secretion markedly depends on the permissive action of glucose (see first section). Very little is known about the cellular mechanisms underlying the changes in β-cell function produced by the combination of physiologic concentrations of glucose and amino acids. On the other hand, studies using high concentrations of individual amino acids have clearly shown that they affect insulin secretion by markedly different mechanisms, which can only be outlined here for representative amino acids.

Leucine is well metabolized in β-cells[150] and induces insulin secretion even in the absence of glucose. Its effects are markedly potentiated by glutamine, which itself is ineffective. This is due to the allosteric activation of glutamate dehydrogenase by leucine and the resulting channelling of glutamate to the citric acid cycle.[151,152] Activation of glutamate dehydrogenase by a nonmetabolized derivative of leucine (BCH or 2-endoaminonorbonane-2-carboxylic acid) accelerates the metabolism of endogenous amino acids and thereby increases insulin secretion.[151,152] The biophysical events linking the metabolism of exogenous or endogenous amino acids and the exocytosis of insulin granules are similar to those involved in the response to glucose[94,153,154] (Fig. 4–5).

Alanine is slowly metabolized in islet cells[150] and only weakly increases insulin secretion.[155] This effect, which requires the presence of glucose, is probably due to the cotransport of alanine with Na^+ in β-cells.[156] The resulting small depolarization slightly augments Ca^{++} influx, while the rise in intracellular Na^+ affects Ca^{++} handling.[155]

Arginine and other cationic amino acids are only poorly metabolized in islet cells.[150,157] Their mode of action markedly differs from that of nutrients that serve as fuels for β-cells. They are thought to depolarize the β-cell membrane because of their transport in the cell in a positively charged form.[153,158] The depolarization then activates voltage-dependent Ca^{++} channels, and Ca^{++} influx ensues (Fig. 4–5). This peculiar mode of action might explain why arginine, unlike glucose, still elicits a rapid secretion of insulin in patients with NIDDM.[159]

Fatty Acids

Exogenous fatty acids are oxidized by islet cells[122,123] and, at physiologic concentrations, slightly increase insulin secretion in the presence of glucose.[123] It is still unclear whether this insulin-releasing action depends more on the esterification[123] or the oxidation of fatty acids.[126]

Ketone Bodies

Acetoacetate and β-hydroxybutyrate are oxidized by islet cells and slightly increase insulin secretion, at least when they are used in high concentrations and when the medium also contains glucose.[1,122,160,161] The available evidence suggests that their effects on insulin secretion are due to their metabolic degradation in β-cells.[161]

PHARMACOLOGIC CONTROL OF INSULIN SECRETION

Many pharmacologic compounds affect insulin secretion in vitro,[162] but the modes of action of only a few of them are summarized here.

Inhibitors of Metabolism

Mannoheptulose and 2-deoxyglucose, which interfere with glucose metabolism in β-cells, and mitochondrial poisons are potent inhibitors of insulin secretion.[2,60,149] The underlying mechanism involves a decrease in the ATP/ADP ratio in the cytoplasm, which leads to opening of ATP-sensitive K^+ channels,[98,100] membrane repolarization,[314] and closure of voltage-dependent Ca^{++} channels (Fig. 4–6). Studies using these substances have been instrumental in the understanding of stimulus-secretion coupling in β-cells. However, no drugs used in therapeutics are known to affect insulin secretion by interfering with glucose metabolism in β-cells. The effects of inhibitors of fatty acid oxidation on insulin release in vitro are still controversial (see previous section), and it is not known whether these compounds affect β-cell function in vivo.

Sulfonylureas

All drugs currently used for the purpose of stimulating insulin secretion in patients with NIDDM belong to the family of sulfonylureas. Numerous studies have concurred to elucidate their mode of action and to show that sulfonylureas of the first (e.g., tolbutamide) and second generation (e.g., glyburide) trigger the same sequence of events in β-cells.[17,26,27,103,163–169] They close ATP-sensitive K^+ channels in the plasma membrane (Fig. 4–6). The resulting decrease in K^+ conductance causes depolarization, with opening of voltage-dependent Ca^{++} channels. The ensuing acceleration of Ca^{++} influx leads to an increase in the concentration of cytoplasmic Ca^{++}, which eventually triggers exocytosis of insulin granules. Unlike glucose, sulfonylureas do not increase β-cell metabolism but block ATP-sensitive K^+ channels by a direct action on a site located at or near the channel (Fig. 4–6). Good correlations exist between the relative potencies of various sulfonylureas on insulin release and their relative affinities for that binding site. Many drugs unrelated to sulfonylureas, several of which also are used for therapeutic purposes, stimulate insulin release by the same mechanisms as does tolbutamide.[162]

Diazoxide

Diazoxide remains the drug of choice for medical treatment of chronic hypoglycemia caused by hyperinsulinemia. The mechanisms by which diazoxide inhibits insulin secretion are well established.[17,27,163,167,170] Diazoxide increases K^+ conductance of the β-cell membrane through a direct opening of ATP-sensitive K^+ channels (Fig. 4–6). Although glucose metabolism is not affected, the membrane repolarizes, voltage-dependent Ca^{++} channels close, Ca^{++} influx decreases, the concentration of cytosolic Ca^{++} drops, and insulin secretion is less or no longer stimulated. Since the primary effect of diazoxide is to open ATP-sensitive K^+ channels, it is obvious why the drug does not interfere with the insulin-releasing action of agents that depolarize the membrane by a mechanism other than a closure of K^+ channels.[171] This is the case of high extracellular K^+ or of arginine (Fig. 4–5). It has long been noted that diazoxide inhibits leucine-stimulated, but not arginine-stimulated, insulin secretion in humans.[172] New drugs with antihypertensive properties (e.g., pinacidil) may open ATP-sensitive K^+ channels in β-cells. However, this side effect requires concentrations higher than those necessary to open K^+ channels in vascular muscle cells.[173]

Ca^{++}-Channel Blockers and Agonists

Blockage of voltage-dependent Ca^{++} channels by dihydropyridines (e.g., nifedipine) or phenylalkylamines (e.g., verapamil) inhibits Ca^{++} influx in β-cells and, therefore, antagonizes the ability of glucose and other

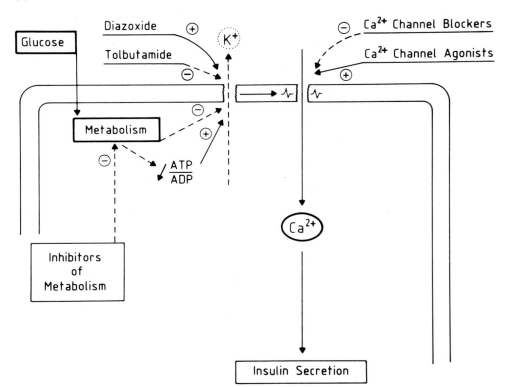

Fig. 4–6. Schematic representation of the mechanisms by which certain pharmacologic agents influence insulin secretion: + = stimulation; − = inhibition.

depolarizing agents to increase cytosolic Ca^{++}[20,83,170,174] (Fig. 4–6). This explains why these drugs nonselectively inhibit the secretion of insulin induced by those agents whose effect depends on Ca^{++} influx, regardless of the mechanisms of depolarization.[171] In vivo, Ca^{++}-channel blockers have no or little deleterious influence on insulin secretion and glucose homeostasis.[175] There also exist dihydropyridine derivatives that do not block Ca^{++} channels but act as agonists at the channel level. They are ineffective in unstimulated β-cells, when the membrane potential is high and the voltage-dependent Ca^{++} channels are closed, but they increase Ca^{++} influx and insulin secretion in the presence of glucose.[162]

NEUROHORMONAL AMPLIFICATION OF INSULIN SECRETION

The amount of insulin that is secreted in response to a given stimulus (e.g., glucose) does not depend simply on the magnitude of the initiating signal (the rise in cytoplasmic Ca^{++}) triggered by that stimulus. It may be amplified by various neurohormonal agents,[176,177] which use two major types of intracellular messengers to affect β-cell function: cAMP or inositol phosphates and diacylglycerol. Before these two pathways are discussed, it is important to emphasize again that the influence of neurohormonal agents on insulin secretion is tightly conditioned by the prevailing concentration of glucose. These agents are ineffective if the concentration of glucose is too low (see first section). It should also be noted that different agents acting through distinct cellular

pathways not only may exert additive or synergistic effects on insulin secretion but also may optimize β-cell responsiveness when applied in sequence.[21]

The cAMP-Protein Kinase A Pathway

Adenylate cyclase, which synthesizes cAMP from ATP, is linked to several membrane receptors by a stimulatory subtype G_s of the guanosine triphosphate (GTP)-binding proteins (G-proteins). Once formed, cAMP binds to its target, protein kinase A, from which it releases the catalytic subunit. The latter catalyzes the phosphorylation of distinct proteins, the nature of which has only been partially identified.[178]

Several mechanisms may underlie the amplification of insulin secretion by cAMP.[81,119,120] The two major ones are depicted in Figure 4–7. cAMP slightly increases Ca^{++} influx triggered by primary secretagogues such as glucose or tolbutamide[179,180] and, hence, accentuates the rise in cytoplasmic Ca^{++} that they produce.[181,182] A second, probably more important, mechanism is a sensitization of the secretory machinery to Ca^{++}. This has been demonstrated by the use of permeabilized β-cells in which cAMP increases the amount of insulin secreted in response to a fixed concentration of cytoplasmic Ca^{++}.[183–185]

The Phosphoinositide-Protein Kinase C Pathway

β-Cells are equipped with different types of receptors that are linked to a phospholipase C by a subtype G_p of the G-proteins.[128] On activation of the receptor, the

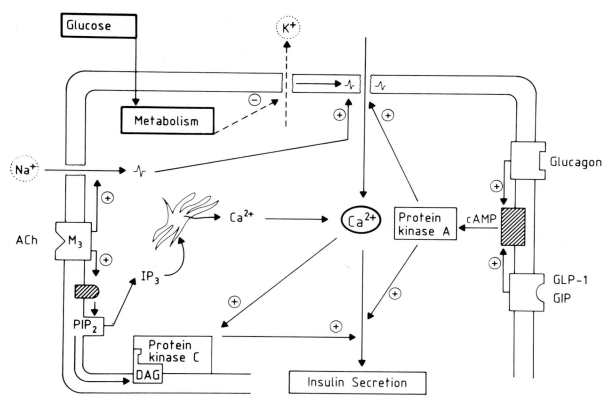

Fig. 4–7. Schematic representation of the major mechanisms by which neurotransmitters and hormones amplify insulin secretion: + = stimulation; − = inhibition; ACh = acetylcholine; M_3 = muscarinic receptor of the M_3 type; PIP_2 = phosphatidylinositol 4,5-biphosphate; IP_3 = inositol 1,4,5-triphosphate; DAG = diacylglycerol; GLP-1 = glucagon-like peptide 1 (7–36 amide); GIP = gastric inhibitory polypeptide, or glucose-dependent insulinotropic polypeptide. Redrawn with permission from reference 93 (Henquin JC. Les mécanismes de contrôle de la sécrétion d'insuline. Arch Int Physiol Biochim 1990;98:A61–80).

enzyme is stimulated to split phosphatidylinositol 4,5-biphosphate (PIP_2), a phospholipid present in small amounts in the plasma membrane, into inositol 1,4,5-triphosphate (IP_3) and diacylglycerol.[128,186]

IP_3, which is hydrosoluble, diffuses in the cytoplasm and releases Ca^{++} from the calciosome, a compartment of the endoplasmic reticulum that sequesters the ion.[81,186] This mobilization is attributed to the opening of a channel through which Ca^{++} diffuses from the organelle to the cytosol. It causes a biphasic change in cytoplasmic Ca^{++} concentration[187]: a large but transient rise, which can trigger a peak of insulin secretion if its amplitude is sufficient,[188] followed by a smaller but sustained increase.

Diacylglycerol, which is liposoluble, remains in the plasma membrane, to which it causes translocation of its target, the protein kinase C[134,189] (Fig. 4–7). This translocation, which also requires Ca^{++} and phosphatidylserine, activates the kinase that can then phosphorylate proteins, the nature of which is still unclear. The result of these phosphorylations is a sensitization of the releasing machinery to Ca^{++}[183,185,190] as after activation of protein kinase A by cAMP. Experiments using phorbol esters, which activate protein kinase C directly, have shown that this pathway does not increase Ca^{++} influx and cytosolic Ca^{++} in normal β-cells.[180,191]

Acetylcholine has a further effect (Fig. 4–7). It depolarizes the β-cell membrane by increasing its Na^+ conductance. The mechanism is still unknown, but the resulting small depolarization augments Ca^{++} influx through voltage-dependent Ca^{++} channels, at least when the membrane is already depolarized by a primary secretagogue.[192]

Physiologic Amplifiers of Insulin Secretion

Amplification of insulin secretion through the cAMP-protein kinase A pathway is physiologically relevant for two gastrointestinal hormones involved in the entero-insular axis.

Gastric inhibitory polypeptide (GIP, also known as glucose-dependent insulinotropic polypeptide), is synthesized by cells from the duodenojejunal mucosa. It acts on specific receptors in β-cells.[193]

Glucagon-like peptide 1 [7–36 amide] (GLP-1) is a product of post-translational processing of proglucagon in cells from the mucosa of the ileum and colon. It acts on specific receptors present in islet cells, mainly β-cells.[194]

These two hormones markedly increase insulin secretion in the presence of glucose.[5,7] They are released following ingestion of nutrients and probably are responsible for the "incretin" effect, i.e., the larger rise in plasma insulin levels observed for a given rise in plasma glucose levels when the sugar is absorbed orally rather than administered intravenously.[195-198]

Amplification of insulin secretion through the phosphoinositide-protein kinase C pathway is physiologically relevant for acetylcholine and cholecystokinin.

Acetylcholine is released by parasympathetic nerve endings in the islets during both the cephalic and intestinal phases of feeding.[177,197] It acts on muscarinic receptors of the M_3 type according to the latest nomenclature.[199,200]

Cholecystokinin is released from the duodenum and proximal jejunum during meals but mainly acts as a neurotransmitter at peptidergic synapses present in the islets.[177,197] It activates specific receptors in β-cells.[201] It is not known whether cholecystokinin, like acetylcholine, depolarizes the membrane by increasing Na^+ conductance.

Putative Amplifiers of Insulin Secretion

Glucagon raises cAMP levels in β-cells and amplifies the secretion of insulin induced by various primary secretagogues.[117,119] Whereas this effect is clear for exogenous glucagon,[202] it is not certain that glucagon released by α-cells of the islets exerts any paracrine action on the neighboring β-cells[47] (See Chapter 2).

Catecholamines have the net effect of inhibiting insulin secretion, but β-adrenergic agonists increase plasma insulin levels in vivo.[177] They have, however, little or no effect in vitro. Functional studies with purified islet cells have suggested that rat β-cells are devoid of β-adrenergic receptors.[203] It is not known whether this is true in all species.

Gastrin and secretin increase insulin secretion only weakly even when they are used at pharmacologic concentrations.[197,204]

Vasoactive intestinal polypeptide (VIP) and gastrin-releasing peptide (GRP) are present in nerve fibers of the pancreas.[205,206] They amplify glucose-induced insulin secretion, but the physiologic significance of this effect is not known.[177,197]

Vasopressin (AVP) and oxytocin (OT) increase glucose-induced insulin secretion in vitro through a stimulation of phosphoinositide metabolism.[207,208] This effect does not occur at physiologic concentrations of AVP and OT in plasma but is compatible with a local control of β-cell function by AVP and OT, which are present in the pancreas.[209]

The purine nucleotides ATP and ADP amplify insulin secretion, at least in certain species, by activating extracellular P_{2y}-purinergic receptors in β-cells.[210] It is unclear whether ATP released with insulin during exocytosis exerts a direct influence on β-cell function by this mechanism.

NEUROHORMONAL ATTENUATION OF INSULIN SECRETION

Cellular Mechanisms

Attenuation of insulin secretion may be achieved by the activation of various types of membrane receptors, which exert their effects by multiple similar mechanisms, the exact nature and relative contribution of which are not completely established[211] (Fig. 4-8).

These receptors are linked to the adenylate cyclase by an inhibitory subtype (G_i) of the G-proteins. Activation of

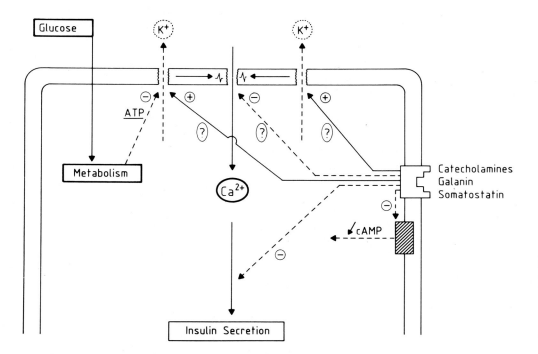

Fig. 4-8. Schematic representation of the major mechanisms by which neurotransmitters and hormones attenuate insulin secretion; + = stimulation; - = inhibition.

the receptor thus leads to a decrease in the concentration of cAMP in β-cells, with consequences opposite to those described above for an increase in cAMP. This, however, cannot fully account for the attenuation of secretion.[119,212] Activation of the receptor also causes partial repolarization of the β-cell membrane, by a mechanism that is still disputed. There is good evidence that opening of K^+ channels is involved,[92,213-215] but it has not been conclusively established whether these are the ATP-sensitive K^+ channels or other K^+ channels.[216] Direct inhibition of Ca^{++} channels has also been envisaged.[211] This partial repolarization of the β-cell membrane reduces the influx of Ca^{++} through voltage-dependent Ca^{++} channels and thus leads to a lowering of cytoplasmic free Ca^{++} in β-cells.[211,214] Experiments using permeabilized β-cells,[217,218] in which the composition of the cytoplasm can be controlled, have established the existence of an inhibitory step distal to the generation of cellular messengers (Ca^{++}, cAMP, DAG). It could involve a GTP-binding protein implicated in the exocytotic process.[219]

Physiologic Attenuators of Insulin Secretion

These complex mechanisms are likely to underlie the physiologically relevant decreases in insulin secretion brought about by catecholamines, galanin, and somatostatin (Fig. 4–8).

Catecholamines are released under stress conditions by the adrenal medulla (epinephrine) or by sympathetic nerve terminals in the pancreas (norepinephrine). They exert their inhibitory effect by activating α_2-adrenoceptors in β-cells.[220]

Galanin is a 29-residue peptide that is also released by sympathetic nerve endings in the pancreas.[221] It acts on specific receptors in β-cells.[222]

Somatostatin-28 is released by the gut during absorption of fat-rich meals,[223] whereas somatostatin-14 is secreted by islet δ-cells. β-Cells preferentially bind somatostatin-28,[224] which is a more potent inhibitor of insulin secretion than is somatostatin-14.[225] The role of somatostatin-14 in the control of β-cell function is probably less important than previously thought[46,47] (see Chapter 2).

Putative Attenuators of Insulin Secretion

Several other hormones or neuropeptides may attenuate insulin secretion. However, the physiologic relevance of the effects observed in vitro has yet to be established, and the cellular mechanisms involved are largely unknown.

Insulin-like growth factor I (IGF-I) inhibits glucose- and arginine-induced insulin secretion from the perfused rat pancreas.[226] This effect occurs at physiologic concentrations and is probably mediated by specific receptors for IGF-I in β-cells.[227]

Pancreastatin is a 49-residue peptide isolated from pancreatic extracts that is structurally similar to chromogranin A.[228,229] It causes a modest inhibition of insulin secretion induced by glucose and other secretagogues.[228]

Opioid peptides have inhibitory and stimulatory effects on insulin secretion, depending on the agent used (β-endorphin, type of enkephalin) and on the concentration.[230] This may be due to the existence of various types of opioid receptors in β-cells.[231]

Calcitonin gene-related peptide (CGRP) is a 37-residue peptide present in intrapancreatic nerve fibers and in a few islet cells.[232] It inhibits stimulated insulin secretion by a direct action on β-cells.[38,232]

Islet amyloid polypeptide (IAPP, also known as amylin) is a 37-residue peptide structurally related to CGRP. It is synthesized in β-cells[233] and is secreted with, but in much smaller amounts (<1%) than insulin.[234,235] IAPP has been reported to inhibit insulin secretion in high concentrations,[236] but this effect is unlikely to have any physiologic significance.[237]

POTENTIATION, DESENSITIZATION, AND PRIMING OF INSULIN SECRETION

Potentiation

Those agents that are ineffective alone, but increase insulin secretion in the presence of a primary stimulus, are named "potentiators" (see first section). This potentiation may result from an increase in the efficacy of the triggering signal (the rise in cytoplasmic Ca^{++}) by mechanisms of amplification described in the section "Neurohormonal Amplification of Insulin Secretion." It also may result from an increase in the amplitude of the triggering signal.

A substrate may be unable to induce insulin secretion when used alone because its metabolism in β-cells is insufficient to depolarize the membrane to the threshold potential at which Ca^{++} channels open. Ca^{++} influx and, hence, insulin release cannot be stimulated. In the presence of glucose, however, the substrate potentiator increases β-cell metabolism, as if the concentration of glucose had been raised; hence, the larger secretory response. This type of potentiating action has been well characterized for fructose and other sugars.[149] It probably also explains the potentiation by other fuels, with the reservation that the metabolic usage rates of different types of substrates are not always simply additive.[65]

When used at low concentrations, nonmetabolized agents such as tolbutamide or arginine do not depolarize the β-cell membrane enough to open voltage-dependent Ca^{++} channels. However, their small effect on the membrane potential is sufficient to increase Ca^{++} influx and to potentiate insulin release in the presence of a threshold or stimulatory concentration of glucose.[238]

It is thus evident that the permissive action of glucose (see first section) depends largely on the depolarization of the β-cell membrane. This depolarization permits the small depolarizing action of the potentiators to activate Ca^{++} channels.[238] However, a membrane potential-independent mechanism also appears to be involved.[22] Its nature is not firmly established, but there are indications suggesting that the efficacy of the Ca^{++} signal might be amplified,[315] perhaps through changes in the activity of protein kinases.[138,178,239]

Desensitization

Prolonged stimulation of β-cells with a high concentration of glucose leads to a progressive decrease in the rate of insulin secretion in vitro.[28,29] This "third phase" of secretion (see section "General Characteristics of Glucose-Induced Insulin Secretion") reflects desensitization of β-cells to glucose. Its possible mechanisms are still disputed.[21,30,240] It should also be noted that several secretagogues other than glucose can cause a similar desensitization in vitro.[30] Moreover, acute stimulation of β-cells by arginine[241,242] or by relatively high concentrations of tolbutamide[26] impair the insulin response to a subsequent or superimposed glucose challenge. The paradoxical "inhibitory" effect of tolbutamide has been ascribed to clamping of the membrane potential at a depolarized levels with inactivation of Ca^{++} channels.[26]

Priming and Proemial Sensitization

Prior exposure of β-cells to a stimulatory concentration of glucose increases their secretory response to a subsequent challenge by glucose or another secretagogue.[243,244] This phenomenon has been called "priming," "memory," or "time-dependent potentiation." It requires glucose metabolism, does not involve redistribution of insulin granules in β-cells,[245] and is not dependent on cAMP[243,244]; its dependence on Ca^{++} is controversial.[243,246] It is perhaps linked to phosphoinositide metabolism.[138]

A related phenomenon has been called "proemial sensitization." It consists of the enhancement of the β-cell response to glucose by a previous exposure to a neurotransmitter or a hormone under conditions in which the latter agents have little or no effect on insulin release.[247] Thus far, this proemial sensitization has been described for acetylcholine and cholecystokinin,[21] two agents that activate the protein kinase C pathway. It has been ascribed to a persistent translocation of protein kinase C to the plasma membrane, where the enzyme can be readily activated by the rise in cytoplasmic Ca^{++} that occurs on glucose stimulation. This phenomenon could be important to the optimization of the β-cell response to nutrients during a meal.[21]

THE EFFECTOR SYSTEM

The mechanism by which the increase in cytoplasmic Ca^{++} eventually leads to the liberation of insulin into the extracellular space is one of the least well understood aspects of stimulus-secretion coupling in β-cells.[2,127,248–252]

The Targets of Calcium

Calmodulin (CM) is a ubiquitous target of Ca^{++}. In β-cells, the Ca^{++}-CM complex activates the Ca^{++}-ATPase (Ca^{++} pump) of the plasma membrane, adenylate cyclase (at least in certain species), and cAMP-phosphodiesterase,[249–251] but these effects cannot account for the increase in insulin secretion. The Ca^{++}-CM complex also may activate protein kinases (Fig. 4–5) that phosphorylate proteins of the cytoskeleton. It should, however, be noted that the available evidence supporting a role of calmodulin in insulin secretion is, at most, suggestive. An important target of Ca^{++} is the protein kinase C.[127,128,134,249] It has also been suggested that a transglutaminase, activated by Ca^{++} and causing polymerization of proteins by incorporation of polyamines, is involved in insulin release.[253,254] Finally, Ca^{++} could neutralize negative charges present on the surface of insulin granules and, hence, facilitate their fusion with the plasma membrane.[255]

Protein Kinases

Intracellular second messengers often act by stimulating a protein kinase. Three major classes of protein kinases have been identified in β-cells: Ca^{++}-CM-dependent protein kinases, the cAMP-dependent protein kinases A, and the Ca^{++}- and phospholipid-dependent protein kinases C.[127,178,249,252] β-Cells also contain several soluble or membrane-bound proteins that can be phosphorylated by these kinases. Unfortunately, neither the nature nor the role of these proteins in the secretory process is clearly established.[178,252]

The Cytoskeleton

Experiments using drugs capable of interfering with the functioning of distinct elements of the cytoskeleton have established that the latter plays a role in the late steps of insulin secretion.[14,15,250,256] This cytoskeleton comprises microfilaments, microtubules, and several types of intermediary filaments (e.g., vimentin, cytokeratin). How these elements interact with one another is not well known.[250] The Ca^{++}-CM complex and cAMP appear to stimulate tubulin polymerization and, thus, formation of microtubules, which could guide the granules towards the sites of exocytosis. Upon stimulation of insulin secretion, there also occurs a polymerization of globular actin with formation of microfilaments. In addition, a myosin light-chain kinase could phosphorylate myosin present in the granular membrane. The progression of the granules could thus result from an interaction with the microfilaments, actomyosin providing the motile forces.[250]

Exocytosis

Release of the granular content into the extracellular space involves a classical process of exocytosis. The physical mechanisms responsible for the fusion of the granules with the plasma membrane, and for the subsequent fission of the granules, are still controversial. Increasing evidence suggests that a G-protein (Ge) could be involved in these most distal steps of stimulus-secretion coupling.[185,257]

LONG-TERM INFLUENCES ON INSULIN SECRETION

Neonatal Maturation

Numerous in vitro studies have shown that fetal and neonatal islets secrete insulin at a lower rate than adult islets.[258,259] The most striking feature of the functional maturation that β-cells undergo during the perinatal period is the acquisition of a normal responsiveness to glucose in terms of both magnitude and kinetics.[260,261] A defect in generation of cAMP has often been thought to contribute to the poor secretory response of fetal and neonatal β-cells.[262] However, stimulation of protein kinase A and protein kinase C pathways increases glucose-induced insulin secretion but does not lead to appearance of an adult-type, biphasic pattern of release.[263] Patch-clamp recordings have conclusively shown that glucose fails to close ATP-sensitive K[+] channels in fetal β-cells and that this is not due to intrinsic abnormalities of the channels, which normally respond to tolbutamide and diazoxide.[264] The available evidence suggests that the defect in nutrient-induced insulin secretion in fetal and neonatal β-cells could be due to an immature oxidative metabolism with insufficient production of ATP.[259,264,265]

Aging

In the rat, the β-cell mass and the insulin content of the pancreas increase with age.[266] When these changes are taken into account, it is obvious that the acute in vitro effects of glucose on insulin secretion are impaired in old age.[266–270] Alterations of glucose metabolism,[268] adenylate cyclase activity,[267] and ionic fluxes[269] have been observed in islets of old rats. It is unlikely that the primary cause of all changes in β-cell function during aging is a defect in the early steps of glycolysis,[267] since insulin secretion in response to amino acids or tolbutamide (in absence of glucose) is also decreased.[271] The contribution of impaired insulin secretion to the glucose intolerance of the aged is not entirely clear.[272,273]

Starvation

During starvation, basal plasma insulin levels are lowered and the β-cell secretory response to glucose is impaired. Many in vitro studies have shown that glucose-induced insulin secretion is more severely impaired than the secretion induced by other fuel or non-fuel secretagogues.[274,275] This selective change is generally attributed to a decreased glycolytic rate in β-cells.[2,274,276] However, the decrease in secretion that can already be observed after 24 hours of food deprivation might be due to reduced levels of cAMP rather than to an alteration of glucose metabolism, which would occur only later.[275,276] It remains unclear whether the inhibition of glucose metabolism by islet cells is exclusively or only partially due to a decrease in glucokinase activity.[66,67,77] It is still disputed whether starvation lowers[277] or does not lower[278] the levels of glucokinase mRNA and glucokinase protein in islet cells. The ability of glucose to shift the metabolism of fatty acids from oxidation to esterification is also impaired in islets from starved rats.[123] The abnormality could contribute to the alteration of β-cell function, since its correction by 2-bromostearate (an inhibitor of fatty acid oxidation) restores glucose-induced insulin secretion.[123]

Exercise Training

Exercise training increases peripheral insulin sensitivity and lowers plasma insulin levels.[279] The mechanisms of this adaptation of β-cells are still unclear. Isolated islets and the perfused pancreas obtained from trained rats exhibit a diminished glucose- or arginine-induced insulin secretion.[280,281] A decrease in islet glucokinase mRNA has been found in islets from trained rats,[282] but it is uncertain whether this explains the lower insulin responses, because such islets were found to metabolize glucose at a rate similar to that of islets from sedentary animals.[280]

Pregnancy

Hyperinsulinemia is a common feature of pregnancy. Islets from pregnant rats are more sensitive to glucose stimulation of insulin secretion and biosynthesis than are islets of control rats.[283–286] The dose-response relationship is shifted to the left. This has been attributed to increased adenylate cyclase activity, cAMP levels, and protein kinase A activity.[283,285] It has also been shown, by dye-transfer experiments, that β-cell coupling is enhanced during pregnancy.[287] Both dietary (increase in food consumption) and hormonal (prolactin and placental lactogen) factors probably are involved in this functional adaptation of β-cells.[288,289]

Lactation

Plasma glucose and insulin levels are relatively low during lactation. Islets from lactating rats have been found to secrete less insulin than islets from nonlactating animals during in vitro stimulation with glucose or leucine.[290] This decrease in β-cell secretory activity is paradoxically associated with increased activity of adenylate cyclase, protein kinase A, and protein kinase C and increased oxidation of glucose and leucine.[290] The β-cell coupling is also increased in lactating rats.[291] It should be noted, however, that the suggestion that β-cells of lactating rats have an intrinsically low secretory activity has been challenged.[292]

Hormones

Growth Hormone

Glucose metabolism and glucose-induced insulin secretion are lower in islets from hypophysectomized rats than in islets from control animals.[293] In most in vitro studies, growth hormone has no acute effect on β-cell function.[289,294] On the other hand, delayed stimulation of β-cell growth, insulin biosynthesis, and insulin release is well established. It appears to be due to a direct action of growth hormone on somatogenic and lactogenic receptors in β-cells rather than to an indirect action mediated by insulin-like growth factors.[289,295]

Thyroid Hormones

In the rat, hyperthyroidism decreases the insulin content of the pancreas and causes a slight and delayed inhibition of insulin secretion in response to glucose but not to other secretagogues. These changes do not seem to be due to alterations of glucose metabolism in islet cells.[296]

Steroid Hormones

There is no convincing evidence that gonadal steroids exert direct effects on the endocrine pancreas.[296] Adrenocortical steroids may have a marked indirect influence on β-cells through their effects on glucose production and their antagonism of insulin action. It is much less clear whether their allegedly direct rapid inhibitory and delayed stimulatory effects on insulin secretion are physiologically relevant.[296] It is of interest, however, that glucocorticoid receptors have been identified in the nuclei of β-cells.[297]

1,25-Dihydroxyvitamin D₃

The isolated and perfused pancreas from vitamin D-deficient rats secretes less insulin than the pancreas of control rats.[298] This decrease may reflect, at least in part, a direct action of vitamin D on β-cells.[298,299] Such a direct effect has been observed in vitro on insulin production by neonatal rat islets.[300] The underlying mechanisms are still unknown.

STIMULUS-SECRETION COUPLING IN HUMAN β-CELLS

Studies with human islets are important in validating the implicit extrapolation that the information gained from experiments in animal models is relevant to human physiology or pathophysiology. It has long been demonstrated that human, like rodent, fetal β-cells do not release insulin when stimulated by glucose alone but respond to amino acids.[301,302] Although biochemical and biophysical studies on normal adult human islets are still few, they have shown that there are no marked differences between the properties of human and rodent β-cells.[303–313]

Like rodent β-cells, human β-cells are equipped with a high K_m glucose transporter (GLUT-2) similar to that present in liver cells.[312] Glucokinase also is present in human islets and has a K_m value (5 mM) somewhat lower than that in rat islets.[307] The concentration dependency of glucose-induced insulin secretion is sigmoidal, with a threshold value between 2 and 4 mM and a half-maximal response between 4 and 6 mM.[305] There is thus a leftward shift of the curve compared with that of rat or mouse islets. This is understandable, since plasma glucose concentrations are lower in humans than in rodents.

Glucose stimulation of insulin secretion correlates well with the rate of glucose oxidation by isolated human islets,[305] is potentiated by inhibitors of the cAMP-phosphodiesterase,[303,305,306] is inhibited by epinephrine,[306] and displays a biphasic pattern in dynamic experiments.[309] It is unlikely that de novo synthesis of DAG is important for the stimulation of insulin secretion by glucose in human islets.[133] On the other hand, these islets convert endogenous arachidonate to both cyclooxygenase and 12-lipoxygenase products, which may modulate insulin secretion.[309]

Patch-clamp experiments have identified ATP-sensitive K^+ channels in human β-cells.[308,310,311] These channels are open in unstimulated β-cells and close on exposure to low concentrations of glucose. This closure, which requires glucose metabolism and can be mimicked by other fuels, is followed by appearance of Ca^{++}-dependent action potentials.[310] The sensitivity of ATP-sensitive K^+ channels to tolbutamide, diazoxide, and intracellular ATP is essentially similar in human and rodent β-cells.[310,311] This stimulation of insulin release by glucose or tolbutamide is dependent on extracellular Ca^{++} and is associated with an increase in cytosolic Ca^{++}.[313]

In conclusion, the available evidence indicates that the models of stimulus-secretion coupling based on studies in normal rat or mouse β-cells are likely to be largely applicable to normal human β-cells.

REFERENCES

1. Matschinsky FM, Ellerman J, Stillings S, et al. Hexoses and insulin secretion. In: Hasselblatt A, Bruchhausen FV, eds. Handbook of experimental pharmacology. Vol 32. Insulin II. New York: Springer-Verlag, 1975:79–114.
2. Hedeskov CJ. Mechanism of glucose-induced insulin secretion. Physiol Rev 1980;60:442–509.
3. Pagliara AS, Stillings SN, Hover B, et al. Glucose modulation of amino acid-induced glucagon and insulin release in the isolated perfused rat pancreas. J Clin Invest 1974;54:819–32.
4. Gerich JE, Charles MA, Grodsky GM. Characterization of the effects of arginine and glucose on glucagon and insulin release from the perfused rat pancreas. J Clin Invest 1974;54:833–41.
5. Pederson RA, Brown JC. The insulinotropic action of gastric inhibitory polypeptide in the perfused isolated rat pancreas. Endocrinology 1976;99:780–5.
6. Joost HG, Hasselblatt A. Insulin release by tolbutamide and glibenclamide: comparative study on the perfused rat pancreas. Naunyn-Schmiedeberg's Arch Pharmacol 1979;306:185–8.
7. Weir GC, Mojsov S, Hendrick GK, Habener JF. Glucagon-like peptide I (7–37) actions on endocrine pancreas. Diabetes 1989;38:338–42.
8. Halter JB, Graf RJ, Porte D Jr. Potentiation of insulin secretory responses by plasma glucose levels in man: evidence that hyperglycemia in diabetes compensates for impaired glucose potentiation. J Clin Endocrinol Metab 1979;48:946–54.
9. Curry DL, Bennett LL, Grodsky GM. Dynamics of insulin secretion by the perfused rat pancreas. Endocrinology 1968;83:572–84.
10. Cerasi E, Luft R, Efendic S. Decreased sensitivity of the pancreatic beta cells to glucose in prediabetic and

diabetic subjects. A glucose dose-response study. Diabetes 1972;21:224–34.

11. Brunzell JD, Robertson RP, Lerner RL, et al. Relationships between fasting plasma glucose levels and insulin secretion during intravenous glucose tolerance tests. J Clin Endocrinol Metab 1976;42:222–9.

12. Grodsky GM. A threshold distribution hypothesis for packet storage of insulin and its mathematical modeling. J Clin Invest 1972;51:2047–59.

13. O'Connor MDL, Landahl H, Grodsky GM. Comparison of storage- and signal-limited models of pancreatic insulin secretion. Am J Physiol 1980;238:R378–89.

14. Lacy PE, Walker MM, Fink CJ. Perifusion of isolated rat islets in vitro: participation of the microtubular system in the biphasic release of insulin. Diabetes 1972; 21:987–98.

15. Malaisse WJ, Malaisse-Lagae F, van Obberghen E, et al. Role of microtubules in the phasic pattern of insulin release. Ann NY Acad Sci 1975;253:630–52.

16. Cerasi E, Fick G, Rudemo M. A mathematical model for the glucose induced insulin release in man Eur J Clin Invest 1974;4:267–78.

17. Gilon P, Henquin JC. Influence of membrane potential changes on cytoplasmic Ca^{2+} concentration in an electrically excitable cell, the insulin-secreting pancreatic B-cell. J Biol Chem 1992;267:20713–20.

18. Grapengiesser E, Gylfe E, Hellman B. Glucose-induced oscillations of cytoplasmic Ca^{2+} in the pancreatic β-cell. Biochem Biophys Res Commun 1988;151:1299–304.

19. Wang J-L, McDaniel ML. Secretagogue-induced oscillations of cytoplasmic Ca^{2+} in single α- and β-cells obtained from pancreatic islets by fluorescence-activated cell sorting. Biochem Biophys Res Commun 1990;166:813–8.

20. Pralong W-F, Bartley C, Wollheim CB. Single islet β-cell stimulation by nutrients: relationship between pyridine nucleotides, cytosolic Ca^{2+} and secretion. EMBO J 1990;9:53–60.

21. Rasmussen H, Zawalich KC, Ganesan S, et al. Physiology and pathophysiology of insulin secretion. Diabetes Care 1990;13:655–66.

22. Gembal M, Gilon P, Henquin JC. Evidence that glucose can control insulin release independently from its action on ATP-sensitive K^+ channels in mouse B-cells. J Clin Invest 1992;89:1288–95.

23. Nilsson T, Arkhammar P, Berggren PO. Dual effect of glucose on cytoplasmic free Ca^{2+} concentration and insulin release reflects the β-cell being deprived of fuel. Biochem Biophys Res Commun 1988;153:984–91.

24. Metz SA, Halter JB, Robertson RP. Paradoxical inhibition of insulin secretion by glucose in human diabetes mellitus. J Clin Endocrinol Metab 1979;48:827–35.

25. Hellman B. Calcium transport in pancreatic β-cells: implications for glucose regulation of insulin release. Diabetes Metab Rev 1986;2:215–41.

26. Henquin JC. Tolbutamide stimulation and inhibition of insulin release: studies of the underlying ionic mechanisms in isolated rat islets. Diabetologia 1980;18:151–60.

27. Panten U, Burgfeld J, Goerke F, et al. Control of insulin secretion by sulfonylureas, meglitinide and diazoxide in relation to their binding to the sulfonylurea receptor in pancreatic islets. Biochem Pharmacol 1989;38:1217–29.

28. Bolaffi JL, Heldt A, Lewis LD, Grodsky GM. The third phase of in vitro insulin secretion: evidence for glucose insensitivity. Diabetes 1986;35:370–3.

29. Hoenig M, MacGregor LC, Matschinsky FM. In vitro exhaustion of pancreatic β-cells. Am J Physiol 1986; 250:E502–11.

30. Grodsky GM. A new phase of insulin secretion: how will it contribute to our understanding of β-cell function? Diabetes 1989;38:673–8.

31. Malaisse W, Malaisse-Lagae F, Wright PH. A new method for the measurement in vitro of pancreatic insulin secretion. Endocrinology 1967;80:99–108.

32. Meglasson MD, Matschinsky FM. New perspectives on pancreatic islet glucokinase. Am J Physiol 1984; 246:E1–13.

33. Henquin JC. D-glucose inhibits potassium efflux from pancreatic islet cells. Nature 1978;271:271–3.

34. Malaisse WJ, Sener A. Glucose-induced changes in cytosolic ATP content in pancreatic islets. Biochim Biophys Acta 1987;927:190–5.

35. Stefan Y, Meda P, Neufeld M, Orci L. Stimulation of insulin secretion reveals heterogeneity of pancreatic B cells in vivo. J Clin Invest 1987;80:175–83.

36. Salomon D, Meda P. Heterogeneity and contact-dependent regulation of hormone secretion by individual B cells. Exp Cell Res 1986;162:507–20.

37. Hiriart M, Ramirez-Mendeles MC. Functional subpopulations of individual pancreatic B-cells in culture. Endocrinology 1991;128:3193–8.

38. Lewis CE, Clark A, Ashcroft SJH, et al. Calcitonin gene-related peptide and somatostatin inhibit insulin release from individual rat B cells. Mol Cell Endocrinol 1988; 57:41–9.

39. Meissner HP. Electrophysiological evidence for coupling between β-cells of pancreatic islets. Nature 1976;262:502–4.

40. Meda P, Perrelet A, Orci L. Gap junctions and cell-to-cell coupling in endocrine glands. Mod Cell Biol 1984; 3:131–96.

41. Lernmark A. The preparation of, and studies on, free cell suspensions from mouse pancreatic islets. Diabetologia 1974;10:431–8.

42. Pipeleers D, in't Veld P, Maes E, Van de Winkel M. Glucose-induced insulin release depends on functional cooperation between islet cells. Proc Natl Acad Sci USA 1982;79:7322–5.

43. Halban PA, Wollheim CB, Blondel B, et al. The possible importance of contact between pancreatic islet cells for the control of insulin release. Endocrinology 1982; 111:86–94.

44. Pipeleers D. The biosociology of pancreatic B cells. Diabetologia 1987;30:277–91.

45. Bosco D, Orci L, Meda P. Homologous but not heterologous contact increases the insulin secretion of individual pancreatic B-cells. Exp Cell Res 1989;184:72–80.

46. Weir GC, Bonner-Weir S. Islets of Langerhans: the puzzle of intraislet interactions and their relevance to diabetes. J Clin Invest 1990;85:983–7.

47. Marks V, Samols E, Stagner J. Intra-islet interactions. In: Flatt PR, ed. Nutrient regulation of insulin secretion. London: Portland Press 1992:41–57.

48. Chan SJ, Keim P, Steiner DF. Cell-free synthesis of rat preproinsulins: characterization and partial amino acid sequence determination. Proc Natl Acad Sci USA 1976;73:1964–8.

49. Orci L. The insulin factory: a tour of the plant surroundings and a visit to the assembly line. Diabetologia 1985:28:528–46.

50. Steiner DF, Bell GI, Tager HS. Chemistry and biosynthesis of pancreatic protein hormones. In: De Groot LJ, ed. Endocrinology. 2nd ed. Vol 2. Philadelphia: WB Saunders, 1989:1263–89.

51. Davidson HW, Rhodes CJ, Hutton JC. Intraorganellar

calcium and pH control of proinsulin cleavage in the pancreatic β cell via two distinct site-specific endopeptidases. Nature 1988;333:93–6.

52. Orci L, Ravazzola M, Amherdt M, et al. Conversion of proinsulin to insulin occurs coordinately with acidification of maturing secretory vesicles. J Cell Biol 1986;103:2273–81.

53. Emdin SO, Dodson GG, Cutfield JM, et al. Role of zinc in insulin biosynthesis: some possible zinc-insulin interactions in the pancreatic B-cell. Diabetologia 1980;19:174–82.

54. Hutton JC. The insulin secretory granule. Diabetologia 1989;32:271–81.

55. Rhodes CJ, Halban PA. Newly synthesized proinsulin/insulin and stored insulin are released from pancreatic B cells predominantly via a regulated, rather than a constitutive, pathway. J Cell Biol 1987;105:145–53.

56. Permutt MA, Kipnis DM. Insulin biosynthesis. I. On the mechanism of glucose stimulation. J Biol Chem 1972;247:1194–9.

57. Giddings SJ, Chirgwin J, Permutt MA. Effects of glucose on proinsulin messenger RNA in rats in vivo. Diabetes 1982;31:624–9.

58. Welsh M, Brunstedt J, Hellerström C. Effects of D-glucose, L-leucine, and 2-ketoisocaproate on insulin mRNA levels in mouse pancreatic islets. Diabetes 1986;35:228–31.

59. Schuit FC, in't Veld PA, Pipeleers DG. Glucose stimulates proinsulin biosynthesis by a dose-dependent recruitment of pancreatic beta cells. Proc Natl Acad Sci USA 1988;85:3865–9.

60. Ashcroft SJH. Glucoreceptor mechanisms and the control of insulin release and biosynthesis. Diabetologia 1980;18:5–15.

61. Permutt MA. Biosynthesis of insulin. In: Cooperstein SJ, Watkins D, eds. The islets of Langerhans: biochemistry, physiology, and pathology. New York: Academic Press, 1981:75–95.

62. Sando H, Borg J, Steiner DF. Studies on the secretion of newly synthesized proinsulin and insulin from isolated rat islets of Langerhans. J Clin Invest 1972;51:76–85.

63. Gold G, Grodsky GM. Kinetic aspects of compartmental storage and secretion of insulin and zinc. Experientia 1984;40:1105–14.

64. Halban PA. Differential rates of release of newly synthesized and of stored insulin from pancreatic islets. Endocrinology 1982;110:1183–8.

65. Sener A, Malaisse WJ. Nutrient metabolism in islet cells. Experientia 1984;40:1026–35.

66. Meglasson MD, Matschinsky FM. Pancreatic islet glucose metabolism and regulation of insulin secretion. Diabetes Metab Rev 1986;2:163–214.

67. Lenzen S, Panten U. Signal recognition by pancreatic B-cells. Biochem Pharmacol 1988;37:371–8.

68. Malaisse WJ. Regulation of insulin secretion by nutrients: the fuel concept: In: Flatt PR, ed. Nutrient regulation of insulin secretion. London: Portland Press 1992:83–100.

69. Niki A, Niki H, Miwa I, Okuda J. Insulin secretion by anomers of D-glucose. Science 1974;186:150–1.

70. Malaisse WJ, Malaisse-Lagae F, Sener A. Anomeric specificity of hexose metabolism in pancreatic islets. Physiol Rev 1983;63:773–86.

71. Thorens B, Sarkar HK, Kaback HR, Lodish HF. Cloning and functional expression in bacteria of a novel glucose transporter present in liver, intestine, kidney, and β-pancreatic islet cells. Cell 1988;55:281–90.

72. Johnson JH, Newgard CB, Milburn JL, et al. The high Km glucose transporter of islets of Langerhans is functionally similar to the low affinity transporter of liver and has an identical primary sequence. J Biol Chem 1990;265:6548–51.

73. Matschinsky FM, Ellerman JE. Metabolism of glucose in the islets of Langerhans. J Biol Chem 1968;243:2730–6.

74. Hellman B, Sehlin J, Täljedal I-B. Evidence for mediated transport of glucose in mammalian pancreatic β-cells. Biochim Biophys Acta 1971;241:147–54.

75. Meglasson MD, Burch PT, Berner DK, et al. Chromatographic resolution and kinetic characterization of glucokinase from islets of Langerhans. Proc Natl Acad Sci USA 1983;80:85–90.

76. Iynedjian PB, Möbius G, Seitz HJ, et al. Tissue-specific expression of glucokinase: identification of the gene product in liver and pancreatic islets. Proc Natl Acad Sci USA 1986;83:1998–2001.

77. Malaisse WJ, Sener A. Glucokinase is not the pancreatic B-cell glucoreceptor. Diabetologia 1985;28:520–7.

78. Meglasson MD, Smith KM, Nelson D, Erecinska M. α-Glycerophosphate shuttle in a clonal β-cell line. Am J Physiol 1989;256:E173–8.

79. Panten U, Lenzen S. Alterations in energy metabolism of secretory cells. In: Akkerman JWN, ed. Energetics of secretion responses. Boca Raton: CRC Press, 1988:109–23.

80. Wollheim CB, Sharp GWG. Regulation of insulin release by calcium. Physiol Rev 1981;61:914–73.

81. Prentki M, Matschinsky FM. Ca^{2+}, cAMP, and phospholipid-derived messengers in coupling mechanisms of insulin secretion. Physiol Rev 1987;67:1185–248.

82. Wolf BA, Colca JR, Turk J, et al. Regulation of Ca^{2+} homeostasis by islet endoplasmic reticulum and its role in insulin secretion. Am J Physiol 1988;254:E121–36.

83. Hellman B, Gylfe E, Grapengiesser E, et al. Cytoplasmic calcium and insulin secretion. In: Flatt PR, ed. Nutrient regulation of insulin secretion. London: Portland Press 1992:213–46.

84. Henquin JC. Relative importance of extracellular and intracellular calcium for the two phases of glucose-stimulated insulin release: studies with theophylline. Endocrinology 1978;102:723–30.

85. Herchuelz A, Malaisse WJ. Calcium and insulin release. In: Anghileri LJ, Anghileri-Truffet L, eds. The role of calcium in biological systems. Boca Raton: CRC Press, 1982:17–32.

86. Dean PM, Matthews EK. Glucose-induced electrical activity in pancreatic islet cells. J Physiol 1970;210:255–64.

87. Meissner HP, Schmelz H. Membrane potential of beta cells in pancreatic islets. Pflügers Arch 1974;351:195–206.

88. Henquin JC, Meissner HP. Significance of ionic fluxes and changes in membrane potential for stimulus-secretion coupling in pancreatic B-cells. Experientia 1984;40:1043–52.

89. Matthews EK. Electrophysiology of pancreatic islet β-cells. In: Poisner AM. Trifaro JM, eds. The electrophysiology of the secretory cell. Amsterdam: Elsevier, 1985:93–112.

90. Henquin JC. Regulation of insulin release by ionic and electrical events in B-cells. Horm Res 1987;27:168–78.

91. Atwater I, Carroll P, Li MX. Electrophysiology of the pancreatic B-cell. In: Draznin B, Melmed S, Leroith D, eds. Insulin secretion. New York: Alan R Liss, 1989:49–68.

92. Henquin JC, Debuyser A, Drews G, Plant TD. Regulation of K^+ permeability and membrane potential in insulin-secreting cells. In: Flatt PR, ed. Nutrient regulation of insulin secretion. London: Portland Press 1992:173–91.

93. Henquin JC. Les mécanismes de contrôle de la sécrétion d'insuline. Arch Int Physiol Biochim 1990;98:A61−80.

94. Gylfe E. Nutrient secretagogues induce bimodal early changes in cytoplasmic calcium of insulin-releasing ob/ob mouse β-cells. J Biol Chem 1988;263:13750-4.

95. Sehlin J, Täljedal I-B. Glucose-induced decrease in Rb^+ permeability in pancreatic B-cells. Nature 1975; 253:635−6.

96. Atwater I, Ribalet B, Rojas E. Cyclic changes in potential and resistance of the β-cell membrane induced by glucose in islets of Langerhans from mouse. J Physiol 1978;278:117−39.

97. Cook DL, Hales CN. Intracellular ATP directly blocks K^+ channels in pancreatic B-cells. Nature 1984;311:271−3.

98. Ashcroft FM, Harrison DE, Ashcroft SJH. Glucose induces closure of single potassium channels in isolated rat pancreatic β-cells. Nature 1984;312:446−8.

99. Rorsman P, Trube G. Glucose dependent K^+-channels in pancreatic β-cells are regulated by intracellular ATP. Pflügers Arch 1985;405:305−9.

100. Misler S, Falke LC, Gillis K, McDaniel ML. A metabolite-regulated potassium channel in rat pancreatic B-cells. Proc Natl Acad Sci USA 1986;83:7119−23.

101. Rorsman P, Trube G. Biophysics and physiology of ATP-regulated K^+ channels. In: Cook NS, ed. Potassium channels: structure, classification, function and therapeutic potential. Chichester: Ellis Horwood, 1990:96−116.

102. Ashcroft FM, Rorsman P. Electrophysiology of the pancreatic β-cell. Prog Biophys Molec Biol 1989; 54:87−143.

103. Ashford ML. Potassium channels and modulation of insulin secretion. In: Cook NS, ed. Potassium channels: structure, classification, function and therapeutic potential. Chichester: Ellis Horwood, 1990:300−25.

104. Dunne MJ, Petersen OH. Potassium selective ion channels in insulin-secreting cells: physiology, pharmacology and their role in stimulus-secretion coupling. Biochim Biophys Acta 1991;1071:67−82.

105. Cook DL, Satin LS, Ashford MLJ, Hales CN. ATP-sensitive K^+ channels in pancreatic β-cells: spare-channel hypothesis. Diabetes 1988;37:495−8.

106. Satin LS, Cook DL. Voltage-gated Ca^{2+} current in pancreatic B-cells. Pflügers Arch 1985;404:385−7.

107. Plant TD. Properties and calcium-dependent inactivation of calcium currents in cultured mouse pancreatic B-cells. J Physiol 1988;404:731−47.

108. Henquin JC. ATP-sensitive K^+ channels may control glucose-induced electrical activity in pancreatic B-cells. Biochem Biophys Res Commun 1988;156:769−75.

109. Cook DL, Ikeuchi M. Tolbutamide as mimic of glucose on β-cell electrical activity: ATP-sensitive K^+ channels as common pathway for both stimuli. Diabetes 1989;38:416−21.

110. Malaisse WJ, Malaisse-Lagae F, Sener A. Coupling factors in nutrient-induced insulin release. Experientia 1984;40:1035−43.

111. Ammon HPT, Mark M. Thiols and pancreatic β-cell function: a review. Cell Biochem Funct 1985;3:157−71.

112. Matschinsky FM, Gosh AK, Meglasson MD, et al. Metabolic concomitants in pure, pancreatic beta cells during glucose-stimulated insulin secretion. J Biol Chem 1986; 261:14057−61.

113. Hedeskov CJ, Capito K, Thams P. Cytosolic ratios of free [NADPH]/[NADP$^+$] and [NADH/NAD$^+$] in mouse pancreatic islets, and nutrient-induced insulin secretion. Biochem J 1987;241:161−7.

114. Lindström P, Sehlin J. Effect of glucose on the intra-

115. cellular pH of pancreatic islet cells. Biochem J 1984; 218:887−92.

115. Grapengiesser E, Gylfe E. Hellman B. Regulation of pH in individual pancreatic β-cells as evaluated by fluorescence ratio microscopy. Biochim Biophys Acta 1989;1014: 219−24.

116. Best L. Intracellular pH and B-cell function. In: Flatt PR, ed. Nutrient regulation of insulin secetion. London: Portland Press 1992:157−171.

117. Sharp GWG. The adenylate cyclase-cyclic AMP system in islets of Langerhans and its role in the control of insulin release. Diabetologia 1979;16:287−96.

118. Thams P, Capito K, Hedeskov CJ. Stimulation by glucose of cyclic AMP accumulation in mouse pancreatic islets is mediated by protein kinase C. Biochem J 1988;253: 229−34.

119. Malaisse WJ, Malaisse-Lagae F. The role of cyclic AMP in insulin release. Experientia 1984;40:1068−75.

120. Henquin JC. The interplay between cyclic AMP and ions in the stimulus-secretion coupling in pancreatic B-cells. Arch Int Physiol Biochim 1985;93:37−48.

121. Persaud SJ, Jones PM, Howell SL. Glucose-stimulated insulin secretion is not dependent on activation of protein kinase A. Biochem Biophys Res Commun 1990; 173: 833−9.

122. Berne C. The metabolism of lipids in mouse pancreatic islets: the oxidation of fatty acids and ketone bodies. Biochem J 1975;152:661−6.

123. Tamarit-Rodriguez J, Vara E, Tamarit J. Starvation-induced changes of palmitate metabolism and insulin secretion in isolated rat islets stimulated by glucose. Biochem J 1984;221:317−24.

124. Corkey BE, Glennon MC, Chen KS, et al. A role for malonyl-CoA in glucose-stimulated insulin secretion from clonal pancreatic β-cells. J Biol Chem 1989;264: 21608−12.

125. Liang Y, Matschinsky FM. Content of CoA-esters in perifused rat islets stimulated by glucose and other fuels. Diabetes 1991;40:327−33.

126. Malaisse WJ, Malaisse-Lagae F, Sener A, Hellerström C. Participation of endogenous fatty acids in the secretory activity of the pancreatic B-cell. Biochem J 1985; 227:995−1002.

127. Turk J, Wolf BA, McDaniel ML. The role of phospholipid-derived mediators including arachidonic acid, its metabolites, and inositoltriphosphate and of intracellular Ca^{2+} in glucose-induced insulin secretion by pancreatic islets. Prog Lipid Res 1987;26:125−81.

128. Biden TJ, Wollheim CB. Generation, metabolism and function of inositol phosphates during nutrient- and neurotransmitter-induced insulin secretion. In: Michell RH, Drummond AH, Downes CP, eds. Inositol lipids in cell signalling. San Diego: Academic Press, 1989:405−25.

129. Morgan NG, Montague W. Phospholipids and insulin secretion. In: Flatt PR, ed. Nutrient regulation of insulin secretion. London: Portland Press 1992:125−55.

130. Laychock SG. Identification and metabolism of polyphosphoinositides in isolated islets of Langerhans. Biochem J 1983;216:101−6.

131. Dunlop ME, Larkins RG. Pancreatic islets synthesize phospholipids de novo from glucose via acyl-dihydroxyacetone phosphate. Biochem Biophys Res Commun 1985;132:467−73.

132. Peter-Riesch B, Fathi M, Schlegel W, Wollheim CB. Glucose and carbachol generate 1,2-diacylglycerols by different mechanisms in pancreatic islets. J Clin Invest 1988;81:1154−61.

133. Wolf BA, Easom RA, McDaniel ML, Turk J. Diacylglycerol synthesis de novo from glucose by pancreatic islets isolated from rats and humans. J Clin Invest 1990;85: 482–90.

134. Wollheim CB, Regazzi R. Protein kinase C in insulin releasing cells: putative role in stimulus secretion coupling. FEBS Lett 1990;268:376–80.

135. Persaud SJ, Jones PM, Howell SL. The role of protein kinase C in insulin secretion. In: Flatt PR, ed. Nutrient regulation of insulin secretion. London: Portland Press 1992: 247–69.

136. Ganesan S, Calle R, Zawalich K, et al. Glucose-induced translocation of protein kinase C in rat pancreatic islets. Proc Natl Acad Sci USA 1990;87:9893–7.

137. Metz SA. Is protein kinase C required for physiologic insulin release? Diabetes 1988;37:3–7.

138. Zawalich WS, Rasmussen H. Control of insulin secretion: a model involving Ca^{2+}, cAMP and diacylglycerol. Mol Cell Endocrinol 1990;70:119–37.

139. Metz SA. The pancreatic islet as Rubik's cube: is phospholipid hydrolysis a piece of the puzzle? Diabetes 1991; 40:1565–73.

140. Robertson RP. Arachidonic acid metabolite regulation of insulin secretion. Diabetes Metab Rev 1986;2:261–6.

141. Santos RM, Rosario LM, Nadal A, et al. Widespread synchronous $[Ca^{2+}]_i$ oscillations due to bursting electrical activity in single pancreatic islets. Pflügers Arch 1991;418:417–22.

142. Gilon P, Shepherd RM, Henquin JC. Oscillations of cytoplasmic Ca^{2+} in pancreatic B-cells trigger synchronous oscillations of insulin secretion (in preparation).

143. Longo EA, Tornheim K, Deeney JT, et al. Oscillations in cytosolic free Ca^{2+}, oxygen consumption, and insulin secretion in glucose-stimulated rat pancreatic islets. J Biol Chem 1991;266:9314–9.

144. Bergstrom RW, Fujimoto WY, Teller DC, De Haën C. Oscillatory insulin secretion in perifused isolated rat islets. Am J Physiol 1989;257:E479–85.

145. Chou H-F, Ipp E. Pulsatile insulin secretion in isolated rat islets. Diabetes 1990;39:112–7.

146. Stagner JI, Samols E, Weir GC. Sustained oscillations of insulin, glucagon, and somatostatin from the isolated canine pancreas during exposure to a constant glucose concentration. J Clin Invest 1980;65:939–42.

147. Lefèbvre PJ, Paolisso G, Scheen AJ, Henquin JC. Pulsatility of insulin and glucagon release: physiological significance and pharmacological implications. Diabetologia 1987; 30:443–52.

148. Weigle DS. Pulsatile secretion of fuel-regulatory hormones. Diabetes 1987;36:764–75.

149. Zawalich WS. Intermediary metabolism and insulin secretion from isolated rat islets of Langerhans. Diabetes 1979;28:252–60.

150. Hellman B, Sehlin J, Täljedal I-B. Effects of glucose and other modifiers of insulin release on the oxidative metabolism of amino acids in micro-dissected pancreatic islets. Biochem J 1971;123:513–21.

151. Panten U. Zielmann S, Joost H-G, Lenzen S. Branched chain amino and keto acids: tools for the investigation of fuel recognition mechanism in pancreatic B-cells. In: Adibi SA, Fekl W, Langenbeck U, Schauder P, eds. Branched chain amino and keto acids in health and disease. Basel: Karger, 1984:134–46.

152. Malaisse WJ. Branched-chain amino and keto acid metabolism in pancreatic islets. Adv Enzyme Regul 1986; 25:203–17.

153. Henquin JC, Meissner HP. Effects of amino acids on membrane potential and $^{86}Rb^+$ fluxes in pancreatic β-cells. Am J Physiol 1981;240:E245–52.

154. Ashcroft FM, Ashcroft SJH, Harrison DE. Effects of 2-ketoisocaproate on insulin release and single potassium channel activity in dispersed rat pancreatic β-cells. J Physiol 1987;385:517–29.

155. Henquin JC, Meissner HP. Cyclic adenosine monophosphate differently affects the response of mouse pancreatic β-cells to various amino acids. J Physiol 1986;381:77–93.

156. Prentki M, Renold AE. Neutral amino acid transport in isolated rat pancreatic islets. J Biol Chem 1983; 258:14239–44.

157. Blachier F, Mourtada A, Sener A, Malaisse WJ. Stimulus-secretion coupling of arginine-induced insulin release: uptake of metabolized and nonmetabolized cationic amino acids by pancreatic islets. Endocrinology 1989;124:134–41.

158. Charles S, Tamagawa T, Henquin JC. A single mechanism for the stimulation of insulin release and $^{86}Rb^+$ efflux from rat islets by cationic amino acids. Biochem J 1982;208:301–8.

159. Palmer JP, Benson JW, Walter RM, Ensinck JW. Arginine-stimulated acute phase of insulin and glucagon secretion in diabetic subjects. J Clin Invest 1976;58:565–70.

160. Biden TJ, Taylor KW. Effects of ketone bodies on insulin release and islet-cell metabolism in the rat. Biochem J 1983;212:371–7.

161. Malaisse WJ, Lebrun P, Rasschaert J, et al. Ketone bodies and islet function: ^{86}Rb handling and metabolic data. Am J Physiol 1990;259:E123–30.

162. Henquin JC. Established, unsuspected and novel pharmacological insulin secretagogues. In: Bailey CJ, Flatt PR, eds. New antidiabetic drugs. London: Smith-Gordon and Co, 1990:93–106.

163. Henquin JC, Meissner HP. Opposite effects of tolbutamide and diazoxide on $^{86}Rb^+$ fluxes and membrane potential in pancreatic B cells. Biochem Pharmacol 1982;31:1407–15.

164. Gylfe E, Hellman B, Sehlin J, Täljedal I-B. Interaction of sulfonylurea with the pancreatic B-cell. Experientia 1984;40:1126–34.

165. Sturgess NC, Ashford MLJ, Cook DL, Hales CN. The sulphonylurea receptor may be an ATP-sensitive potassium channel. Lancet 1985;2:474–5.

166. Abrahamsson H, Berggren P-O, Rorsman P. Direct measurements of increased free cytoplasmic Ca^{2+} in mouse pancreatic β-cells following stimulation by hypoglycemic sulfonylureas. FEBS Lett 1985;190:21–4.

167. Trube G, Rorsman P, Ohno-Shosaku T. Opposite effects of tolbutamide and diazoxide on the ATP-dependent K^+ channel in mouse pancreatic β-cells. Pflügers Arch 1986;407:493–9.

168. Boyd AE III. Sulfonylurea receptors, ion channels, and fruit flies. Diabetes 1988;37:847–50.

169. de Weille JR, Fosset M, Mourre C, et al. Pharmacology and regulation of ATP-sensitive K^+ channels. Pflügers Arch 1989;414(Suppl 1):S80–7.

170. Arkhammar P, Nilsson T, Rorsman P, Berggren P-O. Inhibition of ATP-regulated K^+ channels precedes depolarization-induced increase in cytoplasmic free Ca^{2+} concentration in pancreatic β-cells. J Biol Chem 1987;262:5448–54.

171. Henquin JC, Charles S, Nenquin M, et al. Diazoxide and D600 inhibition of insulin release: distinct mechanisms explain the specificity for different stimuli. Diabetes 1982;31:776–83.

172. Fajans SS, Floyd JC Jr, Knopff RF, et al. A difference in mechanism by which leucine and other amino acids induce insulin release. J Clin Endocrinol Metab 1967;27:1600–6.

173. Garrino MG, Plant TD, Henquin JC. Effects of putative activators of K^+ channels in mouse pancreatic β-cells. Br J Pharmacol 1989;98:957–65.

174. Malaisse WJ, Sener A. Calcium-antagonists and islet function. XII. Comparison between nifedipine and chemically related drugs. Biochem Pharmacol 1981;30:1039–41.

175. Trost BN, Weidmann P. Effects of calcium antagonists on glucose homeostasis and serum lipids in non-diabetic and diabetic subjects: a review. J Hypertension 1987;5(Suppl 4):S81–104.

176. Miller RE. Pancreatic neuroendocrinology: peripheral neural mechanisms in the regulation of the islets of Langerhans. Endocrinol Rev 1981;12:471–94.

177. Ahren B, Taborsky GJ Jr, Porte D Jr. Neuropeptidergic versus cholinergic and adrenergic regulation of islet hormone secretion. Diabetologia 1986;29:827–36.

178. Hughes SJ, Ashcroft SJH. Cyclic AMP, protein phosphorylation and insulin secretion. In: Flatt PR, ed. Nutrient regulation of insulin secretion. London: Portland Press 1992:271–88.

179. Henquin JC, Meissner HP. The ionic, electrical, and secretory effects of endogenous cyclic adenosine monophosphate in mouse pancreatic B cells: studies with forskolin. Endocrinology 1984;115:1125–34.

180. Henquin JC, Bozem M, Schmeer W, Nenquin M. Distinct mechanisms for two amplification systems of insulin release. Biochem J 1987;246:393–9.

181. Prentki M, Glennon MC, Geschwind J-F, et al. Cyclic AMP raises cytosolic Ca^{2+} and promotes Ca^{2+} influx in a clonal pancreatic β-cell line (HIT T-15). FEBS Lett 1987;220:103–7.

182. Rajan AS, Hill RS, Boyd AE. Effect of rise in cAMP levels on Ca^{2+} influx through voltage-dependent Ca^{2+} channels in HIT cells: second-messenger synarchy in β-cells. Diabetes 1989;38:874–80.

183. Tamagawa T, Niki H, Niki A. Insulin release independent of a rise in cytosolic free Ca^{2+} by forskolin and phorbol ester. FEBS Lett 1985;183:430–2.

184. Jones PM, Fyles JM, Howell SL. Regulation of insulin secretion by cAMP in rat islets of Langerhans permeabilised by high-voltage discharge. FEBS Lett 1986;205:205–9.

185. Vallar L, Biden TJ, Wollheim CB. Guanine nucleotides induce Ca^{2+}-independent insulin secretion from permeabilized RINm5F cells. J Biol Chem 1987;262:5049–56.

186. Berridge MJ, Irvine RF. Inositol phosphates and cell signalling. Nature 1989;341:197–205.

187. Prentki M, Glennon MC, Thomas AP, et al. Cell-specific patterns of oscillating free Ca^{2+} in carbamylcholine-stimulated insulinoma cells. J Biol Chem 1988;263:11044–7.

188. Garcia MC, Hermans MP, Henquin JC. Glucose-, calcium- and concentration-dependence of acetylcholine stimulation of insulin release and ionic fluxes in mouse islets. Biochem J 1988;254:211–8.

189. Nishizuka Y. Studies and perspectives of protein kinase C. Science 1986;233:305–12.

190. Jones PM, Stutchfield J, Howell SL. Effects of Ca^{2+} and a phorbol ester on insulin secretion from islets of Langerhans permeabilised by high-voltage discharge. FEBS Lett 1985;191:102–6.

191. Arkhammar P, Nilsson T, Welsh M, et al. Effects of protein kinase C activation on the regulation of the stimulus-secretion coupling in pancreatic β-cells. Biochem J 1989;264:207–15.

192. Henquin JC, Garcia MC, Bozem M, et al. Muscarinic control of pancreatic B cell function involves sodium-dependent depolarization and calcium influx. Endocrinology 1988;122:2134–42.

193. Maletti M, Portha B, Carlquist M, et al. Evidence for and characterization of specific high affinity binding sites for the gastric inhibitory polypeptide in pancreatic β-cells. Endocrinology 1984;115:1324–31.

194. Orskov C, Poulsen SS. Glucagonlike peptide-I-(7–36)-amide receptors only in islets of Langerhans: autoradiographic survey of extracerebral tissues in rats. Diabetes 1991;40:1292–6.

195. McIntyre N, Holdsworth DC, Turner DS. New interpretation of oral glucose tolerance. Lancet 1964;2:20–1.

196. Elrick H, Stimmler L, Hlad CJ Jr, Arai Y. Plasma insulin response to oral and intravenous glucose administration. J Clin Endocrinol Metab 1964;24:1076–82.

197. Ebert R, Creutzfeldt W. Gastrointestinal peptides and insulin secretion. Diabetes Metab Rev 1987;3:1–26.

198. Morgan LM. Insulin secretion and the entero-insular axis. In: Flatt PR, ed. Nutrient regulation of insulin secretion. London: Portland Press 1992:1–22.

199. Henquin JC, Nenquin M. The muscarinic receptor subtype in mouse pancreatic B-cells. FEBS Lett 1988;236:89–92.

200. Verspohl EJ, Tacke R, Mutschler E, Lambrecht G. Muscarinic receptor subtypes in rat pancreatic islets: binding and functional studies. Eur J Pharmacol 1990;178:303–11.

201. Verspohl EJ, Ammon HPT, Williams JA, Goldfine ID. Evidence that cholecystokinin interacts with specific receptors and regulates insulin release in isolated rat islets of Langerhans. Diabetes 1986;35:38–43.

202. Samols E, Marri G, Marks V. Promotion of insulin secretion by glucagon. Lancet 1965;2:415–6.

203. Schuit FC, Pipeleers DG. Differences in adrenergic recognition by pancreatic A and B cells. Science 1986;232:875–7.

204. Kofod H, Andreu D, Thams P, et al. Insulin release by glucagon and secretin: studies with secretin-glucagon hybrids. Am J Physiol 1988;254:E454–8.

205. Bishop AE, Polak JM, Green IC, et al. The location of VIP in the pancreas of man and rat. Diabetologia 1980;18:73–8.

206. Knuhtsen S, Holst JJ, Baldissera FGA, et al. Gastrin-releasing peptide in the porcine pancreas. Gastroenterology 1987;92:1153–8.

207. Dunning BE, Moltz JH, Fawcett CP. Modulation of insulin and glucagon secretion from the perfused rat pancreas by the neurohypophysial hormones and by desamino-D-arginine vasopressin (DDAVP). Peptides 1984;5:871–5.

208. Gao ZY, Drews G, Nenquin M, et al. Mechanisms of the stimulation of insulin release by arginine-vasopressin in normal mouse islets. J Biol Chem 1990;265:15724–30.

209. Amico JA, Finn FM, Haldar J. Oxytocin and vasopressin are present in human and rat pancreas. Am J Med Sci 1988;296:303–7.

210. Loubatières-Mariani MM, Chapal J. Purinergic receptors involved in the stimulation of insulin and glucagon secretion. Diabete Metab 1988;14:119–26.

211. Berggren P-O, Rorsman P, Efendic S, et al. Mechanisms of action of entero-insular hormones, islet peptides and

neural input on the insulin secretory process. In: Flatt PR, ed. Nutrient regulation of insulin secretion. London: Portland Press 1992:289–318.

212. Morgan NG. Regulation of insulin secretion by α_2-adrenergic agonists. Trends Pharmacol Sci 1987;8: 369–70.

213. De Weille J, Schmid-Antomarchi H, Fosset M, Lazdunski M. ATP-sensitive K^+ channels that are blocked by hypoglycemia-inducing sulfonylureas in insulin-secreting cells are activated by galanin, a hyperglycemia-inducing hormone. Proc Natl Acad Sci USA 1988;85:1312–6.

214. Nilsson T, Arkhammar P, Rorsman P, Berggren P-O. Suppression of insulin release by galanin and somatostatin is mediated by a G-protein: an effect involving repolarization and reduction in cytoplasmic free Ca^{2+} concentration. J Biol Chem 1989;264:973–80.

215. Drews G, Debuyser A, Nenquin M, Henquin JC. Galanin and epinephrine act on distinct receptors to inhibit insulin release by the same mechanisms including an increase in K^+ permeability of the B-cell membrane. Endocrinology 1990;126:1646–53.

216. Rorsman P, Bokvist K, Ämmälä C, et al. Activation by adrenaline of a low-conductance G protein-dependent K^+ channel in mouse pancreatic B cells. Nature 1991; 349:77–9.

217. Tamagawa T, Niki I, Niki H, Niki A. Catecholamines inhibit insulin release independently of changes in cytosolic free Ca^{2+}. Biomed Res 1985;6:429–32.

218. Ullrich S, Wollheim CB. Galanin inhibits insulin secretion by direct interference with exocytosis. FEBS Lett 1989;247:401–4.

219. Ullrich S, Wollheim CB. GTP-dependent inhibition of insulin secretion by epinephrine in permeabilized RINm5F cells: lack of correlation between insulin secretion and cyclic AMP levels. J Biol Chem 1988;263: 8615–20.

220. Nakaki T, Nakadate T, Kato R. α_2-Adrenoceptors modulating insulin release from isolated pancreatic islets. Naunyn-Schmiedeberg's Arch Pharmacol 1980;313:151–3.

221. Dunning BE, Taborsky GJ Jr. Galanin—sympathetic neurotransmitter in endocrine pancreas? Diabetes 1988; 37:1157–62.

222. Amiranoff B, Servin AL, Rouyer-Fessard C, et al. Galanin receptors in a hamster pancreatic β-cell tumor: identification and molecular characterization. Endocrinology 1987;121:284–9.

223. D'Alessio DA, Sieber C, Beglinger C, Ensinck JW. A physiologic role for somatostatin 28 as a regulator of insulin secretion. J Clin Invest 1989;84:857–62.

224. Amherdt M, Patel YC, Orci L. Selective binding of somatostatin-14 and somatostatin-28 to islet cells revealed by quantitative electron microscopic autoradiography. J Clin Invest 1987;80:1455–8.

225. Mandarino L, Stenner D, Blanchard W, et al. Selective effects of somatostatin-14, -25 and -28 on in vitro insulin and glucagon secretion. Nature 1981;291:76–7.

226. Leahy JL, Vandekerkhove KM. Insulin-like growth factor-I at physiological concentrations is a potent inhibitor of insulin secretion. Endocrinology 1990;126:1593–8.

227. Van Schravendijk CFH, Foriers A, Van den Brande JL, Pipeleers DG. Evidence for the presence of type I insulin-like growth factor receptors on rat pancreatic A and B cells. Endocrinology 1987;121:1784–6.

228. Efendic S, Tatemoto K, Mutt V, et al. Pancreastatin and islet hormone release. Proc Natl Acad Sci USA 1987; 84:7257–60.

229. Eiden LE. Is chromogranin a prohormone? Nature 1987;325:301.

230. Giugliano D, Torella R, Lefèbvre PJ, D'Onofrio F. Opioid peptides and metabolic regulation. Diabetologia 1988; 31:3–15.

231. Verspohl EJ, Berger U, Ammon HPT. The significance of μ- and δ-receptors in rat pancreatic islets for the opioid-mediated insulin release. Biochim Biophys Acta 1986;888:217–24.

232. Ahren B, Pettersson M. Calcitonin gene-related peptide (CGRP) and amylin and the endocrine pancreas. Int J Pancreatol 1990;6:1.

233. Nishi M, Sanke T, Nagamatsu S, et al. Islet amyloid polypeptide: a new β-cell secretory product related to islet amyloid deposits. J Biol Chem 1990;265:4173–6.

234. Kanatsuka A, Makino H, Ohsawa H, et al. Secretion of islet amyloid polypeptide in response to glucose. FEBS Lett 1989;259:199–201.

235. Kahn SE, D'Alessio DA, Schwartz MW, et al. Evidence of cosecretion of islet amyloid polypeptide and insulin by β-cells. Diabetes 1990;39:634–8.

236. Ohsawa H, Kanatsuka A, Yamaguchi T, et al. Islet amyloid polypeptide inhibits glucose-stimulated insulin secretion from isolated rat pancreatic islets. Biochem Biophys Res Commun 1989;160:961–7.

237. Nagamatsu S, Carroll RJ, Grodsky GM, Steiner DF. Lack of islet amyloid polypeptide regulation of insulin biosynthesis or secretion in normal rat islets. Diabetes 1990; 39:871–4.

238. Hermans MP, Schmeer W, Henquin JC. The permissive effect of glucose, tolbutamide and high K^+ on arginine stimulation of insulin release in isolated mouse islets. Diabetologia 1987;30:659–65.

239. Easom RA, Landt M, Colca JR, et al. Effects of insulin secretagogues on protein kinase C-catalyzed phosphorylation of an endogenous substrate in isolated pancreatic islets. J Biol Chem 1990;265:14938–46.

240. Bolaffi JL, Rodd GG, Ma YH, et al. The role of Ca^{2+}-related events in glucose-stimulated desensitization of insulin secretion. Endocrinology 1991;129:2131–8.

241. Levin SR, Grodsky GM, Hagura R, et al. Relationships between arginine and glucose in the induction of insulin secretion from the isolated perfused rat pancreas. Endocrinology 1972;90:624–31.

242. Nesher R, Waldman L, Cerasi E. Time-dependent inhibition of insulin release: glucose-arginine interactions in the perfused rat pancreas. Diabetologia 1984;26:146–9.

243. Grill V, Adamson U, Cerasi E. Immediate and time-dependent effects of glucose on insulin release from rat pancreatic tissue. J Clin Invest 1978;61:1034–43.

244. Grill V, Rundfeldt M. Effects of priming with D-glucose on insulin secretion from rat pancreatic islets: increased responsiveness to other secretagogues. Endocrinology 1979;105:980–7.

245. Borg LAH, Westberg M, Grill V. The priming effect of glucose on insulin release does not involve redistribution of secretory granules within the pancreatic B-cell. Mol Cell Endocrinol 1988;56:219–25.

246. Chalmers JA, Sharp GWG. The importance of Ca^{2+} for glucose-induced priming in pancreatic islets. Biochim Biophys Acta 1989;1011:46–51.

247. Zawalich WS, Zawalich KC, Rasmussen H. Cholinergic agonists prime the β-cell to glucose stimulation. Endocrinology 1989;125:2400–6.

248. Schubart UK, Erlichman J, Fleischer N. Regulation of insulin release and protein phosphorylation by calcium

and cyclic AMP: possible role for calmodulin. In: Cheung WY, ed. Calcium and cell function. Vol 3. New York: Academic Press, 1982:381–407.

249. Harrison DE, Ashcroft SJH, Christie MR, Lord JM. Protein phosphorylation in the pancreatic B-cell. Experientia 1984;40:1075–84.

250. Howell SL. The mechanism of insulin secretion. Diabetologia 1984;26:319–27.

251. Valverde I, Malaisse WJ. Calmodulin and pancreatic B-cell function. Experientia 1984;40:1061–8.

252. Fleischer N, Erlichman J. Intracellular signals and protein phosphorylation: regulatory mechanisms in the control of insulin secretion from the pancreatic beta cell. In: Draznin B, Melmed S, Leroith D, eds. Insulin secretion. New York: Alan R Liss, 1989:107–16.

253. Sener A, Dunlop ME, Gomis R, et al. Role of transglutaminase in insulin release: study with glycine and sarcosine methylesters. Endocrinology 1985;117:237–42.

254. Bungay PJ, Owen RA, Coutts IC, Griffin M. A role for transglutaminase in glucose-stimulated insulin release from the pancreatic β-cell. Biochem J 1986;235:269–78.

255. Matthews EK. Calcium translocation and control mechanisms for endocrine secretion. In: Hopkins CR, Duncan CJ, eds. Secretory mechanisms. Symp Soc Exp Biol 1979; 33:225–49.

256. Lacy PE, Howell SL, Young DA, Fink CJ. New hypothesis of insulin secretion. Nature 1968;219:1177–9.

257. Gomperts BD. Ge: a GTP-binding protein mediating exocytosis. Annu Rev Physiol 1990;52:591–606.

258. Lambert AE, Kanazawa Y, Burr IM, et al. On the role of cyclic AMP in insulin release: overall effects in cultured fetal rat pancreas. Ann NY Acad Sci 1971;185:232–44.

259. Asplund K, Andersson A, Jarousse C, Hellerström C. Function of the fetal endocrine pancreas. Isr J Med Sci 1975;11:581–90.

260. Kervran A, Randon J. Development of insulin release by fetal rat pancreas in vitro. Effects of glucose, amino acids, and theophylline. Diabetes 1980;29:673–8.

261. Hole RL, Pian-Smith MCM, Sharp GWG. Development of the biphasic response to glucose in fetal and neonatal rat pancreas. Am J Physiol 1988;254:E167–74.

262. Grill V, Lake W, Freinkel N. Generalized diminution in the response to nutrients as insulin-releasing agents during the early neonatal period in the rat. Diabetes 1981; 30:56–63.

263. Mourmeaux JL, Remacle C, Henquin JC. Effects of stimulation of adenylate cyclase and protein kinase-C on cultured fetal rat B-cells. Endocrinology 1989;125: 2536–44.

264. Rorsman P, Arkhammar P, Bokvist K, et al. Failure of glucose to elicit a normal secretory response in fetal pancreatic beta cells results from glucose insensitivity of the ATP-regulated K$^+$ channels. Proc Natl Acad Sci USA 1989;86:4505–9.

265. Freinkel N, Lewis NJ, Johnson R, et al. Differential effects of age versus glycemic stimulation on the maturation of insulin stimulus-secretion coupling during culture of fetal rat islets. Diabetes 1984;33:1028–38.

266. Reaven EP, Gold G, Reaven GM. Effects of age on glucose-stimulated insulin release by the β-cell of the rat. J Clin Invest 1979;64:591–9.

267. Molina JM, Premdas FH, Lipson LG. Insulin release in aging: dynamic response of isolated islets of Langerhans of the rat to D-glucose and D-glyceraldehyde. Endocrinology 1985:116:821–6.

268. Sartin JL. Chaudhuri M, Farina S, Adelman RC. Regulation of insulin secretion by glucose during aging. J Gerontol 1986;41:30–5.

269. Ammon HPT, Fahmy A, Mark M, et al. The effect of glucose on insulin release and ion movements in isolated pancreatic islets of rats in old age. J Physiol 1987;384:347–54.

270. Wang SY, Halban PA, Rowe JW. Effects of aging on insulin synthesis and secretion: differential effects on preproinsulin messenger RNA levels, proinsulin biosynthesis, and secretion of newly made and preformed insulin in the rat. J Clin Invest 1988;81:176–84.

271. Curry DL, Safarik RH, Reaven E. Effect of age on the insulin secretory response of perfused rat pancreas to arginine and tolbutamide. Horm Metab Res 1987;19:453–7.

272. Chen M, Bergman RN, Pacini G, Porte D Jr. Pathogenesis of age-related glucose intolerance in man: insulin resistance and decreased β-cell function. J Clin Endocrinol Metab 1985;60:13–20.

273. Gumbiner B, Polonsky KS, Beltz WF, et al. Effects of aging on insulin secretion. Diabetes 1989;38:1549–56.

274. Levy J, Herchuelz A, Sener A, Malaisse WJ. The stimulus-secretion coupling of glucose-induced insulin release. XX. Fasting: a model for altered glucose recognition by the B-cell. Metabolism 1976;25:583–91.

275. Zawalich WS, Dye ES, Pagliara AS, et al. Starvation diabetes in the rat: onset, recovery, and specificity of reduced responsiveness of pancreatic β-cells. Endocrinology 1979;104:1344–51.

276. Wolters GHJ, Konijnendijk W, Bouman PR. Effects of fasting on insulin secretion, islet glucose metabolism, and the cyclic adenosine 3′,5′-monophosphate content of rat pancreatic islets in vitro. Diabetes 1977; 26:530–7.

277. Tiedge M, Lenzen S. Regulation of glucokinase and GLUT-2 glucose-transporter gene expression in pancreatic B-cells. Biochem J 1991;279:899–901.

278. Iynedjian PB, Pilot P-R, Nouspikel T, et al. Differential expression and regulation of the glucokinase gene in liver and islets of Langerhans. Proc Natl Acad Sci USA 1989;86:7838–42.

279. Mikines KJ, Sonne B, Farrell PA, et al. Effect of training on the dose-response relationship for insulin action in men. J Appl Physiol 1989;66:695–703.

280. Zawalich W, Maturo S, Felig P. Influence of physical training on insulin release and glucose utilization by islet cells and liver glucokinase activity in the rat. Am J Physiol 1982;243:E464–9.

281. Shima K, Hirota M, Sato M, et al. Effect of exercise training on insulin and glucagon release from perfused rat pancreas. Horm Metab Res 1987;19:395–9.

282. Koranyi LI, Bourey RE, Slentz CA, et al. Coordinate reduction of rat pancreatic islet glucokinase and proinsulin mRNA by exercise training. Diabetes 1991;40:401–4.

283. Green IC, Howell SL, Montague W, Taylor KW. Regulation of insulin release from isolated islets of Langerhans of the rat in pregnancy. Biochem J 1973;134:481–7.

284. Bone AJ, Howell SL. Alterations in regulation of insulin biosynthesis in pregnancy and starvation studied in isolated rat islets of Langerhans. Biochem J 1977;166:501–7.

285. Lipson LG, Sharp GWG. Insulin release in pregnancy: studies on adenylate cyclase, phosphodiesterase, protein kinase, and phosphoprotein phosphatase in isolated rat islets of Langerhans. Endocrinology 1978;103:1272–80.

286. Kalkhoff RK, Kim HJ. Effects of pregnancy on insulin and glucagon secretion by perifused rat pancreatic islets. Endocrinology 1978;102:623–31.

287. Sheridan JD, Anaya PA, Parsons JA, Sorenson RL. Increased

dye coupling in pancreatic islets from rats in late-term pregnancy. Diabetes 1988;37:908–11.

288. Green IC, Taylor KW. Insulin secretory response of isolated islets of Langerhans in pregnant rats: effects of dietary restriction. J Endocrinol 1974;62:137–43.

289. Brelje TC, Sorenson RL. Role of prolactin versus growth hormone on islet B-cell proliferation in vitro: implications for pregnancy. Endocrinology 1991;128:45–57.

290. Hubinont CJ, Dufrane SP, Garcia-Morales P, et al. Influence of lactation upon pancreatic islet function. Endocrinology 1986;118:687–94.

291. Michaels RL, Sorenson RL, Parsons JA, Sheridan JD. Prolactin enhances cell-to-cell communication among β-cells in pancreatic islets. Diabetes 1987;36:1098–103.

292. Madon RJ, Ensor DM, Flint DJ. Hypoinsulinaemia in the lactating rat is caused by a decreased glycaemic stimulus to the pancreas. J Endocrinol 1990;125:81–8.

293. Parman AU. Effects of hypophysectomy and short-term growth hormone replacement on insulin release from and glucose metabolism in isolated rat islets of Langerhans. J Endocrinol 1975;67:1–8.

294. Whittaker PG, Taylor KW. Direct effects of growth hormone on rat islets of Langerhans in tissue culture. Diabetologia 1980;18:323–8.

295. Billestrup N, Nielsen JH. The stimulatory effect of growth hormone, prolactin, and placental lactogen on β-cell proliferation is not mediated by insulin-like growth factor-I. Endocrinology 1991;129:883–8.

296. Lenzen S, Bailey CJ. Thyroid hormones, gonadal and adrenocortical steroids and the function of the islets of Langerhans. Endocrine Rev 1984;5:411–34.

297. Fischer B, Rausch U, Wollny P, et al. Immunohistochemical localization of the glucocorticoid receptor in pancreatic β-cells of the rat. Endocrinology 1990;126:2635–41.

298. Kadowaki S, Norman AW. Dietary vitamin D is essential for normal insulin secretion from the perfused rat pancreas. J Clin Invest 1984;73:759–66.

299. Tanaka Y, Seino Y, Ishida M, et al. Effect of 1,25-dihydroxyvitamin D_3 on insulin secretion: direct or mediated? Endocrinology 1986;118:1971–6.

300. d'Emden MC, Dunlop M, Larkins RG, Wark JD. The in vitro effect of 1α,25-dihydroxyvitamin D_3 on insulin production by neonatal rat islets. Biochem Biophys Res Commun 1989;164:413–8.

301. Espinosa de los Monteros AM, Driscoll SG, Steinke J. Insulin release from isolated human fetal pancreatic islets. Science 1970;168:1111–2.

302. Milner RDG, Ashworth MA, Barson AJ. Insulin release from human foetal pancreas in response to glucose, leucine and arginine. J Endocrinol 1972;52:497–505.

303. Andersson A, Borg H, Groth C-G, et al. Survival of isolated human islets of Langerhans maintained in tissue culture. J Clin Invest 1976;57:1295–301.

304. Grant AM, Christie MR, Ashcroft SJH. Insulin release from human pancreatic islets in vitro. Diabetologia 1980;19:114–7.

305. Harrison DE, Christie MR, Gray DWR. Properties of isolated human islets of Langerhans: insulin secretion, glucose oxidation and protein phosphorylation. Diabetologia 1985;28:99–103.

306. Rhodes CJ, Campbell IL, Szopa TM, et al. Effects of glucose and D-3-hydroxybutyrate on human pancreatic islet cell function. Clin Sci 1985;68:567–72.

307. Bedoya FJ, Wilson JM, Ghosh AK, et al. The glucokinase glucose sensor in human pancreatic islet tissue. Diabetes 1986;35:61–70.

308. Ashcroft FM, Kakei M, Kelly RP, et al. ATP-sensitive K channels in isolated human pancreatic β-cells. FEBS Lett 1987;215:9–12.

309. Turk J, Hughes JH, Easom RA, et al. Arachidonic acid metabolism and insulin secretion by isolated human pancreatic islets. Diabetes 1988;37:992–6.

310. Misler S, Gee WM, Gillis KD, et al. Metabolite-regulated ATP-sensitive K^+ channel in human pancreatic islet cells. Diabetes 1989;38:422–7.

311. Ashcroft FM, Kakei M, Gibson JS, et al. The ATP- and tolbutamide-sensitivity of the ATP-sensitive K-channel from human pancreatic B cells. Diabetologia 1989;32:591–8.

312. Permutt MA, Koranyi L, Keller K, et al. Cloning and functional expression of a human pancreatic islet glucose-transporter cDNA. Proc Natl Acad Sci USA 1989;86:8688–92.

313. Misler S, Barnett DW, Pressel DM, et al. Stimulus secretion coupling in beta-cells of transplantable human islets of Langerhans. Evidence for a role of Ca^{2+}. Diabetes 1992;41:662–70.

314. Henquin JC. Adenosine triphosphate sensitive K^+ channels may not be the sole regulators of glucose-induced electrical activity in pancreatic B-cells. Endocrinology 1992;131:127–31.

315. Gembal M, Detimary P, Gilon P, et al. Mechanisms by which glucose can control insulin release independently from its action on ATP-sensitive K^+ channels in mouse B-cells. J Clin Invest 1993;91:871–80.

Chapter 5

INSULIN SECRETION IN VIVO

NIALL M. O'MEARA
KENNETH S. POLONSKY

The classic experiments of Von Mering and Minkowski at the turn of the last century demonstrating that pancreatectomy in dogs resulted in hyperglycemia[1] focused attention on the important role of the pancreas in maintaining glucose homeostasis in vivo. Banting and Best,[2] by reversing this hyperglycemia with internal secretions of the pancreas, confirmed the belief that the islets of Langerhans were the key cells within the pancreas responsible for maintaining normal blood glucose levels. Although the isolation and purification of insulin rapidly followed, many years passed before sensitive techniques for evaluating β-cell function were devised. Since these techniques are critical to the analysis of insulin secretion in vivo, they will be discussed at the outset.

METHODS OF QUANTITATING β-CELL FUNCTION

The development of a sensitive radioimmunoassay for the measurement of insulin levels was the first major advance in our attempts to understand how the β-cell functions in vivo.[3] For many years afterwards, the measurement of peripheral levels of insulin was the gold standard used to evaluate β-cell secretory activity.[4-7] This approach, however, is limited by the fact that 50 to 60% of the insulin produced by the pancreas is extracted by the liver without ever reaching the systemic circulation.[8,9] While these problems can, in fact, be overcome by hepatic vein catheterization allied to intraportal infusion of insulin, these techniques can only be applied in an investigational setting and, even then, are only of value under steady-state conditions.[10] The standard radioimmunoassay for the measurement of insulin concentrations is also limited by its inability to distinguish between endogenous and exogenous insulin, making it ineffective as a measure of endogenous β-cell reserve in the

insulin-treated diabetic patient. The problem is further compounded by the development in many of these patients of antibodies to insulin, which interfere in the interpretation of serum levels of immunoreactive insulin. Another disadvantage of the conventional insulin radioimmunoassay is its inability to distinguish between levels of circulating proinsulin and true levels of circulating insulin.

Following the discovery of proinsulin, the single-chain precursor of insulin,[11] and the identification of the biosynthetic pathway of insulin within the β-cell,[12] β-cell secretory products in addition to insulin were found in the circulation. These included proinsulin, proinsulin conversion intermediates (split proinsulins), and connecting peptide (C-peptide). Within the islet cells, proinsulin undergoes cleavage at the Golgi apparatus,[13] a reaction that leads to the formation of insulin, C-peptide, and two pairs of basic amino acids. Insulin is subsequently released into the circulation at concentrations equimolar to those of C-peptide.[12-14] In addition, small amounts of intact proinsulin and proinsulin conversion intermediates are released. Although these molecules constitute 20% of the total circulating insulin-like immunoreactivity,[15] they are much less potent than insulin biologically. It has been estimated that the biologic potency of proinsulin in vivo is only 10% of that of insulin,[16,17] whereas the potency of split proinsulin is between that of proinsulin and insulin.[18,19] The low concentrations of proinsulin and split proinsulins in serum, however, ensure that in vivo, under normal physiologic conditions, their effects are negligible. In contrast to insulin and proinsulin, C-peptide has no known metabolic effects.[20,21] Unlike insulin, C-peptide is not extracted by the liver[9,22,23] and is excreted almost exclusively by the kidneys. Its plasma half-life of approximately 30 minutes[24] contrasts sharply with that of insulin, which is approximately 4 minutes.

Since C-peptide is secreted in equimolar concentrations with insulin and is not extracted by the liver, many investigators have used levels of C-peptide as a marker of β-cell function. While C-peptide levels are usually measured in plasma, C-peptide levels in urine have also been used to evaluate endogenous insulin secretion.[25–28] This approach is limited, however, since the fraction of the secreted C-peptide that appears in the urine varies considerably among subjects and even in the same subject studied on different occasions.[29] The use of plasma C-peptide levels as an index of β-cell function is dependent on the critical assumption that the mean clearance rates of C-peptide are constant over the range of C-peptide levels observed under normal physiologic conditions. This assumption has been shown to be valid for both dogs and humans[9,30] and this approach can be used to derive rates of insulin secretion from plasma concentrations of C-peptide under steady-state conditions.[30] Because of the long plasma half-life of C-peptide, under non-steady-state conditions (e.g., following a glucose infusion) peripheral plasma levels of C-peptide do not change in proportion to the changing insulin secretory rate.[30,31] Thus, under these conditions, insulin secretion rates are best calculated with use of the two-compartment model initially proposed by Eaton and co-workers.[32] This approach involves nonlinear least-squares regression analysis of C-peptide decay curves to derive model parameters in individual subjects. Once the fractional rate constants and distribution volume are known, the peripheral concentrations of C-peptide can be analyzed mathematically and the corresponding secretion rates derived. Estimates of the secretion rate of insulin in human subjects determined by this method are quite accurate—reportedly 98 ± 3% of the actual rate as rates of insulin secretion are increasing and 100 ± 2% as they are decreasing.[30] Similar findings have been reported for dogs.[33]

Rates of insulin secretion have also been measured by calculating the difference between arterial and hepatic venous C-peptide and by multiplying this difference by the estimated hepatic plasma flow,[34,35] an approach designed to overcome the inherent difficulty of performing portal venous cannulation in humans. Rates of insulin secretion determined by this method are similar to those obtained with other methods, but the technique is invasive and by its nature can only be applied in an investigational setting.

In summary, under steady-state conditions, levels of C-peptide in whole plasma provide an accurate index of the insulin secretory rate, while under non-steady-state conditions, rates of β-cell secretion of insulin can be derived more accurately and easily from mathematical analysis of peripheral C-peptide concentrations with use of a two-compartment model. In interpreting the validity of experimental results evaluating insulin secretion in vivo, one should always take into account the limitations of the method used to assess β-cell function.

REGULATION OF INSULIN SECRETION

Carbohydrate Nutrients

The most important physiologic substance involved in the regulation of insulin release is glucose.[36–38] The effect of glucose on the β-cell is dose-related. Dose-dependent increases in concentrations of insulin and C-peptide and in rates of insulin secretion have been observed following oral and intravenous glucose loads, with 1.4 units (about 50 μg) of insulin, on average, being secreted in response to an oral glucose load as small as 12 g [34,39–41] (Fig. 5–1). The insulin secretory response is greater after oral than after intravenous glucose administration.[41–44] Known as the incretin effect,[40,45] this enhanced response to oral glucose has been interpreted as an indication that absorption of glucose by way of the gastrointestinal tract stimulates the release of hormones and other mechanisms that ultimately enhance the sensitivity of the β-cell to glucose (see section on hormonal factors below). In a recent study involving nine volunteers in whom glucose was infused at a rate designed to achieve levels previously attained following an oral glucose load, the amount of insulin secreted in response to the intravenous load was 26% less than that secreted in response to the oral load.[44]

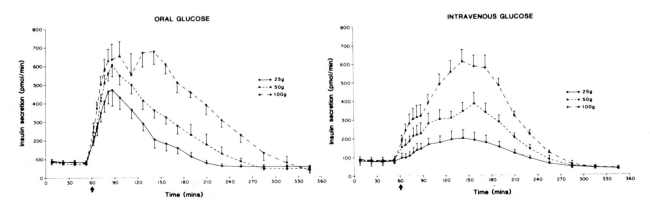

Fig. 5–1.   Insulin secretory responses to graded glucose doses following oral (left) and intravenous (right) administration. Reprinted with permission from reference 41 (Tillel H, Shapiro ET, Miller MA, et al. Dose-dependent effects of oral and intravenous glucose on insulin secretion and clearance in normal humans. Am J Physiol 1988;254:E349–57).

Insulin secretion does not respond as a linear function of glucose concentration. The relationship of glucose concentration to the rate of insulin release follows a sigmoidal curve, with a threshold corresponding to the glucose levels normally seen under fasting conditions and with the steep portion of the dose-response curve corresponding to the range of glucose levels normally achieved postprandially.[46-48] The sigmoidal nature of the dose-response curve has been attributed to a Gaussian distribution of thresholds for stimulation among the individual β-cells.[48-50]

When glucose is infused intravenously at a constant rate, an initial biphasic secretory response is observed that consists of a rapid, early insulin peak followed by a second, more slowly rising, peak.[36,51,52] The significance of the first-phase insulin release is unclear but may reflect the existence of a compartment of readily releasable insulin within the β-cell or a transient rise and fall of a metabolic signal for insulin secretion.[53] Despite earlier suggestions to the contrary,[54,55] a recent report has demonstrated that the first-phase response to intravenous glucose is highly reproducible within subjects.[56] Following the acute response, a second phase of insulin release occurs that is directly related to the level of glucose elevation. Recent in vitro studies of isolated islet cells and the perfused pancreas have identified a third phase of insulin secretion commencing 1.5 to 3.0 hours after exposure to glucose and characterized by a spontaneous decline in secretion to 15 to 25% of the amount released during peak secretion—a level subsequently maintained for more than 48 hours.[57-60]

The effects of a variety of other sugars, sugar derivatives, and sugar alcohols on the β-cell have also been examined.[61] D-glucose, D-mannose, D-glyceraldehyde, dihydroxyacetone, D-glucosamine, N-acetylglucosamine, fructose, and galactose have all been shown to be stimulators or potentiators of insulin secretion in vitro. In vivo studies in dogs and humans suggest that xylitol and sorbitol also enhance β-cell function.

The insulin secretory response to glucose exhibits anomeric specificity, the α-anomer being a more potent stimulator of insulin release than the β-anomer.[62] Similar results have been obtained with mannose.[63] Since α-anomers are more readily metabolized by the glycolytic pathway than are β-anomers,[64,65] it has been suggested that the metabolism of glucose and mannose within the β-cell is a prerequisite for the production of intracellular signals that trigger insulin release in response to these secretagogues. In support of this suggestion is the observation that mannoheptulose, an inhibitor of the glycolytic enzyme glucokinase, blocks the insulin secretory response to glucose. Similarly, iodoacetate, an inhibitor of glyceraldehyde dehydrogenase, blocks the β-cell response to hexoses.[66]

Noncarbohydrate Nutrients

Amino acids have been shown to stimulate insulin release in the absence of glucose, the most potent secretagogues being the essential amino acids leucine, arginine, and lysine.[67,68] Although leucine was the first amino acid to be studied, experiments with high-protein meals showed that the observed β-cell stimulation could not be attributed solely to the leucine content of the meals. Indeed, the effects of arginine and lysine on the β-cell appear to be more potent than that of leucine. Although the effects of amino acids on insulin secretion are independent of concomitant changes in glucose levels, the effects are potentiated by glucose.[68-70] The response of the islet cells to a series of amino acid metabolites has also been evaluated. Phenylpyruvate, α-ketoiscaproate, α-keto-β-methylvalerate, and α-ketocaproate are potent stimulators of insulin release, and most are effective in the absence of glucose.[61,71]

In contrast to amino acids, various lipids and their metabolites appear to have only minor effects on insulin release. Although carbohydrate-rich fat meals stimulate insulin secretion, carbohydrate-free fat meals have minimal effects on β-cell function.[72] Thus, while ketone bodies, as well as short- and long-chain fatty acids, have been shown to potentiate the insulin secretory response in islet cells, their exact role under physiologic conditions remains to be elucidated.

Hormonal Factors

The release of insulin from the β-cell following a meal is facilitated by a number of gastrointestinal peptide hormones, including glucose-dependent insulinotropic peptide (GIP), cholecystokinin (CCK), and glucagon-like peptide 1 (GLP-1).[45,73-80] These hormones are released from intestinal endocrine cells postprandially and travel in the bloodstream to reach the β-cells, where they act through second messengers to increase the sensitivity of these islet cells to glucose. In general, these hormones are not of themselves secretagogues, and their effects are only evident in the presence of hyperglycemia.[73-75] The release of these peptides may explain why the modest postprandial glucose levels achieved in normal subjects in vivo have such a dramatic effect on insulin production whereas similar glucose concentrations in vitro elicit a much smaller response.[80] Similarly, it could account for the greater β-cell response observed following oral as opposed to intravenous glucose administration. The postprandial insulin secretory response may also be influenced by other intestinal peptide hormones, including vasoactive intestinal polypeptide (VIP),[81] secretin,[82,83] and gastrin,[82,84] but the precise role of these hormones remains to be elucidated.

The hormones produced by the α- and δ-cells also modulate insulin release. While glucagon has a stimulatory effect on the β-cell,[85] somatostatin suppresses insulin release.[86] It is currently unclear whether these hormones reach the β-cell by traveling through the islet cell interstitium (thus exerting a paracrine effect) or through islet cell capillaries. Indeed, the importance of these two hormones in regulating basal and postprandial insulin levels under normal physiologic circumstances is in doubt. Paradoxically, the low insulin levels observed during prolonged periods of starvation have been attributed to the elevated glucagon concentrations seen in this setting.[72,87–90] Whether glucagon acts through its own receptor or through the GLP-1 receptor remains to be determined.

Other hormones that exert a stimulatory role on insulin secretion include growth hormone,[91] glucocorticoids,[92] prolactin,[93–95] placental lactogen,[96] and the sex steroids.[97] While all of the above hormones may stimulate insulin secretion indirectly by inducing a state of insulin resistance, some also may act directly on the β-cell, possibly to augment its sensitivity to glucose. Thus, hyperinsulinemia is associated with conditions in which these hormones are present in excess, such as acromegaly, Cushing's syndrome, and the second half of pregnancy. Furthermore, treatment with placental lactogen,[98] hydrocortisone,[99] or growth hormone[99,100] are all effective in reversing the reduction in insulin response to glucose that is observed in vitro after hypophysectomy. Although hyperinsulinemia following an oral glucose load has been observed in patients with hyperthyroidism,[101,102] the increased concentration of immunoreactive insulin in this setting may reflect elevations in serum proinsulin rather than a true increase in serum insulin.[103]

Neural Factors

The islets are innervated by both the cholinergic and adrenergic limbs of the autonomic nervous system. While both sympathetic and parasympathetic stimulation enhance secretion of glucagon and suppress secretion of somatostatin,[104,105] the secretion of insulin is stimulated by vagal nerve fibers and inhibited by sympathetic nerve fibers.[104–109] This adrenergic inhibition of the β-cell appears to be mediated by the α adrenoceptor since it may be attenuated by the α antagonist phentolamine.[105] While the effects of parasympathetic and sympathetic stimulation on islet cell function may be direct, it is possible that stimulation of these fibers may simply activate (or suppress) intrinsic pancreatic peptidergic nerves that in turn modulate the release of insulin.[45]

The importance of the autonomic nervous system in regulating insulin secretion in vivo is unclear. Studies in animals[110,111] and humans[112,113] have emphasized the importance of the cephalic phase of insulin release—that occurring at the sight, smell, and expectation of food—in regulating the postprandial glucose response. It has been suggested that this reflex, which is under vagal control,[80,114] may have a key role in minimizing the early rise in glucose levels following meals.[113] Since cholinergic agonists increase the response of the β-cell to glucose in vitro,[115] this may be the mechanism by which vagal stimulation achieves its effect. Decreased glucose tolerance following vagotomy has been reported in human subjects[116,117] and following islet denervation in rats,[118,119] whereas the insulin secretory response to meals is delayed in patients who have undergone pancreatic transplantation.[120] However, many of these patients remain euglycemic without therapy following transplantation.[120–123] Therefore, the importance of the parasympathetic nervous system in maintaining glucose tolerance is unclear. For similar reasons, doubts exist about whether the sympathetic nerve fibers innervating the islets exert a major influence on the basal or postprandial insulin secretory responses. It is possible, however, that inhibition of insulin secretion mediated by the sympathetic nervous system could in part account for the deteriorating glycemic control reported in individuals with diabetes who are under severe stress.[106,124,125]

The neural effects on β-cell function cannot be entirely dissociated from the hormonal effects, since some of the neurotransmitters of the autonomic nervous system are in fact hormones. Furthermore, the secretion of insulinotropic hormones such as GIP postprandially has been shown to be under vagal[126] and adrenergic[127] control.

TEMPORAL PATTERN OF INSULIN SECRETION

It has been estimated that, in any 24-hour period, 50% of the total insulin secreted by the pancreas is secreted under basal conditions and that the remainder is secreted in response to meals.[128,129] The estimated basal insulin secretion rates range from 18 to 32 units/24 hours (0.7 to 1.3 mg).[30,32,34,128] Moreover, the secretion of insulin is pulsatile, with major pulses being observed every 1.5 to 2 hours[129–133] (Fig. 5–2). These ultradian pulses are present in the basal state but are amplified postprandially.[129,130] These pulses have also been observed in subjects receiving glucose intravenously,[132,133] suggesting that they are not dependent on food ingestion and are not generated by intermittent absorption of nutrients from the gut. Furthermore, they do not appear to be related to fluctuations in glucagon or cortisol levels.[132] Many of these insulin and C-peptide pulses are synchronous with pulses in glucose levels,[129,132,133] and recent evidence suggests that these insulin secretory pulses may actually be entrained by glucose.[134]

Experimental evidence from studies of animals and humans suggests that superimposed on these large-amplitude ultradian pulses are more-rapid oscillations in β-cell activity that occur at a periodicity of 8 to 16 minutes.[135–141] These rapid oscillations in insulin and C-peptide levels do not appear to be coupled as tightly as the ultradian pulses to changes in glucose levels.[138,140,142,143] The frequency of these rapid oscillations varies from study to study, and wide variability between subjects is seen even within studies. Accordingly, the physiologic significance of these rapid oscillations in the peripheral circulation is unclear. Although the amplitude of the rapid oscillations is very low in the peripheral circulation, it is much greater in the portal circulation (Fig. 5–3), where these rapid oscillations may have an important biologic function.[143] In this regard, it is possible that the liver responds more favorably to insulin delivered in a pulsatile fashion than to insulin delivered at a constant rate.[144–146]

Circadian variations in the secretion of insulin have also been reported. When insulin secretory responses are measured during a 24-hour period during which subjects receive three standard meals, the maximal postprandial responses are observed after breakfast.[6,129,147] These findings are mirrored by the results of studies in which subjects were tested for oral glucose tolerance at different times of the day and were found to exhibit maximal

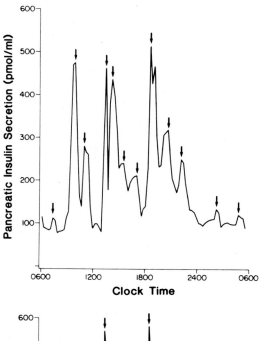

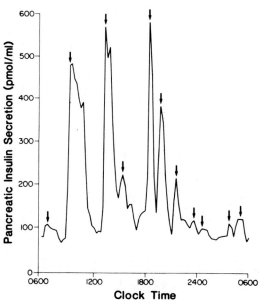

Fig. 5–2. Two 24-hour profiles of insulin secretion from normal-weight subjects. Meals were eaten at 0900, 1300, and 1800. Statistically significant pulses of secretion are shown by the arrows. Reprinted with permission of the American Society of Clinical Investigation from reference 129 (Polonsky KS, Given BD, Van Cauter E. Twenty-four-hour profiles and pulsatile patterns of insulin secretion in normal and obese subjects. J Clin Invest 1988;81:442–8).

insulin secretory responses in the morning and lower responses in the afternoon and evening.[148–150] These diurnal differences are also noted in tests for intravenous glucose tolerance. Furthermore, although ultradian glucose and insulin oscillations are closely correlated during a constant 24-hour glucose infusion, the nocturnal rise in mean glucose levels is not accompanied by a similar increase in the insulin secretory rate.[133] It has been

postulated that these diurnal differences may reflect a diminished responsiveness of the β-cell to glucose in the afternoon and evening.[150]

INSULIN SECRETION FOLLOWING EXERCISE

The effects of exercise on β-cell function have also been evaluated extensively. Individuals who exercise regularly have reduced fasting levels of insulin and C-peptide[151–153] and also exhibit a reduction in the release of these hormones following a carbohydrate load. This reduction has been seen following a 100-g oral glucose load[154,155] and during hyperglycemic clamping, during which reductions in both first-phase and second-phase secretory responses have been described.[151–154,156] Despite these changes, these subjects have normal or even improved glucose tolerance,[151,156] suggesting that insulin sensitivity is improved in those who exercise regularly. This finding has been confirmed by the observation of increased rates of glucose disposal in athletes during hyperinsulinemic euglycemic clamping.[151,156]

Altered β-cell responses to glucose are apparent even after short periods of exercise and have been observed in

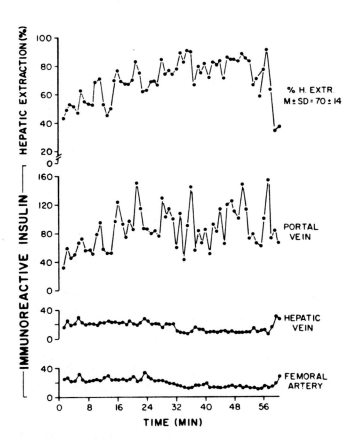

Fig. 5–3. Simultaneous minute-to-minute insulin levels in portal vein, hepatic vein, femoral artery, and derived hepatic insulin extraction in one dog. Because of substantial hepatic extraction of insulin, pulsatility in posthepatic circulation is markedly dampened. Reprinted with permission from reference 143 (Jaspan JB, Lever E, Polonsky KS, Van Cauter E. In vivo pulsatility of pancreatic islet peptides. Am J Physiol 1986;251:E215–26).

individuals subjected to as little as 1 hour of exercise, 24 hours before being tested for oral glucose tolerance.[157] Similarly, even in well-trained athletes, insulin responses to glucose increase dramatically within 2 weeks of cessation of exercise.[152] In this latter study, rates of glucose disposal both before and after cessation of exercise were similar, supporting the view that those who exercise regularly are more sensitive to the action of insulin. The altered β-cell responses to glucose observed in athletic subjects may therefore be a compensatory response to the increased sensitivity to insulin in the periphery. Whatever the mechanism, lack of exercise could be a key factor in the pathogenesis of the insulin resistance associated with aging, since fasting insulin levels and insulin secretory responses to glucose in athletes older and younger than 60 years are similar, the responses in both groups being lower than the corresponding responses in young untrained subjects.[154]

INSULIN SECRETION IN THE ELDERLY

Peripheral insulin resistance, impaired glucose tolerance, and postprandial hyperinsulinemia are metabolic changes associated with aging.[158-160] Although insulin secretion is reduced in aging rats,[161-163] the results of studies of elderly human subjects have conflicted—with increased, normal, and decreased β-cell responses having been reported.[164-170] These discrepancies may in part be a reflection of the indirect methods employed to quantitate insulin secretion in some of these studies. In recent experiments, which used a direct approach to quantitation of insulin secretory rates from peripheral C-peptide levels by means of the two-compartment model,[32] 10 elderly subjects demonstrated enhanced insulin secretion under basal conditions, with an accentuation of this response seen postprandially.[171] Plotted as a percentage of the basal secretory rate, the secretory response to meals in these elderly subjects was no different from that of younger controls. However, when glucose levels are matched during hyperglycemic clamping, the insulin secretory response—although normal in absolute terms—is disproportionately low in the elderly patients, especially when viewed in relation to the degree of insulin resistance associated with aging. Thus, while elderly subjects have enhanced rates of insulin secretion, the β-cell responses are lower than those predicted when one takes into account the insulin insensitivity associated with this population subgroup. Diminished insulin clearance does not appear to be a contributory factor to the observed hyperinsulinemia in the elderly.[170,171]

INSULIN SECRETION IN OBESITY

The insulin resistance of obesity is characterized by hyperinsulinemia.[172-177] While hyperinsulinemia in this setting could be a reflection of increased insulin production,[178,179] decreased insulin clearance,[176-180] or a combination, most evidence suggests that increased insulin secretion is the predominant factor.[181] Both basal and 24-hour insulin secretory rates are enhanced in obese

subjects and are strongly correlated with body mass index (Fig. 5–4). The temporal pattern of insulin secretion is not altered in obesity. As in normal subjects, the basal insulin secretion in the obese accounts for 50% of the total daily production of insulin and secretory pulses of insulin occur every 1.5 to 2 hours.[129,181] However, the amplitude of these pulses postprandially is greater in obese subjects. Nevertheless, when these postprandial secretory responses are expressed as a percentage of the basal secretory rate, the postprandial responses in obese and normal subjects are identical (Fig. 5–5). These findings suggest that the increase in insulin secretion in the obese is due not to a hyperresponsiveness to secretory stimuli but rather to the presence of an abnormally large functional β-cell mass. This suggestion is thus consistent with the earlier pathologic observations of Ogilvie, who described an increased number of islet

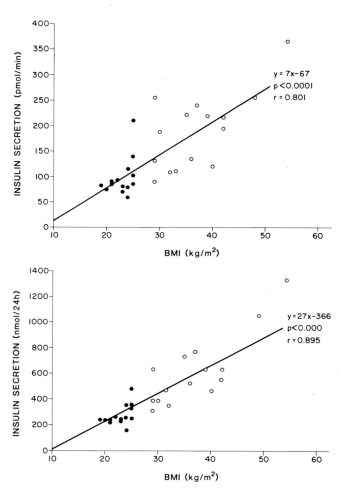

Fig. 5–4. The relationship between body mass index (BMI) and basal (top) or total 24-hour rates of insulin secretion (bottom) in normal (solid circles) and obese (open circles) subjects. Reprinted with permission of the American Society of Clinical Investigation from reference 181 (Polonsky KS, Given BD, Hirsch L, et al. Quantitative study of insulin secretion and clearance in normal and obese subjects. J Clin Invest 1988;81:435–41).

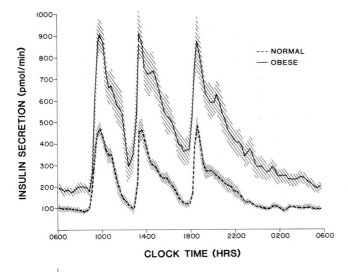

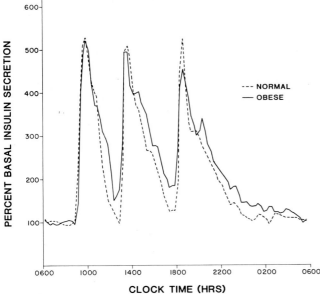

Fig. 5–5. Mean 24-hour profiles of insulin secretion rates in normal and obese subjects (top). The hatched areas represent ±SEM. The curves in the lower panel were derived by dividing the insulin secretion rate measured in each subject by the basal secretion rate derived in the same subject. Mean data for normal and obese subjects are shown. Reprinted with permission of the American Society of Clinical Investigation from reference 129 (Polonsky KS, Given BD, Van Cauter E. Twenty-four-hour profiles and pulsatile patterns of insulin secretion in normal and obese subjects. J Clin Invest 1988;81:442–8).

cells in obese subjects.[182] Rapid oscillations in insulin secretion that occur every 10 to 12 minutes and are similar to those in non-obese subjects have also been found in obese patients, although of an amplitude that tended to be lower than that of the corresponding pulses in the non-obese.[140] It appears, therefore, that the normal regulatory mechanisms controlling insulin secretion in non-obese controls are still operative in hyperinsulinemic obese subjects and that β-cell function is intrinsically normal in this setting.

INSULIN SECRETION IN DIABETES MELLITUS

Patients with Type I diabetes mellitus are insulin-deficient and have practically no β-cell response to glucose and non-glucose stimuli.[125] However, the initial period following diagnosis often is associated with an improvement in glucose tolerance to a degree permitting the maintenance of normoglycemia for a self-limiting duration in some patients in the absence of any definitive therapy.[183] This so-called honeymoon period is associated with increases in the C-peptide and insulin responses to glucose.[7,184–187] Although the secretory capacity of β-cells is improved during this period, it is still less than that observed in normal subjects. A qualitative defect also is present and is manifested in serum by an increased molar ratio of proinsulin to C-peptide.[188–190] Thus, during the honeymoon phase, in addition to secreting less insulin, the pancreas releases greater quantities of immature β-cell granules into the circulation. The subsequent and inevitable deterioration in glycemic control that heralds the end of the honeymoon period is preceded by a gradual reduction in the secretory capacity of the β-cell.[7] The assessment of β-cell function in patients with recently diagnosed Type I diabetes mellitus may be of clinical relevance, in view of the evidence suggesting that the degree of residual β-cell function at this stage is an important prognostic indicator of which patients are most likely to benefit from a period of immunosuppression.[191]

The β-cell secretory responses during the period prior to the onset of Type I diabetes mellitus are also of interest. Studies in normoglycemic, islet cell antibody-positive monozygotic twins in which one twin is already insulinopenic have demonstrated a progressive diminution in the first-phase insulin response to glucose over a number of years before the development of overt diabetes mellitus.[192] During this "early" diabetic phase, the β-cell response to other secretagogues, including arginine, tolbutamide, and glucagon, is also impaired, but to a much smaller extent.[193] In the future, this identification of β-cell dysfunction in response to intravenous glucose in those at high risk for the development of Type I diabetes some years before clinical onset may be of value therapeutically in preventing the onset of Type I diabetes in susceptible individuals.

In contrast to those patients with Type I diabetes, those with Type II diabetes are often hyperinsulinemic but have a degree of hyperinsulinemia inappropriately low for the prevailing glucose concentrations. Nevertheless, many of these patients have sufficient β-cell reserve to maintain a euglycemic state by dietary restriction with or without therapy with an oral agent. It is currently unclear whether insulin resistance or a defect in the β-cell is the primary lesion in Type II diabetes.[194–196] The latter defect is characterized by an attenuated or absent first-phase insulin and C-peptide response to an intravenous glucose load and by a reduced second-phase response.[69,125,197–199]

(Fig. 5–6). This attenuated β-cell response is not confined to glucose; diminished responses to non-glucose secretagogues such as arginine and isoproterenol have also been observed, although again, the reduction is of a lesser magnitude.[69,125] In vitro studies using the isolated perfused pancreas have emphasized the importance of hyperglycemia in the mediation of these changes.[70,200] However, the abnormal first-phase response to intravenous glucose persists in patients whose diabetic control has been markedly improved,[125,197] suggesting that patients with Type II diabetes may have an intrinsic defect in the β-cell. Furthermore, abnormalities in first-phase insulin secretion have also been observed in first-degree relatives of patients with Type II diabetes who exhibit only mild intolerance to glucose,[201] and an attenuated insulin response to oral glucose has been observed in normoglycemic co-twins of patients with Type II diabetes[202]—a group at high risk for Type II diabetes[203] and who can legitimately be classified as being "prediabetic." This pattern of insulin secretion during the so-called prediabetic phase is also seen in subjects with impaired glucose tolerance who later develop Type II diabetes[204–206] and in normoglycemic obese subjects with a recent history of gestational diabetes,[207] another group at high risk for Type II diabetes.[208] β-Cell abnormalities may therefore precede the development of overt Type II diabetes by many years.

Many studies in recent years have examined the effects of Type II diabetes on levels of proinsulin in serum. These studies have consistently demonstrated elevated levels of proinsulin in association with increases in the molar ratio of proinsulin to insulin,[209–214] suggesting that the β-cells of patients with Type II diabetes release an excess of immature secretory granules into the circulation. The amount of proinsulin produced in these patients appears to be related to the degree of glycemic control rather than to the duration of the diabetic state. In one series, proinsulin levels contributed almost 50% of the total insulin immunoreactivity in patients with Type II diabetes who had marked hyperglycemia.[214] Since conventional assays of levels of immunoreactive insulin also measure levels of proinsulin,[213] it is possible that the hyperinsulinemia reported in many studies of patients with Type II diabetes to some degree represents hyperproinsulinemia rather than true hyperinsulinemia. In support of this view, a recent study in which a sensitive insulin assay was used that did not cross-react with proinsulin reported that insulin levels in both obese and non-obese patients with Type II diabetes were lower than those in weight-matched control subjects.[213] Furthermore, the patients with diabetes in this series had elevated levels of both circulating proinsulin and 32–33 split proinsulin (a proinsulin conversion intermediate molecule). When insulin levels in this study population were measured using a conventional insulin assay, the differences between patients with diabetes and control subjects were less apparent. Proinsulin levels have also been measured in subjects with impaired glucose toler-

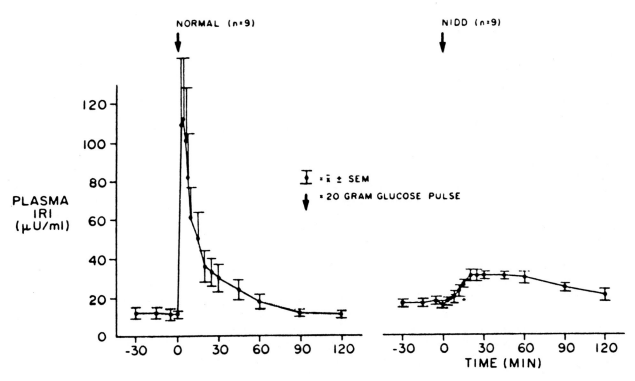

Fig. 5–6. Insulin release in response to the intravenous administration of glucose in normal subjects and in patients with non-insulin-dependent diabetes (NIDD; Type II). Note the lack of first-phase insulin response (IRI) in the diabetic subjects. Reprinted with permission from reference 125 (Pfeifer MA, Halter JB, Porte D Jr. Insulin secretion in diabetes mellitus. Am J Med 1981;70:579–88).

ance. The data here are conflicting since both elevated[212] and normal[214] levels of proinsulin have been observed in this setting.

Abnormalities in the temporal pattern of insulin secretion in patients with Type II diabetes have also been demonstrated. In contrast to normal subjects, who secrete equal amounts of insulin basally and postprandially in a given 24-hour period, patients with Type II diabetes secrete a greater proportion of their daily insulin under basal conditions.[215] This reduction in the proportion of insulin secreted postprandially appears to be related in part to a reduction in the amplitude of the secretory pulses of insulin that occur after meals rather than to a reduction in the number of pulses. The rapid oscillatory pattern of insulin production by the β-cells is also altered in patients with Type II diabetes, who exhibit cycles that are shorter and more irregular than the persistent, regular, rapid oscillations present in normal subjects.[138] Similar findings have been observed in first-degree relatives of patients with Type II diabetes who have only mild glucose intolerance,[216] an observation that suggests abnormalities in oscillatory activity may be an early manifestation of β-cell dysfunction in Type II diabetes.

The effects of therapy on β-cell function in patients with Type II diabetes have also been investigated. While interpretation of the results frequently is limited because β-cell function was not always studied at comparable glucose levels before and during therapy,[217] the majority of the studies indicate that improvements in diabetic control are associated with an enhancement of β-cell secretory activity.[197,218-222] This increased endogenous production of insulin appears to be independent of the mode of treatment and shows a particular association with increases in the amount of insulin secreted postprandially.[197,222] The enhanced β-cell secretory activity following meals reflects an increase in the amplitude of existing secretory pulses rather than an increased number of pulses.[222] Despite improvements in glycemic control, β-cell function is not normalized with therapy,[197,219,222] suggesting that there may be a persistent intrinsic defect in the β-cell in patients with Type II diabetes (Fig. 5–7).

A number of studies evaluating β-cell function in the transplanted pancreas are currently in progress.[120-123,223,224] Since many of those patients who have undergone pancreatic transplantation remain euglycemic without therapy during the post-transplantation period, the β-cell appears to be functional despite denervation. However, marked alterations in the temporal pattern of insulin secretion have been reported. Although the overall daily number of insulin secretory pulses is not altered following transplantation, basal insulin secretion accounts for up to 75% of the total insulin produced by these patients in a given 24-hour period. Postprandial insulin responses are therefore markedly attenuated.[121] Detailed analysis of these postprandial secretory pulses suggests that they are both reduced in amplitude and occur later after meals. This latter factor supports the view that the cephalic phase of insulin secretion mediated by the vagus is an important component of the

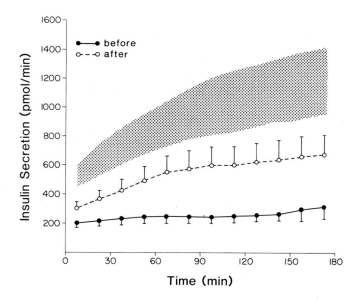

Fig. 5–7. Insulin secretion rates (±SEM) during hyperglycemic clamping at 300 mg/dL (16.7 mmol/L) in patients with non-insulin-dependent diabetes mellitus (NIDDM; Type II) before and during therapy with glyburide. The shaded area represents the secretion rates (±SEM) in a group of nondiabetic subjects. Reprinted with permission from reference 222 (Shapiro ET, Van Cauter E, Tillil H, et al. Glyburide enhances the responsiveness of the β-cell to glucose but does not correct the abnormal patterns of insulin secretion in noninsulin-dependent diabetes mellitus. J Clin Endocrinol Metab 1989;569:571–6; © The Endocrine Society).

prompt insulin response to meals usually observed in normal subjects.[80,113] In addition to quantitative abnormalities in insulin secretion, qualitative defects in the transplanted β-cell have also been reported, with increased proinsulin to C-peptide ratios under fasting conditions and a further accentuation of these abnormalities in the postprandial period.[122]

INSULIN SECRETION IN PATIENTS WITH INSULINOMA

In the diagnosis of insulinoma, a detailed knowledge and a correct interpretation of the β-cell secretory responses are critical. In distinguishing hypoglycemia caused by an islet cell tumor from hypoglycemia caused by other factors, the measurement of plasma levels of insulin alone may not be sufficient. Under normal physiologic circumstances, β-cell secretion is reduced as glucose levels fall. The hypoglycemia seen in patients with an insulinoma, however, is characterized by low glucose levels with inappropriate levels of insulin (which may be normal or elevated).[225,226] Although hypoglycemia induced by the surreptitious administration of insulin may also be associated with hyperinsulinemia, C-peptide levels will be elevated in patients with an insulinoma whereas administration of exogenous insulin usually suppresses the release of C-peptide from the β-cell.[227] Moreover, in patients with an insulinoma, a greater proportion of proinsulin is released into the circulation.[228,229] This latter factor could prove to be important in distinguishing patients with an insulinoma from those rare patients with hypoglycemia caused by surreptitious ingestion of oral hypoglycemic agents. Thus, the simultaneous measurement of proinsulin, insulin, and C-peptide levels can be of value in excluding or confirming the presence of an insulinoma in patients who present with hypoglycemia.

EFFECT OF DRUGS ON INSULIN SECRETION

Many pharmacologic agents other than hypoglycemic agents alter insulin secretion in vivo. In many instances, the effects of these agents on insulin secretion are associated with a deterioration in glucose tolerance. Some of these agents (e.g., phenytoin, verapamil, diazoxide, pentamidine) exert direct effects on the β-cell to suppress insulin release.[230-233] The indirect effects of other drugs may be mediated through alterations in insulin sensitivity (e.g., glucocorticoids) or through potassium depletion (e.g., thiazides), which secondarily alters the resting membrane potential of the β-cell.[234,235] Still other pharmacologic agents modulate both insulin secretion and insulin action. Both α- and β-adrenoceptor antagonists are included in this category. Indeed, the effects of this group of drugs on the rapid insulin secretory oscillations (those that occur every 8 to 16 minutes) have also been characterized. α-Adrenoreceptor blocking agents appear to enhance insulin secretion by increasing the amplitude of these rapid pulses, whereas the reduced insulin secretory response in patients receiving α-adrenergic antagonists appears to be in part a reflection of a smaller pulse amplitude.[141] Neither α- or β-adrenoceptor antagonists alter the frequency of these rapid oscillations. Other pharmacologic agents that affect both insulin secretion and insulin action include clonidine, prazosin, the benzodiazepine and phenothiazine groups of drugs, as well as the opiates. In relation to the latter, hyperglycemia has been observed in subjects receiving morphine,[236] and hyperinsulinemia has been reported in heroin addicts, who also demonstrate insulin secretory responses to intravenous glucose lower than those in age- and weight-matched control subjects.[237]

CONCLUDING REMARKS

The study of insulin secretion in vivo is greatly facilitated by a clear knowledge of the biosynthetic pathway of insulin within the β-cell and of the factors regulating insulin production and clearance from the circulation. In many clinical situations, the simultaneous measurement of proinsulin and C-peptide levels provides information on β-cell secretory function not possible to obtain by measurement of insulin levels in isolation. In interpreting the concentrations of these peptides, it is necessary to take into account the age and weight of the subjects as well as the glucose level at the time of sampling. The presence of any factor likely to alter insulin sensitivity should also be noted. While glucose is the key stimulus regulating insulin secretion in vivo, other nutri-

ents, as well as neural and hormonal factors, interact to modify this response, thus helping to maintain glucose levels within the physiologic range during fasting and postprandial states. This complex regulatory system is disrupted in the early stages of Type I diabetes before absolute insulinopenia develops and also in Type II diabetes. In both cases, the β-cell is unable to respond appropriately to the prevailing glucose concentration. Future studies of β-cell secretory function in vivo are likely to concentrate on the secretory defects present in the β-cell early in the evolutionary phase of diabetes before the clinical manifestations become apparent. The study of β-cell function and reserve during this period could make a major contribution to our understanding of the pathogenesis of diabetes and may ultimately lead to the development of suitable approaches for its prevention.

REFERENCES

1. Von Mering J, Minkowski O. Diabetes Mellitus nach Pankreasextirpation. Arch Exp Pathol Pharmacol (Leipzig) 1890;26:371–87.
2. Banting FG, Best CH. The internal secretion of the pancreas. J Lab Clin Med 1922;7:251–66.
3. Yalow RS, Berson SA. Immunoassay of endogenous plasma insulin in man. J Clin Invest 1960;39:1157–75.
4. Cerasi E, Luft R. Insulin response to glucose infusion in diabetic and non-diabetic monozygotic twin pairs. Genetic control of insulin response? Acta Endocrinol 1967;55:330–45.
5. Taylor KW, Sheldon J, Pyke DA, Oakley WG. Glucose tolerance and serum insulin in the unaffected first-degree relatives of diabetics. BMJ 1967;4:22–4.
6. Malherbe C, De Gasparo M, De Hertogh R, Hoett JJ. Circadian variations of blood sugar and plasma insulin levels in man. Diabetologia 1969;5:397–404.
7. Weber B. Glucose-stimulated insulin secretion during "remission" of juvenile diabetes. Diabetologia 1972;8:189–95.
8. Polonsky K, Jaspan J, Emmanouel D, et al. Differences in the hepatic and renal extraction of insulin and glucagon in the dog: evidence for saturability of insulin metabolism. Acta Endocrinol 1983;102:420–7.
9. Polonsky KS, Jaspan J, Pugh W, et al. Metabolism of C-peptide in the dog: in vivo demonstration of the absence of hepatic extraction. J Clin Invest 1983;72:1114–23.
10. Ferrannini E, Cobelli C. The kinetics of insulin in man. II. Role of the liver. Diabetes Metab Rev 1987;3:365–97.
11. Steiner DF, Oyer PE. The biosynthesis of insulin and a probable precursor of insulin by a human islet cell adenoma. Proc Natl Acad Sci USA 1967;57:473–80.
12. Rubenstein AH, Clark JL, Melani F, Steiner DF. Secretion of proinsulin, C-peptide by pancreatic cells and its circulation in blood. Nature 1969;224:697–9.
13. Steiner DF. On the role of proinsulin C-peptide. Diabetes 1978;27(Suppl 1):145–8.
14. Horwitz DL, Starr JI, Mako ME, et al. Proinsulin, insulin, and C-peptide concentrations in human portal and peripheral blood. J Clin Invest 1975;55:1278–83.
15. Melani F, Rubenstein AH, Steiner DF. Human serum proinsulin. J Clin Invest 1970;49:497–507.
16. Bergenstal RM, Cohen RM, Lever E, et al. The metabolic effects of biosynthetic human proinsulin in individuals

with Type I diabetes. J Clin Endocrinol Metab 1984;58:973–9.

17. Revers RR, Henry R, Schmeiser L, et al. The effects of biosynthetic human proinsulin on carbohydrate metabolism. Diabetes 1984;33:762–70.

18. Peavy DE, Brunner MR, Duckworth WC, et al. Receptor binding and biological potency of several split forms (conversion intermediates) of human proinsulin: studies in cultured IM-9 lymphocytes and in vivo and in vitro in rats. J Biol Chem 1985;260:13989–94.

19. Gruppuso PA, Frank BH, Schwartz, R. Binding of proinsulin and proinsulin conversion intermediates to human placental insulin-like growth factor 1 receptors. J Clin Endocrinol Metab 1988;67:194–7.

20. Polonsky KS, Rubenstein AH. C-peptide as a measure of the secretion and hepatic extraction of insulin: pitfalls and limitations. Diabetes 1984;33:486–94.

21. Wojcikowski C, Blackman J, Ostrega D, et al. Lack of effect of high-dose biosynthetic human C-peptide on pancreatic hormone release in normal subjects. Metabolism 1990;39:827–32.

22. Polonsky KS, Pugh W, Jaspan JB, et al. C-peptide and insulin secretion: relationship between peripheral concentrations of C-peptide and insulin and their secretion rates in the dog. J Clin Invest 1984;74:1821–9.

23. Bratusch-Marrain PR, Waldhäusl WK, Gasić S, Hofer A. Hepatic disposal of biosynthetic human insulin and porcine C-peptide in humans. Metabolism 1984;33:151–7.

24. Faber OK, Hagen C, Binder C, et al. Kinetics of human connecting peptide in normal and diabetic subjects. J Clin Invest 1978;62:197–203.

25. Blix PM, Boddie-Willis C, Landau RL, et al. Urinary C-peptide: an indicator of cell secretion under different metabolic conditions. J Clin Endocrinol Metab 1982;54:574–80.

26. Gero L, Koranyi L, Tamas GJ Jr. Residual β-cell function in insulin dependent (type 1) and non-insulin-dependent (type 2) diabetics (relationship between 24-hour C-peptide excretion and the clinical features of diabetes). Diabetes Metab 1983;9:183–90.

27. Aurbach-Klipper J, Sharph-Dor R, Heding LG, et al. Residual β cell function in diabetic children as determined by urinary C-peptide. Diabetologia 1983;24:88–90.

28. Hoogwerf BF, Goetz FC. Urinary C-peptide: a simple measure of integrated insulin production with emphasis on the effects of body size, diet and corticosteroids. J Clin Endocrinol Metab 1983;56:60–7.

29. Tillil H, Shapiro ET, Given BD, et al. Reevaluation of urine C-peptide as measure of insulin secretion. Diabetes 1988;37:1195–1201.

30. Polonsky KS, Licinio-Paixao J, Given BD, et al. Use of biosynthetic human C-peptide in the measurement of insulin secretion rates in normal volunteers and Type I diabetic patients. J Clin Invest 1986;77:98–105.

31. Shapiro ET, Tillil H, Rubenstein AH, Polonsky KS. Peripheral insulin parallels changes in insulin secretion more closely than C-peptide after bolus intravenous glucose administration. J Clin Endocrinol Metab 1988;67:1094–9.

32. Eaton RP, Allen RC, Shade DS, et al. Prehepatic insulin production in man: kinetic analysis using peripheral connecting peptide behavior. J Clin Endocrinol Metab 1980;51:520–8.

33. Polonsky K, Frank B, Pugh W, et al. The limitations to and valid use of C-peptide as a marker of the secretion of insulin. Diabetes 1986;35:379–86.

34. Waldhäusl W, Bratusch-Marrain P, Gasic S, et al. Insulin production rate following glucose ingestion estimated by splanchnic C-peptide output in normal man. Diabetologia 1979;17:221–7.

35. Waldhäusl W, Bratusch-Marrain P, Gasic S, et al. Insulin production rate, hepatic insulin retention and splanchnic carbohydrate metabolism after oral glucose ingestion in hyperinsulinaemic type 2 (non-insulin-dependent) diabetes mellitus. Diabetologia 1982;23:6–15.

36. Porte D Jr, Pupo AA. Insulin responses to glucose: evidence for a two-pool system in man. J Clin Invest 1969;48:2309–19.

37. Chen M, Porte D Jr. The effect of rate and dose of glucose infusion on the acute insulin response in man. J Clin Endocrinol Metab 1976;42:1168–75.

38. Ward WK, Beard JC, Halter JB, et al. Pathophysiology of insulin secretion in non-insulin dependent diabetes mellitus. Diabetes Care 1984;7:491–502.

39. Eaton RP, Allen RC, Schade DS. Hepatic removal of insulin in normal man: dose response to endogenous insulin secretion J Clin Endocrinol Metab 1983;56:1294–300.

40. Nauck MA, Homberger E, Siegel EG, et al. Incretin effects of increasing glucose loads in man calculated from venous insulin and C-peptide responses. J Clin Endocrinol Metab 1986;63:492–8.

41. Tillil H, Shapiro ET, Miller MA, et al. Dose-dependent effects of oral and intravenous glucose on insulin secretion and clearance in normal humans. Am J Physiol 1988;254:E349–57.

42. Faber OK, Madsbad S, Kehlet H, Binder, C. Pancreatic beta cell secretion during oral and intravenous glucose administration. Acta Med Scand Suppl 1979;624:61–4.

43. Madsbad S, Kehlet H, Hilsted J, Tronier B. Discrepancy between plasma C-peptide and insulin response to oral and intravenous glucose. Diabetes 1983;32:436–8.

44. Shapiro ET, Tillil H, Miller MA, et al. Insulin secretion and clearance: comparison after oral and intravenous glucose. Diabetes 1987;36:1365–71.

45. Creutzfeldt W, Ebert R. New developments in the incretin concept. Diabetologia 1985;28:565–76.

46. Pagliara AS, Stillings SN, Hover B, et al. Glucose modulation of amino acid-induced glucagon and insulin release in the isolated perfused rat pancreas. J Clin Invest 1974;54:819–32.

47. Gerich JE, Charles MA, Grodsky GM. Characterization of the effects of arginine and glucose on glucagon and insulin release from the perfused rat pancreas. J Clin Invest 1974;54:833–41.

48. Grodsky GM. The kinetics of insulin release. In: Hasselblatt A, Bruchhausen FV, eds. Handbook of experimental pharmacology. Vol 32. Insulin II. Berlin: Springer-Verlag, 1975:1–19.

49. Salomon D, Meda P. Heterogeneity and contact-dependent regulation of hormone secretion by individual β cells. Exp Cell Res 1986;162:507–20.

50. Schuit FC, In't Veld PA, Pipeleers DG. Glucose stimulates proinsulin biosynthesis by a dose-dependent recruitment of pancreatic beta cells. Proc Natl Acad Sci USA 1988;85:3865–9.

51. Cerasi E, Luft R. The plasma insulin response to glucose infusion in healthy subjects and in diabetes mellitus. Acta Endocrinol 1967;55:278–304.

52. Bennett L, Grodsky GM. Multiphasic aspects of insulin release after glucose and glucagon. In: Ostman J, Milner RDG, eds. Diabetes. Proceedings of the Sixth Congress of the International Diabetes Federation-1967. Amsterdam: Excerpta Medica, 1969:462–9.

53. Grodsky GM. A threshold distribution hypothesis for packet storage of insulin and its mathematical modeling. J Clin Invest 1972;51:2047–59.

54. Smith CP, Tarn AC, Thomas JM, et al. Between and within subject variation of the first phase insulin response to intravenous glucose. Diabetologia 1988;31:123–5.

55. Bardet S, Pasqual C, Maugendre D, et al. Inter and intra individual variability of acute insulin response during intravenous glucose tolerance tests. Diabetes Metab 1989;15:224–32.

56. Rayman G, Clark P, Schneider AE, Hales CN. The first phase insulin response to intravenous glucose is highly reproducible. Diabetologia 1990;33:631–4.

57. Bolaffi JL, Heldt A, Lewis LD, Grodsky GM. The third phase of in vitro insulin secretion: evidence for glucose insensitivity. Diabetes 1986;35:370–3.

58. Curry DL. Insulin content and insulinogenesis by the perfused rat pancreas: effects of long term glucose stimulation. Endocrinology 1986;118:170–5.

59. Hoenig M, MacGregor LC, Matschinsky FM. In vitro exhaustion of pancreatic β-cells. Am J Physiol 1986;250:E502–11.

60. Grodsky GM. A new phase of insulin secretion: how will it contribute to our understanding of β-cell function? Diabetes 1989;38:673–8.

61. Matschinsky FM, Ellerman J, Stillings S, et al. Hexoses and insulin secretion. In: Hasselblatt A, Bruchhausen FV, eds. Handbook of experimental pharmacology. Vol 32. Insulin II. Berlin: Springer-Verlag, 1975:79–114.

62. Grodsky GM, Fanska R, Lundquist I. Interrelationship between and β anomers of glucose affecting both insulin and glucagon secretion in the perfused rat pancreas. II. Endocrinology 1975;97:573–80.

63. Niki A, Niki H, Miwa I. Effect of anomers of d-mannose on insulin release from perfused rat pancreas. Endocrinology 1979;105:1051–4.

64. Malaisse WJ, Sener A, Koser M, Herchuelz A. Stimulus-secretion coupling of glucose-induced insulin release. Metabolism of α- and β-D-glucose in isolated islets. J Biol Chem 1976;251:5936-42.

65. Malaisse WJ, Malaisse-Lagae F, Lebrun P, et al. Metabolic response of pancreatic islets of the rat to the anomers of d-mannose [Abstract no. 198]. Diabetologia 1982;23:185.

66. Zawalich WS, Pagliara AS, Matschinsky FM. Effects of iodoacetate, mannoheptulose and 3-o-methyl glucose on the secretory function and metabolism of isolated pancreatic islets. Endocrinology 1977;100:1276–83.

67. Levin SR, Karam JH, Hane S, et al. Enhancement of arginine-induced insulin secretion in man by prior administration of glucose. Diabetes 1971;20:171–6.

68. Fajans SS, Floyd JC. Stimulation of islet cell secretion by nutrients and by gastrointestinal hormones released during digestion. In: Steiner DF, Freinkel N, eds. Handbook of physiology. Section 7. Endocrinology. Vol 1. Washington DC: American Physiological Society, 1972:473–93.

69. Ward WK, Bolgiano DC, McKnight B, et al. Diminished cell secretory capacity in patients with noninsulin-dependent diabetes mellitus. J Clin Invest 1984;74:1318–38.

70. Leahy JL, Bonner-Weir S, Weir GC. Minimal chronic hyperglycemia is a critical determinant of impaired insulin secretion after an incomplete pancreatectomy. J Clin Invest 1988;81:1407–14.

71. Matschinsky FM, Fertel R, Kotler-Brajtburg K. et al. Factors governing the action of small calorigenic molecules on the islets of Langerhans. In: Mussacchia XJ, Breitenbach KP, eds. Proceedings of the 8th Midwest Conference on Endocrinology and Metabolism. Columbia, University of Missouri Press, 1973:63–86.

72. Muller WA, Faloona GR, Unger RH. The influence of the antecedent diet upon glucagon and insulin secretion. N Engl J Med 1971;285:1450–4.

73. Dupre J, Ross SA, Watson D, Brown JC. Stimulation of insulin secretion by gastric inhibitory polypeptide in man. J Clin Endocrinol Metab 1973;37:826–8.

74. Andersen DK, Elahi D, Brown JC, et al. Oral glucose augmentation of insulin secretion: interactions of gastric inhibitory polypeptide with ambient glucose and insulin levels. J Clin Invest 1978;62:152–61.

75. Schmidt WE, Siegel EG, Creutzfeldt W. Glucagon-like peptide-1 but not glucagon-like peptide-2 stimulates insulin release from isolated rat pancreatic islets. Diabetologia 1985;28:704–7.

76. Kreymann B, Ghatei MA, Williams G, Bloom SR. Glucagon-like peptide-1 7-36: a physiological incretin in man. Lancet 1987;2:1300–4.

77. Zawalich WS, Diaz VA. Prior cholecystokinin exposure sensitizes islets of Langerhans to glucose stimulation. Diabetes 1987;36:118–227.

78. Zawalich WS. Synergistic impact of cholecystokinin and gastric inhibitory polypeptide on the regulation of insulin secretion. Metabolism 1988;37:778–81.

79. Weir GC, Mojsov S, Hendrick GK, Habener JF. Glucagon-like peptide 1(7–37) actions on endocrine pancreas. Diabetes 1989;38:338–42.

80. Rasmussen H, Zawalich KC, Ganesan S, et al. Physiology and pathophysiology of insulin secretion. Diabetes Care 1990;13:655–66.

81. Schebalin M, Said SI, Makhlouf GM. Stimulation of insulin and glucagon secretion by vasoactive intestinal peptide. Am J Physiol 1977;232:E197–200.

82. Dupre J, Curtis JD, Unger RH, et al. Effects of secretin, pancreozymin, gastrin on the response of the endocrine pancreas to administration of glucose or arginine in man. J Clin Invest 1969;48:745–57.

83. Halter J, Porte D Jr. Mechanisms of impaired acute insulin release in adult onset diabetes: studies with isoproterenol and secretin. J Clin Endocrinol Metab 1978;46:952–60.

84. Rehfeld JF, Stadil F. The effect of gastrin on basal- and glucose-stimulated insulin secretion in man. J Clin Invest 1973;52:1415–26.

85. Samols E, Marri G, Marks V. Promotion of insulin secretion by glucagon. Lancet 1965;2:415–6.

86. Alberti KGMM, Christensen NJ, Christensen SE, et al. Inhibition of insulin secretion by somatostatin. Lancet 1973;2:1299–301.

87. Aguilar-Parada E, Eisentraut AM, Unger RH. Effects of starvation on plasma pancreatic glucagon in normal man. Diabetes 1969;18:717–23.

88. Marliss EB, Aoki TT, Unger RH, et al. Glucagon levels and metabolic effects in fasting man. J Clin Invest 1970;49:2256–70.

89. Malaisse WJ, Malaisse-Lagae F, Wright PH. Effect of fasting upon insulin secretion in the rat. Am J Physiol 1967;213:843–48.

90. Zawalich WS, Dye ES, Pagliara AS, et al. Starvation diabetes in the rat: onset, recovery and specificity of reduced responsiveness of pancreatic β-cells. Endocrinology 1979;104:1344–51.

91. Felig P, Marliss EB, Cahill GF Jr. Metabolic response to human growth hormone during prolonged starvation. J Clin Invest 1971;50:411–21.

92. Kalhan SC, Adam PAJ. Inhibitory effect of prednisone on

insulin secretion in man: model for duplication of blood glucose concentration. J Clin Endocrinol Metab 1975; 41:600–10.

93. Landgraf R, Landgraf-Leurs MMC, Weissmann A, et al. Prolactin: a diabetogenic hormone. Diabetologia 1977; 13:99–104.

94. Gustafson AB, Banasiak MF, Kalkhoff RK, et al. Correlation of hyperprolactinemia with altered plasma insulin and glucagon: similarity to effects of late human pregnancy. J Clin Endocrinol Metab 1980;51:242–6.

95. Brelje TC, Sorenson RL. Nutrient and hormonal regulation of the threshold of glucose-stimulated insulin secretion in isolated rat pancreases. Endocrinology 1988;123:1582–90.

96. Beck P, Daughaday WH. Human placental lactogen: studies of its acute metabolic effects and disposition in normal man. J Clin Invest 1967;46:103–10.

97. Ensinck JW, Williams RH. Hormonal and nonhormonal factors modifying man's response to insulin. In: Steiner DF, Freinkel N, eds. Handbook of physiology. Section 7. Endocrinology. Vol 1. Washington DC: American Physiological Society, 1972:665–9.

98. Martin JM, Friesen H. Effect of human placental lactogen on the isolated islets of Langerhans in vitro. Endocrinology 1969;84:619–21.

99. Curry DL, Bennett LL. Dynamics of insulin release by perfused rat pancreases: effects of hypophysectomy, growth hormone, adrenocorticotropic hormone and hydrocortisone. Endocrinology 1973;93:602–9.

100. Malaisse WJ, Malaisse-Lagae F, King S, Wright PH. Effect of growth hormone on insulin secretion. Am J Physiol 1968;215:423–8.

101. Randin JP, Scazziga B, Jequier E, Felber JP. Study of glucose and lipid metabolism by continuous indirect calorimetry in Graves' disease: effect of an oral glucose load. J Clin Endocrinol Metab 1985;61:1165–71.

102. Foss MC, Paccola GMGF, Saad MJA, et al. Peripheral glucose metabolism in human hyperthyroidism. J Clin Endocrinol Metab 1990;70:1167–72.

103. Sestoft L, Heding LG. Hypersecretion of proinsulin in thyrotoxicosis. Diabetologia 1981;21:103–7.

104. Nishi S, Seino Y, Ishida H, et al. Vagal regulation of insulin, glucagon and somatostatin secretion in vitro in the rat. J Clin Invest 1987;79:1191–6.

105. Kurose T, Seino Y, Nishi S, et al. Mechanism of sympathetic neural regulation of insulin, somatostatin and glucagon secretion. Am J Physiol 1990;258:E220–7.

106. Woods SC, Porte D Jr. Neural control of the endocrine pancreas. Physiol Rev 1974;54:596–619.

107. Bloom SR, Edwards AV. Certain pharmacological characteristics of the release of pancreatic glucagon in response to stimulation of the splanchnic nerves. J Physiol (Lond) 1978;280:25–35.

108. Porte D Jr, Girardier L, Seydoux J, et al. Neural regulation of insulin secretion in the dog. J Clin Invest 1973; 52:210–4.

109. Roy MW, Lee KC, Jones MS, Miller RE. Neural control of pancreatic insulin and somatostatin secretion. Endocrinology 1984;115:770–5.

110. Hommel H, Fischer U, Retzlaff K, Knofler H. The mechanism of insulin secretion after oral glucose administration. II. Reflex insulin secretion in conscious dogs bearing fistulas of the digestive tract by sham-feeding of glucose or tap water. Diabetologia 1972;8:111–6.

111. Berthoud HR, Trimble ER, Siegel EG, et al. Cephalic-phase insulin secretion in normal and pancreatic islet-transplanted rats. Am J Physiol 1980;238:E336–40.

112. Taylor IL, Feldman M. Effect of cephalic-vagal stimulation on insulin, gastric inhibitory polypeptide and pancreatic polypeptide release in humans. J Clin Endocrinol Metab 1982;55:1114–7.

113. Bruce DG, Storlien LH, Furler SM, Chrisholm DJ. Cephalic phase metabolic responses in normal weight adults. Metabolism 1987;36:721–5.

114. Berthoud H-R, Bereiter DA, Trimble ER, et al. Cephalic-phase, reflex insulin secretion: neuroanatomical and physiological characterization. Diabetologia 1981; 20:393–401.

115. Zawalich WS, Zawalich KC, Rasmussen H. Cholinergic agonists prime the β-cell to glucose stimulation. Endocrinology 1989;125:2400–6.

116. Håkanson R, Liedberg G, Lundquist I. Effect of vagal denervation on insulin release after oral and intravenous glucose. Experientia 1971;27:460–1.

117. Linquette M, Fourlinnie JC, Lagache G. Etude de la glycemie et de l'insulinemie apres vagotomie et pylorplastie chez l'homme. Ann Endocrinol (Paris) 1969; 30:96–102.

118. Louis-Sylvestre J. Relationship between two stages of prandial insulin release in rats. Am J Physiol 1978; 235:E103–11.

119. Trimble ER, Siegel EG, Berthoud H-R, Renold AE. Intraportal islet transplantation: functional assessment in conscious unrestrained rats. Endocrinology 1980;106:791–7.

120. Pozza G, Bosi E, Secchi A, et al. Metabolic control of Type I (insulin dependent) diabetes after pancreas transplantation. BMJ 1985;291:510–3.

121. Polonsky K, Jaspan J, Woodle L, Thistlethwaite R. Alterations in the pattern of insulin secretion and C-peptide kinetics post pancreas transplantation [Abstract no. 59]. Diabetes 1990;39(Suppl 1):15A.

122. Madsbad S, Christiansen E, Andersen HB, et al. β Cell defects after pancreas transplantation in Type I patients [Abstract no. 58]. Diabetes 39(Suppl 1):15A.

123. Diem P, Abid M, Redmon JB, et al. Systemic venous drainage of pancreas allografts as independent cause of hyperinsulinemia in Type I diabetic recipients. Diabetes 1990;39:534–40.

124. Treuting TF. The role of emotional factors in the etiology and course of diabetes mellitus: a review of the recent literature. Am J Med Sci 1962;244:93–109.

125. Pfeifer MA, Halter JB, Porte D Jr. Insulin secretion in diabetes mellitus. Am J Med 1981;70:579–88.

126. Larrimer JN, Mazzaferri EL, Cataland S, Mekhjian HS. Effect of atropine on glucose-stimulated gastric inhibitory polypeptide. Diabetes 1978;27:638–42.

127. Flaten O, Sand T, Myren J. Beta-adrenergic stimulation and blockade of the release of gastric inhibitory polypeptide and insulin in man. Scand J Gastroenterol 1982;17:283–8.

128. Kruszynska YT, Home PD, Hanning I, Alberti KGMM. Basal and 24-h C-peptide and insulin secretion rate in normal man. Diabetologia 1987;30:16–21.

129. Polonsky KS, Given BD, Van Cauter E. Twenty-four-hour profiles and pulsatile patterns of insulin secretion in normal and obese subjects. J Clin Invest 1988;81:442–8.

130. Simon C, Follenius M, Brandenberger G. Postprandial oscillations of plasma glucose, insulin and C-peptide in man. Diabetologia 1987;30:769–73.

131. Simon C, Brandenberger G, Follenius M. Ultradian oscillations of plasma glucose, insulin and C-peptide in man during continuous enteral nutrition. J Clin Endocrinol Metab 1987;64:669–74.

132. Shapiro ET, Tillil H, Polonsky KS, et al. Oscillations in

insulin secretion during constant glucose infusion in normal man: relationship to changes in plasma glucose. J Clin Endocrinol Metab 1988;67:307–14.

133. Van Cauter E, Desir D, Decoster C, et al. Nocturnal decrease in glucose tolerance during constant glucose infusion. J Clin Endocrinol Metab 1989;69:604–11.

134. Sturis J, Van Cauter E, Blackman JD, Polonsky KS. Entrainment of pulsatile insulin secretion by oscillatory glucose infusion. J Clin Invest 1991;87:439–45.

135. Goodner CJ, Walike BC, Koerker DJ, et al. Insulin, glucagon and glucose exhibit synchronous sustained oscillations in fasting monkeys. Science 1977;195:177–9.

136. Lang DA, Matthews DR, Peto J, Turner RC. Cyclic oscillations of basal plasma glucose and insulin concentrations in human beings. N Engl J Med 1979;301:1023–7.

137. Hansen BC, Pek S, Koerker DJ, et al. Neural influences on oscillations in basal plasma levels of insulin in monkeys. Am J Physiol 1981;240:E5–11.

138. Lang DA, Matthews DR, Burnett M, Turner RC. Brief, irregular oscillations of basal plasma insulin and glucose concentrations in diabetic man. Diabetes 1981;30:435–9.

139. Lang DA, Matthews DR, Burnett M, et al. Pulsatile, synchronous basal insulin and glucagon secretion in man. Diabetes 1982;31:22–6.

140. Hansen BC, Jen K-LC, Pek SB, Wolfe RA. Rapid oscillations in plasma insulin, glucagon and glucose in obese and normal weight humans. J Clin Endocrinol Metab 1982;54:785–92.

141. Matthews DR, Lang DA, Burnett MA, Turner RC. Control of pulsatile insulin secretion in man. Diabetologia 1983;24:231–7.

142. Stagner JI, Samols E, Weir GC. Sustained oscillations of insulin, glucagon and somatostatin from the isolated canine pancreas during exposure to a constant glucose concentration. J Clin Invest 1980;65:939–42.

143. Jaspan JB, Lever E, Polonsky KS, Van Cauter E. In vivo pulsatility of pancreatic islet peptides. Am J Physiol 1986;251:E215–26.

144. Matthews DR, Naylor BA, Jones RG, et al. Pulsatile insulin has greater hypoglycemic effect than continuous delivery. Diabetes 1983;32:617–21.

145. Bratusch-Marrain PR, Komjati M, Waldhäusl WK. Efficacy of pulsatile versus continuous insulin administration on hepatic glucose production and glucose utilization in type I diabetic humans. Diabetes 1986;35:922–6.

146. Ward GM, Walters JM, Aitken PM, et al. Effects of prolonged pulsatile hyperinsulinemia in humans. Enhancement of insulin sensitivity. Diabetes 1990;39:501–7.

147. Tasaka Y, Sekine M, Wakatsuki M, et al. Levels of pancreatic glucagon, insulin and glucose during twenty-four hours of the day in normal subjects. Horm Metab Res 1975;7:205–6.

148. Jarrett RJ, Baker IA, Keen H, Oakley NW. Diurnal variation in oral glucose tolerance: blood sugar and plasma insulin levels morning, afternoon and evening. BMJ 1972;1:199–201.

149. Carroll KF, Nestel PJ. Diurnal variation in glucose tolerance and in insulin secretion in man. Diabetes 1973;22:333–48.

150. Alparicio NJ, Puchulu FE, Gagliardino JJ, et al. Circadian variation of the blood glucose, plasma insulin and human growth hormone levels in response to an oral glucose load in normal subjects. Diabetes 1974;23:132–7.

151. King DS, Dalsky GP, Staten MA, et al. Insulin action and secretion in endurance-trained and untrained humans. J Appl Physiol 1987;63:2247–52.

152. King DS, Dalsky GP, Clutter WE, et al. Effects of lack of exercise on insulin secretion and action in trained subjects. Am J Physiol 1988;254:E537–42.

153. King DS, Staten MA, Kohrt W, et al. Insulin secretory capacity in endurance-trained and untrained young men. Am J Physiol 1990;259:E155–61.

154. Seals DR, Hagberg JM, Allen WK, et al. Glucose tolerance in young and older athletes and sedentary men. J Appl Physiol 1984;56:1521–5.

155. Heath GW, Gavin JR III, Hinderliter JM, et al. Effects of exercise and lack of exercise on glucose tolerance and insulin sensitivity. J Appl Physiol 1983;55:512–7.

156. King DS, Dalsky GP, Clutter WE, et al. Effects of exercise and lack of exercise on insulin sensitivity and responsiveness. J Appl Physiol 1988;64:1942–6.

157. LeBlanc J, Nadeau A, Richard D, Tremblay A. Studies on the sparing effect of exercise on insulin requirements in human subjects. Metabolism 1981;30:1119–24.

158. Davidson MB. The effect of aging on carbohydrate metabolism: a review of the English literature and a practical approach to the diagnosis of diabetes mellitus in the elderly. Metabolism 1979;28:688–705.

159. DeFronzo RA. Glucose intolerance and aging: evidence for tissue insensitivity to insulin. Diabetes 1979;28:1095–101.

160. Fink RI, Kolterman OG, Olefsky JM. The physiological significance of the glucose intolerance of aging. J Gerontol 1984;39:273–8.

161. Reaven EP, Gold G, Reaven GM. Effect of age on glucose-stimulated insulin release by the beta cell of the rat. J Clin Invest 1979;64:591–9.

162. Reaven E, Wright D, Mondon CE, et al. Effect of age and diet on insulin secretion and insulin action in the rat. Diabetes 1983;32:175–80.

163. Swenne I. Effects of aging on the regenerative capacity of the pancreatic beta-cell of the rat. Diabetes 1983;32:14–9.

164. DeFronzo RA. Glucose intolerance and aging. Diabetes Care 1981;4:493–501.

165. Palmer JP, Ensinck JW. Acute-phase insulin secretion and glucose tolerance in young and aged normal men and diabetic patients. J Clin Endocrinol Metab 1975;41:498–503.

166. Dudl RJ, Ensinck JW. Insulin and glucagon relationships during aging in man. Metabolism 1977;26:33–41.

167. Schreuder HB. Influence of age on insulin secretion and lipid mobilization after glucose stimulation. Isr J Med 1972;8:832–4.

168. Crockford PM, Harbeck RJ, Williams RH. Influence of age on intravenous glucose tolerance and serum immunoreactive insulin. Lancet 1966;1:465–7.

169. Barbagallo-Sangiorgi G, Laudicina E, Bompiani GD, Durante F. The pancreatic beta-cell response to intravenous administration of glucose in elderly subjects. J Am Geriat Soc 1970;18:529–38.

170. Chen M, Bergman RN, Pacini G, Porte D Jr. Pathogenesis of age-related glucose intolerance in man: insulin resistance and decreased β-cell function. J Clin Endocrinol Metab 1985;60:13–20.

171. Gumbiner B, Polonsky KS, Beltz WF, et al. Effects of aging on insulin secretion. Diabetes 1989;38:1549–56.

172. Olefsky JM, Farquhar JW, Reaven GM. Reappraisal of the role of insulin in hypertriglyceridemia. Am J Med 1974;57:551–60.

173. Kissebah AH, Vydelingum N, Murray R, et al. Relation of body fat distribution to metabolic complications of obesity. J Clin Endocrinol Metab 1982;54:254–60.

174. Peiris AN, Mueller RA, Smith GA, et al. Splanchnic insulin metabolism in obesity: influence of body fat distribution. J Clin Invest 1986;78:1648–57.

175. Meistas MT, Rendell M, Margolis S, Kowarski AA. Estimation of the secretion rate of insulin from the urinary excretion rate of C-peptide: study in obese and diabetic subjects. Diabetes 1982;31:449–53.

176. Faber OK, Christensen K, Kehlet H, et al. Decreased insulin removal contributes to hyperinsulinemia in obesity. J Clin Endocrinol Metab 1981;53:618–21.

177. Savage PJ, Flock EV, Mako ME, et al. C-peptide and insulin secretion in Pima Indians and caucasians: constant fractional hepatic extraction over a wide range of insulin concentrations and in obesity. J Clin Endocrinol Metab 1979;48:594–8.

178. Meistas MT, Foster GV, Margolis S, Kowarski AA. Integrated concentrations of growth hormone, insulin, C-peptide and prolactin in human obesity. Metabolism 1982;31:1224–8.

179. DeFronzo RA. Insulin secretion, insulin resistance and obesity. Int J Obesity 1982;6(Suppl 1):73–82.

180. Rossell R, Gomis R, Casamitjana R, et al. Reduced hepatic insulin extraction in obesity: relationship with plasma insulin levels. J Clin Endocrinol Metab 1983;56:608–11.

181. Polonsky KS, Given BD, Hirsch L, et al. Quantitative study of insulin secretion and clearance in normal and obese subjects. J Clin Invest 1988;81:435–41.

182. Ogilvie RF. The islets of Langerhans in 19 cases of obesity. J Pathol Bacteriol 1933;37:473–81.

183. Carlstrom S, Ingemanson CA. Juvenile diabetes with long-standing remission. A case report. Diabetologia 1967;3:465–7.

184. Johansen K, Orskov H. Plasma insulin during remission in juvenile diabetes mellitus. BMJ 1969;1:676–8.

185. Block MB, Rosenfield RL, Mako ME, et al. Sequential changes in beta-cell function in insulin-treated diabetic patients assessed by C-peptide immunoreactivity. N Engl J Med 1973;288:1144–8.

186. Park BN, Soeldner JS, Gleason RE. Diabetes in remission. Insulin secretory dynamics. Diabetes 1974;23:616–23.

187. Ludvigsson J, Heding LG. Beta-cell function in children with diabetes. Diabetes 1978;27(Suppl 1):230–4.

188. Heding LG, Ludvigsson J, Kasperska-Czyzykowa T. β-cell secretion in non-diabetics and insulin-dependent-diabetics. Acta Med Scand Suppl 1981;656:5–9.

189. Ludvigsson J, Heding L. Abnormal proinsulin/C-peptide ratio in juvenile diabetes. Acta Diabet Lat 1982;19:351–8.

190. Snorgaard O, Hartling SG, Binder C. Proinsulin and C-peptide at onset and during 12 months cyclosporin treatment of type 1 (insulin-dependent) diabetes mellitus. Diabetologia 1990;33:36–42.

191. Bougneres PF, Carel JC, Castano L, et al. Factors associated with early remission of type 1 diabetes in children treated with cyclosporine. N Engl J Med 1988;318:663–70.

192. Srikanta S, Ganda OP, Jackson RA, et al. Type I diabetes mellitus in monozygotic twins: chronic progressive beta cell dysfunction. Ann Intern Med 1983;99:320–6.

193. Ganda OP, Srikanta S, Brink SJ, et al. Differential sensitivity to β-cell secretagogues in "early" type 1 diabetes mellitus. Diabetes 1984;33:516–21.

194. Weir GC. Non-insulin-dependent diabetes mellitus: interplay between β-cell inadequacy and insulin resistance. [Editorial]. Am J Med 1982;73:461–4.

195. Reaven GM. Insulin secretion and insulin action in non-insulin-dependent diabetes mellitus: which defect is primary? Diabetes Care 1984;7(Suppl 1):17–24.

196. Cahil GF Jr. Beta-cell deficiency, insulin resistance, or both? [Editorial] N Engl J Med 1988;318:1268–70.

197. Garvey WT, Olefsky JM, Griffin J, et al. The effect of insulin treatment on insulin secretion and insulin action in Type II diabetes mellitus. Diabetes 1985;34:222–34.

198. Ferner RE, Ashworth RL, Tronier B, Alberti KGMM. Effects of short-term hyperglycemia on insulin secretion in normal humans. Am J Physiol 1986;250:E655–61.

199. Nesher R, Della Casa L, Litvin Y, et al. Insulin deficiency and insulin resistance in type 2 (non-insulin-dependent) diabetes: quantitative contributions of pancreatic and peripheral responses to glucose homeostasis. Eur J Clin Invest 1987;17:266–74.

200. Leahy JL, Weir GC. Evolution of abnormal insulin secretory responses during 48-h in vivo hyperglycemia. Diabetes 1988;37:217–22.

201. O'Rahilly SP, Nugent Z, Rudensky AS, et al. Beta-cell dysfunction rather than insulin insensitivity, is the primary defect in familial type 2 diabetes. Lancet 1986;2:360–4.

202. Barnett AH, Spiliopoulos AJ, Pyke DA, et al. Metabolic studies in unaffected co-twins of non-insulin-dependent diabetics. BMJ 1981;282:1656–8.

203. Barnett AH, Eff C, Leslie RDG, Pyke DA. Diabetes in identical twins: a study of 200 pairs. Diabetologia 1981;20:87–93.

204. Kosaka K, Hagura R, Kuzuya T. Insulin responses in equivocal and definite diabetes with special reference to subjects who had mild glucose intolerance but later developed definite diabetes. Diabetes 1977;26:944–52.

205. Kadowaki T, Miyake Y, Hagura R, et al. Risk factors for worsening to diabetes in subjects with impaired glucose tolerance. Diabetologia 1984;26:44–9.

206. Efendic S, Luft R, Wajngot A. Aspects of the pathogenesis of type 2 diabetes. Endocrine Rev 1984;5:395–410.

207. Ward WK, Johnston CLW, Beard JC, et al. Insulin resistance and impaired insulin secretion in subjects with histories of gestational diabetes. Diabetes 1985;34:861–9.

208. O'Sullivan JB. Body weight and subsequent diabetes mellitus. JAMA 1982;248:949–52.

209. Duckworth WC, Kitabachi AE. Direct measurement of plasma proinsulin in normal and diabetic subjects. Am J Med 1972;53:418–27.

210. Mako ME, Starr JI, Rubenstein AH. Circulating proinsulin in patients with maturity onset diabetes. Am J Med 1977;63:865–9.

211. Ward WK, LaCava EC, Paquette TL, et al. Disproportionate elevation of immunoreactive proinsulin in type 2 (non-insulin-dependent) diabetes mellitus and in experimental insulin resistance. Diabetologia 1987;30:698–702.

212. Yoshioka N, Kuzuya T, Matsuda A, et al. Serum proinsulin levels at fasting and after oral glucose load in patients with type 2 (non-insulin-dependent) diabetes mellitus. Diabetologia 1988;31:355–60.

213. Temple RC, Carrington CA, Luzio SD, et al. Insulin deficiency in non-insulin-dependent diabetes. Lancet 1989;1:293–5.

214. Saad MF, Kahn SE, Nelson RG, et al. Disproportionately elevated proinsulin in Pima Indians with noninsulin-dependent diabetes mellitus. J Clin Endocrinol Metab 1990;70:1247–53.

215. Polonsky KS, Given BD, Hirsch LJ, et al. Abnormal patterns of insulin secretion in non-insulin-dependent diabetes mellitus. N Engl J Med 1988;318:1231–9.

216. O'Rahilly S, Turner RC, Matthews DR. Impaired pulsatile secretion of insulin in relatives of patients with non-insulin-dependent diabetes. N Engl J Med 1988;318:1225–30.

217. O'Meara NM, Shapiro ET, Van Cauter E, Polonsky KS. Effect of glyburide on beta cell responsiveness to glucose in non-insulin-dependent diabetes mellitus. Am J Med 1990;89(Suppl 2A):11−16S.

218. Turner RC, Holman RR. Beta cell function during insulin or chlorpropamide treatment of maturity-onset diabetes mellitus. Diabetes 1978;27(Suppl 1):241−6.

219. Kosaka K, Kuzuya T, Akanuma Y, Hagura R. Increase in insulin response after treatment of overt maturity-onset diabetes is independent of the mode of treatment. Diabetologia 1980;18:23−8.

220. Hidaka H, Nagulesparan M, Klimes I, et al. Improvement of insulin secretion but not insulin resistance after short term control of plasma glucose in obese Type II diabetics. J Clin Endocrinol Metab 1982;54:217−22.

221. Karam JH, Sanz N, Salamon E, Nolte MS. Selective unresponsiveness of pancreatic β-cells to acute sulfonylurea stimulation during sulfonylurea therapy in NIDDM. Diabetes 1986;35:1314−20.

222. Shapiro ET, Van Cauter E, Tillil H, et al. Glyburide enhances the responsiveness of the β-cell to glucose but does not correct the abnormal patterns of insulin secretion in noninsulin-dependent diabetes mellitus. J Clin Endocrinol Metab 1989;69:571−6.

223. Osei K, Henry ML, O'Dorisio TM, et al. Physiological and pharmacological stimulation of pancreatic islet hormone secretion in type 1 diabetic pancreas allograft recipients. Diabetes 1990;39:1235−42.

224. Östman J, Bolinder J, Gunnarsson R, et al. Metabolic effects of pancreas transplantation: effects of pancreas transplantation on metabolic and hormonal profiles in IDDM patients. Diabetes 1989;38(Suppl 1):88−93.

225. Grunt JA, Pallotta JA, Soeldner JS. Blood sugar, serum insulin and free fatty acid interrelationships during intravenous tolbutamide testing in normal young adults and in patients with insulinoma. Diabetes 1970;19:122−6.

226. Marks V. Progress report: diagnosis of insulinoma. Gut 1971;12:835−43.

227. Service FJ, Horwitz DL, Rubenstein AH, et al. C-peptide suppression test for insulinoma. J Lab Clin Med 1977;90:180−6.

228. Alsever RN, Roberts JP, Gerber JG, et al. Insulinoma with low circulating insulin levels: the diagnostic value of proinsulin measurements. Ann Intern Med 1975; 82:347−50.

229. Cohen RM, Given BD, Licinio-Paixao J, et al. Proinsulin radioimmunoassay in the evaluation of insulinomas and familial hyperproinsulinemia. Metabolism 1986; 35:1137−46.

230. Malherbe C, Burrill KC, Levin SR, et al. Effect of diphenylhydantoin on insulin secretion in man. N Engl J Med 1972;286:339−42.

231. Pace CS, Livingston E. Ionic basis of phenytoin sodium inhibition of insulin secretion in pancreatic islets. Diabetes 1979;28:1077−82.

232. De Marinis L, Barbarino A. Calcium antagonists and hormone release. I. Effects of verapamil on insulin release in normal subjects and patients with islet-cell tumor. Metabolism 1980;29:599−604.

233. Henquin JC, Meissner HP. Opposite effects of tolbutamide and diazoxide on $^{86}Rb^+$ fluxes and membrane potential in pancreatic β-cells. Biochem Pharmacol 1982; 31:1407−14.

234. Gorden P. Glucose intolerance with hypokalemia: failure of short-term potassium depletion in normal subjects to reproduce the glucose and insulin abnormalities of clinical hypokalemia. Diabetes 1973;22:544−51.

235. Helderman JH, Elahi D, Andersen DK, et al. Prevention of the glucose intolerance of thiazide diuretics by maintenance of body potassium. Diabetes 1983;32:106−11.

236. Feldberg W, Shaligram SV. The hyperglycemic effect of morphine. Br J Pharmacol 1972;46:602−18.

237. Passariello N, Giugliano D, Quatraro A, et al. Glucose tolerance and hormonal responses in heroin addicts: a possible role for endogenous opiates in the pathogenesis of non-insulin-dependent diabetes. Metabolism 1983; 32:1163−5.

Chapter 6

HORMONE-FUEL INTERRELATIONSHIPS: FED STATE, STARVATION, AND DIABETES MELLITUS

STUART R. CHIPKIN
KATHLEEN L. KELLY
NEIL B. RUDERMAN

BASIC PRINCIPLES

Fuel Reservoirs

Humans have a constant requirement for energy, but eat only intermittently. To cope with this problem, we usually ingest food in excess of the immediate caloric needs of our vital organs and store the extra calories in the form of hepatic and muscle glycogen, adipose tissue triglyceride, and to a certain extent as muscle protein. In turn, during starvation and in response to various stresses, we break down these fuel reservoirs to provide energy for organ metabolism and function (Fig. 6–1).

The two principal circulating fuels in humans, glucose and free fatty acids (FFA), are stored intracellularly as glycogen and triglycerides, respectively. The largest reservoir of glycogen (300 to 500 g) is in skeletal muscle.[1] However, the principal reservoir of glycogen from which free glucose can be released into the circulation is in the liver (see Table 6–1).[1] The major site of triglyceride storage is adipose tissue. Adipose tissue triglyceride is the most efficient form of energy storage in humans. Triglyceride contains 9.5 kilocalories (kcal)/g and, the average caloric content of an adipocyte, including its cytosol, is approximately 8 kcal/g.[2] In contrast,

glycogen contains 4 kcal/g. Furthermore, because 3 mL of water is needed to maintain the intracellular osmolality of each gram of glycogen in vivo,[3] in reality glycogen provides only 1 kcal/g. Thus, if the 15 kg of adipose tissue triglyceride in a normal 70-kg man were replaced with an equicaloric quantity of glycogen, the individual would weigh an additional 120 kg!

Body protein, although of considerable mass (Table 6–1), is not, strictly speaking, a fuel reservoir. Protein molecules serve specific roles in maintaining organ structure and function and are less expendable than glycogen or triglycerides. On the other hand, a portion of body protein (e.g., some of the contractile protein of muscle) is degraded during starvation and other periods of stress and provides amino acid substrate for gluconeogenesis.

The Brain and Other Vital Organs

The brain has a continuous need for fuel but stores almost no energy as glycogen or fat. Instead, it utilizes glucose derived from the liver either directly from glycogen or indirectly from other fuel reservoirs via gluconeogenesis. The brain does not utilize FFA directly. During prolonged starvation, however, it is able to use

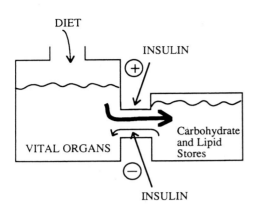

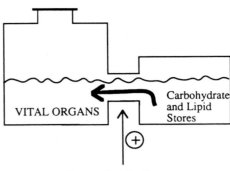

Fig. 6–1. Fuel homeostasis in humans. In the fed state, fuels in excess of the needs of vital organs are stored in carbohydrate and lipid reservoirs, i.e., as glycogen and triglycerides and to some extent as protein. During starvation these stores are broken down to provide fuel for other organs. Changes in circulating levels of insulin and counter-insulin hormones modulate these transitions.

Table 6–1. Fuel Reservoirs in Humans

Source	Grams	Kilocalories
Liver glycogen	75	300
Muscle glycogen	400	1600
Blood glucose	20	80
Adipose tissue triglyceride	15000	141000
Protein	6000	24000

Data are estimates for an overnight-fasted man weighing 70 kg.

energy derived from FFA after their conversion to ketone bodies. Other vital organs, such as liver, heart, and skeletal muscle, also have a continuous requirement for fuels (Table 6–2), but unlike the brain, these organs can utilize fatty acids directly to meet their energy needs.[1,3]

Hormonal Regulators of Fuel Homeostasis

Energy reservoirs in humans are built up and broken down in response to hormonal messages. The principal hormonal messenger is insulin. In the fed state, insulin levels increase, promoting glycogen synthesis in liver and muscle, lipid formation in adipocytes, and amino acid uptake and protein synthesis in most cells. In the postabsorptive state, during starvation and in response to many stresses, decreased insulin levels contribute to

Table 6-2. Typical Daily Fuel Requirements of Liver, Muscle, and Brain of a Physically Active, Normally Fed Human

Organ	Fuel	~kcal/day
Liver	Amino acids, fat, glucose	280
Muscle	Glucose, fat	880
Brain	Glucose	480

glycogen breakdown, lipolysis, hepatic ketogenesis, and decreased synthesis and increased degradation of protein. In the latter situations a major role of insulin is to act as a restraint on these catabolic events (Fig. 6–1).

Multiple hormones counter the effects of insulin. Glucagon stimulates glycogenolysis, gluconeogenesis, and ketogenesis in the liver[4–7] and also can stimulate lipolysis in adipose tissue, although the physiologic relevance of this latter effect is unclear. Catecholamines have effects similar to those of glucagon on the liver and are key regulators of lipolysis in adipose tissue and glycogenolysis in muscle and other tissues. In general, the counter-insulin hormones (also called counterregulatory hormones) liberate energy from fuel reservoirs by actions opposite to those of insulin (Fig. 6–1). However, not all of the actions of these counter-insulin hormones are catabolic. For instance, growth hormone, although catabolic in the sense that it stimulates lipolysis in adipose tissue, also has significant anabolic effects and enhances cell growth.[8] Similarly, glucagon has the anabolic property of stimulating amino acid uptake by the liver.[6]

Glucose Homeostasis

A principal objective of the interplay between insulin and the counter-insulin hormones in humans is the maintenance of normoglycemia. The concentration of glucose in the circulation is more closely controlled than any other fuel. Thus, plasma glucose levels are maintained between 4 and 7 mM in normal humans despite varying rates of glucose utilization (Table 6–3), whereas levels of FFA and ketone bodies may range from 10- to more than a 100-fold, respectively.[9,10] Prevention of hypoglycemia is important because central nervous system function is impaired at low plasma glucose concentrations. Likewise, significant hyperglycemia resulting in glycosuria causes a loss of fuel and may contribute to the complications of

Table 6-3. Rates of Glucose Utilization in the Fed and Fasted State

Tissue	Glucose utilization (g/day)		
	12-hr fast	8-day fast	Marathon run
Brain	120	45	120
Muscle	30	Very low	500

diabetes mellitus. Whether plasma glucose levels modestly above or below the "normal" range are undesirable remains to be determined.

Insulin lowers plasma glucose levels both by stimulating glucose uptake into muscle and adipose tissue and by inhibiting hepatic glycogen breakdown and gluconeogenesis. The different counter-insulin hormones balance these effects of insulin in order to maintain normoglycemia. Thus, glucagon, epinephrine, and norepinephrine all are released into the circulation in response to hypoglycemia[7] and during stresses such as exercise, when glucose utilization is altered by other factors.[11,12] In addition to stimulating hepatic glycogenolysis and gluconeogenesis, the catecholamines inhibit insulin-stimulated glucose utilization in muscle and promote lipolysis in adipose tissue,[13] thereby providing tissues with an alternative fuel to glucose. Glucocorticoids also are released into the circulation in increased quantities in response to hypoglycemia and other stresses.[11,12] Glucocorticoids appear to be necessary for the mobilization of energy stores by catecholamines and glucagon; however, their role may be permissive rather than regulatory.[14]

FIVE PHASES OF FUEL HOMEOSTASIS

Immediately after a carbohydrate or mixed meal has been ingested, the concentrations of insulin, glucose, and glucagon in plasma favor fuel storage. Once absorption of the ingested food is complete, the concentrations of these and other hormones and substrates change, causing a shift from energy storage in fuel reservoirs to energy production. Further alterations in fuel homeostasis occur with more prolonged food deprivation. These changes can be broken down into five phases on the basis of the source and quantity of the glucose entering the circulation. Figure 6–2 illustrates these changes in a hypothetical human who ingests 100 g of glucose and then begins a prolonged fast.[10]

Fed State

During the first few hours after a carbohydrate meal, glucose absorbed from the gastrointestinal tract provides for the metabolic needs of the brain and other organs (Fig. 6–2, phase I). The absorbed glucose in excess of these needs is used to rebuild fuel reservoirs in liver, muscle, and fat and presumably in other tissues (Fig. 6–3). In this setting, plasma insulin levels are high, plasma glucagon levels are low, and glycogen synthesis is stimulated in liver and muscle. Approximately 75 g of carbohydrate is stored as glycogen in liver, and 300 to

500 g is stored in muscle in an overnight-fasted human[1] (Table 6–1).

As noted earlier, the major form of lipid storage in humans is triglyceride and the major site for triglyceride storage is adipose tissue.[2] Smaller amounts of triglyceride are stored in muscle, liver, and other tissues. Triglycerides also are present in the circulation as constituents of lipoproteins. However, the major circulating lipid fuels are the FFA. After a carbohydrate meal, high concentrations of insulin favor the use of both glucose and lipoprotein triglycerides for triglyceride synthesis in adipose tissue.

In addition to promoting the synthesis of glycogen and triglycerides in the fed state, insulin inhibits the breakdown of these fuel reservoirs[15] (i.e., it is anticatabolic). The concentrations of insulin that inhibit lipolysis appear to be lower than those that stimulate glucose transport in muscle. Presumably, it is for this reason that patients with mild Type II diabetes and glucose intolerance are hyperglycemic in the absence of significant elevations of plasma FFA or ketone bodies.

Starvation

With the decrease in plasma insulin levels and the increase in plasma glucagon levels that accompany an overnight fast, fuel homeostasis shifts from energy storage to energy production (Fig. 6–4). At this stage, glucose no longer enters the circulation from the gastrointestinal tract but is derived principally from the breakdown of liver glycogen and, via hepatic gluconeogenesis, from lactate, amino acids, and glycerol.[1] In addition, circulat-

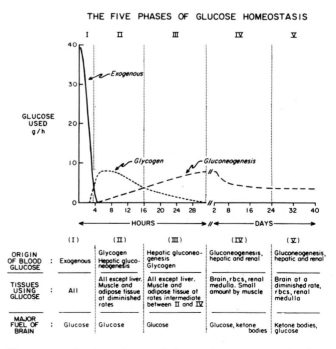

Fig. 6–2. The five phases of glucose homeostasis. The figure depicts rates of glucose utilization and the source of glucose entering the circulation in a 70-kg man who ingests 100 g of glucose and then fasts for 40 days.

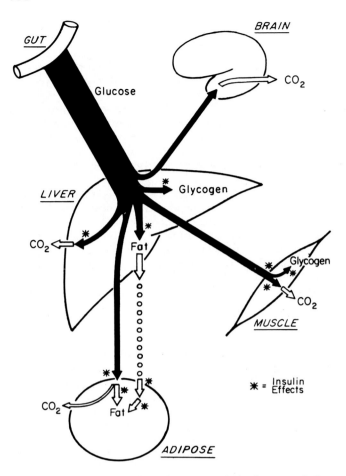

Fig. 6–3. Fuel metabolism during a carbohydrate meal. Soon after the ingestion of carbohydrate, insulin levels rise and stimulate the uptake of glucose. Glucose is the major oxidative fuel of all major tissues at this time. Glucose that is present in excess of the oxidative needs of tissues is stored as glycogen or lipid. Asterisks indicate steps enhanced by insulin.

ing FFA, derived from the hydrolysis of adipocyte triglycerides, become a major source of fuel.[16] As will be discussed later, by using FFA, muscle and liver decrease their oxidation of glucose as a fuel, thereby conserving it for the brain.

Mobilization of Carbohydrate and Lipid Stores

In the earliest phase of starvation, i.e., the postabsorptive state, hepatic glycogen is a major source of the glucose entering the circulation and remains so for 12 to 24 hours.[17,18] Glucagon seems to be necessary for hepatic glycogenolysis during this period, although an increase in the level of plasma glucagon does not appear to be the primary stimulus.[19–21] After an overnight fast, the average rate of glucose utilization by a normal human is approximately 7 g/hour (Table 6–3).[1] By extrapolation, the 70 to 80 g of glycogen present in the liver can provide glucose to the brain and peripheral tissues for 12 to 16 hours. Two events allow for the maintenance of blood glucose levels beyond this time: 1) muscle and other

tissues begin to oxidize lipid-derived fuels in place of glucose and 2) hepatic gluconeogenesis replaces glycogenolysis as the principal source of glucose entering the circulation (Fig. 6–4). As will be discussed later, glycogen breakdown in muscle does not yield significant quantities of free glucose, and after an overnight fast, gluconeogenesis by the kidney is of minor importance.

Two factors stimulate the breakdown of adipocyte triglyceride during starvation. First, the concentration of circulating insulin diminishes and, as a consequence, triglyceride synthesis is decreased and lipolysis is enhanced.[2,22] Second, norepinephrine is released from sympathetic nerve endings and directly stimulates lipolysis by raising levels of cyclic adenosine monophosphate (cAMP) in adipocytes.[2,22] Epinephrine, which is secreted from the adrenal medulla, appears to play a lesser role. The mechanisms by which FFA are released into the circulation are discussed in the section on adipose tissue (see below). The principal users of FFA during the early phases of starvation are skeletal muscle and liver.

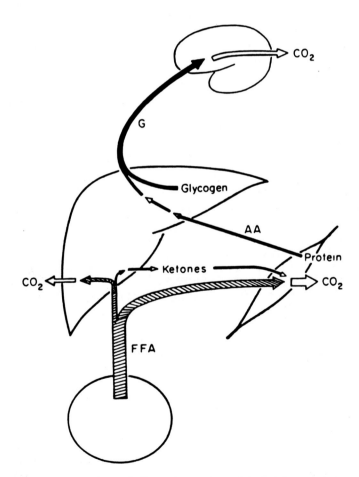

Fig. 6–4. Fuel metabolism after an overnight fast (postabsorptive). After approximately 12 hours of starvation, insulin concentrations have returned to basal levels and glucose entering the circulation is derived from both hepatic glycogen and gluconeogenesis. Free fatty acids (FFA) produced from adipocyte lipolysis have become a principal fuel for skeletal muscle.

Gluconeogenesis

Since the brain is unable to use FFA as a fuel, it must continue to use glucose during the early phases of starvation. Gluconeogenesis is an important source of the glucose entering the circulation even after an overnight fast and becomes the major source as hepatic glycogen stores become depleted (Fig. 6–2, phase III).[18] Gluconeogenesis is responsible for approximately 35 to 60% of the hepatic glucose output after an overnight fast (12 to 15 hours postabsorptive) and for more than 97% the output by 60 hours of starvation.[18,23,24] At 60 hours, glucose production is limited not by the enzymatic capacity of the liver but by the concentration of gluconeogenic substrate in the circulation.[25] During the early phases of starvation, the two principal gluconeogenic precursors are lactate and alanine (Table 6–4).[14,26–28]

Lactate comprises 50% of the gluconeogenic substrate of liver in an overnight-fasted human and is the major gluconeogenic substrate throughout starvation (Table 6–4).[26] When glucose cannot be metabolized beyond pyruvate in peripheral tissues, much of the pyruvate is reduced to lactate, which is then released into the circulation (Fig. 6–5). In red blood cells and renal medulla, this reduction occurs because there are no mitochondria in which pyruvate can be oxidized. In muscle and other tissues, lactate and pyruvate are released during starvation because the activity of pyruvate dehydrogenase, the enzyme that converts pyruvate to acetyl CoA, is decreased.[29] For the most part, lactate generated from glucose in this way is taken up by the liver and reconverted to glucose by the gluconeogenic pathway.[27] This recycling of glucose between liver and peripheral tissues via lactate is referred to as the Cori cycle.

A second major group of gluconeogenic substrates is that of the amino acids. Skeletal muscle is the principal reservoir of amino acids in humans.[28] During early starvation, however, the gut and liver also appear to be important sources of the amino acids entering the circulation.[30] A major stimulus to protein catabolism (both decreased synthesis and increased degradation) during starvation is the decrease in plasma insulin concentrations.[31–33] Glucagon stimulates protein degradation in liver, and glucocorticoids inhibit protein synthesis in muscle and other tissues.[28] Although increases in the plasma levels of these counter-insulin hormones almost certainly play a role in modulating protein catabolism in stressful states (e.g., diabetic ketoacidosis and trauma), their concentrations are not dramatically altered during starvation, and their role here is thought to be limited.

The principal amino acids released into the circulation from muscle are alanine and glutamine (Fig. 6–6). Most of the alanine is taken up directly by the liver, whereas glutamine is metabolized in the gastrointestinal tract, which in turn releases alanine. Glutamine also is taken up directly by the kidney, when it is the principal gluconeogenic substrate. Glutamine and alanine, despite comprising only 15 to 20% of muscle protein,[28,33–35] account for 50% of the amino acids released by muscle because these amino acids can be generated from other constituents in muscle as well as from the degradation of protein. Alanine is formed by the transamination of pyruvate by alanine

Table 6-4. Gluconeogenic Substrates in Humans Starved for 24 Hours

Substrate	Amount generated (g/day)
Lactate	60
Amino acids except alanine	25
Alanine only	25
Glycerol	14
Pyruvate	5
Total	129

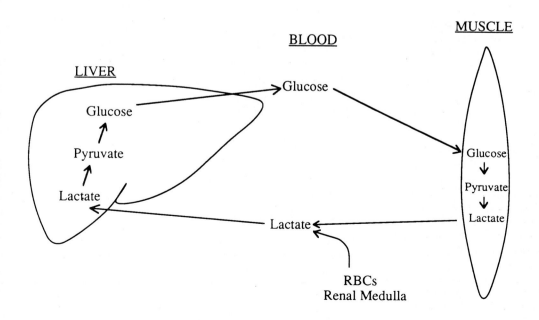

Fig. 6–5. The Cori cycle. Lactate derived from glycolysis in skeletal muscle, red blood cells (RBCs), renal medulla, and other tissues is taken up by the liver, which uses it to synthesize glucose. The glucose can then be reused by these same tissues.

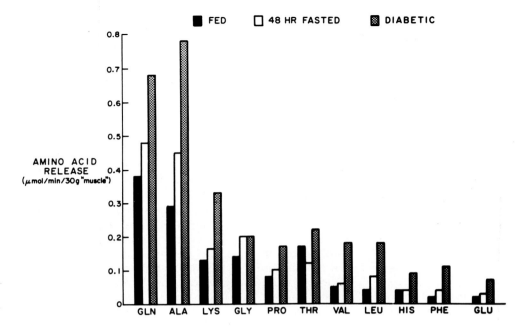

Fig. 6–6. Release of amino acids from hindlimb muscle of fed, fasted, and streptozotocin-diabetic rats perfused with an amino acid-free medium. The amino acids released in greatest amount are glutamine and alanine. In humans the pattern of amino acid release is similar except that glutamine is taken up from the circulation.

aminotransferase and glutamine by the amidation of glutamate by free ammonia, a reaction catalyzed by glutamine synthetase.[35]

The rate of release of alanine increases markedly during starvation and other insulin-deficient states.[28,36] Despite this, its concentration in plasma is usually diminished in these situations because the uptake of alanine by the liver is stimulated to an even greater extent. Since the interorgan relationships of alanine are very much like those of lactate, a "glucose-alanine cycle" similar to the Cori cycle has been proposed.[17] Impaired release of alanine from muscle has been postulated as a contributor to impaired gluconeogenesis and hypoglycemia in patients with uremia, maple syrup urine disease, ketotic hypoglycemia of infancy, and in starved women during pregnancy.[37]

The other major gluconeogenic substrate is glycerol, which is derived principally from the hydrolysis of adipose tissue triglyceride. In nondiabetic subjects the rate with which glycerol appears in the circulation correlates with adipose mass[38] and increases during starvation.

Prolonged Starvation

Ketone Bodies and the Brain

With the prolongation of starvation, several events occur that limit the need for gluconeogenesis and thereby conserve body protein (Fig. 6–7). The first of these, as already noted, is an increase in the reliance of muscle and other peripheral tissues on lipid-derived fuels: initially FFA and later both FFA and the ketone bodies, acetoacetate and β-hydroxybutyrate. The second is a change in the fuels used by the brain. During early starvation, the central nervous system continues to use glucose as its exclusive fuel. However, as starvation is prolonged, plasma levels of the ketone bodies increase to

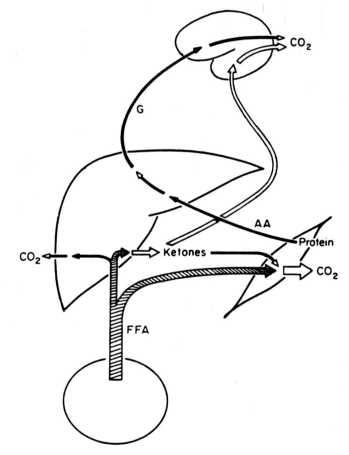

Fig. 6–7. Fuel metabolism during prolonged starvation. As fasting continues, insulin levels remain suppressed and the principal source of hepatic glucose production is gluconeogenesis. Skeletal muscle continues to use free fatty acids (FFA) for fuel but also uses ketone bodies produced in the liver. Ketone bodies may also be used by the brain.

values even greater than that of glucose (Fig. 6−8). Under these circumstances, the brain, or at least parts of it, increases its use of these lipid-derived fuels.[1,39,40]

Ketone bodies are produced from acetyl CoA via the β-oxidation of fatty acids in the liver (Fig. 6−9). This process, termed ketogenesis, is enhanced by glucagon and inhibited by insulin. In contrast to long-chain FFA, the ketone bodies are water-soluble and cross the blood-brain barrier via specific carrier proteins.[41−43] Furthermore, the activity of these carriers is increased in physiologic states associated with sustained hyperketonemia such as diabetic ketoacidosis and starvation.[44,45] These physiologic adaptations enhance the use of ketone bodies by the brain in place of glucose and diminish the need to degrade proteins for gluconeogenesis. It is because of these adaptations that humans of normal weight are able to survive fasts of up to 60 to 70 days.

Gluconeogenesis and Protein Catabolism

The decreased use of glucose by the brain during prolonged starvation is accompanied by a diminished rate of gluconeogenesis in the liver (Fig. 6−2 and Table 6−3). The latter appears to be due to decreases in protein catabolism and secondarily the release of gluconeogenic amino acids (mostly alanine) from muscle.[16,28] Some studies suggest that these adaptations in protein metabolism are related to the increased use of lipid fuels during prolonged starvation.[27,46,47] Whatever the mechanism, as one proceeds from early to prolonged starvation, urinary excretion of nitrogen decreases from 12 g/day to 3 to 4 g/day, indicating a decrease in protein catabolism from 75 g/day to 12 to 20 g/day.[1]

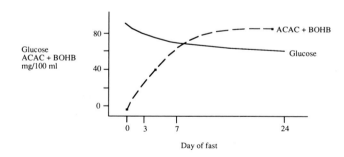

Tissue	Fuel	Quantity Used (g/day)			
Brain	Glucose	120	100		50
	K.B.	0	20		70
Muscle	K.B.	0	100		50
Liver	Glucose	-210	-150	-100	-80

Fig. 6−8. Changes in plasma concentrations of fuels during starvation. Blood glucose concentrations decrease during the first 7 days of a fast but then remain relatively stable. As glucose utilization decreases, the concentration and use of ketone bodies (K.B.) increases (ACAC = acetoacetate; BOHB = β-hydroxybutyrate). After a week of starvation the concentration of ketone bodies in blood is equal to or greater than glucose level.

The relative contribution of the kidney to gluconeogenesis increases from 5 to 10% after an overnight fast to 50% after 3 to 4 weeks of starvation.[1,48] However, in absolute amounts, renal production of glucose is still much lower than hepatic production of glucose after 1 to 2 days of fasting. The increase in renal gluconeogenesis during prolonged starvation is linked to an increase in NH_3 generation from glutamine.

Unlike amino acids, the relative importance of glycerol as a gluconeogenic precursor increases during prolonged starvation. This reflects the fact that the release of glycerol from fat is approximately 14 g/day and remains nearly constant during early and late starvation.[48] After several weeks of starvation, gluconeogenesis from glycerol hypothetically provides upwards of half of the glucose oxidized by the brain.

Hormonal Controls

The gradual decrease in plasma insulin modulates the orderly breakdown of fuel reservoirs during the early phases of starvation. However, during prolonged starvation, the decreases in protein degradation and in glucose and ketone-body use in muscle (see below) occur in the absence of further changes in plasma insulin. Some studies suggest that a decrease in thyroid hormone activity contributes to these adaptations.[47] Presumably the low levels of insulin present during prolonged starvation are needed for these adaptations to occur. Thus, patients without any insulin (e.g., during diabetic ketoacidosis) have an impaired ability both to limit the breakdown of their fuel reservoirs and to use glucose and ketone bodies in peripheral tissues. The precise connection between the presence of insulin and these adaptations remains to be determined.

HORMONE-FUEL INTERRELATIONS AT AN ORGAN LEVEL

Adipose Tissue

Triglyceride Synthesis and Lipolysis

The major function of adipose tissue in fuel homeostasis is to store energy as triglycerides in the fed state, when insulin levels are high, and to release it in the form of FFA and glycerol during starvation and in states when levels of counter-insulin hormones are increased and those of insulin are diminished (Fig. 6−10). Triglyceride metabolism involves the coordinated regulation of various transport processes and enzymes by these hormones. How insulin works in this setting will be discussed to illustrate some of the known and proposed mechanisms of insulin action. Insulin action is discussed in more detail in Chapter 8.

Mechanisms of Insulin Action

The first regulated event in insulin signaling is activation of the tyrosine kinase encoded by the subunit of the insulin receptor.[49,50] Insulin binding stimulates the activity of the receptor kinase, which phosphorylates itself exclusively on tyrosine residues.[50,51] This autophospho-

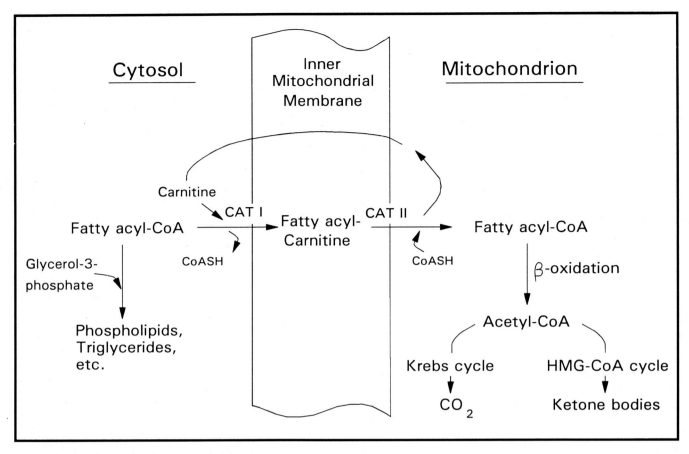

Fig. 6–9. Mitochondrial fatty acid transport. Fatty acyl CoA is transported from the cytosol into mitochondria by a series of steps that involves carnitine acyltransferase (CAT) I and II and a carnitine acyltranslocase (not shown). When rates of fatty acid transport into liver mitochondria are high, the hepatocyte obtains most of its fuel needs from the β-oxidation of the fatty acyl CoA and the Krebs (tricarboxylic acid) cycle is inhibited. By generating malonyl CoA, an inhibitor of CAT I, insulin inhibits fatty acid transport and, secondarily, ketogenesis. Glucagon has the opposite effect.

rylation leads to enhanced protein tyrosine kinase activity toward exogenous substrates.[49,52] Shortly thereafter, following a sequence of events that remains only loosely defined, glucose transport is enhanced and the activity of hormone-sensitive lipase is inhibited.[53,54] In addition, the secretion of lipoprotein lipase[55] and apparently the activity of glycerol phosphate acyltransferase are increased.[56]

Hormone-sensitive lipase is only one of a large number of proteins that are phosphorylated or dephosphorylated on serine and/or threonine residues in response to insulin.[57] On the basis of these and other findings, it has been suggested that insulin action may involve a phosphorylation cascade triggered by activation of the insulin receptor tyrosine kinase. According to this theory, the key event following activation of the insulin receptor is the phosphorylation of one or more pivotal kinases and/or phosphatases, which in turn regulate the activity of insulin target proteins. Several regulatory kinases have recently been shown to be activated by tyrosine phosphorylation in response to insulin,[58–60] thus lending support to this hypothesis.

Lipoprotein lipase, on the other hand, is representative of those proteins for which phosphorylation or dephos-

phorylation has yet to be implicated in their regulation by insulin. One theory suggests that insulin stimulates the generation of second messengers, analogous to cAMP, that could act independently or in concert with a phosphorylation cascade. The compounds proposed as insulin second messengers include diacylglycerol[61] and inositol-phosphoglycans.[62,63] The data to support their role in insulin action are still sketchy, and nothing is known about their effect on lipoprotein lipase.

Glucose Transport

Before glucose enters an intracellular metabolic pathway, it must first be transported across the plasma membrane. Glucose can be actively cotransported with Na^+ in kidney and intestine. However, most cells transport glucose via a facilitated diffusion mechanism that does not require energy.[64] For this purpose they use a specialized family of glucose-transport proteins. Adipose tissue, skeletal muscle, and heart muscle have an abundance of a specific glucose-transport protein (GLUT-4 or insulin-responsive glucose transporter) that is extremely sensitive to the effects of insulin.[65] Exposure of fat cells to insulin causes a translocation of GLUT-4 proteins from a

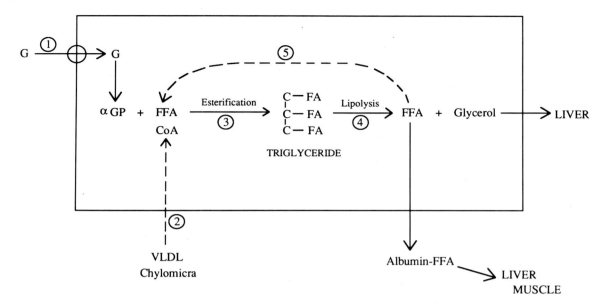

Fig. 6–10. Triglyceride metabolism in adipose tissue. Insulin stimulates triglyceride accumulation by enhancing glucose (G) transport (1), activating lipoprotein lipase (2) and glycerol phosphate (GP) acyltransferase (3), and inhibiting hormone-sensitive lipase (4). By virtue of its effects on (1) and (3), insulin also stimulates the reesterification of free fatty acids (FFA) (5) derived from the lipolysis of intracellular triglyceride. Counter-insulin hormones, such as norepinephrine, stimulate lipolysis by activating hormone-sensitive lipase. In addition, counter-insulin hormones appear to inhibit the three processes, i.e., (1–3), stimulated by insulin. FFA that are released from the adipocyte are carried complexed to albumin in the circulation. Principal sites at which FFA are utilized include muscle and liver (see Fig. 6–11). The glycerol released during lipolysis is not metabolized in the adipocyte, which lacks glycerol kinase. Most of this glycerol appears to be used by the liver for gluconeogenesis. VLDL = very-low-density lipoprotein.

low-density microsomal fraction to the plasma membrane[66] and also may increase their intrinsic activity.[67] During starvation and in insulin-dependent diabetes, the total amount of GLUT-4 in adipocytes decreases,[68] as does the amount of GLUT-4 mRNA,[69] possibly contributing to the decrease in insulin-stimulated glucose transport in these conditions.

Lipoprotein Lipase

Lipoprotein lipase is an N-linked glycoprotein that is synthesized and secreted by a variety of extrahepatic tissues, principally adipose tissue and muscle.[70] In adipose tissue, it is synthesized as an inactive precursor in the endoplasmic reticulum.[71,72] In response to insulin and in the presence of glucose,[73] a high-mannose form of lipoprotein lipase is directed from the endoplasmic reticulum to the Golgi apparatus, where mannose units are trimmed, N-linked glycosylation occurs, and lipoprotein lipase is sorted into a secretory pathway.[72] At this stage, lipoprotein lipase undergoes an undefined "activation" event, after which it moves to the plasma membrane. From the plasma membrane, it is either secreted or diverted into a lysosomal degradative pathway.[72,74,75] Secreted lipoprotein lipase acts at the endothelial cell surface in the presence of apolipoprotein C_{II} to hydrolyze the triglyceride core of chylomicrons and very-low-density lipoproteins (VLDL). The FFA released by this reaction are taken up by the adipocyte, where they are esterified with glycerol-3-phosphate to form triglycerides.

The ability of insulin to stimulate acutely the secretion of lipoprotein lipase is dependent on the presence of glucose.[73] In contrast, the ability of insulin to stimulate lipoprotein lipase synthesis does not show such a dependence.[73] A working model suggests that in adipose tissue in the fed state the majority of lipoprotein lipase is expressed as functional enzyme at the endothelial cell surface or in a secretable Golgi/post-Golgi pool. A smaller fraction is present in a precursor pool associated with the endoplasmic reticulum.[72] During starvation, there is no acute change in the total mass of lipoprotein lipase. However, the enzyme is redistributed, so that the functional pool at the endothelial cell surface is diminished and the majority of enzyme is present in the inactive form associated with the endoplasmic reticulum. As a consequence, the secretion of lipoprotein lipase from adipose tissue is decreased during starvation and the ability of adipose tissue to utilize chylomicron and VLDL triglyceride is depressed. In contrast, the secretion of lipoprotein lipase by heart and skeletal muscle is increased during starvation. Teleologically, this would assist the transition of these tissues to a lipid fuel economy, since the liberated fatty acids are oxidized by these tissues to generate adenosine triphosphate (ATP).[76]

Hormone-Sensitive Lipase

The hydrolysis of adipose tissue triglyceride is catalyzed by hormone-sensitive lipase (Fig. 6–10). The latter is a soluble enzyme that associates with the lipid droplet[77] and bears no structural homology to lipoprotein lipase.[78] Hormone-sensitive lipase specifically catalyzes the conversion of triglycerides to diglycerides. Other lipases complete the degradation process; ultimately, three molecules of fatty acid plus one molecule of glycerol are formed. The initial cleavage catalyzed by the hormone-sensitive lipase is the rate-limiting step in the sequence and is about 10 times slower than the breakdown of diglyceride to monoglyceride.[79] In general, once triglyceride hydrolysis is initiated, FFA are released, with very little accumulation of diglycerides and other intermediates. As shown in Figure 6−10, the FFA can be released into the circulation, where they are transported to other tissues in a complex with albumin. Alternatively, they can be re-esterified with glycerol-3-phosphate derived from glucose to re-form triglycerides. The latter process is favored by insulin and presumably contributes to the high rate of triglyceride synthesis and the low rate of FFA release in the fed state. The glycerol formed during triglyceride breakdown is not used for re-esterification since adipose tissue possesses little, if any, glycerol kinase.

Hormone-sensitive lipase is a classic example of an enzyme regulated by covalent modification. Catecholamines, glucagon, and other hormones that increase cAMP by activating adenylate cyclase activate hormone-sensitive lipase via a phosphorylation of serine and threonine residues on the enzyme.[80] Insulin decreases the activity of hormone-sensitive lipase by promoting its dephosphorylation, either by lowering cAMP levels[81] and/or by activating a phosphoprotein phosphatase.[82,83] Insulin diminishes cAMP by increasing the activity of a phosphodiesterase that converts cAMP to AMP[84] or may decrease the activity of adenylate cyclase directly.[85]

Glycerol Phosphate Acyltransferase

Relatively little is known about the rate-limiting enzyme for triglyceride formation, α-glycerol phosphate acyltransferase. This enzyme appears to become inactive when phosphorylated by a cAMP-dependent protein kinase (catecholamine-stimulated)[86] and to become activated when dephosphorylated by a phosphoprotein phosphatase[87] in response to insulin.[56,88] The regulation therefore is opposite that of triglyceride lipase and should permit a tight control of triglyceride formation and breakdown.

Muscle

Fiber Types

Muscle comprises approximately 40% of body mass in a man of normal weight. It accounts for 20 to 30% of the body's oxygen consumption at rest and for up to 90% during exercise.[89] Muscle fibers in the rat are classified as slow-twitch red (type 1), fast-twitch red (type 2a), and fast-twitch white (type 2b) according to their contractile characteristics and their capacity for oxidative metabo-

A. After a carbohydrate meal (high insulin)

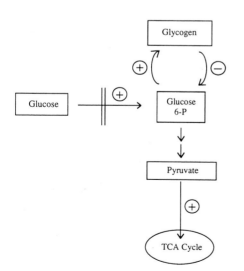

B. After 24-28 hrs. of starvation (low insulin)

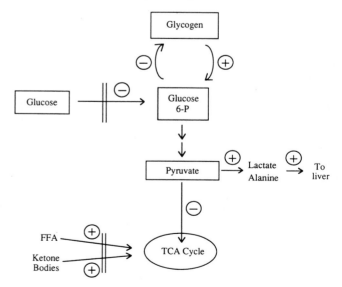

Fig. 6−11. Muscle fuel metabolism. A: After a carbohydrate meal (high insulin), glucose uptake by the muscle is increased. Within the cell, glycogen synthesis is increased, as is use of glucose by the tricarboxylic acid (TCA) cycle. B: After 24 to 48 hours of starvation, muscle glucose uptake is inhibited and glycogen is broken down. Pyruvate dehydrogenase is inhibited, and pyruvate is converted to free fatty acids (FFA) and, to a lesser extent, to ketone bodies. The (+) symbols indicate steps enhanced and the (−) symbols indicate steps diminished in comparison to rates following an overnight fast.

lism.[90,91] The same fiber types are found in human muscle.[90] In general, the red fibers have a high oxidative capacity and oxidize fatty acids and other fuels in addition to glucose. White fibers have a lesser ability to oxidize fuels and generate a greater portion of their ATP from glycolysis. With respect to exercise, white fibers are those principally recruited during brief periods of intense exercise such as sprinting or weight-lifting and red fibers are those recruited during endurance-type activities of low-to-moderate intensity such as walking and running.[17,90,92]

All of the fiber types in muscle respond to insulin. However, red fibers have a greater number of insulin receptors[93] and GLUT-4 glucose transporters[94] than do white fibers. In addition, muscles rich in red fibers have more capillaries per mass,[90,92] which could enhance diffusion of insulin and glucose from the plasma to the muscle cell.[95] Perhaps for all of these reasons, glucose uptake in red muscle is more sensitive to insulin than is white muscle, both in vivo and in vitro.[96-98] Physical training, which causes white fibers to assume some of the characteristics of red fibers, is associated with an increase in their GLUT-4 content.[99,100]

Muscle Fuel Reservoirs

Glycogen. Glycogen in muscle is synthesized from circulating glucose following meals and exercise and is broken down during exercise and starvation. Glycogenolysis in muscle does not result in the release of free glucose into the circulation, since muscle cells are deficient in glucose-6-phosphatase. As a result, the 300 to 500 g of carbohydrate stored as glycogen in muscle is used solely for its own energy needs and for generating lactate and other gluconeogenic substrates for the liver (Fig. 6–11).

The importance of glycogen as a fuel in contracting muscle is underscored by the association of glycogen depletion with the phenomenon of "hitting the wall" in runners.[101] Likewise, patients with McCardle's syndrome, a hereditary deficiency of muscle phosphorylase, are unable to maintain high-energy phosphate stores during exercise.[102] During starvation, muscle glycogen in normal individuals diminishes by approximately 33% after 2 to 3 days and then remains constant as muscle switches over more completely to a lipid fuel economy.[3,17] During early starvation (phases I and II) and exercise, a considerable portion of the lactate, pyruvate, and alanine released by muscle is presumably derived from this glycogen breakdown.[28]

The regulation of glycogen synthesis and degradation in muscle by insulin is similar to its regulation of adipocyte triglyceride. Insulin stimulates glycogen synthesis by enhancing glucose transport and activating (dephosphorylating) a key regulatory enzyme, glycogen synthase[103] (Fig. 6–12). Likewise, it concurrently diminishes the breakdown of glycogen by inhibiting the conversion (phosphorylation) of phosphorylase b to phosphorylase a.[104] These effects of insulin are mediated by specific phosphatases that both activate glycogen synthase and eventually inhibit phosphorylase b kinase. Somewhat analogous changes occur in muscle after

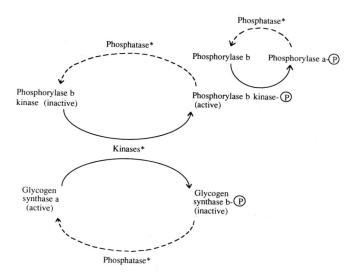

Fig. 6–12. Regulation of glycogen synthase and phosphorylase in skeletal muscle. Asterisks indicate reactions affected by insulin. P = phosphate that alters activity.

exercise, when glycogen synthesis is also increased (see Chapter 26 on exercise). Catecholamines and exercise per se both stimulate the breakdown of muscle glycogen (Fig. 6–13). As in adipose tissue, catecholamines (epinephrine) act by increasing cAMP and secondarily by increasing cAMP-dependent protein kinase, which in turn activates (phosphorylates) phosphorylase b kinase.[15,105,106]

Lipids. Red muscle fibers, in particular, store some energy as triglycerides, and triglyceride hydrolysis may provide a portion of their fuel needs during exercise.[107] The question of whether the synthesis and breakdown of triglycerides in muscle are regulated by the same mechanisms as in adipose tissue has not been intensively studied. The activities of lipoprotein lipase in muscle and adipose tissue go in opposite directions during feeding and starvation, suggesting differences between the two tissues with respect to their use of circulating triglycerides.[76]

Protein. The synthesis and degradation of protein in muscle also are regulated by insulin. Insulin promotes protein synthesis in the fed state and probably acts as a brake on protein degradation during starvation. The mechanisms by which insulin acts on protein metabolism are more complex than its actions on carbohydrate and fat metabolism and have been reviewed elsewhere.[108]

Starvation. Following a carbohydrate meal or insulin administration, glucose derived from the circulation is the principal oxidative fuel of muscle.[109] During early starvation, however, fatty acids are the principle fuel of muscle[109,110] (Fig. 6–11B). As noted earlier, this transition to a lipid fuel conserves glucose for use by the brain and conserves protein by reducing the need for gluconeogenesis. The precise mechanism by which these events are modulated has not been resolved but is almost certainly related initially to a decrease in circulating insulin levels to values lower than those in the fed state.

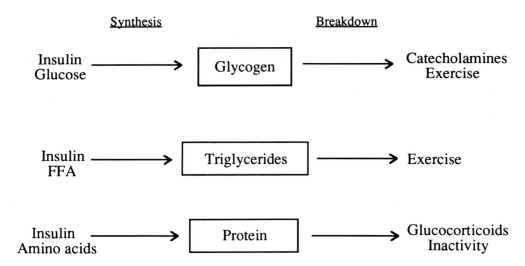

Fig. 6–13. Muscle fuel reservoirs and their regulation. Insulin stimulates the synthesis of glycogen triglycerides and protein. The breakdown of glycogen and triglycerides is stimulated by catecholamines and by exercise. The breakdown of protein is enhanced by glucocorticoids and inactivity. FFA = free fatty acids.

Among the changes attributable to the lowered insulin levels during starvation are 1) diminished glucose transport into muscle; 2) higher plasma levels of FFA; and 3) inhibition of pyruvate dehydrogenase in muscle, resulting in a decrease in glucose oxidation and an increase in release of lactate and pyruvate and, secondarily, of alanine. Whether low levels of plasma insulin activate carnitine palmitoyltransferase (CPT), the enzyme that transports long-chain fatty acyl CoA into the mitochondria of muscle (Fig. 6–9) and thereby regulates its rate of fatty acid oxidation, is not clear. Such activation seems likely since the concentration of malonyl CoA, a metabolite that inhibits CPT, is diminished in the muscle of starved rats.[111]

Another group of fuels used by muscle during starvation are the ketone bodies. Acetoacetate and β-hydroxybutyrate are oxidized by muscle more or less as a function of their concentration in plasma. In rats starved for 48 hours[112] and in humans starved for 1 to 2 weeks,[113] the metabolism of these ketone bodies may account for upwards of 70% of the oxygen consumed by muscle. A role for insulin in regulating the utilization of ketone bodies by muscle has been suggested by studies in rats[114] and humans.[115,116]

It is interesting that during prolonged starvation the use of ketone bodies by muscle diminishes and FFA once again become the principal oxidative fuel[16] (Fig. 6–8). This fuel switch in muscle occurs at a time the when brain is increasing its utilization of acetoacetate and β-hydroxybutyrate, thus permitting the liver to provide these ketone bodies without markedly increasing the rate of ketogenesis. The mechanism responsible for the switch in fuels is not known. From the perspective of total body fuel economy, however, the switch is clearly advantageous because during prolonged starvation the liver is already obtaining most of its energy from the β-oxidation of fatty acids to acetyl CoA (Fig. 6–9). Thus, to increase ketogenesis further would require the liver to oxidize more fatty acid than required for its own needs and would cause an unnecessary waste of body lipid (FFA).

Liver

The liver is the key regulatory site of glucose homeostasis. Blood glucose levels are maintained in a narrow range in great measure because the liver has the ability to take up glucose in the fed state and to release it in varying amounts into the circulation during starvation, exercise, and other situations in which the ratio of insulin to counter-insulin factors is decreased (Fig. 6–13). Although it does not play a key role in determining the rate at which FFA enter the circulation, the liver does appear to play a major role in their disposition. Thus, the liver either can oxidize FFA for its own energy needs or for production of ketone bodies or it can utilize FFA for the synthesis of triglycerides and phospholipids, which it can export as constituents of VLDL.

Fed State

High levels of circulating insulin and decreased levels of glucagon, such as occur after a carbohydrate meal, stimulate glycogen synthase and inhibit glycogen phosphorylase in liver.[15,117] These changes in insulin and glucagon also inhibit hepatic gluconeogenesis.[20,21,118] However, gluconeogenesis does not appear to cease immediately but may continue for several hours after a fast is terminated with a meal. This persistence of gluconeogenesis after a meal may allow hepatic glycogen synthesis to continue when glucose absorption by the gut is no longer in excess of the needs of other organs. According to this glucose paradox hypothesis,[119] dietary glucose is metabolized initially to pyruvate or lactate in peripheral cells; the liver then takes up these gluconeogenic precursors and resynthesizes glucose-6-phosphate, which can be used to synthesize glycogen. Studies in humans suggest that glucose is incorporated into glycogen by this indirect route as well as by the classical direct pathway.[120,121] Recent studies using ^{13}C nuclear magnetic resonance (NMR) spectroscopy suggest that glucose conversion to glycogen via the direct pathway predominates immediately after a standard meal.[121]

Starvation

As starvation proceeds through its different phases (Fig. 6–2), the liver releases fuels into the circulation by three distinct processes: glycogenolysis, gluconeogenesis, and ketone-body formation. The breakdown of glycogen in the liver is essentially regulated by insulin and counter-insulin hormones in a manner analogous to that in skeletal muscle.[117] A major difference between the two tissues, as previously stated, is that liver can generate free glucose, which is released into the circulation, because of the presence of glucose-6-phosphatase. Another difference is that a primary stimulus of hepatic glycogenolysis is glucagon, which does not act on muscle.

Binding of glucagon to its receptor activates adenyl cyclase in liver, producing cAMP from ATP.[122] Besides initiating glycogenolysis, an increase in liver cAMP suppresses glycogen synthesis and increases gluconeogenesis.[4,17,117,122] As noted earlier, liver glycogenolysis is critical in meeting the body's energy requirements in the early stages of starvation. Between one-third and two-thirds of the glucose released by the liver after an overnight fast is derived from hepatic glycogen.[18] Several inherited metabolic disorders of glycogen storage or breakdown have been described. These include von Gierke's disease (type I glycogen storage disease), in which glucose-6-phosphatase is deficient and the liver cannot release free glucose into the circulation, and Cori's disease (type III glycogen storage disease), in which the debranching enzyme that hydrolyzes the 1,6 linkage of the glycogen molecule is absent.[123]

Gluconeogenesis

In humans the maintenance of euglycemia during starvation depends on the ability of the liver to synthesize glucose from non-hexose precursors, i.e., gluconeogenesis (Table 6–4 and Fig. 6–14). The molecular mechanisms regulating gluconeogenesis[17,118,124] and the disorders of this pathway in humans have been reviewed elsewhere.[10,28,118] Gluconeogenesis uses many of the enzymes involved in glycolysis but requires unique enzymes to circumvent the reactions catalyzed by phosphofructokinase and pyruvate kinase (Fig. 6–14). As with glycogenolysis, glucagon is a major positive hormonal modulator of gluconeogenesis and insulin is the primary inhibitor. Catecholamines also stimulate gluconeogenesis and may be the principal positive regulator in some patients with long-standing Type I diabetes in whom glucagon secretion is impaired.[7] Glucocorticoids appear to play an important permissive role, since the stimulation of gluconeogenesis by glucagon and catecholamines is diminished in their absence.[14]

Ketone-Body Formation

Ketone-body synthesis occurs exclusively within the liver. Mitochondrial acetyl CoA produced from oxidation of fatty acids either can combine with oxaloacetate and enter the tricarboxylic acid (TCA) cycle or can be used for the synthesis of acetoacetate and β-hydroxybutyrate within the mitochondrion.[17,124–127] When rates of FFA-

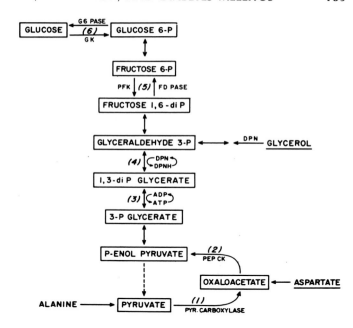

Fig. 6–14. Glucose metabolism in liver during starvation. The reactions in parentheses are altered to favor gluconeogenesis at the expense of glycolysis. PEPCK = phosphoenolpyruvate carboxykinase; PFK = phosphofructokinase; FD PASE = fructose-1,6-diphosphate; DPN = NAD (nicotinamide adenine dinucleotide); DPNH = NADH.

CoA uptake by mitochondria are high, much of the energy needs of the liver are generated by their β-oxidation to CoA. Under these conditions acetyl CoA preferentially enters the pathway for ketone-body formation and its oxidation in the TCA cycle is diminished (Fig. 6–9). The high ratio of glucagon to insulin and the increase in intrahepatic fatty acids during prolonged starvation stimulate the enzyme carnitine acyltransferase I, which is located within the outer leaflet of the inner mitochondrial membrane (Fig. 6–9).[126,127] Carnitine acyltransferase I facilitates the transport of long-chain fatty acyl carnitine across the outer membrane, and its activation is rate-limiting for fatty acid oxidation.

TYPE I DIABETES MELLITUS

The hormone-fuel interrelationships described in normal humans are abnormal in patients with untreated insulin-dependent diabetes mellitus (IDDM) because of the lack of insulin. The precise manifestations of this lack depend on its severity. During the period before the onset of overt IDDM and during the "honeymoon" phase following its diagnosis, patients may have sufficiently high plasma insulin levels to maintain a normal fasting glucose concentration.[128,129] Hyperglycemia may be manifest only postprandially, when higher rates of insulin secretion are required to maintain euglycemia. As β-cell destruction progresses, plasma insulin levels fall even during the fasted state, hepatic glucose production increases, and the patient requires insulin therapy.[129,130] With more severe insulin deficiency, plasma FFA levels

12. Galbo H. Hormonal and metabolic adaptation to exercise. New York: Thieme-Stratton, 1983.

13. Goldstein DS. Physiology of the adrenal medulla and the sympathetic nervous system. In: Becker KL, Bilezikian JP, Bremner WJ, et al, eds. Principles and practice of endocrinology and metabolism. Philadelphia: JB Lippincott, 1990:668–76.

14. Exton JH, Friedmann N, Wong EH-A. Interaction of glucocorticoids with glucagon and epinephrine in the control of gluconeogenesis and glycogenolysis in liver and of lipolysis in adipose tissue. J Biol Chem 1972; 247:3579–88.

15. Newsholme EA, Leech AR. Hormones and metabolism. In: Newsholme EA, Leech AR. Biochemistry for the medical sciences. New York: John Wiley & Sons, 1983:813–912.

16. Owen OE, Reichard GA Jr. Human forearm metabolism during progressive starvation. J Clin Invest 1971; 50:1536–45.

17. Felig P. Amino acid metabolism in man. Annu Rev Biochem 1975;44:933–55.

18. Rothman DL, Magnusson I, Katz LD. Quantitation of hepatic glycogenolysis and gluconeogenesis in fasting humans with ^{13}C NMR. Science 1991;254:573–6.

19. Sherwin RS, Fisher M, Hendler R, Felig P. Hyperglucagonemia and blood glucose regulation in normal, obese and diabetic subjects. N Engl J Med 1976;294:455–61.

20. Gerich JE, Lorenzi M, Hane S, et al. Evidence for a physiologic role of pancreatic glucagon in human glucose homeostasis: studies with somatostatin. Metabolism 1975;24:175–82.

21. Cherrington A, Vranic M. Hormonal control of gluconeogenesis in vivo. In: Krauss-Friedman, ed. Hormonal control of gluconeogenesis. Boca Raton: FL: CRC Press, 1986:15–37.

22. Cahill GF Jr, Aoki TT, Rossini AA. Metabolism in obesity and anorexia nervosa. In: Wurtman RJ, Wurtman JJ, eds. Nutrition and the brain. Vol 3. New York: Raven Press, 1979:1–70.

23. Wahren J, Felig P, Cerasi E, Luft R. Splanchnic and peripheral glucose and amino acid metabolism in diabetes mellitus. J Clin Invest 1972;51:1870–78.

24. Consoli A, Kennedy F, Miles J, Gerich J. Determination of Krebs cycle metabolic carbon exchange in vivo and its use to estimate the individual contributions of gluconeogenesis and glycogenolysis to overall glucose output in man. J Clin Invest 1987;80:1303–10.

25. Katz H, Homan M, Velosa J, et al. Effects of pancreas transplantation on postprandial glucose metabolism. N Engl J Med 1991;325:1278–83.

26. Ross BD, Hems R, Krebs HA. The rate of gluconeogenesis from various precursors in the perfused rat liver. Biochem J 1967;102:942–51.

27. Aoki TT, Toews CJ, Rossini AA, et al. Glucogenic substrate levels in fasting man. Adv Enzyme Regul 1975;13:329–36.

28. Ruderman NB. Muscle amino acid metabolism and gluconeogenesis. Annu Rev Med 1975;26:245–58.

29. Hagg SA, Taylor SI, Ruderman NB. Glucose metabolism in perfused skeletal muscle: pyruvate dehydrogenase activity in starvation, diabetes and exercise. Biochem J 1976; 158:203–10.

30. Goodman MN, Ruderman NB. Starvation in the rat. I. Effect of age and obesity on organ weights, RNA, DNA and protein. Am J Physiol 1980;239:E269–76.

31. Jefferson LS, Rannels DE, Munger BL, Morgan HE. Insulin in the regulation of protein turnover in heart and skeletal muscle. Fed Proc 1974;33:1098–104.

32. Fulks RM, Li JB, Goldberg AL. Effects of insulin, glucose and amino acids on protein turnover in rat diaphragm. J Biol Chem 1975;250:290–8.

33. London DR, Foley TH, Webb CG. Evidence for the release of individual amino-acids from the resting human forearm [Letter]. Nature 1965;208:588–9.

34. Pozefsky T, Felig P, Tobin JD, et al. Amino acid balance across tissues of the forearm in postabsorptive man. Effects of insulin at two dose levels. J Clin Invest 1969;48:2273–82.

35. Ruderman NB, Berger M. The formation of glutamine and alanine in skeletal muscle. J Biol Chem 1974;249:5500–6.

36. Felig P, Marliss E, Pozefsky T, Cahill GF Jr. Amino acid metabolism in the regulation of gluconeogenesis in man. Am J Clin Nutr 1970;23:986–92.

37. Pagliara AS, Karl IE, Haymond M, Kipnis OM. Hypoglycemia in infancy and childhood. Parts I and II. J Pediatr 1973;82:365–79, 558–77.

38. Nurjhan N, Consoli A, Gerich J. Increased lipolysis and its consequences on gluconeogenesis in non-insulin-dependent diabetes mellitus. J Clin Invest 1992;89:169–75.

39. Owen OE, Morgan AP, Kemp HG, et al. Brain metabolism during fasting. J Clin Invest 1967;46:1589–95.

40. Bjorkman O, Ahlborg G, Wahren J, Felig P. Changing patterns of brain ketone, glucose and lactate metabolism within 60 hours of fasting in man [Abstract no. 248]. Diabetes 1982;31(Suppl 2):62A.

41. Gjedde A, Crone C. Induction processes in blood-brain transfer of ketone bodies during starvation. Am J Physiol 1975;229:1165–9.

42. Hawkins RA, Biebuyck JF. Ketone bodies are selectively used by individual brain regions. Science 1979:205; 325–7.

43. Conn AR, Fell DI, Steele RD. Characterization of α-keto acid transport across blood-brain barrier in rats. Am J Physiol 1983;245:E253–60.

44. Oldendorf WH. Carrier-medicated blood-brain barrier transport of short-chain monocarboxylic organic acids. Am J Physiol 1973;224:1450–3.

45. McCall AL, Millington WR, Wurtman RJ. Metabolic fuel and amino acid transport into the brain in experimental diabetes mellitus. Proc Natl Acad Sci USA 1982; 79:5406–10.

46. Sherwin RS, Hendler RG, Felig P. Effect of ketone infusions on amino acid and nitrogen metabolism in man. J Clin Invest 1975;55:1382–90.

47. Owen OE, Felig P, Morgan AP, et al. Liver and kidney metabolism during prolonged starvation. J Clin Invest 1969;48:574–83.

48. Goodman MN, Larsen PR, Kaplan MM, et al. Starvation in the rat. II. Effect of age and obesity on protein sparing and fuel metabolism. Am J Physiol 1980;239:E277–86.

49. Rosen OM. After insulin binds. Science 1987;237:1452–8.

50. Kasuga M, Zick Y, Blithe DL, et al. Insulin stimulates tyrosine phosphorylation of the insulin receptor in a cell-free system. Nature 1982;298:667–9.

51. Petruzzelli LM, Ganguly S, Smith CJ, et al. Insulin activates a tyrosine-specific protein kinase in extracts of 3T3-L1 adipocytes and human placenta. Proc Natl Acad Sci USA 1982;79:6792–6.

52. Rosen OM, Herrera R, Olowe Y, et al. Phosphorylation activates the insulin receptor tyrosine protein kinase. Proc Natl Acad Sci USA 1983;80:3237–40.

53. Crofford OB, Renold AE. Glucose uptake by incubated rat epididymal adipose tissue: rate-limiting steps and site of insulin action. J Biol Chem 1965;240:14–21.

54. Nilsson NÖ, Strålfors P, Fredrikson G, Belfrage P. Regulation of adipose tissue lipolysis: effects of noradrenaline and insulin on phosphorylation of hormone-sensitive lipase and on lipolysis in intact rat adipocytes. FEBS Lett 1980;111:125–30.

55. Spooner PM, Chernick SS, Garrison MM, Scow RO. Insulin regulation of lipoprotein lipase activity and release in 3T3-L1 adipocytes: separation and dependence of hormonal effects on hexose metabolism and synthesis of RNA and protein. J Biol Chem 1979;254:10021–9.

56. Sooranna SR, Saggerson ED. Interactions of insulin and adrenaline with glycerol phosphate acylation processes in fat-cells from rat. FEBS Lett 1976;64:36–9.

57. Cohen P, Parker PJ, Woodgett JR. The molecular mechanism by which insulin activates glycogen synthase in mammalian skeletal muscle. In: Czech MP, ed. Molecular basis of insulin action. New York: Plenum Press, 1985:213–33.

58. Ray LB, Sturgill TW. Insulin-stimulated microtubule-associated protein kinase is phosphorylated on tyrosine and threonine in vivo. Proc Natl Acad Sci USA 1985; 85:3753–7.

59. Boulton TG, Nye SH, Robbins DJ, et al. ERK's: a family of protein-serine/threonine kinases that are activated and tyrosine phosphorylated in response to insulin and NGF. Cell 1991;65:663–75.

60. Kelly KL, Ruderman NB, Chen KS. Phosphatidylinositol-3-kinase in isolated rat adipocytes: activation by insulin and subcellular distribution. J Biol Chem 1992;267:3423–8.

61. Strålfors P. Insulin stimulation of glucose uptake can be mediated by diacylglycerol in adipocytes. Nature 1988; 335:554–6.

62. Saltiel AR, Fox JA, Sherline P, Cuatrecasas P. Insulin-stimulated hydrolysis of a novel glycolipid generates modulators of cAMP phosphodiesterase. Science 1986;233:967–72.

63. Kelly KL, Mato JM, Merida I, Jarett L. Glucose transport and antilipolysis are differentially regulated by the polar head group of an insulin-sensitive glycophospholipid. Proc Natl Acad Sci USA 1987;84:6404–7.

64. Crofford OB, Renold AE. Glucose uptake by incubated rat epididymal adipose tissue: characteristics of the glucose transport system and action of insulin. J Biol Chem 1965;240:3237–44.

65. Mueckler M. Family of glucose-transporter genes: implications for glucose homeostasis and diabetes. Diabetes 1990;39:6–11.

66. James DE, Brown R, Navarro J, Pilch PF. Insulin-regulatable tissues express a unique insulin-sensitive glucose transport protein. Nature 1988;333:183–5.

67. Calderhead DM, Lienhard GE. Labeling of glucose transporters at the cell surface in 3T3-L1 adipocytes: evidence for both translocation and a second mechanism in the insulin stimulation of transport. J Biol Chem 1988; 263:12171–4.

68. Berger J, Biswas C, Vicario PP, et al. Decreased expression of the insulin-responsive glucose transporter in diabetes and fasting. Nature 1989;340:70–2.

69. Sivitz WI, DeSautel SL, Kayano T, et al. Regulation of glucose transporter messenger RNA in insulin-deficient states. Nature 1989;340:72–4.

70. Kirchgessner TG, Svenson KL, Lusis AJ, Schotz MC. The sequence of cDNA encoding lipoprotein lipase: a member of a lipase gene family. J Biol Chem 1987;262:8463–6.

71. Vannier C, Ailhaud G. Biosynthesis of lipoprotein lipase in cultured mouse adipocytes. II. Processing, subunit assembly, and intracellular transport. J Biol Chem 1989; 264:13206–16.

72. Doolittle MH, Ben-Zeev O, Elovson J, et al. The response of lipoprotein lipase to feeding and fasting: evidence for posttranslational regulation. J Biol Chem 1990; 265:4570–7.

73. Ong JM, Kern PA. The role of glucose and glycosylation in the regulation of lipoprotein lipase synthesis and secretion in rat adipocytes. J Biol Chem 1989;264:3177–82.

74. Olivecrona T, Chernick SS, Bengtssen-Olivecrona G, et al. Synthesis and secretion of lipoprotein lipase in 3T3-L1 adipocytes: demonstration of inactive forms of lipase in cells. J Biol Chem 1987;262:10748–59.

75. Cisar LA, Hoogewerf AJ, Cupp M, et al. Secretion and degradation of lipoprotein lipase in cultured adipocytes: binding of lipoprotein lipase to membrane heparan sulfate proteoglycans is necessary for degradation. J Biol Chem 1989;264:1767–74.

76. Borensztajn J. Heart and skeletal muscle lipoprotein lipase. In: Borensztajn J, ed. Lipoprotein lipase. Chicago: Evener, 1987:133–48.

77. Fredrikson G, Strålfors P, Nilsson NÖ, Belfrage P. Hormone-sensitive lipase of rat adipose tissue: purification and some properties. J Biol Chem 1981;256:6311–20.

78. Wion KL, Kerchgessner TG, Lusis AJ, et al. Human lipoprotein lipase complementary DNA sequence. Science 1987;235:1638–41.

79. Fredrikson G, Tornqvist H, Belfrage P. Hormone-sensitive lipase and monoacylglycerol lipase are both required for complete degradation of adipocyte triacylglycerol. Biochim Biophys Acta 1986;876:288–93.

80. Strålfors P, Belfrage P. Phosphorylation of hormone-sensitive lipase by cyclic AMP-dependent protein kinase. J Biol Chem 1983;258:15146–52.

81. Hepp KD, Renner R. Insulin action on the adenyl cyclase system: antagonism to activation by lipolytic hormones. FEBS Lett 1972;20:191–4.

82. Parker PJ, Embi N, Caudwell FB, Cohen P. Glycogen synthase from rabbit skeletal muscle: state of phosphorylation of the seven phosphoserine residues in vivo in the presence and absence of adrenaline. Eur J Biochem 1982;124:47–55.

83. Denton RM, Hughes WA. Pyruvate dehydrogenase and the hormonal regulation of fat synthesis in mammalian tissues. Int J Biochem 1978;9:545–52.

84. Loten EG, Sneyd JGT. An effect of insulin on adipose-tissue adenosine 3':5'-cyclic monophosphate phosphodiesterase. Biochem J 1970;120:187–93.

85. Illiano G, Cuatrecasas P. Modulation of adenylate cyclase activity in liver and fat cell membranes by insulin. Science 1972;175:906–8.

86. Nimmo HG, Houston B. Rat adipose-tissue phosphate glycerol acyltransferase can be inactivated by cyclic AMP-dependent protein kinase. Biochem J 1978; 176:607–10.

87. Vila MC, Milligan G, Standaert ML, Farese RV. Insulin Activates glycerol-3-phosphate acyltransferase (de novo phosphatidic acid synthesis) through a phospholipid-derived mediator. Apparent involvement of Giα and activation of a phospholipase C. Biochemistry 1990; 29:8735–40.

88. Stevens EVJ, Husbands DR. Stimulation of rat liver glycerol-3-phosphate acyltransferase activity by acid- and heat-stable low-molecular-weight substances from skeletal muscle of rats treated with insulin. Arch Biochem Biophys 1987;58:361–4.

89. Astrand PO. Whole body metabolism in exercise. In: Horton ES, Terjung RL. Exercise, nutrition and energy metabolism. New York: Macmillan and Company, 1988:1–8.

90. Armstrong RB. Muscle fiber recruitment patterns and their metabolic correlates. In: Horton ES, Terjung RL, eds. Exercise, nutrition and energy metabolism. New York: Macmillan and Company, 1988:9–26.

91. Armstrong RB, Phelps RO. Muscle fiber type composition of rat hindlimb. Am J Anat 1984;171:259–72.

92. Saltin B, Gollnick PD. Skeletal muscle adaptability: significance for metabolism and performance. In: Peachy LD, Adrian RH, Geiger SR, eds. Handbook of physiology. Section 10. Skeletal muscle. Bethesda, MD: American Physiological Society. 1983:555–631.

93. Bonen A, Tan MH, Watson-Wright WM. Insulin binding and glucose uptake differences in rodent skeletal muscles. Diabetes 1981;30:702–4.

94. Henriksen EJ, Bourey RE, Rodnick KJ, et al. Glucose transporter protein content and glucose transport capacity in rat skeletal muscles. Am J Physiol 1990;259:E593–8.

95. Ader M, Poulin RA, Yang YJ, Bergman RN. Dose-response relationship between lymph insulin and glucose uptake reveals enhanced insulin sensitivity of peripheral tissues. Diabetes 1992;41:241–53.

96. Maizels EZ, Ruderman NB, Goodman MN, Lau D. Effect of acetoacetate on glucose metabolism in the soleus and extensor digitorum longus muscles of the rat. Biochem J 1977;162:557–68.

97. Richter EA, Garetto LP, Goodman MN, Ruderman NB. Muscle glucose metabolism following exercise in the rat: increased sensitivity to insulin. J Clin Invest 1982;69:785–93.

98. James DE, Jenkins AB, Kraegen EW. Heterogeneity of insulin action in individual muscles in vivo: euglycemic clamp studies in rats. Am J Physiol 1985;248:E567–74.

99. Rodnick KJ, Holloszy JO, Mondon CE, James DE. Effects of exercise training on insulin-regulatable glucose-transporter protein levels in rat skeletal muscle. Diabetes 1990;39:1425–9.

100. Houmard JA, Egan PC, Neufer PK, et al. Elevated skeletal muscle glucose transporter levels in exercise-trained middle-aged men. Am J Physiol 1991;261:E437–43.

101. Bergström J, Hermansen L, Hultman E, Saltin B. Diet, muscle glycogen and physical performance. Acta Physiol Scand 1967;71:140–50.

102. Lewis SF, Haller RG. Skeletal muscle disorders and associated factors that limit exercise performance. Exerc Sport Sci Rev 1989;17:67–113.

103. Roach PJ. Glycogen synthase and glycogen synthase kinases. Curr Top Cell Regul 1981;20:45–105.

104. Chock PB, Rhee SG, Stadtman ER. Interconvertible enzyme cascades in cellular regulation. Annu Rev Biochem 1980;49:813–43.

105. Exton JH. Mechanisms involved in α-adrenergic phenomena: role of calcium ions in actions of catecholamines in liver and other tissues. Am J Physiol 1980;238:E3–12.

106. Cohen P. Signal integration at the level of protein kinases, protein phosphatases and their substrates. Trends Biochem Sci 1992;17:408–13.

107. Gollnick PD, Saltin B. Fuel for muscular exercise: role of fat. In: Horton ES, Terjung RL. Exercise, nutrition and energy metabolism. New York: Macmillan and Company, 1988:72–88.

108. Kimball SR, Flaim KE, Peavy DE, Jefferson LS. Protein metabolism. In: Rifkin H, Porte D Jr, eds. Ellenberg and Rifkin's diabetes mellitus: theory and practice. 4th ed. New York: Elsevier, 1990:41–50.

109. Kelley DE, Reilly JP, Veneman T, Mandarino LJ. Effects of insulin on skeletal muscle glucose storage, oxidation and glycolysis in humans. Am J Physiol 1990;258:E923–9.

110. Andres R, Cader G, Zierler KL. The quantitatively minor role of carbohydrate in oxidative metabolism by skeletal muscle in intact man in the basal state. Measurements of oxygen and glucose uptake and carbon dioxide and lactate production in the forearm. J Clin Invest 1956; 35:671–82.

111. McGarry JD, Mills SE, Long CS, Foster DW. Observations on the affinity for carnitine and malonyl-CoA sensitivity, of carnitine palmitoyltransferase I in animal and human tissues: demonstration of the presence of malonyl-CoA in no-hepatic tissues of the rat. Biochem J 1983;214:21–8.

112. Ruderman NB, Houghton CRS, Hems R. Evaluation of the isolated perfused rat hindquarter for the study of muscle metabolism. Biochem J 1971;124:639–51.

113. Gammeltoft D. The significance of ketone bodies in fat metabolism. I. Concentration of ketone bodies in the arterial and venous blood in human subjects during starvation. Acta Physiol Scand 1950;19:270–9.

114. Ruderman NB, Goodman MN. Inhibition of muscle acetoacetate utilization during diabetic ketoacidosis. Am J Physiol 1974;226:136–43.

115. Sherwin RS, Hendler RG, Felig P. Effect of diabetes mellitus and insulin on the turnover and metabolic response to ketones in man. Diabetes 1976;25:776–84.

116. Fery F, Balasse EO. Ketone body production and disposal in diabetic ketosis: a comparison with fasting ketosis. Diabetes 1985;34:326–32.

117. Stalmans W, Bollen M, Mvumbi L. Control of glycogen synthesis in health and disease. Diabetes Metab Rev 1987;3:127–61.

118. Kraus-Friedmann N. Hormonal regulation of hepatic gluconeogenesis. Physiol Rev 1984;64:170–259.

119. Katz J, McGarry JD. The glucose paradox: is glucose a substrate for liver metabolism? J Clin Invest 1981; 74:1901–9.

120. McGarry JD, Kuwajima M, Newgard CB, et al. From dietary glucose to liver glycogen: the full circle round. Annu Rev Nutr 1987;7:51–73.

121. Shulman GI, Cline G, Schumann WC, et al. Quantitative comparison of pathways of hepatic glycogen repletion in fed and fasted humans. Am J Physiol 1990;259:E335–41.

122. Exton JH. Mechanisms of hormonal regulation of hepatic glucose metabolism. Diabetes Metab Rev 1987;3:163–83.

123. Beaudet AL. The glycogen storage diseases. In: Wilson JD, Braunwald E, Isselbacher KJ, eds. Harrison's principles of internal medicine. 12th ed. New York: McGraw-Hill, 1991:1854–60.

124. Hue L. Gluconeogenesis and its regulation. Diabetes Metab Rev 1987;3:111–26.

125. McGilvery RW, Goldstein GW. Biochemistry, a functional approach. 3rd ed. Philadelphia: WB Saunders, 1983.

126. McGarry JD, Foster DW. Regulation of hepatic fatty acid oxidation and ketone body production. Annu Rev Biochem 1980;49:395–420.

127. McGarry J, Foster D. Ketogenesis. In: Rifkin H, Porte D, eds. Ellenberg and Rifkin's diabetes mellitus: theory and practice. 4th ed. New York: Elsevier, 1990:292–8.

128. Srikanta S, Ganda OP, Rabizadeh A, et al. First-degree relatives of patients with Type I diabetes mellitus: islet-cell antibodies and abnormal insulin secretion. N Engl J Med 1985;313:461–4.

129. Palmer JP, Lernmark A. Pathophysiology of Type I (insulin-dependent) diabetes. In: Rifkin H, Porte D, eds. Ellenberg and Rifkin's diabetes mellitus: theory and practice. 4th ed. New York: Elsevier, 1990:414–35.

130. Eisenbarth GS, Connelly J, Soeldner JS. The "natural" history of Type I diabetes. Diabetes Metab Rev 1987; 3:873–91.

131. Lillioja S, Mott DM, Zawadzki JK, et al. In vivo insulin action is familial characteristic in nondiabetic Pima Indians. Diabetes 1987;36:1329–35.

132. Eriksson J, Franssila-Kallunki A, Ekstrand A, et al. Early metabolic defects in persons at increased risk for non-insulated diabetes mellitus. N Engl J Med 1989;321: 337–43.

133. Warram JH, Martin BC, Krolewski AS, et al. Slow glucose removal rate and hyperinsulinemia precede the development of Type II diabetes in the offspring of diabetic parents. Ann Intern Med 1990;113:909–15.

134. Björntorp P. Abdominal obesity and the development of noninsulin-dependent diabetes mellitus. Diabetes Metab Rev 1988;4:622–27.

135. Bergstrom RW, Newell-Morris LL, Leonett DL, et al. Association of elevated fasting C-peptide level and increased intra-abdominal fat distribution with development of NIDDM in Japanese-American men. Diabetes 1990; 39:104–11.

136. Ruderman NB, Schneider SH, Berchtold P. The metabolically obese normal weight individual. Am J Clin Nutr 1981;34:1617–21.

137. Reaven GM. Role of insulin resistance in human diabetes. Diabetes 1988;37:1595–607.

138. DeFronzo RA, Ferrannini E. Insulin resistance: a multifaceted syndrome responsible for NIDDM, obesity, hypertension, dyslipidemia and atherosclerotic cardiovascular disease. Diabetes Care 1991;14:173–94.

139. Ruderman NB, Schneider SH. Exercise in type 2 diabetes. In: Saltin B, Galba H, Richter EA, eds. Biochemistry of exercise. Vol 6. Champaign, IL: Human Kinetics Publishers, 1986:255–65.

140. Ruderman NB, Apelian AZ, Schneider SH. Exercise in therapy and prevention of Type II diabetes: implications for blacks. Diabetes Care 1990;13(Suppl 4):1163–8.

141. Helmrich SP, Ragland DR, Leung RW, Paffenbarger RS Jr. Physical activity and reduced occurrence of non-insulin-dependent diabetes mellitus. N Engl J Med 1991;325:147–52.

142. DeFronzo RA. Tobin JD, Andres R. Glucose clamp technique: a method for quantifying insulin secretion and resistance. Am J Physiol 1979;237:E214–23.

143. DeFronzo RA. Pathogenesis of type 2 (non-insulin dependent) diabetes mellitus: a balanced overview. Diabetologia 1992;35:389–97.

144. DeFronzo RA, Gunnarsson R, Björkman O, et al. Effects of insulin on peripheral and splanchnic glucose metabolism in noninsulin-dependent (Type II) diabetes mellitus. J Clin Invest 1985;76:149–55.

145. Bogardus C, Lillioja S, Stone K, Mott D. Correlation between muscle glycogen synthase activity and in vivo insulin action in man. J Clin Invest 1984;73:1185–90.

146. Roch-Norlund AE, Bergström J, Castenfors H, Hultman E. Muscle glycogen in patients with diabetes mellitus: glycogen content before treatment and the effect of insulin. Acta Med Scand 1970;187:445–53.

147. Schalin-Jäntti C, Härkönen M, Groop LC. Impaired activation of glycogen-synthase in people at increased risk for developing NIDDM. Diabetes 1992;41:598–604.

148. Vaag A, Henriksen JE, Beck-Nielsen H. Decreased insulin activation of glycogen synthase in skeletal muscles in young nonobese caucasian first-degree relatives of patients with non-insulin-dependent diabetes mellitus. J Clin Invest 89:782–8.

149. Rothman DL, Shulman RG, Shulman GI. ^{31}P nuclear magnetic resonance measurements of muscle glucose-6-phosphate: evidence for reduced insulin-dependent muscle glucose transport or phosphorylation activity in non-insulin-dependent diabetes mellitus. J Clin Invest 1992;89:1069–75.

150. Mandarino LJ, Madar Z, Kolterman OG, et al. Adipocyte glycogen synthase and pyruvate dehydrogenase in obese and Type II diabetic subjects. Am J Physiol 1986; 251:E489–96.

151. Unger RH, Grundy S. Hyperglycaemia as an inducer as well as a consequence of impaired islet cell function and insulin resistance: implications for the management of diabetes. Diabetologia 1985;28:119–21.

152. Rossetti L, Giaccari A, DeFronzo RA. Glucose toxicity. Diabetes Care 1990;13:610–30.

153. Kahn BB, Shulman GI, DeFronzo RA, et al. Normalization of blood glucose in diabetic rats with Phlorizin treatment reverses insulin-resistant glucose transport in adipose cells without restoring glucose transporter gene expression. J Clin Invest 1991;87:561–70.

154. Rossetti L, Smith D, Shulman GI, et al. Correction of hyperglycemia with Phlorizin normalizes tissue sensitivity to insulin in diabetic rats. J Clin Invest 1987;79:1510–5.

Chapter 7

ALTERATIONS IN PROTEIN METABOLISM IN DIABETES MELLITUS

ANNE M. KARINCH
SCOT R. KIMBALL
LEONARD S. JEFFERSON, JR.

Centuries ago it was recognized that the disease whose hallmark was excessive flow of sweet, sticky urine, i.e., diabetes mellitus, was accompanied by severe muscle wasting. Early in this century it was found that a pancreatic extract that controlled the symptoms of diabetes also reversed this wasting of muscle. The active agent was identified as insulin, and today we know that in diabetes the metabolism of protein is in some way impaired and that the return of insulin to the system can correct the defect.

Net gain or loss of protein is ultimately determined by a balance between two opposing processes, protein synthesis and protein degradation. To examine the effect of insulin (or other agents or conditions that disturb the normal balance), researchers have developed both in vivo and in vitro techniques for assessing rates of protein synthesis and breakdown. These techniques have evolved over the years as both the complexity of the processes under investigation and the limitations of the earlier investigative methods have become more thoroughly appreciated. As will be described in some detail, new protein is synthesized by way of a complex series of reactions. The synthetic rate can be increased or decreased by a change either in the overall efficiency of the process or in the amount of protein synthetic "machinery" available. Efficiency is reflected by the amount of protein synthesized per unit of total RNA and is affected by the rates of peptide chain initiation and elongation/termination. The synthetic machinery includes all ribosomes, mRNA, tRNA, and catalytic factors and defines the capacity of the tissue for synthesis. Early studies designed to examine the effect of the presence or absence of insulin on protein synthesis simply recorded changes in synthetic rate. However, with the evolution of techniques that permit identification of the points at which regulation occurs, it has become clear that both the efficiency of and capacity for protein synthesis can be changed by insulin and that all tissues do not respond in the same way. The number of examples of the ability of insulin to alter the synthetic rate of specific proteins by acting directly on genes—either stimulating or inhibiting their rate of transcription—has increased steadily. The techniques of molecular biology are being applied to define the regions of the genes responsive to insulin and to discover the mechanism by which insulin influences transcription. The regulation of protein degradation by insulin, beyond the observation that insulin inhibits tissue protein breakdown by deactivating the lysosomal system, is more poorly understood. More progress toward determining the role of insulin in regulating protein degradation may be made in the near future now that distinct proteolytic pathways are being defined more clearly.

PROTEIN METABOLISM IN MAMMALIAN CELLS

Pathway of Protein Synthesis

Synthesis of new protein in eukaryotic cells is achieved via a complex series of discrete reactions, beginning with the aminoacylation of transfer RNA (tRNA) and ending with the release of a completed peptide chain. For convenience of discussion, the pathway usually is divided into three phases: 1) initiation, during which the initiator methionyl-tRNA is bound to messenger RNA (mRNA), which in turn binds first to a 40S ribosomal subunit and subsequently to a 60S subunit, thus forming a translationally competent ribosome; 2) elongation, during which tRNA-bound amino acids are incorporated into a growing peptide chain in the order specified by the mRNA to which the ribosome is bound; and 3) termination, the phase at which the completed peptide chain is released from the ribosome. Each of these steps requires the intervention of protein factors known collectively as eukaryotic initiation factors (eIF), elongation factors (eEF), and releasing factor (RF). A brief description of these steps follows. More detailed information is available in recent reviews.[1,2]

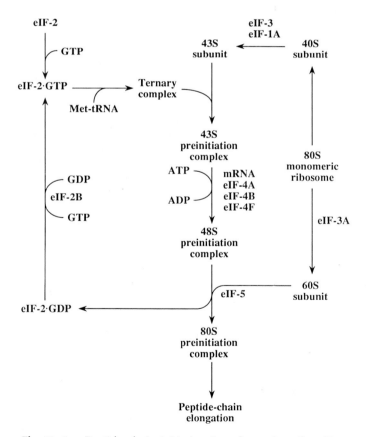

Fig. 7–1. Peptide-chain initiation in eukaryotic cells; eIF = eukaryotic initiation factor; GTP = guanosine triphosphate; GDP = guanosine diphosphate; ATP = adenosine triphosphate; ADP = adenosine diphosphate; tRNA = transfer RNA. A detailed description of the process is presented in the text.

Initiation of Translation

The sequence of events constituting initiation (Fig. 7–1) results in the assembly, piece by piece, of the translation machinery. The final structure, poised to enter the elongation phase of translation, consists of a ribosome bound to a molecule of mRNA that has initiator methionyl-tRNA (met-tRNA$_i$) occupying its AUG start codon. Initiation can be viewed as beginning with the formation of a ternary complex consisting of the initiation factor eIF-2, guanosine triphosphate (GTP), and met-tRNA$_i$. This ternary complex then binds to a small (40S) ribosomal subunit to which the initiation factor eIF-3 is bound, resulting in the formation of a 43S initiation complex. Another group of initiation factors, eIF-4A, eIF-4B, and eIF-4F, along with the ribosome-bound eIF-3 and the hydrolysis of ATP, assist in the recognition of the 5′ cap of mRNA, the binding of the 43S complex to the mRNA cap, and the unwinding of mRNA secondary structure in the cap region. In some as yet unknown way, perhaps by scanning down the 5′ untranslated region of the mRNA molecule, the 43S complex finds the AUG start codon to which the met-tRNA$_i$ then binds. Yet another initiation factor, eIF-5, promotes the release of bound factors, accompanied by the hydrolysis of GTP, so that eIF-2 is released as a binary complex with guanosine diphosphate (GDP). This leaves the 40S·mRNA complex free to join a 60S large ribosomal subunit, forming an 80S ribosomal preinitiation complex ready to enter elongation. As noted above, eIF-2 is released in complex with GDP. For eIF-2 to be used in another round of initiation, this GDP must be replaced by GTP. The exchange of GDP bound to eIF-2 for free GTP is brought about by the intervention of eIF-2B, a guanine nucleotide exchange factor.

Elongation

An 80S ribosome contains two binding sites for aminoacyl-tRNA, the P (donor) site and, adjacent to it, the A (acceptor) site. The initiator met-tRNA, bound to the AUG start codon of mRNA and thereby to a ribosome during initiation, occupies the P site. The A site, initially unoccupied, contains the codon for the first internal amino acid. This site is subsequently filled by the aminoacyl-tRNA specified by the mRNA codon via the codon-anticodon interaction. Both the presence of the elongation factor eEF-1 and the hydrolysis of GTP are necessary for the completion of this step. Then, without the intervention of protein factors or nucleotides, a peptide bond is formed between the methionine of the met-tRNA$_i$ and the tRNA-bound amino acid in the A site, resulting in a deacylated tRNA in the P site and dipeptidyl-tRNA in the A site. A translocation step follows in which the mRNA and ribosome shift relative to each other by the length of one codon. This movement is catalyzed by a second elongation factor, eEF-2, and requires GTP hydrolysis. This shifts the peptidyl-tRNA from the A to the P site, displacing the deacylated tRNA from the P site and leaving the A site open to receive the tRNA-bound amino acid specified by the codon that now occupies the A site. Elongation proceeds by repeated cycles of aminoacyl-tRNA binding, peptide bond formation, peptidyl-tRNA translocation, and deacylated tRNA release from the P site.

Termination

Peptide chain elongation proceeds until all the codons that encode amino acids have been traversed and a termination codon (UAA, UAG, or UGA) enters the A site after translocation of the peptidyl-tRNA carrying the completed peptide chain. In the presence of GTP, the termination factor, RF, binds to the A site and, with the hydrolysis of GTP, catalyzes the termination reaction. The completed peptide chain is released by hydrolysis of the peptide-tRNA ester linkage, and the deacylated tRNA and ribosome both separate from mRNA. After its release from the mRNA molecule, a 80S monomeric ribosome dissociates into 40S and 60S subunits. Initiation factors eIF-3A and eIF-3 bind to the 60S and 40S subunits, respectively, preventing their reassociation. This leaves the subunits available to recycle in another round of translation.

Pathways of Protein Degradation

At least three different proteolytic pathways are involved in protein degradation, but little is known about their mechanisms of action or regulation. These are 1) the lysosomal pathway,[3-5] which is regulated by physiologic conditions that cause changes in protein turnover, although its relative importance varies from tissue to tissue; 2) the ubiquitin-dependent pathway,[4,6] and 3) proteolysis by Ca^{++}-dependent proteases.[4,7] Other important mechanisms for intracellular protein breakdown are known to exist, although they have been even less well described. These include other cytosolic adenosine triphosphate (ATP)-dependent and ATP-independent pathways and some pathways that occur within various cellular organelles.

MEASUREMENT OF PROTEIN TURNOVER

Important to an understanding of the potential role of insulin on protein synthesis and degradation and of the impact of diabetes on protein metabolism is an understanding of some of the methods used to estimate these parameters. The earliest methods for monitoring changes in protein metabolism measured whole-body nitrogen balance,[8] comparing dietary nitrogen intake with nitrogen losses to the urine and feces. Valuable observations have been made with the use of this technique, but a number of problems are associated with it. For example, nitrogen losses tend to be underestimated because of the difficulty involved in accounting for nitrogen eliminated by all routes and intake tends to be overestimated because of food adherence to plates and utensils. Small errors in these measurements can result in large errors when net nitrogen balance is calculated by difference. A more important limitation from the standpoint of furthering the understanding of protein metabolism is the inability of measurements of nitrogen balance at the level of the whole body to tell anything about the underlying changes that have resulted in the new balance. A negative

balance could result from decreased protein synthesis, increased degradation, or both. Furthermore, measurement of change in whole-body nitrogen balance in response to changing physiologic stimuli gives no clue to the site of action of the stimulus and lends no insight into adaptive mechanisms brought into play. A number of different in vitro and in vivo approaches have been taken to measure protein turnover in individual tissues and to study the effects on protein metabolism of a variety of physiologic interventions, including the presence or absence of insulin.

Methods of Measuring Protein Synthesis

Most frequently, protein synthesis has been studied both in vivo and in vitro by following the accumulation of a radiolabeled amino acid in cellular protein. Amino acids used as tracers in studies involving animals or isolated tissues or cells are labeled with radioactive isotopes, while stable isotopes, for example, ^{13}C and ^{15}N, are most often used for human studies. The amino acid to be used as the tracer must be chosen carefully. It should be one of the essential amino acids, thereby eliminating the complication of de novo synthesis (neither alanine nor glutamine would be suitable since large amounts of both are synthesized in muscle[9]), it should not be metabolized to any large extent by the tissue to be studied, it should be an amino acid widely represented in protein, and it should enter the cell and the precursor pool rapidly. Frequently used amino acids that fulfill most of these requirements under specific conditions are valine and leucine in liver and phenylalanine and tyrosine in cardiac and skeletal muscle.

Two conditions must be fulfilled if the synthesis rate is to be calculated accurately. The specific radioactivity of the immediate precursor of the new peptide (tRNA-bound amino acid) must be known and the radiolabeled protein must not degrade during the labeling interval. In practice, however, these conditions are rarely met. It is difficult to measure the specific radioactivity of the tRNA-bound amino acid as it makes up a very small percentage of the cellular content of amino acid. The specific radioactivities of the tRNA-bound amino acid and the total cellular amino acid do not necessarily reach equilibrium during the period of labeling. In tissues in which these parameters have been measured[10-13] the specific radioactivity of the tRNA-bound amino acid has been found to be higher than that of the intracellular free amino acid. This failure to equilibrate may be due to the presence of discrete amino acid compartments that exchange slowly with total free intracellular amino acids.[13-15] However, the situation in heart seems to be somewhat different. In isolated rat heart perfused with physiologic concentrations of phenylalanine, the specific radioactivity of tRNA-bound phenylalanine was more than 80% of that of plasma phenylalanine.[10] A similar result was obtained in vivo with the use of leucine as the radiolabeled tracer. In these studies, the specific radioactivities of the plasma leucine and the heart tRNA-bound leucine equilibrated rapidly, and within 5 minutes[11] or 30 minutes[16] were almost identical. However, the relationship between the specific radioactivity of tRNA-bound amino acid and the intracellular and extracellular amino acid-specific radioactivities varies with different amino acids,[17] and thus estimates of the rate of protein synthesis may differ depending on the amino acid used as tracer.

The second major factor to be considered when measuring protein synthesis is that as the labeling period increases the probability that incorporated labeled tracer will be released and recycled into newly synthesized protein also increases. Significant recycling will lead to an overestimation of the rate of synthesis unless the appropriate correction is made. Over a labeling period of several hours, the recycling of labeled amino acids derived from the breakdown of labeled protein can be ignored without serious error. However, significant recycling of labeled amino acid from short-lived proteins can occur if the labeling period extends beyond approximately 8 hours.[18]

Radiolabeled tracer may be added by infusion over a period of time or injected in a bolus. As implied by its name, the "continuous infusion" technique[19] employs the former approach. Labeled amino acid is infused at a constant rate until the specific radioactivities of the labeled tracer amino acid in the plasma and in the cellular free amino acid compartments of the various tissues have stabilized. Under these conditions it has been shown that the specific radioactivity of the tissue free amino acid can be used as precursor specific radioactivity for calculation of protein synthetic rate in that tissue.[20] Because of the relatively long labeling period, a considerable amount of radiolabeled tracer can be incorporated into cellular protein, permitting, in some cases, the study of the synthesis of specific proteins as well as that of total protein.[21-23] This technique was used to study the in vivo synthesis of myofibrillar proteins in cardiac[21] and skeletal muscle in the rabbit.[22] It has also been employed to label ribosomal proteins of diabetic and insulin-treated rats, permitting the study of ribosome turnover in various tissues.[23,24]

It is technically difficult to measure the specific radioactivity of tRNA-bound amino acid because of the small amount present in tissue and its short half-life. The "flooding-dose" technique was developed to circumvent these problems.[10,25-27] In this approach, a large dose of radiolabeled tracer amino acid is injected as a bolus along with a high concentration of unlabeled tracer, effectively flooding the intracellular amino acid compartment so that the specific radioactivity of the precursor tRNA-bound amino acid approaches that of the free extracellular tracer.[10,27] A short labeling period is used to minimize the loss of incorporated label from rapidly turning over protein. Because of the short labeling interval, this technique has the advantage of permitting incorporation of tracer amino acid into protein in an unrestrained animal, as opposed to the lengthy infusion protocols, which require animal restraint. Limb immobilization per se can cause decreased synthesis of protein.[28] One drawback of the flooding-dose technique is that the specific radioactivity of the extracellular tracer declines over time,[27] making it

necessary to sample plasma periodically and to use an averaged specific radioactivity for the estimation of precursor specific radioactivity. An additional concern is that the short labeling period will result in a bias favoring proteins with a rapid turnover. Finally, an assumption inherent in the use of this method is that the synthetic rate during the short labeling period in fact reflects synthesis as it occurs over the longer term.

Constant infusion and flooding-dose methods have been applied to both in vitro and in vivo systems. In the simplest in vitro experiments, small pieces of tissue, e.g., liver slices,[29] diaphragm,[30] atrial strips,[31] and skeletal muscle,[32] are incubated in medium containing a radiolabeled tracer amino acid. Because the label must diffuse into the tissue, it is not delivered uniformly to all cells and specific radioactivity of the precursor tRNA-bound amino acid is likely to vary throughout the sample, making accurate measurements of protein synthetic rate difficult. However, this method allows relative changes in synthesis to be seen and has the significant advantage of allowing control and treated samples to be taken from the same animal.

Perfusion systems have been developed for a number of tissues and organs, including the isolated rat heart,[33] rat liver,[34] and, for the study of skeletal muscle, rat hind limb[35] and hemicorpus.[36] Tissue or organ perfusion allows controlled delivery of labeled tracer to the cells via the microcirculation, and studies can be carried out without the wide, incompletely described range of hormones and growth factors present in vivo. With the use of the flooding-dose technique with phenylalanine in isolated perfused rat heart[10] and perfused skeletal muscle[37] and valine or leucine in perfused rat liver,[38,39] the specific radioactivity of the precursor tRNA-bound amino acid in the tissue approaches or is identical to the specific radioactivity of the tracer in the perfusing medium. Leucine may not be an ideal tracer to use in this type of experiment because at high concentrations leucine and other branched-chain amino acids may themselves affect protein metabolism[40,41]; however, 5 mM leucine has no effect on protein synthesis in perfused rat liver.[39] Phenylalanine, in a flooding dose, has been widely used for the study of muscle protein synthesis in vivo,[23,24,42,43] although the specific activities of the plasma phenylalanine and the muscle tRNA-bound phenylalanine have not been shown to equilibrate under these conditions in all cases.

Protein synthesis has also been studied in cells in culture; primary hepatocytes,[44-46] fibroblasts,[47,48] cardiac and skeletal myocytes,[49,50] and myotubes[51] have all been used. An attractive feature of cell culture is that it provides a homogeneous population of cells for study, as compared with whole tissues, which contain a variety of cell types. In addition, all cells are equally and simultaneously exposed to the labeled tracer during turnover experiments. However, one must be cautious when extrapolating from results obtained in these experiments, as the response of cells in culture to physiologic stimuli may not reflect their behavior in vivo or in other in vitro systems. For example, no effect of insulin on protein synthesis can be demonstrated in vivo in the liver of the fed rat[52] or in vitro in perfused liver of the normal rat,[53] whereas insulin stimulates protein synthesis in primary cultures of hepatocytes.[45,54]

In vitro techniques have been designed to allow examination of changes in messenger RNA (mRNA) isolated from cells or tissue from control and experimental animals. The amount of total[55,56] or specific[57] mRNAs may be quantified, or alternatively, the mRNA may be translated in an in vitro cell-free system.[55,56,58] Total protein synthesis is represented by the incorporation of a radiolabeled amino acid into total expressed protein. Any changes in the expression of a particular protein, or group of proteins, can be detected by further fractionation of the translation products of the cell-free system by immunologic[21] or electrophoretic methods.[55] Since amino acids labeled to a very high specific radioactivity can be used for the in vitro translation and because two-dimensional gel electrophoresis allows high-resolution separation of proteins, the expression of several hundred proteins can be followed.[56] An obvious, untested assumption underlying this analysis is that the in vitro translation of message accurately reflects its translation in vivo; in other words, the ratio of each mRNA to its expressed protein is the same in vitro as in vivo.

Animal studies of protein synthesis use radioactive isotopes and often require the sampling of quite large amounts of tissue. Such experiments are not usually carried out on human subjects. The availability of amino acids labeled with stable isotopes, e.g., ^{15}N and ^{13}C, has permitted the development of methods that make the study of protein turnover in humans possible, although tracer doses of ^3H- and ^{14}C-labeled amino acids are sometimes used. The exchange (uptake and release) of [^{13}C]leucine is frequently used for study of whole-body protein turnover. After a primed continuous infusion of the labeled tracer, total leucine flux, leucine oxidation, nonoxidative leucine flux (an index of whole-body synthesis), and endogenous leucine flux (an index of whole-body degradation) are commonly measured. Similar measurements can also be made across discrete muscle beds, e.g., the forearm,[59,60] as an indication of the turnover of skeletal muscle. This involves the placement of a catheter deep in a forearm vein that drains primarily muscle tissue. An arterial catheter is positioned in the ipsilateral brachial artery so both blood entering and blood leaving the muscle can be sampled. Tracer and any other additives are infused via the brachial artery or a contralateral vein. However, because 36% of forearm volume is made up of tissues other than muscle,[61] their contribution to [^{13}C]leucine exchange cannot be discounted. The constant-infusion technique has been adapted to permit the study of skeletal muscle protein synthesis in human subjects.[62,63] A modification of the flooding-dose technique has been developed for measuring the rate of protein synthesis in tissues in vivo in humans.[64] The specific radioactivity of plasma [^{13}C]α-ketoisocaproate, the transamination metabolite of leucine, is often used as an index of the intracellular precursor-specific radioactivity[65] when incorporation of [^{13}C]leucine into protein in biopsy samples of muscle is used to measure protein synthesis.[63]

Methods of Studying Control Points in Protein Synthesis

Techniques have been developed that permit identification of control points in translation or examination of certain steps of the translation pathway in some detail. One of the former is the use of sucrose-density gradients for obtaining ribosomal subunit and polysome profiles based on density differences. Ribosomes, isolated from tissue or cell homogenates, are separated into 40S or 60S subunits, 80S monomers, or polysomes containing one or more ribosomes bound to an mRNA molecule. The ratio of unbound (40S, 60S, 80S) vs. bound ribosomes gives an indication of the proportion of ribosomes actively involved in translation of messenger RNA into protein. This ratio reflects the efficiency with which the synthetic machinery is being utilized and also can provide useful information about potential control points.[66] For instance, a decrease in protein synthesis coupled with an increase in the proportion or amount of free subunits suggests that initiation is inhibited relative to elongation and, therefore, that a defect in initiation may be responsible for the inhibition of synthesis.

Several reactions within initiation can be studied with currently available methods: formation of the eIF-2·GTP·met-tRNA$_i$ ternary complex[67]; binding of this complex to the 40S ribosomal subunit[68,69]; and GDP/GTP exchange activity of eIF-2B.[70] Assays have also been developed for a number of other initiation factors, e.g., eIF-3, eIF-4A, eIF-4C, eIF-4D, and eIF-4B.[71] The rate of peptide chain elongation can also be measured by comparison of the amount of newly synthesized, labeled protein free in the cytoplasm with the amount still bound in polysomes. This allows the calculation of the transit time of ribosomes translating mRNA.[72]

Methods of Measuring Protein Degradation

All protein synthesis proceeds along the same reaction pathway, although the synthetic rates for individual proteins may vary. Degradation, on the other hand, is not so straightforward since proteins may be broken down by one or more of a number of different pathways.[4,73,74] Most studies measure total protein breakdown regardless of the proteolytic route.

In vivo estimates of protein degradation often are obtained indirectly by calculation from measured rates of protein synthesis and changes in protein content,[75,76] as these measurements can usually be made with relative accuracy. In such studies, synthesis is measured over a short time interval (10 minutes to a few hours), as compared with the measurement of total protein content, which is made over one to several days. An important underlying assumption is that the measured synthetic rate is representative of the average rate over the longer period during which the change in protein content is measured. For this reason, the indirect technique is not suited to the study of acute changes in degradation. An additional drawback is that an estimate of degradation, made by difference, is subject to compounding of errors incurred in the determination of the rate of synthesis and change in protein content.

Accurate measurement of the rate of protein breakdown requires carefully controlled in vitro experimentation. Many of the in vitro systems used in the study of protein synthesis have been employed in protein degradation studies. Incubated muscle strips,[77] perfused rat heart,[78] liver,[79] hemicorpus,[80] and cells in culture[49,51,81] are some examples. Degradation usually is measured by following the release of a labeled or unlabeled tracer amino acid into the incubation medium or perfusate. The considerations governing the choice of amino acid are the same as those listed previously for synthesis studies. Absolute degradation rates can be obtained by measuring the release of a nonmetabolized amino acid, such as phenylalanine or tyrosine in muscle, in the presence of an inhibitor of protein synthesis, such as cycloheximide. The degradation rate must be measured 5 to 15 minutes after addition of the inhibitor because cycloheximide has an inhibitory effect on protein degradation that becomes apparent after approximately 15 minutes.[73,82]

A commonly used isotopic technique is pulse-labeling, in which a tissue or organism is exposed for a short time to a radiolabeled amino acid to prelabel cellular proteins. Protein degradation is estimated from the rate of loss of label from the previously labeled protein. Reutilization of label released by protein degradation is minimized by using a large excess of the unlabeled amino acid as a "chase" effectively blocking the reincorporation of labeled tracer into newly synthesized protein.[73] When applied to total cellular protein, the decay of label obtained from this type of experiment does not follow a simple exponential curve since total tissue protein is not a homogeneous mixture but contains rapidly and slowly turning over populations. The initial rapid decay reflects primarily the turnover of short-lived proteins, while the later decay is mainly from longer-lived proteins. "Pulse-chase" experiments can therefore be used to study the breakdown of short- and long-lived populations of proteins and have been applied to cells in culture and in vivo.[73] With additional electrophoretic and immunologic techniques, it is possible to follow the degradation of specific proteins labeled in vitro or in vivo.

Degradation has also been measured in vitro by an isotope dilution technique.[80,83] A labeled amino acid is added to the perfusate or incubation medium, and the rate of dilution of the specific radioactivity of the tracer is recorded. Since the dilution must be caused by the addition of unlabeled tracer from the breakdown of unlabeled protein, the rate of proteolysis can be calculated. This principle has been used in studies of degradation in dogs in vivo in skeletal[84] and heart muscle[85] isolated from other tissues by selective catheterization. As noted above, protein degradation, as well as protein synthesis, can be measured in human subjects by determination of whole-body or limb [13C]leucine turnover. In these experiments, endogenous leucine flux is an index of protein breakdown.

Studies in which protein degradation is measured in whole tissues are complicated by the contribution of all cell types represented within the tissue to the measured release of amino acid. In muscle it has been possible, to some degree, to separate the degradation of myofibrillar proteins from that of nonmyofibrillar proteins. Tyrosine is widely distributed in proteins, and its release from muscle has been used as an indicator of whole-tissue proteolysis. 3-Methylhistidine is an amino acid formed by post-translational modification of histidine. 3-Methylhistidine occurs in all actins[86] and in the myosin of fast-twitch white muscle fibers,[87] and since it is neither reincorporated into new protein nor further metabolized after release by proteolysis,[88] its release from the cell is considered an index of myofibrillar protein breakdown. Because actin is prominent not only in muscle but in many types of cells,[89] excretion of 3-methylhistidine in the urine should not be used as a reflection whole-body muscle degradation but should only be used for isolated muscle preparations.[90]

The degree to which the lysosomal pathway contributes to protein degradation under different physiologic conditions can be estimated by the addition of a weak base, e.g., chloroquine or methylamine, which blocks lysosomal function by preventing lysosome acidification, or by addition of inhibitors of thiol proteases, e.g., leupeptin AC-LL. The reduction in proteolysis observed is an indication of lysosome-mediated degradation.[91]

EFFECT OF DIABETES AND INSULIN ON PROTEIN TURNOVER IN ANIMAL MODELS

Insulin is an anabolic hormone, and its presence in the blood during the absorptive state promotes the storage of fuels that are present in excess of immediate need. Glucose is stored as glycogen in the liver and in muscle tissue, glucose and fatty acids are stored as triglycerides in adipose tissue, and amino acids are stored as protein in many tissues, including muscle, liver, and adipose tissue. Insulin increases the uptake of amino acids into these tissues but also stimulates protein synthesis and inhibits protein degradation via mechanisms independent of amino acid transport described in detail in the following sections. Under conditions in which the blood level of insulin is depressed, e.g., diabetes mellitus and starvation, the storage of protein ceases and protein stores, particularly those in muscle, are reduced. Under these conditions, amino acids released from protein are used as fuel; alanine and glutamine released to the blood become substrates for gluconeogenesis in the liver and kidney, respectively, and the oxidation of other amino acids is increased. Figure 7–2 depicts the disposition of amino acids in the diabetic state compared with conditions of normal blood insulin levels.

The loss of protein that accompanies uncontrolled diabetes must result from an overall disruption of the normal balance between protein synthesis and degradation in favor of degradation. However, comparison of the protein content of various tissues taken from control and diabetic animals shows that individual tissues do not

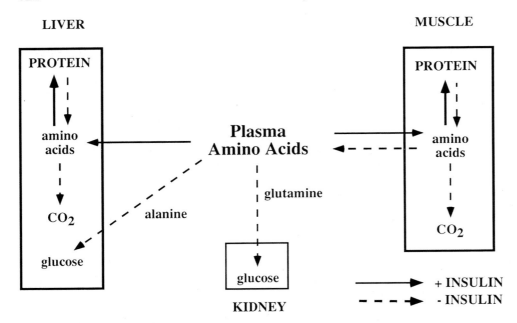

Fig. 7-2. Overview of amino acid disposition under conditions of insulin sufficiency or insulin deficiency. Solid arrows indicate net amino acid flux when insulin is present, e.g., the absorptive state in normal animals; dashed arrows indicate flux in insulin-deficient states, e.g., diabetes mellitus.

respond uniformly to diabetes. The protein content is unchanged[92,93] or increased[94] in liver of diabetic animals, increased in jejunal mucosa and kidney,[93-95] and markedly decreased in skeletal and cardiac muscle.[92]

Protein Synthesis

The observation that the protein content of muscle decreases in diabetes and the results of experiments using eviscerated animals[96-98] suggested that muscle was most likely the major site of net protein loss during diabetes. Evisceration, in which most of the internal organs are literally or functionally removed, leads to a gradual increase in plasma amino acid concentration, which can be reversed in a dose-dependent way by the administration of insulin.[98] In these animals, insulin either inhibited release of amino acids from muscle to the plasma or stimulated the uptake of amino acids by muscle, or both.

Both in vitro and in vivo studies have demonstrated that insulin can stimulate protein synthesis in muscle. Addition of insulin to a variety of muscles isolated from normal animals, including rat diaphragm,[30,99] rat soleus and epitrochlearis muscle,[32] and rabbit atrial strips[31] stimulated the incorporation of labeled amino acids into newly synthesized protein. Insulin has also been readily shown to stimulate protein synthesis in isolated, perfused rat heart[100,101] and hemicorpus.[80,83,102] The rate of protein synthesis in cardiac and skeletal muscle of diabetic animals, when measured in vivo, is consistently inhibited relative to that in control animals. This has been observed in alloxan-diabetic rats,[103] in streptozotocin-diabetic rats,[24,52,76,104] and in eviscerated dogs.[105] Treatment of these animals with insulin resulted in reversal of the inhibition,[24,52,104,105] so that protein synthetic rates approached or regained control rates. Insulin treatment also partially relieved the inhibition of protein synthesis

observed in postabsorptive rats,[106] another condition in which the level of circulating insulin is low.

As observed in the in vitro studies previously described, insulin treatment stimulated protein synthesis in muscle of normal, fed rats. However, attempts to show such an effect of insulin in normal animals in vivo have usually been unsuccessful.[52,106-108] A number of possible explanations for this apparent lack of effect of insulin have been proposed. First, compared with intact tissues in situ, isolated heart and muscle preparations are in a catabolic state, with depressed rates of synthesis exceeded by the overall rate of degradation.[43,100] Inclusion of insulin in the perfusate or incubation medium corrects the negative nitrogen balance. This finding leads to the suggestion that insulin may be important in maintaining nitrogen balance per se.[28] If this is so, since tissue in vivo in normal animals is already in balance, addition of insulin would have no stimulatory effect on protein synthesis. In heart, the addition of alternative oxidative substrates, e.g., fatty acids, or the imposition of a work load have an effect on protein synthesis similar to that of insulin.[40,83,109] These conditions occur in vivo, and it may be that insulin has no further effect in their presence. Another factor that may contribute to the failure of insulin to stimulate protein synthesis in vivo is the hypoaminoacidemia that follows insulin treatment. Hyperinsulinemia decreases the release of amino acids from muscle in animals[98] and stimulates amino acid transport into cells[110]; the resultant decline in plasma amino acids may limit the substrate available for protein synthesis. Studies in dogs[108] and rats[111] confirmed the need to maintain the concentration of plasma amino acids at or above normal levels to demonstrate the stimulation of protein synthesis by insulin. In a recent study in postabsorptive rats, infusion of various concentrations of insulin stimulated protein synthesis.[111] This stimulation was greatly increased by simultaneous infusion of amino acids, whereas the infusion of amino acids alone did not increase protein synthesis above control rates.

On the basis of the observation of a positive correlation between intramuscular glutamine concentration and the rate of protein synthesis in perfused rat hind limb,[112] it has been proposed that the maintenance of intramuscular glutamine levels is involved in control of muscle protein synthesis. Variation of glutamine and insulin concentrations in the perfusate indicates that glutamine can regulate the rate of skeletal muscle protein synthesis but that both glutamine and insulin are required for maximal stimulation.[112] However, this has not been confirmed in all studies.[111]

Extensive studies on the effect of diabetes and insulin on protein synthesis in liver have also been conducted. In early studies using incubated slices of liver[29] or isolated perfused liver from diabetic rats,[79,113] it was reported that less ^{14}C-labeled amino acid was incorporated into protein of diabetic than normal rats. Addition of insulin to the perfusion medium stimulated protein synthesis in livers from mildly diabetic rats but had no effect on the rate of synthesis in livers from more severely diabetic animals.[113] In vivo, liver protein synthesis was unchanged[52] or decreased[23,94,114,115] in alloxan-diabetic or spontaneously diabetic BB/W rats and restored toward control levels with insulin.[114,115] In contrast, no stimulatory effect of insulin could be demonstrated in the perfused liver of normal rats[53] or in vivo in normal rats.[52]

Diabetes and insulin influence the synthesis of hepatic secretory, as well as intracellular, proteins. Thus, albumin secretion is reduced in perfused livers of alloxan-diabetic and fasted rats.[116] Electron micrographs of liver sections of diabetic rats show extensive distortion and disruption of the rough endoplasmic reticulum,[54,117–119] which vary in degree with the severity of the diabetes.[117] These changes are reversed after insulin treatment of diabetic animals.[54,117–119] Since proteins destined for secretion are synthesized primarily by ribosomes of the rough endoplasmic reticulum, the apparent disruption of this organelle in the absence of insulin is consistent with the reduction in albumin secretion by livers of diabetic rats[114–116] and by hepatocytes in culture.[120] Secretion of both albumin and total exported proteins is inhibited by diabetes.[114,115,121,122] Indeed, in alloxan-diabetic and BB/W rats,[114,115] the synthesis of total liver protein is inhibited to a lesser extent than that of total secretory proteins and the synthesis of albumin is more markedly depressed than that of other secreted proteins. Again, insulin treatment increases albumin and total protein secretion, restoring them to nearly normal levels.[114,115] A selective effect of diabetes on other secreted hepatic proteins has also been reported.[45,121,122] These observations are compatible with the disproportionate changes in concentration found in specific serum proteins of diabetic patients.[123]

Isolated hepatocytes in culture have been used as a model system for studying the effects of various interventions on liver cells. A number of studies have shown that protein synthesis in hepatocytes isolated from normal rats is stimulated by addition of insulin to the incubation medium.[45,46,54,120] Protein synthesis in parenchymal liver cells isolated from insulin-maintained alloxan-diabetic rats decreased with time after insulin withdrawal.[124]

Protein Degradation

Insulin promotes positive nitrogen balance in tissues not only by enhancing protein synthesis, as discussed above, but also by suppressing proteolysis. Clear evidence for this anticatabolic effect of insulin in muscle has been obtained from in vitro experiments using isolated muscles of normal rats in which inclusion of insulin in the incubation or perfusion medium resulted in decreased protein degradation. The muscles studied included isolated diaphragm,[99] isolated heart,[49,78,125] skeletal muscle,[80,83] and cultured myoblasts[81] and myotubes.[51] Supraphysiologic concentrations of insulin were required to inhibit proteolysis in the cell culture systems,[49,51,81] suggesting that insulin may not be the natural regulator of muscle growth during the fetal and neonatal periods. The insulin-like growth factors 1 and 2 may be more important at these stages.[51] (Myotubes display incomplete differentiation in culture and possess many embryonic/neonatal characteristics.[126])

Since insulin has been demonstrated to have an inhibitory effect on proteolysis, it is reasonable to predict that accelerated protein degradation would occur under conditions of depressed circulating levels of insulin, such as in diabetes or fasting.[9,127] And indeed, increased proteolysis has been observed in vitro and in vivo in muscle of fasted[99] and diabetic rats[23,128,129] and Type I diabetic patients.[130] Treatment with insulin inhibits this enhanced breakdown of protein. However, in some in vivo studies, there may no change,[131] or even decreased proteolysis[76] in diabetes. Thus, while in vitro studies show a definite antiproteolytic action of insulin, the situation in vivo is somewhat less clear.

There is evidence that all proteins are not affected equally by the antiproteolytic action of insulin. In heart and skeletal muscle of 2-day streptozotocin-diabetic rats, total tissue protein is decreased compared with that in normal rats, and this decrease can be attributed to both reduced protein synthesis and a slight increase in protein degradation.[23] However, over the same period, the animals experience a large decrease in the amount of ribosomal protein in these tissues that is caused by a reduction in ribosomal protein synthesis in concert with a marked increase in ribosomal protein degradation.[23] Clearly, the effect of diabetes on breakdown of muscle ribosomal protein was distinct from that on degradation of total tissue protein. Another example of the selective antiproteolytic action of insulin is seen in muscle. Overall protein degradation in isolated, perfused skeletal muscle[132,133] and heart[134] from starved rats, as measured by tyrosine or phenylalanine release, is reduced by addition of insulin, while degradation of myofibrillar proteins, estimated from release of 3-methylhistidine, is unchanged.[132–134]

In perfused rat hind limb, glutamine inhibited protein degradation.[135] The effects of insulin and glutamine on proteolysis are not additive, suggesting that they may act through a common mechanism.[135] This inhibition of breakdown primarily affects soluble sarcoplasmic proteins, rather than myofibrillar proteins,[135] consistent with studies showing that inhibition of protein degradation in muscle by insulin does not involve myofibrillar proteins.[133,134]

Insulin has also been clearly implicated in the regulation of degradation of hepatic protein. An early study showed that both intracellular and plasma proteins degrade more rapidly in the perfused livers of diabetic rats than of normal rats.[79] In perfused normal liver, addition of insulin or amino acids to the perfusate suppresses the spontaneous breakdown of intracellular protein.[53,136] This reversal of degradation occurred without an appreciable effect on protein synthesis. Similar results have been obtained in livers of starved and refed rats in which protein synthesis was not altered.[137,138] Thus, under these conditions, alterations in protein content of the liver during starvation and refeeding must be primarily the consequence of changes in protein degradation.[137,138] In perfused liver, maximal inhibition of proteolysis is achieved at high physiologic concentrations of amino acids, and addition of insulin to the perfusate causes no further decrease in protein breakdown,[139,140] suggesting that a common mechanism may be regulated by the hormone and amino acids.

One final important consideration is the presence in vivo of other hormones, particularly thyroid and corticosteroid hormones, that can affect protein turnover[141,142] either alone or in concert with insulin. While there are clearly physiologically important interactions, the effects of each hormone alone can be isolated when studies are carried out in vitro or in perfused systems.

EFFECT OF DIABETES AND INSULIN ON PROTEIN TURNOVER IN HUMANS

Insulin treatment rapidly reverses the negative nitrogen balance in patients with insulin-dependent diabetes (IDDM or Type I).[8] Radiolabeled leucine has been used extensively to measure protein turnover in human subjects. Leucine is an essential amino acid, so body protein is the only source of leucine in the postabsorptive state. As a result, changes in the rate of appearance of leucine or its transamination metabolite, α-ketoisocaproate, in the plasma reflect changes in the release of leucine from protein, or proteolysis.

Whole-body proteolysis is significantly increased by withdrawal of insulin from postabsorptive patients with IDDM.[143] Treatment of either control or diabetic subjects with insulin reduces whole-body proteolysis, as shown by a reduction in whole-body leucine flux,[144-149] although insulin is less effective in inhibiting protein breakdown in patients with IDDM than in control subjects.[145] These observations are consistent with an earlier study of forearm perfusion in normal postabsorptive males, in which elevation of insulin to high physiologic levels inhibited the net release of amino acids from the forearm[59] and promoted a more positive nitrogen balance across the limb. However, insulin-induced changes in whole-body protein synthesis, as reflected by nonoxidative leucine flux, have varied. Insulin has been reported to have no effect on whole-body protein synthesis[145-147] or to have an inhibitory effect.[149] The insulin-induced enhancement of protein synthesis demonstrated in numerous in vitro systems and in vivo in animal muscle has been difficult to demonstrate in human studies.[150-153]

A study that measured the kinetics of amino acid exchange across forearm muscle in fasted normal males showed that the net amino acid release that occurs during fasting is reversed to net uptake by infusion of insulin.[60] However, this positive balance is the result of strongly inhibited amino acid release in the presence of unchanged uptake,[60] a finding that implies the anabolic effect of insulin is caused by inhibition of protein degradation rather than by stimulation of synthesis. Insulin infusion does not stimulate protein synthesis in muscle of postabsorptive patients with IDDM[154] but does strongly inhibit proteolysis. Therefore, insulin does not appear to stimulate protein synthesis in either the whole body or muscle tissue. It has been suggested that this may reflect compromised substrate availability, since the plasma concentration of amino acids decreases during insulin infusion.[155] Attempts have been made to address this possibility in studies of leucine kinetics in normal subjects[150,151,153] and patients with IDDM[156] infused with insulin and/or amino acids. These studies suggest an interaction between insulin and substrate concentration. Thus, whole-body protein synthesis is decreased[150,151] by infusion of insulin alone, unchanged by infusion of insulin plus glucose with amino acids sufficient only to maintain plasma levels,[150,156] but increased with combined hyperinsulinemia and hyperaminoacidemia.[150,151,153] Hyperaminoacidemia in the presence of basal insulin also stimulated whole-body protein synthesis, and increasing the concentration of insulin had no further stimulatory effect.[150,151] A study comparing whole-body leucine metabolism in healthy young and old men found that in both groups an increase in incorporation of leucine into protein produced by infusion of an amino acid mixture was not further enhanced by an almost tenfold increase in insulin concentration.[152] In one study, however, insulin appeared to stimulate protein synthesis over and above the effect of hyperaminoacidemia.[153] Protein synthesis in skeletal muscle of patients with IDDM also fails to respond to insulin infusion with maintained amino acids,[156] but insulin stimulates protein synthesis in leg tissues of healthy subjects when a higher level of amino acids is maintained.[153] On balance it appears that in humans the availability of amino acids is more important than insulin in maintaining skeletal muscle protein synthesis[152,153,156] and that the major role of insulin in vivo is the suppression of protein breakdown.

A recent study suggested that skeletal muscle is not the major site at which insulin exerts its inhibition of whole-body proteolysis.[157] The effects of insulin on whole-body and forearm leucine metabolism in patients with IDDM were studied. Infusion of insulin reduced whole-body protein degradation, as indicated by a decrease in the appearance of leucine and α-ketoisocap-roate in the plasma, while uptake and release of leucine and α-ketoisocaproate by the forearm did not change. This result differs from those of earlier studies of forearm perfusion[59,60] which found that insulin infusion inhibited amino acid release. The reason for the lack of agreement is unclear but may be due to experimental differences. In particular, the earlier studies used normal individuals whereas the more recent study used patients with IDDM.

MECHANISMS OF INSULIN ACTION IN REGULATION OF PROTEIN TURNOVER

There are many steps in the life cycle of a protein—from transcription of its gene to its eventual proteolytic degradation—that may be targets for regulation by insulin. Overall protein synthesis can be enhanced by increased efficiency of translation or increased capacity for synthesis via production of new ribosomes, while the rate of synthesis of individual proteins can be altered through increased or decreased transcription of their genes or by preferential translation of specific mRNAs. Table 7–1 summarizes the steps in protein metabolism that have been shown to be regulated by insulin.

Regulation of Translation of Messenger RNA

A number of steps within the process of translation could be regulated by insulin, but the bulk of evidence indicates that peptide-chain initiation is the principal site of action. Elongation/termination appears to be affected in a limited number of instances.

Initiation

When hearts from normal rats are perfused with physiologic concentrations of amino acids and glucose, there is a decline in the rate of protein synthesis after the first hour. An increase in free ribosomal subunits and a decrease in polysomes accompany this decrease in protein synthesis, suggesting that the inhibition of synthesis is caused by a block in peptide-chain initiation.[83] Addition of insulin to the perfusate maintains synthesis at close to the initial rate and maintains ribosome subunits and polysomes at the levels in unperfused hearts.[83] Perfusion of rat skeletal muscle in the presence and absence of insulin produces almost identical effects on protein synthesis and initiation.[80,83] In cardiac and skeletal muscle, actinomycin D does not block the ability of insulin to alter peptide-chain initiation, suggesting that

Table 7–1. Effects of Insulin on Protein Metabolism

Stimulates transcription of ribosomal RNA
Stimulates or inhibits transcription of specific mRNAs
Preferentially recruits ribosomal protein mRNAs into polysomes
Increases ternary complex formation in peptide-chain initiation
Stimulates preferential translation of specific mRNAs
Increases the stability of specific mRNAs
Inhibits protein degradation
Inhibits ribosome degradation
Inhibits lysosomal degradation of macromolecules

the effect of the hormone is independent of RNA synthesis.[158] Although insulin is known to stimulate the transport of amino acids into muscle cells, the effects in heart are not due simply to an increased supply of intracellular amino acids[83] or to some effect that elevates levels of high-energy phosphates.[78,83,158]

Perfusion-induced insulin deficiency causes a depression in protein synthesis and ribosomal disaggregation in both cardiac and skeletal muscle. This leads to the prediction that a similar effect would be seen in muscle from diabetic animals; in fact, diabetes of 2 days' duration results in reduced rates of protein synthesis in perfused gastrocnemius muscle[159] caused both by loss of tissue RNA, which reflects loss of capacity for synthesis, and by decreased translational efficiency, as would result from defective initiation.[159] Inclusion of insulin in the perfusate restores the efficiency to levels seen in normal rats. Protein synthesis is reduced to a much lesser extent in the soleus muscle, in which the reduction in the rate of synthesis is due entirely to a decrease in the concentration of RNA. In this case, addition of insulin to the perfusion medium has no stimulatory effect on protein synthesis. The explanation for this difference in response to diabetes and insulin lies in the different fiber-type composition of these two muscles.

Muscles are composed of three types of fibers: fast-twitch white fibers, which have high glycolytic and low oxidative capacity; fast-twitch red fibers, which have high glycolytic and high oxidative capacity; and slow-twitch red fibers, which have low glycolytic capacity and high oxidative capacity. Gastrocnemius muscle contains both glycolytic and oxidative fast-twitch fibers, while soleus muscle comprises mainly slow-twitch red fibers. Cardiac muscle is also primarily oxidative, and in keeping with the observations in soleus muscle, neither protein synthesis nor the concentration of ribosomal subunits is altered in isolated perfused heart from 2-day alloxan-diabetic rats.[109] It appears that muscles with more oxidative fibers, e.g., heart and soleus, are less susceptible to a block in peptide-chain initiation caused by the insulin deficiency of diabetes. The different responses of fast-twitch glycolytic and slow-twitch oxidative muscles to diabetes noted in the in vitro studies have also been observed in vivo.[42,52]

The resistance of cardiac muscle to the inhibitory effect of diabetes on protein synthesis has been attributed to a protective effect of the high levels of fatty acids present in the circulation of diabetic animals.[83,109] In perfused heart, insulin, fatty acids, or other noncarbohydrate substrates can reverse the block in initiation caused by perfusions lasting more than 1 hour[109,160] and restore normal rates of protein synthesis. The insensitivity to short-term diabetes of slow-twitch muscles like the soleus that have, like the heart, a high capacity to utilize fatty acids may also be caused by a protective action of circulating fatty acids. However, the effect of fatty acids on the rate of protein synthesis and level of ribosomal subunits in slow-twitch skeletal muscle has yet to be determined. Fatty acids do not change the rate of protein synthesis or the state of polysomal aggregation in perfused skeletal muscle of mixed fiber type.[83,102]

The disaggregation of polysomes observed in tissues of diabetic animals and their reassembly following insulin administration suggest that insulin is involved in the control of peptide-chain initiation. Initiation encompasses a number of steps (Fig. 7–1), any one of which could be responsible for the initiation block observed in muscle of diabetic animals. Efforts at identifying the defective step in skeletal muscle have included examination of the formation of 43S initiation complex by the binding of initiator met-tRNA (as part of the ternary complex with eIF-2·GTP) to 40S subunits.[69] Hemicorpus preparations of diabetic rats were perfused with [^{35}S]methionine in the presence or absence of insulin, and 40S subunits were isolated on sucrose density gradients.[69] The presence of insulin in the perfusion medium resulted in a 1.5-fold increase in the amount of ternary complex bound to 40S subunits.[69] Qualitatively similar results were obtained in cell-free extracts prepared from gastrocnemius muscle of normal, diabetic, and fasted rats.[161] Binding of met-tRNA to 40S subunits from extracts of diabetic or fasted animals was increased by treating rats with insulin before killing them or by adding exogenous eIF-2.[161] These findings point to direct involvement of eIF-2 in the inhibition of peptide-chain initiation during insulin deprivation.

A guanine nucleotide exchange factor, eIF-2B, is necessary for recycling eIF-2 at the end of each round of initiation. Defective GDP/GTP exchange would effectively inhibit eIF-2 activity. The exchange activity of eIF-2B has been measured in postmitochondrial supernatants of muscle from normal, 2-day diabetic, and insulin-treated diabetic rats.[162] The eIF-2B activity is decreased in two fast-twitch muscles (gastrocnemius and psoas) and is unchanged in two slow-twitch muscles (heart and soleus). Insulin treatment restores the activity in the fast-twitch muscles and slightly reduces the activity in the slow-twitch muscles.[162] It appears that eIF-2B activity is reduced under the same conditions that result in a decline in protein synthetic rate attributable to a block in peptide-chain initiation. The activity of eIF-2B has been shown, in rabbit reticulocytes, to be inhibited by NADP$^+$.[163] In hearts of both diabetic and starved rats, the NADPH/NADP$^+$ ratio is higher than that in controls,[164] perhaps preserving the eIF-2B activity in this tissue.

In a number of systems in which protein synthesis is impaired, e.g., heme-deprived rabbit reticulocyte lysate, phosphorylation of the α-subunit of eIF-2 results in the formation of a very stable eIF-2α(P)·eIF-2B complex. This effectively eliminates the GDP/GTP exchange activity of eIF-2B and inhibits initiation.[2] Consistent with this mechanism of regulation, protein synthesis in calf chondrocytes is stimulated by insulin, and this stimulation is accompanied by a decrease in eIF-2 phosphorylation.[165] However, the degree of eIF-2α phosphorylation does not appear to change in skeletal muscle of diabetic[166] or starved rats,[167,168] so the observed decrease in eIF-2B activity in insulin-deprived muscle cannot be the result of eIF-2B sequestration by eIF-2α(P). An alternative explanation for a change in eIF-2B activity may lie in direct covalent modification of eIF-2B itself. In rabbit reticulocyte lysate, GDP/GTP exchange activity of eIF-2B can be increased by phosphorylation of eIF-2B by casein kinase II,[169] and dephosphorylation by alkaline phosphatase reduces its activity.[169] Since insulin activates casein kinase II,[170] a sequence of events may be envisaged by which insulin could stimulate protein synthesis by activation of casein kinase II, which in turn could phosphorylate eIF-2B. Phosphorylation, and thus activation, of eIF-2B would enhance the rate of protein synthesis in skeletal muscle. However, no direct evidence for this proposed pathway has been reported.

Approaches similar to those applied to muscle have been employed to identify the site at which insulin acts to alter hepatic protein synthesis. The transport of certain amino acids into the liver is enhanced by insulin,[110] but since insulin does not stimulate protein synthesis in experiments using short-term liver perfusion,[53,171] regulation of amino acid transport is clearly not a major regulatory step in hepatic protein synthesis. Polysome profiles obtained from liver homogenates of both acutely[171–173] and chronically[174,175] diabetic rats have shown that diabetes causes disaggregation of polysomes with a concomitant increase in dimeric and monomeric ribosomes. These changes in polysome profiles suggest that protein synthesis in liver of diabetic rats also is impaired as a result of a block in peptide-chain initiation. In vivo treatment of the diabetic rats with insulin produced a rapid reversal of this effect, with reaggregation of ribosomes into polysomes.[172–175] Disaggregation of polysomes and inhibition of protein synthesis also is observed in perfused livers of diabetic rats.[171] These defects are corrected by perfusion of the liver with high levels of amino acids but not by addition of insulin to the perfusate. These findings are not consistent with the insulin-induced reaggregation of ribosomes observed in vivo[172–175] and suggest that the availability of amino acids rather than the lack of insulin may be important in maintaining protein synthesis in perfused livers of diabetic animals.

Hepatic ribosomes isolated from diabetic rats have diminished protein synthetic activity in a cell-free system as compared with ribosomes from normal animals.[117,174,176–178] Administration of insulin to diabetic rats stimulates incorporation of amino acids into protein in ribosomal[174] and microsomal[176,178] preparations. Insulin treatment of normal rats prior to sacrifice increases incorporation of amino acids into a liver microsomal preparation derived from these animals, whereas addition of insulin to a microsomal preparation from normal animals is without effect.[178] This finding suggests that insulin requires intact cells to initiate its effect and is consistent with action of insulin through its plasma membrane receptor. When poly(U) was added to ribosomes isolated from livers of diabetic and normal rats, the ribosomes from diabetic rats bound more poly(U).[173] This was interpreted as indicating that a greater proportion of ribosomes in normal animals were already bound to endogenous mRNA and were therefore not available to bind to exogenous poly(U). Addition of the initiation inhibitor, poly(I), to a cell-free system based on a postmitochondrial supernatant from liver of diabetic or control rats abolishes the difference in protein synthesis seen in its absence.[177] The translation time for proteins being synthesized was the same for both conditions.[177] These studies suggest that the defect in diabetes involves an inhibition of initiation but does not alter the rate of peptide chain elongation.[177]

Elongation/Termination

Tissues of animals that have been diabetic for relatively short periods display the disaggregation of polysomes indicative of blocked initiation. However, in diabetes of longer duration (10 days for cardiac and 7 days for skeletal muscle), an impairment of translational efficiency is observed in both cardiac and soleus muscle that appears to result from a defect in peptide-chain elongation/termination.[159,179]

Regulation of Protein Degradation

The possibility that the perfusion-induced increase in protein degradation in liver is mediated via a lysosomal mechanism is suggested by a number of changes in lysosomes that are associated with conditions that enhance proteolysis and are reversed by addition of insulin or amino acids to the perfusate. The changes in lysosomes include increased sensitivity to osmotic shock,[180] increased density on isopycnic centrifugation,[139,181] and enlargement.[139,182] Proteolysis is maximally stimulated in livers perfused in the single-pass mode with an amino acid-free perfusate.[182] Electron micrographs of livers perfused under these conditions show large vacuoles, many of which contain organelles such as mitochondria, rough endoplasmic reticulum, and smooth endoplasmic reticulum and glycogen.[182] Similar autophagic vacuoles are observed in the livers of diabetic rats.[119,183] In both in vitro and in vivo experiments, addition of amino acids[182] or insulin[119,183] results in their disappearance.

Amino acids are primary regulators of protein degradation in the liver. In the absence of amino acids, proteolysis rapidly reaches its highest rate, and at physiologic concentrations of amino acids, breakdown is suppressed to basal levels.[182,184] This suppression of proteolysis can also be demonstrated with a group of regulatory amino acids (Leu, Tyr, Gln, Pro, Met, His, Trp). In perfused rat liver, the effect of this regulatory group of amino acids on degradation is multiphasic in that the group optimally inhibits degradation at 0.5 and 4 times ($\times$) normal plasma concentrations but loses its inhibitory effectiveness in a narrow zone around normal plasma concentration ($1\times$).[140] Addition of insulin or alanine to the perfusate with amino acids eliminates the zonal loss of inhibition of proteolysis at $1\times$ amino acids without altering the inhibition observed when regulatory amino acids are absent. The action of alanine appears to be permissive, as $1\times$ alanine alone has no inhibitory effect on degradation. During perfusion with $1\times$ regulatory amino acids, macroautophagy is sharply stimulated, but electron micrographs of liver show that the autophagic vacuoles formed differ from those formed as a result of perfusion in the absence of amino acids. The vacuoles contain less rough endoplasmic reticulum, mitochondria, and other organelles and more smooth endoplasmic reticulum.[140]

This suggests the presence of two separate macroautophagic pathways. The significance of this difference and the role of insulin is unclear at this time.

Electron micrographs of hearts perfused without insulin show the presence of large autophagic vacuoles throughout the cytoplasm,[83,185] whereas hearts perfused with insulin are free of these bodies. The fragility of lysosomes, measured as the loss of latency of lysosomal enzymes, increases as their volume increases. Insulin decreases both the rate of protein degradation and the fragility of lysosomes in perfused rat heart and skeletal muscle.[78,80] As stated previously, the degradation of myofibrillar proteins is neither inhibited by insulin nor reduced by lysosomal inhibitors.[133,186] Taken together, these observations suggest that insulin influences the rate of protein degradation in muscle by altering lysosome function, as it does in liver,[187] although the specific mechanism is unknown at this time.

Diabetes and starvation are associated with enhanced protein degradation differing fundamentally from normal protein catabolism. As a rule, large proteins turn over more rapidly than smaller proteins,[73,74] acidic proteins turn over more rapidly than neutral or basic proteins,[74] and glycoproteins turn over more rapidly than nonglycoproteins.[188,189] In the liver and muscle of diabetic and starved rats these patterns are reduced or completely lost,[4] as would be predicted if the enhanced proteolysis associated with diabetes and starvation results from increased lysosomal autophagy in which all types of proteins are degraded at equivalent rates. In mildly (streptozotocin) diabetic mice, the relative rates of degradation of acidic and basic cytosol proteins are the same as in normal mice and the distribution and activity of lysosome-associated proteinases is unchanged.[190] Furthermore, breakdown of hepatic protein is not enhanced in these mildly diabetic animals. These observations suggest that widespread autophagy is not associated with this mild diabetic condition.[190] This is consistent with morphologic studies that found no change in lysosome size or structure in mildly diabetic rats.[183] Another study in mice showed that, although the rates of protein degradation in perfused livers of fed normal and diabetic animals were the same, after 48 hours of starvation the increase in protein breakdown was much greater in the livers of the diabetic mice than in those of the normal mice.[191] Thus, both the severity of diabetes and the nutritional status of the animal appear to alter hepatic protein breakdown in vivo.

Regulation of Ribosome Turnover

Because ribosomes are the central functional units on which translation occurs, any major change in their cellular content will be accompanied by a parallel change in overall protein synthesis. Since ribosomal RNA makes up approximately 85% of total cellular RNA, changes in total RNA synthesis and content frequently are considered a reflection of changes in ribosomal RNA synthesis and content.

As a means of circumventing difficulties associated with precursor nucleotide compartmentation in the measurement of ribosomal RNA synthesis, frequently ribosome formation is determined from incorporation of radiolabeled amino acids into ribosomal core proteins. Induction of diabetes in rats by injection of streptozotocin inhibits synthesis of ribosomal protein in gastrocnemius and cardiac muscle but has no effect on synthesis of ribosomal proteins in liver. Treatment of diabetic animals with insulin rapidly increases the synthesis of ribosomal proteins in muscle[24,192] and liver,[193] and in skeletal muscle in particular, the rate of increase of ribosomal protein synthesis is more rapid than that of total protein synthesis.[23,24] The content of RNA decreases with induction of diabetes and also rapidly recovers upon administration of insulin. These changes in RNA content are more than could result from changes in ribosome synthesis alone; in fact, diabetes quickly stimulated degradation of ribosomes and the return of insulin as quickly completely suppressed the enhanced degradation.[23,24] Preferential stimulation of ribosomal protein synthesis over total cellular protein synthesis also is observed in chick embryo fibroblasts in culture.[47] In this system, insulin also rapidly (within 10 minutes) stimulates the incorporation of [³H]adenine into preribosomal RNA but has no effect on the speed with which the precursor rRNA is processed or the rate of transport of 60S ribosomal subunits into the cytoplasm. The amount of total RNA is severely reduced in gastrocnemius of 4-day alloxan-diabetic rats, whereas poly(A)⁺RNA is increased relative to total RNA during the induction of diabetes.[56] This suggests that during diabetes poly(A)⁺RNA is more stable than ribosomal RNA and that protein synthesis should not be limited by availability of mRNA for translation. Insulin therapy results in parallel increases in the rates of synthesis of poly(A)⁺RNA and total RNA.[56]

Insight into the mechanism by which insulin stimulates ribosome formation comes from studies of mouse myoblasts.[194] The mRNAs of several ribosomal proteins studied (S16, L18, and L32) that were not being translated prior to treatment with insulin were preferentially recruited into polysomes and actively translated after addition of insulin. Insulin also increases the transcription of rRNA. Both these processes are maximally stimulated within 15 minutes of the administration of insulin and occur with no pronounced effect on ribosomal protein gene transcription or the stability of ribosomal protein mRNAs.[194]

An involvement of prostaglandins in the synthesis of RNA is suggested by the ability of indomethacin to inhibit insulin-induced increases in total RNA synthesis and accumulation in L6 myoblasts.[195] The cyclo-oxygenase inhibitors indomethacin and ibuprofin inhibit the stimulation by insulin of total RNA accumulation and the incorporation of radiolabeled uridine into the ribosomal RNA of L6 myoblasts with little effect on the basal rate of rRNA synthesis.[196] These results suggest that an arachidonate metabolite may be involved in the signal mechanisms through which insulin stimulates RNA synthesis in myoblasts.

As described above, degradation of ribosomes is enhanced in diabetes and is suppressed by addition of insulin.[23,24] Little is known about the degradation of ribosomes or their component proteins and RNA; however, studies with rat liver demonstrated that ribosomal proteins and rRNA have the same apparent half-lives, suggesting that ribosomes are degraded as whole units in the same macroautophagic compartment.[197–199]

Regulation of Gene Expression

Diabetes can inhibit protein synthesis in various tissues by decreasing the number of ribosomes and/or their activity. These changes would be expected to affect the synthesis of all proteins equally, so that the relative rates of synthesis of individual proteins remain constant despite decreased total protein synthesis. Insulin treatment should reverse these effects on translational efficiency and capacity and stimulate the synthesis of all proteins equally. However, the list of proteins whose synthesis (either stimulation or inhibition) is affected disproportionately by insulin is growing steadily, and many insulin-regulated genes have been described.

One of the earliest indications of an effect of insulin on the regulation of a specific protein via regulation of its mRNA concentration is from studies of albumin synthesis in livers of alloxan-diabetic rats, in which changes in the rate of albumin synthesis in the presence and absence of insulin paralleled changes in the abundance of albumin mRNA.[114] Similar results were obtained in studies with the spontaneously diabetic BB/W rat.[115] This change in levels of albumin message was due to a direct effect of insulin on transcription of the albumin gene, a phenomenon demonstrated in primary cultures of rat hepatocytes.[200] Cells in culture have since been used extensively in studies of the regulation of insulin-regulated genes because they allow the actions of insulin to be isolated from those of other counterregulatory hormones or from changes in substrate availability resulting from the insulin-induced hypoglycemia that occurs in intact animals or tissues.

A number of the proteins for which mRNA levels are regulated by insulin have metabolic functions directly connected to the anabolic and anticatabolic functions of insulin. For example, transcription of the genes for the glycolytic enzymes glucokinase[201] and pyruvate kinase[202] and for the lipogenic enzyme fatty acid synthetase[203] is stimulated by insulin, whereas that for the gluconeogenic enzyme PEPCK[204] is inhibited. The insulin-regulated glucose transporter, GLUT-4, is expressed exclusively in muscle and adipose tissue, the major sites of insulin-stimulated glucose uptake. Transcription of the gene encoding this protein is inhibited in muscle and adipose tissue of diabetic rats, resulting in levels of GLUT-4 mRNA lower than those in controls.[205] Insulin therapy in diabetic rats reversed this effect.[205] This action of insulin is clearly compatible with the anabolic function of insulin. Insulin also can regulate the mRNA concentration of a wide range of proteins that carry out many functions and are expressed in a variety of tissues. The mRNA levels of a number of major secretory proteins, including albumin,[114,115,206] amylase,[207] growth hormone,[208] and

$\alpha_{2\mu}$-globulin,[209] are regulated by insulin, as are ovalbumin[210] and casein,[211] which are involved in reproduction, and δ-crystallin,[212] a structural lens protein.

Transcription

In the majority of cases, insulin-induced changes in the synthesis of these proteins reflect corresponding changes in the relative abundance of the mRNAs that encode the proteins. Alteration in the steady-state concentration of a specific message may be achieved by regulation at a number of steps in the pathway that leads from gene transcription to the appearance of mature message in the cytoplasm. The point(s) at which insulin intervenes is still unknown, but for many genes regulation appears to occur at the level of transcription.[213,214] Steroid hormones and cyclic adenosine monophosphate (cAMP), which both influence gene transcription, do so via the mediation of nuclear DNA-binding proteins that bind to cis-acting DNA sequences.[215] There is evidence from the amylase gene in pancreas,[216] the proto-oncogene c-fos in cultures of Chinese hamster ovary (CHO) fibroblasts,[217] the human glyceraldehyde-3-phosphate dehydrogenase (GADPH) gene,[218] the δ-crystallin gene in embryonic lens cells,[219] and the phosphoenolpyruvate carboxykinase (PEPCK) gene in hepatoma H4IIE cells[220] that the 5′ nontranscribed flanking regions of these genes contain insulin-responsive elements (IREs). Evidence of IRE-binding factor(s) in nuclear extracts has been obtained in studies of the GADPH gene in 3T3 adipocytes,[218] the c-fos gene in CHO fibroblasts,[217] and the PEPCK gene in rat liver and hepatoma cells.[221] Transcription of the PEPCK gene, in contrast to that of the amylase, c-fos, and GADPH genes, is inhibited in the presence of insulin. The elongation of PEPCK transcripts is retarded by insulin, but the major effect of insulin is to decrease initiation of transcription.[222] The PEPCK gene contains two IREs in its 5′ nontranscribed region. Since there is no difference in the IRE/nuclear protein binding activity of nuclear extracts from livers of control and streptozotocin-diabetic rats, it is likely that insulin acts through covalent modification, e.g., phosphorylation/dephosphorylation, of the IRE-binding protein.[221,223] PEPCK transcription also is regulated by cAMP and glucocorticoids, which enhance transcription via separate cAMP- and glucocorticoid-responsive elements also located in the 5′ flanking region of the gene. In the presence of all three regulators—insulin, cAMP, and glucocorticoids—the effect of insulin is dominant, resulting in inhibition of PEPCK transcription.[223] The dominant role of insulin is of clinical importance, since insulin is able to inhibit gluconeogenesis in states in which hyperglycemia is related to cAMP and glucocorticoid induction of PEPCK via the action of stress hormones.

Glucokinase, which plays a major role in maintenance of blood glucose concentration, is expressed both in the liver, where its transcription is stimulated by insulin, and in the pancreatic β-cell, where its activity is enhanced by glucose. The glucokinase gene contains two different, separate transcription control sites, one regulating transcription of the gene in the liver and the other regulating β-cell-specific transcription.[224] The glucokinase mRNA in the β-cell is approximately 200 nucleotides longer than that in the liver, and these mRNAs are similar except in their 5′ ends, which are completely different. The transcription control sites of the liver and β-cell mRNAs are structurally dissimilar, suggesting that they may interact with different transcription factors in their respective tissues.[224] The transcription factor(s) in liver may be insulin-responsive.

Messenger RNA Stability

Accumulation of specific mRNAs can also be achieved by enhancement of the stability of the mRNA transcript. The concentration of malic enzyme mRNA in insulin-treated diabetic rats is increased relative to that in untreated diabetic rats, although the transcription rate of the gene is the same in both conditions.[225] Thus, the accumulation of mRNA following insulin treatment must result from regulation of a post-translational step, possibly through an increase in mRNA stability.[225] Insulin and glucose are both necessary for transcription of the L-type pyruvate kinase gene in hepatocytes isolated from adult fasted rats[226] and also have a dramatic effect on the half-life of the L-pyruvate kinase mRNA, increasing it to 24 hours from a half-life of 1 hour in the presence of glucagon, which partially antagonizes the effect of insulin.[226] In human neuroblastoma cells in culture, insulin does not alter the rates of α- or β-tubulin transcription but increases the relative abundance of tubulin mRNA as a result of its stabilization.[227] Tubulin is the major component of microtubules and the cellular content of tubulin may play a major role in axonal and dendritic growth of neurites.

Preferential Translation of Transcripts

Rapid stimulation of protein synthesis by treatment with insulin can be achieved by the recruitment of inactive ribosomal subunits into actively translating polysomes.[228,229] This may take place without concurrent mRNA transcription and allows a rapid response to the hormone. Stimulation occurs at the level of peptide-chain initiation and brings about an increased rate of overall protein synthesis. However, there have been reports of a number of instances in which, following administration of insulin, transcription-independent increases in the synthesis of specific proteins have not been parallel. For example, when pancreatic acini isolated from streptozotocin-diabetic rats are incubated with insulin for 2 hours, the incorporation of [^{35}S]methionine into total cellular proteins increases.[230] Gel electrophoresis reveals that incorporation of label into newly synthesized proteins occurs at varying rates, despite the lack of change in the relative amounts of mRNAs in control diabetic and insulin-treated acini.[230] Insulin also stimulates the translation of fatty acid synthetase mRNA in hepatocytes in culture without affecting the concentration of fatty acid synthetase mRNA.[231] Lipoprotein lipase in differentiated 3T3-LI adipocytes[232] as well as eEF-2 and a number of unidentified proteins in NIH 3T3 cells[233] also exhibit post-transcriptional control in response to insulin. In the latter study,[233] less than 1% of proteins visualized exhibited insulin-sensitive specific translational regulation. The mechanism of action of insulin in the preferential translation of selected mRNAs is unknown but perhaps resembles the scheme described for regulation of translation of ferritin by iron, which involves interaction of an iron-responsive protein(s) with conserved sequences in the 5' untranslated regions of the ferritin heavy- and light-chain mRNAs.[234] Preferential translation of one of a number of mRNAs encoding human insulin-like growth factor II has been shown to involve differences in their 5' untranslated region.[235]

One example of preferential translation is particularly relevant to the ability of insulin to stimulate protein synthesis. In myoblasts, insulin rapidly and selectively increases the translation of ribosomal protein mRNAs by recruiting inactive ribosomal protein mRNAs into actively translating polysomes.[194] In the same study, transcription of ribosomal RNA was enhanced coordinately, so the capacity of the myoblasts to synthesize protein was quickly expanded by the administration of insulin.

INSULIN SIGNAL TRANSDUCTION IN THE REGULATION OF PROTEIN METABOLISM

The series of events that occur between binding of insulin to its plasma membrane receptor and the detection of a physiologic response to insulin have still not been elucidated. The β-subunit of the insulin receptor is a tyrosine protein kinase, and an immediate effect of insulin/receptor binding is activation of the kinase and autophosphorylation of the β-subunit. Activation of the tyrosine kinase seems to be a mandatory step in signal transduction for many, if not all, physiologic actions of insulin. Subsequent events may include activation of serine kinases and/or generation of a second messenger molecule, perhaps an inositol glycan. These possibilities have been discussed in a number of reviews[236-238] and are summarized in Chapter 4 of this volume.

It has been suggested that insulin-induced phosphorylation of ribosomal protein S6 may figure in the stimulation of protein synthesis,[239] although S6 phosphorylation does not always parallel stimulation or inhibition of synthesis.[240-242] Prostaglandins $PGF_{2\alpha}$ and PGE_2 have also been proposed as possible regulators in muscle of protein synthesis[243,244] and degradation,[245] respectively, although they were ineffective in myotubes in culture.[246] The proposed link of prostaglandins to insulin is through alteration of the activity of the plasma membrane phospholipase A2 that releases arachidonic acid, the precursor of prostaglandins, from membrane phospholipids. In addition to its other effects at the plasma membrane, insulin may activate this enzyme.

It is known that cells internalize insulin.[247] Thus, it is possible that insulin plays a direct role in intracellular regulation. Insulin accumulates in the nucleus of 3T3-L1 adipocytes[248] and H35 hepatoma cells[249] and localizes within the matrix fraction.[250] The nuclear matrix appears to be involved with a number of nuclear processes, including RNA transcription,[251] and a variety of putative regulators of gene expression, e.g., steroid hormone receptors,[252] have been shown to be associated with it. Given these facts, it has been suggested that insulin itself may interact directly with some component(s) of the transcription machinery.[250] The effect of intracellular insulin on protein synthesis has been studied in the oocytes of *Xenopus laevis* microinjected with insulin.[253] Both RNA and protein synthesis were stimulated, but since the changes in protein synthesis paralleled those of RNA synthesis, the observed increase in protein synthesis may simply reflect stimulated transcription. Microinjection of isolated nuclei enhanced incorporation of GTP into nuclear RNA, suggesting that insulin interacted directly with some nuclear component.[253]

Since the current understanding of the steps involved between the detection of the presence of insulin and the elicited physiologic response is fragmented, the connections between some of the pathways that appear to play a role in the regulation of protein metabolism are unclear. It is likely that some observed changes in protein turnover attributable to the presence or absence of insulin will prove to be the result of indirect rather than direct actions of insulin.

CONCLUSION

As part of its function as an anabolic hormone, insulin has a profound effect on protein turnover through its dual roles as a stimulator of protein synthesis and an inhibitor of protein degradation (Fig. 7-3). In conditions in which insulin is lacking, as in IDDM, or its plasma concentration is low, as in starvation, total body protein is lost, which is particularly evident as wasting of muscle.

Protein balance, whether net gain or loss, is determined by the opposing processes of protein synthesis and degradation. In vitro studies have clearly demonstrated the ability of insulin to stimulate protein synthesis and suppress proteolysis, and studies in insulin-deficient humans and animals have confirmed these actions of insulin in the intact organism. However, the role of insulin in the control of protein synthesis in healthy humans and animals is less clear. Under these conditions, substrate availability, i.e., the plasma concentration of amino acids, may be more important than insulin as a regulator of protein synthesis. The antiproteolytic action of insulin, on the other hand, can be readily demonstrated in healthy humans and animals, and therefore it appears that under normal circumstances insulin regulates protein balance through its influence on the degradative side of the equation.

In many in vitro systems, insulin can be isolated from other hormones and its specific action observed. However, it is important to remember that in the intact animal insulin does not act in isolation but in a background that includes other regulatory substances, some of which antagonize the action of insulin. The plasma concentration of a number of these substances, e.g., glucagon, glucocorticoids, and branched-chain amino acids, which

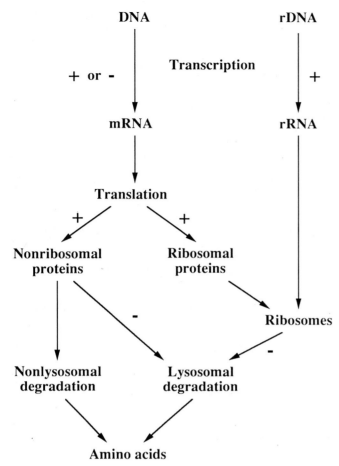

Fig. 7–3. A schematic representation of protein turnover in eukaryotic cells indicating the major steps regulated by insulin. Insulin influences protein metabolism at a number of sites by stimulating some processes while suppressing others. (+) = stimulated by insulin; (−) = inhibited by insulin.

Table 7-2. Important Questions to Be Addressed in the Future

Translation
  What is the defect in ternary complex formation?
  What is the defect in GDP/GTP exchange?
  Why is oxidative muscle resistant to inhibition of peptide-chain initiation?
  What signal marks certain mRNAs for preferential recruitment into polysomes?
Degradation
  How does insulin suppress lysosomal activity?
  How does insulin inhibit the selective degradation of ribosomes?
  Why is the degradation of some proteins inhibited by insulin while that of others is unchanged?
Gene expression
  What is the insulin-responsive element (IRE) in the genes of insulin-responsive proteins?
  Why is the transcription of some genes stimulated by insulin while that of others is inhibited?
  What is the nuclear IRE-binding protein(s)?
  How does insulin modify the activity of the IRE-binding protein?
  How does insulin cause the stabilization of specific mRNAs?
  What is the function of intranuclear insulin and how does it act?

also affect protein metabolism, are altered during the insulin-deficient state, complicating the interpretation of studies of protein metabolism at the level of the whole organism. On the other hand, application of the techniques of the rapidly advancing field of molecular biology has allowed researchers to observe the action of insulin on the gene, from which a picture of control through regulation of transcription factors is emerging.

It has become evident that insulin exerts its influence on protein metabolism not at one site but at multiple sites in the synthetic and degradative pathways. Table 7–2 lists questions, as yet unanswered, that may determine the direction of future research aimed at elucidation of the molecular mechanism of the action of insulin in the regulation of protein turnover. Since the means for discovering the answers to these questions are developing steadily, progress in this important area of research should be significant, resulting in a clearer understanding of the diabetes-induced alterations in protein metabolism.

REFERENCES

1. Moldave K. Eukaryotic protein synthesis. Annu Rev Biochem 1985;54:1109–49.
2. Pain VM. Initiation of protein synthesis in mammalian cells. Biochem J 1986;235:625–37.
3. Mortimore GE, Pösö AR, Lardeux BR. Mechanism and regulation of protein degradation in liver. Diabetes Metab Rev 1989;5:49–70.
4. Dice JF. Molecular determinants of protein half-lives in eukaryotic cells. FASEB J 1987;1:349–57.
5. Glaumann H, Ericsson JLE, Marzella L. Mechanisms of intralysosomal degradation with special reference to autophagocytosis and heterophagocytosis of cell organelles. Int Rev Cytol 1981;73:149–82.
6. Finley D, Varshavsky A. The ubiquitin system: functions and mechanisms. Trends Biochem Sci 1985;10:343–7.
7. Pontremoli S, Melloni E. Extralysosomal protein degradation. Annu Rev Biochem 1986;55:455–81.
8. Atchley DW, Loeb RF, Richards DW Jr, et al. On diabetic acidosis: a detailed study of electrolyte balances following the withdrawal and reestablishment of insulin therapy. J Clin Invest 1933;12:297–326.
9. Felig P. Amino acid metabolism in man. Annu Rev Biochem 1975;44:933–55.
10. McKee EE, Cheung JY, Rannels DE, Morgan HE. Measurement of the rate of protein synthesis and compartmentation of heart phenylalanine. J Biol Chem 1978;253:1030–40.
11. Martin AF, Rabinowitz M, Blough R, et al. Measurements of half-life of rat cardiac myosin heavy chain with leucyl-tRNA used as precursor pool. J Biol Chem 1977;252:3422–9.
12. Airhart J, Vidrich A, Khairallah EA. Compartmentation of free amino acids for protein synthesis in rat liver. Biochem J 1974;140:539–48.
13. Vidrich A, Airhart J, Bruno MK, Khairallah EA. Compartmentation of free amino acids for protein biosynthesis: influence of diurnal changes in hepatic amino acid

concentrations on the composition of the precursor pool charging aminoacyl-transfer ribonucleic acid. Biochem J 1977;162:257–66.

14. Ward WF, Mortimore GE. Compartmentation of intracellular amino acids in rat liver: evidence for an intralysosomal pool derived from protein degradation. J Biol Chem 1978;253:3581–7.

15. Hod Y, Hershko A. Relationship of the pool of intracellular valine to protein synthesis and degradation in cultured cells. J Biol Chem 1976;251:4458–67.

16. Everett AW, Prior G, Zak R. Equilibration of leucine between the plasma compartment and leucyl-tRNA in the heart, and turnover of cardiac myosin heavy chain. Biochem J 1981;194:365–8.

17. Obled C, Barre F, Millward DJ, Arnal M. Whole body protein synthesis: studies with different amino acids in the rat. Am J Physiol 1989;257:E639–46.

18. Melville S, McNurlan MA, McHardy KC, et al. The role of degradation in the acute control of protein balance in adult man: failure of feeding to stimulate protein synthesis as assessed by L-[1-^{13}C]leucine infusion. Metabolism 1989;38:248–55.

19. Waterlow JC, Stephen JML. The effect of low protein diets on the turnover rates of serum, liver and muscle proteins in the rat, measured by continuous infusion of L-[^{14}C]lysine. Clin Sci 1968;35:287–305.

20. Fern EB, Garlick PJ. The specific radioactivity of the tissue free amino acid pool as a basis for measuring the rate of protein synthesis in the rat in vivo. Biochem J 1974;142:413–9.

21. Everett AW, Clark WA, Chizzonite RA, Zak R. Change in synthesis rates of α- and β-myosin heavy chains in rabbit heart after treatment with thyroid hormone. J Biol Chem 1983;258:2421–5.

22. Gregory P, Low RB, Stirewalt WS. Fractional synthesis rates in vivo of skeletal-muscle myosin isoenzymes. Biochem J 1987;245:133–7.

23. Ashford AJ, Pain VM. Effect of diabetes on the rates of synthesis and degradation of ribosomes in rat muscle and liver in vivo. J Biol Chem 1986;261:4059–65.

24. Ashford AJ, Pain VM. Insulin stimulation of growth in diabetic rats: synthesis and degradation of ribosomes and total tissue protein in skeletal muscle and heart. J Biol Chem 1986;261:4066–70.

25. Scornik OA. In vivo rate of translation by ribosomes of normal and regenerating liver. J Biol Chem 1974;249:3876–83.

26. Henshaw EC, Hirsch CA, Morton BE, Hiatt HH. Control of protein synthesis in mammalian tissues through changes in ribosome activity. J Biol Chem 1971;246:436–46.

27. Garlick PJ, McNurlan MA, Preedy VR. A rapid and convenient technique for measuring the rate of protein synthesis in tissues by injection of [^{3}H]phenylalanine. Biochem J 1980;192:719–23.

28. Preedy VR, Garlick PJ. Reduced rates of muscle protein synthesis during tail-vein infusion of rats. Biochem Soc Trans 1984;12:700–1.

29. Krahl ME. Incorporation of C^{14}-amino acids into glutathione and protein fractions of normal and diabetic rat tissues. J Biol Chem 1953;200:99–109.

30. Manchester KL, Young FG. The effect of insulin on incorporation of amino acids into protein of normal rat diaphragm in vitro. Biochem J 1958;70:353–8.

31. Hait G, Kypson J, Massih R. Amino acid incorporation into myocardium: effect of insulin, glucagon, and dibutyryl 3′,5′-AMP. Am J Physiol 1972;222:404–8.

32. Stirewalt WS, Low RB, Slaiby JM. Insulin sensitivity and responsiveness of epitrochlearis and soleus muscles from fed and starved rats: recognition of differential changes in insulin sensitivities of protein synthesis and glucose incorporation into glycogen. Biochem J 1985;227:355–62.

33. Neely JR, Rovetto MJ. Techniques for perfusing isolated rat hearts. Methods Enzymol 1975;39:43–60.

34. Exton JH. The perfused rat liver. Methods Enzymol 1975;39:25–36.

35. Ruderman NB, Houghton CRS, Hems R. Evaluation of the isolated perfused rat hindquarter for the study of muscle metabolism. Biochem J 1971;124:639–51.

36. Jefferson LS. A technique for the perfusion of an isolated preparation of rat hemicorpus. Methods Enzymol 1975;39:73–82.

37. Bylund-Fellenius A-C, Ojamaa KM, Flaim KE, et al. Protein synthesis versus energy state in contracting muscles of perfused rat hindlimb. Am J Physiol 1984;246:E297–305.

38. Mortimore GE, Woodside KH, Henry JE. Compartmentation of free valine and its relation to protein turnover in perfused rat liver. J Biol Chem 1972;247:2776–84.

39. Flaim KE, Peavy DE, Everson WV, Jefferson LS. The role of amino acids in the regulation of protein synthesis in perfused rat liver. I. Reduction in rates of synthesis resulting from amino acid deprivation and recovery during flow-through perfusion. J Biol Chem 1982;257:2932–8.

40. Chua BHL, Siehl DL, Morgan HE. A role for leucine in regulation of protein turnover in working rat hearts. Am J Physiol 1980;239:E510–4.

41. Buse MG, Reid SS. Leucine: a possible regulator of protein turnover in muscle. J Clin Invest 1975;56:1250–61.

42. Pain VM, Albertse EC, Garlick PJ. Protein metabolism in skeletal muscle, diaphragm, and heart of diabetic rats. Am J Physiol 1983;245:E604–10.

43. Preedy VR, Smith DM, Sugden PH. A comparison of rates of protein turnover in rat diaphragm in vivo and in vitro. Biochem J 1986;233:279–82.

44. Feldhoff RC, Taylor JM, Jefferson LS. Synthesis and secretion of rat albumin in vivo, in perfused liver, and in isolated hepatocytes: effects of hypophysectomy and growth hormone treatment. J Biol Chem 1977;252:3611–6.

45. Crane LJ, Miller DL. Plasma protein synthesis by isolated rat hepatocytes. J Cell Biol 1977;72:11–25.

46. Clark RL, Hansen RJ. Insulin stimulates synthesis of soluble proteins in isolated rat hepatocytes. Biochem J 1980;190:615–9.

47. DePhilip RM, Chadwick DE, Ignotz RA, et al. Rapid stimulation by insulin of ribosome synthesis in cultured chick embryo fibroblasts. Biochemistry 1979;18:4812–7.

48. Hesketh JE, Pryme IF. Evidence that insulin increases the proportion of polysomes that are bound to the cytoskeleton in 3T3 fibroblasts. FEBS Lett 1988;231:62–6.

49. Frelin C. The regulation of protein turnover in newborn rat heart cell cultures. J Biol Chem 1980;255:11149–55.

50. Airhart J, Arnold JA, Stirewalt WS, Low RB. Insulin stimulation of protein synthesis in cultured skeletal and cardiac muscle cells. Am J Physiol 1982;243:C81–6.

51. Gulve EA, Dice JF. Regulation of protein synthesis and degradation in L8 myotubes: effects of serum, insulin and insulin-like growth factors. Biochem J 1989;260:377–87.

52. Pain VM, Garlick PJ. Effect of streptozotocin diabetes and insulin treatment on the rate of protein synthesis in tissues of the rat in vivo. J Biol Chem 1974;249:4510–4.

53. Mortimore GE, Mondon CE. Inhibition by insulin of valine turnover in liver: evidence for a general control of proteolysis. J Biol Chem 1970;245:2375–83.

54. Wagle SR, Sampson L. Studies on the differential response to insulin on the stimulation of amino acid incorporation into protein in isolated hepatocytes containing different levels of glycogen. Biochem Biophys Res Commun 1975;64:72–80.

55. Hammond GL, Lai Y-K, Markert CL. The molecules that initiate cardiac hypertrophy are not species-specific. Science 1982;216:529–31.

56. Kent JD, Kimball SR, Jefferson LS. Effect of diabetes and insulin treatment of diabetic rats on total RNA, poly(A)$^+$ RNA, and mRNA in skeletal muscle. Am J Physiol 1991;260:C401–16.

57. Everett AW, Sinha AM, Umeda PK, et al. Regulation of myosin synthesis by thyroid hormone: relative change in the α- and β-myosin heavy chain mRNA levels in rabbit heart. Biochemistry 1984;23:1596–9.

58. Dillmann WH, Barrieux A, Neeley WE, Contreras P. Influence of thyroid hormone on the in vitro translational activity of specific mRNAs in the rat heart. J Biol Chem 1983;258:7738–45.

59. Pozefsky T, Felig P, Tobin JD, et al. Amino acid balance across tissues of the forearm in postabsorptive man. Effects of insulin at two dose levels. J Clin Invest 1969;48:2273–82.

60. Gelfand RA, Barrett EJ. Effect of physiologic hyperinsulinemia on skeletal muscle protein synthesis and breakdown in man. J Clin Invest 1987;80:1–6.

61. Cooper KE, Edholm OG, Mottram RF. The blood flow in skin and muscle of the human forearm. J Physiol (Lond) 1955;128:258–67.

62. Halliday D, McKeran RO. Measurement of muscle protein synthetic rate from serial muscle biopsies and total body protein turnover in man by continuous intravenous infusion of L-[α-^{15}N]lysine. Clin Sci Molec Med 1975;49:581–90.

63. Rennie MJ, Edwards RHT, Halliday D, et al. Muscle protein synthesis measured by stable isotope techniques in man: the effects of feeding and fasting. Clin Sci 1982;63:519–23.

64. Garlick PJ, Wernerman J, McNurlan MA, et al. Measurement of the rate of protein synthesis in muscle of postabsorptive young men by injection of a "flooding dose" of [1-^{13}C]leucine. Clin Sci 1989;77:329–36.

65. Matthews DE, Schwarz HP, Yang RD, et al. Relationship of plasma leucine and α-ketoisocaproate during a L-[1-^{13}C]leucine infusion in man: a method for measuring human intracellular leucine tracer enrichment. Metabolism 1982;31:1105–12.

66. Pain VM. Protein synthesis and its regulation. In: Waterlow JC, Garlick PJ, Millward DJ, eds. Protein turnover in mammalian tissues and in the whole body. Amsterdam: Elsevier North-Holland, 1978:15–54.

67. Smith KE, Henshaw EC. Binding of Met-tRNA$_f$ to native and derived 40S ribosomal subunits. Biochemistry 1975;14:1060–7.

68. Pain VM, Lewis JA, Huvos P, et al. The effects of amino acid starvation on regulation of polypeptide chain initiation in Ehrlich ascites tumor cells. J Biol Chem 1980;255:1486–91.

69. Kelly FJ, Jefferson LS. Control of peptide-chain initiation in rat skeletal muscle: development of methods for preparation of native ribosomal subunits and analysis of the effect of insulin on formation of 40S initiation complexes. J Biol Chem 1985;260:6677–83.

70. Kimball SR, Everson WV, Flaim KE, Jefferson LS. Initiation of protein synthesis in a cell-free system prepared from rat hepatocytes. Am J Physiol 1989;256:C28–34.

71. Voorma HO, Thomas A, Goumans H, et al. Isolation and purification of initiation factors of protein synthesis from rabbit reticulocyte lysate. Methods Enzymol 1979;60:124–35.

72. Fan H, Penman S. Regulation of protein synthesis in mammalian cells. II. Inhibition of protein synthesis at the level of initiation during mitosis. J Mol Biol 1970;50:655–70.

73. Goldberg AL, Dice JF. Intracellular protein degradation in mammalian and bacterial cells. Annu Rev Biochem 1974;43:835–69.

74. Goldberg AL, St John AC. Intracellular protein degradation in mammalian and bacterial cells. Part 2. Annu Rev Biochem 1976;45:747–803.

75. Millward DJ, Garlick PJ, Stewart RJC, et al. Skeletal-muscle growth and protein turnover. Biochem J 1975;150:235–43.

76. Millward DJ, Garlick PJ, Nnanyelugo DO, Waterlow JC. The relative importance of muscle protein synthesis and breakdown in the regulation of muscle mass. Biochem J 1976;156:185–8.

77. Goldberg AL, Martel SB, Kushmerick MJ. In vitro preparations of the diaphragm and other skeletal muscles. Methods Enzymol 1975;39:82–94.

78. Rannels DE, Kao R, Morgan HE. Effect of insulin on protein turnover in heart muscle. J Biol Chem 1975;250:1694–701.

79. Green M, Miller LL. Protein catabolism and protein synthesis in perfused livers of normal and alloxan-diabetic rats. J Biol Chem 1960;235:3202–8.

80. Jefferson LS, Li JB, Rannels SR. Regulation by insulin of amino acid release and protein turnover in the perfused rat hemicorpus. J Biol Chem 1977;252:1476–83.

81. Ballard FJ, Francis GL. Effects of anabolic agents on protein breakdown in L6 myoblasts. Biochem J 1983;210:243–9.

82. Khairallah EA, Mortimore GE. Assessment of protein turnover in perfused rat liver: evidence for amino acid compartmentation from differential labeling of free and tRNA-bound valine. J Biol Chem 1976;251:1375–84.

83. Jefferson LS, Rannels DE, Munger BL, Morgan HE. Insulin in the regulation of protein turnover in heart and skeletal muscle. Fed Proc 1974;33:1098–104.

84. Barrett EJ, Revkin JH, Young LH, et al. An isotopic method for measurement of muscle protein synthesis and degradation in vivo. Biochem J 1987;245:223–8.

85. Revkin J, Young L, Zaret B, et al. A novel isotope dilution technique to measure protein turnover in heart muscle [Abstract]. Clin Res 1986;34:338A.

86. Vandekerckhove J, Weber K. Chordate muscle actins differ distinctly from invertebrate muscle actins: the evolution of the different vertebrate muscle actins. J Mol Biol 1984;179:391–413.

87. Young VR, Munro HN. N$^\tau$-methylhistidine (3-methylhistidine) and muscle protein turnover: an overview. Fed Proc 1978;37:2291–300.

88. Long CL, Haverbert LN, Young VR, et al. Metabolism of 3-methylhistidine in man. Metabolism 1975;24:929–35.

89. Wassner SJ, Li JB. N$^\tau$-methylhistidine release: contributions of rat skeletal muscle, GI tract, and skin. Am J Physiol 1982;243:E293–7.

90. Rennie MJ, Millward DJ. 3-methylhistidine excretion and the urinary 3-methylhistidine/creatinine ratio are poor indicators of skeletal muscle protein breakdown. Clin Sci 1983;65:217–25.

91. Furuno K, Goldberg AL. The activation of protein degradation in muscle by Ca^{2+} or muscle injury does not involve a lysosomal mechanism. Biochem J 1986;237:859–64.

92. Jefferson LS, Flaim KE, Peavy DE. Effect of insulin on protein turnover. In: Brownlee M, ed. Handbook of diabetes mellitus: biochemical pathology. Vol 4. New York: Garland Press, 1981:133–77.

93. Pain VM, McNurlan MA, Albertse EC, et al. Effect of streptozotocin diabetes on protein synthesis in the liver, kidney and intestinal mucosa of young rats [Abstract]. Proc Nutr Soc 1978;37(3):104A.

94. McNurlan MA, Garlick PJ. Protein synthesis in liver and small intestine in protein deprivation and diabetes. Am J Physiol 1981;241:E238–45.

95. Ross J, Goldman JK. Effect of streptozotocin-induced diabetes on kidney weight and compensatory hypertrophy in the rat. Endocrinology 1971;88:1079–82.

96. Mirsky IA. The influence of insulin on the protein metabolism of nephrectomized dogs. Am J Physiol 1938;124:569–75.

97. Frame EG, Russell JA. The effects of insulin and anterior pituitary extract on the blood amino nitrogen in eviscerated rats. Endocrinology 1946;39:420–9.

98. Ingle DJ, Prestrud MC, Nezamis JE. The effect of insulin upon the level of blood amino acids in the eviscerated rat as related to the level of blood glucose. Am J Physiol 1947;150:682–5.

99. Fulks RM, Li JB, Goldberg AL. Effects of insulin, glucose, and amino acids on protein turnover in rat diaphragm. J Biol Chem 1975;250:290–8.

100. Preedy VR, Smith DM, Kearney NF, Sugden PH. Rates of protein turnover in vivo and in vitro in ventricular muscle of hearts from fed and starved rats. Biochem J 1984;222:395–400.

101. Morgan HE, Jefferson LS, Wolpert EB, Rannels DE. Regulation of protein synthesis in heart muscle. II. Effect of amino acid levels and insulin on ribosomal aggregation. J Biol Chem 1971;246:2163–70.

102. Jefferson LS, Koehler JO, Morgan HE. Effect of insulin on protein synthesis in skeletal muscle of an isolated perfused preparation of rat hemicorpus. Proc Natl Acad Sci USA 1972;69:816–20.

103. Hay AM, Waterlow JC. The effect of alloxan diabetes on muscle and liver protein synthesis in the rat, measured by constant infusion of L-[^{14}C]lysine. J Physiol (Lond) 1967;191:111p–12p.

104. Odedra BR, Dalal SS, Millward DJ. Muscle protein synthesis in the streptozotocin-diabetic rat: a possible role for corticosterone in the insensitivity to insulin infusions in vivo. Biochem J 1982;202:363–8.

105. Forker LL, Chaikoff IL, Entenman C, Tarver H. Formation of muscle protein in the diabetic dogs studied with S^{35}-methionine. J Biol Chem 1951;188:37–48.

106. Garlick PJ, Fern M, Preedy VR. The effect of insulin infusion and food intake on muscle protein synthesis in postabsorptive rats. Biochem J 1983;210:669–76.

107. Oddy VH, Lindsay DB, Barker PJ, Northrop AJ. Effect of insulin on hind-limb and whole-body leucine and protein metabolism in fed and fasted lambs. Br J Nutr 1987;58:437–52.

108. Nissen S, Haymond MW. Changes in leucine kinetics during meal absorption: effects of dietary leucine availability. Am J Physiol 1986;250:E695–701.

109. Rannels DE, Hjalmarson AC, Morgan HE. Effects of noncarbohydrate substrates on protein synthesis in muscle. Am J Physiol 1974;226:528–39.

110. Guidotti GG, Borghetti AF, Gazzola GC. The regulation of amino acid transport in animal cells. Biochim Biophys Acta 1978;515:329–66.

111. Garlick PJ, Grant I. Amino acid infusion increases the sensitivity of muscle protein synthesis in vivo to insulin: effect of branched-chain amino acids. Biochem J 1988;254:579–84.

112. MacLennan PA, Brown RA, Rennie MJ. A positive relationship between protein synthetic rate and intracellular glutamine concentration in perfused rat skeletal muscle. FEBS Lett 1987;215:187–91.

113. Penhos JC, Krahl ME. Stimulus of leucine incorporation into perfused liver protein by insulin. Am J Physiol 1963;204:140–2.

114. Peavy DE, Taylor JM, Jefferson LS. Correlation of albumin production rates and albumin mRNA levels in livers of normal, diabetic, and insulin-treated diabetic rats. Proc Natl Acad Sci USA 1978;75:5879–83.

115. Jefferson LS, Liao WSL, Peavy DE, et al. Diabetes-induced alterations in liver protein synthesis: changes in the relative abundance of mRNAs for albumin and other plasma proteins. J Biol Chem 1983;258:1369–75.

116. Marsh JB. Effects of fasting and alloxan diabetes on albumin synthesis by perfused rat liver. Am J Physiol 1961;201:55–7.

117. Reaven EP, Peterson DT, Reaven GM. The effect of experimental diabetes mellitus and insulin replacement on hepatic ultrastructure and protein synthesis. J Clin Invest 1973;52:248–62.

118. Morgan CR, Jersild RA Jr. Alterations in the morphology of rat liver cells influenced by insulin. Anat Rec 1970;166:575–86.

119. Pain VM, Lanoix J, Bergeron JJM, Clemens MJ. Effect of diabetes on the ultrastructure of the hepatocyte and on the distribution and activity of ribosomes in the free and membrane-bound populations. Biochim Biophys Acta 1974;353:487–98.

120. Stanchfield JE, Yager JD Jr. Insulin effects on protein synthesis and secretion in primary cultures of amphibian hepatocytes. J Cell Physiol 1979;100:279–89.

121. Guzdek A, Sarnecka-Keller M, Dubin A. The activities of perfused livers of control and streptozotocin diabetic rats in the synthesis of some plasma proteins and peptides. Horm Metab Res 1979;11:107–11.

122. Berry EM, Ziv E, Bar-On H. Protein and glycoprotein synthesis and secretion by the diabetic liver. Diabetologia 1980;19:535–40.

123. McMillan DE. Changes in serum proteins and protein-bound carbohydrates in diabetes mellitus. Diabetologia 1970;6:597–604.

124. Ingebretsen WR Jr, Moxley MA, Allen DO, Wagle SR. Studies on gluconeogenesis, protein synthesis and cyclic AMP levels in isolated parenchymal cells following insulin withdrawal from alloxan diabetic rats. Biochem Biophys Res Commun 1972;49:601–7.

125. Curfman GD, O'Hara DS, Hopkins BE, Smith TW. Suppression of myocardial protein degradation in the rat during fasting: effects of insulin, glucose, and leucine. Circ Res 1980;46:581–9.

126. Iannaccone ST, Nagy B, Samaha FJ. Partial biochemical maturation of aneurally cultured human skeletal muscle. Neurology 1982;32:846–51.

127. Cahill GF Jr. Starvation in man. N Engl J Med 1970;282:668–75.

128. Dice JF, Walker CD, Byrne B, Cardiel A. General characteristics of protein degradation in diabetes and starvation. Proc Natl Acad Sci USA 1978;75:2093–7.

129. Nakhooda AF, Wei C-N, Marliss EB. Muscle protein catabolism in diabetes: 3-methylhistidine excretion in the spontaneously diabetic "BB" rat. Metabolism 1980; 29:1272–7.

130. Huszar G, Koivisto V, Davis E, Felig P. Urinary 3-methyl-histidine excretion in juvenile-onset diabetics: evidence of increased protein catabolism in the absence of ketoacidosis. Metabolism 1982;31:188–91.

131. Abou-Mourad NN, Jefferson LS, Rannels SR, et al. Effects of acute insulin deficiency on leucine kinetics in conscious dogs [Abstract No. 201]. Diabetes 1980;29(suppl 2):51A.

132. Li JB, Wassner SJ. Effects of food deprivation and refeeding on total protein and actomyosin degradation. Am J Physiol 1984;246:E32–7.

133. Lowell BB, Ruderman NB, Goodman MN. Evidence that lysosomes are not involved in the degradation of myofibrillar proteins in rat skeletal muscle. Biochem J 1986;234:237–40.

134. Smith DM, Sugden PH. Contrasting response of protein degradation to starvation and insulin as measured by release of N^τ-methylhistidine or phenylalanine from the perfused rat heart. Biochem J 1986;237:391–5.

135. MacLennan PA, Smith K, Weryk B, et al. Inhibition of protein breakdown by glutamine in perfused rat skeletal muscle. FEBS Lett 1988;237:133–6.

136. Woodside KH, Mortimore GE. Suppression of protein turnover by amino acids in the perfused rat liver. J Biol Chem 1972;247:6474–81.

137. Garlick PJ, Millward DJ, James WPT. The diurnal response of muscle and liver protein synthesis in vivo in meal-fed rats. Biochem J 1973;136:935–45.

138. Garlick PJ, Millward DJ, James WPT, Waterlow JC. The effect of protein deprivation and starvation on the rate of protein synthesis in tissues of the rat. Biochim Biophys Acta 1975;414:71–84.

139. Neely AN, Cox JR, Fortney JA, et al. Alterations of lysosomal size and density during rat liver perfusion: suppression by insulin and amino acids. J Biol Chem 1977;252:6948–54.

140. Mortimore GE, Pösö AR, Kadowaki M, Wert JJ Jr. Multiphasic control of hepatic protein degradation by regulatory amino acids: general features and hormonal modulation. J Biol Chem 1987;262:16322–7.

141. Millward DJ, Bates PC, Brown JG, et al. Role of thyroid, insulin and corticosteroid hormones in the physiological regulation of proteolysis in muscle. In: Khairallah EA, Bond JS, Bird JWC, eds. Intracellular protein catabolism. New York: Alan R Liss, 1985:531–42.

142. Tischler ME. Hormonal regulation of protein degradation in skeletal and cardiac muscle. Life Sci 1981;28:2569–76.

143. Nair KS, Garrow JS, Ford C, et al. Effect of poor diabetic control and obesity on whole body protein metabolism in man. Diabetologia 1983;25:400–3.

144. Fukagawa NK, Minaker KL, Rowe JW, et al. Insulin-mediated reduction of whole body protein breakdown: dose-response effects on leucine metabolism in postabsorptive men. J Clin Invest 1985;76:2306–11.

145. Tessari P, Nosadini R, Trevisan R, et al. Defective suppression by insulin of leucine-carbon appearance and oxidation in type 1, insulin-dependent diabetes mellitus: evidence for insulin resistance involving glucose and amino acid metabolism. J Clin Invest 1986;77:1797–804.

146. Robert JJ, Beaufrere B, Koziet J, et al. Whole body de novo amino acid synthesis in type 1 (insulin-dependent) diabetes studied with stable isotope-labeled leucine, alanine, and glycine. Diabetes 1985;34:67–73.

147. Umpleby AM, Boroujerdi MA, Brown PM, et al. The effect of metabolic control on leucine metabolism in type 1 (insulin-dependent) diabetic patients. Diabetologia 1986;29:131–41.

148. Tessari P, Trevisan R, Inchiostro S, et al. Dose-response curves of effects of insulin on leucine kinetics in humans. Am J Physiol 1986;251:E334–42.

149. Nair KS, Ford GC, Halliday D. Effect of intravenous insulin treatment on in vivo whole body leucine kinetics and oxygen consumption in insulin-deprived type 1 diabetic patients. Metabolism 1987;36:491–5.

150. Castellino P, Luzi L, Simonson DC, et al. Effect of insulin and plasma amino acid concentrations on leucine metabolism in man: role of substrate availablity on estimates of whole body protein synthesis. J Clin Invest 1987; 80:1784–93.

151. Tessari P, Inchiostro S, Biolo G, et al. Differential effects of hyperinsulinemia and hyperaminoacidemia on leucine carbon metabolism in vivo: evidence for distinct mechanisms in regulation of net amino acid deposition. J Clin Invest 1987;79:1062–9.

152. Fukagawa NK, Minaker KL, Young VR, et al. Leucine metabolism in aging humans: effect of insulin and substrate availability. Am J Physiol 1989;256:E288–94.

153. Bennett WM, Connacher AA, Scrimgeour CM, et al. Euglycemic hyperinsulinemia augments amino acid uptake by human leg tissues during hyperaminoacidemia. Am J Physiol 1990;259:E185–94.

154. Pacy PJ, Nair KS, Ford C, Halliday D. Failure of insulin infusion to stimulate fractional muscle protein synthesis in type 1 diabetic patients: anabolic effect of insulin and decreased proteolysis. Diabetes 1989;38:618–24.

155. Fukagawa NK, Minaker KL, Young VR, Rowe JW. Insulin dose-dependent reductions in plasma amino acids in man. Am J Physiol 1986;250:E13–7.

156. Bennett WM, Connacher AA, Smith K, et al. Inability to stimulate skeletal muscle or whole body protein synthesis in type 1 (insulin-dependent) diabetic patients by insulin-plus-glucose during amino acid infusion: studies of incorporation and turnover of tracer L-[1-^{13}C]leucine. Diabetologia 1990;33:43–51.

157. Tessari P, Biolo G, Inchiostro S, et al. Effects of insulin on whole body and forearm leucine and KIC metabolism in type 1 diabetes. Am J Physiol 1990;259:E96–103.

158. Neely JR, Liebermeister H, Battersby EJ, Morgan HE. Effect of pressure development on oxygen consumption by isolated rat heart. Am J Physiol 1967;212:804–14.

159. Flaim KE, Copenhaver ME, Jefferson LS. Effects of diabetes on protein synthesis in fast- and slow-twitch rat skeletal muscle. Am J Physiol 1980;239:E88–95.

160. Rannels DE, Jefferson LS, Hjalmarson ÅC, et al. Maintenance of protein synthesis in hearts of diabetic animals. Biochem Biophys Res Commun 1970;40:1110–6.

161. Harmon CS, Proud CG, Pain VM. Effects of starvation, diabetes and acute insulin treatment on the regulation of polypeptide-chain initiation in rat skeletal muscle. Biochem J 1984;223:687–96.

162. Kimball SR, Jefferson LS. Effect of diabetes on guanine nucleotide exchange factor activity in skeletal muscle and heart. Biochem Biophys Res Commun 1988; 156:706–96.

163. Dholakia JN, Mueser TC, Woodley CL, et al. The association of NADPH with the guanine nucleotide exchange factor from rabbit reticulocytes: a role of pyridine dinucleotides in eukaryotic polypeptide chain initiation. Proc Natl Acad Sci USA 1986;83:6746–50.

164. Kraupp O, Adler-Kastner L, Niessner H, Plank B. Effects of starvation and of acute and chronic alloxan diabetes on

myocardial substrate levels and on liver glycogen in the rat in vivo. Eur J Biochem 1967;2:197−214.

165. Towle CA, Mankin HJ, Avruch J, Treadwell BV. Insulin promoted decrease in the phosphorylation of protein synthesis initiation factor eIF-2. Biochem Biophys Res Commun 1984;121:134−40.

166. Clemens MJ, Galpine AR, Austin SA, et al. The role of phosphorylation of eIF-2' in translational regulation in nonerythroid cells. In: Mathews MB. Current communications in molecular biology. New York: Cold Spring Harbor Laboratory, 1986:63−9.

167. Cox S, Redpath NT, Proud CG. Regulation of polypeptide-chain initiation in rat skeletal muscle: starvation does not alter the activity or phosphorylation state of initiation factor eIF-2. FEBS Lett 1988;239:333−8.

168. Jeffrey IW, Kelly FJ, Duncan R, et al. Effect of starvation and diabetes on the activity of the eukaryotic initiation factor eIF-2 in rat skeletal muscle. Biochimie 1990;72:751−7.

169. Dholakia JN, Wahba AJ. Phosphorylation of the guanine nucleotide exchange factor from rabbit reticulocytes regulates its activity in polypeptide-chain initiation. Proc Natl Acad Sci USA 1988;85:51−4.

170. Sommercorn J, Mulligan JA, Lozeman FJ, Krebs EG. Activation of casein kinase II in response to insulin and to epidermal growth factor. Proc Natl Acad Sci USA 1987;84:8834−8.

171. Jefferson LS, Robertson JW, Schworer CM. Effects of insulin and diabetes on hepatic protein turnover [Abstract]. Diabetes 1973;22(Suppl 1):321.

172. Peterson DT, Alford FP, Reaven EP, et al. Characteristics of membrane-bound and free hepatic ribosomes from insulin-deficient rats. I. Acute experimental diabetes mellitus. J Clin Invest 1973;52:3201−11.

173. Tragl KH, Reaven GM. Effect of insulin deficiency on hepatic ribosomal aggregation. Diabetes 1972;21:84−8.

174. Pilkis SJ, Korner A. Effect of diabetes and insulin treatment on protein synthetic activity of rat liver ribosomes. Biochim Biophys Acta 1971;247:597−608.

175. Wittman JS III, Lee K-L, Miller ON. Dietary and hormonal influences on rat liver polysome profiles; fat, glucose and insulin. Biochim Biophys Acta 1969;174:536−43.

176. Korner A. Alloxan diabetes and in vitro protein biosynthesis in rat liver microsomes and mitochondria. J Endocrinol 1960;20:256−65.

177. Pain VM. Protein synthesis in a postmitochondrial supernatant system from rat liver. An effect of diabetes at the level of peptide chain initiation. FEBS Lett 1973;35:169−72.

178. Robinson WS. Alloxan diabetes and insulin effects on amino acid incorporating activity of rat liver microsomes. Proc Soc Exp Biol Med 1961;106:115−8.

179. Williams IH, Chua BH, Sahms RH, et al. Effects of diabetes on protein turnover in cardiac muscle. Am J Physiol 1980;239:E178−85.

180. Neely AN, Nelson PB, Mortimore GE. Osmotic alterations of the lysosomal system during rat liver perfusion: reversible suppression by insulin and amino acids. Biochim Biophys Acta 1974;338:458−72.

181. Ward WF, Cox JR, Mortimore GE. Lysosomal sequestration of intracellular protein as a regulatory step in hepatic proteolysis. J Biol Chem 1977;252:6955−61.

182. Mortimore GE, Schworer CM. Induction of autophagy by amino-acid deprivation in perfused rat liver. Nature 1977;270:174−6.

183. Amherdt M, Harris V, Renold AE, et al. Hepatic autophagy in uncontrolled experimental diabetes and its relationships to insulin and glucagon. J Clin Invest 1974;54:188−93.

184. Woodside KH, Ward WF, Mortimore GE. Effects of glucagon on general protein degradation and synthesis in perfused rat liver. J Biol Chem 1974;249:5458−63.

185. Long WM, Chua BHL, Munger BL, Morgan HE. Effects of insulin on cardiac lysosomes and protein degradation. Fed Proc 1984;43:1295−300.

186. Ord JM, Wakeland JR, Crie JS, Wildenthal K. Mechanisms of degradation of myofibrillar and nonmyofibrillar protein in heart. Adv Myocardiol 1983;4:195−9.

187. Mortimore GE, Ward WF, Schworer CM. Lysosomal processing of intracellular protein in rat liver and its general regulation by amino acids and insulin. In: Segal HL, Doyle DJ, eds. Protein turnover and lysosome function. New York: Academic Press, 1978:67−87.

188. Gurd JW, Evans WH. Relative rates of degradation of mouse-liver surface-membrane proteins. Eur J Biochem 1973;36:273−9.

189. Mathews RA, Johnson TC, Hudson JE. Synthesis and turnover of plasma-membrane proteins and glycoproteins in a neuroblastoma cell line. Biochem J 1976;154:57−64.

190. Bond, J.S. Failure to demonstrate increased protein turnover and intracellular proteinase activity in livers of mice with streptozotocin-induced diabetes. Diabetes 1980;29:648−54.

191. Hutson NJ, Lloyd CE, Mortimore GE. Regulation of hepatic protein breakdown by food intake in streptozotocin-diabetic mice [Abstract no. 882]. Fed Proc 1981;40:1692.

192. Kurihara K, Wool IG. Effect of insulin on the synthesis of sarcoplasmic and ribosomal proteins of muscle. Nature 1968;219:721−4.

193. Raw I, Juliani MH, Rocha MC, Maia JCC. Effect of insulin on the synthesis of rat liver ribosomal and endoplasmic reticulum proteins. Braz J Med Biol Res 1985;18:421−6.

194. Hammond ML, Bowman LH. Insulin stimulates the translation of ribosomal proteins and the transcription of rRNA in mouse myoblasts. J Biol Chem 1988;263:17785−91.

195. Palmer RM, Bain PA. Indomethacin inhibits the insulin-induced increases in RNA and protein synthesis in L6 skeletal muscle myoblasts. Prostaglandins 1989;37:193−203.

196. Palmer RM, Campbell GP, Whitelaw PF, et al. The cyclo-oxygenase inhibitors indomethacin and ibuprofen inhibit the insulin-induced stimulation of ribosomal RNA synthesis in L6 myoblasts. Biochem J 1989;264:101−6.

197. Hirsch CA, Hiatt HH. Turnover of liver ribosomes in fed and in fasted rats. J Biol Chem 1966;241:5936−40.

198. Tsurugi K, Morita T, Ogata K. Mode of degradation of ribosomes in regenerating rat liver in vivo. Eur J Biochem 1974;45:119−26.

199. Lardeux BR, Mortimore GE. Amino acid and hormonal control of macromolecular turnover in perfused rat liver: evidence for selective autophagy. J Biol Chem 1987;262:14514−9.

200. Lloyd CE, Kalinyak JE, Hutson SM, Jefferson LS. Stimulation of albumin gene transcription by insulin in primary cultures of rat hepatocytes. Am J Physiol 1987;252:C205−14.

201. Iynedjian PB, Gjinovci A, Renold AE. Stimulation by insulin of glucokinase gene transcription in liver of diabetic rats. J Biol Chem 1988;263:740−4.

202. Noguchi T, Inoue H, Tanaka T. Transcriptional and post-transcriptional regulation of L-type pyruvate kinase in

diabetic rat liver by insulin and dietary fructose. J Biol Chem 1985;260:14393–7.

203. Pry TA, Porter JW. Control of fatty acid synthetase mRNA levels in rat liver by insulin, glucagon, dibutyl cyclic AMP. Biochem Biophys Res Commun 1981;100:1002–9.

204. Granner D, Andreone T, Sasaki K, Beale E. Inhibition of transcription of the phosphoenolpyruvate carboxykinase gene by insulin. Nature 1983;305:549–51.

205. Garvey WT, Huecksteadt TP, Birnbaum MJ. Pretranslational suppression of an insulin-responsive glucose transporter in rats with diabetes mellitus. Science 1989;245:60–3.

206. Plant PW, Deeley RG, Grieninger G. Selective block of albumin gene expression in chick embryo hepatocytes cultured without hormones and its partial reversal by insulin. J Biol Chem 1983;258:15355–60.

207. Korc M, Owerbach D, Quinto C, Rutter WJ. Pancreatic islet-acinar cell interaction: amylase messenger RNA levels are determined by insulin. Science 1981;213:351–3.

208. Melmed S, Neilson L, Slanina S. Insulin suppresses rat growth hormone messenger ribonucleic acid levels in rat pituitary tumor cells. Diabetes 1985;34:409–12.

209. Roy AK, Chatterjee B, Prasad MSK, Unakar NJ. Role of insulin in the regulation of the hepatic messenger RNA for α2μ-globulin in diabetic rats. J Biol Chem 1980;255:11614–8.

210. Evans MI, McKnight GS. Regulation of the ovalbumin gene: effects of insulin, adenosine 3′,5′-monophosphate, estrogen. Endocrinology 1984;115:368–77.

211. Chomczynski P, Qasba P, Topper YJ. Essential role of insulin in transcription of the rat 25,000 molecular weight casein gene. Science 1984;226:1326–8.

212. Milstone LM, Piatigorsky J. k-Crystallin gene expression in embryonic chick lens epithelia cultured in the presence of insulin. Exp Cell Res 1977;105:9–14.

213. Meisler MH, Howard G. Effects of insulin on gene transcription. Annu Rev Physiol 1989;51:701–14.

214. Dillmann WH. Diabetes mellitus-induced changes in the concentration of specific mRNAs and proteins. Diabetes Metab Rev 1988;4:789–97.

215. Maniatis T, Goodbourn S, Fischer JA. Regulation of inducible and tissue-specific gene expression. Science 1987;236:1237–45.

216. Osborn L, Rosenberg MP, Keller SA, et al. Insulin response of a hybrid amylase/CAT gene in transgenic mice. J Biol Chem 1988;263:16519–22.

217. Stumpo DJ, Stewart TN, Gilman MZ, Blackshear PJ. Identification of c-fos sequences involved in induction by insulin and phorbol esters. J Biol Chem 1988;263:1611–4.

218. Nasrin N, Ercolani L, Denaro M, et al. An insulin response element in the glyceraldehyde-3-phosphate dehydrogenase gene binds a nuclear protein induced by insulin in cultured cells and by nutritional manipulations in vivo. Proc Natl Acad Sci USA 1990;87:5273–7.

219. Alemany J, Borras T, de Pablo F. Transcriptional stimulation of the k1-crystallin gene by insulin-like growth factor I and insulin requires DNA cis elements in chicken. Proc Natl Acad Sci USA 1990;87:3353–7.

220. Magnuson MA, Quinn PG, Granner DK. Multihormonal regulation of phosphoenolpyruvate carboxykinase-chloramphenicol acetyltransferase fusion genes: insulin's effects oppose those of cAMP and dexamethasone. J Biol Chem 1987;262:14917–20.

221. O'Brien RM, Lucas PC, Forest CD, et al. Identification of a sequence in the PEPCK gene that mediates a negative

effect of insulin on transcription. Science 1990; 249:533–7.

222. O'Brien RM, Granner DK. PEPCK gene as model of inhibitory effects of insulin on gene transcription. Diabetes Care 1990;13:327–39.

223. Sasaki K, Cripe TP, Koch SR, et al. Multihormonal regulation of phosphoenolpyruvate carboxykinase gene transcription: the dominant role of insulin. J Biol Chem 1984;259:15242–51.

224. Magnuson MA. Glucokinase gene structure: functional implications of molecular genetic studies. Diabetes 1990;39:523–7.

225. Davis BB, Magge S, Mucenski CG, Drake RL. Insulin-mediated post-transcriptional regulation of hepatic malic enzyme and albumin mRNAs. Biochem Biophys Res Commun 1988;154:1081–7.

226. Decaux J-F, Antoine B, Kahn A. Regulation of the expression of the L-type pyruvate kinase gene in adult rat hepatocytes in primary culture. J Biol Chem 1989;264:11584–90.

227. Fernyhough P, Mill JF, Roberts JL, Ishii DN. Stabilization of tubulin mRNAs by insulin and insulin-like growth factor I during neurite formation. Brain Res Mol Brain Res 1989;6:109–20.

228. Lyons RT, Nordeen SK, Young DA. Effects of fasting and insulin administration on polyribosome formation in rat epididymal fat cells. J Biol Chem 1980;255:6330–4.

229. Wool IG, Castles JJ, Leader DP, Fox A. Insulin and the function of muscle ribosomes. In: Steiner DF, Freinkel N, eds. Handbook of physiology, Section 7. Vol 1. Endocrinology. Washington, DC: American Physiological Society, 1972:385–94.

230. Okabayashi Y, Moessner J, Logsdon CD, et al. Insulin and other stimulants have nonparallel translational effects on protein synthesis. Diabetes 1987;36:1054–60.

231. Wilson SB, Back DW, Morris SM Jr, et al. Hormonal regulation of lipogenic enzymes in chick embryo hepatocytes in culture: expression of the fatty acid synthase gene is regulated at both translational and pretranslational steps. J Biol Chem 1986;261:15179–82.

232. Semenkovich CF, Wims M, Noe L, et al. Insulin regulation of lipoprotein lipase activity in 3T3-L1 adipocytes is mediated at posttranscriptional and posttranslational levels. J Biol Chem 1989;264:9030–8.

233. Levenson RM, Nairn AC, Blackshear PJ. Insulin rapidly induces the biosynthesis of elongation factor 2. J Biol Chem 1989;264:11904–11.

234. Leibold EA, Munro HN. Cytoplasmic protein binds in vitro to a highly conserved sequence in the 5′ untranslated region of ferritin heavy- and light-subunit mRNAs. Proc Natl Acad Sci USA 1988;85:2171–5.

235. Nielsen FC, Gammeltoft S, Christiansen J. Translational discrimination of mRNAs coding for human insulin-like growth factor II. J Biol Chem 1990;265:13431–4.

236. Denton RM. Early events in insulin actions. Adv Cyclic Nucleotide Protein Phosphorylation Res 1986;20:293–341.

237. Czech MP, Klarlund JK, Yagaloff KA, et al. Insulin receptor signaling: activation of multiple serine kinases. J Biol Chem 1988;263:11017–20.

238. Rosen OM. After insulin binds. Science 1987;237:1452–8.

239. Traugh JA, Pendergast AM. Regulation of protein synthesis by phosphorylation of ribosomal protein S6 and aminoacyl-tRNA synthetases. Prog Nucleic Acid Res Mol Biol 1986;33:195–230.

240. Gressner AM, Wool IG. The stimulation of the phospho-

rylation of ribosomal protein S6 by cycloheximide and puromycin. Biochem Biophys Res Commun 1974; 60:1482–90.

241. Nielsen PJ, Manchester KL, Towbin H, et al. The phosphorylation of ribosomal protein S6 in rat tissues following cycloheximide injection, in diabetes, and after denervation of diaphragm: a simple immunological determination of the extent of S6 phosphorylation on protein blots. J Biol Chem 1982;257:12316–21.

242. Gressner AM, Wool IG. Effect of experimental diabetes and insulin on phosphorylation of rat liver ribosomal protein S6. Nature 1976;259:148–50.

243. Reeds PJ, Palmer RM. The possible involvement of prostaglandin $F_{2\alpha}$ in the stimulation of muscle protein synthesis by insulin. Biochem Biophys Res Commun 1983;116:1084–90.

244. Reeds PJ, Hay SM, Glennie RT, et al. The effect of indomethacin on the stimulation of protein synthesis by insulin in young post-absorptive rats. Biochem J 1985;227:255–61.

245. Goldberg AL, Baracos V, Rodemann P, et al. Control of protein degradation in muscle by prostaglandins, Ca^{2+}, leukocytic pyrogen (interleukin 1). Fed Proc 1984; 43:1301–6.

246. McElligott MA, Chuang L-Y, Baracos V, Gulve EA. Prostaglandin production in myotube cultures: influence on protein turnover. Biochem J 1988;253:745–9.

247. Goldfine ID. Interaction of insulin, polypeptide hormones, and growth factors with intracellular membranes. Biochim Biophys Acta 1981;650:53–67.

248. Smith RM, Jarett L. Ultrastructural evidence for the accumulation of insulin in nuclei of intact 3T3-L1 adipocytes by an insulin-receptor mediated process. Proc Natl Acad Sci USA 1987;84:459–63.

249. Peralta Soler A, Thompson KA, Smith RM, Jarett L. Immunological demonstration of the accumulation of insulin, but not insulin receptors, in nuclei of insulin-treated cells. Proc Natl Acad Sci USA 1989;86:6640–4.

250. Thompson KA, Peralta Soler A, Smith RM, Jarett L. Intranuclear localization of insulin in rat hepatoma cells: insulin/matrix association. Eur J Cell Biol 1989;50:442–6.

251. Nelson WG, Pienta KJ, Barrack ER, Coffey DS. The role of the nuclear matrix in the organization and function of DNA. Annu Rev Biophys Biophys Chem 1986;15:457–75.

252. Barrack ER, Hawkins EF, Allen SL, et al. Concepts related to salt resistant estradiol receptors in rat uterine nuclei: nuclear matrix. Biochem Biophys Res Commun 1977;79:829–36.

253. Miller DS. Stimulation of RNA and protein synthesis by intracellular insulin. Science 1988;240:506–9.

Chapter 8

MOLECULAR ASPECTS OF INSULIN ACTION

MORRIS F. WHITE
C. RONALD KAHN

Since the discovery of insulin 70 years ago, its effect on carbohydrate, fat, and protein metabolism has been well established.[1] However, the molecular mechanisms of insulin action have been difficult to define.[2] Insulin action begins with the binding of insulin to the α-subunit of the insulin receptor at the surface of the plasma membrane, a process that stimulates the tyrosine kinase in the β-subunit.[3] Most evidence suggests that the tyrosine kinase is essential for insulin action[3,4] via generation of molecular signals that regulate membrane transport processes (glucose, amino acids, and ions), activate and inactivate enzymes, regulate gene expression, and regulate protein and DNA synthesis (Fig. 8–1). However, the nature of these signals has been difficult to determine.

When the insulin signal pathways become resistant to hormonal stimulation, glucose tolerance may become impaired. This type of insulin resistance plays a major pathogenic role in non-insulin-dependent diabetes mellitus (NIDDM).[1] As long as the pancreas sustains insulin secretion sufficient to counterbalance the insulin resistance, glucose tolerance remains normal or only mildly impaired.[1] When insulin secretion is inadequate to compensate for the insulin resistance, the rate of hepatic glucose output increases and the ability of insulin to stimulate glucose uptake in peripheral target tissues decreases, which results in hyperglycemia.[5]

The biochemical problems causing insulin resistance in NIDDM are not well understood. Mutations of the insulin receptor appear to be the culprit in a few cases of severe insulin resistance[6]; however, the underlying molecular defects in the majority of patients with NIDDM are unknown. Approaches that seek to identify marker genes that segregate with NIDDM have succeeded in identifying mutations in some families with maturity-onset diabetes of youth (MODY). The alterations are located on chromosome 20 near the adenosine deaminase gene in some patients[7] and on chromosome 7 in the glucokinase gene in others.[8] However, identification of each element responsible for insulin resistance in NIDDM will arise only from a full characterization of the molecular pathways of insulin signal transmission.

OVERVIEW OF INSULIN ACTION

Insulin is the primary hormone responsible for signaling the storage and utilization of glucose and other nutrients and inhibition of glucose production. Muscle, liver, and fat are the most important target tissues for insulin with respect to glucose homeostasis. Quantitatively, skeletal muscle is the major peripheral site for glucose disposal, but insulin exerts potent regulatory effects on other cell types as well.[1] Hepatic glucose

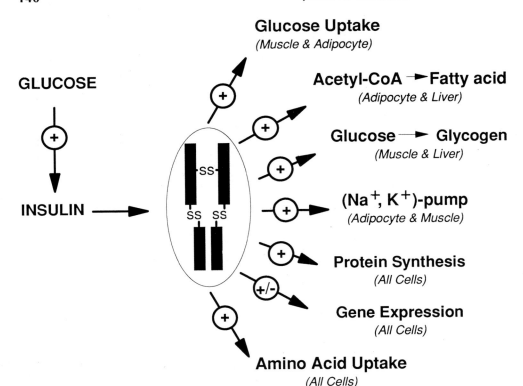

Fig. 8–1. Major insulin responses found in various cell and tissues that are mediated through the binding of insulin to its receptor.

production also contributes significantly to hyperglycemia in NIDDM.[1] In general, insulin activates the transport systems and enzymes involved in intracellular utilization and storage of glucose, amino acids, and fatty acids, while inhibiting gluconeogenesis and catabolic processes evoked by counterregulatory hormones, including the breakdown of glycogen, fat, and protein. However, insulin regulates many other enzymatic and cellular processes as well and is both directly anabolic and anticatabolic.

Insulin evokes immediate, intermediate, and long-term effects on cellular metabolism. The immediate effects occur within seconds or minutes after insulin stimulation and ordinarily involve activation of existing glucose and ion transport systems, recruitment of intracellular transporters to the plasma membrane, and the covalent modification of preexisting enzymes. Insulin stimulates rapid phosphorylation of enzymes thought to mediate insulin signals such as raf-1 kinase, mitogen-activated protein (MAP) kinase, the S6 kinase, and protein phosphatase-1.[9] As a result of these and other changes, certain enzymes controlling the rate-limiting metabolic steps are either activated (pyruvate dehydrogenase, acetyl CoA carboxylase, and glycogen synthase) or inactivated (triacylglycerol lipase, phosphorylase kinase, and glycogen phosphorylase).

The intermediate and long-term effects of insulin usually involve the stimulation or inhibition of specific gene transcription. Various metabolic enzymes are induced during insulin stimulation, including pyruvate kinase, malic enzyme, and glucokinase, whereas others such as phosphoenolpyruvate carboxy kinase (PEPCK), carbamoyl phosphate synthetase-I (CPS-I), and fructose-

1,6-bisphosphatase are inhibited.[10,11] The long-term effects of insulin, which require many hours to several days, include insulin stimulation of DNA synthesis, cell proliferation, and cell differentiation. These effects are likely to be the aggregate result of coordinate changes in the expression of many cellular genes, including the induction of transcription factors such as *srf* (serum response factor), c-*fos*, *egr*-1 (early growth response gene), c-*jun*, and c-*myc*.[11] The rapid, intermediate, and long-term actions of insulin may not share a single common pathway but may be the result of diverging and converging pathways mediated by the insulin and type I insulin-like growth factor (IGF) receptor and insulin/IGF-I hybrid receptors.

THE INSULIN RECEPTOR

Structure

Like all peptide hormones, insulin initiates its action by binding to a cell-surface receptor. The insulin receptor was initially characterized with the use of radio-iodinated insulin.[12,13] These studies revealed that insulin binds to a specific protein or receptor on the surface of most cells, including both the classical target tissues of insulin (liver, muscle, and fat) and nonclassical targets such as circulating blood cells, brain, and gonadal cells. The number of receptors varies among tissues from as few as 40 per cell on circulating erythrocytes to 200,000 to 300,000 per cell on adipocytes and hepatocytes. Covalent labeling of the receptor by cross-linking with ^{125}I-insulin and biosynthetic labeling studies using antibodies to insulin receptor from the serum of patients with severe insulin resistance provided valuable information about the subunit composition of the receptor.[14-16]

The insulin receptor is a large transmembrane glycoprotein of approximately 300 to 400 kilodaltons (kd) as determined by sodium dodecylsulfate-polyacrylamide gel electrophoresis (SDS-PAGE).[17] The receptor is composed of two α-subunits (135 kd) and two β-subunits (95 kd) linked by disulfide bonds to form a β-α-α-β heterotetramer (Fig. 8–2).[3,18] Both subunits are derived from a single-chain precursor molecule or prorecepter that contains the entire sequence of the α- and β-subunits.[19,20] The subunits are obtained from the precursor by proteolytic processing at a site consisting of four basic amino acids (Fig. 8–3). Both subunits contain complex N-linked carbohydrate side chains capped by terminal sialic acid residues.[21] In addition the β-subunit may contain O-linked carbohydrate.[22] Two α-subunits, located entirely outside of the cell, are covalently linked to each other by disulfide bonds. The α-subunits contain the insulin binding site(s). In contrast, the β-subunit is a transmembrane protein that contains the insulin-regulated tyrosine protein kinase activity. One β-subunit is covalently linked to each α-subunit by disulfide bonds minimally requiring cysteine residue 657 in the α-subunit.[23]

The Insulin-Receptor Gene

The insulin-receptor gene is located on the short arm of chromosome 19 near the LDL (low-density lipoprotein)-receptor gene. The insulin-receptor gene itself is more than 150 kilobases (kb) in length and contains 22 exons (Fig. 8–3). Each exon is separated by long introns, so the gene is over 30 times larger (<120 kb pairs) than the 4.2-kb cDNA needed to encode the insulin-receptor molecule.[24] The cDNA encoding the human insulin prorecepter was isolated in 1985, permitting the prediction of the primary amino acid sequence.[25,26] The sequence confirmed all of the previous structural predictions. In addition, analysis of the cDNAs identified alternative splicing of exon 11, to yield two distinct mRNA species that encode α-subunits with different COOH-terminal tails.[27] This variation may account for

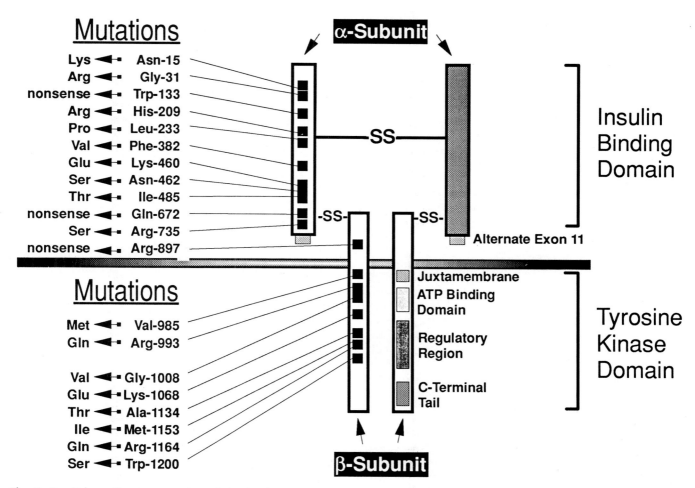

Fig. 8–2. Schematic representation of the insulin-receptor tetramer. Two identical α-subunits are linked together by disulfide bonds, and each α-subunit is covalently linked by another set of disulfide bonds to β-subunits. The β-subunits are transmembrane proteins, whereas the α-subunits are located entirely outside of the cell. Some functional domains identified in the kinase domain are indicated. Point mutations found in patients with severe insulin resistance are indicated.

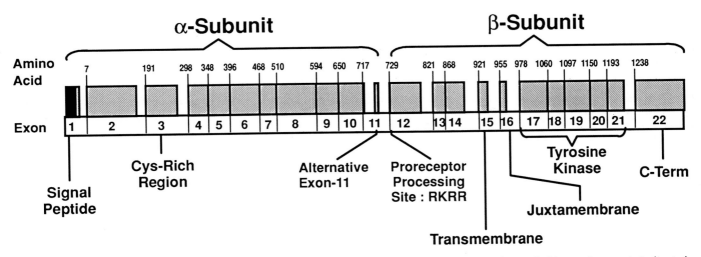

Fig. 8–3. The exon structure of the insulin-receptor gene and precursor. The first amino acid encoded by each exon is indicated. The approximate location of important structural features is also displayed.

some microheterogeneity in insulin binding and suggests that tissue-specific insulin analogues may be found.

The insulin-receptor gene is regulated by the hormonal or metabolic status of the cell and during cell differentiation.[28] Insulin reduces the content of insulin-receptor mRNA in IM-9 lymphocytes, which many contribute partially to the down-regulation of the receptor during prolonged insulin stimulation.[28] In contrast, dexamethasone increases receptor mRNA levels 5- to 10-fold without altering the half-life of the mRNA.[28] During insulin stimulation in the presence of dexamethasone and isobutylmethyxanthine, mouse 3T3-L1 fibroblasts differentiate into adipocytes in a process that results in a large increase in insulin receptors.[29] Differentiation of myoblasts to myocytes also is accompanied by a significant increase of insulin-receptor mRNA.[28] Furthermore, the insulin receptor gene in *Drosophila* is most strongly expressed between 8 and 12 hours of embryogenesis, suggesting that it is developmentally regulated.[30] In some patients, reduced transcription of the insulin-receptor gene may be responsible for insulin resistance.[31,32]

The promoter region of the insulin-receptor gene does not contains a TATA or CAAT box and contains many features of a so-called housekeeping gene. However, it does contain three potential transcription-initiation sites and two clusters of Sp1 regulatory elements (GGGCGGG or CGGCCC) upstream of the translation-initiation site.[24,33] Only one of the potential transcription-start sites (TTTGTAGC, -201 relative to the ATG start site) is utilized in IM-9 lymphocytes.[33] The 5'-untranslated region between -629 and -1 is sufficient for maximal promoter activity in transfected COS or CHO cells, and the cluster of four Sp1 sites between -637 and -594 and two GGGAGG hexamers enhance transcription and probably bind Sp1.[34,35] Two regions, -550 to -530 and -522 to -503, appear to bind two novel nuclear factors (IRNF-I and IRNF-II), which can be identified in nuclear extracts from HepG2 cells and are important for efficient promoter function.[35] Finally, a putative glucocorticoid response element has been identified in the insulin-receptor gene between -345 to -359. This site is not completely homologous to the consensus GRE (glucocorticoid response element), but contains the four guanine residues essential for binding.[28]

Mutation in the Insulin-Receptor Gene

Insulin resistance plays an important role in the pathogenesis of NIDDM. However, mutations in the insulin-receptor gene do not appear to occur in most patients with NIDDM. About 30 patients with syndromes of severe insulin resistance (leprechaunism and type A syndrome) have been reported to have point mutations in at least one insulin-receptor allele.[36] A summary of some of these mutations is given in Figure 8–2. Each mutation is located in the structural gene and results, in one way or another, in a reduction in the ability to mediate the insulin signal. Depending on the location of the mutation, the insulin resistance arises from impaired proreceptor processing, decreased transport of mature receptor to the cell surface, decreased insulin-binding affinity, decreased ATP-binding affinity, or inhibited autophosphorylation and tyrosine kinase activity.[31,36] The presence of naturally occurring mutations that inhibit the tyrosine kinase provides strong evidence that the kinase is essential for normal signal transmission in humans.[37] Although many of these insulin-resistant patients have one normal receptor allele, the insulin resistance is generally more severe than expected for a 50% reduction in functional receptors. This disparity appears to arise from the formation of chimeric receptors composed of a mutant αβ-dimer and a functional αβ-dimer. In certain cases, this completely blocks signal transmission by the functional αβ-dimer. This inhibition of normal receptor function by the abnormal protein has been termed a *trans-dominant-negative phenotype.*[38,39]

The Extracellular Ligand-Binding Domain of the Insulin Receptor

Insulin action begins when insulin binds with high affinity to the α-subunit of the insulin receptor. Insulin binding is a popular target for therapeutic intervention, as it is easily accessible to insulin analogues.[40,41] Since the holoreceptor contains two α-subunits, the receptor is thought to contain two binding sites. However, these sites strongly interact, causing significant negative cooperativity that reduces the affinity of the receptor for the second insulin molecule.[42,43] The apparent stoichiometry of insulin binding lies between one and two insulin molecules per receptor.[42]

A definitive model describing the insulin-binding site has been difficult to deduce from biochemical and genetic analysis. Many amino acid residues throughout the α-subunit have been implicated in insulin binding, but it is not known which ones are directly involved in contacts to the insulin molecule or are important for structural integrity of the receptor. A three-dimensional structure of the receptor:insulin complex will ultimately be required to identify the exact configuration of the insulin-binding domain.

High-affinity insulin binding requires amino acid residues in the NH_2-terminus, cysteine-rich region and in the COOH-terminus of the α-subunit. Photoaffinity insulin analogues have been used to identify regions of the α-subunit that interact directly with the ligand. Modified insulin molecules containing reactive groups have been used to cross-link insulin to the α-subunit. One of these cross-linking reagents, ^{125}I-AZAP[B29]-insulin, labels a fragment of the insulin receptor containing the amino acid sequence 205–316.[44] This domain is derived from exon 3. When a different photolabel is used, Gly^{390} in the region encoded by exon 5 is labeled, suggesting that it is a contact site for insulin.[45] The COOH-terminus of the α-subunit also appears to be involved in insulin binding, as the presence of 12 additional amino acids encoded by exon 11 increases insulin-binding affinity twofold.[46,47] Certain point mutations discovered in the insulin-receptor gene of patients with severe insulin resistance also identify residues important for insulin binding: substitution of Lys^{460} (exon 6) with Glu increases binding affinity

about fivefold and causes accelerated degradation and a decreased steady-state receptor level at the cell surface.[31] Furthermore, monoclonal antibodies that inhibit insulin binding interact with residues 450 to 601 (exons 6 to 9), suggesting that this region is also near the insulin-binding domain.[48]

The IGF-I receptor and the insulin receptor are closely related molecules.[38] Chimeric receptors prepared with the corresponding portions of insulin and IGF-I receptors provide surprising information regarding the location of the ligand-binding domain in these related receptors. A chimeric α-subunit produced by replacing exons 1–3 of the insulin receptor with the corresponding sequences from the cDNA of the IGF-I receptor, reduces high-affinity insulin binding[49] and increases high-affinity IGF-I binding in the chimera, suggesting that the first 298 amino acids of the receptor are important in ligand binding.[50] In contrast, the chimeric receptor obtained by replacing only exon 3 of the insulin receptor with the corresponding portion of the IGF-I receptor retains high-affinity insulin binding and acquires high-affinity IGF-I binding.[50] Moreover, deletion of amino acid residues 1–66 has no inhibitory effect on insulin binding. Therefore, the COOH-terminal portion of exon-2 appears to encode the critical elements for specific insulin binding, whereas exon 3 does not contain elements required for the specific binding site. Within the region encoded by exon 2, residues 83–103 (especially Phe^{89}) appear essential for high-affinity insulin binding.[51] In contrast, the IGF-I-specific binding domain is encoded by a region of IGF-I-receptor cDNA that corresponds to exon 3 of the insulin receptor.[51]

The Tyrosine Kinase of the Insulin Receptor

The tyrosine kinase activity of the insulin receptor was recognized by biochemical studies in 1981.[52] As a tyrosine kinase, the insulin receptor belongs to a family including the tyrosine kinase receptors for platelet-derived growth factor (PDGF), colony-stimulating factor-1 (CSF-1), fibroblast growth factor (FGF), nerve growth factor receptor (NGF), and hepatocyte growth factor, as well as *src*-like oncogene products (Fig. 8–4).[53] Other tyrosine kinase receptors have been identified by molecular cloning, as a high degree of DNA sequence identity exists between the catalytic regions of these homologous molecules.[54] Thus, the insulin receptor is one member of a growing class of protein tyrosine kinases with similar structural features, including an extracellular ligand-binding domain, a single transmembrane-spanning region, and a cytoplasmic kinase domain that transmits regulatory signals to cellular enzymes and organelles (Fig. 8–4).

Protein tyrosine kinases, including the insulin receptor, contain conserved well-defined amino acid sequence motifs, including an ATP-binding site (Gly-X-Gly-X-X-Gly), tyrosine autophosphorylation sites, and COOH-terminal autophosphorylation sites.[53] General structural features are also useful for characterizing receptor tyrosine kinases.[55] Members of the epidermal growth factor (EGF) receptor family are monomeric, with two

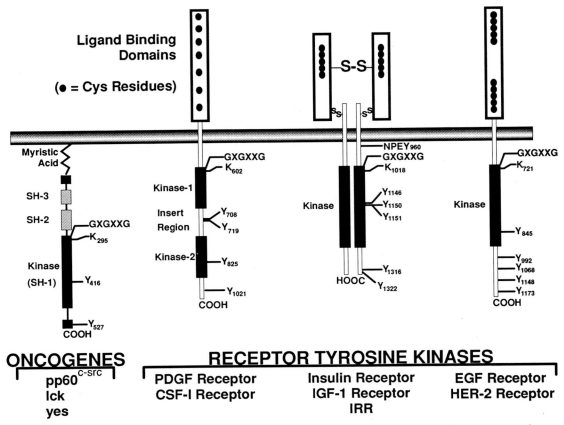

Figure 8–4. A schematic representation of the structure of pp60^{c-src} and the PDGF, insulin, and EGF classes of receptor tyrosine kinases. The approximate location of the extracellular cysteine-rich regions are indicated with closed circles. The conserved kinase domains are displayed as closed rectangles. The position of autophosphorylation sites and the GXGXXG motif and downstream lysine residue of the ATP-binding domain are indicated. (See text for abbreviations.)

clusters of cysteine-rich regions in the extracellular domain and the major autophosphorylation sites in the COOH-terminus.[56] The PDGF receptor family is distinct, as it possesses an immunoglobin-like distribution of cysteine residues in the external domain and a stretch of 100 amino acids that interrupts the kinase domain (Fig. 8–4). This kinase insert domain contains at least two major autophosphorylation sites that are important for signal transmission but not for kinase activity.[57] The insulin receptor represents another family of tyrosine kinase receptor, as it is a tetramer with a single cluster of cysteine residues in the α-subunit (Fig. 8–4). The kinase domain resembles that of the prototype tyrosine kinase, pp60^{c-src}; however, it contains a cluster of three autophosphorylation sites at positions 1146, 1150, and 1151 that activate the kinase after autophosphorylation.[58,59]

The insulin-receptor family has three closely related members: the insulin receptor, the IGF-I receptor, and the insulin receptor-related (IRR) receptor, an orphan receptor for which a ligand has not yet been identified.[60] These receptors share more than 80% amino acid sequence identity in the kinase domain, including all regions thought to be important for signaling: the

intracellular juxtamembrane region, the ATP-binding site, and the major autophosphorylation sites in the regulatory region. However, there is low amino acid sequence homology in the extracellular domain of these receptors, reflecting the fact that they interact with distinct regulatory ligands.

Activation of the Insulin Receptor by Autophosphorylation

The tyrosine kinase of the insulin receptor is initially stimulated by insulin binding and then greatly augmented by insulin-stimulated autophosphorylation.[58,59,61,62] The insulin-binding domain is connected to the catalytic domain by a short α-helical transmembrane segment. Although some mutations in the transmembrane region have no effect on function,[63] other mutations in this region activate the kinase.[64] The unoccupied external domain of the insulin receptor apparently inhibits the kinase, since the kinase is released from this inhibition during insulin binding or after removal of the α-subunits by proteolytic cleavage.[65]

The insulin receptor, like all protein kinases, contains a consensus amino acid sequence encoding an ATP-binding domain including a distinctive glycine-rich motif (Gly-X-Gly-X-X-Gly) followed by a lysine residue (Fig. 8–4) that is covalently cross-linked with ATP-affinity reagents.[53,66] The lysyl residue is absolutely required for insulin action. Substitution with any other amino acid invariably blocks autophosphorylation and kinase activity and biologic responses.[54,67] Although it has been suggested that the kinase-deficient insulin receptor still mediates insulin stimulation of pyruvate dehydrogenase,[68] this has not been confirmed by others.

Three major insulin-stimulated autophosphorylation sites are found about 140 amino acids beyond the ATP-binding site[69] (Fig. 8–4), including Tyr^{1146}, Tyr^{1150}, and Tyr^{1151} (numbered according to the sequence that omits the insert of 12 amino acids at the end of the α-subunit[25]). In the insulin receptor, autophosphorylation of these residues appears to occur through a *trans*-mechanism, in which insulin binding to the α-subunit of one αβ-dimer stimulates the phosphorylation of the adjacent covalently linked β-subunit. A similar mechanism may be employed by the monomeric EGF and PDGF receptors following ligand-induced receptor aggregation.[70–72] Autophosphorylation of these three tyrosine residues inactivates the insulin receptor kinase, which stimulates the phosphorylation of other substrates.[58,62,73] Mutation of a single tyrosine residue in this cluster reduces insulin-stimulated kinase activity more than 50%.[74,75] Autophosphorylation of the homologous residues in the IGF-I receptor, IRR receptor, and the HGF (hepatocyte growth factor) receptor (c-Met) also activates these kinases.[76,77] Thus, a hallmark of the insulin-receptor family of kinases is that autophosphorylation plays a direct stimulatory role on catalytic activity. This feature is not generally observed for other tyrosine kinases.

Autophosphorylation Sites as Binding Domains for Downstream Mediators

In the PDGF and EGF receptors, autophosphorylation creates reversible binding sites for cellular enzymes involved in signal transmission.[78] As noted above, the catalytic region of the PDGF receptor contains an amino acid sequence insert of about 100 residues in the middle of the catalytic region that contains one or more autophosphorylation sites (Fig. 8–4).[55] After phosphorylation, this region provides binding sites for proteins containing a special recognition domain termed the *SH2* (*src* homology-2) domain.[79,80] SH2 domains are structural elements in a variety of proteins involved in cellular signaling that bind with high affinity to phosphotyrosine residues in activated tyrosine kinases.[78] In the PDGF receptor, the autophosphorylation sites bind with high affinity to the SH2 domains of several enzymes, including the phosphatidylinositol (PI) 3′-kinase, the phospholipase C, and the p21^{ras}-activating protein GAP.[81,82] Similar results are observed for the phosphorylation sites in the EGF receptor.[83] The association of signaling molecules with the insulin receptor has not been easily established. However, the PI 3′-kinase associates with the phosphorylated insulin-receptor substrate IRS-1 (see below).

Autophosphorylation of the Intracellular Juxtamembrane Region

In addition to the ATP-binding site and the autophosphorylation sites, the juxtamembrane region of the receptor just inside the membrane is fundamentally important (Fig. 8–5). This region is encoded by exon 16 (Fig. 8–3) of the insulin-receptor gene[24] and probably contains one or two tyrosine autophosphorylation sites, Tyr^{953} and Tyr^{960}.[84–86] Substitution of Tyr^{960} with Phe^{960} or Ala^{960} impairs receptor signal transmission even though activation of kinase occurs normally in vitro.[87–90] This impairment appears to be due to an inability of these receptors to mediate the phosphorylation of endogenous receptor substrates including IRS-1.[90] It is interesting that IRS-1 is also a substrate of the IGF-I receptor.[91,92] The amino acid sequences of the cytoplasmic region of the insulin receptor and the IGF-I receptor are 75% identical in the juxtamembrane region.[93]

Hybrid Insulin-Receptor Molecules

IGF-I and insulin share certain biologic effects, which may be explained in part by cross-reactivity at the level of ligand binding.[94,95] The function of the insulin and the IGF-I receptor in intact cells is further complicated by the fact that these two molecules can form hybrid receptors consisting of one α- and one β-subunit from each receptor.[96,97] In some cells in culture, the hybrid receptor behaves like an IGF-I receptor, as IGF-I, but not insulin, stimulates the autophosphorylation of one insulin receptor β-subunit and one IGF-I receptor β-subunit.[96] The activation of two distinct β-subunits by a single ligand could explain the overlap in the biologic responses triggered by IGF-I and insulin receptors.[96] The consequences of receptor hybrid formation also explains the dominant negative behavior of certain insulin-receptor mutations.

Regulation of the Insulin Receptor by Heterologous Serine/Threonine Phosphorylation

The insulin receptor is under an additional level of regulation other than insulin binding and tyrosine autophosphorylation via phosphorylation on serine and threonine residues.[52] Agents that stimulate serine or threonine kinases, including phorbol esters, cAMP, and insulin itself, increase the Ser/Thr phosphorylation of the β-subunit.[98,99] In hepatoma cells, phorbol ester–stimulated serine phosphorylation inhibits insulin-stimulated autophosphorylation and kinase activity.[100] This inhibition can be reversed by mild trypsinization, which removes the COOH-terminal portion of the receptor, including at least one serine or threonine phosphorylation site.[101] Thr^{1336}, located near the COOH-terminus of the β-subunit, is phosphorylated during phorbol ester stimulation and may be responsible for inhibition of receptor kinase.[102,103] There is also evidence for a tightly associated

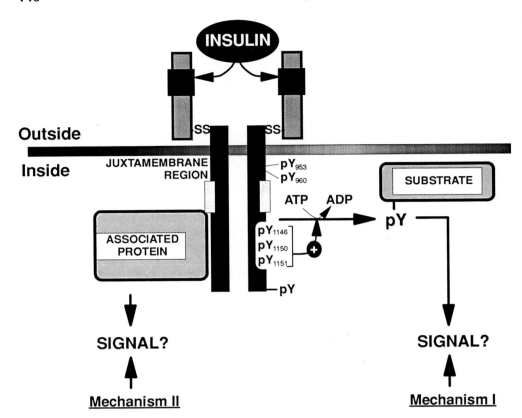

Fig. 8–5. A model of insulin-signal transmission. Mechanism I involves substrate phosphorylation catalyzed by the insulin receptor activated by ligand binding and autophosphorylation. Mechanism II suggests that insulin-stimulated autophosphorylation causes a conformational change that causes the association of cellular signaling molecules, perhaps, but not necessarily, through SH2 domains.

serine kinase that might specifically phosphorylate the insulin receptor.[104]

SIGNAL-TRANSDUCTION MECHANISMS

Although many details of the function of the insulin receptor are understood, the molecular elements that link the receptor to the various downstream components of the action pathway are unknown. Although initial attention focused on classic second-messenger systems that involved cAMP, cGMP, and related small molecules or ion fluxes as mediators of insulin-signal transmission,[105] a complete reorientation of thinking occurred following the discovery of the tyrosine kinase activity of the insulin receptor.[52] Two mechanisms have emerged as the foundation for early steps in the transmission of the insulin-receptor signal. Mechanism I involves tyrosine phosphorylation of cellular proteins by the activated insulin-receptor kinase (Fig. 8–5). Mechanism II is based on the idea that autophosphorylation of the β-subunit mediates noncovalent, but stable, interactions between the receptor and other cellular proteins (Fig. 8–5). Both of these mechanisms require an intact ATP-binding site and receptor autophosphorylation, which is consistent with the majority of current data. Moreover, these mechanisms are not mutually exclusive, as conformational changes are undoubtedly necessary to facilitate interactions between the receptor and cellular substrates and specific association between the receptor and substrates may be essential for subsequent phosphorylation.

Substrates of the Insulin Receptor

Several approaches have been used to identify cellular substrates of the insulin receptor. These include in vitro phosphorylation of candidate proteins in cell-free systems, immunoprecipitation of candidate proteins with specific antibodies, two-dimensional SDS-PAGE separations of [^{32}P]phosphate-labeled cellular proteins, and immunoprecipitation of cellular proteins with antibodies to phosphotyrosine.[106] Although a number of proteins are phosphorylated by the purified insulin receptor in vitro,[107–111] in the intact cell, only a few proteins other than the insulin receptor itself have been shown to undergo insulin-stimulated tyrosine phosphorylation.

The Discovery of pp185[IRS-1]

Immunoprecipitation with antibodies to phosphotyrosine (αPY) provided the first evidence that the insulin receptor has cellular substrates.[106] With the use of this approach with hepatoma cells, a broad-band tyrosine phosphorylated protein with an average molecular mass of 185 kd (pp185) was identified by SDS-PAGE.[112–118] The pp185 is found in most, if not all, cell types studied so far, including hepatoma cells[106]; 3T3-L1 adipocytes[112]; rat-1 fibroblasts[113]; Chinese hamster ovary cells[114]; human epidermal carcinoma cells[115]; mouse neuroblastoma cells[119]; and isolated rat adipocytes,[117] hepatocytes, and skeletal muscle.[118] The pp185 is cytoplasmic[114] and is immediately phosphorylated after insulin stimulation, suggesting that it may play a role in the initial steps of post-receptor insulin signal transduction. The pp185 is also a substrate for the homologous IGF-I receptor,[91] but not for the EGF or the PDGF receptors.[115] Cells that express few insulin receptors (<3000/cell) barely phosphorylate pp185, whereas the expression of more insulin receptors in identical cell backgrounds strongly increases pp185 tyrosine phosphorylation during insulin stimulation.[114,120]

Recently, the major phosphoprotein that migrates in the pp185 band was purified from insulin-stimulated rat liver,[121] and the corresponding cDNA isolated from rat liver cDNA libraries encodes a phosphoprotein called pp185[IRS-1], or just IRS-1 (insulin-receptor substrate-1).[90] IRS-1 shows no overall amino acid sequence identity with currently known proteins. It has a calculated molecular mass of 131 kd but migrates anomalously during SDS-PAGE because of its high level of phosphorylation. IRS-1 is rapidly tyrosine phosphorylated during insulin treatment[90,122] and is a substrate for the IGF-I receptor as well, but not for the PDGF receptor.[123] Thus, IRS-1 may act in the signaling pathways for different tyrosine kinases in the insulin-receptor family.

IRS-1 is highly conserved among rats, mice, and humans. The IRS-1 amino acid sequence of rat is 97% identical to the mouse sequence and 90% identical to the human sequence (Fig. 8–6). IRS-1 contains a potential ATP/GTP binding site and over 30 potential Ser/Thr phosphorylation sites that may serve as targets for casein kinase II; protein kinase C; the MAP kinases; cdc 2; and cAMP- and cGMP-dependent protein kinase. Before insulin stimulation of cells, IRS-1 is phosphorylated on several serine residues and a few threonine residues. Following insulin stimulation there is an increase in serine phosphorylation and the appearance of phosphotyrosine in IRS-1.[122]

There are 14 potential tyrosine phosphorylation sites on IRS-1[90]: six in Tyr-Met-X-Met (YMXM) motifs; three others in YXXM motifs; and single motifs containing YVNI, YIDL, and EYYE (Fig. 8–6). These tyrosine

phosphorylation sites are identical in rat, mouse, and human IRS-1, suggesting some conserved function.[90,124] Synthetic peptides based upon the amino acid sequences of these YMXM and YXXM motifs are excellent substrates of the purified insulin receptor, with K_m values between 20 and 100 mM.[125]

A Mechanism of Insulin-Signal Transmission through IRS-1

The presence of YMXM and YXXM motifs in IRS-1 provides an important key to the understanding of one of the roles of IRS-1 and perhaps defines a new and general mechanism for insulin-signal transmission. On the basis of work with the receptors for PDGF, FGF, CSF-I, and EGF, it appears that autophosphorylation of these motifs by an activated receptor kinase allows binding of other proteins that contain SH2 domains.[82] Phosphorylated IRS-1 binds strongly to the enzyme PI 3'-kinase,[90] which is thought to be an important mediator of cellular growth and metabolism.[82] This enzyme also binds to other phosphotyrosine-containing proteins, including the PDGF receptor and the CSF-I receptor.[82] Although a definitive mechanism whereby the PI 3'-kinase mediates cellular signaling remains to be elucidated, its enzymatic activity is well established.[82] The PI 3'-kinase phosphorylates the lipid PI on the 3' position of the myoinositol ring, yielding PI-3-phosphate.[126] The enzyme can use other phosphorylated forms of PI in vivo, leading to the formation of $PI(3,4)P_2$ and $PI(3,4,5)P_3$.[127,128] In contrast to the "classical" PI pathway, in which $PI(4,5)P_2$ is cleaved by a phospholipase C to diacylglycerol and inositol(1,4,5)-trisphosphate,[129] the lipid products of the PI 3'-kinase are not hydrolyzed by any known phospholipase.[130] Thus, how the PI 3'-kinase products generate a signal is not known.[82]

PI 3'-kinase activity increases severalfold following insulin stimulation in vivo.[131] This stimulation is reconstituted in vitro by adding tyrosine-phosphorylated IRS-1 to PI 3'-kinase from quiescent cells.[131] This activation can

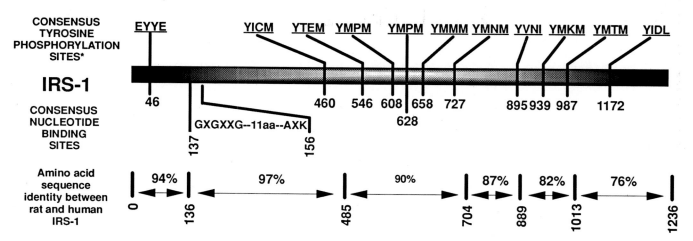

Fig. 8–6. Structural features of IRS-1 (insulin-receptor substrate-1). Predicted tyrosine phosphorylation sites are indicated, along with the downstream tripeptide sequence. The putative protein kinase–like ATP-binding motif and the amino acid sequence identity between rat and human IRS-1 also are shown.

be attributed to the binding of the tyrosine-phosphorylated YMXM motifs of IRS-1 to the SH2 domains in the p85 subunit of the PI 3′-kinase, as synthetic phosphopeptides containing YMXM motifs also activate the enzyme.[131,132] This establishes a new mechanism of allosteric enzyme regulation that may be generalized to other SH2 domain-containing enzymes (Fig. 8–7). Thus, IRS-1 may function as a central molecule in insulin signal transmission that binds to certain SH2 domain-containing proteins during insulin stimulation and regulates the associated catalytic activities that mediate the insulin response (Fig. 8–7). One important future challenge is to identify other cellular elements that may interact with IRS-1 and other molecules that function like IRS-1.

Other Mediators of Insulin Action

Other Insulin-Receptor Substrates

In addition to IRS-1, other proteins have been identified as substrates for the insulin receptor. A 120-kd protein (pp120) was identified by mixing purified insulin receptor with a crude glycoprotein extract from rat liver.[133] The pp120 was subsequently shown to be phosphorylated during insulin stimulation of [^{32}P]phosphate-labeled H35 hepatoma cells.[134] It was identified immunologically as HA4, a 110-kd membrane glycoprotein localized primarily to the bile canalicular region of the plasma membrane.[135] The cDNA clone suggests that HA4 is an ecto-ATPase,[136,137] but the role of this protein in insulin-signal transmission is unknown.

Incubation of cells with general phosphatase inhibitors such as phenylarsine oxide or vanadate increases the detection of Tyr(P)-containing proteins in insulin-stimulated cells, even though the inhibitor increases the risk of detecting nonphysiologic substrates.[138] After treatment with phenylarsine oxide, insulin stimulated the tyrosyl phosphorylation of a 15-kd protein in 3T3-L1 adipocytes.[139] The protein was subsequently identified by sequence analysis as 422(aP2), an abundant protein in 3T3-L1 cells that appears to function as a fatty acid–binding protein in adipocytes.[140] The phosphorylation stoichiometry of 422(aP2) is low[140] but is enhanced by fatty acid binding.[141] It is interesting that phenylarsine oxide also inhibits signal transmission between the insulin receptor and the glucose-transport system,[142] so the flux of phosphate through aP2 may play an important role in the regulation of glucose transport.[141] There is no direct evidence that aP2 plays a role in insulin action.

Generation of the Phosphatidylinositol-Glycan

The search for mediators of insulin-signal transmission has revealed the possible involvement of PI-gly-

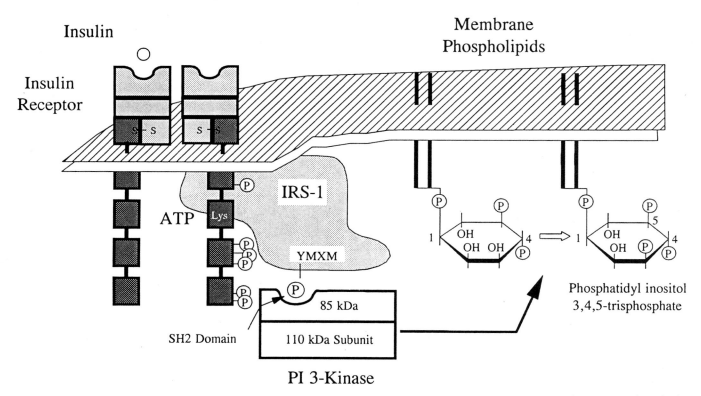

Fig. 8–7. Schematic representation of the activation of the phosphatidylinositol (PI) 3′-kinase by the insulin receptor functioning through the phosphorylation of IRS-1 (insulin-receptor substrate-1). Immediately after insulin stimulation and receptor autophosphorylation, IRS-1 is phosphorylated on multiple tyrosine residues. Phosphorylated YMXM motifs are then thought to bind specifically to the SH2 domains of the 85-kd subunit of the PI 3′-kinase. The association between these molecules activates the kinase in the 110-kd subunit, which increases the cellular levels of phosphatidylinositol-3,4,5-trisphosphate.

cans.[143-146] In this scheme of insulin action, hormonal stimulation causes activation of a phospholipase C specific for PI-glycan through an unknown mechanism.[147] This phospholipase is thought to hydrolyze a membrane-associated substrate to produce the PI-glycan and 1,2-diacylglycerol, both of which could regulate intracellular enzymes. It is further suggested that the insulin mediator is released into the extracellular medium and then taken back up into cells to exert its effect.[148] As the kinase activity of the insulin receptor is required to activate the putative phospholipase C, this pathway may branch off of other pathways proposed for insulin signaling.

Role of p21^{ras} in Insulin-Signal Transmission

The *ras* genes are members of a ubiquitous eukaryotic gene family identified in mammals, birds, insects, plants, and yeast. In mammals, there are at least three distinct *ras* genes, H-*ras*-1, K-*ras*-2, and N-*ras*-2, which encode highly related proteins generally called p21^{ras}. A variety of genes have been identified that display 30 to 55% homology to *ras*, indicating a superfamily of related proteins.[149] The p21^{ras} has been shown to play a role in cell growth and to be the causative agent in certain human tumors. The p21^{ras} binds guanine nucleotides (GTP and GDP) and possesses intrinsic GTPase activity.[149] The biochemical properties of p21^{ras} closely resemble those of G-proteins involved in the modulation of signal transduction through transmembrane signaling systems. The p21^{ras} serves as a biologic switch, which is "on" when GTP is bound and "off" when the GTP is hydrolyzed to GDP. Several observations suggest that the GTP form of p21^{ras} is a positive signal for cell proliferation and differentiation.[150]

The GTPase activity of p21^{ras} is ordinarily regulated by two accessory proteins called *guanine nucleotide-releasing protein* (GNRP) and *GTPase-activating protein* (GAP).[151] GNRP catalyzes the dissociation of GDP from p21^{ras}, whereas GAP catalyzes hydrolysis of GTP to control the GTP/GDP ratio. The potential relevance of this to insulin action is that GAP contains two SH2 domains, suggesting that it is regulated by growth-factor receptors.[78] GAP binds to the activated PDGF and EGF receptors, but it does not appear to associate with IRS-1. During growth-factor stimulation, GAP also associates with two other phosphoproteins, p190 and p62.[152] The p190 is thought to transduce signals from p21^{ras} to the nucleus, perhaps affecting expression of specific cellular genes.[153] The p62 is phosphorylated during insulin stimulation[154] and may regulate GAP by associating with it through its SH2 domains.[155] Recently, another molecule, called *GRB-2/sem-5*, was implicated as an element in the signal pathway between the EGF receptor and p21^{ras}.[156] GRB-2 contains one SH2 domain and two SH3 (*src* homology-3) domains (Fig. 8–8), which mediates its association with the activated EGF and PDGF receptor and other downstream elements, respectively.[156] After injection into rat embryo fibroblasts, GRB-2 and p21^{ras} cooperate to mediate DNA synthesis.[156] GRB-2 may be the molecular link between certain tyrosine kinase receptors and p21^{ras}.

Several recent observations suggest that p21^{ras} may be an integral component of certain insulin signaling pathways. Overexpression in rat-1 fibroblasts of wild-type H-*ras* or the insulin receptor increases the ability of insulin to induce the expression of c-*jun* and p33, suggesting that p21^{ras} lies downstream of the insulin receptor.[157] A dominant negative p21^{ras} (H-*ras*$_{N17}$;

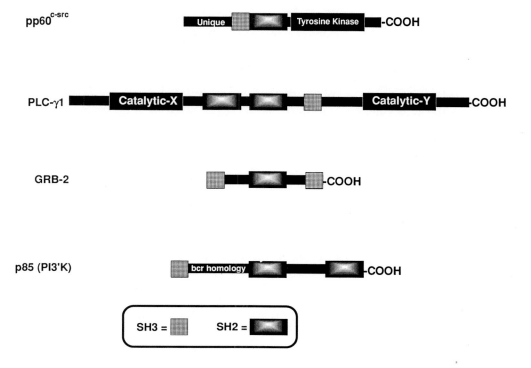

Fig. 8–8. Schematic diagrams of several SH2 domain-containing proteins that may be involved in insulin-signal transmission.

$\text{H-ras}_{L61/S186}$) inhibits the insulin stimulation of gene expression in NIH-3T3 cells and the differentiation of 3T3-L1 fibroblasts to adipocytes.[154,158] Moreover, insulin-stimulated maturation of *Xenopus* oocytes is specifically inhibited by microinjection of antibodies directed against a highly conserved region of p21[ras] required for p21[ras] function.[159] Thus, p21[ras] may function as an intermediate in the insulin-signaling pathway leading to the expression of certain genes.

Insulin-Signal Transmission through Protein Kinase Cascades

Many insulin actions appear to be propagated through an extended network of protein phosphorylation and dephosphorylation on serine residues of proteins.[160] Dephosphorylation is involved in the stimulation of glycogen synthase, pyruvate kinase, and pyruvate dehydrogenase and in the inhibition of triacylglycerol lipase, phosphorylase, and phosphorylase kinase.[160] Phosphorylation of ribosomal protein S6 has been implicated in the stimulation of protein synthesis. Recent evidence suggests that both the phosphorylation and dephosphorylation processes may branch off of a common pathway regulated by an insulin-stimulated protein serine/threonine kinase originally called the *MAP-2 kinase*.[161]

MAP kinases have been implicated in a broad spectrum of biologic responses, including certain insulin-signaling pathways (Fig. 8–9). Originally named *MAP-2 kinase* because it phosphorylates microtubule-associated protein-2 in vitro,[161] the enzyme is now known as *mitogen-activated protein kinase* or as *extracellular signal-regulated kinase* (ERK) because it is activated by a variety of tyrosine kinase receptors, G-protein-coupled receptors, or the protein kinase C.[9,162–164] Two forms of MAP kinase, p42[mapk] (ERK-2) and p44[mapk] (ERK-1), have been purified from fibroblasts and cloned.[165]

MAP kinases were originally thought to be direct substrates for receptor tyrosine kinases,[166] but it is now appreciated that they are intermediate elements in a complicated signal-transduction cascade.[167] Activation of both forms of MAP kinase requires phosphorylation at Thr[183] and Tyr[185].[168] Although MAP kinase undergoes autophosphorylation, this reaction is too slow to account for the rapid phosphorylation during mitogen (insulin) stimulation. Several recent reports suggest that another upstream kinase (~50 kd), provisionally called the *MAP kinase-kinase*, is responsible for activation of MAP kinase.[169,170] This enzyme has dual specificity, as it appears to catalyze the phosphorylation of the threonine and tyrosine residues (Fig. 8–9).

In cells, MAP kinase appears to be an activator of another serine kinase, the 90-kd isoform of the ribosomal protein S6 kinase (p90[rsk]),[162] and also phosphorylates the transcription factors c-*jun*[171] and p62[TCF].[172] This places MAP kinase at a branch point in insulin and mitogen signaling (Fig. 8–9). In skeletal muscle, insulin-stimulated p90[rsk] has been reported to phosphorylate the G-subunit of protein phosphatase-1, which in turn increases the rate of dephosphorylation of glycogen synthase and phosphorylase kinase.[173] Thus, MAP kinase may be a direct intermediate in the regulation of glycogen synthesis by insulin by causing the stimulation of glycogen synthase and the inhibition of glycogen phosphorylase (Fig. 8–9).

The molecular link between the insulin receptor and MAP kinase is an important focus of current studies. Recent evidence suggests that yet another serine kinase, termed *c-raf-1 kinase*, may activate the MAP kinase-kinase through phosphorylation.[174] Although the mechanism of activation of c-*raf*-1 is currently unknown, some reports indicate that it is activated in cells during insulin stimulation.[175,176] The c-*raf*-1 may also have a role downstream of MAP kinase, thus producing a feedback loop at this point in the signaling cascade.[177]

THE INSULIN-SENSITIVE GLUCOSE-TRANSPORT SYSTEM

The Physiology of Glucose-Transport Regulation

Glucose is the major circulating hexose and the major carbohydrate used by the cell for energy. Defining these processes of glucose transport at the cellular and molecular level has progressed remarkably through the application of contemporary techniques of cell and molecular biology. Maintenance of normal glucose homeostasis in the intact animal or human depends on the ability of the body both to absorb glucose from the intestine and to distribute the sugar to all of the cells of the body that use it as a substrate for energy storage and metabolism. These two processes are controlled by two main classes of glucose transporters: the sodium-dependent glucose cotransporters present in the intestine and kidney tubule and the sodium-independent facilitative glucose transporters present in virtually all cells of the body. The Na^+/glucose cotransporters are active transporters that utilize the energy in the sodium gradient to concentrate glucose against its concentration gradient inside of cells. The facilitative transporters are passive and are able to transfer glucose on down a concentration gradient.

Na^+/Glucose Cotransport

Glucose is absorbed from the intestinal tract and reabsorbed from the proximal convoluted tubule in the kidney by Na^+-dependent glucose transporters. These transporters utilize the electrochemical potential created by sodium as their energy source. Following sodium and glucose uptake, the Na^+ inside the cell must be transported out actively by the Na^+/K^+-ATPase also present in the cell membrane, thus keeping the intracellular concentration of Na^+ 10-fold lower than the extracellular concentration. There are at least two transporter proteins involved in this process: a high-affinity ($K_m = 0.3$ mM), relatively low-capacity protein present in the kidney and intestine; and a low-affinity, high-capacity protein ($K_m = 2$ to 6 mM) present primarily in the kidney. These transporters are inhibited by the drug phloridzin. Neither of these transporters is known to be regulated by insulin or altered in diabetes. Phloridzin, however, has been used

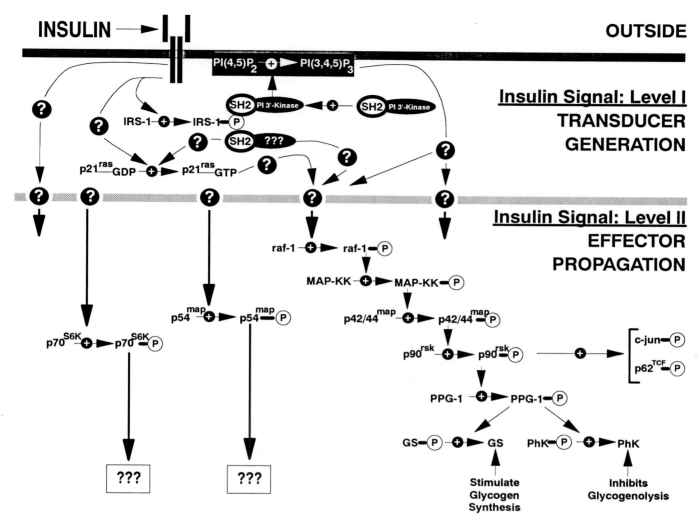

Fig. 8–9. A hypothetical phosphorylation cascade stimulated by insulin binding. The model is divided into two levels. Level I shows the generation of molecular signals that initiate the insulin signal inside of the cells. Level II describes a pathway of signal propagation that most likely emanates from one or more of the initial signals. The molecular link between the two levels is unknown. See the text for an explanation of the various elements.

as a tool in experimental animal models of diabetes to lower blood glucose level (by creating an increased renal leak), making it possible to separate the effects of hyperglycemia from the other metabolic defects in diabetes.[178] Defects in these transporters are present in the heritable disorders of renal and intestinal glucose transport such as renal glycosuria and familial glucose-galactose malabsorption.[179,180]

Facilitative Glucose Transport

The primary pathway for glucose entry into the cell is via the facilitative glucose transporters. These transporters simply facilitate the movement of glucose down a concentration gradient and therefore do not require energy. Facilitative glucose transporters play a role not only in the action of insulin on glucose metabolism but also in the entry of glucose into the β-cell and into tissues

that take up glucose in an insulin-independent fashion, such as brain, erythrocytes, and kidney medulla.

The effect of insulin on glucose influx at the cellular level can be assessed independently of the effect of the hormone on glucose metabolism by using non-metabolizable glucose derivatives, such as 2-deoxy- or 3-O-methylglucose.[181] Insulin increases the rate of 3-O-methylglucose uptake 20- to 30-fold. The effect depends primarily on an increase in the maximal rate of transport with little or no effect on the K_m. The K_m of 3-O-methylglucose transport in adipocytes is in the low physiologic range (2 to 5 mM). Transport is stereospecific and occurs after a short lag period (20 to 45 seconds) following insulin stimulation. Activation and reversal of this process is independent of protein synthesis but requires endogenous ATP. The kinetic behavior is consistent with an insulin-dependent increase in number of active hexose transporters in the plasma

Table 8–1.   Human Glucose Transporters

	Protein (kd)	Amino acids	Chromosomal localization	Expression in tissues and cells	Function	Insulin stimulation
Facilitative						
GLUT-1	55	492	1p35→p31.3	Brain, erythrocyte, fibroblast	Basal glucose transport	+
GLUT-2	58	524	3q26.1→q26.3	Liver, β-cell	Low-affinity glucose transport	−
GLUT-3	54	496	12p13.3	Brain, fibroblast	Basal glucose transport	?
GLUT-4	55	509	17p13	Fat, skeletal muscle, heart	Insulin-stimulated glucose transport	+++
GLUT-5	50	501	1p32→p22	Small intestine	Intestinal absorption (?)	?
Concentrative Na$^+$-dependent						
SGLT-1	75	664	22q11→qter	Intestine, kidney	Intestinal absorption, renal reabsorption	−

membrane. Insulin does not stimulate glucose uptake in liver and several other tissues, despite the sensitivity of these tissues to effects of insulin. This is consistent with the fact that there are several types of glucose transporters differing in their molecular regulation (see below).

Although facilitative transport itself is not energy-dependent, insulin stimulation of glucose transport is a temperature- and energy-dependent process depending largely upon translocation of intracellular vesicles containing the glucose transporter to the plasma membrane.[182–187] This effect is reversible, and on removing insulin, the glucose transporters return to the intracellular pool. There remains considerable debate as to whether translocation accounts for the entire insulin stimulation of glucose uptake; insulin-stimulated translocation causes a 3- to 10-fold increase in membrane transporters, whereas insulin increases glucose influx 20- to 30-fold.[188] In addition, translocation has been difficult to demonstrate in muscle, despite the clear stimulatory effect of insulin on transport in this tissue.[189] These findings have suggested that there may be an activation of plasma membrane glucose transporters in addition to the translocation.[190]

Recent evidence suggests that activation may involve a reversible suppression of intrinsic activity of the transporters residing at the plasma-membrane surface that allows sugar-binding sites on the exofacial surface of the glucose-transporter proteins to be exposed.[190] The notion of regulated intrinsic activity also is supported by the observation that some adrenergic agents and activators of protein kinase C also stimulate glucose transport but have little or no effect on translocation.[185]

Glucose-Transporter Isoforms

Six or more distinct mammalian glucose transporters have been identified at a molecular level by cloning and sequencing (Table 8–1). Five of the glucose transporters are believed to be involved in the Na$^+$-independent facilitative transport of glucose and other hexoses into cells. Two are the Na$^+$/glucose cotransporters involved in absorption of glucose from the intestine and kidney tubule. These glucose transporters are encoded by separate genes and are located on several different chromosomes in the human genome.

The first facilitative transporter cloned (GLUT-1) has been called the *erythroid brain glucose transporter* and is present in large amounts in erythrocytes, in the endothelial cells that form the blood-brain barrier, and in some hepatoma cells in culture. It is not expressed in normal liver and is at low levels in fat and muscle.[187] Proof that this is indeed a glucose transporter came from studies in which the protein was overexpressed in cells and shown to be functional.[191,192] GLUT-1 is located in the cell membranes of most tissues that do not respond to insulin, has a K_m of 1 to 3 mM, and is almost saturated at physiologic concentrations of glucose.

The second (GLUT-2), termed the *liver-glucose transporter*, has a structure similar but not identical to GLUT-1 and is found mainly in liver plasma membranes and pancreatic β-cells. In the β-cells, GLUT-2 may participate in glucose-stimulated insulin secretion.[191,193] This transporter has a slightly higher K_m (5 to 7 mM) for transport, which may account for the difference in β-cell stimulation compared with uptake of glucose by peripheral tissue.

From the standpoint of insulin action, the most important glucose transporter is GLUT-4. This transporter is expressed predominantly in tissues in which glucose transport is sensitive to insulin, including striated muscle, cardiac muscle, and adipose tissue.[194,195] GLUT-4 has a K_m for transport similar to that of GLUT-1. Based on studies using antibodies to GLUT-4 and cell-fractionation techniques, it is clear that in insulin-responsive cells, such as adipocytes, most GLUT-4 is located in an intracellular pool in the basal state. Following insulin stimulation there is a rapid translocation of the GLUT-4 molecules to the plasma membrane of the cell in which they are active in glucose uptake.[190] This agrees well with the observations that glucose-transporter translocation is a major factor in insulin regulation of transport activity.

Two additional types of sugar transporters have been identified, one in fetal muscle, brain, and fibroblasts (GLUT-3) and the other in small intestine (GLUT-5). These are also expressed in many non-muscle adult tissues.[196] It is possible that these transporters, along with GLUT-1, contribute to basal glucose transport. Alternatively, they may be involved in the transport of hexoses other than glucose into the cell.

Glucose-Transporter Structure

All of the facilitative glucose transporters are integral membrane glycoproteins of 45 to 55 kd and have a large degree of sequence identity (50 to 65%) and structural homology. On the basis of sequence analysis, each is thought to contain 12 membrane-spanning α-helical domains (Fig. 8–10). There is an exoplasmic loop between helices 1 and 2 of variable length that bears a single NH_2-terminal-linked oligosaccharide. A long cytoplasmic hydrophilic segment connects helices 6 and 7. The greatest differences in sequence lie in these two loops and in the NH_2- and COOH-terminal intracellular domains. However, whether insulin-stimulated translocation is due to a property of GLUT-4 or to specific insulin receptor–signaling components in adipocytes and muscle is uncertain.[186] In addition to its acute effect on translocation, insulin also stimulates synthesis of glucose transporters. Alterations of this more chronic effect of insulin on the regulation of glucose transport may play a role in the decreased response of the transport system in states of chronic insulin deficiency, such as Type I diabetes mellitus[197] or in the insulin-resistance state of overfeeding[198] (see below).

Exactly how the activation of insulin-receptor kinase is coupled to translocation of the transporter is unknown and one of the most important current questions in insulin action. The transporters themselves are not substrates of the receptor kinase and are not changed in their phosphorylation state upon insulin stimulation. It seems more likely that some protein or proteins involved in the translocation process are involved in the phosphorylation cascade. Further work in this area is extremely important and likely to yield some interesting surprises.

Regulation of Glucose Transporters in Physiologic and Pathologic States

Both Type I and Type II diabetes are characterized by alterations in insulin action. The former is due primarily to insulin deficiency, whereas the latter is due primarily to insulin resistance. Glucose-transporter alterations may contribute to both defective insulin secretion by the β-cell and insulin resistance to glucose uptake by fat and muscle.

In animal models of Type II diabetes, a decrease in the levels of GLUT-2 has been detected in pancreatic β-cells. This defect can be detected before the development of overt diabetes.[199,200] This defect does not appear to be the primary genetic abnormality in any of these animals, as the defect is reversible if islets are transplanted into a

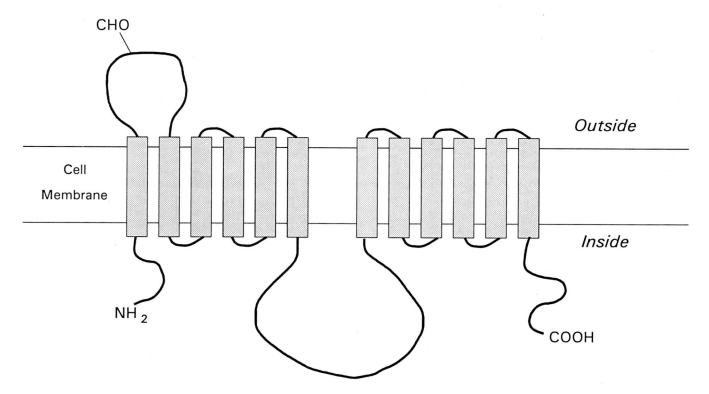

Fig. 8–10. A schematic model of the glucose transporter. The 12 transmembrane-spanning regions are shaded. The site of carbohydrate attachment is shown on the first external loop.

normal animal or if normal islets are transplanted into the diabetic host.[201] The decrease in GLUT-2 transporters is restricted to the pancreatic β-cells and is not present in the liver, the other major site of GLUT-2 expression.[202] The physiologic significance of the decrease in GLUT-2 expression is uncertain. Although it is possible that the decrease in GLUT-2 contributes to a decrease in β-cell response to a glucose stimulus, in some animal models in which there is a decrease in GLUT-2 expression, no defect in glucose-stimulated insulin release has been detected.[203]

Since glucose transport is the rate-limiting step in glucose utilization, at least in adipocytes, some abnormality in either expression or regulation of GLUT-4 transporters probably plays a role in the peripheral insulin resistance observed in various diabetic states. Although, defects in glucose transport have clearly been demonstrated in both human and rodent models of Type II diabetes, the exact nature of the defect is uncertain. The number of GLUT-4 transporters is reduced in adipocytes of patients with NIDDM[204] and in animal models of Type I diabetes.[197,205,206] This is associated with a decrease in the levels of GLUT-4 mRNA, without a change in the level of GLUT-1 mRNA.[207] In the insulin-deficient animal models, normalization of the blood glucose by insulin restores glucose transport and GLUT-4 mRNA to normal or above normal levels. It is interesting that phloridzin treatment, which reduces glucose levels without increasing insulin levels by producing a renal glucose leak, also restores insulin-stimulated glucose transport without increasing the number of GLUT-4 transporters.[178] In the Zucker fatty rat, levels of GLUT-4 mRNA and protein are increased in young animals and then decrease as the animals age. These changes parallel the changes in glucose transport observed in these rodents.[208]

Alterations in GLUT-1 and GLUT-4 expression in skeletal muscle have been much more difficult to demonstrate. Indeed, recent studies in both muscle biopsy specimens from humans with NIDDM, Zucker fatty rats, and rats with streptozotocin-induced Type I diabetes suggest that resistance to insulin-stimulated glucose uptake occurs in muscle without a change in the level of GLUT-4 protein or mRNA.[209,210] Thus, the primary defect appears to be in translocation and/or activation of the existing transporters. In states of prolonged insulin deficiency, there is a decrease in both GLUT-1 and GLUT-4 protein that may further compound the defect in translocation. Mutations in the GLUT-4 transporter have also been suggested to contribute to NIDDM in at least one patient.[211] This point mutation, however, is conservative and may not be of great functional significance. Based on larger screening studies, this type of mutation appears at best to be a rare cause of Type II diabetes.

TERMINATION OF THE INSULIN SIGNAL

Degradation of Insulin

Insulin circulates in blood as the free monomeric hormone. Under basal conditions the pancreas secretes 1 mg of insulin per day, or 40 μg (1 unit) per hour, into the portal vein to give a concentration of insulin in portal blood of 2 to 4 ng/mL (50 to 100 μU/mL). This results in a peripheral circulation of about 0.5 ng/mL (12 μU/mL) or about 10^{-10} M. Following ingestion of a meal, there is a rapid rise in portal insulin level followed by a parallel, but smaller rise, in peripheral insulin level.

The plasma half-life of insulin injected intravenously is about 5 to 6 minutes in humans without diabetes and about the same in humans with uncomplicated diabetes.[212] In a person with diabetes who develops antibodies to insulin, the plasma half-life of insulin may be increased severalfold.[213] The pancreatic content of proinsulin is only about 1 to 3% that of insulin. However, proinsulin has a much longer half-life than insulin (~17 minutes) and therefore may account for 10 to 25% of the immunoreactive "insulin" in plasma.[214] In patients with insulin-secreting islet cell tumors, the percentage of proinsulin in the circulation is usually increased (see Chapter 56). Proinsulin levels are also increased in patients with NIDDM.[215] Since proinsulin has only about 2 to 3% of the intrinsic bioactivity of insulin, the biologically effective concentration of insulin is somewhat lower than that estimated by immunoassay. This has been suggested as a contributing factor in the discordance between circulating insulin levels and insulin action in patients with NIDDM. The C-peptide secreted in equimolar amounts with insulin also has a higher molar concentration in plasma because of its considerably longer half-life (~30 minutes).[214] Levels of C-peptide are also increased in patients with insulin-secreting tumors.

The primary sites for insulin degradation are the liver, kidney, and muscle—in that order.[216] About 50% of the insulin that reaches the liver via the portal vein is taken up in a single passage and never reaches the general circulation. Insulin is filtered by the renal glomerulus, where it also is reabsorbed and degraded by the kidney tubules. Severe impairment of renal function appears to affect the rate of disappearance of circulating insulin to a greater extent than does hepatic disease,[217] presumably because the liver operates closer to its capacity to destroy the hormone and cannot compensate for such loss of renal catabolic function.

Hepatic uptake and degradation of insulin may be altered by a number of factors. In dogs, oral administration of glucose is associated with increased hepatic extraction,[218] whereas in humans oral glucose appears to reduce hepatic extraction.[219] This effect may be mediated by some intestinal hormone such as gastric inhibitory polypeptide. Arginine, cholecystokinin, and a high-protein diet have also been shown to alter hepatic extraction of insulin in animals.[216] Peripheral tissues, such as fat and muscle, also play a role in insulin degradation, but this is of less quantitative significance. Under normal conditions, little, if any, insulin degradation occurs in plasma.

Mechanisms of Insulin Degradation

Proteolytic degradation of insulin in the liver occurs both at the cell surface and after receptor-mediated internalization (Fig. 8–11). Whereas surface degradation

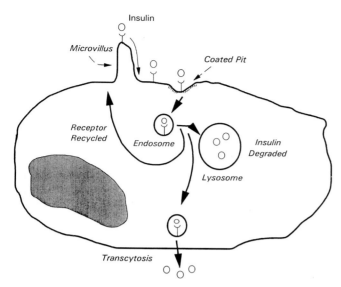

Fig. 8–11. The life cycle of insulin and insulin receptors in cells. Immediately after insulin binding, the receptor is sequestered in coated pits. The pit is internalized and forms an endosome. Depending on the cell type, the receptor recycles to the plasma membrane (recycling), undergoes degradation after fusion with lysosomes, or is transported to the opposite side of a polarized cell (transcytosis).

may account for as much as 50% of total insulin degradation in isolated cellular systems, in intact humans and rodents most degradation follows internalization of insulin.[220–222] The primary pathway for insulin internalization is receptor-mediated uptake. Occupied insulin receptors are internalized in an insulin-stimulated manner into small vesicles termed *endosomes*, the site of initiation of degradation.[216] Some insulin also is delivered to lysosomes or lysosome-related vesicles near the Golgi for degradation. The latter pathway is inhibited by chloroquine or other lysosomotropic agents in isolated cells.[223] Chloroquine, however, has not been shown to inhibit insulin degradation in intact animals.

The extent to which the internalized insulin is degraded by the cell varies considerably depending on the cell type. In hepatocytes more than 50% of the internalized insulin is degraded, whereas in endothelial cells most internalized insulin is released intact. The latter appears to be related to the role of these cells in transport of insulin molecules from the intravascular to the extracellular space.[224] This process has been termed *transcytosis* and is believed to play an important role in the ultimate delivery of the insulin molecule to its target cell in tissues such skeletal muscle and adipose where the capillary endothelial cells have tight junctions. Some internalized insulin also is released by hepatocytes and adipocytes without degradation. This occurs as a result of recycling of the receptor to the plasma membrane and has been termed *retroendocytosis*.[225]

Several enzymes have been suggested to be involved in insulin degradation. One insulin-degrading enzyme sim-

ply termed *IDE* has been purified to homogeneity.[226] The enzyme has a molecular weight of about 300,000 under nonreducing conditions and 110,000 under reducing conditions. It is inhibited by sulfhydryl inhibitors and by chelators such as EDTA, EGTA, and phenanthroline, classifying it as a thiol metaloprotease. IDE is activated by Mn^{++} and low concentrations of Zn^{++}. The apparent K_m of purified IDE for insulin is 20 to 40 nM. IDE may cleave insulin at several sites in the α- and β-chains. The preferential sites appear to be between A13-A14 and B9-B10.[216]

Several lines of evidence have been used to support a major role for IDE in the cellular degradation of insulin. Most important, microinjection of antibodies to IDE have been shown to inhibit insulin degradation by hepatocytes.[226] Immunologically related molecules have also been found in other tissues, including muscle, kidney, and brain.[216] The major portion of IDE appears to be cytosolic. An explanation as to how the internalized insulin, which is presumably isolated in some vesicle or lysosomal structure, becomes associated with the cytosolic IDE is still lacking. IDE is by no means strictly insulin-specific and also may play a role in degradation of other hormones, including glucagon.

A second insulin-degrading enzyme is glutathione-insulin transhydrogenase (GIT).[227] GIT has been identified in liver and is capable of reducing the intra- and interchain disulfide bonds. This would inactivate the insulin molecule or provide the first step in a sequential cascade of degradation. GIT appears to be the same as protein disulfide isomerase (PDI), the enzyme that catalyzes the reactivation of oxidized ribonuclease.[216] It has a relatively high K_m and is of uncertain physiologic significance.

In patients taking insulin, insulin may also be degraded subcutaneously. This appears to be a relatively minor problem in most patients, although several patients have been described in which a presumed increase in subcutaneous destruction is associated with insulin resistance.[228] A few of these patients have even been treated with protease inhibitors, such as aprotinin, with an improvement in insulin sensitivity. Thus far there has been no direct evidence of increased protease activity in subcutaneous extracts from these patients, and many of these individuals have psychosocial disturbances that suggest poor compliance with the insulin regimen. Whether this syndrome truly exists remains controversial.[228]

Phosphotyrosine Phosphatases

In addition to insulin degradation, the signal created by insulin at the cellular level is reversed by dephosphorylation of the receptor, with a decrease in subsequent kinase activity. This dephosphorylation reaction is catalyzed by a class of enzymes called *phosphotyrosine phosphatases* (PTPases). Several members of this class of enzymes have now been defined at the molecular level.[229] These may be divided into two major groups: the large transmembrane PTPases that resemble receptors, with the PTPase domain in the intracellular domain; and

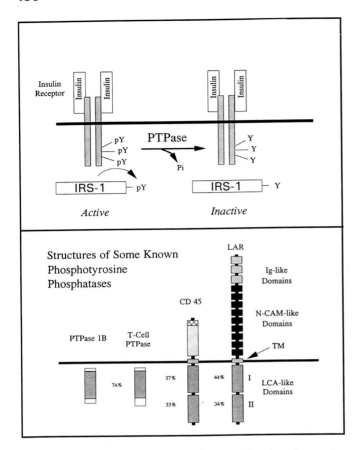

Fig. 8–12. Regulation of the insulin signal by phosphotyrosine phosphatases (PTPase). Phosphatases are important, as they catalyze the dephosphorylation of the insulin receptor and IRS-1 (upper panel). A schematic representation of some known phosphotyrosine phosphatases is shown in the lower panel.

a group of smaller cytoplasmic enzymes (Fig. 8–12). Both classes of PTPases have been shown to be active against the insulin receptor or insulin receptor-related peptides in vitro.[230,231] At present, little is known about which of these enzymes is most important in vivo in turning off the insulin signal.

Cellular PTPases may be regulated in diabetes or other pathophysiologic states. Membrane-associated and cytosolic PTPases increase in streptozotocin-diabetic rats, and cytosolic extracts from liver of streptozotocin-diabetic rats dephosphorylate (and hence inactivate) the insulin receptor more rapidly than do extracts from nondiabetic animals.[231] However, PTPase activity is decreased in the liver of *ob/ob* and *db/db* mice.[232] Insulin has also been suggested to regulate PTPase activity directly,[233,234] although the extent and physiologic significance of this regulation is unknown.

REFERENCES

1. DeFronzo RA, Bonadonna RC, Ferrannini E. Pathogenesis of NIDDM: a balanced overview. Diabetes Care 1992;15:318–68.
2. Rosen OM. After insulin binds. Science 1987;237:1452–8.
3. Kahn CR, White MF. The insulin receptor and the molecular mechanism of insulin action. J Clin Invest 1988;82:1151–6.
4. Ebina Y, Araki E, Taira M, et al. Replacement of lysine residue 1030 in the putative ATP-binding region of the insulin receptor abolishes insulin- and antibody-stimulated glucose uptake and receptor kinase activity. Proc Natl Acad Sci USA 1987;84:704–8.
5. Garvey WT. Glucose transport and NIDDM. Diabetes Care 1992;15:396–417.
6. Moller DE, Flier JS. Insulin resistance—mechanisms, syndromes, and implications. N Engl J Med 1991; 325:938–48.
7. Bell GI, Xiang K-S, Newman MV, et al. Gene for non-insulin-dependent diabetes mellitus (maturity-onset diabetes of the young subtype) is linked to DNA polymorphism on human chromosome 20q. Proc Natl Acad Sci USA 1991;88:1484–8.
8. Vionnet N, Stoffel M, Takeda J, et al. Nonsense mutation in the glucokinase gene causes early-onset non-insulin-dependent diabetes mellitus. Nature 1992; 356:721–2.
9. Blenis J. Growth-regulated signal transduction by the MAP kinases and RSKs. Cancer Cells 1991;3:445–9.
10. Granner DK, O'Brien RM. Molecular physiology and genetics of NIDDM: importance of metabolic staging. Diabetes Care 1992;15:369–95.
11. O'Brien RM, Granner DK. Regulation of gene expression by insulin. Biochem J 1991;278:609–19.
12. Cuatrecasas P. Isolation of the insulin receptor of liver and fat-cell membranes. Proc Natl Acad Sci USA 1972;69: 318–22.
13. Freychet P, Roth J, Neville DM Jr. Insulin receptors in the liver: specific binding of [^{125}I] insulin to the plasma membrane and its relation to insulin bioactvity. Proc Natl Acad Sci USA 1971;68:1833–7.
15. Pilch PF, Czech MP. The subunit structure of the high affinity insulin receptor: evidence for a disulfide-linked receptor complex in fat cell and liver plasma membranes. J Biol Chem 1980;255:1722–31.
16. Kahn CR, Baird KL, Flier JS, et al. Insulin receptors, receptor antibodies, and the mechanism of insulin action. Recent Prog Horm Res 1981;37:477–538.
17. Collier E, Gorden P. O-linked oligosaccharides on insulin receptor. Diabetes 1991;40:197–203.
18. Czech MP. Insulin action. Am J Med 1981;70:142–50.
19. Kasuga M, Hedo JA, Yamada KM, Kahn CR. The structure of insulin receptor and its subunits: evidence for multiple nonreduced forms and a 210,000 possible proreceptor. J Biol Chem 1982;257:10392–9.
20. Ronnett GV, Knutson VP, Kohanski RA, et al. Role of glycosylation in the processing of newly translated insulin proreceptor in 3T3-L1 adipocytes. J Biol Chem 1984; 259:4566–75.
21. Hedo JA, Kahn CR, Hayashi M, et al. Biosynthesis and glycosylation of the insulin receptor: evidence for a single polypeptide precursor of the two major subunits. J Biol Chem 1983;258:10020–6.
22. Herzberg VL, Grigorescu F, Edge ASB, et al. Characterization of insulin receptor carbohydrate by comparison of chemical and enzymatic deglycosylation. Biochem Biophys Res Commun 1985;129:789–96.
23. Cheatham B, Kahn CR. Cysteine 647 in the insulin receptor is required for normal covalent interaction between α- and β-subunits and signal transduction. J Biol Chem 1992;267:7108–15.

24. Seino S, Seino M, Nishi S, Bell GI. Structure of the human insulin receptor gene and characterization of its promoter. Proc Natl Acad Sci USA 1989;86:114–8.

25. Ullrich A, Bell JR, Chen EY, et al. Human insulin receptor and its relationship to the tyrosine kinase family of oncogenes. Nature 1985;313:756–61.

26. Kreig P, Melton D. K/RT Sequencing system manual. Madison, WI: Promega, 1987.

27. Seino S, Bell GI. Alternative splicing of human insulin receptor messenger RNA. Biochem Biophys Res Commun 1989;159:312–6.

28. Mamula PW, McDonald AR, Brunetti A, et al. Regulating insulin-receptor-gene expression by differentiation and hormones. Diabetes Care 1990;13:288–301.

29. Sibley E, Kastelic T, Kelly TJ, Lane MD. Characterization of the mouse insulin receptor gene promoter. Proc Natl Acad Sci USA 1989;86:9732–6.

30. Petruzzelli L, Herrera R, Arenas-Garcia R, et al. Isolation of a *Drosophila* genomic sequence homologous to the kinase domain of the human insulin receptor and detection of the phosphorylated *Drosophila* receptor with an anti-peptide antibody. Proc Natl Acad Sci USA 1986; 83:4710–4.

31. Taylor SI, Kadowaki T, Kadowaki H, et al. Mutations in insulin-receptor gene in insulin-resistant patients. Diabetes Care 1990;13:257–79.

32. Mosthaf L, Vogt B, Häring HU, Ullrich A. Altered expression of insulin receptor types A and B in the skeletal muscle of non-insulin-dependent diabetes mellitus patients. Proc Natl Acad Sci USA 1991;88:4728–30.

33. Araki E, Shimada F, Uzawa H, et al. Characterization of the promoter region of the human insulin receptor gene: evidence for promoter activity. J Biol Chem 1987;262: 16186–91.

34. Araki E, Murakami T, Shirotani T, et al. A cluster of four Sp1 binding sites required for efficient expression of the human insulin receptor gene. J Biol Chem 1991;266: 3944–8.

35. Lee J-K, Tam JWO, Tsai M-J, Tsai SY. Identification of *cis*- and *trans*-acting factors regulating the expression of the human insulin receptor gene. J Biol Chem 1992;267: 4638–45.

36. O'Rahilly S, Moller DE. Mutant insulin receptors in syndromes of insulin resistance. Clin Endocrinol 1992;36: 121–32.

37. Moller DE, Yokota A, White MF, et al. A naturally occurring mutation of insulin receptor alanine 1134 impairs tyrosine kinase function and is associated with dominantly inherited insulin resistance. J Biol Chem 1990;265: 14979–85.

38. Frattali AL, Treadway JL, Pessin JE. Insulin/IGF-1 hybrid receptors: implications for the dominant-negative phenotype in syndromes of insulin resistance. J Cell Biochem 1992;48:43–50.

39. Treadway JL, Morrison BD, Soos MA, et al. Transdominant inhibition of tyrosine kinase activity in mutant insulin/insulin-like growth factor I hybrid receptors. Proc Natl Acad Sci USA 1991;88:214–8.

40. Bornfeldt KE, Gidlöf RA, Wasteson A, et al. Binding and biological effects of insulin, insulin analogues and insulin-like growth factors in rat aortic smooth muscle cells. Comparison of maximal growth promoting activities. Diabetologia 1991;34:307–13.

41. Drejer K, Kruse V, Larsen UD, et al. Receptor binding and tyrosine kinase activation by insulin analogues with extreme affinities studied in human hepatoma HepG2 cells. Diabetes 1991;40:1488–95.

42. Pang DT, Shafer JA. Evidence that insulin receptor from human placenta has a high affinity for only one molecule of insulin. J Biol Chem 1984;259:8589–96.

43. Shymko RM, Gonzales NS, Backer JM, et al. Binding kinetics of mutated insulin receptors in transfected cells grown in suspension culture: application to the Tyr→APhe 960 insulin receptor mutant. Biochem Biophys Res Commun 1989;164:191–8.

44. Yip CC, Hsu H, Patel RG, Hawley DM, et al. Localization of the insulin-binding site to the cysteine-rich region of the insulin receptor α-subunit. Biochem Biophys Res Commun 1988;157:321–9.

45. Fabry M, Schaefer E, Ellis L, et al. Detection of a new hormone contact site within the insulin receptor ectodomain by the use of a novel photoreactive insulin. J Biol Chem 1992;267:8950–6.

46. McClain DA. Different ligand affinities of the two human insulin receptor splice variants are reflected in parallel changes in sensitivity for insulin action. Mol Endocrinol 1991;5:734–9.

47. Kellerer M, Lammers R, Ermel B, et al. Distinct α-subunit structures of human insulin receptor A and B variants determine differences in tyrosine kinase activities. Biochemistry 1992;31:4588–96.

48. Zhang B, Roth RA. A region of the insulin receptor important for ligand binding (residues 450–601) is recognized by patients' autoimmune antibodies and inhibitory monoclonal antibodies. Proc Natl Acad Sci USA 1991;88:9858–62.

49. Andersen AS, Kjeldsen T, Wiberg FC, et al. Changing the insulin receptor to possess insulin-like growth factor I ligand specificity. Biochemistry 1990;29:7363–6.

50. Zhang B, Roth RA. Binding properties of chimeric insulin receptors containing the cysteine-rich domain of either the insulin-like growth factor I receptor or the insulin receptor related receptor. Biochemistry 1991;30:5113–7.

51. De Meyts P, Gu J-L, Shymko RM, et al. Identification of a ligand-binding region of the human insulin receptor encoded by the second exon of the gene. Mol Endocrinol 1990;4:409–16.

52. Kasuga M, Karlsson FA, Kahn CR. Insulin stimulates the phosphorylation of the 95,000-dalton subunit of its own receptor. Science 1982;215:185–7.

53. Hanks SK, Quinn AM, Hunter T. The protein kinase family: conserved features and deduced phylogeny of the catalytic domains. Science 1988;241:42–52.

54. Hunter T, Cooper JA. Viral oncogenes and tyrosine phosphorylation. In: Boyer PD, Krebs EG, eds. The enzymes. eds. 3rd ed. Orlando: Academic Press, 1986:191–246.

55. Yarden Y, Ullrich A. Growth factor receptor tyrosine kinases. Annu Rev Biochem 1988;57:443–78.

56. Margolis BL, Lax I, Kris R, et al. All autophosphorylation sites of epidermal growth factor (EGF) receptor and HER2/*neu* are located in their carboxyl-terminal tails: identification of a novel site in GF receptor. J Biol Chem 1989;264:10667–71.

57. Fantl WJ, Escobedo JA, Martin GA, et al. Distinct phosphotyrosines on a growth factor receptor bind to specific molecules that mediate different signaling pathways. Cell 1992;69:413–23.

58. White MF, Shoelson SE, Keutmann H, Kahn CR. A cascade of tyrosine autophosphorylation in the β-subunit activates the phosphotransferase of the insulin receptor. J Biol Chem 1988;263:2969–80.

59. Wilden PA, Kahn CR, Siddle K, White MF. Insulin receptor kinase domain autophosphorylation regulates receptor enzymatic function. J Biol Chem 1992;267:16660–8.

60. Shier P, Watt VM. Primary structure of a putative receptor for a ligand of the insulin family. J Biol Chem 1989;264:14605–8.

61. Rosen OM, Herrera R, Olowe Y, et al. Phosphorylation activates the insulin receptor tyrosine protein kinase. Proc Natl Acad Sci USA 1983;80:3237–40.

62. Flores-Riveros JR, Sibley E, Kastelic T, Lane MD. Substrate phosphorylation catalyzed by the insulin receptor tyrosine kinase: kinetic correlation to autophosphorylation of specific sites in the β subunit. J Biol Chem 1989; 264:21557–72.

63. Frattali AL, Treadway JL, Pessin JE. Evidence supporting a passive role for the insulin receptor transmembrane domain in insulin-dependent signal transduction. J Biol Chem 1991;266:9829–34.

64. Longo N, Shuster RC, Griffin LD, et al. Activation of insulin receptor signaling by a single amino acid substitution in the transmembrane domain. J Biol Chem 1992;267: 12416–9.

65. Shoelson SE, White MF, Kahn CR. Tryptic activation of the insulin receptor: proteolytic truncation of the α-subunit releases the β-subunit from inhibitory control. J Biol Chem 1988;263:4852–60.

66. Roth RA, Cassell DJ. Insulin receptor: evidence that it is a protein kinase. Science 1983;219:299–301.

67. Chou CK, Dull TJ, Russell DS, et al. Human insulin receptors mutated at the ATP-binding site lack protein tyrosine kinase activity and fail to mediate postreceptor effects of insulin. J Biol Chem 1987;262:1842–7.

68. Wierenga RK, Hol WGJ. Predicted nucleotide-binding properties of p21 protein and its cancer-associated variant. Nature 1983;302:842–4.

69. White MF, Kahn CR. The insulin receptor and tyrosine phosphorylation. In: Boyer PD, Krebs EG, eds. The enzymes. 3rd ed. Orlando: Academic Press, 1986:247–302.

70. Schlessinger J. Signal transduction by allosteric receptor oligomerization. Trends Biochem Sci 1988;13:443–7.

71. Tartare S, Ballotti R, Lammers R, et al. Insulin-EGF receptor chimerae mediate tyrosine phosphorylation and serine/threonine phosphorylation of kinase-deficient EGF receptors. J Biol Chem 1991;266:9900–6.

72. Lammers R, Van Obberghen E, Ballotti R, et al. Transphosphorylation as a possible mechanism for insulin and epidermal growth factor receptor activation. J Biol Chem 1990;265:16886–90.

73. Wilden PA, Backer JM, Kahn CR, et al. The insulin receptor with phenylalanine replacing tyrosine-1146 provides evidence for separate signals regulating cellular metabolism and growth. Proc Natl Acad Sci USA 1990;87: 3358–62.

74. Wilden PA, Siddle K, Haring E, et al. The role of insulin receptor kinase domain autophosphorylation in receptor-mediated activities: analysis with insulin and anti-receptor antibodies. J Biol Chem 1992;267:13719–27.

75. Vogt B, Carrascosa JM, Ermel B, et al. The two isotypes of the human insulin receptor (HIR-A and HIR-B) follow different internalization kinetics. Biochem Biophys Res Commun 1991;177:1013–8.

76. Walker PS, Ramlal T, Sarabia V, et al. Glucose transport activity in L6 muscle cells is regulated by the coordinate control of subcellular glucose transporter distribution, biosynthesis, and mRNA transcription. J Biol Chem 1990;265:1516–23.

77. Zhang B, Roth RA. The insulin receptor-related receptor: tissue expression, ligand binding specificity, and signaling capabilities. J Biol Chem 1992;267:18320–8.

78. Koch CA, Anderson D, Moran MF, et al. SH2 and SH3 domains: elements that control interactions of cytoplasmic signaling proteins. Science 1991;252:668–74.

79. Kazlauskas A, Cooper JA. Autophosphorylation of the PDGF receptor in the kinase insert region regulates interactions with cell proteins. Cell 1989;58:1121–33.

80. Gandino L, Di Renzo MF, Giordano S, et al. Protein kinase-c activation inhibits tyrosine phosphorylation of the c-*met* protein. Oncogene 1990;5:721–5.

81. Escobedo JA, Kaplan DR, Kavanaugh WM, et al. A phosphatidylinositol-3 kinase binds to platelet-derived growth factor receptors through a specific receptor sequence containing phosphotyrosine. Mol Cell Biol 1991;11: 1125–32.

82. Cantley LC, Auger KR, Carpenter C, et al. Oncogenes and signal transduction. Cell 1991;64:281–302.

83. Margolis B, Li N, Koch A, et al. The tyrosine phosphorylated carboxyterminus of the EGF receptor is a binding site for GAP and PLC-γ. EMBO J 1990;9:4375–80.

84. Tornqvist HE, Pierce MW, Frackelton AR, et al. Identification of insulin receptor tyrosine residues autophosphorylated in vitro. J Biol Chem 1987;262:10212--9.

85. Tornqvist HE, Gunsalus JR, Nemenoff RA, et al. Identification of the insulin receptor tyrosine residues undergoing insulin-stimulated phosphorylation in intact rat hepatoma cells. J Biol Chem 1988;263:350–9.

86. Tavaré JM, O'Brien RM, Siddle K, Denton RM. Analysis of insulin-receptor phosphorylation sites in intact cells by two-dimensional phosphopeptide mapping. Biochem J 1988;253:783–8.

87. White MF, Livingston JN, Backer JM, et al. Mutation of the insulin receptor at tyrosine 960 inhibits signal transmission but does not affect its tyrosine kinase activity. Cell 1988;54:641–9.

88. Murakami MS, Rosen OM. The role of insulin receptor autophosphorylation in signal transduction. J Biol Chem 1991;266:22653–60.

89. Backer JM, Schroeder GG, Cahill DA, et al. Cytoplasmic juxtamembrane region of the insulin receptor: a critical role in ATP binding, endogenous substrate phosphorylation, and insulin-stimulated bioeffects in CHO cells. Biochemistry 1991;30:6366–72.

90. Sun XJ, Rothenberg P, Kahn CR, et al. Structure of the insulin receptor substrate IRS-1 defines a unique signal transduction protein. Nature 1991;352:73–7.

91. Izumi T, White MF, Kadowaki T, et al. Insulin-like growth factor I rapidly stimulates tyrosine phosphorylation of a M_r 185,000 protein in intact cells. J Biol Chem 1987; 262:1282–7.

92. Madoff DH, Martensen TM, Lane MD. Insulin and insulin-like growth factor 1 stimulate the phosphorylation on tyrosine of a 160 kDa cytosolic protein in 3T3-L1 adipocytes. Biochem J 1988;252:7–15.

93. Ullrich A, Gray A, Tam AW, et al. Insulin-like growth factor I receptor primary structure: comparison with insulin receptor suggests structural determinants that define functional specificity. EMBO J 1986;5:2503–12.

94. King GL, Kahn CR. The growth promoting effects of insulin. In: Guroff G, ed. Growth and maturation factors. 2nd ed. New York: John Wiley and Sons, 1984: 223–66.

95. King GL, Rechler MM, Kahn CR. Interactions between the receptors for insulin and the insulin-like growth factors on adipocytes. J Biol Chem 1982;257:10001–6.

96. Moxham CP, Duronio V, Jacobs S. Insulin-like growth factor I receptor β-subunit heterogeneity: evidence for hybrid tetramers composed of insulin-like growth factor I

and insulin receptor heterodimers. J Biol Chem 1989; 264:13238–44.

97. Yee D, Lebovic GS, Marcus RR, Rosen N. Identification of an alternate type I insulin-like growth factor receptor β-subunit mRNA transcript. J Biol Chem 1989;264: 21439–41.

98. Takayama S, White MF, Lauris V, Kahn CR. Phorbol esters modulate insulin receptor phosphorylation and insulin action in cultured hepatoma cells. Proc Natl Acad Sci USA 1984;81:7797–801.

99. Kasuga M, Zick Y, Blith DL, et al. Insulin stimulation of phosphorylation of the β-subunit of the insulin receptor: formation of both phosphoserine and phosphotyrosine. J Biol Chem 1982;257:9891–4.

100. Takayama S, White MF, Kahn CR. Phorbol ester-induced serine phosphorylation of the insulin receptor decreases its tyrosine kinase activity. J Biol Chem 1988;263: 3440–7.

101. Karasik A, Rothenberg PL, Yamada K, et al. Increased protein kinase C activity is linked to reduced insulin receptor autophosphorylation in liver of starved rats. J Biol Chem 1990;265:10226–31.

102. Lewis RE, Cao L, Perregaux D, Czech MP. Threonine 1336 of the human insulin receptor is a major target for phosphorylation by protein kinase C. Biochemistry 1990;29:1807–13.

103. Bollag GE, Roth RA, Beaudoin J, et al. Protein kinase C directly phosphorylates the insulin receptor in vitro and reduces its protein-tyrosine kinase activity. Proc Natl Acad Sci USA 1986;83:5822–4.

104. Lewis RE, Wu GP, MacDonald RG, Czech MP. Insulin-sensitive phosphorylation of serine 1293/1294 on the human insulin receptor by a tightly associated serine kinase. J Biol Chem 1990;265:947–54.

105. Czech MP. Molecular basis of insulin action. Annu Rev Biochem 1977;46:359–84.

106. White MF, Maron R, Kahn CR. Insulin rapidly stimulates tyrosine phosphorylation of a M_r 185,000 protein in intact cells. Nature 1985;318:183–6.

107. Kadowaki T, Fujita-Yamaguchi Y, Nishida E, et al. Phosphorylation of tubulin and microtubule-associated proteins by the purified insulin receptor kinase. J Biol Chem 1985;260:4016–20.

108. Kadowaki T, Nishida E, Kasuga M, et al. Phosphorylation of fodrin (nonerythroid spectrin) by the purified insulin receptor kinase. Biochem Biophys Res Commun 1985;127:493–500.

109. Sale EM, White MF, Kahn CR. Phosphorylation of glycolytic and gluconeogenic enzymes by the insulin receptor kinase. J Cell Biochem 1987;33:15–26.

110. Graves CB, Gale RD, Laurino JP, McDonald JM. The insulin receptor and calmodulin: calmodulin enhances insulin-mediated receptor kinase activity and insulin stimulates phosphorylation of calmodulin. J Biol Chem 1986; 261:10429–38.

111. Chen J, Martin BL, Brautigan DL. Regulation of protein serine-threonine phosphatase type-2A by tyrosine phosphorylation. Science 1992;257:1261–4.

112. Gibbs EM, Allard WJ, Lienhard GE. The glucose transporter in 3T3-L1 adipocytes is phosphorylated in response to phorbol ester but not in response to insulin. J Biol Chem 1986;261:16597–603.

113. Maegawa H, Olefsky JM, Thies S, et al. Insulin receptors with defective tyrosine kinase inhibit normal receptor function at the level of substrate phosphorylation. J Biol Chem 1988;263:12629–37.

114. White MF, Stegmann EW, Dull TJ, et al. Characterization of

an endogenous substrate of the insulin receptor in cultured cells. J Biol Chem 1987;262:9769–77.

115. Kadowaki T, Koyasu S, Nishida E, et al. Tyrosine phosphorylation of common and specific sets of cellular proteins rapidly induced by insulin, insulin-like growth factor I, and epidermal growth factor in an intact cell. J Biol Chem 1987;262:7342–50.

116. Shemer J, Perrotti N, Roth J, LeRoith D. Characterization of an endogenous substrate related to insulin and insulin-like growth factor-I receptors in lizard brain. J Biol Chem 1987;262:3436–9.

117. Momomura K, Tobe K, Seyama Y, et al. Insulin-induced tyrosine-phosphorylation in intact rat adipocytes. Biochem Biophys Res Commun 1988;155:1181–6.

118. Tobe K, Koshio O, Tashiro-Hashimoto Y, et al. Immunological detection of phosphotyrosine-containing proteins in rat livers after insulin injection. Diabetes 1990;39: 528–33.

119. Shemer J, Adamo M, Wilson GL, et al. Insulin and insulin-like growth factor-I stimulate a common endogenous phosphoprotein substrate (pp 185) in intact neurobastoma cells. J Biol Chem 1987;262:15476–82.

120. Hofmann C, White MF, Whittaker J. Human insulin receptors expressed in insulin-insensitive mouse fibroblasts couple with extant cellular effector systems to confer insulin-sensitivity and responsiveness. Endocrinology 1989;124:257–64.

121. Rothenberg PL, Lane WS, Karasik A, et al. Purification and partial sequence analysis of pp185, the major cellular substrate of the insulin receptor tyrosine kinase. J Biol Chem 1991;266:8302–11.

122. Sun XJ, Miralpeix M, Myers MG Jr, et al. The expression and function of IRS-1 in insulin signal transmission. J Biol Chem 1992;267:22662–72.

123. Myers MG Jr, Sun XJ, Cheatham B, et al. IRS-1 is a common element in insulin and IGF-1 signaling to the phosphatidylinositol 3′-kinase. Endocrinology 1993 (in press).

124. Nishiyama M, Wands JR. Cloning and increased expression of an insulin receptor substrate-1-like gene in human hepatocellular carcinoma. Biochem Biophys Res Commun 1992;183:280–5.

125. Shoelson SE, Chatterjee S, Chaudhuri M, White MF. YMXM motifs of IRS-1 define substrate specificity of the insulin receptor kinase. Proc Natl Acad Sci USA 1992;89: 2027–31.

126. Whitman M, Downes CP, Keeler M, et al. Type I phosphatidylinositol kinase makes a novel inositol phospholipid, phosphatidylinositol-3-phosphate. Nature 1988;332: 644–6.

127. Ruderman NB, Kapeller R, White MF, Cantley LC. Activation of phosphatidylinositol-3-kinase by insulin. Proc Natl Acad Sci USA 1990;87:1411–5.

128. Hawkins PT, Jackson TR, Stephens LR. Platelet-derived growth factor stimulates synthesis of $PtdIns(3,4,5)P_3$ by activating a $PtdIns(4,5)P_2$ 3-OH kinase. Nature 1992; 358:157–9.

129. Meldrum E, Parker PJ, Carozzi A. The PtdIns-PLC superfamily and signal transduction. Biochim Biophys Acta 1991;1092:49–71.

130. Serunian LA, Haber MT, Fukui T, et al. Polyphosphoinositides produced by phosphatidylinositol 3-kinase are poor substrates for phospholipases C from rat liver and bovine brain. J Biol Chem 1989;264:17809–15.

131. Backer JM, Myers MG Jr, Shoelson SE, et al. The phosphatidylinositol 3′-kinase is activated by association with IRS-1 during insulin stimulation. EMBO J 1992;3469–79.

132. Myers MG Jr, Backer JM, Sun XJ, et al. IRS-1 activates the phosphatidylinositol 3′-kinase by associating with the *src* homology 2 domains of p85. Proc Natl Acad Sci USA 1992;89:10350–4.

133. Rees-Jones RW, Taylor SI. An endogenous substrate for the insulin receptor-associated tyrosine kinase. J Biol Chem 1985;260:4461–7.

134. Perrotti N, Accili D, Marcus-Samuels B, et al. Insulin stimulates phosphorylation of a 120-kDa glycoprotein substrate (pp120) for the receptor-associated protein kinase in intact H-35 hepatoma cells. Proc Natl Acad Sci USA 1987;84:3137–40.

135. Margolis RN, Taylor SI, Seminara D, Hubbard AL. Indentification of pp120, an endogenous substrate for the hepatocyte insulin receptor tyrosine kianse, as an integral membrane glycoprotein of the bile canalicular domain. Proc Natl Acad Sci USA 1988;85:7256–9.

136. Lin S-H. Localization of the ecto-ATPase (ecto-nucleotidease) in the rat hepatocyte plasma membrane: implications for the functions of the ecto-ATPase. J Biol Chem 1989;264:14403–7.

137. Lin S-H, Guidotti G. Cloning and expression of a cDNA coding for a rat liver plasma membrane ecto-ATPase: the primary structure of the ecto-ATP-ase is similar to that of the human biliary glycoprotein I. J Biol Chem 1989; 264:14408–14.

138. Levenson RM, Blackshear PJ. Insulin-stimulated protein tyrosine phosphorylation in intact cells evaluated by giant two-dimensional gel electrophoresis. J Biol Chem 1989;264:19984–93.

139. Bernier M, Laird DM, Lane MD. Insulin-activated tyrosine phosphorylation of a 15-kilodalton protein in intact 3T3-L1 adipocytes. Proc Natl Acad Sci USA 1987;84:1844–8.

140. Hresko RC, Bernier M, Hoffman RD, et al. Identification of phosphorylated 422(aP2) protein as pp15, the 15-kilodalton target of the insulin receptor tyrosine kinase in 3T3-L1 adipocytes. Proc Natl Acad Sci USA 1988;85:8835–9.

141. Hresko RC, Hoffman RD, Flores-Riveros JR, Lane MD. Insulin receptor tyrosine kinase-catalyzed phosphorylation of 422(aP2) protein: substrate activation by long-chain fatty acid. J Biol Chem 1990;265:21075–85.

142. Frost SC, Kohanski RA, Lane MD. Effect of phenylarsine oxide on insulin-dependent protein phosphorylation and glucose transport in 3T3-L1 adipocytes. J Biol Chem 1987;262:9872–6.

143. Saltiel AR, Cuatrecasas P. Insulin stimulates the generation from hepatic plasma membranes of modulators derived from an inositol glycolipid. Proc Natl Acad Sci USA 1986;83:5793–7.

144. Saltiel AR, Fox JA, Sherline P, Cuatrecasas P. Insulin-stimulated hydrolysis of a novel glycolipid generates modulators of cAMP phosphodiesterase. Science 1986; 233:967–72.

145. Kelly KL, Mato JM, Merida I, Jarett L. Glucose transport and antilipolysis are differentially regulated by the polar head group of an insulin-sensitive glycophospholipid. Proc Natl Acad Sci USA 1987;84:6404–7.

146. Gaulton GN, Kelly KL, Pawlowski J, et al. Regulation and function of an insulin-sensitive glycosyl-phosphatidylinositol during T lymphocyte activation. Cell 1988;53:963–70.

147. Fox JA, Soliz NM, Saltiel AR. Purification of a phosphatidylinositol-glycan-specific phospholipase C from liver plasma membranes: a possible target of insulin action. Proc Natl Acad Sci USA 1987;84:2663–7.

148. Alvarez JF, Varela I, Ruiz-Albusac JM, Mato JM. Localisation of the insulinsensitive phosphatidylinositol glycan at the outer surface of the cell membrane. Biochem Biophys Res Commun 1988;152:1455–62.

149. Barbacid M. *ras* Genes. Annu Rev Biochem 1987;56:779–827.

150. Medema RH, Burgering BMT, Bos JL. Insulin-induced p21ras activation does not require protein kinase C, but a protein sensitive to phenylarsine oxide. J Biol Chem 1991;266:21186–9.

151. Haubruck H, McCormick F. *Ras* p21: effects and regulation. Biochim Biophys Acta 1991;1072:215–29.

152. Kazlauskas A, Ellis C, Pawson T, Cooper JA. Binding of GAP to activated PDGF receptors. Science 1990;247:1578–81.

153. Settleman J, Narasimhan V, Foster LC, Weinberg RA. Molecular cloning of cDNAs encoding the GAP-associated protein p190: implications for a signaling pathway from Ras to the nucleus. Cell 1992;69:539–49.

154. Porras A, Nebreda AR, Benito M, Santos E. Activation of Ras by insulin in 3T3 L1 cells does not involve GTPase-activating protein phosphorylation. J Biol Chem 1992;267:21124–31.

155. Wong G, Müller O, Clark R, et al. Molecular cloning and nucleic acid binding properties of the GAP-associated tyrosine phosphoprotein p62. Cell 1992;69:551–8.

156. Towbin H, Staehelin T, Gordon J. Electrophoretic transfer of proteins from polyacrylamide gels to nitrocellulose sheets: procedure and some applications. Proc Natl Acad Sci USA 1979;76:4350–4.

157. Burgering BMT, Medema RH, Maassen JA, et al. Insulin stimulation of gene expression mediated by p21*ras* activation. EMBO J 1991;10:1103–9.

158. Medema RH, Wubbolts R, Bos JL. Two dominant inhibitory mutants of p21*ras* interfere with insulin-induced gene expression. Mol Cell Biol 1991;11:5963–7.

159. Korn LJ, Siebel CW, McCormick F, Roth RA. *Ras* p21 as a potential mediator of insulin action in *Xenopus* oocytes. Science 1987;236:840–1.

160. Denton RM, Brownsey RW, Belsham GJ. A partial view of the mechanism of insulin action. Diabetologia 1981;21:347–62.

161. Sturgill TW, Ray LB. Muscle proteins related to microtubule associated protein-2 are substrates for an insulin-stimulatable kinase. Biochem Biophys Res Commun 1986;134:565–71.

162. Sturgill TW, Ray LB, Erikson E, Maller JL. Insulin-stimulated MAP-2 kinase phosphorylates and activates ribosomal protein S6 kinase II. Nature 1988;334:715–8.

163. Rossomando AJ, Payne DM, Weber MJ, Sturgill TW. Evidence that pp42, a major tyrosine kinase target protein, is a mitogen-activated serine/threonine protein kinase. Proc Natl Acad Sci USA 1989;86:6940–3.

164. Cobb MH, Boulton TG, Robbins DJ. Extracellular signal-regulated kinases: ERKs in progress. Cell Regul 1991; 2:965–78.

165. Boulton TG, Nye SH, Robbins DJ, et al. ERKs: a family of protein-serine/threonine kinases that are activated and tyrosine phosphorylated in response to insulin and NGF. Cell 1991;65:663–75.

166. Ray LB, Sturgill TW. Insulin-stimulated microtubule-associated protein kinase is phosphorylated on tyrosine and threonine in vivo. Proc Natl Acad Sci USA 1988;85:3753–7.

167. Thomas G. MAP kinase by any other name smells just as sweet. Cell 1992;68:3–6.

168. Seger R, Ahn NG, Boulton TG, et al. Microtubule-associated protein 2 kinases, ERK1 and ERK2, undergo autophosphorylation on both tyrosine and threonine

residues: implications for their mechanism of activation. Proc Natl Acad Sci USA 1991;88:6142–6.

169. Ahn NG, Weiel JE, Chan CP, Krebs EG. Identification of multiple epidermal growth factor-stimulated protein serine/threonine kinases from Swiss 3T3 cells. J Biol Chem 1990;265:11487–94.

170. Ahn NG, Seger R, Bratlien RL, et al. Multiple components in an epidermal growth factor-stimulated protein kinase cascade: in vitro activation of a myelin basic protein/microtubule-associated protein 2 kinase. J Biol Chem 1991;266:4220–7.

171. Pulverer BJ, Kyriakis JM, Avruch J, et al. Phosphorylation of c-jun mediated by MAP kinases. Nature 1991; 353:670–4.

172. Gille H, Sharrocks AD, Shaw PE. Phosphorylation of transcription factor p62^{TCF} by MAP kinase stimulates ternary complex formation at c-fos promoter. Nature 1992;358:414–7.

173. Dent P, Lavoinne A, Nakielny S, et al. The molecular mechanism by which insulin stimulates glycogen synthesis in mammalian skeletal muscle. Nature 1990;348: 302–8.

174. Kyriakis JM, App H, Zhang X-F, et al. Raf-1 activates MAP kinase-kinase. Nature 1992;358:417–21.

175. Kovacina KS, Yonezawa K, Brautigan DL, et al. Insulin activates the kinase activity of the raf-1 proto-oncogene by increasing its serine phosphorylation. J Biol Chem 1990; 265:12115–8.

176. Blackshear PJ, Haupt DM, App H, Rapp UR. Insulin activates the raf-1 protein kinase. J Biol Chem 1990; 265:12131–4.

177. Anderson NG, Li P, Marsden LA, et al. Raf-1 is a potential substrate for mitogen-activated protein kinase in vivo. Biochem J 1991;277:573–6.

178. Kahn BB, Shulman GI, DeFronzo RA, et al. Normalization of blood glucose in diabetic rats with phlorizin treatment reverses insulin-resistant glucose transport in adipose cells without restoring glucose transporter gene expression. J Clin Invest 1991;87:561–70.

179. Elsas LJ, Longo N. Glucose transporters. Annu Rev Med 1992;43:377–93.

180. Desjeue JF. Congenital selective Na$^+$, D-glucose transport defects leading to renal glycosuria and congenital selective intestinal malabsorption of glucose and galactase. In: Scriver S, Beandet A, Shy W, Valle D, eds. The metabolic basis of inherited disease. New York: McGraw Hill, 1989:2463–78.

181. Czech MP. Insulin action and the regulation of hexose transport. Diabetes 1980;29:399–409.

182. Suzuki K, Kono T. Evidence that insulin causes translocation of glucose transport activity of the plasma membrane from an intracellular storage site. Proc Natl Acad Sci USA 1980;77:2542–5.

183. Karnieli E, Zarnowski MJ, Hissin PJ, et al. Insulin-stimulated translocation of glucose transport systems in the isolated rat adipose cell: time course, reversal, insulin concentration dependency, and relationship to glucose transport activity. J Biol Chem 1981;256:4772–82.

184. Kono T, Robinson FW, Blevins TL, Ezaki O. Evidence that translocation of the glucose transport activity is the major mechanism of insulin action on glucose transport in fat cells. J Biol Chem 1982;257:10942–7.

185. Simpson IA, Cushman SW. Hormonal regulation of mammalian glucose transport. Annu Rev Biochem 1986; 55:1059–89.

186. James DE, Brown R, Navarro J, Pilch PF. Insulin-regulat-

able tissues express a unique insulin-sensitive glucose transport protein. Nature 1988;333:183–5.

187. Mueckler M, Caruso C, Baldwin SA, et al. Sequence and structure of a human glucose transporter. Science 1985;229:941–5.

188. Harrison SA, Clancy BM, Pessino A, Czech MP. Activation of cell surface glucose transporters measured by photoaffinity labeling of insulin-sensitive 3T3-L1 adipocytes. J Biol Chem 1992;267:3783–8.

189. Marette A, Richardson JM, Ramlal T, et al. Abundance, localization and insulin-induced translocation of glucose transporters in red and white muscle. Am J Physiol 1992;263:c443–52.

190. Czech MP, Clancy BM, Pessino A, et al. Complex regulation of simple sugar transport in insulin-responsive cells. Trends Biochem Sci 1992;17:197–201.

191. Thorens B, Sarkar HK, Kaback HR, Lodish HF. Cloning and functional expression in bacteria of a novel glucose transporter present in liver, intestine, kidney, and β-pancreatic islet cells. Cell 1988;55:281–90.

192. Sarkar HK, Thorens B, Lodish HF, Kaback HR. Expression of the human erythrocyte glucose transporter in Escherichia coli. Proc Natl Acad Sci USA 1988;85:5463–7.

193. Fukumoto H, Seino S, Imura H, et al. Sequence, tissue distribution, and chromosomal localization of mRNA encoding a human glucose transporter-like protein. Proc Natl Acad Sci USA 1988;85:5434–8.

194. Birnbaum MJ. Identification of a novel gene encoding an insulin-responsive glucose transporter protein. Cell 1989;57:305–15.

195. Charron MJ, Fusias FC II, Alper SL, Lodish HF. A glucose transport protein expressed predominantly in insulin-responsive tissues. Proc Natl Acad Sci USA 1989; 86:2535–9.

196. Bell GI, Kayano T, Buse JB, et al. Molecular biology of mammalian glucose transporters. Diabetes Care 1990; 13:198–208.

197. Garvey WT, Huecksteadt TP, Birnbaum MJ. Pretranslational suppression of an insulin-responsive glucose transporter in rats with diabetes mellitus. Science 1989; 245:60–3.

198. Pedersen O, Kahn CR, Flier JS, Kahn BB. High fat feeding causes insulin resistance and a marked decrease in the expression of glucose transporters (GLUT 4) in fat cells of rats. Endocrinology 1992;129:771–7.

199. Johnson JH, Ogawa A, Chen L, et al. Underexpression of β cell high K_m glucose transporters in non-insulin-dependent diabetes. Science 1990;250:546–9.

200. Orci L, Thorens B, Ravazzola M, Lodish HF. Localization of the pancreatic beta cell glucose transporter to specific plasma membrane domains. Science 1989;245: 295–7.

201. Thorens B, Wu Y-J, Leahy JL, Weir GC. The loss of GLUT2 expression by glucose-unresponsive β cells of db/db mice is reversible and is induced by the diabetic environment. J Clin Invest 1992;90:77–85.

202. Oka Y, Asano T, Shibasaki Y, et al. Increased liver glucose-transporter protein and mRNA in streptozocin-induced diabetic rats. Diabetes 1990;39:441–6.

203. Tal M, Wu Y-J, Leiser M, et al. [Val^{12}] HRAS downregulates GLUT2 in β cells of transgenic mice without affecting glucose homeostasis. Proc Natl Acad Sci USA 1992; 89:5744–8.

204. Sinha MK, Raineri-Maldonado C, Buchanan C, et al. Adipose tissue glucose transporters in NIDDM: decreased levels of muscle/fat isoform. Diabetes 1991;40:472–7.

205. Sivitz WI, DeSautel SL, Kayano T, et al. Regulation of glucose transporter messenger RNA in insulin-deficient states. Nature 1989;340:72−4.

206. Berger J, Biswas C, Vicario PP, et al. Decreased expression of the insulin-responsive glucose transporter in diabetes and fasting. Nature 1989;340:70−2.

207. Kahn BB, Charron MJ, Lodish HF, et al. Differential regulation of two glucose transporters and adipose cells from diabetic and insulin-treated diabetic rats. J Clin Invest1989;84:404−11.

208. Pedersen O, Kahn CR, Kahn BB. Divergent regulation of the Glut 1 and Glut 4 glucose transporters in isolated adipocytes from Zucker rats. J Clin Invest 1992;89:1964−73.

209. Pedersen O, Bak JF, Andersen PH, et al. Evidence against altered expression of GLUT 1 or GLUT 4 in skeletal muscle of patients with obesity or NIDDM. Diabetes 1990;39:865−70.

210. Kahn BB, Rossetti L, Lodish HF, Charron MJ. Decreased in vivo glucose uptake but normal expression of GLUT 1 and GLUT 4 in skeletal muscle of diabetic rats. J Clin Invest 1991;87:2197−206.

211. Kusari J, Verma US, Buse JB, et al. Analysis of the gene sequences of the insulin receptor and the insulin-sensitive glucose transporter (GLUT-4) in patients with common-type non-insulin-dependent diabetes mellitus. J Clin Invest1991;88:1323−30.

212. Sodoyez JC, Sodoyez-Goffaux F, Guillaume M, Merchie G. [^{123}I]insulin metabolism in normal rats and humans: external detection by a scintillation camera. Science 1983;219:865−8.

213. Hachiya HL, Treves ST, Kahn CR, et al. Altered insulin distribution and metabolism of type I diabetics assessed by [^{123}I]-insulin scanning. J Clin Endocrinol Metabol 1987;64:801−8.

214. Robbins DC, Tager HS, Rubenstein AH. Biologic and clinical importance of proinsulin. N Engl J Med 1984;310:1165−75.

215. Porte D J, Kahn SE. Hyperproinsulinemia and amyloid in NIDDM: clues to etiology of islet β-cell dysfunction? Diabetes 1989;38:1333−6.

216. Duckworth WC. Insulin degradation: mechanisms, products, and significance. Endocrinol Rev 1988;9:319−45.

217. Rabkin R, Ryan MP, Duckworth WC. The renal metabolism of insulin. Diabetologia 1984;27:351−7.

218. Jaspan J, Polonsky K. Glucose ingestion in dogs alters the hepatic extraction of insulin: in vivo evidence for a relationship between biologic action and extraction of insulin. J Clin Invest 1982;69:516−22.

219. Hanks JB, Andersen DK, Wise JE, et al. The hepatic extraction of gastric inhibitory polypeptide and insulin. Endocrinology 1984;115:1011−8.

220. Caro JF, Muller G, Gennon JA. Insulin processing by the liver. J Biol Chem 1982;257:8459−66.

221. Terris S, Steiner DF. Binding and degradation of ^{125}I-insulin by rat hepatocytes. J Biol Chem 1975;250:8389−98.

222. Berman M, McGuire EA, Roth J, Zeleznik AJ. Kinetic modeling of insulin binding to receptors and degradation in vivo in the rabbit. Diabetes 1980;29:50−9.

223. Posner BI, Patel BA, Khan MN, Bergeron JJM. Effect of chloroquine on the internalization of ^{125}I-insulin into subcellular fractions of rat liver: evidence for an effect of chlorquine on Golgi elements. J Biol Chem 1982;257:5789−99.

224. King GL, Johnson SM. Receptor-mediated transport of insulin across endothelial cells. Science 1985;227:1583−6.

225. Marshall S. Degradative processing of internalized insulin in isolated adipocytes. J Biol Chem 1985;260:13517−22.

226. Shii K, Yokono K, Baba S, Roth RA. Purification and characterization of insulin-degrading enzyme from human erythrocytes. Diabetes 1986;35:675−83.

227. Varandani PT, Shroyer LA, Nafz MA. Sequential degradation of insulin by rat liver homogenates. Proc Natl Acad Sci USA 1972;69:1681−4.

228. Schade DS, Duckworth WC. In search of the subcutaneous-insulin-resistance syndrome. N Engl J Med 1986;315:147−53.

229. Fischer EH, Charbonneau H, Tonks NK. Protein tyrosine phosphatases: a diverse family of intracellular and transmembrane enzymes. Science 1991;253:401−6.

230. Sales GJ. Insulin receptor phosphotyrosyl protein phosphatases and the regulation of insulin receptor tyrosine kinase action. Adv Prot Phosphatases 1991;6:159−86.

231. Meyerovitch J, Backer JM, Kahn CR. Hepatic phosphotyrosine phosphatase activity and its alterations in diabetic rats. J Clin Invest 1989;84:976−83.

232. Meyerovitch J, Rothenberg P, Shechter Y, et al. Vanadate normalizes hyperglycemia in two mouse models of non-insulin dependent diabetes mellitus. J Clin Invest 1991;87:1286−94.

233. Meyerovitch J, Backer JM, Csermely P, et al. Insulin differentially regulates protein phosphotyrosine phosphatase activity in rat hepatoma cells. Biochemistry 1992;31:10338−44.

234. Goldstein BJ, Meyerovitch J, Zhang WR, et al. Hepatic protein-tyrosine phosphatases and their regulation in diabetes. Adv Prot Phosphatases 1991;6:1−17.

Chapter 9

GLUCAGON

ROGER H. UNGER
LELIO ORCI

HISTORY

Glucagon was discovered in 1923 after Kimball and Murlin[1] succeeded in separating the hyperglycemic factor from the hypoglycemic component of the crude extracts of canine pancreas produced by Banting and Best 2 years earlier.[2] Glucagon was purified in crystalline form by Staub et al. in 1955,[3] and the mechanism of its hyperglycemic action was elucidated soon thereafter.[4] However, the polypeptide was not widely accepted as a bona fide hormone until after 1959, when the development of a radioimmunoassay for glucagon[5] made it possible to measure its concentration in the plasma of dogs and humans.[6-8] At this point the metabolic studies of Exton, Park, and Mallette,[9,10] coupled with the physiologic studies of plasma glucagon levels,[6-8] led to the conclusion that glucagon was indeed a second hormone of the pancreas, its principal action being the prevention of hypoglycemia and cerebral neuroglycopenia.[11,12] It is now recognized that coordination of anatomically linked glucagon and insulin-secreting islet cells[13] is required to maintain glucose concentrations within the narrow range that characterizes the normal metabolic state and that this bihormonal unit constitutes one of the important homeostatic systems required for health. The observation that the normal relationship between glucagon and insulin is impaired in all forms of diabetes[8,14-16] led to the hypothesis that absolute or relative hyperglucagonemia is the cause of the hepatic overproduction of glucose and, when insulin is profoundly reduced, of hyperketonemia.[17] Since insulin deficiency in the absence of glucagon is not associated with hepatic overproduction of glucose[16,18] and ketones,[19] glucagon was said to be an essential factor in the metabolic disorder.[17]

More recently, advances in the glucagon field have pinpointed the mechanism by which glucagon induces ketogenesis[20] and elucidated its molecular biology.[21,22]

As a consequence, our understanding of the mechanisms of the major biologic actions of glucagon appears to be more complete than our current knowledge of those of insulin.

THE PREPROGLUCAGON GENE AND ITS PRODUCTS

Located on the long arm of chromosome 2,[23,24] the preproglucagon gene is expressed in pancreatic α-cells, small intestinal L-cells, and certain hypothalamic cells. Preproglucagon consists of a signal peptide, a glicentin-related polypeptide (GRPP) (amino acids 1 through 30), a Lys-Arg doublet, true glucagon (amino acids 32 through 61), an Arg-Arg doublet, glucagon-like peptide-1 (GLP-1), another Lys-Arg doublet, and finally GLP-2[23] (Fig. 9–1). The three dibasic doublets present cleavage sites that make possible the production of multiple forms derived from preproglucagon. The large N-terminal-derived molecules released from the intestinal L-cells contain the full 29 amino acid sequence of pancreatic "true glucagon."[25] This includes glicentin, the 69-amino acid molecule referred to in the earlier literature as "GLI-1" or "enteroglucagon."[26-28] Glicentin is made up of the first 69 amino acid residues of preproglucagon and was shown to be released from the small bowel during the absorption of various food stuffs, including glucose,[26] amino acids,[29] and triglycerides.[30] The 33- through 69-residue segment of glicentin, previously referred to as "GLI-2,"[31] is presumably derived from glicentin and constitutes approximately 40% of the total glucagon-like immunoreactivity of the gut.[32] Now known as oxyntomodulin, it is an inhibitor of gastric HCl secretion and of pancreatic exocrine products.[33] Oxyntomodulin binds to glucagon receptors and activates adenylate cyclase in liver membranes at about 10 to 20% of the potency of glucagon.[34]

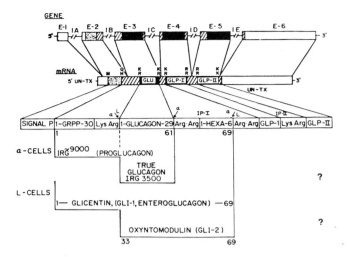

Fig. 9–1. Preproglucagon gene and its products (see text for further explanation).

Antisera directed at the C-terminal residues of glucagon do not react with oxyntomodulin because of interference by its C-terminal extension, whereas antisera directed at its N-terminal or central residues will react. The intestinal L-cells presumably lack enzymes required to cleave the C-terminal extension of oxyntomodulin, as do the hypothalamic neurons that also produce these peptides.[35] The function of these peptides in the hypothalamus is completely unknown, but they are presumably neurotransmitters. Although lacking the enzymes required to produce true glucagon, the L-cells are equipped to produce GLP-1 by cleaving it from the hexapeptide extension of glucagon and from GLP-2. It is secreted by the gut as a 7 to 36 amide, and its concentration rises in the plasma after glucose or food is ingested.[36] Pancreatic α-cells, by contrast, lack the enzymes required to process the GLP precursor to biologically active GLP.[37] The potentiating effect exerted by GLP-1 on glucose-stimulated insulin secretion has suggested that it may be the long-sought physiologic "incretin."[38] The GLPs do not compete with glucagon for liver-cell glucagon receptors and have no stimulatory effect on hepatic cAMP. However, both GLP and glucagon raise cAMP levels in hypothalamic and pituitary cells. The function of GLP-2 in these tissues is entirely unknown.

The pancreatic α-cells are unique among preproglucagon-expressing cells in that late in fetal life they develop the ability to cleave the C-terminal residue of glucagon from the Arg-Arg doublet. In certain species such as the dog, the gastric fundus also contains cells that secrete the pancreatic form of glucagon[39] and resemble pancreatic α-cells both morphologically and immunocytochemically.[40] The glucagon these cells produce is immunochemically, physicochemically, and biologically identical to pancreatic glucagon.[41,42] However, such cells have never been identified in the adult human stomach, although they have been observed in the gastric tissue of human fetuses.[43]

The pancreatic α-cells or A-cells were first discovered in 1907,[44] long before the discovery of glucagon in 1923.

However, it was not until 1962 that α-cells were proven, by immunofluorescent staining, to be the source of glucagon.[45] Today it is recognized that glucagon-secreting α-cells are one of four distinct polypeptide-secreting islet cell types: glucagon-secreting α-cells, insulin- and amylin-secreting β-cells, somatostatin-secreting δ-cells, and pancreatic polypeptide-secreting F-cells. It has been established that these cells are nonrandomly arranged in highly organized patterns that vary from species to species.[46] In the rat islet (Fig. 9–2), the glucagon and somatostatin cells form the outer rim or cortex of each islet, representing approximately 25% of the endocrine pancreas, while the α-cells, which comprise at least 70% of the endocrine pancreas, form the central portion. Pancreatic polypeptide-secreting F cells replace α-cells in a minority of islets located in the duodenal portion of the rat pancreas and in the corresponding posterior portion of the head of the human pancreas.[47] The functional significance of this anatomic arrangement is not understood.

The human islet (Fig. 9–2) appears to be a more complex version of the rat islet in that the α- and δ-cells surround a β-cell core as in the rat but form perivascular septa that subdivide each islet into pseudomicrolobules, each of which has an intercellular arrangement similar to that of a rat islet.[48]

At the electron-microscopic level, α-cell secretory granules are distinctive (Fig. 9–3). Although these granules vary in overall appearance from species to species, they generally have a central core that is more electron dense than the outer region of the granule, giving the appearance of a halo. The electron-dense core contains mature glucagon, with its C-terminal residues available for reaction with C-terminal-directed antiglucagon serum.[12] The halo region does not react with glucagon-specific antisera, suggesting that the C-terminal residues are not available—probably because the C-terminal extension of the glucagon molecule has not yet been cleaved. Since the halo region

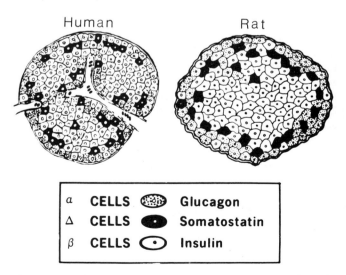

Fig. 9–2. Schematic representations of the human and rat islet showing the topologic distribution of the principal endocrine cell types.

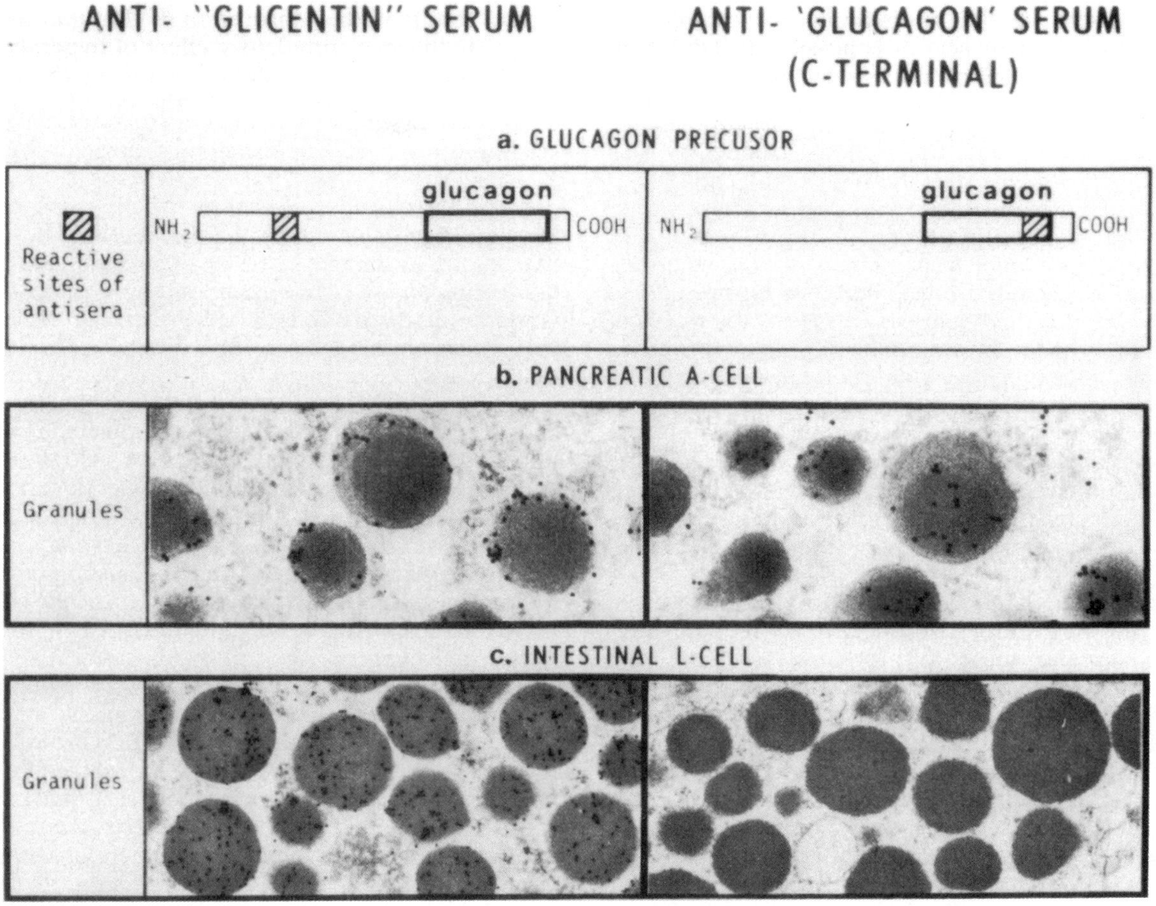

ANTI- "GLICENTIN" SERUM

ANTI- 'GLUCAGON' SERUM
(C-TERMINAL)

a. GLUCAGON PRECUSOR

b. PANCREATIC A-CELL

c. INTESTINAL L-CELL

Fig. 9–3. Electron-microscopic appearance of granules of pancreatic A (α)-cells (b) and intestinal L-cells (c), both of which express the preproglucagon gene. Differential immunocytochemistry by the protein A-gold technique using antisera directed against either an epitope in the glicentin domain of the glucagon precursor (a: left panel) or the C-terminal region of glucagon (a: right panel) reveals the central core of pancreatic '-cells to contain processed glucagon (b: right panel), while the halo of the secretory granule contains precursor (b: left panel). By contrast, the intestinal L-cells (c) contain no glucagon-like immunoreactivity but antiglicentin activity is apparent throughout the homogeneous granules. Not shown here is the reactivity of the latter, if pretreated with trypsin, with antiglucagon serum. Reprinted with permission from reference 12 (Unger RH, Orci L. Glucagon and the A cell: physiology and pathophysiology. N Engl J Med 1981;301:1518–24).

does react with antisera directed against the N-terminal and central regions of the glucagon molecule and with antiserum to glicentin, it has been concluded that the halo region contains unprocessed glucagon precursor. Small amounts of glicentin-like immunoreactivity are released from the pancreas during the secretion of glucagon.[49]

Like other cells of the endocrine pancreas, α-cells have gap junctions best discerned in freeze-fracture replicas, where they appear as patches of closely packed globular particles called "connexons." These are hydrophilic channels that link the cytosol of two contiguous cells.[50] Ions, nucleotides, and other small molecules can thus move from one cell to another without entering the extracellular space. This syncytial arrangement is believed to provide a means of intercellular communication and coordination. Within an islet the gap junctions create distinct syncytial domains or subunits.[51] Gap junctions are most prevalent in the heterocellular cortical region of

the islet, and they connect both the same and different endocrine cells to one another.

Another specialization of plasma membrane that could be important in islet function are the tight junctions, which constitute lines of fusion between the outer leaflets of contiguous cells. These are not static anatomic landmarks but rather are fluid structures that are constantly undergoing remodeling and that vary in abundance with the functional activity of the cells.[52] It has been suggested that tight junctions create domains that govern the direction of flow of the secretion products into the efferent capillaries of the islets rather than into the islet interstitium.[53] If these peptides could flow freely into the islet interstitium, secretory chaos in the endocrine pancreas might result, inasmuch as glucagon is a potent stimulus of both insulin[54] and somatostatin[55] secretion, while somatostatin is a powerful inhibitor of insulin,[56] glucagon,[57] and somatostatin.[58] There are reasons to doubt that interactions of islet hormones occur via the interstitium. For example, in the isolated canine pancreas, it is possible to inhibit the concentration of insulin and glucagon by perfusing somatostatin into the arterial circulation at a concentration that is only 10% of the level of endogenous somatostatin exiting via the venous effluent.[53] This finding strongly implies that the high endogenous concentration of secreted somatostatin did not have direct access to the somatostatin receptors on α- and β-cells. A hormone-poor zone from which locally secreted somatostatin is excluded must therefore be present on islet cells to enable them to respond to the low systemic levels of the hormone. If islet hormones could freely diffuse through the islet interstitium, their very high local concentrations would prevent responses by islet cells to the relatively minute levels of islet hormones in the arterial circulation. The fact that low arterial levels of the hormones influence islet-cell secretion suggests that the newly secreted peptides are excluded from free access to the islet interstitial spaces.

If, in fact, tight junctions constitute a barrier against regurgitation of secretory products into the islet interstitium, a vascular route for interactions of the islet peptides must be the major pathway. If so, the microcirculation of the islets becomes an extraordinarily important system for regulation of normal islet function. It has been demonstrated in the rat that afferent blood vessels penetrate the cortex of the islet into the central β-cell region, where they ramify into smaller capillaries that radiate centrifugally into the heterocellular cortex.[59] More recently, it has been proposed that each islet cell may have both an afferent and efferent capillary in contact with the specialized zones of the cells[60]; the afferent capillary would presumably bring signals to the "sensory pole" of islet cells on which their various receptors are displayed. The efferent capillary would abut on the secretory pole of the islet cell, the region in which exocytosis of secretory granules takes place.[61] The inhibitory effect of insulin on glucagon secretion, perhaps the single most important regulatory interaction between an islet hormone and an islet cell, is believed to take place entirely within the microcirculation of the islets, which flows from centrally located β-cells to the peripherally situated α-cells.[62] Actions of other islet hormones such as glucagon and somatostatin on β-cells would necessarily occur via the systemic circulation, since the direction of blood flow is out of the islets.

GLUCAGON SECRETION

Glucose-Insulin Actions on Glucagon Secretion

In keeping with the role of glucagon as the guarantor of cerebral fuel delivery, glycemia is the primary regulator of α-cell secretion. Glucose acts on α-cells to suppress glucagon release both directly and through insulin.

Ever since the discovery by Samols et al. that insulin is a powerful inhibitor of glucagon secretion,[63] efforts have been made to sort out the relative importance of glucose

versus insulin in the suppression of glucagon secretion in vivo. The normal stimulatory effect of hyperglycemia on β-cells maintains a parallelism between the concentrations of glucose and insulin in the circulation and thus creates an experimental obstacle to dissection of their relative roles in the suppression of glucagon by glucose. In vitro studies of isolated α-cells exhibit glucose suppression of glucagon secretion in the absence of any insulin.[64] However, earlier in vivo studies had indicated that hyperglucagonemia of severe insulin-deprived diabetic dogs could not be suppressed by hyperglycemia but could be dramatically reduced to normal levels by even very small amounts of insulin, a finding that suggested that glucose controlled the glucagon secretion only indirectly via its stimulatory effect on insulin secretion and could not directly suppress glucagon in vivo.[15] Recently, however, it has been demonstrated that the apparent insensitivity of diabetic hyperglucagonemia to a further increase in hyperglycemia is apparent rather than real; in diabetes the α-cells have already been suppressed maximally by the preexisting steady-state hyperglycemia, albeit to concentrations that are still far above normal. This residual hyperglucagonemia is entirely the consequence of insulin deficiency and is completely corrected by repletion with insulin.[65] Thus, in diabetic animals the hyperglucagonemia of the insulin-deficient state represents the hyperglucagonemic effect of insulin deficiency minus the glucagon-lowering effect of the resulting hyperglycemia; if the hyperglycemia is eliminated by means of treatment with the glucuretic agent phloridzin, the hyperglucagonemia becomes far greater than before when hyperglycemia was present.[65] This excess hyperglucagonemia is suppressible with glucose (Fig. 9–4).

Under normal conditions, glycemia and insulinemia are tightly coupled, making it impossible to isolate the two influences from each other. In view of the evidence of morphologic and functional β- and α-cell linkage in rat islets, the influence of insulin would seem transcendent. As mentioned, the microcirculatory pathway from β-cells to the outer rim of the islets makes the α-cells among the first targets of insulin action and exposes them to the highest insulin concentration in the body—estimated to be 1000 times its systemic level.[62] Moreover, as shown in Figure 9–5, there is compelling evidence indicating that insulin within the microcirculation of the islet exerts a tonic suppressive effect upon glucagon secretion. This is based on the report that glucagon secretion rises dramatically the moment the neutralizing anti-insulin serum enters the microcirculation of the islet.[62]

Control by Neurotransmitters

The islets of Langerhans receive endings of adrenergic, cholinergic, peptidergic, and purinergic nerves, which form a virtual "basket" around them.[67,68] Neurotransmitted signals can elicit secretory responses in a matter of seconds and thus have distinct advantages over the slower signals carried via the circulation. For example, if the α-cell response to the increased glucose requirements induced by exercise occurred only after hypoglycemia had occurred, the ability to perform that exertion would be compromised by cerebral neuroglucopenia. Instead the α-cells respond at the very onset of exercise as the result of exercise-induced adrenergic signals originating in the lateral hypothalamus, thereby preventing rather than correcting hypoglycemia.[69] Similarly, the islet hormone response to the ingestion of food begins not after a rise in the concentration of the absorbed nutrient, but rather at the time of food absorption.[70] This is attributed to cholinergic and perhaps peptidergic signals neurotransmitted to the islets, followed by humoral signals from gastrointestinal hormones such as GLP-1, gastric inhibitory peptide (GIP), cholecystokinin, gastrin, secretin, and others released in the course of nutrient absorption. Thus, the initial response of glucagon and insulin is under way before the initial rise in the concentration of the ingested nutrient has occurred. This "anticipatory response" is believed to be an important function of the so-called enteroinsular axis.[71]

Circulating Glucagon

Glucagon is released from the pancreatic α-cells into the plasma predominately as 3485-kilodalton (kd) glucagon.[72] Plasma also contains a 9000-kd moiety that reacts in the radioimmunoassay for glucagon; it is believed to be an incompletely processed intermediate of glucagon biosynthesis and has been shown to be biologically inactive.[72] This fraction is elevated in the plasma of patients with glucagonoma[73,74] and with renal insufficiency.[75] A smaller glucagon immunoreactive fraction of

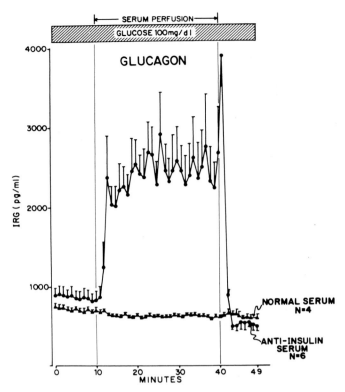

Fig. 9–5. The effect of anti-insulin serum (closed circles) on glucagon secretion (mean ± SEM) in the isolated perfused rat pancreas. Normal guinea pig serum (closed triangles) was used as a control. Reprinted with permission from reference 66 (Unger RH, Orci L. Glucagon. In: Ellenberg M, Rifkin H, eds. Diabetes mellitus. Theory and practice. 4th ed. New York: Elsevier Science Publishing Co, 1990:104–20).

approximately 2000 kd had been considered to be a minor degradation product of glucagon without biologic activity.[72] However, the demonstration that a C-terminal decapeptide derivative of glucagon (residues 19–29) has biologic activity[76] raises the possibility that this fraction may have some physiologic importance.

Glucagon Receptors

The actions of glucagon upon its major target tissue, the liver, begins with binding to the hepatic glucagon receptor. The glucagon receptor is a glycoprotein of 63 kd that is sensitive to GTP and to an excess of unlabeled glucagon.[77] A second 33,000-kd species of glucagon receptor has also been reported. The larger receptor contains a minimum of four N-linked glycans, which make up approximately 18,000 kd of its mass. The 21,000-kd fragment of the receptor contains both the glucagon-binding function and the ability to interact with the guanine nucleotide-binding regulatory protein G_s. This fragment has no N-linked glycans. The hepatocyte glucagon receptor, referred to as GR-2, exists in two functionally distinct forms, a high-affinity form that comprises 1% of the total glucagon-binding sites and a low-affinity form that makes up 99%.[78] At its customary portal-vein concentration, glucagon is equally distrib-

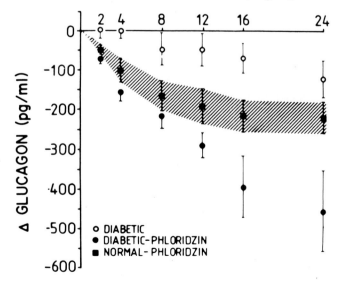

Fig. 9–4. The data from Figure 9–1 replotted to show cumulative reduction in glucagon (mean ± SEM) as a function of glucose infusion rate. The hatched area brackets the normal mean ± SEM. Reprinted from reference 65 (Starke A, Grundy S, McGarry JD, Unger RH. Correction of hyperglycemia with phloridzin restores the glucagon response to glucose in insulindeficient dogs. Proc Natl Acad Sci USA 1985;82:1544–6).

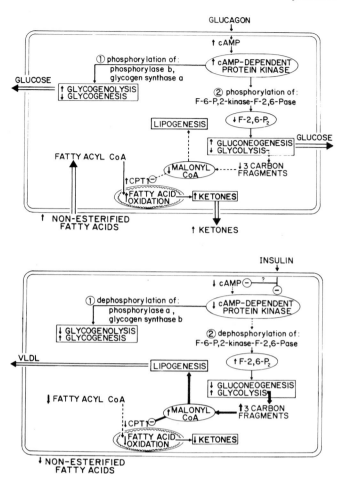

Fig. 9–6. Upper panel: Glucagon-induced catabolic cascade in hepatocytes. Binding of glucagon to the regulatory subunit of its receptor activates adenylate cyclase → increased cAMP. This activates cAMP-dependent protein kinase, which initiates all the known actions of glucagon by phosphorylating certain key enzymes, thereby redirecting their activities toward catabolism. Phosphorylation of inactive phosphorylase b (1) converts it to the active a form, thereby promoting glycogenolysis and enhanced glucose production. Phosphorylation of glycogen synthase a (1) inactivates it to the b form and reduces glycogen formation. Phosphorylation of the bifunctional enzyme (2) that regulates fructose $2,6-P_2$ synthesis and degradation (F-6 P,2-kinase, F-2,6-Pase) lowers its kinase activity and increases its phosphatase action. This depletes $F-2,6-P_2$, a stimulator of glycolysis and inhibitor of gluconeogenesis. The result of $F-2,6-P_2$ depletion is enhanced glucose production from nonglucose precursors and diminished formation of pyruvate, the substrate for lipogenesis. Consequently, levels of malonyl Co-A, the first committed step in lipogenesis, are reduced. This abolishes the inhibitory action of malonyl CoA upon carnitine palmitoyltransferase 1 (CPT-1), the enzyme responsible for transesterification of fatty acyl CoA to fatty acylcarnitine, allowing entry of fatty acids into the mitochondrion, the site of β-oxidation to ketones. Fatty acyl CoA derived from free fatty acids delivered to liver from adipocytes is increased as the consequence of deficiency of insulin, an antilipolytic hormone. Thus, the high glucagon-low insulin mixture induces the full catabolic syndrome of increased glucose production and accelerated ketogenesis. Lower panel: Insulin-induced anabolic cascade. Insulin, when present in sufficient concentration, lowers glucagon release and reverses the glucagon-mediated catabolic cascade. Cyclic AMP is lowered, probably by insulin-mediated increase in phosphodiesterase activity. The major effect of insulin may be to inactivate the cAMP-dependent protein kinase (see text). Dephosphorylation of enzymes at (1) and (2) promotes glycogen formation and increases $F-2, 6-P_2$ levels, thereby stimulating glycolysis and inhibiting gluconeogenesis. Pyruvate becomes available for lipogenesis, increasing malonyl CoA and inhibiting CPT-1. Ketone formation slows and fatty acid synthesis increases. Fatty acids are esterified to triglycerides (TG), which are then packaged and released as VLDL. Plasma-free fatty acids are much lower but continue to contribute to triglyceride and VLDL formation. Modified from reference 84 (Unger RH, Foster DW. Diabetes mellitus. In: Wilson JD, Foster DW, eds. Williams textbook of endocrinology. 6th ed. Philadelphia: WB Saunders, 1985:1018-80).

uted between the high- and low-affinity GR-2 populations. The inhibitory effect of glucagon upon hepatic glycogen formation is attributed to occupancy of the high-affinity GR-2 population.[79] Conversion of GR-2 from one affinity state to another is time- and temperature-dependent.[79]

When glucagon binds with GR-2, it interacts with the stimulatory G_s.[80] This frees the α-subunit of G_s to activate the enzyme adenylate cyclase. Another G protein, G_i, inhibits adenylate cyclase.[80] Activated adenylate cyclase catalyzes the conversion of ATP to cAMP, thus increasing its intracellular level within seconds after the interaction between glucagon and GR-2. The intracellular level of cyclic AMP is lowered by phosphodiesterase. The ret glucagon receptor has now been cloned and expressed in kidney cell lines. The cloned receptor bound glucagon and increased both cAMP and intracellular calcium.[80a]

Glucagon Actions Mediated by cAMP

Cyclic AMP (cAMP) binds to and activates dimeric cAMP-dependent protein kinase in a dose-dependent manner by dissociating its regulatory subunits and thus liberating its catalytic subunits.[81] The activated kinase initiates all known actions of glucagon by promoting phosphorylation of intracellular enzymes with ATP, the phosphoryl donor. Insulin is believed to oppose gluca-

gon action at this site by reducing the dissociation of the regulatory subunits and thereby decreasing its activity.[82,83] As depicted in Figure 9–6A, the glucagon-stimulated increase in cAMP-dependent protein kinase activity enhances glycogenolysis and decreases glycogen synthesis by phosphorylating phosphorylase b kinase, which converts it to active phosphorylase a, the rate-limiting enzyme for hepatic glycogenolysis. Simultaneous phosphorylation of glycogen synthase a converts it to the inactive b form and prevents glycogen formation.[85,86]

At the same time, hepatic gluconeogenesis and ketogenesis are stimulated by glucagon through phosphorylation of at least two critical enzymes, 6-phosphofructo-2-kinase/fructose-2,6-bis phosphatase and L-type pyruvate kinase.[87] The former is a unique bifunctional enzyme that controls both glycolysis and gluconeogenesis, depending upon its phosphorylation state. When unphosphorylated, as in the fed state, the enzyme is a kinase (6-phosphofructo-2-kinase or PFK-2). It thus raises the level of fructose-2,6-biphosphate ($F-2,6-P_2$), a key regulator that allosterically increases 6-phosphofructo-1-kinase (PFK-1), the rate-limiting enzyme for glycolysis, and simultaneously inhibits the rate-limiting enzyme of gluconeogenesis, fructose-1,6-biphosphate (FBPase-1).[88-91] Thus, in the fed state the level of $F-2,6-P_2$ is high, promoting glycolysis and inhibiting gluconeogenesis. When the enzyme is phosphorylated, as in the fasted state or in diabetes, the high levels of glucagon and low levels of insulin result in phosphorylation of the enzyme, which makes it a phosphatase. This lowers $F-2,6-P_2$, thereby inactivating the rate-limiting enzyme of glycolysis, PFK-1, and stimulating the rate-limiting enzyme of gluconeogenesis, FBPase-1. The reduction in $F-2,6-P_2$ decreases glycolytic flux and enhances gluconeogenesis as shown below:

↑ cAMP ↑ cAMP-dependent protein kinase
↓
↑ phosphorylation of the bifunctional enzyme
↓
↓ $F-2,6-P_2$
↓
↓ glycolysis and ↑ gluconeogenesis
(Fig. 9–6, upper panel)

The second important hepatic action of glucagon results in phosphorylation of L-type pyruvate kinase, which inactivates it and spares phospho-enol pyruvate for gluconeogenesis.[92] Glucagon also enhances gluconeogenesis through stimulation of pyruvate carboxylase activity[93] via an unknown mechanism that does not involve phosphorylation.[94]

The antagonistic action of insulin upon these effects of glucagon is believed to be exerted first by enhancing the phosphodiesterase activity of the hepatocyte membrane, which reduces the level of cAMP, and second by opposing the glucagon-mediated activation of cAMP-dependent protein kinase[83] so as to reduce the overall phosphorylation state of the enzymes of glycogenesis and glycogenolysis, as well as of the bifunctional enzyme and the L-type pyruvate kinase (Fig. 9–6, lower panel). The actions of insulin can be depicted as follows:

↓ cAMP ↓ cAMP-dependent kinase,
↓
↑ glycogen synthase a, ↓ phosphorylase a,
↓
↑ $F-2,6-P_2$, ↑ pyruvate kinase
↓
↑ glycolysis and ↓ gluconeogenesis.

As depicted in Figure 9–6 (upper panel), the stimulatory effect of glucagon on hepatic ketone production is linked to its effects on glucose metabolism. However, when insulin is high relative to glucagon, as in the fed state, the bifunctional enzyme is not phosphorylated and thus acts as a kinase, increasing the flow of three-carbon fragments down the glycolytic pathway of the liver and thus providing the substrate for lipogenesis. The resulting glucose-derived fatty acids are esterified to triglycerides and secreted by the liver as very-low-density lipoprotein (VLDL). VLDL is transported to the adipocytes, where the fatty acids are stored. Under such conditions of active lipogenesis, oxidation of newly formed fatty acids to

ketones must be completely blocked so as to avoid a futile cycle. The block is produced by the first committed intermediate in fatty acid synthesis, malonyl CoA, a powerful inhibitor of carnitine palmitoyl transferase-1 (CPT-1), the transesterifying enzyme for fatty acyl CoA to fatty acyl carnitine. This transesterification is required for entry of the fatty acyl into the mitochondria, where oxidation to ketones takes place. The high levels of malonyl CoA that form during lipogenesis block this conversion and hence prevent a futile cycle in which newly formed fatty acids would immediately be oxidized to ketones (see Foster and McGarry[87] for review).

However, in the fasting and diabetic states when glucagon is high relative to insulin, the levels of $F-2,6-P_2$ are reduced. This blocks glycolysis in the liver and reduces the flow of three-carbon fragments, the substrate for lipogenesis. Malonyl CoA levels therefore become vanishingly low, and CPT-1 is released from inhibition. The low levels of insulin in starvation or diabetes increase lipolysis in adipocytes, thereby augmenting the hepatic supply of fatty acids transported via the circulation to the liver. The low hepatic levels of malonyl CoA abolish the normal inhibition of CPT-1, allowing transesterification to fatty acyl carnitine and entry into the mitochondria, where oxidation to ketones takes place.[87]

Glucagon Action Not Mediated by cAMP

The existence of a second glucagon receptor, GR-1, has been postulated because of evidence that glucagon has biologic activity independent of cAMP.[86] The presumption is that glucagon acts through GR-1 to enhance the breakdown of inositol phospholipid and elevate cytosolic Ca^{++} released from the endoplasmic reticulum. In the presence of calcium and phosphytidyl serine, 1,2-diacylglycerol (DAG) activates protein kinase C. It is not yet known which proteins are phosphorylated as a consequence of protein kinase C activation, nor have the metabolic consequences of these events been elucidated. A current assumption, however, is that glucagon acts both via cAMP-mediated and inositol triphosphate (IP_3)-mediated pathways and its effects on glycogenolysis, gluconeogenesis, and ureagenesis are the result of phosphorylation of key enzymes via both pathways. It has been suggested that at low concentrations of glucagon, glucagon activity is largely mediated by GR-1 receptors, while at more elevated concentrations mediation by GR-2 receptors predominates.[95] However, further validation of this concept is required.

Glucagon as a Prohormone

The dibasic doublet in the glucagon molecule (Arg 17-Arg 18) renders glucagon susceptible to tryptic cleavage to form a 19- to 29-residue fragment. This peptide does not activate adenylate cyclase but inhibits the Ca^{++} pump in liver plasma membrane vesicles with an efficiency that is far greater than that of glucagon.[76] This effect is dependent on guanine nucleotides. It remains to be determined if glucagon 19–29 is secreted from the pancreas in this form or if it is generated after release of the full glucagon molecule into plasma—

possibly by proteases in the plasma membranes of liver cells. Neither the glucagon 19–29 receptor nor its metabolic effects have as yet been identified.

THE PHYSIOLOGIC ROLES OF GLUCAGON

The primary function of glucagon is to maintain a rate of glucose production sufficient to meet the glucose requirements of the moment. In the basal state approximately two-thirds of the basal output of glucose by the canine liver is driven by glucagon,[96] and in humans approximately 75% of net glucose production is mediated by glucagon.[97] It has been demonstrated that when glucagon secretion is blocked by somatostatin infusion and hepatic glucose production is thereby reduced, the basal glucose concentration can no longer be maintained within the normal range but declines progressively to hypoglycemia. This occurs even in the total absence of insulin because the brain is the major consumer of glucose and it utilizes glucose independently of insulin. Thus, glucagon, through its ability to maintain glucose production at a rate equal to consumption, is the primary determinant of the postabsorptive glucose concentration. After an overnight fast, glucagon-induced glucose production is primarily the consequence of hepatic glycogenolysis. After a more prolonged fast, hepatic glycogen stores are profoundly reduced and the main source of glucagon-driven glucose production is via enhanced gluconeogenesis.

When the levels of glucagon increase above the basal concentration, without a change in insulin levels, glucose production will rise by more than twofold within 15 minutes.[98] In diabetic patients maintained on a constant basal insulin infusion, the stimulation of endogenous glucagon secretion by the administration of arginine will cause the glucagon concentration to rise by 100 pg/mL, and this is accompanied by a doubling of glucose production.[99] However, these effects of increments in glucagon upon hepatic glucagon production are demonstrable only if the insulin concentration is fixed. In normal individuals given exogenous glucagon, the stimulatory effect upon the secretion of insulin will virtually cancel out the action of glucagon on the liver.

The glycogenolytic action of glucagon begins to diminish after 1 or 2 hours of glucagon infusion, and hepatic glucose production returns to its original level.[98] This waning of glucagon's effect may be due to an inhibitory effect of glucagon-induced hyperglycemia upon glycogenolysis,[100] which persists, but at a lower rate.[101] The gluconeogenic and ketogenic effects of glucagon on the liver do not diminish with time.[102,103] This explains why hyperglucagonemia causes sustained hyperglycemia in insulin-dependent diabetic animals[96,104] and in patients.[18,105] As mentioned above, insulin antagonizes the action of glucagon on the liver by stimulating phosphodiesterase activity and inactivating cAMP-dependent protein kinase. It is therefore the relative concentrations of insulin and glucagon, i.e., the molar ratio of insulin to glucagon, that determines the net effect upon hepatic glucose production.[106] A decline in glucagon without a parallel decline in insulin will result in a prompt decline in glucose production, while a decrease in insulin

without a parallel change in glucagon will rapidly augment hepatic glucose output.

THE PHYSIOLOGY OF GLUCOREGULATION

Resting State

Under normal circumstances, glucose produced by the liver is the only source of cerebral fuels in the fasting state. Normal neurologic function and, indeed, survival of the species require continuous delivery of this fuel to the brain throughout life. The insulin-glucagon system provides a remarkably precise means for maintaining normoglycemia and adequate flow of glucose to the central nervous system during fasting and exercise, while preventing excessive hyperglycemia during meals. In humans the brain requires approximately 6 g of glucose/hour while other tissues use about 4 g/hour in the resting state. Therefore, in the resting/fasting state the liver must produce glucose at a rate of 10 g/hour to avoid hypoglycemia[12] (Fig. 9–7a). As mentioned, glucagon stimulation of glucose production accounts for 75% of hepatic glucose output, evidence that deficiency of glucagon would cause rapid and fatal hypoglycemia.

Fight or Flight

Optimal function during sudden and often intense physical effort required in emergency "fight or flight" circumstances demands an instant increase in fuel supply for muscle without a reduction in cerebral fuel delivery. The skeletal muscles contain a supply of glycogen and lipids that can provide fuel for a limited time, but for sustained muscular activity, a major increase in glucose and free fatty acids is needed. Despite the important role of free fatty acids as a fuel for muscle, they never completely replace glucose, even in highly trained athletes.[107] Indeed, the availability of circulating glucose is a limiting factor for prolonged muscular work, as well as for normal neurologic function. For this reason hepatic glucose production must constantly equal the rate of glucose utilization, no matter how high this may be, to assure optimal performance. Catecholamines and glucagon are the two major mediators of this hepatic adjustment to the "fight or flight" crisis. In humans the contribution of glucagon in exhaustive exercise is believed to be less important than in the dog, in which glucagon exerts a direct influence on the control of glucose production during exercise.[107] The role of catecholamines, however, may be even more important than that of glucagon; in addition to directly enhancing hepatic glucose production, the catecholamines stimulate glucagon secretion[108] and reduce insulin levels during exercise.[109] The reduction in insulin plays a critical role in limiting glucose uptake by tissues that play no role in the "fight or flight" crisis, e.g., adipose tissue. The reduction in plasma insulin levels does not limit glucose uptake by the exercising muscles because the number of insulin receptors exposed to circulating insulin increases as a consequence of the marked increase in blood flow through the active muscles. The net result is a restriction in glucose uptake to the tissues that need it most, i.e., the brain and the exercising muscles (Fig. 9–7b).

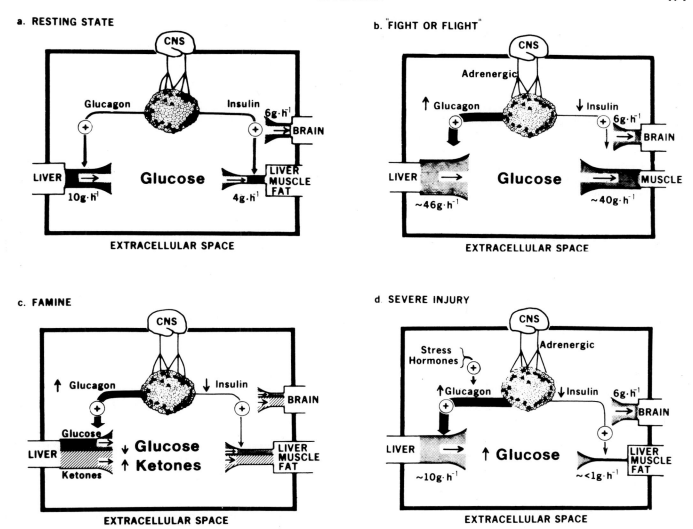

Fig. 9–7. Schematic representation of islet cell role in fuel homeostasis under various circumstances. Extracellular glucose and space is represented by a box. The islet is depicted as being in contact with extracellular fluid and with the central nervous system. Glucagon and insulin are released to stimulate, respectively, hepatic glucose production and uptake by tissues other than the brain (liver, muscle, and fat). The approximate rates of glucose flux into the box from the liver and out of the box into the brain and the insulin-sensitive tissues are indicated whenever possible next to the funnels leading from or to these tissues. a. Resting state: insulin and glucagon secretion occur at a rate required to maintain equality between hepatic glucose production and the sum of insulin-independent uptake by the brain and insulin-mediated uptake by liver, muscle, and fat. b. "Fight or flight": adrenergic effects on the islets enhance glucagon secretion and suppress insulin secretion. The marked increase in glucose uptake by the exercising muscle is precisely matched by an increase in hepatic glucose production mediated both by the higher glucagon levels and direct adrenergic effects on the liver (see also text). c. Famine: a modest increase in glucagon coupled with a decline in insulin enhances hepatic fuel production. Initially, glucose is the major fuel. Within a few days, however, the reduced insulin permits increased release of free fatty acids from adipose tissue (not shown), thereby providing the liver with substrate for ketogenesis. Ketone levels rise to replace glucose as the major cerebral fuel, thereby sparing protein that would otherwise be used for gluconeogenesis. d. Severe injury: adrenergic effects on the islets increase glucagon and suppress insulin secretion. The glucagon-mediated increase in hepatic glucose production is excluded by the decline in insulin levels from the insulin-sensitive tissues, liver, muscle, and fat. This raises arterial glucose concentrations and thus maintains cerebral glucose delivery despite a reduction in cerebral blood flow from the shock. Stress hyperglycemia is abetted by stress hormones such as growth hormone, β-endorphin, catecholamines, and cortisol, all of which increase glucagon secretion. Glucagon's effects on the liver are potentiated by cortisol. Norepinephrine released from adrenergic nerve endings in the liver is also of great importance. Reprinted with permission from reference 12 (Unger RH, Orci L. Glucagon and the A cell: physiology and pathophysiology. N Engl J Med 1981;301:1518–24).

Circulatory Failure

Circulatory failure, irrespective of cause, will be associated with reduction in cerebral glucose delivery as a consequence of hypoperfusion. The islets respond to this life-threatening state by secreting an insulin/glucagon mixture that will increase concentrations of arterial glucose (Fig. 9–7c). By doubling the arterial glucose concentration during a 50% reduction in cerebral blood flow, cerebral glucose delivery would theoretically remain normal.[12] This is usually referred to as "stress hyperglycemia." It is mediated by catecholamine-stimulated hyperglucagonemia and by the direct effect of norepinephrine on hepatic glucose production. In addition, the potentiation of the hepatic effects of glucagon by increased secretion of cortisol,[110] which also enhances glucagon secretion,[111] helps in raising glucose concentrations. Insulin secretion is restricted by catecholamines from rising in response to stress hyperglycemia, which otherwise would result in its correction. By blocking the insulin response to the hyperglycemia, glucose uptake by insulin-requiring tissues of the body such as fat and muscles is inhibited, thus guaranteeing that the circulating glucose will not be squandered for nonessential metabolism. The adrenergic effects upon α- and β-cells are crucially important: the enhancement of glucagon secretion and reduction of insulin secretion prevent the normal islet cell responses to hyperglycemia, i.e., glucose-mediated suppression of glucagon secretion and stimulation of insulin secretion to correct the hyperglycemia.

Meals

The normal coordination of insulin and glucagon secretion maintains nutrient homeostasis during ingestion of various foods (Fig. 9–7d). With a carbohydrate-rich meal, the mission of the islets is to prevent excessive hyperglycemia. The appropriate secretion of insulin is critical in achieving this goal, with the concomitant suppression of glucagon playing a relatively modest role. Inasmuch as the response of islet hormones to the ingestion of food precedes the initial increase in arterial nutrient levels, it is assumed that cholinergic signals and gut hormones such as GLP-1, GIP, and other factors provide the earliest signals to the β-cells, permitting them to prevent, rather than to correct, any major increase in the levels of circulating glucose.

The response to a protein meal also is mediated largely by signals arising from the gastrointestinal tract rather than by the amino acid levels themselves, which at high concentrations are powerful stimuli of both the β- and α-cells. The response to a carbohydrate-free meal is the only physiologic circumstance in which insulin and glucagon levels rise in parallel. Insulin is required for normal utilization of amino acids, while glucagon is needed to replace glucose that is moving into cells as a consequence of the aminogenic increase in insulin levels. Thus, under normal circumstances ingestion of a carbohydrate-free protein meal will not result in hypoglycemia.

GLUCAGON AND DIABETES: PATHOPHYSIOLOGY

The tightly coupled relationships between α- and β-cells described above predict that derangements in β-cell function will be associated with reciprocal changes in α-cell function. An absolute increase in plasma glucagon is invariably present in severe insulin deficiency in every species thus far studied.[12] The hyperglucagonemia of insulin deficiency responds dramatically to replacement doses of insulin.[15] In diabetes without insulin deficiency, glucagon levels may be normal or high in the absolute sense but are always increased relative to the ambient glucose concentration.[112] It is permissible to define overt diabetes (both insulin-dependent and non-insulin-dependent forms) as conditions in which production of endogenous insulin is never sufficient to suppress glucagon secretion and/or to overcome its effects on hepatic glucose production. The former defect is manifested by failure of a carbohydrate meal to suppress glucagon levels in all forms of diabetes and by the exaggerated rise in glucagon levels in response to a protein meal[14] or an arginine infusion.[8] Both these defects are corrected if the meals are accompanied by an infusion of insulin designed to simulate the normal response of endogenous insulin levels to such challenges.[99,113] Is glucagon required for the hepatic abnormalities of diabetes? The "essential" role of glucagon in the overproduction of glucose and ketones that characterizes uncontrolled diabetes is strongly supported by clinical and experimental evidence. No instance of uncontrolled diabetes has yet been reported in which glucagon is absent. Even in totally depancreatized humans, measurable levels of glucagon are present[114] when the patient is hyperglycemic due to poor control with insulin. However, since such patients are extremely sensitive to insulin administration, which promptly reduces glucagon levels to unmeasurable levels, this glucagon presumably being derived from intestinal sources, the reported cases of so-called diabetes without glucagon[115] were studied only while patients were receiving insulin treatment. There is, however, a case report of a totally depancreatized patient in whom discontinuation of insulin was not associated with the presence of measurable glucagon in plasma; this patient did not become hyperglycemic when insulin treatment was discontinued.[116] This clinical experience duplicates the studies in totally depancreatized dogs treated with somatostatin to suppress extrapancreatic glucagon secretion[16]; in these dogs normoglycemia persisted in the absence of insulin treatment. Similarly, deficiency of extrapancreatic glucagon induced in totally depancreatized dogs by hypophysectomy (Houssay animal) permits discontinuation of insulin therapy without the development of hyperglycemia[117]; hyperglycemia rapidly appears if replacement doses of glucagon are administered. In insulin-dependent diabetic patients, the infusion of somatostatin to suppress glucagon secretion makes it possible to discontinue insulin administration without inducing the overproduction of glucose and ketones that occurs in the presence of glucagon[19] (Fig. 9–8). The metabolic syndrome of combined insulin-glucagon deficiency is characterized by impaired glucose utilization and increased lipolysis without the endogenous hyperglycemia and hyperketonemia that would otherwise occur in the presence of glucagon.[17] Finally, the administration of a glucagon antagonist[118] that prevents activation of hepatic adenylate cyclase[116] or a neutralizing antibody to glucagon[119] also prevents the usual effects of insulin deficiency. Thus, insulin deficiency is necessary, but without glucagon it is not sufficient to produce the endogenous hyperglycemia and ketoacidosis of insulin deprivation. It is now clear that the major action of insulin on hepatic glycogenolysis, gluconeogenesis, and

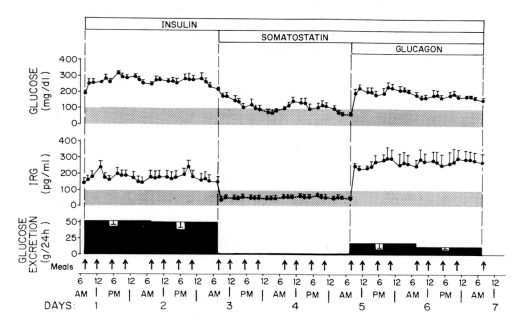

Fig. 9—8. Effects of somatostatin and somatostatin with glucagon (glucagon) on the daily profiles of mean (± SEM). Levels of glucose and glucose immunoreactive glucagon (IRG) on glucose excretion in four patients with Type 1 diabetes receiving a continuous insulin infusion and a diet containing 150 g of carbohydrate per day. Reprinted with permission from reference 18 (Raskin P, Unger RH. Hyperglucagonemia and its suppression: importance in the metabolic control of diabetes. N Engl J Med 1978;299:433–6).

ketogenesis is to oppose glucagon-mediated effects. In the absence of glucagon, hepatic cAMP is low and cAMP-dependent protein kinase is inactive, leaving insulin with no cAMP to reduce or cAMP-dependent kinase to inactivate. Glucagon suppression without impairment of insulin response is therefore a plausible strategy for blood glucose control in the treatment of diabetes.

REFERENCES

1. Kimball CP, Murlin JR. Aqueous extracts of pancreas. III. Some precipitation reactions of insulin. J Biol Chem 1923:58:337–46.
2. Banting FG, Best CH. The internal secretion of the pancreas. J Lab Clin Med 1921;7:251–66.
3. Staub A, Sinn LG, Behrens OK. Purification and crystallization of glucagon. J Biol Chem 1955;214:619–32.
4. Sutherland EW. Studies on the mechanism of hormone action. Science 1972;177:401–8.
5. Unger RH, Eisentraut AM, McCall MS, et al. Glucagon antibodies and their use for immunoassay for glucagon. Proc Soc Exp Biol Med 1959;102:621–3.
6. Unger RH, Eisentraut AM, McCall MS, Madison LL. Demonstration of the hormonal status of endogenous glucagon. In: Wolstenholme GEW, Cameron MP, eds. Immunoassay of hormones. CIBA Foundation Colloquia on Endocrinology. Vol 14. London: J & A Churchill, 1962:212–24.
7. Unger RH, Eisentraut AM, Madison LL. The effects of total starvation upon the levels of circulating glucagon and insulin in man. J Clin Invest 1963;42:1031–9.
8. Unger RH, Aguilar-Parada E, Muller WA, Eisentraut AM. Studies of pancreatic alpha cell function in normal and diabetic subjects. J Clin Invest 1970;49:837–48.
9. Exton JH, Park CR. Control of gluconeogenesis in liver. III. Effects of L-lactate, pyruvate, fructose, glucagon, epinephrine and adenosine 3′,5′-monophosphate on gluconeogenic intermediates in the perfused rat liver.J Biol Chem 1969;244:1424–33.
10. Mallette LE, Exton JH, Park CR. Control of gluconeogenesis from amino acids in the perfused rat liver. J Biol Chem 1969;244:5713–23.
11. Unger RH. Diabetes and the alpha cell. Diabetes 1976;25:136–51.
12. Unger RH, Orci L. Glucagon and the A-cell: physiology and pathophysiology. N Engl J Med 1981;304:1518–24, 1575–80.
13. Orci L, Malaisse-Lagae F, Ravazzola M, et al. A morphologic basis for intercellular communication between α- and β-cells in the endocrine pancreas. J Clin Invest 1975;56:1066–70.
14. Muller WA, Faloona GR, Aguilar-Parada E, Unger RH. Abnormal alpha-cell function in diabetes. Response to carbohydrate and protein ingestion. N Engl J Med 1970;283:109–15.
15. Muller WA, Faloona GR, Unger RH. The effect of experimental insulin deficiency on glucagon secretion. J Clin Invest 1971;50:1992–9.
16. Dobbs RE, Sakurai H, Sasaki H, et al. Glucagon: role in the hyperglycemia of diabetes mellitus. Science 1975;187:544–7.
17. Unger RH, Orci L. The essential role of glucagon in the pathogenesis of diabetes mellitus. Lancet 1975;1:14–6.
18. Raskin P, Unger RH. Hyperglucagonemia and its suppression: importance in the metabolic control of diabetes. N Engl J Med 1978;299:433–6.
19. Gerich JE, Lorenzi M, Bier DM, et al. Prevention of human ketoacidosis by somatostatin: evidence for an essential role of glucagon. N Engl J Med 1975;292:985–9.
20. McGarry JD. New perspectives in the regulation of ketogenesis. Diabetes 1979;28:517–23.
21. Bell GI, Sanchez-Pescador R, Laybourn PJ, Najarian RC. Exon duplication and divergence in the human preproglucagon gene [Letter]. Nature 1983;304:368–71.
22. Lund PK, Goodman RH, Montminy MR, et al. Anglerfish islet pre-proglucagon. II. Nucleotide and corresponding amino acid sequence of the cDNA. J Biol Chem 1983;258:3280–4.
23. Tricoli JV, Bell GI, Shows TB. The human glucagon gene is located on chromosome 2. Diabetes 1984;33:200–2.

24. Schroeder WT, Lopez LC, Harper ME, Saunders GF. Localization of the human glucagon gene (GCG) to chromosome segment 2q36→A37. Cytogenet Cell Genet 1984;38:76–9.

25. Thim L, Moody AJ. The primary structure of porcine glicentin (proglucagon). Regul Pept 1981;2:139–50.

26. Unger RH, Ohneda A, Valverde I, et al. Characterization of the responses of circulating glucagon-like immunoreactivity to intraduodenal and intravenous administration of glucose. J Clin Invest 1968;47:48–65.

27. Valverde I, Rigopoulou D, Exton J, et al. Demonstration and characterization of a second fraction of glucagon-like immunoreactivity in jejunal extracts. Am J Med Sci 1968;255:415–20.

28. Ohneda A, Parada E, Eisentraut A, Unger RH. The physiologic roles of pancreatic glucagon and a gastrointestinal glucagon-like hormone. In: The 14th Symposium of the German Society of Endocrinology: Nebenschilddruse und Regulationen, Heidelberg, Germany, 1968:224.

29. Ohneda A, Parada E, Eisentraut AM, Unger RH. Characterization of response of circulating glucagon to intraduodenal and intravenous administration of amino acids. J Clin Invest 1968;47:2305–22.

30. Bottger I, Dobbs R, Faloona GR, Unger RH. The effects of triglyceride absorption upon glucagon, insulin, and gut glucagon-like immunoreactivity. J Clin Invest 1973; 52:2532–41.

31. Unger RH, Ketterer H, Dupre J, Eisentraut AM. The effects of secretin, pancreozymin, and gastrin on insulin and glucagon secretion in anesthetized dogs. J Clin Invest 1967;46:630–45.

32. Kervran A, Blache P, Bataille D. Distribution of oxyntomodulin and glucagon in the gastrointestinal tract and the plasma of the rat. Endocrinology 1987;121: 704–13.

33. Biedzinski TM, Bataille D, Devaux MA, Sarles H. The effect of oxyntomodulin (glucagon-37) and glucagon on exocrine pancreatic secretion in the conscious rat. Peptides 1987;8:967–72.

34. Bataille D, Coudray AM, Carlqvist M, et al. Isolation of glucagon-37 (bioactive enteroglucagon/oxyntomodulin) from porcine jejuno-ileum: isolation of the peptide. FEBS Lett 1982;146:73–8.

35. Conlon JM, Samson WK, Dobbs RE, et al. Glucagon-like polypeptides in canine brain. Diabetes 1979;28: 700–2.

36. Ørskov C, Holst JJ, Knuhtsen S, et al. Glucagon-like peptides GLP-1 and GLP-2, predicted products of the glucagon gene, are secreted separately from pig small intestine but not pancreas. Endocrinology 1986;119: 1467–75.

37. Ørskov C, Holst JJ, Poulsen SS, Kirkegaard P. Pancreatic and intestinal processing of proglucagon in man. Diabetologia 1987;30:874–81.

38. Kreymann B, Williams G, Ghatei MA, Bloom SR. Glucagon-like peptide-1 7-36: a physiological incretin in man. Lancet 1987;2:1300–4.

39. Munoz-Barragan L, Blazquez E, Patton GS, et al. Gastric A-cell function in normal dogs. Am J Physiol 1976; 231:1057–61.

40. Baetens D, Rufener C, Srikant BC, et al. Identification of glucagon-producing cells (A-cells) in dog gastric mucosa. J Cell Biol 1976;69:455–64.

41. Sasaki H, Rubalcava B, Baetens D, et al. Identification of glucagon in the gastrointestinal tract. J Clin Invest 1975;56:135–45.

42. Srikant CB, McCorkle K, Unger RH. Properties of immu-

43. Munoz-Barragan L, Rufener C, Srikant CB, et al. Immunocytochemical evidence for glucagon-containing cells in the human stomach. Horm Metab Res 1977;9:37–9.

44. Lane MA. The cytological characters of the areas of Langerhans. Am J Anat 1907–08;7:409–22.

45. Baum J, Simons BE Jr, Unger RH, Madison LL. Localization of glucagon in the alpha cells in the pancreatic islet by immunofluorescent technics. Diabetes 1962; 11:371–4.

46. Orci L, Unger RH. Functional subdivisions of islets of Langerhans and possible role of D-cells. Lancet 1975; 2:1243–4.

47. Orci L, Malaisse-Lagae F, Baetens D, Perrelet A. Pancreatic-polypeptide-rich regions in human pancreas [Letter]. Lancet 1978;2:1200–1.

48. Orci L, Baetens D, Rufener C, et al. Hypertrophy and hyperplasia of somatostatin-containing D-cells in diabetes. Proc Natl Acad Sci USA 1976;73:1338–42.

49. Moody AJ, Thim L, Holst JJ, et al. Porcine pancreatic glicentin-related peptide (GRP) [Abstract no. 271]. Diabetologia 1980;19:300.

50. Orci L, Malaisse-Lagae F, Ravazzola M, et al. A morphologic basis for intercellular communication between α- and β-cells in the endocrine pancreas. J Clin Invest 1975; 56:1066–70.

51. Meda P, Kohen E, Kohen C, et al. Direct communication of homologous and heterologous endocrine islet cells in culture. J Cell Biol 1982;92:221–6.

52. Orci L. The microanatomy of the islets of Langerhans. Metabolism 1976;25(Suppl 1):1303–13.

53. Kawai K, Ipp E, Orci L, et al. Circulating somatostatin acts on the islets of Langerhans by way of a somatostatin-poor compartment. Science 1982;218:477–8.

54. Samols E, Marri G, Marks V. Promotion of insulin secretion by glucagon. Lancet 1965;2:415–6.

55. Patton GS, Ipp E, Dobbs RE, et al. Pancreatic immunoreactive somatostatin release. Proc Natl Acad Sci USA 1977;74:2140–3.

56. Alberti KGMM, Christensen NJ, Christensen SE, et al. Inhibition of insulin secretion by somatostatin. Lancet 1973;2:1299–301.

57. Koerker DJ, Ruch W, Chideckel E, et al. Somatostatin: hypothalamic inhibitor of the endocrine pancreas. Science 1974;184:482–4.

58. Ipp E, Rivier J, Dobbs RE, et al. Somatostatin analogs inhibit somatostatin release. Endocrinology 1979; 104:1270–3.

59. Bonner-Weir S, Orci L. New perspectives on the microvasculature of the islets of Langerhans in the rat. Diabetes 1982;31:883–9.

60. Samols E, Stagner JI, Ewart RBL, Marks V. The order of islet microvascular cellular perfusion is B → A A → D in the perfused rat pancreas. J Clin Invest 1988;82: 350–3.

61. Weir GC, Bonner-Weir S. Islets of Langerhans: the puzzle of intraislet interactions and their relevance to diabetes. J Clin Invest 1990;85:983–7.

62. Maruyama H, Hisatomi A, Orci L, et al. Insulin within islets is a physiologic glucagon release inhibitor. J Clin Invest 1984;74:2296–9.

63. Samols E, Marri G, Marks V. The interrelationship of glucagon, insulin and glucose. Diabetes 1965;15: 855–66.

64. Pipeleers DG, Schuit FC, Van Schravendijk CF, Van de Winkel M. Interplay of nutrients and hormones in the

regulation of glucagon release. Endocrinology 1985; 117:817−23.

65. Starke A, Grundy S, McGarry JD, Unger RH. Correction of hyperglycemia with phloridzin restores the glucagon response to glucose in insulin-deficient dogs: implications for human diabetes. Proc Natl Acad Sci USA 1985; 82:1544−6.

66. Unger RH, Orci L. Glucagon. In: Ellenberg M, Rifkin H, eds. Diabetes mellitus. Theory and practice. 4th ed. New York: Elsevier Science Publishing Co, 1990:104−20.

67. Palmer JP, Porte D Jr. Control of glucagon secretion: the central nervous system. In: Unger RH, Orci L, eds. Glucagon: physiology, pathophysiology and morphology of the pancreatic A-cells. New York: Elsevier-North Holland Publishing Co, 1981:133−57.

68. Bloom SR. Control of glucagon secretion: an overview. In: Unger RH, Orci L, eds. Glucagon: physiology, pathophysiology and morphology of the pancreatic A-cells. New York: Elsevier-North Holland Publishing Co, 1981:99−113.

69. Frohman LA, Bernardis LL. Effect of hypothalamic stimulation on plasma glucose, insulin, and glucagon levels. Am J Physiol 1971;221:1596−603.

70. Fischer U, Hommel H, Ziegler M, Michael R. The mechanism of insulin secretion after oral glucose administration. I. multiphasic course of insulin mobilization after oral administration of glucose in conscious dogs. Differences to the behaviour after intravenous administration. Diabetologia 1972;8:104−10.

71. Unger RH, Eisentraut AM. Entero-insular axis. Arch Intern Med 1969;123:261−6.

72. Valverde I, Rigopoulou D, Marco J, et al. Molecular size of extractable glucagon and glucagon-like immunoreactivity (GLI) in plasma. Diabetes 1970;19:624−9.

73. Danforth DN Jr, Tiche T, Doppman JL, et al. Elevated plasma proglucagon-like component with a glucagon-secreting tumor. N Engl J Med 1976;295:242−5.

74. Valverde I, Lemon HM, Kessinger A, Unger RH. Distribution of plasma glucagon immunoreactivity in a patient with suspected glucagonoma. J Clin Endocrinol Metab 1976;42:804−8.

75. Jaspan JB, Rubenstein AH. Circulating glucagon: plasma profiles and metabolism in health and disease. Diabetes 1977;26:887−902.

76. Mallat A, Pavoine C, Dufour M, et al. A glucagon fragment is responsible for the inhibition of the liver Ca^{2+} pump by glucagon. Nature 1987;325:620−2.

77. Iyengar R, Herberg JT. Structural analysis of the hepatic glucagon receptor: identification of a guanine nucleotide-sensitive hormone-binding region. J Biol Chem 1984; 259:5222−9.

78. Musso GF, Assoian RK, Kaiser ET, et al. Heterogeneity of glucagon receptors of rat hepatocytes: a synthetic peptide probe for the high affinity site. Biochem Biophys Res Commun 1984;119:713−9.

79. Bonnevie-Nielsen V, Tager HS. Glucagon receptors on isolated hepatocytes and hepatocyte membrane vesicles: discrete populations with ligand- and environment-dependent affinities. J Biol Chem 1983;258:11313−20.

80. Gilman AG. Guanine nucleotide-binding regulatory proteins and dual control of adenylate cyclase. J Clin Invest 1984;73:1−4.

80a. Jelinek LJ, et al. Expression cloning and signaling properties of the ret glucagon receptor. Science 1993;259:1614−16.

81. Ciudad CJ, Vila J, Mor MA, Guinovart JJ. Effects of glucagon and insulin on the cyclic AMP binding capacity of hepatocyte cyclic AMP-dependent protein kinase. Mol Cell Biochem 1987;73:37−44.

82. Horuk R, Beckner S, Lin M, et al. Purification of the photoaffinity-labeled glucagon receptor by gel electrophoretic methods. Prep Biochem 1984;14:99−121.

83. Gabbay RA, Lardy HA. Site of insulin inhibition of cAMP-stimulated glycogenolysis: cAMP-dependent protein kinase is affected independent of cAMP changes. J Biol Chem 1984;259:6052−55.

84. Unger RH, Foster DW. Diabetes mellitus. In: Wilson JD, Foster DW, eds. Williams textbook of endocrinology. 6th ed. Philadelphia: WB Saunders, 1985:1018−80.

85. Exton JH. Mechanisms of hormonal regulation of hepatic glucose metabolism. Diabetes Metab Rev 1987;3:163−83.

86. Stalmans W. Glucagon and liver glycogen metabolism. In: Lefebvre PJ, ed. Handbook of experimental pharmacology. Vol 66/I. Berlin: Springer-Verlag, 1983:291−314.

87. Foster DW, McGarry JD. The metabolic derangements and treatment of diabetic ketoacidosis. N Engl J Med 1983;309:159−69.

88. Furuya E, Uyeda K. A novel enzyme catalyzes the synthesis of activation factor from ATP and D-fructose-6-P. J Biol Chem 1981;256:7109−12.

89. Van Schaftingen E, Davies DR, Hers H-G. Inactivation of phosphofructokinase 2 by cyclic AMP-dependent protein kinase. Biochem Biophys Res Commun 1981;103:362−8.

90. El-Maghrabi MR, Claus TH, Pilkis J, et al. Regulation of rat liver fructose 2, 6-bisphosphatase. J Biol Chem 1982; 257:7603−7.

91. Hers H-G, Van Schaftingen E. Fructose-2, 6-bisphosphate 2 years after its discovery. Biochem J 1982;1982;206:1−12.

92. Riou JP, Claus TH, Pilkis SJ. Control of pyruvate kinase activity by glucagon in isolated hepatocytes. Biochem Biophys Res Commun 1976;73:591−9.

93. Claus TH, Park CR, Pilkis SJ. Glucagon and gluconeogenesis. In: Lefebvre PJ, ed. Handbook of experimental pharmacology. Vol 66/I. Berlin: Springer-Verlag, 1983: 315−60.

94. Leiter AB, Weinberg M, Isohashi F, Utter MF. Relationship between phosphorylation and activity of pyruvate dehydrogenase in rat liver mitochondria and the absence of such a relationship for pyruvate carboxylase. J Biol Chem 1978;253:2716−23.

95. Wakelam MJO, Murphy GJ, Hruby VJ, Houslay MD. Activation of two signal-transduction systems in hepatocytes by glucagon [Letter]. Nature 1986;323:68−71.

96. Cherrington AD, Lacy WW, Chiasson J-L. Effect of glucagon on glucose production during insulin deficiency in the dog. J Clin Invest 1978;62:664−77.

97. Liljenquist JE, Mueller GL, Cherrington AD, et al. Evidence for an important role of glucagon in the regulation of hepatic glucose production in normal man. J Clin Invest 1977;59:369−74.

98. Felig P, Wahren J, Hendler R. Influence of physiologic hyperglucagonemia on basal and insulin-inhibited splanchnic glucose output in normal man. J Clin Invest 1976;58:761−5.

99. Raskin P, Aydin I, Yamamoto T, Unger RH. Abnormal alpha cell function in human diabetes: the response to oral protein. Am J Med 1978;64:988−97.

100. Liljenquist JE, Mueller GL, Cherrington AD, et al. Hyperglycemia per se (insulin and glucagon withdrawn) can inhibit hepatic glucose production in man. J Clin Endocrinol Metab 1979;48:171−5.

101. Bloomgarden ZT, Liljenquist JE, Cherrington AD, Rabinowitz D. Persistent stimulatory effect of glucagon on

glucose production despite downregulation. J Clin Endocrinol Metab 1978;47:1152–5.

102. Jennings AS, Cherrington AD, Liljenquist JE, et al. The roles of insulin and glucagon in the regulation of gluconeogenesis in the postabsorptive dog. Diabetes 1977; 26:847–56.

103. Keller U, Chiasson J-L, Liljenquist JE, et al. The roles of insulin, glucagon, and free fatty acids in the regulation of ketogenesis in dogs. Diabetes 1977;26:1040–51.

104. Rizza R, Verdonk C, Miles J, et al. Effect of intermittent endogenous hyperglucagonemia on glucose homeostasis in normal and diabetic man. J Clin Invest 1979;63:1119–23.

105. Raskin P, Unger RH. Effects of exogenous hyperglucagonemia in insulin-treated diabetics. Diabetes 1977; 26:1034–9.

106. Unger RH. Glucagon and the insulin:glucagon ratio in diabetes and other catabolic illnesses. Diabetes 1971; 20:834–8.

107. Kemmer FW, Vranic M. The role of glucagon and its relationship to other glucoregulatory hormones in exercise. In: Unger RH, Orci L, eds. Glucagon: physiology, pathophysiology, and morphology of the pancreatic A-cells. New York: Elsevier-North Holland Publishing Co, 1981:297–331.

108. Gerich JE, Langlois M, Noacco C, et al. Adrenergic modulation of pancreatic glucagon secretion in man. J Clin Invest 1974;53:1441–6.

109. Porte D Jr, Robertson RP. Control of insulin secretion by catecholamines stress and the sympathetic nervous system. Fed Proc 1973;32:1792–6.

110. Park CR, Exton JH. Glucagon and the metabolism of glucose. In: Lefebvre PJ, Unger RH, eds. Glucagon: molecular physiology, clinical and therapeutic implications. Oxford: Pergamon Press, 1972:77–108.

111. Marco J, Calle C, Roman D, et al. Hyperglucagonism induced by glucocorticoid treatment in man. N Engl J Med 1973;288:128–31.

112. Unger RH. The influence of gastrointestinal hormones on the secretion of the islets of Langerhans and other hormones of homeostatic regulation. In; Demling L, ed. Gastrointestinal hormones: international symposium at Erlangen, Germany. Stuttgart: George Theime Verlag, 1972:113–7.

113. Raskin P, Aydin I, Unger RH. Effect of insulin on the exaggerated glucagon response to arginine stimulation in diabetes mellitus. Diabetes 1976;25:227–9.

114. Holst JJ, Pedersen JH, Baldissera F. Circulating glucagon after total pancreatectomy in man. Diabetologia 1983; 25:396–9.

115. Barnes AJ, Bloom SR. Pancreatectomized man: a model for diabetes without glucagon. Lancet 1976;1:219–21.

116. Santeusanio F, Massi-Benedetti M, Angeletti G, et al. Glucagon and carbohydrate disorder in a totally pancreatectomized man (a study with the aid of an artificial endocrine pancreas). J Endocrinol Invest 1981;4:93–6.

117. Nakabayashi H, Dobbs RE, Unger RH. The role of glucagon deficiency in the Houssay phenomenon of dogs. J Clin Invest 1978;61:1355–62.

118. Johnson DG, Goebel CU, Hruby VJ, et al. Hyperglycemia of diabetic rats decreased by a glucagon receptor antagonist. Science 1982;215:1115–6.

119. Flatt PR, Swanston-Flatt SK, Bailey CJ. Glucagon antiserum: a tool to investigate the role of circulating glucagon in obese-hyperglycaemic (ob/ob) mice. Biochem Soc Trans 1979;7:911–3.

Chapter 10

PEPTIDE GROWTH FACTORS

DAVID R. CLEMMONS

Peptide growth factors have been defined as small peptides that generally are secreted in a local microenvironment and then stimulate the growth of specific cell types. At least 30 structurally distinct mitogens have been identified (Table 10–1). Peptide growth factors are believed to act in the G1 phase of the cell cycle and to stimulate specific biochemical events that are necessary to prepare a cell to enter the "S" phase. Although several specific growth factors have been identified and studied intensively, this field is evolving rapidly. New growth factors are still being identified, their target cells are still being determined, and the molecular mechanisms by which growth factors act have only been preliminarily defined. Further complicating our ability to determine the alterations that occur in growth-factor function in the diabetic state is the lack of in vitro test systems enabling us to determine how growth factors work in a localized microenvironment. Such model systems could help provide important insights into the role of growth factors in the stimulation of abnormal cell proliferation during the development of atherosclerosis, nephropathy, and retinopathy. Cell-culture systems have provided valuable information regarding the types of growth-factor receptors present on discrete cell types, such as mesangial cells, and on the capacity of these cells to respond to specific mitogens. These systems have significant limitations, the most important being the inability to reproduce a pericellular environment in culture that mimics the in vivo environment. Progress has recently been made in defining the cell types that secrete specific growth factors in vivo. The use of in situ hybridization has enabled investigators to determine the cell type of origin of specific mitogens and the alterations in this pattern of expression that may occur in diabetes. To date, however, these studies have been descriptive and the significance

of alterations in cell type-specific expression of distinct mitogens has not been determined.

An important challenge to our attempts at understanding of growth-factor physiology is our minimal under-

Table 10–1. Growth-Factor Families

1. Insulin-like growth factors
   a. IGF-I
   b. IGF-II
   c. Insulin
2. Epidermal growth factor
   a. EGF
   b. TGF-α
   c. Amphiregulin
3. Transforming growth factor β
   a. TGF-β 1, 2, and 3
   b. Inhibin
   c. Activin
   d. Bone morphogenic proteins
   e. Vg1-oncogene product
   f. Drosophila decaptaplegic product C
   g. Mullerian inhibitory substance
4. Fibroblast growth factor or heparin-binding growth factor
   a. FGF acidic
   b. FGF basic
   c. Oncogene *int*-2
   d. Oncogene *hst*
5. Nerve growth factor
6. Cytokines
   a. Interleukins 1–9
   b. Tumor necrosis factor
   c. Interferons
7. Hematopoietic growth factors
   a. Erythropoietin
   b. Colony-stimulating factors
      1. Granulocyte-macrophage-CSF
      2. Granulocyte CSF
      3. Macrophage CSF
      4. Multi-CSF

standing of how growth factors work together to stimulate cell replication. Recently, there has been much interest in identifying the specific genes induced in cells after their exposure to growth factor. Although it has been determined that specific genes can be induced, the exact roles of these genes in mediating cell proliferation and the other trophic functions of many of these molecules have yet to be determined. For example, one set of growth factors that stimulate early response to genes, including platelet-derived growth factor (PDGF) and fibroblast growth factor (FGF), appear to be able to recruit quiescent cells into the cell cycle.[1] At that point these cells can be stimulated to progress to DNA synthesis by growth factors such as epidermal growth factor and the insulin-like growth factors (IGFs).[2] However, the complex interactions between different growth factors and the interactions between growth factors and hormones that occur in vivo are not well understood. The use of whole animal model test systems often does not permit identification of all the other growth factors involved at the molecular level. Complicating our understanding of this problem is the frequent involvement of autocrine or paracrine mechanisms in growth-factor function. A growth factor may exert all of its target-cell actions in a very discrete area; therefore, in vivo infusion experiments designed to analyze its target-cell actions in whole animals may be inappropriate. Likewise, when growth factors do function by classic endocrine mechanisms it may be difficult to determine whether their target-cell actions are mediated by paracrine or endocrine mechanisms.

An additional problem in investigating how growth factors function has been the identification of structurally distinct subtypes of growth factor receptors. The IGFs, PDGF, transforming growth factor β (TGF-β), and FGF, as well as several other growth factors, have been found to have more than one type of receptor, each capable of transmembrane signaling. Why there should be two or more relatively homologous receptors to mediate growth-factor actions is not clear. How these receptors function together to coordinate signaling for each mitogen is the subject of intensive investigation. A narrow study of growth factors that focuses simply on their stimulation of cell replication may be superficial and inadequate, since it has been shown that most growth factors modulate many other cell processes, including differentiation, matrix protein synthesis, cell adhesion, and release of proteolytic enzymes. Future investigators will be forced to address these additional issues before reaching a complete understanding of molecular mechanisms of action of these mitogens and the molecular pathogenesis of growth abnormalities in disease states such as diabetes.

Finally, the nomenclature for growth factors has become increasingly complex. The naming of particular growth factors has not followed a specific pattern. Often growth factors were assigned names based on cell type of origin, such as "macrophage growth factor," even though the cell type was since shown to contain multiple structurally distinct mitogens. Similarly, factors were named for the cell type they stimulated, such as "endothelial cell growth factor," even though several mitogens have since been shown to stimulate the growth of this cell type. Since bioassays and crude organ or cell extracts were initially used to characterize these substances, it is not surprising that the same substance has been rediscovered several times. Thus FGF has been assigned 30 different names because of its wide distribution. More recent emphasis on determinations of amino acid sequence has permitted classification of growth factors into structurally related superfamilies. This type of classification should help clear up some of the confusion that has existed to date.

INSULIN-LIKE GROWTH FACTORS (IGFs)

Because of their structural relationship to insulin, the IGFs have received a great deal of attention by investigators interested in the pathogenesis of diabetic complications. The IGFs are small peptides of 7600 kilodaltons (kd) whose primary amino acid sequences are strikingly similar to one another as well as to human proinsulin.[3] Both IGF-I and IGF-II are single-chain molecules with three disulfide bridges. IGF-I and IGF-II have a 62% sequence homology and a 43% and 41% amino acid sequence homology, respectively, with proinsulin. Recent studies of IGF mutants have shown that specific amino acids critical for the binding of IGF to its receptors are also required for the binding of insulin to its receptor.[4] For example, tyrosines at amino acid positions 24, 31, and 60 appear to be critical for IGF and insulin and interact with their respective cell-surface receptors. Therefore, the molecular geometry and tertiary structure of the molecules may have to be conserved in such a way as to use a common motif for receptor binding. Similarity of tertiary structure is inferred by the presence of three disulfide linkages in the same position in all three proteins. A major obvious structural difference is found in the connecting peptide region (Fig. 10–1). The connecting peptide of insulin is substantially longer than that of IGF-I and IGF-II, and the amino acid sequences of the three peptides within the connecting peptide region are not conserved.

A substantial difference between proinsulin and IGF-I and IGF-II, only recently analyzed, is in their affinity for IGF-binding proteins. Whereas IGF-I and IGF-II circulate bound to high-affinity carrier proteins, insulin does not. The structural feature that accounts for this difference is localized to the first 16 amino acids of the B-chain region.[5,6] Discrete amino acid substitutions for the amino acids in IGF-I or IGF-II at positions 4,5 and 15,16 of the B chain with amino acids that are present in insulin results in a 400-fold reduction in the affinity of IGF-I and IGF-II for the major IGF-binding protein in serum, IGFBP-3. IGF-I and IGF-II require these amino acids to maintain their high affinity for IGFBP-3, whereas insulin, having distinctly different amino acids at these positions, does not bind to this protein and circulates in blood primarily in a free form. The molecular significance of this difference will be discussed below.

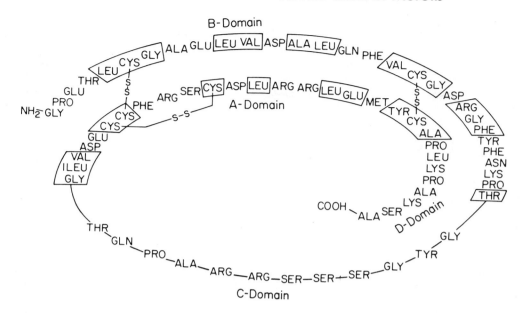

Fig. 10—1. Amino acid sequence of insulin-like growth factor-I (IGF-I). The boxed residues are identical to human proinsulin. Note that the connecting peptide and the D-domain extension contain no homologies.

Control of IGF Secretion

IGF secretion has been analyzed in whole-animal models by determining the factors that control concentrations of IGF-I and IGF-II in serum and at the cellular level by either in situ hybridization or direct measurement of the secretion of IGF by cells in culture. The primary variable controlling serum concentrations of IGF-I is nutrient intake.[7] However, with IGF-I, unlike insulin, there are no acute minute-to-minute fluctuations in serum concentrations based on carbohydrate intake. Rather, the levels are very stable and change only after the intake of either calories and protein has been inadequate for several days.[8] A diet deficient in either total energy or protein will result in significant changes in serum IGF-I concentrations, but a new steady-state level will be reached only after 3 to 5 days. Changes in serum IGF-I concentrations correlate with maintenance of positive nitrogen balance, and at least 1500 kcal/day must be ingested to maintain normal serum IGF-I levels.[8] Ingestion of fewer calories results in major attenuation of responsiveness to administration of growth hormone, and when less than 800 kcal/day is ingested, there is no response to growth hormone.[9] This refractoriness to growth hormone also is noted during severe restriction of dietary protein. The effect appears to be mediated at a post-transcriptional level, since rats fed a protein-restricted diet and then given growth hormone exhibit an appropriate increase in IGF-I mRNA but no increase in IGF-I secretion.[10]

During fasting and refeeding, the degree of decline or increase in IGF-I correlates well with the changes in nitrogen balance.[7] Since IGF-I stimulates the accretion of muscle protein in vitro, it has been predicted that the changes in IGF-I may be the mediators of nutrient-induced changes in nitrogen balance. This hypothesis has recently received major support. If normal subjects are restricted in their caloric intake enter a state of negative nitrogen balance, administration of IGF-I results in a pronounced anabolic response despite continued restriction in caloric intake. Therefore, IGF-I may be an important regulatory signal of the adequacy of protein and energy ingestion for the support of normal rates of protein accretion. These findings suggest that measurement of serum IGF-I may be useful as a predictor of the anabolic state in catabolic patients. Several studies have shown that physiologic stresses that lead to nitrogen wasting, e.g., infection, fever, fractures, wounds, and burns, will lead to decreases in serum IGF-I concentrations. Likewise, when subjects are severely insulin-deficient during the acute diabetic state and enter into a nitrogen-wasting state, their levels of IGF-I also fall.[11] Determination of IGF-I levels can be used to monitor the responses of these patients to nutritional support therapy. Specifically, the levels of IGF-I in patients who are catabolic and are receiving hyperalimentation have been found to correlate with the response to therapy and to predict entry into positive nitrogen balance[12,13] (Fig. 10—2). Two studies have shown that in patients with short-bowel syndromes who are receiving hyperalimentation there is a strong correlation between the daily change in levels of IGF-I and entry into a positive nitrogen balance. Likewise, patients in an intensive care unit receiving intravenous hyperalimentation showed similar responses.[14] Therefore, measurement of serum IGF-I appears to be an excellent index of total protein and energy intake and of whether intake is sufficient to improve nitrogen balance.

IGF-II is much less sensitive than IGF-I to changes in nutrient intake. Fasting for 9 days did not lower IGF-II levels in normal adults.[15] The exact relationship between nutrient intake and IGF-II levels in children has not been determined.

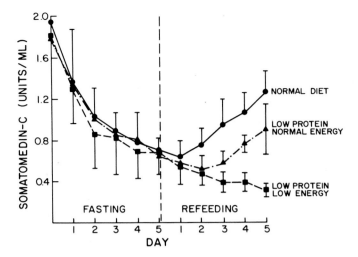

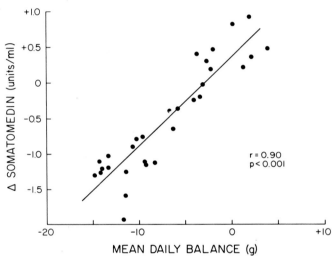

Fig. 10–2. Changes in serum insulin-like growth factor-I (IGF-I; somatomedin-C) concentrations and nitrogen balance. Normal adults were fasted for 5 days and then refed one of three diets containing 35 kcal and 1.0 g protein/kg (normal), 35 kcal and 0.4 g protein/kg (low protein), or 11 kcal and 0.4 g protein (low protein, low energy) for 5 days. Top panel: Serum IGF-I response. Lower panel: Correlation between mean daily nitrogen balance for each day during fasting and refeeding and the change in IGF-I.

Control of Serum IGF-I by Growth Hormone

The initial discovery of the IGFs was based on the observation that serum sulfation factor/somatomedin activity (terms used to describe IGF-I and II) was controlled by the secretion of pituitary growth hormone (GH).[16] Administration of GH to hypophysectomized rats resulted in the induction of a serum factor necessary for optimal stimulation of cartilage sulfation, and incubation of GH directly with the cartilage was not stimulatory. The addition of the GH-inducible serum factor restored cartilage sulfation. In patients with GH deficiency, serum IGF-I concentrations are approximately 5 to 8% of normal values and increase to normal levels with administration of GH.[17] Likewise, serum IGF-I concentrations

are elevated three- to ninefold in individuals with acromegaly.[18] Serum IGF-I concentrations will return to normal values following amelioration of the acromegalic state.[19] Therefore, the serum IGF-I levels can be useful in the diagnosis of GH deficiency or excess. There is a hierarchy of control of IGF-I secretion, with nutritional intake dominant over GH.

The control of the IGF-I synthesis in response to GH appears to occur at several levels. Specifically, increases in serum IGFs and in the secretion of IGF-I by the liver in response to the administration of GH have been documented. These increases appear to be due primarily to an increase in transcription, since hepatic IGF-I mRNA is reduced severalfold in hypophysectomized animals.[20] However, there is a strong interaction between GH and nutritional intake, and nutrient restriction can control the synthesis and secretion of IGF-I at several levels (Fig. 10–3). When young rats are starved, the number of GH receptors in the liver will decrease by approximately 50%.[21] If young, growing rats receive a protein-restricted diet (66% restriction), there are reductions in the baseline level of IGF-I transcription in the liver and in the abundance of IGF-I mRNA.[22] However, if older rats are protein-restricted and then given GH, the induction of IGF-I mRNA proceeds normally but serum IGF-I levels do not increase, a finding that suggests a defect at the level of translation.[10] This defect appears to be due to the binding of IGF-I mRNA to high-molecular-weight polysomes that do not bind to the translational apparatus. There also appear to be changes in the stability of IGF-I mRNA that are induced by changes in dietary intake.[23]

Although pulsatile secretion of GH does not result in concomitant increases in IGF-I synthesis, IGF-I levels do change over time with GH administration. There appears to be no time-dependent loss of IGF-I responsiveness as long as dietary intake continues to be adequate. This observation is useful in monitoring response to GH treatment as well the reversal of GH hypersecretion in acromegaly.

Other hormones appear to control serum IGF-I concentrations. Serum IGF-I concentration in GH-deficient subjects with high prolactin levels are usually within the normal range. Likewise, IGF-I levels in subjects with hypothyroidism are subnormal and increase when thyroxine is administered.[24] Administration of physiologic replacement doses of estrogen or androgen does not lead to changes in serum IGF-I levels attributable directly to these hormones.[25,26] An additional factor required for maintenance of serum IGF-I is a normal complement of GH receptors and GH-receptor responsiveness. This has recently been proven in studies of children with GH insensitivity syndrome. These children have acquired mutations in the GH receptor and do not respond to high serum concentrations of GH with normal IGF-I synthesis.[27] This condition leads to severe growth retardation, confirming that signaling through the GH receptor is necessary to the maintenance of normal serum IGF-I levels and normal rates of growth. Such children recently were shown to respond to the infusion of IGF-I, a finding that suggests this

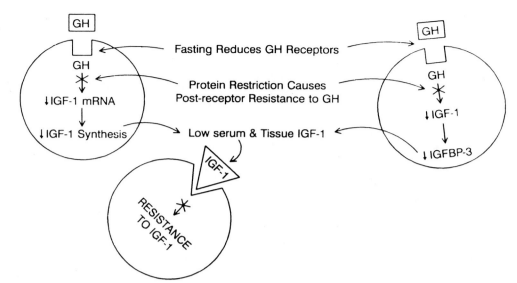

Fig. 10–3. Specific points in the biosynthetic pathway of insulin-like growth factor-I (IGF-I) that are sensitive to changes in nutrient uptake. Extreme changes such as fasting result in a 50% reduction in growth hormone (GH) receptors. Less severe restrictions such as a 66% reduction in protein intake result in impaired GH signaling but in no change in GH receptors. Caloric restriction results in postreceptor resistance to IGF-I actions.

selective defect is a major factor contributing to their growth retardation.[28]

Autocrine/Paracrine Control of Synthesis and Secretion

IGF-I and IGF-II are secreted into blood and appear to function by classic endocrine mechanisms. When IGF-I levels are low, there is balanced growth reduction in multiple organs and tissues; when levels are high, there is overgrowth, particularly of connective tissue. In situ hybridization studies have not revealed a concentrated organ source of IGF-I and IGF-II but have shown that their mRNAs are present in stromal cells within multiple organs and tissues.[29] GH can stimulate synthesis of IGF-I in multiple extrahepatic tissues.[30]

Mechanisms other than GH secretion may control local synthesis of IGF-I. Dermal fibroblasts synthesize and release IGF-I, and secretion can be stimulated by exposure to PDGF or FGF. That this response is linked to increased growth was shown by experiments in which antibodies to IGF or to IGF receptor were used to block binding of secreted IGF-I to IGF receptors.[31] DNA synthesis was inhibited, confirming that the secreted IGF-I was functioning by an autocrine or paracrine mechanism.

Paracrine signaling has been proposed as having a role in breast cancer, wherein IGF-I is synthesized by stromal cells adjacent to the breast tumor tissue but not by the tumor cells themselves, which possess IGF receptors and are presumably capable of responding to the peptide secreted by the stromal cell[32] (Fig. 10–4). The IGF-I that is synthesized by the stromal cells then appears to be transported to the surface of the tumor cells, since IGF-I can be localized there by immunocytochemical assays. Autocrine/paracrine mechanisms may also be important in the regulation of local proliferative responses in tissues such as the ovary, in which ovarian granulosa cells have been shown to produce IGF-I and IGF-II in response to stimulation by follicle-stimulating hormone (FSH).[33] Lo-

cal production may be important in spermatogenesis, since the Sertoli cell appears to be an important source of IGF-I.[26] IGF-I synthesis has also been detected in the thyroid gland and in gastrointestinal epithelium, as well as in fibroblasts located in multiple tissues and organs throughout the body. This stroma-derived IGF-I is believed to be important in the repair process by which fibroblasts respond to injury and has been proposed as an integral part of normal wound-healing mechanisms[34] and possibly in the pathogenesis of fibrotic disorders in which fibroblast proliferation appears to proceed in an unrestrained manner. This mechanism is independent of endocrine regulation, as demonstrated by an increase in the expression of IGF-I mRNA after tissue injury in hypophysectomized animals.[35]

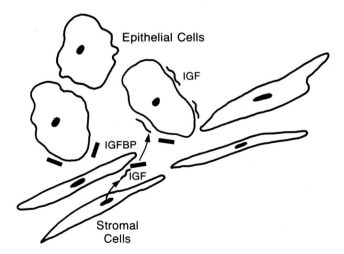

Fig. 10–4. Paracrine signaling between stromal and epithelial cells. Stromal cells synthesize insulin-like growth factor-I (IGF), which is transported to epithelial cell surfaces by IGF-binding proteins (IGFBP). Although epithelial cells often do not synthesize IGF-I, they contain IGF-I receptors and are capable of responding to the paracrine-mediated signal.

Of interest to diabetologists is the finding that both the mesangial cell of the kidney and the retinal pigment epithelial cell synthesize and secrete IGF-I in culture. Thus, these cells are possible sources of IGF-I and IGF-II that could be involved in the development of retinopathy and glomerulosclerosis. The molecular mechanisms that control secretion by these cell types have yet to be defined. Another cell type of interest to diabetologists is the arterial smooth muscle cell. Smooth muscle cells have been shown to synthesize and secrete an IGF-I-like peptide, and synthesis of IGF-I appears to be regulated by PDGF and FGF.[36] There appears to be a clear relationship between IGF-I synthesis and the development of atherosclerosis in acute experimental models. Following balloon-denudation carotid injury and other acute-injury models, there appears to be a proliferative wave of IGF synthesis. In models of chronic lesion induction, such as the hypercholesterolemic pig model, tissue IGF synthesis does not appear to be increased when normalized for changes in total RNA or protein. Thus, the exact role for IGFs in the pathogenesis of atherosclerosis is not completely established. Current interest has focused on the role of IGF-binding proteins in modulating the response to the IGFs (see below).

Although arguments continue about whether IGFs function primarily by endocrine or by autocrine/paracrine mechanisms, it is clear that autocrine/paracrine mechanisms are also under the influence of GH and that the two hypotheses are not mutually exclusive. Isgaard and co-workers have shown that local injection of GH into cartilage results in a proliferative wave of DNA synthesis by the chondrocyte.[37] However, local injection also results in the induction of IGF-I mRNA in chondrocyte precursors.[38] As these cells differentiate into mature chondrocytes, synthesis of IGF-I increases. When these cells cease to proliferate and become hypertrophic chondrocytes, IGF-I synthesis decreases. Therefore, the biosynthesis of IGF-I can be stimulated locally by GH; this correlates with changes in DNA synthesis by the chondrocyte, suggesting that local synthesis of IGF-I mediates the trophic effects of GH. Supporting this hypothesis is the observation that local infusion of antiserum to IGF-I also attenuates IGF-I responsiveness. The relative contribution of both autocrine/paracrine-synthesized IGFs as compared with that of blood-borne IGFs to total body somatic growth is unclear, but both mechanisms appear to contribute to this process.

IGF Receptors

Three distinct receptor subtypes that bind the peptides in the IGF family have been characterized. The insulin and type I IGF receptors have a high degree of structural homology. Their primary amino acid sequences show approximately 38% homology, although certain domains have shown much greater homology.[39] Both receptors are heterotetramers, containing two α subunits that contain the binding region for both IGF and insulin and two β subunits. There is a high degree of specificity of ligand recognition, with the type I receptor binding IGF-I, IGF-II, and insulin—with the affinity decreasing in that

order—but with the insulin receptor binding insulin with a much greater affinity than it binds IGF-I or IGF-II.[40] The affinity of the type I receptor is reduced approximately 3-fold for IGF-II and approximately 800-fold for insulin. The insulin receptor shows 100-fold reduction in affinity for IGF-I. Antibody blocking studies have shown that there is significant receptor specificity. Specifically, antibodies to insulin receptor will block IGF-I binding to the insulin receptor, and a monoclonal antibody to IGF-I receptor will block the binding of supraphysiologic concentrations of insulin to the IGF receptor.[41] This requirement for supraphysiologic concentrations of either insulin or IGF-I for binding to the heterologous receptor shows that the specificity of ligand recognition of the specificity of each receptor confers an important regulatory function. Following the binding of IGF or insulin, the transmembrane signaling mechanisms that are stimulated may show some overlap. Receptor-mediated phosphorylation of intracellular substrates can show some crossover, i.e., the insulin receptor can phosphorylate some proteins that appear to be targets for the IGF receptor and vice versa. The β subunit of each reactor has intrinsic tyrosine kinase activity.[42] Following autophosphorylation of the β subunit, this kinase activity is increased and other intracellular proteins are phosphorylated. The best-described intracellular substrate is a protein termed pp185 that is phosphorylated within 1 minute after IGF-I or insulin binds to its respective specific receptor.[43] The blocking of pp185 phosphorylation has been shown to block insulin action. Receptor number is also regulated at the cell surface. The abundance of both receptors has been shown to be downregulated following binding. Heterologous receptor regulation has also been shown by the demonstration that PDGF can induce changes in the abundance of IGF receptors.[44]

Even though IGF-II can bind to the type-I IGF receptor and the insulin receptor, another type of receptor subtype, the type-II IGF receptor, has been identified. In contrast to the other two receptors, it is a 260,000-kd, single-chain monomeric unit.[45] This receptor binds IGF-II with an affinity approximately three times greater than for IGF-I and does not bind insulin. The structure of this protein has been analyzed and shown to be identical with the cation-independent type-II mannose-6-phosphate receptor.[46] Thus, this is a multifunctional protein that binds not only insulin-like growth factors but also mannose-6-phosphate. Following mannose-6-phosphate binding to this receptor, its affinity for IGF-II increases. It is interesting, however, that mannose-6-phosphate can inhibit IGF-II action.[47] In some test systems that require IGF-II to function, IGF-II actions can be inhibited by the addition of mannose-6-phosphate, a finding that indicates the signaling of type II receptor may be blocked by this factor. Several agents have been shown to stimulate the translocation of this protein from lysosomes to the cell surface. The most interesting of these is insulin, which induces a translocation of approximately 50% of the type-II receptors within 10 minutes.[48] The type-II receptor can be cleaved from the cell surface, producing a 205-kd form of soluble binding protein that circulates in blood. The functional significance of this binding protein has not been determined. Cleavage occurs at the transmembrane junction, and the cleaved fragment has been shown to functionally bind IGFs in rat plasma.[49]

The role of the type-II receptor in regulating IGF-dependent growth has not been established. However, Nishimoto and co-workers recently showed that IGF-induced mobilization of intracellular calcium is mediated by the type-II receptor.[50] This response is dependent on the generation of an inositol triphosphate, and induction of phospholipase C is involved in the transduction of this signal by type-II receptor.[51]

Target-Cell Actions

When IGFs are studied in cell culture, a primary effect of both IGF-I and IGF-II appears to be stimulation of DNA synthesis and cell proliferation. However, in many systems IGF is a relatively weak mitogen and synergism with PDGF or FGF is required for IGF to manifest its full effects as a promotor of cell growth.[52] Whereas PDGF and FGF function to recruit quiescent cells into the cell cycle, IGF-I and IGF-II stimulate progression towards the "S" phase. The IGFs stimulate growth of cell types derived from all three embryonic stem-cell lineages. IGF-I and IGF-II stimulate not only cell growth but also other anabolic processes required for cell growth such as uptake of amino acids[53] and protein synthesis.[54] Insulin-like actions can also be stimulated in target tissues; however, these require significantly higher concentrations of IGF-I capable of binding to the insulin receptor.[55] IGFs are also potent stimulators of cellular differentiation. Myoblasts, osteoblasts, adipocytes, and oligodendrocytes all differentiate under the control of IGF-I. IGF-I and IGF-II have been shown to induce erythropoiesis and granulopoiesis as well as chemotaxis of endothelial cells. Skeletal muscle cells differentiate and fuse into myotubes following stimulation with IGF-I or IGF-II. Epithelium and cartilage cells also undergo significant differentiation in response to IGF-I. These growth factors also potentiate the effects of tissue-specific hormones. For example, IGF-I potentiates the effect of ACTH or FSH on steroidogenesis in the adrenal gland[56] and ovary,[57] respectively. In summary, the IGFs are pluripotent trophic growth factors with a broad spectrum of actions that function to augment the effects of tissue-specific hormones and mitogens on target cells.

IGF-Binding Proteins

Since the IGFs are ubiquitous in extracellular fluids and tissues, a mechanism that mediates their actions in a tissue- or cell type-specific manner is undoubtedly present. IGF-binding proteins have been proposed as providing such a mechanism. High-affinity soluble proteins are also present in all extracellular fluids and tissues, but the type of proteins detected and their specific effects differ markedly among tissues.

At present, six IGF-binding proteins have been cloned and sequenced and their specific structures determined.[58] The major IGF-binding protein in serum is IGFBP-3, a 45,000- to 54,000-kd glycoprotein whose serum concentration is dependent upon GH and IGF-I.[59] IGFBP-3 accounts for binding of 95% or more of the total IGF-I and II in serum binds to an additional 88,000-kd acid-labile protein termed acid-labile subunit. Induction of the acid-labile subunit by GH results in formation of a 150,000-kd complex that acts as the major IGF-binding moiety in serum.[60] This complex cannot permeate capillaries freely and therefore acts as a large reservoir of IGF-I and IGF-II. IGF-binding proteins 1 and 2 also circulate in serum. These binding proteins are lower-molecular-weight, nonglycosylated proteins.[61,62] The serum concentrations of both these proteins vary in response to IGF-I stimulation[63] but are inversely related to growth hormone levels.[64] Likewise, concentrations of IGFBP-1 are tightly regulated by serum insulin levels, being elevated in patients with diabetes and low in patients with insulinomas.[65] Both IGFBP-1 and IGFBP-2 are transported across capillary barriers; the transport of IGFBP-1 is insulin-dependent and therefore may be impaired in those with diabetes. The serum concentrations of IGFBP-4, a 24,000-dalton protein, appear to be unaffected by changes in GH levels.

All forms of IGF-binding protein have a high affinity for IGF-I and IGF-II. With IGFBP-3 and IGFBP-4, the affinity is sufficiently high to result in a significant blockage of binding of IGF-I and II to cell-surface receptors. Therefore, an important function of these proteins may be to control the amount of IGF-I and IGF-II available for binding to IGF-receptor subtypes.[66] The manner in which this control over receptor interaction is regulated is complex. In some cases, coincubation of IGF-binding protein with IGF-I appears to augment the effects of IGF-I in cell growth and differentiation,[67] whereas in other cases, such coincubation is clearly inhibitory.[61] Studies are under way to determine the molecular mechanisms by which these inhibitory and stimulatory effects are mediated.

Different cells secrete different combinations of IGFBPs. For example, human fibroblasts secrete IGFBPs 3, 4, and 5, whereas smooth muscle cells secrete IGFBPs 2 and 4,[68] decidual cells secrete IGFBPs 1, 2, and 4, and breast epithelial cells secrete IGFBPs 2, 3, and 4. How these specific combinations function together to regulate IGF actions is unclear. Likewise, each protein has specific post-translational modifications. IGFBPs 3 and 4 are glycosylated, whereas IGFBPs 1 and 3 are phosphorylated. Phosphorylation has been shown to alter the bioactivity of IGFBP-1,[70] and this IGFBP will potentiate IGF-I actions on cell growth only if it is dephosphorylated. These observations suggest that regulation of IGF actions by IGFBPs is complex, involving multiple specific mechanisms.

OTHER PEPTIDE GROWTH FACTORS

Epidermal Growth Factor

Epidermal growth factor (EGF) was first discovered in connection with its property of stimulating eyelid opening and tooth eruption in newborn mice.[70] The secreted protein is approximately 6000 daltons but arises from a larger precursor of an estimated 122,000 daltons with eight repeating subunits of 40 amino acids. EGF is found in a wide variety of tissues, including the kidney, intestinal tract, and brain. EGF stimulates DNA synthesis in a wide variety of cell types.[71] The name may be somewhat of a misnomer since EGF is a strong mitogen for both epithelial and mesenchymal cells. The EGF precursor has characteristics of a membrane protein, but the role of membrane-associated EGF in stimulating the growth of adjacent cells is not well defined. EGF may be synergistic with other growth factors and hormones in stimulating DNA synthesis; in epithelial cells its effects are often potentiated by insulin and hydrocortisone. EGF has been shown to potentiate the effects of PDGF on replication of fibroblasts.

The EGF receptor is a 170,000-kd protein with three domains: a growth factor-binding domain, a transmembrane domain, and cytosolic domain.[72] The cytosolic domain contains tyrosine kinase activity, which is capable of autophosphorylating the receptor and phosphorylating exogenous substrates in response to EGF stimulation. It has recently been shown that the receptor specifically phosphorylates phospholipase C and that this phosphorylation reaction is critical to the induction of mitogenic actions by EGF.[73] When the growth factor-binding domain of EGF receptor is deleted, the truncated protein has sequence homology with the v-erb-B or avian erythroblastosis virus oncogene.[74] This truncated receptor appears to be constitutively activated in the cells in which it is expressed and can act as a growth regulatory moiety for these cell types. Overexpression and transactivation of this receptor contributes to cell transformation.[75] EGF receptors appear to be localized on the basolateral aspect of epithelial cells, with directional transepithelial transport of EGF from basolateral to apical surfaces. A second EGF-receptor homologue has been identified. It has strong structural homology with the receptor and has been proposed to be the amphiregulin receptor.[76] EGF has been postulated to play a role both in organogenesis in developing embryonic tissues and in the response to tissue injury.[77] EGF mRNA is expressed in several tissues during regeneration following injury and often is accompanied by an increase in EGF receptors. Application of pure EGF to healing wounds has been shown to produce an increase in granulation tissue and in tissue breaking strength.[78] However, a definitive role for EGF during tissue regeneration has not been proven by deletion experiments.

Transforming Growth Factor α

Transforming growth factor α (TGF-α) is a 5600-kd, single-chain polypeptide of 50 amino acids. Its sequence homology to EGF is 42%, including conservation of all six cysteine residues. This close relationship may account for many of the functions, such as organogenesis, that previously were attributed to EGF.[79] Vaccinia virus growth factor is also structurally homologous to EGF. TGF-α mediates its effect through binding to the EGF receptor. There is a highly conserved area of primary amino acid sequence, compared with the EGF sequence, in the membrane receptor-binding domain. TGF-α is produced by embryonic tissues and malignant cells and can be detected by in situ hybridization in keratinocytes of the human fetus.[80] During regeneration, TGF-α is strongly expressed during wound healing or angiogenesis. TGF-α stimulates a wide variety of cell types, including epithelial and mesenchymal cells. It is expressed in macrophages during wound healing and acts as a mitogen for normal fibroblasts, thereby enhancing wound recovery.

Transforming Growth Factor β

Transforming growth factor β (TGF-β) is a 26,500-kd polypeptide that is a disulfide-linked homodimer. It does not bind to EGF receptors and was originally purified from bovine kidney.[81] It is unrelated to TGF-α but is a member of a closely related family of growth factors that includes TGF-β 1, 2 and 3; inhibin; activin; mullerian inhibitory substance; Vg-1 protein produced in Xenopus; and the decapetaplegic gene product of Drosophila. Expression of the TGF-β gene and its receptor is widespread, suggesting that this is an important growth factor functioning at multiple sites of action. TGF-β is an important bifunctional regulator of cell growth. It stimulates anchorage-independent growth of several cell types in soft agar but inhibits the growth of several anchorage-dependent cell types in culture.[82] Whether or not TGF-β is inhibitory or stimulatory depends on the presence of other growth factors or the ability of a particular cell type to synthesize a specific growth factor, such as PDGF, in response to TGF-β and the methods used in the test cell-culture system. In the adult, TGF-β has been detected in lung, liver, heart, kidney, placenta, brain, and bone. One of its most important properties appears to be a potent capacity to stimulate synthesis of matrix proteins such as collagen, laminen, and fibronectin. The stimulation of collagen synthesis by TGF-β is believed to be a major mechanism by which it acts as a growth inhibitor.[83] The TGF-β peptide is released in an inactive form associated with a high-affinity-binding protein. TGF-β purified from human platelets is complexed with the high-molecular-weight binding protein, and exposure to low pH or plasminogen activator is required to free the biologically active moiety from its precursor binding protein.[84] The potential regulatory role of this release reaction is not yet completely defined. Several peptides that regulate bone-cell formation, such as bone morphogenic proteins 2A and 3, have structural similarity to TGF-β, as do the cartilage-inducing factors C, I, A, F, and B. They are homologues of TGF-β 1 and 2. Expression of TGF-β is detected in blood islands and capillaries early in development. In the adult, platelets and bone are the two most abundant sources of this protein. Although TGF-β is expressed in multiple cell types in culture, its expression in vivo is much more limited, suggesting that cell culture deregulates the factors that regulate TGF-β gene expression.

Three distinct forms of TGF-β receptors have been identified.[85] All are high-affinity receptors but differ in their estimated molecular weights. Type I has an estimated molecular weight of 65,000 to 85,000; type II, 115,000 to 140,000; and type III, 280,000 to 330,000. The third type of receptor is heavily glycosylated and sulfated, with long glucosaminoglycan side chains and with heparin as nearly one-half of its mass. TGF-β, like PDGF, is inactivated by binding to α₂-macroglobulin. Closely related to forms of TGF-β 1 are TGF-β 2 and TGF-β 3 also found in platelets. TGF-β 2 is produced by adenocarcinoma cells in culture. TGF-β 1 and 2 appear to have similar spectrums of biologic activity. A TGF-β 3 has been described that has an 80% homology with TGF-β 1 and 2. TGF-β 1 can induce the expression of proto-oncogene c-*myc* in several cell types in culture. Induction of c-*myc* is followed by stimulation of other PDGF-dependent genes such as the c-*fos* proto-oncogene.[86] TGF-β also leads to enhanced expression of proto-oncogenes c-*jun* and c-*jun-B*. One of the major functions of TGF-β appears to be inhibition of cell growth. TGF-β has been shown to have antiproliferative effects on a wide variety of both neoplastic and non-neoplastic cells. Its inhibitory effects are reversible, and it is not cytotoxic. The evidence for TGF-β functioning as a growth inhibitor in vivo is minimal, however. TGF-β is also a potent modulator of cellular differentiation. Both TGF-β 1 and TGF-β 2 stimulate fetal muscle and cartilage cells to differentiate into bone cells,[87] induce terminal differentiation of human bronchial epithelial cells, and act as potent promoters of chondrogenesis, bone formation, and keratinization of epithelial cells.

In addition to accelerating all these differentiated functions, TGF-β inhibits mitogenesis in muscle and differentiation of myoblasts into myocytes.[88] Similarly, it will inhibit insulin-stimulated differentiation of 3T3-L1 cells into adipocytes. TGF-β appears to be an important regulator of wound healing. Large amounts are released directly into the site of injury. Thrombin can stimulate release of TGF-β from platelets. Latent TGF-β that is released appears to be activated by proteinases in healing wounds.[89] TGF-β applied to wound tissue increases the formation of granulation tissue, and it appears to be the most potent growth factor in terms of accelerating wound healing and enhancing wound-breaking strength. The accumulation of collagen in wounds is definitely accelerated by application of TGF-β. Fetal bone cells synthesize TGF-β, and approximately 25% of the released peptide is in the active form.[87] TGF-β increases the synthesis of multiple bone matrix proteins and the differentiation of mesenchymal cells into chondrocytes. Fibronectin, tenacin, and type-I collagen are all synthesized by fibroblasts in response to TGF-β. Type-II collagen is synthesized by bone cells, and chondroitin and dermatan sulfate proteoglycans also are synthesized preferentially after response to this growth factor. TGF-β enhances not only the secretion of these matrix proteins but also the synthesis of their receptors. Specifically, the integrin that accounts for fibronectin receptor binding is

synthesized in response to stimulation by TGF-β.[83] In summary, TGF-β is a potent growth factor and/or inhibitor. It also functions as an inductor of differentiation in tissues.

Fibroblast Growth Factor

The fibroblast growth factor (FGF) family of compounds are characterized by their affinity for heparin and extracellular-matrix proteins.[90] The family encodes five proteins, including acidic and basic FGFs, the *int-2* and *hst* proto-oncogene homologues, and a protein isolated from Kaposi sarcoma cells. An interesting property of the FGFs is that they lack a signal peptide necessary for cellular secretion and probably are released primarily under specialized circumstances during wound healing, tissue remodeling, or during states of cellular injury.[91] They have the distinct property of being angiogenic and of stimulating both endothelial cell division and capillary formation in vitro.[92]

Both basic and acidic FGFs are stored in extracellular matrix of connective tissues. FGF has mitogenic effects on a wide variety of cell types. It stimulates both proliferation and differentiation of a large variety of neuroectoderm and mesodermally derived cells.[93] FGF peptides are between 15,000 and 17,000 kd and are single-chain polypeptides. Acidic FGF has 55% homology with basic FGF. Acidic FGF has a more restrictive pattern of tissue expression, being present primarily in bovine brain and retina. In contrast, basic FGF has been isolated from a wide variety of tissues, including kidney. The FGF receptor is structurally similar to the c-*kit* proto-oncogene. The FGF receptor is between 130,000 and 165,000 daltons. Both acidic and basic FGF bind with high affinity to this receptor. Although it is controversial whether the receptor itself possesses intrinsic tyrosine kinase activity, there is rapid tyrosine phosphorylation of 135,000-kd protein following FGF binding to its receptor. A second receptor has also been identified. It has significant structural homology to the FGF receptor.[94]

The biologic activity of acidic FGF can be enhanced by coincubation with heparin, whereas basic FGF appears to be fully potent without heparin binding.[95] In vivo, FGF appears to play an important role in the induction of mesoderm in the developing embryo, in limb regeneration, in development of the central nervous system, as in vascularization of several organs. Many of the differentiation-dependent functions in embryogenesis that have been attributed to extracellular matrix are now being reassigned to FGF bound to the matrix. FGF is also a potent stimulator of cellular differentiation. It stimulates differentiation of chondrocytes, pre-adipocytes, and astrocytes and delays differentiation or fusion of myoblasts. It also is believed to be a potent stimulant of mesoderm formation in the developing nervous system.[96] It promotes neuronal survival and regulates differentiation of nerve cells, astrocytes, and oligodendrocytes. In addition to being angiogenic, the FGFs are also chemotactic for endothelial cells. They induce the rapid expression of c-*fos* and c-*myc* mRNA, as well as ornithine decarboxylase. Like PDGF, FGF appears to be a competence factor, since it is capable of recruiting quiescent cells into entering the cell cycle. In summary, FGF appears to be a potent growth factor for mesoderm in embryonic tissue and, postnatally, to be an important mitogen for mesodermal and neuroectodermally derived tissues and an important regulator of extracellular matrix protein synthesis and deposition.

Platelet-Derived Growth Factor

Platelet-derived growth factor (PDGF) is the major mitogen in serum accounting for its proliferative effect on cultured cells. As its name implies, PDGF is released from platelets, but it also is released from macrophages.[97] It also is produced by monocytes, endothelial cells, and placental cell types. PDGF is a cationic glycoprotein composed of two chains designated the α and β chains.[98] The PDGF α and β chains can form heterodimers, and the αβ heterodimer is the main isoform of PDGF present in human platelets. However, homodimers of αα and ββ have been identified in osteosarcoma cell lines and porcine platelets, respectively. The amino acid sequence of the β chain is identical with the v-*sis* oncogene product, a finding that has led to the proposal that the transformation by v-*sis* is mediated by an autocrine growth stimulatory mechanism.[99] Two subtypes of PDGF receptor have been described—also designated α and β.[100] The β receptor mediates the major mitogenic actions of PDGF; it binds preferentially to the homodimeric ββ isoform over the αα isoform of PDGF and does not bind the αβ isoform. The α receptor can bind all three isoforms of PDGF. PDGF receptors have been demonstrated to have tyrosine kinase activity. Target cells for PDGF include connective tissue cells, vascular smooth muscle cells, glial cells, and chondrocytes.[101] It is interesting that PDGF has no effect on epithelial cells, which do not appear to express PDGF receptors. PDGF stimulates the synthesis of multiple extracellular-matrix proteins by fibroblasts and smooth muscle cells, including laminen, fibronectin, and type-I collagen. PDGF appears to play a major role in wound healing and repair. PDGF stimulates chemotaxis of fibroblasts into wounds and the synthesis of extracellular matrix proteins, as well as fibroblast division.[102] PDGF has been shown to accelerate wound healing in rodent animal models of wound healing. PDGF mRNA appears to be expressed after injury in multiple wound models, particularly that of balloon denudation of the aorta. This mechanical injury results in the expression of PDGF by smooth muscle cells and endothelial cells.[103] Application of PDGF to healing wounds results in chemotaxis of macrophages, proliferation of fibroblasts, increased collagen formation at the wound, and increased wound-breaking strength.[104] During atherogenesis PDGF is secreted by smooth muscle cells at the site of lesions and is expressed in macrophages near the sites of smooth muscle cell proliferation. Agents that inhibit platelet release have been shown to attenuate atheroma formation in certain experimental model systems. The PDGF-responsive system that has been best characterized is the BALB/c 3T3 fibroblast model. The addition of PDGF to these cultures results in acquisition of competence by the cells and their resulting ability to respond to the combination of EGF and IGF-I and to progress into the "S" phase of the cell cycle. PDGF also induces the rapid synthesis of several oncogene homologues, including c-*fos* and c-*myc*. This action of PDGF is mimicked by a variety of stimuli, including macrophage growth factor, bombesin, and calcium phosphate crystals. PDGF expression has been implicated in the growth of mesenchymal tissues during embryogenesis.[105]

Cytokines

Many other molecules regulate the effects of growth factors in both positive and negative ways. The interleukin family of growth factors comprises molecules with important growth regulatory properties for lymphocyte and monocyte function.[106] Interleukin 1 (IL-1) modulates lymphocytic replication but also stimulates matrix protein synthesis by connective tissue cells. However, this stimulation is selective, since the synthesis of certain types of collagen is actually inhibited. Thus, in tissues undergoing rapid remodeling, such as bone, IL-1 may be a potent stimulator of tissue remodeling by controlling both osteoclast activation and matrix protein synthesis. At least nine structurally distinct interleukins have been identified. All have been reported to modulate immune system function and the growth and differentiation of both lymphocytes and monocytes.

The tumor necrosis factors, TNF-α and TNF-β, are also powerful cytokines.[107] The biologic properties of the TNFs overlap with those of IL-1. They can function as growth factors, growth inhibitors, or modulators of differentiation and are powerful stimulants of bone resorption. The colony-stimulating factors (CSFs) are also a family of growth factors that are important mitogens for cells of granulocytic and monocytic lineages.[108] These factors stimulate monocyte-macrophage-derived and granulocyte-derived progenitor cells. At least four members of this family have been identified in the mouse. CSFs are synthesized not only by cells in bone marrow but also by T cells obtained from the spleen after antigen stimulation. Granulocyte-macrophage CSF (GM-CSF) has a proto-oncogene homologue, as does the CSF receptor. Interferon (IFN) is a multifunctional cytokine produced by T lymphocytes. In many cell-culture systems, it has been shown to inhibit growth. IFN-α and IFN-β have similar spectrums of activity.

An additional important hematopoietic growth factor is erythropoietin (EPO).[109] This is a 39,000-kd sialoprotein. The major site of EPO synthesis is the kidney. Its major stimulus is hypoxia, but it is under the control of GH and its concentration in urine is reduced by hypophysectomy. EPO appears to function by stimulating cell division of erythropoietic stem cells. This expands the population of these cells that go on to differentiate into mature erythrocytes.

Nerve Growth Factor

Nerve growth factor (NGF) is synthesized as a 140-kd precursor, of which the β subunit is the biologically active component.[110] The major biologic function of NGF is the promotion of neurite outgrowth and the maintenance of neuronal survival. Injection of antibodies to NGF into fetal animals results in neuronal degeneration. NGF has also been proposed to have a role in stimulating axonal connections. The NGF receptor is an 80,000-kd protein that is present in neural tissue in a high-affinity form but on lymphocytes in a low-affinity form.

GROWTH FACTORS IN DIABETES

The multitude of growth factors and the relative lack of suitable in vivo models for studying their expression have hampered attempts to identify definitively the specific functions of these factors that may be altered in the diabetic state. For historical reasons, one of the most extensively studied has been IGF-I because of the finding several years ago that some patients with diabetes have increased circulating levels of GH.[111] Likewise, hypophysectomy was shown to improve the diabetic state in dogs, and extraction and injection of pituitary extracts to worsen the diabetic state. Attention was further focused on GH when highly purified GH was found to make normal dogs severely diabetic.[112]

Because of the relationship between GH and the diabetic state, several investigators have focused on the role of IGFs in mediation of some of the complications of diabetes. A major problem encountered has been in determining IGF-I levels in patients with diabetes. Patients with poorly controlled diabetes have been reported to have low-normal or high levels of IGF-I, depending on the type of patients enrolled in the study.[113] No doubt these discrepant findings are due to differences in assay methodology, interference of IGF-binding proteins in IGF radioimmunoassays, and failure to standardize the patient treatment parameters, variations that have made cross-study comparisons difficult. Despite the elevation in GH secretion in patients with poorly controlled diabetes, it appears that their IGF-I levels actually are reduced and that precise control of blood glucose levels may result in normalization of IGF-I.[11] Therefore, it has been proposed that metabolic deterioration first results in decreased biosynthesis of IGF-I and subsequently in decreased serum levels. Secondarily, GH hypersecretion occurs as a result of loss of negative feedback regulation. Tamborlane et al. demonstrated a 70% increase in patients' serum IGF-I levels following chronic insulin infusion therapy.[11] In contrast, Merimee et al. found no change in IGF-I levels in either children or adults with diabetes following improvements in their glucose control.[114] Blethen et al. found a significant correlation between hemoglobin A_{1C} and IGF-I levels in children.[115] Lanes et al. noted a low basal IGF-I level in children whose levels of hemoglobin A_{1C} were greater than 12% and a diminished response to administration of GH.[116] These findings all suggest that patients with poorly controlled diabetes have a blunted hepatic sensitivity to the effects of GH on IGF-I synthesis.

The relationship between retinopathy, GH, and control of the diabetic state is less clear. Several studies have demonstrated that blockage of GH hypersecretion with drugs such as somatostatin may improve retinopathy and that hypophysectomy in diabetic patients results in improved visual acuity.[117,118] Likewise, somatostatin has been found to result in suppressive effects on glomerular filtration rate and renal plasma flow in patients with poorly controlled diabetes.[119] Merimee et al. found high IGF-I levels in seven patient with Type I diabetes who had accelerated retinopathy.[120] However, this study did not rule out an effect of IGF-binding proteins on the IGF assay.

It has been proposed that deterioration of retinopathy during attempts to achieve very tight glucose control is related to a change in serum IGF-I levels.[121] However, contradictory results have also been reported.[122] Interpretation of these studies is complicated by the interference of IGF-binding protein in radioimmunoassays. However, evidence that IGF-I is involved in the development of neovascularization is compelling: IGF-I is GH-dependent, is found in large quantities in capillaries that might leak during lesion development, and directly stimulates the division of endothelial cells as well as the division of retinal pigment epithelial cells.[123] Likewise, IGF-I levels in the vitreous have been found to be elevated in some patients with severe, advanced retinopathy.[124]

There is also compelling evidence implicating IGF-I in renal pathogenesis. GH-deficient patients have low renal plasma flow and glomerular filtration rates (GFRs), both of which normalize after administration of GH.[125] Hirschberg et al. demonstrated that a single muscular injection of GH increases renal plasma flow and GFR within 24 hours, with these increases occurring in parallel with changes in serum IGF-I levels.[126] These authors also directly infused IGF-I into rats and found a 30% increase in GFR. Guler et al. demonstrated that the infusion of IGF-I in humans produces a 30% increase in GFR and renal plasma flow.[127] In rats, the effect of IGF-I on renal plasma flow can be blocked by administration of dexamethasone.

These acute studies point to a possible role of IGF-I in the increase in renal size found in patients with diabetes. Furthermore, 6-day infusion studies in rats have been associated with disproportionately large increases in kidney, spleen, and thymus size in comparison to the increases in other organs.[128] Although transgenic animals expressing the GH genes have typical lesions of diabetic glomerulopathy, animals with IGF-I overexpression do not show similar changes.[129] However, this latter study has been criticized on the basis that the strain of mice expressing IGF-I had serum IGF-I levels only 50% lower than those of the strain expressing GH. Likewise, IGF-I peptide accumulates in kidney during the initial growth phase of experimental streptozotocin-induced diabetes.[130] It is interesting that there is no increase in IGF-I messenger RNA and that the increase in IGF-I appears to be due to changes in IGF-binding protein, with consequently significant accumulation of peptide. Strict insulin treatment abolishes the accumulation of IGF-I and the increase in kidney growth.[131] This finding of IGF-I accumulation during diabetic renal hypertrophy has been confirmed, and the accumulation is apparently greater in postpubertal than in prepubertal rats. Whether the transvascular transport is responsible for the IGF-I that arrives in the kidney is unknown, but clearly the induction of IGF-I mRNA does not occur in streptozotocin diabetes. However, other studies have shown short-term increases in IGF-I levels in the kidney. The pattern of change as determined by immunocytochemical assays is more consistent with an increase in levels of IGF-binding proteins, which have been shown to be present in the proximal and distal tubules as well as in the collecting ducts of normal rats.[132]

FGF may also be involved in the pathogenesis of diabetic complications. It is an important angiogenic factor for retinal capillaries and may be derived from retinal tissue.[133] It also binds to heparin sulfate proteoglycan components of the endothelial cell extracellular matrix. FGF has been shown to act synergistically with IGF-I in stimulating fibroblast growth. Therefore, a coordinate role for both growth factors in the development of retinopathy is an attractive hypothesis. PDGF has been implicated in the pathogenesis of macroangiopathy in diabetes and atherosclerosis. Insulin is believed to accelerate the effects of PDGF on proliferation of smooth muscle cells if present in pharmacologic concentrations, and these levels of insulin can occur in some diabetic patients.[134] The abnormal growth-promoting activity in platelet extracts that has been documented in patients with Type I diabetes normalizes after intensive insulin therapy.[135] This activity appeared to be due to a mixture of growth factors, however, and could not be ascribed solely to PDGF.

EGF may have potent effects on kidneys. It appears to be important in the development of the embryonic kidney. Urinary excretion of EGF is reduced during the development of diabetic nephropathy. Therefore, EGF has been postulated to have a role in the development of diabetic glomerulopathy.[136] Synthesis of EGF increases after unilateral nephrectomy, and transient increases in the secretion of EGF into distal tubules have been observed in patients with diabetes.[137]

The role of other growth factors in the pathogenesis of diabetes and diabetic complications remains to be elucidated. However, it is clear that important roles for these growth factors in the pathogenesis of diabetic complications may be present.

SUMMARY

Definitive determination of the role of specific peptide growth factors in the development of diabetic complications has been hampered by the complexity of the model test systems used for analysis. Current studies that identify the changes in abundance of specific mitogens following the induction of diabetes in experimental animals may provide clues as to which mitogens should receive more extensive study. New techniques involving mutagenesis and expression of mutants in transgenic animals may help provide a better understanding of the role of each of these factors in the pathogenesis of complications involving tissue overgrowth or degeneration.

REFERENCES

1. Pledger WJ, Stiles CD, Antoniades HN, Scher CD. Induction of DNA synthesis and BALB/c 3T3 cells by serum components: a reevaluation of the commitment process. Proc Natl Acad Sci USA 1977;74:4481–5.
2. Leof EB, Wharton W, Van Wyk JJ, Pledger WJ. Epidermal growth factor (EGF) and somatomedin-C regulate G1 progression in competent BALB/c-3T3 cells. Exp Cell Res 1982;141:107–15.
3. Rinderknecht E, Humbel RE. The amino acid sequence of human insulin-like growth factor I and its structural homology with proinsulin. J Biol Chem 1978;253:2769–76.
4. Cascieri MA, Chicchi GG, Applebaum J, et al. Mutants of human insulin-like growth factor I with reduced affinity for the type I insulin-like growth factor receptor. Biochemistry 1988;27:3229–33.
5. Bayne ML, Applebaum J, Chicchi GG, et al. Structural analogs of human insulin-like growth factor-I with reduced affinity for serum binding proteins and the type 2 insulin-like growth factor receptor. J Biol Chem 1988; 263:6233–9.
6. Cascieri MA, Hayes NS, Bayne ML. Characterization of the increased biological potency in BALB/c 3T3 cells of two analogs of human insulin-like growth factor-I which have reduced affinity for the 28 k cell-derived binding protein. J Cell Physiol 1989;139:181–8.
7. Isley WL, Underwood LE, Clemmons DR. Dietary components that regulate serum somatomedin-C concentrations in humans. J Clin Invest 1983;71:175–82.
8. Isley WL, Underwood LE, Clemmons DR. Changes in plasma somatomedin-C in response to ingestion of diets with variable protein and energy content. JPEN J Parenter Enteral Nutr 1984;8:407–11.
9. Merimee TJ, Zapf J, Froesch ER. Insulin-like growth factors in the fed and fasted states. J Clin Endocrinol Metab 1982;55:999–1002.
10. Maes M, Amand Y, Underwood LE, et al. Decreased serum insulin-like growth factor-I response to growth hormone in hypophysectomized rats fed a low protein diet: evidence for a postreceptor defect. Acta Endocrinol 1988; 117:320–6.
11. Tamborlane WV, Hintz RL, Bergman M, et al. Insulin-infusion-pump treatment of diabetes: influence of improved metabolic control on plasma somatomedin levels. N Engl J Med 1981;305:303–7.
12. Clemmons DR, Underwood LE, Dickerson RN, et al. Use of plasma somatomedin-C/insulin-like growth factor I measurements to monitor the response to nutritional repletion in malnourished patients. Am J Clin Nutr 1985; 41:191–8.
13. Hawker FH, Stewart PM, Baxter RC, et al. Relationship of somatomedin-C/insulin-like growth factor-I levels to conventional nutritional indices in critically ill patients. Crit Care Med 1987;15:732–6.
14. Donahue SP, Phillips LS. Response of IGF-I to nutritional support in malnourished hospital patients: a possible indicator of short-term changes in nutritional status. Am J Clin Nutr 1989;50:962–9.
15. Davenport ML, Svoboda ME, Koerber KL, et al. Serum concentrations of insulin-like growth factor II are not changed by short-term fasting and refeeding. J Clin Endocrinol Metab 1988;67:1231–6.

16. Salmon WD Jr, Daughaday WH. A hormonally controlled serum factor which stimulates sulfate incorporation by cartilage in vitro. J Lab Clin Med 1957;49:825–36.

17. Copeland KC, Underwood LE, Van Wyk JJ. Induction of immunoreactive somatomedin-C in human serum by growth hormone: dose-response relationships and effect on chromatographic profiles. J Clin Endocrinol Metab 1980;50:690–7.

18. Clemmons DR, Van Wyk JJ, Ridgway EG, et al. Evaluation of acromegaly by radioimmunoassay of somatomedin-C. N Engl J Med 1979;301:1138–42.

19. Lamberts SWJ, Vitterlinden P, Schuijff PC, Klijn JGM. Therapy of acromegaly with sandostatin: the predictive value of an acute test, the value of serum somatomedin-C measurements in dose adjustment and their definition of a biochemical cure. Clin Endocrinol 1988;29:411–20.

20. Roberts CT Jr, Brown AL, Graham DE, et al. Growth hormone regulates the abundance of insulin-like growth factor-I RNA in adult rat liver. J Biol Chem 1986;261:10025–8.

21. Maes M, Underwood LE, Ketelslegers J-M. Low serum somatomedin-C in protein deficiency: relationship with changes in liver somatogenic and lactogenic binding sites. Mol Cell Endocrinol 1984;37:301–9.

22. Moats-Staats BM, Brady JL Jr, Underwood LE, D'Ercole AJ. Dietary protein restriction in artifically reared neonatal rats causes a reduction of insulin-like growth factor-I gene expression. Endocrinology 1989;125:2368–74.

23. Straus DS, Takemoto CD. Effect of fasting on insulin-like growth factor-I (IGF-I) and growth hormone receptor mRNA levels and IGF-I gene transcription in rat liver. Mol Endocrinol 1990;4:91–100.

24. Chernausek SD, Underwood LE, Utiger RD, Van Wyk JJ. Growth hormone secretion and plasma somatomedin-C in primary hypothyroidism. Clin Endocrinol 1983;19:337–44.

25. Copeland KC, Johnson DM, Kuehl TJ, Castracane VD. Estrogen stimulates growth hormone and somatomedin-C in castrate and intact female baboons. J Clin Endocrinol Metab 1984;58:698–703.

26. Smith EP, Sadler TW, D'Ercole AJ. Somatomedins/insulin-like growth factors, their receptors and binding proteins are present during mouse embryogenesis. Development 1987;101:73–82.

27. Godowski PJ, Leung DW, Meacham LR, et al. Characterization of the human growth hormone receptor gene and demonstration of a partial gene deletion in two patients with Laron-type dwarfism. Proc Natl Acad Sci USA 1989;86:8083–7.

28. Walker JL, Ginalska-Malinowska M, Romer TE, et al. Effects of infusion of insulin-like growth factor I in a child with growth hormone insensitivity syndrome (Laron dwarfism). N Engl J Med 1991;324:1483–8.

29. Han VKM, D'Ercole AJ, Lund PK. Cellular localization of somatomedin (insulin-like growth factor) messenger RNA in the human fetus. Science 1987;236:193–7.

30. Roberts CT Jr, Lasky SR, Lowe WL Jr, et al. Molecular coding of rat insulin-like growth factor-I complementary deoxyribonucleic acids: differential messenger ribonucleic acid processing and regulation by growth hormone in extrahepatic tissues. Mol Endocrinol 1987;1:243–8.

31. Clemmons DR, Van Wyk JJ. Evidence for a functional role of endogenously produced somatomedinlike peptides in the regulation of DNA synthesis in cultured human fibroblasts and porcine smooth muscle cells. J Clin Invest 1985;75:1914–8.

32. Yee D, Favoni RE, Lupu R, et al. The insulin-like growth factor binding protein BP-25 is expressed by human breast cancer cells. Biochem Biophys Res Commun 1989;158:38–44.

33. Adashi EY, Resnick CE, D'Ercole AJ, et al. Insulin-like growth factors as intraovarian regulators of granulosa cell growth and function. Endocrine Rev 1985;6:400–20.

34. Jennische E, and Hansson H-A. Regenerating skeletal muscle cells express insulin-like growth factor I. Acta Physiol Scand 1987;130:327–32.

35. Edwall D, Schalling M, Jennische E, Norstedt G. Induction of insulin-like growth factor-I messenger ribonucleic acid during regeneration of skeletal muscle. Endocrinology 1989;124:820–5.

36. Clemmons DR. Exposure to platelet-derived growth factor modulates the porcine aortic smooth muscle cell response to somatomedin-C. Endocrinology 1985;117:77–83.

37. Isgaard J, Nilsson A, Lindahl A, et al. Effects of local administration of GH and IGF-I on longitudinal bone growth in rats. Am J Physiol 1986;250:E367–72.

38. Nilsson A, Isgaard J, Lindahl A, et al. Regulation by growth hormone of number of chondrocytes containing IGF-I in rat growth plate. Science 1986;233:571–4.

39. Ullrich A, Gray A, Tam AW, et al. Insulin-like growth factor-I receptor primary structure: cmparison with insulin receptor suggests structural determinants that define functional specificity. EMBO J 1986;5:2503–12.

40. Sara VR, Hall K. Insulin-like growth factors and their binding proteins. Physiol Rev 1990;70:591–614.

41. Flier JS, Usher P, Moses AC. Monoclonal antibody to the type I insulin-like growth factor (IGF-I) receptor blocks IGF-I receptor-mediated DNA synthesis: clarification of the mitogenic mechanisms of IGF-I and insulin in human skin fibroblasts. Proc Natl Acad Sci USA 1986;83:664–8.

42. Massague J, Czech MP. The subunit structures of two distinct receptors for insulin-like growth factors I and II and their relationship to the insulin receptor. J Biol Chem 1982;257:5038–45.

43. Kasuga M, Sasaki N, Kahn CR, Nissley SP. Antireceptor antibodies as probes of insulinlike growth factor receptor structure. J Clin Invest 1983;72:1459.

44. Clemmons DR, Van Wyk JJ, Pledger WJ. Sequential addition of platelet factor and plasma to BALB/c 3T3 fibroblast cultures stimulates somatomedin-C binding early in the cell cycle. Proc Natl Acad Sci USA 1980;77:6644–8.

45. Massague J, Guillette BJ, Czech MP. Affinity labeling of multiplication stimulating activity receptors in membranes from rat and human tissues. J Biol Chem 1981;256:2122–5.

46. Oshima A, Nolan CM, Kyle JW, et al. The human cation-independent mannose-6-phosphate receptor: cloning and sequence of the full-length cDNA and expression of functional receptor in COS cells. J Biol Chem 1988;263:2553–62.

47. Nissley SP, Kiess W, Skalar MM. The insulin-like growth factor-II mannose-6-phosphate receptor. In: LeRoith D, ed. Insulin-like growth factors: cellular and molecular aspects. Boca Raton: CRC Press, 1991:111–50.

48. Oppenheimer CL, Pessin JE, Massague J, et al. Insulin action rapidly modulates the apparent affinity of the insulin-like growth factor-II receptor. J Biol Chem 1983;258:4824–30.

49. Kiess W, Greenstein LA, White RM, et al. Type II insulin-like growth factor receptor is present in rat serum. Proc Natl Acad Sci USA 1987;84:7720–4.

50. Nishimoto I, Hata Y, Ogata E, Kojima I. Insulin-like growth factor-II stimulates calcium influx in competent BALB/C 3T3 cells primed with epidermal growth factor: characteristics of calcium influx and involvement of GTP-binding proteins. J Biol Chem 1987;262:12120–6.

51. Nishimoto I, Murayama Y, Katada T, et al. Possible direct linkage of insulin-like growth factor-II receptor with guanine nucleotide-binding proteins. J Biol Chem 1989;264:14029–38.

52. Stiles CD, Capone GT, Scher CD, et al. Dual control of cell growth by somatomedins and platelet-derived growth factor. Proc Natl Acad Sci USA 1979;76:1279–83.

53. Kaplowitz PB, D'Ercole AJ, Underwood LE, Van Wyk JJ. Stimulation by somatomedin-c of aminoisobutyric acid uptake in human fibroblasts: a possible test for cellular responsiveness to somatomedin. J Clin Endocrinol Metab 1984;58:176–81.

54. Salmon WD Jr, DuVall MR. In vitro stimulation of leucine incorporation into muscle and cartilage protein by a serum fraction with sulfation factor activity: differentiation of effects from those of growth hormone and insulin. Endocrinology 1970;87:1168–80.

55. Hintz RL, Clemmons DR, Underwood LE, Van Wyk JJ. Competitive binding of somatomedin to the insulin receptors of adipocytes, chondrocytes, and liver membranes. Proc Natl Acad Sci USA 1972;69:2351–3.

56. Penhoat A, Jiallard C, Saez JM. Synergistic effects of corticotropin and insulin-like growth factor-I on corticotropin receptors and corticotropin responsiveness in cultured bovine adrenocortical cells. Biochem Biophys Res Commun 1989;165:355–9.

57. Adashi EY, Resnick CE, Hernandez ER, et al. Insulin-like growth factor-I as an amplifier of follicle-stimulating hormone action: studies on mechanism(s) and site(s) of action in cultured rat granulosa cells. Endocrinology 1988;122:1583–91.

58. Shimasaki S, Shimonaka M, Zhang H-P, Ling N. Isolation and molecular characterization of three novel insulin-like growth factor binding proteins (IGFBP-4, 5 and 6). In: Spencer EM, ed. Modern concepts of insulin-like growth factors. New York: Elsevier, 1991:343–58.

59. Baxter RC, Martin JL. Radioimmunoassay of growth hormone-dependent insulinlike growth factor binding protein in human plasma. J Clin Invest 1986;78:1504–12.

60. Baxter RC, Martin JL. Structure of the Mr 140,000 growth hormone-dependent insulin-like growth factor binding protein complex: determination by reconstitution and affinity labeling. Proc Natl Acad Sci USA 1989;86:6898–902.

61. Busby WH, Klapper DS, Clemmons DR. Purification of a 31000 dalton somatomedin-C binding protein from human amniotic fluid: isolation of two forms with different biologic actions. J Biol Chem 1988;263:14203–10.

62. Brown AL, Chiariotti L, Orlowski CC, et al. Nucleotide sequence and expression of a cDNA clone encoding a fetal rat binding protein for insulin-like growth factors. J Biol Chem 1989;264:5148–54.

63. Zapf J, Schmid C, Guler HP, et al. Regulation of binding proteins for insulin-like growth factors (IGF) in humans: increased expression of IGF binding protein 2 during IGF I treatment of healthy adults and in patients with extrapancreatic tumor hypoglycemia. J Clin Invest 1990;86:952–61.

64. Hardouin S, Gourmelen M, Noguiez P, et al. Molecular forms of serum insulin-like growth factor (IGF)-binding proteins in man: relationships with growth hormone and

IGFs and physiological significance. J Clin Endocrinol Metab 1989;69:1291–301.

65. Suikkari A-M, Koivisto VA, Koistinen R, et al. Dose-response characteristics for suppression of low molecular weight plasma insulin-like growth factor-binding protein by insulin. J Clin Endocrinol Metab 1989;68:135–40.

66. McCusker RH, Camacho-Hubner C, Bayne ML, et al. Insulin-like growth factor (IGF) binding to human fibroblast and glioblastoma cells: the modulating effect of cell released IGF binding proteins (IGFBPs). J Cell Physiol 1990;144:244–53.

67. Elgin RG, Busby WH, Clemmons DR. An insulin-like growth factor (IGF) binding protein enhances the biologic response to IGF-I. Proc Natl Acad Sci USA 1987;84:3254–8.

68. Clemmons DR, Camacho-Hubner C, Jones JI, et al. Insulin-like growth factor binding proteins: mechanisms of action at the cellular level. In: Spencer EM, ed. Modern concepts of insulin-like growth factors. New York: Elsevier, 1991:475–86.

69. Jones JI, D'Ercole AJ, Clemmons DR. Phosphorylation of insulin-like growth factor binding protein in cell culture and in vivo: effects on affinity for IGF-I. Proc Natl Acad Sci USA 1991;88:7481–5.

70. Cohen S. Isolation of a mouse submaxillary gland protein accelerating incisor eruption and eyelid opening in the new-born animal. J Biol Chem 1962;237:1555–62.

71. Carpenter G, Cohen S. Epidermal growth factor. Annu Rev Biochem 1979;48:193–216.

72. Das M. Epidermal growth factor: mechanisms of action. Int Rev Cytol 1982;78:233–56.

73. Wahl MI, Nishibe S, Kim JW, et al. Identification of two epidermal growth factor sensitive tyrosine phosphorylation sites of phospholipase C- in intact HSC-1 cells. J Biol Chem 1990;265:3944–8.

74. Downward J, Yarden Y, Mayes E, et al. Close similarity of epidermal growth factor receptor and V-erb-B oncogene protein sequences. Nature 1984;307:521–7.

75. Bradshaw TK. Cellular transformation: the role of oncogenes and grwoth factors. Mutagenesis 1986;1:91–7.

76. Plowman GD, Whitney GS, Neubauer MG, et al. Molecular cloning and expression of an additional epidermal growth factor receptor-related gene. Proc Natl Acad Sci USA 1990;87:4905–9.

77. Grotendorst GR, Soma Y, Takehara K, Charette M. EGF and TGF-alpha are potent chemoattractants for endothelial cells and EGF-like peptides are present at sites of tissue regeneration. J Cell Physiol 1989;139:617–23.

78. Pessa ME, Bland KI, Copeland EM III. Growth factors and determinants of wound repair. J Surg Res 1987;42:207–17.

79. Lee DC, Rochford R, Todaro GJ, Villarreal LP. Developmental expression of rat transforming growth factor-' mRNA. Mol Cell Biol 1985;5:3644–6.

80. Gottlieb AB, Chang CK, Posnett DN, et al. Detection of transforming growth factor β in normal, malignant and hyperproliferative human keratinocytes. J Exp Med 1988;167:670–5.

81. Barnard JA, Lyons RM, Moses HL. The cell biology of transforming growth factor β. Biochim Biophys Acta 1990;1032:79–87.

82. Roberts AB, Anzano MA, Wakefield LM, et al. Type β transforming growth factor: a bifunctional regulator of cellular growth. Proc Natl Acad Sci USA 1985;82:119–23.

83. Massague J, Cheifetz S, Boyd FT, Andres JL. Transforming TGF-beta receptors and TGF-beta binding proteoglycans:

recent progress in identifying their functional properties. Ann NY Acad Sci 1990;593:59–72.

84. Sato Y, Rifkin DB. Inhibition of endothelial cell movement by pericytes and smooth muscle cells: activation of latent transforming growth factor-βI-like molecule by plasmin during co-culture. J Cell Biol 1989;109:309–15.

85. Massague J, Cheifetz S, Ignotz RA, Boyd FT. Multiple type-beta transforming growth factors and their receptors. J Cell Physiol Suppl 1987;5:43–7.

86. Pertovaara L, Sistonen L, Bos TJ, et al. Enhanced *jun* gene expression is an early genomic response to transforming growth factor β stimulation. Mol Cell Biol 1989;9:1255–62.

87. Canalis E, McCarthy T, Centrella M. Growth factors and the regulation of bone remodeling. J Clin Invest 1988;81:277–81.

88. Florini JR, Roberts AB, Ewton DZ, et al. Transforming growth factor-β: a very potent inhibitor of myoblast differentiation, identical to the differentiation inhibitor secreted by buffalo rat liver cells. J Biol Chem 1986;261:16509–13.

89. Laiho M, Keski-Oja J. Growth factors in the regulation of pericellular proteolysis. Cancer Res 1989;49:2533–53.

90. Burgess WH, Maciag T. The heparin-binding (fibroblast) growth factor family of proteins. Annu Rev Biochem 1989;58:575–606.

91. Gospodarowicz D, Ferrara N, Schweigerer L, Neufeld G. Structural characterization, and biological functions of fibroblast growth factor. Endocrine Rev 1987;8:95–114.

92. Folkman J, Klagsbrun M. Angiogenic factors. Science 1987;235:442–7.

93. Gospodarowicz D, Bialecki H, Greenburg G. Purification of the fibroblast growth factor activity from bovine brain. J Biol Chem 1970;253:3736–43.

94. Neufeld G, Gospodarowicz D. Basic and acidic fibroblast growth factors interact with the same cell surface receptors. J Biol Chem 1986;261:5631–7.

95. Rifkin DB, Moscatelli D. Recent developments in the cell biology of basic fibroblast growth factor. J Cell Biol 1989;109:1–6.

96. Grunz H, McKeehan Wl, Knöchel W, et al. Induction of mesodermal tissues by acidic and basic heparin binding growth factors. Cell Diff 1988;22:183–90.

97. Heldin C-H, Westermark B. Platelet-derived growth factor: mechanism of action and possible in vivo function. Cell Reg 1990;1:555–66.

98. Deuel TF, Huang JS. Platelet-derived growth factor: structure, function, and roles in normal and transformed cells. J Clin Invest 1984;74:669–76.

99. Deuel TF, Pierce GF, Yeh HJ, et al. Platelet-derived growth factor/sis in normal and neoplastic cell growth. J Cell Physiol Suppl 1987;5:95–9.

100. Heldin C-H, Bäckström G, Östman A. Binding of different dimeric forms of PDGF to human fibroblasts: evidence for two separate receptor types. EMBO J 1988;7:1387–93.

101. Ross R, Raines EW, Bowen-Pope DF. The biology of platelet derived growth factor. Cell 1986;46:155–69.

102. Grotendorst GR, Seppä HEJ, Kleinman HK, Martin G. Attachment of smooth muscle cells to collagen and their migration toward platelet-derived growth factor. Proc Natl Acad Sci USA 1981;78:3669–72.

103. Collins T, Ginsburg D, Boss JM, et al. Cultured human endothelial cells express platelet-derived growth factor B chain: cDNA cloning and structural analysis [Letter]. Nature 1985;316:748–50.

104. Pierce GF, Mustoe TA, Senior RM, et al. In vivo incisional wound healing augmented by platelet-derived growth factor and recombinant c-*sis* gene homodimeric proteins. J Exp Med 1988;167:974–87.

105. Rizzino A, Bowen-Pope DF. Production of PDGF-like growth factors by embryonal carcinoma cells and binding of PDGF to their endoderm-like differentiated cells. Dev Biol 1985;110:15–22.

106. Bendtzen K. Biological properties of interleukins. Allergy 1983;38:219–26.

107. Balkwill FR. Tumour necrosis factor. Br Med Bull 1989;45(2):389–400.

108. Platzer E. Human hemopoietic growth factors. Eur J Haematol 1989;42:1–15.

109. Groopman JE, Molina J-M, Scadden DT. Hematopoietic growth factors: biology and clinical applications. N Engl J Med 1989;321:1449–59.

110. Bradshaw RA. Nerve growth factor. Annu Rev Biochem 1978;47:191–216.

111. Hansen AP, Johansen K. Diurnal patterns of blood glucose, serum free fatty acids, insulin, glucagon and growth hormone in normals and juvenile diabetics. Diabetelogia 1970;6:27–33.

112. Campbell J, Davidson IWF, Lei HP. Production of permanent diabetes by highly purified growth hormone. Endocrinology 1950;46:588–90.

113. Flyvbjerg A. Growth factors and diabetic complications. Diabetic Med 1991;90:387–99.

114. Merimee TJ, Gardner DF, Zapf J, Froesch ER. Effect of glycemic control on serum insulin-like growth factors in diabetes mellitus. Diabetes 1984;33:790–3.

115. Blethen SL, Sargeant DT, Whitlow MG, Santiago JV. Effect of pubertal stage and recent blood glucose control on plasma somatomedin-C in children with insulin-dependent diabetes mellitus. Diabetes 1981;30:868–72.

116. Lanes R, Recker B, Fort P, Lifshitz F. Impaired somatomedin generation test in children with insulin-dependent diabetes mellitus. Diabetes 1985;34:156–60.

117. Fassler JE, Hughes JH, Titterington L. Somatostatin analog: an inhibitor of angiogenesis? Clin Res 1988;36:896A.

118. Lee HK, Suh KU, Koh C-S, et al. Effect of SMS 201–995 in rapidly progressive diabetic retinopathy [Letter]. Diabetes Care 1988;11:441–3.

119. Vora J, Owens DR, Luzio S, et al. Renal response to intravenous somatostatin in insulin-dependent diabetic patients and normal subjects. J Clin Endocrinol Metab 1987;64:975–9.

120. Merimee TJ, Zapf J, Froesch ER. Insulin-like growth factors: studies in diabetics with and without retinopathy. N Engl J Med 1983;309:527–30.

121. Hanssen K, Dahl-Jørgensen K, Lauritzen T, et al. Diabetic control and microvascular complications: the near-normoglycaemic experience. Diabetelogia 1986;29:677–64.

122. Hyer SL, Sharps PS, Brooks RA, et al. A two-year follow-up study of serum insulinlike growth factor-I in diabetics with retinopathy. Metabolism 1989;38:586–9.

123. King GL, Goodman AD, Buzney S, et al. Receptors and growth-promoting effects of insulin and insulinlike growth factors on cells from bovine retinal capillaries and aorta. J Clin Invest 1985;5:1028–36.

124. Grant M, Russell B, Fitzgerald C, Merimee TJ. Insulin-like growth factors in vitreous: studies in control and diabetic subjects with neovascularization. Diabetes 1986;35:416–20.

125. Christiansen JS, Gammelgaard J, Ørskov H, et al. Kidney function and size in normal subjects before and during

growth hormone administration for one week. Eur J Clin Invest 1981;11:487–90.

126. Hirschberg R, Rabb H, Begamo R, Kopple JD. The delayed effect of growth hormone on renal function in humans. Kidney Int 1989;35:865–70.

127. Guler HP, Eckardt KU, Zapf J, et al. Insulin-like growth factor-I increases glomerular filtration rate and renal plasma flow in man. Acta Endocrinol 1989;121:101–6.

128. Guler H-P, Zapf J, Scheiwiller E, Froesch ER. Recombinant human insulin-like growth factor-I stimulates growth and has distinct effects on organ size in hypophysectomized rats. Proc Natl Acad Sci USA 1988;85:4889–93.

129. Quaife CJ, Mathews LS, Pinkert CA, et al. Histopathology associated with elevated levels of growth hormone and insulin-like growth factor I in transgenic mice. Endocrinology 1989;124:40–8.

130. Flyvbjerg A, Ørskov H. Kidney tissue insulin-like growth factor-I and initial renal growth in diabetic rats: relation to severity of diabetes. Acta Endocrinol 1990;122:374–8.

131. Flyvbjerg A, Thorlacius-Ussing O, Naeraa R, et al. Kidney tissue somatomedin C and initial renal growth in diabetic and uninephrectomised rats. Diabetelogia 1988;31: 310–4.

132. Kobayashi S, Clemmons DR, Venkatachalam MA. Co-localization of insulin-like growth factor binding protein with insulin-like growth factor I in rat kidney. Am J Physiol 1991;261:F22–8.

133. Baird A, Esch F, Gospodarowicz D, Guillemin, R. Retina- and eye-derived endothelial cell growth factors: partial molecular characterization and identity with acidic and basic fibroblast growth factors. Biochemistry 1985;24: 7855–60.

134. Ross R. Atherosclerosis: a problem of the biology of arterial wall cells and their interactions with blood components. Arteriosclerosis 1981;1:293–11.

135. Hamet P, Sugimoto H, Umeda F, et al. Abnormalities of platelet-derived growth factors in insulin-dependent diabetes. Metabolism 1985;34(Suppl 1):25–31.

136. Mathiesen ER, Nexø, Hommel E, Parving HH. Reduced urinary excretion of epidermal growth factor in incipient and overt diabetic nephropathy. Diabetic Med 1989; 6:121–6.

137. Jennische E, Andersson G, Hansson H-A. Epidermal growth factor is expressed by cells in the distal tubules during postnephrectomy renal growth. Acta Physiol Scand 1987;129:449–50.

Chapter 11

DEFINITION, DIAGNOSIS, AND CLASSIFICATION OF DIABETES MELLITUS AND IMPAIRED GLUCOSE TOLERANCE

PETER H. BENNETT

Diabetes mellitus represents a heterogenous group of disorders, some of which can be characterized in terms of specific etiology and/or pathogenesis. In many cases, however, such specific pathogenetic characterization is not possible. Consequently, the most widely used classification of diabetes is based primarily upon clinical descriptive criteria and, when possible, on more specific etiologic characterization within these classes.

DEFINITION OF DIABETES MELLITUS

Diabetes mellitus is a syndrome characterized by chronic hyperglycemia and disturbances of carbohydrate, fat, and protein metabolism associated with absolute or relative deficiencies in insulin secretion and/or insulin action. When fully expressed, diabetes is characterized by fasting hyperglycemia, but the disease can also be recognized during less overt stages and before fasting hyperglycemia appears, most usually by the presence of glucose intolerance. Diabetes mellitus may be suspected or recognized clinically by the presence of characteristic symptoms such as excessive thirst, polyuria, pruritus, otherwise unexplained weight loss, or one or more of the many complications associated with or attributable to the disease.

Diabetes, particularly non-insulin-dependent diabetes, however, may be asymptomatic, in which case the diagnosis depends on biochemical investigations. Quite often, however, diabetes is discovered because of an abnormal result of a routine blood or urine glucose test. In some instances diabetes may be present only intermit-tently, as for example, with glucose intolerance in pregnancy, which may reverse after parturition. In some cases the likelihood of the development of diabetes may be recognized even before abnormalities of glucose tolerance are apparent. In the evolution of insulin-dependent diabetes mellitus, immunologic disturbances such as the presence of islet cell and other antibodies may precede the appearance of clinically apparent disease by months or even years. In some families it is possible to detect certain gene mutations that are strongly associated with certain forms of diabetes, e.g., certain insulin-receptor abnormalities, or mutations in the glucokinase gene. Presumably, these abnormalities are detectable at any time in life.

Although a number of specific causes of diabetes mellitus have been elucidated, the etiology and pathogenesis of the more common types of diabetes are poorly understood, and the extent of the heterogeneity among these more common types remains uncertain. Because of these uncertainties, the most widely accepted classification of diabetes mellitus is based primarily on clinical descriptive criteria. Nevertheless, specific etiologic classification is possible in some cases.

CLASSIFICATION OF DIABETES MELLITUS AND ALLIED CATEGORIES OF GLUCOSE INTOLERANCE

The most widely accepted classification of diabetes mellitus was devised initially by the National Diabetes Data Group (NDDG) in the United States[1] and subsequently became the basis for the World Health Organiza-

193

tion (WHO) classification of diabetes.[2,3] This classification was first adopted by WHO in 1980 and modified in 1985 (Table 11−1).

The WHO classification of diabetes mellitus and allied categories of glucose intolerance includes a number of clinical classes and two statistical risk classes. The use of the risk classes permits the classification of individuals who have had an abnormality of glucose tolerance that reverted to normality, i.e., previous abnormality of glucose tolerance, and of individuals who can be designated as having a high likelihood of developing glucose intolerance in the future, i.e., potential abnormality of glucose tolerance.

The WHO classification has become accepted internationally, and although it represents a compromise between a clinical and an etiologic system, it does permit a clinically useful characterization of diabetes mellitus even when the specific cause or etiology is not known.

Clinical Classes

The WHO system of classification contains three major clinical classes: diabetes mellitus, impaired glucose tolerance, and gestational diabetes mellitus. The diagnosis of diabetes mellitus is reserved for those who meet the criteria for diagnosis of diabetes (see below). The designation of impaired glucose tolerance is assigned to persons whose glucose tolerance is above the conventional boundaries of normality but does not meet the criteria for a diagnosis of diabetes. As a group, the persons in this category have a much higher likelihood than the general population of experiencing a progression of their condition, and many ultimately develop and meet the

Table 11−1. World Health Organization Classification of Diabetes Mellitus and Allied Categories of Glucose Intolerance

A. Clinical classes
   Diabetes mellitus
     Insulin-dependent diabetes mellitus
     Non-insulin-dependent diabetes mellitus
       a) Non-obese
       b) Obese
     Malnutrition-related diabetes mellitus
     Other types of diabetes associated with certain conditions and
      syndromes:
       1) pancreatic disease, 2) disease of hormonal etiology, 3)
        drug- or chemical-induced conditions, 4) abnormalities of
        insulin or its receptors, 5) certain genetic syndromes, 6)
        miscellaneous
   Impaired glucose tolerance
       a) Non-obese
       b) Obese
       c) Associated with certain conditions and syndromes
   Gestational diabetes mellitus
B. Statistical risk classes (normal glucose tolerance but substantially
   increased risk of developing diabetes)
   1) Previous abnormality of glucose tolerance
   2) Potential abnormality of glucose tolerance

Data from reference 3.

criteria for diabetes. The third clinical class is gestational diabetes mellitus. Gestational diabetes is defined as diabetes that is first recognized during pregnancy. Both the degree and severity of hyperglycemia in this form of diabetes vary considerably. Following parturition, some women whose glucose intolerance is first recognized in pregnancy will revert to normal glucose tolerance, whereas others may continue to have impaired glucose tolerance or diabetes, which then can be categorized more specifically. Women with gestational diabetes whose glucose tolerance becomes normal after parturition are then reclassified in the statistical risk class of previous abnormality of glucose intolerance. These women have a high likelihood of developing gestational diabetes again during a subsequent pregnancy and a high risk of developing diabetes even when they are not pregnant.

Diabetes Mellitus

The clinical class of diabetes mellitus is divided into four subgroups: insulin-dependent diabetes mellitus; non-insulin-dependent diabetes mellitus; malnutrition-related diabetes mellitus; and other types of diabetes associated with certain conditions and syndromes.

Insulin-Dependent Diabetes Mellitus (IDDM). IDDM is defined by the presence of classical symptoms of diabetes such as thirst, polyuria, wasting, and/or ketoacidosis and the necessity for insulin treatment not only to control the hyperglycemia and symptoms but to prevent the spontaneous occurrence of ketoacidosis. Unless persons with IDDM are already receiving insulin treatment, they usually have markedly elevated fasting glucose levels and raised serum levels of ketone bodies. The diagnosis of IDDM usually is made on the basis of symptoms and these biochemical parameters alone. A glucose tolerance test is seldom required for diagnosis.

IDDM can be a manifestation of several different pathogenetic processes. All of these produce marked deficits in insulin secretion that lead to profound deficits in insulin action. This deficiency in insulin action leads to a variety of metabolic consequences, the more common manifestations of which are severe hyperglycemia and its immediately related symptoms (polyuria, thirst, polyphagia, and weight loss) and poorly regulated lipolysis, producing elevated concentrations of ketone bodies (acetone, acetoacetate, β-hydroxybutyrate) that lead to ketosis and ketonuria. If the blood ketone levels are sufficiently high, they result in metabolic acidosis, which leads to diabetic coma and sometimes death.

IDDM is the most common form of diabetes in children and young adults, particularly those of northern European origin. The disease has a much lower incidence among persons of Oriental or native American heritage. Although the incidence increases with age until adolescence and then declines, the disease can have its onset at any age.

An etiologic classification of IDDM is outlined in Table 11−2. Autoimmune destruction of pancreatic β-cells is the most common cause of IDDM. Evidence of this autoimmune process includes the presence of islet cell antibodies (ICA), insulin autoantibodies (IAA), and anti-

Table 11–2.   Etiologic Classification:
Insulin-Dependent Diabetes Mellitus

Associated with deficient insulin secretion due to
  A. Idiopathic autoimmune pancreatic β-cell destruction
  B. Polyglandular autoimmune syndrome type II (Schmidt syndrome)
  C. Viral infection with β-cell destruction due to
      Congenital rubella
      Coxsackievirus B (especially types B4 and B3?)
      Cytomegalovirus(?)
      Others(?)
  D. Loss of pancreatic mass due to
      Acute pancreatitis
      Chronic relapsing pancreatitis
      Carcinoma of pancreas
      Congenital pancreatic hypoplasia
      Pancreatectomy
  E. Chemical agents leading to β-cell destruction
      N-3-pyridylmethyl-N-p-nitrophenylurea
  F. Genetic syndromes
      DIDMOAD syndrome*
      Friedreich's ataxia
  G. Undetermined: insulin secretion deficient but underlying abnormality undefined or uncertain

*Diabetes insipidus, diabetes mellitus, optic atrophy, and deafness.

bodies to glutamic acid decarboxylase (GAD) or 64-kilodalton protein.[4–7] Abnormal titers of these antibodies may predate the onset of IDDM, but after onset the titers tend to fall, although less for GAD than for ICA or IAA. Thus, verification of the autoimmune nature of the disease by searching for these antibodies in patients who have had IDDM for some time may not be possible.

Autoimmune β-cell destruction is more frequent in patients with certain HLA types, but the particular types associated with the disease vary by racial and ethnic group.[4] IDDM rarely develops in subjects with aspartic acid at the 57 position of the HLA DQβ1 allele.[8] Although this and the other HLA relationships represent risk factors, their sensitivity and specificity for diagnosis are low and therefore not clinically useful.

The factors that initiate autoimmune pancreatic β-cell destruction are unknown. While viruses and chemical toxins have been suggested as initiating agents, specific agents have only rarely been identified as causes of IDDM.

Less common causes of IDDM are conditions that result in a reduction in the mass of functioning islet cell tissue, such as may occur with several types of pancreatitis, pancreatic carcinoma, and pancreatectomy with removal of most of the organ. Only a minority of the unusual genetic syndromes associated with diabetes result in IDDM. It is perhaps surprising that no molecular disorders of insulin structure or processing or of the insulin receptor have yet been associated with IDDM.

IDDM was formerly known as juvenile-onset diabetes; ketosis-prone diabetes; and, more recently, Type I diabetes. However, many authors have used the term Type I to signify a particular etiopathogenesis. As a result the 1985 WHO Study Group recommended that the term IDDM be used to avoid such confusion.[3]

Most patients with IDDM present with one or more symptoms of polyuria, polydipsia, excessive hunger, fatigue, or weight loss. Usually the fasting blood or plasma glucose concentration is unequivocally elevated (≥ 140 mg/dL or ≥ 7.8 mM) and glucose and ketones are present in the urine. If ketones are found in the urine, serum concentrations should be measured to determine the severity of the ketosis. Glucose tolerance testing is rarely necessary to make a diagnosis of IDDM.

Following initial treatment with insulin, some patients experience a temporary improvement in their insulin dependency—the so-called honeymoon period. During this period, which sometimes extends over a few months, exogenous administration of insulin is not necessary to prevent ketosis, but usually insulin dependency returns after only a short interval.

Some patients, especially those with diabetes onset before they are 30 years old, receive insulin treatment on the basis of elevated blood glucose levels without their proneness to development of ketosis having ever been documented. Unless these patients subsequently develop ketosis or have insulin treatment withdrawn, it may be difficult to determine retrospectively whether they are indeed insulin-dependent and, therefore, whether they do have IDDM. Since NIDDM does occur in children and young adults as well as in older persons, at the time of diagnosis, attempts should be made to determine and document proneness to ketosis. Without such documentation, a definitive diagnosis of IDDM may be problematic. In such patients an indication of the extent of the insulin deficiency may be obtained by determining the fasting serum concentration or the urinary excretion of C-peptide. A provocative test with measurement of serum C-peptide after intravenous administration of glucagon probably provides the most sensitive means of determining whether the insulin deficiency in such patients is of the severity characteristic of IDDM.[9] Patients who require insulin treatment for the control of hyperglycemia but not for the prevention of ketosis should not be classified as having IDDM.

Non-Insulin-Dependent Diabetes Mellitus (NIDDM). NIDDM also may present with classical symptoms but often is asymptomatic. Despite the presence of hyperglycemia, the concentrations of ketone bodies in the blood and urine are low. Insulin treatment is not necessary to maintain life or prevent spontaneous ketosis in patients with NIDDM, although many may need it to attain adequate blood glucose control. Diabetic ketoacidosis does not develop spontaneously in such patients, but in rare instances, coma may result from extreme hyperglycemia and hyperosmolarity. Acidosis and ketosis in NIDDM can occur in the presence of serious illnesses or conditions such as severe infection or mesenteric artery thrombosis.

NIDDM is the consequence of a deficiency in insulin action due to abnormalities at the cell surface or within the cell, a deficiency in insulin secretion less severe than that characterizing IDDM, or a combination of these processes. The deficit in insulin action results in hyperglycemia and other metabolic disturbances but not in disturbances of lipolysis severe enough to produce clinical ketonemia or metabolic acidosis. In contrast to IDDM, NIDDM is frequently asymptomatic.

NIDDM can present with classical diabetic symptoms and signs such as thirst, polyuria, polyphagia, pruritus, and weight loss, but these usually appear only after a long asymptomatic period. As a result, other complications of diabetes, such as retinopathy, nephropathy, atherosclerotic heart disease, or neuropathy, may be the first clinical indications of the disease. Conversely, an abnormal urine or blood glucose test, performed as part of health screening or routine medical care in an otherwise asymptomatic individual, may be the first indication that the subject may have NIDDM.

NIDDM is a common disease, and even among persons of northern European origin among whom IDDM is relatively common, NIDDM constitutes 85% or more of all cases of diabetes. Because the natural history of NIDDM is characterized by a prolonged asymptomatic period, in most populations—even those exposed to a high level of medical care—at any point in time at least one-half of the cases are undiagnosed.

Most forms of NIDDM are associated with a positive family history of disease. NIDDM is also commonly associated with obesity. Although obesity may exacerbate insulin resistance and may precipitate hyperglycemia, NIDDM also may develop in the absence of obesity. The extent to which the presence of obesity can be used to differentiate "causes" of NIDDM is debatable. Nevertheless, the NDDG and WHO recommended subdividing NIDDM into non-obese and obese categories. Since obesity represents a continuum, these subcategories have received little attention in research publications.

The understanding of the pathogenesis of NIDDM has advanced considerably in recent years. In some instances, specific pathogenetic mechanisms have been elucidated, yet the most commonly encountered forms are still not defined precisely. However, NIDDM is heterogenous and a specific underlying molecular or biochemical abnormality can be defined in some cases.

An etiologic classification of NIDDM is outlined in Table 11–3. Although NIDDM is subdivided according to those abnormalities attributable to insulin action and those attributable to insulin secretion, fully developed NIDDM displays abnormalities of both insulin secretion and insulin action. Although defects in either insulin secretion or insulin action may be the initial pathogenetic process that ultimately leads to NIDDM, most patients with the fully developed syndrome show impairments both of insulin secretion and insulin-mediated glucose disposal, or insulin resistance. Although for research purposes it is important to attempt to identify the extent to which the initiating cause of the syndrome is inadequate insulin action or inadequate insulin secretion, it is also important to recognize clinically that improvement in either one (or both) may have a beneficial therapeutic effect.

NIDDM may present at any age. Certain forms, however, particularly those in adolescents and young adults, show a dominant form of inheritance. The term maturity-onset diabetes of the young (MODY) has been widely used to describe this form of NIDDM, but this syndrome is also heterogeneous. Recently, some (but not all) patients with MODY were found to have mutations of the

Table 11–3. Etiologic Classification: Non-Insulin-Dependent Diabetes Mellitus (NIDDM)

Associated with underlying abnormalities of
A. Insulin action due to
  1) Intracellular defect of glucose disposal (most common type)
  2) Defects of insulin receptor function due to
    a) Antibodies to insulin receptor
    b) Mutations in insulin receptor (chromosome 19p)
  3) Abnormal insulin structure due to
    a) Mutations in insulin gene (chromosome 11p) with abnormal structure of insulin per se, or incomplete cleavage of proinsulin
  4) Iatrogenic
    a) Glucocorticoids
    b) Growth hormone
    c) Nicotinic acid
    d) Others
  5) Other, e.g., other (rare) specified genetic disorders
B. Insulin secretion due to
  1) Defects of signaling
    a) Glucokinase (hexokinase IV) mutations (chromosome 7p) (variable but often early-adult age of onset)
  2) Partial destruction of β-cell mass due to
    a) Autoimmune β-cell destruction
    b) Pancreatitis (includes fibrocalculous pancreatic diabetes)
    c) Other specified causes, e.g., pancreatectomy (may progress to insulin-dependent diabetes mellitus)
C. Unknown pathogenesis
  Includes NIDDM associated with malnutrition, cystic fibrosis, thalassemia, hemochromatosis, ADA-linked diabetes (chromosome 20q)
D. Unclassified
  Both insulin action and secretion are deficient but the underlying or initiating abnormality is uncertain

glucokinase (hexokinase IV) gene on chromosome 7p, and the primary cause of their NIDDM is presumably the reduction in glucose-stimulated insulin secretion.[10,11] In another family the disease was shown to be linked genetically to the ADA (adenosine deaminase) locus on chromosome 20q.[12] Autoimmune pancreatic β-cell destruction of the type that is well recognized as a major cause of IDDM also can result in NIDDM if the loss of β-cell mass is only partial. Although the extent to which these syndromes account for NIDDM is presently unknown, the possibility of these specific types of NIDDM should be considered, particularly among younger non-obese subjects.

Specific mutations of the insulin receptor gene have now been identified in some persons with NIDDM.[13] Although these are rare causes of NIDDM, they should be considered if circulating insulin levels are exceptionally high or if other clinical characteristics of insulin resistance syndromes are present, e.g., acanthosis nigrans, ovarian dysfunction, lipoatrophy, or extreme hypertriglyceridemia. The possibility of the presence of antibodies to the insulin receptor should be entertained if other autoimmune disease such as systemic lupus erythematosus, Sjögren syndrome, or ataxic telangiectasia are present.

Most often the clinician encounters patients who present with either suggestive symptomatology, i.e., a possible complication of diabetes, or an abnormal blood

Table 11–4. Diagnostic Values for the Oral Glucose Tolerance Test*

| Diagnosis, Test | Glucose Concentration, mmol/L (mg/dL) | | | |
| | Whole Blood | | Plasma | |
	Venous	Capillary	Venous	Capillary
DIABETES MELLITUS				
Fasting value	≥6.7 (≥120)	≥6.7 (≥120)	7.8 (≥140)	≥7.8 (≥140)
or				
2 hr after glucose load	≥10.0 (≥180)	≥11.1 (≥200)	11.1 (≥200)	≥12.2 (≥220)
IMPAIRED GLUCOSE TOLERANCE				
Fasting value	<6.7 (<120)	<6.7 (<120)	<7.8 (<140)	<7.8 (<140)
and				
2 hr after glucose load	6.7–10.0 (120–180)	7.8–11.1 (140–200)	7.8–11.1 (140–200)	8.9–12.2 (160–220)

*For epidemiologic or population-screening purposes, the 2-hour value after a 75-g oral glucose load may be used alone. The fasting value alone is considered less reliable since true fasting cannot be assured and a spurious diagnosis of diabetes may occur. For clinical purposes a diagnosis of diabetes based on a fasting glucose determination should be confirmed by repeating the test. Table is adapted from reference 3.

or urine glucose test. The immediate question is whether they have NIDDM. Diagnosis depends primarily on whether hyperglycemia can be confirmed. In such circumstances the most useful initial test is the measurement of fasting blood or plasma glucose level. If it can be shown and/or confirmed that the fasting glucose concentration is elevated to a level diagnostic of diabetes (Table 11–4) and that ketosis is absent, the diagnosis of NIDDM is established. If the fasting circulating glucose concentration is below these levels, an oral glucose tolerance test is needed to exclude or confirm the diagnosis of NIDDM or to determine whether impaired glucose tolerance is present.

Malnutrition-Related Diabetes. Malnutrition-related diabetes includes two forms of NIDDM that, although quite rare, are well described in developing, tropical countries.[14] The two forms are fibrocalculous pancreatic diabetes and protein-deficient diabetes. Fibrocalculous pancreatic diabetes is characterized by the presence of pancreatic calculi, a history of recurrent abdominal pain, and concomitant evidence of pancreatic exocrine dysfunction. Although the hyperglycemia is usually quite severe, ketosis does not develop, but about 80% of those affected require insulin to control hyperglycemia.

Protein-deficient pancreatic diabetes has no pathognomonic features. It occurs in malnourished young adults, who are said to require large doses of insulin to control hyperglycemia. The implication of this requirement is that this condition is associated with marked insulin resistance. The pathogenetic mechanism and its relationship to protein-calorie malnutrition is unknown.

Other Types of Diabetes. The fourth major subclass of diabetes mellitus designated in the WHO and NDDG classification is that of other types of diabetes associated with certain conditions or syndromes (Table 11–5). The class encompasses a variety of types of diabetes in which the etiology is either secondary to other conditions or the association of diabetes with a specific disease or agent is sufficiently strong to justify a belief in a specific distinctive etiology and that the joint occurrence of diabetes and the other condition is not coincidental. In a therapeutic

sense each of these types of diabetes can also be classified as either insulin-dependent or non-insulin-dependent.

These other types of diabetes and glucose intolerance are recognized primarily by the presence of clinical

Table 11–5. World Health Organization and National Diabetes Data Group Classification of Other Types of Diabetes Mellitus

1. Diabetes due to pancreatic disease
   Chronic or recurrent pancreatitis
   Hemochromatosis
2. Diabetes due to other endocrine disease
   Cushing syndrome
   Hyperaldosteronism
   Acromegaly
   Thyrotoxicosis
   Phaeochromocytoma
   Glucagonoma
   Polyglandular autoimmune syndromes, e.g., Schmidt syndrome
3. Diabetes due to drugs and toxins
   Glucocorticoids and adrenocorticotropic hormone
   Diazoxide
   Phenytoin
   Pentamidine
   Pyriminil (Vacor; a rodenticide)
4. Diabetes due to abnormalities of insulin or its receptor
   Insulinopathies
   Receptor defects
   Circulating antibodies to insulin receptor
   Leprechaunism
   Lipoatrophy
   Lipodystrophies (Rabson-Mendenhall syndrome)
5. Diabetes associated with other genetic syndromes
   DIDMOAD syndrome*
   Myotonic dystrophy and other muscle disorders
   Type 1 glycogen storage disease
   Cystic fibrosis
   Werner syndrome
   Prader-Willi syndrome
   Alström syndrome
6. Diabetes associated with chromosomal defects
   Down syndrome
   Klinefelter syndrome
   Turner syndrome

*Diabetes insipidus, diabetes mellitus, optic atrophy, and deafness.

features not present in the more typical forms of NIDDM or IDDM. The more common diseases and conditions included in this subclass are listed in Table 11–5, and some are discussed in more detail elsewhere (see Chapters 15, 16, 17, 35). Examples include diabetes associated with pancreatic diseases, e.g., chronic pancreatitis or hemochromatosis; diabetes of hormonal etiology, such as that associated with acromegaly, pheochromocytoma, Cushing disease; and cystic fibrosis; a variety of drug- or chemical-induced forms of hyperglycemia; and diabetes associated with abnormalities of insulin or its receptors. Also included in this group is diabetes mellitus associated with certain inborn errors of metabolism such as type 1 glycogen storage disease; certain chromosome abnormalities such as Down, Turner, and Klinefelter syndromes; genetic diseases such as Alström and Prader-Willi syndromes; muscle disorders such as myotonic dystrophy; Werner syndrome; and the polyglandular autoimmune syndromes. Many of these genetic syndromes do not yet have a specific molecular basis, but the likelihood that the diabetes is due to these diseases, rather than to the more usual causes, is inferred from the presence of the other specific features of these syndromes.

Diabetes and impaired glucose tolerance have been associated with therapeutic use of many drugs, but in most cases it is unlikely that these represent a major underlying cause of diabetes and more likely that they aggravate preexisting glucose intolerance. Nevertheless, there are often alternative therapeutic agents available which if substituted may lead to better glycemic control (see reference 1 for an extensive list of such agents).

Impaired Glucose Tolerance

Impaired glucose tolerance is a category that permits classification of individuals whose glucose tolerance is above the conventional normal range but lower than the level considered diagnostic of diabetes. Such persons do have a high risk of developing diabetes mellitus. On the other hand, not all individuals with impaired glucose tolerance will develop diabetes. Some revert to normal glucose tolerance, and others continue to have impaired glucose tolerance for many years. In some populations persons with impaired glucose tolerance appear to have a greater risk than persons of similar age with normal glucose tolerance of developing arterial disease but do not develop the more specific microvascular complications of diabetes unless they develop diabetes.

Impaired glucose tolerance is more frequent in obese than in non-obese persons and is frequently, but not always, associated with hyperinsulinemia and insulin resistance. Impaired glucose tolerance may be attributable to a wide variety of causes, including certain medications, many of the specific genetic syndromes, and other conditions that also are associated with diabetes mellitus (see Table 11–5). In most subjects, however, impaired glucose tolerance represents a transient stage during the development of NIDDM. Impaired glucose tolerance cannot be defined on the basis of fasting glucose concentrations; an oral glucose tolerance test is needed to categorize such individuals.

Gestational Diabetes

Gestational diabetes is a designation specifically for women whose diabetes is first recognized or has its onset during pregnancy. Gestational diabetes may have deleterious consequences for both the fetus and the mother. During pregnancy, however, it is usually impossible to determine whether such glucose intolerance will persist after delivery. In many women with gestational diabetes, glucose tolerance reverts to normal after parturition, but in others, diabetes or impaired glucose tolerance persists. As a group, women with gestational diabetes, even those whose glucose tolerance reverts to normal after parturition, have a high risk of developing diabetes in subsequent years. Such diabetes may be of the insulin-dependent or non-insulin-dependent type. The diagnosis of gestational diabetes serves to alert the physician or obstetrician about the high-risk nature of the pregnancy and at the same time to emphasize the importance of reassessing and classifying the type and severity of the disordered carbohydrate more definitively after parturition.

Statistical Risk Classes

Statistical risk classes are included to enable classification of individuals who exhibited glucose intolerance or diabetes in the past but who presently have normal glucose tolerance as well as others who can be recognized statistically as having a high likelihood of developing diabetes but whose glucose tolerance is currently normal.

Subjects who previously met the criteria for a diagnosis of diabetes or impaired glucose tolerance but who can no longer be so classified are included in the risk class of previous abnormality of glucose tolerance. For example, women who had diabetes or impaired glucose tolerance during pregnancy and who reverted to glucose tolerance after delivery are placed in this category. The category of potential abnormality enables classification of subjects who have not yet developed disease but who are at high risk of developing diabetes or impaired glucose tolerance, such as persons with a high titer of islet cell antibodies or insulin autoantibodies or those whose HLA-identical sibling has IDDM or whose monozygotic twin has NIDDM. Although not widely used, these classes are useful for research purposes and serve to alert the clinician of the high risk of subsequent diabetes.

DIAGNOSTIC CRITERIA FOR DIABETES AND IMPAIRED GLUCOSE TOLERANCE

A diagnosis of diabetes carries considerable and life-long consequences for the patient. If the patient has symptoms such as thirst, polyuria, unexplained weight loss, possibly drowsiness or coma, and marked glucosuria, the diagnosis can be established by demonstrating fasting hyperglycemia. If the fasting glucose concentration alone is in the diagnostic range, a glucose tolerance test is not required for diagnosis. However, in such instances a confirmatory test should be performed since incomplete fasting may result in a spurious diagnosis. On the other hand, if the patient is asymptomatic or has only minimal symptoms and fasting blood or plasma glucose concentrations that are not unequivocally in the diagnostic range (Table 11–4), a glucose tolerance test is required to confirm or exclude the diagnosis of diabetes. Similarly, a glucose tolerance test is necessary to establish the presence of impaired glucose tolerance.

Oral Glucose Tolerance Test

The oral glucose tolerance test should be administered the morning after the patient has had at least 3 days of an unrestricted diet (more than 150 g of carbohydrate daily) and usual physical activity. The test should be preceded by an overnight fast of 10 to 16 hours, during which the patient may drink water. The patient may not smoke during the test. The presence of factors that influence interpretation of the results of the test must be recorded (e.g., medications, inactivity, infection).

After the fasting blood sample is collected, the subject should drink 75 g of glucose (or partial hydrolysates of starch with an equivalent carbohydrate content) in 250 to 300 mL of water over the course of 5 minutes. For children, the glucose test load should be 1.75 g/kg of body weight, up to a total of 75 g of glucose. Blood samples must be collected 2 hours after the test load; if appropriate, samples may also be taken every half hour during this period.

Unless the glucose concentration can be determined immediately, the blood sample should be collected in a tube containing sodium fluoride (6 mg/mL of whole blood) and centrifuged to separate out the plasma. The plasma should be frozen until the glucose measurement can be done.

The results of the glucose tolerance test should be interpreted according to the criteria given in Table 11–4. It is important to note that the diagnostic levels differ to some extent according to whether capillary or venous blood is collected and whether the glucose assay determines plasma or blood glucose concentrations.

The criteria shown in Table 11–4 do not explicitly define a category of normal glucose tolerance, but for research purposes glucose tolerance is usually considered normal if it is below the post-load 2-hour levels used to define the lower boundary of impaired glucose tolerance. The presence of normal glucose tolerance cannot be established on the basis of a fasting blood glucose determination alone. In normal subjects fasting glucose levels are less than 5.5 mmol/L (100 mg/dL) for venous or capillary plasma and less than 5.0 mmol/L (90 mg/dL) in whole blood, but many subjects with fasting levels below these limits exhibit impaired glucose tolerance and some even have diabetes. The much higher fasting glucose levels that are required to meet the criteria for the diagnosis of diabetes represent levels that are highly specific for this diagnosis. Subjects with fasting glucose levels above those that are characteristic for normal subjects but below those diagnostic of diabetes have a very high likelihood of having diabetes or impaired glucose tolerance. Such levels represent a primary indication for the performance of an oral glucose tolerance test to confirm or exclude the diagnosis of diabetes or impaired glucose tolerance.

DIAGNOSTIC CRITERIA FOR GESTATIONAL DIABETES

In the United States screening and diagnosis of gestational diabetes have been conducted primarily using methods first proposed in 1964 (Table 11–6). Between the 24th and 28th week of pregnancy women who are not known to have diabetes and who have not been recognized to have diabetes earlier in pregnancy undergo a screening test with a 50-g oral glucose load. In women whose venous plasma glucose value is 140 mg/dL or higher (7.8 mmol/L), this test is followed by an oral test with 100 g of glucose.

Since 1980 the WHO, on the other hand, has recommended that the diagnosis of gestational diabetes and impaired glucose tolerance in pregnancy be based on the same 75-g oral glucose tolerance test and criteria used in nonpregnant subjects but that the management of the impaired glucose tolerance in pregnancy be similar to

Table 11–6.   Screening Methods and Diagnostic Criteria for Gestational Diabetes Mellitus

Screening for gestational diabetes
  1) By glucose measurement in plasma
  2) Administration of 50-g oral glucose load between the 24th and 28th week, without regard to time of day or time of last meal to all pregnant women who have not been identified before the 24th week as having glucose intolerance
  3) Venous plasma glucose measured 1 hour later
  4) A glucose value of ≥140 mg/dL (7.8 mmol/L) in venous plasma indicates the need for a full diagnostic glucose tolerance test
Diagnosis of gestational diabetes mellitus
  1) Administration of 100-g oral glucose load the morning after overnight fast of at least 8 but no more than 14 hours and after at least 3 days of unrestricted diet (≥150 g of carbohydrate) and physical activity
  2) Plasma glucose is measured fasting and at 1, 2, and 3 hours after the oral glucose load (subject should remain seated and should not smoke throughout the test)
  3) Two or more of the following venous plasma glucose concentrations must be met or exceeded for a positive diagnosis:
    Fasting, 105 mg/dL (5.8 mmol/L)
    1 hour, 190 mg/dL (10.6 mmol/L)
    2 hour, 165 mg/dL (9.2 mmol/L)
    3 hour, 145 mg/dL (8.1 mmol/L)

*Data from reference 15.

that for diabetes. The use of the 75-g test has gained wide acceptance in many parts of the world but not the United States, where the older screening and diagnostic methods were again endorsed in 1991.[15] It seems likely that these recommendations will be reconsidered and revised as more extensive data on prognosis and outcome with tests using the 75-g oral glucose load become available.

CONCLUSIONS

The WHO classification and diagnostic criteria for diabetes have been used and applied widely for over a decade. The WHO criteria differ to some extent from those of the NDDG, insofar as the latter stipulated that one or more intermediate glucose values during the glucose tolerance test be elevated for a diagnosis of diabetes or impaired glucose tolerance. This requirement led to some glucose tolerance test results being designated as "unclassified" or "indeterminate," categories that subsequent studies have shown to have prognostic significance similar to those defined as impaired glucose tolerance by the WHO criteria.

A classification based primarily on etiopathogenesis, although desirable, is still not possible for many patients with diabetes. The present WHO classification does provide a clinically useful framework that can be supplemented by more specific pathogenetic subclasses as knowledge of the pathogenesis of diabetes is further refined. The classification and criteria have served to standardize terminology and definitions and to focus research and investigations in many areas of diabetes and glucose intolerance. Future developments will inevitably lead to a more precise knowledge of the underlying causes of the more common types of diabetes and to the need for periodic revision of the classification.

REFERENCES

1. National Diabetes Data Group. Classification and diagnosis of diabetes mellitus and other categories of glucose intolerance. Diabetes 1979;28:1039–57.

2. WHO Expert Committee on Diabetes Mellitus. Second report. WHO Tech Rep Ser 1980;646:1–80.

3. Diabetes mellitus. Report of WHO study group. Tech Rep Ser 1985;727:1–113.

4. Maclaren NK, Schatz D, Drash A, Grave G. Initial pathogenic events in IDDM. Diabetes 1988;38:534–8.

5. Palmer JP, Asplin CM, Clemons P, et al. Insulin antibodies in insulin-dependent diabetics before insulin treatment. Science 1983;222:1337–9.

6. Baekkeskov S, Aanstoot H-J, Christgau S, et al. Identification of the 64K autoantigen in insulin-dependent diabetes as the GABA-synthesizing enzyme glutamic acid decarboxylase. Nature 1990;347:151–6.

7. Rowley MJ, Mackay IR, Chen Q-Y, et al. Antibodies to glutamic acid decarboxylase discriminate major types of diabetes mellitus. Diabetes 1992;41:548–51.

8. Morel PA, Dorman JS, Todd JA, et al. Aspartic acid at position 57 of the HLA-DQ β-chain protects against Type I diabetes: a family study. Proc Natl Acad Sci USA 1988; 85:8111–5.

9. Hother-Nielsen O, Faber O, Sørensen NS, Beck-Nielsen H. Classification of newly diagnosed diabetes patients as insulin-requiring or non-insulin-requiring based on clinical and biochemical variables. Diabetes Care 1988;11:531–7.

10. Froguel P, Vaxillaire M, Sur F, et al. Cross linkage of glucokinase locus on chromosome 7p to early-onset non-insulin-dependent diabetes mellitus. Nature 1992;356; 162–4.

11. Vionnet N, Stoffel M, Takeda J, et al. Nonsense mutation in the glucokinase gene causes early-onset non-insulin-dependent diabetes mellitus. Nature 1992;356:721–2.

12. Bell GI, Xiang K, Newman MV, et al. Gene for non-insulin-dependent diabetes mellitus (maturity-onset diabetes of the young subtype) is linked to DNA polymorphism on human chromosome 20q. Proc Natl Acad Sci USA 1991; 88:1484–8.

13. Flier JS. Syndromes of insulin resistance: from patient to gene and back again. Diabetes 1992;41:1207–19.

14. Mohan V, Ramachandran A, Viseranathan M. Malnutrition-related diabetes mellitus. In: Pickup J, Williams G, eds. Textbook of diabetes. Vol 1. Oxford: Blackwell Scientific Publications, 1991:247–55.

15. Metzger BE, the Organizing Committee. Summary and recommendations of the Third International Workshop-Conference on Gestational Diabetes Mellitus. Diabetes 1991;40(Suppl 2):197–201.

Chapter 12

EPIDEMIOLOGY AND GENETICS OF DIABETES MELLITUS

JAMES H. WARRAM
STEPHEN S. RICH
ANDRZEJ S. KROLEWSKI

In this chapter, we will review the descriptive epidemiology of insulin-dependent diabetes mellitus (Type I) and non-insulin-dependent diabetes mellitus (Type II) and discuss its relevance to the etiology of the disease.[1] However, it is first necessary to define some of the indices used to estimate diabetes frequency in populations.[2]

SOME USEFUL DEFINITIONS

Prevalence, Incidence Rate, and Cumulative Incidence. The number of persons who have diabetes in a particular place at a particular time (e.g., in Massachusetts on July 1, 1991) is a frequently cited statistic. Expressed as a proportion, this number is commonly called the prevalence rate or, preferably, *prevalence,* so it is not confused with the incidence rate, which is defined below. The prevalence in Massachusetts is the accumulation of persons who acquired diabetes before July 1, 1991, but the size of this collection depends not only on the frequency of new cases but also on how long they remain alive to be counted. For example, a marked increase in the prevalence of insulin-dependent diabetes followed the discovery of insulin, although we have no evidence that the number of new cases that developed each year increased.

To express diabetes frequency in a manner suitable for drawing conclusions regarding etiology of the disease, we use the *incidence rate.* The incidence rate is calculated by dividing the number of *new* cases of diabetes in Massachusetts residents during the 12 months of 1992, for example, by the number of nondiabetic individuals residing in Massachusetts during that year. Typically, the incidence rate is expressed as the number of new cases per 100,000 persons observed for a year (called *person-years*).

When an incidence rate is calculated according to a characteristic such as age, sex, or race, the results are referred to as a *specific rate.* The age-specific incidence rate of diabetes varies enormously across the normal life span, and populations typically have different age distributions. Meaningful comparisons among populations must therefore be based on a particular age-specific rate or, for simplicity, on a summary of age-specific rates determined by a technique that gives each population the same age distribution.[2] This produces age-adjusted or age-standardized rates. Alternatively, one can compare populations that have different age structures by calculating the *cumulative incidence* of diabetes at specific ages in each population.

Cumulative incidence or *cumulative risk* of diabetes is calculated from the age-specific incidence rate by use of life-table methods.[2] One begins with an arbitrary number of births, e.g., 1000 births, and applies the age-specific incidence rate to the number of persons who remain unaffected after each successive year of age. By accumulating the cases from previous ages, one obtains the proportion of the original 1000 children born who would be affected by each successive age in a population. By extending this process to the whole life span, one obtains the lifetime risk of diabetes. In a specific instance, the prevalence of diabetes at a certain age may be a reasonable estimate of cumulative incidence at that age. For example, NIDDM-related mortality before the age of 55 is negligible. Therefore, the prevalence of NIDDM in the age group 45 through 54 is a reasonable estimate of the cumulative incidence at age 50. However, at older ages, prevalence typically underestimates cumulative incidence of diabetes because persons with early-onset of the disease may have died.

DIFFERENCES IN DISTRIBUTION OF INSULIN-DEPENDENT (IDDM) AND NON-INSULIN-DEPENDENT DIABETES MELLITUS (NIDDM)

The incidence rate is the most informative measure of the frequency of diabetes in a population for the study of etiologic factors. For the computation of the incidence rate, new cases of diabetes must be recognized and counted. IDDM is easily recognized, and virtually all new cases are ascertained in a society with access to medical care. Recognition of new cases of non-insulin-dependent diabetes mellitus (NIDDM), however, depends on the severity of symptoms, diagnostic activity of the medical-care system, and the choice of diagnostic criteria. For example, the incidence rate determined by the criteria of the National Diabetes Data Group[3] will be lower than one determined by the World Health Organization (WHO) criteria[4] because the former are more stringent.

Data on the incidence rate of diabetes in Rochester, Minnesota, as ascertained through medical-care institutions, show how the incidence rate of IDDM varies according to age (Table 12–1).[5,6] Among the nondiabetic population of Rochester, IDDM developed in 7 to 27 individuals per 100,000 per year—depending on the age group being counted. The risk increases in the first and second decades of life, levels off in the third and fourth decades, and increases again thereafter, suggesting that there are two peaks of occurrence of IDDM, one centered in the second decade and the other in the sixth and seventh decades. The incidence rate of NIDDM increases steadily with age (Table 12–1), with an almost 100-fold increase from early childhood to old age.

The sets of age-specific incidence rates can be summarized as cumulative incidence rates, i.e., the cumulative risk in a cohort of individuals that is followed from birth and exposed to the age-specific rates. For the age-specific rates in Table 12–1, the cumulative risk by age 70 years would be 1% for IDDM and 11% for NIDDM.

EPIDEMIOLOGY OF IDDM

Any hypothesis put forward regarding the etiology of IDDM must account for characteristics of the distribution of IDDM in human populations that are discussed below.

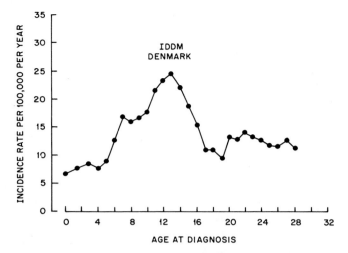

Fig. 12–1. Incidence rate of insulin-dependent diabetes (IDDM) according to individual years of age. Adapted from Christau et al.[8]

Variation in Incidence with Age

IDDM rarely occurs during the first 6 months of life. Gamble found only a few cases in a very large registry of children with diabetes in Great Britain.[7] The incidence begins to increase sharply at about 9 months of age, continues to rise until age 12 to 14 years, and then declines. The relationship with age is clearly seen in Figure 12–1, in which the incidence rate of IDDM in Denmark is presented according to age.[8] A similar pattern is seen in most other countries, regardless of whether their overall incidence of IDDM is high or low.

Data on the incidence of IDDM with onset after the age of 30 years are scarce. In a population study in Copenhagen,[9] the rate was 9.6 per 100,000 when stringent diagnostic criteria for IDDM were used. When the criteria were relaxed to identify all patients treated with insulin from the onset of diabetes as having IDDM, the incidence rate resembled that for IDDM in Rochester, Minnesota (Table 12–1).

Temporal Increase in Incidence

The pattern of occurrence of IDDM over time can be important evidence for discriminating between alternative etiologic hypotheses. Lack of variability from generation to generation is a feature of many genetic traits. If, on the other hand, there is significant variability over time, the particular pattern of variation may suggest specific environmental factors, which can be investigated as components in the etiology of IDDM. Several types of variation over time have been described: long-term trends, a seasonal cycle, and episodic changes over a few years.

The few sources of data that contribute to an analysis of long-term trends in IDDM incidence are summarized in Figure 12–2.[10] During the first 30 years of this century, the incidence rate of IDDM in the white population of the

Table 12–1. Age-Specific Incidence Rates of Insulin-Dependent (IDDM) and Non-Insulin-Dependent Diabetes (NIDDM) per 100,000 person-years in Rochester, Minnesota, 1960 through 1969

Age (yrs)	IDDM	NIDDM
0–9	6.5	0.0
10–19	12.5	7.5
20–29	9.5	9.5
30–39	6.9	66.8
40–49	17.3	155.4
50–59	25.8	322.2
60–69	26.9	612.8
Cumulative incidence rate (%) by age 70	1.05	11.10

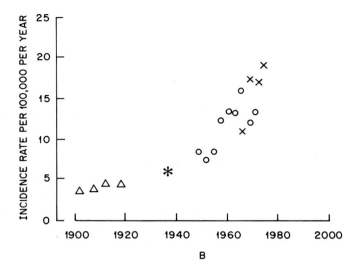

Fig. 12–2. Incidence rate of insulin-dependent diabetes in children in the white population of the United States from 1900 to 1976. Adapted from Krolewski et al.[10]

United States under age 15 years was fairly constant. However, over the past three decades, the rate has almost tripled. Data from several other countries are compatible with those from the United States. The incidence rate for children under age 15 in Oslo, Norway, rose from 6.2 for the years 1925 through 1954 to 10.8 for the years 1956 through 1965[11] and then to 20.5 for the years 1973 through 1982,[12] values quite close to those in the United States. In Finland, where the incidence of IDDM is higher than in the United States, there was a similar increase between 1965 and 1984.[13] Studies in Sweden[14,15] and Scotland[16] have also reported a rising incidence rate for juvenile-onset IDDM during similar calendar periods. In the United Kingdom[17] and Denmark,[18] where it has been possible to compute cumulative risk for birth cohorts, the increase has been steeper than that shown by the cross-sectional data for the United States (Fig. 12–2). The explanation for the secular increase in the incidence of IDDM in so many populations is unclear. In several regards, this long-term trend in the occurrence of IDDM resembles aspects of the emergence of poliomyelitis early in this century. It has been speculated that, by analogy, delayed exposure to a common virus may predispose to autoimmunity involving β-cells.[10]

Seasonal variability in diagnoses of IDDM attracted much attention in the 1970s.[7,19] It has since been established, however, that IDDM has a long subclinical period, so the seasonal pattern in diagnoses presumably results from the seasonal occurrence of factors that precipitate the appearance of symptoms in asymptomatic cases (such as common infections) or result in closer observation of children (such as the return to school).

Recently, some attention has focused on variability in the incidence of IDDM from year to year. Statistically significant year-to-year variation, which affected age groups 0 to 4, 5 to 9, and 10 to 14 in a nonparallel pattern,

was reported from a region of Sweden over the period 1966 through 1986.[20] Moreover, an apparent epidemic during 1982 through 1984 was described in midwestern Poland.[21] The incidence rate in children under 18 years old in those years was double that between 1970 and 1981. Similar "epidemics" in the U.S. Virgin Islands and Jefferson County, Alabama, in 1984 have been described.[22,23] The basis for these variations remains unresolved, but many attempts have been made to link them with epidemics of infectious diseases. However, since the subclinical period for IDDM typically lasts for several years, it is difficult to establish an etiologic link between a specific infection and the diabetes "epidemic," if such a link does exist.

Variation in Incidence among Races and Countries

Interest in the epidemiology of diabetes during the last decade has resulted in the publication of a multitude of papers on the incidence rates in various parts of the world. These data permit an examination of geographic patterns in the occurrence of IDDM. Age-adjusted incidence rates for the population aged 0 to 14 years are lowest in Japan, the Caribbean, and southern Europe, while the highest are in the Scandinavian countries (Fig. 12–3).[24] The incidence rates of IDDM among several white populations studied in the United States are similar. These rates are slightly higher than those in several countries in northern Europe but significantly lower than those in Sweden and Finland.

Data on the occurrence of IDDM among nonwhite populations in the United States have been accumulating during the last decade. Among blacks in Allegheny County, Pennsylvania, the incidence rate for the population aged 0 to 14 years was 11.8 per 100,000 during the 5-year period 1978 to 1983, a rate 73% of that for white children (16.2 per 100,000) in that county during the same period.[25] The rate in children aged 0 to 14 years was much lower in blacks in Jefferson County, Alabama, and San Diego, California, during a similar interval (4.4 and 3.3 per 100,000, respectively).[25] An intermediate rate of 7.5 per 100,000 was found in the U.S. Virgin Islands during the decade 1979 through 1988, and an association was demonstrated between diabetes risk and percentage of white ancestry.[22] The reported rate among Hispanic children aged 0 to 14 years ranges from 9.7 per 100,000 in Colorado to 4.1 per 100,000 in California. In Cuban children, the rate is reported to be only 2.6 per 100,000 (Fig. 12–3).[25]

In summary, the accumulated data on the incidence of IDDM during the last 20 years demonstrate that IDDM occurs in most racial and ethnic groups but that the risk is highest among white populations.[24] While these differences among races may be determined in part by genes, the range of variation within the white population is almost as great as the range among races. Therefore, an important question to be resolved is how much of the variation in white groups is due to genetic differences and how much is due to exposure to different environmental factors.

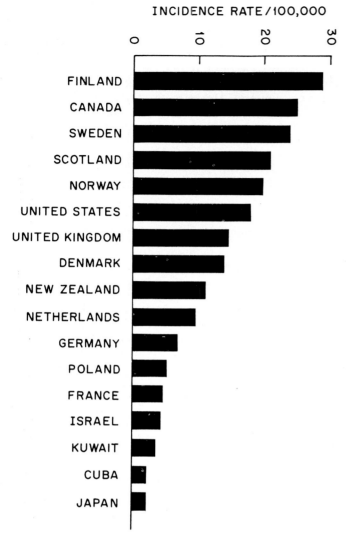

Fig. 12–3. Incidence rate of insulin-dependent diabetes in children less than 15 years old (per 100,000) in various populations. Adapted from Patrick et al.[24]

Clustering in Families

Three studies, two conducted at the Joslin Diabetes Center in Boston and one conducted at the Steno Hospital in Copenhagen, permit computation of the cumulative risk of diabetes up to age 50 years for the siblings of IDDM probands. In the earlier Joslin Diabetes Center study,[26] there were 289 probands (patients with IDDM that brought the family into the study) for whom the diagnosis was made before the age of 20 during the years 1928 through 1938 (1930s cohort). The 589 siblings of these probands were studied in 1968 when their median age was 49 years. In the 168 probands in the later Joslin Diabetes Center study, the diagnosis was made before the age of 21 in the years 1948 through 1960 (1950s cohort).[27] The 335 siblings of these probands were studied in 1981 when their median age was 41 years. In the 187 probands in the Danish study, the

diagnosis was made before the age of 21 during the years 1918 through 1944. The 375 siblings of these probands were studied in 1974 when their median age was 52 years.[28]

The three studies yielded almost identical estimates of the cumulative risks by age 50 years (Fig. 12–4). For comparison, the cumulative risk at age 50 years in the general population was calculated to be 0.5% (Table 12–1). Thus, the risk to siblings by age 50 seems to be approximately 10%, or 20 times the risk in the general population. Despite the close agreement among studies regarding the cumulative risk at age 50, there are interesting and statistically significant differences in the cumulative incidence rates at younger ages. The cumulative percentage affected by the age of 15 was 6.3 for the siblings of the 1950s cohort of the Joslin patients but only 1.7 and 1.9 for the siblings in the earlier Joslin and Danish studies, respectively. Results very similar to those of the recent Joslin study were reported for a study in Wisconsin of 194 probands with IDDM whose diagnosis was made before the age of 30 during the years 1984 through 1987. The cumulative risk of IDDM was 10.5% by age 20 years in the siblings.[29] This three- to fourfold increase in early-onset diabetes in the siblings of recently diagnosed probands suggests that there is a shift toward a younger age at clinical onset of IDDM in a population enriched with susceptible individuals. The secular trend in the incidence rates of IDDM in the general population discussed above might also reflect a shift toward earlier manifestation of IDDM in susceptible individuals.[17]

Studies in twins are the basis for the evaluation of the relative contributions of genetic and environmental factors to familial clustering of diabetes. The premise for

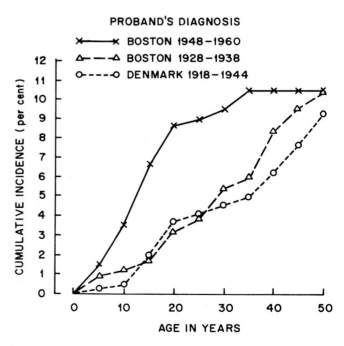

Fig. 12–4. Cumulative incidence of insulin-dependent diabetes (IDDM) in the siblings of probands with IDDM, as estimated in three different studies of families.[27]

this type of study is that monozygotic twins carry identical genotypes but that dizygotic twins are no more similar genotypically than non-twin siblings. A more frequent concordance for diabetes among monozygotic twins than among dizygotic twins therefore favors a greater role of genetic factors. Unfortunately, no twin study of IDDM meets the basic requirements for design and execution permitting inferences regarding the concordance rate.[1] The chief problems have been small sample size or study methods that almost certainly produced an ascertainment bias toward concordant pairs. However, even with this bias, the concordance rate for IDDM in monozygotic twins appears to be only in the neighborhood of 25% to 50%. Thus, although the concordance rate for monozygotic twins is severalfold larger than that for non-twin siblings, it is far from 100%.

Parent-offspring pairs are another type of first-degree familial relationship that can be examined for familial aggregation of IDDM. A few follow-up studies of children of a parent with IDDM permit estimation of the cumulative risk of IDDM in the offspring up to the age of 20 years. As was found for siblings, the risk is much higher than for the general population, but surprisingly, there is a significant difference between the rate for offspring of diabetic fathers and the rate for offspring of diabetic mothers. For the offspring of diabetic fathers, the cumulative incidence of IDDM by age 20 years is 6%, or 20 times that for the general population.[30,31] For the offspring of diabetic mothers, the corresponding cumulative incidence is approximately 2%, which is only seven times that in the general population.[32] In a very small study of offspring born to women who did not develop IDDM until after the birth of the child,[33] the children appeared to have a risk of IDDM similar to that of children of fathers with IDDM. These data suggest that exposure to a diabetic environment in utero may have a protective effect on the offspring, perhaps by inducing immunologic tolerance to the antigen involved in the autoimmune destruction of the pancreatic β-cells.[33]

The risk of IDDM in the offspring of a mother with IDDM is even lower if the child is born after the mother is 25 years old.[33] Only 1% of the children born to mothers age 25 years or older develop diabetes by the age of 20 years, whereas their older siblings born when the mother was younger than 25 years old have a risk of 3.6%. Thus, there is less familial clustering in families in which the mother has IDDM, particularly if she is over the age of 25 at the birth of the children. The 1% risk for her offspring by age 20 is only three times that for the general population.

Another factor that seems to modify the clustering of IDDM in families is the age of the proband at onset of IDDM (M. El Hashimy, M. C. Angelico, J. H. Warram, and A. S. Krolewski, unpublished data). Regardless of the gender of the diabetic parent in the studies just described, the risk for offspring was approximately two times higher if IDDM in the parent was diagnosed before age 11 years rather than later (Fig. 12−5). This finding suggests that environmental factors played a larger role in the etiology of parental diabetes when its onset was at age 11 years or later.

The risk for offspring of mothers with IDDM was lower than that for offspring of fathers with IDDM regardless of the parent's age at diagnosis, and the pattern was the same if the offspring of diabetic mothers were further stratified by maternal age (data not shown). For simplicity, the

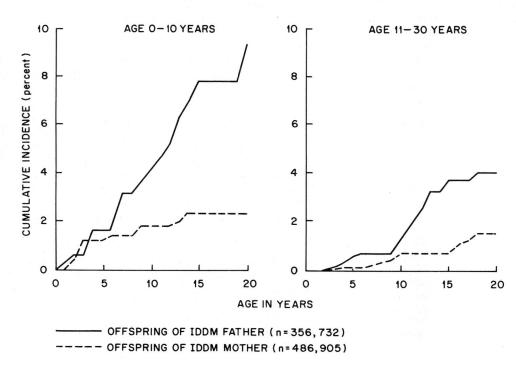

AGE OF DIAGNOSIS IN IDDM PARENT

Fig. 12−5. Cumulative incidence of insulin-dependent diabetes (IDDM) in the offspring of a parent with IDDM according to gender and age at diagnosis of IDDM in the parent proband (M. El Hashimy, M. C. Angelico, J. H. Warram, and A. S. Krolewski, unpublished data).

cumulative-incidence curves in Figure 12–5 have been adjusted for maternal age by the direct method, using the age distribution for the mothers of the total group of children (M. El Hashimy, M. C. Angelico, J. H. Warram, and A. S. Krolewski, unpublished data). Consistent with these results for offspring of IDDM probands are data on siblings of IDDM probands from the Wisconsin study cited above.[29] The cumulative risk at age 26 for siblings of probands whose IDDM diagnosis was made before age 10 was 18.5%, while it was 10.1% and 9.1% for siblings of probands whose diagnosis was made at age 10 to 14 years and 15 to 29 years, respectively. A similar pattern was found in an earlier study of siblings of IDDM probands in Minnesota.[34]

Close Relationship of Occurrence to Certain HLA Antigens

The HLA antigens are encoded by loci on the short arm of chromosome 6. This region contains three groups of closely linked loci: class I loci encode the classic transplantation antigens (HLA-A, -B, and -C); class II loci (HLA-DR, -DQ, and -DP) encode proteins involved in presentation of peptide antigens to helper T lymphocytes; and class III loci encode components of complement, among other proteins. In the early 1970s, certain HLA antigens determined by serologic typing methods were shown to be positively associated with IDDM but not NIDDM (see Chapter 13). Although the first recognized association of IDDM was with HLA-B antigens, DR antigens have since been shown to have a stronger association with the disease. A review of the investigation of HLA and IDDM has been presented elsewhere.[35] In all populations studied, IDDM has been confined largely to individuals who carry HLA-DR3 and/or HLA-DR4.[1,36]

Using the distribution of HLA-DR antigens in the total population and patients with IDDM in the U.S. population,[1] one can estimate the lifetime cumulative risk of IDDM according to various HLA-DR antigens. In such an analysis of a cohort of 10,000 (Table 12–2), there would be 4887 persons who had neither HLA-DR3 nor HLA-DR4. It can be estimated that 5.5 of them would develop IDDM during their lifetime, i.e., a cumulative incidence of .11%. In the cohort, 4577 persons would have either

Table 12-2. Estimated Lifetime Risk of Insulin-Dependent Diabetes (IDDM) According to the Presence of HLA Antigens DR3 or DR4

HLA-DR phenotype	Persons born*	IDDM absent	IDDM present*	Cumulative incidence (%)
DR 3 and DR 4 present	536	508.6	27.4	5.11
DR 3 or DR 4 present	4577	4504.9	72.1	1.58
DR 3 and DR 4 absent	4887	4881.5	5.5	0.11
Total†	10000	9895.0	105.0	1.05

*Distribution calculated according to distribution of the phenotype in whites in the United States.[1]
†Based on the cumulative incidence of IDDM by age 70 in Table 12-1.

HLA-DR3 or HLA-DR4, and 72.1 of them would develop IDDM during their lifetime, i.e., a cumulative incidence of 1.58%. The 536 remaining persons in the cohort would be HLA DR3/DR4 heterozygotes, and 27.4 of them would develop IDDM, i.e., a cumulative incidence of 5.11%. It appears then that although the risk of IDDM is profoundly influenced by HLA-DR antigens, only a small percentage of individuals carrying HLA-DR3 and/or HLA-DR4 ever develop IDDM.

Several explanations can be offered for this observation. One is that these alleles themselves confer genetic susceptibility to IDDM but that some other genetic or nongenetic factor prevents the development of IDDM in all but a small proportion of those with the alleles. Another possibility is that the true susceptibility alleles are near the HLA-DR loci, one in linkage disequilibrium with HLA-DR3 and one in linkage disequilibrium with HLA-DR4.[37] A variation of this hypothesis is that IDDM susceptibility is determined by more than one locus in the HLA region, e.g., DR and the closely linked DQ locus. Finally, the HLA-linked gene that conveys susceptibility to IDDM might not be distinguishable by the available serologic methods.

DR and DQ molecules are heterodimers composed of an α and a β chain. The many conventional DR serologic types are generated by polymorphisms at the DR-B1 locus (the DR-A locus is not polymorphic), while DQ serologic types are generated by polymorphism at both DQ-A and DQ-B loci. HLA typing methods have recently been developed that identify DNA sequence differences in the coding sequences at DR-B1, DQ-B1, and DQ-A1 loci.[37] Application of these methods, i.e., the analysis of nucleotide sequence polymorphism by means of polymerase chain reaction amplification and oligonucleotide probes, has identified specific DR-4 haplotypes defined by DQ-B1 alleles that are strongly associated with IDDM.[38] So far, it has not been possible to subdivide DR-3 haplotypes. In addition, certain DQ-B1 alleles have been found to confer protection against IDDM.[39]

Using the distributions of DQ-B1 alleles in the general population and in a large group of white patients with IDDM,[39] we estimated the lifetime risk of IDDM in a cohort of 10,000 individuals according to their DQ-B1 genotypes (Table 12–3). In the cohort, 3744 individuals would have the DQ-B1 allele 0602, which is described as protective against IDDM because persons carrying it have a low risk of IDDM, regardless of the DQ-B1 with which it is paired. One can estimate that only 2.4 of the individuals in this subgroup will develop IDDM, a lifetime risk of .06%. A large proportion of the cohort has DQ-B1 alleles that carry moderate risk, and 43.4 individuals among them would develop IDDM, giving a lifetime cumulative incidence of .91%. The remainder of the cohort carries the high-risk allele, DQ-B1 0302 and can be subdivided into two groups with somewhat different risks of IDDM. One group consists of 936 individuals who have the DQ-B1 0302 allele in combination with itself or one of various DQ-B1 alleles (exclusive of DQ-B1 0602, the protective allele), and the last group consists of 542 persons with the specific heterozygous

Table 12-3. Estimated Lifetime Risk of Insulin-Dependent Diabetes (IDDM) According to the Presence of HLA DQ-B1 Genotype

HLA DQ-B1 genotype	Persons born*	IDDM absent	IDDM present*	Cumulative incidence (%)
0302/0201	542	515.2	26.8	4.94
0302/X[†]	936	903.6	32.4	3.46
X/X[†]	4778	4734.6	43.4	0.91
0602/X[†]	3744	3741.6	2.4	0.06
Total[‡]	10000	9895.0	105.0	1.05

*Distribution calculated according to distribution of the genotype in whites in the United States.[39]
[†]HLA DQ-B1 allele other than 0302 or 0602.
[‡]Based on cumulative incidence of IDDM by age 70 in Table 12-1.

combination, DQ-B1 0302/0201. The latter allele is linked with DR-3 haplotype. The lifetime risks of IDDM for these two groups are 3.46 and 4.94%, respectively.

As can be seen in Table 12–3, the application of techniques that identify the alleles at the DQ-B1 locus with greater specificity improves the ability to predict low risk of IDDM, but the lifetime risk in the high-risk group is the same as that based on HLA-DR. Thus, one must conclude that other genetic (non-HLA) or nongenetic factors are involved in determining who will and who will not develop IDDM among those who have a susceptible HLA type.

Genetic Models

From the evidence reviewed thus far, it appears that an individual's risk of developing IDDM is determined by an HLA gene or one closely linked to the HLA region. However, most individuals with an at-risk HLA type do not develop IDDM. The challenge is to devise a strategy for studying non-HLA genes or environmental determinants that account for the absence of disease in HLA-susceptible individuals. One approach is to use genetic models. These models can be divided into two groups: parametric and nonparametric models.[40]

In fitting parametric models, one relates the pattern of occurrence of disease among members of a pedigree to the probabilities that these individuals have a disease genotype. The probability that two relatives share an allele at a particular locus is known from their degree of kinship. The probability that each has a disease genotype depends on the number of loci involved in determining disease susceptibility and the mode of inheritance (dominant, recessive, or intermediate) at each locus. By comparing the ability of alternative models to explain the pedigree data, one can choose a "best" model—usually on the basis of parsimony.

Several collections of nuclear families with IDDM have been investigated in this manner. These results are similar in concluding that occurrence of disease in these families is in part governed by a gene with a mode of inheritance that is intermediate between recessive and dominant modes but is close to recessive.[40] In one analysis by Rich

et al., the locus of this IDDM susceptibility gene was shown to be tightly linked to HLA,[41] and there was not strong evidence to support a role for a major genetic factor beyond that played by HLA. This result is appealingly consistent with the findings of the case-control studies of HLA DQ-B1 discussed in the preceding section. The DQ-B1 allele known as 0602 was described as protective in that it is associated with a low risk of disease even when paired with a high-risk DQ-B1 allele.[39] In other words, the susceptibility alleles had to be present in a double dose to convey their effect on risk. In terms of mode of inheritance, this shows closer analogy to a recessive than a dominant mode.

An alternative method of gaining insight into the complexity of the IDDM genotype is based on epidemiologic data regarding variation in risk to relatives according to degree of genetic relationship.[42] This type of genetic modeling is considered "nonparametric" since it is independent of the mode of inheritance at each locus and, therefore, obviates the need to estimate all the parameters associated with specifying the mode of inheritance at each locus. Recently, a series of nonparametric models was evaluated with respect to IDDM susceptibility.[40] On the basis of a variety of single-locus, multiple-locus, and polygenic models, a number of tentative predictions were made. First, a single major locus is not sufficient to explain all susceptibility to IDDM, and second, the effect of the HLA-linked major locus does account for most of the genetic contribution to susceptibility. This much is a repetition of conclusions based on parametric genetic models, but a third prediction is that the model of the non-HLA determinants may be relatively simple. Addition of just one more major locus and polygenes is sufficient to bring the nonparametric model into close agreement with available estimates of risk to relatives.

There are a few clues to the identity of the non-HLA locus involved in the IDDM susceptible genotype. Evidence has been found for a second susceptibility locus near the insulin gene on the short arm of chromosome 11p,[43] and there are hints that susceptibility is influenced by immunoglobulin genes on the long arm of chromosome 14.[44] Animal models of IDDM are another possible source of clues. In the NOD (non-obese diabetic) murine model, breeding experiments indicate that five different genes influence the occurrence and time of onset of disease[45] (see Chapter 18, Table 18–6).

EPIDEMIOLOGY OF NIDDM

In contrast to IDDM, incidence data on NIDDM are scarce, and thus we must rely on prevalence data as estimates of cumulative incidence to describe the occurrence of NIDDM in human populations. Diabetes that occurs in adults will be considered equivalent to NIDDM for these purposes, since new cases of IDDM are rare relative to new cases of NIDDM in adult populations, and cases of early-onset IDDM that remain among the prevalent cases of diabetes among persons over 30 years of age represent only a small percentage of the total.

Occurrence in the United States

The prevalence of diabetes, physician-diagnosed as well as undiagnosed, was estimated for the U.S. population aged 20 through 74 from the 1976 to 1980 National Health and Nutrition Examination Survey, which used National Diabetes Data Group criteria.[45] The overall prevalence of diabetes in the U.S. population aged 20 through 74 was 6.6%, corresponding to more than 8 million people. Diagnosed diabetes accounted for only one-half (3.4%) of these cases. The prevalence of undiagnosed diabetes increased with age, in parallel with that of diagnosed diabetes, so that the prevalence of the two remained approximately equal at all ages. The increase with age was similar for men and women and for blacks and whites, but the prevalence was slightly higher among women than men except in the group 65 through 74 years old. The prevalence among blacks was higher than that among whites at all ages and for both sexes.

The prevalence of diabetes, both diagnosed and undiagnosed, in the U.S. white population aged 20 through 74 is compared with the cumulative incidence of physician-diagnosed diabetes in Rochester, Minnesota, in Figure 12–6. Total prevalence (undiagnosed and diagnosed) of diabetes rose much more steeply with age than did the cumulative incidence of diagnosed diabetes in Rochester, a pattern implying a much higher incidence rate of diabetes in young adults than that generally realized. Even for diagnosed diabetes, the prevalence in 1976 to 1980 was higher at young ages than the cumulative incidence a decade earlier. The difference may reflect a temporal increase in the incidence rate for symptomatic diabetes or merely increased detection of a portion of the large reservoir of undiagnosed diabetes as a result of the screening activity by physicians. The prevalence of diagnosed diabetes after age 50 rose less steeply and

eventually fell below the cumulative incidence rate, a change that presumably reflects the removal of prevalent cases because of excess mortality in persons with diabetes and that illustrates quite graphically how prevalence data underestimate the cumulative incidence in older age groups.

Ethnic and Geographic Differences

The consideration of geographic and ethnic differences in the occurrence of NIDDM is simplified by concentrating on a narrow age range (45 through 54 years) and one sex (men). Since few patients with NIDDM die before the age of 55 years, these prevalence data can be considered reasonable estimates of cumulative incidence as of age 50 years.

Prevalence of diagnosed and undiagnosed NIDDM in various ethnic groups in the United States and around the world are summarized in Figure 12–7. In the examination of a representative sample of the United States population, 1976 to 1980, the prevalence of NIDDM was 7.7% among whites and 11.1% among blacks in the age group 45 through 54.[45] The prevalence in Hispanic minorities (Cubans in Florida and Mexican-Americans in the border states) was even higher[46] but did not approach that among Pima Indians of Arizona.[47]

The prevalence of NIDDM in European populations is rather low compared with the prevalence in these American populations. Several populations in Europe have been subjected to screening for undiagnosed diabetes[48–52] (and P. Garancini, C. Giliola, E. Manara, et al., unpublished data). In each of these populations, the combined prevalence of diagnosed and undiagnosed diabetes is less than half that in American whites even though less stringent diagnostic criteria (WHO) were used. The prevalence of NIDDM in Saudi Arabia[53] was similar to that in the United States,[45] while in central Asia the

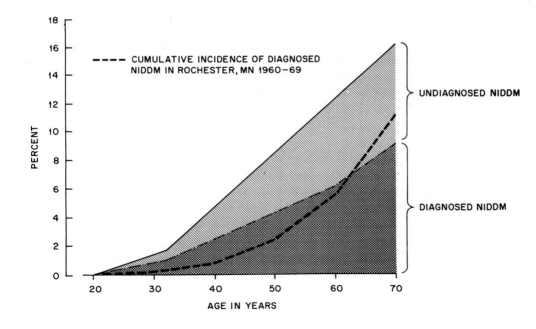

Fig. 12–6. Prevalence of diagnosed and undiagnosed non-insulin-dependent diabetes (NIDDM) in the white population of the United States aged 20 through 74 years, 1976 to 1980 (adapted from data in Harris et al.[45]), and the cumulative incidence of diagnosed NIDDM in Rochester, Minnesota, 1960 through 1969 (adapted from data in Melton et al.[5,6]).

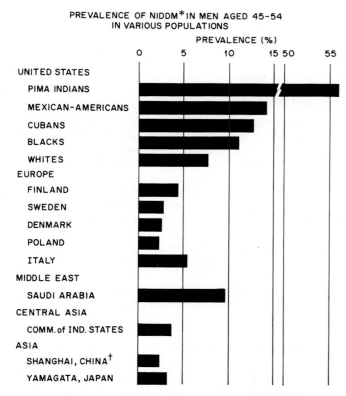

PREVALENCE OF NIDDM* IN MEN AGED 45-54
IN VARIOUS POPULATIONS

*INCLUDES UNDIAGNOSED DIABETES DETECTED BY SCREENING
†AGES 50-59

Fig. 12–7. Prevalence of non-insulin-dependent diabetes (NIDDM) in men 45 to 54 years old in various populations screened for undiagnosed diabetes (data sources: Pima Indians[47]; Hispanic-Americans[46]; black and white Americans[45]; Finland[48]; Sweden[49]; Denmark[50,51]; Poland[52]; Italy (P. Garancini et al., unpublished data); Saudi Arabia[53]; Commonwealth of Independent States[54]; China[55]; and Japan (A. Sekikawa et al., unpublished data).

prevalence among men aged 50 to 59 years[54] is quite similar to that in European men surveyed at a slightly younger age (45 to 54).

The substantial difference in the occurrence of diabetes among white populations, particularly between those in Europe and North America, points to an environmental component in the development of diabetes in whites. The contrast between Asian populations[55] (and A. Sekikawa, M. Tominaga, K. Takahashi, et al., unpublished data) and European white populations is inconsequential in comparison. Moreover, an important role of environment in the development of NIDDM in Asian populations is suggested by data on Chinese living outside of Asia. For example, the prevalence of NIDDM is high (20.8%) among Chinese living on the island of Mauritius in the Indian Ocean.[56] Reports that NIDDM is more common in Japanese living in the United States than in those in Hiroshima, Japan, are also in agreement with this conclusion.[57,58]

In summary, a large variability in the occurrence of NIDDM in different racial groups points to an important

role for environmental factors as determinants of the development of NIDDM.

Variation According to Obesity

As early as 1921, Dr. Elliott P. Joslin published a report in which he provided evidence that obese individuals had a high risk of developing diabetes (NIDDM according to the current classification).[59] Evidence of this association has been found in many subsequent cross-sectional studies, but the strength of the association has been problematic because of the criteria used to classify diabetes or because of ascertainment biases.

Excellent data have recently been obtained on adult height and weight from the participants in the 1976 to 1980 National Health and Nutrition Examination Survey.[60] For each category of glucose tolerance, the survey produced estimates of the average body weight (presented as percent of ideal body weight) at three time points: age 25 years; age at the time of survey (between 25 and 74 years of age); and the maximum body weight between those two ages (Fig. 12–8). There was only a small difference in body weight at age 25 years between the groups who subsequently became glucose intolerant and those whose glucose tolerance remained normal; this was true regardless of gender. However, at later adult ages, there were clear differences between the sexes with regard to the association between glucose tolerance and weight. For men, the largest difference in body weight between the glucose-tolerant and glucose-intolerant groups was in their maximum adult weight, but the difference was small and diminished by the time of survey. Among women, the association between glucose tolerance and body weight was stronger. There was a 20% difference between the maximum weights of the normal and diabetic groups, and this difference was maintained in the weights obtained during the survey.

Another way to examine the relationship between NIDDM and obesity is to group the survey participants according to the increase in percent ideal body weight after age 25 (Fig. 12–9). Even among the groups whose maximal weight gain was no more than 10 or 20%, the prevalence of diabetes was 4%, and this percentage increased little until the weight gain exceeded 40%. Among those with a weight gain greater than 40%, however, the prevalence of NIDDM rose quite steeply. One interpretation of these findings is that obesity is strongly associated with NIDDM in a subgroup of individuals who are particularly prone to gaining large amounts of weight but that in most individuals obesity is a weak discriminator between those who will develop diabetes and those who will not. Similarly, although the prevalence of impaired glucose tolerance increases steadily with weight gain, it varies only twofold over the whole range of weight gains in adults.

In a 10-year follow-up study of over 2000 Israelis aged 40 to 70, Modan et al.[61] found an association between obesity and the incidence rate of NIDDM, which resembles in several regards the survey data on the U.S. population. In both studies, a high body-mass index at

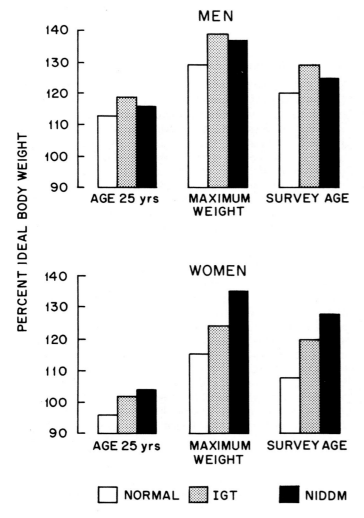

Fig. 12–8. Three measures of body weight according to glucose-tolerance category (IGT = impaired glucose tolerance; NIDDM = non-insulin-dependent diabetes) and gender. Adapted from data in Harris.[60]

a significant determinant of NIDDM risk. There has been much speculation regarding a genetic difference between the Pima Indians and white populations that is responsible for the extremely high risk of diabetes in the Pima Indians.

Familial Occurrence

Another avenue that may be taken in assessing the contribution of genetic factors to the development of NIDDM is the study of risk of diabetes in relatives of NIDDM probands. In such studies, it is informative to consider the age at onset of NIDDM in probands. One may estimate from the data in Table 12–1 and Figure 12–6 that about 20% of patients with NIDDM develop NIDDM before age 40, 40% develop it between the ages of 40 and 59, and 40% develop it at age 60 or later.

Several studies have reported data on the occurrence of diabetes in parents of NIDDM probands. A population-based cohort of NIDDM patients in Warsaw, Poland, was examined regarding occurrence of various noncommunicable diseases in relatives.[64] Patients with NIDDM diagnosed when they were between 30 and 50 years old reported parental diabetes twice as frequently as did those with NIDDM diagnosed when they were between 50 and 64. In a study in France, which compared patients with a diagnosis of NIDDM between the ages of 10 and 44 with a group of patients with a diagnosis between the ages of 45 and 59,[65] parental diabetes was reported by

some point in the past was more predictive of NIDDM than was the body mass at the beginning of the follow-up observation. The findings of an 8-year follow-up study in nurses aged 30 to 55 were similar[62] and also were consistent with the U.S. survey data, in showing that the body-mass index at age 18 was less predictive of NIDDM than was the body-mass index at the beginning of follow-up.

In a prospective study of diabetes in Pima Indians, the incidence of NIDDM was strongly related to preceding obesity, increasing steadily from 3500 cases per 100,000 person-years for women aged 35 to 64 whose body-mass index was 20 to 25 to 11,700 cases per 100,000 person-years for women whose body-mass index was 40 or more.[63] These rates are extraordinarily high—nearly 100 times the rates among white U.S. nurses with the corresponding body-mass index.[62] These differences demonstrate that a factor in addition to age and obesity is

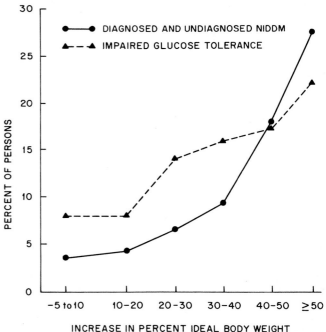

Fig. 12–9. Total prevalence of diagnosed and undiagnosed non-insulin-dependent diabetes and prevalence of impaired glucose tolerance according to percent ideal body weight. Adapted from data in Harris.[60]

66% of the patients with early-onset NIDDM and in only 36% of those with later-onset NIDDM.[65] Similar findings were reported in a smaller study conducted in Great Britain.[67] A very high prevalence of parental diabetes has also been found in individuals with onset of NIDDM before age 25 — the MODY (maturity-onset diabetes of the young)-type families.[67]

These data on parent-offspring pairs suggest a difference between the mode of inheritance of NIDDM with onset early in life and NIDDM with onset late in life. The occurrence of early cases is more consistent with an autosomal dominant disorder, whereas late-occurring NIDDM might be a recessive disorder or, in a large proportion of cases, environmentally determined. This interpretation should, however, be entertained with caution, since such a recessive inheritance pattern can result if a parent had undiagnosed diabetes and died without the diagnosis having been made or lived under conditions in which susceptibility to diabetes was not expressed.

A few studies have attempted to quantify the occurrence of diabetes in siblings of NIDDM probands. The living conditions of probands and siblings should be more similar than those of probands and parents. The most informative study is one conducted in the late 1960s at the Joslin Diabetes Center involving 446 siblings of 137 probands who developed diabetes between ages 30 and 59 years and were treated with oral agents or diet.[26] There was a strong relation between diabetes risk in the sibling and age at diagnosis in the proband. The cumulative incidence estimated by life-table methods was already 20% by age 50 years in the siblings of probands who were diagnosed before age 45 and only reached 17% by age 65 in siblings of probands diagnosed after age 45,[26] whereas in the general population the cumulative incidence was only 11% by age 70[5,6] (Fig. 12—10).

In another study conducted at the Joslin Diabetes Center over a period of 25 years, the risk of NIDDM was determined in 606 offspring of two parents with NIDDM.

The cumulative risk of NIDDM determined by life-table methods was 45% by age 65,[68] i.e., five times that in the general population.[5,6] The interesting observation was that the onset of NIDDM was strikingly earlier in offspring of parents who developed NIDDM before age 50 than in offspring of parents who developed NIDDM after age 50 (Fig. 12—11). If onset of NIDDM occurred before age 50 in one parent and after age 50 in the other, the age at onset in the offspring was intermediate between the ages at onset for the other two groups. Thus, there seems to be a correlation between age at onset in affected offspring and age at onset in their parents.

Studies of twins are another type of investigation that can provide insight into the nature of familial clustering of disease. In a recent study of U.S. veterans, 250 monozygotic and 264 dizygotic white male twins were examined for the presence of NIDDM.[69] For both types of twins, the prevalence of NIDDM in the entire group aged 52 to 65 years was 13%. This approximates the cumulative incidence at this age and is consistent with data for the general U.S. population (Fig. 12—6). The interesting finding was the difference in twin concordance rates. Among monozygotic (genetically identical) twins with at least one NIDDM-affected twin, the second twin also was affected in 41% (concordance rate), whereas in dizygotic twins, NIDDM typically occurred in one but not the other twin (concordance 10%). In the monozygotic twins concordant for NIDDM, the ages of onset of diabetes were closely correlated. Presumably, the determinants of this correlation also are responsible for the correlation between the ages at onset in pairs of affected siblings or in affected parents and children (Fig. 12—10 and Fig. 12—11).

The estimate of 41% for the concordance rate in monozygotic twins may be low; the diabetic twin in many of the discordant monozygotic twin-pairs had recently diagnosed diabetes. The correlation between ages at onset implies that the second twin in these pairs has a higher risk of developing NIDDM within a few years than

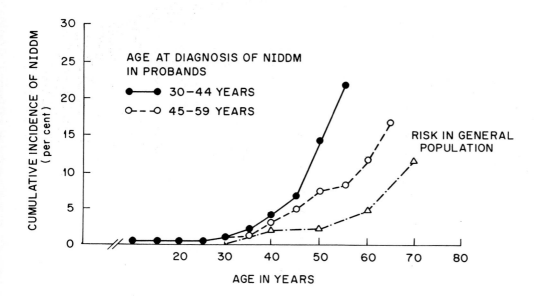

Fig. 12—10. Cumulative incidence of non-insulin-dependent diabetes (NIDDM) in siblings of probands with NIDDM according to the age at diagnosis of NIDDM in the proband (adapted from data in Gottlieb[26]), and cumulative incidence of NIDDM in the general population (adapted from data in Melton et al.[5,6]).

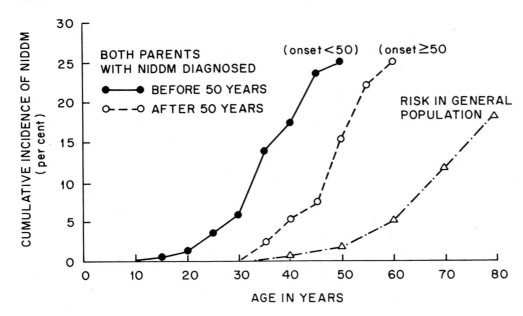

Fig. 12—11. Cumulative incidence of non-insulin-dependent diabetes (NIDDM) in offspring of two parents with NIDDM according to the age at diagnosis of NIDDM in the parents (adapted from data in Warram et al.[68]) and cumulative incidence of NIDDM in the general population (adapted from data in Melton et al.[5,6]).

did individuals in unaffected pairs. If the pairs that had been discordant for a short time were followed for a longer period, the concordance would rise but not likely reach the very high rate of 94% noted in a study conducted in the United Kingdom in the 1970s.[70] Because of ascertainment bias in the study in the United Kingdom, this concordance rate should be considered to be an upper bound to the range of possible values. An analysis of the Danish twin register that included 7000 pairs of twins born between 1870 and 1910[71] avoids ascertainment bias. In the Danish study, 26 (55%) of 47 pairs of presumed monozygotic twins were concordant for "maturity-onset diabetes," whereas only 15% of the dizygotic twins were concordant for this type of diabetes.

Because a substantial number of offspring and siblings of NIDDM probands will themselves develop NIDDM, they have often been studied with the goal of identifying physiologic characteristics distinguishing those who will develop diabetes, i.e., those with "prediabetes," from those who will not. In a follow-up of offspring of two parents with NIDDM, we found that all of the "prediabetic" offspring were insensitive to insulin or had impairment of insulin-independent glucose disposal long before they developed diabetes.[72] However, only half of the offspring with these impairments developed NIDDM during follow-up. Therefore, these characteristics are not the phenotype of "prediabetes" so much as they are the phenotype of a state that confers particular susceptibility to NIDDM. Such physiologic characteristics are sometimes called "intervening phenotypes" since they lie between a genetic determinant and a disease phenotype. We found significant clustering of levels of sensitivity within sibships, a pattern consistent with polygenic inheritance.[73] Thus, a plausible hypothesis is that some polygenic determinants of insulin insensitivity contribute to the correlation of age at onset among relatives. In our follow-up study of offspring of parents with NIDDM, no abnormality of β-cell secretion was detectable at baseline

but all those who progressed to diabetes were ultimately unable to sustain insulin secretion capable of maintaining euglycemia. This susceptibility to failure may be due to a genetic determinant, and the condition of its expression may be the presence of a defect in insulin sensitivity. Alternatively, this β-cell failure may be caused by environmental factors.

Genetic Models

Studies in relatives suggest that more than one genetic determinant contributes to the etiology of NIDDM. The effects of some of them may be additive, each contributing to the total prevalence of NIDDM. Alternatively, the effects may interact (epistasis), as would be the case, for example, if an "insulin resistance gene" could produce NIDDM only when a "β-cell failure gene" also was present. One approach to estimating the complexity of the set of genetic mechanisms involved in the etiology of NIDDM is based on the variation in risk to relatives according to the degree of genetic relatedness to the proband[40] (e.g., identical twins share 100% of genes, first-degree relatives share 50%, second-degree relatives share 25%). If the risk of NIDDM decreases as the proportion of shared genes diminishes, a single-locus model would be sufficient to account for the risk to relatives. However, available data indicate that the risk to relatives decreases more rapidly than the proportion of shared genes. Therefore, involvement of multiple loci must be postulated to mimic the more rapid decrease in risk with increasing genetic distance. This approach to modeling is called *nonparametric* because the evaluation of the model is independent of the mode of inheritance at each locus.

Recently, a series of nonparametric models was evaluated with respect to NIDDM susceptibility.[40] In brief, it was concluded that the pattern of risks to relatives of persons with NIDDM is compatible with inheritance based on only few interacting loci plus polygenes (many genes having small additive effects) or shared family environment. This result is surprising given the clinical heterogeneity of NIDDM, but it suggests that the task of mapping a series of single genes with moderate effects on NIDDM susceptibility may be quite feasible.

In summary, twin studies of NIDDM have shown that genetic or common (familial) environmental factors play a dominant role in defining the risk for development of this disease. Although no single gene locus has been identified that significantly contributes to susceptibility to NIDDM, a number of studies have demonstrated that many of the risk factors for NIDDM (obesity, hyperinsulinemia, and other intermediate phenotypes) may be under genetic control. The risk for NIDDM is likely to be dependent on an individual's having a "diabetogenic" constitution that is expressed only in a given environment. The detection of the NIDDM susceptibility genes, the identification of the modifiable risk factors, and the means by which they interact is the focus of current research.

REFERENCES

1. Krolewski AS, Warram JH. Epidemiology of diabetes mellitus. In: Marble A, Krall LP, Bradley RF, et al., eds. Joslin's diabetes mellitus. 12th ed. Philadelphia: Lea & Febiger, 1985:12–42.
2. Rothman KJ. Measures of disease frequency. In: Rothman KJ. Modern epidemiology. Boston: Little, Brown and Company, 1986:23–49.
3. National Diabetes Data Group. Classification and diagnosis of diabetes mellitus and other categories of glucose intolerance. Diabetes 1979;28:1039–57.
4. World Health Organization. Second report of the Expert Committee on Diabetes Mellitus. WHO Tech Rep Ser 1980;646:7–80.
5. Melton LJ III, Palumbo PJ, Chu C-P. Incidence of diabetes mellitus by clinical type. Diabetes Care 1983;6:75–86.
6. Melton LJ, Palumbo PJ, Dwyer MS, Chu C. Impact of recent changes in diagnostic criteria on the apparent natural history of diabetes mellitus. Am J Epidemiol 1983;117:559–65.
7. Gamble DR. The epidemiology of insulin-dependent diabetes, with particular reference to the relationship of virus infection to its etiology. Epidemiol Rev 1980;2:49–70.
8. Christau B, Kromann H, Christy M, et al. Incidence of insulin-dependent diabetes mellitus (0–29 years at onset) in Denmark. Acta Med Scand Suppl 1979;624:54–60.
9. Christau B, Mølbak AG. Incidence rates for type 1 (insulin-dependent) diabetes and insulin-treated diabetes in age groups over 30 years [Abstract no. 56]. Diabetologia 1982;23:160.
10. Krolewski AS, Warram JH, Rand LI, Kahn CR. Epidemiologic approach to the etiology of Type I diabetes mellitus and its complications. N Engl J Med 1987;317:1390–8.
11. Ustvedt HJ, Olsen E. Incidence of diabetes mellitus in Oslo, Norway 1956–65. Br J Prev Soc Med 1977;31:251–7.
12. Joner G, Søvik O. Incidence, age at onset and seasonal variation of diabetes mellitus in Norwegian children, 1973–1977. Acta Paediatr Scand 1981;70:329–35.
13. Tuomilehto J, Rewers M, Reunanen A, et al. Increasing trend in type 1 (insulin-dependent) diabetes mellitus in childhood in Finland: analysis of age, calendar time and

14. Hägglöf B, Holmgren G, Wall S. Incidence of insulin-dependent diabetes mellitus among children in a North-Swedish population 1938–1977. Hum Hered 1982; 32:408–17.
15. Dahlquist G, Blom L, Holmgren G, et al. The epidemiology of diabetes in Swedish children 0–14 years—a six-year prospective study. Diabetologia 1985;28:802–8.
16. Patterson CC, Thorogood M, Smith PG, et al. Epidemiology of Type I (insulin-dependent) diabetes in Scotland 1968–1976: evidence of an increasing incidence. Diabetologia 1983;24:238–43.
17. Kurtz Z, Peckham CS, Ades AE. Changing prevalence of juvenile-onset diabetes mellitus. Lancet 1988;2:88–90.
18. Green A, Andersen PK, Svendsen AJ, Mortensen K. Increasing incidence of early onset Type I (insulin-dependent) diabetes mellitus: a study of Danish male birth cohorts. Diabetologia 1992;35:178–82.
19. Gleason RE, Kahn CB, Funk IB, Craighead JE. Seasonal incidence of insulin-dependent diabetes (IDDM) in Massachusetts, 1964–1973. Int J Epidemiol 1982;11:39–45.
20. Diabetes Epidemiology Research International Group. Secular trends in incidence of childhood IDDM in 10 countries. Diabetes 1990;39:858–64.
21. Rewers M, LaPorte RE, Walczak M, et al. Apparent epidemic of insulin-dependent diabetes mellitus in midwestern Poland. Diabetes 1987;36:106–13.
22. Tull ES, Roseman JM, Christian CLE. Epidemiology of childhood IDDM in U.S. Virgin Islands from 1979 to 1988: evidence of an epidemic in early 1980s and variation by degree of racial admixture. Diabetes Care 1991;14:558–64.
23. Wagenknecht LE, Roseman JM, Herman WH. Increased incidence of insulin-dependent diabetes mellitus following an epidemic of coxsackievirus B5. Am J Epidemiol 1991;133:1024–31.
24. Patrick SL, Moy CS, LaPorte RE. The world of insulin-dependent diabetes mellitus: what international epidemiologic studies reveal about the etiology and natural history of IDDM. Diabetes Metab Rev 1989;5:571–8.
25. Diabetes Epidemiology Research International Group. Geographic patterns of childhood insulin-dependent diabetes mellitus. Diabetes 1988;37:1113–9.
26. Gottlieb MS. Diabetes in offspring and siblings of juvenile- and maturity-onset-type diabetics. J Chronic Dis 1980; 33:331–9.
27. Warram JH, Krolewski AS. Changing age-at-onset of diabetes in siblings of probands with insulin-dependent diabetes [Abstract no. 617]. Am J Hum Gen 1985;37 (Suppl):A208.
28. Degnbol B, Green A. Diabetes mellitus among first- and second-degree relatives of early onset diabetics. Ann Hum Genet 1978;42:25–47.
29. Allen C, Palta M, D'Alessio DJ. Risk of diabetes in siblings and other relatives of IDDM subjects. Diabetes 1991;40:831–6.
30. Warram JH, Krolewski AS, Gottlieb MS, Kahn CR. Differences in risk of insulin-dependent diabetes in offspring of diabetic mothers and diabetic fathers. N Engl J Med 1984;311:149–52.
31. LaPorte RE, Fishbein HA, Drash AL, et al. The Pittsburgh insulin-dependent diabetes mellitus (IDDM) registry: the incidence of insulin-dependent diabetes mellitus in Allegheny County, Pennsylvania (1965–1976). Diabetes 1981; 30:279–84.

32. Warram JH, Krolewski AS, Kahn CR. Determinants of IDDM and perinatal mortality in children of diabetic mothers. Diabetes 1988;37:1328–34.

33. Warram JH, Martin BC, Krolewski AS. Risk of IDDM in children of diabetic mothers decreases with increasing maternal age at pregnancy. Diabetes 1991;40:1679–84.

34. Chern MM, Anderson VE, Barbosa J. Empirical risk for insulin-dependent diabetes (IDD) in sibs: further definition of genetic heterogeneity. Diabetes 1982;31:1115–8.

35. Svejgaard A, Ryder LP. HLA genotype distribution and genetic models of insulin-dependent diabetes mellitus. Ann Hum Genet 1981;45:293–8.

36. Thomson G, Robinson WP, Kuhner MK, et al. Genetic heterogeneity, modes of inheritance, and risk estimates for a joint study of caucasians with insulin-dependent diabetes mellitus. Am J Hum Genet 1988;43:799–816.

37. Bodmer JG, Marsh SGE, Albert ED, et al. Nomenclature for factors of the HLA system, 1990. Tissue Antigens 1991;37:97–104.

38. Erlich HA, Bugawan TL, Scharf S, et al. HLA-DQβ sequence polymorphism and genetic susceptibility to IDDM. Diabetes 1990;39:96–103.

39. Baisch JM, Weeks T, Giles R, et al. Analysis of HLA-DQ genotypes and susceptibility in insulin-dependent diabetes mellitus. N Engl J Med 1990;322:1836–41.

40. Rich SS. Mapping genes in diabetes: genetic epidemiological perspective. Diabetes 1990;39:1315–9.

41. Rich SS, Green A, Morton NE, Barbosa J. A combined segregation and linkage analysis of insulin-dependent diabetes mellitus. Am J Hum Genet 1987;40:237–49.

42. Risch N. Linkage strategies for genetically complex traits. I. Multilocus models. Am J Hum Genet 1990;46:222–8.

43. Julier C, Hyer RN, Davies J, et al. Insulin-IGF2 region on chromosome 11p encodes a gene implicated in HLA-DR4-dependent diabetes susceptibility. Nature 1991;354:155–9.

44. Rich SS, Weitkamp LR, Guttormsen S, Barbosa J. Gm, Km, and HLA in insulin-dependent Type I diabetes mellitus: a log-linear analysis of association. Diabetes 1986;35:927–32.

45. Harris MI, Hadden WC, Knowler WC, Bennett PH. Prevalence of diabetes and impaired glucose tolerance and plasma glucose levels in U.S. population aged 20–74 yr. Diabetes 1987;36:523–34.

46. Flegal KM, Ezzati TM, Harris MI, et al. Prevalence of diabetes in Mexican Americans, Cubans, and Puerto Ricans from the Hispanic Health and Nutrition Examination Survey, 1982–84. Diabetes Care 1991;14(Suppl 3):628–38.

47. Knowler WC, Pettitt DJ, Saad MF, Bennett PH. Diabetes mellitus in the Pima Indians: incidence, risk factors and pathogenesis. Diabetes Metab Rev 1990;6:1–27.

48. Tuomilehto J, Korhonen H, Kartovaara L, et al. Prevalence of diabetes mellitus and impaired glucose tolerance in the middle-aged population of three areas in Finland. Int J Epidemiol 1991;20:1010–7.

49. Andersson DKG, Svärdsudd K, Tibblin G. Prevalence and incidence of diabetes in a Swedish community 1972–1987. Diabetic Med 1991;8:428–34.

50. Schroll M, Hagerup L. Relationship of fasting blood glucose to prevalence of ECG abnormalities and 10 yr risk of mortality from cardiovascular diseases in men born in 1914: from the Glostrup population studies. J Chronic Dis 1979;32:699–707.

51. Hagerup L, Eriksen M, Schroll M, et al. The Glostrup population studies collection of epidemiologic tables: reference values for use in cardiovascular population studies. Scand J Soc Med Suppl 1981;20:1–112.

52. Mroszczyk M, Gdulewicz T, Torzecka W, et al. Cukrzyca w probie losowej trzech dzielnic Lodzi. Zdrowie Publiczne 1976;87:169. (See also Diabetologia 1981;21:520–4.)

53. Bacchus RA, Bell JL, Madkour M, Kilshaw B. The prevalence of diabetes mellitus in male Saudi Arabs. Diabetologia 1982;23:330–2.

54. Samokhvalova MA, Dzhuraeva-Akhmedova SD, Zhukovsky GS, et al. Study of diabetes mellitus incidence. Probl Endokrinol (Mosk) 1976;22:27–31.

55. Shanghai Diabetes Research Cooperative Group. Diabetes mellitus survey in Shanghai. Chin Med J 1980;93:663–72.

56. Dowse GK, Gareeboo H, Zimmet PZ, et al, for the Mauritius Noncommunicable Disease Study Group. High prevalence of NIDDM and impaired glucose tolerance in Indian, Creole, and Chinese Mauritians. Diabetes 1990;39:390–6.

57. Kawate R, Yamakido M, Nishimoto Y, et al. Diabetes mellitus and its vascular complications in Japanese migrants on the island of Hawaii. Diabetes Care 1979;2:161–70.

58. Kawate R, Yamakido M, Nishimoto Y. Migrant studies among the Japanese in Hiroshima and Hawaii. In: Waldhäusl WK, ed. Diabetes 1979. Proceedings of the 10th Congress of the International Diabetes Federation. Amsterdam: Excerpta Medica, 1980:526–31.

59. Joslin EP. The prevention of diabetes mellitus. JAMA 1921;76:79–84.

60. Harris MI. Impaired glucose tolerance in the U.S. population. Diabetes Care 1989;12:464–74.

61. Modan M, Karasik A, Halkin H, et al. Effect of past and concurrent body mass index on prevalence of glucose intolerance and type 2 (non-insulin-dependent) diabetes and on insulin response: the Israel study of glucose intolerance, obesity and hypertension. Diabetologia 1986;29:82–9.

62. Colditz GA, Willett WC, Stampfer MJ, et al. Weight as a risk factor for clinical diabetes in women. Am J Epidemiol 1990;132:501–13.

63. Knowler WC, Pettitt DJ, Savage PJ, Bennett PH. Diabetes incidence in Pima Indians: contributions of obesity and parental diabetes. Am J Epidemiol 1981;113:144–56.

64. Królewski AS, Czyzyk A, Kopczyński J, Rywik S. Prevalence of diabetes mellitus, coronary heart disease and hypertension in the families of insulin dependent and insulin independent diabetics. Diabetologia 1981;21:520–4.

65. Vague P, Lassmann V, Grosset C, Vialettes B. Type II diabetes in young subjects: a study of 90 unrelated cases. Diabete Metab 1987;13:92–8.

66. O'Rahilly S, Spivey RS, Holman RR, et al. Type II diabetes of early onset: a distinct clinical and genetic syndrome? BMJ 1987;294:923–6.

67. Fajans SS. Scope and heterogeneous nature of MODY. Diabetes Care 1990;13:49–64.

68. Warram JH, Martin BC, Soeldner JS, Krolewski AS. Study of glucose removal rate and first phase insulin secretion in the offspring of two parents with non-insulin-dependent diabetes. In: Camerini-Davalos RA, Cole HS, eds. Advances in experimental medicine and biology. Vol 246. Prediabetes. New York: Plenum Press, 1988:175–83.

69. Newman B, Selby JV, King M-C, et al. Concordance for type 2 (non-insulin-dependent) diabetes mellitus in male twins. Diabetologia 1987;30:763–8.

70. Barnett AH, Eff C, Leslie RDG, Pyke DA. Diabetes in identical twins: a study of 200 pairs. Diabetologia 1981;20:87−93.

71. Harvald B, Hauge M. Selection in diabetes in modern society. Acta Med Scand 1963;173:459−65.

72. Martin BC, Warram JH, Krolewski AS, et al. Role of glucose and insulin resistance in the development of Type II diabetes: results of a 25-year follow up study. Lancet 1992;340:925−29.

73. Martin BC, Warram JH, Rosner B, et al. Familial clustering of insulin sensitivity. Diabetes 1992;41:850−4.

Chapter 13

PATHOGENESIS OF INSULIN-DEPENDENT (TYPE I) DIABETES MELLITUS

GEORGE S. EISENBARTH
ANETTE G. ZIEGLER
PETER A. COLMAN

In parallel with dramatic developments in basic immunology and the techniques for studying genetic diseases, it has become clear that Type I diabetes is an autoimmune disorder in which β-cell destruction occurs in a genetically susceptible host.[1-5] In this chapter on the pathogenesis of Type I diabetes, we will review the changes in basic knowledge concerning Type I diabetes and address areas in which such knowledge has already entered the realm of clinical care or is likely to do so before the next edition of *Joslin's Diabetes Mellitus* is published.

The hallmark of Type I diabetes is an almost complete destruction of β-cells with maintenance of the α- (glucagon-secreting) and δ- (somatostatin-secreting) cells within islets of Langerhans.[6] Thus, given sufficient time after the recognition of overt hyperglycemia, essentially all patients with Type I diabetes become dependent on insulin for maintenance of life.

We will use the term *Type I diabetes* to refer only to the HLA-associated, presumably autoimmune, form of insulin-dependent diabetes mellitus (IDDM). Disorders other than Type I diabetes can result in β-cell destruction. We will not include these other disorders under the term Type I diabetes, including the effects of ingestion of toxins such as pyriminil (Vacor)[7] and the rare Wolfram's (DIDMOAD) syndrome (diabetes insipidus, diabetes mellitus, optic atrophy, and nerve deafness[8]). Wolfram's syndrome is an autosomal recessive disorder in which β-cells of the islets and a variety of neurons are destroyed. In Wolfram's syndrome, as in Type I diabetes, β-cells are selectively lost, with preservation of α- and δ-cells.[9] These individuals typically develop diabetes in infancy and later succumb to a series of diabetic and neuropathic disorders. This disorder is not associated with the HLA alleles (e.g., DR3 and DR4) typically associated with Type I diabetes.

GENETICS OF TYPE I DIABETES

It has long been recognized that Type I diabetes is a familial disorder. Approximately 1 in 20 first-degree relatives of patients with Type I diabetes will develop the disease (vs. 4 per 1000 in the general white population). Approximately 50% of identical twins are concordant for the disease. Table 13-1 lists empiric risks for development of Type I diabetes,[10,11] and Table 13-2 details risks for identical twins and siblings of diabetic persons with specific HLA-DR alleles.

Twins identical to a person with Type I diabetes who have the two high-risk alleles, DR3 and DR4, have a concordance rate of approximately 70%.[12] The maximal estimate of genetic penetrance of diabetes is thus approximately 70%. Despite this strong familial influence, it should be emphasized that 90% of individuals who develop Type I diabetes do not have a first-degree relative with diabetes. Among siblings of diabetic patients, both the specific HLA DR type and the "sharing" of HLA haplotypes with the diabetic sibling influence the risk of diabetes. Siblings who are HLA identical to a diabetic

Table 13–1. Empiric Risk of Type I Diabetes

Relation to diabetic proband	Risk
General population	0.4%
Sibling	5%
Parent	5%
Offspring of diabetic father	6.1%
Offspring of diabetic mother	2%
Mother's age >25 at birth	1.1%
Mother's age <25 at birth	3.6%
Offspring of diabetic mother and father	30%
Monozygotic twin (white)	30–50%
Monozygotic twin (Japanese)	30–50%
Dizygotic twin	5%
Sibling and offspring	30%

sibling (two haplotypes identical to those of sibling) have the highest risk of diabetes for siblings—approaching 20% when they express both DR3 and DR4. In families with two first-degree relatives with diabetes (e.g., both parents, one parent and one sibling, two siblings), risk of diabetes for other first-degree relatives is approximately 30%.

Several of the empiric risks given in Table 13–1 require further study because of the limited number of individuals in various subgroups that have been analyzed. Precise definition of disease prevalence in larger studies (e.g., concordance rates among Japanese identical twins, offspring of parents who both have Type I diabetes, concordance for dizygotic twins, development of diabetes in offspring of diabetic mothers who give birth before or after age 25 years) would be important, as they will influence a number of hypotheses concerning the pathogenesis of Type I diabetes. For example:

1) If the concordance for diabetes of identical twins in Japan equals that in the United States (despite a thirtyfold lower overall incidence of diabetes in Japan than in white Americans), differences between the incidence of diabetes in Japan compared with that in the United States may be the result primarily of differences in the prevalence of susceptibility genes.

2) If the concordance rate for Type I diabetes of dizygotic twins is equal to that of siblings, it is likely that acute environmental factors (which dizygotic twins would share) may not be of major importance for determining which twin develops diabetes.

3) If the risk of diabetes in offspring of two parents with Type I diabetes approaches that of identical twins, genes creating diabetes susceptibility would be expected to be relatively few or to readily complement each other such that offspring of "random-mating" pairs have a high incidence of disease. For comparison, if a DB mouse is mated with an NOD mouse (two strains that spontaneously develop diabetes), none of their offspring would develop diabetes, since distinct recessive genes (which do not complement each other) are responsible for the diabetes of each strain.

4) If the incidence of diabetes in offspring of diabetic mothers who give birth after the age of 25 years[13] is lower than the incidence in offspring of mothers who give birth before the age of 25 years, factors in the maternal diabetic environment may be protective.

Not only is the incidence of Type I diabetes influenced by genetic factors, the age at which Type I diabetes develops also appears to be under genetic control, as illustrated by Figure 13–1, which compares the ages of onset in families with more than one sibling with Type I diabetes. There is an overall correlation in age at onset of diabetes in siblings. The second child in the family to develop diabetes does not have to be born before the first child develops diabetes to experience an early age of diabetes onset similar to that of the first child (Fig. 13–1, right). This suggests that acute environmental factors affecting two siblings simultaneously may not be important with regard to the correlation in timing of diabetes onset.

Essentially everyone who develops Type I diabetes has alleles within the major histocompatibility region associated with the disorder.[14] The ability to identify the same HLA alleles associated with diabetes in both "familial" and "nonfamilial" Type I diabetes suggests that similar genes contribute to disease susceptibility in both groups. The major histocompatibility complex (Fig. 13–2) was so named because genes in this region of the genome in mice (chromosome 17) and humans (chromosome 6) determine the rapidity with which skin grafts or other transplanted tissue is rejected. Approximately 3 billion (3×10^9) nucleotide base-pairs comprise the human genome; of these base-pairs approximately 3 million (3×10^6) make up the major histocompatibility complex. These 3 million base-pairs code for approximately 100 genes, only a portion of which have been identified. Differences in the nucleotide sequences among individuals determine amino acid polymorphisms of histocompatibility molecules such that essentially no two unrelated individuals are identical for all histocompatibility alleles.[14] The classic histocompatibility genes are extremely polymorphic (amino acid sequence differs

Table 13–2. Risk of Type I Diabetes with Known HLA-DR and Haplotype Sharing with Proband

HLA-DR	Identical Twin	Sibling With Indicated No. of HLA Haplotypes Identical to Proband		
		2	1	0
3/4	70.2%	19.2%	3.7%	1.3%
4/4	33%	7.4%	3.5%	1.0%
4/X*	42%	11.1%	6.8%	1.6%
3/3	43%	14.1%	3.9%	2.4%
3/X	38%	11.2%	4.9%	2.8%
X/X	25%	5.7%	3.3%	3.8%

*X = non-3 and non-4.

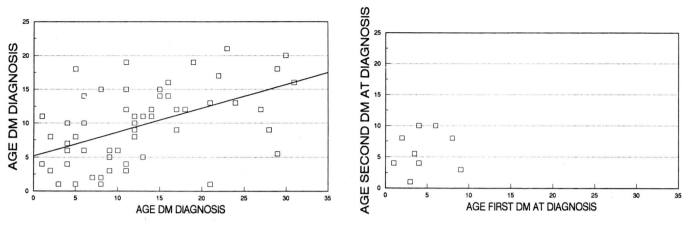

Fig. 13–1. Left: Age of onset of Type I diabetes mellitus (DM) among sibling pairs. Right: Age of onset among sibling pairs for which second child to develop diabetes had not yet been born when the first child developed diabetes. (Data are combined from the Human Biologic Disease Interchange [HBDI] Juvenile Diabetes Foundation initial survey and families followed at the Joslin Diabetes Center.)

among individuals) and include HLA-A, B, and C molecules (class I histocompatibility antigens), and the "immune-response genes" DP, DQ, and DR (class II histocompatibility antigens). Numbers (e.g., DR3, DR4; A1, A2; B1, B8) are given to distinguish different alleles of any given gene. The designation "w" (workshop) with numbers is given for provisionally named alleles (e.g., DQw8, DQw7). In addition to class I and class II molecules, the histocompatibility region contains genes for complement components such as C2 and C4, for tumor necrosis factor, for a 70-kilodalton (kd) heat-shock protein, for the 21 hydroxylase enzyme (abnormalities of which lead to congenital adrenal hyperplasia[15]), and for an unknown recessive gene determining hemochromatosis[16].

The gene for hemochromatosis is relatively common (1 in 15 individuals in the general population are carriers, and approximately 1 in 200 are homozygous; O'Brien and co-workers detected three new cases of hemochromatosis by random screening, e.g., for serum ferritin, in 572 persons with diabetes onset after the age of 30 years[16]). As soon as a person is identified as having hemochromatosis, all first-degree relatives should be screened for the disease (e.g., ferritin levels, HLA typing of siblings), since 25% of siblings of a person with hemochromatosis will be homozygous for the hemochromatosis gene, as will be approximately 6% of offspring. Although class I and class II histocompatibility genes are not the cause of hemochromatosis, at the population level, hemochromatosis is associated with HLA allele A3. The disease gene is in linkage disequilibrium with A3, suggesting that the mutation causing hemochromatosis may have arisen on a chromosome bearing HLA A3 and that the elapsed

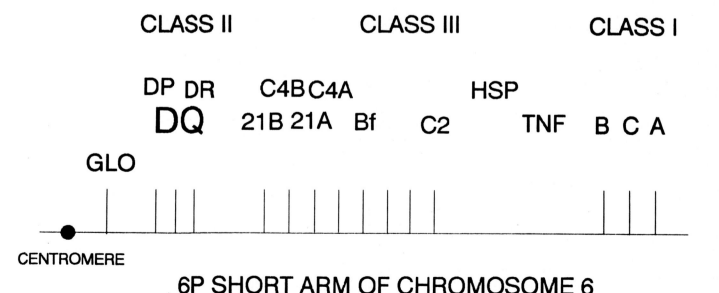

Fig. 13–2. Major histocompatibility complex of humans with class II (immune response genes DP, DQ, DR), class I genes (A,B,C), class III genes (complement), and additional genes such as the 21 hydroxylase gene and the gene for heat-shock protein 70 (HSP 70).

evolutionary time has not been sufficient for the disease gene to dissociate from A3 by crossing-over events. Linkage disequilibrium of many alleles in the HLA region makes it more difficult to pinpoint causative genes, in that an association of alleles with disease is not proof of a causal relationship.

Alleles of class I histocompatibility molecules differ in the amino acid sequences of a 44-kd surface protein.[17] This 44-kd molecule is non-covalently bound to β_2 macroglobulin (which is not polymorphic) to form the complete class I molecule. The class II histocompatibility molecules are made up of an α and a β chain. The β chains of DP, DQ, and DR are all polymorphic. For DQ molecules, but not for DP or DR molecules, the α chain is also polymorphic.

The past decade has seen a tremendous expansion in knowledge concerning class I and class II histocompatibility molecules. Sequences of multiple alleles are now available, and the crystal structure has been obtained for a class I molecule. The manner in which these molecules function to bind peptides and to present peptides to T cells is being defined.[17] In addition, disease associations with histocompatibility alleles have been refined.

According to current evidence, DQ molecules appear to be the major determinant of diabetes susceptibility or resistance for haplotypes bearing the DR4 susceptibility allele or the DR2 protective allele.[18,19] How might these molecules influence the development of diabetes? From the known function of immune response genes and the manner by which T and B lymphocytes recognize antigens, a number of hypotheses have been generated. To a large extent the specificity of the immune system is determined by antigen receptors of both T and B lymphocytes. Each clone of T and B lymphocytes expresses as its antigen receptor a unique T-cell receptor or immunoglobulin molecule, respectively. Activation of either the T-cell receptor or the B-cell receptor (which is surface immunoglobulin) by antigen leads to clonal expansion of the stimulated lymphocytes, to synthesis and secretion of potent effector molecules (lymphokines), and to acquisition of surface receptors (e.g., interleukin-2 receptor, transferrin receptor). Both immunoglobulin and T-cell receptors are produced by a random combinatorial process in which the heavy- and light-chain genes of immunoglobulin or the chains of the T-cell receptor (α and β, or γ, and δ, depending on the class of T cells) are created by combining genetic segments. Thus, one of many variable region gene segments is combined with one or two other short gene segments (depending on the molecule, D [diversity] and J [joining] segments), which are then combined with constant-region gene segments to produce a final molecule. The ability of the immune system by random genetic recombinatorial mechanisms to produce billions of different T-cell receptor and immunoglobulin molecules underlies the immune systems repertoire and enables the immune system to respond to "any" protein.[20]

Despite a similar mechanism for generating the diversity of the immune system, T and B lymphocytes "see" antigen in fundamentally different manners. This difference in recognition of antigen involves the histocompatibility molecules discussed previously. B lymphocytes and the immunoglobulin they produce react directly with soluble antigen. Thus, a B lymphocyte that expresses surface antibody that reacts with insulin can be directly stimulated to divide by the addition of soluble insulin. T lymphocytes are "blind" to antigen unless it is complexed to histocompatibility molecules. In addition, T lymphocytes usually react with processed portions (peptides) of a given antigen. T cells respond to antigens that are bound by histocompatibility molecules on the surface of a variety of antigen-presenting cells (e.g., macrophages, dendritic cells, B lymphocytes).

Recent crystallographic studies indicate that histocompatibility molecules are made up of an antigen-binding groove lined by two domains of α helices. The polymorphic amino acids of histocompatibility molecules making up the α helices and the floor of the peptide binding groove determine which peptides are bound and thus presented to T-cell receptors. Thus, the molecular complex that stimulates T lymphocytes is a ternary complex made up of antigen bound to a histocompatibility molecule interacting with the T-cell receptor. Even this model of the ternary complex is simplified in that accessory surface molecules and lymphokines produced by antigen-presenting cells are essential for T-cell activation. For instance, the CD4 molecule is essential for antigen presentation to T cells by class II histocompatibility molecules (e.g., DP, DQ, and DR), while CD8-positive T cells react with class I (HLA A, B, C)-bound antigen. Not only are T cells restricted to recognizing antigen bound to histocompatibility molecules, they only "see" antigen presented by a person's (or animal's) own histocompatibility molecules. In addition, T cells are not activated unless the antigen-presenting cell produces accessory signals such as the lymphokine interleukin-1. By way of generalization, T lymphocytes are designed to recognize cell-bound antigens, while B lymphocytes respond to free antigens.

From the above brief review of immunologic activation and specificity, it is apparent how important class II molecules are in determining an immune response. Hence their name: immune-response genes. The ability of class II molecules to bind specific antigenic peptides can and does determine the immune response to given antigens. Thus, one manner in which class II molecules such as the DQβ chain of DQw8 associated with DR4 haplotypes may predispose to diabetes is by binding an islet-derived peptide and enhancing a T-cell response to that peptide. For example, DR4-associated class II genes may contribute to diabetes by enhancing the immune response to insulin.[21]

In addition to their effects on antigen presentation, class II molecules have recently been shown to correlate with T-lymphocyte repertoire in normal mice. Thus, mice that express the analogue of DR (termed I-E) delete a series of T lymphocytes bearing specific families of T-cell receptors (e.g., Vβ5, Vβ11, which are named for the variable-region gene used to produce the complete receptor).[18] It is noteworthy that NOD mice that develop Type I diabetes have a deletion of their I-E gene and do not produce I-E molecules. It was hypothesized that such an influence of I-E on the T-cell receptor repertoire might account for the protective effect of the I-E gene in NOD mice. Recent data suggest that the targeting of the islets in these mice is not dependent on limited Vβ T cell–receptor usage, and the potent effect of I-E may be secondary to "protective" antigen presentation. For NOD mice, the introduction of either a transgene replacing the missing I-E gene or a transgene of normal I-A molecules prevents diabetes.[18,19] This is the most direct demonstration of the importance of these specific genes in creating susceptibility to diabetes.

It is noteworthy that in the insulitis process of humans, the BB rat, and the NOD mouse, β-cells show enhanced expression of class I molecules. This may enhance β-cell destruction, since CD8-positive cytotoxic lymphocytes destroy cells that bear antigen bound to class I molecules. In addition, islets expressing class II molecules in insulitis lesions have been described. However, the latter is probably a late event in the development of insulitis and in humans is probably secondary to lymphocytic infiltrates, with interferon-γ plus tumor necrosis factor capable of inducing expression of class II molecules by β-cells.[22] Studies by Foulis and co-workers indicate that islets in which β-cells have enhanced expression of class II antigens have infiltrating lymphocytes. A hypothesis suggesting that β-cells act as their own antigen-presenting cell when they express class II molecules is controversial. Transgenic mice induced to express class II molecules in their β-cells do not develop autoimmunity, although excess production of class II molecules (or other molecules) leads to cell death. In particular, studies of transgenic animals with β-cell expression of class II molecules have shown that this leads to T-cell tolerance rather than to autoimmunity.[23]

Many of the alleles of genes in the major histocompatibility complex are nonrandomly associated. Such nonrandom association of alleles (linkage disequilibrium) of different genes on the same chromosome defines a complete histocompatibility haplotype, which, except for rare crossing-over events (1/100), are inherited as a group. For example, one diabetes-associated haplotype consists of alleles A1, B8, DR3, DQβw2 and a deletion of the C4 complement gene (C4A null).[24] For this haplotype it is not yet certain which gene is responsible for the association of the haplotype with diabetes, and it is likely that the major pathogenic gene of this haplotype has not yet been identified.

Haplotypes that are typed as DR4 by classic serologic methods (typing primarily for the DRβ1 locus) have one of several DQβ gene sequences. In the past the two major sequences were termed DQ3.2 and DQ3.1 (associated with DQw8 and DQw7), and by World Health Organization (WHO) criteria are now called DQB1*0301 and DQB1*0302.[25] The sequences of the two DQβ genes of these alleles differ from each other in four amino acids of the terminal polymorphic portion of the DQβ chain. It is particularly informative that the DQB1*0302 sequence is the gene most associated with Type I diabetes and that the DQB1*0301 sequence appears to increase diabetes risk in only a subset of the white population (Table 13–3). Analysis of such specific DQβ sequences led to the hypothesis that a single amino acid difference at position 57 (namely, lack of aspartic acid) of the DQβ chain would suffice to explain diabetogenicity of HLA haplotypes.[26] For example, both the DQw8 sequence and the DR3 diabetes-associated DQw2 (DQB1*0602) sequence lack an aspartic acid at position 57 and have an alanine at this residue, whereas DQw7 and the protective DQ1.2 (DQB1*0602) of DR2-bearing haplotypes have aspartic acid at position 57 (Table 13–3). This hypothesis is important for calling attention to DQβ sequences, but in its simplest form has not been confirmed. For instance, several diabetes-associated haplotypes have aspartic acid at position 57 of their DQβ chain, such as the DR4-associated DQw4 of Japanese and the Japanese

Table 13–3. Relative Risks Associated with Common HLA-DQ Alleles

	Relative Risk Associated With Allele*				
	DQw1.2 (DQB1*0602) (+)	DQw7 (DQB1*0301) (+)	DQw1.1 (DQB1*0501) (−)	DQw2 (DQB1*0201) (−)	DQw8 (DQB1*0302) (−)
DQw1.2(+) (DQB1*0602)	0.01	0.29	0.09	0.04	0.37
DQw7(+) (DQB1*0301)	...	0.18	1.05	1.10	2.12
DQw1.1(−) (DQB1*0501)	...	...	0.17	1.11	4.29
DQw2(−) (DQB1*0201)	...	...	...	1.35	5.99
DQw8(−) (DQB1*0302)	...	...	...	...	5.62

Table is adapted from Baisch et al.[28]
*The relative risk of the haplotype is given for the combination of DQ haplotypes of each sixth chromosome. The (+) indicates aspartic acid is at position 57 of DQB1 allele; (−) indicates aspartic acid is not at this position. The current WHO terminology for DQB gene sequences is given in parentheses. DQ2w1.2 is associated with DR2. DQw7 and DQw8 are both associated with DR4; DQw2 is associated with DR3; and DQw1.1 is associated with DR1.

DR9 DQw9 allele, which only differs from DQw8 by having aspartic acid at position 57.[26]

Both DQβ and DQα chains combine to form class II immune-response genes, and it appears that multiple amino acid substitutions of both the α and β chains will affect diabetes susceptibility. In fact, for certain haplotypes it is also likely that both DQ and DR molecules influence diabetes susceptibility and that these class II genes are not the only genes of the major histocompatibility complex influencing susceptibility.[27] For instance, the DR3 association with diabetes is not yet explainable by any combination of class II immune response genes (DR7 haplotypes and DR3 have an identical DQβ sequence, but only DR3 haplotypes are diabetogenic). In addition to a permissive class II gene in the DR3 haplotype, the extensive deletions (e.g., complement C4A gene is deleted) found in this haplotype may contribute to diabetes susceptibility.

Not only are there class II genes associated with diabetes susceptibility, there also are haplotypes that confer protection from Type I diabetes. For example, haplotypes bearing DR2 alleles usually protect from diabetes independently of whether the other HLA haplotype contains a high-risk allele (Table 13–3).[28] DR2 haplotypes, like DR4 haplotypes, can be subdivided by sequencing the DQβ alleles associated with them. A rare DR2 haplotype, differing at both DRβ and DQβ from common DR2 haplotypes at both and relatively common on the island of Sardinia, is associated with Type I diabetes.[29] Further evidence that the DQβ alleles and not, for instance, DRβ specifically determine diabetes resistance of DR2 haplotypes comes from the sequencing of DQ and DR genes of a unique family in which three siblings developed Type I diabetes. All three were HLA identical and DR2/DR1. In these three diabetic brothers, the class II gene differed only at DQβ and DQα (the two genes coding for the DQ molecule) from the usual protective DR2 haplotype and were identical at DRβ1 to the usual protective DR2 haplotype ("protective" DR2 haplotype DQB1*0602, DQA*0102, DRB1*1501, families "diabetogenic" DR2 haplotype DQB1*0402, DQA*0402, DRB1*1501). Their DQβ gene differs from all DR2 haplotypes studied to date[30] and, though associated with Type I diabetes, has an aspartic acid at position 57. The findings in this family again suggest that the total sequence of the DQ molecule, and not simply the presence or absence of aspartic acid at position 57, determines susceptibility.

Given the advances in understanding of basic immunology and the sequencing of multiple class II genes associated with diabetes, what is the current status of genetic prediction of Type I diabetes? Direct DNA sequencing of histocompatibility alleles is now possible and relatively simple. Application of a recently developed technique to amplify segments of DNA, termed the *polymerase chain reaction* (PCR), coupled with oligonucleotides specific for histocompatibility gene sequences, now allow rapid determination of class II alleles.[31] Thousands of individuals could be rapidly screened for diabetes-associated alleles with the use of

DNA derived, for instance, from buccal smears. For DR4- and DR2-bearing haplotypes, it is most likely that class II, DQβ chain gene polymorphisms underlie diabetes susceptibility or protection. For the DR3 haplotype, the responsible gene is unknown; we believe that finer mapping of this haplotype, with characterization of deletions, will lead to the discovery of genetic deletions associated with autoimmunity. With current genetic knowledge, it is possible to identify individuals in the general population who have a risk of developing Type I diabetes similar to that of first-degree relatives of patients with Type I diabetes. In particular, individuals in the general population homozygous for DQw8, or heterozygous for DR4/DR3 (DQw8/DQw2), have a calculated risk of developing Type I diabetes of 6%. Such individuals comprise approximately 3% of the general population but make up 40% of whites who develop Type I diabetes! In addition within families, risk of Type I diabetes correlates with the sharing of haplotype with the proband and DR, DQ subtypes. A sibling who is HLA-identical to a diabetic DR3/DR4 sibling has a risk of developing diabetes of approximately 1 in 5, whereas an HLA-nonidentical sibling has a risk of 1 in 100 vs. a risk of 1 in 300 for the general population.[11] In that a DR3/DR4 identical twin has a risk of diabetes of approximately 70%, it is likely that unknown genes outside of the major histocompatibility complex contribute to diabetes.

There are important syndromes associated with Type I diabetes that suggest genetic heterogeneity. Probably the most important from a clinical standpoint are the polyendocrine autoimmune syndromes type I[32] and type II.[33,34] Some of the characteristics of these disorders, including disease associations, are listed in Table 13–4. Approximately 5% of patients with the polyendocrine syndrome type I are reported to develop Type I diabetes (these individuals typically have mucocutaneous candidiasis, hypoparathyroidism, and/or Addison's disease).[32] It is likely that the type I syndrome results from the inheritance of an immunodeficiency gene, with attendant abnormal immunoregulation as evidenced by the presence of mucocutaneous candidiasis. The contribution of

Table 13–4. Polyendocrine Autoimmune Syndromes

Type I	Type II
No HLA association	HLA DR3 and DR4
Autosomal recessive	Autosomal dominant
Mucocutaneous candidiasis	…
Hypoparathyroidism	…
Addison's disease	Addison's disease
Graves disease	Graves disease
Thyroiditis	Thyroiditis
Type I diabetes (5%)	Type I diabetes (50%)
Vitiligo	Vitiligo
Hepatitis	…
Malabsorption	Celiac disease
…	Myasthenia gravis
Pernicious anemia	Pernicious anemia
…	Serositis
…	Parkinson's disease

this to diabetes susceptibility is conceptually similar to the BB rat model of Type I diabetes, with its autosomal recessive T-cell immunodeficiency gene.

The type II polyendocrine syndrome is termed Schmidt's syndrome. Although both patients with type I and type II syndrome have Addison's disease, only the type II syndrome is associated with HLA alleles DR3 and DR4.[33] Components of this syndrome appear to be inherited in an autosomal dominant manner, and approximately 50% of patients with this syndrome develop Type I diabetes. Approximately 10% of individuals who develop Type I diabetes have associated autoimmune disorders. Autoimmune thyroid disease, in particular, is so common (Graves disease or thyroiditis) that routine evaluation of thyroid function is recommended for patients with Type I diabetes. In addition, all first-degree relatives of patients with polyendocrine autoimmunity should be evaluated periodically for thyroid function.[34] Evaluation for Addison's disease with cosyntropin stimulation and cortisol determinations should be considered in patients with Type I diabetes with dramatically decreasing insulin requirements or other signs or symptoms of Addison's disease and in relatives of patients with Addison's disease. Wolfram's syndrome (DIDMOAD) is an autosomal recessive disorder with selected β-cell loss and a series of neuronal deficits.[8] Maturity-onset diabetes of youth (MODY) appears to be a heterogenous group of diabetes syndromes of early onset, usually non-insulin-dependent, and of increased frequency in individuals from India and in black Americans.[35,36] Neither Wolfram's syndrome or MODY are associated with DR3, DR4 or anti-islet autoantibodies.

ENVIRONMENT

Even though considerable advances have been made in our understanding of the genetic predisposition to Type I diabetes, worldwide regional differences in its incidence and the discordance between monozygotic twins suggest a potential role for environmental factors in initiating autoimmune β-cell destruction. In addition, temporal increases in the incidence of Type I diabetes have been described in several countries outside of North America (the incidence of Type I diabetes in North America has not changed in the last two decades[37]). If these studies in several European countries are truly reflective of an increase in the incidence of diabetes of approximately 3% per year (rather than ascertainment bias, genetic drift, or dramatic changes in gene pool resulting from decreasing genetic isolation of communities since World War II), such an increase would not be explainable by a change in gene frequency (too rapid) resulting from the improved survival rate of persons with diabetes. These incidence figures would suggest that something that affects diabetes incidence has either been introduced or removed from the environment.

Viruses

There is evidence that viruses may play a role in the pathogenesis of Type I diabetes. The evidence for virus-induced diabetes comes largely from experiments in animals,[38] but several studies in humans also point to viruses as a potential trigger of the disease. There are three theories as to how viruses might influence diabetes incidence: through direct β-cell cytotoxicity, by triggering autoimmunity to islets by the infection of β-cells or lymphocytes, and by preventing diabetes by effects on the immune system. It was initially proposed that viral infections might cause acute β-cell damage resulting in diabetes. This idea is supported by several case reports and epidemiologic studies that show a high frequency of coxsackievirus B-specific IgM responses at diabetes onset,[39] β-cell damage in children with overwhelming infections with coxsackievirus B,[40] and the isolation of viruses from patients with acute-onset diabetes and the demonstration that these isolated viruses induced diabetes in mice.[41] However, there is now evidence that autoimmunity directed at islets is present long before the clinical onset of diabetes. Therefore, if viruses are involved in pathogenesis, the possibility must be considered that either acute or persistent viral infection could trigger the autoimmune process and render the target cell vulnerable to autoimmune attack without necessarily causing acute cell damage. In humans, the congenital rubella syndrome provides some of the best evidence that viral infection can be associated with subsequent development of Type I diabetes.[42] Approximately 20% of individuals who have had congenital rubella infection, but not those who have had postnatal rubella infection, develop Type I diabetes. Those developing diabetes have high-risk HLA alleles DR3 or DR4. The congenital infection is associated with persistent T-cell abnormalities and thyroid autoimmunity, developments that suggest widespread immunologic abnormalities. Karounos and Thomas have described a monoclonal antibody that reacts with a rubella protein and a 52-kd islet protein.[43] In addition to the congenital rubella syndrome, there is a case-report of a child with congenital cytomegalovirus (CMV) infection who became diabetic at the age of 13 months.[44]

It was recently reported that persistent CMV infections may be relevant to pathogenesis in some cases of Type I diabetes. Pak and co-workers reported that the CMV-specific viral genome was found in 22% of diabetic subjects but in only 2.6% of controls.[45] In a group of multiple-case families tested for the presence of CMV gene segments in lymphocyte DNA, 26% of those with diabetes were CMV-positive, as were 17% of their first-degree relatives. The prevalence of positivity for the CMV genome was thus not significantly greater among those with diabetes than among relatives without diabetes, decreasing the likelihood of a pathogenic role for CMV.

The best experimental evidence indicating that viruses may have an etiologic role in the pathogenesis of Type I diabetes comes from studies of mice infected with different virus strains. Injection of nondiabetic SJL/J mice with a highly diabetogenic encephalomyocarditis (EMC-D) virus results in the development of diabetes in 95% of the animals.[46] In contrast, EMC-B virus does not cause disease. Recently, it has been possible to determine differences in nucleotide sequences of the EMC-B and

EMC-D viruses. It was found that the two viruses differ by only 14 of 7829 nucleotides; therefore, a maximum of 14 nucleotides may be critical in determining the diabetogenicity of the EMC virus.[47] In addition, diabetogenic strains of coxsackievirus B4 (CB4) produce a syndrome in mice resembling Type I diabetes in humans. CB4 infection increases the expression of the 64-kd antigen.[48] Guberski et al. recently reported that infection with Kilham's rat virus induces diabetes in the nonlymphopenic BB-related DR rat strain.[49]

Retrovirus-like particles have been detected in pancreatic islet β-cells of NOD mice.[50] Ciampolillo and co-workers have reported retrovirus-like sequences in patients with Graves disease.[51] DNA extracted from thyroid glands of five patients with Graves disease gave a positive signal for the human immunodeficiency virus (HIV-1), suggesting that the presence of retrovirus-like sequences may be associated with thyroid autoimmunity, but apparently this finding was not confirmed and was the result of a laboratory artefact.

In addition to the attention given viruses as potential triggers of Type I diabetes, there is interest in viruses that can prevent diabetes. Whether viruses can induce selective immunosuppression in an autoimmune disorder was tested by Oldstone in a study of NOD mice.[52] NOD mice usually develop autoimmune IDDM by 6 months of age, with an incidence of ~80% in females by 9 to 12 months of age. Newborn or adult NOD mice infected with a lymphocytic choriomeningitis virus (LCMV), which primarily affects T helper cells, did not develop diabetes. In addition, lymphocytes from infected donor animals failed to transfer disease, as did lymphocytes from age- and sex-matched uninfected donors. Furthermore, lactate dehydrogenase virus (LDV) was shown to suppress the development of diabetes in NOD mice.[53] LDV is believed to bind to I-A and replicate in macrophages, hence presumably interfering with antigen processing. The manner by which infection prevents diabetes is not fully characterized, and it is noteworthy that a single injection of Freund's adjuvant (extract of tuberculous bacilli) will prevent diabetes in NOD mice.

Other Environmental Factors

Various dietary changes have also been shown to alter the incidence of diabetes in both the NOD mouse and the BB rat.[54,55] Replacing proteins with amino acids in the diets of NOD mice decreases the incidence of diabetes. Two recent studies reported a reduced risk of Type I diabetes among children who had been breast fed to an older age,[56,57] suggesting that unknown external factors such as sanitation may play a role in disease susceptibility. Bovine serum albumin has been implicated as a potential triggering factor because of the presence of antibodies to albumin.[58]

It has been reported that the risk for Type I diabetes appears to correlate with average yearly temperature, distance from the equator, and ethnicity of the population at risk.[59] What causes the north to south geographic differences in the distribution of Type I diabetes remains unknown, although it may reflect genetic differences in

populations similar to the postulated influence of settlement patterns on multiple sclerosis. (The higher incidence of diabetes in Sardinia is an important exception to the North/South gradient.) Ziegler and co-workers have evaluated skin pigmentation type and reactivity to ultraviolet (UV) light in association with susceptibility to Type I diabetes.[60] In a study in southern Germany, significantly more Type I diabetic patients than nondiabetic controls exhibited light eye color, fair skin type, and increased sensitivity. This may reflect a direct influence of UV irradiation on systemic immunity or may be secondary to linkage of genes determining skin color or eye color and diabetes.

PRECLINICAL NATURAL HISTORY AND DIAGNOSIS

In the mid-1970s and early 1980s, islet cell autoantibodies (ICA), insulin autoantibodies (IAA), and a 64-kd protein were found to be present in the serum of the majority of patients with Type I diabetes at the time of diagnosis. Subsequently, a number of studies demonstrated that the presence of these antibodies in serum can be used to identify subjects at increased risk of developing Type I diabetes.

This section will summarize the studies of the "preclinical" phase of Type I diabetes that have been performed to date, with special emphasis on the assays used and their predictive power.

The following autoantibodies have been reported in Type I diabetes: cytoplasmic islet cells autoantibodies; insulin autoantibodies; antibodies to glutamic acid decarboxylase (GAD, the 64-kd protein); islet cell surface autoantibodies; and carboxypeptidase H autoantibodies.

Assays Used in Preclinical Studies

Islet Cell Antibodies

Assay Method and Standardization. Assay of ICA by indirect immunofluorescence using frozen human pancreas sections was first described by Bottazzo et al.[61] and MacCuish et al.[62] A number of modifications to the original technique have since been suggested. These modifications involved the use of pancreas from different species and fixation of the substrate pancreas, different incubation times (30 minutes to 24 hours), and different detecting reagents (anti-IgG or protein A conjugated with either fluorescein or peroxidase). These modifications resulted in dramatic variations in both sensitivity and specificity of many different ICA assays. With the increased use of ICA in predictive studies, the Juvenile Diabetes Foundation International sponsored a series of workshops of the Immunology of Diabetes Workshop Committee to standardize the measurement of cytoplasmic ICA. In the first workshop, striking variation in the results of different laboratories was observed, even between apparently identical methods.[63] Subsequently, the second and third workshops[64,65] addressed issues of precision, specificity, and threshold of detection of individual assays. The availability of a standard serum has allowed the reporting of results in standard units (JDF units) based on end-point titrations relative to the standard sera. Thus, measurement of ICA is now standardized to the extent that reports can be issued in JDF units. This has allowed the predictive power of a positive test to be addressed.

ICA assays vary in both sensitivity and specificity. Some assays can reliably detect levels of ICA as low as 2.5 JDF units. Most of these sensitive assays employ a prolonged incubation period with serum, as initially described by Pilcher and Elliott.[66] Although these assays are more sensitive, they may have a lower specificity than the less-sensitive assays. Indeed low-titer ICA have been reported to disappear in many individuals,[67] although some relatives of persons with diabetes with low-titer antibody have progressed to diabetes. Another group of assays have lower sensitivity but higher specificity. These assays include the Joslin Diabetes Center assay,[68] which uses protein A as detecting reagent, and the Barts-Windsor study complement-fixation assay,[69] which uses fluorescinated anticomplement as detecting reagent. Both of these assays have a low sensitivity but a high specificity. Most subjects with such antibodies eventually progress to diabetes. Thus, in assessing the significance of a positive ICA result, it is necessary to consider both the level of antibody and the type of assay used. Furthermore, we have recently found a subset of high-titer ICA that appears not to predict diabetes. These "restricted" or class II antibodies react with human and rat islets but not with mouse islets and are β-cell-specific in contrast to "nonrestricted" class I ICA antibodies, which react with human, rat, and mouse islets[70] and with β- and non-β-cells within the islets. Restricted ICA are autoantibodies that react only with GAD, the 64-kd protein.[71]

A major question that has been raised is whether ICA titers can fluctuate. Early studies suggested that the observed fluctuations were purely an artefact of an imperfect assay system. However, in a recent report, ICA levels were determined for sera of nearly all children who developed diabetes in Sweden during 1 year (389 of 405 were positive) and from 321 controls matched for age, sex, and geographic location.[72] ICA were detected in 9 (3%) of 321 of control children (range, 17 to 1200 JDF units). Subsequently, two of these ICA-positive children developed diabetes, but, more important, the remaining seven all became ICA-negative, and during 20 to 34 months of observation, the fasting blood glucose, glycosylated hemoglobin, and C-peptide levels of these children remained normal. Most of the children who became ICA-negative had ICA levels that were initially lower than 40 JDF units (concordant with a large body of literature indicating that low-titer ICA lack prognostic significance), but one subject had a high ICA level of 470 JDF units. In general, high-titer ICA of greater than 80 JDF units uncommonly fluctuate outside the interassay coefficient of the ICA assay, while low-titer antibodies frequently are negative on repeat evaluation. The accurate quantitation of ICA fluctuation will probably depend on development of a biochemical assay.

All ICA assays are complicated by subjectivity in reading and are cumbersome to use for assaying large numbers of samples. Any laboratory measuring ICA should participate in a proficiency program such as that sponsored by the IDW (Immunology of Diabetes Workshop) and report results in JDF units. There is a critical need for simplification of the ICA assay to a stage at which it can easily be used to test large populations. To this end, many groups are endeavoring to isolate the target antigen of ICA.

It is likely the target antigen for ICA consists of several antigens (e.g., restricted vs. nonrestricted ICA), and a subset of ICA is probably a charged glycolipid (e.g., a ganglioside). Initial biochemical studies suggested that the target of ICA had the biochemical characteristics of a sialic acid-containing lipid, possibly a ganglioside.[73] These studies were extended by the finding that lipid extracts of human pancreas could block the binding of ICA-containing serum to pancreas sections.[74] More-recent studies have identified islet-specific gangliosides.[75] Early studies also suggest that these gangliosides are regulated by the metabolic state of the animal. However, to date it has not been possible to show directly that ICA bind to these molecules. Thus, purified antigen permitting the development of an easily automated assay for ICA is not available, and at this stage the gold-standard assay remains the cumbersome indirect immunofluorescence assay described 16 years ago. In addition, as briefly discussed above (restricted vs. nonrestricted ICA), it is clear that ICA reactivity is due to heterogeneous antibodies. In particular, any antibody reacting more with islet antigens of frozen sections then with acinar tissue will give a positive reading. For example, high-titer GAD antibodies from patients with stiff-man syndrome can give β-cell-specific staining (restricted pattern).

Insulin Autoantibodies

While the development of IAA following insulin therapy is well known to all diabetologists, the finding of IAA in the serum of patients with Type I diabetes before they are first given insulin was first reported by Palmer and colleagues in 1983.[76] Subsequently, a number of groups replicated these findings and also demonstrated the presence of IAA during the "prediabetic" phase of Type I diabetes. To date, these antibodies are the only antibodies whose levels correlate with the rate of progression to diabetes and the age (Fig. 13–3) at which Type I diabetes develops (the younger the age at which diabetes develops and/or the faster the progression to diabetes, the higher the level of IAA).

Assay Method and Standardization. As with ICA, several different assays have been used to measure IAA. The two major assay formats used are radiobinding and enzyme-linked immunosorbent assays (ELISA). Radiobinding assays compare the ability of serum to bind ^{125}I-labeled insulin in the presence and absence of excess unlabeled insulin. The difference in amount of labeled insulin bound in the presence and absence of unlabeled insulin is used to calculate the insulin-binding activity of the sample. In the ELISA, insulin attached to plastic wells is allowed to react with serum. After an incubation period, the amount of antibody bound to the wells is

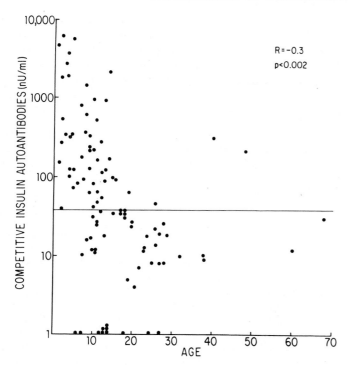

Fig. 13–3. Age of onset of Type I diabetes vs. level of insulin autoantibodies. The y axis is on a log scale, showing extremely high levels of insulin autoantibodies in children who develop diabetes before the age of 5 years. Reprinted with permission from reference 77 (Ziegler AG, Herskowitz RD, Jackson RA, et al. Predicting type I diabetes. Diabetes Care 1990;13:762–75; copyright © 1990 by the American Diabetes Association, Inc.)

determined with methods using anti-antibody detection.

As with ICA, four international workshops have now addressed the standardization of IAA measurement. The first, second, and third workshops suggested strongly that fluid-phase and solid-phase antibody detection assays give discordant results for many sera.[78] In the fourth workshop (Jerusalem, 1990), the disease association of IAA as determined by radiobinding vs. that by ELISA was ascertained. In sera from patients with newly diagnosed Type I diabetes, the radiobinding assays showed dramatically higher specific signals than did those obtained by ELISA (none of the ELISAs detected a positive [exceeding control signals] in new-onset diabetic patients or high-risk relatives). Because of the higher specific signal and the concomitantly higher rate of positivity in patient sera, it was concluded that fluid-phase assays were superior to current solid-phase assays for identifying disease-associated IAA. In the near future efforts will be made to make the IAA results from different laboratories more comparable, possibly by the use of a standard serum.

IAA measured by fluid-phase radiobinding assays have been reported to be associated with ICA results and also to be predictive for later development of Type I diabetes.[78–82] Although differences in the magnitude of the results of several fluid-phase assays occurred in the early IAA workshops, it now appears that these assays can identify a uniform antibody group.

Target Epitopes. Although the exact target-antigen sequence of IAA on the insulin molecule is not known, studies using insulins from different species that compared the binding of IAA from prediabetic individuals suggest that a very limited region of the insulin molecule is a major determinant of binding (B1–3, A11–13).[83] In fact these antibodies bind equally strongly to proinsulin. The region of binding seems similar in all the prediabetic individuals studied to date at the Joslin Diabetes Center.

Autoantibodies to Glutamic Acid Decarboxylase (64-kd Protein)

Antibodies to a 64-kd protein were first described in 1982 by Baekkeskov and colleagues.[84] Subsequently, the same group of investigators showed that these antibodies can also be present in serum several years before the clinical onset of diabetes.[85] Studies by another group have suggested that antibodies to the 64-kd antigen are more consistently associated with the outcome of diabetes in "prediabetic" subjects than are ICA or IAA alone.[86,87] Unfortunately, the assay for antibodies to the 64-kd antigen is cumbersome, and to date the number of reported studies have been too few to allow the full potential of these antibodies to be clarified. At present, the assay requires the purification of large numbers of islets, labeling with [^{35}S]methionine, detergent solubilization and a phase partition step, and finally separation by sodium dodecyl sulfate-polyacrylamide gel electrophoresis (SDS-PAGE) or two-dimensional gels.

Currently, the major problem preventing more generalized use of this assay is the need for purified islets. This problem will almost certainly be circumvented within the next year. DeCamilli and co-workers, following their studies of the rare stiff-man syndrome, in which antibodies to the enzyme GAD are present,[86] made the surprising discovery that the 64-kd antigen is GAD.[86] This enzyme, which produces the neurotransmitter γ-aminobutyric acid (GABA), is found in neurons of the central nervous system and in β-cells of islets. The molecule is located within the cytoplasm of islets; thus, antibodies to GAD may be secondary to β-cell destruction rather than etiologic.

Insulin Receptor Antibodies

Antibodies to insulin receptor have been found in a number of patients with acanthosis and insulin-resistant diabetes.[88] In 1983, Maron and co-workers described antibodies that reacted with the insulin receptor in patients with newly diagnosed Type I diabetes.[89] In a study using a lipogenesis assay, they found IgM insulin receptor antibodies were found in the sera of 10 of 22 patients with Type I diabetes before their treatment with exogenous insulin and in none of 20 healthy volunteer blood donors. Several other studies using assays of the inhibition of insulin binding to insulin receptor-positive cells have shown a similar incidence of positivity for insulin receptor antibodies in patients with newly diagnosed Type I diabetes patients before institution of insulin therapy.[90,91] Nevertheless, direct biochemical evidence (e.g., precipitation of labeled purified insulin receptors) is lacking, and it has not been clarified whether the described antibodies actually react with the insulin receptor.

Islet Cell Surface Antibodies

Antibodies to the islet cell surface were initially described by Lernmark and colleagues in 1978.[92] Subsequent studies suggested these antibodies were both specific and weakly cytotoxic for β-cells.[90] Few reports characterizing these antibodies have emerged over the past decade, and studies are lacking in large control and diabetes-related populations. It is thus difficult to make a judgment as to whether the use of assays for islet cell surface antibodies is useful in identifying subjects at risk of developing diabetes. Against the use of such assays is a high false-positive rate in first-degree relatives of patients with Type I diabetes. Furthermore, this assay requires large numbers of purified islet cells. To date there is no general agreement as to the most suitable cellular substrate to use for the assays, although assays using human and animal pancreatic islets and various β-cell lines have been reported.[93]

Carboxypeptidase H

In a recent study, serum from a prediabetic subject was used to screen an islet λgt11 expression library in which islet genes are expressed by bacterial colonies. A positive colony was obtained and sequenced and identified to be a 136-amino acid fragment of carboxypeptidase H.[94] Approximately 30% of prediabetic subjects express antibodies to this islet granule enzyme involved in proinsulin. The use of expression libraries to identify more autoantigens will certainly lead to the identification of additional target molecules. As the list of islet autoantigens associated with Type I diabetes grows,[94] it is likely that the prediction of diabetes will improve. Different prediabetic subjects express different autoantibodies, often in stable patterns; thus, a series of assays will likely be combined to increase specificity and sensitivity of detecting prediabetics.

DIAGNOSIS OF "PREDIABETES"

Twin Studies

Several studies of sets of identical twins and triplets initially discordant for Type I diabetes have been reported. Johnston et al. pioneered the distinction between Type I and Type II diabetes by defining concordance among identical twins, with a higher concordance for Type I diabetes.[95] Monozygotic twins initially discordant for Type I diabetes at the Joslin Clinic were followed with metabolic testing, and their sera were tested for ICA with up to a 21-year follow-up period.[96,97] Diabetes developed in four twins during this period, and in three of these four twins, antibodies to islet cells preceded the diagnosis by more than 8, 5, and 7 years, respectively. During the prediabetic phase, the presence of ICA was temporally associated with a decline in first-phase insulin secretion as measured by the intravenous glucose tolerance test.

Thus, a prolonged prediabetic phase of β-cell dysfunction with associated immunologic dysfunction was observed. As we will review, these observations were subsequently extended to first-degree relatives of patients with Type I diabetes patients and to the general population. It is now agreed that the majority of cases of Type I diabetes are preceded by a long prediabetic phase, with active β-cell destruction rather than a long "latency period" preceding acute destruction. Data from several of the largest prediabetes screening studies will be summarized.

The Joslin-Sacramento Study

Since the beginning of the Joslin-Sacramento study in 1983, well over 8000 first-degree relatives have been tested either for ICA alone or for both ICA and IAA (with a fluid-phase radioimmunoassay). In the initial report of the study, the prevalence of ICA positivity in relatives was 0.9% (16/1723).[97] ICA were detected with use of a low-sensitivity assay, so all those who were identified as ICA-positive had levels of at least 40 JDF units. Over a maximal follow-up period of 2 years, Type I diabetes developed in 2 of 16 relatives with ICA and in 1 of 1707 without ICA.[97] Currently, more than 23 antibody-positive relatives have been followed to the development of diabetes.[77] Approximately, 10% of ICA-positive (>40 JDF units consistently present) relatives progress to overt diabetes per year.

Recently, data on the prevalence and predictive value of IAA in this group have been published.[77] Serum samples from 1670 relatives (628 offspring, 689 siblings, 353 parents) who were ICA-negative and from 42 relatives (11 offspring, 25 siblings, 6 parents), who were ICA-positive were assayed for IAA with use of a fluid-phase radiobinding assay. The prevalence of IAA exceeding the normal range was 2.7% (45/1670) among ICA-negative (i.e., <20 JDF units) subjects (20 offspring, 22 siblings, 3 parents) and 45% (19/42) among ICA-positive relatives. After 2 years of follow-up, diabetes had developed in 4 (9%) of 45 of the ICA-negative/IAA-positive relatives, 5 (22%) of 23 ICA-positive/IAA-negative relatives, and 12 (63%) 19 ICA-positive/IAA-positive relatives. Two (0.1%) of 1625 relatives who were negative for both ICA and IAA developed diabetes. By life-table analysis the predicted risk for progression to diabetes after 5 years of follow-up is 17% for IAA-positive/ICA-negative relatives, 42% for IAA-negative/ICA-positive relatives, and 77% for IAA-positive/ICA-positive relatives.

The Joslin-Sacramento twin and family studies have led to the use of the intravenous glucose tolerance test (IVGTT) in the assessment of ICA-positive subjects.[77,96–100] In the IVGTT, the sum of the insulin levels at 1 and 3 minutes after an intravenous bolus of glucose (0.5 g/kg body weight) is used as a measure of first-phase insulin secretion. Table 13–5 lists a consensus for IVGTT testing of a committee (ICARUS) establishing an international data base for prediction of diabetes. To date in our studies more than 20 relatives have had one or more IVGTTs before the development of overt diabetes, with some relatives having had more than 20 IVGTTs before overt diabetes.[100] In ICA-positive relatives with first-

Table 13–5. Protocol for Intravenous Glucose Tolerance Test

PREPARATION: As recommended by the National Diabetes Data Group for oral glucose tolerance test, i.e., 3 days of unrestricted diet (containing at least 150 g carbohydrate) and normal physical activity. Unusual physical exertion should be avoided for 1 day prior to test. Test should be deferred if subject has intercurrent illness.
FAST: At least 10 hours but not more than 16 hours. Water permitted but subject should not smoke.
TIME OF START OF TEST (GLUCOSE INFUSION): 0730–1000
GLUCOSE DOSE: 0.5 g/kg up to 35 g maximum
GLUCOSE CONCENTRATION INFUSED: 25%
DILUENT: Normal saline
INFUSION: Manual or pump-driven syringe, timed to ensure steady rate of infusion
DURATION OF INFUSION: 3 min ± 15 sec
TIME ZERO: End of infusion
MINIMUM NUMBER OF SAMPLES TO BE COLLECTED: 2 baseline samples, +1, +3, +5, +10 min
CANNULA: A single forearm vein cannula may be used but should be flushed with saline after glucose infused. Dead space should be cleared before samples drawn.

Table is modified from Bingley et al.[101] on behalf of the ICARUS group.

phase insulin secretion below the first percentile of normal values, the relative risk of progression to overt diabetes was 41 compared with the risk for antibody-positive relatives with IVGTT values greater than 48 μU/mL (sum of 1- plus 3-minute insulin level after glucose infusion). In some relatives, the profound loss of insulin secretion preceded diabetes by up to 4 years. A subset of individuals, particularly children, progressed rapidly to overt diabetes, and in these individuals the loss of first-phase insulin secretion was occasionally not observed with tests up to 6 months before onset of overt diabetes. In addition, in some children the conversion from an IVGTT response in the normal range to a markedly abnormal IVGTT response occurred within months.

Smith and colleagues[102] have determined the within- and between-subject variation for the first-phase response in normal subjects. The sum of 1- plus 3-minute insulin values showed a coefficient of variation of 72% between subjects and of 36% within subjects, leading the authors to advise "appropriate restraint" in the interpretation of these tests. In a further study the same group showed relatively small (compared with the intersubject variation) increases in basal and stimulated insulin responses throughout puberty (associated with an increase in insulin resistance), a decline following puberty until the third decade, and thereafter a constant insulin release.[103] Studies at the Joslin Diabetes Center do not confirm a pubertal increase of IVGTT results among antibody-positive relatives. Although a pubertal rise was not observed in autoantibody-positive or autoantibody-negative relatives, on average the IVGTT responses of relatives younger than 6 years were approximately one-half of those of relatives older than 6 years, with no consistent change thereafter to ages as old as 80 years. Some of these differences between IVGTT results may be related to the use of different protocols; thus, the adoption of a standard ICARUS protocol is recommended (pending studies

indicating whether a modified technique would improve either the coefficient of variation for normal subjects on repeat measurements (~36%) or the prediction of diabetes onset). The variation of IVGTT response is primarily a problem when insulin secretion is in the normal range. Thus changes of 1- plus 3-minute insulin secretion within the normal range (>5th percentile) cannot be interpreted as disease progression.[100]

In addition to changes in insulin secretion on IVGTT, it is evident that during a variable period (as long as 1 to 2 years before the diagnosis of diabetes) blood glucose levels rise gradually. In our studies some individuals had as many as 40 determinations of fasting blood glucose levels before the development of diabetes.[100] For all relatives studied to date, fasting blood glucose levels remained stable until approximately 1.5 years before the development of overt diabetes. For most, but not all prediabetic subjects, a progressive intermittent subclinical rise in fasting blood glucose level during the last 1.5 years was seen.[104] When fasting glucose levels greater than 6 mmol/L (108 mg/dL) were observed, diabetes occurred within 1 year. This experience confirms that seen in the Barts-Windsor study.

The level of insulin autoantibodies and first-phase insulin secretion (Fig. 13–4) are major determinants of the time to development of diabetes. In ICA-positive relatives, the initial IVGTT results divided by the IAA level was strongly correlated with the time to development of diabetes. These findings have led to a dual-parameter model for the prediction of time to diabetes.[105] This model is being used as entry criteria for the

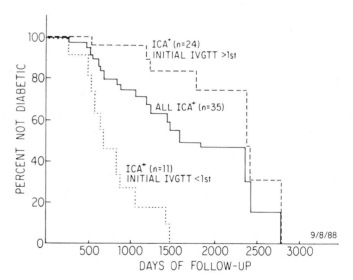

Fig. 13–4. Life-table analysis of progression to diabetes in islet cell antibody (ICA)-positive relatives subdivided according to whether their initial 1- plus 3-minute insulin value following intravenous glucose tolerance testing was below or above the first percentile (<48 and >48 μU/mL, respectively). Reprinted with permission from reference 100 (Vardi P, Crisa L, Jackson RA, et al. Predictive value of intravenous glucose tolerance test insulin secretion less than or greater than the first percentile in islet cell antibody positive relatives of type I (insulin-dependent) diabetic patients. Diabetologia 1991;34:93–102).

selection of subjects for intervention trials aimed at preventing Type I diabetes. The model appears particularly useful for distinguishing ICA-positive (>40 JDF units) relatives who will develop diabetes within 3 years (diabetes in >90% within 3 years) vs. those who will not (diabetes in <10%). For example, no ICA-positive relative studied who had an initial IVGTT (1- plus 3-minute insulin level) greater than 48 μU/mL and who lacked IAA has developed diabetes in less than 7 years. Among ICA-positive relatives with an IVGTT greater than 48 μU/mL but positive for IAA, approximately one-third have progressed to diabetes. The influence of level of IAA on progression to overt diabetes is independent of age (e.g., no ICA-positive child younger than 5 years old lacking IAA has yet progressed to diabetes with up to 3 years of follow-up).

It is likely that the dual-parameter model does not distinguish individuals who will develop diabetes in 5 years vs. those who will develop it in 10 or more years. Random fluctuations of the insulin secretion on IVGTT when it is the normal range limit the ability to predict time to diabetes. For example, we have now followed many ICA-positive relatives (usually lacking IAA) who have had more than 5 years of stable first-phase insulin secretion. As will be discussed later, a significant proportion of these relatives have the restricted pattern of ICA. Thus, the major utility of the model is in defining relatives who have a high risk vs. those who have a low risk of developing diabetes over the next 3 years. We currently have evaluated approximately 250 IVGTTs in ICA-positive relatives No relative with a predicted time to development of diabetes of less than 2.5 years has not developed diabetes within 5 years.

The Barts-Windsor Family Study

This study was begun in 1978 and drew its subjects from clinics in southern England. Recruitment was limited to white families with a diabetic proband diagnosed before the age of 21 years and at least one unaffected sibling under that age. A total of 198 families with 376 unaffected parents and 343 unaffected siblings were followed prospectively.[106,107] Blood for ICA assay was taken at 4- to 6-monthly intervals. Since entry into the study, 5 parents and 11 siblings have developed Type I diabetes. Of the 15 subjects who subsequently became insulin-dependent, 14 were ICA-positive before diagnosis. In all, 54 (7.5%) of 719 were positive for any titer of ICA; 14 (26%) of the 54 ICA-positive subjects developed diabetes as compared with 2 (0.3%) of 665 who developed diabetes despite their being ICA-negative. Of the ICA-positive subjects, 24 of 54 were positive for complement-fixing ICA (high-titer ICA); 13 of these 24 developed diabetes. In contrast, 30 subjects had non-complement-fixing ICA (i.e., low titer); of these only 1 developed diabetes. Clearly, the high-titer ICA proved the best predictor of Type I diabetes.

The Barts-Windsor study also followed metabolic profiles. A normal range for random blood glucose values was obtained from over 800 samples from nondiabetic family members in the study. The 97.5th percentile for these

samples was 6.3 mmol/L. Of the 15 ICA-positive subjects, 11 were found to have had random blood glucose levels above the 97.5th percentile 26 to 364 weeks before they started taking insulin. Thus, the majority of subjects who eventually developed diabetes showed intermittent development of hyperglycemia over many months and also nonspecific symptoms over a long period before becoming insulin-dependent.[108,109]

In summary, in the Barts-Windsor study, relative risks for the development of Type I diabetes according to ICA status were 341 for subjects with complement-fixing ICA (i.e., high titer) and 14 for those with non-complement-fixing ICA (including low- and high-titer ICA). Risk of diabetes was minimal for relatives with only low-titer ICA. By current workshop comparisons with a Juvenile Diabetes Foundation standard, it is likely that low-titer ICA would be less than 20 JDF units. By life-table analysis, the risk of diabetes after 8 years of known ICA positivity was 42.3% compared with 0.6% for the ICA-negative group. Subdivision of the ICA-positive group gave a risk of 76% for complement-fixing ICA (high-titer) positivity and 3.4% for non-complement-fixing positivity.

Gainesville Studies

The Gainesville group has now assayed serum for ICA from over 11,000 subjects with no family history of Type I diabetes and for over 6000 first-degree relatives of patients with Type I diabetes. The ICA-positivity rate in control subjects was 0.32%, and the rate in relatives was 2.33%.[110] As in the Barts-Windsor study, titer of ICA clearly correlated with development of Type I diabetes, with those with higher-titer antibodies being most likely to develop diabetes. The cut-off point for high risk appears to be at approximately 40 JDF units. In relatives of subjects with Type I diabetes, the risk of development of diabetes was dependent on the age and the actual relationship to the proband. If the relative of the proband was younger than 20 years or if the individual was a sibling, the relative risk was significantly higher.

IAA have also been measured, with use of a radiobinding assay, in selected groups of controls, first-degree relatives, and subjects with newly diagnosed Type I diabetes. IAA positivity was found in 4 (1.4%) of 292 controls, 9 (4.0%) of 225 relatives, and 14 (37%) of 38 newly diagnosed patients. A strong positive correlation between ICA and IAA was observed. Furthermore, after intravenous glucose stimulation, insulinopenia was present in 70% of ICA-positive/IAA-positive individuals in contrast to only 23% of ICA-positive/IAA-negative subjects.[111] IAA predict Type I diabetes in ICA-positive relatives, especially in those destined to develop diabetes before puberty.

The Gainesville group also used the IVGTT as a predictor of impending development of diabetes and pointed out that the applicability of this test may be affected by the age of the subject. As was seen in prior studies, in adult patients, the insulin responses were near or below the first or fifth percentile months to years before overt disease. On the other hand, children were less likely to have insulin responses below the first percentile 6 to 8 months before clinical symptoms and presumably passed through this phase more quickly.

A major contribution of this group has been in the assessment of the predictive ability of ICA in nonrelatives. Testing of the first 5000 normal schoolchildren aged 6 to 14 years showed that 1 in 300 children were ICA-positive. Two children with high-titer ICA developed Type I diabetes during the 2- to 3-year follow-up. Thus, the autoantibody markers for IDDM so far appear to be holding up for the low-risk general population as for high-risk relatives. One of the problems with screening for ICA is the question of when ICA will first be detectable in these prediabetic individuals. One subject converted to ICA positivity in this study in the 12 months prior to development of diabetes after having had two negative samples previously. Sera from two other patients with initially positive samples were negative on at least two occasions before the development of diabetes.[112]

In the Gainesville study the relative risk of development of Type I diabetes in an ICA-positive relative of a proband with Type I diabetes was 82.3. The actuarial estimate of the probability of developing Type I diabetes at 5 years was approximately 35% for any ICA-positive relative of a person with Type I diabetes and 57% in siblings.

Auckland Studies

The Auckland group has carried out large screening studies on both first-degree relatives of persons with diabetes and normal children. In their most recent update, 1765 first-degree relatives and 84 normal schoolchildren had been tested for ICA with a very sensitive 24-hour incubation assay.[113] Fifty-nine (3.3%) of the relatives and two (2.4%) of normal children had ICA values greater than 10 JDF units. Of these children, 19 showed first-phase insulin release on IVGTT that was below the 10th percentile. Some of the group have been treated with nicotinamide, but of 13 untreated subjects whose IVGTT values were below the 10th percentile, six developed diabetes within 15 months. These studies are consistent with those already cited but suggest a lower level of ICA might also be associated with a somewhat increased risk of progression to diabetes.

Denver Studies

Chase and colleagues[114] found ICA in 71 of 1169 first-degree relatives from 448 families who had a proband with Type I diabetes. In the follow-up period of 2 years, seven children became insulin-dependent. All had IAA and were followed with IVGTT testing. Subjects progressing to diabetes had low first-phase insulin release as shown by IVGTT.

SUMMARY OF PREDICTION

High-titer ICA are predictive of Type I diabetes, with between 8 and 10% of such relatives with high-titer ICA progressing to diabetes per year. For ICA values greater than 40 to 80 JDF units, the Barts-Windsor, Joslin-Sacramento, and Gainesville studies report similar data with respect to risk, particularly in relatives who are consistently ICA-positive. However, the question as to whether diabetes is inevitable once high-titer ICA appears cannot yet be answered. Our recent finding of a subset of high-titer ICA (restricted, or GAD ICA) that can be distinguished by β-cell specificity and the species specificity of the antibodies (react with human and rat islets but not with mouse islets) and adsorption with GAD that appear not to presage diabetes suggests that heterogeneity of ICA must be addressed in assessing risk.

All the studies have a group of "survivors" representing almost one-half of the total number of individuals identified to be at high risk who have normal glucose tolerance up to 7 years after the first detection of ICA. It is noteworthy that most of these individuals can be predicted at initial evaluation (normal IVGTT, lack of IAA, and restricted ICA). These individuals are unlikely to develop diabetes in their lifetime. For example, we are following a 57-year-old parent of three children with Type I diabetes. The parent has had high-titer (complement-fixing) restricted ICA for 7 years. She has stable first-phase insulin secretion, no IAA, and is DR2-positive (with the "protective" DQB1*0602 allele). It is likely that she will not develop diabetes despite her having three offspring with the disorder. Her diabetic offspring did not inherit her "protective" DR2 haplotype.

The presence of IAA, particularly with ICA, identifies individuals with an increased risk of developing diabetes. IAA may be predictive in the absence of ICA, but it is clear that rate of progression to diabetes of relatives who are IAA-positive but with low titers (<40 JDF units) or ICA-negative is slow. The Majority (80%) do not progress with up to 7 years of follow-up. An issue regarding which IAA assay—radiobinding vs. current ELISAs—provides the most predictive information has now been largely settled, with ELISAs unable to detect disease-related antibodies in the 1990 Jerusalem workshop.

The Barts-Windsor and Joslin-Sacramento studies have both found that blood glucose levels rise progressively prior to clinical diagnosis of diabetes in most subjects. In addition, the Joslin-Sacramento, Barts-Windsor, Gainesville, and Denver studies have all found that a very low first-phase insulin response to intravenous glucose makes progression to diabetes a virtual certainty for the ICA-positive individual. The conventional IVGTT has a coefficient of variation of approximately 30%, which precludes its ability to identify changes in β-cell function within the normal range early in the disease.

A recent policy statement of the American Diabetes Association,[115] recommends screening of first-degree relatives of patients with Type I diabetes for potential entry into trials for diabetes prevention. This statement reflects the concordant results of the studies reviewed. Nevertheless, a number of significant problems remain to be resolved before clinically useful and convenient assays become available. The data reviewed apply only to research laboratories. Each of the variables used in prediction (including insulin determinations) vary significantly between laboratories. The precision, sensitivity, and specificity of the determinations by laboratories participating in IDW proficiency testing vary widely, and most commercial laboratories have not participated in proficiency testing at all. Commercial anti-insulin assays have been designed to detect the antibodies associated with insulin therapy and insulin resistance, and to date, ELISA anti-insulin assays have failed to detect relevant antibodies. A clinician ordering a test for ICA or IAA should use characterized laboratories (laboratories participating in IDW proficiency testing programs) and, at a minimum, have the results reported in standard units (e.g., JDF units). Low-titer ICA (<40 JDF units) has minimal prognostic significance, while absence of high-titer ICA in a person with diabetes does not rule out Type I diabetes, since at least 30% of relatives who develop diabetes lack such antibodies. Some centers, such as the Joslin Diabetes Center and the Barbara Davis Center for Childhood Diabetes in Denver, will assay the sera of first-degree relatives without charge.

With the feasibility of diabetes prediction comes the question of when such testing is warranted. Table 13−6 lists a number of indications that will almost certainly be better defined and expanded over the next decade. Development of Type I diabetes after kidney donation is unusual, but the ideal donor (HLA identical sibling) has the highest genetic risk. Riley and co-workers have described one such ICA-positive patient who developed diabetes following kidney donation.[116] The major current limitation to trials for the prevention of Type I diabetes is the identification of at-risk individuals. Approximately 1 of 150 first-degree relatives are strongly ICA-positive and by analysis of first-phase insulin secretion and IAA are at highest risk of developing diabetes (90% within 3 years). In the absence of a prevention trial, indications for screening are less certain. A potential for increased anxiety in response to being identified as autoantibody-positive would have to be balanced against the use of prognostic information to prevent presentation with ketoacidosis. Formal studies to date suggest only mild anxiety and good coping among autoantibody-positive individuals,[117] but no trials are available that compare, for example, long-term coping after diagnosis of diabetes in those identified vs. those not identified as prediabetic.

Transient hyperglycemia is a relatively common diagnosis in referral pediatric diabetology centers. Approximately 10% of such children develop diabetes within 2 years. In the past 4 years, Herskowitz and colleagues at the Joslin Diabetes Center have evaluated approximately 100 such children.[118] Presence of autoantibodies presages diabetes but misses a significant percentage of prediabetic children. Loss of first-phase insulin secretion had the best overall accuracy in defining prediabetic

Table 13−6. Indications for Autoantibody/Intravenous Glucose Tolerance Determinations

1. Potential renal transplant donor
2. First-degree relative screened for entry into research trial of prevention of Type I diabetes
3. First-degree relative requesting prognostic information
4. Patient with history of transient hyperglycemia
5. To aid in diagnosis of Type I vs. Type II diabetes

status. Normal first-phase secretion (48 μU/mL) had a greater than 98% negative predictive value. If first-phase secretion (1- plus 3-minute insulin on IVGTT) is less than 48 μU/mL in the setting of transient hyperglycemia, the IVGTT should be repeated approximately 1 month later. Restoration of insulin secretion has been observed, particularly in children younger than 5 years old. Children with consistent loss of first-phase secretion should be monitored closely for development of overt diabetes, as severe hyperglycemia can develop rapidly.

Approximately 10% of adults presenting with what appears clinically to be Type II diabetes are ICA-positive. These individuals have HLA alleles DR3 and DR4 and behave like patients with Type I diabetes, with accelerated failure of oral hypoglycemic agents. The clinical management of such patients has not been addressed in formal trials. Given the data that "resting" of β-cells may preserve β-cell function, it is not known whether ICA-positive patients with non-insulin-dependent diabetes should be treated with insulin rather than oral hypoglycemic agents.

IMMUNOTHERAPY

Immunosuppressive therapy for patients with recently diagnosed Type I diabetes was begun with the assumption that the destructive process is immune-mediated and that sufficient β-cell secretory capacity remained to permit normal glucose metabolism to be restored once the destructive immune process was suppressed. Since the early 1980s various forms of immunotherapy, ranging from aggressive immunosuppression to mild immunomodulation, have been tried. Cyclosporin A (CsA) has been most intensively studied, and when administered after onset of diabetes but within 6 weeks of onset, it increases the rate and duration of remission in patients with recent-onset Type I diabetes.[119−121] In a double-blind trial of the French Multicenter Group, the rate of complete remission after 9 months of treatment with CsA was 24% vs. 6% in the placebo group. Similar results were reported by the Canadian/European Diabetes Study Group. The maximal benefit of immunosuppression was observed in patients who had the largest residual insulin secretion when first treated. There is thus no doubt that CsA enhances β-cell function during the first year of Type I diabetes. However, almost all patients reverted to insulin dependence within 1 to 3 years of treatment even if CsA was continued. In the French trial, 50% of the children remained in remission for more than 12 months, 30% for more than 18 months, but fewer than 10% for more than 24 months.[112] A high fasting ratio of proinsulin to C-peptide levels at diagnosis was shown to be of value in predicting remission in patients treated with CsA. Of importance, the absence of a decline in basal or stimulated C-peptide levels was associated with occurrence of relapse, a finding suggesting that loss of metabolic remission in these patients is probably due not to the progression of β-cell destruction but rather to an increase in insulin resistance.

What of the complications of CsA treatment in these trials? The most relevant side effect of CsA is nephrotoxicity, which presents both as functional, acute toxicity with dose-dependent and reversible increase in serum creatinine and as chronic toxicity with interstitial fibrosis, tubular atrophy, and arteriolopathy. Renal biopsy specimens from 40 patients (11 clinical centers) treated long-term and continuously with CsA (6 to 29 months) in the Canadian/European Study or French Study were evaluated. The serum creatinine level increased from a mean baseline value of 74 μmol/L to a value of 104 μmol/L at time of biopsy. Histopathologic changes characteristic of CsA-mediated chronic nephrotoxicity (arteriolopathy, tubular atrophy, and interstitial fibrosis) were rated on a five-point scale (absent, minimal, slight, moderate, severe). In the majority of patients, lesions were only minimal or slight; however, in 10 patients (25%), lesions were of moderate intensity. In the mean, arteriolopathy was minimal. The highest rating was of moderate arteriolopathy and was found in two patients. The mean scores for tubular atrophy and interstitial fibrosis were both slight; however, moderate lesions were found in seven and eight patients, respectively. Trough CsA levels correlated significantly with the extent of tubular atrophy. No correlation was found between histopathologic alterations and duration of therapy, dose of CsA, or increase of creatinine values. Thus, it was concluded that irreversible renal changes did occur in some patients.

In addition to the adverse effect of CsA on the kidney, a number of investigators have suggested that CsA causes glucose intolerance and inhibits pancreatic islet β-cell function. Consequently, concern has been raised that the beneficial effects of immunosuppression may be offset by the adverse metabolic effects of the drug. Robertson and colleagues, therefore, examined intravenous glucose tolerance and β-cell function before and during a 2-year course of CsA or placebo therapy in a group of nondiabetic patients with multiple sclerosis. Fortunately, no abnormalities of basal and stimulated glucose values, insulin levels, and C-peptide were observed in the CsA-treated group, implying that CsA can be given in conventional doses for as long as 2 years without patients showing evidence of impaired glucose homeostasis.[122]

Therapy with azathioprine and prednisone in combination also extends metabolic remission.[123] Three of 20 immunosuppressed patients, but no nonimmunosuppressed control patients, were insulin-independent at 1 year, and 50% had a satisfactory metabolic outcome as compared with controls. Older age, better initial metabolic status, and lymphopenia were predictive of a favorable response to immunosuppression.

Several groups are conducting trials of nicotinamide in both persons with newly diagnosed diabetes and prediabetic individuals. Animals given nicotinamide after streptozotocin show an increase in intracellular nicotinamide adenine dinucleotide content, which may protect the β-cells by limiting the damage by free radicals. Nicotinamide has been shown to weakly delay development of diabetes in the NOD mouse[124,125] but not in the BB rat. In addition, several groups, but not all, found that nicotinamide increases C-peptide secretory function in patients with newly diagnosed IDDM but has no effect on clinical remission or insulin requirements in these patients.[126] Herskowitz and co-workers at the Joslin Diabetes Clinic have studied three ICA-positive first-degree relatives whose levels of insulin secretion are below the first percentile. No losses of ICA, losses of IAA, or improvements in IVGTT results were observed with nicotinamide therapy. All three of these individuals progressed to overt diabetes while receiving nicotinamide.[127] In contrast, Elliott and Chase,[113] in a trial without concurrent controls, reported that ICA-positive children (>10 JDF units) with insulin secretion below the 10th percentile who were treated with nicotinamide remained free of diabetes for 6 to 40 months. This study suggests that nicotinamide treatment of children whose insulin release is impaired but has not yet declined to the first percentile may delay the onset of Type I diabetes. Evaluation of the results of the trial is difficult because of the absence of concurrent controls and follow-up data indicating that three-fourths of the children treated with nicotinamide in Denver are now diabetic.

Recently, a randomized trial assessed whether the use of intensive insulin therapy during the first 2 weeks after diagnosis in patients with newly diagnosed Type I diabetes would preserve β-cell function.[128] Continuous insulin infusion was delivered by an external artificial pancreas (Biostator), and blood glucose levels were maintained at 3.3 to 4.4 mmol/L for 2 weeks, the control group receiving conventional treatment of two injections of NPH insulin per day. During the intervention the experimental group received four times more insulin than the conventionally treated group. After the first 2 weeks, the two groups were treated similarly and received similar amounts of insulin. Surprisingly, at 1 year the experimental group had significantly higher C-peptide levels and better metabolic control. These data suggest that suppression of endogenous insulin by intensive continuous insulin treatment may improve β-cell function for one full year. Diabetes and insulitis is prevented in both the BB rat and NOD mouse by insulin therapy. A trial of insulin for high-risk nondiabetic relatives of patients with Type I diabetes has been initiated with promising preliminary data.[129]

It has thus been shown definitively that with CsA or azathioprine and steroids it is possible to change the natural history of β-cell destruction in patients with newly diagnosed Type I diabetes. The failure of any of these protocols to prevent diabetes over the long-term and the attendant side effects of these agents makes the use of such immunotherapy after the onset of diabetes onset problematic. Until trials demonstrate a clear clinical benefit of the preservation of C-peptide secretion—greater than attendant adverse effects of such therapy—in patients treated after the onset of diabetes, we believe that such therapy is not clinically warranted and that it likely will not be clinically warranted for drugs such as cyclosporin A or azathioprine unless they actually cure diabetes.

Immunotherapy at the time of onset of diabetes is limited by the marked β-cell destruction that has already occurred. The question therefore arises as to whether treatment should be initiated in asymptomatic individuals before development of diabetes. We believe that with selective current autoantibody assays and metabolic testing, the development of Type I diabetes can be predicted. For the moment, at least four ongoing trials in nondiabetic, ICA-positive subjects ICA have been reported to the International Diabetes Immunotherapy Group (IDIG): 1) one study carried out in Dusseldorf, Germany, with ketotifen, an antihistamine; 2) one study using insulin therapy at the Joslin Diabetes Center, Boston, MA; and the Barbara Davis Center for Childhood Diabetes, Denver, CO, USA; and 3) three studies using nicotinamide (Auckland, New Zealand; Rome, Italy; and Marseille, France). In several years we hope to know whether such treatment will be beneficial in preventing the development of overt diabetes in nondiabetic autoantibody-positive relatives.

In addition, possible future immune interventions are being identified through studies in the animal models of IDDM. Administration of monoclonal antibodies specific for some lymphocyte surface markers can block function or destroy the corresponding cell subset.[130] Thus, murine IDDM can be prevented by monoclonal antibody therapy directed against different T-lymphocyte subsets. Treatment with an anti-Thy1.2 monoclonal antibody prevents diabetes but does not influence the progression of insulitis. However, administration of L3T4 monoclonal antibody abolishes insulitis and diabetes. Cyclophosphamide-induced diabetes in NOD/Wehi mice is prevented by administration of monoclonal antibody to the VβB T-lymphocyte receptor.[131] These mice exhibit a low incidence of spontaneous diabetes, but one large dose of cyclophosphamide can lead to a rapid progression of overt diabetes. The monoclonal antibody recognizes a specific subset of T lymphocytes that express one particular segment of the T-lymphocyte receptor. Furthermore, treatment with either an antibody to interleukin-2 or interleukin-2-diphtheria toxin conjugate suppresses autoimmune insulitis in non-obese diabetic mice and BB rats.[132,133] T-cell lines responding to autologous cells or a heat-shock protein[134] prevent diabetes in NOD mice, and a single injection of Freund's adjuvant at a young age prevents diabetes in these animals.[135]

INSULIN AUTOIMMUNE SYNDROME

Insulin autoimmune syndrome is characterized by the presence of circulating antibodies to insulin in patients who have never received insulin. Its most definitive symptom is recurrent episodes of spontaneous hypoglycemia.[136] However, the clinical course and presentation vary, depending in part on the characteristics of the insulin antibodies. This syndrome was first described and is most common in patients from Japan and has been associated with methimazole treatment of patients with Graves disease. Recently, Wasada and co-workers described an unusual case of insulin autoimmune syndrome in a patient with benign monoclonal gammopathy.[137] Scatchard analysis of the antibodies in this patient revealed antibodies to insulin of the IgG1 type with low affinity, high capacity, and a single binding site. With use of competitive inhibition analysis with various insulins,

the epitope of human insulin recognized by the patient's antibodies was tentatively mapped; it was suggested that this patient's antibodies are directed against a determinant at B-3 (asparagine) on the human insulin B-chain.[137] This is of interest because anti-insulin antibodies in Type I diabetes, even though they differ in affinity and capacity (high-affinity, low-capacity), might recognize a similar epitope.

EXTRA-ISLET AUTOIMMUNITY AND TYPE I DIABETES

As discussed previously, Type I diabetes is associated with both the polyendocrine syndromes type I and type II. In patients with Addison's disease and these syndromes, approximately 50% of those with the type II syndrome develop diabetes as approximately 5% of patients with the type I syndrome. In addition to its association with these two syndromes, Type I diabetes is frequently associated with thyroid autoimmunity (e.g., Graves disease, hypothyroidism, and thyroid autoantibodies). Both persons with trisomy 21 and those with congenital rubella develop thyroid autoimmunity more frequently than they develop Type I diabetes. Such a common association of Type I diabetes with thyroid disease has led to periodic (e.g., every 5 years) screening (e.g., with sensitive thyroid-stimulating hormone [TSH] assay) of thyroid function in patients with Type I diabetes. The association of these disorders implies that the loss of immune tolerance to β-cells is a more general phenomenon, with the potential for loss of tolerance to a series of unrelated molecules (e.g., TSH receptor in Graves disease, acetylcholine receptor in myasthenia gravis, thyroid peroxidase in thyroiditis). In sequentially followed patients, the appearance of autoantibodies to different organs often occurs at different times, suggesting independent activation of the different autoimmune disorders.

Islets share with neurons a large series of differentiation molecules, including cell-surface molecules such as "neuronal" gangliosides, which are cell-surface receptors for tetanus toxin (GT1) and monoclonal antibodies A2B5, 3G5, and R2D6.[138–140] The latter monoclonal antibody is reported to be specific for β-cells. Islets and neurons express certain enzymes in common, such as GAD and carboxypeptidase H. Carboxypeptidase H within islets apparently functions in the processing of proinsulin to insulin, whereas in the central nervous system it functions in processing peptides such as enkephalin. The enzyme GAD produces GABA and is expressed within cells of the islets and within the central nervous system. Chromogranins of secretory granules are found in both islets and neurons. The sharing of differentiation antigens by neurons and islets raises the possibility that neuroendocrine autoimmunity would overlap with Type I diabetes.

A fascinating example of the overlap of neuroendocrine autoimmunity with Type I diabetes is stiff-man syndrome. This syndrome is characterized by involuntary muscle contractions. The great majority of patients with stiff-man syndrome express autoantibodies to GAD, which, as discussed previously, is the 64-kd antigen to which most prediabetic individuals produce autoantibodies. Approximately one-third of patients with stiff-man syndrome have Type I diabetes. It was the association of the syndrome with diabetes that led eventually to the discovery of the identity of the 64-kd antigen and GAD. Titers of antibody to the 64-kd antigen are extremely high in patients with stiff-man syndrome—much lower than the titers in prediabetic individuals. The pathogenic relationship between stiff-man syndrome, which is extremely rare, and Type I diabetes, which is common, is not understood. For example, the extremely high titers of autoantibodies to GAD predispose only one-third of patients with stiff-man syndrome to the development of IAA and Type I diabetes. Fewer than 1 per 10,000 patients who develop Type I diabetes with associated antibodies to GAD go on to develop higher titers of antibodies to GAD and autoimmunity directed against GABAergic neurons.

A much more common association of neuroendocrine autoimmunity with Type I diabetes is the occurrence of autoantibodies to peripheral nerves and the adrenal medulla. Antibodies detected by indirect immunofluorescence are found that react with adrenal medulla, sympathetic ganglia, and the vagus nerve.[141-143] Such antibodies are frequent not only in patients with Type I diabetes but also in persons with pre–Type I diabetes and in more than 20% of "normal" first-degree relatives of patients with Type I diabetes. A recent study of the adrenal medulla of patients with Type I diabetes indicates that destruction of the adrenal medulla with fibrosis affects more than one-third of patients, and several patients show marked T-lymphocyte infiltrates in the adrenal medulla. Studies are just beginning to correlate the presence of autoantibodies with autonomic dysfunction. These studies suggest that anti-neuronal autoimmunity is widespread in patients with Type I diabetes, raising the possibility that in the setting of hyperglycemia such autoimmunity may predispose to selected neuropathic syndromes.

Necrobiosis lipoidica is a vasculitic skin lesion affecting approximately 1% of patients with Type I diabetes.[144] It is well recognized that such lesions frequently precede the development of Type I diabetes. We have observed this lesion in several autoantibody-positive first-degree relatives of patients with Type I diabetes. The relationship between necrobiosis lipoidica and β-cell destruction is unknown.

Pericytes of the retinal microvasculature are lost early in the development of diabetic retinopathy. This loss is most likely due to the effects of hyperglycemia. Nevertheless, it is of interest that pericytes react with anti-neuronal monoclonal antibody 3G5, which also reacts with islet cells.[145] This monoclonal antibody appears to react with the acylated ganglioside GD3.

PATHOPHYSIOLOGIC HYPOTHESES

Despite a long prodromal phase preceding Type I diabetes (Fig. 13–5), characterization of two animal models, and recent studies of transgenic mouse models of

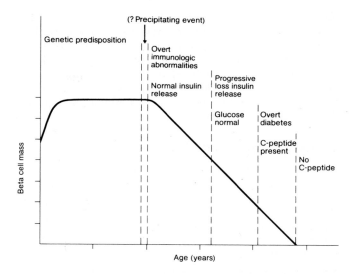

Fig. 13–5. Hypothetical stages in the development of Type I diabetes beginning with genetic susceptibility and ending with complete β-cell destruction. Reprinted with permission from reference 146 (Eisenbarth GS. Type I diabetes mellitus: a chronic autoimmune disease. N Engl J Med 1986;314:1360–8).

diabetes, no unitary, accepted hypothesis of diabetes pathogenesis is available.

Current hypotheses concerning the development of Type I diabetes must account for the long prodromal phase preceding the development of overt diabetes in the great majority of patients. Genetic susceptibility is required for diabetes development in humans and the animal models. The chronicity of the process leading to diabetes appears to be secondary to T cell-dependent destruction of β-cells in genetically susceptible individuals. T cells appear to destroy different islets over time in a plaque-like process similar, in concept, to the brain lesions of multiple sclerosis. Thus, within the same pancreas, islets at different stages of destruction can be found, with overt diabetes developing only after extensive β-cell destruction.

Ongoing studies in humans suggest that humoral tolerance to different islet antigens can be independently broken in a quantitative manner and that the pattern of autoantibodies expressed profoundly influences progression to diabetes. For example, relatives whose IVGTT results are normal at the time they are found to be autoantibody-positive (and the autoantibodies indicated persist) can be subdivided after just two antibody assays into three groups according to their approximate risk of developing diabetes within 6 years:

1) Those with ICA values >40 JDF units who are IAA-negative have a risk of <10%.
2) Those with ICA values >40 JDF units and IAA levels >80 nU/mL have a risk of >90%.
3) Those with ICA values <40 JDF units and IAA levels >80 nU/mL have a risk of <10%.

Thus, it appears that breaking of immune tolerance in Type I diabetes is not simply an all-or-none phenomenon but is both quantitative and antigen selective. Each of the steps in the pathogenesis of Type I diabetes is defined only partially, and many of the genes that create diabetes susceptibility have not been defined. Thus, at present any pathogenic scheme is speculative and incomplete. Nevertheless, as a means of summarizing a large body of data, we will outline one of many pathogenic schemes (Table 13-7).

Genetic Susceptibility/Resistance

Essentially everyone who develops Type I diabetes is genetically susceptible. Genes creating diabetes susceptibility appear to act at the level of the immune system (Table 13-8). In NOD mice and BB rats, lymphoid cells transfer diabetes susceptibility and resistance. Thus, NOD lymphocytes can destroy normal islets, and NOD bone-marrow stem cells transplanted into normal mice produce diabetes. Genetic susceptibility can be divided into several interrelated components: 1) probability of breaking tolerance and initiating autoimmunity; 2) recognition of specific islet target antigens, with recognition of multiple islet target antigens appearing to result in accelerated destruction and increased progression to diabetes; 3) suppression of anti-islet autoimmunity.

Immune-response or class II genes probably determine lymphocyte targeting of islet antigens and thus, in part, diabetes susceptibility. For the two animal models of spontaneous development of Type I diabetes (NOD mouse and BB rat), class II or immune-response genes are

Table 13-8. Known Genetic Abnormalities and Environmental Factors that Promote or Suppress Development of Type I Diabetes

KNOWN GENETIC ABNORMALITIES
a. Class II genes
   1. Promote
      DR4, DQw8   (human)
      RT_1-U   (BB rat)
      I-A-NOD   (NOD mouse)
   2. Suppress
      DR2, DQw1.2   (human)
      I-E   (NOD mouse)
      I-A^k (NOD mouse)
b. Immunodeficiency genes
   1. RT6 T-cell deficiency gene   (BB rat)
   2. Polyendocrine type I syndrome   (human)
      (mucocutaneous candidiasis)
c. Chromosomal abnormalities
   1. Trisomy 21
      Thyroiditis and Type I diabetes
KNOWN ENVIRONMENTAL FACTORS
a. Promote
   Congenital rubella   (human)
   Wheat proteins   (NOD mouse)
b. Suppress
   LCMV   (NOD mouse)
   LDV   (NOD mouse)
   Freund's adjuvant   (NOD mouse)

LCMV = lymphocytic choriomeningitis virus; LDV = lactic dehydrogenase virus.

essential for susceptibility. As was discussed, class II molecules bind antigens for presentation to T cells. In Type I diabetes, class II molecules may function to target unique islet molecules to enhance autoimmunity and also may suppress autoimmunity. Such suppression by class II genes has been directly tested with transgenic NOD mice. Injection of isolated class II genes into fertilized eggs of mice and expression of the products of these genes on lymphoid tissue (but not islets) can suppress anti-islet autoimmunity. Breaking of immune tolerance to islets can also be determined by genes outside of the major histocompatibility complex. This is most evident in BB rats, with their gene for profound T-cell immunodeficiency (autosomal recessive), and in patients with the type I polyendocrine autoimmune syndrome, with its associated mucocutaneous candidiasis. The specific genes leading to immunodeficiency in the type I syndrome and loss of tolerance maintenance in Type I diabetes of humans are unknown. Potential candidate genes may influence cytokine production, thymic development, T-cell subsets, lymphocyte trafficking, antigen processing, immunoglobulin gene mutation rates, somatic mutation rates, and other lymphocyte functions. The molecular definition of such non-major histocompatibility complex genes will be essential for refining pathogenic hypotheses.

Triggering of Autoimmunity

There are relatively few well-defined mechanisms for activating autoimmunity. Among the best defined are the autoimmunities occurring with B-cell malignancies with

Table 13-7. Pathogenesis of Type I Diabetes

Event	Potential determinants
Altered T-cell/B-cell repertoire	Class II genes/ immunoregulatory genes
Altered T-cell regulation ↓	Congenital/neonatal infection Somatic mutations Non-MHC genes Class II genes
Antigen presentation by B lymphocytes and monocytes ↓	
Expansion anti-islet CD4 T lymphocytes ↓	Islet damage/β-cell secretion Immunoglobulin gene mutations
Perpetuation/regulation autoimmunity	DR4 haplotypes: high-response insulin Local lymphokine production Enhanced vascular permeability Enhanced class I, class II expression
β-cell toxicity ↓	Lymphokines Free radicals CD8 T cells NK cells Macrophages
Progressive plaque-like destruction ↓	B-cell activity
Diabetes	

MHC = major histocompatibility complex; NK cells = natural killer.

polyclonal B-cell stimulation following infection with Epstein-Barr virus, in response to malignancy (paraneoplastic syndromes), following infections (e.g., rheumatic fever), and with specific drugs. The trigger for the autoimmunity of Type I diabetes is unknown.

The process leading to autoimmunity in Type I diabetes appears to be stochastic. We therefore favor the hypotheses that, given genetic susceptibility, there may be many environmental triggers or that random events such as mutations in the immunoglobulin gene or development of subclinical tumor transformation (?lymphoid) may be sufficient for triggering. Once autoimmunity is initiated, the seeding of islets by autoreactive B lymphocytes and T lymphocytes and attendant β-cell death would lead to loss of tolerance to multiple islet antigens.

Studies of the pancreas of nondiabetic identical twins of patients with Type I diabetes by Sutherland and co-workers indicate that the pancreas is normal in long-term discordant twins.[147] In addition, we rarely (<2/1,000 relatives of patients with Type I diabetes) detect transient IAA. This suggests that insulitis even in genetically susceptible individuals is rare or rarely leads to detectable lesions.

With activation of autoimmunity, a self-regenerating and regulated process of β-cell destruction may ensue. Once insulitis has become self-regenerating (even at the stage in humans of five to six lymphocytes per islet), expression of islet class II antigen is enhanced. In addition, enhanced expression of islet class I antigen is found in the NOD mouse, BB rat, and humans during the process of β-cell destruction. Enhanced expression of class I antigens may facilitate CD8 T lymphocyte-mediated cytotoxicity. Alternative hypotheses for activation of autoimmunity are that viral infection of β-cells initiates islet destruction or that cross-reactive environmental antigens (e.g., antigenic mimicry) initiate autoimmunity. It is noteworthy that the drug penicillamine (dimethylcysteine) frequently induces the development of IAA without progression to diabetes. This suggests that loss of tolerance to a single islet antigen is usually insufficient for progressive β-cell destruction.

β-Cell Destruction

The final destruction of β-cells is probably the result of many factors, being dependent on multiple cell types (e.g., macrophages, CD4- and CD8-positive T lymphocytes) and multiple mechanisms (free-radical damage, interleukin-1, CD8 T cell-mediated toxicity). Specific targeting of islet antigens by immunoglobulin and T-cell receptors almost certainly underlies the tissue specificity of β-cell destruction. Once activated, the autoimmunity is in many respects similar to a regulated immune response to a pathogen, and it is unlikely that blocking of a single peripheral destructive mechanisms will prevent disease progression, although removal of essential classes of cells responsible for initiating immune responses (e.g., CD4 T lymphocytes, macrophages) could prevent diabetes. An important question not yet addressed in detail is whether the disease process depends on oligoclonal or monoclonal lymphocytes. Cytoplasmic ICA (all IgG) are polyclonal, while IAA have not been subtyped. In the NOD mouse, T cell–receptor usage, including clones of cells that can transfer diabetes, is polyclonal, despite an initial report suggesting the use of a single Vβ gene (Vβ5) by such T lymphocytes.

At present, the pathogenesis of Type I diabetes is only partially understood, but prediction of the disorder is feasible, and with potent, nonspecific immunosuppressive drugs, prevention of diabetes is a possibility. The basic questions being addressed concerning Type I diabetes are identical to questions about other autoimmune disorders, such as lupus erythematosus and myasthenia gravis. In all autoimmune disorders, fewer than 100% of identical twins are concordant, while disease is strongly dependent on largely undefined genetic abnormalities. Only in a few disorders have events triggering autoimmunity been identified (e.g., paraneoplastic autoimmunity, drug-induced autoimmunity), but it is clear that multiple pathways can induce autoimmunity. It is likely that, as the basic pathogenesis of Type I diabetes is better defined, elegant strategies for preventing the disorder will be developed. Pending such strategies, we believe—given the morbidity and mortality of Type I diabetes—that immunotherapy for pre–Type I diabetes will become a clinical option. The rational development of such therapies must include careful clinical trials to define both who might benefit from therapy and what its risks are. This will require cooperation of multiple centers worldwide and of multiple disciplines within the diabetes and immunologic community. The cooperation of the past decade bodes well for the future prevention of Type I diabetes.

Despite the significant gaps in our knowledge of the pathogenesis of Type I diabetes, we believe that the many steps involved in β-cell destruction and the chronicity of the process make it likely that effective and safe therapies will be developed for the prevention of this disease. With the recent adoption by the American Diabetes Association of a policy statement that recommends screening of first-degree relatives of patients with Type I diabetes for potential participation in preventive trials, such attempts at preventing diabetes are entering the clinical-trial stage. At present, such therapy should be considered only in the research setting.

REFERENCES

1. Castano L, Eisenbarth GS. Type-I diabetes: a chronic autoimmune disease of human, mouse and rat. Ann Rev Immunol 1990;8:647−79.
2. Nerup J, Mandrup-Poulsen T, Mølvig J, et al. Mechanisms of pancreatic β-cell destruction in type I diabetes. Diabetes Care 1988;11(Suppl 1):16−22.
3. Bach J-F. Mechanisms of autoimmunity in insulin-dependent diabetes mellitus. Clin Exp Immunol 1988;2:1−8.
4. Pujol-Borrell R, Soldevila G, Buscema M, et al. Inappropriate expression of HLA class II molecules in endocrine epithelial cells: the phenomenon, the new experimental data and comparison with animal models. J Autoimmune 1989;2(Suppl):163−9.
5. Rossini AA, Mordes JP, Greiner DL. The pathogenesis of autoimmune diabetes. Curr Opin Immunol 1989−90; 2:598−603.

6. Foulis AK, Liddle CN, Farquharson MA, et al. The histopathology of the pancreas in Type I (insulin-dependent) diabetes mellitus: a 25-year review of deaths in patients under 20 years of age in the United Kingdom. Diabetologia 1986;29:267–74.

7. Prosser PR, Karam JH. Diabetes mellitus following rodenticide ingestion in man. JAMA 1978;239:1148–50.

8. Van Haeften TW, Razenberg PPA. DIDMOAD syndrome and HLA-DR haplotypes. Horm Metab Res 1989; 21:214–5.

9. Karasik A, O'Hara C, Srikanta S, et al. Genetically programmed selective islet beta-cell loss in diabetic subjects with Wolfram's syndrome. Diabetes Care 1989;12: 135–8.

10. Spielman RS, Bair MP, Clerget-Darpoux F. Genetic analysis of IDDM: summary of GAW5 IDDM results. Genet Epidemiol 1989;6:43–58.

11. Thomson G, Robinson WP, Kuhner MK, et al. Genetic heterogeneity, modes of inheritance and risk estimates for a joint study of caucasians with insulin-dependent diabetes mellitus. Am J Hum Genet 1988;43:799–816.

12. Johnston C, Pyke DA, Cudworth AG, Wolf E. HLA-DR typing inidentical twins with insulin-dependent diabetes: differences between concordant and discordant pairs. BMJ 1983;286:253–5.

13. Warram JH, Krolewski AS, Kahn CR. Determinants of IDDM and perinatal mortality in children of diabetic mothers. Diabetes 1988;37:1328–34.

14. The WHO Nomenclature Committee for Factors of the HLA System. Nomenclature for factors of the HLA system, 1989. Immunogenetics 1990;31:131–40.

15. Morel Y, David M, Forest MG, et al. Gene conversions and rearrangements cause discordance between inheritance of forms of 21-hydroxylase deficiency and HLA types. J Clin Endocrinol Metab 1989;68:592–9.

16. O'Brien T, Barrett B, Murray DM, et al. Usefulness of biochemical screening of diabetic patients for hemochromatosis. Diabetes Care 1990;13:532–4.

17. Bjorkman PJ, Saper MA, Samraoui B, et al. The foreign antigen binding site and T cell recognition regions of class I histocompatibility antigens. Nature 1987;329:512–8.

18. Nishimoto H, Kikutani H, Yamamura K, Kishimoto T. Prevention of autoimmune insulitis by expression of I-E molecules in NOD mice [Letter]. Nature 1987;328: 432–4.

19. Miyazaki T, Uno M, Uehira M, et al. Direct evidence for the contribution of the unique I-A NOD to the development of insulitis in non-obese diabetic mice [Letter]. Nature 1990;345:722–4.

20. Strominger JL. Biology of the human histocompatibility leukocyte antigen (HLA) system and a hypothesis regarding the generation of autoimmune diseases. J Clin Invest 1986;77:1411–5.

21. Ziegler R, Alper CA, Awdeh ZL, et al. Specific association of HLA-DR4 with increased prevalence and level of insulin autoantibodies in first-degree relatives of patients with Type I diabetes. Diabetes 1991;40:709–14.

22. Pujol-Borrell R, Todd I, Doshi M, et al. HLA class II induction in human islet cells by interferon-γ plus tumour necrosis factor or lymphotoxin. Nature 1987;326:304–6.

23. Miller J, Daitch L, Rath S, Selsing E. Tissue-specific expression of allogeneic class II MHC molecules induces neither tissue rejection nor clonal inactivation of alloreactive T cells. J Immunol 1990;144:334–41.

24. Raum D, Awdeh Z, Yunis EJ, et al. Extended major histocompatibility complex haplotypes in Type I diabetes mellitus. J Clin Invest 1984;74:449–54.

25. Todd JA, Bell JI, McDevitt HO. A molecular basis for genetic susceptibility to insulin-dependent diabetes mellitus. Trends Genet 1988;4:129–34.

26. Todd JA, Mijovic C, Fletcher J, et al. Identification of susceptibility loci for insulin-dependent diabetes mellitus by trans-racial gene mapping [Letter]. Nature 1989; 338:587–9.

27. Sheehy MJ, Scharf SJ, Rowe JR, et al. A diabetes-susceptible HLA haplotype is best defined by a combination of HLA-DR and-DQ alleles. J Clin Invest 1989;83:830–5.

28. Baisch JM, Weeks T, Giles R, et al. Analysis of HLA-DQ genotypes and susceptibility in insulin-dependent diabetes mellitus. N Engl J Med 1990;322:1836–41.

29. Horn GT, Bugawan TL, Long CM, Erlich HA. Allelic sequence variation of the HLA-DQ loci relationship to serology and to insulin-dependent diabetes susceptibility. Proc Natl Acad Sci USA 1988;85:6012–6.

30. Erlich HA, Griffith RL, Bugawan TL, et al. Implication of specific DQB1 alleles in genetic susceptibility and resistance by identification of IDDM siblings with novel HLA-DZB1 allele and unusual DR2 and DR1 haplotypes. Diabetes 1991;40:478–81.

31. Erlich HA, Bugawan TL. HLA class II gene polymorphism: DNA typing, evolution and relationship to disease susceptibility. In: Erlich HA, ed. PCR technology: principles and applications for DNA amplification. New York: Stockton Press, 1989:193–208.

32. Ahonen P, Myllarniemi S, Sipila I, Perheentupa J. Clinical variation of autoimmune polyendocrinopathy-candidiasis-ectodermal dystrophy (apeced) in a series of 68 patients. N Engl J Med 1990;322:26:1829–6.

33. Maclaren NK, Riley WJ. Inherited susceptibility to autoimmune Addison's disease is linked to human leukocyte antigens-DR3 and/or DR4 except when associated with Type I autoimmune polyglandular syndrome. J Clin Endocrinol Metab 1986;62:455–9.

34. Eisenbarth GS, Wilson PW, Ward F, et al. The polyglandular failure syndrome: disease inheritance, HLA-type and immune function: studies in patients and families. Ann Intern Med 1979;91:528–33.

35. Fajans SS. Scope and heterogeneous nature of MODY. Diabetes Care 1990;13:49–64.

36. Winter WE, Maclaren NK, Riley WJ, et al. Maturity-onset diabetes of youth in black Americans. N Engl J Med 1987;316:285–91.

37. Patrick SL, Moy CS, LaPorte RE. The world of insulin-dependent diabetes mellitus: what international epidemiologic studies reveal about the etiology and natural history of IDDM. Diabetes Metab Rev 1989;5:571–8.

38. Yoon JW, McClintock PR, Bachurski CJ, et al. Virus-induced diabetes mellitus: no evidence for immune mechanisms in the destruction of β-cells by the D-variant of encephalomyocarditis virus. Diabetes 1985;34: 922–5.

39. King ML, Shaikh A, Bidwell D, et al. Coxsackie-B-virus specific IgM responses in children with insulin-dependent (juvenile-onset; Type I) diabetes mellitus. Lancet 1983; 1:1397–9.

40. Jenson AB, Rosenberg HS, Notkins AL. Pancreatic islet-cell damage in children with fatal viral infections. Lancet 1980;2:354–8.

41. Yoon J-W, Austin M, Onodera T, Notkins AL. Virus-induced diabetes mellitus: isolation of a virus from pancreas of a child with diabetic ketoacidosis. N Engl J Med 1979; 300:1173–9.

42. Ginsberg-Fellner F, Witt ME, Yagihasi S, et al. Congenital rubella syndrome as a model for Type I (insulin-depen-

dent) diabetes mellitus: increased prevalence of islet cell surface antibodies. Diabetologia 1984;27:87−9.

43. Karounos DG, Thomas JW. Recognition of common islet antigen by autoantibodies from NOD mice and humans with IDDM. Diabetes 1990;39:1085−90.

44. Ward KP, Galloway WH, Auchterlonie IA. Congenital cytomegalovirus infection and diabetes [Letter]. Lancet 1979;1:497.

45. Pak C-Y, Eun H-M, McArthur RG, Yoon J-W. Association of cytomegalovirus infection with autoimmune Type I diabetes. Lancet 1988;2:1−4.

46. Hellqvist LNB, Rhodes CJ, Taylor KW. Long-term biochemical changes in the islets of Langerhans in mice following infection with encephalomyocarditis virus. Diabetologia 1984;26:370−4.

47. Bae Y-S, Eun H-M, Yoon J-W. Molecular identification of diabetogenic viral gene. Diabetes 1989;38:316−20.

48. Gerling I, Nejman C, Chatterjee NK. Effect of coxsackievirus B4 infection in mice on expression of 64,000-Mr autoantigen and glucose sensitivity of islets before development of hyperglycemia. Diabetes 1988;37:1419−25.

49. Guberski DL, Thomas VA, Shek WR, et al. Induction of type 1 diabetes by Kilham's rat virus in diabetes-resistant BB/Wor rats. Science 1991;254:1010−3.

50. Suenaga K, Yoon J-W. Association of β-cell-specific expression of endogenous retrovirus with development of insulitis and diabetes in NOD mouse. Diabetes 1988;37:1722−6.

51. Ciampolillo A, Marini V, Mirakian R, et al. Retrovirus-like sequences in Graves' disease: implications for human autoimmunity. Lancet 1989;1:1096−9.

52. Oldstone MBA. Prevention of Type I diabetes in nonobese diabetic mice by virus infection. Science 1988;239:500−2.

53. Oldstone MBA. Prevention of Type I diabetes in nonobese diabetic mice by virus infection. Science 1988;239:500−2.

54. Coleman DL, Kuzava JE, Leiter EH. Effect of diet on incidence of diabetes in nonobese diabetic mice. Diabetes 1990;39:432−6.

55. Elliott RB, Martin JM. Dietary protein: a trigger of insulin-dependent diabetes in the BB rat? Diabetologia 1984;26:297−9.

56. Mayer EJ, Hamman RH, Gay EC, et al. Reduced risk of IDDM among breast-fed children: the Colorado IDDM registry. Diabetes 1988;37:1625−32.

57. Siemiatycki J, Colle E, Campbell S, et al. Case-control study of IDDM. Diabetes Care 1989;12:209−16.

58. Martin JM, Trink B, Daneman D, et al. Milk proteins in the etiology of insulin-dependent diabetes mellitus (IDDM). Ann Med 1991;23:447−52.

59. Diabetes Epidemiology Research International Group. Geographic patterns of childhood insulin-dependent diabetes mellitus. Diabetes 1988;37:1113−9.

60. Ziegler AG, Baumgartl HJ, Ede G, et al. Low-pigment skin type and predisposition for development of Type I diabetes. Diabetes Care 1990;13:529−31.

61. Bottazzo GF, Florin-Christensen A, Doniach D. Islet-cell antibodies in diabetes mellitus with autoimmune polyendocrine deficiencies. Lancet 1974;2:1279−83.

62. MacCuish AC, Barnes EW, Irvine WJ, Duncan LJP. Antibodies to pancreatic islet cells in insulin-dependent diabetics with coexistent autoimmune disease. Lancet 1974;2:1529−31.

63. Gleichmann H, Bottazzo GF. Progress toward standardization of cytoplasmic islet cell-antibody assay. Diabetes 1987;36:578−84.

64. Bonifacio E, Lernmark A, Dawkins RL, et al. Serum exchange and use of dilutions have improved precision of measurement of islet cell antibodies. J Immunol Methods 1988;106:83−8.

65. Boitard C, Bonifacio F, Bottazzo GF, et al. Immunology and Diabetes Workshop: report on the third international (stage 3) workshop on the standardization of cytoplasmic islet cell antibodies. Diabetologia 1988;31:451−2.

66. Pilcher C, Elliott RB. Improved sensitivity of islet cell cytoplasmic antibody assay in diabetics [Letter]. Lancet 1984;1:1352.

67. Spencer KM, Tarn A, Dean BM, et al. Fluctuating islet-cell autoimmunity in unaffected relatives of patients with insulin-dependent diabetes. Lancet 1984;1:764−6.

68. Colman PG, Tautkus M, Rabizadeh A, et al. Assay for islet cell antibodies with rat pancreas and peroxidase protein A [Letter]. Diabetes Care 1988;11:367−8.

69. Bottazzo GF, Dean BM, Gorsuch AN, et al. Complement-fixing islet-cell antibodies in Type I-diabetes: possible monitors of active beta-cell damage. Lancet 1980;1:668−72.

70. Gianani R, Rabizadeh A, Jackson R, et al. Heterogeneity of cytoplasmic islet cell autoantibodies. Diabetes 1992;41:347−53.

71. Pugliese A, Gianani R, Alper CA, et al. Class II determinants of restricted islet cell antibodies (stiff-man syndrome like anti-GAD ICA) and protection from Type I diabetes. Clin Res 1992;40:299A.

72. Landin-Olsson M, Karlsson A, Dahlquist G, et al. Islet cell and other organ-specific autoantibodies in all children developing Type I (insulin-dependent) diabetes mellitus in Sweden during one year and in matched control children. Diabetologia 1989;32:387−95.

73. Nayak RC, Omar MAK, Rabizadeh A, et al. "Cytoplasmic" islet cell antibodies: evidence that the target antigen is a sialoglycoconjugate. Diabetes 1985;34:617−9.

74. Colman PG, Nayak RC, Campbell IL, Eisenbarth GS. Binding of cytoplasmic islet cell antibodies is blocked by human pancreatic glycolipid extracts. Diabetes 1988;37:645−52.

75. Dotta F, Colman PG, Lombardi D, et al. Ganglioside expression in human pancreatic islets. Diabetes 1989;38:1478−83.

76. Palmer JP, Asplin CM, Clemons P, et al. Insulin antibodies in insulin-dependent diabetics before insulin treatment. Science 1983;222:1337−9.

77. Ziegler AG, Herskowitz RD, Jackson RA, et al. Predicting Type I diabetes. Diabetes Care 1990;13:762−75.

78. Wilkin T, Palmer J, Bonifacio E, et al. First international workshop on the standardization of insulin autoantibodies. Diabetologia 1987;30:676−7.

79. Ziegler AG, Ziegler R, Vardi P, et al. Life-table analysis of progression to diabetes of anti-insulin autoantibody-positive relatives of individuals with Type I diabetes. Diabetes 1989;38:1320−5.

80. Atkinson MA, Maclaren NK, Riley WJ, et al. Are insulin autoantibodies markers for insulin-dependent diabetes mellitus? Diabetes 1986;35:894−8.

81. Ziegler AG, Ziegler R, Jackson RA, Eisenbarth GS. Testing the linear destruction hypothesis in Type I diabetes: the Joslin study. In: Andreani D, Kolb H, Pozzilli P, eds. Immunotherapy of Type I diabetes. Chichester: John Wiley & Sons, 1989:155−67.

82. Wilkin TJ, Schoenfeld SL, Diaz J-L, et al. Systematic variation and differences in insulin-autoantibody measurements. Diabetes 1989;38:172−81.

83. Castano L, Ziegler R, Reske I, Eisenbarth GS. Proinsulin autoantibodies (PIAA) in prediabetics and autoantibody positive relatives of patients with Type I diabetes [Abstract no. 961]. Diabetes 1990;39(Suppl 1):247A.

84. Baekkeskov S, Nielsen JH, Marner B, et al. Autoantibodies in newly diagnosed diabetic children immunoprecipitate human pancreatic islet cel proteins. Nature 1982; 298:167–9.

85. Baekkeskov S, Landin M, Kristensen JK, et al. Antibodies to a 64,000 Mr human islet cell antigen precede the clinical onset of insulin dependent diabetes. J Clin Invest 1987; 79:926–34.

86. Solimena M, Folli F, Denis-Donini S, et al. Autoantibodies to glutamic acid decarboxylase in a patient with stiff-man syndrome, epilepsy, and Type I diabetes mellitus. N Engl J Med 1988;318:1012–20.

87. Baekkeskov S, Aanstoot H-J, Christgaus S, et al. Identification of the 64k autoantigen in insulin-dependent diabetes as the GABA-synthesizing enzyme glutamic acid decarboxylase. Nature 1990;347:151–6.

88. Flier JS, Bar RS, Muggeo M, et al. The evolving clinical course of patients with insulin receptor autoantibodies: spontaneous remission or receptor proliferation with hypoglycemia. J Clin Endocrinol Metab 1978;47: 985–95.

89. Maron R, Elias D, de Jongh BM, et al. Autoantibodies to the insulin receptor in juvenile onset insulin-dependent diabetes [Letter]. Nature 1983;303:817–8.

90. Ludwig SM, Faiman C, Dean HJ. Insulin and insulin-receptor autoantibodies in children with newly diagnosed IDDM before insulin therapy. Diabetes 1987;36:420–5.

91. Batarseh H, Thompson RA, Odugbesan O, Barnett AH. Insulin receptor antibodies in diabetes mellitus. Clin Exp Immunol 1988;71:85–90.

92. Lernmark A, Freedman ZR, Hofmann C, et al. Islet-cell-surface antibodies in juvenile diabetes mellitus. N Engl J Med 1978;299:375–80.

93. Cavender DE, Virji MA, Holze-Joost S. Presence of complement-dependent cytotoxic activity against clonally-derived rat islet tumour cells in sera from Type I (insulin-dependent) diabetic patients and control subjects. Diabetologia 1986;29:616–22.

94. Pietropaolo M, Castano L, Russo E, et al. Utilization of a rat λGT11 islet library to identify novel autoantigens associated with Type I diabetes. Diabetes 1991 (in press).

95. Tattersall RB, Pyke DA. Diabetes in identical twins. Lancet 1975;2:1120–5.

96. Srikanta S, Ganda OP, Jackson RA, et al. Type I diabetes mellitus in monozygotic twins: chronic progressive beta cell dysfunction. Ann Intern Med 1983;99:320–6.

97. Srikanta S, Ganda OP, Rabizadeh A, et al. First-degree relatives of patients with Type I diabetes mellitus: islet-cell antibodies and abnormal insulin secretion. N Engl J Med 1985;313:461–4.

98. Herskowitz RD, Jackson RA, Soeldner JS, Eisenbarth GS. Pilot trial to prevent Type I diabetes: progression to overt IDDM despite oral nicotinamide. J Autoimmun 1989; 2:733–7.

99. Eisenbarth GS, Srikanta S, Fleischnick E, et al. Progressive autoimmune beta cell insufficiency: occurrence in the absence of high-risk HLA alleles DR3, DR4. Diabetes Care 1985;8:477–80.

100. Vardi P, Crisa L, Jackson RA, et al. Predictive value of intravenous glucose tolerance test insulin secretion less than or greater than the first percentile in islet cell antibody positive relatives of Type I (insulin-dependent) diabetic patients. Diabetologia 1991;34:93–102.

101. Bingley PJ, Colman P, Eisenbarth GS, et al. Standardization of the intravenous glucose tolerance test for use in prediction of insulin-dependent diabetes. Diabetes Care 1992 (in press).

102. Smith CP, Tarn AC, Thomas JM, et al. Between and within subject variation of the first phase insulin response to intravenous glucose. Diabetologia 1988;31:123–5.

103. Smith CP, Williams AJK, Thomas JM, et al. The pattern of basal and stimulated insulin responses to intravenous glucose in first degree relatives of Type I (insulin-dependent) diabetic children and unrelated adults aged 5 to 50 years. Diabetologia 1988;31:430–4.

104. Bleich D, Jackson RA, Soeldner JS, Eisenbarth GS. Analysis of metabolic progression to Type I diabetes in ICA⁺ relatives of patients with Type I diabetes. Diabetes Care 1990;13:111–8.

105. Jackson R, Vardi P, Herskowitz R, et al. Dual parameter linear model for prediction of onset of Type I diabetes in islet cell antibody positive relatives. Clin Res 1988; 36:484A.

106. Gorsuch AN, Spencer KM, Lister J, et al. Evidence for a long prediabetic period in Type I (insulin-dependent) diabetes mellitus. Lancet 1981;2:1363–5.

107. Tarn AC, Thomas JM, Dean BM, et al. Predicting insulin-dependent diabetes. Lancet 1988;1:845–50.

108. Tarn AC, Smith CP, Spencer KM, et al. Type I (insulin-dependent) diabetes: a disease of slow clinical onset? BMJ 1987;294:342–5.

109. Bingley PJ, Gale EAM. Prediction of Type I diabetes: the Barts-Windsor family study. In: Andreani D, Kolb H, Pozzilli P, eds. Immunotherapy of Type I diabetes. Chichester: John Wiley & Sons, 1989:137–45.

110. Maclaren N, Riley W, Silverstein J, et al. Progress towards the prevention of insulin-dependent diabetes: the Gainesville studies. In: Andreani D, Kolb H, Pozzilli P, eds. Immunotherapy of Type I diabetes. Chichester: John Wiley & Sons, 1989:147–54.

111. Atkinson MA, Maclaren NK, Riley WJ, et al. Are insulin autoantibodies markers for insulin-dependent diabetes mellitus? Diabetes 1986;35:894–8.

112. Riley WJ, Maclaren NK, Spillar RP, et al. The use of islet cell autoantibodies in identifying "prediabetes." In: Larkins RG, Zimmet PZ, Chisolm DJ, eds. Diabetes 1988. New York: Excerpta Medica, 1989;263–7.

113. Elliott RB, Chase HP. Prevention or delay of Type I (insulin-dependent) diabetes mellitus in children using nicotinamide. Diabetologia 1991;34:362–5.

114. Chase HP, Voss Ma, Butler-Simon N, et al. Diagnosis of pre-Type I diabetes. J Pediatr 1987;111:807–12.

115. American Diabetes Association Position Statement. Prevention of Type I diabetes mellitus. Diabetes 1990; 39:1151–2.

116. Riley WJ, Maclaren NK, Spillar RP. The development of insulin dependent diabetes after donating kidney to diabetic sibling. Diabetes Care 1990;13:883–5.

117. Johnson SB, Riley WJ, Hansen CA, Nurick MA. Psychological impact of islet cell antibody screening: preliminary results. Diabetes Care 1990;13:93–7.

118. Herskowitz RD, Wolfsdorf JI, Ricker AT, et al. Transient hyperglycemia in childhood: identification of a subgroup with imminent diabetes mellitus. Diabetes Res 1988; 9:161–7

119. Dupré J, Stiller CR, Gent M, et al. Clinical trials of cyclosporin in IDDM. Diabetes Care 1988;11(Suppl 1): 37–44.

120. Bougneres PF, Carel JC, Castano L, et al. Factors associated with early remission of Type I diabetes in children

treated with cyclosporine. N Engl J Med 1988;318: 663–70.

121. Marks JB, Skyler S. Immunotherapy of Type I diabetes. J Clin Endocrinol Metab 1991;72:3–9.

122. Robertson RB, Franklin G, Nelson L. Intravenous glucose tolerance and pancreatic islet β-cell function in patients with multiple sclerosis during 2-year treatment with cyclosporin. Diabetes 1989;38:58–64.

123. Silverstein J, Maclaren N, Riley W, et al. Immunosuppression with azathioprine and prednisone in recent-onset insulin-dependent diabetes mellitus. N Engl J Med 1988; 319:599–604.

124. Tochino Y. The NOD mouse as a model of Type I diabetes. Crit Rev Immunol 1987;8:49–81.

125. Nomikos IN, Prowse SJ, Carotenuto P, Lafferty KJ. Combined treatment with nicotinamide and desferrioxamine prevents islet allograft destruction in NOD mice. Diabetes 1986;35:1302–4.

126. Pozzilli P, Visalli N, Ghirlanda G, et al. Nicotinamide increases C-peptide secretion in patients with recent onset Type I diabetes. Diabetic Med 1989;6:568–72.

127. Herskowitz R, Jackson RA. Pilot trial of preventive therapy: progression to overt hyperglycemia by 3/3 "prediabetics" despite oral nicotinamide [Abstract no. 233]. Diabetes 1988;37(Suppl 1):59A.

128. Shah SC, Malone JI, Simpson NE. A randomized trial of intensive insulin therapy in newly diagnosed insulin-dependent diabetes mellitus. N Engl J Med 1989; 320:550–4.

129. Keller RJ, Jackson RA, Eisenbarth GS. Preservation of beta cell function in islet cell antibody (ICA) positive first degreee relatives treated with insulin [Abstract]. Diabetes 1992;41(Suppl 1):50A.

130. Shizuru JA, Taylor-Edwards C, Banks BA, et al. Immunotherapy of the nonobese diabetic mouse: treatment with an antibody to T-helper lymphocytes. Science 1988; 240:659–62.

131. Schwartz S, Skyler J, Einhorn D, et al. Treatment of new onset Type I diabetics with a Pan T lymphocyte immunoconjugate H65-RTA. Diabetes 1991;40(Suppl 1):229A.

132. Pankewycz O, Mackie J, Hassarjion R, et al. Interleukin-2-diphtheria toxin fusion protein prolongs murine islet cell engraftment. Transplantation 1989;47:318–22.

133. Hahn HJ, Lucke S, Klöting I, et al. Curing BB rats of freshly manifested diabetes by short-term treatment with a combination of a monoclonal anti-interleukin 2 receptor anitbody and a subtherapeutic dose of cyclosporin A. Eur J Immunol 1987;17:1075–8.

134. Cohen IR. Autoimmunity to chaperonins in the pathogenesis of arthritis and diabetes. Ann Rev Immunol 1991; 9:567–89.

135. Sadelain MW, Qin HY, Lauzon J, Singh B. Prevention of Type I diabetes in NOD mice by adjuvant immunotherapy. Diabetes 1990;39:583–9.

136. Goldman J, Baldwin D, Rubenstein AH, et al. Characterization of circulating insulin and proinsulin-binding antibodies in autoimmune hypoglycemia. J Clin Invest 1979; 63:1050–9.

137. Wasada T, Eguchi Y, Takayama S, et al. Insulin autoimmune syndrome associated with benign monoclonal gammopathy. Evidence for monoclonal insulin autoantibodies. Diabetes Care 1989;12:147–50.

138. Eisenbarth GS, Shimizu K, Bowring MA, Wells S. Expression of receptors for tetanus toxin and monoclonal antibody A2B5 by pancreatic islet cells. Proc Natl Acad Sci USA 1982;79:5066–70.

139. Powers AC, Rabizadeh A, Akeson R, Eisenbarth GS. Characterization of monocolonal antibody 3G5 and utilization of this antibody to immobilize pancreatic islet cell gangliosides in a solid phase radioassay. Endocrinology 1984;114:1338–43.

140. Alejandro R, Shienvold FL, Hajek SAV, et al. A ganglioside antigen on the rat pancreatic B cell surface identified by monoclonal antibody R2D6. J Clin Invest 1984;74:25–38.

141. Brown FM, Smith AM, Longway S, Rabinowe SL. Adrenal medullitis in Type I diabetes. J Clin Endocrinol Metab 1990;71:1491–5.

142. Rabinowe SL, Brown FM, Watts M, Smith AM. Complement-fixing antibodies to sympathetic and parasympathetic tissues in IDDM: autonomic brake index and heart-rate variation. Diabetes Care 1990;13:1084–8.

143. Brown FM, Vinik AI, Ganda OP, et al. Different effects of duration on prevalence of anti-adrenal medullary and pancreatic islet cell antibodies in Type I diabetes mellitus. Horm Metab Res 1989;21:434–7.

144. Quimby SR, Muller SA, Schroeter AL. The cutaneous immunopathology of necrobiosis lipoidica diabeticorum. Arch Dermatol 1988;124:1364–71.

145. Nayak RC, Berman AB, George KL, et al. A monoclonal antibody (3G5) defined ganglioside antigen is expressed on the cell surface of microvascular pericytes. J Exp Med 1988;167:1003–15.

146. Eisenbarth GS. Type I diabetes mellitus: a chronic autoimmune disease. N Engl J Med 1986;314:1360–8.

147. Sutherland DE, Sibley R, Xu X, et al. Twin to twin pancreas transplantation: reversal and reenactment of the pathogenesis of Type I diabetes. Trans Assoc Am Physicians 1984;97:80–7.

Chapter 14

PATHOGENESIS OF NON-INSULIN-DEPENDENT (TYPE II) DIABETES MELLITUS

GORDON C. WEIR
JACK L. LEAHY

Non-insulin-dependent diabetes mellitus (NIDDM) accounts for over 85% of diabetes worldwide and is associated with an enormous amount of morbidity and mortality resulting from its microvascular, macrovascular, and neuropathic complications. In the United States alone, the financial costs of NIDDM probably exceed $30 billion,[1] and the suffering incurred is enormous. The prevalence of NIDDM is closely linked to industrialization, affluence, and increased life expectancy, a combination of factors that has allowed the problem to grow at a frightening rate during the past few decades. One must reluctantly predict that the number of individuals afflicted with this disease will increase at an even faster rate in the foreseeable future.

Descriptions of NIDDM have been available for many years. In 1893 William Osler wrote: "Hereditary influences play an important role. . . . It is a disease of adult life; a majority of the cases occur from the third to the sixth decade. . . . In a considerable proportion of the cases of diabetes the subjects have been excessively fat at the beginning of, or prior to, the onset of the disease. . . . The combination of . . . over-indulgence in food and drink, with a sedentary life, seem particularly prone to

induce the disease."[2] This description summarizes the fundamental elements of NIDDM.

The environmental factors that contribute to the development of NIDDM are partially understood, but the important genetic basis of the disease remains to be defined. The superficial phenotypic aspects of the syndrome have been described in detail, and much has been learned about some aspects of its pathogenesis. The disease is characterized by abnormalities of insulin secretion and resistance of tissues to the action of insulin, with muscle and liver being particularly important. The relative contributions of these two abnormalities in established NIDDM are now reasonably well understood, but the early pathogenetic events continue to be poorly defined. NIDDM has always been assumed to be a heterogeneous disease. In the past 10 years individuals, who have fulfilled the definition for NIDDM, have been found to have specific mutations of the insulin molecule, the insulin receptor, and the enzyme glucokinase, accounting for their hyperglycemia. The conditions stemming from these different mutations are now considered to be separate diseases. Undoubtedly, other types of mutations will continue to emerge from the enormous pool of individuals with NIDDM. Because so little is known about the genetic basis of NIDDM, the focus of this chapter will be the metabolic changes that underlie the pathogenesis of this important disease.

DEFINITION AND EPIDEMIOLOGY OF NON-INSULIN-DEPENDENT DIABETES (NIDDM)

The definition of NIDDM and the criteria for diagnosis are discussed in detail in Chapter 11. The term *non-insulin-dependent diabetes mellitus,* which is synonymous with Type II diabetes mellitus, became widely used after the publication of the report of the National Diabetes Data Group in 1979.[3] A similar classification was developed by the World Health Organization.[4] This disease was previously called maturity-onset or adult-onset diabetes mellitus. The entity of impaired glucose tolerance (IGT), a condition of glucose intolerance not severe enough to satisfy the criteria for the diagnosis of diabetes, also was defined by the National Diabetes Data Group and has proven to be a useful category. IGT is associated with relatively little microvascular disease but with an increased risk of macrovascular disease,[5,6] and 5% or more of these patients per year go on to develop NIDDM.[7-9] Thus, people with IGT probably can benefit from weight loss and exercise, as well as from other steps to reduce cardiovascular risk factors. Furthermore, IGT has been a useful category for investigators attempting to learn more about the early events in the pathogenesis of NIDDM.

Unfortunately, the term NIDDM has weaknesses—particularly in its focus on severity and phenotype rather than on etiology and genotype. One can make an analogy between NIDDM and anemia, in that many pathways can lead to each condition. Thus, individuals with moderate rather than severe chronic pancreatitis might be diagnosed as having NIDDM; likewise, people with autoimmune β-cell destruction might be at an early or incomplete stage of the disease. In Finland 10% of a group of subjects with NIDDM were found to have antibodies to islet cells.[10] This figure may have been an underestimate of the prevalence of autoimmune diabetes, since others with this condition may have been antibody-negative. Another diabetic state that frequently fits the criteria for NIDDM is so-called malnutrition-related diabetes, also known as tropical diabetes, pancreatic diabetes, or J-type diabetes.[11] There is a fibrocalcific form of diabetes that may be associated with eating the root of cassava and another form that is more closely related to protein deficiency. In any case, because so little is known about the causes of NIDDM, use of the term often leads to confusion. For example, it is difficult to categorize the patients who have mild diabetes, are thin, and are 30 to 50 years old. In addition, it is often difficult to make a confident diagnosis of IDDM or NIDDM in the older patient who is taking insulin. These uncertainties create problems for investigators studying NIDDM, because subjects within any experimental group are likely to have different underlying causes for their diabetes.

A subset of NIDDM is called maturity-onset diabetes of the young (MODY). In these individuals, the diagnosis of diabetes is usually made before the age of 25 years, with the diabetes being nonketotic and typically responsive to diet and/or sulfonylurea therapy. MODY is familial, and in some families the inheritance pattern is consistent with an autosomal dominant defect.[12] Recently it has been found that many families, perhaps over half, have mutations in the enzyme glucokinase.[13,14] This enzyme is thought to serve as the glucose sensor of the β-cell and, in addition, to be important for optimal hepatic glucose uptake, making these mutations highly likely to be the cause of diabetes in this syndrome. Indeed, one would predict that such a defect in the β-cell would lead to a higher set-point for glucose-induced insulin secretion, and this has been found in several kindreds. Some other families have been found to show close linkage to the gene locus of adenosine deaminase on chromosome 20,[15] but there is no particular reason to think this enzyme is involved in the pathogenesis. There must be other heterogeneity among MODY families because in several parts of the world families have been identified in which the inheritance is not consistent with an autosomal dominant pattern.[16] In addition, a syndrome has been described in young black Americans who presented with severe symptoms necessitating insulin therapy but whose course was much milder than that seen in typical IDDM.[17] The inheritance pattern of this group was consistent with a dominant gene defect, and none of the immune markers normally found in IDDM were present.

With regard to the heterogeneity of NIDDM, much remains to be learned about the genetic and environmental factors accounting for the marked differences in prevalence seen throughout the world (see Chapter 12 on epidemiology). For example, among the Pima Indians of Arizona, the prevalence of NIDDM is about 50% in adults over the age of 35 years.[18] Among the Nauruans of Micronesia, the prevalence is only modestly lower.[19] In contrast, whites in Australia, Bantus in Tanzania, and rural Polynesians show a prevalence that is only about one-tenth of these high rates.[20] In addition, striking changes in prevalence rates can be found when racial groups move to different parts of the world. Two well-studied examples are Asian Indians living in the United Kingdom[21] and Japanese living in the United States.[22]

The many other epidemiologic factors relevant to the pathogenesis of NIDDM are discussed in more detail in Chapter 12. Increases in both incidence and prevalence rates of NIDDM with age have been documented in many population groups.[23] Changes in carbohydrate metabolism occur with normal aging that differ from those in NIDDM, with many individuals showing normal fasting glucose concentrations but glucose intolerance after an oral glucose challenge.[24] The gender differences in prevalence of NIDDM that have been observed in some groups are minor and suggest that gender is not an important factor in pathogenesis. Uterine environment may be important. Studies of Pima Indians indicate that the prevalence of diabetes is considerably higher in the offspring of diabetic mothers than in the offspring of diabetic fathers.[25] Questions have been raised, but remain unsettled, about whether multiparity increases the risk of NIDDM in the offspring.[26-28] Recently, an interesting hypothesis was advanced suggesting that low weight at birth and at 1 year of age is associated with diabetes and glucose intolerance later in life, with questions being raised about impaired early growth somehow being related to diminished insulin production many years later.[29] Many studies have examined the impact of nutrition on the incidence of NIDDM; the most obvious conclusion is that diets leading to obesity are strongly associated with NIDDM. Furthermore, it has been shown that a "Western diet" with a high fat content can worsen glucose tolerance in Pima Indians.[31] Exercise is known to improve insulin action, and there are data consistent with the hypothesis that a long-term increase in physical activity is associated with a reduced prevalence of NIDDM.[31,32]

ALTERED FUEL METABOLISM IN NIDDM

Fasting Hyperglycemia

NIDDM is characterized by both fasting and postprandial hyperglycemia. In the fasting (postabsorptive) state, plasma glucose concentrations are maintained by a balance between hepatic glucose production (HGP) and glucose uptake by peripheral tissues.[33,34] Hormonal regulation of HGP is provided primarily by the combined effects of insulin and glucagon secretion, whereas glucose

disposal is regulated by insulin and various other insulin-independent mechanisms. In nondiabetic individuals, after an overnight fast the rate of glucose release by liver is about 8 g/hour, 70% of which originates from glycogenolysis and the rest from gluconeogenesis.[35] About 25% of this glucose is taken up by neural tissue through insulin-independent mechanisms, about 10% by splanchnic and adipose tissue, and the major share—about 60%—by muscle.[36-38] Once frank NIDDM is present, with fasting plasma glucose values greater than 140 mg/dL (7.7 mM), HGP is usually elevated and continues to increase as the diabetic state worsens (Fig. 14-1), even in the face of a suppressive effect of hyperglycemia on the glucose output of the liver.[38,39] Glucose uptake by neural tissue is thought to remain stable, and glucose disposal by muscle is actually increased,[40,41] being accomplished by the combination of an insulin-stimulated uptake and a concentration-dependent mass-action effect of glucose.[42,43]

Insight into the contribution of insulin resistance to the abnormalities in glucose disposal in NIDDM can be fully appreciated only by maintaining the same glucose concentration in diabetic and control subjects so that the mass-action effect of glucose on uptake is normalized. This is best accomplished with the euglycemic insulin-clamp, which holds glucose levels at 100 mg/dL (5.5 mM) and plasma insulin concentrations at about 100 μU/mL. In patients with NIDDM, glucose disposal by muscle is then found to be about 60% of normal[38] (Fig. 14-2). Thus, the most obvious site of insulin resistance in NIDDM is in muscle; the liver defect is more complicated.[44-46] The liver was thought to be more sensitive than muscle to the

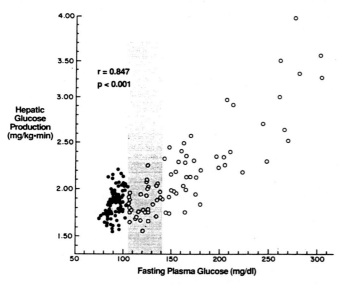

Fig. 14-1. Depiction of hepatic glucose production and rising fasting plasma glucose levels in 77 non-obese subjects with non-insulin-dependent diabetes (open circles) and 73 age- and weight-matched controls (closed circles). In those subjects with fasting glucose levels greater than 140 mg/dL, there was a close correlation between increasing HGP and rising glucose levels. Reprinted with permission from reference 38 (DeFronzo RA. The triumvirate: β-cell, muscle, liver: a collusion responsible for NIDDM. Diabetes 1988;37:667-87; copyright © of the American Diabetes Association).

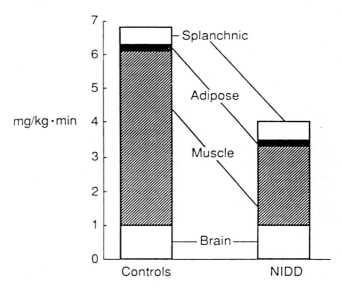

Fig. 14-2. Glucose uptake by various tissues during euglycemic insulin (100 μU/mL)-clamp studies in 38 normal-weight subjects with non-insulin-dependent diabetes (NIDD) and 33 matched controls. Reprinted with permission from reference 38 (DeFronzo RA. The triumvirate: β-cell, muscle, liver: a collusion responsible for NIDDM. Diabetes 1988;37:667-87; copyright © of the American Diabetes Association).

effects of insulin,[38] but this conclusion must be revised now that an artefact in the glucose-clamp technique has been identified.[47] It now appears that the dose-response curves for insulin effects on uptake of glucose by muscle and HGP in NIDDM show comparable degrees of insulin resistance.[47] Further evidence for impaired insulin action on HGP is provided by the observation that, in the fasting state, subjects with NIDDM usually will have either normal or elevated levels of plasma insulin and increased HGP. This finding, by definition, tells us that the liver is resistant to insulin.

States of Impaired Glucose Tolerance and Mild NIDDM

The pathophysiology of IGT and mild NIDDM is similar to that found in more severe NIDDM. Fasting glucose concentrations are higher than normal, but HGP is normal. Fasting plasma insulin concentrations are typically elevated in these milder forms of diabetes, and HGP would be expected to be suppressed if hepatic insulin resistance were not present. This is currently the strongest argument for the presence of hepatic insulin resistance in these states. Yet, with HGP being normal, there must be a defect in glucose disposal to account for the hyperglycemia, and such a defect has been found in the early stages of diabetes.[44,48] Therefore, in IGT and mild NIDDM, fasting HGP is increased in either a relative or absolute sense and glucose uptake by muscle is impaired.

Glucose Metabolism in Muscle

The major uptake mechanism for glucose in muscle is the insulin-sensitive glucose transporter GLUT-4.[49,50] Once inside the cell, glucose is for the most part stored as glycogen, with the key enzymatic step being glycogen synthase (nonoxidative glucose metabolism), or oxidized to carbon dioxide and water by pyruvate dehydrogenase and the Krebs cycle; very little is converted to lactate or lipid.[36] In an insulin-stimulated state, such as that produced by euglycemic insulin-clamping, during which events resemble those during a meal, total glucose metabolism by muscle is about 25 g/hour; 60% is nonoxidative and 40% is oxidative.[48,51] In moderately severe NIDDM, insulin-stimulated glucose metabolism is reduced by about 45%, with about 35% accounted for by nonoxidative metabolism and the remaining 10% by oxidative metabolism.[38,48,51] In milder diabetic states such as IGT, only the reduction of nonoxidative metabolism is measurable.[48] Important questions in relation to NIDDM are how much of the defect in muscle glucose uptake can be accounted for by glucose transport alone and to what extent post-transport pathways can be rate-limiting.[52] Considerable attention has therefore focused on glycogen synthase, and the responsiveness of the enzyme to insulin has been found to be decreased in subjects with NIDDM.[53,54] There is less reason to think that the oxidative pathway of glucose is rate-limiting, but the insulin responsiveness of pyruvate dehydrogenase has been found to be impaired in NIDDM.[55]

Lipid Oxidation

There has been considerable interest in the possibility of a deleterious influence of free fatty acids (FFA) on glucose metabolism in NIDDM. Oxidation of FFA in muscle can inhibit glucose oxidation, as well as glucose transport and glycogen synthesis, thus potentially reducing glucose disposal through a complex set of mechanisms found in the "glucose-fatty acid cycle."[56] Correlative relationships suggest that such mechanisms may be important in obesity and in obese subjects with NIDDM.[57,58] However, studies suggest that FFA metabolism is not significantly altered in persons with mild NIDDM or in individuals at risk of developing NIDDM.[59] There are no convincing reports of clearly important effects of FFA on glucose uptake by muscle in persons with full-blown NIDDM, although infusions of Intralipid have been found to reduce both the oxidative and nonoxidative pathways of glucose metabolism.[60,61] A more important contribution of FFA to the hyperglycemia of NIDDM may be accomplished through the enhancement of HGP by FFA-induced stimulation of gluconeogenesis, a hypothesis that has been strengthened by the finding that inhibitors of FFA release lead to a profound reduction in HGP.[62,63]

Glucose Metabolism in the Fed State

NIDDM is characterized by excessive increases in plasma glucose levels after ingestion of either glucose or meals, elevations superimposed on fasting hyperglycemia. These large glycemic excursions result from a failure in inhibition of HGP in combination with a reduction in glucose uptake by muscle.[41,64] In moderately severe NIDDM, these abnormalities result from a combination of inadequate insulin secretion and insulin resistance by both liver and muscle. The failure to appropriately suppress plasma glucagon levels probably contributes to persistently elevated HGP. In addition, failure to suppress FFA levels may play a role. A less-straightforward situation is that of very mild NIDDM or IGT, in which excessive increases in glucose concentrations may be associated with insulin levels that are considerably higher than normal. A failure of early insulin release, coupled with poor suppression of glucagon secretion, within the first 30 minutes of an oral glucose tolerance test (OGTT) probably leads to enhanced HGP and resultant hyperglycemia, which feeds back to stimulate insulin secretion.[65,66] Thus, the insulin levels seen at 90 or 120 minutes after an oral glucose challenge are higher than those found in subjects with normal glucose tolerance but are inadequate when the level of hyperglycemia is taken into account. Considerable attention is paid to the excessive postprandial glycemic excursions found in NIDDM and the interesting pathophysiology that underlies this abnormality. However, in the pathogenesis of NIDDM, the fundamental metabolic abnormalities probably lie in whatever factors are responsible for fasting hyperglycemia, in that fasting hyperglycemia is inevitably accompanied by glucose intolerance. Perhaps more attention should be focused on the abnormalities of the postabsorptive state in NIDDM and IGT.

INSULIN SECRETION IN NIDDM

The function of pancreatic β-cells in NIDDM has been studied intensively since the development of the insulin radioimmunoassay by Yalow and Berson in 1959. Their first studies produced the startling results that the plasma insulin concentrations in subjects with typical NIDDM were higher or equal to those in nondiabetic controls.[67] This finding led to the conclusion that NIDDM is caused not by insulin deficiency but by an inability of insulin to lower plasma glucose levels effectively—an abnormality termed *insulin resistance*. The situation has turned out to be far more complicated than initially thought, because it is now clear that NIDDM is characterized by insulin resistance and a myriad of abnormalities of islet function. Insight into this puzzle was provided by Karam and co-workers, who found that obese individuals have hyperinsulinemia, which compensates for their insulin resistance.[68] Indeed, it has since been found that in nondiabetic subjects fasting and postprandial insulin concentrations correlate well with the severity of insulin resistance. Studies by Perley and Kipnis then demonstrated that normal-weight subjects with diabetes secreted less insulin than did weight-matched normoglycemic controls and that obese subjects with diabetes secreted less insulin than did obese controls.[69,70] In addition, these authors showed, in a study in which plasma glucose concentrations were matched in diabetic and nondiabetic subjects of similar weight, that the diabetic subjects secreted less insulin than did the controls. These important studies highlight a recurrent theme in the evaluation of studies of insulin secretion in NIDDM: plasma insulin levels can be interpreted only in

the context of the degree of insulin resistance and the concentration of plasma glucose. For example, in a normoglycemic population, fasting plasma insulin levels are quite variable and are a much better indicator of the severity of insulin resistance than of the functional capacity of β-cells. Thus, a low fasting plasma insulin level does not in any way indicate β-cell inadequacy, but instead reflects insulin sensitivity. In contrast, a high insulin level indicates the presence of insulin resistance, except for the rare patient with hyperproinsulinemia or a mutation of the insulin molecule for whom the immunoreactivity of circulating insulin is not accompanied by commensurate biologic activity. In hyperglycemic states the situation is more complicated; insulin concentrations may be high, with the level depending on the extent of insulin resistance, but no matter how high these concentrations are, the β-cells do not compensate sufficiently.

Insulin Secretion during 24 Hours

During a typical 24-hour day, plasma glucose concentrations in persons with NIDDM remain elevated throughout, with excessive glycemic excursions after each meal. In the state of IGT, and even in mild to moderately severe NIDDM, the plasma insulin concentrations look similar to those for weight-matched controls (Fig. 14–3).[71,72] Closer inspection shows that the early insulin responses to meals tend to be lower than normal and that the later plasma levels are higher, findings reflecting what is seen during OGTTs.

Although the ability of β-cells to respond to glucose as a primary stimulus is profoundly impaired, the combination of stimuli associated with meals somehow produces these seemingly normal patterns—these stimuli probably being gastrointestinal hormones, increased vagal activity, amino acids, and glucose. Nonetheless, the amount of

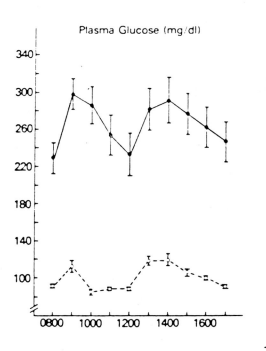

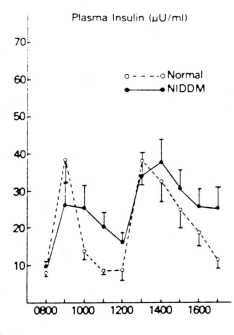

Fig. 14–3. Plasma glucose and insulin responses to two mixed meals in 15 subjects with non-insulin-dependent diabetes (NIDDM) and 15 normal subjects. Reprinted with permission from reference 72 (Liu G, Couston A, Chen Y-DI, Reaven GM. Does day-long absolute hypoinsulinemia characterize the patient with non-insulin-dependent diabetes mellitus? Metabolism 1983; 32:754–6).

insulin released is clearly inadequate to control the hyperglycemia. The nearly normal insulin profiles found over a considerable range of severity of NIDDM are a puzzling adaption of β-cell function.

Circulating Proinsulin-Related Peptides

Proinsulin and its related peptides (partially cleaved proinsulin) circulate in plasma and have less than 5% of the biologic activity of insulin on glucose clearance and hepatic glucose output.[73-75] Although the proinsulin-related peptides account for only about 2 to 4% of the total amount of insulin immunoreactivity secreted from β-cells, the circulating proportion of these peptides is far higher—10 to 40% of insulin immunoreactivity—because of the slow clearance of the prohormone. Intact proinsulin makes up about one-third of the component attributed to proinsulin-related peptides. The des 32–33 split proinsulin makes up about two-thirds, and des 65–66 split proinsulin is present in only very small amounts.[76] Since the 1970s it has been known that the plasma of subjects with NIDDM contains a disproportionate amount of proinsulin-like immunoreactivity.[77-79] Recently, these findings were confirmed and clarified with improved assays, and the ratio of proinsulin-related peptide to insulin was found to be two to four times higher in subjects with NIDDM than in controls.[76,80-82] Although the influence of these peptides on glucose metabolism appears to be trivial, the recent appreciation of their elevated levels in NIDDM leads to the assessment that past measurements of insulin immunoreactivity overestimated circulating insulin levels and thus underestimated the role of insulin deficiency in the pathogenesis of NIDDM. The mechanisms responsible for these increased concentrations of proinsulin-related peptides are unknown, but in animal models of hyperglycemia, proinsulin-related peptides have been found to be secreted in disproportionate amounts, suggesting that increased demand for insulin leads to the release of relatively immature granules.[83] Alternatively, there could be a problem with the mechanisms responsible for proinsulin processing. The value of these measurements as a marker for strain on β-cells or early diabetes remains to be defined. Nonetheless, when plasma insulin immunoreactivity in established NIDDM is assessed, particularly that present during OGTTs or meals, the substantial contribution of proinsulin-like molecules must be taken into account.

Pulsatile Insulin Secretion

Insulin is secreted in a pulsatile fashion in humans and other mammals.[84-86] In the fasting state, humans show oscillations of plasma insulin levels that have a periodicity of 11 to 13 minutes and are synchronous with oscillations of glucose concentration.[86,87] The mechanisms responsible for these oscillations are unknown, but they are found as insulin is secreted from the isolated perfused canine pancreas when perfusate glucose concentrations are held constant, suggesting that the pancreas exhibits a neural or metabolic rhythm that is synchronized with β-cell function.[88] Oscillations of insulin release can also be found in perifused isolated rat islets,[89] findings that make a metabolic explanation more attractive than a neural explanation. In addition, humans have several large-amplitude pulses of insulin secretion 10 to 15 times per day, with greater frequency after meals.[90] Even less is known about the mechanisms responsible for these spikes.

The rapid oscillations of insulin secretion are lost in NIDDM,[90,92] and although the number of large-amplitude pulses remains normal, their amplitude is reduced.[93] This loss seems to occur in the early stages of NIDDM, and there is obvious interest in knowing whether the defect is genetic or acquired. The importance of these changes is unknown. However, when insulin is delivered in a pulsatile fashion that mimics the normal rapid oscillations, its hypoglycemic effect is greater, with hepatic glucose output being more efficiently suppressed, than when delivery is continuous.[94,95] Thus, the loss of these oscillations not only may be a marker of early NIDDM but may also contribute to the hyperglycemia by decreasing the efficiency of the action of insulin on the liver and muscle. This speculation about a potential mechanism for some of the insulin resistance of early NIDDM remains to be proven. Of interest is the finding that glucagon concentrations in plasma also oscillate and that pulsatile delivery of glucagon to the liver in vitro results in more efficient hepatic glucose output.[96]

Oral Glucose Tolerance Test

The OGTT has often been used in studies of insulin secretion in diabetes. In 1968 Reaven and Miller demonstrated that individuals with what is now known as impaired glucose tolerance have a greater insulin response after a glucose challenge than do either nondiabetic or frankly diabetic subjects.[97] This phenomenon has been called the "inverted U-shaped curve."[38] Most subjects with even moderately severe diabetes have responses that are lower than those of nondiabetic subjects.[81] The same general relationship holds true for fasting plasma insulin concentrations.[98,99] The situation is made more complex, however, by the responsibility of proinsulin and its conversion intermediates—which have less than 5% of the biologic activity of insulin itself—for anywhere from 10 to 49% of the total amount of insulin immunoreactivity.[73-75] Thus, the levels of these proinsulin-like peptides are disproportionately elevated in NIDDM, reducing the relative contribution of true insulin to the total amount of insulin immunoreactivity.

In addition to the abnormalities in the magnitude of insulin secretion during OGTTs in NIDDM, there are alterations in the patterns of insulin release.[65,66,100-103] The early insulin responses—those measured at 30 minutes—of subjects with even mild NIDDM are often lower than those of normal controls. This is thought to contribute to the inefficient suppression of hepatic glucose output found in NIDDM.[65,66] At the later time points of 60 to 120 minutes, the insulin responses may be higher than those of normal controls, but this result must be interpreted in light of the different plasma glucose concentrations. Thus, the late hyperinsulinemia, which is usually seen in IGT and often in mild NIDDM, occurs in the presence of hyperglycemia and is at least partially dependent on it. Therefore, the inverted U-shaped curve seen during OGTTs is, at least in part, secondary to a deficiency in early insulin secretion. However, it is important to note that the phenomenon of hyperinsulinemia in states of mild glucose intolerance is not just an artefact of the fed state, because an inverted U-shaped curve has also been found with fasting plasma insulin concentrations (Fig. 14–4).[46] Finally, in severe NIDDM the insulin responses during an OGTT are lower than normal at all time points in spite of high plasma glucose levels.[101]

Role of Incretin in Pathogenesis

When glucose is ingested orally, insulin secretion is potentiated by still-undefined alimentary factors included under the term *incretin*. Neural mechanisms may be involved, and gastrointestinal hormones have been implicated, with the most attractive candidates being gastric inhibitory peptide (GIP)[104] and the truncated forms of glucagon-like peptide I (GLP-I).[105] Cholecystokinin (CCK) has also been a candidate, but recent studies suggest that it is probably not an important incretin in humans.[106] An incretin effect can be measured by comparing insulin responses to oral and intravenous glucose, and subjects with NIDDM have been found to

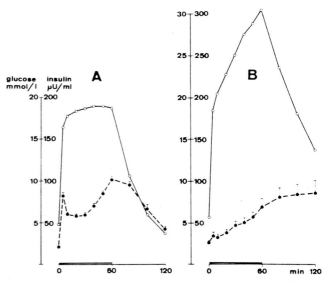

Fig. 14–5. Blood glucose (open circles) and plasma insulin (closed circles) levels during intravenous glucose infusion in 226 control subjects and 25 subjects with mild non-insulin-dependent diabetes mellitus (NIDDM). Reprinted with permission from reference 102 (Cerasi E, Efendić S, Luft R. Dose-responses in equivocal and definite diabetes, with special reference to subjects who had mild glucose intolerance but later developed definite diabetes. Diabetes 1977;26:944–52; copyright © of the American Diabetes Association).

have a relatively reduced response to oral glucose.[107] However, the increases in GIP during an OGTT are comparable in the NIDDM and control groups.[107] These data suggest that the effect of GIP on insulin release is impaired or that other incretin factors are important in NIDDM. A loss of an incretin effect could account for some degree of glucose intolerance in NIDDM. Furthermore, an incretin defect in a prediabetic stage could contribute to the complex multifactorial process that culminates in NIDDM.

Insulin Secretion in Response to Intravenous Glucose

The loss of early, or "first-phase," glucose-induced insulin secretion in NIDDM is a striking abnormality. Normally, pancreatic islets respond rapidly to an intravenous glucose challenge with a first phase of insulin secretion that lasts for about 4 to 5 minutes and produces a spike-like pattern of insulin immunoreactivity in plasma that lasts for about 10 minutes[103,108,109] (Fig. 14–5). A nadir of secretion ensues, which is followed immediately by a gradually increasing second phase of insulin release. When glucose is administered intravenously as an intravenous glucose tolerance test (IVGTT) or as a constant infusion to subjects with NIDDM, first-phase insulin secretion is absent.[103,110–113] Sometimes a paradoxical fall in plasma insulin concentration is noted.[114] A second phase of insulin secretion can be seen in all but the most severe cases of NIDDM.[110] These insulin responses, which can be identical to those of normal weight-

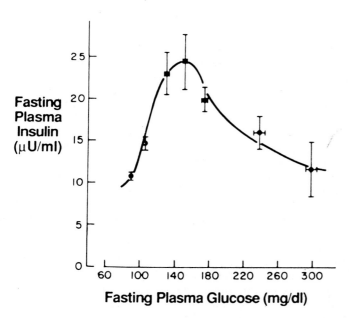

Fig. 14–4. Fasting immunoreactive plasma insulin levels in non-obese subjects stratified by the level of glycemia. Reprinted with permission from reference 46 (DeFronzo RA, Ferrannini E, Simonson DC. Fasting hyperglycemia in non-insulin-dependent diabetes mellitus: contributions of excessive hepatic glucose production and impaired tissue glucose uptake. Metabolism 1989;38:387–95).

matched control subjects, must be regarded as impaired when hyperglycemia is taken into account. A person without diabetes would secrete much more insulin when challenged with a similar glucose concentration. The first phase of insulin release, also referred to as *acute insulin release* (AIR), has been thoroughly studied by Porte and co-workers using rapid intravenous boluses of 20 g of glucose.[111–113] Insight into the development of the defect was obtained by studying subjects who had a variety of fasting plasma glucose concentrations (Fig. 14–6).[112] Thus, when the fasting glucose level is only 100 to 114 mg/dL (5.5 to 6.3 mM) in persons who might not even be diagnosed as having IGT, AIR is one-half that of subjects with fasting levels below 5.5 mM. When the fasting glucose level is above 114 mg/dL (6.3 mM), the AIR response to glucose is absent. The findings of these cross-sectional studies are in basic agreement with those of longitudinal studies of a group of Pima Indians who progressed from nondiabetic status, to IGT, and then to NIDDM.[115] An obvious question is whether this loss of first-phase secretion is important. The deficient early insulin responses seen during OGTTs and meals probably represent the same phenomenon, and intravenous administration of small amounts of insulin to replace this deficit results in marked improvement in the exaggerated postprandial rise in glucose level seen in persons with NIDDM.[116]

Not only do β-cells fail to respond to increases in glucose concentration, but plasma insulin concentrations do not decrease properly in response to hypoglycemia.[117] This phenomenon may contribute to the delayed decline in insulin levels during glucose tolerance tests or during the later stages of a meal, as noted in 24-hour profiles of insulin levels.[72] Furthermore, inappropriate insulin suppression may be responsible for the reactive hypoglycemia often found in conjunction with states of IGT or mild NIDDM.

Insulin Responses to Non-Glucose Secretagogues and Glucose Potentiation

In contrast to their loss of responsiveness to glucose in NIDDM, the β-cells can respond to a variety of other secretagogues, such as arginine, isoproterenol, secretin, and tolbutamide[118–123] (Fig. 14–7). Even in moderately severe NIDDM, the magnitude and pattern of the insulin response to these agents is virtually identical to those found in people without diabetes. However, this apparently normal response is dependent on hyperglycemia. For example, when glucose infusions are used to raise glucose levels in euglycemic subjects, the insulin responses to an acute arginine challenge are far higher than those found in NIDDM.[124,125] When glucose levels in both groups are brought to concentrations of about 600 mg/dL (33 mM), the insulin responses in the nondiabetic subjects are seven times higher than those in the diabetic subjects (Fig. 14–8). This poor insulin response to arginine in NIDDM is noteworthy because pathologic studies indicate that the β-cell mass in NIDDM is on average 60% of normal values, thus highlighting the severe impairment of function in whatever β-cells are present.

Insulin responses to many non-glucose secretagogues are normally quite dependent on glucose concentrations. For example, arginine-induced insulin secretion is far higher at glucose concentrations of 20 mM than at 4 mM, showing a potentiating effect of glucose. This potentiation is impaired in NIDDM; indeed, the abnormality has been quantified by determining the slope of various insulin responses at different experimentally induced glucose levels.[113,126] The slope in NIDDM is not as steep as that found normally. This so-called slope of potentiation test is thought to show abnormalities in the earliest stages of the pathogenesis of diabetes, even before impairments in glucose tolerance or glucose-induced insulin secretion are found.[126,127] On the other hand, in healthy subjects the induction of insulin resistance with dexamethasone or nicotinic acid or with prolonged infusion of glucose will produce a steeper slope of potentiation.[113,128,129] The changes in the slope of potentiation during longitudinal studies of the evolution from normal carbohydrate tolerance to NIDDM are not known.

Adverse Influence of Chronic Hyperglycemia on β-Cell Function

A hypothesis has been advanced that chronic hyperglycemia causes alterations in β-cell function.[130–132] In the normal nondiabetic state, the plasma glucose concentration is maintained within a narrow range—usually between 4.5 and 8.0 mM (82 to 145 mg/dL). Glucose levels higher than this present β-cells with an unnatural environment that results in abnormal function. This hypothesis has been tested extensively in models in

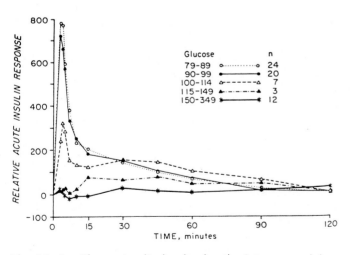

Fig. 14–6. Plasma insulin levels after the intravenous injection of 20 g of glucose in subjects with various fasting plasma glucose levels. Acute insulin responses are already reduced in subjects with fasting glucose concentrations of 100 to 114 mg/dL. Reprinted with permission from reference 112 (Brunzell JD, Roberson RP, Lerner RL, et al. Relationships between fasting plasma glucose levels and insulin secretion during intravenous glucose tolerance tests. J Clin Endocrinol Metab 1976;42:222–9).

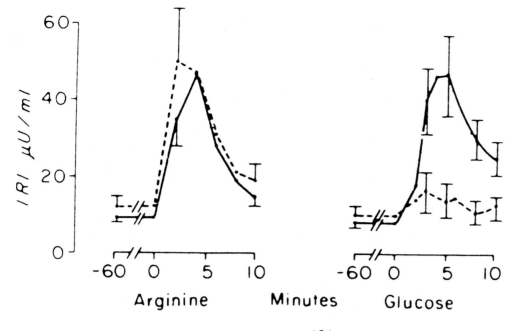

Fig. 14–7. Acute responses of immunoreactive insulin (IRI) to intravenous injections of arginine or glucose in control subjects (solid line) and subjects with non-insulin-dependent diabetes (NIDDM) (dashed line). Note that arginine causes a brisk insulin response in subjects with NIDDM, whereas glucose is without effect. Reprinted with permission of the American Society of Clinical Investigation from reference 120 (Palmer JP, Benson JW, Walter RM, Ensinck JW. Arginine-stimulated acute phase of insulin and glucagon secretion in diabetic subjects. J Clin Invest 1976;58:565–70).

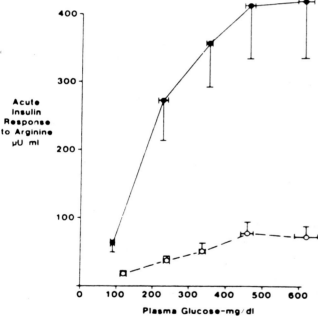

Fig. 14–8. Insulin secretory response to glucose and arginine in the perfused pancreatic remnant of 90% pancreatectomized diabetic rats (solid line) and controls (dotted line). Studies were performed 8 to 11 weeks after pancreatectomy or sham surgery. Reprinted with permission of the American Society of Clinical Investigation from reference 138 (Bonner-Weir S, Trent DF, Weir GC. Partial pancreatectomy in the rat and subsequent defect in glucose-induced insulin release. J Clin Invest 1983; 1544–53).

rats,[143] and *db/db* mice.[144] Insulin secretion has been characterized primarily in the perfused rat pancreas but also in vivo. The most obvious lesion found in all of these models is a specific blindness of β-cells to glucose, as evidenced by their not being acutely stimulated by high concentrations of glucose or turned off by low levels.[135,145] Hypersecretion of insulin can even be found in the absence of extracellular glucose.[146] In contrast, insulin secretion can be stimulated by non-glucose secretagogues such as arginine, glucagon, or tolbutamide and inhibited by somatostatin and epinephrine. Some of these abnormalities can be reversed in less than an hour by simply exposing the β-cells to buffer solutions that contain no glucose.[147,148] In addition, insulin stores are reduced in the β-cells of these models and proinsulin secretion is disproportionately increased, findings that provide a potential explanation for the altered plasma proinsulin concentrations found in NIDDM.[83]

The secretory abnormalities found in experimental animals closely resemble those seen in humans with NIDDM. The hypothesis is further strengthened by the finding that glucose-induced insulin secretion can be partially restored in NIDDM by normalization of glucose concentrations for 20 hours with insulin infusions.[149] In addition, in the earliest stages of IDDM, a similar loss of glucose-induced insulin secretion with preservation of responses to non-glucose secretagogues is seen, a finding consistent with the hypothesis.[150] Of note, the fasting glucose concentrations have been found to be slightly elevated in these individuals with pre-IDDM.[151] One important aspect of the question of the effects of hyperglycemia on β-cell function concerns the set point for glucose-induced insulin secretion. As the concentration of glucose creeps up, does the threshold or set point for β-cell secretion change? For example, when a group of normal subjects are given dexamethasone, their fasting glucose concentrations increase slightly.[128] This would

which rats are made hyperglycemic by the administration of streptozotocin during the neonatal period,[133–137] by partial pancreatectomy[138,139] (Fig. 14–9), or by glucose infusions.[140,141] Studies have also been carried out in GK rats,[142] the glucose-intolerant Zucker fatty (*fa/fa*)

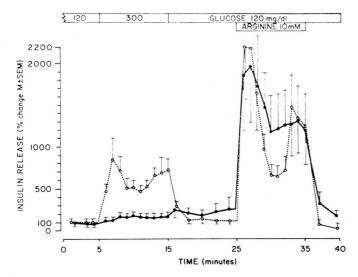

Fig. 14–9. Acute insulin responses to intravenous arginine at 5 different glucose levels in eight subjects with non-insulin-dependent diabetes (NIDDM) (open circles) and eight control subjects (closed circles). Note that the maximal response is markedly attenuated in subjects with NIDDM. Reprinted with permission of the American Society of Clinical Investigation from reference 124 (Ward WK, Bolgiano DC, McNight B, et al. Diminished β cell secretory capacity in patients with noninsulin-dependent diabetes mellitus. J. Clin Invest 1984;1318–28).

not happen if the β-cells were functioning perfectly as a homeostatic force because insulin secretion would increase until the fasting glucose level was normalized. Perhaps such "slippage" serves a yet uncertain adaptive function. Data from experimental animal systems support this concept of an altered set point for glucose-induced insulin secretion.[152]

The mechanisms responsible for these defects are unknown. Because of the complexity of the mechanisms of insulin secretion, multiple abnormalities can be expected. To understand glucose-induced insulin secretion, it is necessary to remember that the rate of glucose metabolism in β-cells is closely coupled to the rate of insulin secretion, with the rate-limiting step in metabolism being the phosphorylation of glucose by glucokinase[153] (see Chapter 4). A potential explanation for the hypersecretion of insulin found in the absence of extracellular glucose is that glycogen stores are abnormally increased in the β-cells of some models, providing an endogenous fuel source that could supply metabolism-dependent secretory mechanisms.[154] Another potential trouble spot is glucose oxidation, which is reduced in islets obtained from these rats[155] and could contribute to the loss of glucose-induced insulin secretion. Biochemical studies suggest that this abnormality in oxidation could be due, at least in part, to impairment of the glycerol phosphate shuttle.[155] In addition, there could be a problem with glucose transport, which under normal circumstances is not rate-limiting for glucose metabolism. Indeed, in multiple rodent models of NIDDM, the expression of the glucose transporter GLUT-2 is markedly reduced.[143,144,156] The significance of this finding is not

known, but there are reasons to think that a second (or more), as yet unidentified, glucose transporter is present on β-cells, thus further complicating the situation.[143] Although it is difficult to fully understand the cause and significance of this change in GLUT-2, which has not yet been confirmed in human diabetes, the profound reduction in glucose transporters appears to provide a good explanation for the reduction in first-phase glucose-induced insulin secretion. A complete reduction of transport would be incompatible with continued insulin secretion, so presumably there are enough GLUT-2 transporters, or some other transporters, to allow relatively slow equilibration of extracellular and intracellular glucose concentrations. Therefore, in the diabetic state there could be enough intracellular glucose in β-cells to account for the hyperinsulinemia that is often seen in NIDDM. However, because of the reduction in transporters, the β-cell is unable to react quickly to a sudden increase in glucose, explaining deficient early insulin release. A reduced GLUT-2 also could provide an explanation for the reactive hypoglycemia of early diabetes. As plasma glucose levels fall after a meal, glucose may not be able to leave β-cells rapidly enough because of an inadequate number of transporters. Then continued metabolism of glucose in the β-cell could lead to insulin secretion in the face of hypoglycemia, which normally would have efficiently shut off secretion Provision of glucose from β-cell glycogen stores could also contribute to an inappropriately high rate of insulin secretion.

The Concept of β-Cell Exhaustion

It is often assumed that β-cells can become exhausted after prolonged periods of increased demand. This phenomenon has been poorly delineated, and a precise definition is necessary. There could be a structural exhaustion in which hyperglycemia leads to premature death of β-cells. On the other hand, the life span of individual cells might be normal but the overall replicative capacity of β-cells might be used up by excessive demand. Some insights have been provided by animal experiments. Although the β-cells of some animal species seem resistant to structural exhaustion, those of dogs and cats have been found to be vulnerable.[157–159] Functional exhaustion can also exist. The loss of glucose-induced insulin secretion by the experimental production of chronic hyperglycemia is a functional abnormality.[131] A more relevant example is found in NIDDM; when hyperglycemia is reduced by diet, sulfonylurea treatment, or insulin treatment, insulin secretion increases after challenges with meals or oral glucose[1608] (Fig. 14–10). Whatever loss of β-cell function results from something other than excessive demand must be due to processes other than exhaustion. The issue of exhaustion is important to the understanding of the pathogenesis of NIDDM, because during the development of NIDDM β-cell failure is inevitable. The mechanisms behind this failure are obviously complex, but at least some of what happens must fall into the general set of events called exhaustion.

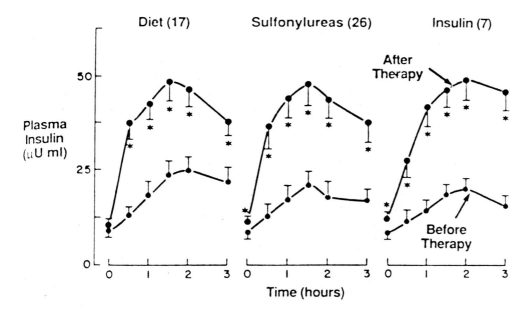

Fig. 14–10. Plasma insulin responses in non-insulin-dependent diabetes after the institution of glycemic control with diet, sulfonylureas, or insulin. Note the increased insulin response following therapy in each case. Reprinted with permission from reference 160 (Kosaka K, Kuzuya T, Akanuma Y, Hagura R. Increase in insulin response after treatment of overt maturity-onset diabetes is independent of the mode of treatment. Diabetologia 1980;18:23–8).

The Insulin Gene in NIDDM

Because NIDDM results from an insufficiency in insulin secretion, the limiting steps could be an inadequacy in the number of β-cells, a problem with proinsulin biosynthesis, or a block in the processing and secretion pathways. In fact, a combination of all of these may be responsible. In any case, little is known about proinsulin biosynthesis in NIDDM. Considerable attention has been paid to the possibility that mutations in the insulin gene play a key role in the pathogenesis of NIDDM. The insulin gene is on the short arm of chromosome 11, and restriction fragment length polymorphism (RFLP) analysis has been used extensively in the analysis of this gene.[161] Two kinds of RFLPs have been found, those that result from a single base-pair difference in the promoter region and those characterized by areas with a variable number of repetitive DNA sequences, otherwise known as variable-number tandem repeats (VNTRs). These analyses have been carried out in African-American, white, Chinese, and Pima Indian populations, and no convincing linkage between polymorphism and NIDDM has materialized. The case is not closed, however, because further analysis of the promoter region could lead to the identification of mutations that account for some cases of NIDDM. A single base-pair change on even one allele could lead to NIDDM. In the future, considerable attention will be devoted to the genes of the proteins that regulate insulin gene expression through interaction with the *cis*-regulatory elements of the 5′ flanking region. There are many ways in which disordered expression of the insulin gene could lead to critical limitations in insulin production.

Mutations of the Proinsulin Gene and NIDDM

As is discussed elsewhere (Chapter 12), mutations of the insulin gene have been identified that are associated with, but do not necessarily cause, NIDDM.[162] Amino acid substitutions have been found in parts of the insulin molecule that lead to a marked loss of biologic activity—typically to levels 2% of normal values. Three mutations have been found in six families; these are known as insulin Chicago (Phe-B25-Leu), insulin Los Angeles (Phe-B24-Ser), and insulin Wakayama (Val-A3-Leu). These mutant insulins exhibit a marked loss of biologic activity because they can no longer bind effectively to the insulin receptor, a property that also accounts for their markedly reduced clearance in plasma. Only heterozygotes for these mutations have been found, suggesting that mutations in both alleles may be incompatible with fetal survival. The question is why diabetes develops in persons with these mutations, since normal insulin can be produced by one normal allele. A likely explanation, although not proven, is that an inborn limitation in synthetic capacity makes adequate insulin secretion over a lifetime unsustainable, thus resulting in a state that, without molecular analysis, would be diagnosed as NIDDM. Mutations in less essential parts of the insulin molecule have not yet been found, which is not surprising because those with such mutations would be less likely to have diabetes and therefore be difficult to identify.

Other mutations have been found that cause problems with proinsulin processing and lead to hyperproinsulinemia. They also may or may not be associated with diabetes.[162] The first mutation was found in one of the dibasic cleavage sites of proinsulin, with the C65 arginine being replaced by histidine, making the site resistant to endopeptidase activity. Three families thought to have this or a similar defect have been found. This cleavage abnormality creates a situation much like that of the insulin mutations described above; one allele produces an abnormal product with markedly reduced biologic activity, while the other produces normal insulin. This leads to the prediction that affected individuals are at greater risk for developing diabetes. A second mutation has been found in which the B10 histidine is replaced by aspartic acid, producing a complicated situation in which this abnormal proinsulin is incompletely cleaved to insulin and partially secreted through the normally inactive constitutive secretory pathway (see Chapter 3).

Glucagon Secretion in NIDDM

As a result of an explosive expansion in research focused on glucagon secretion in the 1970s, the role of glucagon in diabetes has been defined almost completely[163,164] (see Chapter 9). In individuals with NIDDM, plasma glucagon levels are inappropriately elevated in either an absolute or a relative sense, in that they are not suppressed by hyperglycemia, as would occur in individuals without diabetes. In addition, glucagon secretion is increased after meals and most clearly in experimental situations with the intravenous infusion of arginine.[163] Glucagon, by enhancing hepatic glucose output, is undoubtedly responsible for some of the hyperglycemia of NIDDM. This is important in the fasting state, but also during meals, with the increased insulin/glucagon ratio restraining glycogenolysis and gluconeogenesis.[65] Another abnormality of glucagon in NIDDM is the lack of an appropriate increase in its secretion in response to hypoglycemia. During experimental insulin-induced hypoglycemia in subjects with NIDDM, plasma glucagon concentrations increase more than in subjects with IDDM but not as much as in normal subjects.[165] This impairment of a potentially important counterregulatory mechanism for hypoglycemia may have clinical relevance for insulin-requiring patients with NIDDM. The mechanisms responsible for the failure of glucagon secretion to respond appropriately to changes in glucose concentration in NIDDM have not been completely defined. A leading hypothesis is that inhibition of glucagon secretion by glucose is largely dependent on the suppression of pancreatic α-cells by intra-islet insulin.[166] Therefore, in NIDDM β-cells do not respond appropriately to either hypo- or hyperglycemia, and the blunted changes in the intra-islet concentration of insulin lead to similar unresponsiveness of glucagon secretion.

ISLET PATHOLOGY IN NIDDM

β-Cell Mass

Although the pathologic features of the islets of Langerhans in diabetes are covered in detail in Chapter 2, several points must be reinforced to provide a complete picture of the pathogenesis of NIDDM. Perhaps the most important finding is the reduction in β-cell mass noted in all available large autopsy studies.[167–173] There has been general agreement that β-cell mass is about 60% of normal. Unfortunately, these autopsy studies are accompanied by little clinical information, particularly about the degree of obesity of the individuals studied. In obese persons without diabetes, β-cell mass is thought to be increased,[172,174] as is expected from the increase in insulin secretion in this group.[68] Ideally, one would like to have more comparisons of β-cell mass in obese diabetic persons vs. obese nondiabetic persons and in

thin diabetic persons vs. thin nondiabetic persons.[175] One would also like to have more information about the degree of insulin resistance not related to obesity. It is not certain what β-cell mass is required to prevent hyperglycemia, and the amount necessary must depend on many factors.[176] Some insight is provided by the developments in donors who provided the distal half of their pancreas for transplantation into a diabetic family member.[177] Within a year many of the donors had glucose intolerance and some had diabetes.

Little is known about the longitudinal changes that occur during the development of NIDDM. In the early stages most subjects are obese and insulin-resistant. Thus, there may be a stage of β-cell hypertrophy preceding an end-stage stable reduction of mass. In any event, studies of insulin secretion in subjects with moderately severe NIDDM indicate that even during maximal stimulation with high glucose concentrations and either arginine or isoproterenol, insulin responses are only about 15% of those found in controls without diabetes.[124,178] These findings suggest that in NIDDM the insulin output for a given β-cell mass that might be 60% of the normal value is considerably lower than expected. Some of this discordance may be explained by chronic hyperglycemia, which is associated with potentially reversible suppression of stimulated insulin secretion.[160]

The importance of β-cell mass in the pathogenesis of all forms of diabetes should not be underestimated.[176] In the nondiabetic state, the amount of β-cell tissue is obviously tightly regulated and may be the main factor responsible for the maintenance of euglycemia. Investigators focus on the characteristics of insulin secretion, paying particular attention to the abnormalities found in diabetes. Perhaps all of the characterized secretory abnormalities, such as the loss of glucose-induced insulin secretion and the problems with potentiation, are secondary to inadequate β-cell mass, i.e., a inadequate for whatever degree of insulin resistance is present. This concept may be critical to our understanding of the pathogenesis of NIDDM. It is now accepted that diabetes does not occur unless insulin secretion can no longer compensate for a given amount of insulin resistance. The key point is that this progression to NIDDM should perhaps be viewed less as a failure to secrete insulin and more as a failure to maintain adequate β-cell mass. Thus, a critical loss in β-cell mass may lead to a complex series of pathogenetic events that produce all of the observed defects in insulin secretion as well as an important component of the insulin resistance found in diabetes.[130,179,180] This is obviously an important point in considering the therapeutic options for all forms of diabetes. Obviously, restoration of normal β-cell mass would be the ideal therapy.

Amyloid Deposition in Islets

The amyloid deposits found in the islets of most subjects with NIDDM are of considerable interest.[169,181] Described for the first time in 1900 by Opie,[182] the material was isolated and purified only in 1986[183,184] and found to consist of fibrils formed by a 37-amino-acid peptide, now called islet-amyloid polypeptide (IAPP), diabetes-associated polypeptide (DAP), or amylin. This peptide has structural homology with the neuroendocrine peptide calcitonin gene-related peptide (CGRP). The formation of amyloid is thought to depend on the amino acid sequence between positions 20 and 29, with position 25 being particularly important, a finding that helps explain why islet amyloid is found in primates and cats but not in many other species.[185,186] The IAPP gene is expressed in β-cells, and the precursor contains 89 amino acids. Within the β-cell the precursor is cleaved to IAPP, which is contained in secretory granules and then co-secreted with insulin.[187,188] The IAPP content of β-cells is only about 1% that of insulin on a molar basis, and this ratio is reflected in the secreted peptides.[189]

The role of IAPP in the pathogenesis of NIDDM is unknown. It has been suggested that the extracellular amyloid deposits have a toxic effect on residual β-cells or that intracellular IAPP somehow exerts an adverse effect on β-cell function.[190] On the other hand, the amyloid could merely be a marker of the disease process—perhaps an insoluble residue from dead β-cells. Evidence that β-cell turnover is a much more dynamic process than previously thought and almost like a slow-motion version of the turnover of intestinal epithelial cells gives this possibility some support.[191] Throughout a person's life, a substantial β-cell birth rate is balanced by an equally substantial death rate. Perhaps NIDDM develops only after a great number of cells have died—a number larger than that what may occur in insulin-resistant states as obesity or acromegaly. This could explain why amyloid deposits are not very prominent in situations accompanied by insulin resistance.[192] The possibility that circulating IAPP contributes to the insulin resistance of NIDDM has also been raised,[193] but the concentrations of IAPP in plasma are so low that this has become a less attractive hypothesis.[188,194]

INSULIN RESISTANCE IN NIDDM

Insulin resistance is a cardinal feature of NIDDM. Himsworth and Kerr, in 1936, may have been the first to appreciate this, having described groups of patients who were either insulin-insensitive or insulin-sensitive.[195] The insensitive group probably was made up of subjects who would now be considered to have NIDDM. This finding has been made in many population groups and with many techniques. Insulin resistance can be estimated clinically by the insulin requirements of individuals with diabetes, although the presence or absence of endogenous insulin secretion is a confounding variable. Another approach is to measure the effect of a given amount of exogenous insulin on the rate of decline in plasma glucose levels.[196] The forearm perfusion technique has been used to correlate glucose uptake across tissue beds with plasma insulin concentrations.[197] Fat tissue obtained by biopsy has been used for studies of insulin action, and the results are often in agreement with the results in vivo.[198,199] The simple measurement of fasting or stimulated plasma insulin concentrations correlates well with insulin resistance, although interpretation becomes more difficult if subjects are not euglycemic. Some of the complexity

stems from the fact that glucose itself can influence glucose uptake by muscle and liver.[39,42,43]

The problem of this influence of glucose has been partially circumvented with the euglycemic insulin-clamp, which has become the "gold standard" for measuring insulin sensitivity.[42,200,201] Infusion of labeled glucose by this technique permits estimation of glucose disposal and endogenous glucose production. An alternative approach is that of the Bergman minimal model.[202] This method uses the frequently sampled intravenous glucose tolerance test (FSIGT), in which glucose is injected intravenously. Insulin sensitivity (Si) is then derived from measurements of glucose clearance and the concentration of endogenous insulin. In addition, the effect of glucose on its own uptake can be estimated (Sg). Both Si and Sg are found to be reduced in NIDDM. There are variations of this approach in which tolbutamide is used to stimulate endogenous insulin secretion or exogenous insulin is injected along with glucose. It is important to remember that insulin has many effects in addition to those on glucose uptake and metabolism. Thus, what is measured as insulin resistance in the handling of glucose by muscle may not be true for lipolysis, amino acid uptake, gene expression, or ion transport. Furthermore, all of these techniques have important limitations.

FACTORS INFLUENCING INSULIN SENSITIVITY

Obesity

The most common and important cause of insulin resistance is obesity, yet little is known about the underlying mechanisms. There are at least two components. Hyperphagia itself produces some degree of resistance, as is suggested by the dramatic declines in plasma glucose levels seen in NIDDM following moderate caloric reduction.[203,204] Obese individuals are still thought to be insulin resistant even when their food intake is controlled, although this has not yet been rigorously quantitated. In assessments of whole-body glucose metabolism in obese subjects, the insulin resistance of muscle and liver is quantitatively more important than that of adipose tissue.

Considerable attention has focused recently on the pattern of fat distribution. The central pattern of distribution, with its increased waist/hip ratio, is associated with more insulin resistance than is the peripheral pattern of distribution, in which fat is more plentiful in the buttock and upper leg areas.[205-207] This is an important issue, because individuals with the central pattern are more likely to have glucose intolerance, hypertension, hyperlipidemia, and vascular disease, a constellation of features that has been termed "syndrome X."[63] The mechanisms through which central obesity causes insulin resistance are unknown, but one hypothesis suggests that release of free fatty acids by omental fat into the portal circulation enhances gluconeogenesis and interferes with insulin action on the liver.[62] Another possible explanation for the insulin resistance of obesity is the reduced binding of insulin to target tissues that has been found[199,208] but it has been difficult to quantitate the impact of this change in binding. In addition, there is clearly an important post-receptor contribution to the resistance, for which countless mechanisms could be responsible. Blunting of insulin-induced increases of muscle blood flow in obese subjects, leading to reduced uptake of glucose, could also be of some importance.[209] In addition, evidence for a reduction in the capillary density of muscle in obese subjects has been found.[63] Questions have also been raised about the contribution of elevated plasma levels of free fatty acids[56,59] and about altered androgen metabolism.[210] There are obvious difficulties involved in trying to sift through multiple potential mechanisms in a heterogeneous populations of overweight individuals.

Physical Activity

An individual's level of physical activity has profound effects on insulin sensitivity, as has been documented by the finding that trained athletes have very low plasma insulin responses to an intravenous glucose challenge.[211] Much of this insulin sensitivity appears to be related temporally to a particular bout of exercise, with the sensitivity waning sharply within 24 to 36 hours.[211] Some of this sensitivity is thought to be due to the repletion of muscle glycogen stores that is linked to enhanced glucose uptake.[213] Conversely, individuals consigned to bed rest for 7 days have shown an increase in their level of insulin resistance.[214]

Age

Insulin sensitivity varies with age; for example, the onset of adolescence is marked by an increase in insulin resistance, the cause of which is unknown, but it may be related, at least in part, to increased caloric intake.[215] Advanced age is also associated with insulin resistance, but it has proven difficult to determine how much of this is independent of inactivity and obesity.[24]

Phenotypic Aspects of Insulin Resistance in NIDDM

Insulin resistance is almost always found in NIDDM. Because of the confounding influence of obesity, efforts have been made to study thin individuals with NIDDM. In attempts to understand the mechanisms of insulin resistance, a distinction has been made between insulin sensitivity and insulin responsiveness.[216] A loss in sensitivity would be reflected by a rightward shift of a dose-response curve and could be caused by a problem with receptor binding. A loss in responsiveness would be reflected in a reduction in the maximal response and would be consistent with a post-binding abnormality. Although this approach is most appropriately used with studies of homogeneous cell populations in vitro, it has also been employed for in vivo studies in humans.

Dose-response curves have been constructed from data obtained in euglycemic insulin-clamp studies of obese and non-obese subjects with NIDDM[44,217,218] (Fig. 14–11). With regard to the rate of insulin-stimulated glucose disposal, the most striking finding is a marked

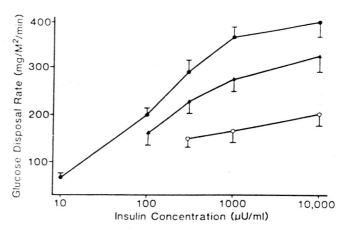

Fig. 14–11. Insulin dose-response curves during euglycemic glucose-clamp studies in control subjects (closed circles), subjects with non-insulin-dependent diabetes (NIDDM) (open circles), and subjects with NIDDM who have been aggressively treated with insulin (closed triangles). Note that improvement in insulin resistance after treatment is only partial. Reprinted with permission from reference 217 (Scarlett JA, Gray RS, Griffin J, et al. Insulin treatment reverses the insulin resistance of type II diabetes mellitus. Diabetes Care 1982;5:353–63; copyright © of the American Diabetes Association).

reduction in maximal response, indicating the presence of a severe problem with the post-binding mechanisms of insulin action. Similar studies also were performed in subjects with IGT, with the results considered compatible with a decrease in insulin sensitivity.[44] However, the patterns of the individual subjects are heterogeneous enough to suggest that this conclusion be made with caution. Although it is generally assumed that target hepatocytes and myocytes are the most important sites of insulin resistance, Bergman has suggested that a component of insulin resistance may be impedance to the departure of insulin from the vascular compartment, a process known as transcapillary insulin transport[202]; however, further exploration of this hypothesis is necessary.

Insulin action has been assessed in vitro in many tissues obtained from human subjects and experimental animals with diabetes. Some of the clearest results were from studies of adipocytes from human subjects that assessed the transport of insulin-stimulated 3-O-methylglucose, deoxyglucose, and labeled D-glucose.[198,199] The adipocytes of subjects with NIDDM and of some obese subjects show a marked reduction in responsiveness that resembles the reduction noted in glucose-clamp studies (Fig. 14–12). The adipocytes of subjects with IGT show a pattern of decreased sensitivity in vitro that could be related to a problem in the insulin receptor. The reduction of glucose transport found in NIDDM can be correlated to some degree with a reduction of GLUT-4 transporters (also called the muscle/fat glucose transporter isoform) in the plasma membrane of adipocytes.[219,220] The reduction in transporter protein, as determined by immunoblotting, was quantitatively similar to the decline in GLUT-4 mRNA. Results obtained in

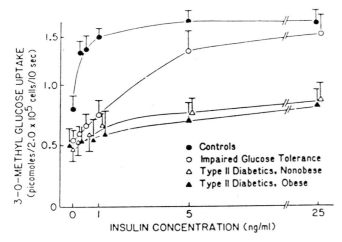

Fig. 14–12. Dose-response curves of insulin-stimulated glucose transport (3-O-methylglucose uptake) in isolated adipocytes in controls, subjects with impaired glucose tolerance, and non-obese and obese subjects with non-insulin-dependent diabetes (NIDDM). Note the markedly reduced responsiveness of the adipocytes of subjects with NIDDM. Reprinted with permission from reference 199 (Olefsky JM, Molin JM. Insulin resistance in man. In: Rifkin H, Porte D Jr, eds. Ellenberg and Rifkin's diabetes mellitus: theory and practice. New York: Elsevier, 1989:121–53).

studies of adipocytes in rodents are in general agreement with those from studies in humans.[221,222] However, the reduction in glucose transport does not necessarily correlate with the amount of GLUT-4 protein in the plasma membrane, in that normalization of plasma glucose levels with phloridzin in partially pancreatized rats resulted in improved glucose transport of fat cells without any increase in the amount of transport protein, a finding that suggests hyperglycemia may have a direct influence on the intrinsic activity of GLUT-4 that is independent of insulin.[223]

Because most insulin-stimulated glucose clearance from plasma is accounted for by muscle, there is great interest in understanding the mechanisms of insulin resistance in this tissue. Muscle is more difficult to study than fat, but measurements of 3-O-methylglucose uptake in muscle strips taken from subjects with NIDDM do reveal a reduction in insulin-stimulated uptake.[224] However, the results of studies of the expression of GLUT-4 protein and mRNA in muscle have not been as clearcut as those in studies of adipocytes. Some workers find no difference in diabetes[225,226]; others obtain results that resemble those from studies of fat cells.[227–231] Evidence of variability in the intrinsic activity of transporters is increasing[223]; thus, the amount of GLUT-4 transporter in the plasma membrane certainly cannot be expected to correlate perfectly with transport activity. This situation should be clarified within the next few years.

Some studies have found that the number of insulin receptors on the adipocytes, monocytes, and other cells of subjects with NIDDM is reduced.[38,198,199,232,233] On the other hand, both the number and affinity of insulin receptors on liver membranes were found to be in-

creased in patients with NIDDM[234] but decreased in hyperinsulinemic obese subjects. The discrepancies found in NIDDM may depend in part on circulating insulin concentrations, with "down-regulation" being seen in hyperinsulinemic patients and "up-regulation" in those with absolute insulin deficiency. Hyperinsulinemic subjects with IGT should be expected to have reduced binding. The contributions of alterations of insulin binding to the insulin resistance of NIDDM and obesity are still not well quantitated. Several groups have been unable to find good correlations between insulin binding and insulin resistance in NIDDM.[235,236]

The insulin receptor has tyrosine kinase activity, such that the receptor can phosphorylate itself and other substrates.[237] Reduced tyrosine kinase activity of the receptor at multiple insulin concentrations has been found in NIDDM.[199,238] Reduced phosphorylation activity has also been found in subjects with IDDM and in animal models of clear insulin deficiency.[239] In nondiabetic obese subjects, the tyrosine kinase activity of the insulin receptor is generally found not to be reduced, but this question needs further clarification.[240] The cause and impact of this altered insulin-receptor phosphorylation has not yet been determined, but it correlates with reduced insulin action and is reversible.[241–242]

Genetic Differences in Insulin Action

Certainly, important genetic differences in insulin action exist that are independent of obesity and of critical importance to the pathogenesis of NIDDM.[243–246] There has been recent interest in the insulin resistance noted in the nondiabetic population because of its possible link to hypertension and cardiovascular disease.[63,243,247] It has been estimated that 25% of the population are insulin resistant,[63] but one must be cautious about accepting this number because of the lack of agreement on the criteria for insulin resistance. Nonetheless, many people without diabetes undoubtedly have genetically determined insulin resistance and increased risk for developing NIDDM.

Much is being learned about the genetic syndromes of extreme insulin resistance such as type A insulin resistance and leprechaunism,[248] as is detailed in Chapter 16. As of early 1991, 14 different genetic defects had been found in 14 patients.[185] The relevance of these well-defined, rare gene defects to the molecular basis of the insulin resistance of NIDDM is uncertain, but the methodologic advances attained through work in this field should serve as important building blocks for future studies. The mechanisms of insulin action have turned out to be extremely complicated, and probably many pathways are influenced by genetic factors (Chapter 8). Particular attention is being given to the insulin receptor and the insulin-responsive GLUT-4 glucose transporter, in part because the steps in between these processes have not yet been fully elucidated.

With regard to the insulin receptor, the search continues for abnormalities that could account for a proportion of the population with NIDDM. Relatives of patients with the type A syndrome or leprechaunism can be heterozygous for the defect and manifest mild degrees of insulin resistance.[248] However, the known number of individuals with severe insulin resistance is not high enough to support a hypothesis that heterozygosity accounts for much of the existing NIDDM.[248] Nonetheless, there could be as yet unidentified mutations that produce subtle, but important, binding defects. In addition, problems with the promoter of the insulin-receptor gene or in processing mechanisms could lead to insulin resistance. Many of the complexities involved in the study of this problem have been outlined by Taylor et al.[248] For example, NIDDM typically develops when people are relatively old; thus, many individuals may have the required gene(s) but may have not yet developed diabetes, thus making it difficult to establish a cause-and-effect relationship. Furthermore, a critical mutation of the insulin-receptor gene may lead to diabetes only if certain other genes are present, such as those responsible for obesity or β-cell growth. Once an important lesion is found it can be expected to be present in some proportion of the NIDDM population but also both in people destined to develop NIDDM and in others who will never have NIDDM.

The insulin-receptor gene is very large, consisting of more than 120 kilobases (kb) with 22 exons on chromosome 19.[185] Considerable polymorphism has already been described in population studies, although efforts to use RFLP analysis in families with NIDDM to identify alleles linked to diabetes have to date been unsuccessful.[185,248–252] Other approaches that will be used more in the future are RNA heteroduplex mapping and direct determination of mutations by nucleotide sequence analysis. Analysis of genomic DNA in two studies of Pima Indians, in whom the prevalence of NIDDM is extremely high, led to the conclusion that the amino acid sequence of the insulin-receptor gene was normal.[253,254] The available data suggest that a structural abnormality of the insulin receptor itself is unlikely to account for a large proportion of cases of NIDDM.[255,256]

The insulin-responsive GLUT-4 glucose transporter in muscle is another attractive candidate for explaining, at least in part, the genetic basis for NIDDM. The human GLUT-4 protein consists of 509 amino acids and is a product of a 8-kb gene on chromosome 17.[50] Initial reports based on genomic studies indicate that the amino acid sequence of this transporter protein is normal in some subjects with NIDDM.[256] There are also early suggestions that polymorphism of this gene may be present in some individuals with NIDDM,[257] and such a defect could lead to a reduction in the expression of structurally normal transporter.

The Diabetic State

Hyperglycemia itself is associated with insulin resistance, as has been clearly demonstrated in IDDM and in animal models of insulin-deficient hyperglycemia.[130,179,180,258,259] This resistance can be improved by insulin treatment in humans with IDDM[180] and even by lowering glucose levels with phloridzin without changing plasma insulin concentrations in partially pancreatectomized rats.[260] Furthermore, the insulin resistance of

NIDDM can be at least partially normalized by lowering plasma glucose levels with aggressive insulin treatment.[217] Reduced glucose transport across the blood-brain barrier has also been found in hyperglycemic states.[261,262] This phenomenon is often referred to as "glucose toxicity;" the responsible mechanisms have not yet been defined. Hyperglycemia has been associated with reductions in the amount of the GLUT-4 in adipocytes,[220,222] but workers have been able to partially dissociate the amount of transporter in the plasma membrane from the rate of glucose transport.[223] In muscle, as noted above, transport is decreased, but reductions in GLUT-4 have been more difficult to define. All of this leads to the assumption that hyperglycemia can somehow cause alterations in the intrinsic activity of the glucose transporter, as well as to produce a reduction in transporter protein. Indeed, in studies using cultured adipocytes and muscle cells, high glucose concentrations were found to induce resistance to insulin-stimulated glucose uptake.[263–265] Therefore, the hyperglycemic state appears to be able to induce insulin resistance and defects in insulin secretion, both of which are at least partially reversible. It is still not fully accepted that these abnormalities are caused by hyperglycemia itself, although this remains the most attractive hypothesis. Nonetheless, this concept has important implications for all forms of diabetes, in that even mild hyperglycemia, once it develops, adversely affects both insulin action and insulin secretion; the interplay of the two exerts a deleterious influence on the progression toward frank diabetes.[130–132,266]

Interplay between Insulin Resistance and Inadequate Insulin Secretion: A Pathogenetic Final Common Pathway

There are similarities in the pathophysiology of IDDM and NIDDM. Once even mild hyperglycemia develops, a final common pathway is entered that can lead toward further metabolic deterioration[130–132,266] (Fig. 14–13). The term "glucose toxicity," which has been used to describe this situation, may give the inappropriate impression that the process is simple. As has been discussed, chronic hyperglycemia appears to lead directly to a loss of normal pulsatile secretion, a loss of glucose-induced insulin release, and a lowered overall rate of secretion throughout the day. Furthermore, hyperglycemia—whether in the presence of absolute or relative insulin deficiency—is associated with an impairment in glucose disposal that can be considered a form of insulin resistance. To make matters worse, the development of insulin deficiency leads to enhanced lipolysis and increased levels of free fatty acids, which can lead to increase hepatic glucose production and perhaps even contribute to the impairment in glucose disposal.[62,63] A vicious cycle may ensue, but obviously there are brakes on the process, because many people have mild NIDDM that remains stable for years. This deleterious interplay has theoretical implications for treatment, because lowering glucose concentrations with any form of treatment can improve both insulin secretion and insulin action.

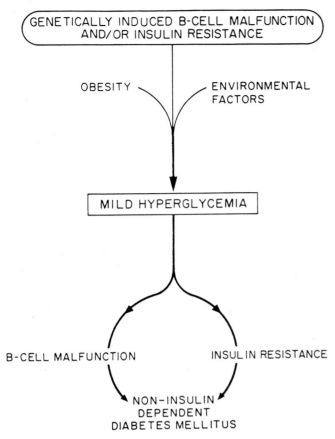

Fig. 14–13. Schematic representation of the pathogenesis of non-insulin-dependent diabetes mellitus. Note the final common pathway in which hyperglycemia is thought to have a deleterious influence upon both insulin secretion and insulin action. Reprinted with permission from reference 266 (Leahy JL, Bonner-Weir S, Weir GC. Beta-cell dysfunction induced by chronic hyperglycemia: current ideas on mechanism of impaired glucose-induced insulin secretion. Diabetes Care 1992;15:442–55; copyright © of the American Diabetes Association).

Contributions of Insulin Resistance and β-Cell Failure to the Development of NIDDM

Populations with a high prevalence of insulin resistance also have a high prevalence of NIDDM. The Nauruans from Micronesia are a particularly good example. When affluence led to obesity and physical inactivity, the prevalence of NIDDM increased dramatically.[19] The Pima Indians are an even more extreme example of this phenomenon.[18] In a mostly white population at the Joslin Diabetes Center, among offspring of two parents with NIDDM, the presence of insulin resistance greatly increases the risk of developing diabetes.[245] A similar result was seen in the Paris Prospective Study.[45] Therefore, a combination of environmental and genetic factors leads to a degree of insulin resistance that often results in NIDDM. Nonetheless, a critical point is that diabetes does not usually accompany insulin resistance. Although no definition of insulin resistance has been agreed upon,

insulin resistance is certainly far more common in populations of developed countries, with a prevalence possibly greater than 25%.[63] Because only a small proportion of such individuals have NIDDM, insulin resistance should be thought of as a risk factor. An important distinction to make, however, is between the proportion of individuals with insulin resistance in a population of varying ages who have NIDDM and the proportion who will develop the disease if they live long enough. Populations with obesity are also instructive. The majority of such individuals are insulin resistant, but only about 10 to 15% have diabetes.[243] Likewise, fewer than 20% of subjects with the severe insulin resistance of acromegaly or Cushing disease have diabetes.[63,130,243] Frequently, even individuals with the rare syndromes of extreme insulin resistance do not have diabetes.[267] Therefore, frank diabetes will develop only when insulin secretion is unable to compensate for whatever degree of insulin resistance is present; β-cell failure can therefore be considered the sine qua non for diabetes. This then raises the critical question: In the face of severe insulin resistance, how much β-cell capacity is required to compensate and maintain normal glucose levels for 75 years?

Another important question is how often NIDDM will develop in individuals who are insulin sensitive. There are reports of a substantial number of individuals with IGT and first-degree relatives of people with NIDDM who are considered to have a normal degree of insulin resistance.[65,268] Population differences seem to be important. Studies from Japan suggest that NIDDM commonly develops in subjects without insulin resistance,[101] whereas in Pima Indians NIDDM hardly ever evolves without insulin resistance. There are few longitudinal data about individuals who are truly insulin sensitive. The study of offspring of two parents with NIDDM described above found that insulin sensitivity greatly reduced the likelihood of a child's developing NIDDM.[245] Therefore, it appears that individuals who are very insulin-sensitive as well as those with a good capacity for β-cell compensation are unlikely to develop diabetes.

The Search for a Primary Defect in NIDDM

Considerable effort has been devoted to the search for the earliest identifiable metabolic defect in NIDDM. The most common approaches have been to study offspring or first-degree relatives of persons with diabetes or subjects with IGT. Much of the data are cross-sectional, although the most rigorous and valuable are longitudinal. In individuals who are truly normoglycemic, insulin resistance is the best predictor of the development of NIDDM.[45,245] This insulin resistance can be accounted for only partially by obesity. Much of it seems to have a genetic basis, and the quantitative contributions of physical inactivity are unknown. Once IGT develops, evidence of insufficient insulin secretion usually is found, suggesting that some kind of β-cell inadequacy is a prerequisite for progression to hyperglycemia.[98,99,131,266] It should not be assumed that the β-cells are normal in the normoglycemic prediabetic state with insulin resistance. The presence of normoglycemia indicates that the insulin resistance is completely compensated for by hyperinsulinemia. Thus, in the presence of true euglycemia, insulin resistance will always be associated with hyperinsulinemia, and individuals destined to develop diabetes should not be expected to have decreased insulin secretion. Perhaps some nonphysiologic challenge to β-cells, such as a slope of potentiation test[113] or an analysis of oscillation patterns,[92] could identify an underlying inadequacy in insulin secretory function. But at present, there is no test that measures the long-term secretory capacity of β-cells. Indeed, as discussed earlier, the critical defect allowing progression to NIDDM may be a failure to maintain β-cell mass, either because of a reduction in capacity for replication or because of an acceleration in the rate of cell death. At present there are no ways to measure these phenomena. Thus, in the absence of definitive genetic information about the true cause of NIDDM, one can only conclude that no primary lesion can be identified at present, that individuals destined to progress to NIDDM usually have insulin resistance, and that a failure of β-cell compensation is a requirement for actual progression to hyperglycemia.

The Search for the Genetic Cause of NIDDM

The genetic contributions to NIDDM appear to be strong. Concordance is found in 60 to 90% of identical twins, and in some families the frequency of NIDDM even suggests autosomal dominant inheritance (see Chapter 12). Some progress is being made in the identification of the genes responsible for NIDDM, with the focus being upon those candidate genes that are involved with insulin action and production. On the insulin-action side, a variety of mutations of the insulin receptor have been described, but these may account for as little as 1% of cases of NIDDM. The GLUT-4 glucose-transporter gene is an attractive candidate, but so far, little has turned up to suggest an important etiologic role. Other genes connected with the mechanisms of insulin action, such as the insulin receptor substrate-1 (IRS-1), will no doubt be scrutinized in the near future. Choosing promising genes that might be responsible for reduced β-cell secretory capacity is also difficult. The recent identification of mutations in the glucokinase gene in MODY kindreds has been a major discovery, but the contribution of this to typical NIDDM is uncertain, accounting at most for 5% of cases. Rare mutations of the insulin gene have been identified, but in most people with NIDDM, the structure of this gene is normal. The GLUT-2 glucose transporter and IAPP genes will be closely examined. Unfortunately, the genes responsible for β-cell replicative capacity and senescence have not yet been identified. One can predict that an abnormality in only one allele of the genes that control insulin synthesis or secretion or β-cell growth could lead to a diminished insulin output that might become quantitatively important only later in life. The genes that predispose people to obesity will no doubt turn out to be part of the genetic etiology of NIDDM. The era of the genetic analysis of NIDDM will certainly produce many interesting and complicated results. Certainly some important single abnormal genes will be identified, but probably most cases of NIDDM will be found to have a polygenic basis.

REFERENCES

1. Huse DM, Oster G, Killen AR, Lacey MJ, Golditz GA. The economic costs of non-insulin-dependent diabetes mellitus. JAMA 1989;262:2708–13.
2. Osler W. The principles and practice of medicine. New York: Appleton and Co, 1893:295.
3. National Diabetes Data Group. Classification and diagnosis of diabetes mellitus and other categories of glucose intolerance. Diabetes 1979:1039–57.
4. World Health Organization Study Group. Diabetes mellitus. WHO Tech Rep Ser 1985;727:1–113.
5. Fuller JH, Shipley MJ, Rose G, et al. Coronary heart disease risk and impaired glucose tolerance: the Whitehall study. Lancet 1980;1:1373–6.
6. Pyörälä K, Laakso M, Uusitupa M. Diabetes and atherosclerosis: an epidemiologic view. Diabetes Metab Rev 1987; 3:463–524.
7. Bennett PH, Knowler WC, Pettitt DJ, et al. Longitudinal studies of the development of diabetes in the Pima Indians. In: Eschewege E, ed. Advances in diabetes epidemiology: Inserm Symposium 22. Elsevier Biomedical Press: New York, 1982:65–74.
8. Kadowaki T, Miyake Y, Hagura R, et al. Risk factors for worsening to diabetes in subjects with impaired glucose tolerance. Diabetologia 1984;26:44–9.
9. Keen H, Jarrett RJ, McCartney P. The ten-year follow-up of the Bedford Survey (1962–1972): glucose tolerance and diabetes. Diabetologia 1982;22:73–8.
10. Groop LC, Bottazzo GF, Doniach D. Islet cell antibodies identify latent Type I diabetes in patients aged 35–75 years at diagnosis. Diabetes 1986;35:237–41.
11. Abu-Bakare A, Taylor R, Gill GV, Alberti KGMM. Tropical or malnutrition-related diabetes: a real syndrome? Lancet 1986;1:1135–8.
12. Fajans SS. Maturity-onset diabetes of the young (MODY). Diabetes Metab Rev 1989;5:579–606.
13. Froguel Ph, Vaxillaire M, Sun F, et al. Close linkage of glucokinase locus on chromosome 7p to early-onset non-insulin-dependent diabetes mellitus. Nature 1992; 356:162–4.
14. Velho G. Froguel P, Clement K, et al. Primary beta-cell secretory defect caused by mutations in glucokinase gene of chromosome 7 in kindreds of maturity onset diabetes of the young. Lancet 1992;340:444–8.
15. Bell GI, Xiang K-S, Newman MV, et al. Gene for non-insulin-dependent diabetes mellitus (maturity-onset diabetes of the young subtype) is linked to DNA polymorphism on human chromosome 20q. Proc Natl Acad Sci USA 1991;88:1484–8.
16. Mohan V, Ramachandran A, Snehalatha C, et al. High prevalence of maturity-onset diabetes of the young (MODY) among Indians. Diabetes Care 1985;8:371–4.
17. Winter WE, Maclaren NK, Riley WJ, et al. Maturity-onset diabetes of youth in black Americans. N Engl J Med 1987;316:285–91.
18. Knowler WC, Bennett PH, Hamman RF, Miller M. Diabetes incidence and prevalence in Pima Indians: a 19-fold greater incidence than in Rochester, Minnesota. Am J Epidemiol 1978;108:497–505.
19. Zimmet P, King H, Taylor R, et al. The high prevalence of diabetes mellitus, impaired glucose tolerance and diabetic

retinopathy in Nauru—the 1982 Survey. Diabetes Res 1984;1:13−8.

20. King H, Zimmet P. Trends in the prevalence and incidence of diabetes: non-insulin-dependent diabetes mellitus. WHO Health Stat Q 1988;41:190−6.

21. Mather HM, Keen H. The Southall Diabetes Survey: prevalence of known diabetes in Asians and Europeans. BMJ 1985;291:1081−4.

22. Kawate R, Yamakido M, Nishimoto Y, et al. Diabetes mellitus and its vascular complications in Japanese migrants on the island of Hawaii. Diabetes Care 1979; 2:161−70.

23. Palumbo PJ, Elveback LR, Chu C-P, et al. Diabetes mellitus: incidence, prevalence, survivorship, and causes of death in Rochester, Minnesota, 1945-1970. Diabetes 1976; 25:566−73.

24. Jackson RA. Mechanisms of age-related glucose intolerance. Diabetes Care 1990;13(Suppl 2):9−19.

25. Pettitt DJ, Aleck KA, Baird HR, et al. Congenital susceptibility to NIDDM role of intrauterine environment. Diabetes 1988;37:622−8.

26. Keen H. The Bedford survey: a critique of methods and findings. Proc R Soc Med 1964;57:200−2.

27. O'Sullivan JB, Mahan CM. Prospective study of 352 young patients with chemical diabetes. N Engl J Med 1969; 278:1038−41.

28. Kritz-Silverstein D, Barrett-Connor E, Wingard DL. The effect of parity on the later development of non-insulin-dependent diabetes mellitus or impaired glucose tolerance. N Engl J Med 1989;321:1214−9.

29. Hales CN, Barker DJP, Clark PMS, et al. Fetal and infant growth and impaired glucose tolerance at age 64. BMJ 1991;303:1−19−22.

30. Swinburn BA, Boyce VL, Bergman RN, et al. Deterioration in carbohydrate metabolism and lipoprotein changes induced by modern, high fat diet in Pima Indians and caucasians. J Clin Endocrinol Metab 1991;73: 156−65.

31. Frisch RE, Wyshak G, Albright TE, et al. Lower prevalence of diabetes in female former college athletes compared with nonathletes. Diabetes 1986;35:1101−5.

32. Helmrich SP, Ragland DR, Leung RW, Paffenbarger RS Jr. Physical activity and reduced occurrence of non-insulin-dependent diabetes mellitus. N Engl J Med 1991; 325:147−52.

33. DeFronzo RA, Ferrannini E. Regulation of hepatic glucose metabolism in humans. Diabetes Metab Rev 1987; 3:415−59.

34. Cherrington AD, Stevenson RW, Steiner KE, et al. Insulin, glucagon and glucose as regulators of hepatic glucose uptake and production in vivo. Diabetes Metab Rev 1987;3:307−32.

35. Consoli A, Kennedy F, Miles J, Gerich J. Determination of Krebs cycle metabolic carbon exhange in vivo and its use to estimate the individual contributions of gluconeogenesis and glycogenolysis to overall glucose output in man. J Clin Invest 80:1303, 1987.

36. DeFronzo RA, Gunnarsson R, Björkman O, et al. Effects of insulin on peripheral and splanchnic glucose metabolism in noninsulin-dependent (Type II) diabetes mellitus. J Clin Invest 1985;76:149−55.

37. Björntorp P, Sjöström L. Carbohydrate storage in man: speculations and some quantitative considerations. Metabolism 1978;27(Suppl 2):1853−65.

38. DeFronzo RA. The triumvirate: β-cell, muscle, liver: a collusion responsible for NIDDM. Diabetes 1988; 37:667−87.

39. Revers RR, Fink R, Griffin J, et al. Influence of hyperglycemia on insulin's in vivo effects in Type II diabetes. J Clin Invest 1984;73:664−72.

40. Bogardus C, Lillioja S, Howard BV, et al. Relationships between insulin secretion, insulin action and fasting plasma glucose concentration in nondiabetic and noninsulin-dependent diabetic subjects. J Clin Invest 1984; 74:1238−46.

41. Firth RG, Bell PM, Marsh HM, et al. Postprandial hyperglycemia in patients with noninsulin-dependent diabetes mellitus: role of hepatic and extrahepatic tissues. J Clin Invest 1986;77:1525−32.

42. DeFronzo RA, Ferrannini E, Hendler R, et al. Regulation of splanchnic and peripheral glucose uptake by insulin and hyperglycemia in man. Diabetes 1983;32:35−45.

43. Klauser R, Prager R, Schernthaner G, Olefsky JM. Contribution of postprandial insulin and glucose to glucose disposal in normal and insulin resistant obese subjects. J Clin Endocrinol Metab 1991;73:758−64.

44. Kolterman OG, Gray RS, Griffin J, et al. Receptor and postreceptor defects contribute to the insulin resistance in noninsulin-dependent diabetes mellitus. J Clin Invest 1981;68:957−69.

45. Charles MA, Fontbonne A, Thibult N, et al. Risk factors for NIDDM in white population: Paris prospective study. Diabetes 1991;40:796−9.

46. DeFronzo RA, Ferrannini E, Simonson DC. Fasting hyperglycemia in noninsulin-dependent diabetes mellitus: contributions of excessive hepatic glucose production and impaired tissue glucose uptake. Metabolism 1989; 38:387−95.

47. Butler PC, Kryshak EJ, Schwenk WF, et al. Hepatic and extrahepatic responses to insulin in NIDDM and nondiabetic humans: assessments in absence of artifact introduced by tritiated nonglucose contaminants. Diabetes 1990;39:217−25.

48. Eriksson J, Franssila-Kallunki A, Ekstrand A, et al. Early metabolic defects in persons at increased risk for non-insulin-dependent diabetes mellitus. N Engl J Med 1989; 321:337−43.

49. Mueckler M. Family of glucose-transporter genes implications for glucose homeostasis and diabetes. Diabetes 1990;39:6−11.

50. Bell GI, Kayano T, Buse JB, et al. Molecular biology of mammalian glucose transporters. Diabetes Care 13:198, 1990.

51. Shulman GI, Rothman DL, Jue T, et al. Quantitation of muscle glycogen synthesis in normal subjects and subjects with non-insulin-dependent diabetes by ^{13}C nuclear magnetic resonance spectroscopy. N Engl J Med 1990; 322:223−8.

52. Thorburn AW, Gumbiner B, Bulacan F, et al. Intracellular glucose oxidation and glycogen synthase activity are reduced in non-insulin-dependent (Type II) diabetes independent of impaired glucose uptake. J Clin Invest 1990;85:522−9.

53. Bogardus C, Lillioja S, Stone K, Mott D. Correlation between muscle glycogen synthase activity and in vivo insulin action in man. J Clin Invest 1984;73:1185−90.

54. Thorburn AW, Gumbiner B, Bulacan F. Multiple defects in muscle glycogen synthase activity contribute to reduced glycogen synthesis in non-insulin-dependent diabetes mellitus. J Clin Invest 1991;87:489−95.

55. Mandarino LJ, Madar Z, Kolterman OG, et al. Adipocyte glycogen synthase and pyruvate dehydrogenase in obese and Type II diabetic subjects. Am J Physiol 1986; 251:E489−96.

56. Randle PJ, Garland PB, Hales CN, Newsholme EA. The glucose fatty-acid cycle: its role in insulin sensitivity and the metabolic disturbances of diabetes mellitus. Lancet 1963;1:785–9.

57. Lillioja S, Bogardus C, Mott DM, et al. Relationship between insulin-mediated glucose disposal and lipid metabolism in man. J Clin Invest 1985;75:1106–15.

58. Felber J-P, Ferrannini E, Golay A, et al. Role of lipid oxidation in pathogenesis of insulin resistance of obesity and Type II diabetes. Diabetes 1987;36:1341–50.

59. Eriksson J, Saloranta C, Widén E, et al. Non-esterified fatty acids do not contribute to insulin resistance in persons at increased risk of developing Type 2 (non-insulin-dependent) diabetes mellitus. Diabetologia 1991; 34:192–7.

60. Ferrannini E, Barrett EJ, Bevilacqua S, DeFronzo RA. Effect of fatty acids on glucose production and utilization in man. J Clin Invest 1983;72:1737–47.

61. Thiébaud D, DeFronzo RA, Jacot E, et al. Effect of long chain triglyceride infusion on glucose metabolism in man. Metabolism 1982;31:1128–36.

62. Saloranta C, Franssila-Kallunki A, Ekstrand A, et al. Modulation of hepatic glucose production by non-esterified fatty acids in Type 2 (non-insulin-dependent) diabetes mellitus. Diabetologia 1991;34:409–15.

63. Reaven GM. Banting Lecture 1988: role of insulin resistance in human disease. Diabetes 1988;37:1595–607.

64. Ferrannini E, Simonson DC, Katz LD, et al. The disposal of an oral glucose load in patients with non-insulin-dependent diabetes. Metabolism 1988;37:79–85.

65. Evron W, Mitrakou A, Jenssen T, et al. Impaired glucose tolerance—a disorder of the pancreatic B-cell [Abstract no. 87]. Diabetes 1990;39(Suppl 1):22A.

66. Mitrakou A, Evron W, Jenssen T, et al. Hyperinsulinemia as a consequence of impaired insulin secretion rather than insulin resistance [Abstract no. 122]. Diabetes 1991;40 (Suppl 1):31A.

67. Yalow RS, Berson SA. Plasma insulin concentrations in nondiabetic and early diabetic subjects: determinations by a new sensitive immuno-assay technic. Diabetes 1960; 9:254–60.

68. Karam JH, Grodsky GM, Forsham PH. Excessive insulin response to glucose in obese subjects as measured by immunochemical assay. Diabetes 1963;12:197–204.

69. Perley M, Kipnis DM. Plasma insulin responses to glucose and tolbutamide of normal weight and obese diabetic and nondiabetic subjects. Diabetes 1966;15:867–74.

70. Perley MJ, Kipnis DM. Plasma insulin responses to oral and intravenous glucose: studies in normal and diabetic subjects. J Clin Invest 1967;46:1954–62.

71. Turner RC, Mann JI, Simpson RD, et al. Fasting hyperglycaemia and relatively unimpaired meal responses in mild diabetes. Clin Endocrinol 1977;6:253–64.

72. Liu G, Coulston A, Chen Y-DI, Reaven GM. Does day-long absolute hypoinsulinemia characterize the patient with non-insulin-dependent diabetes mellitus? Metabolism 1983;32:754–6.

73. Peavy DE, Brunner MR, Duckworth WC, et al. Receptor binding and biological potency of several split forms (conversion intermediates) of human proinsulin: studies in cultured Im-9 lymphocytes and in vivo and in vitro in rats. J Biol Chem 1985;260:13989–94.

74. Cohen RM, Licinio J, Polonsky KS, et al. The effect of biosynthetic human proinsulin on the hepatic response to glucagon in insulin-deficient diabetes. J Clin Endocrinol Metab 1987;64:476–81.

75. Kitabchi AE, Duckworth WC, Stentz FB. In: Rifkin H, Porte D Jr, eds. Ellenberg and Rifkin's diabetes mellitus: theory and practice. New York: Elsevier, 1989:71–88.

76. Temple RC, Carrington CA, Luzio SD, et al. Insulin deficiency in non-insulin-dependent diabetes. Lancet 1989;1:293–5.

77. Duckworth WC, Kitabchi AE, Heinemann M. Direct measurement of plasma proinsulin in normal and diabetic subjects. Am J Med 1972;53:418–27.

78. Gorden P, Hendricks CM, Roth J. Circulating proinsulin-like component in man: increased proportion in hypoinsulinemic states. Diabetologia 1974;10:469–74.

79. Mako ME, Starr JI, Rubenstein AH. Circulating proinsulin in patients with maturity onset diabetes. Am J Med 1977;63:865–9.

80. Deacon CF, Schleser-Mohr S, Ballmann M, et al. Preferential release of proinsulin relative to insulin in non-insulin-dependent diabetes mellitus. Acta Endocrinol (Copenh) 1988;119:549–54.

81. Yoshioka N, Kuzuya T, Matsuda A, et al. Serum proinsulin levels at fasting and after oral glucose load in patients with Type 2 (non-insulin-dependent) diabetes mellitus. Diabetologia 1988;31:355–60.

82. Yoshioka N, Kuzuya T, Matsuda A, Iwamoto Y. Effects of dietary treatment on serum insulin and proinsulin response in newly diagnosed NIDDM. Diabetes 1989; 38:262–6.

83. Leahy JL, Halban PA, Weir GC. Relative hypersecretion of proinsulin in rat model of NIDDM. Diabetes 1991; 40:985–9.

84. Goodner CJ, Walike BC, Koerker DJ, et al. Insulin, glucagon, and glucose exhibit synchronous, sustained oscillations in fasting monkeys. Science 1977;195:177–9.

85. Weigle, D.S. Pulsatile secretion of fuel-regulatory hormones. Diabetes 1987;36:764–5.

86. Lang DA, Matthews DR, Peto J, Turner RC. Cyclic oscillations of basal plasma glucose and insulin concentrations in human beings. N Engl J Med 1979;301:1023–7.

87. Hansen BC, Jen K-LC, Pek SB, Wolfe RA. Rapid oscillations in plasma insulin, glucagon, and glucose in obese and normal weight humans. J Clin Endocrinol Metab 1982; 54:785–92.

88. Stagner JI, Samols E, Weir GC. Sustained oscillations of insulin, glucagon, and somatostatin from the isolated canine pancreas during exposure to a constant glucose concentration. J Clin Invest 1980;65:939–42.

89. Chou H-F, Ipp E. Pulsatile insulin secretion in isolated rat islets. Diabetes 1990;39:112–7.

90. Polonsky KS, Given BD, Van Cauter E. Twenty-four-hour profiles and pulsatile patterns of insulin secretion in normal and obese subjects. J Clin Invest 1988;81:442–8.

91. Lang DA, Matthews DR, Burnett M, Turner RC. Brief, irregular oscillations of basal insulin and glucose concentrations in diabetic man. Diabetes 1981;30:435–9.

92. O'Rahilly S, Turner RC, Matthews DR. Impaired pulsatile secretion of insulin in relatives of patients with non-insulin-dependent diabetes. N Engl J Med 1988; 318:1225–30.

93. Polonsky KS, Given BD, Hirsch LJ, et al. Abnormal patterns of insulin secretion in non-insulin-dependent diabetes mellitus. N Engl J Med 1988;318:1231–9.

94. Paolisso G, Scheen AJ, Giugliano D, et al. Pulsatile insulin delivery has greater metabolic effects than continuous hormone administration in man: importance of pulse frequency. J Clin Endocrinol Metab 1991;72:607–15.

95. Bratusch-Marrain PR, Komjati M, Waldhäusl WK. Efficacy of pulsatile versus continuous insulin administration on

hepatic glucose production and glucose utilization in Type I diabetic humans. Diabetes 1986;35:922–6.

96. Weigle DS, Rumbaoa AV, Goodner CJ. Lack of evidence for improvement in long-term glycemic control by pulsatile insulin infusion in streptozocin-induced diabetic baboon. Diabetes 1991;40:349–57.

97. Reaven G, Miller R. Study of the relationship between glucose and insulin responses to an oral glucose load in man. Diabetes 1968;17:560–9.

98. Saad MF, Knowler WC, Pettitt DJ, et al. Sequential changes in serum insulin concentration during development of non-insulin-dependent diabetes. Lancet 1989;1:1356–9.

99. Saad MF, Knowler WC, Pettitt DJ, et al. The natural history of impaired glucose tolerance in the Pima Indians. N Engl J Med 1988;319:1500–6.

100. Bergstrom RW, Wahl PW, Leonetti DL, Fujimoto WY. Association of fasting glucose levels with a delayed secretion of insulin after oral glucose in subjects with glucose intolerance. J Clin Endocrinol Metab 1990; 71:1447–53.

101. Kosaka K, Hagura R, Kuzuya T. Insulin responses in equivocal and definite diabetes, with special reference to subjects who had mild glucose intolerance but later developed definite diabetes. Diabetes 1977;26:944–52.

102. Cerasi E, Efendić S, Luft R. Dose-response relation between plasma-insulin and blood-glucose levels during oral glucose loads in prediabetic and diabetic subjects. Lancet 1973; 1:794–7.

103. Cerasi E. Insulin secretion in diabetes mellitus. In: Lefebvre PJ, Pipeleers DG, eds. The pathology of the endocrine pancreas in diabetes. Heidelberg: Springer-Verlag, 1988; 191–218.

104. Creutzfeldt W. The incretin concept today. Diabetologia 1979;16:75–85.

105. Kreymann B, Williams G, Ghatei MA, Bloom SR. Glucagon-like peptide-I 7–36: a physiological incretin in man. Lancet 1987;2:1300–4.

106. Reimers J, Nauck M, Creutzfeldt W, et al. Lack of insulinotropic effect of endogenous and exogenous cholecystokinin in man. Diabetologia 1988;31:271–80.

107. Nauck, M, Stöckmann F, Ebert R, Creutzfeldt W. Reduced incretin effect in type 2 (non-insulin-dependent) diabetes. Diabetologia 1986;29:46–52.

108. Curry DL, Bennett LL, Grodsky GM. Dynamics of insulin secretion by the perfused rat pancreas. Endocrinology 1968;83:572–84.

109. Simpson RG, Benedetti A, Grodsky GM, et al. Early phase of insulin release. Diabetes 1968;17:684–92.

110. Seltzer HS, Allen EW, Herron AL Jr, Brennan MT. Insulin secretion in response to glycemic stimulus: relation of delayed initial release to carbohydrate intolerance in mild diabetes mellitus. J Clin Invest 1967;46:323–5.

111. Pfeifer MA, Halter JB, Porte D Jr. Insulin secretion in diabetes mellitus. Am J Med 1981;70:579–88.

112. Brunzell JD, Robertson RP, Lerner RL, et al. Relationships between fasting plasma glucose levels and insulin secretion during intravenous glucose tolerance tests. J Clin Endocrinol Metab 1976;42:222–9.

113. Porte D Jr. β-Cells in Type II diabetes mellitus. Diabetes 1991;40:166–80.

114. Metz SA, Halter JB, Robertson RP. Paradoxical inhibition of insulin secretion by glucose in human diabetes mellitus. J Clin Endocrinol Metab 1979;48:827–35.

115. Lillioja S, Mott DM, Howard BV, et al. Impaired glucose-tolerance as a disorder of insulin action: longitudinal and cross-sectional studies in Pima Indians. N Engl J Med 1988;318:1217–25.

116. Bruce DG, Chisholm DJ, Storlien LH, Kraegen EW. Physiological importance of deficiency in early prandial insulin secretion in non-insulin-dependent diabetes. Diabetes 1988;37:736–44.

117. Hosker JP, Burnett MA, Matthews DR, Turner RC. Suppression of insulin secretion by falling plasma glucose levels is impaired in type 2 diabetes. Diabetic Med 1988; 5:856–60.

118. Deckert T. Insulin secretion following administration of secretin in patients with diabetes mellitus. Acta Endocrinol 1968;59:150–8.

119. Deckert T, Lauridsen UB, Madsen SN, Mogensen P. Insulin responses to glucose, tolbutamide, secretin, and isoprenaline in maturity-onset diabetes mellitus. Dan Med Bull 1972;19:222–6.

120. Palmer JP, Benson JW, Walter RM, Ensinck JW. Arginine-stimulated acute phase of insulin and glucagon secretion in diabetic subjects. J Clin Invest 1976;58:565–70.

121. Robertson RP, Halter JB, Porte D Jr. A role for alpha-adrenergic receptors in abnormal insulin secretion in diabetes mellitus. J Clin Invest 1976;57:791–5.

122. Lerner RL, Porte D Jr. Studies of secretin-stimulated insulin responses in man. J Clin Invest 1972;51:2205–10.

123. Varsano-Aharon N, Echemendia E, Yalow RS, Berson SA. Early insulin responses to glucose and to tolbutamide in maturity-onset diabetes. Metabolism 1970;19:409–17.

124. Ward WK, Bolgiano DC, McKnight B, et al. Diminished β cell secretory capacity in patients with noninsulin-dependent diabetes mellitus. J Clin Invest 1984;74:1318–28.

125. Dimitriadis GD, Pehling GB, Gerich JE. Abnormal glucose modulation of islet A- and B- cell responses to arginine in non-insulin-dependent diabetes mellitus. Diabetes 1985; 34:541–7.

126. McCulloch DK, Klaff LJ, Kahn SE, et al. Nonprogression of subclinical beta-cell dysfunction among first-degree relatives of IDDM patients: 5-yr follow-up of the Seattle Family Study. Diabetes 1990;39:549–56.

127. McCulloch DK, Raghu PK, Johnston C, et al. Defects in β-cell function and insulin sensitivity in normoglycemic streptozocin-treated baboons: a model of preclinical insulin-dependent diabetes. J Clin Endocrinol Metab 1988; 67:785–92.

128. Beard JC, Halter JB, Best JD, et al. Dexamethasone-induced insulin resistance enhances B-cell responsiveness to glucose level in normal men. Am J Physiol 1984;247:E592–6.

129. Kahn SE, Beard JC, Schwartz MW, et al. Increased β-cell secretory capacity as mechanism for islet adaptation to nicotinic acid-induced insulin resistance. Diabetes 1989; 38:562–8.

130. Weir GC. Non-insulin-dependent diabetes mellitus: interplay between B-cell inadequacy and insulin resistance. Am J Med 1982;73:461–4.

131. Weir GC, Leahy JL, Bonner-Weir S. Experimental reduction of B-cell mass: implications for the pathogenesis of diabetes. Diabetes Metab Rev 1986;2:125–61.

132. Leahy JL. Natural history of β-cell dysfunction in NIDDM. Diabetes Care 1990;13:992–1010.

133. Bonner-Weir S, Trent DF, Honey RN, Weir GC. Responses of neonatal rat islets to streptozotocin: limited B-cell regeneration and hyperglycemia. Diabetes 1981;30:64–9.

134. Weir GC, Clore ET, Zmachinski CJ, Bonner-Weir S. Islet secretion in a new experimental model for non-insulin-dependent diabetes. Diabetes 1981;30:590–5.

135. Giroix MH, Portha B, Kergoat M, et al. Glucose insensitivity and amino acid hypersensitivity of insulin release in rats with non-insulin-dependent diabetes: a study with the perfused pancreas. Diabetes 1983;32:445–51.

136. Portha B, Blondel O, Serradas P, et al. The rat models of non-insulin dependent diabetes induced by neonatal streptozotocin. Diabete Metab 1989;15:61–75.

137. Grill V, Sako Y, Östenson C-G, Jalkanen P. Multiple abnormalities in insulin responses to nonglucose nutrients in neonatally streptozotocin diabetic rats. Endocrinology 1991;128:2195–203.

138. Bonner-Weir S, Trent DF, Weir GC. Partial pancreatectomy in the rat and subsequent defect in glucose-induced insulin release. J Clin Invest 1983;71:1544–53.

139. Rossetti L, Shulman GI, Zawalich W, DeFronzo RA. Effect of chronic hyperglycemia on in vivo insulin secretion in partially pancreatectomized rats. J Clin Invest 1987; 80:1037–44.

140. Leahy JL, Cooper HE, Deal DA, Weir G.C. Chronic hyperglycemia is associated with impaired glucose influence on insulin secretion: a study in normal rats using chronic in vivo glucose infusions. J Clin Invest 1986; 77:908–15.

141. Leahy JL, Cooper HE, Weir GC. Impaired insulin secretion associated with near normoglycemia: study in normal rats with 96-h in vivo glucose infusions. Diabetes 1987; 36:459–64.

142. Portha B, Serradas P, Bailbé D, et al. β-Cell insensitivity to glucose in the GK rat a spontaneous nonobese model for Type II diabetes. Diabetes 1991;40:486–91.

143. Unger RH. Diabetic hyperglycemia: link to impaired glucose transport in pancreatic β cells. Science 1991; 251:1200–5.

144. Wu Y-J, Thorens B, Leahy JL, et al. Increased basal and normal glucose-potentiated arginine-induced insulin secretion in the presence of reduced GLUT-2 expression in the db/db mouse [Abstract]. Clin Res 1991;39: 307A.

145. Leahy JL, Weir GC. Unresponsiveness to glucose in a streptozocin model of diabetes: inappropriate insulin and glucagon responses to a reduction of glucose concentration. Diabetes 1985;34:653–9.

146. Portha B, Blondel O, Serradas P, et al. The rat models of non-insulin-dependent diabetes induced by neonatal streptozotocin. Diabete Metab 1989;15:61–75.

147. Grill V, Westberg M, Östenson C-G. B cell insensitivity in a rat model of non-insulin-dependent diabetes: evidence for a rapidly reversible effect of previous hyperglycemia. J Clin Invest 1987;80:664–9.

148. Leahy JL, Weir GC. B-cell dysfunction in hyperglycemic rat models: recovery of glucose-induced insulin secretion with lowering of the ambient glucose level. Diabetologia 1991;34:640–7.

149. Vague P, Moulin J-P. The defective glucose sensitivity of the B cell in non insulin dependent diabetes: improvement after twenty hours of normoglycaemia. Metabolism 1982;31:139–42.

150. Ganda OP, Srikanta S, Brink SJ, et al. Differential sensitivity to β-cell secretagogues in "early," Type I diabetes mellitus. Diabetes 1984;33:516–21.

151. Bleich D, Jackson RA, Soeldner JS, Eisenbarth GS. Analysis of metabolic progression to Type I diabetes in ICA+ relatives of patients with Type I diabetes. Diabetes Care 1990;13:111–8.

152. Sorenson RL, Parsons JA. Insulin secretion in mammosomatotropic tumor-bearing and pregnant rats: a role for lactogens. Diabetes 1985;34:337–41.

153. Meglasson MD, Matschinsky FM. Pancreatic islet glucose metabolism and regulation of insulin secretion. Diabetes Metab Rev 1986;2:163–214.

154. Marynissen G, Leclercg-Meyer V, Sener A, Malaisse WJ. Perturbation of pancreatic islet function in glucose-infused rats. Metabolism 1990;39:87–95.

155. Giroix M-H, Rasschaert J, Bailbe D, et al. Impairment of glycerol phosphate shuttle in islets from rats with diabetes induced by neonatal streptozocin. Diabetes 1991; 40:227–32.

156. Thorens B, Weir GC, Leahy JL, et al. Reduced expression of the liver/beta-cell glucose transporter isoform in glucose-insensitive pancreatic beta cells of diabetic rats. Proc Natl Acad Sci USA 1990;87:6492–6.

157. Richardson KC, Young FG. Histology of diabetes induced in dogs by injection of anterior-pituitary extracts. Lancet 1938;1:1098–101.

158. Imamura T, Koffler M, Helderman JH, et al. Severe diabetes induced in subtotally depancreatized dogs by sustained hyperglycemia. Diabetes 1988;37:600–9.

159. Lukens FDW, Dohan FC. Pituitary-diabetes in the cat: recovery following insulin or dietary treatment. Endocrinology 1942;30:175–202.

160. Kosaka K, Kuzuya T, Akanuma Y, Hagura R. Increase in insulin response after treatment of overt maturity-onset diabetes is independent of the mode of treatment. Diabetologia 1980;18:23–8.

161. Permutt MA, Elbein SC. Insulin gene in diabetes: analysis through RFLP. Diabetes Care 1990;13:364–74.

162. Steiner DF, Tager HS, Chan SJ, et al. Lessons learned from molecular biology of insulin-gene mutations. Diabetes Care 1990;13:600–9.

163. Samols E, Bonner-Weir S, Weir GC. Intra-islet insulin-glucagon-somatostatin relationships. Clin Endocrinol Metab 1986;15:33–56.

164. Unger RH. Glucagon physiology and pathophysiology in the light of new advances. Diabetologia 1985;28: 574–8.

165. Bolli GB, Tsalikian E, Haymond MW, et al. Defective glucose counterregulation after subcutaneous insulin in noninsulin-dependent diabetes mellitus. J Clin Invest 1984;73:1532–41.

166. Weir GC, Bonner-Weir S. Islets of Langerhans: the puzzle of intraislet interactions and their relevance to diabetes. J Clin Invest 1990;85:983–7.

167. Maclean N, Ogilvie RF. Quantitative estimation of the pancreatic islet tissue in diabetic subjects. Diabetes 1955;4:367–76.

168. Saito K, Yaginuma N, Takahashi T. Differential volumetry of A, B, and D cells in the pancreatic islets of diabetic and nondiabetic subjects. Tohoku J Exp Med 1979; 129:273–83.

169. Westermark P, Wilander E. The influence of amyloid deposits on the islet volume in maturity onset diabetes mellitus. Diabetologia 1978;15:417–21.

170. Gepts W, Lecompte PM. The pancreatic islets in diabetes. Am J Med 1981;70:105–15.

171. Stefan Y, Orci L, Malaisse-Lagae F, et al. Quantitation of endocrine cell content in the pancreas of nondiabetic and diabetic humans. Diabetes 1982;31:694–700.

172. Klöppel G, Löhr M, Habich K, et al. Islet pathology and the pathogenesis of type 1 and type 2 diabetes mellitus revisited. Surv Synth Pathol Res 1985;4:110–25.

173. Clark A, Wells CA, Buley ID, et al. Islet amyloid, increased A-cells, reduced B-cells and exocrine fibrosis: quantitative changes in the pancreas in type 2 diabetes. Diabetes Res 1988;9:151–9.

174. Ogilvie RF. The islands of Langerhans in 19 cases of obesity. J Pathol Bacteriol 1933;37:473–81.

175. Bonner-Weir S. Pancreatic islets: morphology, organization, and physiological implications. In: Draznin B,

Melmed S, LeRoith D, eds. Insulin secretion. New York: Alan R. Liss, 1989:1–11.

176. Weir GC, Bonner-Weir S, Leahy JL. Islet mass and function in diabetes and transplantation. Diabetes 1990;39: 401–5.

177. Kendall DM, Sutherland DER, Najarian JS, et al. Effects of hemipancreatectomy on insulin secretion and glucose tolerance in healthy humans. N Engl J Med 1990; 322:898–93.

178. Halter JB, Graf RJ, Porte D Jr. Potentiation of insulinecretory responses by plasma glucose levels in man: evidence that hyperglycemia in diabetes compensates for impaired glucose potentiation. J Clin Endocrinol Metab 1979; 48:946–54.

179. Unger RH, Grundy S. Hyperglycemia as an inducer as well as a consequence of impaired islet cell function and insulin resistance: implications for the management of diabetes. Diabetologia 1985;28:119–21.

180. Rossetti L, Giaccari A, DeFronzo RA. Glucose toxicity. Diabetes Care 1990;13:610–30.

181. Johnson KH, O'Brien TD, Betsholtz C, Westermark P. Islet amyloid, islet-amyloid polypeptide and diabets mellitus. N Engl J Med 1989;321:513–8.

182. Opie EL. The relation of diabetes mellitus to lesions of the pancreas: hyaline degeneration of the islands of Langerhans. J Exp Med 1900–1901;5:527–40.

183. Westermark P, Wernstedt C, Wilander E, et al. Amyloid fibrils in human insulinoma and islets of Langerhans of the diabetic cat are derived from a neuropeptide-like protein also present in normal islet cells. Proc Natl Acad Sci USA 1987;84:3881–5.

184. Cooper GJS, Willis AC, Clark A, et al. Purification and characterization of a peptide from amyloid-rich pancreases of type 2 diabetic patients. Proc Natl Acad Sci USA 1987; 84:8628–32.

185. Bell GI. Molecular defects in diabetes mellitus. Diabetes 1991;40:413–22.

186. Steiner DF, Ohagi S, Nagamatsu S, et al. Perspectives in diabetes: is islet amyloid polypeptide a significant factor in pathogenesis or pathophysiology of diabetes? Diabetes 1991;40:305–9.

187. Clark A, Lloyd J, Novials A, et al. Localisation of islet amyloid polypeptide and its carboxyl terminal flanking peptide in islets of diabetic man and monkey. Diabetologia 1991;34:449–51.

188. Johnson KH, O'Brien TD, Westermark P. Newly identified pancreatic protein islet amyloid polypeptide: what is its relationship to diabetes? Diabetes 1991;40:310–4.

189. Ogawa A, Harris V, McCorkle SK, et al. Amylin secretion from the rat pancreas and its selective loss after streptozotocin treatment. J Clin Invest 1990;85:973–6.

190. Clark A. Islet amyloid and type 2 diabetes. Diabetic Med 1989;6:561–7.

191. Brockenbrough JS, Weir GC, Bonner-Weir S. Discordance of exocrine and endocrine growth after 90% pancreatectomy in rats. Diabetes 1988;37:232–6.

192. Butler PC, Butler AE, Roche PC. Islet-associated polypeptide (IAPP) deposits in noninsulin dependent diabetes mellitus (NIDDM): cause or effect? [Abstract] Clin Res 1991;39:306A.

193. Cooper GJS, Leighton B, Dimitriadis GD, et al. Amylin found in amyloid deposits in human type 2 diabetes mellitus may be a hormone that regulates glycogen metabolism in skeletal muscle. Proc Natl Acad Sci USA 1988;85:7763–6.

194. Sanke T, Hanabusa T, Nakano Y, et al. Plasma islet amyloid polypeptide (amylin) levels and their responses to oral glucose in type 2 (non-insulin-dependent) diabetic patients. Diabetologia 1991;34:129–32.

195. Himsworth HP, Kerr RB. Insulin-sensitive and insulin-insensitive types of diabetes mellitus. Clin Sci 1942; 4:120.

196. Beck-Nielsen H, Pedersen O, Sørensen NS. Effects of dietary changes on cellular insulin binding and in vivo insulin sensitivity. Metabolism 1980;29:482–7.

197. Zierler KL, Rabinowitz D. Roles of insulin and growth hormone, based on studies of forearm metabolism in man. Medicine (Baltimore) 1963;42:385–402.

198. Foley JE. Mechanisms of impaired insulin action in isolated adipocytes from obese and diabetic subjects. Diabetes Metab Rev 1988;4:487–505.

199. Olefsky JM, Molina JM. Insulin resistance in man. In: Rifkin H, Porte D Jr, eds. Ellenberg and Rifkin's diabetes mellitus: theory and practice. New York: Elsevier, 1989: 121–53.

200. DeFronzo RA, Tobin JD, Andres R. Glucose clamp technique: a method for quantifying insulin secretion and resistance. Am J Physiol 1979;237:E214–23.

201. DeFronzo RA, Simonson D, Ferrannini E. Hepatic and peripheral insulin resistance: a common feature of type 2 (non-insulin-dependent), type 1 (insulin-dependent) diabetes mellitus. Diabetologia 1982;23:313–9.

202. Bergman RN. Toward physiological understanding of glucose-tolerance: minimal-model approach. Diabetes 1989;38:1512–27.

203. Campbell PJ, Gerich JE. Impact of obesity on insulin action in volunteers with normal glucose tolerance: demonstration of a threshold for the adverse effect of obesity. J Clin Endocrinol Metab 1990;70:1114–8.

204. Henry RR, Wallace P, Olefsky JM. Effects of weight loss on mechanisms of hyperglycemia in obese non-insulin-dependent diabetes mellitus. Diabetes 1986;35:990–8.

205. Vague J. The degree of masculine differentiation of obesities: a factor determining predisposition to diabetes, atheriosclerosis, gout, and uric calculous disease. Am J Clin Nutr 1956;4:20–34.

206. Kissebah AH, Vydelingum N, Murray R, et al. Relation of body fat distribution to metabolic complications of obesity. J Clin Endocrinol Metab 1982;54:254–60.

207. Krotkiewski M, Björntorp P, Sjöström L, Smith U. Impact of obesity on metabolism in men and women: importance of regional adipose tissue distribution. J Clin Invest 1983; 72:1150–62.

208. Kolterman OG, Insel J, Seakow M, Olefsky JM. Mechanisms of insulin resistance in human obesity: evidence of receptor and postreceptor defects. J Clin Invest 1980; 65:1272–84.

209. Laakso M, Edelman SV, Brechtel G, Baron AD. Decreased effect of insulin to stimulate skeletal muscle blood flow in obese man: a novel mechanism for insulin resistance. J Clin Invest 1990;85:1844–52.

210. Björntorp P. The associations between obesity, adipose tissue distribution and disease. Acta Med Scand Suppl 1988;723:121–34.

211. Lohmann D, Liebold F, Heilmann W, et al. Diminished insulin response in highly trained athletes. Metabolism 1978;27:521–4.

212. Devlin JT, Hirshman M, Horton ED, Horton ES. Enhanced peripheral and splanchnic insulin sensitivity in NIDDM men after single bout of exercise. Diabetes 1987; 36:434–9.

213. Bogardus C, Thuillez P, Revussin E, et al. Effect of muscle glycogen depletion on in vivo insulin action in man. Clin Invest 1983;72:1605–10.

214. King DS, Dalsky GP, Clutter WE, et al. Effects of lack of exercise on insulin secretion and action in trained subjects. Am J Physiol 1988;254:E537–42.

215. Amiel SA, Sherwin RS, Simonson DC, et al. Impaired insuin action in puberty, a contributing factor to poor glycemic control in adolescents with diabetes. N Engl J Med 1986;315:215–9.

216. Kahn CR. Insulin resistance, insulin insensitivity, and insulin unresponsiveness: a necessary distinction. Metabolism 1978;27(Suppl 2):1893–902.

217. Scarlett JA, Gray RS, Griffin J, et al. Insulin treatment reverses the insulin resistance of Type II diabetes mellitus. Diabetes Care 1982;5:353–63.

218. Groop LC, Bonadonna RC, DelPrato S, et al. Glucose and free fatty acid metabolism in non-insulin-dependent diabetes mellitus: evidence for multiple sites of insulin resistance. J Clin Invest 1989;84:205–13.

219. Sinha MK, Raineri-Maldonado C, Buchanan C, et al. Adipose tissue glucose transporters in NIDDM: decreased levels of muscle/fat isoform. Diabetes 1991;40:472–7.

220. Garvey WT, Maianu L, Huecksteadt TP, et al. Pretranslational suppression of a glucose transporter protein causes insulin resistance in adipocytes from patients with non-insulin-dependent diabetes mellitus and obesity. J Clin Invest 1991;87:1072–81.

221. Kahn BB, Flier JS. Regulation of glucose-transporter gene expression in vitro and in vivo. Diabetes Care 1990;13:548–64.

222. Garvey WT, Huecksteadt TP, Birnbaum MJ. Pretranslational suppression of an insulin-responsive glucose transporter in rats with diabetes mellitus. Science 1989;245:60–3.

223. Kahn BB, Shulman GI, DeFronzo RA, et al. Normalization of blood glucose in diabetic rats with phlorizin treatment reverses insulin-resistant glucose transport in adipose cells without restoring glucose transporter gene expression. J Clin Invest 1991;87:561–70.

224. Dohm GL, Tapscott EB, Pories WJ, et al. An in vitro human muscle preparation suitable for metabolic studies: decreased insulin stimulation of glucose transport in muscle from morbidly obese and diabetic subjects. J Clin Invest 1988;82:486–94.

225. Pedersen O, Bak JF, Andersen PH, et al. Evidence against altered expression of GLUT 1 or GLUT 4 in skeletal muscle of patients with obesity or NIDDM. Diabetes 1990;39:865–70.

226. Kahn BB, Rossetti L, Lodish HF, Charron MJ. Decreased in vivo glucose uptake but normal expression of GLUT 1 and GLUT 4 in skeletal muscle of diabetic rats. J Clin Invest 1991;87:2197–206.

227. Bourey RE, Koranyi L, James DE, et al. Effects of altered glucose homeostasis on glucose transporter expression in skeletal muscle of the rat. J Clin Invest 1990;86:542–7.

228. Vogt B, Carrascosa JM, Mushak J, et al. Altered distribution of GLUT 4 and GLUT 1 in plasma membranes of skeletal muscle from NIDDM patients [Abstract no. 629]. Diabetes 1991;40(Suppl 1):151A.

229. Friedman JE, Pories WJ, Leggett-Frazier N, et al. Evidence for decreased insulin sensitive glucose transporters (GLUT4) in skeletal muscle from a large sample of obese and obese-NIDDM patients [Abstract no. 630]. Diabetes 1991;40(Suppl 1):158A.

230. Dimitrakoudis D, Ramlal T, Rastogi S, et al. Hyperglycemia alters the subcellular distribution of the GLUT-1 and GLUT-4 glucose transporters differentially [Abstract no. 1165]. Diabetes 1991;40(Suppl 1):292A.

231. Hardin D, Dominguez J, Garvey WT. Expression of GLUT-4 glucose transporters varies as a function of skeletal muscle group in control and diabetic rats [Abstract no. 1166. Diabetes 1991;40(Suppl 1):292A.

232. DeFronzo RA, Bonadonna RC, Ferrannini E. Pathogenesis of NIDDM: a balanced overview. Diabetes Care 1992;15:318–68.

233. Comi RJ, Brunberger G, Gorden P. Relationship of insulin binding and insulin-stimulated tyrosine kinase activity is altered in Type II diabetes. J Clin Invest 1987;79:432–62.

234. Arner P, Einarsson K, Backman L, et al. Studies of liver insulin receptors in non-obese and obese human subjects. J Clin Invest 1983;72:1729–6.

235. Lönnroth P, Digirolamo M, Krotkiewski M, Smith U. Insulin binding and responsiveness in fat cells from patients with reduced glucose tolerance and Type II diabetes. Diabetes 1983;32:748–54.

236. Bolinder J, Östman J, Arner P. Postreceptor defects causing insulin resistance in normoinsulinemic non-insulin-dependent diabetes mellitus. Diabetes 1982;31:911–6.

237. Häring H, Obermaier-Kusser B. Insulin receptor kinase defects in insulin-resistant tissues and their role in the pathogenesis of NIDDM. Diabetes Metab Rev 1989;5:431–41.

238. Burant CF, Treutelaar MK, Buse MG. Diabetes-induced functional and structural changes in insulin receptors from rat skeletal muscle. J Clin Invest 1986;77:260–70.

239. Freidenberg GR, Henry RR, Klein HH, et al. Decreased kinase activity of insulin receptors from adipocytes of non-insulin-dependent diabetic subjects. J Clin Invest 1987;79:240–50.

240. Takayama S, Kahn CR, Kubo KK, Foley JE. Alterations in insulin receptor autophosphorylation in insulin resistance: correlation with altered sensitivity to glucose transport and antilipolysis to insulin. J Clin Endocrinol Metab 1988;66:992–9.

241. Freidenberg GR, Suter SL, Henry RR, et al. In vivo stimulation of the insulin receptor kinase in human skeletal muscle: correlation with insulin-stimulated glucose disposal during euglycemic clamp studies. J Clin Invest 1991;87:2222–9.

242. Freidenberg GR, Reichart D, Olefsky JM, Henry RR. Reversibility of defective adipocyte insulin receptor kinase activity in non-insulin-dependent diabetes mellitus: effect of weight loss. J Clin Invest 1988;82:1398–406.

243. DeFronzo RA, Ferrannini E. Insulin resistance: a multifaceted syndrome responsible for NIDDM, obesity, hypertension, dyslipidemia, and atherosclerotic cardiovascular disease. Diabetes Care 1991;14:173–94.

244. Haffner SM, Stern MP, Hazuda HP, et al. Increased insulin concentrations in nondiabetic offspring of diabetic parents. N Engl J Med 1988;319:1297–301.

245. Warram JH, Martin BC, Krolewski AS, et al. Slow glucose removal rate and hyperinsulinemia precede the development of Type II diabetes in the offspring of diabetic parents. Ann Intern Med 1990;113:909–15.

246. Bogardus C, Lillioja S, Nyomba BL, et al. Distribution of in vivo insulin action in Pima Indians as mixture of three normal distributions. Diabetes 1989;38:1423–32.

247. Stout RW. Insulin and atheroma: 20-yr perspective. Diabetes Care 1990;13:631–54.

248. Taylor SI, Kadowaki T, Kadowaki H, et al. Mutations in insulin-receptor gene in insulin-resistant patients. Diabetes Care 1990;13:257–79.

249. Elbein SC, Borecki I, Corsetti L, et al. Linkage analysis of the human insulin receptor gene and maturity onset diabetes of the young. Diabetologia 1987;30:641–7.

250. O'Rahilly S, Trembath RC, Patel P, et al. Linkage analysis of the human insulin receptor gene in type 2 (non-insulin-dependent) diabetic families and a family with maturity onset diabetes of the young. Diabetologia 1988;31:792–7.

251. Cox NJ, Epstein PA, Spielman RS. Linkage studies on NIDDM and the insulin and insulin-receptor genes. Diabetes 1989;38:653–8.

252. O'Rahilly S, Woong HC, Patel P, et al. Detection of mutations in insulin-receptor gene in NIDDM patients by analysis of single-stranded conformation polymorphisms. Diabetes 1991;40:777–82.

253. Moller DE, Yokota A, Flier JS. Normal insulin-receptor cDNA sequence in Pima Indians with NIDDM. Diabetes 1989;38:1496–500.

254. Cama A, Patterson AP, Kadowaki T, et al. The amino acid sequence of the insulin receptor is normal in an insulin-resistant Pima Indian. J Clin Endocrinol Metab 1990; 70:1155–61.

255. Kusari J, Olefsky JM, Strahl C, McClain DA. Insulin-receptor cDNA sequence in NIDDM patient homozygous for insulin-receptor gene RFLP. Diabetes 1991; 40:249–54.

256. Kusari J, Verma US, Olefsky JM. Analysis of insulin receptor and insulin responsive glucose transporter gene sequences in patients with common type non-insulin dependent diabetes mellitus (NIDDM) [Abstract no. 631]. Diabetes 1991;40(Suppl 1):158A.

257. Goldfine A, Magre J, Goldstein BJ, et al. Denaturing gradient gel electrophoresis of glucose transporter and insulin receptor genes [Abstract]. Clin Res 1991;39: 383A.

258. Yki-Järvinen H, Koivisto VA. Natural course of insulin resistance in Type I diabetes. N Engl J Med 1986; 315:224–30.

259. Finegood DT, Hramiak IM, Dupre J. A modified protocol for estimation of insulin sensitivity with the minimal model of glucose kinetics in patients with insulin-dependent diabetes. J Clin Endocrinol Metab 1990;70:1538–49.

260. Rossetti L, Smith D, Shulman GI, et al. Correction of hyperglycemia with phorizin normalizes tissue sensitivity to insulin in diabetic rats. J Clin Invest 1987;79:1510–5.

261. Gjedde A, Crone C. Blood-brain glucose transfer: repression in chronic hyperglycemia. Science 1981;214:456–7.

262. McCall AL, Millington WR, Wurtman RJ. Metabolic fuel and amino acid transport into the brain in experimental diabetes mellitus. Proc Natl Acad Sci USA 1982; 79:5406–10.

263. Van Putten JPM, Krans HMJ. Glucose as a regulator of insulin-sensitive hexose uptake in 3T3 adipocytes. J Biol Chem 1985;260:7996–8001.

264. Traxinger RR, Marshall S. Recovery of maximal insulin responsiveness and insulin sensitivity after induction of insulin resistance in primary cultured adipocytes. J Biol Chem 1989;264:8156–63.

265. Sasson S, Edelson D, Cerasi E. In vitro autoregulation of glucose utilization in rat soleus muscle. Diabetes 1987;36:1041–6.

266. Leahy JL, Bonner-Weir S, Weir GC. Beta-cell dysfunction induced by chronic hyperglycemia: current ideas on mechanism of impaired glucose-induced insulin secretion. Diabetes Care 1992;15:442–55.

267. Kahn CR, Flier JS, Bar RS, et al. The syndrome of insulin resistance and acanthosis nigricans: insulin receptor disorders in man. N Engl J Med 1976;294:739–45.

268. O'Rahilly SP, Nugent Z, Rudenski AS, et al. Beta-cell dysfunction, rather than insulin insensitivity, is the primary defect in familial type 2 diabetes. Lancet 1986;2:360–4.

Chapter 15

PATHOLOGY OF THE PANCREAS IN DIABETES MELLITUS

ALAN K. FOULIS
ANNE CLARK

The different diseases that cause the syndrome of diabetes have been defined largely from a clinical point of view. Most of these diseases can also be recognized as entities on histologic examination of the pancreas. It is the purpose of this chapter to describe the morphologic changes that occur in the pancreas in the various forms of diabetes and to show how the study of the pancreas in these situations has helped elucidate some aspects of the pathogenesis of the diseases concerned.

NORMAL HUMAN PANCREAS

To appreciate the changes found in the endocrine pancreas in the various forms of diabetes, a basic knowledge of normal anatomy is required.

The pancreatic islets in humans differ from the much-studied rodent islets in some important features. The islets occupy approximately 1 to 5% of the total pancreatic mass in adults[1,2] and are randomly distributed in the exocrine pancreas, with a slightly increased density in the head of the organ.[2] The endocrine-cell content of the islets is not uniform throughout the pancreas and is related to the embryologic development of the gland. The pancreas is derived from two primordial pouches of the foregut,[3-5] the dorsal and ventral primordia, which come together to form a single structure. Exocrine and endocrine cells arise from stem cells in the ductular epithelium during fetal development,[3,4] with neoformed primitive islets being apparent by 10 weeks' gestation.[6-8] In the normal adult pancreas, islets in that part of the organ derived from the dorsal bud (superior anterior part of

head, and all of the body and tail of pancreas), consist of 82% insulin-secreting β-cells, 13% glucagon-secreting α-cells, 4% somatostatin-secreting δ-cells, and 1% pancreatic polypeptide (PP)-secreting cells (Fig. 15–1). In contrast, islets in the part derived from the ventral bud are composed of 18% β-cells, 1% α-cells, 2% δ-cells, and 79% PP cells.[8] The former area is known as the PP-poor lobe, and the latter, as the PP-rich lobe.

Human islets are more irregular in shape than the ovoid and spherical rodent islets. β-Cells are located largely in the central portion of the islet, whereas the other cell types line the islet capillaries that run around the periphery of the islet and penetrate the islet core. Hence, in cross-section, many non-β-cells are found in the center of the islet situated adjacent to the capillaries.

TYPE I DIABETES MELLITUS

Type I diabetes usually occurs in young people and is characterized by progressive loss of insulin-secreting β-cells from the islets of Langerhans. The destruction of these cells appears to be the result of an autoimmune reaction directed against them.[9] The vast majority of patients with insulin-dependent diabetes mellitus (IDDM or Type I) in Western countries have this disease.

Morphologic Changes in Pancreatic Islets

In Type I diabetes there is selective destruction of β-cells within islets. At the same time there seems to be relatively little alteration in the numbers of α, δ, and PP

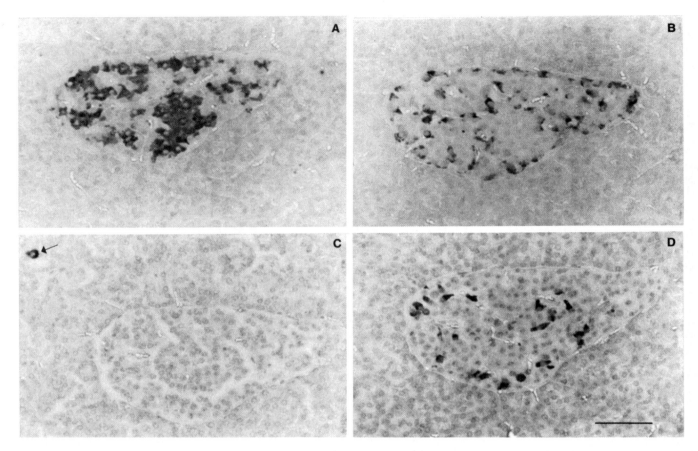

Fig. 15–1.   Serial 5-μm sections of an islet from the body region of the pancreas of a nondiabetic subject. Sections were stained with immunoperoxidase to demonstrate the distribution of islet cells. A: β-Cells immunoreactive for insulin. B: α-Cells lining the capillaries. C: Absence of pancreatic peptide–secreting cells in the islet section but presence of a positively staining cell in a duct (arrow). D: δ-Cells containing somatostatin. Scale bar = 50μm.

cells. Although patients with this disease may present clinically with a relatively acute illness, there is evidence that the destruction of β-cells proceeds very slowly and that it may well have been occurring for years before diagnosis.[10] There is a considerable reserve within the endocrine pancreas, and it has been estimated that it is not until patients have lost approximately 80% of their β-cell mass that they decompensate and present with clinical diabetes.[11]

In patients with Type I diabetes of many years' duration, very few residual β-cells, if any, will be found in the pancreas.[12,13] In the PP-poor lobe, these "insulin-deficient islets" consist almost entirely of α- and δ-cells (Fig. 15–2). Similarly, islets in the PP-rich lobe will have lost their β-cells and will consist virtually exclusively of PP cells.[13]

In contrast, at clinical presentation of the disease, there are essentially three morphologic types of islet. First, approximately 70% of the islets are insulin-deficient. Second, there are islets that are histologically normal and have a normal complement of β-cells. Third, there are islets that are inflamed and exhibit a variable reduction in the number of β-cells.[14]

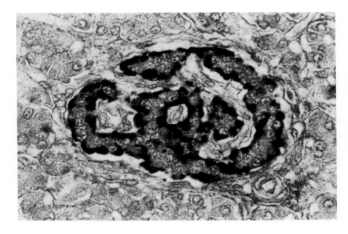

Fig. 15–2.   Insulin-deficient islet. This section has been immunostained simultaneously for glucagon, somatostatin, and pancreatic polypeptide. All of the endocrine cells are stained, indicating that all the β-cells have been destroyed (original magnification ×400).

Insulitis

The classic work of Gepts[12] can be said to be the foundation of modern studies of autoimmune Type I diabetes. He described the appearance of islets in pancreases obtained at autopsy from 22 patients who had died within 6 months of first experiencing diabetic symptoms. He noted that in 15 of these pancreases, a proportion of the islets were inflamed. The inflammation consisted primarily of lymphocytes, with very few polymorphs and no plasma cells (Fig. 15–3). There is controversy in the literature concerning the frequency of insulitis in autoimmune Type I diabetes,[14-16] with one study denying its very existence.[17] Several factors probably contribute to these differences. First, tissue sampling is important. If a renal biopsy is done in a patient who is developing diabetic nephropathy, examination of the 20 or so glomeruli obtained will provide a representative picture of the changes taking place in the other million glomeruli. By contrast, in patients who are developing diabetes, the islet changes in the pancreas are not uniform at any moment in time. Thus, in some islets the β-cells have been destroyed while in others they have yet to be destroyed. Residual insulin-containing islets tend to be grouped together, in a nonrandom way, and these groups tend to be defined by exocrine pancreatic lobules.[12,14] Thus, in one lobule all islets may be insulin-deficient while in an adjacent lobule all islets will contain β-cells (Fig. 15–4). Islets with β-cells are 23 times more likely to be inflamed than are insulin-deficient islets.[14] All the studies on insulitis have been retrospective examinations of autopsy tissues, and the amount of pancreatic tissue sampled post-mortem was often very small. If such a specimen contained only insulin-deficient islets (as seen in some of the published cases[17]), the chances of observing insulitis would be greatly diminished.

In addition, there is evidence that the speed of destruction of β-cells is slower in patients presenting with Type I diabetes at an older age, with fewer

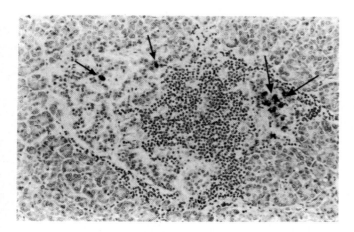

Fig. 15–3. Insulitis. Islet shows a marked lymphocytic infiltrate. The arrows indicate the few residual β-cells that are present (indirect immunoperoxidase staining for insulin; original magnification ×220).

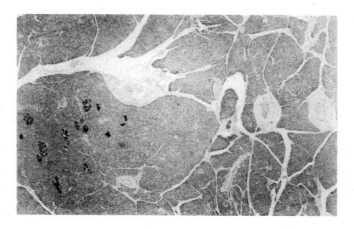

Fig. 15–4. Pancreas in recent-onset diabetes. Residual insulin–containing islets are grouped together in a nonrandom fashion. There are many insulin-deficient islets in the right half of the photograph (indirect immunoperoxidase staining for insulin; original magnification ×24).

insulin-containing islets being affected by insulitis.[14] This, plus the increased sampling error involved in examining an adult-sized pancreas, may have contributed to the difficulty encountered in observing this lesion in older patients with recent-onset Type I diabetes.[17]

Finally, there is the problem of defining insulitis. All authors, including the present ones, illustrate insulitis by showing islets that contain vast numbers of lymphocytes. However, the islet illustrated in Figure 15–5 is probably also affected by insulitis, although this could be proven satisfactorily only by examining the entire islet in serial sections. In a retrospective study of pancreases from 60 patients with recent-onset Type I diabetes, obvious insulitis was seen in 47 (78%) without resorting to examination of serial sections.[14] Since this study included all the problems of sampling error that have been discussed, it seems likely that insulitis is a feature of all cases of autoimmune Type I diabetes.

If insulitis is the pathognomonic lesion of autoimmune diabetes, what process does it represent? In a study of a single case, in which frozen material was available, the majority of lymphocytes in the islets were T cells, with a predominance of cells of the CD8 phenotype (cytotoxic/suppressor cells). While helper T lymphocytes and natural killer cells also were present in small numbers, macrophages were inconspicuous.[18] These findings, taken in conjunction with the preferential effects of insulitis on islets that contain residual β-cells, make it likely that insulitis represents the immunologically mediated, selective destruction of β-cells.[12,14] Given the fact that the loss of β-cells seems to be a very slow process, one would expect to find insulitis before and after clinical presentation. This is indeed the case. Insulitis was seen in a patient thought to be prediabetic[19] and also was found to be affecting insulin-containing islets in the pancreas of a child who had had clinical diabetes for 6 years.[14]

Since the destructive process affecting β-cells is a chronic one, it is not surprising that evidence of regen-

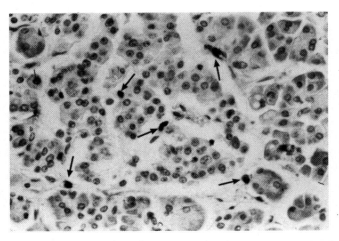

Fig. 15–5. Minimal insulitis. Section has been immunostained to show lymphocytes (arrows). Approximately 60 lymphocytes were present on the serial sections of this islet (original magnification ×490).

eration of residual β-cells may be present at clinical presentation. In many cases, some insulin-containing islets are enlarged and contain an increased number of β-cells, some of which have polyploid nuclei.[12,14] However, there is little convincing evidence of neoformation of islets from ductal elements, and the fact that diabetes actually occurs following such a slow disease process implies that the regenerative capacity of β-cells is limited.

Immunologic Events in Islets

The pancreas at clinical presentation of Type I diabetes contains 1) islets in which β-cells have not been destroyed (histologically normal), 2) islets in which β-cells are being destroyed (insulitis), and 3) islets in which β-cells have been destroyed (insulin-deficient islets). Use can be made of this observation to predict the sequence of immunologic events that may occur within an individual islet over time. Different factors, within or on the surface of β-cells, can be identified by immunocytochemical staining in these specimens.

Aberrant Expression of Class II MHC Molecules by β-Cells

There is a marked genetic component to the development of diabetes that is linked to the class II major histocompatibility complex (MHC) genes (HLA-DR, HLA-DP, and HLA-DQ) in humans.[20] The proteins coded by these genes are expressed on the cell surface of certain cells and are intimately involved in antigen presentation. Normally, helper T lymphocytes, the cells that initiate the immune response, only recognize the antigen to which they are directed if the antigen is presented to them by cells that express class II MHC molecules.[21,22] Thus, even if potentially autoreactive T lymphocytes that could recognize antigens on these cells were present, they would not react because the antigens would not be "presented" to them in the context of class II MHC. This may be one mechanism of tolerance.[23] Bottazzo et al.[24] proposed that one event that might provoke organ-specific autoimmunity could be the aberrant expression of class II MHC by target cells, such as thyroid epithelial cells or pancreatic β-cells. This aberration theoretically could convert these into antigen-presenting cells, capable of presenting their own surface antigens to potentially autoreactive T lymphocytes. The pancreas in autoimmune Type I diabetes seems to be designed to test this hypothesis, since only the β-cells in the islets are destroyed. Support for the hypothesis would be forthcoming only if β-cells, but not α, δ, and PP cells, expressed class II MHC in those with the disease. This specific expression is exactly what has been observed. In 22 of 24 cases of recent-onset diabetes, aberrant expression of class II MHC has been found and has been confined to β-cells[18,25,26] (Fig. 15–6). Such expression has not been found in normal or chronically inflamed

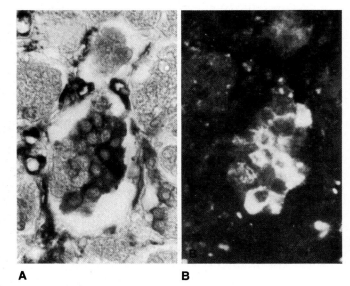

A   **B**

Fig. 15–6. Aberrant expression of class II MHC on β-cells in patient with recent-onset Type I diabetes. The section has been double-stained for class II MHC by immunoperoxidase (A) and for insulin by immunofluorescence (B) (original magnification ×490).

pancreases or in pancreases affected by graft-vs.-host disease, Type II diabetes, or viral pancreatitis. This finding is as unique to Type I diabetes as is the presence of insulitis.

Hyperexpression of Class I MHC Molecules

Whereas helper T lymphocytes can only recognize the antigen to which they are directed in the context of class II MHC molecules, cytotoxic T lymphocytes, which are the cells most likely to be responsible for destroying islet β-cells, recognize antigen only in the presence of class I MHC (HLA-A, HLA-B, and HLA-C in humans). Islet β-cells, in common with most nucleated cells in the body, normally express these molecules. However, hyperexpression of class I MHC molecules by these cells may make them more susceptible to the action of cytotoxic T lymphocytes. In a preliminary report, Bottazzo et al. noted that some islets in a diabetic pancreas hyperexpressed class I MHC molecules.[18] Further analysis of this phenomenon in a large number of cases showed that, in the pancreases from patients with recent-onset diabetes, 92% of insulin-containing islets hyperexpressed class I MHC molecules but only 1% of insulin-deficient islets displayed this phenomenon[26] (Fig. 15–7). Within affected islets, β, δ, and PP cells, as well as β-cells, hyperexpressed class I MHC molecules. Hyperexpression of this product by endocrine cells in islets also appeared to be a finding characteristic of Type I diabetes, being absent in more than 90 control pancreases from nondiabetic subjects or patients with Type II diabetes.

Interferon-α in β-Cells

As has been described above, when α- and δ-cells were adjacent to β-cells in insulin-containing islets, they hyperexpressed class I MHC molecules. However, when they were physically divorced from β-cells, in insulin-deficient islets, they ceased to hyperexpress this product. This, in conjunction with the lack of apparent inflammation in many islets that hyperexpressed class I MHC molecules, suggested that the β-cells may be secreting some factor that causes hyperexpression of class I MHC molecules by adjacent endocrine cells. Substances that are known to be able to cause hyperexpression in cultured islet endocrine cells in vitro included interferons-α, β, and γ.[27] Interferon-γ is produced only by T lymphocytes, and the presence of interferon-β cannot yet be reliably studied in autopsy-fixed tissues. In an immunohistochemical study of 37 pancreases from patients with Type I diabetes, immunoreactive interferon-α, confined to β-cells, was found in 93% of islets that hyperexpressed class I MHC molecules but in only 0.4% of those showing no hyperexpression (Fig. 15–7). Among 80 pancreases from nondiabetic patients or from patients with Type II diabetes, significant numbers of β-cells containing interferon-α were present only in the pancreases of four patients who had acute infantile coxsackie

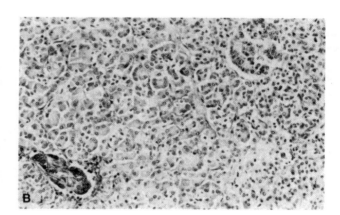

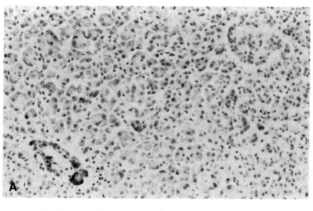

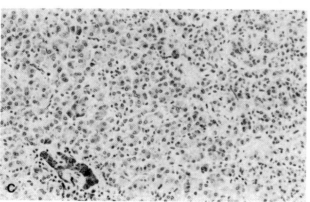

Fig. 15–7. Insulin-containing islets that hyperexpress class I MHC contain interferon-α. A: Section has been immunostained for insulin. The islet in the bottom left of the photograph contains β-cells, and the islet in the top right does not. B: Section has been immunostained for class I MHC molecules. The insulin-containing islet hyperexpresses class I MHC molecules. This islet also contains interferon-α, as seen C, that has been immunostained for this cytokine (original magnification ×160).

viral pancreatitis. This finding raised the possibility that β-cells in diabetes are infected by a virus.[28] Serologic studies of patients with newly diagnosed Type I diabetes also have suggested that viral infection could be implicated in the pathogenesis of the disease.[29–31]

The Sequence of Immunologic Events within a Given Islet

In the pancreas at clinical presentation of Type I diabetes, many histologically normal islets, which show no loss of β-cells or evidence of insulitis, hyperexpress class I MHC.[26] At least one likely reason for the hyperexpression of class I MHC by islet endocrine cells is secretion of interferon-α by β-cells; thus, both these phenomena are likely to precede insulitis and destruction of β-cells. Both probably also occur before aberrant expression of class II MHC by β-cells within the islet. This probable sequence is deduced from the fact that all islets in which β-cell expression of class II MHC was observed also hyperexpressed class I MHC. By contrast, islets could be found that hyperexpressed class I MHC but in which β-cells did not display class II MHC molecules.[26] Whether aberrant expression of class II MHC is a consequence of insulitis or precedes it remains uncertain (Fig. 15–8).

Insights into the Pathogenesis of Type I Diabetes

The concordance rate in monozygotic twins for autoimmune diabetes is no more than 50%,[32] indicating that environmental factors as well as genetic susceptibility play a role in the pathogenesis of the disease. Chief among the environmental suspects are viruses, particularly coxsackie, mumps, and rubella viruses.[29,31,33] The finding that β-cells in both diabetes and coxsackie viral pancre-

atitis express interferon-α raises the possibility that in patients with Type I diabetes β-cells are chronically infected by a virus. This infection is not likely to be cytopathic, given the long time required for destruction of β-cells in the disease. However, if a "slow" viral infection provoked secretion of interferon-α by the β-cells, hyperexpression of class I MHC by islet endocrine cells might result. In the absence of a genetic predisposition, perhaps nothing further would happen. However, it is conceivable that either the virus alone or the virus plus cytokines, such as interferon-γ and tumor necrosis factor released in an inflammatory infiltrate, may cause β-cells to express class II MHC in persons carrying the genetic susceptibility for diabetes. Support for this idea comes from the finding that patients with congenital rubella who develop diabetes carry the class II MHC alleles DR3 and/or DR4.[34] It is proposed that aberrant expression of class II MHC by β-cells is a crucial pathogenic event in diabetes, causing induction of autoimmunity and eventually the destruction of the insulin-secreting cells in a cell-mediated fashion. This hypothesis suggests that the development of diabetes is a "multistep" process involving both environmental and genetic components.[35]

It has been proposed above that viruses may act as a trigger to the development of autoimmunity directed at β-cells. The question arises whether viral infection of β-cells alone can cause diabetes. Coxsackievirus B is known to show tropism for the endocrine pancreas and for β-cells in particular.[36–38] In neonates such infection can cause a widespread necrosis of islet β-cells associated with marked inflammation. There have been scattered case reports suggesting that similar infection may cause diabetes in an acute fashion by causing widespread β-cell necrosis in older children or adults.[33,39,40] However, it should be emphasized that all these patients were atypical clinically and that there is little to suggest that more than a very few cases of Type I diabetes result from this mechanism.[38]

Changes in the Exocrine Pancreas

The pancreas in patients who have had diabetes for many years is often reduced in weight.[12] A moderate degree of acinar atrophy is associated with periacinar and perilobular fibrosis. In recent-onset diabetes, acini around insulin-deficient islets are atrophic whereas those around insulin-containing islets appear normal.[41] The explanation for these findings probably lies in an understanding of the islet blood supply. Islets generally are supplied by a single arteriole but are drained, not by a vein, but by a series of capillaries that ramify in the surrounding exocrine acinar tissue[42] (Fig. 15–9). Thus, peri-islet acini are supplied by blood containing high levels of all islet hormones—possibly several hundred times greater than levels in the general circulation. Insulin is a trophic hormone to the exocrine pancreas, whereas glucagon and somatostatin are inhibitory. Acini around insulin-deficient islets will thus be supplied by blood containing high levels of only inhibitory hormones—thus causing atrophy; however, acini around insulin-containing islets will

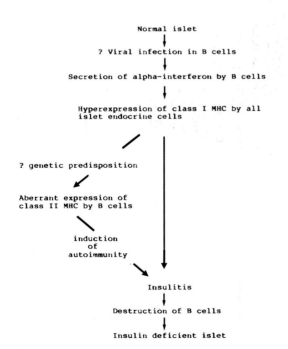

Fig. 15–8. Possible sequence of events in islets in Type I diabetes.

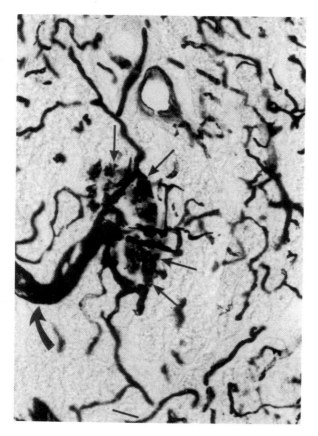

Fig. 15–9. Islet blood supply. The blood vessels of this normal pancreas at autopsy were injected with india ink. The β-cells were immunostained black, and the periphery of the islet is marked by straight arrows. An arteriole (curved arrow) enters the islet and breaks up into sinusoids that supply the islet and drain into capillaries that supply the surrounding exocrine tissue (original magnification ×120).

contain a balance of trophic and nontrophic hormones. Not surprisingly, patients with long-standing Type I diabetes have measurable malfunction of the exocrine pancreas,[43,44] although the malfunction is not sufficient to manifest as steatorrhea. These findings point to the importance of the islets of Langerhans in normal exocrine pancreatic function.[45,56]

TYPE II DIABETES MELLITUS

The etiopathology of Type II diabetes is unknown. Both increased peripheral insulin resistance and decreased β-cell function are involved in the pathophysiology of the disease. However, it is unlikely that a single factor is the cause of this heterogeneous disease. Clinical presentation is usually in patients over the age of 40 years; hence, the former name of maturity-onset diabetes. Initially, the clinical features are associated with poorly regulated insulin secretion but not with the total loss that is characteristic of Type I diabetes. Inadequate insulin secretion may result from progression of the disease over 30 to 40 years. Pathologic evidence visible in the islets could explain a gradual deterioration of islet function.

Quantitative Changes of Islet Cells in Type II Diabetes

The random arrangement of islets within the exocrine lobules and their nonspherical shape have created difficulties for quantitative morphometry. In the early quantitative studies,[47-49] data on islet and cellular volume were derived from mathematical conversions of point-counting measurements, which assumed spherical or ovoid islets. The results indicated little change in the islet size in Type II diabetes[48,50] but a 30 to 50% reduction in the amount of islet tissue.[48,51] Later studies had the benefit of improved clinical diagnosis of Type II diabetes and sensitive immunocytochemical techniques that could identify individual cell types. More accurate morphometric methods indicated only a small reduction (up to 30%) in the β-cell population of the islets, together with an increase of glucagon-producing α-cells.[1,2,52,53] The increase in α-cells may be related to the hyperglucagonemia found in some patients with Type II diabetes,[54] but the decrease in β-cells is relatively insignificant compared with the decrease in insulin secretion in patients with Type II diabetes. As in Type I diabetes, in Type II diabetes there is little evidence of β-cell regeneration.

Islet Amyloid

Amyloid (originally described as *hyaline substance*) is the term given to amorphous deposits of fibrillar material formed from polymerized peptides that stain with congo red dye in histologic sections. The name *amyloid*, meaning "starch-like,"[55] derives from the presence of polysaccharides (e.g., heparan sulfate proteoglycans) in the amyloid deposits.[56] Amyloidoses are associated with many pathologic conditions, the constituent peptide being specific for each disease state.[56,57]

Quantitative histochemical analysis has shown that deposition of amyloid in the islets is a consistent pathologic feature in Type II diabetes. Islet amyloid ("hyalinization") associated with diabetes was first described by Opie in 1900.[58] Large postmortem studies that included both individuals with Type I and Type II diabetes showed that the prevalence of amyloid in islets was higher in subjects with diabetes than in age-matched subjects without diabetes (Table 15–1) and that the prevalence increased with age.[48,59-61] More recent postmortem studies, excluding subjects with Type I diabetes, have shown a prevalence of amyloid in islets of up to 90% in groups with Type II diabetes as compared with a prevalence of 12% in elderly subjects without diabetes.[66] The prevalence is high in patients with diabetes in Japan[64] and India[62] and in North American Pima Indians with diabetes,[68] suggesting that this pathologic feature is a characteristic of Type II diabetes and is not a nonspecific feature of aging as originally thought.

The extracellular masses of amyloid are found only within the islets and are unrelated to other systemic forms of amyloidosis[69,70] (Fig. 15–10). The deposits may be found in 0.5% to 80% of islets in diabetic subjects.[2,51,63] Islets affected by amyloidosis are distributed in a nonrandom fashion within the pancreas; the deposits are rarely found in the PP-rich islets of the caput region that contain few β-cells,[71] a finding that implicates β-cells

Table 15–1.   Historical Review of the Prevalence of Islet Amyloid as Determined from Postmortem Examination

	Diabetic patients				Nondiabetic subjects		
Author (year)	*n*	Age (yr)	% with amyloid	Diabetes type	*n*	Age (yr)	% with amyloid
Cecil[59] (1909)	61	>40	39	I, II			
Bell[60] (1952)	159	<40	5.9	I, II	535	<40	0.2
	1525	>40	28.4	I, II	3424	>40	8.2
Maclean and Oglivie[48] (1955)	72	>40	39	I, II			
Erlich and Ratner[61] (1961)	91	>50	49.5	II	178	>60	3.9
Vishwanathan et al.[62] (1972)	16	NA*	56	II	20	NA*	0
Westermark and Grimelius[63] (1973)	11	66–82	91	I, II	16	60–87	0
Saito et al.[64] (1978)	26	42–85	76.9	II	18	21–81	27
Schneider et al.[65] (1980)	60	40–90	72	II	60	40–90	18
Maloy et al.[66] (1981)	27	6–98	59	II	142	6–98	11.9
Westermark et al.[67] (1987)	13	60–81	92	II	11	56–90	54.5
Clark et al.[2] (1988)	15	48–86	87	II	10	56–79	0
Clark et al.[68] (1990)	26	41–89	77	II	14	27–87	7

*Ages not given.

in amyloid formation. In mild amyloidosis, all islets in one or two exocrine lobules may be affected without involvement of the remainder of the organ. Examination of tissue from several regions of the pancreas is thus required to make an accurate diagnosis of islet amyloidosis.[66] It will be appreciated that this "lobular" distribution of islet cell changes in Type II diabetes is reminiscent of the distribution of insulitis and β-cell destruction in Type I diabetes. One could speculate that these phenomena indicate a hitherto unexplored hierarchy of endocrine function or cellular susceptibility defined within the lobular unit, originating from the vascular or nerve supply or from the embryologic origin of the lobules.

The peptide of amyloid in pancreatic islets and insulinomas is very insoluble but was identified by two independent groups in 1987.[72,73] Islet amyloid polypeptide (IAPP) (also known as amylin)[74] is a 37-amino acid peptide with structural homology to calcitonin gene-related peptide (CGRP), which is a product of the C-cells of the thyroid and some peripheral nerves[75–79] (Fig. 15–11).

Immunohistochemical studies showed that the peptide is a normal constituent of β-cells located in the insulin granules and lysosomes of humans with and without diabetes[80] (Fig. 15–12) and in the insulin granules of cats.[81,82] Examination of cDNA libraries has identified the

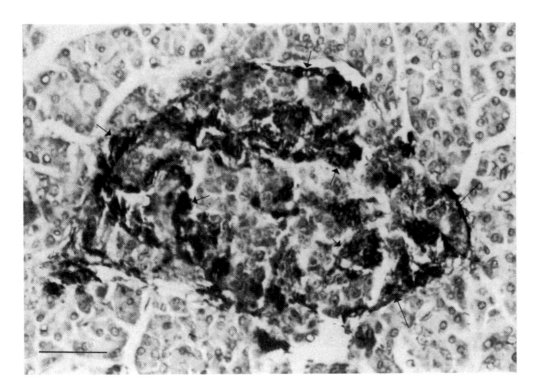

Fig. 15–10. Amyloid in an islet from a subject with Type II diabetes. The amorphous masses of amyloid are stained with immunoperoxidase for islet amyloid polypeptide. Amyloid is present around the periphery of the islet (arrows) and in the center of the islet (arrowheads). Scale bar = 50 μm.

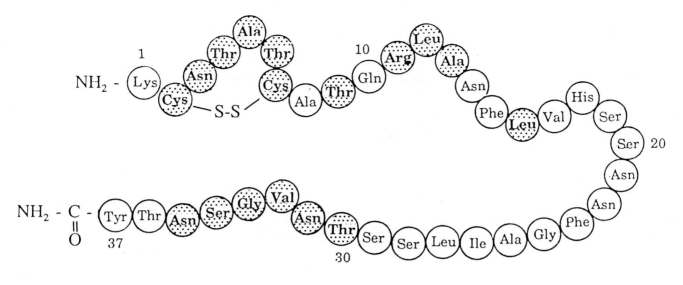

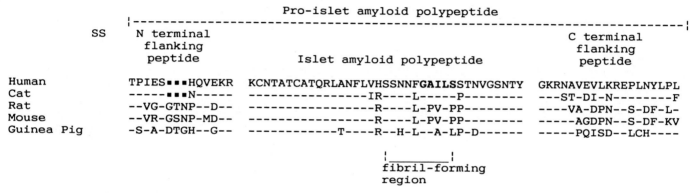

	SS	N terminal flanking peptide	Islet amyloid polypeptide	C terminal flanking peptide
Human		TPIES■■■HQVEKR	KCNTATCATQRLANFLVHSSNNF**GAILS**STNVGSNTY	GKRNAVEVLKREPLNYLPL
Cat		-----■■■N-----	----------------IR----L-----P--------	---ST-DI-N--------F
Rat		--VG-GTNP--D--	----------------R----L-PV-PP--------	----VA-DPN--S-DF-L-
Mouse		--VR-GSNP-MD--	----------------R----L-PV-PP--------	-----AGDPN--S-DF-KV
Guinea Pig		-S-A-DTGH--G--	------------T----R--H-L--A-LP-D------	-----PQISD--LCH----

Fig. 15—11. Top: Amino acid sequence of human islet amyloid polypeptide (IAPP), with shading indicating amino acids in common with calcitonin gene–related polypeptide (CGRP). Predictions from cDNA indicate C-terminal amidation. (Adapted from Nishi et al.[83]) Bottom: Amino acid sequences of pro-IAPP from humans, cats, rats, mice, and guinea pigs. Amino acids are indicated by single-letter code, and species-specific differences in the sequence are indicated by the appropriate letter. IAPP is flanked by an N-terminal peptide (14 residues in rodents, 11 residues in humans and cats) and a C-terminal peptide (19 amino acids). Fibril formation is dependent upon amino acids IAPP$_{20-29}$, particularly the sequence GAILS (IAPP$_{24-28}$).

peptide in several species, including rats, mice, cats, and guinea pigs.[83–85] However, species-specific differences in the amino acid sequence of IAPP, particularly in the region of IAPP$_{24-28}$, appear to be critical determinants of the tendency for the molecule to form fibrils in vitro[86,87] (Fig. 15–11). Thus, rodents that have amino acid sequences in this region that differ from those in primates and cats do not develop diabetic amyloid, whereas the development of islet amyloid is a feature of spontaneous diabetes in primates and cats of advanced age.[88–90]

The amyloid in Type II diabetes is situated between the endocrine cells and the islet capillaries either in the islet core or on the periphery. The deposits can occupy up to 80% of the islet space and are associated with a reduction in islet endocrine cells. In severe islet amyloidosis, fewer than 10% of the islet β-cells remain.[91] The factors responsible for conversion of the intracellular form of IAPP to the insoluble extracellular amyloid fibrils are unknown.

Abnormal biosynthesis and/or catabolism of the peptide at intra- or extracellular sites may be important.[92,93] IAPP is derived from pro-IAPP by proteolytic cleavage that releases small N- and C-terminal flanking peptides[84,85,94,95] (Fig. 15–11); therefore, abnormal proteolysis could result in fibril formation.[96] The margins of the β-cells adjacent to the deposits show deep irregular invaginations filled with fibrils; furthermore, cellular debris may be present within the amyloid masses (Fig. 15–13). However, the site of fibril formation could be either outside the cell (arising from accumulated IAPP secreted from the cell) or at an intracellular location. Membrane-bound vesicles containing fibrils are found in β-cells of diabetic cats, and intracellular amyloid fibrils formed from IAPP have been identified in insulinoma β-cells. Islet amyloidosis is unlikely to be caused by production of a genetically determined abnormal variant of IAPP; the molecular structure predicted by the cDNA for IAPP is identical to that found in the amyloid

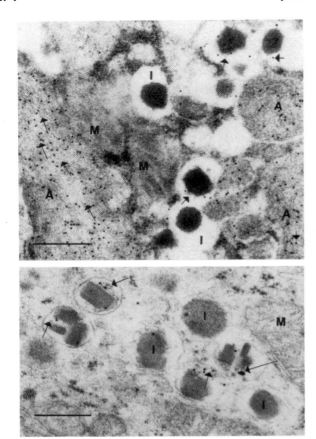

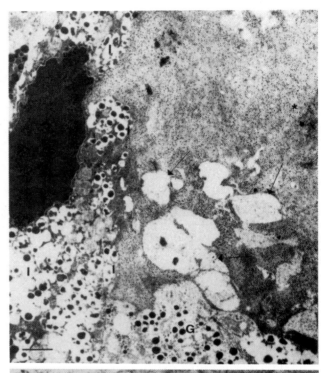

Fig. 15–12. Top: Immunoreactivity for islet amyloid polypeptide (IAPP) in an islet from a patient with diabetes. Immunogold labeling for IAPP of granules (arrowheads) and amyloid fibrils (arrows). Bottom: IAPP colocalized with insulin (arrows) in islet from a patient without diabetes. I = insulin granule; M = mitochondrion; A = amyloid. Scale bars = 0.5 μm.

extracts.[83,85] Also, linkage analyses with a cDNA probe for IAPP have shown no association of IAPP polymorphisms with diabetes in family or population studies.[97]

The role of amyloid in the etiopathology of Type II diabetes is unclear. Amyloid deposition precedes the onset of diabetic symptoms in spontaneous feline and primate diabetes. Deposits have been identified in glucose-intolerant cats[98] and in obese, insulin-resistant, and hyperinsulinemic monkeys with normal fasting glucose levels[99–100] (Fig. 15–14). In spite of the presence of amyloid at early stages of the disease, it is unlikely that amyloidosis alone is the primary initiating factor for the development of the glucose intolerance of prediabetes. In prediabetic cats and monkeys, the deposits are small initially and few islets are affected,[91,101] so that the β-cell reserve is relatively normal (Fig. 15–14). The anatomic disruption of the islet may not be of major importance to islet function in mild amyloidosis. Islets with other types of amyloid deposits are present in some cases of systemic amyloidosis without symptoms of diabetes. Amyloid also is found in the islets of older patients with cystic fibrosis who have developed diabetes as a secondary complica-

tion.[102,103] However, the degree of amyloidosis in humans increases with the severity of diabetic symptoms, as demonstrated by the need for insulin therapy,[65] and severe amyloidosis is associated with presentation of diabetic symptoms in cats and monkeys.[98,100] Progressive deposition of amyloid associated with islet-cell destruction could be a major factor in the gradual deterioration of islet function in patients with Type II diabetes. In severe amyloidosis the normal architecture of the islets

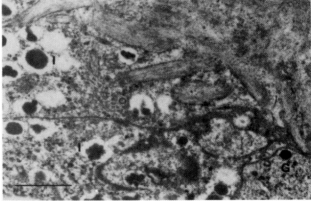

Fig. 15–13. Amyloid in an islet from a patient with Type II diabetes. Top: Amyloid immunolabeled with islet amyloid polypeptide and immunogold (asterisks). Cellular debris is present within the amyloid (arrows). Adjacent β-cell has pyknotic nucleus adjacent to the amyloid, and many granules appear to be surrounded by amyloid. I = insulin; G = glucagon. Bottom: Amyloid fibrils in invaginations into the margins of β-cells. I = insulin; G = glucagon granules. Scale bars = 1.0 μm.

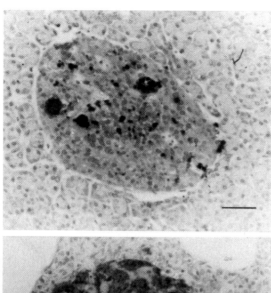

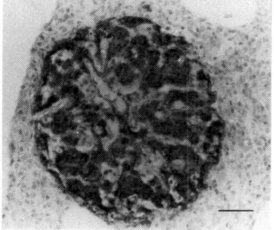

Fig. 15–14. Islet amyloid in spontaneous diabetes in the monkey species *Macaca mulatta*. Top: Islet amyloid polypeptide–immunoreactive amyloid in an islet from a hyperinsulinemic, obese, normoglycemic animal. Small deposits of amyloid are scattered throughout the islet. Bottom: Amyloid in islet from a diabetic animal that almost fills the islet, with less than 15% of islet β-cells remaining. Scale bars = 50 μm.

is destroyed, disrupting the intra-islet network of communications via gap junctions and paracrine hormones.[104,105] In addition, large amyloid masses situated between the capillaries and endocrine cells could affect transfer of glucose and insulin between the circulation and endocrine cells. Thus, amyloid may represent a secondary phenomenon to an aberrant biochemical mechanism that is related to the cause of Type II diabetes.

IAPP secreted from the β-cells[106,110] may have a hormonal role in the body related to the action or secretion of insulin. IAPP reduces the glycogenic action of insulin on skeletal muscle in vitro,[74,108] suggesting that the peptide is involved in the increased insulin resistance in Type II diabetes.[109,110] However, this hypothesis has yet to be confirmed in vivo since higher concentrations of the peptide are required to elicit an effect than have been identified in the peripheral circulation.[110–112] Further studies are required to resolve this question.

Changes in the Exocrine Pancreas

Ultrasound scanning studies have shown a 30% reduction in pancreatic size in patients with Type II diabetes compared with patients without diabetes.[113] This difference is comparable to the small decrease of 27% in exocrine function determined by serum immunoreactive trypsin measurements in subjects with Type II diabetes compared with a control group.[114] Diminished pancreatic size and function in diabetes may be related to several factors, including the lack of the trophic effect of high local concentrations of insulin on exocrine function[115,116] and inadequate perfusion of the organ as a result of arteriosclerosis.[117] These factors probably lead to mild atrophy of exocrine pancreatic tissue and to a degree of perilobular and intralobular fibrosis. Many patients with Type II diabetes are overweight, and obesity is associated with deposition of excess adipose tissue among pancreatic acinar cells (lipomatosis). Less fat is deposited in the PP-rich, caput region of the pancreas than in the remainder of the pancreas.[118] In extreme obesity, acinar tissue is replaced by swollen adiposites, and the islets, although unaffected, become isolated within the adipose tissue attached to vascular bundles or ducts.

Acinar atrophy, lipomatosis, and fibrosis in the exocrine pancreas are also characteristics of aging,[119] but in Type II diabetes, they appear at an earlier age.[2,52] Measurable exocrine function is more severely abnormal in patients with Type I diabetes than in those with Type II diabetes,[114] but exocrine pancreatic failure is not a clinical feature of either condition.

SECONDARY DIABETES

Diabetes complicates several primarily exocrine pancreatic diseases and is also a feature of several systemic diseases. However, it is worth emphasizing that secondary diabetes accounts for only about 0.2% of all cases of diabetes in Western countries.

Diabetes Complicating Primary Exocrine Pancreatic Disease

Chronic Calcifying Pancreatitis

In white populations, chronic calcifying pancreatitis occurs primarily in alcoholics, particularly in wine-drinking countries. Diabetes is found in about one-third of cases. It usually begins within a decade of the onset of abdominal pain but can be the presenting problem in patients with painless chronic pancreatitis.

Histologically, the pancreatic ducts become filled with proteinaceous concretions, which calcify, causing ulceration of the duct mucosa with resulting strictures. The stones and strictures obstruct the drainage of the exocrine pancreas in a patchy manner. The acini in obstructed areas of the pancreas atrophy and finally disappear. However, the islets remain and become embedded in fibrous tissue (Fig. 15–15). The ratio of β-cells to α-cells in these "sclerosed" islets is different from that found in

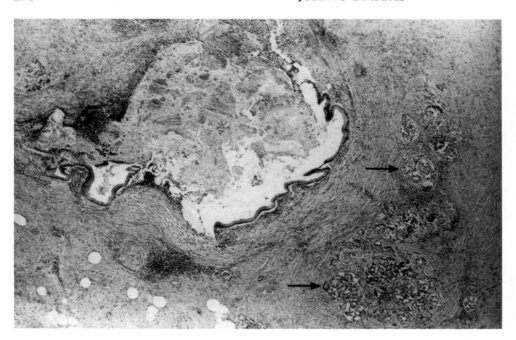

Fig. 15–15. Chronic pancreatitis showing ulceration and dilatation of a duct and periductal fibrosis. Note the loss of acini but preservation of islets (arrows), which are embedded in fibrous tissue (original magnification ×25).

islets still embedded in acinar tissue, there being a relative reduction in the number of β-cells.[117] Since the vascular drainage of these islets may be severely disturbed, this loss of β-cells may be the result of ischemia.

Diabetes in Tropical Regions

Although both Type I and Type II diabetes occur in developing countries, a World Health Organization study group[120] has defined a third major cause of diabetes that has a high prevalence in tropical regions as "malnutrition-related diabetes mellitus" (MRDM). This classification includes the condition known as fibrocalculus pancreatic diabetes (FCPD) and protein-deficient diabetes mellitus (PDDM). However, clinical and pathologic separation of these two latter subgroups remains a contentious issue.[121]

The spectrum of histologic changes seen in the pancreas in these diseases is virtually identical to that observed in chronic pancreatitis in Western countries. Just as cirrhosis can be the final outcome of many forms of hepatitis, so this appearance in the pancreas is probably the end result of several different diseases that cause chronic damage to the epithelial lining of the pancreatic ducts. Consumption of various toxins has been implicated, including cassava (*Maniot esculenta*), which contains many cyanogens,[122,123] but the etiology remains unknown.

Clinically, malnutrition-related diabetes differs from chronic alcoholic pancreatitis in several respects. The disease occurs at an earlier age (usually before age 30)) and is related to malnutrition, particularly in childhood, rather than to alcoholism. The pancreatitis is progressive and may eventually involve the whole pancreas. In FCPD the calcification of the ductal precipitates is massive, and diagnosis can readily be made from visualization of the calculi on an abdominal x-ray film.[124] There is clinical

exocrine insufficiency, which often correlates with the severity of the diabetes.[125,126] There is little histologic evidence to identify PDDM as a separate entity; patients develop diabetes at a younger age, and pancreatic calculi are rarely present.[121,124]

Diabetes Secondary to Cystic Fibrosis

Diabetes is a well-recognized complication of cystic fibrosis now that improved therapy has permitted survival into the third and fourth decade. Fewer than 1% of children with cystic fibrosis have symptomatic hyperglycemia,[127] but the prevalence of diabetes is approximately 10% in adults with cystic fibrosis. Treatment with insulin is usual, but ketoacidosis is rare,[128] and the condition is not similar to Type I diabetes since a large number of β-cells are retained.[103,129,130]

Cystic fibrosis is an autosomal recessive condition, the involved gene being on chromosome 7.[131] The protein encoded by this gene is expressed in secretory cells, including the exocrine acinar cells, and is likely to be involved in transmembrane ionic exchange. This may explain the extremely viscid secretions from some glands, including the pancreatic exocrine tissue.

Although the pancreas may appear normal at birth,[132] ductal obstruction results in a progressive diffuse atrophy of the acinar cells.[129,132] The viscid pancreatic secretions precipitate to form proteinaceous concretions, which accumulate within the ducts. Unlike the concretions in chronic pancreatitis, these concretions rarely calcify or cause ulceration or stricture of the ducts.[130,133] The exocrine atrophy is initially associated with fibrosis, but in some patients the pancreas is progressively replaced by fat so that macroscopically it resembles a piece of adipose tissue.

Pancreatic islets do not disappear as a result of the exocrine atrophy; scattered islets become embedded in

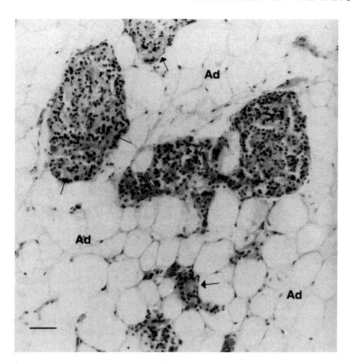

Fig. 15–16. Pancreas from a diabetic patient with cystic fibrosis. Islets are surrounded by adipose tissue (Ad). Amorphous areas (arrows) in the islets are stained with congo red dye, which identifies islet amyloid (stain: hematoxylin and congo red). Scale bar = 50 μm.

fibrous or adipose tissue (Fig. 15–16). Semiquantitative studies suggest that fatty replacement is more characteristic of nondiabetic patients with cystic fibrosis, whereas more extensive fibrosis is found in those who become diabetic.[102,103,129] The density of the islets in the pancreas (including the adipose or fibrous tissue) is similar to that of the islets in subjects without cystic fibrosis, and all the islet cell types are preserved, with a distribution similar to that found in unaffected subjects.[102,129] An increase in the ratio of α- to β-cells has been found but is not correlated with glucose intolerance or diabetes.[129] Islet amyloid has been detected in a group of diabetic patients older than 30 years with cystic fibrosis, implying abnormalities in β-cell function in these patients similar to those found in patients with Type II diabetes.[102,103] Neoformation of islets from ductular epithelium in patients with cystic fibrosis has been reported,[134] and in a few patients the fibrotic lesions may extend within the islets.[129]

The Causes of Diabetes in Chronic Pancreatitis, Malnutrition-Related Diabetes, and Cystic Fibrosis

In chronic pancreatitis, malnutrition-related diabetes, and cystic fibrosis, the end-stage pancreases are similar. Almost all of the exocrine pancreas is lost, islets are preserved but may be embedded in fibrous tissue, and the relative loss of β-cells may be greater than that of α-cells. Thus, the mechanisms of development of diabetes in these diseases are likely to be similar.

At least two factors are likely to be involved. First, islets surrounded by fibrous tissue may have suffered from ischemia as a result of the disruption of their normal vasculature during the preceding inflammatory damage. Second, endocrine failure (diabetes) usually occurs when there is also exocrine failure (steatorrhea). Intestinal malabsorption due to pancreatic failure may result in decreased secretion of "incretins" such as glucose-dependent insulinotropic peptide, with a resultant diminution in insulin release from islets.[135,136]

Hemochromatosis

Approximately 50% of patients with hemochromatosis develop diabetes. The changes seen in the pancreas are the same in both primary and secondary hemochromatosis. Early in the disease hemosiderin is deposited in acini, particularly in those surrounding islets. In a painstaking analysis of the hemochromatotic pancreas, Rahier et al.[137] found that iron in the islets of patients with diabetes is found almost exclusively in the β-cells—α, δ, and PP cells being virtually free of hemosiderin. Many of the β-cells contained little immunoreactive insulin. Amyloid was not present in the islets. These findings strongly support the conclusion that diabetes in hemochromatosis is quite distinct from Types I and II diabetes. The pathogenesis of diabetes appears to involve selective uptake of hemosiderin by β-cells, with resulting toxic damage and impairment of their ability to synthesize and secrete insulin.

Diabetes without Significant Pancreatic Histopathology

In patients with excess counterregulatory hormone secretion, such as patients with acromegaly or Cushing syndrome, islets are usually normal. Islet hypertrophy is seen in only a few cases.[52] Similarly, no consistent islet abnormality is seen in patients with insulin receptor-blocking antibodies, such as those patients with insulin-resistant diabetes associated with acanthosis nigricans. Finally, several cases of insulin-dependent diabetes in children less than 18 months old whose islet histologic features were normal have been described.[14] While these infants died of ketoacidosis, there was little else to suggest that they were particularly atypical from a clinical point of view. Nothing is known of the pathogenesis of this disease, but it must be very rare.

REFERENCES

1. Rahier J, Goebbels RM, Henquin JC. Cellular composition of the human diabetic pancreas. Diabetologia 1983; 24:366–71.
2. Clark A, Wells CA, Buley ID, et al. Islet amyloid, increased A-cells, reduced B-cells and exocrine fibrosis: quantitative changes in the pancreas in type 2 diabetes. Diabetes Res 1988;6:151–9.
3. Like AA, Orci L. Embryogenesis of the human pancreatic islets: a light and electron microscopic study. Diabetes 1972;21:511–37.
4. Falin LI. The development and cytodifferentiation of the islets of Langerhans in human embryos and foetuses. Acta Anat 1967;68:147–68.

5. Spooner BS, Walther BT, Rutter WJ. The development of the dorsal and ventral mammalian pancreas in vivo and in vitro. J Cell Biol 1970;47:235−46.

6. Clark A, Grant AM. Quantitative morphology of endocrine cells in human fetal pancreas. Diabetologia 1983;25:31−5.

7. Pictet RL, Rall L, de Gasparo M, Rutter WJ. Regulation of differentiation of endocrine cells during pancreatic development in vitro. In: Camerini-Davalos RA, Cole HS, eds. Early diabetes in early life. New York: Academic Press, 1975:25−39.

8. Stefan Y, Orci L, Malaisse-Lagae F, et al. Quantitation of endocrine cell content in the pancreas of nondiabetic and diabetic humans. Diabetes 1982;31:694−700.

9. Bottazzo GF. β-Cell damage in diabetic insulitis: are we approaching a solution? Diabetologia 1984;26:241−9.

10. Tarn AC, Smith CP, Spencer KM, et al. Type 1 (insulin dependent) diabetes: a disease of slow clinical onset? BMJ 1987;294:342−5.

11. Klöppel G, Drenck CR, Oberholzer M, et al. Morphometric evidence for a striking B-cell reduction at the clinical onset of type 1 diabetes. Virchows Arch [A] 1984; 403;441−52.

12. Gepts W. Pathologic anatomy of the pancreas in juvenile diabetes mellitus. Diabetes 1965;14:619−33.

13. Gepts W, De Mey J. Islet cell survival determined by morphology: an immunocytochemical study of the islets of Langerhans in juvenile diabetes mellitus. Diabetes 1978;27(Suppl 1):251−61.

14. Foulis AK, Liddle CN, Farquharson MA, et al. The histopathology of the pancreas in type 1 (insulin-dependent) diabetes mellitus: a 25-year review of deaths in patients under 20 years of age in the United Kingdom. Diabetologia 1986;29:267−74.

15. Maclean N, Ogilvie RF. Observations on the pancreatic islet tissue of young diabetic subjects. Diabetes 1959; 8:83−91.

16. Junker K, Egeberg J, Kromann H, et al. An autopsy study of the islets of Langerhans in acute-onset juvenile diabetes mellitus. Acta Pathol Microbiol Scand [A] 1977; 85:699−706.

17. Doniach I, Morgan AG. Islets of Langerhans in juvenile diabetes mellitus. Clin Endocrinol 1973;2:233−48.

18. Bottazzo GF, Dean BM, McNally JM, et al. In situ characterization of autoimmune phenomena and expression of HLA molecules in the pancreas in diabetic insulitis. N Engl J Med 1985;313:353−60.

19. Foulis AK, Jackson R, Farquharson MA. The pancreas in idiopathic Addison's disease—a search for a prediabetic pancreas. Histopathology 1988;12:481−90.

20. Wolf E, Spencer KM, Cudworth AG, et al. The genetic susceptibility to type 1 (insulin-dependent) diabetes: analysis of the HLA-DR association. Diabetologia 1983; 24:224−30.

21. Natali PG, DeMartino C, Quaranta V, et al. Expression of Ia-like antigens in normal human nonlymphoid tissues. Transplantation 1981;31;75−8.

22. Alejandro R, Shienvold FL, Hajek SV, et al. Immunocytochemical localization of HLA-DR in human islets of Langerhans. Diabetes 1982;31(Suppl 4):17−22.

23. Cowing G. Does T-cell restriction to Ia limit the need for self-tolerance? Immunol Today 1985;6:72−4.

24. Bottazzo GF, Pujol-Borrell R, Hanafusa T. Role of aberrant HLA-DR expression and antigen presentation in induction of endocrine autoimmunity. Lancet 1983;2:1115−9.

25. Foulis AK, Farquharson MA. Aberrant expression of HLA-DR antigens by insulin containing β-cells in recent-onset type 1 diabetes mellitus. Diabetes 1986; 35:1215−24.

26. Foulis AK, Farquharson MA, Hardman R. Aberrant expression of class II major histocompatibility complex molecules by B cells and hyperexpression of class I major histocompatibility complex molecules by insulin containing islets in type 1 (insulin-dependent) diabetes mellitus. Diabetologia 1987;30:333−43.

27. Pujol-Borrell R, Todd I, Doshi M, et al. Differential expression and regulation of MHC products in the endocrine and exocrine cells of the human pancreas. Clin Exp Immunol 1986;65:128−39.

28. Foulis AK, Farquharson MA, Meager A. Immunoreactive alpha-interferon in insulin-secreting β cells in type 1 diabetes mellitus. Lancet 1987;2:1423−7.

29. Banatvala JE, Bryant J, Schernthaner G, et al. Coxsackie B, mumps, rubella, and cytomegalovirus specific IgM responses in patients with juvenile-onset insulin-dependent diabetes mellitus in Britain, Austria and Australia. Lancet 1985;1:1409−12.

30. Mueller-Eckhardt G, Stief T, Otten A, et al. Complications of mumps infection, islet-cell antibodies, and HLA. Immunobiology 1984;167:338−44.

31. Forrest JM, Menser MA, Burgess JA. HIgh frequency of diabetes mellitus in young adults with congenital rubella. Lancet 1971;2:332−4.

32. Tattersall RB, Pyke DA. Diabetes in identical twins. Lancet 1972;2:1120−1.

33. Yoon J-W, Austin M, Ondera T, et al. Virus induced diabetes mellitus: isolation of a virus from the pancreas of a child with diabetic ketoacidosis. N Engl J Med 1979; 300:1173−9.

34. Rubinstein P, Walker ME, Fedun B, et al. The HLA system in congenital rubella in patients with and without diabetes. Diabetes 1982;31:1088−91.

35. Foulis AK. In type 1 diabetes, does a non-cytopathic viral infection of insulin-secreting B-cells initiate the disease process leading to their autoimmune destruction. Diabetic Med 1989;6:666−74.

36. Ujevich MM, Jaffe R. Pancreatic islet cell damage. Its occurrence in neonatal coxsackievirus encephalomyocarditis. Arch Pathol Lab Med 1980;104:438−41.

37. Jenson AB, Rosenberg HS, Notkins AL. Pancreatic islet-cell damage in children with fatal viral infections. Lancet 1980;2:354−58.

38. Foulis AK, Farquharson MA, Cameron SO, et al. A search for the presence of the enteroviral capsid protein VP1 in pancreases of patients with type 1 (insulin dependent) diabetes and pancreases and hearts of infants who died of coxsackieviral myocarditis. Diabetologia 1990; 33:290−8.

39. Gladisch R, Hofmann W, Waldherr R. Mykarditis und Insulitis nach Coxsackie-Virus-Infect. Z Kardiol 1976; 65:837−49.

40. Foulis AK, Francis ND, Farquharson MA, et al. Massive synchronous B cell necrosis causing type 1 (insulin-dependent) diabetes: a unique histopathological case report. Diabetologia 1988;31:46−50.

41. Foulis AK, Steward JA. The pancreas in recent-onset type 1 (insulin-dependent) diabetes mellitus: insulin content of islets, insulitis and associated changes in the exocrine acinar tissue. Diabetologia 1984;26:456−61.

42. Yaginuma N, Takahashi T, Saito K, et al. The microvasculature of the human pancreas and its relation to Langerhans islets and lobules. Pathol Res Pract 1986;181:77−84.

43. Frier BM, Saunders JHB, Wormsley KG, et al. Exocrine

pancreatic function in juvenile-onset diabetes mellitus. Gut 1976;17:685–91.

44. Frier BM, Faber OK, Binder C, et al. The effect of residual insulin secretion on exocrine pancreatic function in juvenile-onset diabetes mellitus. Diabetologia 1978; 14:301–4.

45. Henderson JR. Why are the islets of Langerhans? Lancet 1969;2:469–70.

46. Foulis AK, Frier BM. Pancreatic endocrine-exocrine function in diabetes: an old alliance disturbed. Diabetic Med 1984;1:263–6.

47. Hellman B. Actual distribution of the number and volume of the islets of Langerhans in different size classes in non-diabetic humans of varying ages. Nature 1959; 184:1498–9.

48. Maclean N, Ogilvie RF. Quantitative estimation of the pancreatic islet tissue in diabetic subjects. Diabetes 1955;4:367–76.

49. Saito K, Yaginuma N, Takahashi T. Differential volumetry of A, B and D cells in the pancreatic islets of diabetic and non-diabetic subjects. Toholi J Exp Med 1979; 129:273–83.

50. Hellman B. The frequency distribution of the number and volume of the islets of Langerhans in man. 2. Studies in diabetes of adult onset. Acta Pathol Microbiol Scand 1961;51:95–102.

51. Westermark P, Wilander E. The influence of amyloid deposits on the islet volume in maturity-onset diabetes mellitus. Diabetologia 1978;15;417–21.

52. Klöppel G, Drenck CR. Immunzytochemische Morphometrie beim Typ-I Diabetes Mellitus. Dtsch Med Wochenschr 1983;108:188–9.

53. Klöppel G. Islet histopathology in diabetes mellitus. In: Klöppel G, Heitz PU, eds. Pancreatic pathology. New York: Churchill Livingston, 1984:154–92.

54. Unger RH, Orci L. Glucagon and the A cell: physiology and pathophysiology. N Engl J Med 1981;304:1575–80.

55. Puchtler H, Sweat F. A review of early concepts of amyloid in context with contemporary chemical literature from 1839–1859. J Histochem Cytochem 1966;14:123–34.

56. Pepys MB. Amyloidosis: some recent developments. Q J Med [NS] 1988;67:283–98.

57. Glenner GG. Amyloid deposits and amyloidosis: the β-fibrilloses. N Engl J Med 1980;302:1333–43.

58. Opie EL. On the relation of chronic interstitial pancreatitis to the islands of Langerhans and to diabetes mellitus. J Exp Med 1901;5:397–428.

59. Cecil RL. A study of the pathological anatomy of the pancreas in ninety cases of diabetes mellitus. J Exp Med 1909;11:266–90.

60. Bell ET. Hyalinization of the islets of Langerhans in diabetes mellitus. Diabetes 1952;1:341–4.

61. Erlich JC, Ratner IM. Amyloidosis of the islets of Langerhans: a restudy of islet hyalin in diabetic and nondiabetic individuals. Am J Pathol 1961;38:49–59.

62. Vishwanathan KA, Bazaz-Malik G, Dandekar J, Vaishnava H. A qualitative and quantitative histologic study of the islets of Langerhans in diabetes mellitus. Indian J Med Sci 1972;26:807–12.

63. Westermark P, Grimelius L. The pancreatic islet cells in insular amyloidosis in human diabetic and non-diabetic adults. Acta Pathol Microbiol Scand [A] 1973; 81:291–300.

64. Saito K, Takahashi T, Yaginuma N, Iwama N. Islet morphometry in the diabetic pancreas of man. Tohoku J Exp Med 1978;125:185–97.

65. Schneider H-M, Störkel S, Will W. Das Amyloid der Langerhansschen Inseln und seine beziehung zum Diabetes Mellitus. Dtsch Med Wochenschr 1980;105:1143–7.

66. Maloy AL, Longnecker DS, Greenberg ER. The relation of islet amyloid to the clinical type of diabetes. Hum Pathol 1981;12:917–22.

67. Westermark P, Wilander E, Westermark GT, Johnson KH. Islet amyloid polypeptide-like immunoreactivity in the islet B cells of type 2 (non-insulin-dependent) diabetic and non-diabetic individuals. Diabetologia 1987; 30:887–92.

68. Clark A, Saad MF, Nezzer T, et al. Islet amyloid polypeptide in diabetic and non-diabetic Pima Indians. Diabetologia 1990;33:285–9.

69. Pearse AGP, Ewen SWB, Polak JM. The genesis of apudamyloid in endocrine polypeptide tumours: histochemical distinction from immunoamyloid. Virchows Arch [B] 1972;10:93–107.

70. Westermark P. Amyloid of human islets of Langerhans. 1. Isolation and some characteristics. Acta Pathol Microbiol Scand [C] 1975;83:439–46.

71. Clark A, Holman RR, Matthews DR, et al. Non-uniform distribution of islet amyloid in the pancreas of 'maturity-onset' diabetic patients. Diabetologia 1984;27:527–8.

72. Westermark P, Wernstedt C, Wilander E, et al. Amyloid fibrils in human insulinoma and islets of Langerhans of the diabetic cat are derived from a neuropeptide-like protein also present in normal islet cells. Proc Natl Acad Sci USA 1987;84:3881–5.

73. Clark A, Cooper GJS, Lewis CE, et al. Islet amyloid formed from diabetes-associated peptide may be pathogenic in type-2 diabetes. Lancet 1987;2:231–4.

74. Cooper GJS, Leighton B, Dimitriadis GD, et al. Amylin found in amyloid deposits in human type 2 diabetes mellitus may be a hormone that regulates glycogen metabolism in skeletal muscle. Proc Natl Acad Sci USA 1988;85:7763–6.

75. Cooper GJS, Willis AC, Clark A, et al. Purification and characterization of a peptide from amyloid-rich pancreases of type 2 diabetic patients. Proc Natl Acad Sci USA 1987;84:8628–32.

76. Rosenfeld MG, Mermod J-J, Amara SG, et al. Production of a novel neuropeptide encoded by the calcitonin gene via tissue-specific RNA processing. Nature 1983;304:129–35.

77. Morris HR, Panico M, Etienne T, et al. Isolation and characterization of human calcitonin gene-related peptide. Nature 1984;308:746–8.

78. Pettersson M, Ahren B, Böttcher, G, Sundler F. Calcitonin-gene-related peptide: occurrence in pancreatic islets in the mouse and the rat and inhibition of insulin secretion in the mouse. Endocrinology 1986;119:865–9.

79. Sternini C, Brecha N. Immunocytochemical identification of islet cells and nerve fibers containing calcitonin-gene-related peptide-like immunoreactivity in the rat pancreas. Gastroenterology 1986;90:1155–63.

80. Clark A, Edwards CA, Ostle LR, et al. Localisation of islet amyloid peptide in lipofuscin bodies and secretory granules of human B-cells and in islets of type-2 diabetic subjects. Cell Tissue Res 1989;257:179–85.

81. Lukinius A, Wilander E, Westermark GT, et al. Co-localization of islet amyloid polypeptide and insulin in the B-cell secretory granules of the human pancreatic islets. Diabetologia 1989;32:240–4.

82. Johnson KH, O'Brien TD, Hayden DW, et al. Immunlocalization of islet amyloid polypeptide (IAPP) in pancreatic beta cells by means of peroxidase-antiperoxidase (PAP)

and protein A-gold techniques. Am J Pathol 1988; 130:1–8.

83. Mosselman S, Höppener JWM, Zandberg J, et al. Islet amyloid polypeptide: Identfication and chromosomal localization of the human gene. FEBS Lett 1988; 239:227–32.

84. Nishi M, Sanke T, Nagamatsu S, et al. Islet amyloid polypeptide: a new β-cell secretory product related to islet amyloid deposits. J Biol Chem 1990;265:4173–6.

85. Sanke T, Bell GI, Sample C, et al. An islet amyloid peptide is derived from an 89-amino acid precursor by proteolytic processing. J Biol Chem 1988;263:17243–6.

86. Betsholtz C, Christmansson L, et al. Structure of cat islet amyloid polypeptide and identification of amino acid residues of potential significance for islet amyloid formation. Diabetes 1990;39:118–22.

87. Betsholtz C, Christmansson L, Engström U, et al. Sequence divergence in a specific region of islet amyloid polypeptide (IAPP) explains differences in islet amyloid formation between species. FEBS Lett 1989;251:261–4.

88. Howard CF Jr. Diabetes in macaca nigra: metabolic and histologic changes. Diabetologia 1974;10:671–7.

89. Yano BL, Hayden DW, Johnson KH. Feline insular amyloid: ultrastructural evidence for intracellular formation by nonendocrine cells. Lab Invest 1981;45:149–56.

90. Johnson KH, Stevens JB. Light and electron microscopic studies of islet amyloid in diabetic cats. Diabetes 1973;22:81–90.

91. de Koning EJP, Clark A, Bodkin N, Hansen BC. Correlation of islet amyloid and reduced B-cell mass with B-cell function in diabetic monkeys [Abstract no. P397]. Diabetologia 1990;33(Suppl):A111.

92. Johnson KH, O'Brien TD, Betsholtz C, Westermark P. Islet amyloid, islet-amyloid polypeptide, and diabetes mellitus. N Engl J Med 1989;321:513–8.

93. Clark A. Islet amyloid and type 2 diabetes. Diabetic Med 1989;6:561–7.

94. Mosselman S, Höppener JWM, Lips CJM, Jansz HS. The complete islet amyloid polypeptide precursor is encoded by two exons. FEBS Lett 1989;247:154–8.

95. Nishi M, Sanke T, Seino S, et al. Human islet amyloid polypeptide gene: complete nucleotide sequence, chromosomal localization and evolutionary history. Mol Endocrinol 1989;3:1775–81.

96. Westermark P, Engström U, Westermark GT, et al. Islet amyloid polypeptide (IAPP) and pro-IAPP immunoreactivity in human islets of Langerhans. Diabetes Res Clin Pract 1989;7:219–26.

97. Cook JTE, Patel PP, Clark A, et al. Non-linkage of the islet amyloid polypeptide gene with type II diabetes. Diabetologia 1990;34:103–8.

98. Johnson KH, O'Brien TD, Jordan K, Westermark P. Impaired glucose tolerance is associated with increased islet amyloid polypeptide (IAPP) immunoreactivity in pancreatic beta-cells. Am J Pathol 1989;135:245–50.

99. Hansen BC, Bodkin NL. Heterogeneity of insulin responses: phases leading to type 2 (non-insulin-dependent) diabetes mellitus in the rhesus monkey. Diabetologia 1986;29:713–9.

100. Howard CF Jr. Longitudinal studies on the development of diabetes in individual *Macaca nigra*. Diabetologia 1986;29:301–6.

101. Clark A, de Koning EJ, Hansen B, et al. Islet amyloid in glucose intolerant and spontaneous diabetic "Macaca mulatta" monkeys. In: Shafrir E, ed. Frontiers in diabetic research II. Lessons in animal diabetes III. London: Smith-Gordon, 1990:502–6.

102. Clark A, et al. Quantitative morphometry of pancreatic islet cells in cystic fibrosis. Diabetic Med 1985;2:514A.

103. Iannuci A, Mukai K, Johnson D, Burke B. Endocrine pancreas in cystic fibrosis: an immunohistochemical study. Hum Pathol 1984;15:278–84.

104. Matthews DR, Clark A. Neural control of the endocrine pancreas. Proc Nutr Soc 1987;46:89–95.

105. Orci L. Macro- and micro-domains in the endocrine pancreas. Diabetes 1982;31:538–65.

106. Mitsukawa T, Takemura J, Asai J, et al. Islet amyloid polypeptide response to glucose insulin and somatostatin analogue administration. Diabetes 1990;39:639–42.

107. Butler PC, Chou J, Carter WB, et al. Effects of meal ingestion on plasma amylin concentration in NIDDM and nondiabetic humans. Diabetes 1990;39:752–6.

108. Leighton B, Cooper GJS. Pancreatic amylin and calcitonin gene-related peptide cause resistance to insulin in skeletal muscle in vitro [Letter]. Nature 1988;335:632–5.

109. Sowa R, Sanke T, Hirayama J. Islet amyloid polypeptide amide causes peripheral insulin resistance in vivo in dogs. Diabetologia 1990;33:118–20.

110. Molina JM, Cooper GJS, Leighton B, Olefsky JM. Induction of insulin resistance in vivo by amylin and calcitonin gene-related peptide. Diabetes 1990;39:260–5.

111. Bretherton-Watt D, Gilbey SG, Ghatei MA, et al. Failure to establish islet amyloid polypeptide (amylin as a circulating beta-cell inhibiting hormone in man. Diabetologia 1990;33:115–7.

112. Tedstone AE, Nezzer T, Hughes SJ, et al. The effect of islet amyloid polypeptide (amylin) and calcitonin-gene-related peptide on glucose removal in the anaesthetised rat and on insulin secretion from rat islets in vitro. Biosci Rep 1990;10:339–45.

113. Fonseca V, Berger LA, Beckett AG, Dandona P. Size of the pancreas in diabetes mellitus: a study based on ultrasound. BMJ 1985;291:1240–1.

114. Dandona P, Freedman DB, Foo Y, et al. Exocrine pancreatic function in diabetes mellitus. J Clin Pathol 1984; 37:302–6.

115. Korc M, Owerbach D, Quinto C, Rutter WJ. Pancreatic islet-acinar cell interaction: amylase messenger RNA levels are determined by insulin. Science 1981;213:351–3.

116. Williams JA, Goldfine ID. The insulin-pancreatic axis. Diabetes 1985;34:980–6.

117. Klöppel G, Bommer G, Commandeur G, Heitz P. The endocrine pancreas in chronic pancreatitis: immunocytochemical and ultrastructural studies. Virchows Arch [A] 1978;377:157–74.

118. Orci L, Stefan Y, Malaisse-Lagae F, et al. Pancreatic fat [Letter]. N Engl J Med 1979;301:1292.

119. Olsen TS. Lipomatosis of the pancreas in autopsy material and its relation to age and overweight. Acta Pathol Microbiol Scand [A] 1978;86:367–73.

120. WHO Study Group on Diabetes Mellitus. WHO Tech Rep Ser 1985:725.

121. Mohan R, Rachandran A, Viswanathan M. Other malnutrition-related diabetes mellitus. In: Krall LP, Alberti KGMN, Turtle JR, eds. World book of diabetes in practice, 3. New York: Elsevier Science Publishers, 1988.

122. Bajaj JS, Subba Rao G. Malnutrition-related diabetes mellitus. In: Krall LP, Alberti KGMN, Turtle JR, eds. World book of diabetes in practice, 3. New York: Elsevier Science Publishing, 1988.

123. McLarty DG, Swai ABM, Mlingi N, et al. Glucose tolerance in a Tanzanian community chronically exposed to cassava toxicity [Abstract no. 272]. Diabetologia 1990;33(Suppl):A79.

124. Nagalotimath SJ. Pancreatic pathology in pancreatic calcification with diabetes. In: Podolsky S, Viswanathan M, eds. Secondary diabetes: the spectrum of the diabetic syndromes. New York: Raven Press, 1980;117–45.

125. Yajnik CS, Shelgikar KM, Sahasrabudhe RA, et al. The spectrum of pancreatic exocrine and endocrine (beta-cell) function in tropical calcific pancreatitis. Diabetologia 1990;33:417–21.

126. Mohan V, Mohan R, Susheela L, et al. Tropical pancreatic diabetes in South India:. heterogeneity in clinical and biochemical profile. Diabetologia 1985;28:229–32.

127. Stead RJ, Hodson ME, Batten JC. Diabetes mellitus (DM) associated with cystic fibrosis (CF) in adolescents and adults. In: Lennis G, ed. Proceedings of the 12th Annual European Working Group on Cystic Fibrosis, Athens, 1983.

128. Handwerger S, Roth J, Gordon P, et al. Glucose intolerance in cystic fibrosis. N Engl J Med 1969;281:451–61.

129. Löhr M, Goertchen P, Nizze H, et al. Cystic fibrosis associated with islet changes may provide a basis for diabetes: an immunocytochemical and morphometrical study. Virchows Arch [A] 1989;414:179–85.

130. Klöppel G. Development of pathological lesions in cystic fibrosis. In: Kaiser D, ed. Approaches to cystic fibrosis research. Heilbronn: Maisena Diat Gmbh, 1983.

131. Rommens JM, Ianuzzi MC, Kerem B-S, et al. Identification of the cystic fibrosis gene: chromosome walking and jumping. Science 1989;245:1059–65.

132. Sturgess JM. Structural and developmental abnormalities of the exocrine pancreas in cystic fibrosis. J Pediatr Gastroenterol Nutr 1984;3(Suppl 1):S55–6.

133. Kopito LE, Shwachman H, Vawter GF, Edlow J. The pancreas in cystic fibrosis: chemical composition and comparative morphology. Pediatr Res 1976;10:742–9.

134. Brown RE, Madge GE. Cystic fibrosis and nesidioblastosis. Arch Pathol 1971;92:53–7.

135. Marks V. The enteroinsular axis. J Clin Pathol 1978; 33(Suppl 8):38–42.

136. Ebert R, Creutzfeldt W. Reversal of impaired GIP and insulin secretion in patients with pancreatogenic steatorrhea following enzyme substitution. Diabetologia 1980;19:198–204.

137. Rahier J, Loozen S, Goebbels RM, Abrahem M. The haemochromatotic human pancreas: a quantitative immunohistochemical and ultrastructural study. Diabetologia 1987;30:5–12.

Chapter 16

SYNDROMES OF EXTREME INSULIN RESISTANCE

BARRY J. GOLDSTEIN

GENERAL CONSIDERATIONS

Insulin resistance of a mild to moderate degree is frequently observed in several clinical settings (Table 16–1). In all of these conditions but non-insulin-dependent diabetes mellitus (Type II), the defective physiologic responses to insulin may be considered to be regulatory abnormalities since they are acquired and usually reversible.[1] The most severe defects in insulin action, however, are encountered in the several rare syndromes that will be discussed in this chapter. These syndromes are distinct clinical entities with several features in common, including extreme hyperinsulinemia and severe target-cell resistance to insulin.[2,3]

In general, the syndromes of extreme insulin resistance are caused by genetic defects in the insulin action pathway or by the presence of autoantibodies to the insulin receptor that affect receptor function (Table 16–2). The hyperinsulinemia commonly observed in these patients develops by two complementary mechanisms. One is an increase in insulin secretion by the pancreatic β-cell in response to persistent elevations in fasting or postprandial glucose levels, and the other—the result of defects in the peripheral action of insulin—is a

Table 16–1. Conditions Frequently Associated with Clinical Insulin Resistance

Obesity
Non-insulin-dependent diabetes mellitus
Insulin-dependent diabetes mellitus
Physiologic states (puberty, pregnancy)
Severe illness (sepsis)
Metabolic derangement (e.g., acidosis, uremia)
Endocrinopathies (Cushing syndrome, acromegaly)

Table 16–2. Classification of Syndromes of Severe Insulin Resistance

Genetic defects in insulin receptor
  Type A syndrome
  Rabson-Mendenhall Syndrome
  Leprechaunism
Immunologic, autoimmune
  Antibodies to the insulin receptor
    Type B syndrome
    Ataxia-telangiectasia
  Antibodies to insulin
Disorders of unknown etiology: lipotrophic diabetes
  Congenital
    Dominant inheritance (Köbberling-Dunnigan syndrome)
    Autosomal recessive inheritance (Seip syndrome)
  Acquired
    Generalized (Lawrence syndrome)
    Partial lipoatrophy

striking reduction in the metabolic clearance of circulating insulin.[4]

Syndromes of Severe Insulin Resistance

Dramatic insights into the pathophysiology and classification of the syndromes of severe insulin resistance have been provided by clinical, biochemical, and genetic studies carried out over the past several years. In the type A syndrome and leprechaunism, intrinsic abnormalities in the structure or genetic expression of the insulin receptor have been shown to be key pathogenetic factors. The type B syndrome of severe insulin resistance is caused by circulating antibodies that disrupt the normal functions of the insulin receptor. In lipoatrophic diabetes, cellular defects in the insulin-action pathway have been found, but the etiology of this condition remains obscure.

In most cases, the syndromes of extreme insulin resistance have been categorized as separate disease states that may be distinguished by appropriate clinical and laboratory evaluation (Table 16–3). As more individuals with severe insulin resistance have been studied, however, they have frequently been found to have overlapping clinical and pathogenetic features. These observations suggest, for example, that the type A syndrome and leprechaunism may actually represent varying degrees of severity of similar underlying defects in the structure and function of the insulin receptor (see below).

Clinical Findings Associated with Extreme Insulin Resistance

Acanthosis Nigricans

One clinical feature common to many of the syndromes of extreme insulin resistance is acanthosis nigricans, a velvety rash characterized by papillomatosis, hyperkeratosis, and hyperpigmentation in the epidermis (Fig. 16–1). Lesions are commonly found at the neck and axillae and occasionally in the antecubital fossae and other areas. Acanthosis nigricans has been observed in a variety of clinical settings, including several endocrinopathies and internal malignancies, particularly gastrointestinal cancer.[6] However, when present, acanthosis nigricans typically indicates at least a moderate degree of underlying insulin resistance.

When specifically searched for, acanthosis nigricans may be found to occur more frequently than previously thought. In an unselected population of 1412 schoolchildren in Texas, acanthosis nigricans was present equally among boys and girls with a prevalence of 7.1%.[7] The acanthosis nigricans was more frequently noted in obese children, and its severity was correlated with the fasting plasma insulin level. Acanthosis nigricans is even more common in selected groups of patients and was shown to affect up to 29% of women with hyperandrogenism referred to a subspecialty clinic and up to 50% of obese women with polycystic ovarian disease.[8] Many of these patients have variants of the type A syndrome with moderate insulin resistance that at least partially reverts with weight loss (see below).

The development of acanthosis nigricans in patients with extreme insulin resistance has been attributed to direct effects of the hyperinsulinemia on skin tissue that result in epidermal hypertrophy. In these individuals, circulating levels of insulin can become high enough to promote binding of insulin to insulin-like growth factor 1 (IGF-1) receptors. IGF-1 receptors have a substantially lower affinity for insulin than do insulin receptors themselves, but when the ambient concentration of insulin is high enough, IGF-1 receptors may become activated by a mechanism that has been called "specificity spillover."[9,10] Increased stimulation of the IGF-1 receptor by hyperinsulinemia may be an important mechanism for

Table 16–3. Clinical Findings in the Syndromes of Extreme Insulin Resistance

	Type A	Type A variant	Type B	Generalized lipoatrophy	Leprechaunism
CLINICAL FEATURES					
Peak age of onset (y)	10–20	12–28	30–60	10–20	0–1
Obesity	+/−	++	+/−	−	−
Hirsutism, PCO*	+	+	+	+	+
Hepatomegaly	−	−	−	+++	+
LABORATORY FINDINGS					
Hyperandrogenemia	+	+	+	+	+
Insulin-receptor antibodies	−	−	+++	−	−
Antinuclear antibodies	−	−	+	−	−
Hyperlipidemia	−	−	−	+++	+
Fasting hypoglycemia	−	−	+/−	−	+
Insulin resistance in cultured cells	+++	+	−	+	+++
Pathogenesis	Insulin-receptor mutation	Regulatory or mild fixed insulin-receptor defect	Circulating antibodies to the insulin receptor	Unknown (?post-insulin-binding defect)	Insulin-receptor mutation (? + associated defects)

*Polycystic ovarian syndrome.

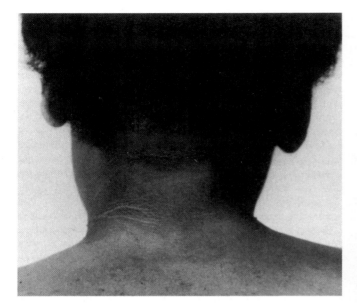

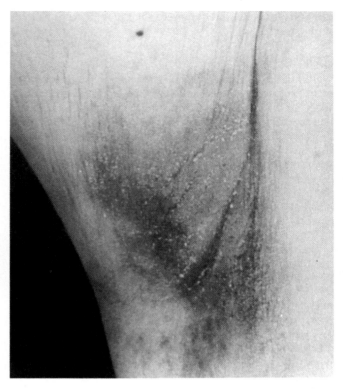

Fig. 16–1. Acanthosis nigricans in two patients with extreme insulin resistance. This skin condition is characterized by a velvety rash with epidermal hyperkeratosis and hyperpigmentation. Lesions are commonly found at the neck (left) and axilla (right). Figure on the left is reprinted with permission from reference 5 (Kahn CR, Goldstein BJ, Reddy SSK. Hereditary and acquired syndromes of insulin resistance. In: Pickup J, Williams G, eds. Textbook of diabetes. Oxford: Blackwell Scientific Publications, 1991:276–85).

the stimulation of epidermal growth in acanthosis nigricans. In addition, this mechanism may play an important role in the increased production of ovarian androgens in insulin-resistant states.

Hyperandrogenism and Ovarian Dysfunction

Ovarian dysfunction, presenting as primary or secondary amenorrhea, is very common in female patients with syndromes of extreme insulin resistance.[3] The menstrual irregularity is associated with an increased production of ovarian androgens leading to moderately elevated serum testosterone levels and various degrees of hirsutism and virilization.[11] The ovaries are typically polycystic and hyperthecotic. Although the exact pathophysiology of such ovarian dysfunction is not known, insulin may cause ovarian hyperstimulation via its own receptor or by cross-reacting with the receptors for IGF-1, which also are present in the ovary. Luteinizing hormone (LH) has also been shown to act synergistically with insulin to promote the production of androgen by the ovaries.[12]

Lipoatrophy

Lipoatrophy, a marked reduction in subcutaneous adipose tissue that occurs in a segmental or generalized distribution, is an additional clinical sign associated with the insulin-resistance syndromes of leprechaunism and lipoatrophic diabetes. If lipoatrophy is localized to sites of

insulin injection, it can be the result of a form of insulin allergy in individuals without marked insulin resistance. Total or generalized loss of subcutaneous fat tissue, however, is commonly associated with extreme insulin resistance and occurs as either an acquired or a congenital variant of lipoatrophic diabetes. Partial lipoatrophy, affecting localized regions of the body, may also occur as a distinct syndrome.

EVALUATION OF INSULIN RESISTANCE

When confronted with a patient with diabetes who, in attempts to establish glycemic control, requires high doses of insulin, the physician must determine if the patient has a defined form of extreme insulin resistance that may require special management. This assessment is made by first estimating the magnitude of the underlying insulin resistance and then evaluating the possible occurrence of an underlying pathogenetic mechanism. This evaluation scheme is summarized in Figure 16–2.

Initial Clinical Features

A convenient, arbitrary indicator that suggests a need for further evaluation is the use by the patient, whether an adult or a child, of a daily insulin dose of greater than 1.5 to 2.0 U/kg of body weight. Behavioral problems or improper diabetes management should be excluded as causes for the "insulin resistance" by a careful evaluation

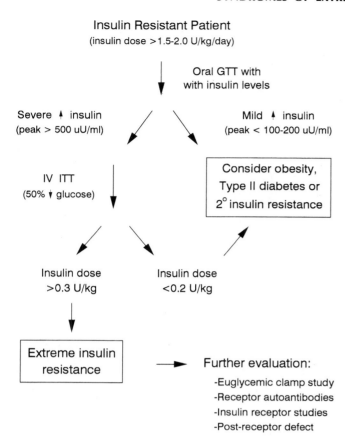

Fig. 16–2. Clinical evaluation scheme for the diagnosis of extreme insulin resistance in a patient with a high insulin requirement. GTT = glucose tolerance test; IV ITT = intravenous insulin tolerance test.

of the patient's dietary and drug history and understanding of insulin therapy. Occasionally, the patient may need to be hospitalized for close monitoring and careful assessment of the magnitude of the insulin requirement. On examination, the patient should be carefully evaluated for clinical signs and symptoms suggestive of marked insulin resistance such as acanthosis nigricans, hirsutism, and lipoatrophy. Secondary causes of worsening insulin resistance, such as superimposed severe illness, metabolic acidosis, acromegaly, hypercortisolism, etc., should be excluded.

Physiologic Resistance to Endogenous Insulin

If further investigation is warranted, laboratory studies should begin with a standard oral glucose tolerance test with measurement of serum insulin levels as well as blood glucose levels. The blood glucose level alone is a poor indicator of insulin resistance since the response of the β-cell to insulin together with the magnitude of the peripheral insulin resistance will determine the overall degree of glucose tolerance. An insulin-resistant patient thus may present with overt diabetes mellitus or may compensate for this defect and have only impaired postprandial tolerance to glucose or even euglycemia.

Serum insulin values are more useful measures since profoundly elevated fasting and/or postprandial insulin levels are the laboratory hallmarks of severe resistance to circulating insulin.

Representative oral glucose tolerance tests from patients with clinical insulin resistance are shown in Figure 16–3. As mentioned above, the glucose profile provides less diagnostic information and is helpful only in documenting the severity of the diabetes. On the other hand, with normally functioning pancreatic β-cells, the fasting and peak plasma insulin concentrations are directly related to the degree of peripheral insulin resistance. With conditions of mild to moderate insulin resistance, such as in simple obesity, the fasting plasma insulin level rarely exceeds 50 μU/mL. The peak insulin level in obese subjects after an oral 100-g glucose load may rise to 100 to 200 μU/mL, although there is marked variation among individuals. In individuals with extreme insulin resistance, the fasting insulin level may be close to normal or markedly elevated, ranging from 200 to 400 μU/mL. After a glucose load, however, these patients exhibit a striking hyperinsulinemia that typically climbs to a level higher than 1000 μU/mL.

Assessment of Response to Exogenous Insulin

Resistance to the physiologic action of insulin can be further documented by testing for tolerance to intravenous insulin, administering insulin at gradually increasing doses.[10] After an overnight fast, in a normal individual, an intravenous bolus injection of a dose of regular insulin of 0.1 U/kg of body weight will reduce the blood glucose level to a value 50% or less of the initial value. A patient with peripheral insulin resistance will require a higher dose of injected insulin (≥0.2 U/kg) to produce this reduction in the fasting glucose level. If the patient requires an insulin bolus of ≥0.3 U/kg to induce hypoglycemia, the diagnosis of extreme insulin resistance is certain (Fig. 16–2).

A more quantitative assessment of peripheral resistance to injected insulin can be made by euglycemic clamp studies.[13,14] With this technique, insulin is infused in gradually increasing amounts with concomitant administration of glucose to prevent a fall in the plasma glucose concentration. The steady-state rate of peripheral glucose utilization (M value) at several insulin levels is then measured as milligrams of glucose used per kilogram of body weight per minute. The M value provides an estimate of the sensitivity of peripheral tissues, primarily skeletal muscle, to exogenous insulin administration. This test is performed only at specialized medical centers and is not usually required for clinical evaluation.

Evaluation of Pathogenetic Mechanisms

At this stage in the diagnostic evaluation, the physician will have determined whether or not the patient has severe peripheral insulin resistance. Additional tests and studies may be indicated to establish a firm diagnosis of one of the defined syndromes discussed in this chapter (Table 16–4). For example, if the patient has associated autoimmune features and is suspected of having the type

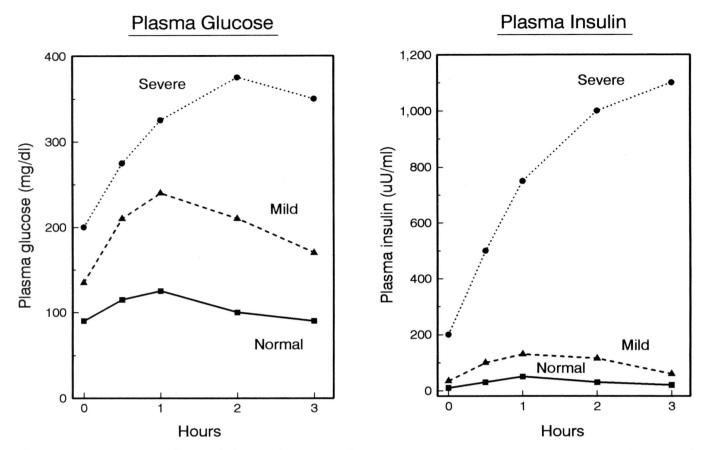

Fig. 16–3. Representative 3-hour oral glucose tolerance tests showing plasma glucose levels and plasma insulin levels for normal individuals and patients with mild and severe peripheral insulin resistance.

B syndrome, an assay for antibodies to the insulin receptor should be done (see below). These tests can be ordered from certain clinical laboratories.

If the patient is believed to have a genetic abnormality of the insulin receptor or of the insulin-action pathway, further studies can be performed on tissue or blood samples. Freshly isolated peripheral blood cells, including erythrocytes and monocytes, have often been used for evaluation of the insulin-binding properties and tyrosine

Table 16–4. Evaluation of Pathogenetic Mechanism in Patients with Extreme Insulin Resistance

Patient with associated autoimmune features: suspect type B syndrome:
   Measurement of anti-insulin receptor antibodies:
      Insulin receptor binding-inhibition assay
      Insulin receptor immunoprecipitation assay
   Assay of serum insulin-like activity
   Flow cytometry
Patient with suspected antibodies to insulin:
   Quantitative measurement of antibodies to insulin by competitive protein-binding assay
Patient with clinical features of type A syndrome or leprechaunism:
   Biochemical studies of insulin-receptor function
   Molecular analysis of insulin-receptor gene
   Assay of post-receptor defect in cultured cells

kinase activity of the patient's insulin receptors.[10] An assessment for possible post-receptor defects in the insulin-action pathway may be done with use of insulin-sensitive cultured cells such as skin fibroblasts or subcutaneous adipocytes obtained by biopsy for measurements of cellular pathways stimulated by insulin. If necessary, peripheral B-lymphocytes from the patient can be immortalized by transformation with Epstein-Barr virus and grown in the laboratory to provide larger quantities of cells for study. One limitation of the use of transformed lymphocytes, however, is that they do not exhibit measurable physiologic responses to insulin and cannot be used for evaluation of post-receptor defects in insulin pathways. Molecular genetic analyses of the insulin receptor can be performed on genomic DNA or mRNA isolated from peripheral blood or cultured cells from affected patients.[15–17]

DISORDERS ASSOCIATED WITH GENETIC DEFECTS IN INSULIN RECEPTOR

Type A Syndrome

The type A syndrome of severe insulin resistance is typically recognized in adolescent girls who are seen for evaluation of hirsutism or menstrual irregularities. This syndrome was first identified in three thin young women with marked glucose intolerance, severe target-cell insulin resistance, acanthosis nigricans, and hyperandrogenism.[2] Subsequent reports have broadened the clinical spectrum of the type A syndrome, describing its occurrence in men, in patients with mild obesity, and in some individuals with normal glucose tolerance.[18,19] The insulin resistance can be profound, and patients have been treated with more than 100,000 U of insulin daily with little effect. Some patients have histories of accelerated growth in childhood or acromegalic features, possibly as a result of cross-reaction of the elevated circulating insulin levels with tissue IGF-1 receptors, as discussed above. Although most patients with the type A syndrome are first identified as isolated cases, familial inheritance has been observed in some kindreds, and a history of parental consanguinity is found in some cases.

Variants of Type A Syndrome

Since the original description of the type A syndrome of severe insulin resistance, several variant forms have been reported. The designation of classical type A syndrome might best be limited to patients with the typical clinical findings as well as specific laboratory abnormalities, including a biochemical defect in the function of the insulin receptor and, ultimately, the finding of a genetic defect in the receptor structure or in the expression of the receptor mRNA. Patients with clinical features of the type A syndrome but a biochemically normal insulin receptor constitute one variant group.[20] These patients may have post-receptor defects that alter the signal transduction system for insulin action rather than abnormalities that directly affect the synthesis or structure of the insulin receptor itself.

The Rabson-Mendenhall syndrome[21,22] is similar to the type A syndrome with regard to the presence of acanthosis nigricans, virilization, and insulin resistance. Additional clinical features associated with this syndrome include precocious puberty, hyperplasia of the pineal body, and dystrophic nails and teeth. An additional variant of the type A syndrome, reported in one kindred, also includes the associated features of acral hypertrophy and recurrent muscle cramps.[18,23]

Several features of the type A syndrome are seen in a subset of patients who present initially with polycystic ovarian disease and hyperandrogenism.[14,24,25] These patients frequently are seen in endocrine clinics for evaluation of infertility or hirsutism. Typically, they do not have overt diabetes mellitus, although they are commonly overweight. In this setting, patients with acanthosis nigricans have been found to be more hyperinsulinemic and insulin resistant than a matched cohort of hyperandrogenized women with simple obesity. The receptor defect in these patients is less marked than that seen in patients with type A syndrome, and in some cases the defect may be secondary to the down-regulation of insulin receptors that occurs with the hyperinsulinemia of obesity. This is further supported by the observation in a few patients that insulin binding increases towards the normal range with dietary restriction, a finding suggesting

an acquired rather than a fixed genetic defect in the insulin receptor.[14]

A similar condition has been described in a cross-sectional study of a nondiabetic pediatric population with acanthosis nigricans, hyperandrogenism, and obesity in whom the degree of insulin resistance was much greater than that found in a control group with simple obesity alone.[26] It is of interest that in each case acanthosis nigricans and hyperinsulinemia appeared after the onset of obesity, a course suggesting that the increased insulin resistance associated with the weight gain may be a reversible component of this type A syndrome variant.

Pathogenesis

A variety of structural and functional defects in the insulin receptor have been demonstrated in patients with type A severe insulin resistance.[10,15,27] Many patients exhibit a marked decrease in cellular insulin binding in both freshly isolated and cultured cells related either to a reduction in the number of receptors or to an alteration in receptor affinity. Unlike the decreased insulin binding seen in obese patients, which improves with caloric restriction, in patients with classical type A insulin resistance, dietary manipulation has little or no effect. The cellular abnormalities occur in the absence of antibodies to insulin receptor (which are found in the type B syndrome) or other circulating inhibitors of receptor function.

The cultured fibroblasts of some patients with less severe forms of insulin resistance, such as the type A variant syndromes, have been shown to have a mild decrement in insulin binding and/or an additional defect in the autophosphorylation activity of the insulin receptor.[25,28] Some of these individuals may thus have relatively milder underlying genetic or regulatory defects in the insulin receptor that result in less tissue insulin resistance than that found in patients with the overt type A syndrome.

Recent studies have shown that type A severe insulin resistance is caused by genetic abnormalities in the insulin receptor that can affect various aspects of its cellular expression or function.[15,29] Some patients have a decreased number of apparently normal receptors as the result of a defect in receptor biosynthesis at the level of gene transcription or a genetic abnormality that affects either the stability of the insulin receptor mRNA or the post-translational processing of the receptor protein precursor. Other patients with a similar clinical presentation may have a normal abundance of receptor protein but have receptors that harbor molecular defects affecting the activation of the tyrosine kinase activity of the receptor β-subunit.

Specific mutations that alter the protein coding region of the insulin-receptor gene have now been elucidated by several laboratories in a number of patients with the type A syndrome (Table 16–5). Some of these mutations occur as homozygous alterations that affect both copies of the insulin-receptor gene. In other individuals, however, heterozygous changes in the insulin-receptor alleles

Table 16–5. Genetic Mutations in the Insulin Receptor

Position	Amino acid alteration*	Receptor defect†	Clinical Phenotype
Homozygous defects			
1. 209	his→arg	↓ insulin binding	Leprechaunism
2. 233	leu→pro	↓ insulin binding	Leprechaunism
3. 382	phe→val	↓ receptor on cell surface	Type A syndrome
4. 735	arg→ser	Uncleaved receptor precursor	Type A syndrome
Heterozygous defects (one normal allele)			
1. 1008	gly→val	↓ tyrosine kinase	Type A syndrome
2. 1013	Deletion	↓ tyrosine kinase	Type A syndrome
3. 1200	trp→ser	↓ tyrosine kinase	Type A syndrome
Compound heterozygotes			
1. 15	asn→lys	↓ insulin binding	
1000	arg→STOP	Truncated receptor protein	Rabson-Mendenhall
2. 133	trp→STOP	Truncated receptor protein	
462	asn→ser	↓ insulin binding	Type A syndrome
3. 460	lys→glu	↓ receptor degradation	
672	gln→STOP	Truncated receptor protein	Leprechaunism
4. 867	→STOP	Truncated receptor protein	
?	Presumed	Mutation in second allele	Type A syndrome
5. 897	arg→STOP	Truncated receptor protein	
?	Presumed	↓ receptor mRNA levels	Leprechaunism

See Taylor et al.[14]
*STOP indicates nonsense mutation.
† ↑ and ↓ indicate increase and decrease, respectively.

have been found. The mutations affecting the structure of the receptor protein occur at a variety of locations along the insulin-receptor sequence, affecting the insulin-binding subunit of the receptor as well as the intracellular tyrosine kinase domain in different patients (Fig. 16–4). Each distinctive mutation is associated with specific molecular defects that appear to account for the biochemical alterations of the insulin receptors and for the tissue resistance to insulin in these patients. In addition, other defects associated with the expression of the insulin receptor gene and the processing of its mRNA can cause insulin resistance (Table 16–6).

One of the first patients with type A insulin resistance in whom a specific genetic abnormality in the insulin receptor was found was the product of a consanguineous marriage. This individual is homozygous for a single point mutation in the insulin receptor gene that changes the arginine residue at position 735 to a serine and effectively prevents cleavage of the insulin precursor (proreceptor) into its α- and β-subunits.[30] The high-molecular-weight proreceptor is expressed at a low level on the cell surface and binds insulin with a reduced affinity. There is also decreased stimulation by insulin of the tyrosine kinase activity of the receptor that is associated with insulin resistance in the patient's tissues.

Additional examples of genetic defects in the type A syndrome include those affecting two sisters from a consanguineous marriage who were found to be homozygous for a point mutation at the insulin-binding subunit of the insulin receptor that altered the phenylalanine at position 382 to a valine residue.[31] It is interesting that this mutation affects the biosynthesis and delivery of the processed precursor of the insulin receptor to the cell surface, an effect that results in a decrease of 80 to 90% in the number of insulin receptors available to bind circulating insulin. Other patients have mutations in the

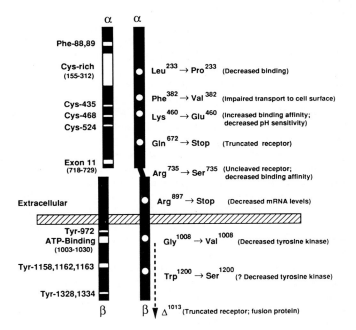

Fig. 16–4. Mutations of the insulin-receptor gene in patients with insulin resistance. The insulin-receptor structure is depicted as a tetramer consisting of two extracellular α-subunits that are responsible for insulin binding and two β-subunits that span the plasma membrane and encode the tyrosine kinase activity of the receptor. Key structural landmarks at certain amino acid positions are shown on the left. Several of the reported mutations in the insulin-receptor gene are indicated on the right, with the amino acid alteration and effect on receptor structure or function in parentheses. Reprinted with permission from reference 15 (Taylor SI, Kadowaki T, Kadowaki H, et al. Mutations in insulin-receptor gene in insulin-resistant patients. Diabetes Care 1990;13:257–79; copyright © of the American Diabetes Association).

Table 16–6. Mechanisms of Insulin Resistance Caused by Mutations in the Insulin Receptor Gene

Decreased number of insulin receptors on surface of target cells:
  Reduced abundance of insulin receptor mRNA
    Receptor gene promoter abnormality
    Impaired processing (splicing) of pre-mRNA
    Some nonsense mutations in coding region
    Accelerated receptor mRNA degradation
  Impaired transport of receptors to cell surface
  Truncated receptor protein due to nonsense mutation
  Accelerated receptor degradation
    Impaired receptor recycling to plasma membrane
Defects in receptor function:
  Decreased binding affinity for insulin
  Decreased insulin-stimulated tyrosine kinase activity of receptor

Adapted from Taylor et al.[14]

cytoplasmic domain of the insulin receptor that affect the tyrosine kinase activity of the receptor or harbor nonsense mutations that prematurely terminate the synthesis of the receptor and lead to truncated forms of the receptor protein (Table 16–5).

Analysis of the insulin-receptor genes in one patient with the Rabson-Mendenhall syndrome revealed that the patient was a compound heterozygote for two alleles with different insulin-receptor mutations.[32] One mutation altered the α-subunit sequence and caused abnormal receptor biosynthesis and decreased insulin binding. A nonsense mutation was present in the other insulin-receptor allele that caused the synthesis of a truncated receptor precursor.

Some individuals with the type A syndrome are heterozygous at the insulin-receptor locus and carry one normal allele for the receptor gene do not appear to be able to express a sufficient amount of structurally normal insulin receptors at the surface of target cells to allow their tissues to respond appropriately to insulin. This observation suggests that the presence of the mutant insulin receptor has an adverse effect on the synthesis or functional activity of the normal receptor protein in the target cell.[33] Since the mature insulin receptor exists as a heterodimer in the plasma membrane, mutant receptor subunits can actually combine with the subunits from the normal allele during receptor biosynthesis to form inactive receptor heterotetramers. In addition to specific alterations in the amino acid sequence of individual receptors, interactions between normal and mutant receptors also can play an important role in the heterogeneity and severity of the cellular defect in insulin action that is observed clinically in various kindreds with insulin-receptor defects.

Leprechaunism

Leprechaunism[34] is a rare congenital syndrome characterized by elfin-like facies, decreased subcutaneous adipose tissue, hirsutism, acanthosis nigricans, and intrauterine and neonatal growth retardation (Fig. 16–5). The metabolic abnormalities include severe insulin resistance with hyperinsulinemia that is associated with postprandial glucose intolerance. These patients also are subject to episodes of paradoxical fasting hypoglycemia, which

may be due to poor availability of gluconeogenic substrates. Affected infants often die within the first year or two of life.

Since the first report of leprechaunism in 1948 by Donohue and Uchida,[34] only a few patients with the syndrome have been studied extensively. The syndrome is both phenotypically and biochemically heterogeneous. There is a 2:1 ratio between affected girls and boys, and approximately one-third of the patients are known to be the products of a consanguineous marriage. Four patients were found to have abnormal karyotypes, but no consistent patterns have been evident.

Pathogenesis

Early laboratory studies demonstrated that insulin resistance persists in cultured cells from patients with leprechaunism, a finding providing strong evidence of an inherited defect in insulin action.[35] Most often there is decreased insulin binding caused by either reduced

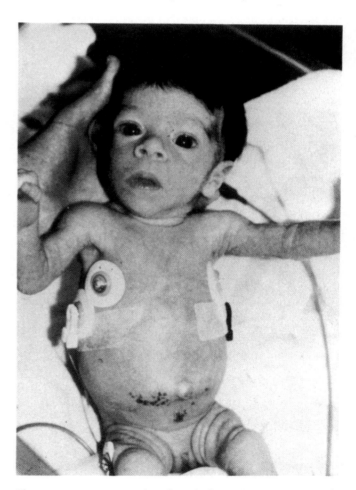

Fig. 16–5. A neonatal girl with leprechaunism. Note the characteristic elfin-like facies; marked loss of subcutaneous adipose tissue, especially in the thighs and upper arms; and increased facial hair. Reprinted with permission from reference 5 (Kahn CR, Goldstein BJ, Reddy SSK. Hereditary and acquired syndromes of insulin resistance. In: Pickup J, Williams G, eds. Textbook of diabetes. Oxford: Blackwell Scientific Publications, 1991:276–85).

receptor affinity or diminished receptor number. In some patients there appears to be reduced insulin-stimulated kinase activity of the receptor, which may play a role in the insulin resistance.[36] One unusual patient with leprechaunism was reported to have a constitutive increase in the autophosphorylation of the insulin receptor associated with an elevated basal level of glucose transport in cultured fibroblasts that was not sensitive to further stimulation by insulin treatment.[37] This continuous activation of the receptor kinase may trigger an unknown regulatory mechanism in the insulin-action pathway that is the ultimate cause of the severe insulin resistance observed in this patient.

The parents of several patients with leprechaunism have been studied with respect to insulin binding by the receptor as well as insulin-stimulated kinase activity.[38] In one family, both the mother and father were found to have mild abnormalities in receptor kinase activity. In another pedigree, insulin receptors on cells of both parents had different defects in receptor affinity and number. Thus, in some cases it appeared that the proband may have inherited two different insulin-receptor defects (compound heterozygote), resulting in a more severe global defect in insulin action.

This possibility was proven to be correct in 1988, when a patient with leprechaunism was shown, by sequence analysis of the insulin-receptor cDNA, to have inherited two abnormal insulin receptor alleles.[39] The paternal allele coded for a truncated receptor protein apparently not expressed at the cell surface. The maternal allele had a single point mutation in the α-subunit of the insulin receptor that causes biochemical abnormalities in the binding of insulin by the mutant receptor and that also may increase the rate of insulin-receptor degradation in target cells. Other genetic defects that have recently been found in patients with leprechaunism are summarized in Table 16–5.

One puzzling question about the pathogenesis of these syndromes is how various mutations in the insulin-receptor gene may ultimately lead to the disparate phenotypes of the type A syndrome in one individual and to the Rabson-Mendenhall syndrome or leprechaunism in another. The combined effect of mutations that cause more profound defects in the cellular function of the insulin receptor might be responsible for the clinically more severe syndrome of leprechaunism. On the other hand, insulin-receptor mutations that have less severe effects on receptor function might lead to the type A syndrome or to one of the variant type A syndromes with a milder clinical phenotype. In accordance with this spectrum of genetic defects in insulin-receptor function, milder insulin resistance has been documented in genetically affected family members of some probands with leprechaunism or the type A syndrome.[40,41] These findings suggest that more subtle, heterozygous mutations in the insulin-receptor gene are likely to contribute to clinically imperceptible insulin resistance that occurs in the general population. Furthermore, while most individuals with Type II diabetes apparently have a normal gene sequence for the insulin receptor, some patients with Type II diabetes may actually have a receptor mutation as a component of the etiology of their diabetes.[17]

In vitro studies of insulin-receptor function have shown that some patients with the type A syndrome have a degree of biochemical dysfunction of the insulin receptor similar to that observed in leprechaunism, which is clinically much more severe. These observations have also questioned whether insulin resistance alone can explain the clinical manifestations of leprechaunism, including the usually rapid death of those with this syndrome. Some patients with leprechaunism have been found to be resistant to the action of several growth factors, including epidermal growth factor and IGF-1, as well as to insulin.[42,43] Although the biochemical basis for this resistance to various hormones is unknown, these studies have provided evidence for a more generalized defect that may contribute to the clinical severity of the disease.

Management

Dermatologic Manifestations

Although the dermatologic complications of the genetic defects in the insulin receptor may be mild, in some patients severe acanthosis nigricans or hirsutism is the primary reason for their seeking medical attention. The acanthosis nigricans and hirsutism frequently will respond to successful treatment directed at the underlying cause, i.e., hyperinsulinemia and hyperandrogenemia, respectively. In many patients with extreme insulin resistance, however, the severe, fixed genetic defect cannot be ameliorated with any currently available therapy. No controlled studies on the treatment of acanthosis nigricans in insulin-resistant states have been reported. However, some control of the hyperpigmentation may be achieved with local application of tretinoin cream or gel.

Hyperandrogenism

The elevated levels of ovarian androgens that cause hirsutism are typically associated with polycystic ovarian disease and may respond to oral contraceptive estrogen preparations. However, in some patients with insulin resistance, these agents might be contraindicated because they have been associated with a further worsening of glucose tolerance, hypertension, and hyperlipidemia. Alternatively, spironolactone or ketoconazole has been used in a few cases with good results.[44] In accordance with recent studies showing that LH acts synergistically with insulin to promote ovarian androgen production, one report demonstrated the successful treatment of virilization in two sisters with severe insulin resistance with an agonist of gonadotropin-releasing hormone (leuprolide acetate), which suppressed LH secretion and normalized serum testosterone levels within 2 to 4 months.[45] In these patients, the addition of dexamethasone—to suppress adrenal androgen production—and the anti-androgen compound cyproterone acetate resulted in regression of the hirsutism to normal at 12 months. In patients with severe virilization, ovarian wedge resection or oophorectomy has occasionally been helpful in reducing the degree of hyperandrogenism.

Insulin Resistance

In patients with classical type A syndrome and a severe, fixed defect in the expression or function of the insulin receptor, the extreme insulin resistance has generally not responded to therapeutic maneuvers, and no remissions of the insulin resistance have been observed. The goals of therapy must therefore be individualized according to the level of glucose intolerance. Titration of the administered insulin dose to the glucose level may be attempted, but because of the intrinsic abnormalities in the cellular insulin-action pathway in these patients, the blood glucose level may be difficult to regulate. When extremely high doses of insulin must be given, U500 insulin may be more effective than equivalent doses of U100, for reasons that are not clear.[46]

In individuals with the type A syndrome variant of moderate insulin resistance who have acanthosis nigricans and obesity, weight loss may ameliorate the peripheral insulin resistance to some degree. This may reduce the level of hyperinsulinemia and, in turn, lead to a regression in the severity of the acanthosis nigricans or hyperandrogenism. With regard to blood glucose control, however, it is important to keep in mind that many of these patients have only a mild intolerance to glucose that should respond to dietary control.

In the type A syndrome variant with the additional features of muscle cramps and acral hypertrophy, three patients have had a beneficial clinical response to phenytoin.[47] In two patients with mild abnormalities of carbohydrate metabolism, some improvement in glycemic control was observed. Phenytoin also was found to be of some benefit in alleviating muscle pain.

Without knowledge about the exact pathophysiology of leprechaunism, management is directed at the symptoms only. The most important facets of therapy include close surveillance of blood sugar level and the judicious use of insulin. Frequent small feedings are useful since these patients are subject to fasting hypoglycemia as a result of diminished fuel storage as well as to postprandial glucose intolerance. Despite these measures, the illness is typically fatal early in infancy, although some exceptions have been observed.

Prenatal Diagnosis of Severe Insulin Resistance

Techniques for the biochemical characterization of the insulin receptor have recently become refined to a degree that permits careful analysis of the tyrosine kinase activity of the receptor in a small tissue sample obtained by a chorionic villus biopsy or by culture of amniotic fluid cells. This methodology was recently used to analyze a pregnancy at risk for fetal leprechaunism in which the unaffected status of the child was correctly predicted.[48] Although not yet reported for syndromes of insulin resistance, specific DNA sequence alterations known to occur in the insulin-receptor gene within a given pedigree might also be detected in a fetus at risk with the use of sensitive molecular genetic techniques such as allele-specific oligonucleotide hybridization.[15]

AUTOIMMUNE AND IMMUNOLOGIC DISORDERS

In several syndromes of extreme insulin resistance, the insulin action pathway in target cells is intact but the effectiveness of circulating insulin is blocked by the presence of antibodies that react with the insulin receptor or the insulin molecule itself.

Autoantibodies to the Insulin Receptor

The Type B Syndrome

The type B syndrome of severe insulin resistance is an autoimmune syndrome caused by circulating antibodies directed at the insulin receptor.[2,49,50] This condition has a female preponderance (female-to-male ratio 2:1) and most often presents in the fourth to sixth decade of life. Because of the target-cell insulin resistance and endogenous hyperinsulinemia, patients with type B syndrome have some clinical features in common with patients with type A syndrome, including acanthosis nigricans, hirsutism, oligomenorrhea, and hyperandrogenism. However, one important distinguishing typical feature in patients with type B syndrome is evidence of other autoimmune phenomena such as an increased erythrocyte sedimentation rate, elevated levels of γ-globulins, and autoantibodies to nuclear antigens or DNA. In fact, up to one-third of the patients satisfy criteria for the diagnosis of systemic lupus erythematosus or Sjögren's syndrome.[51] As with other autoimmune disorders, a waxing and waning of symptoms over time is frequently observed, and a fraction of these patients have experienced a spontaneous remission of their hyperinsulinemia over a 2- to 3-year period. Some of the clinical features of this disorder, such as the severity of the acanthosis nigricans, tend to follow the severity of the underlying insulin resistance.

Pathogenesis. Laboratory studies of antibodies to the insulin receptor isolated from patients with extreme type B insulin resistance have shown that the antibodies can affect any of several vital aspects of the insulin-action pathway (Fig. 16–6). Most often, the antibodies to the insulin receptor cause a decrease in the affinity of the insulin receptor for insulin and lead to peripheral insulin resistance by acting as competitive antagonists of insulin binding. Other receptor antibodies that do not affect hormone binding can interfere with signal transduction by the insulin receptor, accelerate turnover of the insulin receptor, or lead to post-receptor desensitization of the insulin-action pathway. Since the antibodies are typically polyclonal, several types of biochemical effects may be elicited by different classes of antibodies to receptor even in an individual patient.[52]

Further clinical heterogeneity of the type B syndrome has been observed in several patients who have developed or have presented with fasting hypoglycemia in association with the presence of circulating antibodies to the insulin receptor.[53] In contrast to the patients with severe insulin resistance, these patients exhibit antibodies to the insulin receptor that can interact with the

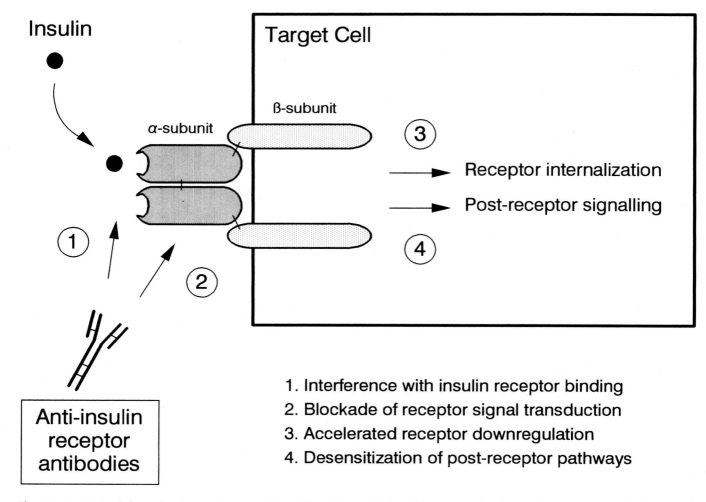

Fig. 16—6. Potential mechanisms of target-cell insulin resistance induced by autoantibodies to insulin receptor in the type B syndrome of severe insulin resistance. The α- and β-subunits of the insulin receptor are shown in the plasma membrane of a target cell.

insulin-binding domain of the receptor in a positive manner and actually mimic the actions of insulin. In these individuals, the insulin-like activity of the antibodies is clinically manifest as an erratic hypoglycemic syndrome that may be confused with an islet-cell tumor.

The clinical severity of the type B syndrome can wax and wane with variation in the titer and properties of the circulating autoantibodies, as in other autoimmune disease states. Remarkable clinical heterogeneity has been observed in some patients with type B syndrome whose condition has actually evolved from one of severe insulin resistance to a hypoglycemic state. This development may occur because of changes in the abundance or activity of free autoantibodies in the circulation, which can produce variable effects on insulin action in target tissues. These combined effects can obviously complicate the precise management of blood glucose control in these patients.

In laboratory studies, the chronicity of exposure has also been shown to play an important role in the cellular effects of particular antibodies to the receptor.[54] Thus,

acute exposure of cultured cells to receptor antibodies may demonstrate insulinomimetic effects, whereas exposure for several hours may result in insulin resistance as a result of accelerated internalization and degradation of the receptors in the target cells.[55] As in other autoimmune disorders, the type B syndrome arises from a defect in the regulation of the immune system rather than from an abnormality of the tissue insulin receptors. This conclusion is supported by the observation that insulin sensitivity appears to be normal in patients with the type B syndrome during periods of antibody remission. Furthermore, normal function of insulin receptors has been demonstrated in cultured cells from patients with type B syndrome, and insulin resistance can be mimicked by incubating the patient's cells with serum containing the receptor antibodies.

Several methods are used by specialized clinical laboratories to detect the presence of antibodies to the insulin receptor, which are typically polyclonal and of the IgG class.[56,57] These include the binding-inhibition assay, the immunoprecipitation assay, and an assay of insulin-like activity in the γ-globulin fraction of the patient's serum (Table 16–4). The first method, which depends on the ability of the antibody to inhibit the binding of insulin to its receptor on cultured human lymphoblastoid cells, is the method most commonly used. However, the specificity of this technique may be affected by the presence of nonspecific inhibitors of insulin binding that may be found in the plasma of individuals without receptor antibodies.

The immunoprecipitation assay is performed by incubating the patient's serum with affinity-labeled insulin receptors and isolating the immune complexes that result in a positive test.[57] This assay is somewhat more difficult to perform but is more sensitive than the binding-inhibition assay and can detect antibodies directed at sites other than the insulin-binding domain of the receptor. Flow cytometry has also been used to demonstrate the presence of antibodies to insulin receptor in the serum of patients with the type B syndrome.[58] Assays based on the insulin-like activity of the antibodies are sensitive but are not specific for antibodies to insulin receptor and may give a positive response to other factors in the patient's circulation.

Ataxia-Telangiectasia

In several patients with ataxia telangiectasia, low-molecular-weight IgM antibodies to insulin receptors have been described.[59] Ataxia telangiectasia is a rare recessive syndrome characterized by progressive cerebellar ataxia, oculocutaneous telangiectasia, recurrent upper and lower respiratory tract infections, and a variety of immunologic abnormalities. About 60% of patients with this syndrome have glucose intolerance, hyperinsulinemia, and a decreased sensitivity to exogenous insulin. As in the typical type B syndrome, the insulin receptors on cultured fibroblasts are normal, indicating that there is no underlying defect in the insulin receptor itself.

Antibodies to Insulin

Circulating antibodies to insulin may rarely lead to significant clinical insulin resistance.[60] Patients with Type I diabetes often have low titers of antibodies to insulin before insulin therapy that are associated with autoimmune attack on the pancreatic β-cells. Low-titer IgG antibodies to insulin also are found in virtually all insulin-requiring patients, and the physiologic action of insulin administered to these patients is usually normal. However, in a Joslin Clinic series of patients between 1940 and 1960, about 0.01% of all insulin-treated patients had significant insulin resistance.[61] In general, insulin resistance in these patients has a gradual onset over a period of weeks to months and often is associated with a history of intermittent or interrupted insulin therapy. Allergic reactions to insulin are found in 25 to 35% of the insulin-resistant patients. Many patients also have a history of treatment with outdated formulations of less highly purified pork or beef insulins.

The diagnosis of insulin resistance caused by antibodies to insulin relies on the exclusion of other causes of peripheral insulin resistance, as summarized above. Since virtually all insulin-treated patients develop antibodies to insulin, especially those treated with older insulin formulations, a quantitative measurement of antibody by a competitive protein-binding assay is necessary to confirm the presence of a high titer of antibodies to insulin.[60] In most patients, the insulin-binding capacity is less than 10 U/L of plasma. Patients with significant circulating titers of insulin antibodies typically have a much higher serum insulin-binding capacity, which in some cases can exceed 500 U/L.

Of interest is the demonstration of insulin-receptor autoantibodies in some patients with insulin-dependent diabetes, which possibly arise as anti-idiotypes.[62] In this setting, which is quite rare, the patient's antibodies to insulin may actually serve as antigens for the generation of a new complement of autoantibodies. If these anti-idiotypes are directed against the insulin-binding domain of the antibodies to insulin, they may, in turn, cross-react with the patient's insulin receptors. Antibodies to receptor have been similarly observed in laboratory animals injected with antibodies to insulin or with insulin only.

Management

In many patients with autoimmune insulin resistance, the glucose intolerance is only a minor component of their overall symptomatology, and management should be planned accordingly. Furthermore, many patients with the type B syndrome have experienced a gradual reduction in the titer of receptor antibody, with a spontaneous remission of insulin resistance and diabetes over a 2- to 3-year period. For these patients, the efficacy of any therapy is thus confounded by the cyclical nature of the autoimmune disease, and thus it has been difficult to evaluate whether a particular therapeutic intervention has led directly to clinical improvement.

In attempts to reduce the antibody titer more rapidly, several approaches have been used, including plasmapheresis and immunosuppressive therapy with corticosteroids and/or antimetabolite compounds.[63–65] Typical initial therapy might consist of prednisone (60 to 80 mg/day) or cyclophosphamide (1 mg/kg body weight per day). Plasmapheresis produces only a transient fall in antibody levels and needs to be combined with other immunosuppressive therapy. After therapy to reduce the titer of antibody to the insulin receptor has been instituted, careful follow-up of diabetes status and rapid adjustment of the insulin dosage is mandatory.

For patients with insulin resistance caused by antibodies to insulin, it is important to note that the disorder tends to be self-limited and will remit within 6 months in about 60% of patients.[61] The mainstay of therapy is the substitution of less antigenic forms of insulin, such as highly purified pork or recombinant human insulin, for an older preparation that the patient may be using.[66] Since the pre-existing antibodies will typically bind purified insulins with a lower affinity than they bind the less purified preparation, this maneuver may achieve adequate control in up to 50% of patients. Other less immunogenic insulins that might be considered include fish insulin, desalanine pork insulin (a chemically modified insulin), and sulfated insulin.[60] Since the antibody titer will fall with removal of the antigenic stimulus, the patient must be closely monitored and the physician should anticipate further reductions in the insulin dosage to avoid hypoglycemia. Glucocorticoids may also be required in the treatment of patients with autoantibodies to insulin, starting with a moderately high dose of prednisone (60 to 80 mg/day), with a therapeutic response anticipated in up to 75% of patients within several days.[60,61] Patients receiving glucocorticoids need to be monitored for potential worsening of glucose tolerance related to the countering effects of glucocorticoids on insulin action as well as for the precipitous fall in the blood glucose level and insulin requirement as the effect of the circulating antibodies is mitigated.

DISORDERS OF UNKNOWN ETIOLOGY: LIPOTROPHIC DIABETES

Lipoatrophic diabetes encompasses a genetically heterogeneous group of rare syndromes characterized by insulin-resistant diabetes mellitus associated with an absence of subcutaneous adipose tissue (Fig. 16−7). Several forms of this condition have been reported according to mode of inheritance and extent and regional distribution of the lipoatrophy.[67] These include congenital types of generalized lipoatrophic diabetes, which may exhibit either dominant (Köbberling-Dunnigan syndrome) or recessive inheritance (Seip syndrome). In addition, syndromes of acquired total lipoatrophy (Lawrence syndrome) and various types of acquired partial lipoatrophy have been described.

Clinical Syndromes

Congenital Lipoatrophy

Dominant Inheritance. By studying pedigrees of congenital lipoatrophy with dominant inheritance in Scotland and Germany, Köbberling and Dunnigan delineated two clinical subtypes with characteristic distributions of subcutaneous fat that appear to be consistent within each pedigree.[68−70] In type 1 familial lipodystrophy, the loss of subcutaneous fat is confined to the limbs, sparing the face and trunk. In the type 2 syndrome, the trunk is also affected with the exception of the vulva, giving the impression of labial hypertrophy. Associated clinical features variably expressed in the pedigrees included severe hyperlipidemia, acanthosis nigricans, hepatosplenomegaly, tubero-eruptive xanthomata, elevated basal metabolic rate, and insulin-resistant diabetes without ketoacidosis. The pedigrees of five families with these lipodystrophic disorders revealed that only females were affected, suggesting an X-linked dominant mode of inheritance that may be lethal in the hemizygous (XY) state.

Recessive Inheritance. The autosomal recessive form of congenital generalized lipoatrophy (Seip syndrome) has been reported to occur more widely.[71,72] Parental consanguinity is frequent, and cases are equally distributed among males and females. The absence of subcutaneous fat is noted in early infancy, although the

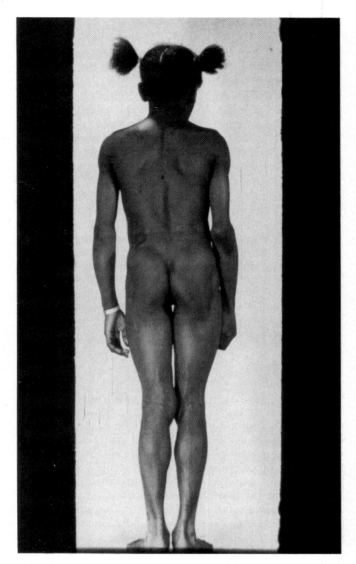

Fig. 16−7. Congenital lipoatrophic diabetes in an adolescent girl. Note the generalized loss of subcutaneous adipose tissue, which gives the appearance of muscular hypertrophy, especially in the lower extremities.

diabetes typically appears later, with a mean onset of 12 years. In addition to the absence of subcutaneous adipose tissue is an absence of fat in perirenal, retroperitoneal, and epicardial locations. In these syndromes, unlike the dominantly inherited Köbberling-Dunnigan syndromes, facial and buccal fat is also affected. Mammary fat tissue may be spared in some cases. Loss of subcutaneous adipose tissue causes the thyroid, peripheral veins, and skeletal muscles to appear more prominent, and actual muscular hypertrophy may also occur (Fig. 16−7).

Growth and maturation of bone during the first 4 to 5 years of life are frequently accelerated.[71] Acromegalic facies along with thick skin and large hands and feet may also be present in association with normal levels of circulating growth hormone, characteristics suggesting that in this syndrome, as in other states of severe insulin resistance, the degree of hyperinsulinemia may lead to cross-stimulation of IGF-1 receptors. Hepatomegaly, resulting from increased stores of lipid and glycogen, is observed frequently and can be massive. Hypertriglyceridemia with eruptive xanthomas, lipemia retinalis, and episodic pancreatitis also may occur. Polycystic ovaries and menstrual irregularity are common in affected females. Mental retardation, psychiatric disturbances, and intracerebral disorders localized to the region of the third ventricle have also been associated with congenital lipoatrophy.

Laboratory studies of patients with recessive, congenital lipoatrophic diabetes have demonstrated a striking elevation of the basal metabolic rate with normal thyroid function. A striking type IV or type V hyperlipoproteinemia is typically present and appears to be due to increased synthesis as well as to decreased clearance of lipoproteins.[73] When diabetes has been present for years, long-term diabetic complications have been known to occur, including nephropathy with proteinuria and hypertension, peripheral neuropathy, and diabetic retinopathy. The hepatomegaly often leads to portal hypertension and irreversible cirrhosis, which is commonly the cause of death in this patients with this disorder.

Acquired Lipoatrophy

Generalized Form. Acquired, generalized lipoatrophy was first described by Lawrence in 1946.[74] Affected patients exhibit a generalized absence of body fat, insulin-resistant nonketotic diabetes mellitus, an elevated basal metabolic rate with hyperhidrosis, and hyperlipidemia with hepatosplenomegaly. The occurrence of this condition is sporadic, without familial inheritance. In many cases, a viral illness precedes the development of lipoatrophy, but a direct viral etiology has not been demonstrated. The onset is usually in childhood or shortly after puberty, and this condition has a 2:1 preponderance in females. Clinical diabetes typically follows the onset of lipoatrophy by an average of 4 years. In the Lawrence syndrome, as in the congenital form of lipoatrophic diabetes, hepatomegaly can lead to cirrhosis, which may be the ultimate cause of death. Accelerated atherosclerosis also may occur and contribute to premature coronary artery disease.

Partial Lipoatrophy. Several forms of acquired, partial loss of subcutaneous adipose tissue have been described.[75] In partial lipoatrophy, the most common pattern is loss of fat from the face and trunk with normal or actually increased fat deposition below the waist. Occasionally, only the lower half of the body is affected or lipodystrophy is segmental in a dermatomal distribution.

Familial occurrence of partial lipoatrophy has also been described, although the mode of inheritance is not clearly Mendelian. Acquired partial lipoatrophy may represent a less severe variant of the generalized disorder (Lawrence syndrome), and families have been described in which both forms of the disease occur. In rare cases, the partial form may develop into generalized total lipoatrophy. Like acquired generalized lipoatrophy, in this syndrome females are predominantly affected, the onset of partial lipoatrophy usually occurs in childhood, and in some cases onset has been preceded by an infectious illness.

Patients with partial lipoatrophy frequently have hypocomplementemia, which has also been associated with membranoproliferative (mesangiocapillary) glomerulonephritis in some individuals.[76,77] These alterations have not been observed in the congenital lipoatrophic disorders. The reduction in levels of serum complement is due to the presence of an IgG autoantibody that binds to and stabilizes the C3 convertase enzyme. The result of this antibody action is an increase in the splitting of complement factor C3 and the activation of the alternative pathway of complement. This autoantibody is indistinguishable from the C3 nephritic factor observed in patients with membranoproliferative glomerulonephritis who do not have partial lipodystrophy, and the relationship between the complement system defect and the clinical lipodystrophy remains obscure.

A potential association between the immune system and disorders of adiposity and energy balance may ultimately be found in a serum protein named *adipsin,* which is secreted by adipocytes into the bloodstream. Adipsin has recently been shown to have serine protease activity identical to that of complement factor D, a process that is the initial step in the activation of the alternative pathway.[78] It is interesting that both factor D activity and levels of adipsin mRNA are dramatically reduced in several models of genetic obesity in mice, a finding suggesting a possible role for adipsin in the energy balance of certain states of obesity.[79] Further studies of adipsin expression in patients with partial lipoatrophy may help define a potential role for this protein not only in the loss of adipose tissue mass and increased metabolic rate observed in the lipoatrophic syndromes but also in the occurrence of complement activation and glomerulonephritis.

Pathogenesis

Although many theories about the etiology of lipoatrophic diabetes have appeared over the years, the underlying cause of this disorder remains enigmatic. While subcutaneous adipose tissue appears to be absent on gross examination, histologic evidence has revealed that in congenital lipoatrophy fat cells are present but appear to be immature, containing little intracellular lipid. Recently, in a case of partial lipoatrophy affecting the upper body, measurement of substrate kinetics demonstrated directly that the remaining adipose tissue in the forearm was capable of releasing substantial amounts of free fatty acids.[80]

The elevated metabolic rate, hyperlipidemia, and insulin resistance suggests hyperactivity of the sympathetic nervous system, but catecholamine tests have not been consistently elevated in the patients studied.[80,81] However, segmental dysfunction of the adrenergic nervous system or regional differences in the response of adipose tissue to circulating hormones may be etiologic factors in the unique distribution of affected adipose tissue in partial lipodystrophy.[82,83]

Early studies suggested that at least some of the metabolic disturbances in lipoatrophic diabetes might be caused by a decreased binding of insulin to its receptor. This was not a fixed receptor abnormality, however, and was reversible by a 60-hour fast.[84] Additional studies revealed a marked heterogeneity in insulin-receptor binding, with some individuals, even within the same kindred, exhibiting normal or actually increased levels of insulin binding.[85,86]

Studies on several siblings in a pedigree with recessive congenital lipodystrophy revealed heterogeneity in the function and expression of the insulin receptor in cultured cells as well as a variant sequence of the insulin-receptor gene in the family members.[87] The abnormalities were not fully linked to the clinical expression of the lipodystrophy, a finding that supports a complex nature of the genetic and metabolic defects in this syndrome that may lead to secondary effects on the insulin receptor.

No circulating insulin inhibitors or antibodies directed at insulin or the insulin receptor have been found that account for the insulin resistance in patients with lipoatrophic diabetes. However, one case of total acquired lipodystrophy with diabetes but normal circulating insulin levels was associated with increased clearance of circulating insulin or accelerated degradation of insulin at target tissues.[88]

Direct examination of cultured fibroblasts from several patients with generalized lipodystrophy has suggested that the severe insulin resistance in this syndrome may actually be due to a post-binding defect in insulin action that affects primarily glucose uptake or glucose metabolism.[89] Furthermore, both insulin and IGF-1 receptors from these fibroblasts were found to have defects in their tyrosine kinase activity, suggesting that a signaling abnormality common to these related receptors may play a role in the pathogenesis of the insulin resistance.[90]

Some years ago the presence of a circulating lipid-mobilizing factor was thought to be causally associated with lipoatrophic diabetes, but this component remains poorly characterized. This factor was initially isolated from the urine of lipoatrophic patients and, when injected into animals, produced insulin resistance and lipolysis of fat stores.[91] The factor was not specific for this syndrome, since it was later found in the urine of diabetic patients with proteinuria.[92]

The association of increased hypothalamic releasing factors in the circulation of lipoatrophic patients has raised the possibility of a hypothalamic role in the etiology of these conditions. Since an accumulation of dopamine within the hypothalamus might lead to accelerated release of hypothalamic hormones, drugs that affect dopamine synthesis or action were tested in lipoatrophic patients. The neuroleptic agent pimozide, which reduces levels of hypothalamic dopamine, was initially described as producing dramatic clinical improvement in several prepubertal or peripubertal patients with lipoatrophy.[93] However, subsequent reports demonstrated no clinical benefit from pimozide and diminish the practical therapeutic value of this drug.[94,95] Fenfluramine, a dopamine-blocking agent that also lowers serotonin

levels, has also been used in a few patients with lipoatrophic diabetes. This agent was initially found to increase the sensitivity of a few patients to exogenous insulin and to improve the hyperhidrosis and hyperlipidemia; however, no consistent long-term beneficial effect has been observed in other studies.[96-98]

The possibility that a hypothalamic lesion might play a role in these disorders is suggested by the frequent occurrence of tumors of the third ventricle in patients with congenital lipoatrophic diabetes.[99] It is of interest that in the diencephalic syndrome of infancy, anterior hypothalamic tumors have also been found to occur in association with diminished body fat, elevated metabolic rate, and accelerated growth. A boy with acquired lipoatrophic diabetes associated with stenosis of the aqueduct of Sylvius showed dramatic clinical improvement after placement of a ventriculocisternal shunt, providing further evidence that hypothalamic dysfunction may contribute to the perturbed metabolic state.[95]

Management

Since the etiology of insulin-resistant diabetes in the lipoatrophic syndromes is enigmatic, therapy has consisted of attempts at maintaining the blood glucose level within a reasonable range. Caloric restriction may improve the hyperlipemia and carbohydrate tolerance in patients with lipoatrophic diabetes.[98,100] Good control of blood glucose levels may be difficult to achieve in patients with lipodystrophy because of the fixed nature of the underlying abnormalities in peripheral insulin action found in many of these patients. Attempts at dietary therapy for lipoatrophic diabetes with omega-3 fatty acids demonstrated a reduction in serum triglyceride levels and an amelioration of pancreatitis in at least one patient but at the expense of more severe glucose intolerance caused by an inhibition of insulin secretion.[101] As described above, neuroleptic agents have been used in the treatment of lipoatrophic diabetes, with transient or no improvement noted in most cases.

Medical or dietary therapy has not accomplished a reversal of the lipoatrophy with the reappearance of subcutaneous fat tissue. In a case of acquired partial lipodystrophy, however, transplantation of autologous adipose tissue to the face was recently reported to provide a favorable cosmetic improvement.[102]

REFERENCES

1. Reddy SSK, Kahn CR. Insulin resistance: a look at the role of insulin receptor kinase. Diabetic Med 1988;5:621–9.
2. Kahn CR, Flier JS, Bar RS, et al. The syndromes of insulin resistance and acanthosis nigricans: insulin-receptor disorders in man. N Engl J Med 1976;294:739–45.
3. Flier JS, Kahn CR, Roth J. Receptors, antireceptor antibodies and mechanisms of insulin resistance. N Engl J Med 1979;300:413–9.
4. Flier JS, Minaker KL, Landsberg L, et al. Impaired in vivo insulin clearance in patients with severe target-cell resistance to insulin. Diabetes 1982;31:132–5.
5. Kahn CR, Goldstein BJ, Reddy SSK. Hereditary and acquired syndromes of insulin resistance. In: Pickup J,

Williams G, eds. Textbook of diabetes. Oxford: Blackwell Scientific Publications, 1991:276–854.

6. Brown J, Winkelmann RK. Acanthosis nigricans: a study of 90 cases. Medicine (Baltimore) 1968;47:33–51.

7. Stuart CA, Pate CJ, Peters EJ. Prevalence of acanthosis nigricans in an unselected population. Am J Med 1989; 87:269–72.

8. Dunaif A, Graf M, Maneli J, et al. Characterization of groups of hyperandrogenic women with acanthosis nigricans, impaired glucose tolerance, and/or hyperinsulinemia. J Clin Endocrinol Metab 1987;65:499–507.

9. Fradkin JE, Eastman RC, Lesniak MA, Roth J. Specificity spillover at the hormone receptor—exploring its role in human disease. N Engl J Med 1989;320:640–5.

10. Taylor SI. Receptor defects in patients with extreme insulin resistance. Diabetes Metab Rev 1985;1:171–202.

11. DeClue TJ, Shah SC, Marchese M, Malone JI. Insulin resistance and hyperinsulinemia induce hyperandrogenism in a young type B insulin-resistant female. J Clin Endocrinol Metab 1991;72:1308–11.

12. Poretsky L, Kalin MF. The gonadotropic function of insulin. Endocr Rev 1987;8:132–41.

13. DeFronzo RA, Tobin JD, Andres R. Glucose clamp technique: a method for quantifying insulin secretion and resistance. Am J Physiol 1979;237:E214–23.

14. Flier JS, Eastman RC, Minaker KL, et al. Acanthosis nigricans in obese women with hyperandrogenism. Characterization of an insulin-resistant state distinct from the type A and B syndromes. Diabetes 1985;34: 101–7.

15. Taylor SI, Kadowaki T, Kadowaki H, et al. Mutations in insulin-receptor gene in insulin-resistant patients. Diabetes Care 1990;13:257–79.

16. Goldstein BJ, Kahn CR. Insulin receptor messenger ribonucleic acid sequence alterations detected by ribonuclease cleavage in patients with syndromes of insulin resistance. J Clin Endocrinol Metab 1989;69:15–24.

17. O'Rahilly S, Choi WH, Patel P, et al. Detection of mutations in insulin-receptor gene in NIDDM patients by analysis of single-stranded conformation polymorphisms. Diabetes 1991;40:777–82.

18. Flier JS, Young JB, Landsberg L. Familial insulin resistance with acanthosis nigricans, acral hypertrophy and muscle cramps. N Engl J Med 1980;303:970–3.

19. Flier JS. Insulin receptors and insulin resistance. Annu Rev Med 1983;34:145–60.

20. Bar RS, Muggeo M, Roth J, et al. Insulin resistance, acanthosis nigricans, and normal insulin receptors in a young woman: evidence for a postreceptor defect. J Clin Endocrinol Metab 1978;47:620–5.

21. Rabson SM, Mendenhall EN. Familial hypertrophy of pineal body, hyperplasia of adrenal cortex and diabetes mellitus: report of 3 cases. Am J Clin Pathol 1956;26:283–90.

22. West RJ, Leonard JV. Familial insulin resistance with pineal hyperplasia: metabolic studies and effects of hypophysectomy. Arch Dis Child 1980;55:619–21.

23. Holdaway IM, Frengley PA, Graham FM, et al. Insulin resistance with acanthosis nigricans and acral hypertrophy. N Z Med J 1984;97:286–8.

24. Stuart CA, Peters EJ, Prince MJ, et al. Insulin resistance with acanthosis nigricans: the roles of obesity and androgen excess. Metabolism 1986;35:197–205.

25. Peters EJ, Stuart CA, Prince MJ. Acanthosis nigricans and obesity: acquired and intrinsic defects in insulin action. Metabolism 1986;35:807–13.

26. Richards GE, Cavallo A, Meyer WJ III, et al. Obesity, acanthosis nigricans, insulin resistance, and hyperandrogenemia: pediatric perspective and natural history. J Pediatr 1985;107:893–7.

27. Bar RS, Muggeo M, Kahn CR, et al. Characterization of insulin receptors in patients with the syndromes of insulin resistance and acanthosis nigricans. Diabetologia 1980; 18: 209–16.

28. Stuart CA, Pietrzyk RA, Peters, EJ, et al. Autophosphorylation of cultured skin fibroblast insulin receptors from patients with severe insulin resistance and acanthosis nigricans. Diabetes 1989;38:328–32.

29. Taylor SI, Kadowaki T, Accili D, et al. Mutations in the insulin receptor gene in genetic forms of insulin resistance. Recent Prog Horm Res 1990;46:185–213.

30. Yoshimasa Y, Seino S, Whittaker J, et al. Insulin-resistant diabetes due to a point mutation that prevents insulin proreceptor processing. Science 1988;240:784–7.

31. Accili D, Frapier C, Mosthaf L, et al. A mutation in the insulin receptor gene that impairs transport of the receptor to the plasma membrane and causes insulin-resistant diabetes. EMBO J 1989;8:2509–17.

32. Kadowaki T, Kadowaki H, Rechler MM, et al. Five mutant alleles of the insulin receptor gene in patients with genetic forms of insulin resistance. J Clin Invest 1990; 86:254–64.

33. Whittaker J, Soos MA, Siddle K. Hybrid insulin receptors: molecular mechanisms of negative-dominant mutations in receptor-mediated insulin resistance. Diabetes Care 1990;13:576–81.

34. Donohue WL, Uchida I. Leprechaunism: a euphemism for a rare familial disorder. J Pediatr 1954;45:505–19.

35. Kobayashi M, Olefsky JM, Elders J, et al. Insulin resistance due to a defect distal to the insulin receptor: demonstration in a patient with leprechaunism. Proc Natl Acad Sci USA 1978;75:3469–73.

36. Reddy SS-K, Lauris V, Kahn CR. Insulin receptor function in fibroblasts from patients with leprechaunism: differential alterations in binding, autophosphorylation, kinase activity and receptor-mediated internalization. J Clin Invest 1988;82:1359–65.

37. Longo N, Shuster RC, Griffin LD, Elsas IJ. Insulin-receptor autophosphorylation and kinase activity are constitutively increased in fibroblasts cultured from a patient with heritable insulin-resistance. Biochem Biophys Res Commun 1990;167:1229–34.

38. Reddy SS-K, Müller-Wieland D, Kriauciunas KM, Kahn CR. Molecular defects in the insulin receptor in patients with leprechaunism and in their parents. J Lab Clin Med 1989;114:165–70.

39. Kadowaki T, Bevins CL, Cama A, et al. Two mutant alleles of the insulin receptor gene in a patient with extreme insulin resistance. Science 1988;240:787–90.

40. Deprez RHL, van Loon BJP, van der Zon GCM, et al. Individuals with only one allele for a functional insulin receptor have a tendency to hyperinsulinaemia but not to hyperglycaemia. Diabetologia 1989;32:740–4.

41. Moller DE, Yokota A, White MF, et al. A naturally occurring mutation of insulin receptor alanine 1134 impairs tyrosine kinase function and is associated with dominantly inherited insulin resistance. J Biol Chem 1990;265:14979–85.

42. Kaplowitz PB, D'Ercole AJ. Fibroblasts from a patient with leprechaunism are resistant to insulin, epidermal growth factor and somatomedin C. J Clin Endocrinol Metab 1982;55:741–8.

43. Reddy SS-K, Kahn CR. Epidermal growth factor receptor defects in leprechaunism: a multiple growth factor-resistant syndrome. J Clin Invest 1989;84:1569–76.

44. Pepper GM, Poretsky L, Gabrilove JL, Ariton MM. Keto-conazole reverses hyperandrogenism in a patient with insulin resistance and acanthosis nigricans. J Clin Endocrinol Metab 1987;65:1047–52.

45. Corenblum B, Baylis BW. Medical therapy for the syndrome of familial virilization, insulin resistance, and acanthosis nigricans. Fertil Steril 1990;53:421–5.

46. Nathan DM, Axelrod L, Flier JS, et al. U-500 insulin in the treatment of antibody-mediated insulin resistance. Ann Intern Med 1981;94:653–6.

47. Minaker KL, Flier JS, Landsberg L, et al. Phenytoin-induced improvement in muscle cramping and insulin action in three patients with the syndrome of insulin resistance, acanthosis nigricans, and acral hypertrophy. Arch Neurol 1989;46:981–5.

48. Maassen JA, Lindhout D, Reuss A, Kleijer WJ. Prenatal analysis of insulin receptor autophosphorylation in a family with leprechaunism. Prenat Diagn 1990;10:13–6.

49. Kahn CR, Flier JS, Muggeo M, Harrison LC. Autoantibodies to the insulin receptor in insulin resistant diabetes. In: Irvine J, ed. Immunology of diabetes. Edinburgh: Teviot Scientific Publications, 1980:205–19.

50. Taylor SI, Barbetti F, Accili D, et al. Syndromes of autoimmunity and hypoglycemia: autoantibodies directed against insulin and its receptor. Endocrinol Metab Clin North Am 1989;18:123–43.

51. Tsokos GC, Gorden P, Antonovych T, et al. Lupus nephritis and other autoimmune features in patients with diabetes mellitus due to autoantibody to insulin receptors. Ann Intern Med 1985;102:176–81.

52. De Pirro R, Roth RA, Rossetti L, Goldfine ID. Characterization of the serum from a patient with insulin resistance and hypoglycemia: evidence for multiple populations of insulin receptor antibodies with different receptor binding and insulin-mimicking activities. Diabetes 1984;33:301–4.

53. Taylor SI, Grunberger G, Marcus-Samuels B, et al. Hypoglycemia associated with antibodies to the insulin receptor. N Engl J Med 1982;307:1422–6.

54. Grunfeld C, Van Obberghen E, Karlsson FA, Kahn CR. Antibody-induced desensitization of the insulin receptor: studies on the mechanism of desensitization in 3T3-L1 fatty fibroblasts. J Clin Invest 1980;66:1124–34.

55. Taylor SI, Marcus-Samuels B. Anti-receptor antibodies mimic the effect of insulin to down-regulate insulin receptors in cultured human lymphoblastoid (IM-9) cells. J Clin Endocrinol Metab 1984;58:182–86.

56. Flier JS, Kahn CR, Jarrett DB, Roth J. Characterization of antibodies to the insulin receptor: a cause of insulin-resistant diabetes in man. J Clin Invest 1976;58:1442–9.

57. Taylor SI, Underhill LH, Marcus-Samuels B. Assay of antibodies directed against cell surface receptors. Methods Enzymol 1985;109:656–67.

58. Maron R, Jackson RA, Jacobs S, et al. Analysis of the insulin receptor by anti-receptor antibodies and flow cytometry. Proc Natl Acad Sci USA 1984;81:7446–50.

59. Bar RS, Levis WR, Rechler MM, et al. Extreme insulin resistance in ataxia telangiectasia: defect in affinity of insulin receptors. N Engl J Med 1978;298:1164–71.

60. Kahn CR, Rosenthal AS. Immunologic reactions to insulin: insulin allergy, insulin resistance, and the autoimmune insulin syndrome. Diabetes Care 1979;2:283–95.

61. Shipp JC, Cunningham RW, Russell RO, Marble A. Insulin resistance: clinical features natural course and effects of adrenal steroid treatment. Medicine (Baltimore) 1965;44:165–86.

62. Shoelson SE, Marshal S, Horkoshi H, et al. Antiinsulin receptor antibodies in an insulin-dependent diabetic may arise as autoantiidiotypes. J Clin Endocrinol Metab 1986;63:56–61.

63. Muggeo M, Flier JS, Abrams RA, et al. Treatment with plasma exchange of a patient with autoantibodies to the insulin receptor. N Engl J Med 1979;300:477–80.

64. Kawanishi K, Kawamura K, Nishina Y, et al. Successful immunosuppressive therapy in insulin resistant diabetes caused by anti-insulin receptor autoantibodies. J Clin Endocrinol Metab 1977;44:15–21.

65. Sims RE, Rushford FE, Huston DP, Cunningham GR. Successful immunosuppressive therapy in a patient with autoantibodies to insulin receptors and immune complex glomerulonephritis. South Med J 1987;80:903–6.

66. Goldstein BJ, Kahn CR. Insulin allergy and insulin resistance. In: Lichtenstein LM, Fauci AS, eds. Current therapy in allergy, immunology and rheumatology. Lewiston, NY: BC Decker, 1988:327–30.

67. Podolsky S. Lipoatrophic diabetes and leprechaunism. In: Podolsky S, Viswanathan M, eds. Secondary diabetes: the spectrum of the diabetic syndromes. New York: Raven Press, 1980:335–52.

68. Dunnigan MG, Cochrane MA, Kelly A, Scott JW. Familial lipoatrophic diabetes with dominant transmission: a new syndrome. Q J Med (New Series) 1974;43:33–48.

69. Köbberling J, Willms B, Kattermann R, Creutzfeldt W. Lipodystrophy of the extremities. A dominantly inherited syndrome associated with lipoatrophic diabetes. Humangenetik 1975;29:111–20.

70. Köbberling J, Dunnigan MG. Familial partial lipodystrophy: two types of an X-linked dominant syndrome, lethal in the hemizygous state. J Med Genet 1986;23:120–7.

71. Seip M, Trygstad O. Generalized lipodystrophy. Arch Dis Child 1963;38:447–53.

72. Berardinelli W. An undiagnosed endocrinometabolic syndrome: report of 2 cases. J Clin Endocrinol 1954;14:193–204.

73. Enzi G, Digito M, Baldo-Enzi G, et al. Lipid metabolism in lipoatrophic diabetes. Horm Metab Res 1988;20:587–91.

74. Lawrence RD. Lipodystrophy and hepatomegaly with diabetes, lipaemia, and other metabolic disturbances: a case throwing new light on the action of insulin. Lancet 1946;1:724–31.

75. Senior B, Gellis SS. The syndromes of total lipodystrophy and of partial lipodystrophy. Pediatrics 1964;33:593–612.

76. Ipp MM, Minta JO, Gelfand EW. Disorders of the complement system in lipodystrophy. Clin Immunol Immunopathol 1977;7:281–7.

77. Sissons JGP, West RJ, Fallows J, et al. The complement abnormalities of lipodystrophy. N Engl J Med 1976;294:461–65.

78. Rosen BS, Cool KS, Yaglom J, et al. Adipsin and complement factor D activity: an immune-related defect in obesity. Science 1989;244:1483–7.

79. Flier JS, Cook KS, Usher P, Spiegelman BM. Severely impaired adipsin expression in genetic and acquired obesity. Science 1987;237:405–8.

80. Jensen MD. Adrenergic regulation of lipolysis in a patient with lipoatrophy of the upper body. Mayo Clin Proc 1991;66:704–10.

81. Huseman C, Johanson A, Varma M, Blizzard RM. Congenital lipodystrophy: an endocrine study of three siblings. I. Disorders of carbohydrate metabolism. J Pediatr 1978;93:221–6.

82. Steinberg T, Gwinup G. Lipodystrophy: a variant of lipoatrophic diabetes. Diabetes 1967;16:715–21.

83. Davidson MB, Young RT. Metabolic studies in familial partial lipodystrophy of the lower trunk and extremities. Diabetologia 1975;11:561–8.

84. Oseid S, Beck-Nielsen H, Pedersen O, Søvik O. Decreased binding of insulin to its receptor in patients with congenital generalized lipodystrophy. N Engl J Med 1977;296:245–8.

85. Wachslicht-Rodbard H, Muggeo M, Kahn CR, et al. Heterogeneity of the insulin-receptor interaction in lipoatrophic diabetes. J Clin Endocrinol Metab 1981;52:416–25.

86. Rosenbloom AL, Goldstein S, Yip CC. Normal insulin binding to cultured fibroblasts from patients with lipoatrophic diabetes. J Clin Endocrinol Metab 1977;44:803–6.

87. Kriauciunas KM, Kahn CR, Muller-Wieland D, et al. Altered expression and function of the insulin receptor in a family with lipoatrophic diabetes. J Clin Endocrinol Metab 1988;67:1284–93.

88. Golden MP, Charles MA, Arquilla ER, et al. Insulin resistance in total lipodystrophy: evidence for a prereceptor defect in insulin action. Metabolism 1985;34:330–5.

89. Magré J, Reynet C, Capeau J, et al. In vitro studies of insulin resistance in patients with lipoatrophic diabetes. Evidence for heterogeneous postbinding defects. Diabetes 1988;37:421–8.

90. Magré J, Grigorescu F, Reynet C, et al. Tyrosine-kinase defect of the insulin receptor in cultured fibroblasts from patients with lipoatrophic diabetes. J Clin Endocrinol Metab 1989;69:142–50.

91. Foss I, Trygstad O. Lipoatrophy produced in mice and rabbits by a fraction prepared from the urine from patients with congenital generalized lipodystrophy. Acta Endocrinol 1975;80:398–416.

92. Louis LH, Conn JW. A urinary diabetogenic peptide in proteinuric diabetic patients. Metabolism 1969;18:556–63.

93. Corbin A, Upton GV, Mabry CC, et al. Diencephalic involvement in generalized lipodystrophy: rationale and treatment with the neuroleptic agent, pimozide. Acta Endocrinol 1974;77:209–20.

94. Rossini AA, Self J, Aoki TT, et al. Metabolic and endocrine studies in a case of lipoatrophic diabetes. Metabolism 1977;26:637–50.

95. Häger A, Heding LG, Larsson Y, et al. Pancreatic β-cell function and abnormal urinary peptides in a boy with lipoatrophic diabetes and stenosis of the aqueduct of Sylvius. Acta Paediatr Scand 1980;69:537–45.

96. Trygstad O, Foss I. Congenital generalized lipodystrophy and experimental lipoatrophic diabetes in rabbits treated successfully with fenfluramine. Acta Endocrinol 1977;85:436–48.

97. Trygstad O, Seip M, Oseid S. Lipodystrophic diabetes treated with fenfluramine. Int J Obesity 1977;1:287–92.

98. Wilson TA, Melton T, Clarke WL. The effect of fenfluramine and caloric restriction on carbohydrate homeostasis in patients with lipodystrophy. Diabetes Care 1983;6:160–5.

99. Rossini AA. Lipoatrophic diabetes. In: Marble A, Krall LP, Bradley RF, et al, eds. Joslin's diabetes mellitus. 12th ed. Philadelphia: Lea & Febiger, 1985:834–42.

100. Schwartz R, Schafer IA, Renold AE. Generalized lipoatrophy, hepatic cirrhosis, disturbed carbohydrate metabolism and accelerated growth (lipoatrophic diabetes): longitudinal observations and metabolic studies. Am J Med 1960;28:973–85.

101. Stacpoole PW, Alig J, Kilgore LL, et al. Lipodystrophic diabetes mellitus. Investigations of lipoprotein metabolism and the effects of omega-3 fatty acid administration in two patients. Metabolism 1988;37:944–51.

102. Hurwitz PJ, Sarel R. Facial reconstruction in partial lipodystrophy. Ann Plast Surg 1982;8:253–7.

Chapter 17

SECONDARY FORMS OF DIABETES

OM P. GANDA

The term *secondary diabetes* generally refers to diabetes or glucose intolerance that develops in association with disorders (or factors) other than those currently defined as Type I or Type II diabetes mellitus or gestational diabetes mellitus. According to the classification system developed by the National Institutes of Health international work group, the subclass "secondary diabetes" contains "a variety of types of diabetes, in some of which the etiologic relationship is known (e.g., diabetes secondary to pancreatic disease, endocrine disease, or administration of certain drugs). In others, an etiologic relationship is suspected because of a higher frequency of association of diabetes with a syndrome or condition (e.g., a number of genetic syndromes)."[1] The extent of glucose intolerance in patients with secondary forms of diabetes varies widely, presenting as insulin-requiring or non-insulin-requiring overt diabetes, simulating Type I (insulin-dependent diabetes mellitus; IDDM) or Type II diabetes (non-insulin-dependent diabetes mellitus; NIDDM) or as milder forms such as impaired glucose tolerance or minimally abnormal glucose tolerance, considered nondiagnostic. Another complexity in the evolution of secondary diabetes is that an underlying coexisting predisposition to primary diabetes might be unmasked, a not uncommon occurrence, considering the prevalence of diabetes gene(s) in the population.

Table 17–1 presents a classification of various forms of secondary diabetes. When diabetes is secondary to pancreatic disorders, particularly when β-cell mass is greatly reduced, e.g., by malignancy or pancreatectomy, or when diabetes is due to chemical agents toxic to the β-cell, e.g., pentamidine or pyriminil (Vacor), overt diabetes with or without ketoacidosis often will result, depending on the extent of β-cell loss. On the other hand, when diabetes is secondary to endocrinopathies leading to counterregulatory hormone production (e.g., acromegaly, Cushing syndrome, hyperthyroidism), overt diabetes or ketoacidosis are unusual, thanks to the amazing potential of the normal β-cell reserve.[2,3] Thus, the net metabolic outcome in patients with secondary diabetes depends on the direct or indirect impact of the underlying disorders on 1) insulin secretion, i.e., inhibition or compensatory hyperinsulinemia; 2) insulin sensitivity, i.e., glucose utilization; and 3) hepatic glucose output.

PANCREATIC DIABETES

Pancreatectomy

Diabetes that results from pancreatectomy is, in a mechanistic sense, the prototype of insulin-deficient secondary diabetes. The amount of human pancreas that must be surgically removed or pathologically destroyed

Table 17–1. A Classification of Secondary Forms of Diabetes or Impaired Glucose Tolerance

A. Pancreatic disorders
   a. Pancreatectomy
   b. Pancreatitis
   c. Malnutrition-related pancreatic diabetes
   d. Hemochromatosis
B. Endocrinopathies
   a. Disorders of growth-hormone secretion
      1. Acromegaly
      2. Growth hormone-deficiency states
   b. Hyperprolactinemic states
   c. Glucocorticoid excess (Cushing syndrome)
   d. Catecholamine excess (pheochromocytoma)
   e. Primary hyperaldosteronism
   f. Hyperthyroidism
   g. Disorders of calcium and/or phosphorus metabolism
   h. Tumors of endocrine pancreas or gut (see Chapter 56)
      1. Glucagonoma
      2. Somatostatinoma
      3. Pancreatic cholera syndrome
      4. Carcinoid syndrome
      5. Multiple endocrine neoplasia (MEN) syndromes
   i. Polyglandular deficiency syndromes (see Chapter 55)
   j. Polyneuropathy, organomegaly, endocrinopathy, monoclonal gammopathy, skin changes (POEMS) syndrome
C. Drugs, chemical agents, and toxins
   a. Diuretics and antihypertensive agents
     Thiazides; chlorthalidone; loop diuretics (furosemide, ethacrynic acid, metolazone); diazoxide; clonidine; β-adrenergic antagonists
   b. Hormones
     Glucocorticoids, adrenocorticotropic hormone, α-adrenergic agonists, growth hormone, glucagon, oral contraceptives, progestational agents
   c. Psychoactive agents
     Lithium, opiates, ethanol, phenothiazines
   d. Anticonvulsants
     Diphenylhydantoins (Dilantin)
   e. Antineoplastic agents
     Streptozotocin, L-asparaginase, mithramycin
   f. Antiprotozoal agents
     Pentamidine
   g. Rodenticides
     Pyriminil (Vacor)
   h. Miscellaneous
     Nicotinic acid
     Cyclosporine
     N-Nitrosamines
     Theophylline
D. Genetic syndromes
   a. Pancreatic deficiencies
      1. Congenital absence of pancreatic islets
      2. Cystic fibrosis
      3. Hereditary relapsing pancreatitis
   b. Inborn errors of metabolism
      1. Glycogen-storage disease type
      2. Acute intermittent porphyria
      3. Hyperlipidemias
   c. Severe to extreme insulin resistance syndromes (see Chapter 16)
      1. Type A syndrome: classic and variants
      2. Type B syndrome: associated with autoantibodies to insulin receptor
      3. Leprechaunism
      4. Lipodystrophic syndromes
      5. Rabson-Mendenhall syndrome
        (precocious puberty, dental dysplasia, dystrophic nails)
      6. Ataxia-telangiectasia
      7. Alström syndrome
        (obesity, retinitis pigmentosa, deafness)
      8. Dystrophia myotonica
   d. Obesity-associated insulin resistance
      1. Laurence-Moon-Biedl syndrome
      2. Bardet-Biedl syndrome
      3. Prader-Willi syndrome
      4. Achondroplasia
   e. Progeroid syndromes
      1. Werner syndrome

Table Continued

Table 17−1. Continued

2. Cockayne syndrome
(microcephaly, dwarfism, deafness, nephropathy)
f. Chromosomal defects
1. Down syndrome (trisomy 21)
2. Klinefelter syndrome (47, XXY)
3. Turner syndrome (45, XO)
g. Hereditary neuromuscular disorders
1. Muscular dystrophy
2. Huntington's chorea
3. Friedreich's ataxia (spinocerebellar ataxia)
4. Machado disease (ataxia, dysarthria, nystagmus)
5. Herrmann syndrome (photomyoclonus, dementia, deafness, nephropathy)
6. Stiff-man syndrome
7. DIDMOAD syndrome (diabetes insipidus, diabetes mellitus, optic atrophy, deafness), or Wolfram's syndrome, and variants

before the development of fasting hyperglycemia is a matter of some debate. Of interest, recent elegant studies in baboons revealed that after induction of diabetes with streptozotocin the animals developed fasting hyperglycemia and a reduction in β-cell function in vivo when 40 to 50% of the β-cell mass was still detectable by islet morphometric assessment.[4] Furthermore, of 28 healthy human donors who underwent ~50% pancreatectomy, seven (25%) developed glucose intolerance and a deterioration in insulin secretion after 8 to 15 months[5] (Fig. 17−1). However, none of these individuals developed

overt diabetes during this time. It has been suggested that development of diabetes in partially pancreatectomized humans depends on several additional factors, such as rate of regeneration of β-cells, changes in nutritional status caused by weight loss and concomitant exocrine insufficiency, and the glucagon deficiency resulting from loss of α-cells.[6]

Subtotal or total pancreatectomy provides a model for diabetes without pancreatic glucagon.[7] However, there are many reports of normal or elevated levels of immunoreactive glucagon (IRG), originating from extrapancre-

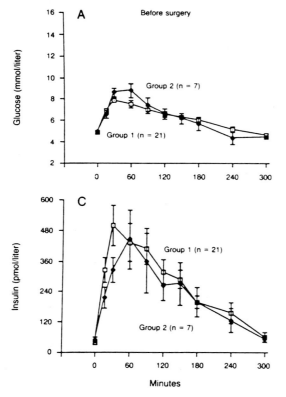
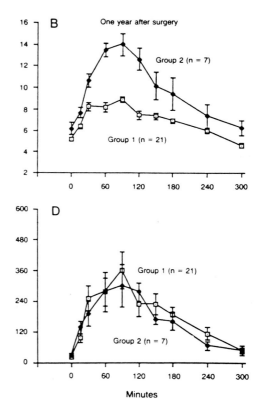

Fig. 17−1. Mean (± SEM) serum glucose levels (A and B) and serum insulin levels (C and D), measured before and 1 year after hemipancreatectomy during 5-hour oral glucose-tolerance tests in 21 transplant donors with normal glucose tolerance at 1 year (group 1; open squares) and 7 donors with abnormal glucose tolerance at 1 year (group 2; closed circles). Reprinted with permission from reference 5 (Kendall DM, Sutherland DER, Najarian JS, et al. Effects of hemipancreatectomy on insulin secretion and glucose tolerance in healthy humans. N Engl J Med 1990;322:898−903).

atic sources (gastrointestinal), in such patients.[8-10] In most studies, the majority of this IRG comprised larger-molecular-weight material, which does not have biologic activity, but small quantities of 3500-kilodalton pancreatic glucagon may also be detectable.[8] The biologic significance of extrapancreatic glucagon in these patients is not known, and their levels of IRG do not respond to arginine administration, although paradoxical stimulation in response to oral glucose or mixed meals has been reported.[8,10]

The clinical presentation of diabetes in pancreatectomized humans differs from that of Type I diabetes in several respects:

1. Because of coexisting exocrine deficiency, pancreatectomized individuals present a nutritional challenge. They tend to be leaner than patients with Type I diabetes and present with various degrees of malabsorption despite treatment with pancreatic enzyme supplements. Consequently, their insulin requirements are lower than those of weight-matched patients with Type I diabetes.[11]

2. Pancreatectomized patients are more prone to hypoglycemia and may have a more sluggish and delayed recovery from hypoglycemia. The reasons for these differences are multiple. Glucose turnover and gluconeogenesis are considerably diminished, and levels of gluconeogenic precursors (alanine, lactate, pyruvate) are markedly increased[12,13]; these changes are reversible by physiologic replacement of glucagon. Furthermore, epinephrine release in response to hypoglycemia may be markedly blunted,[14] but the mechanism is unclear. Thus, combined defects in glucagon and epinephrine may underlie prolonged and delayed recovery from hypoglycemia in such patients.

3. Ketonemia and ketoacidosis are less severe in pancreatectomized patients despite comparable stimulation of lipolysis. As shown in Figure 17–2, withdrawal of insulin for 12 hours from totally pancreatectomized subjects ($n = 4$) and age- and weight-matched patients with Type I diabetes ($n = 6$) resulted in about a 50% reduction in the magnitude of hyperglycemia and hyperketonemia in the former.[15] There were no significant differences in levels of free fatty acids and glycerol. Glucagon was undetectable before and after insulin withdrawal in pancreatectomized subjects.[7,15] These studies strongly support the important role of glucagon in the promotion of ketogenesis but also argue against a primary role of glucagon in the induction of ketoacidosis.

4. The issue of insulin sensitivity and peripheral glucose utilization following pancreatectomy is controversial. While some reported increased cellular insulin binding and enhanced hepatic and extrahepatic insulin sensitivity,[16] others observed a state of peripheral insulin resistance[17] that was further impaired by glucagon replacement.[18] Some of these discrepancies may be explained by differences in patient characteristics and alcohol intake and by the lack of consistent control for the induction of insulin resistance by antecedent hyperglycemia, per se.

Pancreatitis

Diabetes secondary to pancreatitis accounts for less than 1% of cases of diabetes in the United States and other Western countries. However, in many parts of the world (especially tropical countries), the proportion is much higher.

Diabetic ●——●
Pancreatectomized ○——○

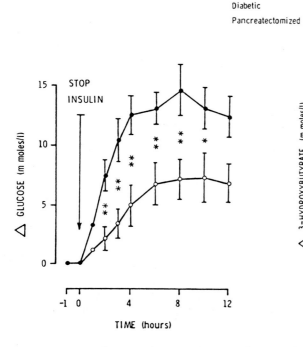

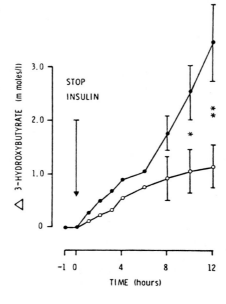

Fig. 17–2. Changes in blood concentrations (mean ± SEM) of glucose and 3-hydroxybutyrate in patients with Type I diabetes ($n = 6$) and pancreatectomized subjects ($n = 4$) after withdrawal of insulin. $*P < .05; **P < .02$. Reprinted with permission from reference 15 (Barnes AT, Bloom SR, Alberti KGMM, et al. Ketoacidosis in pancreatectomized man. N Engl J Med 1977;296: 1250–3).

Transient hyperglycemia may be seen in up to 50% of patients with acute pancreatitis in the absence of further attacks, but persistent diabetes develops—presumably as a result of ongoing chronic, painless pancreatitis—in fewer than 5% of such individuals during long-term follow-up in the absence of further attacks.[19] On the other hand, in patients with chronic pancreatitis, the incidence of diabetes increases over the years, being present in about 40 to 50% of patients after 20 years, with an additional 25 to 30% having impaired glucose tolerance.[19,20] Among patients with fibrocalcific pancreatitis, up to 80 to 90% have overt diabetes or impaired glucose tolerance.[19,20] In Western societies, the etiology of chronic pancreatitis is largely alcohol related, in both patients with and without biliary disease. As the number of patients with cystic fibrosis who survive into adulthood has increased, the prevalence of overt diabetes in this group has reached 10 to 15% and that of impaired glucose tolerance in those older than 12 years ranges from 27 to 57%.[21]

The precise mechanisms by which chronic pancreatic inflammation leads to glucose intolerance are not established, but compromised blood flow to islets from fibrotic scarring of exocrine pancreas may play a role. Insulin and C-peptide secretory responses to various secretagogues, including orally and intravenously administered glucose, sulfonylureas, glucagon, and amino acids, are impaired, and these abnormalities are correlated with the magnitude of exocrine pancreatic dysfunction.[19,22,23] Glucagon levels are markedly increased in acute pancreatitis, both in the basal state and following stimulation with alanine. This increase may contribute to the transient hyperglycemia frequently seen in this situation.[24] In chronic pancreatitis, the basal glucagon levels are normal or elevated, but the responses to amino acids[9,24] or to insulin-induced hypoglycemia[25,26] are usually found to be blunted. In some studies, however, levels of glucagon-like immunoreactivity were increased after stimulation,[20,27] perhaps due to glucagon derived from extrapancreatic sources, but the significance of this observation is uncertain.

Patients with diabetes secondary to chronic pancreatitis may show a delayed recovery from hypoglycemia, a situation similar to that seen in pancreatectomized subjects. However, the incidence and severity of hypoglycemia in these patients is influenced by a number of other factors, e.g., alcohol intake, nutritional status, and state of malabsorption.

Subtle abnormalities of pancreatic exocrine function may sometimes be seen in patients with Type I or Type II diabetes,[28,29] a finding that suggests the loss of a trophic effect of islet cell secretion on acinar cell function. These abnormalities, usually asymptomatic, may occasionally be difficult to differentiate from chronic, painless pancreatitis and may make additional diagnostic work-up necessary.

Malnutrition-Related Pancreatic Diabetes

In many tropical countries, extending from West Indies and Latin America to Africa to the Indian subcontinent and Southeast Asia, diabetes presents with many atypical clinical features.[30,31] The features of this presentation of diabetes, initially characterized by Hugh-Jones in Jamaica and termed *J-type diabetes,*[32] include early onset, resistance to the development of ketosis, relatively large insulin requirement, and lean body habitus. A number of variants have since been described in many tropical countries. With all the variants reported, malnutrition and protein deficiency are the common features in those affected, and the estimated prevalence, although not adequately studied in all areas, ranges from less than 10% to greater than 75% among all persons younger than 40 years old with diabetes.[31]

Recently, the World Health Organization study group identified two main subgroups of pancreatic diabetes: protein-deficient pancreatic diabetes (or J-type diabetes); and fibrocalculous pancreatic diabetes.[33] In patients with fibrocalculous pancreatic diabetes, no history of alcohol, biliary disease, or other known cause of pancreatitis exists. However, loss of β-cell function appears to be correlated with loss of exocrine function,[34] a situation similar to that with chronic pancreatitis in general.[19,22,23] However, the etiology of both forms of malnutrition-related diabetes and their relationship, if any, to conventional Type I or Type II diabetes remain enigmatic.[31,35-37] Theories relating malnutrition to diabetes abound,[38] none having been proven. Perhaps protein deficiency renders β-cells susceptible to damage by toxic, viral, or autoimmune factors. It has been observed that tropical diabetes is endemic where cassava (tapioca) is the staple food.[38,39] Cassava (95% starch) contains a cyanogenic glycoside that is normally inactivated by conjugation with S-H radicals derived from amino acids, yielding thiocyanate. Oral or intraperitoneal administration of cyanide in rats can produce transient hyperglycemia. However, the causal relationship is far from having been proven, and there are many weaknesses in the association between cassava consumption and diabetes.[40]

Hemochromatosis

Prevalence and Clinical Features

Hemochromatosis is an autosomal recessive disorder for which the gene frequency is 7 to 10% among white populations and the disease prevalence is 2 to 4 per 1000 population.[41-43] The disease is expressed three to five times more frequently in men than in women, since about 80% of homozygous women do not accumulate iron significantly because of menstrual blood loss. About 70% of patients have antigen HLA-A3, the frequency of which ranges from 22 to 28% in the general white populations.[43]

Iron deposition occurs primarily in parenchymal cells of liver, pancreas, adrenals, anterior pituitary, myocardium, and skeletal muscle. The classic triad of hepatomegaly, diabetes, and skin pigmentation ("bronze diabetes") once considered common is in fact not a frequent association, considering the changing clinical presentation associated with early diagnosis and earlier treatment.[43,44] Some of the common presenting symptoms are hepatomegaly with or without abdominal pain, arthralgias, fatigue, and impotence. Presence of symptoms usually correlates with the severity of iron accumulation as documented by liver biopsy and with the presence of cirrhosis. Cirrhosis is present at diagnosis in about 70% of patients.[45] Hepatocellular carcinoma develops in about 15 to 30% of patients, depending on patients' longevity, despite the successful removal of iron.

Hemochromatosis may have a number of secondary causes, including sideroblastic anemias (chiefly thalassemia major), chronic hemolytic anemias, multiple blood transfusions, porphyria cutanea tarda, and dietary or medical iron overload, e.g., consumption of iron-rich beer among the Bantus.[41] The severity of total-body iron load produced by these states is variable but is usually less than the loads of 30 g or more seen in primary (idiopathic) hemochromatosis. Alcohol promotes iron absorption but does not, by itself, result in hemochromatosis.

Diabetes in Hemochromatosis

Abnormal glucose tolerance occurs in up to 75 to 80% of patients with hemochromatosis; of these, 50 to 60% have overt diabetes.[45-47] Similarly, glucose intolerance was present in about 50% of patients with thalassemia major following chronic transfusion therapy.[48,49] In a large series of patients with hemochromatosis, 25% had first-degree relatives with diabetes.[46] The pathogenesis of glucose intolerance in iron-overload states remains controversial, since multiple factors, including cirrhosis, pancreatic iron deposition, and underlying primary diabetes, can be involved. However, the severity of cirrhosis and iron load are correlated with the degree of glucose intolerance, and the control of diabetes improves in 35 to 45% of patients following iron depletion.[41,45]

Studies of β-cell and α-cell function in hemochromatosis have revealed several interesting features. Patients who develop overt diabetes usually have impaired β-cell function,[46-48] and about 40 to 50% of them require insulin therapy. However, in patients studied in a precirrhotic stage and in those who have not developed overt diabetes, significant hyperinsulinemia was observed in response to oral glucose[50,51] and during a hyperglycemic clamp.[51] Furthermore, rates of insulin-mediated glucose disposal were impaired in patients with transfusion-induced iron overload in the latter study.[51] These observations suggest that insulin resistance secondary to hepatic or extrahepatic iron deposition (muscle ?) precedes the β-cell dysfunction and overt diabetes that eventually develops. However, the mechanism of insulin resistance produced by iron overload remains unknown. In histopathologic studies, an increase in β-cell mass was demonstrated in a small number of nondiabetic or mildly diabetic patients with iron overload.[52] However, whether iron infiltration of pancreatic islets explains the later β-cell dysfunction remains controversial. In patients with hemochromatosis, glucagon secretion was augmented by arginine and was not suppressed by oral glucose,[53,54] responses similar to those seen in primary diabetes. In this respect, the α-cell responses seem to differ from those seen in patients with chronic pancreatitis[22,23] and are in keeping with the observation that iron deposition in islets, albeit variable, is restricted to β-cells.[52]

In making the diagnosis of hemochromatosis, it should be noted that biochemical tests of iron metabolism, i.e., determinations of serum iron, transferrin saturation, and ferritin levels, are helpful but are not as specific for the diagnosis as the hepatic histology.[41,43] Recently, attention was drawn to the presence of hyperferritinemia in 6.6% of unselected patients with Type II diabetes. In most cases, this hyperferritinemia had resolved spontaneously or proved to be due to other causes when follow-up studies were done.[55] Such studies underscore the need for confirmation of results, particularly when patients with diabetes are being screened for hemochromatosis.

Management and Prognosis

Regular phlebotomy treatment, often lifelong, remains the treatment of choice in hemochromatosis. Successful iron depletion, initiated early in the course of disease, clearly reduces the incidence and progression of cirrhosis, improves diabetes control, and frequently reduces damage to other target organs and overall morbidity and mortality.[43,45] In a large prospective study of 163 patients, with a mean follow-up period of 10.5 ± 5.6 years, the major determinants of reduced survival included the presence of cirrhosis, diabetes, and failure of iron depletion[45] (Fig. 17-3). Mortality ratios (observed/expected) for liver cancer, cardiomyopathy, cirrhosis, and diabetes were 219, 306, 13 and 7, respectively, for patients with hematochromatosis as compared with those for the general population in this study. Successful iron depletion, however, did not protect from the development of liver cancer.

In patients unable to undergo phlebotomy, such as those with thalassemia or other forms of anemia, chelation therapy with deferoxamine is an alternative for which the outcome is often successful,[56,57] although the effects of this regimen on diabetes control have not been studied.

ENDOCRINOPATHIES

The major sites of action of various counterregulatory hormones on target organs and the principal mechanisms of their diabetogenic effects are listed in Table 17-2.

Disorders of Growth-Hormone Secretion

Classic experiments, using crude pituitary extracts, performed more than 50 years ago showed a relationship between the anterior pituitary and diabetes.[58] In rat pancreatic monolayer cultures derived from an islet tumor cell line[59] or neonatal pancreas,[60] growth hormone (GH) stimulated β-cell replication, an effect that was shown to be independent of GH-induced insulin-like growth factors.[60] However, chronic administration of GH in experimental animals over prolonged periods has been shown to result in hypersecretion of insulin followed by eventual loss of β-cells and permanent diabetes.[61]

Secretion and Metabolic Effects of Growth Hormone

The physiology of GH secretion and its diverse metabolic effects in humans have been studied extensively.[62,63] In normal subjects GH release is stimulated by

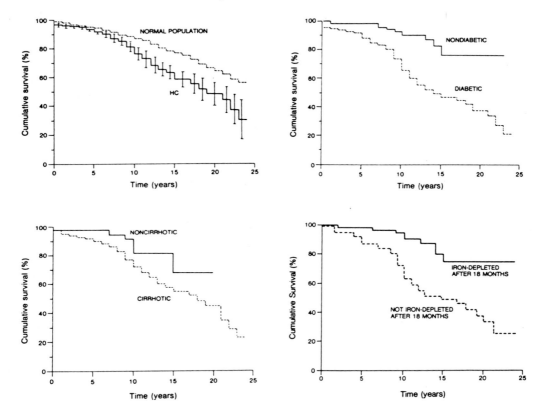

Fig. 17–3. Cumulative survival in 163 patients with hemochromatosis compared with normal population and in the same patients with (*n* = 112) or without (*n* = 51) cirrhosis; with (*n* = 89) or without (*n* = 74) diabetes; and depleted (*n* = 77) or not depleted (*n* = 75) of iron during the first 18 months of venesection (see text for details). All differences were statistically significant (*P* < .05 to < .002 by log-rank test). Reprinted with permission from reference 45 (Niederau C, Fischer R, Sonnenberg A, et al. Survival and causes of death in cirrhotic and noncirrhotic patients with primary hemochromatosis. N Engl J Med 1985;313:1256–62).

hypoglycemia, sleep, exercise, stress, and amino acids and is inhibited by hyperglycemia. Infusions of GH in normal subjects that produce increments in plasma GH levels within the supraphysiologic range (up to 30 to 50 ng/mL) initially result in acute but transient (2 to 4 hours) insulin-like effects, i.e., suppression of hepatic glucose production and enhancement of peripheral glucose clearance.[64–66] In fact, insulin levels increase over this period, offering an explanation for some portion of these effects. Subsequently, over a 2- to 12-hour period, similar increments or increments closer to the physiologic range,[67] are associated with the "delayed" insulin-antagonistic effects. The primary site of GH-induced insulin resistance resides at the level of peripheral tissues,[66,67] as first suggested by the elegant studies of forearm perfusion by Zierler and Rabinowitz.[68] Although an effect of GH on inhibition of peripheral glucose uptake is well established, the lipolytic effect has not always been confirmed.[69]

The understanding of the cellular site of insulin resistance induced by GH is complicated; multiple coexisting factors are involved, including GH concentrations, presence of hyperinsulinemia, and glucose intolerance. In most studies of normal subjects given GH infusions or in patients with acromegaly, binding of insulin to receptors on circulating monocytes or hepatocytes was found to be little affected, as a result of

Table 17-2. Sites of Actions of Major Diabetogenic Hormones in Humans

Hormone	β-Cell secretion	Liver		Muscle		Adipose Tissue	
		Glycogen*	Gluco-neogenesis	Glucose	Amino acid release	Glucose uptake	Lipolysis
Growth hormone	+	+	+	−	?	−	+
Glucocorticoids	+	+	+	−	+	−	+
Catecholamines	−	−	+	−	−	?	+
Glucagon	+	−	+	0	?	0	?
Thyroid hormones	+	−	+	0	0	?	+

+ = stimulation; − = inhibition; O = no effect; ? = uncertain.
*Net effect on glycogen content via glycogen synthesis or glycogenolysis.

reciprocal effects on receptor number and affinity.[66,67,70,71] However, in acromegalic patients with fasting hyperglycemia, the compensatory increase in receptor affinity that occurs in such patients with normoglycemia may fail to occur, a factor contributing to glucose intolerance.[72] In cultured adipocytes, GH was shown to inhibit the expression of the gene for the glucose transporters GLUT-1 but not that for the GLUT-4 transporter.[72] Thus, probably both postreceptor and receptor defects in insulin action underlie the diabetogenic effects of GH excess.

Diabetes in Acromegaly

Anterior pituitary adenomas that hypersecrete GH account for more than 90% of cases of acromegaly.[73] Other causes include ectopic (nonpituitary) sources of GH or growth hormone-releasing hormone (GHRH), e.g., pancreatic islet cell tumors, carcinoid tumors, and hypothalamic hamartomas.

Glucose intolerance is prevalent in patients with acromegaly, affecting about 60 to 70%. However, overt diabetes requiring treatment occurs in only 10 to 15% of patients.[72a,73,74] Even more frequent than glucose intolerance is evidence of insulin resistance, which is manifested by a striking hyperinsulinemia in response to orally or intravenously administered glucose and other secretagogues, as well as markedly attenuated responses to exogenous insulin.[74–76] Furthermore, in acromegalic patients with normal glucose tolerance but with hyperinsulinemia, glucose uptake by muscle is impaired as a result of diminished nonoxidative metabolism of glucose.[77] Overall, GH levels in individual patients correlate poorly with both hyperinsulinemia and the severity of glucose intolerance. A better correlation of disease activity and glucose intolerance is found with serum levels of insulin-like growth factor 1 (IGF-1).[73,78] In contrast to patients with normal or impaired glucose tolerance, in patients with acromegaly the insulin reserve is quite blunted by the time overt diabetes develops, with or without ketosis,[74,76] a finding reminiscent of that in animal models of metasomatotrophic diabetes.[61] However, coexistent primary diabetes (Type I or Type II) may also be present, particularly if diabetes persists after successful treatment of acromegaly in such patients. Considerable evidence exists from studies of somatostatin infusion that lipolytic and ketogenic effects of GH supervene only after significant insulinopenia.[65,79]

Successful treatment of acromegaly, with normalization of GH and IGF-1, is usually accompanied by striking improvements in glucose tolerance and a reversal of hyperinsulinemia, as well as by normalization of insulin sensitivity.[73,76,78] However, the results are unpredictable in those with overt, symptomatic diabetes.[76,80]

Diabetes Associated with Isolated Growth-Hormone Deficiency

It has long been appreciated that GH has cytotrophic effects on β-cells in vitro.[59,60,81] In addition, exogenous GH administration, both in normal subjects and in subjects with hypopituitarism, augments insulin responses to a variety of secretagogues before any significant change in blood glucose level is noted.[82] In light of these observations, it is of interest that patients with monotropic GH deficiency (sexual ateliotic dwarfs) have been found to have mild to moderately severe glucose intolerance and insulin deficiency.[83] In the majority of these patients, insulin responses to glucose or arginine were impaired, and treatment with GH resulted in augmented insulin release.[84] These findings further support the role of GH in the maintenance of β-cell growth and maturation.

Hyperprolactinemia

The human prolactin molecule shares considerable homology with the human GH molecule, and an even greater homology exists between their respective mRNAs,[73] similarities that suggest a common evolutionary origin. The precise role of prolactin in human physiology is poorly understood.[85] A diabetogenic effect of prolactin has been suggested but has not been established in humans. Hyperprolactinemic states are sometimes associated with mild glucose intolerance; however, the difference is of only marginal statistical significance when compared with controls.[86,87] In one study of 26 patients with prolactinomas, basal levels of glucose and insulin were comparable to those for controls, despite the presence of chronic endogenous hyperprolactinemia in these patients.[86] However, oral glucose tolerance was significantly impaired and associated with insulin insensitivity, as reflected by hyperinsulinemia. It is interesting that both glucose intolerance and hyperinsulinism improved after treatment with bromocriptine, which reduced levels of prolactin. Similarly, in a group of nine patients with hyperprolactinemia and the amenorrhea-galactorrhea syndrome, four of whom had pituitary tumors, mild impairment in glucose tolerance associated with elevated basal levels and postglucose insulin levels was found in comparisons with matched controls.[87] These changes were similar in some ways to those normally seen in late pregnancy. Whether prolactin causes insulin resistance leading to hyperinsulinemia or exerts direct effects on the β-cell, or both, is not known.

Cushing Syndrome

Metabolic Effects of Glucocorticoids

Glucocorticoids like growth hormone are the principal insulin-antagonistic hormones. They have diverse metabolic effects on liver, adipose tissue, and muscle.[88,89] In the liver, glucocorticoids serve as the key gluconeogenic agents by accelerating the biochemical events at every rate-limiting step. Specifically, glucocorticoids stimulate 1) hepatic uptake of amino acids; 2) activation of pyruvate carboxylase in generating pyruvate from amino acids; and 3) activation of phosphoenolpyruvate carboxykinase (PEPCK), the unidirectional rate-limiting enzyme in the initiation of the cascade of gluconeogenesis from pyruvate. Insulin antagonizes by glucocorticoid and cyclic adenosine monophosphate (cAMP) stimulation of PEPCK gene transcription.[90] Paradoxically, glucocorticoids enhance glycogen deposition and insulin-like effect. It has been proposed that glycogenesis in response to glucocorticoids may be mediated by insulin.[88] However, this effect may well be a direct consequence of activation of glycogen synthetase by glucocorticoids.[89]

At the level of adipose tissue and muscle, glucocorticoids antagonize insulin-mediated uptake and utilization of glucose.[91,92] This effect is mediated at the cellular level by multiple mechanisms, including a decrease in insulin-receptor affinity[70,93] and defects at the postreceptor level.[91–94] Dexamethasone was shown to inhibit glucose transport by causing translocation of glucose transporters from the plasma membrane, an effect reversible by insulin.[92] Glucocorticoids also exert a permissive effect on lipolysis by promoting the activation of cAMP-dependent hormone-sensitive lipase, a key enzyme inhibited by insulin.[88] The net clinical effect of glucocorticoid excess in humans is a relocation of fat depots, which results in the typical truncal obesity of Cushing syndrome. The precise mechanism by which this unique pattern of fat redistribution develops remains unexplained. However, adipose tissues from various sites do show metabolic differences. Lipoprotein lipase activity is increased and lipolytic activity is decreased in abdominal adipose tissue in comparison to that in femoral adipose tissue in patients with Cushing syndrome.[95] Finally, glucocorticoids augment proteolysis in skeletal muscle,[88,89] and the relative distribution of types of muscle fibers may be altered.[95]

Glucocorticoid-Induced Diabetes

In normal humans, short-term increments in levels of plasma cortisol levels within the range seen in moderate stress situations ($\sim$40 μg/dL) result in only a slight increase in levels of glucose, which is mediated by both hepatic and extrahepatic effects,[94,96] as well as in a significant increase in levels of ketones and branched-chain amino acids.[96] However, the effects of chronic administration of moderate doses of glucocorticoids to normal humans are usually compensated for by increased insulin release, which results in minimal changes in glucose levels. Thus, the spectrum of glucose intolerance in patients with Cushing syndrome or exogenous steroid use depends in large part on endogenous β-cell reserve, a situation similar to that in acromegaly. Glucose intolerance occurs in 75 to 80% of patients with Cushing syndrome, but only 10 to 15% of patients develop overt diabetes.[74,97] Almost all patients, however, manifest basal and stimulated hyperinsulinemia and insulin resistance.

A contributory diabetogenic effect of glucocorticoid excess is stimulation of glucagon secretion. Glucocorticoid administration over 3 to 4 days in normal subjects induced an augmented α-cell responsiveness both during the basal state and following protein ingestion or amino acid infusion.[98,99] This effect may be mediated by hyperaminoacidemia brought about by augmented proteolysis and perhaps by decreased glucose utilization by α-cells or some other direct effect of corticosteroids on α-cells.

Pheochromocytoma

Metabolic Effects of Catecholamines

Catecholamines influence insulin secretion directly and produce anti-insulin effects at several loci in intermediary metabolism.[100,101] In the human, basal insulin secretion is inhibited by α$_2$-adrenergic and augmented by β$_2$-adrenergic stimulation.[101,102] The net effect on insulin secretion is governed by the relative local concentrations of epinephrine, norepinephrine, and various other secretagogues. However, the inhibitory effects on the α-receptor generally predominate over the stimulatory effects on the β-receptor. Stimulation of the α-receptor also may promote glucagon secretion. The role of catecholamines in the physiologic regulation of insulin secretion is still uncertain. Recently, a 29-amino-acid polypeptide, galanin, was shown to be contained in sympathetic nerve endings in the islets and is proposed to be an additional mediator of insulin inhibition by sympathetic activation.[103] In patients with pre-existing glucose intolerance, the acute effects of physiologic increments in epinephrine levels on β-cell inhibition are exaggerated, producing greater hyperglycemia than in controls.[104]

Catecholamines stimulate hepatic glucose output by promoting glycogenolysis and gluconeogenesis, the former being the predominant immediate effect.[101] Glycogenolysis results from the β-adrenergic stimulation of adenyl cyclase, which leads to the release of cAMP. In addition, epinephrine also stimulates hepatic glycogenolysis via a cAMP-independent, Ca^{++}-dependent pathway involving the α$_1$-adrenergic pathway.[105] The effects of catecholamines (mainly epinephrine) on adipose tissue (lipolysis) and muscle (glycogenolysis) are mediated primarily via β-adrenergic receptors. In response to β-adrenergic agonists, proteolysis is inhibited[106] but oxidation of branched-chain amino acids is enhanced.[107] However, the effects of catecholamines on muscle nitrogen balance require further elucidation.

Diabetes in Pheochromocytoma

Glucose intolerance occurs in about 30% of patients with pheochromocytoma.[101,108] Multiple mechanisms may contribute to this intolerance, including 1) the α$_2$-adrenergic inhibition of insulin secretion, 2) β-adrenergic stimulation of hepatic glycogenolysis and gluconeogenesis, and 3) enhanced lipolysis. Overt diabetes and ketoacidosis are distinctly unusual. Administration of α-adrenergic blocking agents, e.g., phentolamine or phenoxybenzamine, characteristically improves insulin secretion and glucose tolerance.[109,110] Glucagon levels were surprisingly normal in the basal state[109,110] and markedly suppressed in response to arginine[111] or hypoglycemia,[112] findings suggesting normal regulation by hyperglycemia despite an enormous increase in circulating catecholamine levels. Surgical removal of the tumor usually restores or improves glucose tolerance within several weeks[108,111]; however, in some cases, it may take up to several months. The responsiveness of the α-cell to arginine also was restored to normal after tumor resection.[111]

Primary Hyperaldosteronism

The triad of hypertension, hypokalemia, and glucose intolerance (Conn syndrome) was described in 1955.[113] Contrary to previous estimates, this syndrome accounts for more than 2% of cases of hypertension.[114,115] Glucose intolerance, previously thought to be present in about 50% of patients with Conn syndrome, is somewhat less common and is usually mild. It probably is the result, to a variable degree, of K^+ depletion, which may be responsible for blunted insulin secretion[113,116] and perhaps for increased glycogenolysis. In normal men, K^+ depletion of 200 to 500 mEq ($\sim$10% of total total body K^+, during 5- to 14-day periods was shown to result in mild glucose intolerance, while insulin sensitivity remained essentially unchanged.[115,118] However, it is not certain if the glucose intolerance seen in Conn syndrome is completely explained by K^+ depletion.

Hyperthyroidism

Hyperthyroidism is associated with significant aberrations of carbohydrate, lipid, and protein metabolism.[119] This state is characterized by increased oxygen consumption, rapid gastric emptying, enhanced gluconeogenesis and glycogenolysis, increased lipolysis and ketogenesis, and increased proteolysis. Many of these effects are reproducible in experimental hyperthyroidism induced in nondiabetic[120] or diabetic[121] individuals. The insulin clearance rate was found to be increased by about 40%.[122] The data on peripheral glucose disposal and insulin sensitivity are controversial, perhaps because of differences in the methods used. Some studies reported a decreased peripheral insulin sensitivity,[123] whereas most others found it to be normal[122] or increased[120,124] compared with that in controls, primarily because of enhanced rates of glucose oxidation as determined by indirect calorimetry.

An increased incidence of glucose intolerance, usually of mild to moderate severity, was documented in 30 to 50% of patients with hyperthyroidism.[125–127] Increased sympathetic sensitivity mediated via a β-adrenergic mechanism[101] probably contributes to the increased propensity to lipolysis and ketogenesis in such patients.[120,128] In patients with pre-existing diabetes, the metabolic consequences of untreated hyperthyroidism on hepatic glucose production, lipolysis, and insulin clearance would facilitate the deterioration of glycemic control and even the development of recurrent ketoacidosis.[129] In previously nondiabetic individuals, glucose intolerance persisted in 32% (7 of 22) of patients with hyperthyroidism after 12 years of follow-up following treatment.[127] This may be explained, at least in part, on the basis of common autoimmune mechanisms underlying Graves disease and Type I diabetes.

Disorders of Calcium and/or Phosphorus Metabolism

Disorders of calcium and phosphorus metabolism may occasionally be associated with significant changes in insulin secretion and/or sensitivity. Hyperinsulinemia in primary hyperparathyroidism has been reported[130–133]

and found to correlate with calcium levels,[131] whereas glucose tolerance was preserved. On the other hand, experimental hypophosphatemia was shown to produce insulin insensitivity in dogs[134] and humans[135] and may thus be a possible mediator of insulin resistance in primary hyperparathyroidism. In secondary hyperparathyroidism induced by diet in dogs[134] or in patients with renal insufficiency who had undergone parathyroidectomy,[136] no evidence was noted of any direct effects of parathyroid hormone itself on glucose disposal or insulin secretion. However, two diabetic patients who underwent parathyroidectomy for primary hyperparathyroidism showed an increased sensitivity to endogenous and exogenous insulin postoperatively.[137] The α-cell responses to arginine, or to protein meal, and to glucose were found to be normal before and after removal of the parathyroid adenoma.[133]

For discussions of tumors of the endocrine pancreas or gut and of polyglandular deficiency syndromes see Chapters 55 and 56.

POEMS Syndrome (Polyneuropathy, Organomegaly, Endocrinopathy, Monoclonal Gammopathy, Skin Changes)

POEMS syndrome is a rare form of plasma-cell disorder associated with an osteosclerotic type of myeloma and several systemic features. About 100 cases have been reported.[138,139] In most cases (>90%), the M-component is of the λ-light chain type. Other eponyms of this entity include "Takatsuki syndrome," and "Crow-Fukase syndrome." A relationship of this syndrome to multicentric angiofollicular lymph node hyperplasia (Castleman's disease) has also been suggested.[140] The etiology of these entities is obscure, but they appear to be secondary to a defect in immunoglobulin synthesis.

Glucose intolerance has been reported in 30% of cases.[138,139] Other endocrine features include hypogonadism, hypothyroidism, hyperprolactinemia, and adrenal insufficiency.

DRUGS, CHEMICAL AGENTS, AND TOXINS

Administration of a variety of drugs or chemical agents (Table 17–1) is known to produce glucose intolerance or diabetes in previously nondiabetic subjects or to exacerbate hyperglycemia in previously diabetic patients. The diabetogenic effects may be brought about by effects on islet-cell secretion, either directly or indirectly, or on insulin action at hepatic or extrahepatic sites or may be due to variable combinations of these factors. Table 17–3 presents the principal mechanisms of effects of certain therapeutic agents more commonly associated with glucose intolerance or diabetes.

Diuretics and β-Adrenergic Antagonists

The diabetogenic effects of diuretics, particularly thiazides and chlorthalidone, and β-adrenergic antagonists have been well recognized in clinical practice. A 12-year follow-up epidemiologic study revealed that the increase in the risk of developing diabetes over the risk in controls

Table 17-3. Sites of Action of Drugs or Agents More Commonly Associated with Diabetes or Glucose Intolerance

	Impaired insulin secretion	Impaired insulin action	Comments
Diuretics			
Thiazide	+	±	Effects primarily mediated
Loop diuretics	+	0	by K$^+$ depletion
Diphenylhydantoin	+	0	Direct β-cell effects
Pentamidine	+	0	Structurally similar to
Pyriminil (Vacor)	+	±	streptozotocin and alloxan
Glucocorticoids	0	+	Also cause hyperglucagonemia
Oral contraceptives	0	+	Effects less prominent than glucocorticoids
Nicotinic acid	0	+	Minimal effects in normal subjects
β-Adrenergic antagonists	+	+	Effects more common with nonselective agents
Diazoxide	+	+	A nondiuretic thiazide
Cyclosporine	+	+	Often used in combination with glucocorticoids
Opiates	+	±	Also stimulate glucagon secretion

was three- to fourfold in subjects receiving thiazides, five- to sixfold in those receiving β-adrenergic blockers, and 11-fold in subjects receiving both drugs.[141] For thiazides, most studies have indicated the mechanism involved in this increased risk is an insulin secretory defect caused by hypokalemia and that the defect can be corrected by K$^+$ replacement.[118,142] However, others have found evidence for extrapancreatic effects.[143,144] For β-blockers, an inhibitory effect on β-cell secretion would be anticipated. Indeed, in some cases, drugs such as propranolol precipitated hyperglycemic, hyperosmolar, nonketotic coma.[145] Moreover, evidence of peripheral effects of propranolol resulting in insulin resistance has also been reported.[143,144] Diazoxide, a nondiuretic thiazide, has pronounced inhibitory effects on the β-cell as well as peripheral effects.[146]

Diphenylhydantoins

Phenytoin (Dilantin) has direct inhibitory effects on β-cell secretion.[147] This effect appears to be dose-related, and hyperglycemic, nonketotic coma precipitated by phenytoin have been reported.[148]

Glucocorticoids

Glucocorticoid-induced glucose intolerance is characterized by insulin resistance and hyperinsulinemia. As discussed earlier, as in patients with Cushing syndrome, chronic administration of glucocorticoids induces distinct effects on hepatic and extrahepatic sites.

Pentamidine and Pyriminil

Pentamidine, an antiprotozoal agent, and pyriminil (Vacor), a nitrosourea-derived rodenticide, resemble streptozotocin and alloxan chemically. Pentamidine is being used increasingly in prophylaxis and treatment of *Pneumocystis carinii* infection in patients with acquired immunodeficiency syndrome (AIDS), and an increasing incidence of insulin-dependent diabetes following its use

is being reported.[149] Similarly, accidental or intentional ingestion of pyriminil may result in the development of insulin-dependent diabetes with or without ketoacidosis as a result of β-cell destruction.[150,151] The sequence of events leading to diabetes following use of these agents is similar to that seen with streptozotocin and initially involves a release of insulin from lysed β-cells that lasts for hours and is frequently associated with hypoglycemia and a delayed persistent hyperglycemia caused by β-cell loss after days to weeks.[150,152]

Nicotinic Acid

Nicotinic acid causes glucose intolerance by inducing peripheral insulin insensitivity.[153] In normal individuals this is accompanied by minimal changes in glucose tolerance because of adaptive hyperinsulinemia. However, significant hyperglycemia or deterioration in glucose tolerance may result in patients with limited a β-cell reserve or pre-existing diabetes.[154]

Cyclosporine

An increased incidence of diabetes has been reported in renal transplant recipients receiving cyclosporine.[155,156] This increase is probably independent of the concomitant diabetogenic effects of corticosteroids in these patients. Direct inhibitory effects of cyclosporine on β-cells have been found in studies of isolated islets.[157] Moreover, a peripheral effect on muscle glucose transport also may occur.[158]

Opiates

A hyperglycemic effect of morphine and other opiates has been recognized. Human islets produce β-endorphins and enkephalins. In normal and diabetic subjects, infusions of β-endorphin resulted in hyperglycemia accompanied by hyperglucagonemia.[159] These results are in keeping with the observation of impaired β-cell responsiveness to glucose in subjects addicted to narcotics.[160]

GENETIC SYNDROMES

There are about 50 distinct rare genetic syndromes associated with glucose intolerance.[161] Some of these represent chromosomal defects such as Down syndrome (trisomy 21), Klinefelter syndrome, and Turner syndrome, whereas many others are single-gene defects (Table 17–1). In addition to congenital pancreatic disorders and certain inborn errors of metabolism, a variety of disorders characterized by severe or extreme insulin resistance caused by structural or functional abnormalities of the insulin receptor may produce glucose intolerance or non-insulin-dependent diabetes (see Chapter 14). Examples of genetic disorders associated with obesity-associated insulin resistance include Prader-Willi syndrome,[162] Laurence-Moon-Biedl syndrome, and its variant, Bardet-Biedl syndrome.[163] About 45% of patients with the Bardet-Biedl syndrome are glucose intolerant.

In a few of these genetic syndromes, a striking incidence of insulin-dependent diabetes, simulating typical autoimmune Type I diabetes, is an integral feature. These examples include stiff-man syndrome, an autoimmune disorder (see Chapter 13), and two other hereditary neurologic disorders, Friedrich's ataxia[164] and DIDMOAD (diabetes insipidus, diabetes mellitus, optic atrophy, sensoryneural deafness), also known as Wolfram's syndrome, and its variants.[165] In Friedrich's ataxia, up to 20% of patients have diabetes, although some may be non-insulin-dependent for variable periods. In contrast, in Wolfram's syndrome, autopsy studies show a selective loss of islet β-cells,[166] a finding explaining the onset of diabetes in early childhood and the absolute insulin requirement in these patients.

CHRONIC COMPLICATIONS IN SECONDARY FORMS OF DIABETES

Whether chronic complications of diabetes (microangiopathy, neuropathy, macroangiopathy) are a consequence of long-term hyperglycemia per se or require additional metabolic, hormonal, or genetic factor(s) is a controversial issue. If hyperglycemia per se is the most important factor, one would expect an equivalent incidence and prevalence of these complications in secondary forms of diabetes. However, in practical terms, such comparisons of complications in primary vs. secondary diabetes are difficult in view of 1) the milder severity of hyperglycemia in most patients with secondary diabetes,

2) the relatively shorter durations of follow-up in patients with secondary diabetes either because of poor prognosis of underlying disease or of adequate treatment of the disorder with amelioration of hyperglycemia, and 3) lack of genetic markers for the detection of primary diabetes in association with secondary diabetes.

Despite these limitations, there is evidence that diabetic microvascular disease and neuropathy are mainly a function of severity and duration of hyperglycemia, and this view is strengthened by the demonstration of microangiopathic lesions in animal models of diabetes induced by alloxan or streptozotocin and of amelioration of these lesions by insulin treatment. In diabetes secondary to chronic pancreatitis or pancreatectomy, careful comparisons with patients with IDDM matched for age, sex, and duration and treatment of diabetes revealed a similar prevalence of retinopathy in the two groups.[167,168] In another human model, pyriminil-induced insulin-dependent diabetes,[150,151] a striking prevalence of diabetic retinopathy, overt proteinuria, and thickened muscle-capillary basement membranes was observed that was equal to or even greater than that in matched patients with IDDM[169] (Table 17–4). This form of diabetes is akin to chemically induced diabetes in animals and excludes the potentially confounding variable of genetic factor(s).

In one respect, however, the type of retinopathy in secondary forms of diabetes differs from that in genetic diabetes, i.e., severe or proliferative retinopathy is rare or quite infrequent. This difference may in part be due to a lack the concomitant increase in growth hormone or related growth factors that may be involved in the progression of proliferative retinopathy in patients with genetic diabetes.[170,171] Growth hormone at physiologic concentrations was shown to enhance proliferation of human retinal microvascular endothelial cells in cultures.[172] Dwarfs with isolated growth-hormone deficiency and glucose intolerance do not develop retinopathy (or macrovascular disease),[173] and pituitary ablation was shown to arrest or retard the progression of proliferative retinopathy.[174] Similarly, in patients with hemochromatosis, a blunted growth hormone responsiveness was associated with only a mild, background retinopathy.[175] On the other hand, background retinopathy was reported in the absence of growth hormone in a patient with diabetes following pancreatectomy.[176] However, no proliferative retinopathy was observed in this patient despite 24 years of diabetes and the presence

Table 17–4. Pyriminil (Vacor)-Induced Diabetes and Microangiopathy

Group	n	Age (yr)	Duration (yr)	HbA$_1$ (%)	QCBM (A)	DR (%)	Proteinuria (%)
IDDM	16	27 ± 2	6.2 ± 0.3	11.9	2287 ± 144*	25	6
Vacor	18	28 ± 2	4.7 ± 1.5	12.1	2320 ± 149*	44	28
Control	20	28 ± 2	. . .	. . .	1781 ± 46	0	0

Data are from Feingold et al.[169]
DR = diabetic retinopathy; QCBM = quadriceps capillary basement membrane width.
*P < .001 vs. controls.

of severe nephropathy and neuropathy. Proliferative retinopathy is also rare in patients with acromegaly, despite their having marked elevations in levels of growth hormone for many years. Overall, the available evidence supports the concept that growth hormone is involved in the progression, but not in the initiation, of at least some of the long-term diabetic vascular complications.

REFERENCES

1. National Diabetes Data Group. Classification and diagnosis of diabetes mellitus and other categories of glucose intolerance. Diabetes 1979;28:1039–57.
2. Seldin DW, Tarail R. Effect of hypertonic solutions on metabolism and excretion of electrolytes. Am J Physiol 1949;159:160–74.
3. Seltzer HS, Harris VL. Exhaustion of insulogenic reserve in maturity-onset diabetic patients during prolonged and continuous hyperglycemic stress. Diabetes 1964; 13:6–13.
4. McCulloch DK, Koerker DJ, Kahn SE, et al. Correlations of in vivo β-cell function tests with β-cell mass and pancreatic insulin content in streptozocin-administered baboons. Diabetes 1991;40:673–9.
5. Kendall DM, Sutherland DER, Najarian JS, et al. Effects of hemipancreatectomy on insulin secretion and glucose tolerance in healthy humans. N Engl J Med 1990;322:898–903.
6. Weir GC, Bonner-Weir S, Leahy JL. Islet mass and function in diabetes and transplantation. Diabetes 1990;39:401–5.
7. Barnes AJ, Bloom SR. Pancreatectomised man: a model for diabetes without glucagon. Lancet 1976;1:219–21.
8. Boden G. Extrapancreatic glucagon in human subjects. In: Unger RH, Orci L, eds. Glucagon: physiology, pathophysiology, and morphology of the pancreatic A-cells. New York: Elsevier, 1981:349–57.
9. Tiengo A, Bessioud M, Valverde I, et al. Absence of islet alpha cell function in pancreatectomized patients. Diabetologia 1982;22:25–32.
10. Holst JJ, Pedersen JH, Baldissera F, Stadil F. Circulating glucagon after total pancreatectomy in man. Diabetologia 1983;25:396–9.
11. Del Prato S, Tiengo A, Baccaglini U, et al. Effect of insulin replacement on intermediary metabolism in diabetes secondary to pancreatectomy. Diabetologia 1983; 25:252–9.
12. Bajorunas DR, Fortner JG, Jaspan J, Sherwin RS. Total pancreatectomy increases the metabolic response to glucagon in humans. J Clin Endocrinol Metab 1986;63:439–46.
13. de Kreutzenberg SV, Maifreni L, LiSato G, et al. Glucose turnover and recycling in diabetes secondary to total pancreatectomy: effect of glucagon infusion. J Clin Endocrinol Metab 1990;70:1023–9.
14. Polonsky KS, Herold KC, Gilden JL, et al. Glucose counterregulation in patients after pancreatectomy: comparison with other clinical forms of diabetes. Diabetes 1984;33:1112–9.
15. Barnes AJ, Bloom SR, Alberti KGMM, et al. Ketoacidosis in pancreatectomized man. N Engl J Med 1977;296:1250–3.
16. Nosadini R, Del Prato S, Tiengo A, et al. Insulin sensitivity, binding, and kinetics in pancreatogenic and Type I diabetes. Diabetes 1982;31:346–55.
17. Yki-Järvinen H, Kiviluoto T, Taskinen M-R. Insulin re-

18. Bajorunas DR, Dresler CM, Horowitz GD, et al. Basal glucagon replacement in chronic glucagon deficiency increases insulin resistance. Diabetes 1986;35:556–62.
19. Bank S. Chronic pancreatitis: clinical features and medical management. Am J Gastroenterol 1986;81:153–67.
20. Vinik AI, Jackson WPU. Endocrine secretions in chronic pancreatitis. In: Podolsky S, Viswanathan M, eds. Secondary diabetes: the spectrum of the diabetic syndromes. New York: Raven Press, 1980:165–89.
21. Boat TF, Welsh MJ, Beaudet AL. Cystic fibrosis. In: Scriver CR, Beaudet AL, Sly WS, Valle D, eds. The metabolic basis of inherited disease. 6th ed. New York: McGraw-Hill, 1989:2649–80.
22. Kalk WJ, Vinik AI, Jackson WPU, Bank S. Insulin secretion and pancreatic exocrine function in patients with chronic pancreatitis. Diabetologia 1979;16:355–8.
23. Andersen BN, Krarup T, Pedersen NT, et al. B cell function in patients with chronic pancreatitis and its relation to exocrine pancreatic function. Diabetologia 1982;23:86–9.
24. Donowitz M, Hendler R, Spiro HM, et al. Glucagon secretion in acute and chronic pancreatitis. Ann Intern Med 1975;83:778–81.
25. Persson I, Gyntelberg F, Heding LG, Boss-Nielsen J. Pancreatic-glucagon-like immunoreactivity after intravenous insulin in normals and chronic-pancreatitis patients. Acta Endocrinologica 1971;67:401–4.
26. Larsen S, Hilsted J, Philipsen EK, et al. Glucose counterregulation in diabetes secondary to chronic pancreatitis. Metabolism 1990;39:138–143.
27. Kalk WJ, Vinik AI, Paul M, et al. Immunoreactive glucagon responses to intravenous tolbutamide in chronic pancreatitis. Diabetes 1975;24:851–5.
28. Williams JA, Goldfine ID. The insulin-pancreatic acinar axis. Diabetes 1985;34:980–6.
29. Baron JH, Nabarro JDN. Pancreatic exocrine function in maturity-onset diabetes mellitus. BMJ 1973;4:25–7.
30. Ekoe JM. Recent trends in prevalence and incidence of diabetes mellitus syndrome in the world. Diabetes Res Clin Pract 1985–86;1:249–64.
31. Abu-Bakare A, Taylor R, Gill GV, Alberti KGMM. Tropical or malnutrition-related diabetes: a real syndrome? Lancet 1986;1:1135–8.
32. Hugh-Jones P. Diabetes in Jamaica. Lancet 1955;2:891–7.
33. World Health Organization. Report of a WHO study group: diabetes mellitus. WHO Tech Rep Ser 1985;727:7–12.
34. Yajnik CS, Shelgikar KM, Sahasrabudhe RA, et al. The spectrum of pancreatic exocrine and endocrine (beta-cell) function in tropical calcific pancreatitis. Diabetologia 1990;33:417–21.
35. Ahuja MMS. Profile of young Indian diabetics: biochemical studies. Acta Diabetol Lat 1973;10:439–53.
36. Bajaj JS. Malnutrition-related, ketosis-resistant diabetes mellitus: classification, causes and mechanisms. In: Krall LP, ed. World book of diabetes in practice. Amsterdam: Elsevier Science Publishers, 1986:276–80.
37. Ramachandran A, Mohan V, Snehalatha C, et al. Clinical features of diabetes in the young as seen at a diabetes centre in South India. Diabetes Res Clin Pract 1988;4:117–25.
38. Rao RH. Diabetes in the undernourished: coincidence or consequence? Endocrine Rev 1988;9:67–87.
39. McMillan DE, Geevarghese PJ. Dietary cyanide and tropical malnutrition diabetes. Diabetes Care 1979;2:202–8.

40. Teuscher T, Baillod P, Rosman JB, Teuscher A. Absence of diabetes in a rural west African population with a high carbohydrate/cassava diet. Lancet 1987;1:765–8.

41. Crosby WH. Hemochromatosis: current concepts and management. Hosp Practice 1987;22(2):173–92.

42. Edwards CQ, Griffen LM, Goldgar D, et al. Prevalence of hemochromatosis among 11,065 presumably healthy blood donors. N Engl J Med 1988;318:1355–62.

43. Edwards CQ, Griffen LM, Kushner JP. Disorders of excess iron. Hosp Pract [Off] 1991;26(Suppl 3):30–6.

44. Adams PC, Kertesz AE, Valberg LS. Clinical presentation of hemochromatosis: a changing scene. Am J Med 1991; 90:445–9.

45. Niederau C, Fischer R, Sonnenberg A, et al. Survival and causes of death in cirrhotic and in noncirrhotic patients with primary hemochromatosis. N Engl J Med 1985; 313:1256–62.

46. Dymock IW, Cassar J, Pyke DA, et al. Observations on the pathogenesis complications and treatment of diabetes in 115 cases of haemochromatosis. Am J Med 1972; 52:203–10.

47. Rowe JW, Wands JR, Mezey E, et al. Familial hemochromatosis: characteristics of the pre-cirrhotic stage in a large kindred. Medicine (Baltimore) 1977;56:197–211.

48. Lassman MN, Genel M, Wise JK, et al. Carbohydrate homeostasis and pancreatic islet cell function in thalassemia. Ann Intern Med 1974;80:65–9.

49. Saudek CD, Hemm RM, Peterson CM. Abnormal glucose tolerance in β-thalassemia major. Metabolism 1977; 26:43–52.

50. Niederau C, Berger M, Stremmel W, et al. Hyperinsulinaemia in non-cirrhotic haemochromatosis: impaired hepatic insulin degradation? Diabetologia 1984;26:441–4.

51. Merkel PA, Simonson DC, Amiel SA, et al. Insulin resistance and hyperinsulinemia in patients with thalassemia major treated by hypertransfusion. N Engl J Med 1988;318:809–14.

52. Rahier JR, Loozen S, Goebbels RM, Abrahem M. The hemochromatotic human pancreas: a quantitative immunohistoche mical and ultrastructural study. Diabetologia 1987;30:5–12.

53. Passa P, Luyckx AS, Carpentier JL, et al. Glucagon secretion in diabetic patients with idiopathic haemochromatosis. Diabetologia 1977;13:509–13.

54. Nelson RL, Baldus WD, Rubenstein AH, et al. Pancreatic α-cell function in diabetic hemochromatotic subjects. J Clin Endocrinol Metab 1979;49:412–6.

55. O'Brien T, Bassett B, Burray DM, et al. Usefulness of biochemical screening of diabetic patients for hemochromatosis. Diabetes Care 1990;13:532–4.

56. Schafer AI, Rabinowe S, LeBoff MS, et al. Long-term efficacy of deferoxamine iron chelation therapy in adults with acquired transfusional iron overload. Arch Intern Med 1985;145:1217–21.

57. Bronspiegel-Weintrob N, Olivieri NF, Tyler B, et al. Effect of age at the start of iron chelation therapy on gonadal function in β-thalassemia major. N Engl J Med 1990; 323:713–9.

58. Young FG. The relation of the anterior pituitary gland to carbohydrate metabolism. BMJ 1939;2:393–6.

59. Fong HKW, Chick WL, Sato GH. Hormones and factors that stimulate growth of a rat islet tumor cell line in serum-free medium. Diabetes 1981;30:1022–8.

60. Rabinovitch A, Quigley C, Rechler MW. Growth hormone stimulates islet B-cell replication in neonatal rat pancreatic monolayer cultures. Diabetes 1983;32:307–12.

61. Pierluissi J, Campbell J. Metasomatotrophic diabetes and its induction: basal insulin secretion and insulin release responses to glucose, glucagon, arginine and meals. Diabetologia 1980;18:223–8.

62. Press M. Growth hormone and metabolism. Diab Metab Rev 1988;4:391–414.

63. Daughaday WH. Growth hormone: normal synthesis, secretion, control and mechanisms of action. In: DeGroot LJ, Besser GM, Cahill GF, Jr, et al, eds. Endocrinology. Vol 1. 2nd ed. Philadelphia: WB Saunders, 1989:318–29.

64. Hansen I, Taslikian E, Beaufrere B, et al. Insulin resistance in acromegaly: defects in both hepatic and extrahepatic insulin action. Am J Physiol 1986;250:E269–73.

65. Metcalfe P, Johnston DG, Nosadini R, et al. Metabolic effects of acute and prolonged growth hormone excess in normal and insulin-deficient man. Diabetologia 1981; 20:123–8.

66. Bratusch-Marrian PR, Smith D, DeFronzo RA. The effect of growth hormone on glucose metabolism and insulin secretion in man. J Clin Endocrinol Metab 1982; 55:973–82.

67. Rizza RA, Mandarino LJ, Gerich JE. Effects of growth hormone on insulin action in man: mechanisms of insulin resistance, impaired suppression of glucose production, and impaired stimulation of glucose utilization. Diabetes 1982;31:663–9.

68. Zierler KL, Rabinowitz D. Roles of insulin and growth hormone, based on studies of forearm metabolism in man. Medicine (Baltimore) 1963;42:385–402.

69. Fineberg SE, Merimee TJ. Acute metabolic effects of human growth hormone. Diabetes 1974;23:499–504.

70. Kahn CR, Goldfine ID, Neville DM Jr, De Meyts P. Alterations in insulin binding induced by changes in vivo in the levels of glucocorticoids and growth hormone. Endocrinology 1978;103:1054–66.

71. Muggeo M, Saviolakis GA, Businaro V, et al. Insulin receptor on monocytes from patients with acromegaly and fasting hyperglycemia. J Clin Endocrinol Metab 1983;56:733–8.

72. Tai PK, Liao J-F, Chen EH, et al. Differential regulation of two glucose transporters by chronic growth hormone treatment of cultured 3T3-F442A adipose cells. J Biol Chem 1990; 265:21828–34.

72a. Jadresic A, Banks LM, Child DF, et al. The acromegaly syndrome: relation between clinical features, growth hormone values, and radiologic characteristics. Q J Med 1982;202:189–204.

73. Melmed S, Braunstein GD, Chang RJ, Becker DP. Pituitary tumors secreting growth hormone and prolactin. Ann Intern Med 1986;105:238–53.

74. Kahn CR, Catanese VM. Secondary forms of diabetes mellitus. In: Becker KL, et al. eds. Principles and practice of endocrinology and metabolism. Philadelphia: JB Lippincott, 1990:1087–93.

75. Beck P, Schalch DS, Parker ML, et al. Correlative studies of growth hormone and insulin plasma concentrations with metabolic abnormalities in acromegaly. J Lab Clin Med 1965;66:366–79.

76. Sönksen PH, Greenwood FC, Ellis JP, et al. Changes of carbohydrate tolerance in acromegaly with progress of the disease and in response to treatment. J Clin Endocrinol Metab 1967;27:1418–30.

77. Foss MC, Saad MJA, Paccola GMGF, et al. Peripheral glucose metabolism in acromegaly. J Clin Endocrinol Metab 1991;72:1048–53.

78. Rieu M, Girard F, Bricaire H, Binoux M. The importance of

insulin-like growth factor (somatomedin) measurements in the diagnosis and surveillance of acromegaly. J Clin Endocrinol Metab 1982;55:147–53.

79. Gerich JE, Lorenzi M, Bier DM, et al. Effects of physiologic levels of glucagon and growth hormone on human carbohydrate and lipid metabolism: studies involving administration of exogenous hormone during suppression of endogenous hormone secretion with somatostatin. J Clin Invest 1976;57:875–84.

80. Boden G, Soeldner JS, Steinke J, Thorn GW. Serum human growth-hormone (HGH) response to IV glucose: diagnosis of acromegaly in females and males. Metabolism 1968; 17:1–9.

81. Martin JM, Gagliardino JJ. Effect of growth hormone on the isolated pancreatic islets of rat in vitro. Nature 1967;213:630–1.

82. Daughaday WH, Kipnis DM. The growth-promoting and anti-insulin actions of somatotropin. Recent Prog Horm Res 1966;22:49–99.

83. Merimee TJ, Fineberg SE, McKusick VA, Hall J. Diabetes mellitus and sexual ateliotic dwarfism: a comparative study. J Clin Invest 1970;49:1096–102.

84. Merimee TJ, Rabinowitz D, Rimoin DL, McKusick VA. Isolated human growth hormone deficiency. III. Insulin secretion in sexual ateliotic dwarfism. Metabolism 1968;17:1005–11.

85. Evans WS, Carlsen E, Ho KY. Prolactin and its disorders. In: Becker KL, ed. Principles and practice of endocrinology and metabolism. New York: JB Lippincott, 1990:134–9.

86. Landgraf R, Landgraf-Leurs MMC, Weissmann A, et al. Prolactin: a diabetogenic hormone. Diabetologia 1977; 13:99–104.

87. Gustafson AB, Banasiak MF, Kalkhoff RK, et al. Correlation of hyperprolactinemia with altered plasma insulin and glucagon: similarity to effects of late human pregnancy. J Clin Endocrinol Metab 1980;51:242–6.

88. Cahill GF Jr. Action of adrenal cortical steroids on carbohydrate metabolism. In: Christy NP, ed. The human adrenal cortex. New York: Harper and Row, 1971: 205–38.

89. Exton JH, Miller TB, Jr, Harper SC, Park CR. Carbohydrate metabolism in perfused livers of adrenalectomized and steroid-replaced rats. Am J Physiol 1976;230:163–70.

90. O'Brien RM, Lucas PC, Forest CD, et al. Identification of a sequence in the PEPCK gene that mediates a negative effect of insulin on transcription. Science 1990;249: 533–7.

91. Olefsky JM. Effect of dexamethasone on insulin binding, glucose transport and glucose oxidation of isolated rat adipocytes. J Clin Invest 1975;56:1499–508.

92. Horner HC, Munck A, Lienhard GE. Dexamethasone causes translocation of glucose transporters from the plasma membrane to an intracellular site in human fibroblasts. J Biol Chem 1987;262:17696–702.

93. Yasuda K, Hines E III, Kitabchi AE. Hypercortisolism and insulin resistance: comparative effects of prednisone, hydrocortisone, and dexamethasone on insulin binding of human erythrocytes. J Clin Endocrinol Metab 1982; 55:910–5.

94. Rizza RA, Mandarino LJ, Gerich JE. Cortisol-induced insulin resistance in man: impaired suppression of glucose production and stimulation of glucose utilization due to a postreceptor defect of insulin action. J Clin Endocrinol Metab 1982;54:131–8.

95. Rebuffé-Scrive M, Krotkiewski M, Elfverson J, Björntorp P. Muscle and adipose tissue morphology and metabolism in

Cushing's syndrome. J Clin Endocrinol Metab 1988; 67:1122–8.

96. Shamoon H, Soman V, Sherwin RS. The influence of acute physiological increments of cortisol on fuel metabolism and insulin binding to monocytes in normal humans. J Clin Endocrinol Metab 1980;50:495–501.

97. Pupo AA, Wajchenberg BL, Schnaider J. Carbohydrate metabolism in hyperadrenocorticism. Diabetes 1966; 15:24–9.

98. Marco J, Calle C, Rom n D, et al. Hyperglucagonism induced by glucocorticoid treatment in man. N Engl J Med 1973;288:128–31.

99. Wise JK, Hendler R, Felig P. Influence of glucocorticoids on glucagon secretion and plasma amino acid concentrations in man. J Clin Invest 1973;52:2774–82.

100. Cryer PE Physiology and pathophysiology of the human sympathoadrenal neuroendocrine system. N Engl J Med 1980;303:436–44.

101. Landsberg L, Young JB. Catecholamines and the adrenal medulla. In: Wilson JD, Foster DW, eds. Williams textbook of endocrinology. 7th ed. Philadelphia: WB Saunders, 1985:891–965.

102. Robertson RP, Halter JB, Porte D Jr. A role for alpha-adrenergic receptors in abnormal insulin secretion in diabetes mellitus. J Clin Invest 1976;57:791–5.

103. Dunning BE, Taborsky GJ Jr. Galanin—sympathetic neurotransmitter in endocrine pancreas? Diabetes 1988; 37:1157–62.

104. Ortiz-Alonso FJ, Herman WH, Zobel DL, et al. Effect of epinephrine on pancreatic β-cell and α-cell function in patients with NIDDM. Diabetes 1991;40:1194–202.

105. Strickland WG, Blackmore PF, Exton JH. The role of calcium in alpha-adrenergic inactivation of glycogen synthase in rat hepatocytes and its inhibition by insulin. Diabetes 1980;29:617–22.

106. Garber AJ, Karl IE, Kipnis DM. Alanine and glutamine synthesis and release from skeletal muscle. IV. β-Adrenergic inhibition of amino acid release. J Biol Chem 1976;251:851–7.

107. Shamoon H, Jacob R, Sherwin RS. Epinephrine-induced hypoaminoacidemia in normal and diabetic human subjects: effect of beta blockade. Diabetes 1980;29:875–81.

108. Stenström G, Sjöström L, Smith U. Diabetes mellitus in phaeochromocytoma: fasting blood glucose levels before and after surgery in 60 patients with phaeochromocytoma. Acta Endocrinol 1984;106:511–5.

109. Vance JE, Buchanan KD, O'Hara D, et al. Insulin and glucagon responses in subjects with pheochromocytoma: effect of alpha adrenergic blockade. J Clin Endocrinol Metab 1969;29:911–6.

110. Turnbull DM, Johnston DG, Alberti KGMM, Hall R. Hormonal and metabolic studies in a patient with a pheochromocytoma. J Clin Endocrinol Metab 1980; 51:930–3.

111. Hamaji M. Pancreatic α- and β-cell function in pheochromocytoma. J Clin Endocrinol Metab 1979;49:322–5.

112. Bolli G, DeFeo P, Massi-Benedetti M, et al. Circulating catecholamine and glucagon responses to insulin-induced blood glucose decrement in a patient with pheochromocytoma. J Clin Endocrinol Metab 1982;54:447–9.

113. Conn JW. Hypertension, the potassium ion and impaired carbohydrate tolerance. N Engl J Med 1965; 273:1135–43.

114. Kotchen TA, Guthrie GP Jr. Renin-angiotensin-aldosterone and hypertension. Endocrinol Rev 1980;1:78–99.

115. Young WF Jr, Hogan MJ, Klee GG, et al. Primary aldoste-

ronism: diagnosis and treatment. Mayo Clin Proc 1990; 65:96–110.

116. Podolsky S, Melby JC. Improvement of growth-hormone response to stimulation in primary aldosteronism with correction of potassium deficiency. Metabolism 1976; 25:1027–32.

117. Sagild U, Andersen V, Andreasen PB. Glucose tolerance and insulin responsiveness in experimental potassium depletion. Acta Med Scand 1961;169:243–51.

118. Gorden P. Glucose intolerance with hypokalemia: failure of short-term potassium depletion in normal subjects to reproduce the glucose and insulin abnormalities of clinical hypokalemia. Diabetes 1973;22:544–51.

119. Loeb JN. Metabolic changes. In: Werner SC, Ingbar SH, eds. The thyroid: a fundamental and clinical text. 4th ed. New York: Harper and Row, 1978:705–11.

120. Sandler MP, Robinson RP, Rabin D, et al. The effect of thyroid hormones on gluconeogenesis and forearm metabolism in man. J Clin Endocrinol Metab 1983; 56:479–85.

121. Bratusch-Marrain PR, Komjati M, Waldhäusl WK. Glucose metabolism in noninsulin-dependent diabetic patients with experimental hyperthyroidism. J Clin Endocrinol Metab 1985;60:1063–8.

122. Randin J-P, Tappy L, Scazziga B, et al. Insulin sensitivity and exogenous insulin clearance in Graves' disease: measurement by the glucose clamp technique and continuous indirect calorimetry. Diabetes 1986;35:178–81.

123. Shen D-C, Davidson MB, Kuo S-W, Sheu WH-H. Peripheral and hepatic insulin antagonism in hyperthyroidism. J Clin Endocrinol Metab 1988;66:565–9.

124. Foss MC, Paccola GMGF, Saad MJA, et al. Peripheral glucose metabolism in human hyperthyroidism. J Clin Endocrinol Metab 1990;70:1167–72.

125. Kreines K, Jett M, Knowles HC, Jr. Observations in hyperthyroidism of abnormal glucose tolerance and other traits related to diabetes mellitus. Diabetes 1965; 14:740–4.

126. Doar JWH, Stamp TCB, Wynn V, Audhya TK. Effects of oral and intravenous glucose loading in thyrotoxicosis: studies of plasma glucose, free fatty acid, plasma insulin and blood pyruvate levels. Diabetes 1969;18:633–9.

127. Maxon HR, Kreines KW, Goldsmith RE, Knowles HC Jr. Long-term observations of glucose tolerance in thyrotoxic patients. Arch Intern Med 1975;135:1477–80.

128. Beylot M, Riou JP, Bienvenu F, Mornex R. Increased ketonaemia in hyperthyroidism: evidence for a β-adrenergic mechanism. Diabetologia 1980;19:505–10.

129. Cooppan R, Kozak GP. Hyperthyroidism and diabetes mellitus: an analysis of 70 patients. Arch Intern Med 1980;140:370–3.

130. Kim H, Kalkhoff RK, Costrini NV, et al. Plasma insulin disturbances in primary hyperparathyroidism. J Clin Invest 1971;50:2596–605.

131. Yasuda K, Hurukawa Y, Okuyama M, et al. Glucose tolerance and insulin secretion in patients with parathyroid disorders: effect of serum calcium on insulin release. N Engl J Med 1975;292:501–4.

132. Ginsberg H, Olefsky JM, Reaven GM. Evaluation of insulin resistance in patients with primary hyperparathyroidism. Proc Soc Exp Biol Med 1975;148:942–5.

133. Kalkhoff RK, Gossain VV, Matute ML, Wilson SD. Plasma alpha-cell glucagon in primary hyperparathyroidism. Metabolism 1976;25:769–75.

134. Harter HR, Santiago JV, Rutherford WE, et al. The relative roles of calcium, phosphorus, and parathyroid hormone in glucose- and tolbutamide-mediated insulin release. J Clin Invest 1976;58:359–67.

135. DeFronzo RA, Lang R. Hypophosphatemia and glucose intolerance: evidence for tissue insensitivity to insulin. N Engl J Med 1980;303:1259–63.

136. Amend WJC Jr, Steinberg SM, Lowrie EG, et al. The influence of serum calcium and parathyroid hormone upon glucose metabolism in uremia. J Lab Clin Med 1975;86:435–44.

137. Akgun S, Ertel NH. Hyperparathyroidism and coexisting diabetes mellitus: altered carbohydrate metabolism. Arch Intern Med 1978;138:1500–2.

138. Bardwick PA, Zvaifler NJ, Gill GN, et al. Plasma cell dyscrasia with polyneuropathy, organomegaly, endocrinopathy, M-protein, and skin changes: the POEMS syndrome. Report on two cases and a review of the literature. Medicine (Baltimore) 1980;59:311–22.

139. Viard J-P, Lesavre P, Boitard C, et al. POEMS syndrome presenting as systemic sclerosis: clinical and pathologic study of a case with microangiopathic glomerular lesions. Am J Med 1988;84:524–8.

140. Feigert JM, Sweet DL, Coleman M, et al. Multicentric angiofollicular lymph node hyperplasia with peripheral neuropathy, pseudotumor cerebri, IgA dysproteinemia, and thrombocytosis in women: a distinct syndrome. Ann Intern Med 1990;113:362–7.

141. Bengtsson C, Blohmé G, Lapidus L, et al. Do antihypertensive drugs precipitate diabetes? BMJ 1984;289:1495–7.

142. Grunfeld C, Chappell DA. Hypokalemia and diabetes mellitus [Editorial]. Am J Med 1983;75:553–4.

143. Dornhorst A, Powell SH, Pensky J. Aggravation by propranolol of hyperglycaemic effect of hydrochlorothiazide in Type II diabetics without alteration of insulin secretion. Lancet 1985;1:123–6.

144. Swislocki ALM, Hoffman BB, Reaven GM. Insulin resistance, glucose intolerance and hyperinsulinemia in patients with hypertension. Am J Hypertens 1989; 2:419–23.

145. Podolsky S, Pattavina CG. Hyperosmolar nonketotic diabetic coma: a complication of propranolol therapy. Metabolism 1973;22:685–93.

146. Fajans SS, Floyd JC Jr, Thiffault CA, et al. Further studies on diazoxide suppression of insulin release from abnormal and normal islet tissue in man. Ann NY Acad Sci 1968;150:261–80.

147. Pace CS, Livingston E. Ionic basis of phenytoin sodium inhibition of insulin secretion in pancreatic islets. Diabetes 1979;28:1077–82.

148. Goldberg EM, Sanbar SS. Hyperglycemic, nonketotic coma following administration of dilantin (diphenylhydantoin). Diabetes 1969;18:101–6.

149. Bouchard P, Sai P, Reach G, et al. Diabetes mellitus following pentamidine-induced hypoglycemia in humans. Diabetes 1982;31:40–5.

150. LeWitt PA. The neurotoxicity of the rat poison vacor: a clinical study of 12 cases. N Engl J Med 1980;302:73–7.

151. Karam JH, Lewitt PA, Young CW, et al. Insulinopenic diabetes after rodenticide (vacor) ingestion: a unique model of acquired diabetes in man. Diabetes 1980;29:971–8.

152. Osei K, Falko JM, Nelson KP, Stephens R. Diabetogenic effect of pentamidine: in vitro and in vivo studies in a patient with malignant insulinoma. Am J Med 1984;77:41–6.

153. Kahn SE, Beard JC, Schwartz MW, et al. Increased β-cell secretory capacity as mechanism for islet adaptation to

nicotinic acid-induced insulin resistance. Diabetes 1989;38:562–8.

154. Garg A, Grundy SM. Nicotinic acid as therapy for dyslipidemia in non-insulin-dependent diabetes. JAMA 1990;264:723–6.

155. Sumrani NB, Delaney V, Daskalakis P, et al. Retrospective analysis of posttransplantation diabetes mellitus in black renal allograft recipients. Diabetes Care 1991;14:760–2.

156. Yamamoto H, Akazawa S, Yamaguchi Y, et al. Effects of cyclosporin A and low dosages of steroid on posttransplantation diabetes in kidney transplant recipients. Diabetes Care 1991;14:867–70.

157. Martin F, Bedoya F. Effects of cyclosporin A on the cAMP system in pancreatic islets [Abstract no. 713]. Diabetes 1991;40(Suppl 1):179A.

158. Kida K, Ikeuchi M, Goto Y, et al. The effect of cyclosporin A on glucose transport by muscles in vivo and in vitro [Abstract no. 361]. Diabetes 1991;40(Suppl 1):91A.

159. Feldman M, Kiser RS, Unger RH, Li CH. Beta-endorphin and the endocrine pancreas: studies in healthy and diabetic human beings. N Engl J Med 1983;308:349–53.

160. Giugliano D. Morphine, opioid peptides, and pancreatic islet function. Diabetes Care 1984;7:92–8.

161. Rotter JI, Vadheim CM, Rimoin DL. Genetics of diabetes mellitus. In: Rifkin H, Porte H, eds. Diabetes mellitus: theory and practice. New York: Elsevier, 1990:378–413.

162. Bray GA, Dahms WT, Swerdloff, RS, et al. The Prader-Willi syndrome: a study of 40 patients and a review of the literature. Medicine (Baltimore) 1983;62:59–80.

163. Green JS, Parfrey PS, Harnett JD, et al. The cardinal manifestations of Bardet-Biedl syndrome, a form of Laurence-Moon-Biedl syndrome. N Engl J Med 1989; 321:1002–9.

164. Schoenle EJ, Boltshauser EJ, Baekkeskov S, et al. Preclinical and manifest diabetes mellitus in young patients with Friedreich's ataxia: no evidence of immune process behind the islet cell destruction. Diabetologia 1989; 32:378–81.

165. Blasi C, Pierelli F, Rispoli E, et al. Wolfram's syndrome: a clinical, diagnostic, and interpretative contribution. Diabetes Care 1986;9:521–8.

166. Karasik A, O'Hara C, Srikanta S, et al. Genetically programmed selective islet β-cell loss in diabetic subjects with Wolfram's syndrome. Diabetes Care 1989;12:135–8.

167. Tiengo A, Segato T, Briani C, et al. The presence of retinopathy in patients with secondary diabetes following pancreatectomy or chronic pancreatitis. Diabetes Care 1983;6:570–4.

168. Couet C, Genton P, Pointel JP, et al. The prevalence of retinopathy is similar in diabetes mellitus secondary to chronic pancreatitis with or without pancreatectomy and in idiopathic diabetes mellitus. Diabetes Care 1985;8:323–8.

169. Feingold KR, Lee TH, Chung MY, Siperstein MD. Muscle capillary basement membrane width in patients with vacor-induced diabetes mellitus. J Clin Invest 1986;78:102–7.

170. Passa P, Gauville C, Canivet J. Influence of muscular exercise on plasma levels of growth hormone in diabetics with and without retinopathy. Lancet 1974;2:72–4.

171. Merimee TJ, Zapf J, Froesch ER. Insulin-like growth factors: studies in diabetes with or without retinopathy. N Engl J Med 1983;309:527–30.

172. Rymaszewski Z, Cohen RM, Chomczynski P. Human growth hormone stimulates proliferation of human retinal microvascular endothelial cells in vitro. Proc Natl Acad Sci USA 1991;88:617–21.

173. Merimee TJ. A follow-up study of vascular disease in growth-hormone-deficient dwarfs with diabetes. N Engl J Med 1978;298:1217–22.

174. Sharp PS, Fallon TJ, Brazier OJ, et al. Long-term follow-up of patients who underwent Yttrium-90 pituitary implantation for treatment of proliferative diabetic retinopathy. Diabetologia 1987;30:199–207.

175. Passa P, Rousselie F, Gauville C, Canivet J. Retinopathy and plasma growth hormone levels in idiopathic hemochromatosis with diabetes. Diabetes 1977;26:113–20.

176. Rabin D, Bloomgarden ZT, Feman SS, Davis TQ. Development of diabetic complications despite the absence of growth hormone in a patient with post-pancreatectomy diabetes. N Engl J Med 1984;310:837–9.

Chapter 18

USE OF ANIMAL MODELS IN THE STUDY OF DIABETES

AVRAHAM KARASIK
MASAKAZU HATTORI

Our understanding of the complex pathogenesis of diabetes mellitus has progressed greatly through the use of animal models of this disease. The benefits of animal studies in diabetes research are illustrated most dramatically by the early studies of the dog over a century ago in which the induction of diabetes by pancreatectomy led to a realization of the role of the pancreas in insulin secretion. The successful extraction of insulin from the canine pancreas began the modern era in our understanding and treatment of diabetes. Multiple other aspects of diabetes, including the genetics, physiology, biochemistry, and development of complications and their prevention, as well as trials of new forms of therapy, have also been greatly aided by studies in animal models.

The use of animals, rather than humans, in diabetes research has multiple advantages. Study of the multifactorial genetics of diabetes is feasible in animals since inbreeding, maintenance of accurate genealogies, and observation of multiple generations in a short period are all possible. Some animals, such as the autosomal recessive *db/db* mouse, develop different degrees of diabetes when bred on different genetic backgrounds,[1] permitting a better understanding of the role of a single mutation and of polygenic factors in the production of the diabetes syndrome. In addition, careful inbreeding studies of diabetic animals, such as the NOD (non-obese diabetic) mouse, have permitted recognition of the multiple genes controlling expression of the diabetic syndrome in these animals.[2] In the exploration of the pathogenesis of diabetes, animal models permit a better analysis of the biochemical and anatomic alterations in organs inaccessible in humans.

The etiology of diabetes in many animal models is homogeneous, permitting the isolation of one of the many different pathogenetic factors that influence the development of diabetes in humans. Moreover, a selected etiologic factor can be induced and studied in depth by a specific manipulation. Diabetes may be induced by viruses,[3,4] chemical agents,[5,6] or partial pancreatectomy.[7] Use of transgenic mice allows an even finer experimental focus and targeting of etiologic factors that induce diabetes. Animal models also provide unique opportunities for investigating the toxicity and efficiency of therapeutic measures developed for the prevention and cure of diabetes and its complications.

The major limitation in the use of animal models is the lack of a perfect correlation between animal and human disease. No animal model has characteristics of diabetes identical to those in humans. Nevertheless, once a specific pathologic mechanism is fully understood in the diabetic animal, a similar defect may be found in diabetic humans, contributing to our knowledge of this disease in humans. Careful selection of the appropriate animal model, accurate characterization of the specific animals studied, and a cautious approach to interpreting the data when making inferences about human disease are critical for the investigator using animal models in the study of diabetes mellitus.

CLASSIFICATION OF ANIMAL MODELS OF DIABETES MELLITUS

A large array of animal models are available for experimentation relevant to the study of diabetes. Although all models manifest hyperglycemia, the degrees of glucose intolerance and the etiologies differ. The animal models of diabetes can be classified according to causative factor, pathogenesis, nature of the diabetic syndrome, or other characteristics of the disease. In this chapter we have classified the different animal models by their clinical resemblance to human disease (Table 18–1). The first criterion for classification of an animal model is its resemblance to insulin-dependent diabetes (IDDM) or non-insulin-dependent diabetes (NIDDM).

Table 18–1.   Animal Models for Diabetes

SYNDROMES RESEMBLING NON-INSULIN-DEPENDENT DIABETES
A. Obese rodents with severe diabetes
    db/db mouse (diabetes mouse)
B. Obese rodents with mild diabetes
    Mice
        ob/ob mouse (obese mouse)
        Obese yellow mouse
        KK mouse
        New Zealand obese mouse (NZO mouse)
        PPB/Ld mouse
        Wellesley hybrid mouse
    Rats
        Fatty "Zucker" rat
        BHE rat
        Hypertensive SHR/N-cp rat
        WKY fatty rat
C. Nutrition-induced diabetes
    Sand rat (*Psammomys obesus*)
    Spiny mouse (*Acomys cahirinus*)
    Mongolian gerbil (*Meriones unguiculatus*)
    Tuco-tuco (*Ctenomys talarum*)
D. Rodents with a decrease in β-cell mass
    Neonatal streptozotocin-induced diabetes
    Rats with partial pancreatectomy
E. Diabetes developed by selective inbreeding in rodents
    Swiss-Hauschka mice
    Cohen diabetic rat
    Goto-Kakizaki rat
SYNDROMES RESEMBLING HUMAN INSULIN-DEPENDENT DIABETES
A. Spontaneous diabetes
    NOD mouse
    BB rat
    LETL rat
    Chinese hamster
    Keeshond dog
B. Experimental diabetes
    Streptozotocin-induced diabetes
    Virus-induced diabetes
    Suppression of diabetes by viral infection
    (transgenic diabetes: overexpression of MHC class I and II molecules and interferon-γ)

ANIMAL MODELS OF NON-INSULIN-DEPENDENT DIABETES

Hyperglycemia is a consequence of an imbalance between two factors that govern glucose metabolism: insulin production and insulin sensitivity (Fig. 18–1). In NIDDM, insulin resistance is a major pathophysiologic element influencing glucose hemostasis but cannot by itself create hyperglycemia. Only when the pancreatic β-cells fail to secrete enough insulin to overcome the resistance is diabetes expressed.[8,9] Because the etiology of NIDDM in humans is heterogeneous and the two major pathogenetic factors influence one another, it is often difficult to determine which of the two is the initiating factor and what is their relative contributions to the development of glucose intolerance.

Each animal model for NIDDM exhibits the interplay between peripheral insulin resistance and compromised β-cell potential. Different models exhibit several facets of this interplay. For example, in the "Zucker" diabetic fat (ZDF) rat, insulin resistance is the major initial pathogenetic mechanism. While β-cells in these animals are

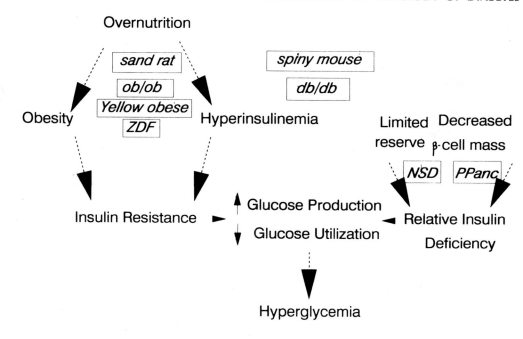

Fig. 18–1. A schematic diagram of the pathogenesis of non-insulin-dependent diabetes (NIDDM), showing the factors that lead to hyperglycemia in NIDDM by altering either insulin resistance or pancreatic β-cell capacity. Names of animals are localized on the scheme by the relative effect of these factors in the pathogenesis of hyperglycemia in each animal model. ZDF = "Zucker" diabetes fatty rat; NSD = neonatal streptozotocin rat; PPanc = partial pancreatectomy.

robust, this combination leads to hyperinsulinemia with mild glucose intolerance,[10] and only a subgroup of these animals with "weak" β-cells develops hyperglycemia. On the other hand, in the neonatal streptozotocin model, compromised insulin secretion leads to a degree of glucose intolerance similar to that in the ZDF rat, with insulin resistance only a minor contributor to glucose intolerance.[11] Thus, each animal model portrays a subgroup of patients with NIDDM and delineates a specific aspect of the pathophysiology of NIDDM. Figure 18–1 illustrates where in this interplay each animal model lies.

Several pathophysiologic facets of NIDDM are represented to different extents in the different animal models. The first is the concurrence of NIDDM and obesity. Obesity is prevalent in patients with NIDDM and contributes to the expression of insulin resistance and diabetes in this group.[12] Certain subgroups of persons with NIDDM, such as the Pima Indians, show a high prevalence of both diabetes and obesity, despite the genetic separation of the two conditions.[13] Many animal models, such as db/db mice and yellow obese mice, show a genetic concurrence of diabetes and obesity.[14] These animals manifest hyperglycemia as a result of overeating and weight gain. The converging appearance of obesity and diabetes may be the result of a purely genetic defect but is usually the result of a genetic predisposition unmasked by environmental factors. In human NIDDM, changes in diet unmask diabetes. In several societies, such as the Australian aborigines and Pima Indians, the prevalence of NIDDM surged when these individuals were exposed to a more abundant diet of "Western"-type food.[15] A similar phenomenon is exhibited in the sand rat. This desert inhabitant is euglycemic in its original environment, where it eats a low-calorie plant diet. When transferred to a captive environment and fed a calorie-rich laboratory

chow ad libitum, the sand rat becomes obese and develops diabetes.[16]

Development of glucose intolerance in NIDDM, both in humans and in animal models of the disease, follows a horseshoe-shaped pattern (Fig. 18–2).[17] In the initial phase, the individual develops hyperinsulinemia to compensate for the insulin resistance (stage A), a mechanism that allows for normoglycemia (stage B). At later stages, although hyperinsulinemia continues to prevail, the increased resistance is not overcome and hyperglycemia develops (stage C). The ability of the pancreas to overproduce insulin eventually is lost, and the relative hypoinsulinemia leads to a decline in glucose tolerance (stage D). This continuum in the development of diabetes from normal glucose tolerance to overt diabetes can be observed in the sand rat as well as in the db/db mouse.[1,18] In contrast, the ob/ob mouse does not progress into the more severe stages but remains hyperinsulinemic and moderately glucose-intolerant,[14] as do many obese patients with insulin resistance. The factor that determines the degree to which hyperglycemia will develop in a certain animal is the β-cell reserve. In human NIDDM, weight gain has a regulatory effect on insulin resistance and glucose tolerance.[12] Likewise, the sand rat and the ob/ob mouse show an improvement in glucose tolerance when they resume a low-calorie diet.[18] Choice of the relevant aspects in each phase of disease and the animal model that expresses this facet permits the study of the various factors of importance in the development of NIDDM in humans.

All of the animal models described in this chapter are rodent models. Diabetes that resembles NIDDM, however, has been described in subhuman primates, cows, and pigs,[19–22] but none is as well characterized as the rodent models. The technical difficulties involved in cultivating large colonies and the high maintenance costs

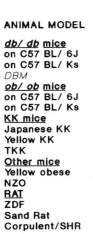

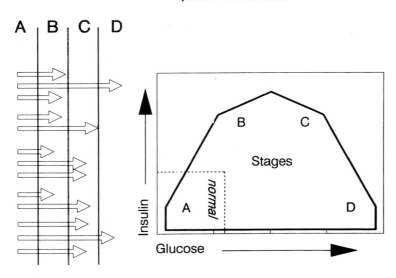

Fig. 18–2. A scheme of the different stages of glucose intolerance in the development of non-insulin-dependent diabetes showing the horseshoe-like development of the hyperinsulinemic, hyperglycemic syndrome. The maximal degree of glucose intolerance reached by each animal is depicted.

limits the characterization of diabetes in these larger animals. They are used primarily for studies of the physiology and metabolic aspects of diabetes because vessel catheterization and multiple blood sampling are possible in these animals.

An NIDDM-like picture can also be induced in rodents by pharmacologic intervention. Insulin counterregulatory hormones and extreme changes in dietary composition induce insulin resistance and glucose intolerance. Steroid hormones introduced parenterally in pharmacologic doses or increased levels of growth hormone induced by implanting growth hormone-producing tumors or by feeding animals diets high in fat interfere with insulin action and mimic aspects of NIDDM.[23–28] Description of these animal models of secondary diabetes is beyond the scope of this chapter (see Chapter 17).

Animal models of NIDDM may be divided into four categories (Table 18–1). The first two categories include animals that exhibit obesity before developing diabetes.[29] The *db/db* mouse, the only animal model in the first category, develops a severe form of diabetes caused by the inability of the β-cells to compensate for the increased demand for insulin. The second category, which includes several models, is characterized by obesity and mild glucose intolerance such as that in the majority of patients with NIDDM. The third category includes animals that display diabetes only when they are exposed to a high-calorie diet and includes non-obese animals that have a decreased β-cell mass.

Obese Rodents with Severe Diabetes

The db/db Mouse

Genetics. The *db* mutation leading to diabetes in mice is a single gene mutation on chromosome 4 at linkage group VIII, close to the misty (*m*) gene for coat color.[14,30,31] The *db* mutant gene is flanked by several genes that, in the human genome, are located on human chromosome 1p31–36.[32] The mutation was first recognized and well characterized at the Jackson Laboratories

in Bar Harbor, Maine. This mutation is inherited as an autosomal recessive gene with full penetrance. Homozygotes for the *db* mutation are infertile, and the parental heterozygotes are required to continue the line. When this gene is bred on the C57BL/6J background, animals develop obesity with mild hyperglycemia. When the gene is bred on the C57BL/Ks background, expression is more vigorous, creating a syndrome of obesity with severe hyperglycemia and diabetes.[33] The major difference between the two phenotypes is that the pancreatic β-cells of mice with the C57BL/Ks background lose much of their ability to synthesize insulin as the animals grow older, whereas mice with the C57BL/6J background manifest a non-exhaustive insulin supply. This decline in β-cell function associated with the Ks background leads to a NIDDM-like picture that culminates in a severe form of ketotic diabetes that shortens the life-span. Analysis shows that allelic differences at two or more loci, rather than a single mutation, act as gene modifiers that determine the phenotypic outcome and the severity of disease.[34]

Some genetic modifiers of *db* gene expression are related to gender.[35] These modifiers act through the ratio of androgens, which may impair glucose tolerance, to estrogens, which may promote glucose tolerance.[36] The ratio is governed both by the rate of production of the hormones and by their inactivation through sulfation by the steroid sulfotransferase (ST), a hepatic enzyme, which by means of its differential affinity for estrogens and androgens exerts differential control on hormone levels. On the C57BL/Ks background, diabetes is present in both sexes because of the increased ability of the enzyme to inactivate estrogens with the minimal androgen sulfation activity.[36] On other backgrounds, only males are affected since estrogen protects the females. Other gene expression modifiers lead to a spectrum of hyperglycemic syndromes in animals carrying the *db/db* gene. For example, expression of *db* on the combined B6 and BL/Ks genetic pools leads to the mild form of diabetes known as DBM.[37] In this genetically non-inbred model, the animal develops obesity and insulin resistance, but because the pancreatic β-cells overcome the resistance, the animal develops only a mild form of diabetes. The *db* mutation illustrates how the mode of expression of a single mutation is contingent on interaction with the genetic background in the creation of a NIDDM-like syndrome in rodents. In humans, NIDDM is believed to stem from similar interactions between several diabetes genes and gene modifiers.

Development of Obesity and Diabetes. Development of diabetes in animals with the *db* mutation on the C57BL/Ks background follows the "classic" horseshoe-shaped pattern described in Figure 18–2. When these animals are as young as 10 to 14 days old, normoglycemic mice become hyperinsulinemic.[29] During their first month of life, they are not obese but increase their food intake and show a moderate weight gain. In their second month of life, the *db/db* animals become hyperglycemic, with blood glucose levels reaching as high as 300 mg/dL. In parallel, insulin levels increase, reaching up to 10 times normal values when the animals are 3 months old.[38,39] In this period the mice gain weight and become markedly obese, reaching a maximal body weight of 50 to 60 g.[29] When the mice are 3 to 6 months old, hyperinsulinemia diminishes and the animals manifest symptoms of insulin deficiency. They lose weight, develop severe diabetes with ketosis, and die at the age of 5 to 8 months.

Mass and Function of Pancreatic Islet Cells. The stepped alterations in plasma insulin levels in the *db/db* mice are mirrored in the pancreatic β-cell morphology and insulin biosynthesis.[40] Young mice have normal-size islets, which show a progressive increase in degranulation. With progression of the disease, the islet tissue enlarges markedly, the cells become more degranulated, and the boundaries with the acinar cells of the exocrine pancreas are less clear.[41,42] Degeneration and necrosis follow, resulting in reduced β-cell mass and atrophic islets.[43]

Increased insulin production in the initial hyperinsulinemic phases of the disease, a decline in plasma insulin levels, and an elevation in glucose levels are accompanied by parallel changes in proinsulin synthesis and proinsulin mRNA.[44] The mechanisms leading to the deterioration in the islet β-cells are not clear: both an inability of β-cells to replicate and retroviral A infection have been suggested as possible etiologic factors.[45,46] Restriction of carbohydrate intake and control of blood glucose levels will influence the rate of β-cell deterioration.[47,48]

Glucagon has been implicated as a possible factor in the development of hyperglycemia in the initial phases.[49] The α-cells manifest an increase in glucagon content, an augmentation of arginine stimulation of glucagon release, and a lack of suppression by glucose. Various changes in somatostatin content of the islets have been reported, although the role of somatostatin in β-cell failure in this syndrome is not clear.[50,51]

Insulin Resistance. Obese hyperglycemic mice are insulin-resistant, as manifest by the high levels of endogenous insulin in the face of hyperglycemia and by the weak effect of exogenous insulin in reducing blood glucose levels.[14] The site of resistance is primarily the liver, which is enlarged in relation to other organs.[52]

Glycogen metabolism and gluconeogenesis, as well as their corresponding enzymes, are hyperactive. Increased glucose production occurs at 4 weeks of age despite the hyperinsulinemia. Lack of suppression of the gluconeogenetic enzymes by insulin is a major component contributing to hyperglycemia in all stages of the disease in the mouse.[53] Studies in isolated muscle and adipose tissue in vitro confirm the existence of insulin resistance in peripheral tissues.[54] As for the mechanism of resistance, both the glucose transporter and the insulin receptor systems have been studied in this animal model. Although muscle glucose transport is impaired in the *db/db* mouse,[55] the insulin-sensitive glucose transporter (GLUT-4) does not appear to be expressed differently in the muscle tissue of obese *db/db* mice and lean *db/+* control mice.[56] The number of insulin receptors in liver, muscle, and fat cells is decreased and correlates with the degree of hyperinsulinemia.[57] It is not clear, however, whether this decrease causes resistance or is a result of insulin-induced down-regulation of the receptor. Beyond the binding defect, there is also a decrease in the tyrosine kinase activity of the insulin receptor.[58] The changes observed in the receptor are not due to a defect in the genome of the receptor but to a post-translation alteration in receptor expression.[59]

Obesity and Hyperphagia. A defect in the satiety center is believed to be involved in the hyperphagia and obesity in the *db/db* mice. This was first suggested by parabiosis experiments,[60] in which a diabetic mouse and a nondiabetic mouse were joined by a cutaneous bridge along the animals' abdomens, allowing the exchange of 1 to 2% of the blood volume hourly. In these experiments the nondiabetic mice died of starvation within 2 to 4 weeks of surgery, an outcome suggesting that the diabetic mice produced a circulating satiety factor but were insensitive to it. In investigations of the importance of the satiety center in the production of the syndrome, lesions were preformed in the ventromedial nucleus. This manipulation did not abolish hyperphagia or fat-cell mass but produced a milder form of diabetes.[61]

The nature of the overproduced satiety factor is not clear. Adipsin, a serine protease homologue synthesized and secreted by adipose cells, may play a role in regulation of food intake and expenditure of energy.[62] In normal rodents, levels of adipsin in blood and tissues correlate with the energy balance of the organism. In *ob/ob* and *db/db* mice, a hundredfold decrease in tissue mRNA and blood adipsin levels has been found. The role of adipsin, however, is questionable, as the impairment seems to develop after obesity has already been established,[63] and thus far no reports have appeared that indicate adipsin replacement will reverse this syndrome.

Obese Rodents with Milder Forms of Diabetes

The ob/ob Mouse

Genetics and Animal Profile. The *ob/ob* mouse develops only a mild diabetic syndrome that includes obesity, hyperinsulinemia, and mild hyperglycemia. The pathophysiology of the disease and its development are similar to the first stages observed in the *db/db* mice.[14,29] The *ob* mutation is a single autosomal recessive mutation on chromosome 6, linkage group XI.[64] The classic description relates to the expression of the mutation on the C57BL/6J background. Mildly different phenotypes are produced when the mutation is expressed on different backgrounds.[65] For example, animals with the C57BL/Ks background become more hyperglycemic and exhibit a picture similar to that of the *db/db* mouse. Obesity is expressed early and is apparent in the first month of life, reaching a climax at the age of 6 months. The mice may weigh up to 90 g. The weight increase is accounted for by hyperplasia and hypertrophy of the fat cells in the adipose tissue.[66-68] During this period of weight gain, the animals manifest hyperphagia and increasing degrees of hyperinsulinemia.[69] Insulin levels can be as high as 10 to 50 times those in control mice.[70] During this dynamic phase, mice may show a mild degree of hyperglycemia. Unlike *db/db* mice, *ob/ob* mice do not progress further on the horseshoe-shaped course but either remain mildly hyperglycemic and hyperinsulinemic or reestablish euglycemia.[29]

Pancreatic Islets and Insulin Resistance. In this animal model the increased demand for insulin is met by an increased effort by the islets. Histologically, islets are large and contain mainly hyperplastic β-cells.[71] Among animals in a specific colony of obese mice bred in Sweden, islet mass was found to be 10 times higher than in controls.[72] Insulin biosynthesis is increased, and cells are degranulated as a result of their hypersecretory state. This hypertrophy-hyperplasia of the β-cells secures a non-exhaustive insulin supply. The number of α-cells is also increased, but the ratio between α- and β-cells is low in the *ob/ob* mice, in parallel with the ratio of the respective hormones in plasma.

The markedly high ratio of insulin to glucose in the plasma of these mice suggests an extreme degree of insulin resistance.[73] Insulin resistance appears only after the onset of obesity, a course implying that resistance is not the basic defect.[70] Moreover, several reports describe hypoglycemia as a reaction to the first stages of hyperinsulinemia, which would point to appropriate insulin sensitivity in the earliest phases.[74] Insulin resistance is manifest in muscle, where insulin-induced glucose uptake is reduced.[70] Excessive hepatic production of glucose is observed despite hyperinsulinemia. The excess is due both to lack of activation of glycogen synthesis and to failure of gluconeogenesis suppression in the fasted and the postprandial state.[75] Insulin-receptor number is decreased in all tissues in animals as young as 6 weeks of age.[74] The number of receptors is negatively correlated with plasma insulin levels, a relationship suggesting that down-regulation caused by the excessive insulin levels is the mechanism leading to the decreased receptor number. Receptor autophosphorylation and kinase activity are reduced beyond the decrease expected by the decrease in receptor number.[76]

Obesity and Hyperphagia. The similarity in pathophysiologic aspects of the diabetic syndrome in *ob/ob* and *db/db* mice does not extend to the causes of hyperphagia. When experiments involving parabiosis between the *ob/ob* and *db/db* mice are carried out, the *ob/ob* mouse dies of starvation, as is the case for a normal animal in parabiosis with a *db/db* mouse. An *ob/ob* mouse in parabiosis with a normal lean mouse eats less and gains weight less rapidly.[77] After the animals are separated, the obese partner gains weight rapidly. These experiments suggest that the *ob/ob* mouse lacks a humoral satiety factor but is capable of responding to it. Levels of blood adipsin and of adipose tissue adipsin mRNA in *ob/ob* mice are decreased to the same extent as in *db/db* mice,[62] making it unlikely that adipsin is the mediator of these two very different, but closely related, models of obesity and NIDDM.

The defect in fat metabolism extends beyond the hypothalamic appetite-control centers. There is a primary change in lipid metabolism. Food-restricted *ob/ob* mice gain weight less rapidly, but still accumulate larger fat deposits, than parallel-fed controls.[68,78] Lipogenesis in liver, increased turnover of free fatty acids, and increased lipoprotein lipase activity in the peripheral adipose tissue all contribute to fat accumulation.[79,80] Metabolism is normal in adipocytes from *ob/ob* mice. Moreover, when fat cells from *ob/ob* mice are transplanted to a normal host, they behave like fat cells of the host.[81] Surgical removal of large amounts of fat tissue leads to regeneration of the tissue to its former size, pointing to the presence of a factor that regulates the size of fat tissue.[82] Insulin is possibly one hormone that mediates these anabolic phenomena in fat.[83] There also is evidence of a role of adrenal steroids in the induction of obesity, since levels of adrenal steroids are increased in *ob/ob* mice and some reports show that adrenalectomy ameliorates obesity and hyperinsulinemia.[84,85] A pituitary β-cell tropin similar to adrenocorticotropic hormone (ACTH), as well as some of the neuropeptides found in the brain and gastrointestinal tract (cholecystokinin, somatostatin, and pancreatic polypeptide), have been mentioned as possible hyperphagia- and obesity-inducing factors in this animal model.[86,87] Decreased physical activity, increased efficiency of food absorption and utilization, and decreased energy consumption have all been suggested as contributors to the tendency for animals to become obese.[88,89]

Yellow Obese Mouse

The yellow obese mouse, originally described over a century ago, develops a mild form of glucose intolerance, obesity, and hyperinsulinemia. The insulin levels and the degree of insulin resistance are lower than those in the *ob/ob* mouse.[29]

Genetics. The mutation leading to this syndrome was established as an allele at the agouti locus. The original dominant allele, designated A^Y, was found to be lethal in homozygotes. Another dominant allele at the agouti locus, labeled A^{vy} for viable yellow, arose spontaneously in C3H/HeJ mice at the Bar Harbor Jackson Laboratory. Additional alleles leading to different phenotypes have been described.[90] The yellow skin pigmentation and obesity are interconnected, and the amount of weight gain is related to the percentage of yellow in the animal's coat.[91] Expression of these alleles also depends on background genome and gender.[92]

Animal Characteristics. The main feature of the yellow obese mouse is obesity, which results from an impressive hyperphagia in young mice.[93] Older animals eat less and lose weight.[94] Parabiosis experiments suggest that lack of a circulating satiety factor causes hyperphagia. The ensuing obesity is a result of fat-cell hypertrophy and is more pronounced in males and in the yellower animals.[95] Changes in lipogenetic enzymes occur during the period of weight gain.[96,97] Insulin levels are increased and mirror the increase in β-cell mass in the pancreas.[98] An exaggerated sensitivity to counterregulatory hormones such as glucagon and glucocorticoids is observed, whereas adrenalectomy partially prevents the development of obesity.[99] Glucose intolerance is expressed as postprandial hyperglycemia in the obese rats, while their fasting blood glucose levels are normal.

KK Mouse

Japanese KK mice, originally described by Kondo et al.,[100] were bred for their large size. The product of this breeding is a hyperphagic, moderately obese animal with hyperglycemia. KK mice weigh up to 50 g,[101] as compared with weights as high as 100 g in other obese strains of mice, such as *ob/ob* mice. Breeding of the KK mice with different strains resulted in several phenotypes with various degrees of obesity, insulin resistance, hyperinsulinemia, and hypertrophy of the islets of Langerhans.[102] Breeding of KK mice with BL/6 mice produced the Toronto-KK hybrid mouse (T-KK).[101] Transfer of the gene of the yellow mouse to the Japanese KK mouse produced the KKA^y mouse.[103]

Japanese KK mice manifest moderate obesity and hyperinsulinemia. Only animals fed a high-calorie diet become hyperglycemic, while food-restricted animals remain euglycemic.[104] A peak in the metabolic derangements is seen at age of 4 to 6 months, with obesity, insulin levels of over 1200 μU/mL, and hyperglycemia with glucose levels of less than 300 mg/dL. The obesity and hyperinsulinemic-hyperglycemic syndrome, which is more pronounced in males, fades with advancing age. Blood glucose levels approach normal with successive generations of consecutive inbreeding, as penetrance of the dominant diabetes mutation is influenced by the expression of gene modifiers that are inherited independently.[105] The degree of hyperglycemia is more severe in the T-KK hybrids and the yellow KK mice, both of which display overt diabetes.

The primary defect leading to diabetes in these animal models has not yet been elucidated. Defects in insulin sensitivity in both the liver and peripheral tissues have been found to contribute to the development of hyperglycemia.[106] Islet function is almost normal, and changes in the pituitary-adrenal axis are secondary to the development of the diabetic syndrome.

NZO Mouse

Selective inbreeding of obese mice from a mixed colony led to a New Zealand obese (NZO) strain characterized by obesity, hyperglycemia, and hyperinsulinemia.[107] Neither the mode of inheritance nor the pathogenetic mechanisms of this syndrome are understood.

As in the other animal models, insulin resistance, hyperinsulinemia, and glucose intolerance develop in parallel with hyperphagia and obesity.[29] Development of obesity and deterioration of glucose tolerance is most pronounced in animals on high-fat diets, and both phenomena are responsive to dietary manipulations.[108] The degree of obesity is comparable to that in the yellow, *ob/ob*, and *db/db* mice; however, hyperglycemia and hyperinsulinemia are less pronounced.[109] Weight gain is gradual, and mice weigh up 100 g and have blood glucose levels of 250 mg/dL at 4 to 6 months of age.[108] Males have a higher blood glucose level as a reflection of peripheral and hepatic insulin resistance. Gluconeogenetic enzyme activity in the liver is increased despite hyperinsulinemia, while glucose uptake by muscle and adipose tissue is low.[110,111]

Unlike other obese hyperglycemic rodents, NZO mice respond to long-term administration of sulfonylurea with an increase in insulin secretion and a decrease in blood glucose level.[112] Insulin levels are three to four times higher than in controls but show a blunted first-phase response.[113] The β-cell mass is increased in pancreases from these mice.[114] Several autoimmune phenomena, such as the presence of antibodies to the insulin receptor and the islet cell, have also been described, but their importance in the pathogenesis of the disease remains obscure.[115]

PPB/Ld Mouse

The PPB/Ld (Paul Bailey black) mouse is another inbred model of obesity and diabetes with polygenic inheritance.[116] Animals show a mild form of the obese hyperglycemia-hyperinsulinemia syndrome. Of special interest is the hyperlipidemia they develop, which can be modified by various diets.[117]

Wellesley Hybrid Mouse

The Wellesley hybrid mouse was developed by crossing the inbred I and C3Hf lines.[118] About 50% of males and 5% of females on an ad libitum diet develop the triad of obesity, hyperinsulinemia, and hyperglycemia. Diabetes is reversible with dietary restriction and may also reverse spontaneously.[119]

"Zucker" Fatty (fa/fa) Rat

Animal Profile. The Zucker diabetic rat (ZDF), first described by Zucker in 1965, is a result of cross-breeding Sherman and Merck Stock M rats.[120] Obesity is inherited as an autosomal recessive mutation assigned the name *fa*. Homozygous rats develop hyperphagia and extreme obesity. Obesity is evident at 4 weeks of age, but many of the biochemical abnormalities and the size and metabolism of the fat tissue are already altered in the preweaning period.[121] Hyperphagia, low physical activity, and increased efficiency of energy utilization all lead to a positive energy balance in these animals. The excess energy is stored in the adipose tissue, which manifests abnormal metabolism. Fat-cell mass increases by both cellular hypertrophy and hyperplasia. Unlike other animals, the ZDF rat can increase the number of fat cells even when older.[122] ZDF rats develop insulin resistance, hyperinsulinemia, glucose intolerance, and hyperlipidemia along with their obesity.[123] On the hyperinsulinemia-hyperglycemia curve, the ZDF rat resembles the *ob/ob* mouse, as it maintains hyperinsulinemia and demonstrates only mild hyperglycemia without progression to overt diabetes.[124] When the *fa* gene from the ZDF is transferred to the Kyoto Wistar rat, a more glucose-intolerant strain emerges.[125] The manifestations expressed in this strain, referred to as the Wistar fatty rat, underscore the importance of the genetic background in effecting the expression of a mutation.[126] The ZDF rat is an excellent model for the commonly occurring impaired glucose tolerance associated with insulin resistance in humans.

Insulin Resistance. Insulin resistance is a major feature of the *fa/fa* rat.[127] It has been documented both in vivo and in vitro in isolated organs and cells. Resistance is found in the muscle of animals as young as 4 weeks old. In animals this age, liver enzymes show normal insulin sensitivity,[124] while the sensitivity of adipose tissue in vitro is increased—consistent with the accelerated growth of this tissue.[120] Tracer studies confirm the low insulin sensitivity of muscle and the high sensitivity of fat tissue in these young animals. In older animals, both muscle and hepatic resistance are present. Glucose-clamp studies performed on 11-week-old obese *fa/fa* rats show that peripheral glucose utilization is decreased as a result of insulin resistance in muscle and unrestrained hepatic glucose production.[127] In other studies hepatic glucose production was not suppressed in these animals even during the ingestion of glucose.[128] The increased and unsuppressed gluconeogenesis correlates with enhanced phosphoenolpyruvate carboxykinase (PEPCK) activity in the liver of *fa/fa* rats.[129] Studies in vitro confirm the observations in vivo; a decrease in insulin sensitivity in muscle was documented in isolated muscle preparations[130] and eviscerated rats,[131] and a low sensitivity to insulin was found in isolated hepatocytes.[132]

Insulin-receptor number and tyrosine kinase activity have been studied in adipose, muscle, and liver cells of these animals. The results differ with differences in the age, tissue, glucose levels, and dietary status of the animal.[133–135] Defects at post-receptor steps in insulin action contribute to insulin resistance.[136] Changes in levels of glucose transporter are found to parallel the physiologic observations of glucose metabolism. A decrease in glucose-transporter number and alterations in regulation have been demonstrated in heart muscle with the use of cytochalasin B, while the level of insulin-dependent glucose transporter (GLUT-4) mRNA in adipose tissue is increased fourfold even before obesity is expressed.[137]

Islet-Cell Function and Mass. Islet cells of the pancreas in ZDF rats do not deteriorate with time but continue to secrete insulin. In this regard these animals resemble *ob/ob* mice. Constant hyperinsulinemia is exaggerated with meal loading and does not decrease with food and carbohydrate restriction, a result of the presence of this robust β-cell mass.[138] Anatomically, the pancreatic islets are large because of both hyperplasia and hypertrophy of β-cells.[139] It has even been suggested that the abnormal insulin secretion is the primary defect in the obesity syndrome in ZDF rats. According to this hypothesis, increased insulin secretion initiates and causes preservation of fat deposition in these animals, as well as the evolution towards insulin resistance. This hypothesis is supported by the finding of insulin hypersecretion in the youngest animals and of autonomic oversecretion of isolated islet cells of the ZDF rat, which show prolonged oversecretion even in culture.[140] Insulin-secreting β-cells, glucagon-secreting α-cells, and somatostatin-secreting d-cells all react abnormally to secretagogues.[141–143] Insulin has an anoretic effect in lean rats but not in ZDF rats.[144] Hypothalamic levels of neuropeptide Y, an appetite-inducing neurotransmitter, are high in ZDF rats[145] and are not suppressed by insulin as they are in lean animals.[146] Thus, in this animal, appetite is not suppressed despite the hyperinsulinemia, a condition allowing for continuous and uninhibited food intake. An alternative connection between hyperinsulinemia and the hypothalamus suggests that the primary defect in the ZDF rats is a central one. According to this hypothesis a central defect, transmitted via the vagus nerve, leads to increased insulin secretion and hyperinsulinemia, which in turn cause obesity and insulin resistance.[129] This hypothesis is supported by the similarity in the characteristics of the ZDF rat and animals with obesity caused by a ventromedial hypothalamic lesion. In contrast, other studies suggest that some of the changes in fat tissues in the *fa/fa* rat are independent of insulin. Thus, streptozotocin-treated ZDF rats show increased fat deposition even in the absence of insulin.[147] A third hypothesis points to anatomic and physiologic aberrations in the pituitary-adrenal axis as the potential basic defect.[148] This suggestion is based on the observation that adrenalectomy leads to reduced hyperinsulinemia and diminished fat-tissue metabolism and deposition in the rat.[149] Although each of these hypotheses has some basis, none can explain all the metabolic facets of disease in this animal. It can therefore be concluded that the alterations seen in adrenal and islet hormones have a permissive but not a primary causative role in the development of the obesity hyperinsulinemic syndrome in the ZDF rat.

A recent finding in a subgroup of the ZDF rats that develop hyperglycemia may unravel the discriminating characteristic that leads to β-cell failure in several diabetic animals. The islets of these diabetes-prone animals have been found to have a low level of the high K_m glucose transporter (GLUT-2) even before the animals develop diabetes.[150] Further depletion of GLUT-2 was seen in the islets of fully diabetic rats.

Nutritionally Evoked Diabetes

Sand Rat (Psammomys obesus)

In humans, the highest prevalence of diabetes is found in societies that subsisted on low-calorie restricted diets before being exposed to an abundance of food in the last century. These groups, such as the Pima Indians in North America and the Australian aborigine, when shifted to the conditions and diet of a "Western" society, manifest a high prevalence of obesity, insulin resistance, and glucose intolerance.[13,16] This phenomenon has been attributed to the "thrifty genotype," a genetically inherited evolutionary metabolic phenomenon that serves peoples living under meager conditions but causes a positive energy balance under conditions of food abundance leading to obesity and diabetes.

The sand rat is a model for this subgroup of patients with NIDDM. The sand rat is really a gerbil. In its natural habitat in the deserts of North Africa and the Middle East, it feeds on a low-caloric vegetable diet and is non-obese, normoglycemic, and normoinsulinemic. Once in captivity and eating a regular laboratory chow diet ad libitum, the sand rat becomes obese and develops mild to severe hyperglycemia.[16,151]

Animal Profile. Several colonies of sand rats trapped in their habitat have been bred and studied in Europe and North America. These colonies differ in disease profile, depending on dietary and environmental conditions.[16,151,152] A colony of sand rats trapped in the Dead Sea region and bred since 1968 by Adler and colleagues at the Hebrew University in Jerusalem maintained their fertility when fed a mix of regular laboratory chow and the native diet of the salt bush.[153] The development of diabetes in this colony has been documented in detail. The members of the sand rat colony divide equally into those in stage A (normoglycemic-normoinsulinemic), stage B (normoglycemic-hyperinsulinemic), and stage C (hyperglycemic-hyperinsulinemic) of the horseshoe curve, with 30% in each stage in cross-section. The remaining 10% develop stage D disease with hypoinsulinemia and ketosis. In the individual sand rat, the development of the different stages is not gradual or predetermined, as is the case in some of the purely genetic forms of diabetes in rodents. The clinical picture of diabetes will develop only in animals that receive the appropriate diet, and the ingredients and quantity of food determine the pace of deterioration to diabetes. In animals eating a diet rich in lipids, the development of diabetes is more rapid and pronounced.[154] With food restriction or with a return to a low-calorie, high-fiber diet, the animals can revert back from stage C to normality. Animals in group D who have already lost part of their insulin reserve cannot recover to normoglycemia. The metabolic status of these animals is determined by an interplay between a genetic adaptive change in metabolism and environmental nutritional factors.[155]

Insulin Resistance. When animals are on a high-calorie diet, the insulin resistance is evident from the elevated blood glucose level in the face of hyperinsulinemia. Further documentation of insulin resistance has been demonstrated in isolated hepatocytes and muscle fibers.[17] In isolated hepatocytes from normoglycemic-normoinsulinemic sand rats in group A, gluconeogenesis is twice as high as in hepatocytes from albino rat controls in both the fasted and fed state and is correlated with an increased level of PEPCK in the liver.[154] The soleus muscle of animals in stage B shows decreased insulin-stimulated

uptake of deoxyglucose, with a further gradual decrease seen in the diabetic animals in group C. On the other hand, the lipoprotein lipase level, which is insulin-dependent, is increased in adipocytes of sand rats, being maximally active in animals in group C.[156] Elevated levels of lipoprotein lipase parallel the rate of uptake of very-low-density lipoprotein triglycerides by adipose tissue.

Receptor studies reveal extremely low hepatic insulin binding in the normoglycemic, normoinsulinemic sand rat as compared with that in the albino rat, a defect that leads to low hepatic extraction of insulin.[157,158] The tyrosine kinase activity per receptor is normal in stage A animals but deteriorates with the development of hyperinsulinemia. The primary defect in the hepatic insulin receptor could form the basis for the hyperinsulinemic, hyperglycemic syndrome in this animal. When the sand rat is exposed to a diet of affluence, it reacts appropriately by secreting more insulin. The receptor defect in liver could account for both the low sensitivity to insulin of glucose metabolism in the liver and, through low extraction of insulin, to peripheral hyperinsulinemia. In turn, hyperinsulinemia may lead to the development of insulin resistance in the periphery, a process culminating in diabetes.

Islet-Cell Function and Mass. Before the sand rat develops diabetes, the islet β-cells show characteristics under light microscopy and patterns of insulin secretion similar to those of normal animals.[152,159] It seems that the primary defect does not lie in the islet cells in this group of animals. Furthermore, in animals in stages B and C, β-cells show enhanced protein synthesis and hypertrophy in an effort to compensate for the resistance. Only in the later phases of the development of the syndrome (stage D) do the islets undergo degranulation and lysis of the β cells.

Corpulent/SHR Rat

The corpulent rat arose spontaneously as an autosomal recessive mutation, *cp* (corpulent), in a stock derived from a SHR/N (spontaneous hypertensive rat) female crossed with a normotensive Sprague-Dawley male.[160] The breeding stock of this model was eventually transferred to the National Institutes of Health, where the mutant strain was backcrossed onto three inbred strains: SHR, WKY, and LA. The *cp* gene on the SHR background gave rise to an interesting model of NIDDM and hypertension. Different stages of inbreeding led to a diversity of syndromes that differ in the severity of the hypertension and diabetes.[161]

Because the *cp* gene is an autosomal recessive, the colony of the SHR/NIH-cp contains both lean and obese animals. Hyperinsulinemia followed by glucose intolerance and frank diabetes is seen in these animals once they are fed a high-carbohydrate diet. Insulin levels are three times higher than in controls, and postprandial plasma glucose levels are over 300 mg/dL. Deterioration in glucose metabolism is more pronounced in obese than in lean animals and occurs more rapidly when the proportion of simple carbohydrates in the diet is increased. Glucose intolerance is more pronounced in male than in female SHR/NIH-cp rats. Islets of obese SHR/NIH-cp rats show a marked β-cell hypertrophy, and cells demonstrate multiple alterations in response to stimuli by secretagogues.[162]

Spiny Mouse (Acomys cahirinus)

The spiny mouse is a large desert mouse that originated in the Middle East. Colonies originating in Israel were characterized in Geneva by Gonet and Renold and colleagues[163] and in Jerusalem by Gutman et al.[164] In a recent review, Shafrir describes the history of the development of the model and the sources of differences between the two colonies.[154] In Switzerland the animals were fed a diet with an extremely high fat content; many became obese and 15% manifested diabetes. In Jerusalem, mice fed a regular chow showed no obesity or hyperglycemia. Challenge with a high-sucrose diet caused mild glucose intolerance and hyperinsulinemia but no obesity. A fat-rich diet similar to that fed the animals in Geneva led to obesity and diabetes. Both obesity and hyperglycemia are reversible with dietary restriction. Exchange of mice and diets between the two colonies substantiated the role of diet in the induction of the diabetic state.[164]

Islet cells in the spiny mouse exhibit a decreased insulin response to stimulation with glucose and other secretagogues, despite a normal and even supernormal insulin content. The defect in insulin response is improved by priming with glucose and stems from a problem in coupling between glucose recognition and the elicited increase in the cyclic adenosine monophosphate (cAMP) that mediates insulin secretion.[165]

The situation in the spiny mouse emphasizes the role of a primary defect in the islets in the development of a NIDDM-like condition. This islet defect is unmasked by a high-calorie diet and a deposition of fat that augments insulin requirements, which cannot be met.[166]

Other Models with Nutritionally Induced Diabetes

All animals grown in captivity on high-fat, high-carbohydrate, low-fiber diets will become obese. Several genetically susceptible strains also will develop glucose intolerance and diabetes. Among them are the C57/6J mice,[167] the Argentinean tuco-tuco,[168] and the Mongolian gerbil bred in both Japan[169] and Sweden.[170]

Rodent Models with a Decrease in β-Cell Mass

Hyperglycemia in NIDDM is a result of an interplay between peripheral insulin resistance and the ability of β-cells to secrete insulin. In most animal models of NIDDM described above, obesity and insulin resistance are the primary determining factors in the development of hyperglycemia. The role of pancreatic reserve in the pathogenesis of NIDDM has been investigated through the development of animal models in which the primary defect lies primarily in the β-cells. This can be achieved by chemical or surgical destruction of the endocrine pancreas. The metabolic consequences of this insult allowed for a detailed study of the effect of reduced β-cell mass on the development of NIDDM.

Neonatal Streptozotocin Model

Partial β-cell destruction induced by streptozotocin given to neonatal mice, followed by regeneration of the β-cells, leads to a clinical syndrome resembling NIDDM. Two versions of this model have been developed. In one, streptozotocin, 100 mg/kg, is given intravenously to female neonatal Wistar rats at birth.[171] This manipulation results in a transient 2-day increase of blood glucose levels followed by a return to normoglycemia. As adults, these animals manifest a low insulin response to glucose stimuli and impaired glucose tolerance. In the second version, β-cells are injured by administration of streptozotocin, 90 mg/kg, given to 2-day-old male Sprague-Dawley rats.[12] The pups develop a transient hyperglycemia for 2 to 4 days, followed by recovery. At 4 to 6 weeks of age, these animals manifest mild fasting and postprandial hyperglycemia as well as oral glucose tolerance in the diabetic range. The second version leads to a more severe form of diabetes because of the timing of injection. The later that streptozotocin is given, the more severe the diabetes, as injured cells of younger animals demonstrate a better ability to regenerate. Both forms of this model can be used to evaluate the effect of reduced β-cell mass on the development of NIDDM.

A model intended to mimic the combined effect between hypertension and NIDDM was recently developed by the injection of streptozotocin in neonates of the spontaneous hypertensive rat.[172] In this model spontaneous recovery occurs after a few weeks in some diabetic animals as a result of the development of insulinomas.[173]

Islet-Cell Mass and Function. The streptozotocin insult to 2-day-old rats leads to a reduction of the β-cell number to 23% that in the controls is followed by an increase in cell number through regeneration to about one-half that in the control adults.[12] Beyond the reduced mass, the islet cells are hyporesponsive to glucose stimuli. This has been shown in vivo after an oral glucose challenge, as well as in vitro in the perfused pancreas or in isolated islet preparations.[174] Normalization of blood glucose levels by insulin treatment improves insulin response to glucose stimuli by the islets, a response suggesting that cells are normal and that the altered response to secretagogues is a result of the noxious effect of glucose.[175] The amplification effects of glucose on arginine secretion that are initially lost also recover after insulin therapy.[176] A secretory defect for the glucagon- and somatostatin-producing cells also is seen secondary to the β-cell insult.[177]

In this model of NIDDM, it is clear that β-cell deficiency is the primary defect. In the milder form of the model, neither peripheral nor hepatic insulin resistance is found, but in the more severe forms, hepatic and peripheral tissues have a reduced response to insulin.[178] No defects in insulin binding or insulin receptor tyrosine kinase activity are observed in this model.[179]

Partial Pancreatectomy in the Rat

A more precise evaluation of the consequences of reduced β-cell mass in rats can be achieved by partial pancreatectomy.[7,180] After 90% of the pancreas is removed, animals maintain moderate hyperglycemia in the fed state but show no differences in body weight and plasma insulin concentrations as compared with sham-operated control animals. Loss of glucose-stimulated insulin secretion was documented in the whole animal after oral or intravenous glucose challenge. No glucose-stimulated insulin release can be seen in perfused pancreases from these animals. In contrast, the reaction to other secretagogues is retained.[7]

Use of such models and a comparison between them and the results of different degrees of pancreatectomy in animals permits a dissection of the role of a reduction in β-cell mass from the consequences of hyperglycemia and hypoinsulinemia.[180] For example, insulin resistance found in these animals can be reversed by the use of phloridzin. The latter agent normalized blood glucose levels by increasing renal glucose loss. This produces a decrease in insulin resistance without altering insulin levels, proving that in this case insulin resistance is a result, rather than a cause, of the hyperglycemia.[181]

Production of NIDDM by Selective Inbreeding

In most animals models described above, a specific mutation or insult leads to NIDDM. Selective inbreeding for glucose intolerance leads to a NIDDM-like picture in rodents. These animals manifest both insulin resistance and reduced insulin reserve but do not have a localized mutation or a specific defect as the basis for diabetes. In Israel, Cohen et al., using an oral glucose tolerance test for selection and four to five generations of breeding, produced a diabetic rat with fasting blood glucose levels above 280 mg/dL.[182] These diabetic rats are not obese and show hepatic insulin resistance and a defective insulin reserve. In Japan, the inbreeding of rats for 35 generations, with blood glucose level following a glucose load used for selection, has led to the development of the diabetic Goto-Kakizaki rat (GK).[183] Another model, developed in a similar fashion in mice, is called the Swiss-Hauschka mouse.[784]

ANIMAL MODELS OF INSULIN-DEPENDENT DIABETES MELLITUS

Insulin-dependent diabetes mellitus (IDDM or Type I) both in humans and in animals models is a multifactorial disease resulting from destruction of islet β-cells that leads to an absence of intrinsic insulin secretion. The destruction of islet β-cells may be caused by autoimmune mechanisms, viral infection, chemicals, or introduction of transgenes into the β-cell, each in a setting of some genetic predisposition. Animal models of spontaneous IDDM include the non-obese diabetic (NOD) mouse, the BioBreeding (BB) rat, the Long-Evans Tokushima Lean rat (LETL), and the Chinese hamster (Table 18–1). These animals become incapable of intrinsic insulin secretion and develop hyperglycemia, polyuria, and weight loss. Although there is considerable heterogeneity in the pathologic and clinical features of these animal models, in all of them IDDM appears to result from autoimmune destruction of islet β-cells. Dietary and other environmental factors also contribute to the development of diabetes. Viral infection, chemicals such as streptozotocin and alloxan, and overexpression of major histocompatibility class I and II molecules or interferon-γ (INF-γ) by transgenes can induce the development of IDDM. However, the pathologic and clinical features of virus-, chemical-, and transgene-induced diabetes are quite readily distinguished from those in animal models of spontaneous diabetes. These animal models provide tools to understand some aspects of IDDM in humans.

Spontaneous Diabetes

NOD Mouse

IDDM in the NOD mouse appears to be the result of autoimmune β-cell destruction in a setting of genetic predisposition. Makino and co-workers established the NOD strain of mice in 1984.[185] The characteristics of the NOD mouse are summarized in Table 18–2.

Table 18–2. Summary of the Characteristics of the DP-BB and NLD-BB Rat, LETL Rat, and NOD Mouse Models of Insulin-Dependent Diabetes

	DP-BB Rat	NLD-BB Rat	LETL Rat	NOD Mouse
Incidence of diabetes	50–80%	<3%	(15–21%) (23–64%)	Female: 80–90% Male: 20–50%
Age at onset	55–120 days	53 days	3–4 months	3–6 months
Sex predominance	1:1	1:1	1:1	Female > male
Insulitis	+	+	+	+
Susceptible genes	Recessive	Recessive	Recessive	Recessive
MHC-linked	RT1ᵘ (chrom. 9)	RT1ᵘ (chrom. 9)	RT1ᵘ (chrom. 9)	Unique I-A (chrom. 17),lack of I-E
Non-MHC-linked	Unknown	Unknown	Unknown	Chrom. 1, 3, 11
Lymphopenia	+ (recessive)	–	–	–
CD4, CD8 T cells	Decreased	Normal number	Normal number	Normal number
RT6⁺ T cells	Absent or very low	Present (RT6.1)	Present (RT6.2)	Reduced (Rt-6)
NK cells	Increased	Not available	Unknown	Unknown
Polyglandular autoimmune diseases	Thyroiditis (+) Sjögren's syndrome (–)	Thyroiditis (–) Sjögren's syndrome (–)	Thyroiditis (–) Sjögren's syndrome (+)	Thyroiditis (±) Sjögren's syndrome (+)

*In offspring of diabetic parents, the incidence of diabetes is 64%; in offspring of a diabetic father and nondiabetic mother, it is 42%; and in offspring of a diabetic mother and nondiabetic father, it is 23.5%.

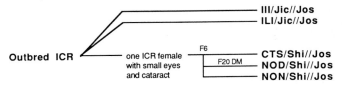

Fig. 18–3. Genealogy of the non-obese diabetic (NOD) mouse and several related strains: the Institute of Cancer Research (ICR) strains ICR-L-Ishibe (ILI) and ICR-I-Ishibe (III); the non-obese nondiabetic (NON) mouse; and the cataract Shionogi (CTS) mouse.

In the NOD mouse, IDDM develops secondary to the destruction of islet β-cells by infiltrating monocytic and lymphocytic cells (insulitis) (Plate I, A to D). Insulitis appears in animals as young as 5 weeks old. The lymphoid cells invade islets and often are seen adjacent to the ducts and blood vessels. The incidence of insulitis is 90% in NOD female mice and 70% in NOD male mice at 9 weeks of age. The incidence and degree of insulitis increase with age, resulting in β-cell destruction, loss of insulin secretion, hyperglycemia, a catabolic state, and ketosis similar to that seen in humans with uncontrolled IDDM. The female NOD mouse usually develops diabetes by the age of 6 months.

The incidence of diabetes varies depending on the colony. There are two sublines of the NOD mouse colony at Joslin (NOD/Shi//Jos). The high-incidence NOD subline shows a diabetes incidence of 90 to 100% in females and 50% in males. The medium-incidence NOD subline shows a diabetes incidence of 70 to 80% in NOD females and less than 20% in NOD males at 7 months of age. By comparison, the incidence of diabetes is less than 20% in NOD/Wehi females at the Walter and Eliza Hall Institute in Melbourne, Australia. These differences may be due to differences in diet, environment, or other features of each NOD subline.

Genealogy and Related Strains. The NOD mouse was originally derived from outbred mice from the Institute of Cancer Research (ICR).[185] Figure 18–3 shows the genealogy of the NOD mouse and several related strains: the ICR mice ICR-L-Ishibe (ILI) and ICR-I-Ishibe (III), the non-obese nondiabetic (NON) mouse, and the cataract Shionogi (CTS) mouse. One mouse with cataracts and small eyes was found in outbred ICR mice at Shionogi Pharmaceutical Company in Japan,

and an inbred cataract Shionogi (CTS) strain characterized by cataracts and microphthalmia was established.[186] Since cataracts often are observed in diabetic patients, two sublines were separated at the sixth generation, according to fasting blood glucose levels, during the process of establishing the CTS strain. The subline with euglycemia (fasting blood glucose level ~100 mg/dL) eventually became the NOD strain, whereas the subline with slight hyperglycemia (fasting blood glucose level ~150 mg/dL) eventually became the NON strain. The ILI mouse and the III mouse are inbred and derived directly from outbred ICR mice.

Clinical Course of IDDM. The NOD mouse develops insulitis as early as 5 weeks of age and IDDM as early as 2 months of age. The animals develop clinical symptoms such as polyuria, glycosuria, and weight loss. The clinical signs include hyperglycemia, increased hemoglobin A_1 (glycosylated hemoglobin), and a deficit of intrinsic insulin secretion. Diabetic animals are easily found by checking for wet bedding, glycosuria (with a test tape), leanness, and dark tail vein (increased HbA_1). The animals are diagnosed as diabetic by the continued presence of glycosuria and hyperglycemia (250 mg of glucose/dL). The diabetic animals usually can survive 3 to 4 weeks without insulin treatment and then develop ketosis.

Control of Blood Glucose Levels in Diabetic Mice with Insulin. Hyperglycemia is one of the major risks contributing to the development of diabetic nephropathy. Therefore, it is important to monitor or control the level of hyperglycemia during insulin treatment. Diabetic NOD mice in the Joslin colony are treated with insulin (a 1:1 mixture of regular and NPH insulin) injected subcutaneously twice a day (7:30 a.m. and 4:00 p.m.). The dose of insulin can be determined prior to each insulin injection according to the degree of glycosuria (grade of glycosuria, insulin dose: − to ±, 0 U; + to ++, 0.5 U; +++, 1.0 U). Table 18–3 shows random glucose and HbA_1 measurements in diabetic animals with and without insulin treatment.

It is also possible to use intensive insulin treatment in some diabetic NOD mice. In this protocol, blood glucose levels are measured before insulin is injected and the dose is adjusted accordingly (blood glucose level, insulin dose: 200 to 300 mg/dL, 0.5 U; 301 to >500 mg/dL, 1.0 U; 500 mg/dL, 1.5 U). A mixture of regular and NPH insulin (1:1) is used for the injection at 7:30 a.m., and only NPH

Table 18–3. Hemoglobin A_1 Levels in Diabetic NOD Mice with and without Insulin Treatment

Mice (n)	Age at HbA_1 assay (mo)	Duration of Diabetes at HbA_1 assay (wk)	HbA_1 (%)	Blood Glucose (mg/dL)
Diabetic NOD				
Insulin (9)	7.0 ± 0.9	6.0 ± 1.5	6.4 ± 0.5*	370 ± 27*
No insulin (6)	5.8 ± 0.7	4.7 ± 0.4	9.2 ± 0.5*	439 ± 26*†
Nondiabetic NOD (6)	3.9 ± 0.7	—	3.3 ± 0.2	73 ± 4
C57BL/6 (4)	6–7	—	3.6 ± 0.1	120 ± 2

Values are mean ± SEM.
*$P < .002$ (Student's t-test, two-tailed).
†Two of the six mice showed blood glucose levels of >500 mg/dL (the upper limit of the glucometer).

insulin is used for the injection at 4:00 p.m. With this intensive regimen, a diabetic NOD mouse showed a decrease in the HbA_1 level from 8.8 to 3.4% in 5 weeks. Although it requires an extensive effort to maintain the HbA_1 levels within a normal range, this intensive regimen provides an approach to the study of the effects of diabetes control on susceptibility to diabetic nephropathy.

Glucose Tolerance Test. Glucose tolerance in diabetic and nondiabetic NOD mice usually is assessed by an intraperitoneal glucose tolerance test (GTT) (Table 18–4). Prior to the GTT, the animals are fasted overnight and given water ad libitum. Overnight fasting brings blood glucose levels to approximately 100 mg/dL (5.6 mM) in nondiabetic animals. A 5% glucose solution (1 to 2 mg of glucose per gram of body weight) is then injected intraperitoneally. Blood samples are collected at 0, 30, 60, 120 and 180 minutes after the injection from the retro-orbital plexus of animals lightly anesthetized with ether or methoxyflurane. Blood glucose levels can be measured by the glucose oxidase method. Some nondiabetic NOD female mice show glucose levels higher than those in other nondiabetic NOD mice 30 and 60 minutes after glucose administration. This impaired glucose tolerance usually precedes by days the development of overt diabetes. Strandell and associates have observed clearly such a disturbance in intravenous glucose tolerance in nondiabetic 12- to 13-week-old NOD mice.[187]

Insulitis and T Cells. Infiltration of the islets of Langerhans by lymphoid and monocytic cells (insulitis) is a well-recognized feature of Type I diabetes both in humans[188] and in rodents with spontaneous diabetes.[185,189] This insulitis lesion indicates a cell-mediated immune process is responsible for the destruction of islet β-cells.

Studies by Harada and Makino indicate that T cells play an important role in the development of insulitis and diabetes.[190] Nude NOD mice that receive splenocytes from adult NOD mice will develop insulitis but not diabetes. Administration of human interleukin (IL)-2 following the transfer of the adult NOD splenocytes can induce diabetes in nude NOD mice. By contrast, antibody to IL-2 receptor suppresses the development of insulitis in NOD mice.[191] Wicker and associates have demonstrated the successful transfer of diabetes from diabetic NOD mice into irradiated young NOD mice by the injection of splenocytes.[192] More recent studies suggest that induction of insulitis and diabetes in NOD mice is mediated by $CD4^+$ (L3T4, helper/inducer) T cells[193] and $CD4^+$ and $CD8^+$ (suppressor/cytotoxic) T cells.[194]

T-Cell Clones and T-Cell Receptor Function in Development of Insulitis and Diabetes. The T-cell receptor (TcR) consists of two polypeptide chains, α and β, and is responsible for recognition of antigen associated with major histocompatibility complex (MHC). The variable region of the β chain of TcR ($TcR V_\beta$) constitutes the major component leading to diversity in immune recognition. In T cell-mediated immune processes, the immune responses to self-antigens are dependent on certain combinations of MHC and $TcR V_\beta$ family.[195,196] The use of TcR in autoimmune mice differs from that of normal mice, a difference suggesting that only certain TcR may be selected for autoimmunity. Restricted TcR usage has been reported in some T cell-dependent autoimmune diseases. For example, the $TcR V_\beta8$ is used preferentially in experimental allergic encephalomyelitis[195] and systemic lupus erythematosus-like disease in MRL-*lpr/lpr* lupus mice.[197]

Haskins and associates established islet-specific $CD4^+$ T-cell clones from the splenic lymphocytes of the diabetic NOD mice and succeeded in inducing insulitis in young NOD mice and in irradiated F_1 (CBA×NOD) mice and diabetes in the NOD mice by transferring the T-cell clones.[198,199] F_1 (CBA×NOD) mice do not develop insulitis and diabetes. These islet-specific T-cell clones are $CD4^+$ T cells but do not bear antigen receptors of any particular $TcR V_\beta$ type. Nakano et al. established five islet-reactive $CD4^+$ T-cell clones from islet-infiltrating T cells.[200] All clones are $CD4^+$ but not $CD8^+$. Like the T-cell clones established by Haskins and associates, in these clones the usage of TcR V and J segments is not restricted, but rather diverse. The islet-reactive T-cell clones can transfer insulitis into I-E transgenic NOD mice that are disease-resistant. The NOD mouse lacks MHC class II I-E molecules,[2] and the development of insulitis can be prevented by expressing I-E molecules with a transgene.[201]

Shizuru et al. recently reported that intercross animals (F_1) of BC2[(NOD×SWR)×NOD] develop insulitis and diabetes regardless of homozygosity or heterozygosity for SWR TcR usage.[202] SWR mice have an extensive deletion of $TcR V_\beta$ gene segments ($TcR V_\beta$5, 8, 9, 11, 12, and 13).

Table 18–4. Blood Glucose Levels During the Intraperitoneal Glucose Tolerance Test in 4-Month-Old Diabetic and Nondiabetic NOD Mice and ILI Female Mice

Strain	Body Weight (kg)	Mean Glucose Level ± SEM (mg/dL) at Indicated Time (min)				
		0	30	60	120	180
NOD						
Diabetic	22.5 ± 0.8	343 ± 58	502 ± 83	549 ± 46	540 ± 61	497 ± 79
Nondiabetic	22.6 ± 0.4	71 ± 5	126 ± 6	118 ± 2	112 ± 6	101 ± 4
[F5280]*	23.5	91	419	228	127	110
[F5281]*	21.2	115	195	177	125	120
ILI	32.1 ± 1.6	84 ± 9	138 ± 9	99 ± 5	89 ± 8	Not tested

Each group included 4 to 15 animals.
*These two mice developed overt diabetes 2 days after the glucose tolerance test.

McDuffie made a similar observation in the intercross animals of BC2[(NOD×C57L/J)×NOD].[203] These observations suggest that 1) the inductive pathologic T cells may not demonstrate predominant TcR V_β gene usage, 2) initiation of the diabetogenic events in NOD mice may depend on the utilization by T cells of particular V_β gene segments shared by both V_β^{nod} and V_β^{swr} or V_β^{c57l}, and 3) in NOD mice, disease is indeed triggered by the use by T cells of a TcR V_β gene segment(s) that maps within the region deleted in the V_β^{swr} haplotype (such as $V_\beta 5$ or $V_\beta 8$), but NOD V_β^{swr} and V_β^{c57l4} mice (BC$_2$-F$_1$), in the absence of this gene segment, might compensate for the deletion(s) by shifting V_β usage without affecting recognition of the autoantigen.[203]

Genetic Susceptibility to Diabetes.

MHC-Linked Diabetogenic Gene(s). The development of diabetes is controlled by at least two, and probably more, genes.[2,204] Environmental factors such as viruses, diet, and hormones also can influence the development of diabetes. One of the recessive diabetogenic genes is tightly linked to the MHC on chromosome 17.[2,204] With the use of a panel of monoclonal antibodies and restriction fragment length polymorphism (RFLP) analysis, it has been shown that the NOD mouse possesses a recombinant MHC class I (K^d, D^b: H-2^g) and unique MHC class II molecules. There is no expression of surface I-E molecules because of the absence of messenger RNA for I-E$_\alpha$.[3] Sequence studies indicate that the I-A$_\beta$ chain in NOD mice is also unique.[205] The amino acid residue at position 57 of the I-A$_\beta$ chain is serine in NOD mice and aspartic acid in nondiabetic inbred laboratory mouse strains. It is suggested that the unique sequence of the I-A$_\beta$ allele in NOD mice makes them susceptible to diabetes.

Breeding studies in crosses of NOD mice with C57BL/6 [B6(I-E$_\alpha$ of d)] transgenic mice expressing I-E suggest that I-E$_\alpha$ gene expression prevents the development of insulitis.[201] Recent studies of transgenic mice indicate that introduction of normal I-A$_\alpha$ and I-A$_\beta$ of k into NOD mice can prevent the development of insulitis.[206-208] These studies indicate that both the unique I-A molecules and the lack of I-E expression in NOD mice are essential for the development of insulitis and diabetes.

Incidence of Diabetes and Insulitis in F$_1$ and Back- *cross Animals of NOD and Nondiabetic Inbred Strains.* To determine the number of genes that contribute to the development of diabetes in NOD mice, we studied the inheritance of insulitis and diabetes in backcrosses of NOD with NON, BALB/c, C3H/He, and C57BL/6 mice. NOD males were mated with nondiabetic females to produce F$_1$ animals, and the F$_1$ animals were mated with NOD mice reciprocally to produce backcrosses. The backcrosses were screened for the development of diabetes over a 1-year period. Nondiabetic backcross animals were examined for histologic evidence of insulitis. In the NOD/Shi//Jos colony, the incidence of diabetes is 70 to 80% in NOD females and less than 20% in NOD males at 12 months of age. As shown in Table 18–5, the incidence of diabetes was 0% in the F$_1$, 12.1 to 15.6% in female backcross, and 1.7 to 3.4% in male backcross offspring of NOD with NON, BALB/c, and C3H/He females. These data on incidence of diabetes indicate that two (or three) recessive genes contribute to the development of diabetes in NOD mice. Female backcross offspring of NOD with C57BL/6 mice had a 3.3% incidence of diabetes, and none of the male backcross and F$_1$ animals developed diabetes, indicating suppression of the development of diabetes.

The incidence of insulitis over a 1-year period in backcrosses of NOD with NON, BALB/c, and C3H/He mice was 42 to 50%. Among the F$_1$ animals, none developed insulitis. The incidence of insulitis suggests that a single recessive non-MHC gene determines the development of insulitis regardless of MHC haplotypes. The incidence of insulitis among backcrosses of NOD with C57BL/6 was 24%—half the incidence in the other backcross groups, a decrease indicating a suppressed development of insulitis. Female offspring of backcrosses of NOD with C57BL/6 mice show a lower incidence of insulitis (24%) and diabetes (3.3%) than female offspring of backcrosses of NOD with NON, BALB/c, and C3H/He. The present data suggest that two genes for susceptibility and one gene for resistance contribute to susceptibility to IDDM in the NOD mouse.

Primary Destruction of Islet β-Cells Caused by Single Recessive "Non-MHC" and Enhancement of Immune Reaction by an MHC-Linked Diabetogenic Gene. Insulitis in offspring of the backcross of NOD mice with NON,

Table 18–5. Incidence of Diabetes and Insulitis at 12 Months of Age in F$_1$ and Backcross Animals of NOD Mice with Nondiabetic Laboratory Mouse Strains

| Cross | Sex | Diabetes (%) | | Insulitis (%) | |
		F$_1$	Backcross to NOD	F$_1$	Backcross to NOD
NON×NOD	F	0	12.1	0	50
	M	0	3.4	—	50
BALB/c×NOD	F	0	12.1	0	42
	M	0	2.0	—	—
C3H/He×NOD	F	0	15.6	0	48
	M	0	1.7	—	—
C57BL/6×NOD	F	0	3.3	0	24
	M	0	0	—	—

C3H/He, BALB/c, and ILI mice is controlled by a single recessive non-MHC diabetogenic gene regardless of homozygosity or heterozygosity of the NOD MHC.[209] In first-backcross animals of [(NOD×NON)F$_1$×NOD], all diabetic animals are homozygous for the NOD MHC. One-half of the nondiabetic backcross offspring develop insulitis regardless of the homozygosity or heterozygosity of the MHC, an observation indicating that one-half of the nondiabetic backcross animals possess a non-MHC diabetogenic gene. Among the nondiabetic backcross mice with insulitis, the number of islets with insulitis is higher in the animals homozygous for the NOD MHC than in the animals heterozygous for NOD/NON MHC. Furthermore, the relative volume and the absolute islet mass of the undamaged islets is smaller in the MHC homozygous animals than in the heterozygous animals. These observations suggest more severe islet damage in the animals homozygous for NOD MHC. Nondiabetic backcross mice without insulitis lack the non-MHC diabetogenic gene and have well-conserved intact islets.

The exact site(s) of the non-MHC-linked gene(s) is uncertain. Prochazka et al. reported a Thy 1-linked diabetogenic gene (*idd-2*) on chromosome 9 in animals from the backcross of NOD with NON.[210] Todd et al., Garchon et al., and Cornall et al. have recently reported that the non-MHC diabetogenic genes are located on chromosomes 3 and 11[211] and chromosome 1[212,213] (Table 18–6).

Is a Unique Antigenic Determinant a Target on Islet β-Cells of the NOD Mouse? To determine whether any of the diabetogenic loci exert their effects through the immune system, the islets, or both, Wicker and associates constructed irradiated bone marrow chimeric F$_1$(NOD×B10) mice that were reconstituted with NOD bone-marrow cells.[214] The majority of the recipient animals developed insulitis, and 21% of the mice developed diabetes. The irradiated F$_1$(NOD×B10) reconstituted animals not only developed insulitis and diabetes but also rejected β-cells within pancreas transplants from newborn B10 mice. In contrast, unmanipulated F$_1$ mice or irradiated F$_1$ mice reconstituted with F$_1$ or B10 bone marrow did not display insulitis or diabetes. These data demonstrate that expression of the diabetic phenotype in

Table 18–6. Type I Diabetogenic Genes of the NOD Mouse

MHC-linked gene(s)
  idd-1: MHC-linked gene on chromosome 17
    MHC class II: Unique I-AB, lack of I-E molecules
    The exact localization of the MHC-linked diabetogenic gene(s) is still unknown
Non-MHC-linked genes
  idd-2: Thy-1-linked gene on chromosome 9
  idd-3 on chromosome 3 implicated in development of insulitis
  idd-4 on chromosome 11 implicated in aging factor for development of diabetes
  idd-5 on chromosome 1 implicated in development of peri-insulitis, insulitis, and diabetes

---

Recent reports have suggested that MHC class I is also important for the development of diabetes. The existence of a Thy-1-linked gene (on chromosome 11) in humans with Type I diabetes has been excluded.

the NOD mouse is dependent on NOD-derived hematopoietic stem cells. Similar experiments performed with F$_1$(NOD×NON) mice suggested that diabetogenic genes in the NOD mouse do not function at the level of the insulin-producing β-cells.[215] Thus, there appears to be no unique antigen expressed on islet β cells of the NOD mouse as compared with the β-cells of nondiabetic mouse strains. Several other studies suggest that β-cells of the NOD mouse are not antigenically unique. For example, when bone marrow cells from diabetic NOD mice were transferred into diabetes-resistant NOD mice with B10 or NON F$_1$ hybrids, the recipient animals developed insulitis and diabetes. However, these F$_1$ hybrids always carry the genetic background of the NOD mouse. In another report, when bone marrow cells from diabetic NOD mice were transferred into nondiabetic and MHC-incompatible mice (C57BL/6 and B10.BR strains), the recipient mice developed insulitis. Ihm and colleagues recently presented evidence that neonatal islets of BB rats do not express the same target antigens as adult islets transplanted into diabetic BB rats.[216] This suggests that islet cells also contribute to the susceptibility to Type I diabetes; however, it is still unclear exactly how islet cells contribute to the susceptibility to autoimmune Type I diabetes.

To pursue the same question, we transferred bone narrow cells from diabetic NOD mice into irradiated ILI mice. The ILI mice and the NOD mice are MHC identical from the K through D regions (serologic typing). The irradiated ILI mice that received the NOD bone marrow cells developed insulitis and diabetes.[217] However, the bone marrow cells from 3-week-old NOD mice failed to induce diabetes in the irradiated ILI mice, although insulitis appears in NOD mice as young as 4 to 5 weeks old. Likewise, Wicker et al.[192] found that splenic lymphocytes from diabetic NOD mice did not induce diabetes in young NOD mice (<6 week of age). This does not appear to be due to insufficient expression of antigenic determinants on islet β-cells in the young NOD mice.[198] Splenic lymphocytes from 3-week-old NOD mice also fail to induce diabetes in 12-week-old irradiated NOD mice. These observations suggest that β-cells of the NOD mouse express a unique antigenic determinant as a target for the autoimmune response.

Autoantibodies to Islet β-Cells. The NOD mouse spontaneously develops autoimmune Type I diabetes. Consequent to this observation, several autoantibodies were found in the sera from the NOD mouse. These autoantibodies are useful markers for predicting the development of diabetes and identifying a target antigen(s) in the β-cell destruction.

Cytoplasmic Islet Cell Antibodies. Cytoplasmic islet cell antibodies (ICAs) are markers for autoimmune β-cell destruction in human IDDM.[218] High titers of ICAs have been observed in over 60% of patients with new-onset Type I diabetes and in approximately 5% of initially nondiabetic first-degree relatives of patients with Type I diabetes. The presence of ICAs in NOD mice has been reported in studies using Bouin's-fixed pancreatic tissues[219,220] but not in those using frozen pancreatic tissues. Bouin's fixation may alter the antigenic properties of islet tissues. The properties of the islet cell antigen and antigens for ICA on frozen sections are not fully understood. The autoantigens on frozen sections have the properties of a sialic acid-containing glycolipid.[221]

Antibodies to Glutamic Acid Decarboxylase. Antibodies to an islet β-cell glycoprotein with a molecular weight of 64,000 (64-kd relative molecular mass) have been found in approximately 70% of patients with new-onset Type I diabetes.[222] The enzyme glutamic acid decarboxylase (GAD) has been identified as the antigen to the 64-kd glycoprotein.[223] Autoantibodies to the 64-kd autoantigen have been found in NOD mice[224] and BB rats,[225] precede the onset of diabetes, and disappear within weeks after the onset of diabetes. The 64-kd protein is now recognized to be GAD and has been proposed as a potential autoantigen in humans, as well in animals with autoimmune diabetes.[223,225]

Other Autoantibodies. Autoantibodies to insulin are detectable in patients with newly diagnosed diabetes before they are treated with insulin.[226] NOD mice also produce low levels of autoantibodies to insulin.[227]

Elias et al.[228] and Cohen[229] have reported that a β-cell target antigen in NOD mice is cross-reactive with the 65-kd heat-shock protein (hsp65) of *Mycobacterium tuberculosis.* The onset of β-cell destruction is associated with the spontaneous development of anti-hsp65 T lymphocytes. Subsequently, hsp65 cross-reactive antigen becomes detectable in the sera of the prediabetic mice.

Boitard and associates detected autoantibodies to a 58-kd islet cell antigen in NOD mice but not in other strains, including lupus-prone mice.[230] The 58-kd antigen was found to be expressed only by neuroblastoma cells and was identified as peripherin. This autoantigen cross-reacted with I-A^{nod} class II antigens, suggesting that it contributed to defective self-tolerance of islet β-cells in the NOD mouse.

Role of Macrophages and Cytokines in Islet β-Cell Destruction. The cells infiltrating into the islets of the NOD mouse consist of T cells (~50%), macrophages (18%), plasma cells (3%), and unidentified cells—possibly natural killer (NK) cells (25%). In addition to the role of the T cell discussed above, recent studies indicate that macrophages also may play an important role in the initiation of islet β-cell destruction. Silica particles selectively inhibit macrophage function in vivo[231] and have been shown to prevent the development of diabetes in BB rats.[232] Administration of silica particles prevents the development of insulitis and diabetes in NOD mice.[233,234] Administration of monoclonal antibody to the adhesion-promoting receptor on macrophages also prevents the development of diabetes.[225]

Macrophages appear to exert their functions in at least two ways: as antigen-presenting cells and as effector cells. An antigen(s) on islet β-cells may be processed by macrophages and presented to CD4$^+$ helper T cells in an MHC-restricted manner.[236] After antigen presentation by the macrophages, the CD4$^+$ helper T cells may be activated by the antigen-presenting cells and secrete cytokines such as IL-1[237,238] and tumor necrosis factor (TNF)[239] and lymphokines such as INF-γ, resulting in

activation of macrophages.[240] Activated macrophages may secrete IL-1 and produce free-radical oxygen.[241] IL-1, TNF, and INF-γ have synergistically cytotoxic effects on islet cells in vitro.[242] In addition, IL-1 can impair the islet β-cell activity in vitro.[243,244]

Polyglandular Autoimmunity and Other Complications. The NOD mouse develops lymphoid cell infiltration of the salivary, lacrimal, and parotid glands resembling human Sjögren's syndrome. The cell infiltration in these organs is not linked to the MHC. A high frequency of thyroiditis in the NOD mouse has also been reported.[245] This may be subline-specific, since thyroiditis is rarely seen in the NOD/Shi colony (Susumu Makino, personal communication).

The NOD mouse develops renal lesions that consist of diffuse mesangial sclerosis associated with glomerular hypertrophy, thickening of glomerular basement membrane, accumulation of type IV collagen in mesangial areas, and the development of albuminuria[246] (Plate I, E and F). These findings closely mimic those in human diabetic patients. The lesions of glomerulosclerosis are detected even in nondiabetic NOD adult mice but are not seen in 3-week-old NOD mice. The degree of the glomerular lesion, however, is much less pronounced in nondiabetic NOD mice than in diabetic NOD mice. The NOD mouse provides a model for investigating the pathogenesis of the early events of diabetic glomerulosclerosis. Diabetic NOD mice also develop muscular atrophy, diarrhea, abnormal gas production in the intestine, and atrophy of upper and lower extremities.

Control Animals. Several different mice have been used as controls for the NOD mouse, including the ICR, NON, ILI, and NOD congenic mice. The NOD mouse is derived from outbred ICR mice that have a heterogeneous genetic background. The NON mouse is a sister strain of the NOD mouse but is not MHC-identical. The NON mouse tends to become obese and develops impaired glucose tolerance (Fig. 18–4) and lipoprotein glomerulopathy (Plate I, G).[247,248] The ILI mouse is serologically MHC-identical to the NOD mouse and does not develop insulitis and diabetes.

Induction of Diabetes in Mice by Transgenes

Overexpression of MHC Class I and II Molecules and INF-γ in Islets. Since IDDM is an autoimmune disease secondary to islet β-cell destruction by infiltrating immune cells, it has been postulated that aberrant expression of MHC class II molecules on islet β-cells may stimulate this autoimmune attack on β-cell antigens. Although the significance of the aberrant expression of MHC class II molecules is unclear, it is speculated that the MHC class II expression could cause presentation of islet antigens to CD4 T cells (helper T cells) and initiate β-cell destruction. Islet β-cells do not express MHC class II molecules in healthy human subjects and animals. Patients with newly diagnosed Type I diabetes have been found to have aberrant expression of MHC class II molecules on the surface of islet β-cells fixed in formalin.[249] However, the aberrant expression of the MHC class II molecules on islet β-cells appears to be a rare

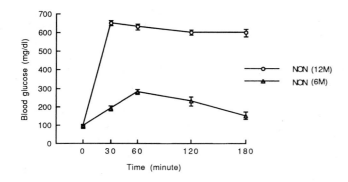

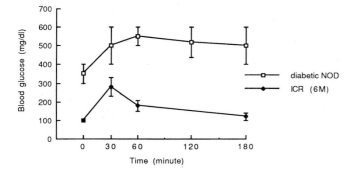

Fig. 18–4. Glucose tolerance test in non-obese nondiabetic (NON), non-obese diabetic (NOD), and control ICR mice at 6 and 12 months of age. Glucose solution (5%, 1 mg/g body weight) was given intraperitoneally. Animals were fasted overnight before the test.

phenomenon in fresh-frozen pancreas.[250] MHC class II molecules also are detectable on islet β-cells of NOD pancreases fixed in Bouin's solution,[220] while the molecules are undetectable on the β-cells of fresh-frozen NOD pancreases.[251] Thus, it is still controversial whether the NOD mouse expresses MHC class II molecules on islet β-cells during the development of diabetes.

As a means of testing whether aberrant expression of MHC class II molecules stimulates the autoimmune process in islet β-cell destruction, transgenic mice that express MHC class II molecules on β-cells have been generated with the use of a hybrid gene with the rat insulin gene II as promoter and the structural part of the MHC genes. The murine MHC molecules consist of class I K and D (HLA-A, B, and C in humans) and class II I-A (HLA-DQ) and I-E (HLA-DR). Hybrid gene fragments of rat insulin gene II and MHC-K gene,[252] MHC-A gene,[253] and MHC-E gene[254] have been used. The transgenic progeny showed overexpression of the MHC class I-K and class II I-A and I-E molecules on islet β-cells. Diabetes was found in 100% of transgenic progeny. However, histologic examination revealed no evidence of insulitis lesions in the three transgenic mouse strains at any time during the development of diabetes, suggesting a nonimmune mechanism. Instead, islet cells were degranulated, had pleomorphic nuclei, and were unevenly distributed.[253] Furthermore, the transgenic mice acquired tolerance to the transgene I-E molecules despite the

absence of expression of I-E in the thymus or any other lymphoid tissues, also suggesting a nonimmune mechanism.[254] One possible explanation for the dysfunction of β-cells is that the presence of large amounts of MHC molecules might interfere physically with insulin secretory machinery.

Sarvetnick and associates produced transgenic mice with the INF-γ gene.[253] The transgenic mice expressing INF-γ in islet β-cells developed diabetes and severe lymphocytic infiltration of islets. This is one of the few transgenic models that appears to have an "autoimmune" type of diabetes.

BB Rat

The BioBreeding (BB) rat develops IDDM resembling human Type I diabetes spontaneously secondary to islet β-cell destruction by infiltrating immune cells.[255,256] The BB rat develops hyperglycemia, lack of intrinsic insulin secretion, glycosuria, ketosis, and weight loss. The incidence of diabetes is 40 to 80%, depending on the family lines and environmental factors at individual colonies. The University of Massachusetts colony of BB/Wor rats is made up of diabetes-prone (DP) and diabetes-resistant (DR) family lines. These lines have been raised by brother-sister matings and have reached more than the 30th generation.[257] The cumulative incidence of diabetes is 40 to 80% in the DP-BB rats and is less than 1% in the DR-BB rats.[257,258] Eighty-five percent of the diabetic DP-BB rats show the symptoms by 120 days of age.[259] The DP-BB rat has T-cell lymphopenia[260–262] with reduced levels of CD4+ (helper/inducer) T cells and near or complete absence of both the CD8+ (suppressor/cytotoxic) T-cell and RT6+ (differentiation alloantigen) T-cell subsets.[263] The DR-BB rat is histocompatible with the DP-BB rat and has normal numbers of all lymphocyte phenotypes, including the RT6+ subset.[257] Although the DP-BB rat has lymphocytopenia, one of the diabetic BB/Wor lines develops diabetes but is not lymphopenic (nonlymphopenic diabetic, NLD). The diabetic W-line (NLD) rats possess normal percentages of phenotypic T-cell subsets.[264] The incidence of diabetes, however, is less than 3% in the diabetic W-line. The characteristics of the BB and NLD rat are listed in Table 18–2. An outstanding review of the BB rat by Crisa et al. contains most of the latest information.[265]

Genetic Susceptibility.

MHC-linked Diabetogenic Gene. The major histocompatibility complex of the rat is referred to as the RT1 complex and consists of class I antigens (RT1A, RT1E, RT1C) and class II antigens (RT1B and RT1D).[266] RT1B and RT1D are identical to the mouse I-A and I-E, respectively. The RT1 complex of the BB rat is *u* haplotype (RT1u/u). Breeding studies of the BB rat with the Lewis rat (RT1l/l) and Buffalo rat (RT1b/b) showed that all the diabetic offspring in the F₂ generation carried at least one *u* haplotype.[267,268]

MHC class II *u* alleles of several origins can contribute the permissive MHC genetic susceptibility. MHC class II *u* alleles derived from a non-BB-related strain (RT1BuDu) are permissive for the development of diabetes, indicating that the diabetogenic potential is not restricted to the BB-derived class II genes.[269,270] A normal MHC class II *u* allele product is responsible for the MHC association of diabetes in the BB rat. As noted above, it has been postulated that the identity of amino acid residue 57 of the β-chain of I-A in the NOD mouse and DQ in human Type I diabetes confers risk or protection from diabetes depending on whether it is aspartic acid (protective) or some other amino acid (high risk).[205,271] The codon 57 theory, however, does not apply to the BB rat.[272] The Wistar-Furth (WF) rat and the Yoshida rat are MHC-compatible with the BB rat and often are used as control strains.

Non-MHC-Linked Diabetogenic Gene. In the BB rat, insulitis occurs before overt diabetes and can be seen in the F_1 generation of crosses between diabetic and nondiabetic strains.[273] The insulitis trait appears to be independent of the MHC and behaves as a Mendelian dominant.

The DP-BB rat has severe lymphopenia characterized by a substantial reduction in W3/25[+] (CD5[+]) helper/inducer T cells and a nearly complete absence of OX8[+] (CD8[+]) cytotoxic/suppressor T cells. The relative number of OX19[−]/OX8[+] T cells, however, is increased in the DP-BB rat, suggesting that NK cells are relatively over-represented.[274] The T-cell lymphopenia of the BB rat also segregates independently of the MHC. Linkage studies to assign the lymphopenia gene are under way.

Regulatory Role of RT6[+] T-Cell Subset in Pathogenesis of Diabetes.

Absence of RT6.1[+] T Cells in DP-BB Rats. As described above, the BB rat colony at the University of Massachusetts has been bred into diabetes-prone (DP) and diabetes-resistant (DR) subgroups. The diabetes-prone BB/Wor rats lack the RT6[+] peripheral T-cell subset, whereas the diabetes-resistant BB/Wor rats have normal numbers of RT6[+] T-cells.[275] The RT6 alloantigenic system consists of two known antigens, RT6.1 and RT6.2[276] and is not linked to the MHC.[277,278] Approximately 50% of W3/25[+] (CD4, helper/inducer) and 70% of OX8[+] (CD8) peripheral T cells express RT6.[279] Lymphocyte transfusion from RT6.1[+] DR or WF rats protects RT6-deficient DP-BB rats from diabetes.[280] In vivo depletion of RT6.1[+] T cells in 30-day-old DR-BB rats induces diabetes in approximately 50% of the treated animals within 2 to 4 weeks and removes the cell population capable of protecting DP-BB rats from diabetes in lymphocytic transfusion experiments.[281] Thus, RT6[+] T cells play an important regulatory role in the pathogenesis of IDDM in BB/Wor rats.

Absence of RT6[+] T Cells in DP-BB Rats Caused by Genetic and Cell Developmental Defects. Although DP-BB rats lack RT6[+] T-cells, they possess the RT6 gene (RT6[a]). T cells from DP-BB rats fail to express RT6 antigen during ontogeny.[258] The genetic basis for the lack of RT6[+] T cells in DP-BB rats was investigated by generating three combinations of F_1 hybrids between DP-BB (RT6[−]), DR-BB (RT6.1[+]), and WF (RT6.2[+]) rats. On the basis of studies of expression of the RT6.1 and RT6.2 antigens in the T cells from lymph nodes from the F_1, Angelillo et al.[282] concluded that the DP-BB rat has the RT6.1 (RT6[a]) and not the RT6.2 (RT6[b]) gene. The

absence of RT6[+] T cells in DP-BB rats is not due to the absence of a functional RT6 gene but to intrinsic defects in the development of prothymocytes into RT6[+] cells.

RT6.1 and RT6.2 molecules appear to be anchored to the cell membrane through a phosphatidylinositol linkage. Treatment with phosphatidylinositol-phospholipase C can release the molecules into solution.[283] RT6.1 molecules consist of a 24- to 26-kd nonglycosylated peptide plus at least five additional glycosylated polypeptides of 30 to 35 kd.[284] The RT6 gene is located on rat chromosome 1, which is equivalent to mouse chromosome 7. Rt-6 (homologous to rat RT-6) molecules are less expressed in the mature splenic T cells of the NOD mouse than in those of the NON mouse.[285]

Role of Natural Killer Cells in Islet β-Cell Destruction.
In addition to a role of regulatory T cells in the pathogenesis of islet β-cell destruction, studies of the effector phase have suggested that NK cells may play a role in β-cell destruction in the DP-BB rat. Treatment of DB-BB rats with monoclonal antibody (MAb) OX8, an antibody to the CD8 antigens expressed on the surface of cytotoxic/suppressor T cells and NK cells, or with MAb OX19, an antibody to CD5 that reduces all T-cell populations (NK cells and helper/inducer T-cells) prevents insulitis and thyroiditis.[286] Injections of MAbs W3/25 (anti-CD4), OX35 (CD4), and OX38 (CD4) to antigens expressed on the surface of helper/inducer T cells resulted in marginal protection against diabetes without a reduction in phenotypic subsets. The absence of cytotoxic/suppressor T cells and the results of in vivo injections of monoclonal antibodies suggest that islet β-cell destruction in the DP-BB rat is mediated by the combined action of NK and helper/inducer T cells. Treatment with anti-asialo GM1 (NK cell marker) also prevented the disease in the DP-BB rat.[274,287]

Complications.
The BB rat develops lymphocytic thyroiditis resembling human Hashimoto's thyroiditis[288,289] and testicular atrophy.[290] However, the BB rat does not develop the lymphocytic infiltration into the salivary, lacrimal, and parotid glands that is seen in the NOD mouse.

LETL Rat

The Long-Evans Tokushima Lean (LETL) rat develops polyuria, polyphagia, hyperglycemia, and a lack of intrinsic insulin secretion secondary to the destruction of islet β-cells by infiltrating lymphocytes (insulitis) resembling human type I diabetes.[291,292] The insulitis gradually regresses after the onset of diabetes. The infiltrating immune cells leave the insulitis lesion after completing β-cell destruction, and atrophic islets remain as in the NOD mouse and the BB rat. The animals have been raised by brother-sister matings and have reached more than the 20th generation. The incidence of diabetes averages 15 to 21% and is the same in both sexes. The mean time of diabetes onset after birth is 3 to 4 months. The incidence of diabetes depends on the mating conditions, and 64% of the offspring of diabetic parents, 14% of those of nondiabetic parents, 42% of those of a diabetic father and a nondiabetic mother, and 24% of those of a diabetic mother and a nondiabetic father are diabetic.

The Long-Evans Tokushima Otsuka (LETO) rat was established as a control strain from the same colony. The LETO rat does not develop diabetes and insulitis throughout the 20th generation. The LETL rat and the LETO rat are MHC-identical ($RT1.A^uH^uB^uD^u$). Of the 22 biochemical markers examined, only the Ahd-2 allele is different in the diabetic and the control rats ($Ahd-2^b$ in the LETL rat; $Ahd-2^c$ in the LETO rat).[291]

The most striking characteristic of this new animal model for Type I diabetes is the normal levels of all T cells and T-cell subpopulations, including helper/inducer and cytotoxic/suppressor T cells. Thus, the LETL rat is not lymphopenic at any time during the disease process.[292] Some of the characteristics of the LETL rat are listed in Table 18–2.

Genetics. Breeding studies of LETL with F344/Ducrj and WKAH/Hkm strains have been performed. In the F_1 generations of both these crosses, the incidence of insulitis was 0%. The incidence of insulitis was 3 to 6% in the F_2 generations and 6.6 to 26.3% in the first backcross generation.[292] These data suggest that at least two recessive genes are involved in the development of insulitis in the LETL rat.

Complications. The LETL rat develops infiltration of lymphoid cells into the salivary gland (21.4%) and lacrimal glands (30%) but not into the thyroid gland and reproductive organs. It does not develop glomerular lesions.

Chinese Hamster and Keeshond Dog

The Chinese hamster develops diabetes spontaneously.[293] The animals develop diabetes as early as 1 month of age and usually before 4 months of age. The cumulative incidence of glycosuria is close to 100% at 4 months of age. However, the incidence of severe diabetes is low. If 10 Chinese hamsters with severe ketoacidic diabetes are needed, a minimum of 500 animals must be produced.[294] It is still uncertain whether diabetes in the Chinese hamster is autoimmune Type I diabetes. The most notable change in the islets is degranulation of β-cells. Lymphocytic infiltration has occasionally been observed in islets of diabetic Chinese hamsters soon after the onset of diabetes. The diabetic Chinese hamsters in the Asahikawa colony show an incidence of insulitis of only 4%. The mode of genetic inheritance is autosomal recessive, and at least two genes contribute to the susceptibility.

The Keeshond dog develops IDDM spontaneously by 6 months of age. Insulinopenia is caused by hypoplasia of the islets. The remnant β-cells are without cytoplasmic vacuolation. There are no primary exocrine pancreatic lesions. The mode of genetic inheritance is autosomal recessive.[295]

Experimental Diabetes

Streptozotocin-Induced Diabetes

Streptozotocin is a naturally occurring nitrosoamide that has been used extensively to produce diabetes in experimental models.[296] In rodents, streptozotocin is cytotoxic to islet β-cells. A single large injection of streptozotocin (200 to 250 mg/kg body weight, intraperitoneally or intravenously) can induce diabetes in mice, rats, guinea pigs, hamsters, and rabbits within 1 to 7 days. Islet β-cell necrosis is detectable by electron microscopic examination after 2 to 4 hours and by light microscopic examination within 24 hours.[297] Streptozotocin alkylates DNA, resulting in the cessation of functions of islet β-cells, eventual cell death, and diabetes.[298] Islet β-cells are most sensitive to streptozotocin, presumably because of a glucose moiety in its structure.[299,300]

Multiple- and Low-Dose Injection of Streptozotocin. Multiple and low-dose injection of streptozotocin can cause β-cell destruction and insulitis leading to IDDM. Like and Rossini demonstrated that five daily intraperitoneal or intravenous injections of streptozotocin (40 mg/kg dissolved in a citrate buffer, pH 4.2, just before injection) induced diabetes in CD-1 male mice.[301] Plasma glucose concentrations were increased significantly after the fourth injection. Histologic examination revealed large numbers of lymphocytes, moderate numbers of macrophages, and rare neutrophils surrounding and permeating the islets, with distortion of the islet architecture and β-cell necrosis. Islet inflammation gradually diminished in animals killed 12, 16, and 25 days after the completion of injections, and the remaining islets were small and composed almost exclusively of α- and δ-cells. Ultrastructural studies of the islets revealed occasional necrotic β-cells and numerous infiltrating lymphocytes and macrophages and, unexpectedly, large numbers of type C virus particles within many intact, partially degranulated β-cells. Islet β- and δ-cells were normal. The pancreatic islets of uninjected mice and mice injected with citrate buffer appeared normal. Only an occasional virus particle was observed within the well-granulated β-cells. Viruses were not observed in the α- and δ-cells and in the inflammatory cells. The same dose schedule, route of the administration, and timing of sacrifice failed to produce similar lesions in Charles River rats despite their development of marked hyperglycemia after a single injection of a large dose of streptozotocin.

Although insulitis is present in the mouse with diabetes induced by low-dose streptozotocin, this diabetes should be distinguished from the autoimmune Type I diabetes seen in the BB rat, the LETL rat, and the NOD mouse. Splenocytes from male C57BL/6 mice with streptozotocin-induced diabetes fail to transfer diabetes into syngeneic recipients.[302] Furthermore, transplantation of C57BL/KsJ islets into C57BL/KsJ mice with streptozotocin-induced diabetes does not result in an autoimmune elimination of the transplanted islets.[303]

The susceptibility of animals to diabetes induced by multiple and low doses of streptozotocin is dependent on sex and strains. Male mice are more susceptible to diabetes. Male C57BL/KsJ mice are highly susceptible to diabetes. C57BL/6, A/J, AKR/J, BALB/cJ, CBA/J, C3H/HeJ, and DBA/2J show various degrees of resistance to insulitis and diabetes induced by multiple- and low-dose injections of streptozotocin.[304] The sensitivity to the diabetes is controlled by at least one non-MHC gene.[305,306]

Mechanism of Action of Streptozotocin in Diabetes. At least two models of the mechanism of streptozotocin induction of β-cell damage have been proposed.

Okamoto and co-workers have suggested that streptozotocin and alloxan break nuclear DNA strands of islet β-cells by generating free-radical oxygen.[298,299] The breakage of the DNA strands activates nuclear poly (adenosine diphosphate [ADP]-ribose) synthetase. This enzyme uses cellular nicotinamide adenine dinucleotide (NAD) as a source of ADP-ribose for DNA repair. The decline in cellular NAD concentration ultimately results in the death of the β-cells. The administration of inhibitors of poly (ADP-ribose) synthetase inhibitors such as nicotinamide and 3-aminobenzamide suppresses the consumption of NAD and consequently prevents the development of streptozotocin- and alloxan-induced diabetes.[307] A lethal concentration of streptozotocin and a nonlethal concentration of its nitrosoamide moiety methylnitrosourea alkylate the DNA of β-cells at the N7 position of guanine to the same extent and cause comparable amounts of DNA strand breakage. This finding suggests that factors in addition to the activation of poly (ADP-ribose) synthetase contribute to the specific toxicity of streptozotocin to β-cells.

Wilson and co-workers have proposed that streptozotocin alkylates not only DNA but also other key cellular components, such as glycolytic or mitochondrial enzymes necessary for the generation of adenosine triphosphate (ATP).[300] This decline in the generation of ATP would impair the resynthesis of NAD, causing the levels of this cellular component to drop below critical levels. In β-cells, which are very sensitive to the toxic effects of streptozotocin, many more of the reactive carbonium ions bind to protein.

Influence of Streptozotocin on the Immune System.

In studies of streptozotocin-induced diabetes, suppression of T-cell function associated with atrophy of the thymus and peripheral lymph lymphoid tissues are universal observations.[308,309] Direct toxic effects of streptozotocin on the immune system have been reported.[310-312] A large dose (250 mg) of streptozotocin can induce a brief inhibition of DNA synthesis in bone marrow and thymus, a transient selective depletion of circulating lymphocytes, and a transient selective depletion (CD8$^+$) of cortical thymocytes. Even a single subdiabetogenic dose (50 mg/kg body weight) depletes circulating thymocytes.

Viral Induction and Suppression of Diabetes

Type I diabetes is a multifactorial disease, and its development appears to be influenced by genetic and environmental factors. Viruses have been implicated in the pathogenesis of β-cell destruction in Type I diabetes. In the early studies on the association of viruses with diabetes, viruses were regarded as agents causing diabetes.[313] However, the appearance of animal models for spontaneous Type I diabetes, such as the BB rat and the NOD mouse raised under virus-free conditions, has changed the concept of the role of viruses in the development of Type I diabetes. Thus, viruses may be divided into two groups, those that induce or accelerate the development of Type I diabetes and those that suppress its development.

Viruses Inducing Type I Diabetes.

Extensive studies have shown that the development of virus-induced Type I diabetes in mice depends on the genetic background of the host and the genetic make-up of the virus[313-315] (Table 18–7). While the diabetes that develops spontaneously in the NOD mouse, the BB rat, and the LETL rat is permanent and severe, virus-induced diabetes is transient and mild in most mice.[313] For example, encephalomyocarditis virus multiplies in the islets of Langerhans after subcutaneous inoculation and promptly causes lesions of the β-cells. During the early stages of infection, these cells are degranulated and the pancreatic insulin concentrations decrease markedly. Hyperglycemia appears concomitantly. With persistence of the infection, a mononuclear cell infiltrate appears in and around the islets. The insulitis is transient and rarely observed after the second week of infection. Virus persists in detectable quantities in the islets for 2 to 3 weeks.[313] During the course of recovery from the viral infection, the individual animals show a variety of clinical courses. Some develop profound hyperglycemia and ketoacidosis; they lose weight and die several months after inoculation. Other animals exhibit chronic hyperglycemia of a less severe degree for extended periods and even diabetic nephropathy[316]; some of these animals recover after several months, apparently in response to the regeneration of islet tissues. Finally, a number of animals have normal fasting blood glucose levels and still exhibit impaired glucose tolerance. In addition to genetic susceptibility of the host strains and viral make-up, steroid hormones, obesity, and irradiation influence the severity of the β-cell damage in the infected animals.[313]

Reovirus type I can induce Type I diabetes in SJL/J mice. Reovirus-infected mice develop autoantibodies that react with antigens on the surface of islet cells, thymocytes, and a growth hormone-producing cell line.[317]

Table 18–7. Viruses Inducing and Suppressing Type I Diabetes and Animals Susceptible to These Effects

A. Mode of induction of islet damage
   1. Direct β-cell infection with virus
       M-variant of encephalomyocarditis (EMC) viruses: M variant is subdivided into D (diabetogenic) and B (nondiabetogenic) variants
       Variants of coxsackie B viruses
       Reoviruses
       Mengo virus
       Cytomegaloviruses
       Rubella
       Lymphocytic choriomeningitis virus (LCMV) in transgenic mice expressing viral antigens of LCMV glycoprotein and nucleoprotein on islet β-cells
   2. Immune cells infected with virus
       Kilham's rat virus in diabetes-resistant (DR)-BB rat
   3. Susceptible animals
       Mouse: SJK/J; C57BL/6-ob/ob; CD1; SWR/J; DBA/1J; DBA/2J
       Hamster: Golden Syrian hamsters
       Rabbit
B. Suppression of development of diabetes
   LCMV in BB rat and NOD mouse
   Pichinde virus, lactate dehydrogenase virus, vaccinia virus, Sendai virus, and mouse hepatitis virus in NOD mouse

Coxsackievirus B4 can induce type I diabetes in SJL/J and CD1 mice and increase expression of the 64-kd autoantigen in the islets, suggesting initiation or enhancement of an autoimmune reaction by this virus.[318]

It has been reported that lymphocytic choriomeningitis viruses (LCMV) (strains Armstrong 1371 and WE) cause abnormal glucose tolerance in BALB/Wehi mice[319] and C3H/St mice.[320] The islets from the virus-infected animals hypertrophy and secrete significantly more insulin than islets from uninfected mice. This abnormal glucose metabolism appears to be due to insulin resistance in the target tissues such as liver and muscle rather than to defects in islet cells. However, recent studies in which transgenic mice were produced that expressed viral antigens of LCMV glycoprotein and nucleoprotein on islet β-cells have demonstrated that LCMV infection induces severe autoimmune Type I diabetes mediated by CD8+ T cells.[321,322]

Mumps and rubella viruses have been implicated in the pathogenesis of Type I diabetes in humans. Human viruses have been shown to cause islet damage in laboratory animals that leads to impaired glucose tolerance. These viruses include Venezuelan encephalitis virus in hamsters and subhuman primates,[323] rubella viruses in infant rabbits[324] and neonatal hamsters,[325] reoviruses in infant mice,[326] and cytomegaloviruses in mice.[313] Reovirus infection increases expression of MHC class I molecules on human islet β-cells and rat RINm5F cells.[327] In addition to direct effects on β-cells, reovirus infection may contribute to β-cell destruction by increasing the expression of MHC class I molecules and therefore to reactivity of β-cells with cytotoxic T-cells.

Role of Viral Pathogens in Development of Diabetes in BB Rat.
Viruses have been implicated in the etiology of IDDM. Environmental pathogens, and probably viral pathogens, may modulate the immune system so as to exacerbate or dampen a genetically programmed process of target-cell destruction. The previous studies on the role of viruses in the development of diabetes have revealed that islet β-cells are directly infected and damaged by the viruses, resulting in diabetes and impaired glucose tolerance. Since facilities for maintaining virus antibody-free animals have become available, studies on the role of viruses have made remarkable progress, opening up a new vista on the pathogenesis of Type I diabetes in animal models, especially the BB rat.[328–330] Without having virus particles in their islet β-cells, virus-infected animals develop Type I diabetes.

Induction of Diabetes by Kilham's Rat Virus in DR-BB Rats. Evidence for a role of virus in the pathogenesis of diabetes in the BB rat became apparent when an outbreak of spontaneous diabetes among diabetes-resistant BB rats was found to coincide with serologic evidence of the onset of infection with Kilham's rat virus (KRV). The investigators followed these findings with an attempt to isolate the responsible viruses from the seropositive DR-BB rats. Viruses were isolated from the spleen, bone marrow, lymph nodes, and pancreases of several diabetic and nondiabetic DR rats and identified serologically as KRV. KRV infection reproducibly induced lymphocytic insulitis and diabetes in naive DR-BB rats.[328] No viral

antigen was identified in islet β-cells, and no β-cell cytolysis was seen until after lymphocytic insulitis was observed. KRV did not induce diabetes in MHC-concordant and MHC-discordant non-BB rats and did not accelerate onset of diabetes in DP-BB/Wor rats unless the rats had been reconstituted with spleen cells from DR-BB rats. There were no significant changes in the percentages of peripheral CD4+ and CD8+ T-cells or NK cells in the diabetic and control animals after infection with KRV. RT6.1+ lymph node cells also were unchanged.

Induction of Diabetes in DR-BB Rats by Increased Cytokines Caused by Viral Pathogens and Polyinosinic-Polycytidylic Acid. Polyinosinic-polycytidylic acid is known to increase levels of INF-α and to accelerate the onset of diabetes in DP-BB rats,[331] and viral infection increases levels of interferon. Injections of various cytokines (IL-1 and IL-2, INF-α, INF-γ) also alter the frequency and tempo of the diabetes syndrome.[242,243] Although depletion of the RT6.1+ T-cell population by administration of anti-RT6.1 has been shown to induce diabetes and thyroiditis in DR-BB rats,[281] this treatment did not induce diabetes in DR-BB rats seronegative for viral antibody. Administration of polyinosinic-polycytidylic acid was weakly effective in inducing diabetes in DR-BB rats. When both anti-RT6 and polyinosinic-polycytidylic acid were administered to seronegative DR-BB rats, nearly all animals became diabetic. Either agent alone induced diabetes in seropositive DR-BB rats (infected with Sendai virus, KRV, sialodacryoadenitis virus, and Toolan's H-1 virus). Administration of polyinosinic-polycytidylic acid produced a more rapid acceleration of the onset of diabetes in seropositive than in seronegative DR-BB rats despite its controversial effect in DP-BB rats.

Increase in Frequency and Tempo of Diabetes in DP-BB Rat under Viral Antibody-Free Conditions. Elimination of environmental viral pathogens (Sendai and sialodacryoadenitis viruses) has been found to increase the incidence and accelerate the tempo of diabetes development in DP-BB rats.[330,331] In contrast, seropositive DR-BB rats did not develop diabetes when raised under a viral antibody-free environment after cesarean delivery and depletion of RT6+ T cells. Germ-free conditions have also been reported to increase the frequency of diabetes in the NOD mouse in comparison to that seen under specific pathogen-free conditions.[332] However, this observation has not been confirmed in the original NOD/Shi colony under gnotobiotic and specific pathogen-free conditions (S. Makino, personal communication).

Suppression of Autoimmune Type I Diabetes by Viruses in NOD Mouse and BB Rat. Newborn and adult NOD mice infected with a variant of LCMV, called ARM 53b or clone 13, did not develop diabetes.[333] In most murine strains, injection at birth (immunoincompetent host) or in adulthood (immunocompetent host) with a lymphotropic variant of LCMV results in infection of lymphocytes—primarily CD4+ T cells. The injection with LCMV variant resulted in infection of a subset of CD4+ T cells and a mild reduction in CD4+ T cells, and this was associated with prevention of the development of diabetes in NOD mice.[334] Ablation of this autoimmune

Type I diabetes did not significantly change immune responses to a variety of non-LCMV antigens that require the participation of CD4$^+$ T cells. The prevention of Type I diabetes associated with the viral infection is maintained throughout the life of the NOD mouse. Similarly, the injection with LCMV (ARM 53b) reduced the incidence of diabetes in DP-BB rats.[335] The number of T cells, including both helper/inducer and cytotoxic/suppressor T cells, decreased significantly 4 and 7 days after viral inoculation of DP-BB rats. The number of T cells in LCMV-infected DP-BB rats returned to control levels by 14 days after inoculation and remained at normal levels thereafter. In contrast, LCMV-infected DR-BB rats did not show marked changes in the number of T cells.

Mouse hepatitis virus,[336] lactate dehydrogenase virus, Pichinde virus, vaccinia virus, and Sendai virus have also been reported to suppress the development of diabetes in NOD mice. Lactate dehydrogenase virus preferentially infects macrophages and alters accompanying T-cell functions.[337–339] MHC class II molecules serve as receptors for lactate dehydrogenase virus,[338] and infection with this virus aborts experimental allergic encephalitis.[339]

Mechanisms of Action of Virus-Induced Diabetes. Mechanisms by which viruses may induce diabetes include the modification of β-cell antigens, molecular mimicry, direct lysis of β-cells, and virus-induced functional changes in effector or regulatory lymphocytes.[315,329,330] There has been no direct demonstration that viruses induce diabetes in experimental animals without extensive β-cell infection or lysis.[315,321,322] Most hypotheses assume that immune destruction of the β-cells follows direct interaction between virus and β-cell (infection), with resulting alteration of β-cell antigenicity. However, this has not been confirmed, and it is likely that the etiology of virus-induced diabetes is more complicated.

Environmental viral pathogens enhance or inhibit the process of islet-cell destruction depending on the immunologic surroundings of the host.[330] Experimental LCMV infections protect against diabetes in BB rats and NOD mice by directly infecting and down-regulating a subset of helper T cells.[333–335] Environmental viruses may have infected and down-regulated effector cell function in seropositive diabetes-prone animals, while infecting suppressor cells, with a resultant up-regulation of effector cells, in seropositive diabetes-resistant animals.

Thus, environmental organisms may induce diabetes in susceptible humans by stimulating genetically programmed effector cells or by disrupting a balanced network of autoreactive and regulatory cells. In addition to the viral factors, environmental bacteria, especially intestinal bacteria, need to be considered in the pathogenesis of autoimmune Type I diabetes.

Influence of Diet and Chronic Stress on Development of IDDM

Semisynthetic diets in which natural proteins were replaced by L-amino acids prevented the development of diabetes in the DP-BB rat.[340,341] More animals that received the semisynthetic diet plus 1% skim milk or 1%

gliadin developed diabetes than did animals fed the semisynthetic diet alone, suggesting the precipitation of diabetes by dietary protein.[340] A semipurified diet (AIN-76) also could prevent the development of diabetes in the BB rat[341] and the NOD mouse.[342] The AIN-76 diet increased the weight of the thymus and the total number of white blood cells, doubled the ratio of thymic helper T cells to suppressor T cells, and decreased the proportion of suppressor T cells in the spleen and thymus in the DP-BB rat.[341] Pregestimil is a hypoallergenic infant formula based on enzymically hydrolysed casein from cow's milk further treated with charcoal to remove antigenic peptides. Pregestimil ingestion by NOD mice reduced islet damage[342] and completely prevented the development of diabetes in animals up to 40 weeks of age.[343] When a chloroform-methanol extract of the natural-ingredient Old Guilford 96 (OG96) mouse diet was added to Pregestimil, the incidence of diabetes in the NOD mice reached 75%.[342] The effect of dietary factors on the development of Type I diabetes is summarized in Table 18–8.

Environmental stress, especially chronic moderate stress, can accelerate the development of diabetes in the BB rat.[344] BB rats exposed to daily chronic moderate stress (rotation, vibration, restraint) over a 14-week period developed diabetes more often than did control animals (70 to 80% in the stressed group vs. 50% in the control group). The BB rats exposed to the stress showed larger adrenal glands and smaller thymuses and spleens than the control animals.

Immune Modulation and Immunotherapy for IDDM

Type I diabetes is a chronic autoimmune disease. It may be possible to halt destruction of islet β-cells with immune intervention during the long prediabetic period. Islet transplantation into the neonatal thymus; administration of insulin; oral tolerance (to insulin); bone marrow transplantation; thymectomy; and administration of cytokines, antibodies to lymphocytes and to MHC class

Table 18–8. Dietary and Other Environmental Factors in the Development of Diabetes in NOD Mice and BB Rats

Acceleration	Suppression
Diet	Diet
Unknown dietary protein	Semipurified AIN-76 diet in both DP-BB rats and NOD mice (20% casein or 20% soy protein)
Unknown extract of natural-ingredient OG96 mouse diet by chloroform-methanol	Hypoallergenic infant formula (Pregestimil, a casein hydrolysate)
Chronic stress in BB rats (rotation, vibration, restraint)	Lactalbumin hydrolysate
	Sorbose (reducing 2-ketohexose)
	Temperature 24 ± 1.5° C (vs. 20 ± 1.7° C)

All effects observed in NOD mice unless otherwise indicated.

II molecules, and immunosuppressive drugs have been demonstrated to prevent the development of diabetes and insulitis in NOD mice and BB rats (Table 18–9). These forms of immunotherapy are nonspecific and suppress the entire immune system rather than the responsible regulatory or effector immune cells. Since these therapies may affect nontarget organs, they also may lead to drug-induced complications. The ideal approach to the prevention of the development of Type I diabetes should be specific for blocking regulatory or effector immune cells (antigen-specific) and have few side effects.

Prevention of Diabetes by Intrathymic Islet Implantation. Posselt et al. have demonstrated the prevention of diabetes by intrathymic islet implantation in the DP-BB rat.[345,346] Rat pancreatic islet allografts transplanted into the thymuses of allogenic hosts survive indefinitely without chronic immunosuppression. Recipients of these grafts are unresponsive to transplanted extrathymic islets from the same strain, possibly as a result of the deletion or functional inactivation of donor-specific alloreactive clones.[345]

None of the newborn BB rats (within 24 hours of birth) given an intrathymic inoculum of 60 to 80 islets isolated from MHC-identical (RT1^u) adult WF male donors developed diabetes. In contrast, one-half of the control animals given an intrathymic injection of saline developed diabetes between 55 and 121 days.[385] Histologic examination revealed that all rats that received intrathymic islets at birth possessed healthy islets in their native pancreas and no signs of insulitis. The excised thymus showed small clusters of healthy, insulin-containing islet endocrine cells within the thymic parenchyma. Despite the prevention of diabetes in recipients of intrathymic islets, the incidence of thyroiditis in these animals was not reduced. The possibility that the transplanted intrathymic islets rather than the native islets were producing insulin was ruled out by thymectomizing the adult recipients. The animals whose transplanted intrathymic islets were removed still maintained normoglycemia.

To determine whether the prevention of autoimmune insulitis by neonatal islet tissue requires that the implant be situated in the thymus, neonatal BB rats were inoculated with WF islets beneath the renal capsule. Fifty percent of these rats developed diabetes and insulitis in their native pancreas. The interpretation of these findings by Posselt et al. was that intrathymic transplantation of islets into neonatal BB rats alters T-cell development by promoting the deletion or functional inactivation of antigen-specific clones before they migrate to the periphery.

Insulin Therapy. The loss of first-phase insulin secretion in response to glucose is one of the earlier signs of the ongoing damage of pancreatic islets in IDDM both in humans[383,385] and in animal models.[386] These functional abnormalities correlate with the loss of a significant proportion of β-cell mass.[387]

Chronic administration of insulin in young DP-BB rats[355–357] and NOD mice[358] significantly decreases the incidence of diabetes and insulitis. Despite the discontinuation of insulin administration at 140 days of age, most of the treated DP-BB rats remained normoglycemic until 230 days of age.[355] NOD mice that received insulin therapy from weaning until 180 days of age showed significantly lower frequencies of diabetes and insulitis.[358]

Some explanations of the protective effect of insulin treatment in BB rats and NOD mice are 1) that the β-cells are put to rest by rendering the endogenous islets metabolically inactive and decreasing their expression of the β-cell-specific autoantigens and 2) that the suscepti-

Table 18–9. Immune Modulation and Immunotherapy for Insulin-Dependent Diabetes in Diabetes-Prone (BB) Rats and NOD Mice

	DP-BB rat	NOD Mouse
Islet transplantation into the neonatal thymus	Prevents[345,346]	Not known
Neonatal thymectomy	Prevents[347]	Prevents*[348,349]
Bone marrow transplantation	WF, DR-BB marrow prevents[350,351]	BALB/c or ILI marrow prevents[352–354]
Insulin therapy	Prevents[355–357]	Prevents[358]
Oral tolerance (insulin)	Not known	Prevents[359]
Interferon-γ	Prevents[360]	Prevents[361]
Tumor necrosis factor-α	Prevents[362]	Prevents[363,364]
Interleukin-2 (IL-2)	Controversial[365,366]	—
Antilymphocyte serum	Prevents[367]	Prevents[368]
Anti-IL-2 receptor	Prevents†[369]	Prevents[370]
Anti-MHC class II antigens	Prevents[371]	Prevents[372]
Anti-CD4$^+$ T cells	—	Prevents[373–375]
Anti-CD8$^+$ T cells	Prevents‡[286]	Prevents[376]
CD4$^+$ T-cell transfusion	Prevents[377]	
Cyclophosphamide	Accelerates§[378]	Accelerates[379]
Cyclosporin A	Prevents[380]	Prevents[381]
FK 506	Prevents[382]	Prevents[383]

*Thymectomy at weaning accelerates diabetes.
†In addition to cyclosporin A.
‡Depletion of CD8$^+$ and NK cells.
§In (DR×DP) F$_1$.

bility of islets to toxic cytokines is decreased. For example, the islet cytotoxic effects of IL-1 in vivo are enhanced by high ambient glucose concentrations and decreased by the inhibition of β-cell secretory activity.[388,389] Decreasing glycemia and insulin secretory activity may enhance the resistance of β-cells to the cytotoxic mediators of immune cells.[265]

Oral Tolerance. Oral administration of autoantigens suppresses autoimmunity in animal models, including experimental autoimmune encephalomyelitis,[390] adjuvant- and collagen-induced arthritis,[391] and experimental autoimmune uveitis.[392] Oral administration of insulin also delayed the onset and reduced the incidence of diabetes in NOD mice over a 1-year period. The protocol involves the administration of 1 mg of porcine monocomponent insulin orally twice a week for 5 weeks and then weekly until the animal is a year old.[359] One possible explanation for this oral tolerance is that insulin is not a pathogenic autoantigen in the NOD mouse but that the regulatory cells generated in the gut by feeding the animal insulin migrate to the pancreas and are triggered by insulin to release transforming growth factor β, which downregulates the local inflammatory processes in the pancreas.[359]

REFERENCES

1. Coleman DL, Hummel KP. Studies with the mutation, diabetes, in the mouse. Diabetologia 1967;3:238−48.
2. Hattori M, Buse JB, Jackson RA, et al. The NOD mouse: recessive diabetogenic gene in the major histocompatibility complex. Science 1986;231:733−5.
3. Craighead JE, McLane MF. Diabetes mellitus: induction in mice by encephalomyocarditis virus. Science 1968;162:913−4.
4. Hayashi K, Boucher DW, Notkins AL. Virus-induced diabetes mellitus. II. Relationship between beta cell damage and hyperglycemia in mice infected with encephalomyocarditis virus. Am J Pathol 1974;75:91−104.
5. Dunn JS, Sheehan HL, McLetchie NGB. Necrosis of the islets of Langerhans produced experimentally. Lancet 1943;1:484−7.
6. Rerup CC. Drugs producing diabetes through damage of the insulin secreting cells. Pharmacol Rev 1970;22:485−515.
7. Bonner-Weir S, Trent DF, Weir GC. Partial pancreatectomy in the rat and subsequent defect in glucose-induced insulin release. J Clin Invest 1983;71:1544−53.
8. Weir GC. Non-insulin-dependent diabetes mellitus: interplay between B-cells inadequacy and insulin resistance [Editorial]. Am J Med 1962;73:461−4.
9. Reaven GM. Non-insulin-dependent diabetes mellitus (NIDDM): speculation on etiology. In: Alberti KGMM, Krall LP, eds. The diabetes annual/5. New York: Elsevier, 1990.
10. Bray GA. The Zucker-fatty rat: a review. Fed Proc 1977;36:148−53.
11. Bonner-Weir S, Trent DF, Honey RN, Weir GC. Responses of neonatal rat islets to streptozotocin: limited B-cell regeneration and hyperglycemia. Diabetes 1981;30:64−9.
12. DeFronzo RA, Soman V, Sherwin RS, Hendler R. Insulin binding to monocytes and insulin action in human obesity, starvation, and refeeding. J Clin Invest 1978;62:204−13.
13. Knowler WC, Bennett PH, Hamman RF, Miller M. Diabetes incidence and prevalence in Pima Indians: a 19-fold greater incidence than in Rochester, Minnesota. Am J Epidemiol 1978;108:497−505.
14. Coleman DL. Diabetes-obesity syndromes in mice. Diabetes 31(Suppl 1):1−6.
15. Zimmet P, Pinkstone G, Whitehouse S, Thoma K. The high incidence of diabetes mellitus in the Micronesian population of Nauru. Acta Diab Lat 1982;19:75−9.
16. Schmidt-Nielsen K, Haines HB, Hackel DB. Diabetes mellitus in the sand rat induced by standard laboratory diets. Science 1964;143:689−90.
17. Reaven GM. Insulin-independent diabetes mellitus: metabolic characteristics. Metabolism 1980;29:445−54.
18. Kalderon B, Gutman A, Levy E, et al. Characterization of stages in the development of obesity-diabetes syndrome in the sand rat (*Psammomys obesus*). Diabetes 1986;35:717−24.
19. Hamilton CL, Ciaccia P. The course of development of glucose intolerance in the monkey (*Macaca mulatta*). J Med Primatol 1978;7:165−73.
20. Dunaif A, Tattersall I. Prevalence of glucose intolerance in free-ranging *Macaca fascicularis* of Mauritius. Am J Primatol 1987;13:435−42.
21. Phillips RW, Westmoreland N, Panepinto L, Case GL. Dietary effects on metabolism of Yucatan miniature swine selected for low and high glucose utilization. J Nutr 1982;112:104−11.
22. Phillips RW, Panepinto LM, Will DH. Genetic selection for diabetogenic traits in Yucatan miniature swine. Diabetes 1979;28:1102−7.
23. Kahn CR, Goldfine ID, Neville DM Jr, De Meyts P. Alterations in insulin binding induced by changes in vivo in the levels of glucocorticoids and growth hormone. Endocrinology 1978;103:1054−66.
24. Karasik A, Kahn CR. Dexamethasone-induced changes in phosphorylation of the insulin and epidermal growth factor receptors and their substrates in intact rat hepatocytes. Endocrinology 1988;123:2214−22.
25. Frigeri LG, Teguh C, Ling N, et al. Increased sensitivity of adipose tissue to insulin after in vivo treatment of yellow A^vy/A obese mice with amino-terminal peptides of human growth hormone. Endocrinology 1988;122:2940−5.
26. Pascoe WS, Storlien LH. Inducement by fat feeding of basal hyperglycemia in rats with abnormal β-cell function: model for study of etiology and pathogenesis of NIDDM. Diabetes 1990;39:226−33.
27. Kraegen EW, James DE, Storlien LH, et al. In vivo insulin resistance in individual peripheral tissues of the high fat fed rat: assessment by euglycaemic clamp plus deoxyglucose administration. Diabetologia 1986;29:192−8.
28. Kraegan EW, Storlien LH, Jenkins AB, Chisholm DJ. Factors influencing the etiology and amelioration of high fat diet induced insulin resistance in the rat. In: Shafrir E, ed. Lessons from animal diabetes III. London: Libbey Publishers, 1991.
29. Herberg L, Coleman DL. Laboratory animals exhibiting obesity and diabetes syndromes. Metabolism 1977;26:59−99.
30. Coleman DL, Hummel KP. Influence of genetic background on the expressions of mutation at the diabetes locus in the mouse. II. Studies on background modifiers. Isr J Med Sci 1975;11:708−13.
31. Hummel KP, Dickie MM, Coleman DL. Diabetes, a new mutation in the mouse. Science 1966;153:1127−8.

32. Bahary N, Leibel RL, Joseph L, Friedman JM. Molecular mapping of the mouse *db* mutation. Proc Natl Acad Sci USA 87:1990;8642–6.

33. Kaku K, Province M, Permutt MA. Genetic analysis of obesity-induced diabetes associated with a limited capacity to synthesize insulin in C57BL/KS mice: evidence for polygenic control. Diabetologia 1989;32:636–43.

34. Leiter EH, Coleman DL, Hummel KP. The influence of genetic background on the expression of mutations at the diabetes locus in the mouse. III. Effect of H-2 haplotype and sex. Diabetes 1981;30:1029–34.

35. Leiter EH. The genetics of diabetes susceptibility in mice. FASEB J 1989;3:2231–41.

36. Leiter EH, Chapman HD, Coleman DL. The influence of genetic background on the expression of mutations at the diabetes locus in the mouse. V. Interaction between the *db* gene and hepatic sex steroid sulfotransferases correlates with gender-dependent susceptibility to hyperglycemia. Endocrinology 1989;124:912–22.

37. Chick WL, Like AA. Studies in the diabetic mutant mouse. IV. DBM, a modified diabetic mutant produced by outcrossing of the original strain. Diabetologia 1970; 6:252–6.

38. Coleman DL. Obese and diabetes: two mutant genes causing diabetes-obesity syndromes in mice. Diabetologia 1978;14:141–8.

39. Coleman DL, Hummel KP. Hyperinsulinemia in preweaning diabetes (*db*) mice. Diabetologia 1974;10: 607–10.

40. Bergland O, Frankel BJ, Hellman B. Development of the insulin secretory defect in genetically diabetic (*db/db*) mouse. Acta Endocrinol 1978;87:543–51.

41. Chick WL, Like AA. Studies in the diabetic mutant mouse. III. Physiological factors associated with alterations in beta cell proliferation. Diabetologia 1970;6:243–51.

42. Like AA, Chick WL. Studies in the diabetic mutant mouse. I. Light microscopy and radioautography of pancreatic islets. Diabetologia 1970;6:207–15.

43. Like AA, Coleman DL, Hummel KP. Pancreatic islet studies in diabetic mutant mice [Abstract no. 1754]. Fed Proc 1969;28:574.

44. Orland MJ, Permutt MA. Quantitative analysis of pancreatic proinsulin mRNA in genetically diabetic (*db/db*) mice. Diabetes 1987;36:341–7.

45. Swenne I, Andersson A. Effect of genetic background on the capacity for islet cell replication in mice. Diabetologia 1984;27:464–7.

46. Leiter EH, Bedigian HG. Intracisternal A-particles in genetically diabetic mice: identification in pancreas and induction in cultured beta cells. Diabetologia 1979; 17:175–85.

47. Leiter EH, Coleman DL, Eisenstein AB, Strack I. Dietary control of pathogenesis in C57BL/KsJ *db/db* diabetes mice. Metabolism 1981;30:554–62.

48. Leiter EH, Coleman DL, Ingram DK, Reynolds MA. Influence of dietary carbohydrate on the induction of diabetes in C57BL/KsJ-*db/db* diabetes mice. J Nutr 1983;113: 184–95.

49. Stearns SB, Benzo CA. Glucagon and insulin relationships in genetically diabetic (*db/db*) and in streptozotocin-induced diabetic mice. Horm Metab Res 1978;10: 20–3.

50. Patel YC, Orci L, Bankier A, Cameron DP. Decreased pancreatic somatostatin (SRIF) concentration in spontaneously diabetic mice. Endocrinology 1976;99:1415–8.

51. Makino H, Matsushima Y, Kanatsuka A, et al. Changes in pancreatic somatostatin content in spontaneously diabetic mice, as determined by radioimmunoassay and immunohistochemical methods. Endocrinology 1979;104: 243–7.

52. Chan TM, Young KM, Huston MJ, et al. Hepatic metabolism of genetically diabetic (*db/db*) mice. I. Carbohydrate metabolism. Am J Physiol 1975;229:1702–12.

53. Shafrir E. Nonrecognition of insulin as a glucose suppressant—a manifestation of selective hepatic insulin resistance in several animal species with type II diabetes: sand rats, spiny mice and (*db/db*) mice. In: Shafrir E, Renold AE, eds. Lessons from animal diabetes II. London, Libbey Publishers, 1988:304.

54. Chan TM, Dehaye JP. Hormone regulation of glucose metabolism in the genetically obese-diabetic mouse (*db/db*): glucose metabolism in the perfused hindquarters of lean and obese mice. Diabetes 1981;30:211–8.

55. Cuendet GS, Loten EG, Jeanrenaud B, et al. Decreased basal noninsulin-stimulated glucose uptake and metabolism by skeletal soleus muscle isolated from obese-hyperglycemic (*ob/ob*) mice. J Clin Invest 1976;58: 1078–88.

56. Koranyi L, James D, Mueckler M, Permutt MA. Glucose transporter levels in spontaneously obese (*db/db*) insulin-resistant mice. J Clin Invest 1990;85:962–7.

57. Soll AH, Kahn CR, Neville DM Jr, Roth J. Insulin receptor deficiency in genetic and acquired obesity. J Clin Invest 1975;56:769–80.

58. Shargill NS, Tatoyan A, El-Rafai MF, et al. Impaired insulin receptor phosphorylation in skeletal muscle membranes of *db/db* mice: the use of a novel skeletal muscle plasma preparation to compare insulin binding and stimulation of receptor phosphorylation. Biochem Biophys Res Commun 1986;137:286–94.

59. Ludwig S, Muller-Wieland D, Goldstein BJ, Kahn CR. The insulin receptor gene and its expression in insulin-resistant mice. Endocrinology 1988;123:594–600.

60. Coleman DL, Hummel KP. Effects of parabiosis of normal with genetically diabetic mice. Am J Physiol 1969; 217:1298–304.

61. Coleman DL, Hummel KP. The effects of hypothalamic lesions in genetically diabetic mice. Diabetologia 1970; 6:263–7.

62. Flier JS, Usher P, Spiegelman BM. Severely impaired adipsin expression in genetic and acquired obesity. Science 1987;237:405–8.

63. Dugail, I, Quingnard-Boulangé A, LeLiepvre X, Lavau M. Impairment of adipsin expression is secondary to the onset of obesity in *db/db* mice. J Biol Chem 1990; 265:1831–3.

64. Bray GA, York DA. Hypothalamic and genetic obesity in experimental animals: an autonomic and endocrine hypothesis. Physiol Rev 1979;59:719–809.

65. Coleman DL, Hummel KP. The influence of genetic background on the expression of the obese (*ob*) gene in the mouse. Diabetologia 1973;9:287–93.

66. Bates MW, Nauss SF, Hagman NC, Mayer J. Fat metabolism in three forms of experimental obesity. I. Body composition. Am J Physiol 1955;180:301–3.

67. Thurlby PL, Trayhurn P. The development of obesity in preweaning *ob/ob* mice. Br J Nutr 1978;39:397–402.

68. Herberg L, Gries FA, Hesese-Wortmann C. Effect of weight and cell size on hormone-induced lipolysis in New Zealand obese hyperglycemic mice and American obese hyperglycemic mice. Diabetologia 1970;6:300–5.

69. Chlouverakis C. Induction of obesity in obese-hyperglycaemic mice on normal food intake. Experientia 1970;26:1262–3.

70. Genuth SM, Przybylski RJ, Rosenberg DM. Insulin resistance in genetically obese, hyperglycemic mice. Endocrinology 1971;88:1230−8.

71. Wrenshall GA, Andrus SB, Mayer J. High levels of pancreatic insulin coexistent with hyperplasia and degranulation of beta cells in mice with the hereditary obese-hyperglycemic syndrome. Endocrinology 1955;56:335−91.

72. Petersson B, Hellman B. Long-term effects of restricted caloric intake on pancreatic islet tissue in obese-hyperglycemic mice. Metabolism 1962;11:342−8.

73. Genuth SM. Hyperinsulinism in mice with genetically determined obesity. Endocrinology 1969;84:386−91.

74. Grundleger ML, Godbole VY, Thenen SW. Age-dependent development of insulin resistance of soleus muscle in genetically obese (ob/ob) mice. Am J Physiol 1980; 239:E365−71.

75. Kreutner W, Springer SC, Sherwood JE. Resistance of gluconeogenic and glycogenic pathways in obese-hyperglycemic mice. Am J Physiol 1975;228:663−71.

76. Le Marchand-Brustel Y, Grémeaux T, Ballotti R, Van Obberghen I. Insulin receptor tyrosine kinase is defective in skeletal muscle of insulin-resistant obese mice. Nature 1985;315:676−9.

77. Coleman DL. Effects of parabiosis of obese with diabetes and normal mice. Diabetologia 1973;9:294−8.

78. Boozer CN, Mayer J. Effects of long-term restricted insulin production in obese-hyperglycemic (genotype ob/ob) mice. Diabetologia 1976;12:181−7.

79. Hollifield G, Parson W, Ayers CR. In vitro synthesis of lipids from C-14 acetate by adipose tissue from four types of obese mice. Am J Physiol 1960;198:37−8.

80. Renold AE, Christophe J, Jeanrenaud B. The obese hyperglycemic syndrome in mice: metabolism of isolated adipose tissue in vitro. Am J Clin Nutr 1960;8: 719−27.

81. Assimacopoulos-Jeannet F, Singh A, Le Marchand Y, et al. Abnormalities in lipogenesis and triglyceride secretion by perfused livers of obese-hyperglycemic (ob/ob) mice: relationship with hyperinsulinaemia. Diabetologia 1974; 10:155−62.

82. Ashwell M, Meade CJ. Obesity: do fat cells from genetically obese mice (C57BL/6J ob/ob) have an innate capacity for increased fat storage? Diabetologia 1978;15:465−70.

83. Chlouverakis CL, White PA. Obesity and insulin resistance in obese hyperglycemic mouse. Metabolism 1969;18: 998−1006.

84. Loten EG, Le Marchand Y, Assimacopoulos-Jeannet F, et al. Does hyperinsulinemia in ob/ob mice cause an insulin stimulated adipose tissue? Am J Physiol 1976;230: 602−7.

85. Edwardson JA, Hough CAM. The pituitary-adrenal system of the genetically obese (ob/ob) mouse. J Endocrinol 1975;65:99−107.

86. Solomon J, Mayer J. The effect of adrenalectomy on the development of the obese-hyperglycemic syndrome in ob/ob mice. Endocrinology 1973;93:510−3.

87. Flatt PR, Bailey CJ, Kwasowk P, et al. Plasma immunoreactive gastric inhibitory polypeptide in obese hyperglycaemic (ob/ob) mice. J Endocrinol 1984;101:249−56.

88. Mayer J, Yannoni CZ. Increased intestinal absorption of glucose in three forms of obesity in the mouse. Am J Physiol 1956;185:49−53.

89. Yen TTT, Acton JM. Locomotor activity of various types of genetically obese mice. Proc Soc Exp Biol Med 1972;140:647−50.

90. Dickie MM. A new viable yellow mutation in the house mouse. J Hered 1962;53:84−6.

91. Wolff GL. Body composition and coat color correlation in different phenotypes of "viable yellow" mice. Science 1965;147:1145−7.

92. Wolff GL, Pitot HC. Influence of background genome on enzymatic characteristics of yellow (A^y/-,A^{vy}/-) mice. Genetics 1973;73:109−23.

93. Hollifield G, Parson W. Food drive and satiety in yellow mice. Am J Physiol 1957;189:36−8.

94. Dickie MM, Woolley GW. The age factor in weight of yellow mice: weight reducing of ageing yellows and "thin-yellows" revealed in littermate comparisons. J Hered 1946;37:365−8.

95. Johnson PR, Hirsch J. Cellularity of adipose depots of six strains of genetically obese mice. J Lipid Res 1972;13: 2−11.

96. Zomzely C, Mayer J. Fat metabolism in experimental obesities. IX. Lipogenesis and cholesterogenesis in yellow obese mice. Am J Physiol 1959;196:611−3.

97. Yen TTT, Steinmetz J, Wolff GL. Lipolysis in genetically obese and diabetes-prone mice. Horm Metab Res 1970;2:200−3.

98. Carpenter KJ, Mayer J. Physiologic observations on yellow obesity in the mouse. Am J Physiol 1958;193: 499−504.

99. Hausberger FX, Hausberger BC. The etiologic mechanism of some forms of hormonally induced obesity. Am J Clin Nutr 1960;8:671−81.

100. Kondo ZK, Nozawa K, Tomito T, Ezaki K. Inbred strains resulting from Japanese mice. Bull Exp Anim 1957;6: 107−16.

101. Dulin WE, Wyse BM. Diabetes in the KK mouse. Diabetologia 1970;6:317−23.

102. Chang AY, Wyse BM, Copeland EJ, et al. The Upjohn colony of KKA^y mice: a model for obese type II diabetes. In: Serrano-Rios M, Lefèbvre PJ, eds. Diabetes 1985. Amsterdam: Elsevier, 1986:466−70.

103. Iwatsuka H, Shino A, Suzuoki Z. General survey of diabetic features of yellow KK mice. Endocrinol Jpn 1970;17: 23−35.

104. Matsuo T, Shino A, Iwatsuka H, Suzuoki Z. Induction of overt diabetes in KK mice by dietary means. Endocrinol Jpn 1970;17:477−88.

105. Nakamura M, Yamada K. Studies on a diabetic (KK) strain of the mouse. Diabetologia 1967;3:212−21.

106. Wyse BM, Dulin WE. Further characterization of diabetes-like abnormalities in the T-KK mouse. Diabetologia 1974;10:617−23.

107. Bielschowsky M, Goodall CM. Origin of inbred NZ mouse strains. Cancer Res 1970;30:834−6.

108. Bielschowsky M, Bielschowsky F. The New Zealand strain of obese mice: their response to stilboestrol and to insulin. Aust J Exp Biol Med Sci 1956;34:181−98.

109. Crofford OB, Davis CK Jr. Growth characteristics, glucose tolerance and insulin sensitivity of New Zealand obese mice. Metabolism 1965;14:271−80.

110. Willms B, Ben-Ami P, Sling HD. Hepatic enzyme activities of glycolysis and gluconeogenesis in diabetes of man and laboratory animals. Horm Metab Res 1970;2:135−41.

111. Veroni MC, Larkins RG. Evolution of insulin resistance in isolated soleus muscle of the NZO mouse. Horm Metab Res 1986;18:299−302.

112. Borgalound E, Brolin SE, Ohlsson A. On the long-term effects of chlorpentazide in mice with hereditary hyperglycemia. In: International Diabetes Federation, 1967. International Congress Series, no. 172. Amsterdam: Excerpta Medica, 1969:747.

113. Cameron DP, Opat F, Insch S. Studies of immunoreactive

insulin secretion in NZO mice in vivo. Diabetologia 1974;10:649–54.

114. Sneyd JGT. Pancreatic and serum insulin in the New Zealand strain of obese mice. J Endocrinol 1964;28:163–72.

115. Melez KA, Harrison LC, Gilliam JN, Steinberg AD. Diabetes is associated with autoimmunity in the New Zealand obese (NZO) mouse. Diabetes 1980;29:835–40.

116. Hunt CE, Lindsey JR, Walkley SU. Animal models of diabetes and obesity, including the PBB/Ld mouse. Fed Proc 1976;35:1206–17.

117. Walkely SU, Hunt CE, Clements RS, Lindsey JR. Description of obesity in the PBB/Ld mouse. J Lipid Res 1978;19:335–41.

118. Cahill GF Jr, Jones EE, Lauris V, et al. Studies on experimental diabetes in the Wellesley hybrid mouse. II. Serum insulin levels and response of peripheral tissues. Diabetologia 1967;3:171–4.

119. Gleason RE, Lauris V, Soeldner JS. Studies on experimental diabetes in the Wellesley hybrid mouse. IV. Dietary effects and similar changes in a commercial Swiss-Hauschka strain. Diabetologia 1967;3:175–8.

120. Zucker LM. Hereditary obesity in the rat associated with hyperlipemia. Ann NY Acad Sci 1965;131:447–58.

121. Bray GA. The Zucker-fatty rat: a review. Fed Proc 1977;36:148–53.

122. Rohner-Jeanrenaud F, Bobbioni F, Ionsescu E, et al. Central nervous system regulation of insulin secretion. In: Szabo AJ, ed. Advances of metabolic disorders. New York: Academic Press, 1983:193–209.

123. Ionescu E, Sauter JF, Jeanrenaud B. Abnormal oral glucose tolerance in genetically obese (fa/fa) rats. Am J Physiol 1985;248:E500–6.

124. Penicaud L, Ferré P, Terretaz J, et al. Development of obesity in Zucker rats: early insulin resistance in muscles but normal sensitivity in white adipose tissue. Diabetes 1987;36:626–31.

125. Ikeda H, Shino A, Matsuo T, et al. A new genetically obese-hyperglycemic rat (Wistar fatty). Diabetes 1981;30:1045–50.

126. Kava RA, West DB, Lukasik VA, Greenwood MRC. Sexual dimorphism of hyperglycemia and glucose tolerance in Wistar fatty rats. Diabetes 1989;38:159–63.

127. Terrettaz J, Jeanrenaud B. In vivo and peripheral insulin resistance in genetically obese (fa/fa) rats. Endocrinology 1983;112:1346–51.

128. Rohner-Jeanrenaud F, Proietto J, Ionescu E, Jeanrenaud, B. Mechanism of abnormal oral glucose tolerance of genetically obese fa/fa rats. Diabetes 1986;35:1350–5.

129. Terrettaz J, Assimacopoulus-Jeannet F, Jeanrenaud B. Severe hepatic and peripheral insulin resistance as evidenced by euglycemic clamps in genetically obese fa/fa rats. Endocrinology 1986;118:674–8.

130. Crettaz M, Prentki M, Zaninetti D, Jeanrenaud B. Insulin resistance in soleus muscle from obese Zucker rats: involvement of several defective sites. Biochem J 1980;186: 525–34.

131. Smith OLK, Czech MP. Insulin sensitivity and response in eviscerated obese Zucker rats. Metabolism 1983;32:597–602.

132. Poole GP, Pogson CI, O'Connor KJ, Lazarus NR. The metabolism of ^{125}I-labelled insulin by isolated Zucker rat hepatocytes. Biosci Rep 1981;1:903–6.

133. Hurrell DG, Pedersen O, Kahn CR. Alterations in the hepatic insulin receptor kinase in genetic and acquired obesity in rats. Endocrinology 1989;125:2454–62.

134. Slieker LJ, Roberts EF, Shaw WN, Johnson WT. Effect of streptozocin-induced diabetes on insulin-receptor tyrosine kinase activity in obese Zucker rats. Diabetes 1990;39:619–25.

135. Shemer J, Ota A, Adamo M, LeRoith D. Insulin-sensitive tyrosine kinase is increased in livers of adult obese Zucker rats: correction with prolonged fasting. Endocrinology 1988;123:140–8.

136. Rösen P, Herberg L, Reinauer H. Different types of postinsulin receptor defects contribute to insulin resistance in hearts of obese Zucker rats. Endocrinology 1986;119:1285–91.

137. Hainault I, Guerre-Millo M, Guichard C, Lavau M. Differential regulation of adipose tissue glucose transporters in genetic obesity (fatty rat): selective increase in the adipose cell/muscle glucose transporter GLUT 4) expression. J Clin Invest 1991;87:1127–31.

138. Stern JS, Johnson PR, Batchelor BR, et al. Pancreatic insulin release and peripheral tissue resistance in Zucker obese rats fed high- and low-carbohydrate diets. Am J Physiol 1975;228:543–8.

139. Shino A, Matsuo T, Iwatsuka H, Suzuoki Z. Structural changes of pancreatic islets in genetically obese rats. Diabetologia 1973;9:413–21.

140. Hayek H. Insulin release in long-term culture from isolated islets of obese and lean Zucker rats. Horm Metab Res 1980;12:85–6.

141. Nishikawa K, Ikeda H, Matsuo T. Abnormal glucagon secretion in Zucker fatty rats. Horm Metab Res 1981;13:259–63.

142. Rohner-Jeanrenaud F, Jeanrenaud B. Abnormal regulation of pancreatic glucagon secretion in obese fa/fa rats. Diabetologia 1988;31:235–40.

143. Trimble ER, Herberg L, Renold AE. Hypersecretion of pancreatic somatostatin in the obese Zucker rat: effects of food restriction and age. Diabetes 1988;29:889–94.

144. Ikeda H, West DB, Pustek JJ, et al. Intraventricular insulin reduces food intake and body weight of lean but not obese Zucker rats. Appetite 1986;7:381–6.

145. Beck B, Burlet A, Nicolas JP, Burlet C. Hypothalamic neuropeptide Y (NPY) in obese Zucker rats: implications in feeding and sexual behaviors. Physiol Behav 1990;47:449–53.

146. Schwartz MW, Marks JL, Sipols AJ, et al. Central insulin administration reduces neuropeptide Y mRNA expression in the arcuate nucleus of food-deprived lean (Fa/Fa) but not obese (fa/fa) Zucker rats. Endocrinology 1991;128:2645–7.

147. Stolz DJ, Martin RJ. Role of insulin in food intake, weight gain and lipid deposition in the Zucker obese rat. J Nutr 1982;112:997–1002.

148. Bestetti GE, Abramo F, Guillaume-Gentil C, et al. Changes in the hypothalamo-pituitary-adrenal axis of genetically obese fa/fa rats: a structural, immunocytochemical, and morphometrical study. Endocrinology 1990;126:1880–7.

149. Freedman MR, Stern JS, Reaven GM, Mondon CE. Effect of adrenalectomy on in vivo glucose metabolism in insulin resistant zucker obese rats. Horm Metab Res 1986;18:296–8.

150. Orci L, Ravazzola M, Baetens D, et al. Evidence that down regulation of β-cell glucose transporters in non-insulin dependent diabetes may be the cause of diabetic hyperglycemia. Proc Natl Acad Sci USA 1990;187:9953–7.

151. Miki E, Like AA, Steinke J, Soeldner JS. Diabetic syndrome in sand rats. II. Variability and association with diet. Diabetologia 1967;3:135–9.

152. Rice MG, Robertson RP. Reevaluation of the sand rat as a model for diabetes mellitus. Am J Physiol 1980;239: E340–5.

153. Aharonson Z, Shani (Mishkinsky) J, Sulman FG. Hypoglycemic effect of the salt bush (*Atriplex halimus*)—a feeding source of the sand rat (*Psammomys obesus*). Diabetologia 1969;5:379–83.

154. Shafrir E. Diabetes in animals. In: Rifkin H, Porte D, eds. Diabetes mellitus: theory and practice. New York: Elsevier, 1990.

155. Adler JH, Lazarovici G, Marton M, Levy E. The diabetic response of weanling sand rats (*Psammomys obesus*) to diets containing different concentrations of salt bush (*Atriplex halimus*). Diabetes Res 1986;3:169–71.

156. Kalderon B, Adler JH, Levy E, Gutman A. Lipogenesis in the sand rat (*Psammomys obesus*). Am J Physiol 1983; 244:E480–6.

157. Kanety H, Goldstein BJ, Shafrir E, Karasik A. Characteristics of the sand rat insulin receptor: the basis for diabetes in this animal model of NIDDM. Proc Natl Acad Sci USA (in press).

158. Ziv E, Adler JH, Lior O, Bar-On H. Insulin uptake by the liver of sand rat [Abstract no. 610]. Diabetes 1986; 35(Suppl 1):158A.

159. Petkov P, Hadjiisky P, Marquie G. Pancreatic islets histochemistry in normal sand rats (*Psammomys obesus*). Cell Mol Biol 1981;27:655–65.

160. Michaelis OE, Patrick DH, Hansen CT, et al. Insulin-independent diabetes mellitus (type II): spontaneous hypertensive/NIH-corpulent rat. Am J Pathol 1986; 123:398–400.

161. Greenhouse DD, Michaelis OE, McCune SA. The development of corpulent rat strains. In: Shafrir E, ed. Frontiers in diabetes research: lessons from animal diabetes III. London: John Libbey, 1991:375–7.

162. Recant L, et al. Islets from genetically obese diabetic rats (SHR/N-CP) show multiple abnormalities of insulin secretion in response to glucose. In: Shafrir E, ed. Frontiers in diabetes research: lessons from animal diabetes III. London: John Libbey, 1991:350–4.

163. Gonet AE, Stauffacher W, Pictet R, Renold AE. Obesity and diabetes mellitus with striking congenital hyperplasia of the islets of Langerhans in spiny mice (*Acomys cahirinus*). I. Histological findings and preliminary metabolic observations. Diabetologia 1965;1:162–71.

164. Gutman A, Hasin M, Shafrir E. Adaptive responses in enzyme activities of Israeli spiny mice (*Acomys cahirinus*). Isr J Med Sci 1972;8:364–71.

165. Nesher R, Abramovitch E, Cerasi E. Reduced early and late phase insulin response to glucose in isolated spiny mouse (*Acomys cahirinus*) islets: a defective link between glycolysis and adenylate cyclase. Diabetologia 1989;32: 644–8.

166. Rabinovitch A, Gutzeit A, Grill V, et al. Defective insulin secretion in the spiny mouse (*Acomys cahirinus*): possible value in the study of the pathophysiology of diabetes. Isr J Med Sci 1975;11:730–7.

167. Surwit RS, Kuhn CM, Cochrane C, et al. Diet-induced type II diabetes in C57BL/6J mice. Diabetes 1988;37: 1163–7.

168. Wise PH, Weir BJ, Hime JM, Forrest E. The diabetic syndrome in the tuco-tuco (*Ctenomys talarum*). Diabetologia 1972;8:165–72.

169. Nakama K. Studies on diabetic syndrome and influences of long-term tolbutamide administration in Mongolian gerbils (*Meriones unguiculatus*). Endocrinol Jpn 1977;24: 421–33.

170. Boquist L. Obesity and pancreatic islet hyperplasia in the Mongolian gerbil. Diabetologia 1972;8:274–82.

171. Portha B, Picon L. Rosselin G. Chemical diabetes in the adult rat as the spontaneous evolution of neonatal diabetes. Diabetologia 1979;17:371–7.

172. Iwase M, Kikuchi M, Nunoi K, et al. A new model of type 2 (non-insulin-dependent) diabetes mellitus in spontaneously hypertensive rats: diabetes induced by neonatal streptozotocin treatment. Diabetologia 1986;29:808–11.

173. Iwase M, Nunoi K, Wakisaka M, et al. Spontaneous recovery from non-insulin-dependent diabetes mellitus induced by neonatal streptozotocin treatment in spontaneously hypertensive rats. Metabolism 1991;40:10–4.

174. Trent DF, Fletcher DJ, May JM. Abnormal islet and adipocyte function in young β-cell-deficient rats with near-normoglycemia. Diabetes 1984;33:170–5.

175. Portha B, Giroix M-H, Serradas P, et al. Insulin production and glucose metabolism in isolated pancreatic islets of rats with NIDDM. Diabetes 1988;37:1226–33.

176. Kergoat M, Bailbe D, Portha B. Insulin treatment improves glucose-induced insulin release in rats with NIDDM induced by streptozocin. Diabetes 1987;36:971–7.

177. Weir GC, Clore ET, Zmachinski CJ, Bonner-Weir S. Islet secretion in a new experimental model for non-insulin-dependent diabetes. Diabetes 1981;30:590–5.

178. Blondel O, Bailbé D, Portha B. Relation of insulin deficiency to impaired insulin action in NIDDM adult rats given streptozocin as neonates. Diabetes 1989;38:610–7.

179. Fantus IG, Chayoth R, O'Dea L, et al. Insulin binding and glucose transport in adipocytes in neonatal streptozotocin-injected rat model of diabetes mellitus. Diabetes 1987;36:654–60.

180. Leahy JL. Bonner-Weir S, Weir GC. Minimal chronic hyperglycemia is a critical determinant of impaired insulin secretion after an incomplete pancreatectomy. J Clin Invest 1988;81:1407–14.

181. Rossetti L, Smith D, Shulman GI, et al. Correction of hyperglycemia with phlorizin normalizes tissue sensitivity to insulin in diabetic rats. J Clin Invest 1987;79–5.

182. Cohen AM, Teitelbaum A, Saliternik R. Genetics and diet as factors in development of diabetes mellitus. Metabolism 1972;21:235–40.

183. Goto Y, Suzuki KI, Sazaki M, et al. GK rat as a model of non-obese, non-insulin-dependent diabetes. Selective breeding over 35 generations. In: Shafrir E, Renold AE, eds. Lessons from animal diabetes. London: John Libbey, 1988:301–30.

184. Gleason RE, Poffenbarger PL, Lavine RL. Genetic selection for high and low fasting blood glucose levels in mice. I. Fasting blood glucose levels, glucose tolerance and isolated tissue studies. Diabetologia 1973;9:268–73.

185. Makino S, Kunimoto K, Muraoka Y, et al. Breeding of a non-obese diabetic strain of mice. Exp Anim (Tokyo) 1980;29:1–13.

186. Ohtori H, Yoshida T, Inuta T. "Small eye and cataract", a new dominant mutation in the mouse. Exp Anim (Tokyo) 1968;17:91–6.

187. Strandell E, Eizirik DL, Sandler S. Reversal of β-cell suppression in vitro in pancreatic islets isolated from nonobese diabetic mice during the phase preceding insulin-dependent diabetes mellitus. J Clin Invest 1990; 85:1944–50.

188. Gepts W. Pathologic anatomy of the pancreas in juvenile diabetes mellitus. Diabetes 1965;14:619–33.

189. Like AA, Rossini AA. Spontaneous autoimmune diabetes mellitus in the Biobreeding/Worcester rat. Surv Synth Pathol Res 1984;3:131–8.

190. Harada M, Makino S. Absence of insulitis and overt diabetes in athymic nude mice with NOD genetic background. Exp Anim (Tokyo) 1986;35:495–8.

191. Kelley V, Gaulton GN, Hattori M, et al. Anti-interleukin 2 receptor antibody suppresses murine diabetic insulitis and lupus nephritis. J Immunol 1988;140:59–61.

192. Wicker LS, Miller BJ, Mullen Y. Transfer of autoimmune diabetes mellitus with splenocytes from nonobese diabetic (NOD) mice. Diabetes 1986;35:855–60.

193. Wang Y, Hao L, Gill RG, Lafferty KJ. Autoimmune diabetes in NOD mouse is L3T4 T-lymphocyte dependent. Diabetes 1987;36: 535–8.

194. Miller BJ, Appel MC, O'Neil JJ, Wicker LS. Both the Lyt2$^+$ and L3T4$^+$ T cell subsets are required for the transfer of diabetes in nonobese diabetic mice. J Immunol 1988;140:52–8.

195. Acha-Orbea H, Mitchell DJ, Timmermann L, et al. Limited heterogeneity of T cell receptors from lymphocytes mediating autoimmune encephalomyelitis allows specific immune intervention. Cell 1988;54:263–73.

196. Banerjee S, Haqqi TM, Luthra HS, et al. Possible role of Vβ T cell receptor genes in susceptibility to collagen-induced arthritis in mice. J Exp Med 1988;167:832–9.

197. Singer PA, McEvilly RJ, Noonan DJ, et al. Clonal diversity and T-cell receptor β-chain variable gene expression in enlarged lymph nodes of MRL-lpr/lpr lupus mice. Proc Natl Acad Sci USA 1986;83:7018–22.

198. Haskins K, Portas M, Bergman B, et al. Pancreatic islet-specific T-cell clones from nonobese diabetic mice. Proc Natl Acad Sci USA 1989;86:8000–4.

199. Haskins K, McDuffie M. Acceleration of diabetes in young NOD mice with a CD4$^+$ islet-specific T cell clone. Science 1990;49:1433–6.

200. Nakano N, Kikutani H, Nishimoto H, Kishimoto T. T cell receptor V gene usage of islet β cell-reactive T cells is not restricted in non-obese diabetic mice. J Exp Med 1991;173:1091–7.

201. Nishimoto H, Kikutani H, Yamamura K, Kishimoto T. Prevention of autoimmune insulitis by expression of I-E molecules in NOD mice. Nature 1987;328:432–34.

202. Shizuru JA, Taylor-Edwards C, Livingstone A, Fathman CG. Genetic dissection of T cell receptor V$_β$ gene requirements for spontaneous murine diabetes. J Exp Med 1991;174:633–8.

203. McDuffie M. Diabetes in NOD mice does not require T-lymphocytes expressing of V$_{β8}$ or V$_{β5}$. Diabetes 1991;40:1555–9.

204. Wicker LS, Miller BJ, Coker LZ, et al. Genetic control of diabetes and insulitis in the nonobese diabetic (NOD) mouse. J Exp Med 1987;165:1639–54.

205. Acha-Orbea H, McDevitt HO. The first external domain of the nonobese diabetic mouse class II I-Aβ chain is unique. Proc Natl Acad Sci USA 1987;84:2435–9.

206. Miyazaki T, Uno M, Uehira M, et al. Direct evidence for the contribution of the unique I-A^{nod} to the development of insulitis in non-obese diabetic mice. Nature 1990;345:722–4.

207. Slattery RM, Kjer-Nielsen L, Allison J. et al. Prevention of diabetes in non-obese diabetic I-A^k transgenic mice. Nature 1990;345:724–6.

208. Lund T, O'Reilly L, Hutchings P, et al. Prevention of insulin-dependent diabetes mellitus in non-obese diabetic mice by transgenes encoding modified I-A β-chain or normal I-E α-chain. Nature 1990;345:727–9.

209. Hattori M, Fukuda M, Ichikawa T, et al. A single recessive non-MHC diabetogenic gene determines the development of insulitis in the presence of an MHC-linked diabetogenic gene in NOD mice. J Autoimmun 1990;3:1–10.

210. Prochazka M, Leiter EH, Serreze DV, Coleman DL. Three recessive loci required for insulin-dependent diabetes in nonobese diabetic mice. Science 1987;237:286–9.

211. Todd JA, Aitman TJ, Cornall RJ, et al. Genetic analysis of autoimmune type 1 diabetes mellitus in mice. Nature 1991;351:542–7.

212. Garchon H-J, Bedossa P, Eloy L, Bach J-F. Identification and mapping to chromosome 1 of a susceptibility locus for periinsulitis in non-obese diabetic mice. Nature 1991;353:260–2.

213. Cornall RJ, Prins J-B, Todd JA, et al. Type I diabetes in mice is linked to the interleukin-1 receptor and Lsh/Ity/Bcg genes on chromosome 1. Nature 1991;353:262–5.

214. Wicker LS, Miller BJ, Chai A, et al. Expression of genetically determined diabetes and insulitis in the nonobese diabetic (NOD) mouse at the level of bone marrow-derived cells. Transfer of diabetes and insulitis to nondiabetic (NOD×B10)F1 mice with bone marrow cells from NOD mice. J Exp Med 1988;167:1801–10.

215. Serreze DV, Leiter EH, Worthen SM, Shultz LD. NOD marrow stem cells adoptively transfer diabetes to resistant (NOD×NON)F1 mice. Diabetes 1988;37:252–5.

216. Ihm S-H, Lee K-U, Yoon J-W. Studies on autoimmunity for initiation of β-cell destruction. VII. Evidence for antigenic changes on β-cells leading to autoimmune destruction of β-cells in BB rats. Diabetes 1991;40:269–74.

217. Yamato E, Hirokawa KJ, Minoshima T, et al. Both islet β cells and the immune system are responsible for the development of diabetes in NOD mice [Abstract]. Clin Res 1992;40:210A.

218. Bottazzo GF, Florin-Christensen A, Doniach D. Islet-cell antibodies in diabetes mellitus with autoimmune polyendocrine deficiencies. Lancet 1974;2:1279–82.

219. Reddy S, Bibby NJ, Elliott RB. Ontogeny of islet cell antibodies, insulin autoantibodies and insulitis in the non-obese diabetic mouse. Diabetologia 1988;31:322–8.

220. Hanafusa T, Fujino-Kurihara H, Miyazaki A, et al. Expression of class II major histocompatibility complex antigens on pancreatic B cells in the NOD mouse. Diabetologia 1987;30:104–8.

221. Nayak RC, Omar MAK, Rabizadeh A, et al. "Cytoplasmic" islet cell antibodies: evidence that the target antigen is a sialoglycoconjugate. Diabetes 1985;34:617–9.

222. Lernmark Å, Freedman ZR, Hofmann C, et al. Islet-cell-surface antibodies in juvenile diabetes mellitus. N Engl J Med 1978;299:375–80.

223. Baekkeskov S, Aanstoot H-J, Christgau S, et al. Identification of the 64K autoantigen in insulin-dependent diabetes as the GABA-synthesizing enzyme glutamic acid decarboxylase. Nature 1990;347:151–6.

224. Atkinson MA, Maclaren NK. Autoantibodies in nonobese diabetic mice immunoprecipitate 64,000-Mr islet antigen. Diabetes 1988:37:1587–90.

225. Baekkeskov S, Dryberg T, Lernmark A. Autoantibodies to a 64-kilodalton islet cell protein precede the onset of spontaneous diabetes in the BB rat. Science 1984;224:1348–50.

226. Palmer JP, Asplin CM, Clemons P, et al. Insulin antibodies in insulin-dependent diabetics before insulin treatment. Science 1983;222:1337–9.

227. Ziegler AG, Vardi P, Ricker AT, et al. Radioassay determination of insulin autoantibodies in NOD mice: correlation with increased risk of progression to overt diabetes. Diabetes 1989;38:358–63.

228. Elias D, Markovits D, Reshef T, et al. Induction and therapy of autoimmune diabetes in the non-obese diabetic (NOD/Lt) mouse by a 65-kDa heat shock protein. Proc Natl Acad Sci USA 1990;87:1576–80.

229. Cohen IR. Autoimmunity to chaperonins in the pathogenesis of arthritis and diabetes. Annu Rev Immunol 1991;9:567–89.

230. Boitard C, Villa MC, Becourt C, et al. Peripherin: an islet antigen that is cross-reactive with nonobese diabetic mouse class II gene products. Proc Natl Acad Sci USA 1992;89:172–6.

231. Brosnan CF, Bornstein MB, Bloom BR. The effects of macrophage depletion on the clinical and pathologic expression of experimental allergic encephalomyelitis. J Immunol 1981;126:614–20.

232. Oschilewski U, Kiesel U, Kolb H. Administration of silica prevents diabetes in BB-rats. Diabetes 1985;34:197–9.

233. Charlton B, Bacelj A, Mandel TE. Administration of silica particles or anti-Lyt2 antibody prevents β-cell destruction in NOD mice given cyclophosphamide. Diabetes 1988;37:930–5.

234. Lee K-U, Amano K, Yoon J-W. Evidence for initial involvement of macrophage in development of insulitis in NOD mice. Diabetes 1988;37:989–91.

235. Hutchings P, Rosen H, O'Reilly L, et al. Transfer of diabetes in mice prevented by blockade of adhesion-promoting receptor on macrophages. Nature 1990;348:639–42.

236. Ziegler K, Unanue ER. Identification of a macrophage antigen-processing event required for I-region-restricted antigen presentation to T lymphocytes. J Immunol 1981;127:1869–75.

237. Adams D. Molecules, membranes and macrophage activation. Immunol Today 1982;3:285–7.

238. Durum SK, Schmidt JA, Oppenheim JJ. Interleukin 1: an immunological perspective. Annu Rev Immunol 1985;3:263–87.

239. Beutler B, Greenwald D, Hulmes JD, et al. Identity of tumour necrosis factor and the macrophage-secreted factor cachectin. Nature 1985;316:552–4.

240. Murray HW, Spitalny GL, Nathan CF. Activation of mouse peritoneal macrophages in vitro and in vivo by interferon-γ. J Immunol 1985;134:1619–22.

241. Horio F, Fukuda M, Bonner-Weir S, Hattori M. Free radical oxygen scavengers (superoxide dismutase and catalase) prevent the development of insulitis in NOD mice [Abstract]. Clin Res 1989;37:451A.

242. Pukel C, Baquerizo H, Rabinovitch A. Destruction of rat islet cell monolayers by cytokines: synergistic interactions of interferon-γ, tumor necrosis factor, lymphotoxin, and interleukin-1. Diabetes 1988;37:133–6.

243. Bendtzen K, Mandrup-Poulsen T, Nerup J, et al. Cytotoxicity of human pI7 interleukin-1 for pancreatic islets of Langerhans. Science 1986;232:1545–47.

244. Palmer JP, Helqvist S, Spinas GA, et al. Interaction of β-cell activity and IL-1 concentration and exposure time in isolated rat islets of Langerhans. Diabetes 1989;38:1211–6.

245. Bernard NF, Ertug F, Margolese H. High incidence of thyroiditis and anti-thyroid autoantibodies in NOD mice. Diabetes 1992;41:40–6.

246. Doi T, Hattori M, Agodoa LYC, et al. Glomerular lesions in nonobese diabetic mouse: before and after the onset of hyperglycemia. Lab Invest 1990;63:204–12.

247. Muraoka Y, Matsui N, Makino S. Renal lesions in NON mice. Jin To Toseki (Kidney and Dialysis) (Tokyo) 1991;31:70–4.

248. Watanabe Y, Itoh Y, Yoshida F, et al. Unique glomerular lesion with spontaneous lipid deposition in glomerular capillary lumina in the NON strain of mice. Nephron 1991;58:210–8.

249. Foulis AK, Farquharson MA, Hardman R. Aberrant expression of class-II major histocompatibility complex molecules by B cells and hyperexpression of class I major histocompatibility complex molecules by insulin containing islets in type I (insulin-dependent) diabetes mellitus. Diabetologia 1987;30:333–43.

250. Bottazzo GF, Dean BM, McNally JM, et al. In situ characterization of autoimmune phenomena and expression of HLA molecules in the pancreas in diabetic insulitis. N Engl J Med 1985;313:353–60.

251. Signore A, Cooke A, Pozzilli P, et al. Class-II and IL 2 receptor positive cells in the pancreas of NOD mice. Diabetologia 1987;30:902–5.

252. Allison J, Campbell IL, Morahan G, et al. Diabetes in transgenic mice resulting from over-expression of class I histocompatibility molecules in pancreatic β cells. Nature 1988;333:529–33.

253. Sarvetnick N, Liggitt D, Pitts SL, et al. Insulin-dependent diabetes mellitus induced in transgenic mice by ectopic expression of class II MHC and interferon-gamma. Cell 1988;52:773–82.

254. Lo D, Burkly LC, Widera G, et al. Diabetes and tolerance in transgenic mice expressing class II MHC molecules in pancreatic beta cells. Cell 1988;53:159–68.

255. Nakhooda AF, Like AA, Chappel CI, et al. The spontaneously diabetic Wistar rat: metabolic and morphologic studies. Diabetes 1977;26:100–12.

256. Nakhooda AF, Like AA, Chappel CI, et al. The spontaneously diabetic Wistar rat (the "BB" rat); studies prior to and during development of the overt syndrome. Diabetologia 1978;14:199–207.

257. Like AA. Depletion of RT6.1+ T lymphocytes alone is insufficient to induce diabetes in diabetes-resistant BB/Wor rats. Am J Pathol 1990;136:565–74.

258. Crisa L, Greiner DL, Mordes JP, et al. Biochemical studies of RT6 alloantigens in BB/Wor and normal rats: evidence for intact unexpressed RT6ᵃ structural gene in diabetes-prone BB rats. Diabetes 1990;39:1279–88.

259. Butler L, Guberski DL, Like AA. Genetics of diabetes production in the Worcester colony of the BB rat. In: Shafrir E, Renold AE, eds. Frontiers in diabetes research: lessons from animal diabetes II. London: John Libbey, 1988:74–8.

260. Jackson R, Rassi N, Crump T, et al. The BB diabetic rat: profound T-cell lymphocytopenia. Diabetes 1981;30:887–9.

261. Poussier P, Nakhooda AF, Falk JA, et al. Lymphopenia and abnormal lymphocyte subsets in the "BB" rat: relationship to the diabetic syndrome. Endocrinology 1982;110:1825–7.

262. Elder ME, Maclaren NK. Identification of profound peripheral T lymphocyte immunodeficiencies in the spontaneously diabetic BB rat. J Immunol 1983;130:1723–31.

263. Woda BA, Like AA, Padden C, McFadden ML. Deficiency of phenotypic cytotoxic-suppressor T lymphocytes in the BB/W rat. J Immunol 1986;136:856–9.

264. Like AA, Guberski DL, Butler L. Diabetic Biobreeding/Worcester (BB/Wor) rats need not be lymphopenic. J Immunol 1986;136:3254–8.

265. Crisa L, Mordes JP, Rossini AA. Autoimmune diabetes mellitus in the BB rat. Diabetes Metab Rev 1993 (in press).

266. Gill TJ III, Kunz HW, Misra DN, Cortese Hassett AL. The

major histocompatibility complex of the rat. Transplantation 1987;43:773–85.

267. Colle E, Guttmann RD, Seemayer T. Spontaneous diabetes mellitus syndrome in the rat. I. Association with the major histocompatibility complex. J Exp Med 1981;154:1237–42.

268. Jackson RA, Buse JB, Rifai R, et al. Two genes required for diabetes in BB rats: evidence from cyclical intercrosses and backcrosses. J Exp Med 1984;159:1629–36.

269. Colle ER, Guttmann RD, Fuks A. Insulin-dependent diabetes mellitus is associated with genes that map to the right of the class I RT1.A locus of the major histocompatibility complex of the rat. Diabetes 1986;35:454–8.

270. Parfrey NA, Prud'homme GJ, Colle E, et al. Immunologic and genetic studies of diabetes in the BB rat. CRC Crit Rev Immunol 1989;9:45–65.

271. Todd JA, Bell JI, McDevitt HO. HLA DQ_β gene contributes to susceptibility and resistance to insulin-dependent diabetes mellitus. Nature 1987;329:599–604.

272. Chao NJ, Timmerman L, McDevitt HO, Jacob CO. Molecular characterization of MHC class II antigens (β1 domain) in the BB diabetes-prone and -resistant rat. Immunogenetics 1989;29:231–4.

273. Guttmann RD, Colle E, Michel F, Seemayer T. Spontaneous diabetes mellitus syndrome in the rat. II. T lymphopenia and its association with clinical disease and pancreatic lymphocytic infiltration. J Immunol 1983;130:1732–5.

274. Woda BA, Biron CA. Natural killer cell number and function in the spontaneously diabetic BB/W rat. J Immunol 1986;137:1860–6.

275. Greiner DL, Handler ES, Nakano K, et al. Absence of the RT-6 T cell subset in diabetes-prone BB/W rats. J Immunol 1986;136:148–51.

276. Fourth International Workshop on Alloantigenic Systems in the Rat. Standardized nomenclature for the rat T-cell alloantigens: report of the committee. Transplant Proc 1983;15:1683.

277. Butcher GW, Clarke S, Tucker EM. Close linkage of peripheral T-lymphocyte antigen A (PtaA) to the hemoglobin variant Hbb on linkage group I of the rat. Transplant Proc 1979;11:29–30.

278. Greiner DL, Barton RW, Goldschneider I, Lubaroff DM. Genetic linkage and cell distribution analysis of T cell alloantigens in the rat. J Immunogenet 1982;9:43–50.

279. Mojcik CF, Greiner DL, Medlock ES, et al. Characterization of RT6 bearing rat lymphocytes. I. Ontogeny of the RT6+ subset. Cell Immunol 1988;114:336–46.

280. Mordes JP, Gallina DL, Handler ES, et al. Transfusions enriched for W3/25+ helper/inducer T lymphocytes prevent spontaneous diabetes in the BB/W rat. Diabetologia 1987;30:22–6.

281. Greiner DL, Mordes JP, Handler ES, et al. Depletion of RT.6.1+ T lymphocytes induces diabetes in resistant Biobreeding/Worcester (BB/W) rats. J Exp Med 1987;166:461–75.

282. Angelillo M, Greiner DL, Mordes JP, et al. Absence of RT6+ T cells in diabetes-prone Biobreeding/Worcester rats is due to genetic and cell developmental defects. J Immunol 1988;141:4146–51.

283. Koch F, Thiele H-G, Low MG. Release of the rat T cell alloantigen RT-6.2 from cell membranes by phosphatidylinositol-specific phospholipase C. J Exp Med 1986;164:1338–43.

284. Koch F, Kashan A, Thiele H-G. The rat T-cell differentiation marker RT6.1 is more polymorphic than its alloantigenic counterpart RT6.2. Immunology 1988;65:259–65.

285. Prochazka M, Gaskins HR, Leiter EH, et al. Chromosomal localization, DNA polymorphism, and expression of Rt-6, the mouse homologue of rat T-lymphocyte differentiation marker RT6. Immunogenetics 1991;33:152–6.

286. Like AA, Biron CA, Weringer EJ, et al. Prevention of diabetes in Biobreeding/Worcester rats with monoclonal antibodies that recognize T lymphocytes or natural killer cells. J Exp Med 1986;164:1145–59.

287. Pukel C, Baquerizo H, Rabinovitch A. Interleukin-2 activates BB/W diabetic rat lymphoid cells cytotoxic to islet cells. Diabetes 1987;36:1217–22.

288. Sternthal E, Like AA, Sarantis K, Braverman LE. Lymphocytic thyroiditis and diabetes in the BB/W rat: a new model of autoimmune endocrinopathy. Diabetes 1981;30:1058–61.

289. Colle E, Guttmann RD, Seemayer TA. Association of spontaneous thyroiditis with the major histocompatibility complex of the rat. Endocrinology 1985;116:1243–7.

290. Wright JR Jr, Yates AJ, Sharma HM, et al. Testicular atrophy in the spontaneously diabetic BB Wistar rat. Am J Pathol 1982;108:72–9.

291. Kawano K, Hirashima T, Mori S, et al. A new rat strain with insulin-dependent diabetes mellitus, "LETL". Rat News Letter 1989;22:14–5.

292. Kawano K, Hirashima T, Mori S, et al. New inbred strain of Long-Evans Tokushima Lean rats with IDDM without lymphopenia. Diabetes 1991;40:1375-81.

293. Meier H, Yerganian GA. Spontaneous hereditary diabetes mellitus in Chinese hamster (Cricetulus griseus). 1. Pathological findings. Proc Soc Exp Biol Med 1959;100:810–5.

294. Gerritsen GC. The Chinese hamster as a model for the study of diabetes mellitus. Diabetes 1982;31(Suppl 1):14–21.

295. Kramer JW, Klaassen JK, Baskin DG, et al. Inheritance of diabetes mellitus in Keeshond dogs. Am J Vet Res 1988;49:428–31.

296. Rakieten N, Rakieten ML, Nadkarni MV. Studies on the diabetogenic action of streptozotocin (NSC-37917). Cancer Chemother Rep 1963;29:91–8.

297. Junod A, Lambert AE, Orci L, et al. Studies of the diabetogenic action of streptozotocin. Proc Soc Exp Biol Med 1967;126:201–5.

298. Yamamoto H, Uchigata Y, Okamoto H. Streptozotocin and alloxan induce DNA strand breaks and poly(ADP-ribose) synthetase in pancreatic islets. Nature 1981;294:284–6.

299. Uchigata Y, Yamamoto H, Kawamura A, Okamoto H. Protection by superoxide dismutase, catalase, and poly (ADP-ribose) synthetase inhibitors against alloxan- and streptozotocin-induced islet DNA strand breaks and against the inhibition of proinsulin synthesis. J Biol Chem 1982;257:6084–8.

300. Wilson GL, Hartig PC, Patton NJ, LeDoux SP. Mechanisms of nitrosourea-induced β-cell damage: activation of poly-(ADP-ribose) synthetase and cellular distribution. Diabetes 1988;37:213–6.

301. Like AA, Rossini AA. Streptozotocin-induced pancreatic insulitis: new model of diabetes mellitus. Science 1976;193:415–7.

302. Kim YT, Steinberg C. Immunologic studies on the induction of diabetes in experimental animals. Cellular basis for the induction of diabetes by streptozotocin. Diabetes 1984;33:771–7.

303. Andersson A. Islet implantation normalises hyperglycaemia caused by streptozotocin-induced insulitis: experiments in mice. Lancet 1979;1:581–4.

304. Rossini AA, Appel MC, Williams RM, Like AA. Genetic influence of the streptozotocin-induced insulitis and hyperglycemia. Diabetes 1977;26:916–20.

305. Kiesel U, Falkenberg FW, Kolb H. Genetic control of low-dose streptozotocin-induced autoimmune diabetes in mice. J Immunol 1983;130:1719–22.

306. Wolf J, Lilly F, Shin SI. The influence of genetic background on the susceptibility of inbred mice to streptozotocin-induced diabetes. Diabetes 1984;33:567–71.

307. Uchigata Y, Yamamoto H, Nagai H, Okamoto H. Effect of poly (ADP-ribose) synthetase inhibitor administration to rats before and after injection of alloxan and streptozotocin on islet proinsulin synthesis. Diabetes 1983;32:316–8.

308. Nichols WK, Spellman JB, Daynes RA. Immune responses of diabetic animals: comparison of genetically obese and streptozotocin-diabetic mice. Diabetologia 1978;14:343–9.

309. Mahmoud AA, Rodman HM, Mandel MA, Warren KS. Induced and spontaneous diabetes mellitus and suppression of cell-mediated immunologic responses: granuloma formation, delayed dermal reactivity and allograft rejection. J Clin Invest 1976;57:362–7.

310. Nichols WK, Vann LL, Spellman JB. Streptozotocin effects on T lymphocytes and bone marrow cells. Clin Exp Immunol 1981;46:627–32.

311. Nichols WK, Spellman JB, Vann LL, Daynes RA. Immune responses of diabetic animals: direct immunosuppressant effects of streptozotocin in mice. Diabetologia 1979;16:51–7.

312. Wellhausen SR. Definition of streptozocin toxicity for primary lymphoidal tissues. Diabetes 1986;35:1404–11.

313. Craighead JE. Viral diabetes mellitus in man and experimental animals. Am J Med 1981;70:127–34.

314. Notkins AL, Yoon J-W. Virus-induced diabetes mellitus. In: Notkins AL, Oldstone MBA, eds. Concepts in viral pathogenesis. New York: Springer-Verlag, 1984:241–7.

315. Yoon JW. The role of viruses and environmental factors in the induction of diabetes. Curr Top Microbiol Immunol 1990;164:95–123.

316. Yoon J-W, Rodrigues MM, Currier C, Notkins AL. Long-term complications of virus-induced diabetes mellitus in mice. Nature 296;1982:566–9.

317. Onodera T, Ray UR, Melez KA, et al. Virus-induced diabetes mellitus: autoimmunity and polyendocrine disease prevented by immunosuppression. Nature 1982;297:66–8.

318. Gerling I, Nejman C, Chatterjee NK. Effect of coxsackievirus B4 infection in mice on expression of 64,000-Mr autoantigen and glucose sensitivity of islets before development of hyperglycemia. Diabetes 1988;37:1419–25.

319. Oldstone MBA, Southern P, Rodriguez M, Lampert P. Virus persists in β cells of islets of Langerhans and is associated with chemical manifestations of diabetes. Science 1984;224:1440–3.

320. Oldstone MBA, Rodriguez M, Daughaday WH, Lampert PW. Viral perturbation of endocrine function: disordered cell function leads to disturbed homeostasis and disease. Nature 1984;307:278–81.

321. Ohashi PS, Oehen S, Buerki K, et al. Ablation of "tolerance" and induction of diabetes by virus infection in viral antigen transgenic mice. Cell 1991;65:305–17.

322. Oldstone MBA, Nerenberg M, Southern P, Price J, Lewicki H. Virus infection triggers insulin-dependent diabetes mellitus in a transgenic model: role of anti-self (virus) immune response. Cell 1991;65:319–31.

323. Rayfield EJ, Gorelkin L, Curnow RT, Jahrling PB. Virus-induced pancreatic disease by Venezuelan encephalitis virus: alterations in glucose tolerance and insulin release. Diabetes 1976;25:623–31.

324. Menser MA, Forrest JM, Bransby RD. Rubella infection and diabetes mellitus. Lancet 1978;1:57–60.

325. Rayfield EJ. Effects of rubella virus infection on islet function. Curr Top Microbiol Immunol 1990;156:63–74.

326. Onodera T, Jenson AB, Yoon J-W, Notkins AL. Virus-induced diabetes mellitus: reovirus infection of pancreatic β cells in mice. Science 1978;201:529–31.

327. Campbell IL, Harrison LC, Ashcroft RG, Jack I. Reovirus infection enhances expression of class I MHC proteins on human β-cell and rat RINm5F cell. Diabetes 1988;37:362–5.

328. Guberski DL, Thomas VA, Shek WR, Like AA, Handler ES, Rossini AA, Wallace JE, Welsh RM. Induction of type I diabetes by Kilham's rat virus in diabetes-resistant BB/Wor rats. Science 1991;254:1010–3.

329. Thomas VA, Woda BA, Handler ES, Greiner DL, Mordes JP, Rossini AA. Altered expression of diabetes in BB/Wor rats by exposure to viral pathogens. Diabetes 1991;40:255–8.

330. Like AA, Guberski DL, Butler L. Influence of environmental viral agents on frequency and tempo of diabetes mellitus in BB/Wor rats. Diabetes 1991;40:259–62.

331. Ewel C, Sobel DO, Zeligs B, et al. The role of alpha interferon in the pathogenesis of diabetes mellitus [Abstract no. 292]. Diabetes 1989;38(Suppl 2):73A.

332. Suzuki T, Yamada T, Fujumura T, Kawamura E, Shimizu M, Yamashita R, Nomoto K. Diabetogenic effects of lymphocyte transfusion on the NOD or NOD nude mouse. In: Rygaard J, Brunner N, Graem N, Sprang-Thomsen M, eds. Immune-deficient animals in biomedical research. Fifth International Workshop on Immune-Deficient Animals. Basel: Karger, 1987:112–6.

333. Oldstone MBA. Prevention of type I diabetes in nonobese diabetic mice by virus infection. Science 1988;239:500–2.

334. Oldstone MBA. Viruses as therapeutic agents. I. Treatment of nonobese insulin-dependent diabetes mice with virus prevents insulin-dependent diabetes mellitus while maintaining general immune competence. J Exp Med 1990;171:2077–89.

335. Dyrberg T, Schwimmbeck PL, Oldstone MBA. Inhibition of diabetes in BB rats by virus infection. J Clin Invest 1988;81:928–31.

336. Wilberz S, Partke HJ, Dagnaes-Hansen F, Herberg L. Persistent MHV (mouse hepatitis virus) infection reduces the incidence of diabetes mellitus in non-obese diabetic mice. Diabetologia 1991;34:2–5.

337. Oldstone MBA, Yamazaki S, Niwa A, Notkins AL. In vitro detection of cells infected with lactic dehydrogenase virus (LDV) by fluorescein-labeled antibody to LDV. Intervirology 1973/74;2:261–5.

338. Inada T, Mims CA. Mouse Ia antigens are receptors for lactate dehydrogenase virus. Nature 1984;309:59–61.

339. Inada T, Mims CA. Infection of mice with lactic dehydrogenase virus prevents development of experimental allergic encephalomyelitis. J Neuroimmunol 1986;11:53–6.

340. Elliott RB, Martin JM. Dietary protein: a trigger of insulin-dependent diabetes in the BB rat? Diabetologia 1984;26:297–9.

341. Scott FW, Mongeau R, Kardish M, et al. Diet can prevent diabetes in the BB rat. Diabetes 1985;34:1059–62.

342. Elliott RB, Reddy SN, Bibby NJ, Kida K. Dietary prevention of diabetes in the non-obese diabetic mouse. Diabetologia 1988;31:62–4.

343. Coleman DL, Kuzava JE, Leiter EH. Effect of diet on incidence of diabetes in nonobese diabetic mice. Diabetes 1990;39:432–6.

344. Lehman CD, Rodin J, McEwen B, Brinton R. Impact of environmental stress on the expression of insulin-dependent diabetes mellitus. Behav Neurosci 1991;105:241–5.

345. Posselt AM, Barker CF, Tomaszewski JE, et al. Induction of donor-specific unresponsiveness by intrathymic islet transplantation. Science 1990;249:1293–5.

346. Posselt AM, Barker CF, Friedman AL, Naji A. Prevention of autoimmune diabetes in the BB rat by intrathymic islet transplantation at birth. Science 1992;256:1321–4.

347. Like AA, Kislauskis E, Williams RM, Rossini AA. Neonatal thymectomy prevents spontaneous diabetes mellitus in the BB/W rat. Science 1982;216:644–6.

348. Ogawa M, Maruyama T, Hasegawa T, et al. The inhibitory effect of neonatal thymectomy on the incidence of insulitis in non-obese diabetes (NOD) mice. Biomed Res 1985;6:103–5.

349. Dardenne M, Lepault F, Bendelac A, Bach J-F. Acceleration of the onset of diabetes in NOD mice by thymectomy at weaning. Eur J Immunol 1989;19:889–95.

350. Naji A, Silvers WK, Bellgrau D, Barker CF. Spontaneous diabetes in rats: destruction of islets is prevented by immunological tolerance. Science 1981;213:1390–2.

351. Nakano K, Mordes JP, Handler ES, et al. Role of host immune system in BB/Wor rat: predisposition to diabetes resides in bone marrow. Diabetes 1988;37:520–5.

352. Ikehara S, Ohtsuki H, Good RA, et al. Prevention of type I diabetes in nonobese diabetic mice by allogeneic bone marrow transplantation. Proc Natl Acad Sci USA 1985;82:7743–7.

353. Yasumizu R, Sugiura K, Iwai H, et al. Treatment of type I diabetes mellitus in non-obese mice by transplantion of allogeneic bone marrow and pancreatic tissue. Proc Natl Acad Sci USA 1987;84:6555–7.

354. Yamato E, Hirokawa KJ, Minoshima T, et al. Both islet β cells and the immune system are responsible for the development of diabetes in NOD mice [Abstract]. Clin Res 1992;40:210A.

355. Gotfredsen CF, Buschard K, Frandsen EK. Reduction of diabetes incidence of BB Wistar rats by early prophylactic insulin treatment of diabetes-prone animals. Diabetologia 1985;28:933–5.

356. Like AA. Insulin injections prevent diabetes (DB) in Bio-Breeding/Worcester (BB/Wor) rats [Abstract no. 295]. Diabetes 1986;35(Suppl 1):74A.

357. Appel MC, O'Neil JJ. Prevention of spontaneous diabetes in the BB/W rat by insulin treatment. Pancreas 1986;1:356.

358. Atkinson MA, Maclaren NK, Luchetta R. Insulitis and diabetes in NOD mice reduced by prophylactic insulin therapy. Diabetes 1990;39:933–7.

359. Zhang ZJ, Davidson L, Eisenbarth G, Weiner HL. Suppression of diabetes in nonobese diabetic mice by oral administration of porcine insulin. Proc Natl Acad Sci USA 1991;88:10252–6.

360. Nicoletti F, Mughini L, Landolfo S, et al. Prevention of diabetes in BB/Wor rats treated with monoclonal antibodies to interferon-gamma. Lancet 1990;336:319.

361. Campbell IL, Oxbrow L, Harrison LC. Reduction in insulitis following administration of IFN-γ and TNF-α. J Autoimmun 1991;4:249–62.

362. Satoh J, Seino H, Shintani S, et al. Inhibition of type I diabetes in BB rats with recombinant human tumor necrosis factor-α. J Immunol 1990;145:1395–9.

363. Satoh J, Seino H, Abo T, et al. Recombinant human tumor necrosis factor-α suppresses autoimmune diabetes in nonobese diabetic mice. J Clin Invest 1989;84:1345–8.

364. Campbell IL, Oxbrow L, Harrison LC. Reduction in insulitis following administration of IFN-γ and TNF-α. J Autoimmun 1991;4:249–62.

365. Zielasek J, Burkart V, Naylor P, et al. Interleukin-2-dependent control of disease development in spontaneously diabetic BB rats. Immunology 1990;69:209–14.

366. Burstein D, Handler ES, Schindler J, et al. Effect of interleukin-2 on diabetes in the BB/Wor rat. Diabetes Res 1987;5:163–7.

367. Like AA, Rossini AA, Guberski DL, et al. Spontaneous diabetes mellitus: reversal and prevention in the BB/WW rat with antisera to rat lymphocytes. Science 1979;206:1421–3.

368. Harada M, Makino S. Suppression of overt diabetes in NOD mice by anti-thymocyte serum or anti-Thy 1.2 antibody. Exp Anim 1986;35:501–4.

369. Hahn HJ, Lucke W, Kloting I, et al. Curing BB rats of freshly manifested diabetes by short-term treatment with a combination of a monoclonal anti-interleukin 2 receptor antibody and a subtherapeutic dose of cyclosporin A. Eur J Immunol 1987;40:825–9.

370. Kelly V, Gaulton GN, Hattori M, et al. Anti-interleukin 2 receptor suppresses murine diabetic insulitis and lupus nephritis. J Immunol 1988;140:59–61.

371. Boitard C, Michie S, Serrurier P, et al. In vivo prevention of thyroid and pancreatic autoimmunity in the BB rat by antibody to class II major histocompatibility complex gene products. Proc Natl Acad Sci USA 1985;82:6627–31.

372. Boitard C, Bendelac A, Richard M, et al. Prevention of diabetes in nonobese diabetic mice by anti-I-A monoclonal antibodies: transfer of protection by splenic T cells. Proc Natl Acad Sci USA 1988;85:9719–23.

373. Koike T, Itoh Y, Ishi T, et al. Preventive effect of monoclonal anti-L3T4 antibody on development of diabetes in NOD mice. Diabetes 1987;36:539–41.

374. Wang Y, Hao L, Gill RG, Lafferty KJ. Autoimmune diabetes in NOD mouse is L3T4 T-lymphocyte dependent. Diabetes 1987;35:535–8.

375. Shizuru JA, Taylor Edwards C, Banks BA, et al. Immunotherapy of the non-obese diabetic mouse: treatment with an antibody to T-helper lymphocytes. Science 1988;240:659–62.

376. Hutchings PR, Simpson E, O'Reilly LA, et al. The involvement of Ly2+ cells in beta cell destruction. J Autoimmun 1990;3:101–9.

377. Mordes JP, Gallina DL, Handler ES, et al. Tranfusions enriched for W3/25+ helper/inducer T lymphocytes prevent spontaneous diabetes in the BB/W rat. Diabetologia 1987;30:22–6.

378. Like AA, Weringer EJ, Holdash A, et al. Adoptive transfer of autoimmune diabetes mellitus in BioBreeding/Worcester (BB/W) inbred and hybrid rats. J Immunol 1985;134:1583–7.

379. Harada M, Makino S. Promotion of spontaneous diabetes in nonobese diabetes-prone mice by cyclophosphamide. Diabetologia 1982;27:604–6.

380. Like AA, Dirodi V, Thomas S, et al. Prevention of diabetes mellitus in the BB/W rat with cyclosporin-A. Am J Pathol 1984;117:92–7.

381. Mori Y, Suko M, Okudaira H, et al. Preventive effects of cyclosporin on diabetes in NOD mice. Diabetologia 1986;29:244–7.

382. Murase N, Lieberman I, Nalesnik MA, et al. Effect of FK 506 on spontaneous diabetes in BB rats. Diabetes 1990;39:1584–6.

383. Miyagawa J, Yamamoto K, Hanafusa T, et al. Preventive effect of a new immunosuppressant FK-506 on insulitis and diabetes in non-obese diabetic mice. Diabetologia 1990;33:503−5.

384. Eisenbarth GS. Type I diabetes mellitus: a chronic autoimmune disease. N Engl J Med 1986;314:1360−8.

385. Srikanta S, Ganda OP, Gleason RE, et al. Pre-type I diabetes: linear loss of beta cell response to intravenous glucose. Diabetes 1984;33:717−20.

386. Rossini AA, Mordes JP, Like AA. Immunology of insulin-dependent diabetes mellitus. Annu Rev Immunol 1985;3:289−320.

387. Tominaga M, Komiya I, Johnson JH, et al. Loss of insulin response to glucose but not arginine during the development of autoimmune diabetes in BB/W rats: relationships to islet volume and glucose transport rate. Proc Natl Acad Sci USA 1986;83:9749−53.

388. Spinas GA, Palmer JP, Mandrup-Poulsen T, et al. The bimodal effect of interleukin-1 on rat pancreatic beta-cells—stimulation followed by inhibition—depends upon dose, duration of exposure, and ambient glucose concentration. Acta Endocrinol 1988; 119:307−11.

389. Palmer JP, Helqvist S, Spinas GA, et al. Interaction of β-cell activity and IL-1 concentration and exposure time in isolated rat islets of Langerhans. Diabetes 1989;38: 1211−6.

390. Higgins PJ, Weiner HL. Suppression of experimental autoimmune encephalomyelitis by oral administration of myelin basic protein and its fragments. J Immunol 1988;140:440−5.

391. Zhang ZJ, Lee CSY, Lider O, Weiner HL. Suppression of adjuvant arthritis in Lewis rats by oral administration of type II collagen. J Immunol 1990;145:2489−93.

392. Nussenblatt RB, Caspi RR, Mahdi R, et al. Inhibition of S-antigen induced experimental autoimmune uveoretinitis by oral induction of tolerance with S-antigen. J Immunol 1990;144:1689−95.

Chapter 19

OBESITY

JEFFREY S. FLIER

Adipose tissue has two primary functions: to serve as the site for storage of energy-rich fatty acids in the form of triglyceride and to effect the controlled release of the constituent fatty acids and glycerol in response to neural, endocrine, and local signals for metabolism at distant sites. Obesity is defined as a state of excessive adipose-tissue mass and is best viewed as a symptom or group of diseases rather than as a single disease entity. The importance of this state derives from its high prevalence in our society and its association with serious morbidity, not the least of which is a marked increase in the prevalence of non-insulin-dependent diabetes mellitus (NIDDM). Specific syndromes of obesity both in animal models and in humans are associated with identified neural, endocrine, or genetic causes. However, the pathogenesis of obesity in the vast majority of humans is unknown, apart from the fact of an unexplained chronic excess in caloric intake relative to energy needs. An understanding of obesity and its consequences therefore requires the investigation of the many factors that control energy intake and energy expenditure, the two interrelated components of the energy-balance equation. As with our understanding of pathogenesis, our understanding of the molecular connection between obesity and its most important complications is limited, and our approach to therapy, as defined by clinical success rate, is extremely poor. In this chapter, I will review our current understanding of the pathogenesis, complications, and treatment of obesity.

DEFINITION AND INDICES OF OBESITY

The distribution of body weight in the population is a continuous function without a clear separation between lean and obese. As a result, the selection of such a cut-off is somewhat arbitrary. A number of different criteria have been used. The most medically relevant criterion relates to the identification of a weight that confers morbidity. The most influential application of this approach has been through the use of life-insurance data (Metropolitan Life) that assesses mortality as a function of body weight per height, adjusted for frame size, with obesity defined on purely statistical grounds as a weight that is 20% or more above the average weight per height.[1] This approach can be criticized on many grounds, including the nonrepresentative nature of the insured group, the absence of a correction for age or race, and a number of other methodologic issues. Nonetheless, data such as these based on populations in the millions have demonstrated excess mortality in men who are more than 15 to 20% heavier than the average weight for age and in women who are more than 45% heavier than the average weight for age. Whether obesity is tolerated better by women than by men, as is suggested by such numbers, has not been established.

A second approach to defining the obese state involves quantitation of adipose tissue, either directly or indirectly. Values are obtained for a reference group viewed as normal, and obesity is defined in statistical terms by comparisons to that group. The methods that have been used to quantitate adipose tissue are listed in Table 19–1.[2] The direct methods are viewed as accurate but generally are used as research tools. Of the indirect methods, determination of weight/height ratios is the one used most widely. The body-mass index (BMI), defined as the weight in kilograms divided by the height in meters squared, has been shown to correlate well with definitions based on measurements of body fat by densitometry. A BMI of 25 is generally considered the upper limit of normal, with BMIs of 25 to 30 being defined as overweight and of those in excess of 30 being defined as obesity.[3]

The definition of obesity can be refined on the basis of the realization that the accumulation of adipose tissue in different depots has distinct consequences. Thus, many of the most important complications of obesity, including insulin resistance, diabetes, hypertension, and hyperlipidemia, are linked to the amount of intra-abdominal fat, rather than to lower-body fat (i.e., buttocks and leg) or subcutaneous abdominal fat.[4,5] This parameter, typically evident on physical examination, can be quantitated by determining the waist-to-hip circumference ratio (with a ratio greater than 0.72 considered abnormal) or, more accurately, by computed tomography.

PREVALENCE OF OBESITY

It is obvious from casual inspection of the population that obesity is prevalent in the United States, although the precise prevalence figures vary considerably, depending on the nature of the population surveyed and the definition of obesity used. When one uses data from the 1979 Build Study and the cut-off point of 20% or more above the average weight as representing obesity, 4 to 14% of men and 10 to 24% of women will be considered obese.[1] The lower figures in these ranges are based on the assumption that the age-related increase in body weight is normal, and the higher figures are based, more appropriately, on the assumption that the proper standards are the weights of the population between 20 and 29 years of age. It seems clear that obesity is more prevalent in women than in men and that black women, particularly those between the ages of 45 and 65, are at especially high risk (49%).[6] Whether the prevalence of obesity is increasing in the population at large in recent years has not been clearly established.

CELL BIOLOGY AND METABOLISM OF THE ADIPOSE CELL

Seen in terms of cellular and molecular biology, the development of adipose tissue requires the replication of

Table 19–1. Methods Used to Quantitate Adipose Mass

1. Densitometry: underwater weighing
2. Estimate of total body water: tritiated or deuterated water
3. Total body potassium: isotope dilution or whole-body counter
4. Computed tomographic or magnetic resonance imaging
5. Electrical impedance
6. Dual photon beam absorptiometry

fibroblast-like precursor cells, or preadipocytes, and their subsequent differentiation into adipocytes, defined by their ability to express and regulate an array of adipose-specific mRNAs. These mRNAs in turn encode the characteristic protein machinery of the adipocyte. In recent years, much has been learned about the regulated expression of adipocyte-specific genes.[7] For example, genes that encode metabolic enzymes such as glycerophosphate dehydrogenase or fatty acid-binding proteins such as adipocyte protein 2 (AP-2) have been intensively investigated, and the nuclear proteins that interact with specific regulatory elements in the 5′-flanking region of such genes have been defined.[8] However, the key transcription factors and DNA elements that must interact to establish a cell as a preadipocyte, i.e., a cell that will express adipocyte-specific genes under appropriate conditions, are not known. Neither are the extracellular factors, apart from insulin and insulin-like growth factor-I (IGF-I),[9] that regulate the proliferation and differentiated expression of such cells. Such information is likely to be obtained in the next several years and will allow investigators to account more completely for the differences found in the number and distribution of adipose cells in different individuals. It has been known for many years that the adipocytes of individuals who have been obese from childhood or who are severely obese at any age are not only bigger but more numerous than those in non-obese individuals.[10] Hyperplasia of adipocytes has been suggested to increase—through an unclear mechanism—the difficulty of losing and keeping off weight.[10]

The source of most fatty acids stored in adipose tissue are circulating triglyceride-rich lipoproteins. Triglycerides contained in chylomicrons and very-low-density lipoproteins (VLDL) are hydrolyzed on the capillary endothelium by the enzyme lipoprotein lipase (LPL) to produce fatty acids that are transported into adipocytes.[11] Insulin plays a key role in this process, both by activating LPL in adipose tissue and by facilitating glucose transport into adipocytes, where conversion to α-glycerol phosphate provides the backbone for esterification of free fatty acids (FFA) to triglyceride. LPL activity is influenced by nutrition, and the nature of this regulation differs in adipose tissue and muscle, reflecting the different roles (i.e., energy storage vs. use) of FFA in these tissues. Abnormal regulation of adipose tissue LPL, with a resultant increase in activity, has been observed in obese individuals by some investigators.[12] Glucose- and ethanol-derived acetate contribute, to a limited extent, to fatty acid synthesis.

Hydrolysis of stored triglyceride to yield FFA and glycerol is brought about by hormone-sensitive lipase, an enzyme that is activated through phosphorylation via cyclic adenosine monophosphate (cAMP)-mediated activation of protein kinase A. Positive effectors of the lipase include epinephrine, norepinephrine, glucagon, adrenocorticotropic hormone (ACTH), and growth hormone. Thyroxine and cortisol exert permissive effects. These neural and hormonal actions are opposed by insulin, which is the dominant anabolic hormone in fat.

Recent studies indicate that adipose cells may be regulated in ways other than these classic hormonal actions. Thus, blood flow to fat appears to be a highly regulated process that may play an important role in the net amount of lipolysis through effects on the rate of reesterification that takes place.[13] The mechanism of this regulation and its possible role in disease are not known. It has also become apparent that the adipocyte is capable of producing and secreting an array of proteins not previously thought to be associated with this cell. These include a variety of complement proteins (factor D),[14] cytokines (tumor necrosis factor), and hormones or hormone precursors (angiotensinogen)[15] that may influence adipocyte function and/or systemic processes in unanticipated ways.

ETIOLOGY OF OBESITY

On one level, the pathophysiology of obesity is straightforward: a sustained excess of nutrient intake over expenditure. The interrelated systems that regulate energy intake and expenditure are complex and only partially understood, and it has proven difficult to define and quantitate all of the relevant parameters over appropriate time periods in human subjects. It is clear, however, that obesity can be caused by a variety of specific lesions acting at different physiologic sites, in both animals and humans. These lesions may involve neural and endocrine pathways and, as seen in animal models, can be caused by a number of distinct single gene defects. At this time, such specific disorders causing obesity account for only a small percentage of persons with obesity (see below), with the vast majority having no defined basis for their obesity.

General Considerations Related to Energy Balance

Two major processes comprise the regulators of energy balance in vivo: nutrient intake and energy expenditure. Chronic excess of intake over expenditure necessitates storage, which is accomplished primarily through accumulation of fat; storage of energy as glycogen is extremely limited. Energy may also be stored in the form of an increased lean body mass, which is evident in individuals with major obesity.[16] Several questions emerge from this formulation. Is obesity (or are individual syndromes of obesity), either during its development or in the established state, associated with excessive food intake, diminished energy expenditure, or both? If it is, what molecular mechanisms are responsible for the defects?

Several methodologic issues have hampered progress in this regard, including 1) potential etiologic heterogeneity of the obese population; 2) fundamental differences between established obesity and the pre-obese state; 3) difficulties in obtaining accurate assessments of food intake under free-living conditions; 4) difficulties in obtaining accurate measurements of energy expenditure under free-living conditions; and 5) insufficient understanding of the critical molecular and neuroendocrine factors that control and integrate these systems. Despite these difficulties, progress has been made over the past several years and will be discussed in the sections that follow.

Abnormal Regulation of Food Intake

The mechanisms responsible for regulation of food intake are complex and not completely understood, and a detailed discussion is beyond the scope of this chapter. In brief, regulation involves both internal signals that govern hunger and satiety and external factors that relate to availability and palatability of food, as well as numerous cultural, psychological, and environmental influences.[17] The physiologic basis for hunger and satiety has been studied extensively. Much is known about the role of specific hypothalamic centers in this process, in part through the study of animals with chemical or surgical lesions.[18] Many hormones, substrates, and neurotransmitters have been and continue to be studied as putative hunger or satiety factors, although no dominant factors have emerged to date. Among the best-studied candidates are cholecystokinin (CCK) and neuropeptide Y.[19,20] CCK is a gastrointestinal hormone that may play a role in induction of satiety via vagal afferent nerves, whereas administration of neuropeptide Y,[21] induces food intake.

It has been speculated for many years that a regulatory loop might exist for the purpose of maintaining a desired stable weight, or "set point," at least in part by down-regulating food intake in response to increases in adipose mass.[22] The "set point" hypothesis postulates an afferent signal responsive to energy stores, one or more efferent signals to regulate appetite and energy expenditure, and a center for the integration of these components. Physiologic proof of the existence of an afferent signal from adipose tissue, the biochemical basis for such a signal, and the identity of a central "lipostat" are presently lacking.

Regardless of the mechanism of food intake, do obese individuals, as they frequently claim, ingest fewer calories than their lean counterparts or do they have an absolute increase in caloric intake? Many different answers, each based on attempts to estimate food ingestion per se, have been found, the variability presumably reflecting the methodologic difficulties inherent to such estimates. More definitive answers have emerged from studies of energy expenditure, which, under conditions of stable weight, must equal energy intake. These studies, which are discussed in more detail below, reveal that obese individuals (or at least the great majority of them), have increased 24-hour energy expenditure compared with lean sedentary individuals.[23–28] This increase in energy expenditure is due to the increase in lean body mass in these individuals, as well as to an increase in the energy required for weight-bearing activities. Thus, the proposition that patients with established obesity maintain their excess weight despite low-calorie intake is without support. It is less clear whether some individuals in the pre-obese or post-reduced state are predisposed to the development of obesity and a positive energy balance when their energy intake is relatively low. This notion appears to be supported by some studies.[29,30] The period during the dynamic state of weight gain is an important time since it is clear that overeating and resultant obesity themselves result in secondary increases in energy expenditure.

Abnormal Regulation of Energy Expenditure

Energy expenditure can be divided into four components: the resting metabolic rate (RMR), the thermic effect of food (TEF), the thermic effect of exercise (TEE), and adaptive thermogenesis.[23] The RMR normally accounts for between 65 and 75% of the total daily energy expenditure. RMR measures the energy expended for maintenance of normal body functions at rest and is obtained by taking measurements several hours remote from food intake or exercise. The rate is determined in large part by fat-free mass but also is influenced by sex, age, physical conditioning, and genetic factors. RMR in absolute terms is almost always increased in obese individuals; however, when RMR is expressed in terms of fat-free mass, it is typically normal.[23,25-28] These two expressions of RMR have different applications. RMR expressed in absolute terms is most relevant to the question of total energy expenditure (and by inference, if weight is stable, to food intake) in obese individuals. RMR expressed per lean body mass is most relevant to the question of possible biochemical differences between lean and obese individuals that might predispose to efficient energy metabolism and weight gain. It is possible that some obese individuals in the so-called pre-obese state or after weight reduction have a reduction in RMR per lean body mass. The molecular/physiologic basis for such a potential defect is not clear, but abnormalities of futile cycling[31] and/or energy-expensive processes such as ion pumping[32,33] have been proposed. It has been calculated that a low RMR by itself, i.e., in the absence of hyperphagia, would contribute only modestly to the tendency to gain weight, since the increased total RMR consequent to weight gain would counter any earlier reduction in RMR. That is, in the absence of hyperphagia, an increased RMR would result in equilibration at a new, modestly increased weight. Thus, for major obesity to develop, dysregulation of food intake must coexist with any possible thermogenic defect.

The TEF, also referred to as dietary induced thermogenesis, accounts for approximately 10% of energy ingested. It consists of the energy costs of absorbing and processing food, as well as the consequences of certain post-meal events such as activation of sympathetic nervous system activity.[34] The possible involvement of TEF in the genesis of obesity has engendered much controversy, with numerous studies supporting either a defect or a normal energy expenditure in obese individuals after meals or glucose ingestion.[35,36] It is clear that under conditions of euglycemic clamping at comparable insulin infusion rates, obesity is associated with reduced levels of insulin-stimulated energy expenditure, and this defect is even more apparent as glucose intolerance supervenes.[35,36] It is likely that this reduction is a consequence of a reduction in the capacity of insulin to promote glucose storage, an energy-requiring process.

The thermic effect of exercise is the most variable component of energy expenditure, and a possible causative role for this component in obesity has been studied. As with studies of food intake, methodologic issues have limited progress. There is little reason to believe that a reduction in the energy expended during exercise is an important cause of obesity,[57] although some studies have supported this notion.[29,30]

Adaptive thermogenesis refers to that component of energy expenditure that develops over time in response to changes in environmental temperature or chronic modulation of caloric intake. It is distinguished from the change in thermogenesis consequent to changes in lean body mass or the cost of exercise and is viewed as purely regulatory. In rodents, a major share of this process occurs in a particular anatomic site, the brown adipose tissue (BAT).[38,39] Under stimulation of the sympathetic nervous system that occurs in response to ambient cold temperature or overfeeding, BAT undergoes marked hypertrophy. The mitochondrial uncoupling protein, thermogenin,[40] is induced; as a result this tissue functions to increase the generation of heat. Thus, white and brown adipose tissue have opposite functional roles: white adipose tissue functions to store energy, and BAT functions to dissipate energy. Although brown adipose tissue does exist in humans[41] and is capable of undergoing marked hypertrophy in response to adrenergic stimulation, as seen in pheochromocytoma,[42] its physiologic role, if any, in the regulation of energy expenditure and body weight in humans is not yet clear.[39] Independent of the possible role of BAT, the existence or importance of adaptive thermogenesis in humans in the response to overeating has not yet been settled.

In summary, most or all patients with established obesity have an increased rate of total energy expenditure, implying that their total energy intake is also increased in absolute terms. Some evidence supports the claim, frequently encountered in clinical practice, that individuals destined to become obese but who are not yet obese (or after massive weight loss[43]) may have modest reductions in energy expenditure that would permit the development of obesity despite an absolutely low energy intake. However, even if such a defect is present, its basis is unknown, and it is unlikely, on the basis of current knowledge, that efficient energy metabolism on its own plays a major role in the generation or maintenance of the obese state.

Endocrine Factors

There is no established endocrine cause for most cases of obesity. However, endocrinologists frequently are consulted because of concern that the patient may have Cushing syndrome or hypothyroidism. Endocrine syndromes that may be associated with obesity are listed in Table 19-2. Although obese patients may have central

Table 19-2. Endocrine Syndromes Associated with Obesity

---

1. Cushing syndrome
2. Hypothyroidism
3. Insulinoma
4. Craniopharyngioma
5. Turner syndrome
6. Male hypogonadism

obesity, hypertension, and glucose tolerance, they are free of most other stigmata of Cushing syndrome, and for the most part this can be ruled out as a cause of obesity by the use of dexamethasone suppression testing.[44,45] Some individuals with hypothyroidism become obese. This probably results from the decrease in metabolic rate and lipolysis brought about by hypothyroidism. However, much of the weight gain in hypothyroidism is due to myxedema, and tests of thyroid function rule out the diagnosis. Other endocrine disorders that may be associated with obesity include insulinoma, male hypogonadism, growth hormone deficiency, and Turner syndrome. The consequences of obesity for endocrine function are discussed below.

Neurologic Factors

Animals with ventromedial hypothalamic lesions develop obesity associated with hyperinsulinemia and hyperphagia.[46] In rare instances, tumors (especially craniopharyngioma), trauma, or inflammation produce a similar picture in humans.[47] Although hypothalamic dysfunction is postulated to be responsible for obesity in certain unusual syndromes, the plausible notion that subtle variants of such problems exist in certain cases of typical obesity has not been validated.

Genetic Factors

Obesity commonly is seen in families. The inheritance pattern is not Mendelian, and making a distinction between environmental and genetic influences is difficult. In the past several years, a number of twin and adoption studies have provided strong evidence for a heritable component of human obesity, potentially involving a limited number of genes.[48–50] One explanation for the heritable component of body composition may be a familial determination of energy expenditure, both basally and in response to overeeding. It is likely that the genetic contribution to obesity will prove to be complex.[51]

A genetic basis for obesity is clear in a number of distinct syndromes that have obesity as a characteristic feature[52–57] (Table 19–3). In no case is the identity of the responsible gene known. It is likely, however, that identification of the genes involved in human obesity or of any of the genes that cause obesity in mice will advance the search for the genetic factors that contribute to the common varieties of human obesity.

PATHOLOGIC CONSEQUENCES OF OBESITY

Obesity has psychological, behavioral, and medical consequences, the nature and severity of which are influenced by the degree of obesity. The health consequences of massive obesity are clearly evident, with as much as a 12-fold increase in the rate of death from cardiovascular disease in men aged 25 to 34 with this condition.[4] However, the point along the spectrum between normal weight and severe obesity at which various complications first arise is difficult to define, even in large epidemiologic studies. It is likely that better

Table 19-3. Genetic Syndromes Associated with Obesity

1. Prader-Willi syndrome
   Short stature, mental retardation, hypogonadotropic hypogonadism, hypotonia, small hands and feet, fish-shaped mouth
   Hyperphagia, progressive generalized obesity
   Deletion on chromosome 15
2. Laurence-Moon-Biedl syndrome
   Mental retardation, retinitis pigmentosa
   Polydactyly, hypogonadotropic hypogonadism
   Progressive generalized obesity
3. Alström syndrome
   Retinal degeneration, nerve deafness
   Testicular failure
   Insulin-resistant diabetes, acanthosis nigricans
4. Cohen syndrome
   Microcephaly, facial abnormalities, mental retardation
   Short stature, hypogonadism
5. Carpenter syndrome
   Retardation, male hypogonadism
   Polydactyly, syndactyly, acrocephaly

insight into the mechanisms that link obesity to various outcomes would allow better assessments of the health risks of obesity in individual cases. The recent realization that intra-abdominal obesity, rather than total increase in body fat, is the parameter that correlates best with several of the key morbid consequences of obesity (diabetes, hypertension, cardiovascular disease) is an excellent example.[4] Although the mechanism for this association remains uncertain, testable hypotheses are readily generated from this observation.

In considering the complications of obesity, it is often not clear which complications are due to obesity per se, i.e., direct consequences of increased weight or altered body composition; which are due to a metabolic concomitant of obesity (i.e., increased levels of FFA); and which may be due to common underlying pathogenetic factors, i.e., hyperinsulinemia or a possible defect in the central nervous system. Weight reduction brings about improvement or reversal of most of the obesity-related complications that have been well studied. It is virtually certain, however, that certain morbid consequences of obesity, such as diabetes, are critically influenced by independent genetic factors, without which specific adverse consequences may never occur.

Non-Insulin-Dependent Diabetes

Despite being insulin-resistant, the majority of obese individuals do not develop diabetes. It is clear, however, that obesity is a major risk factor for NIDDM, and as many as 80% of patients with NIDDM are obese. Presumably, the passage of an obese patient from insulin resistance and a normal state of glucose tolerance to diabetes is determined by factors independent of the obesity itself, including, most importantly, the presence of genes that influence the adequacy of compensatory insulin secretion. Apart from the fact that weight loss can ameliorate the diabetes in obese subjects with NIDDM, no fundamental differences between the clinical characteristics of

NIDDM in obese vs. non-obese individuals have emerged. The most common view of the basis for an increased risk of NIDDM in obesity is that obesity-induced insulin resistance is the responsible factor.[58] Physiologic studies have revealed that insulin resistance varies over a broad range of severity in obese subjects and may be seen in each of the major organs and tissues responsible for regulated glucose homeostasis, including liver, muscle, and fat. In studies of weight-matched individuals, the severity of insulin resistance has in most instances been found to increase when individuals proceed from normal to increasingly abnormal glucose homeostasis.[58] It is commonly overlooked that insulin has a wide variety of actions that need not be equally affected in states of insulin resistance. For example, following down-regulation brought about by exposure of isolated hepatocytes to insulin, the effect of insulin on the promotion of their amino acid uptake is decreased whereas the action of insulin on lipogenesis in the same cells is increased. Most studies of insulin resistance in obesity have focused on glucoregulatory actions of the hormone. In the face of insulin-resistant glucose metabolism, some actions of insulin may be relatively or completely preserved.

The cellular and biochemical basis for tissue resistance to insulin in established obesity has received much attention over the years. A number of potentially contributory abnormalities have been described. A decrease in the number of insulin receptors has been observed in a wide variety of tissues in most studies. It appears, however, that a defect in receptor expression cannot fully account for the insulin resistance that is seen, particularly in those with greater degrees of resistance.[59] A decrease in insulin receptor kinase activity has been observed in a number of tissues[60] as have decreases in the activity of the glucose transport system[61] and in the number of GLUT-4 glucose transporters in adipocytes.[62] Considerable heterogeneity in the results of various studies and for different tissues has been observed. In addition, the molecular basis for these established defects at the level of the insulin receptor and GLUT-4 has not been defined. Two factors have received attention as proximal mediators of at least some of these defects. The first is insulin itself. Insulin has been shown to cause receptor down-regulation and certain post-receptor desensitizing effects. It is therefore possible that hyperinsulinemia, whether simply a result of overeating or caused by something else, might bring about some of these effects.[58] FFA are the second potential molecular mediators of insulin resistance. It now seems clear that obesity is associated with increased levels of FFA,[63] which probably are due in large measure to the presence of more lipolytically active intra-abdominal adipocytes.[63] There are several potential adverse consequences of increased levels of FFA, including inhibition of insulin-stimulated glucose utilization in muscle via the "Randle effect"[64] and inhibition of hepatic clearance of insulin.[5] The improvement in the utilization of glucose that may be seen when FFA levels are reduced through pharmacologic means[65] is consistent with this hypothesis, thus increasing the importance of determining the basis for intra-abdominal obesity and its consequences.

Cardiovascular Disease

Epidemiologic studies reveal that obesity is associated with an increased mortality and morbidity from cardiovascular disease, and the association persists even when age, blood pressure, smoking history, cholesterol, and diabetes are factored out.[66] Since obesity is clearly associated with known cardiovascular risk factors such as diabetes and hypertension, these contribute additionally to the risk of cardiovascular disease.

Obesity per se, through the need for perfusion through an increased mass of tissue, results in increased cardiac work. Blood volume, stroke volume, and cardiac output are all increased.[67] These physiologic changes, and the resultant increased ventricular mass, are reversible with weight loss.[68] Obesity also is associated with an atherogenic lipid profile, i.e., increased low-density lipoprotein (LDL) cholesterol, increased VLDL and triglyceride, and decreased high-density lipoprotein (HDL) cholesterol.[66] This profile tends to occur in persons with abdominal obesity[69,70] and appears to result at least in part from overproduction of VLDL, perhaps through the effects of insulin on the liver.[71,72]

Obesity is a cause of reversible hypertension[73] that is typically associated with increases in both peripheral resistance and cardiac output.[74] Several possible causes for this association have been put forward. There is evidence to support an increased output of the sympathetic nervous system in obesity,[75] as assessed imperfectly through determination of norepinephrine levels, and these do decrease with weight loss, suggesting a role for dietary regulation of activity of the sympathetic nervous system. Enhanced sensitivity to the effect of dietary salt on blood pressure has also been seen in certain groups.[76]

Currently, there is strong interest in the possible role of insulin as a pathophysiologic factor in the hypertension of obesity as well as in the hypertension in some subjects without obesity.[77,78] This interest is based on the observation that hyperinsulinemia is found in hypertensive subjects with or without obesity and on the ability of insulin to exert actions on the kidney (i.e., salt retention), vasculature, and possibly other sites that could elevate systemic blood pressure. A major challenge over the next several years will be to identify molecular mechanisms for insulin resistance at the level of glucose homeostasis that will permit insulin to exert specific actions on blood pressure control.

Pulmonary Disease

Abnormalities in pulmonary function may be seen in obese patients.[67,79,80] These range from quantitative abnormalities in pulmonary function tests that have no clinical significance to major dysfunction replete with symptoms and morbid consequences. The increased metabolic rate in obese subjects increases oxygen consumption and CO_2 production, and these changes result in increased minute ventilation. In subjects with marked obesity, compliance of the chest wall is reduced, the work of breathing is increased, and the respiratory reserve volume and vital capacity are reduced; a resultant mismatch between ventilation and perfusion may result in hypoxemia. Severe obesity may cause hypoventilation, defined by the development of CO_2 retention. The full designation of the obesity-hypoventilation or pickwickian syndrome includes somnolence, lethargy, and respiratory acidosis and typically includes sleep apnea as part of the picture. Such patients may have reduced ventilatory drive to hypoxia and hypercapnia, as well as obstructive/mechanical causes of hypoventilation, and sleep studies may be necessary to distinguish between these.

Gallstones

Obesity is associated with enhanced biliary secretion of cholesterol. This results in supersaturation of bile and a higher incidence of gallstones—particularly cholesterol gallstones.[81] Fasting, as opposed to more-limited caloric restriction, increases the saturation of bile by reducing the phospholipid component, and cholecystitis induced by fasting is a well recognized problem in obese individuals.

Endocrine Consequences

Many changes in endocrine function can be seen in patients with established obesity.[44] These changes can be induced by overeating, and normal function resumes after weight loss. Therefore, these changes are viewed as being secondary to the obese state. A possible causal link has been sought between some of these changes and the pathogenesis of obesity, and thus they have undergone considerable scrutiny.

Endocrine Pancreas

As discussed earlier, hyperinsulinemia is a pervasive concomitant of obesity. Hyperinsulinemia results from an increased rate of insulin secretion,[82] although decreased hepatic clearance of insulin may also be seen in patients with intra-abdominal obesity.[82,83] Hyperinsulinemia follows weight gain and reverses with weight loss and is most likely a consequence of insulin resistance that accompanies the obese state. Given the fact that, in the animal model of ventromedial hypothalamic lesions, hyperinsulinism driven by the vagus nerve may precede and possibly induce obesity,[84] the possibility that a defect in central control of insulin secretion exists in a subset of persons with obesity should be considered. Studies of glucagon, somatostatin, pancreatic polypeptide, and amylin secretion in obesity have not been particularly revealing.

Thyroid

Given the known effect of thyroid hormone on the basal metabolic rate, it is reasonable to wonder whether defects in this axis might be a factor in obesity. In general, studies of obese individuals have revealed normal levels of thyroxine (T_4) and thyroid-stimulating hormone (TSH) and increased levels of triiodothyronine (T_3) in a minority of subjects. The increased T_3 levels are probably secondary to increased carbohydrate intake, and they fall, as do values in non-obese subjects, in response to caloric restriction.[85]

Gonadal Function

Marked obesity in men is associated with changes in both testosterone and estrogen metabolism, although these are usually without clinical consequences. Rates of estrogen production, primarily from androgen precursors, are increased, as are levels of estradiol.[44] Decreased total testosterone levels are common but usually are due to diminished levels of sex hormone-binding globulin (SHBG), with a preservation of normal levels of free testosterone. Levels of free testosterone may, however, be reduced in men with massive obesity.[86,87] Gynecomastia may result from these changes.

In women, marked obesity is associated with increased androgen production, increased peripheral conversion of androgen to estrogen, an increased rate of estrogen production and, decreased levels of SHBG. The specific findings in women with upper-body obesity differ from those in women with lower-body obesity.[88–90] Thus, upper-body obesity is associated with increased testosterone production, decreased SHBG, and increased levels of free testosterone in comparison to levels in obese women with lower-body or gynoid obesity. This constellation may be a major cause of the amenorrhea not infrequently seen in morbidly obese women. The fact that upper-body obesity also is associated with hyperinsulinemia has led to the hypothesis that insulin may be a factor that contributes to hyperandrogenism through actions on the ovary, as seems to be the case in syndromes of extreme insulin resistance.[91] The increased peripheral production of estrogen from androstenedione, which occurs to a greater degree in women with lower-body obesity, may contribute to the increased incidence of uterine cancer in postmenopausal women with obesity.

Adrenal Function

The relationship between obesity and altered adrenal function can be addressed from a number of perspectives. The first relates to the clinical issue of whether a given patient with obesity, particularly one with hypertension and glucose intolerance, has Cushing syndrome. As discussed earlier, in 90% of obese individuals, the overnight cortisol response to 1 mg of dexamethasone given at midnight is normal, a finding sufficient to rule out Cushing syndrome. The 10% of individuals who fail to suppress cortisol production adequately on this test will suppress cortisol production normally in the formal 2-day low-dose dexamethasone test.[45]

It should be emphasized, however, that obesity is associated with abnormalities of the cortisol axis, with increases in the rates of cortisol production and levels of urinary 17-hydroxy-steroids typically observed. Despite these findings, serum cortisol levels—including their diurnal variation—appear to be normal, and no clear defects in ACTH secretion have been observed.[44] Thus, the precise basis for the increased cortisol production is unclear. One reason for interest in this area is the finding that cortisol is overproduced in a number of animal models of obesity such as the *ob/ob* mouse and *fa/fa* rat and that removal of the adrenal gland markedly ameliorates many of the phenotypic and biochemical findings in these animals.[92] The role, if any, of increased cortisol production in the syndromes of human obesity is not established.

Pituitary Function

Obesity is clearly associated with defects in growth-hormone secretion.[44,93] Levels of growth hormone are reduced in response to many stimuli, including insulin hypoglycemia, arginine, levodopa, exercise, sleep, and the physiologic regulator growth hormone-releasing hormone (GRH). Treatment with cholinergic antagonists may reverse this defect.[94] Since administration of growth hormone will reduce the percentage of body fat,[95] these observations raise the obvious question of whether functional growth hormone deficiency is present in obesity. On the basis of levels of IGF-I, this would appear not to be the case. Many other investigations of pituitary adrenal function in obesity have been carried out, in part because of the persistent interest in whether subtle hypothalamic dysfunction might be present in this disorder. A variety of findings that have no obvious clinical relevance have been made.[44]

TREATMENT OF OBESITY

Successful treatment of obesity, defined as treatment that results in sustained attainment of normal body weight and composition without producing unacceptable treatment-induced morbidity, is rarely achievable in clinical practice.[96] Many therapeutic approaches can bring about short-term weight loss, but long-term success is infrequent regardless of the approach. Nevertheless, billions of dollars are spent annually in the United States in pursuit of this goal. Although many individuals diet in pursuit of cosmetic goals unrelated to any medically relevant definition of obesity, the need for effective and safe therapies for those individuals in whom obesity represents a major health risk is great.

Given the limitations, discomforts, and potential risks of available therapy, it is necessary to consider the risks of obesity-related morbidity in any individual. It is clear that the morbidity of obesity increases with body-mass index and that for any body-mass index, greater waist/hip ratios confer greater risk. Moderate risk begins at a body-mass index of 30, and doubles with a body-mass index between 30 and 40.[3] In addition to the risk conferred by an increased body-mass index, the presence of diabetes, hypertension, and an atherogenic lipid profile each increase the impact of obesity on health. Through evaluation of these factors and assessment of the likelihood that an individual patient will respond to a particular therapeutic regimen, an individualized and, it is hoped, a long-term treatment plan must be developed.

Diet

Reduction of caloric intake is the cornerstone of any therapy for obesity and is discussed extensively in Chapter 20. The fundamental goal is the reduction of energy intake to a level substantially below that of energy expenditure. This simple prescription is difficult to accomplish despite a wide variety of specific dietary approaches. A number of factors complicate the ability to predict the result of any given diet.[96-98] Since energy expenditure increases with increasing obesity, at any given level of caloric intake, those individuals who are most obese will lose weight more rapidly than those who are less obese. The rate of weight loss at any level of energy intake is also influenced by factors that increase energy expenditure, such as exercise and thyroid function, and by gender and age, since women and persons of advancing age have lower metabolic rates for any body weight. As discussed below, there are claims that specific features of a diet, i.e., level of carbohydrate or protein, may influence the efficacy of a diet. Importantly, many obese individuals believe that they are resistant to weight loss despite severe caloric restriction. The issues related to energy expenditure in obesity and the possibility that some individuals have a metabolic predisposition to efficient metabolism were discussed earlier. Whatever the answer to that question, it must be emphasized that there are no reliable demonstrations of failure of weight loss among obese individuals placed on diets of 1200 kilocalories (kcal) or less while under strict observation. On the other hand, diets that produce weight loss for inpatients are frequently unsuccessful when applied to outpatients, indicating the problems with compliance with dietary regimens.

Apart from the initial weight loss consequent to natriuresis and fluid shifts, a deficit of 7500 kcal is predicted to produce a weight loss of 1 kg.[98] Therefore, a reduction in food intake by as little as 100 kcal per day should bring about a 5-kg weight loss over 1 year. It is clear from common experience, however, that attempts at dieting that rely on such small reductions in food intake are rarely successful. Thus, more severe reductions in energy intake are typically prescribed. Three general categories of calorie-restricted diets have been used.[96] Total starvation will produce the most rapid weight loss, although a greater fraction of the lost weight is from fluid losses than is found with other approaches. The extreme nature of the therapy, the need for close inpatient supervision, the excessive loss of lean body mass, and the occurrence of complications such as gout, renal stones, and hypotension have led to the virtual disappearance of this approach.

So-called very-low-calorie diets of 200 to 600 kcal were initially designed to supplement fasting, primarily with protein, with the goal being the prevention of protein loss.[99] During the 1970s, the use of formula supplements that contained low-quality protein derived largely from collagen and were deficient in essential amino acids led to excessive cardiovascular deaths.[100] Contemporary versions of such diets use high-quality protein derived from soy, casein, egg, or lean fish or fowl and adequate quantities of other nutrients, including unsaturated fatty acids, potassium, magnesium, vitamins, and minerals. Whether or not carbohydrate should be a component of such diets, with the goal of minimizing ketosis and reducing the decrease in T_3 but with the possible side effect of reducing conservation of lean body mass, is a subject of debate and is discussed more fully in Chapter 20. Recent application of such diets under medical supervision has not been associated with unexpected deaths.[101,102] Indeed, institution of such therapy virtually always has beneficial effects: a prompt reduction in blood pressure in hypertensive patients and in blood glucose levels in diabetic patients, typically allowing the discontinuation of medication, at least for the duration of the diet. The average weight loss is 1.5 kg per week, although the rate of loss diminishes as weight is lost as a result of several factors, including the decline in metabolic rate that follows loss of lean body mass.[103,104] Since regaining weight after cessation of dieting is extremely common, such diets make sense only as part of an overall plan to modify food intake chronically.

Many different diets that provide 800 to 1000 kcal/day are in common use, and with adequate compliance by the patient, these diets should produce weight loss. Balanced low-calorie diets, as well as those that feature low amounts of carbohydrate or protein have been advocated by different authorities. There are also many programs that recommend specific foods or combinations of foods or unusual sequences for eating, but none of these approaches has any proven merit.

Exercise

It is appropriate to consider the therapeutic use of exercise for any patient with obesity. Since exercise increases energy expenditure, the most obvious purpose of exercise in obesity is to shift the energy balance equation towards a negative balance. Unfortunately, long-term compliance is limited. This, and the relatively small impact of moderate exercise on net energy balance, combine to explain the view that exercise is at best a small aid to weight loss in clinical practice.[105] Nevertheless, given the potential benefit of exercise on blood pressure, lipids, cardiovascular fitness, insulin sensitivity, and sense of well-being, attempts should be made to incorporate it into the therapeutic approach.

Drugs

In this author's opinion, at present there are no drugs that can be recommended for the treatment of the obese patient, apart from those used to treat patients with established disorders (i.e., thyroid hormone in hypothyroidism) that might contribute to obesity. Although T_3 levels decline with caloric restriction in euthyroid individuals and T_3 supplementation during a diet will increase rate of weight loss, 75% of the weight lost is from lean body mass, and thus T_3 or T_4 treatment of euthyroid obese individuals seems inappropriate. Central nervous system stimulants that are analogues of amphetamine and certain inhibitors of serotonin re-uptake have received much attention for their appetite-suppressing effects. Although short-term weight loss has been seen in double-blind studies of several of these analogues, the effects are lost after drug withdrawal and thus it is difficult to recommend their use. Studies of certain adrenergic agonists, such as ephedrine, have shown some efficacy in animal studies,[106] and agonists of the β_3 class that may be particularly capable of stimulating energy expenditure[92] are under development by several pharmaceutical companies.

Surgery

A number of surgical procedures have been devised in an attempt to treat those individuals with massive obesity who are refractory to therapy and subject to major morbidity from their disease. Good reviews of these procedures are found in references 107 and 108. It is clear, however, that no surgical procedure is sufficiently successful or free of complications to be recommended except as a last resort in patients with the greatest degrees of obesity.

REFERENCES

1. Build study, 1979. Society of Actuaries and Association of Life Insurance Medical Directors of America, Chicago, 1980.
2. Lukaski HC. Methods for the assessment of human body composition: traditional and new. Am J Clin Nutr 1987;46:537–6.
3. Bray GA. Overweight is risking fate: definition, classification, prevalence, and risks. Ann NY Acad Sci 1987; 499:14–28.
4. Kissebah AH, Vydelingum N, Murray R, et al. Relation of body fat distribution to metabolic complications of obesity. J Clin Endocrinol Metab 1982;54:254–60.
5. Kissebah AH, Peiris AN. Biology of regional body fat distribution; relationship to non-insulin-dependent diabetes mellitus. Diabetes Metab Rev 1989;5:83–109.
6. Health, United States, 1978. National Center for Health Services Research, US Department of Health Education and Welfare. DHEW Publication No. (PHS) 78–1232. Washington DC: Government Printing Office, 1978:215.
7. Spiegelman BM. Regulation of gene expression in the adipocyte: implications for obesity and proto-oncogene function. Trends Genet 1988;4:203–7.
8. Ross SR, Graves RA, Greenstein A, et al. A fat-specific enhancer is the primary determinant of gene expression for adipocyte P2 in vivo. Proc Natl Acad Sci USA 1990;87:9590–4.
9. Lowell BB, Flier JS. Differentiation dependent biphasic regulation of adipsin gene expression by insulin and insulin-like growth factor-1 in 3T3-F442A adipocytes. Endocrinology 1990;127:2898–906.
10. Knittle JL, Timmers K, Ginsberg-Fellner F, et al. The growth of adipose tissue in children and adolescents. Cross-sectional and longitudinal studies of adipose cell number and size. J Clin Invest 1979;63:239–246.
11. Eckel RH. Lipoprotein lipase: a multifunctional enzyme relevant to common metabolic diseases. N Engl J Med 1989;320:1060–8.
12. Kern PA, Ong JM Saffari B, Arty J. The effects of weight loss on the activity and expression of adipose-tissue lipoprotein lipase in very obese humans. N Engl J Med 1990;322:1053–9.
13. Edens NK, Leibel RL Hirsch J. Mechanism of free fatty acid re-esterification in human adipocytes in vitro. J Lipid Res 1990:1423–31.
14. Rosen BS, Cook KS, Yaglom J et al. Adipsin and comple-

ment factor D activity: an immune-related defect in obesity. Science 1989;244:1483–7.

15. Frederich RC Jr, Kahn BB, Peach MJ, Flier JS. Tissue-specific nutritional regulation of angiotensinogen in adipose tissue. Hypertension 1992:19:339–44.

16. Forbes GB Welle SL. Lean body mass in obesity. Int J Obes 1983;7:99–107.

17. Sahakian BJ. The interaction of psychological and metabolic factors in the control of eating and obesity. Hum Nutr Appl Nutr 1982;36A:262–71.

18. Keesey RE. Physiological regulation of body weight and the issue of obesity. Med Clin North Am 1989;73:15–27.

19. Weller A, Smith GP, Gibbs J. Endogenous cholecystokinin reduces feeding in young rats. Science 1990; 247:1589–91.

20. Dourish CT, Rycroft W, Iversen SD. Postponement of satiety by blockade of brain cholecystokinin (CCK-B) receptors. Science 1989;245:1509–11.

21. Morley JE. Neuropeptide regulation of appetite and weight. Endocr Rev 1987;8:256–87.

22. Harris RBS. Role of set-point theory in regulation of body weight. FASEB J 1990;4:3310–8.

23. James WPT Trayhurn P. Thermogenesis and obesity. Br Med Bull 1981;37:43–8.

24. Coleman DL. Diabetes and obesity: thrifty mutants? Nutr Rev 1978;36:129–32.

25. Blaza S, Garrow JS. Thermogenic response to temperature, exercise and food stimuli in lean and obese women, studied by 24 h direct calorimetry. Br J Nutr 1983; 49:171–80.

26. Dauncey MJ. Metabolic effects of altering the 24 h energy intake in man, using direct and indirect calorimetry. Br J Nutr 1980;43:257–69.

27. James WPT, Davies HL, Bailes J, Dauncey MJ. Elevated metabolic rates in obesity. Lancet 1978;1:1122–5.

28. Feurer ID, Crosby LO, Buzby GP, et al. Resting energy expenditure in morbid obesity. Ann Surg 1983; 197:17–21.

29. Ravussin E, Lillioja S, Anderson TE, et al. Determinants of 24-hour energy expenditure in man: methods and results using a respiratory chamber. J Clin Invest 1986; 78:1568–78.

30. Griffiths M, Payne PR. Energy expenditure in small children of obese and non-obese parents. Nature 1976;260:698–700.

31. Newsholme EA. A possible metabolic basis for the control of body weight. N Engl J Med 1980;302:400–5.

32. Bray GA, York DA, Yukimura Y. Activity of (Na^+ + K^+)-ATPase in the liver of animals with experimental obesity. Life Sci 1978;22:1637–42.

33. DeLuise M, Blackburn GL Flier JS. Reduced activity of the red cell sodium-potassium pump in human obesity. N Engl J Med 1980;303:1017–22.

34. Berne C, Fagius J, Niklasson F. Sympathetic response to oral carbohydrate administration: evidence from micro-electrode nerve recordings. J Clin Invest 1989; 84:1403–9.

35. Jéquier E, Schutz Y. Energy expenditure in obesity and diabetes. Diabetes Metab Rev 1988;4:583–93.

36. Tappy L, Felber JP, Jéquier E. Energy and substrate metabolism in obesity and postobese state. Diabetes Care 1991;14:1180–8.

37. Black D, James WPT, Besser GM, et al. Obesity: a report of the Royal College of Physicians. J R Coll Physicians Lond 1983;17:5–65.

38. Himms-Hagen J. Thermogenesis in brown adipose tissue

39. Rothwell NJ, Stock MJ. Brown adipose tissue: does it play a role in the development of obesity? Diabetes Metab Rev 1988;4:595–601.

40. Ricquier D, Bouillaud F, Toumelin P, et al. Expression of uncoupling protein mRNA in thermogenic or weakly thermogenic brown adipose tissue: evidence for a rapid β-adrenoreceptor-mediated and transcriptionally regulated step during activation of thermogenesis. J Biol Chem 1986;261:13905–10.

41. Heaton JM. The distribution of brown adipose tissue in the human. J Anat 1972;112:35–39.

42. Ricquier D, Nechad M, Mory G. Ultrastructural and biochemical characterization of human brown adipose tissue in pheochromocytoma. J Clin Endocrinol Metab 1982;54:803–7.

43. Leibel RL, Hirsch J. Diminished energy requirements in reduced-obese patients. Metabolism 1984;33:164–70.

44. Glass AR. Endocrine aspects of obesity. Med Clin North Am 1989;73:139–60.

45. Crapo L. Cushing's syndrome: a review of diagnostic tests. Metabolism 1979;28:955–77.

46. Jeanrenaud B, Assimocopoulos JF, Crettaz M, et al. Experimental obesities: a progressive pathology with reference to the potential importance of the CNS in hyperinsulinemia. In: Bjorntorp P, Cairella M Howard AN, eds. Recent advances in obesity research. London: Libbey, 1981:159–96.

47. Bray GA, Gallagher TF Jr. Manifestations of hypothalamic obesity in man; a comprehensive investigation of eight patients and a review of the literature. Medicine (Baltimore) 1975;54:301–30.

48. Stunkard AJ, Sørensen TIA, Hanis C, et al. An adoption study of human obesity. N Engl J Med 1986;314:193–8.

49. Stunkard AJ, Harris JR Pedersen NL, McClearn GE. The body-mass index of twins who have been reared apart. N Engl J Med 1990;322:1483–7.

50. Bouchard C, Tremblay A Després J-P, et al. The response to long-term overfeeding in identical twins. N Engl J Med 1990 322:1477–82.

51. Friedman JM, Leibel RL. Tackling a weighty problem. Cell 1992;69:217–20.

52. Rimoin DL, Schimke RN. Genetic disorders of the endocrine glands. St Louis: CV Mosby, 1971.

53. Goecke T, Majewski F, Kauther KD, et al. Mental retardation, hypotonia, obesity, ocular, facial, dental, and limb abnormalities (Cohen syndrome). Eur J Pediatr 1982; 138:338–40.

54. Dietz WH Jr, Gross WL, Kirkpatrick JA Jr. Blount disease (tibia vara): another skeletal disorder associated with childhood obesity. J Pediatr 1982;101:735–7.

55. Goldstein JL, Fialkow PJ. The Alström syndrome: report of three cases with further delineation of the clinical, pathophysiological, and genetic aspects of the disorder. Medicine (Baltimore) 1973;52:53–71.

56. Ledbetter DH, Riccardi VM, Airhart SD, et al. Deletions of chromosome 15 as a cause of the Prader-Willi syndrome. N Engl J Med 1981;304:325–9.

57. Norio R, Raitta C Lindahl E. Further delineation of the Cohen syndrome: report on chorioretinal dystrophy, leukopenia, and consanguinity. Clin Genet 1984;25:1–14.

58. Olefsky JM. Insulin resistance and insulin action: an in vitro and in vivo perspective. Diabetes 1981;30:148–62.

59. Kolterman OG, Insel J, Saekow M, Olefsy JM. Mechanisms of insulin resistance in human obesity: evidence for

receptor and postreceptor defects. J Clin Invest 1980; 65:1272–84.

60. Caro JF, Dohm LG, Pories WJ, Sinha MK. Cellular alterations in liver, skeletal muscle, and adipose tissue responsible for insulin resistance in obesity and Type II diabetes. Diabetes Metab Rev 1989;5:665–89.

61. Ciaraldi TP, Kolterman OG, Olefsky JM. Mechanism of the postreceptor defect in insulin action in human obesity: decrease in glucose transport system activity. J Clin Invest 1981;68:875–80.

62. Garvey WT, Maianu L, Huecksteadt TP, et al. Pretranslational suppression of a glucose transporter protein causes insulin resistance in adipocytes from patients with non-insulin-dependent diabetes mellitus and obesity. J Clin Invest 1991;87:1072–81.

63. Björntorp P. Metabolic implications of body fat distribution. Diabetes Care 1991;14:1132–43.

64. Randle PJ, Kerbey AL, Espinal J. Mechanisms decreasing glucose oxidation in diabetes and starvation: role of lipid fuels and hormones. Diabetes Metab Rev 1988;4:623–38.

65. Meylan M, Henny C, Temler E, et al. Metabolic factors in the insulin resistance in human obesity. Metabolism 1987;36:256–61.

66. Hubert HB, Feinleib M, McNamara PM, Castelli WP. Obesity as an independent risk factor for cardiovascular disease: a 26-year follow-up of participants in the Framingham Heart Study. Circulation 1983;67:968–77.

67. Vaughan RW Conahan TJ III. Part I: Cardiopulmonary consequences of morbid obesity. Life Sci 1980; 26:2119–27.

68. MacMahon SW, Wilcken DEL, MacDonald GJ. The effect of weight reduction on left ventricular mass: a randomized controlled trial in young, overweight hypertensive patients. N Engl J Med 1986;314:334–9.

69. Peeples LH, Carpenter JW, Israel RG, Barakat HA. Alterations in low-density lipoproteins in subjects with abdominal adiposity. Metabolism 1989;38:1029–36.

70. Ostlund RE Jr, Staten M, Kohrt WM, et al. The ratio of waist-to-hip circumference, plasma insulin level, and glucose intolerance as independent predictors of the HDL_2 cholesterol level in older adults. N Engl J Med 1990;322:229–234.

71. Wolf RN, Grundy SM. Influence of weight reduction on plasma lipoproteins in obese patients. Arterioscleroisis 1983;3:160–9.

72. Reaven GM Chen D. Role of insulin in regulation of lipoprotein metabolism in diabetes. Diabetes Metab Rev 1988;4:639–52.

73. Tuck ML, Sowers J, Dornfeld L, et al. The effect of weight reduction on blood pressure, plasma renin activity, and plasma aldosterone levels in obese patients. N Engl J Med 1981;304:930–3.

74. Messerli FH, Ventura HO, Reisin E. et al. Borderline hypertension and obesity: two prehypertensive states with elevated cardiac output. Circulation 1982;66:55–60.

75. Landsberg L Krieger DR. Obesity, metabolism, and the sympathetic nervous system. Am J Hypertens 1989;2(Suppl 3):125S–32S.

76. Rocchini AP, Key J, Bondie D, et al. The effect of weight loss on the sensitivity of blood pressure to sodium in obese adolescents. N Engl J Med 1989;321:580–5.

77. Kaplan NM. The deadly quartet: upper-body obesity, glucose intolerance, hypertriglyceridemia, and hypertension. Arch Intern Med 1989;149:1514–20.

78. Zavaroni I, Bonora E, Pagliara M, et al. Risk factors for coronary artery disease in healthy persons with hyperin-sulinemia and normal glucose tolerance. N Engl J Med 1989;320:702–6.

79. Luce JM. Respiratory complications of obesity. Chest 1980;78:626–31.

80. Kryger M, Quesney LF, Holder D, et al. The sleep deprivation syndrome of the obese patient: a problem of periodic nocturnal upper airway obstruction. Am J Med 1974;56:531–39.

81. Grundy SM. Mechanism of cholesterol gallstones formation. Semin Liver Dis 1983;3:97–111.

82. Polonsky KS, Given BD, Hirsch L, et al. Quantitative study of insulin secretion and clearance in normal and obese subjects. J Clin Invest 1988;81:435–41.

83. Peiris AN, Mueller RA, Smith GA, et al. Splanchnic insulin metabolism in obesity: influence of body-fat distribution. J Clin Invest 1986;78:1648–57.

84. Bray GA, York DA. Hypothalamic and genetic obesity in experimental animals: an autonomic and endocrine hypothesis. Physiol Rev 1979;59:719–809.

85. Danforth E Jr, Horton ES, O'Connell M, et al. Dietary-induced alterations in thyroid hormone metabolism during overnutrition. J Clin Invest 1979;64:1336–47.

86. Glass AR, Swerdloff RS, Bray GA, et al. Low serum testosterone and sex-hormone-binding-globulin in massively obese men. J Clin Endocrinol Metab 1977; 45:1211–9.

87. Stanik S, Dornfeld LP, Maxwell MH, et al. The effect of weight loss on reproductive hormones in obese men. J Clin Endocrinol Metab 1981;53:828–32.

88. Kirschner MA, Samojlik E, Drejka M, et al. Androgen-estrogen metabolism in women with upper body versus lower body obesity. J Clin Endocrinol Metab 1990; 70:473–9.

89. Glass AR, Dahms WT, Abraham G, et al. Secondary amenorrhea in obesity: etiologic role of weight-related androgen excess. Fertil Steril 1978;30:243–4.

90. Pasquali R, Antenucci D, Casimirri F, et al. Clinical and hormonal characteristics of obese amenorrheic hyperandrogenic women before and after weight loss. J Clin Endocrinol Metab 1989;68:173–9.

91. Poretsky L. On the paradox of insulin-induced hyperandrogenism in insulin-resistant states. Endocr Rev 1991; 12:3–13.

92. Arch JRS, Ainsworth AT, Cawthorne MA, et al. Atypical β-adrenoceptor on brown adipocytes as target for anti-obesity drugs. Nature 1984;309:163–5.

93. Meistas MT, Foster GV, Margolis S, Kowarski AA. Integrated concentrations of growth hormone, insulin, C-peptide and prolactin in human obesity. Metabolism 1982;31:1224–8.

94. Ghigo E, Mazza E, Corrias A, et al. Effect of cholinergic enhancement by pyridostigmine on growth hormone secretion in obese adults and children. Metabolism 1989;38:631–3.

95. Rudman D, Feller AG, Nagraj HS, et al. Effects of human growth hormone in men over 60 years old. N Engl J Med 1990;323:1–6.

96. Bray GA, Gray DS. Treatment of obesity: an overview. Diabetes Metab Rev 1988;4:653–79.

97. Yang M-U, Van Itallie TB. Composition of weight lost during short-term weight reduction: metabolic responses of obese subjects to starvation and low-calorie ketogenic and nonketogenic diets. J Clin Invest 1976;58:722–30.

98. Passmore R, Strong JA Ritchie FJ. The chemical composition of the tissue lost by obese patients on a reducing regimen. Br J Nutr 1958;12:113–22.

99. Howard AN. The historical development, efficacy and safety of very-low-calorie diets. Int J Obes 1981;5:195–208.

100. Sours HE, Frattali VP, Brand CD, et al. Sudden death associated with very low calorie weight reduction regimens. Am J Clin Nutr 1981;34:453–61.

101. Vertes V, Genuth SM Hazelton IM. Supplemented fasting as a large scale outpatient program. JAMA 1977;238:2151–3.

102. Amatruda JM, Richeson JF, Welle SL, et al. The safety and efficacy of a controlled low energy (very-low-calorie) diet in the treatment of non-insulin dependent diabetes and obesity. Arch Intern Med 1988;148:873–7.

103. Miller DS, Parsonage S. Resistance to slimming: adaptation or illusion?. Lancet 1975;1:773–5.

104. Wadden TA, Foster GD, Letizia KA, Mullen JL. Long-term effects of dieting on resting metabolic rate in obese outpatients. JAMA 1990;264:707–11.

105. Segal KR, Pi-Sunyer FX. Exercise and obesity. Med Clin North Am 1989;73:217–36.

106. Dullo AG, Miller DS. The thermogenic properties of ephedrine/methylxanthine mixtures: animal studies. Am J Clin Nutr 1986;43:388–94.

107. Kral JG. Surgical treatment of obesity. Med Clin North Am 1989;73:251–64.

108. Alpers DH. Surgical therapy for obesity [Editorial]. N Engl J Med 1983;308:1026–7.

Chapter 20

TREATMENT OF OBESITY

EDWARD A. MASCIOLI
BRUCE R. BISTRIAN

This chapter focuses on the therapeutic aspects of obesity. The significant medical risks associated with obesity, as well as the pathogenic relationship between obesity and diabetes, are well-discussed in Chapter 19 on obesity and Chapter 14 on the pathogenesis of non-insulin-dependent diabetes. A reduction in adipose-tissue mass in the patient with diabetes generally leads to significantly improved glycemic control, which often permits a reduction in dosage or cessation of therapy with oral hypoglycemic drugs and insulin. Obesity can be a difficult disease to treat; nonetheless, because of the close linkage of adipose tissue mass with control of diabetes, treatment should be a mainstay of proper management of the patient with diabetes who has excess adipose tissue.

We will first outline weight criteria upon which recommendations for treatment are based and then discuss several different approaches to the treatment of the obese patient.

TREATABLE OBESITY

In 1985, a summary statement from a National Institutes of Health (NIH) Consensus Development Conference on the Health Implications of Obesity concluded, "Thirty-four million adult Americans have a body mass index of 27.8 (men) or 27.3 (women); at this level of obesity, which is very close to a weight increase of 20% above desirable, treatment is strongly advised. When diabetes, hypertension, or a family history for these diseases is present, treatment will lead to benefit even when lesser degrees of obesity are present."[1] Body mass index (BMI) is defined as the body weight in kilograms divided by the square of the height in meters. Table 20–1 gives the corresponding weights in pounds and the corresponding heights in feet and inches for men and

Table 20–1. Medically Significant Body Weights: Weights That Correspond to a Body Mass Index of 27.8 for Men and 27.3 for Women

Height	Men	Women
5'0"	142	139
5'1"	147	144
5'2"	152	149
5'3"	157	154
5'4"	162	159
5'5"	167	164
5'6"	172	169
5'7"	177	174
5'8"	182	179
5'9"	188	185
5'10"	193	190
5'11"	199	195
6'0"	205	201
6'1"	210	206
6'2"	216	212
6'3"	222	218

women. It must be emphasized that the panel recommended weight-loss therapy for persons at weights lower than those given in Table 20–1 who had comorbid conditions, such as diabetes. In addition, tables of simply body weight for height or BMI fail to incorporate the added risks of an upper body distribution of adipose tissue.[2] This is most easily assessed clinically with the waist-to-hip ratio, which is determined by dividing the patient's waist circumference by the maximal circumference at the hip level. In men, metabolic risk from obesity—including the risk of diabetes—is increased when this ratio exceeds 1.0. In women, this risk is increased when the ratio is greater than 0.8.[3] The potential mechanism(s) for the particularly deleterious effects of intra-abdominal fat, as indirectly measured by the waist-to-hip ratio, are discussed in Chapters 14 and 19.

DIETARY TREATMENTS

Total Fasts

Some years ago, total fasts were commonly employed as a means of achieving weight loss.[4] Advantages were rapid loss of weight, most of which was fat, and starvation-induced anorexia. Serious disadvantages of this draconian therapy included vitamin and mineral deficiencies; loss of lean tissue, which led in some cases, to death during treatment; and rapid weight regain on restoration of dietary intake. Although relative protein losses in the dieting individual decrease during the first 3 to 4 weeks of the hypocaloric diet, if the diet is lacking in protein, some net body protein is oxidized for the duration of the hypocaloric diet. The source of lean tissue is derived from all sites, including the heart. Ventricular arrhythmias are a common mode of death in obese patients who die of starvation. Because of both limited short-term effectiveness and the significant risks involved, total fasting as therapy for obesity has fallen into disfavor and has largely been abandoned.

Balanced-Deficit Diets

Balanced-deficit diets (BDDs) are reduced in calories in comparison to the patient's previous diet but contain foods from all major food groups. By conventional definition these diets include more then 800 kilocalories (kcal) and generally less than 1500 kcal/day. In practice these diets initially result in a relatively small average weight loss—on the order of 10 to 20 pounds. For most patients such a weight loss is too small and too temporary to be of much medical benefit. The principal therapeutic value of a BDD lies in its influence on reorienting the patient towards a maintenance diet. Educating patients about lower-calorie and especially lower-fat diets increases the potential for successful maintenance of weight loss. Because of the risks of total fasting and of the relative ineffectiveness of BDDs in achieving major weight loss, the very-low-calorie diets or supplemented fasts were developed.

Very-Low-Calorie Diets

Very-low-calorie diets (VLCDs), or semistarvation supplemented fasts, had their beginnings with early work focused on minimizing the losses of lean tissue from total starvation. In the 1920s and 1930s, workers showed that retention of body protein, as reflected in nitrogen balance studies, was greater when total starvation was modified by the addition of small amounts of dietary protein.[5,6] Supplementation with dietary protein in fasting patients was further advanced by other workers.[7–10] A definitive study by Hoffer et al. showed that the provision of 1.5 g of high-quality dietary protein per kilogram of ideal body weight (IBW) in conjunction with other essential micro-nutrients, and particularly with supplemental potassium as a base, permitted the establishment of protein equilibrium by week 3 of the supplemented fast in overweight women, whereas the comparison group, fed an equal number of calories but half protein (0.8 g/kg IBW) and half carbohydrate (0.7 g/kg IBW), stabilized at a nitrogen balance of -2 g/day and had approximately 25% of their weight loss from lean tissue.[11] This study clearly demonstrates that dietary carbohydrate is not equivalent to dietary protein in sparing loss of lean tissue during semistarvation, reemphasizing the need to provide more than the usual 0.8 g of protein/kg IBW to those ingesting a hypocaloric diet. This lack of equivalency is at least intuitively obvious given the interaction between protein and carbohydrate calories in a weight-maintaining diet. Clearly, many people consume and are prescribed diets that contain inadequate amounts of dietary protein. Most patients escape deleterious clinical consequences because of the limited time they spend dieting.

Liquid-Protein Diets

A major setback to the further development and acceptance of VLCDs occurred in 1977 and 1978 in response to adverse outcomes related to the use of over-the-counter liquid-protein products. These preparations were composed of partially hydrolyzed collagen, sometimes supplemented with tryptophan, a protein that is of very low quality for human nutrition, and were seriously deficient in most essential minerals. It was estimated that approximately 100,000 people subsisted on these products as their only form of nutrition for at least 1 month. During 1977 and 1978, 58 deaths associated with the use of these products were reported.[12] Seventeen of those who died had been well, without comorbid sequelae of their obesity.

Deaths were described as sudden and usually occurred during fasting rather than during refeeding.[13,14] In patients who were being closely observed just before their death, syncope was a common presenting symptom and the electrocardiogram often revealed low QRS voltage and a prolonged QTc interval (QT interval corrected for heart rate). Many patients developed refractory ventricular tachycardia and fibrillation, and several patients had an unusual ventricular tachycardia termed *torsade de pointes.*[15]

Vitamin and mineral supplementation during weight loss was variable in the patients reported, as were the serum electrolyte levels upon presentation. Cardiac histologic studies at autopsy showed atrophy and fragmentation of the myofibers.[16] This mode of sudden death—cardiac arrhythmias in a setting of cardiac atrophy due to prolonged semistarvation—is reminiscent of the findings in earlier cases of total starvation.[17] A common thread in these cases is the similar degree of protein wasting—around 25% of the weight loss was from lean tissue whether the patients were on a total fast, were receiving an inadequate amount of good-quality protein, or were receiving an adequate amount of poor-quality protein. In subsequent studies, 24-hour cardiac rhythm monitoring was performed in patients consuming a variety of low-calorie diets, including formulas containing protein only, protein plus carbohydrate, or meat only—all with nutritionally complete supplementation, without their developing ventricular arrhythmias.[18,19] This unfortunate, unnecessary, and unplanned nutritional experiment in human starvation did, for a time, foster a reluctance in some patients to try VLCDs and for many physicians to recommend them. Public and medical acceptance did return over time, although recently there has been concern about the long-term success of these diets. The lesson learned from the liquid-protein fiasco is that an incompletely supplemented weight-loss diet can produce weight and protein losses sufficient to pose a cardiac risk but that a prudently supplemented fast can be safe in the medically supervised setting. The contraindications to a VLCD are listed in Table 20–2.

Protein-Sparing Modified Fast

There are basically two types of semistarvation, ketogenic regimens: food-based and formula-based. The one that is food-based, the so-called protein-sparing modified fast (PSMF), contains 400 to 800 kcal. The formula-based regimens contain protein and some carbohydrate but a very limited amount of fat and are in the 300- to 500-kcal range, hence the generic designation *very-low-calorie diet*. The PSMF is a fast that is modified to deliver adequate amounts of all noncaloric nutrients.[20] *Protein sparing* refers to the ability of the diet to minimize the dieter's losses of lean tissue. Although the protein-sparing feature of the PSMF is principally a consequence of the quality and quantity of dietary protein prescribed, supplementation of potassium in basic form as bicarbonate or citrate also is essential for optimal protein sparing. The only foods given are lean muscle meats from animal, fish, or fowl as sources of protein. The amount of protein prescribed is 1.5 g/kg of desirable body weight per day, taken in three meals. Since most lean muscle meats have 7 or 8 g of protein per ounce, this amount of protein is equivalent to approximately 12 to 15 ounces per day, in three meals, for most women and men, respectively. The number of calories delivered is variable, depending on the type of meat chosen. Lean meats, such as a white fish like cod, would deliver fewer than 400 calories per day for a woman, but a fatty cut of beef could easily deliver in excess of 1000 calories. The fat included does not perform any essential metabolic role and thus should be minimized. Preparation methods include all routine ones except frying, to avoid added fat.

Fat intake is limited to that from the meat. Carbohydrate intake is essentially zero except for the clinically insignificant amounts of glycogen in meat. Hoffer et al. demonstrated that such an intake of protein resulted in nitrogen equilibrium after 4 weeks, in contrast to an equicaloric diet containing 0.8 g of protein and 0.7 g of carbohydrate per kilogram of IBW, which resulted in continued loss of lean tissue.[11] Furthermore, improved aerobic and anaerobic performance was demonstrated in a comparison of a PSMF with a VLCD containing 70 g of protein with added carbohydrate.[21] Studies that have not shown the nitrogen-sparing benefit of a protein intake of 1.5 g/kg have frequently had some identifiable defect in design. In one study that compared 100 g of turkey meat with 50 g of turkey meat plus 50 g of carbohydrate, the turkey was boiled, which removed virtually all of the potassium.[22] It should be stated that with lesser amounts of protein, i.e., ≤0.8 g/kg IBW, added carbohydrate will have an additional protein-sparing effect not seen with added fat, but given that the recommended dietary allowance for protein is 0.8 g/kg when the energy intake is adequate, it is not reasonable to expect that protein requirements will be less or the same when the caloric intake is so significantly reduced.

Other nutrients that need to be included are water and salt because of the diuretic effect of a low-carbohydrate diet.[23] A minimum of 2 L of noncaloric beverages and 2.5 g of salt (1 g of sodium) as bouillon is prescribed to nonhypertensive patients. Potassium, in the amount of 25 mEq, is required. Because of the small risk of gastrointestinal ulcerations and perforation from swallowed potassium pills and the decreased gastrointestinal motility when food intake is decreased, it is preferable to give the potassium as a liquid when swallowed. In addition, the bicarbonate and citrate salts are preferred since administration of some base, as well as administration of potassium, has been shown to decrease ammoniagenesis and thereby to improve protein utilization.[24]

Vitamins and minerals in quantities that meet the respective recommended dietary allowances are given. These include supplements of 800 mg of calcium and 300 mg of magnesium per day. The nutritional components of the PSMF are listed in Table 20–3.

Physician-supervised, nationally marketed VLCD programs include Health Management Resources, Medifast, New Direction, and Optifast. The nutritional supplements vary somewhat, but most preparations are powders composed principally of protein and generally similar in nutritional content to the food-based VLCD outlined above. An important clinical consideration is the adequacy of protein intake. Too often the same daily amount of these protein powders is prescribed to fasting patients even though their desirable body weights may be quite different because of differences in sex and height. As discussed earlier, the prescribed daily amount may not supply a sufficient amount of protein for taller patients,

Table 20-2. Contraindications to a Very-Low-Calorie Diet

Advanced age
Cerebrovascular disease
Recent myocardial infarction (within 3 months)
Type I diabetes mellitus
Young age
Malignancy
Severe hepatic disease
Severe renal disease
Mild obesity (<20% above desirable weight)

Table 20-3. Daily Nutritional Components of the Protein-Sparing Modified Fast

Component	Daily Requirement
Protein	1.5 g/kg of desirable body weight in 3 meals, using mostly lean fish and poultry
Water	2 L of noncaloric beverages, minimum
Sodium	2.5 g of salt, minimum
Potassium	25 mEq potassium as citrate, bicarbonate salts
Micronutrients	Multivitamin and multimineral tablet to fully meet recommended daily allowances
Calcium	800 mg as the carbonate or citrate salt
Magnesium	300 mg as the gluconate or hydroxide salt

particularly men. Emphasis needs to be placed on the target amount of protein of 1.5 g/kg of desirable body weight, especially for patients who will be fasting for a prolonged period.

Side Effects of VLCDs

Side effects of VLCDs are generally minor and preventable. The most common serious one is orthostatic hypotension secondary to hypovolemia due to a diet-induced diuresis. Since dietary carbohydrate is significantly reduced in comparison to the amount supplied by maintenance feeding, the combination of reduced insulin and catecholamine levels and increased glucagon levels promotes diuresis.[23] This loss can amount to several liters in excess of intake during the first week in morbidly obese patients. Symptoms are prevented in most patients by the routine, prophylactic prescription of a minimum of 2 L of water and by the daily administration of 1000 mg of sodium, as contained in a bouillon cube. Some patients may require a second daily bouillon cube during the first or second week, when the diuretic effect is maximal.

Because of this diet-induced diuresis, diuretics should be discontinued or their dosage decreased when the fast is initiated, aiming for the ultimate elimination of diuretics early in the fasting period. The dosage of other antihypertensive agents may also need to be reduced, but these changes can usually be done on a weekly basis, as determined by blood-pressure readings.

Constipation can be a troubling side effect, given the inadequacy or absence of dietary fiber in the supplemented fast. Patients should be advised to take, either from the beginning of the fast if they have a history of constipation or when the problem arises during the fast, over-the-counter, sugar-free, fiber preparations. Given the limited amounts of dietary fiber included in the patient's supplements, emphasis must be placed on their ingesting adequate amounts of the fiber supplement, which for most fasting patients is more than that usually recommended. In general, patients should be counseled that their frequency of defecation will decrease when they are on the supplemented fast.

Acute attacks of gout are occasionally seen. These occur because ketoacids that are formed during the first 6 to 8 weeks of a fast as a result of increased ketogenesis during fasting successfully compete with uric acid for renal tubular secretion.[25] The increase in serum urate can precipitate an acute attack of gout, but clinical experience shows that this occurs almost exclusively in patients who have a history of gouty attacks and conversely can regularly be expected to occur in patients who have had prior gouty attacks. Allopurinol works well as prophylaxis. Acute attacks are treated in the normal fashion with either anti-inflammatory agents or colchicine. Over time, weight loss will result in levels of uric acid lower than those before the diet, another metabolic benefit of therapy for obesity.[26]

Anorexia is quite common in patients on VLCDs. The mechanism is uncertain, but it is associated with constant, low intake of dietary carbohydrates. Hunger often returns if the patient does not adhere to the diet, even if the intake of dietary carbohydrate is relatively small. The diet-induced anorexia is beneficial for two reasons: it enhances adherence to the diet and allows the patient to discriminate between internal and external cues for hunger—often the first time the patient has appreciated the difference.

Increased loss of scalp hairs in the resting phase (telogen effluvium) occurs in a small minority of patients undergoing major weight loss, as it does in other clinical situations such as pregnancy, emotional stress, and surgery. The effluvium is seen following a greater than normal shift of growing hair follicles, or those in the anagen phase, to the telogen, or resting, phase. Since follicles remain in the telogen phase for approximately 3 months, increased hair loss in telogen effluvium is seen much later than the initial clinical event that caused it. The loss is temporary; hair does grow back, but often only during weight maintenance. Since hair growth is normally slow (1 cm/month), it may be several months before the appearance of the scalp is restored to its previous state. It has been noted that women account almost exclusively for those with weight loss-associated telogen effluvium.

Lately, considerable attention has been directed to the increased risk for development of cholesterol gallstones in patients who are losing weight. It is well-established that the risk for development of gallstones is much greater in obese patients than in individuals of normal weight.[27] One mechanism appears to be increased cholesterol secretion into bile.[28] In a study in which weight loss was induced with a 1000-calorie balanced diet, the secretion of cholesterol decreased but the proportional decreases in the secretion of phospholipid and bile acid were even greater. Thus, cholesterol saturation was even higher than in the weight-maintaining obese state.[28] Other workers, using cholesterol precipitation within the gallbladder as end points, showed that a high proportion of patients on VLCDs exhibit some manifestation of cholesterol precipitation (stones, crystals) within 1 to 2 months.[29,30] Pharmacologic treatment with either aspirin or ursodiol was successful in preventing much of the cholesterol precipitation, with the bile acid, ursodiol, being most potent.[29] Given the increased cholesterol saturation seen in the bile of subjects on a 1000-kcal diet,[28] it is not clear whether the incidence of gallstone formation is actually higher in those on VLCDs or that they only appear to be so because of the popularity of VLCDs and their widespread use. An additional factor may be related to stasis of the gallbladder, since hormonal stimulation of gallbladder contraction is diminished as compared with the stimulation with a maintenance diet simply because the patient eats less fat-containing food.[31] The usually higher protein and fat intake of a patient on a PSMF may explain the absence of overt clinical gallbladder disease in a large series of such patients.[32]

Most patients who develop sludge or small gallstones while dieting remain asymptomatic. Presumably, most pass the sludge and recently formed stones when they resume a maintenance diet that includes more protein and fat. Overall, weight reduction is clearly beneficial in lowering the risk of developing gallstones as a result of reduced cholesterol secretion, with resultant reduction in biliary cholesterol saturation.[28]

It has long been known that resting metabolic rate varies with feeding. In a teleologic sense the phenomenon can be seen as the alteration in energy requirements necessary to minimize fluctuations in body weight when caloric intake changes. Medical practitioners are quite familiar on clinical grounds with the decrease in metabolic rate that occurs when caloric intake is decreased.[33] However, the reverse also occurs during overfeeding, most identifiably among the lean, when energy needs are seen to increase.[34] The mechanism of this decrease during fasting or reduced caloric intake was first thought to be a reduction in energy needs per unit of metabolically active tissue, mediated by a decrease in levels of catecholamines and the active form of thyroid hormone liothyronine (triiodothyronine).[33-35] More recent work attributes the decrease in total energy needs, as well as the decrease in resting needs, to a combination of a loss of lean tissue common to all dieters during early weight loss, a decrease in diet-induced thermogenesis because fewer calories are being consumed, and a decrease in spontaneous physical activity—not to a diminution in energy consumption per given amount of lean body mass.[36,37] This distinction may be largely a semantic one, since diet-induced thermogenesis is in part a consequence of changes in activity of the sympathetic nervous system and in part a consequence of inefficient metabolic pathways, both processes that occur in lean tissue.

Since the reduction in energy needs can be quite substantial—up to 25% in many patients after a month of a VLCD—the concern arose that maintenance of the lost weight would be especially difficult because of much-reduced energy needs. A recent study addressed this issue and noted that although the diet-induced reduction in energy needs is roughly proportionate to the decrease in caloric intake, the metabolic rate recovers when a maintenance diet is introduced. It may be several weeks before the new rate is reached, but this delay does not differ from that seen after a less-strict diet.[38] Furthermore, it is not the level of energy expenditure that determines obesity, since overweight individuals expend more energy than their lean counterparts. Rather, it is the imbalance between intake and expenditure that leads to a new steady state at an excessive weight that is the root of obesity. In other words, whereas the energy intake of normal-weight individuals is regulated by energy expenditure, in obese individuals, energy expenditure is regulated in large part by intake. It must be further emphasized that the decrease in metabolic rate that occurs during dieting is far less than the decrease in caloric intake that caused it. Many patients and medical practitioners alike believe, erroneously, that this is not the case. This point was illustrated in a study in which 29 women who claimed to be unable to lose weight were placed in a controlled environment on a diet of 1500 kcal (well more than in VLCDs).[39] More than two-thirds of the women lost weight, confirming that underestimation of dietary intake was the major cause for lack of weight loss. Of note was the lack of weight loss in nine of the 29 women; these women were found to have lower energy needs.

Weight loss has an early hypotensive effect, which is especially prominent in obese hypertensive patients. Hypertension is present in up to 40% of patients who attend organized VLCD programs; approximately 75% of these obese hypertensive patients experience a normalization of blood pressure during weight loss—usually without pharmacologic therapy.[40,41] Most of this decrease in blood pressure occurs early during weight reduction in association with the diet-induced diuresis.[42] A hormonal contribution to the hypotensive effect is made through a decrease in catecholamine levels as well as in aldosterone and plasma renin activity.[43,44] The reduction in blood pressure tends to be maintained if weight is not regained. However, there is a small hypotensive effect attributable to on-going weight reduction; blood pressure is somewhat higher at a given weight when weight is stable than when body weight is decreasing.[45]

Clinically significant changes in blood lipid levels occur with weight loss. Triglyceride levels are generally very sensitive to weight loss, decreasing early and staying at reduced levels as long as weight loss is maintained.[46] The response of cholesterol levels is more complex, varying according to when, in relation to weight loss, measurement occurs. Decreases in total, high-density lipoprotein (HDL), and low-density lipoprotein (LDL) cholesterol occur early—generally by 1 to 2 months. Thereafter, despite continued weight loss, the levels of these cholesterol fractions rise, but generally do not reach baseline values, with the exception of HDL cholesterol.[46] Therefore, weight loss is beneficial in reducing the cardiovascular risk associated with high blood lipid levels. The time-related changes in lipid levels is probably a major reason for the wide discrepancies in the literature on the effects of weight loss on blood lipids. The beneficial effects of weight loss on blood lipid levels are similar to those of exercise, but the effects of the two modalities are synergistic.[47,48]

Diabetes Mellitus and VLCDs

Patients with Type II diabetes mellitus will have substantial improvements in glycemic control, with concomitant decreases in their dependence on insulin or oral agents, with weight loss. VLCDs thus offer significant clinical benefit in the patient with Type II diabetes. Since patients with Type I diabetes must continue to take insulin and to ingest a reasonable amount of carbohydrate to minimize the risk of hypoglycemia, a strict VLCD is not advised for these patients. Many obese patients with Type I diabetes have been taking excessive amounts of insulin; thus, intensive education and training regarding diabetes should be the primary focus of their therapy.

When the patient with Type II diabetes, who does not have a risk of ketoacidosis, initiates a VLCD, rapid reduction in pharmacologic hypoglycemic therapy is warranted to prevent hypoglycemia. If hypoglycemia occurs, the diet needs to be interrupted (at least temporarily) to permit treatment, and the patient's confidence in following the VLCD can be seriously weakened.

The general rule is to discontinue the use of all oral hypoglycemic agents at the start of the VLCD. Endogenous insulin production in these patients allows them to adequately dispose of the small amount of dietary glucose consumed and the 100 to 200 g of endogenously synthesized glucose during the dietary program. Patients who are taking either oral agents or insulin should perform their own capillary blood sugar determinations at least twice a day and as necessary during the first week or two, until the blood sugar level is stable. The importance of the patient's self-monitoring must be stressed so as to avoid dietary noncompliance without documented hypoglycemia.

The approach to the patient who is using insulin is slightly more involved. Since there is some endogenous release of insulin, some investigators have discontinued insulin therapy completely when the VLCD is initiated, with only a transient period of diminishing hyperglycemia.[49] Another, more conservative, approach is to discontinue insulin therapy only if the total daily requirement is 30 units or less. If the patient is taking more than 30 units/day, on the first day of the VLCD, he or she should take one-half the normal daily dose, as a long-acting insulin preparation. If the blood glucose remains below 200 mg/dL, on the following day the patient's dose of insulin should be one-half the dose taken the previous day (or one-fourth of the regular, pre-VLCD, total daily insulin dose). These guidelines are continued daily until the total daily dose is less than 30 units, when insulin can be discontinued altogether. While losing weight during a VLCD, all patients were able to discontinue their regular oral hypoglycemic therapy and nearly 90% of insulin-requiring patients were able to discontinue insulin completely, with the rest able to decrease their dose substantially.[40] During a PSMF all insulin-taking patients were able to discontinue insulin within 2 weeks.[50] Obviously, long-term weight maintenance is crucial if this improved glycemic control is to continue.

Results of Weight Loss

Many different groups, using different VLCDs with variable protein and carbohydrate content, have been able to show an average short-term weight loss of approximately 40 to 50 pounds for women and 50 to 60 pounds for men.[32,40,51] These weight losses, occurring

after 3 to 4 months of dieting, are a substantial improvement over the results with treatments for obesity that have been reported in the medical literature over nearly 50 years and reviewed in two articles.[52,53] The average weight loss achieved in the majority of evaluable studies was less than 20 pounds. Given the relatively small short-term weight loss expected with diets other than VLCDs, and the substantial amounts of weight that many patients have to lose, it is easy to explain the rapid acceptance of VLCDs as the primary dietary means of obtaining short-term weight loss.

The maintenance of weight loss remains a challenge. Many studies attest to the short-term nature of weight loss, especially when a patient is given a VLCD without being trained in behavior modification. Two-thirds of the lost weight is regained at 1 year in patients without training, and only one-third of the weight is regained at 1 year in patients given behavioral training during the course of the VLCD.[40,51,54]

Longer-term follow-up—at 5 years—shows that essentially all weight is regained,[55] although much more optimistic results were found in a small study of a largely young adult population of volunteers, with 20% maintaining 40 pounds of their weight loss and 50% being 20 pounds lighter at 4 years.[56] These data indicate either that obesity is a chronic disorder requiring on-going treatment or that the published studies have a preselected subpopulation. This latter point is supported by the fact that the average dieter on a VLCD has tried and failed to lose weight approximately four or five times. Clearly, results of weight-loss programs in this subgroup can be expected to be poorer than the results for all obese individuals or for those who are dieting for the first time. Additional support for a selection bias comes from a survey of two groups of individuals selected on the basis of their location of employment for a history of obesity.[57] The survey yielded the interesting finding that 50 to 70% of the people surveyed who had a history of obesity had lost at least 10% of their heaviest weight, achieved a body weight no more than 10% above the desirable weight for their height and sex, and kept this weight off for several years. These data are clearly at odds with the general perception among medical professionals regarding the futility of treatment for obesity. It is only common sense to appreciate that patients whose treatment for obesity is successful will not need to re-enter treatment programs and therefore that most will not be included in the populations of patients in programs for obesity treatment, which will thus have an overrepresentation of patients with multiple previous failures.

BEHAVIOR MODIFICATION

Behavior modification is an essential component of a responsible obesity treatment program. It should be thought of as a means of training patients to be able to live without being obese in a society in which they have been susceptible, prior to their training, to factors that contributed to weight gain. There are different components of behavior therapy. Many people include nutrition education and exercise. Other, more traditional, components include control of eating stimuli, changing and slowing of direct eating behaviors, rewarding (in some noncaloric fashion!) positive changes in life-style, monitoring their body weight and food intake, and cognitive restructuring—i.e., producing alterations in dieters' thinking that will improve their confidence in the possibility of successful weight loss.[58] Clearly, the components included in behavioral therapy and the relative emphasis given vary from group to group, but overall, such behavioral modification is very important for weight maintenance.[54] The emphasis is not on the necessity for behavioral change regarding food consumption but on the means by which the patient can accomplish this task. There is agreement on the need for behavioral change but less certainty about whether our present methods are sufficiently effective at accomplishing this goal.

EXERCISE

One could easily argue that in our society, obesity is a disease that is due not to overconsumption of food but to underexpenditure of energy. Despite the prevalence of obesity in our society, Americans eat far fewer calories today than they consumed at the turn of the century because the present physical demands of daily life are lower. This societal and cultural standard of low energy expenditure, as well as the ready availability of calorically dense, fatty foods in the environment, may play a role in the disordered energy regulation of obesity and make it difficult for obese patients to treat their disease or to prevent relapse.

Exercise has been shown to be a potent factor of weight-loss maintenance.[59] Patients who persisted with regular exercise were better able to maintain their weight loss, whereas the subgroup that did not continue to exercise after losing weight regained weight rapidly. A survey done of women who were divided into three groups on the basis of their weight history (those without a history of obesity, those with a previous history of obesity, and those who had only temporary success at losing weight) showed that those women who maintained a near-normal weight were far more likely to exercise regularly than were women whose obesity had relapsed.[60] One must be cautious not to draw a conclusion as to causation from an association, but the consistency of this association is certainly compelling.

The type of exercise taught to obese patients is generally aerobic. A benefit is the preservation of lean body mass during dieting, especially with diets that are inadequate in protein, in addition to enhancement of aerobic conditioning, which can contribute to an improved sense of well-being. There are data to support the use of anaerobic or resistance strength training in obesity therapy. The benefits are related to its ability to increase the patient's lean body mass during a period of reduced intake.[61] Theoretically, the use of strength training, because it can preserve and increase lean body mass more effectively than aerobic exercise, could have significant value in helping the obese patient maintain

weight, because resting energy needs are directly related to amount of lean body mass. By increasing resting energy needs, the net amount of adipose tissue can increase only after greater amounts of overeating.

COMPREHENSIVE MEDICAL PROGRAMS

Given the large number of different commercial programs using formula-based VLCDs and the present emphasis on the importance of multifaceted programs including diet, behavior therapy, and exercise counseling, it is important to state that present evidence indicates that practitioner-based programs can be as effective. All components of responsible weight control therapy must be included. Much of the education in behavior and nutrition can be done in a group format. The use of formulas can be replaced by the conventional food option of the PSMF. The PSMF was found to be as effective for short-term weight loss and better tolerated by the patient in one randomized study[62] and to lead to better aerobic and anaerobic exercise performance in another.[21]

SURGERY

Surgical operations for obesity have a long history and are still evolving. The two classes of procedures used most recently include small-intestinal bypass and gastric-restriction operations. Because of a substantial number of long-term complications, largely the result of malabsorption, intestinal procedures have been abandoned in favor of gastric procedures, which produce comparable weight losses with little malabsorption. Reserved usually for patients who are morbidly obese, or 200% of desirable weight, losses of 100 pounds or one-third of preoperative weight are achieved at 1 year.[63] Some weight is regained over the subsequent years, and in some patients technical failures allow full weight regain. For optimal results, the surgery should be done by a multidisciplinary team of professionals who are experienced in surgery for obesity and only in patients who have been carefully screened and are committed to altering their life-style to foster weight maintenance, as should any patient using a diet as the primary weight-loss therapy. Despite the significant benefits of these procedures for many patients, they will gain wider acceptance by both patients and physicians only if risks are minimized. Given the data on long-term success of dietary therapy, the greater severity of the medical complications and the premature mortality in the morbidly obese as compared with the less severely obese, and the reasonable success of surgery, surgical therapy has become indicated therapy for morbid obesity, and an NIH Consensus Conference held in March 1991 adopted this position.[64]

REFERENCES

1. National Institute Health Consensus Development Panel on the Health Implications of Obesity. Health implications of obesity: National Institutes of Health Consensus Development Conference statement. Ann Intern Med 1985;103(6 Suppl, Part 2):1073-7.

2. Krotkiewski M, Björntorp P, Sjöström L, Smith U. Impact of obesity on metabolism in men and women: importance of regional adipose tissue distribution. J Clin Invest 1983;72:1150–62.

3. Björntorp P. Regional patterns of fat distribution. Ann Intern Med 1985;103(Suppl 6, Part 2):994–5.

4. Johnson D, Drenick EJ. Therapeutic fasting in morbid obesity: long-term follow-up. Arch Intern Med 1977; 137:1381–2.

5. Mason EH. The treatment of obesity. Can Med Assoc J 1924;14:1052–6.

6. Evans FA, Strang JM. The treatment of obesity with low caloric diets. JAMA 1931;97:1063–9.

7. Apfelbaum M. The effects of very restrictive high protein diets. Clin Endocrinol Metab 1976;5:417–30.

8. Bistrian BR, Winterer J, Blackburn GL, et al. Effect of a protein-sparing diet and brief fast on nitrogen metabolism in mildly obese subjects. J Lab Clin Med 1977;89:1030–5.

9. Genuth SM, Castro JH, Vertes V. Weight reduction in obesity by outpatient semistarvation. JAMA 1974; 230:987–91.

10. Vertes V, Genuth SM, Hazelton IM. Supplemented fasting as a large-scale outpatient program. JAMA 1977; 238:2151–3.

11. Hoffer LJ, Bistrian BR, Young VR, et al. Metabolic effects of very low calorie weight reduction diets. J Clin Invest 1984;73:750–8.

12. Sours HE, Frattali VP, Brand CD, et al. Sudden death associated with very low-calorie weight reduction regimens. Am J Clin Nutr 1981;34:453–61.

13. Brown JM, Yetter JF, Spicer MJ, Jones JD. Cardiac complications of protein sparing modified fasting. JAMA 1978;240:120–2.

14. Lantigua RA, Amatruda JM, Biddle TL, et al. Cardiac arrhythmias associated with a liquid protein diet for the treatment of obesity. N Engl J Med 1980;303:735–8.

15. Singh BN, Gaarder TD, Kanegae T, et al. Liquid protein diets and torsade de pointes. JAMA 1978;240:115–9.

16. Michiel RR, Sneider JS, Dickstein RA, et al. Sudden death in a patient on a liquid protein diet. N Engl J Med 1978;298:1005–7.

17. Garnett ES, Barnard DL, Ford J, et al. Gross fragmentation of cardiac myofibrils after therapeutic starvation for obesity. Lancet 1969;1:914–6.

18. Phinney SD, Bistrian BR, Kosinski E, et al. Normal cardiac rhythm during hypocaloric diets of varying carbohydrate content. Arch Intern Med 1983;143:2258–61.

19. Amatruda JM, Biddle TL, Patton ML, Lockwood DH. Vigorous supplementation of a hypocaloric diet prevents cardiac arrhythmias and mineral depletion. Am J Med 1983; 74:1016–22.

20. Bistrian BR. Clinical use of a protein-sparing modified fast. JAMA 1978;240:2299–302.

21. Davis PG, Phinney SD. Differential effects of two very low calorie diets on aerobic and anaerobic performance. Int J Obes 1990;14:779–87.

22. De Haven J, Sherwin R, Hendler R, Felig P. Nitrogen and sodium balance and sympathetic-nervous-system activity in obese subjects treated with a low-calorie protein or mixed diet. N Engl J Med 1980;302:477–82.

23. Sigler MH. The mechanism of the natriuresis of fasting. J Clin Invest 1975;55:377–87.

24. Gougeon-Reyburn R, Marliss EB. Effects of sodium bicarbonate on nitrogen metabolism and ketone bodies during very low energy protein diets in obese subjects. Metabolism 1989;38:1222–30.

25. Lecoq FR, McPhaul JJ Jr. The effects of starvation, high fat diets, and ketone infusions on uric acid balance. Metabolism 1965;14:186–97.

26. Nicholls A, Scott JT. Effect of weight loss on plasma and urinary levels of uric acid. Lancet 1972;2:1223–4.

27. Maclure KM, Hayes KC, Colditz GA, et al. Weight, diet, and the risk of symptomatic gallstones in middle-aged women. N Engl J Med 1989;321:563–9.

28. Bennion LJ, Grundy SM. Effects of obesity and caloric intake on biliary lipid metabolism in man. J Clin Invest 1975;56:996–1011.

29. Broomfield PH, Chopra R, Sheinbaum RC, et al. Effects of ursodeoxycholic acid and aspirin on the formation of lithogenic bile and gallstones during loss of weight. N Engl J Med 1988;319:1567–72.

30. Liddle RA, Goldstein RB, Saxton J. Gallstone formation during weight-reduction dieting. Arch Intern Med 1989;149:1750–3.

31. Gebhard RL, Ansel HJ, Peterson FJ, Stone BG. Gallbladder emptying stimuli in obese and normal weight subjects [Abstract no. 244]. Hepatology 1990;12:898.

32. Palgi A, Read JL, Greenberg I, et al. Multidisciplinary treatment of obesity with a protein-sparing modified fast: results in 668 outpatients. Am J Public Health 1985; 75:1190–4.

33. Welle SL, Amatruda JM, Forbes GB, Lockwood DH. Resting metabolic rates of obese women after rapid weight loss. J Clin Endocrinol Metab 1984;59:41–4.

34. Landsberg L, Young JB. Fasting, feeding, and regulation of the sympathetic nervous system. N Engl J Med 1978; 298:1295–301.

35. Mathieson RA, Walberg JL, Gwazdauskas FC, et al. The effect of varying carbohydrate content of a very-low-caloric diet on resting metabolic rate and thyroid hormones. Metabolism 1986;35:394–8.

36. Ravussin E, Burnand B, Schutz Y, Jequier E. Energy expenditure before and during energy restriction in obese patients. Am J Clin Nutr 1985;41:753–9.

37. de Groot LCPGM, Van Es AJH, van Raaij JMA, et al. Adaptation of energy metabolism of overweight women to alternating and continuous low energy intake. Am J Clin Nutr 1989;50:1314–23.

38. Wadden TA, Foster GD, Letizia KA, Mullen JL. Long-term effects of dieting on resting metabolic rate in obese outpatients. JAMA 1990;264:707–11.

39. Miller DS, Parsonage S. Resistance to slimming: adaptation or illusion? Lancet 1975;1:773–5.

40. Kirschner MA, Schneider G, Ertel NH, Gorman J. An eight-year experience with a very-low-calorie formula diet for control of major obesity. Int J Obes 1988; 12:69–80.

41. Reisin E, Abel R, Modan M, et al. Effect of weight loss without salt restriction on the reduction of blood pressure in overweight hypertensive patients. N Engl J Med 1978;298:1–6.

42. Maxwell MH, Kushiro T, Dornfeld LP, et al. BP changes in obese hypertensive subjects during rapid weight loss: comparison of restricted versus unchanged salt intake. Arch Intern Med 1984;144:1581–4.

43. Tuck ML, Sowers JR, Dornfeld L, et al. The effect of weight reduction on blood pressure, plasma renin activity, and plasma aldosterone levels in obese patients. N Engl J Med 1981;304:930–3.

44. Tuck ML, Sowers JR, Dornfeld L, et al. Reductions in plasma catecholamines and blood pressure during weight loss in obese subjects. Acta Endocrinol 1983;102:252–7.

45. Dornfeld LP, Maxwell MH, Waks AU, et al. Obesity and hypertension: long-term effects of weight reduction on blood pressure. Int J Obes 1985;9:381–9.

46. Ellis RW, Darga LL, Lucas CP. The short- and long-term effects of a low-fat, cholesterol-free, hypocaloric diet on serum triglyceride and cholesterol distribution in severely obese humans. Int J Obes 1987;11:29–40.

47. Wood PD, Stefanick ML, Dreon DM, et al. Changes in plasma lipids and lipoproteins in overweight men during weight loss through dieting as compared with exercise. N Engl J Med 1988;319:1173–9.

48. Tran ZV, Weltman A. Differential effects of exercise on serum lipid and lipoprotein levels seen with changes in body weight: a meta-analysis. JAMA 1985;254:919–24.

49. Henry RR, Scheaffer L, Olefsky JM. Glycemic effects of intensive caloric restriction and isocaloric refeeding in noninsulin-dependent diabetes mellitus. J Clin Endocrinol Metab 1985;61:917–25.

50. Bistrian BR, Blackburn GL, Flatt JP, et al. Nitrogen metabolism and insulin requirements in obese diabetic adults on a protein-sparing modified fast. Diabetes 1976;25:494–504.

51. Hovell MF, Koch A, Hofstetter CR, et al. Long-term weight loss maintenance: assessment of a behavioral and supplemented fasting regimen. Am J Public Health 1988;78:663–6.

52. Stunkard A, McLaren-Hume M. The results of treatment for obesity: a review of the literature and report of a series. Arch Intern Med 1959;103:79–85.

53. Wing RR, Jeffery RW. Outpatient treatment of obesity: a comparison of methodology and clinical results. Int J Obes 1979;3:261–79.

54. Wadden TA, Stunkard AJ. Controlled trial of very low calorie diet, behavior therapy, and their combination in the treatment of obesity. J Consult Clin Psychol 1986; 54:482–8.

55. Wadden TA, Sternberg JA, Letizia KA, et al. Treatment of obesity by very low-calorie diet, behavior therapy, and their combination: a five-year perspective. Int J Obes 1989; 13(Suppl 2):39–46.

56. Bistrian BR, Sherman M. Results of the treatment of obesity with a protein-sparing modified fast. Int J Obes 1978; 2:143–8.

57. Schachter S. Recidivism and self-cure of smoking and obesity. Am Psychol 1982;37:436–44.

58. Stunkard AJ, Berthold HC. What is behavior therapy? A very short description of behavioral weight control. Am J Clin Nutr 1985;41:821–3.

59. Pavlou KN, Krey S, Steffee WP. Exercise as an adjunct to weight loss and maintenance in moderately obese subjects. Am J Clin Nutr 1989;49:1115–23.

60. Kayman S, Bruvold W, Stern JS. Maintenance and relapse after weight loss in women: behavioral aspects. Am J Clin Nutr 1990;52:800–7.

61. Ballor DL, Katch VL, Becque MD, Marks CR. Resistance weight training during caloric restriction enhances lean body weight maintenance. Am J Clin Nutr 1988;47:19–25.

62. Wadden TA, Stunkard AJ, Brownell KD, Day SC. A comparison of two very-low-calorie diets: protein-sparing-modified fast versus protein-formula-liquid diet. Am J Clin Nutr 1985;41:533–9.

63. Benotti PN, Hollingshead J, Mascioli EA, et al. Gastric restrictive operations for morbid obesity. Am J Surg 1989;157:150–5.

64. Consensus Development Conference Panel. Gastrointestinal surgery for severe obesity: Consensus Development Conference statement. Ann Intern Med 1991;115:956–61.

Chapter 21

THE PATHOPHYSIOLOGY AND TREATMENT OF LIPID DISORDERS IN DIABETES MELLITUS

BARBARA V. HOWARD
WM. JAMES HOWARD

An understanding of lipoprotein metabolism and how it influences diabetes is of particular importance because of the association of lipoproteins with cardiovascular disease, presently the leading cause of death among persons with diabetes.[1] Abnormalities in lipoproteins are very common in both individuals with non-insulin-dependent diabetes (NIDDM) and those with insulin-dependent diabetes (IDDM). Although lipoprotein alterations appear to be an intrinsic part of these disorders, such alterations also are induced by diabetes-associated complications such as obesity and renal disease and are sometimes exacerbated by therapeutic regimens associated with the management of diabetic patients. A recent report by the National Cholesterol Education Program (NCEP)[2] has focused attention on the necessity for managing lipid disorders. However, in applying the guidelines to lipid abnormalities and their treatment among persons with diabetes, several additional issues must be considered, including the relationship between glycemic control and lipoproteins and the potential for a different response by persons with diabetes to lipid-lowering agents. This chapter will review the basics of lipoprotein composition and metabolism, review the alterations in lipoprotein composition and metabolism that occur in diabetes, and then outline potential therapeutic approaches to management of lipid disorders in diabetic patients.

LIPOPROTEIN METABOLISM

Structure and Classification

Lipoproteins are microemulsions composed of lipids (cholesterol, cholesteryl ester, triglyceride, and phospholipid) and proteins (apoproteins). Their function is to transport non-water-soluble cholesterol and triglycerides in plasma. Lipoproteins are spherical particles containing a central core of non-polar lipids (primarily triglycerides and cholesteryl ester) and a surface monolayer of phospholipids ˙and apoproteins. Free cholesterol is present primarily in the surface monolayer. For a detailed review of lipoprotein structure and metabolism, the reader is referred to references 3–10.

Lipoproteins have been classified on the basis of their densities during ultracentrifugation (Table 21–1). Chylomicrons, particles that are primarily triglyceride-bearing, are produced by the intestine after exogenous fat undergoes digestion.[11] Very-low-density lipoproteins (VLDL), also triglyceride-bearing lipoproteins, are secreted by the liver and carry endogenously produced triglyceride.[11] Intermediate-density lipoproteins (IDL) represent remnants of the metabolism of triglyceride-rich lipoproteins and are also intermediates in the conversion of VLDL to low-density lipoproteins (LDL).[11] LDL are the major cholesterol-bearing lipoproteins and are those most strongly related to the occurrence of cardiovascular disease.[12] Lp(a) is a subclass of the LDL fraction that consists of LDL complexed to a large glycoprotein resembling plasminogen; this complex has also been associated with atherosclerosis.[13] High-density lipoproteins (HDL) are the smallest and densest of the lipoproteins. Although HDL also transport substantial amounts of cholesterol, they are negatively associated with cardiovascular disease.[14] HDL can be divided into subfractions, the most abundant of which are HDL$_2$ (between densities 1.063 and 1.125) and HDL$_3$ (between densities 1.125 and 1.210).[15]

The metabolism and production of all lipoproteins are controlled primarily by the apoproteins contained within the complex (Table 21–2). All of these apoproteins have been sequenced and their genes localized.[16] Most are hydrophobic proteins and serve as ligands for specific receptors involved in the metabolism of the various lipoproteins and as cofactors for enzymatic activities involved in lipoprotein metabolism. Several other proteins and enzymes play key roles in plasma lipoprotein transport (Table 21–2), including lipoprotein lipase[17] and hepatic lipase,[18] which catalyze the delipidation of triglyceride rich particles; lecithin-cholesterol acyltransferase (LCAT),[19] which is responsible for the synthesis of virtually all cholesteryl esters in plasma lipoproteins; and cholesterol ester transfer protein (CETP),[20] which facilitates the transfer of cholesterol and cholesteryl ester between lipoproteins during their metabolism.

Formation and Metabolism of Chylomicrons

Chylomicrons are responsible for the transport of dietary triglycerides and cholesterol. Dietary triglycerides are hydrolyzed in the gut, releasing fatty acids that are then re-esterified to form triglycerides in the intestinal mucosal cell. These triglycerides are assembled with newly absorbed cholesterol, apoprotein (apo) B$_{48}$, and the A apoproteins. Upon secretion from the enterocyte, these assembled particles enter the lymphatic circulation and then the bloodstream, where they acquire C apoproteins and apoE by transfer from HDL. As chylomicrons enter the plasma, the triglyceride is rapidly hydrolyzed by the enzyme lipoprotein lipase, which resides on the surface of capillary endothelial cells. Lipoprotein lipase is synthesized primarily in adipose tissue and striated muscle. It is secreted and transported to the endothelial surface, where it acts on triglyceride-rich particles. Its action requires the presence of ApoC$_{II}$ on the surface of the lipoprotein, while apoC$_{III}$ inhibits lipoprotein lipase. Lipoprotein lipase is induced in adipose tissue by insulin.[21] The liberated free fatty acids are available for oxidative needs of peripheral cells, and excess free fatty acids are stored mainly in triglycerides in adipose tissue to serve as a future source of free fatty acids.

As triglyceride is depleted from the chylomicrons, phospholipids and A and C apoproteins are transferred to HDL. The residual chylomicron particle, which has lost 80% to 90% of its triglyceride and is now relatively cholesterol-enriched, is called a chylomicron remnant. These remnants are believed to be cleared by the liver via a specific receptor that probably recognizes apoE.[22] The remnants thus enter lysosomes in the liver, from which cholesterol can enter metabolic pathways in the hepatocytes, including excretion into the bile. The remaining triglyceride enters the hepatic triglyceride stores. Figure 21–1 summarizes the various steps of lipoprotein metabolism.

Very-Low-Density Lipoproteins

VLDL are synthesized in the endoplasmic reticulum of hepatocytes and are composed of endogenous triglyceride derived from plasma-free fatty acids, from chylomi-

Table 21–1. Human Plasma Lipoproteins

Lipoprotein	Density (g/mL)	Electrophoretic Mobility	Diameter (nm)	Chol/CE (%)	Triglyceride (%)*	Protein (%)
Chylomicrons	0.95	Origin	75–1200	5	86	2
VLDL	<1.006	Pre-β	30–80	15	55	10
IDL	1.006–1.019	Preβ-β	25–35	38	23	19
LDL	1.019–1.063	β	18–25	50	5	22
Lp(a)	1.040–1.063	β	25–35	50	5	36
HDL	1.063–1.210	α	5–12	19	3	48

VLDL, LDL, and HDL = very-low-density, intermediate-density, low-density, and high-density lipoproteins, respectively; Lp(a) = lipoprotein a; Chol = cholesterol; and CE = cholesteryl ester.
*Approximate value

Table 21–2. Major Apoproteins Associated with Plasma Lipoproteins

Apoprotein	Chylomicrons	VLDL	IDL	LDL	HDL	Lp(a)	Function
						Association	
ApoA$_I$	x				x		Binds to HDL receptor
ApoA$_{II}$					x		Binds to HDL receptor
ApoB$_{48}$	x						Structure & clearance of chylomicrons
ApoB$_{100}$		x	x	x		x	Binds to apoB/E receptor
ApoC$_{II}$	x	x	x		x		Activates LPL
ApoC$_{III}$	x	x	x		x		Inhibits LPL
ApoE	x	x	x		x		Binds to apoB/E and remnant receptors
Apo(a)						x	Plasminogen antagonist

LPL = lipoprotein lipase. See Table 21–1 for other abbreviations.

cron remnants, and from de novo lipogenesis (Fig. 21–1).

VLDL production is influenced by glucose, fatty acids, and insulin. The concentration of circulating free fatty acids governs the rate of triglyceride esterification in the liver, and glucose—especially when glycogen synthesis is impeded—may stimulate de novo production of free fatty acid and thus triglycerides. Insulin is required for VLDL production, both for apoprotein synthesis and because it regulates several enzymes involved in lipogenesis.[23] On the other hand, increases in insulin have been shown to inhibit VLDL secretion in hepatocytes by phosphorylating apoB, which impedes the assembly of apoB with lipids.[24]

Nascent VLDL, as secreted into the circulation, contain apoB$_{100}$ and small amounts of apoC and apoE. After VLDL enter the circulation, they are metabolized in the same manner as chylomicrons by the enzyme lipoprotein lipase, with the fatty acids that are liberated following the same fate as those liberated from chylomicrons. After secretion, VLDL acquire more C and E apoproteins by transfer from HDL. In addition, free cholesterol is progressively exchanged to HDL, where it is esterified and the cholesteryl ester is returned to VLDL. As VLDL become progressively depleted of triglyceride, a portion of the surface, including apolipoproteins C and E and phospholipids, is transferred to HDL.[15] The enzyme hepatic lipase also plays a role in the metabolism of smaller VLDL particles during the latter stages of the VLDL catabolic cascade.[25] The smaller remnants of VLDL are triglyceride-depleted, cholesterol-rich particles, some of which are isolated in the IDL compartment but some of which still remain in the VLDL compartment. These remnant particles are cleared from the circulation primarily by receptors in the liver. These receptors include both the B/E receptor (see below) and possibly a remnant receptor, which acts on chylomicron remnants. A portion of VLDL remnants is further metabolized, possibly by a process involving hepatic lipase, to form LDL. During this process, the remainder of apoproteins other than apoE are lost.

The mechanisms that determine which and how much VLDL are converted to LDL are not clearly understood.

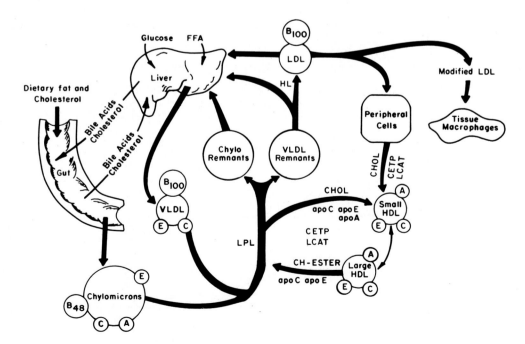

Fig. 21–1. Summary of lipoprotein metabolism. HDL = high-density lipoproteins; LDL = low-density lipoproteins; VLDL = very-low-density lipoproteins; CHOL = cholesterol; FFA = free fatty acids; CETP = cholesteryl ester transfer protein; LCAT = lecithin-cholesterol acyltransferase; HL = hepatic lipase; A, C, and E are the respective apoproteins (apo).

VLDL particles are believed to be secreted in a spectrum of sizes with various degrees of triglyceride enrichment. The larger VLDL particles appear to be more rapidly cleared and less likely to be converted to LDL.[26] On the other hand, smaller VLDL particles that are richer in cholesterol may be preferentially converted to LDL. When apoE is missing or defective (as in type III hyperlipidemia), clearance of chylomicron remnants and VLDL remnants is much slower than normal. These remnants accumulate in plasma and are not readily converted to LDL.

Low-Density Lipoproteins

As indicated above, LDL are products of the metabolism of VLDL. The only apolipoprotein in LDL is apoB, and only one molecule of apoB is present per particle of LDL. Clearance of LDL is mediated by a specific receptor (the B/E receptor) present on the surface of both liver and peripheral cells.[10] Once it is bound to the receptor, the lipoprotein is internalized by an endocytotic process. The vesicle then fuses with a lysosome, where enzymes degrade the apoB and hydrolyze the cholesteryl ester to free cholesterol. Triglycerides and phospholipids may also be hydrolyzed. The influx of free cholesterol from LDL sets into motion a cascade of regulatory events aimed at controlling the cell's cholesterol content. Esterification of cholesterol is stimulated by activation of acyl CoA cholesterol acyltransferase (ACAT). Simultaneously, de novo cholesterol production is inhibited by the inhibition of 3-hydroxy-3-methyl-glutaryl (HMG)-CoA reductase, the rate-limiting enzyme in cholesterol biosynthesis. Finally, accumulation of intracellular cholesterol limits the further uptake of cholesterol-rich lipoproteins by inhibiting synthesis of the B/E receptor.

LDL may also be cleared by clearance mechanisms mediated not by the B/E receptor but by phagocytic cells; such mechanisms include both nonspecific endocytotic uptake and a receptor-mediated process in which macrophages recognize altered LDL.[27] These phagocytic processes, thought to be responsible for cholesterol deposition in the vessel wall, become increasingly important when either defects in the LDL receptor or abnormalities in LDL composition are present (Figs. 21-1 and 21-2).

High-Density Lipoproteins

HDL are secreted by the hepatocyte as cholesterol-poor/protein-rich particles that contain the A apoproteins

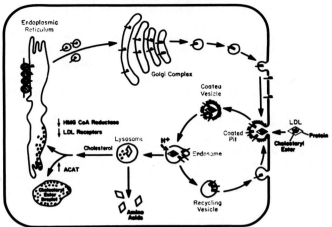

THE LDL RECEPTOR PATHWAY

Fig. 21-2. Binding and cellular metabolism of low-density lipoprotein (LDL). HMG = 3-hydroxy-3-methyl-glutaryl; ACAT = acyl CoA cholesterol acyltransferase. Reprinted with permission from reference 10 (Brown MS, Goldstein JL. The LDL receptor and HMG-CoA reductase—two membrane molecules that regulate cholesterol homeostasis. Curr Top Cell Regul 1985;26:3-15).

as well as apoE; HDL also are produced by the intestine. Some HDL particles contain both apoA$_I$ and apoA$_{II}$, whereas others contain only apoA$_I$. In the plasma, surface components of triglyceride-rich lipoproteins are transferred to HDL during lipolysis. In addition, HDL are the sites of synthesis of cholesteryl ester from free cholesterol and lecithin through the enzyme LCAT, which circulates in association with HDL particles. HDL participates in the catabolism of triglyceride-rich lipoproteins, serving as a source for cholesteryl esters and the C and E apoproteins and ultimately as the receptacle for surface components. During the lipolytic process, the size of the HDL particle increases. Larger particles are referred to as HDL$_2$ and the smaller HDL precursors, as HDL$_3$.

HDL along with LCAT and CETP (Table 21-3) are also involved in the flux of cholesterol between cells and plasma lipoproteins.[20,28] Cholesterol substrate for LCAT can be derived from cell membranes, especially when HDL is relatively depleted of cholesterol and/or when cell cholesterol content is elevated. Excess free cholesterol can be transferred from cells to HDL particles in a process mediated by CETP. After action by LCAT, the free

Table 21-3. Important Plasma Regulators of Lipoprotein Metabolism

Plasma Regulator	Major Source	Function
Lipoprotein lipase (LPL)	Adipose tissue Muscle Heart	Hydrolyzes TG and PL in chylomicrons and large VLDL
Hepatic lipase (HL)	Liver	Hydrolyzes TG and PL in small VLDL and HDL
Lecithin-cholesterol acyltransferase (LCAT)	Liver	Esterifies free cholesterol
Cholesteryl ester transfer protein (CETP)	Liver	Transfers CE and C between lipoproteins and cells

TG = triglycerides; PL = phospholipids; VLDL and LDL = high-density and low-density lipoproteins; CE = cholesteryl ester; C = cholesterol.

cholesterol then becomes trapped within the nonpolar center of the HDL; this cholesteryl ester can subsequently be transferred to triglyceride-rich lipoproteins. Since triglyceride-rich lipoprotein remnants are cleared by the liver, as HDL may be to some extent, this process represents a pathway for "reverse cholesterol transport," by which cholesterol from peripheral cells can be removed and transported to the liver for excretion in bile.

The mechanisms that control clearance of HDL are not well understood. Cholesteryl esters from HDL may be taken up by hepatic cells without endocytosis of the HDL particles per se. In addition, hepatic lipase may hydrolyze HDL phospholipids, which in turn may promote net transfer of cholesterol from the surface of HDL to the liver. Finally, there may be specific HDL receptors on peripheral cells that may be involved not only in the cholesterol efflux process but also in specific uptake and degradation of the HDL particles.[29]

LIPOPROTEIN ALTERATIONS IN NON-INSULIN-DEPENDENT DIABETES MELLITUS (NIDDM)

The following will summarize commonly observed lipoprotein changes and their possible metabolic determinants in patients with NIDDM (Table 21–4) (for additional details, see references 23 and 30–36).

Triglycerides and VLDL

The most common alteration of lipoproteins in NIDDM is hypertriglyceridemia caused by an elevation in VLDL. In earlier descriptions of diabetic hypertriglyceridemia, an emphasis was placed on individuals with extremely high levels of plasma and VLDL triglycerides. It is clear, however, from population-based studies that NIDDM generally is associated with only a 50 to 100% elevation in the plasma levels of total and VLDL triglycerides. Thus, it is likely that NIDDM subjects with concentrations of total triglycerides greater than 350 to 400 mg/dL also have genetic defects in lipoprotein metabolism, the

Table 21–4. Lipoprotein Alterations in Non-Insulin-Dependent Diabetes Mellitus

Lipoprotein	Alterations
VLDL ↑	Increased production of Tg and apoB
	Decreased clearance of Tg and apoB
	Increased Tg/apoB ratio
LDL ↑→	Increased production of LDL apoB
	Decreased receptor-mediated clearance
	Tg enrichment
	Glycation
	Oxidation
HDL ↓	Increased clearance of apoA
	Decreased proportion of HDL$_2$
	Tg enrichment
	Glycation
	Diminished reverse cholesterol transport

VLDL, LDL, and HDL = very-density, low-density, and high-density lipoprotein; Tg = triglycerides; and apo = apoprotein.

expression of which may be exacerbated by hyperglycemia[37] (see below).

Metabolic Determinants

One of the determinants of diabetic hypertriglyceridemia is the overproduction of VLDL triglyceride.[38–41] This increase in the production of VLDL triglycerides is more pronounced in diabetic patients whose triglyceride values are very high. The most likely explanation for the overproduction of VLDL triglycerides is the increased flow of substrates, particularly glucose and free fatty acids, to the liver. In addition, individuals with NIDDM appear to have a defect in clearance of VLDL triglyceride,[38,39,41,42] that parallels the degree of hyperglycemia. Studies to date (reviewed by Taskinen[43]) suggest that lipoprotein lipase activity is decreased in individuals with NIDDM, especially those with moderate to severe hyperglycemia who exhibit both an insulin deficiency and insulin resistance. However, clearance defects have not been consistently observed in patients with NIDDM, especially in those with greatly elevated triglyceride levels.

The metabolism of VLDL apoB may also be altered in NIDDM. Subjects with NIDDM have a decreased fractional catabolic rate for VLDL apoB[38,42] similar to that for VLDL triglyceride. Overproduction of VLDL apoB occurs in NIDDM. It has also been suggested that this overproduction is further increased by obesity.[38,42] Although obese diabetic subjects have a higher VLDL-B production than do lean individuals, in obese nondiabetic subjects, VLDL-B production may already be maximally stimulated.[42] Thus, the extent of overproduction of VLDL triglyceride may be greater than that of apoB in NIDDM, a situation that results in the production on larger triglyceride-rich VLDL particles.

The overproduction of VLDL in NIDDM may be related to hyperinsulinemia. Some studies,[44,45] but not others,[46] have noted a correlation between VLDL production and insulin concentrations. On the other hand, studies of isolated hepatocytes have demonstrated an inhibitory effect of insulin on VLDL and apoB production.[47,48] Insulin may have a permissive effect on VLDL production, in that some insulin is necessary for protein biosynthesis; however, VLDL production or secretion may be inhibited when insulin concentrations are raised above a threshold level. Significant relationships have been observed between VLDL and insulin resistance, as measured by euglycemic clamp techniques, independent of insulin concentrations.[49,50] These relationships suggest that the elevated VLDL in NIDDM may be directly related to insulin resistance rather than to insulin concentrations per se.

VLDL Composition

In addition to increases in the amount of VLDL, there may be changes in the composition of VLDL in NIDDM that either may reflect or be the cause of alterations in VLDL metabolism. Several studies suggest that individuals with diabetes, especially those with more severe hyperglycemia, may have larger triglyceride-rich VLDL.[42,51] This increased ratio of triglyceride to apoB may be a reflection of a disproportionate influence of NIDDM on VLDL triglyceride production (see above). Subfractions of VLDL have been found to be enriched in the proportion of smaller particles.[52] These compositional changes may have implications for the increased propensity for atherosclerosis among individuals with NIDDM, since cholesterol-enriched VLDL or VLDL remnants may be atherogenic. Changes in the distribution of apoE would have important implications for VLDL metabolism in NIDDM since apoE influences the affinity of binding to receptors. An increased proportion of apoE in the VLDL of NIDDM has been reported.[53] Although diabetics have not been shown to have differences in distribution of apoE phenotypes, apoE sialation has been reported to be higher in diabetics than nondiabetics, a change that also may affect binding to the B/E receptor.[54]

Additional evidence for abnormal VLDL in NIDDM is that VLDL from persons with NIDDM have altered metabolic properties in vitro. VLDL isolated from normotriglyceridemic patients with NIDDM produced a greater cellular accumulation of lipids in mouse peritoneal macrophages than did VLDL isolated from either normotriglyceridemic or hypertriglyceridemic nondiabetic control subjects.[55] Thus, altered VLDL composition may contribute to metabolic abnormalities as well as to the atherosclerotic propensity of the VLDL particles. Finally, although it has been suggested that insulin resistance induces hypertriglyceridemia, it is also possible that hypertriglyceridemia per se, especially when VLDL particles are altered, may impair insulin activity and lead to insulin resistance.[56]

LDL

Studies examining plasma concentrations of total and LDL cholesterol in NIDDM have been contradictory, with some showing higher and some showing lower levels in NIDDM than in control subjects. Recent data from Study II of the National Health and Nutrition Examination Survey (NHANES) indicate that levels of LDL-cholesterol that are greater than 160 mg/dL occur in 40% of patients with NIDDM as compared with 25% of adult nondiabetic patients, confirming that elevations in LDL, although common in the population in general, are even more frequent in individuals with NIDDM.[57] It should be pointed out that in most population studies, the density ranges chosen for quantitation of LDL (1.006 to 1.063) result in the inclusion of the IDL fraction. In some studies, the increase in LDL in NIDDM has been shown to be the result of an increase in this IDL fraction.[58]

Metabolism

Few reports on LDL metabolism in NIDDM have been published. In NIDDM subjects with relatively severe hyperglycemia, the clearance rate for LDL apoB is reduced.[42,59] Mildly hyperglycemic NIDDM individuals may have increased LDL production as well.[59] Since LDL binding has been shown to be stimulated by insulin,[60]

defects in LDL clearance in NIDDM may be due to insulin resistance or relative insulin deficiency. This possibility is supported by the observation that clearance of LDL in NIDDM is positively related to plasma insulin levels and to the insulin response from oral glucose challenge.[59] If a clearance defect is a characteristic of NIDDM, why is it that many diabetics do not show increases in the concentration of LDL? The answer may be found in the observation that direct removal of VLDL apoB is increased in those individuals with NIDDM with large, triglyceride-rich VLDL.[42] Thus, the concentrations of LDL in NIDDM may be influenced by two opposing phenomena. On the one hand, decreased clearance in NIDDM may lead to increased LDL; on the other hand, increased direct removal tends to lower production. The resultant concentration may thus be dependent on the relative magnitude of these two processes, and the net result may be a lack of significant change in LDL concentrations. Nevertheless, these alterations in the flux of both VLDL remnants and LDL particles may have atherogenic potential.

Composition

The composition of LDL in NIDDM appears to be altered, and these alterations also may contribute to abnormal metabolism and atherosclerosis. An increase in the proportion of triglyceride in LDL has been consistently observed,[51,61] and in some diabetic patients, LDL particles may have greater density.[62] LDL from individuals with diabetes have a decreased ability to bind to receptors on skin fibroblasts, and this decrease in binding is inversely related to the ratio of triglyceride to protein in LDL.[63] This finding suggests that triglyceride-enriched LDL in NIDDM can result in altered metabolism. An abnormal lipoprotein in the LDL range that contains apoE has been demonstrated in NIDDM, and it appears to stimulate cholesteryl ester accumulation in mouse peritoneal macrophages.[53]

Nonenzymatic glycation (or glycosylation) of apoB also may influence LDL metabolism in diabetes. The extent of glycation of LDL in patients with NIDDM with moderate hyperglycemia is approximately 2 to 5%,[64] and this degree of glycation of lysine residues has been shown to decrease LDL catabolism in vivo by 5 to 25%.[65] Glycated LDL also appear to exhibit altered interactions with endothelial cells and to enhance cholesteryl ester synthesis in human macrophages.[66] Thus, the glycation of LDL may represent an important mechanism by which atherogenesis is increased in NIDDM.

Finally, a pattern of abnormal cholesterol transport and transfer has been shown in the plasma of patients with NIDDM. The transfer of LCAT-synthesized cholesteryl esters to VLDL and LDL is inhibited, with a concomitant increase in their transfer to HDL; this abnormal metabolic pattern is reversed by insulin therapy.[67] The block in cholesteryl ester transfer activity in patients in NIDDM is correlated with an increase in free cholesterol content of both LDL and VLDL. Therefore, in NIDDM this abnormal cholesteryl ester transfer may be related to an increased risk for atherosclerosis.

HDL

Almost as common as the observation of increased VLDL concentrations in NIDDM is the finding of decreased HDL cholesterol concentrations in individuals with NIDDM.

Metabolism

To date there has been only one report on HDL metabolism in NIDDM that showed an increased rate of HDL clearance, as measured by apoA$_I$ kinetics.[68] Significant correlations were found between HDL clearance and plasma concentrations of HDL cholesterol and apoA$_I$, and the increase in HDL clearance was directly related to plasma glucose levels. The finding of increased HDL clearance is consistent with lower VLDL clearance and lower lipoprotein lipase activity. Since HDL concentrations, especially of HDL$_2$, increase during the lipolytic process, lipoprotein lipase activity has been shown to correlate significantly with HDL concentrations in patients with NIDDM. Elevated hepatic lipase activity also may contribute to the decrease in HDL concentrations in NIDDM, since this enzyme also plays a key role in the metabolism of HDL. The changes in lipoprotein and hepatic lipases may act in concert to decrease HDL levels in NIDDM.[69]

Composition

There are several indications that the composition of HDL in NIDDM may be altered.[30] These differences may in part be a reflection of alterations in the delipidation cascade. Decreased HDL in NIDDM is reflected most in decreases in the HDL$_2$ subfraction. As with LDL, in NIDDM an increased proportion of triglyceride in HDL has been observed. An increase in the ratio of cholesterol to protein in HDL has been reported, with a preferential depletion of apoA$_I$. These compositional changes appear to correlate with the degree of stimulation of adipose tissue lipoprotein lipase, since LPL deficiency may be a factor responsible for the altered distribution of HDL

particles in untreated NIDDM. Nonenzymatic glycation of HDL appears to interfere with HDL receptor binding.[70] Thus glycation of HDL may also play a role in producing the lower levels of HDL observed in diabetes. Finally, abnormalities in HDL composition have been noted even in individuals with optimal glycemic control.[71] All of these alterations in HDL composition may impair the role of HDL in reverse cholesterol transport.

Significant negative relationships between plasma concentrations of insulin and HDL have been observed in subjects with NIDDM as well as a negative relationship between insulin resistance and HDL cholesterol that is independent of VLDL concentrations.[49,50] These observations raise the possibility that insulin or insulin resistance in some way influences the concentration or composition of HDL. This would suggest that either insulin or insulin resistance is involved in the control of apoA$_I$ metabolism or in mechanisms of HDL removal.

LIPOPROTEINS IN INSULIN-DEPENDENT DIABETES MELLITUS (IDDM)

The consideration of lipoprotein metabolism in IDDM is influenced by the obligatory requirement for insulin therapy. Thus, a spectrum of situations is possible, from the insulin-deficient ketoacidotic state with greatly elevated glucose, free fatty acids, ketones, and lipolytic hormones such as glucagon and epinephrine to that seen when continuous insulin infusion therapy is administered, in which an excess of insulin in peripheral plasma is found, and glucose and fatty acid levels are close to normal (Fig. 21–3).[30–36] In the following sections, an attempt will be made to differentiate between these various degrees of control.

VLDL

Extreme elevations in VLDL levels have been recognized as being a common occurrence in diabetic ketoacidosis (DKA),[72] the stage at which insulin concentrations are minimal. On the other hand, VLDL levels in individ-

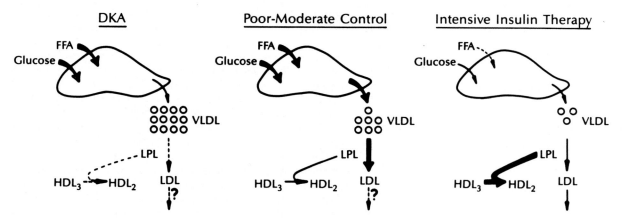

Fig. 21–3. Spectrum of lipoprotein changes in insulin-dependent diabetes mellitus with various degrees of control. DKA = diabetic ketoacidosis; see legend to Figure 21–1 for other abbreviations. Reprinted with permission from reference 30 (Howard BV. Lipoprotein metabolism in diabetes mellitus. J Lipid Res 1987;28:613–28).

uals with IDDM who are receiving adequate therapy may not be elevated. It is now well established that elevations in VLDL triglycerides in IDDM are often correlated with the degree of diabetic control.[73,74]

Metabolism

In untreated IDDM subjects, the fractional catabolic rate for endogenous triglyceride is decreased[75] and the clearance rate for exogenous triglyceride also is lower.[76] Thus, when insulin deficiency is extreme, clearance is impaired because the activity of lipoprotein lipase is dependent on insulin. In the early stages of insulin deficiency, production of VLDL is increased, probably because of the increase in mobilization of free fatty acids. This enhanced hepatic VLDL secretion falls off in the later stages of ketoacidosis because of the decrease in hepatic protein synthesis secondary to the insulin deficiency. In poorly controlled but non-ketotic patients with IDDM, both overproduction and decreased clearance are observed.[77] Kinetic studies of VLDL triglyceride in a group of IDDM subjects receiving adequate conventional insulin therapy showed that the production rates and fractional catabolic rates (FCR) of VLDL triglycerides were normal when compared with those of weight- and age-matched controls.[78] Institution of continuous subcutaneous insulin infusion resulted in a significant fall in the rates of VLDL triglyceride production to levels below those observed in the nondiabetic subjects. There was no change in the mean FCR for VLDL triglyceride after insulin infusion. A similar decrease in plasma VLDL triglyceride production was observed after treatment with the artificial β-cell in a group of patients with IDDM.[79] These latter studies indicate that rigorous insulin therapy can result in decreased rates of VLDL production and subnormal levels of VLDL triglyceride.

During severe ketoacidosis when there is a definite insulin deficiency, hypertriglyceridemia is caused primarily by a deficiency in lipoprotein lipase activity, and overproduction of triglycerides might not occur despite elevated levels of free fatty acids. As insulin therapy is instituted, the situation changes. With moderate control, i.e., when insulin administration is suboptimal, there is both an overproduction of VLDL because of an increase in level of free fatty acids and some deficiency in VLDL clearance because of the continued limitation in lipoprotein lipase. As stringent control is instituted with the administration of large amounts of peripheral insulin, clearance is normal. VLDL production rates may fall to subnormal levels since excess insulin may suppress hepatic VLDL formation. IDDM subjects in this situation will have normal or even low-normal levels of circulating VLDL triglyceride.

LDL

The concentration of LDL appears to vary directly with the extent of hyperglycemia. LDL levels are increased in poorly controlled IDDM subjects. However, in many individuals with IDDM, LDL concentrations are not different from those of age- and weight-matched controls,

and some IDDM subjects receiving insulin by means of a pump exhibit LDL concentrations considerably below those of controls.

Metabolism

Fractional catabolic rates for LDL in subjects receiving conventional therapy or who have received 3 weeks of continuous subcutaneous insulin infusion are similar to those for nondiabetic controls. Improvement in glycemic control results in a decrease in the production for LDL apoB to levels below those of nondiabetic subjects. In uncontrolled Type I diabetes, LDL fractional clearance is probably decreased, since insulin appears to potentiate LDL binding to its receptor. With increased control, LDL metabolism may return to normal.[80] It is also plausible that insulin deficiency may lead to overproduction of LDL in response to an increased influx of VLDL or its precursor or to impaired removal of VLDL remnants by the liver. Abnormalities in the VLDL particle also may influence conversion to LDL.

Composition

The LDL of individuals with IDDM also may exhibit an increase in the ratio of cholesterol to apoB,[73] that has not been related to any metabolic parameter. LDL isolated from patients with poorly controlled IDDM are taken up and degraded by fibroblasts at a lower rate than LDL isolated from normal subjects; when glucose concentrations are lowered by insulin therapy, the binding properties of LDL return to normal.[81] Glycated LDL and defects in cholesteryl ester transfer may also be found in individuals with IDDM, as in those with NIDDM, but to date no studies on glycation in IDDM have been performed. Exposure of cells to lipoprotein-deficient serum obtained from poorly controlled patients with IDDM enhances the efficiency of LDL binding.[82] It has been postulated that in IDDM membrane changes may be induced that result in altered LDL binding.

HDL

A number of observations have suggested that concentrations of HDL may be low in untreated, insulin-deficient diabetics. Response of HDL to insulin therapy is slower than that of VLDL, but HDL increases with the degree of glycemic control. In many studies of IDDM, HDL concentration have been shown to be normal or higher than normal than the concentrations in age-, sex-, and weight-matched controls. HDL levels may also be higher in those who are receiving insulin-pump therapy.[74,80]

Metabolism

One factor responsible for the decrease in HDL in poorly controlled IDDM subjects is low lipoprotein lipase activity. The reduced activity, because it results in an impairment in lipolysis of VLDL, leads to a reduction in the formation of HDL particles.[43] In insulin-treated diabetics, levels of both HDL-cholesterol and phospholipids have been shown to correlate positively with lipoprotein lipase activity; thus, greatly increased catabolism of triglyceride-rich lipoproteins in the presence of excess insulin might augment the HDL compartment. An inverse correlation has been observed between HDL and hepatic lipase activity in the plasma of IDDM subjects. Hepatic lipase activity may be lower in well-controlled IDDM subjects and associated with a high ratio of HDL_2 to HDL_3; thus, the role of this enzyme in regulating HDL levels and the possible influence of insulin on this process are similar to those postulated for NIDDM.[83]

Composition

When HDL is elevated in well-controlled IDDM subjects, it is generally due to an increase in the HDL_2 subfraction. These observations confirm the hypothesis that the action of insulin, whether it occurs through the activity of lipoprotein lipase or by means of some other process, results in an increased transfer of material to the HDL_2 compartment. As for NIDDM, data indicate that alterations in HDL composition may be found in IDDM. HDL_3 is smaller and richer in triglycerides in those who have lower concentrations of HDL. Abnormalities in both the triglyceride and $apoA_I$ content have been observed in the HDL in IDDM,[84] and $apoA_I$ and $apoA_{II}$ content may also be decreased. ApoA has also been reported to be glycated in patients with IDDM.[85]

RATIONALE FOR THERAPY FOR LIPID ABNORMALITIES IN DIABETES

The concern about lipid abnormalities in patients with diabetes mellitus is a response to an accumulating body of data that implicate abnormal lipids as significant risk factors for arteriosclerotic vascular disease (ASCVD).[86] In recent years it has become clearer that arteriosclerosis is the predominant cause of both morbidity and mortality in patients with diabetes.[1] Multiple studies have shown that the prevalence of ASCVD is significantly higher in individuals with diabetes than in the general population[87] (see Chapter 38). The accumulation of evidence that modification of risk factors can lower mortality related to cardiovascular disease in the general population[88-90] has brought with it an increased enthusiasm for managing all the cardiovascular risk factors in people with diabetes as well as controlling their blood sugar. Hypertension must be effectively controlled, and smoking is contraindicated in the patient with diabetes. Thus, in the individual with diabetes, it is extremely important to consider total risk-factor management as well as the management of the lipid abnormalities frequently found in these patients.

Total Cholesterol and LDL-Cholesterol

Multiple clinical trials have proven conclusively that the risk of cardiovascular disease can be prevented by lowering levels of serum lipids[91-93] and that the prognosis for individuals with pre-existing cardiovascular disease can be significantly improved by lipid-lowering therapy.[94-99] Both the Lipid Research Clinics-Coronary Primary Prevention Trial (LRC-CPPT)[91] and the Helsinki Heart Study[93] demonstrated that the lowering of LDL-cholesterol is associated with a significant reduction in values of all end points of cardiovascular morbidity and mortality. In addition, the Helsinki Heart Study showed that the diminution in the rate of cardiovascular disease that results from lowering serum LDL concentrations could be further enhanced by also increasing the concentration of HDL-cholesterol. Among a series of recent clinical trials showing the benefits of aggressive lipid-lowering therapy in patients with pre-existing cardiovascular disease,[94-99] were several trials suggesting that significantly decreasing LDL-cholesterol and increasing the HDL-cholesterol fraction could produce a regression in arteriosclerotic lesions.[95,96,99] In addition to the trials showing decreased ASCVD-related mortality and morbidity, some showed that reduction in cholesterol levels decreases mortality due to all causes.[92,94] At the end of 15 years, the niacin-treated group in the Coronary Drug Project demonstrated an 11% decrease in mortality from any cause.[92] At the end of 5 years the Stockholm Study has shown a decrease in both ASCVD-related mortality and total mortality in the group that received cholesterol-lowering therapy.[94]

Although there are no comparable studies in patients with diabetes mellitus, there is no reason to believe that elevated total or LDL-cholesterol levels are of less atherogenic potential in diabetic than in nondiabetic subjects. In fact, as the previous discussion has demonstrated, abnormalities in lipid composition in diabetics—even those whose absolute lipid levels are normal—may accentuate atherosclerosis.[30,42,51-56,61-66,70,71,100] These factors led the American Diabetes Association to convene a special consensus conference in 1989 to discuss the role of modification of cardiovascular risk factors in the prevention and treatment of macrovascular disease in patients with diabetes mellitus.[101] In considering all of the data, this group concluded it was reasonable to assume that lowering cholesterol in patients with diabetes would have beneficial effects on cardiovascular events and recommended that clinical trials similar to the LRC[91] and the Cholesterol-Lowering Atherosclerosis Study (CLAS)[95] be conducted in diabetic populations.

Triglycerides

In patients with diabetes, lipid abnormalities other than elevations of LDL cholesterol must also be considered potentially atherogenic. For patients with diabetes, unlike the general population, hypertriglyceridemia has been implicated as an important contributor to ASCVD.[102,103] Both the World Health Organization Multi-National Trial[102] and the Paris Prospective Study[103] have shown that hypertriglyceridemia is a significant predictor of subsequent cardiovascular mortality in persons with diabetes. Finally, the Stockholm Study[94] demonstrated that a reduction in triglyceride levels was the most important factor in the decrease observed in the total and cardiovascular mortality in this study. As discussed previously, abnormalities in VLDL composition and the delayed clearance of chylomicron remnants may contribute to the accelerated ASCVD in patients with diabetes. In addition, diabetics are known to accumulate IDL or remnants of VLDL, which are definitely known to be atherogenic.[39,40]

HDL

Epidemiologic studies have shown an inverse relationship between the concentration of HDL-cholesterol and ASCVD.[104] As stated previously, the Helsinki Heart Study[94] demonstrated a significant effect of a therapeutically induced increase in HDL in the prevention of ASCVD, and the CLAS[95] and Familial Atherosclerosis Treatment Study (FATS)[96] trials have suggested that increases in HDL also play a role in slowing the progression of ASCVD. Although no definitive studies involving diabetic patients have been performed, the frequent occurrence of low HDL levels in persons with diabetes is probably also a contributing factor in the increased frequency and severity of ASCVD in these patients.[35,36,70]

GOALS OF THERAPY

Despite a growing awareness of the importance of ASCVD in the morbidity and mortality of diabetes, it appears that little attention is being paid to the management of hyperlipidemia in diabetic patients. In a recent community survey of more than 450 non-Hispanic whites and Mexican-Americans with Type II diabetes randomly selected from over 5000 diabetics residing in San Antonio, Texas, it was found that only 25% of non-Hispanic whites with diabetes were aware of their hyperlipidemia and that fewer than 10% were receiving treatment.[105] Both the awareness and treatment of lipid disorders were even less frequent among the Mexican-Americans with diabetes.

In 1988, the Adult Treatment Panel of the National Cholesterol Education Program (NCEP) released its recommendations concerning the diagnosis and management of hyperlipidemia in adults in the United States.[2] This group recommended that total cholesterol be measured in every patient older than 20 years of age and that individuals be classified as having "desirable cholesterol" levels if their serum cholesterol level was lower than 200 mg/dL, "borderline high cholesterol" levels if values were between 200 and 239 mg/dL, and "high cholesterol" levels if values were greater than 240 mg/dL (Table 21–5). If an individual has a desirable cholesterol level, no further therapeutic intervention is indicated and a repeat cholesterol determination should be performed in approximately 5 years because of the tendency of

Table 21–5.   Initial Classification Based on Serum Levels of Total Cholesterol

Classification	Cholesterol Level (mg/dL)
Desirable	<200
Borderline high	200–239
High	≥240

Data from the report of the NCEP Expert Panel.[2]

Table 21–6.   Risk Factors Other than LDL-Cholesterol for Coronary Artery Disease

Male gender
Family history of premature coronary heart disease
Cigarette smoking (>10 cigarettes/day)
Hypertension
Glucose intolerance/diabetes mellitus
HDL-cholesterol <35 mg/dL
History of other arteriosclerotic vascular diseases
Significant obesity (>30% overweight)

Data from the report of the NCEP Expert Panel.[2]
LDL and HDL = low-density and high-density lipoprotein.

cholesterol levels to rise with age in the United States. All individuals with cholesterol levels higher than 200 mg/dL should have these levels confirmed by repeat testing, and those with total cholesterol levels in the high range should have a full lipoprotein profile performed. Individuals with borderline high cholesterol who have pre-existing cardiovascular disease or who have two additional risk factors should also have a lipoprotein profile performed. Table 21–6 gives the risk factors delineated by the NCEP that should be considered in deciding on further testing for individuals with borderline high cholesterol levels. Although the screening measurements of total cholesterol can be done on nonfasting blood specimens, specimens used for a lipoprotein profile should be obtained after a 12-hour fast. The lipoprotein profile consists of measurements of total cholesterol, HDL-cholesterol, and triglycerides and a calculation of the LDL-cholesterol according to the Friedewald equation (Table 21–7). The NCEP recommends that all further therapeutic decisions be based on the LDL-cholesterol value. Dietary therapy is instituted when the LDL-cholesterol level exceeds 130 mg/dL in individuals with heart disease or two other risk factors and when the level is greater than 160 mg/dL in individuals who do not have these pre-existing conditions. When 6 months of dietary intervention has not been successful in reducing the LDL cholesterol to goal levels, pharmacologic therapy is then recommended for individuals who have LDL levels greater than 160 mg/dL and existing cardiovascular disease or two other risk factors and for those with levels greater than 190 mg/dL who do not have these accompanying conditions.

The recommendations of the NCEP are based on studies in the general population. Although diabetes and impaired glucose tolerance are listed as risk factors by the NCEP, no specific recommendations are given concerning the special therapeutic requirements of patients with diabetic dyslipidemia. Strict application of the criteria suggested by the NCEP to males with diabetes would dictate that all diabetic males with LDL-cholesterol levels greater than 130 mg/dL should receive diet therapy and that those with LDL levels greater than 160 mg/dL after 6 months of diet therapy should be treated pharmacologically. Since some studies have shown that females with diabetes demonstrate an even greater relative acceleration of atherosclerosis than do males,[106,107] most investigators would now agree that for both male and female

Table 21–7.   Lipoprotein Analysis

Confirm elevated total cholesterol
12-hour fast
Measure total cholesterol (TC), HDL-cholesterol (HDL), and
  triglycerides (TG)
Estimate LDL-cholesterol by Friedewald formula:
  LDL = TC − HDL − Tg/5

HDL and LDL = high-density and low-density lipoprotein.

patients with diabetes these maximal levels of LDL-cholesterol should be cut-off points for the institution of dietary and pharmacologic therapy. Since populations of diabetics with low LDL values (100 to 130 mg/dL) have lower levels of ASCVD than diabetics whose LDL values are above 130 mg/dL,[101] an even more aggressive approach to the treatment of elevated LDL levels can be recommended for patients with diabetes.

In a recent review of diabetic dyslipidemia, Garg and Grundy proposed that an LDL level of 100 mg/dL is a more appropriate goal for patients with NIDDM.[108] They further suggested that since cholesterol is abnormally distributed in various lipoprotein fractions in patients with NIDDM and since hypertriglyceridemia is often accompanied by an elevated level of VLDL-cholesterol, a more appropriate parameter for setting therapeutic goals in patients with diabetes would be the sum of the VLDL-cholesterol and LDL-cholesterol. This combined fraction of the VLDL-cholesterol plus the LDL-cholesterol is also known as the non-HDL-cholesterol fraction. Garg and Grundy proposed a minimal goal of less than 160 mg/dL for the non-HDL-cholesterol component in patients with NIDDM and an ideal goal of approximately 130 mg/dL or lower (Table 21–8). The non-HDL-cholesterol value is computed by subtracting the HDL-cholesterol concentration from the total cholesterol concentration, a calculation that can readily be made from the data obtained from a standard lipoprotein profile.

Although no recommendations were made by the NCEP for lowering triglyceride levels to prevent heart disease,[2] there is little doubt that significantly elevated triglyceride concentrations can produce pancreatitis. In 1984, a National Institutes of Health (NIH) Consensus Conference considered the problem of hypertriglyceridemia in nondiabetics and concluded that those whose triglyceride levels are higher than 500 mg/dL should receive careful consideration for drug therapy when non-pharmacologic measures are unsuccessful.[109] Individuals with triglyceride levels higher than 1000 mg/dL should definitely be treated with hypotriglyceridemic drugs to prevent the occurrence of pancreatitis. As stated previously, a number of studies have suggested that elevated triglycerides are an independent risk factor for ASCVD in patients with diabetes.[102,103] For this reason, the recent American Diabetes Association (ADA) consensus panel on cardiovascular disease in diabetics recommended that patients with triglyceride concentrations greater than 250 mg/dL receive effective therapy.[101]

The NCEP also made no recommendations regarding HDL levels.[2] Although a low HDL concentration (<35 mg/dL) was listed as one of the risk factors that influences whether further therapy should be instituted in individuals with borderline high total and LDL-cholesterol levels, the NCEP did not feel justified in recommending guidelines for treatment of patients with reduced levels of HDL-cholesterol. However, significant new data have since accumulated implicating HDL as an important independent risk factor in the genesis of cardiovascular disease. Epidemiologic studies such as the Framingham study[104] have long shown that HDL plays an important role in the prevention of heart disease. The Helsinki Heart Study[93] and the CLAS[54] and FATS[76] regression trials have all indicated that increasing low HDL levels results in a favorable outcome. Recent studies of patients with proven ASCVD in the presence of "desirable" plasma levels of both total cholesterol and LDL have shown that a significant prevalence of low HDL is the only identifiable risk factor in many of these patients.[110]

As has been demonstrated in the previous discussion, a low HDL level is a common abnormality in patients with diabetes and often does not respond to the usual methods for managing hyperglycemia. Although data are still insufficient to permit a recommendation of more exact criteria for the consideration of pharmacologic treatment of patients with low HDL levels as an isolated abnormality, the HDL profile certainly should be considered in decisions regarding the institution of non-pharmacologic therapy for patients with diabetes and should decrease the cut-off point for treatment with lipid-lowering drugs when non-pharmacologic therapy for diabetic dyslipidemia fails.

TREATMENT OF HYPERGLYCEMIA IN PATIENTS WITH DIABETIC DYSLIPIDEMIA

Nonpharmacologic Therapy

In considerations regarding therapy for diabetic dyslipidemia, the control of plasma glucose is of primary importance. As pointed out previously, there is abundant evidence that lipid abnormalities often are related to the degree of hyperglycemia.[30–36,108] Diet and exercise have long been advocated as important components of the therapeutic regimen for diabetes. Although

Table 21–8.   Proposed Therapeutic Goals for Men and Women with Non-Insulin-Dependent Diabetes Mellitus

Lipid fractions	Minimal Goal (mg/dL)	Ideal Goal (mg/dL)*
Total cholesterol	<200	170
LDL-cholesterol	<130	100
Non-HDL-cholesterol	<160	130

From Garg and Grundy.[107]
LDL and HDL = low-density and high-density lipoprotein.
*Approximate value.

these two areas are more completely covered in other chapters of this text, their importance will briefly be discussed in relation to the therapy for dyslipidemia in diabetes.

Exercise

Although exercise programs have not been shown to consistently improve glycemic control in patients with IDDM, exercise has long been advocated for Type I diabetics for its other beneficial effects.[111] A recent position statement from the Council on Exercise of the ADA advocates exercise for patients with IDDM because of its potential to improve cardiovascular fitness.[112] Several studies have shown that exercise in IDDM patients both decreases triglyceride levels and increases HDL-cholesterol levels.[111] The ADA Council on Exercise also has pointed out possible risks of exercise for individuals with IDDM: hyperglycemia, hypoglycemia, ketosis, cardiovascular ischemia and arrhythmias, exacerbation of proliferative retinopathy, and injury to the lower extremities.[112]

In NIDDM, exercise may be even more important than in IDDM in the management of both hyperglycemia and dyslipidemia.[110,112] In considering the appropriate role of exercise in patients with NIDDM, The ADA Council on Exercise emphasized the reduction of ASCVD risk factors in their position statement.[112] Again, however, the Council on Exercise points out risks of exercise in patients with NIDDM, which are the same as those outlined for patients with IDDM. They also strongly recommend that before beginning an exercise program individuals with NIDDM undergo an evaluation specifically designed to diagnose previously unknown hypertension, nephropathy, retinopathy, neuropathy, and silent ischemic heart disease, which would include an exercise stress cardiogram for all subjects older than 35 years of age.

Exercise has several potential benefits for patients with NIDDM.[111,113] First, there is some evidence that weight-loss programs that incorporate exercise will be more successful in maintaining weight reduction, with a resulting beneficial effect on lipid levels. In addition, there are direct effects of exercise training on reducing insulin resistance, a factor that may contribute to dyslipidemia, as discussed previously. Exercise has also been shown to increase HDL-cholesterol levels and lower triglycerides in individuals with NIDDM.

Diet Therapy

Weight Loss. Weight loss is the conservative form of therapy for NIDDM and has been discussed in Chapter 20. As has been stated previously, weight reduction in patients with NIDDM has multiple benefits.[113] A decrease in insulin resistance and hyperinsulinemia would be expected to have beneficial effects on hyperglycemia and hyperlipidemia. Weight reduction in NIDDM has been shown to lower concentrations of triglycerides and increase those of HDL-cholesterol and, in some studies, to lower LDL-cholesterol levels.[40] Even when hypoglycemic drug therapy is necessary, an appropriate diet will minimize the dose of drug required to control glucose levels.

Diet Composition. The dietary management of diabetes is discussed further in Chapter 24. The diet for diabetic patients recommended by both the ADA and the NCEP Expert Panel (Table 21–9) includes a reduction in the amount of total fat to less than 30% of the total calories and of saturated fat to less than 10% of total calories.[2,113,114] Cholesterol intake should be reduced to less than 300 mg/day, and the rest of the diet should consist of 15 to 20% of calories from protein, with complex carbohydrates accounting for 50 to 60% of total calories consumed. In addition, it is emphasized that this increase in the amount of complex carbohydrates in the diet will result in a concomitant increase in fiber intake.[2,113,114] Both the ADA and the NCEP have a second level of dietary recommendation for those with more severe hyperlipidemia,[2,114] that of reducing total fat to less than 20% of total calories and cholesterol to less than 200 mg/day (<150 mg/day for the ADA). Nevertheless, there has been considerable controversy concerning the wisom of these dietary recommendations.[115–118] For many years, it was believed that dietary carbohydrate should be restricted to prevent diabetic complications. In addition, studies in nondiabetics have suggested that diets high in carbohydrate, especially those containing simple sugars, lead to increases in triglyceride levels and decreases in HDL levels, both of which will exaggerate the pattern of dyslipidemia already present in diabetes.[2,113] Finally, there was some concern that metabolic control might deteriorate with the increased consumption of carbohydrates,[115,117] although this has not been borne out in clinical studies comparing high- and low-carbohydrate diets.

Table 21–9. Dietary Guidelines of the American Diabetes Association[2] and the National Cholesterol Education Program[113]

Nutrient	Step 1 Diet	Step 2 Diet
Total fat	<30% of total calories	<30% of total calories
Saturated fat	<10% of total calories	<7% of total calories
Polyunsaturated fat	Up to 10% of total calories	Up to 10% of total calories
Monounsaturated fat	10–15% of total calories	10–15% of total calories
Carbohydrates	50–60% of total calories	50–60% of total calories
Protein	10–20% of total calories	10–20% of total calories
Cholesterol	<300 mg/day	<200 mg/day
Total calories	To achieve and maintain desirable body weight	

The majority of studies of both patients with NIDDM and those with IDDM have shown that replacing foods high in saturated fat with foods containing predominantly complex carbohydrate lowers both total and LDL-cholesterol levels.[118-123] This response has been noted in both lean and obese NIDDM subjects as well as in subjects with IDDM. Lowering of LDL levels is not observed in situations in which the ratio of polyunsaturated to saturated fat has been held constant and in which carbohydrates have replaced primarily polyunsaturated fat.[115] Decreases in HDL-cholesterol concentrations have been observed in some[117] but not other studies in which complex carbohydrate replaced saturated fat.[119,120] Decreases in HDL concentrations appear to be less pronounced in those diabetics with lower initial HDL concentrations. Significant increases in fasting triglyceride concentrations have not been seen in most studies of NIDDM patients on various solid-food, high-carbohydrate diets either with or without an additional increase in the amount of fiber.[118,120-122] Three studies that measured postprandial triglyceride concentrations also found no change.[120-121,124] However, increased triglyceride concentrations have been found in studies of diabetic subjects for whom the ratio of polyunsaturated to saturated fat has been constant[116] or in studies in which carbohydrates have replaced primarily unsaturated fats.[115] An additional advantage of diets that are higher in complex carbohydrates is that they are lower in calories for comparable portion sizes and thus may promote weight reduction.

Another dietary approach that appears promising for the treatment of dyslipidemia in patients with NIDDM who cannot or will not follow a high-carbohydrate diet is a diet high in monounsaturated fatty acids.[108,117] Diets high in monounsaturated fatty acids result in a reduction in triglyceride and LDL concentrations and appear to produce less of a lowering in HDL concentrations than a high-carbohydrate diet.

Finally, another suggested dietary approach for diabetic patients concerns increases in n-3 polyunsaturated fatty acids. These fatty acids, which are found predominantly in fish oils, have a hypotriglyceridemic action in nondiabetic persons.[125] Numerous epidemiologic studies have provided evidence that diets high in fatty fish may be beneficial in preventing cardiovascular disease, and this effect has been attributed to the presence of n-3 polyunsaturated fatty acids.[126] Fish oil supplements have been shown to reduce serum triglyceride levels in some studies of NIDDM patients.[127,128] However, increases in LDL-cholesterol and apoB concentrations may occur in hypertriglyceridemic subjects given fish oil, a situation often observed in diabetic subjects.[129,130] In addition, in at least half of the studies of diabetic patients, fish oil supplementation has had an adverse effect on glycemic control.[130,131] Thus, the use of such supplements in diabetic patients is probably contraindicated, although they should be encouraged to eat fish.

In summary, on the basis of the NCEP and ADA recommendations, several changes to typical American diets should be made, including decreases in saturated fat, increases in complex carbohydrates, increases in dietary fiber, and an exchange of vegetable protein for animal protein. Although a mild propensity for triglyceride elevations may be seen in metabolic ward studies in which only the carbohydrate content of the food is altered without any change being made in the content of fiber, the ratio of unsaturated to saturated fat, and in the amount of animal protein, most studies have not shown significant increases in triglyceride levels when the NCEP or the ADA dietary recommendations are followed. It is clear that the ADA/NCEP diet can lower both the levels of LDL-cholesterol and blood sugar in individuals with diabetes without exacerbating hypertriglyceridemia, although it has still not been determined which aspect(s) of this diet is responsible for the observed metabolic change.

PHARMACOLOGIC THERAPY FOR IDDM AND ITS RELATION TO DYSLIPIDEMIA

As discussed above, the absolute insulin deficiency of IDDM results in multiple lipid abnormalities. In IDDM patients with pure diabetic dyslipidemia (i.e., patients who do not have underlying primary abnormalities of lipid metabolism in addition to IDDM), adequate insulin therapy often completely corrects all the diabetes-associated lipid abnormalities.[73,74,132] In patients with poorly controlled IDDM, both the clearance of chylomicrons and of VLDL are accelerated by the stimulatory effect of insulin therapy on lipoprotein lipase activity, with a resulting resolution of hypertriglyceridemia within several days.[72,132] Overproduction of VLDL and the subsequent abnormal composition of VLDL, VLDL remnants, and LDL will often respond to adequate control of glucose with insulin therapy. Finally, HDL levels are often increased to normal or even supranormal levels with insulin therapy. It has also been shown by numerous investigators that the degree of glucose control has a direct effect on the normalization of lipids. When standard insulin therapy is unsuccessful, tight control with multiple subcutaneous insulin injections or with subcutaneous insulin infusion via an insulin pump will often result in near normalization of glucose levels and in significant improvement in the diabetic dyslipidemia.[78,79,133,134] In some cases of resistance to glycemic control, studies have suggested that intraperitoneal infusion of insulin is more effective in controlling glucose than is peripheral subcutaneous administration of insulin. Clinical trials are ongoing that are designed to assess the efficacy and long-term safety of intraperitoneal insulin infusion.[135]

PHARMACOLOGIC THERAPY FOR NIDDM AND ITS RELATION TO DYSLIPIDEMIA

Current evidence indicates that insulin resistance and hyperinsulinemia play a significant role in the lipid abnormalities of patients with NIDDM; thus, treatment of hyperglycemia in NIDDM patients with lipid disorders is more complex than that in patient with IDDM.[136,137] When the "ideal" therapy for reducing insulin resistance and hyperinsulinemia by diet and exercise is unsuccessful either because of the severity of the diabetes or because of the lack of patient compliance, hypoglycemic pharmacologic therapy should be undertaken, but with significant concern for its potential to aggravate the underlying hyperinsulinemia.[138] Numerous epidemiologic studies have demonstrated an association between the presence of hyperinsulinemia and accelerated atherosclerotic disease.[136,137] Insulin may play a role through direct effects on the cells of the arterial wall, the aggravation of hypertension, and/or its effects on lipid metabolism.

Sulfonylurea Therapy

The acute effects of sulfonylureas are principally mediated by an increase in the pancreatic secretion of insulin.[139,140] However, some studies have suggested that chronic therapy with these oral hypoglycemic agents produces extrapancreatic effects that result in a decrease in insulin resistance (i.e., increased insulin action) in addition to the augmentation of insulin secretion[141] (also see Chapter 29). When sulfonylurea therapy is effective in lowering glucose levels, the accompanying elevated lipid levels often are significantly reduced as well.[35,36,139] An improvement in glycemic control is usually accompanied by decreases in plasma levels of total cholesterol, triglycerides, VLDL-cholesterol, and apolipoprotein B. The effects of improved glycemic control on HDL-cholesterol levels are variable, with some studies showing no change and others demonstrating a moderate increase. However, HDL levels are often not completely normalized, even when levels of other lipids are brought within the normal range. When comparable levels of glycemic control are achieved with either insulin or sulfonylurea therapy, little difference is seen in the resulting levels of cholesterol and triglycerides. However, some studies have shown that levels of HDL-cholesterol are more responsive to insulin therapy.[36,142] One of the major drawbacks of sulfonylurea therapy is the significant rate of primary and secondary failure.[140,141] Often when patients are not motivated to follow a diet or are unable to lose weight when on a diet, the period of efficacy of sulfonylurea therapy is limited.

Insulin Therapy

In patients with NIDDM and hyperlipidemia, all other measures for the control of hyperglycemia should be utilized before insulin therapy is considered.[138] Some studies have suggested that the administration of exogenous insulin aggravates the underlying hyperinsulinemia of NIDDM and may accelerate the progression of atherosclerosis.[143,144] As commonly practiced, insulin therapy is often ineffective in controlling the hyperglycemia of patients with NIDDM. In patients who are unable to lose weight with diet and exercise, insulin therapy may also result in an additional weight gain.[145,146] On the other hand, insulin therapy in NIDDM patients with significant dyslipidemia helps control the accompanying lipid abnormalities.[35,36,145–148] Just as in Type I diabetes, efficacy of insulin therapy in achieving anti-atherogenic changes in serum lipoproteins in NIDDM patients may require the use of home glucose monitoring and multiple insulin injections with both short-acting and intermediate or long-acting insulin preparations. In patients with diabetic dyslipidemia, the goal of insulin therapy is to control hyperglycemia. As large doses of insulin often are required to control hyperglycemia in patients with NIDDM, studies are currently being conducted to determine whether aggressive insulin therapy in patients with NIDDM offers advantages as compared with those of other forms of management in the long-term reduction of macrovascular disease.[149] When their blood glucose level is effectively controlled, many Type II diabetics will have a normalization of their triglyceride concentrations and a decrease in their total cholesterol values.[35,36,148,150,151] HDL measurements, however, frequently do not return to a desirable range. In addition, patients with NIDDM may have additional underlying primary abnormalities of lipid metabolism. Insulin therapy alone, even when glucose is successfully controlled, may improve but not normalize levels of triglycerides and other lipid subfractions in these patients.[152]

A great deal of recent interest has focused on combination therapy with sulfonylurea and insulin as a way of improving the control of hyperglycemia and at the same time diminishing insulin dosage.[153,154] When this form of therapy is effective, both glucose and lipid levels can be positively influenced with a decreased contribution of exogenous insulin to underlying hyperinsulinemia. Even when glucose control is inadequate, when sulfonylurea is added to insulin therapy, there may be a diminution in the resultant hyperinsulinemia.[153,154] This form of therapy is only effective in approximately 30% of patients, and its drawbacks include increased cost and the known adverse effects of sulfonylureas. In addition, data on long-term efficacy of combined sulfonylurea-insulin therapy are limited. In most patients, the reduction in insulin dosage with combined therapy is only modest, and concentrations of circulating insulin may not be reduced, as endogenous insulin secretion increases to compensate for the decrease in exogenous insulin. However, combined therapy is worth considering in patients whose hyperglycemia is not controlled by sulfonylurea or insulin therapy alone.

DRUG THERAPY FOR DIABETIC DYSLIPIDEMIA

When the goal levels for cholesterol and triglycerides are not met by the control of hyperglycemia, other factors contributing to hyperlipidemia should be sought. Diabetics are subject to a number of accompanying diseases that result in secondary hyperlipidemia. The prevalence of hypothyroidism is increased both in individuals with Type I diabetes and in elderly patients with Type II diabetes. The nephrotic syndrome and renal failure are frequent long-term sequelae of both Type I and Type II diabetes. Liver disease may result either from metabolic factors or factors associated with therapy for diabetes. Antihypertensive therapy with thiazide diuretics or β-adrenergic blocking agents may aggravate both the hyperglycemia and the dyslipidemia of diabetes.[155] Alcohol consumption may contribute to the presence of significant hypertriglyceridemia and should be assessed and corrected before hypolipidemic drug therapy is initiated. All attempts to control the hyperglycemia and dyslipidemia of NIDDM through diet should be maximized by effective patient education. The NCEP recommends that at least 6 months of dietary therapy be attempted before drug therapy for hyperlipidemia is initiated. Such attempts at successful dietary therapy should include consultation and followup with a registered dietician if dietary counseling by personnel at the physician's office is not successful.[2] However, when goals for cholesterol levels are not met, effective hypolipidemic drug therapy should be instituted.

The NCEP recognizes five classes of hypolipidemic agents as being useful in the treatment of lipid disorders.[2] Although these recommendations are made without regard to the status of a patient's carbohydrate tolerance, each of these classes of drugs is potentially applicable to the treatment of diabetic dyslipidemia. The five types of drugs currently employed and their effects on each lipid fraction are listed in Table 21–10. The effectiveness of each class of drug in lowering the various lipid fractions varies considerably. All of these recommended drugs are potentially useful for patients with diabetic dyslipidemia. The specific choice of drug should be determined by the lipid pattern exhibited by the individual patient and by the known effects of these drugs on diabetes and its complications. Dosing information for each drug is provided in Table 21–11.

Nicotinic Acid

Nicotinic acid (niacin) is a cofactor for intermediary metabolism at physiologic doses of less than 20 mg/day; however, when doses of 1000 mg/day or greater are used, this agent has profound lipid-lowering effects.[156–157] The NCEP recommends nicotinic acid as one of the first-line drugs for the treatment of hyperlipidemia, and it is the oldest available hypolipidemic agent currently utilized. Both short-acting and long-acting forms of the drug are available as either over-the-counter or prescription preparations. Although the exact mechanism of action of nicotinic acid is unknown, there is considerable evidence that this agent decreases the hepatic synthesis of VLDL, with a resultant decrease in both concentrations of triglyceride and LDL-cholesterol. It also has a significant effect on HDL concentrations, producing increases even at doses ineffective in lowering concentrations of the other lipid subfractions.[159] The drug is also known to inhibit lipolysis; however, this action is extremely short-lived, and the role of this effect in the hypolipidemic action of nicotinic acid is questionable.

The clinical utility of nicotinic acid has been diminished by the frequent occurrence of side effects, particularly with higher doses.[156–158] Cutaneous flushing, usually beginning within 15 to 120 minutes of ingestion, is extremely common. Gastrointestinal side effects of nausea, abdominal discomfort, and diarrhea are also common. Itching is an occasional problem; rash and hyperpigmentation occur less frequently. Nicotinic acid therapy may result in the activation of peptic ulcer disease, inflammatory bowel disease, and asthma. Hepatic dysfunction is another potentially serious side effect of nicotinic acid therapy, particularly when one of the long-acting preparations is employed.[160] Of particular concern when nicotinic acid is used in patients with impaired glucose tolerance or diabetes is its propensity to increase insulin resistance, which often results in further deterioration of carbohydrate tolerance.[156–158,161]

Some of the adverse effects of nicotinic acid can be avoided or minimized with appropriate usage.[157,158] At initiation of therapy doses of nicotinic acid should be low—50 to 100 mg daily—and then slowly increased until a therapeutically effective level is reached (usually $\geq$500 mg tid). Blood sugar, liver enzymes, and uric acid should be monitored during this period of dosage adjustment. A once-daily dose of aspirin or another prostaglandin inhibitor may reduce the frequency and severity of flushing episodes. Although lipid disorders in most patients can be controlled with a daily dose of nicotinic acid of 3 g or less, some patients may require as much as 6 to 9 g for normalization of lipid levels. With these higher doses, the incidence of side effects is significantly increased. In this situation, other drugs, either alone or in combination with nicotinic acid, should be considered.

At the 15th year of follow-up of the Coronary Drug Project, nicotinic acid was shown to have reduced both cardiovascular and total mortality[92] and consequently has

Table 21–10.   Effect of Hypolipidemic Drugs on Lipid Fractions

Drug Class	Lipoprotein fractions (% change)			
	Cholesterol			Triglycerides
	Total	LDL	HDL	
Bile acid sequestrant	↓ 10–25	↓ 15–30	↑ 0–5	↑ 0–15*
Nicotinic acid	↓ 10–25	↓ 20–30	↑ 10–35	↓ 30–50
Fibric acid derivatives	↓ 10–25	↓ 5–25†	↑ 10–25	↓ 20–50
HMG CoA reductase inhibitor	↓ 25–30	↓ 30–40	↑ 5–15	↓ 20–25
Probucol	↓ 10–30	↓ 10–20	↓ 15–30	↔

LDL and HDL = low-density and high-density lipoproteins; HMG CoA = 3-hydroxy-3-methyl-glutaryl CoA.
*Triglyceride levels may increase by $\geq$100% in patients with pre-existing hypertriglyceridemia.
†LDL levels may increase significantly in patients with hypertriglyceridemia.

Table 21–11. Hypercholesterolemic Drugs

Drug Class	Generic Name	Tradename	Usual Effective Dose	Maximal Dose
Bile acid sequestrants	Cholestyramine	Questran	8–12 g	24 g
		Questran Light		
		Colybar		
	Colistipol	Colistid	10–15 g	30 g
Nicotinic acid	Niacin	Niacin	1500–3000 mg	9 g
		Lipo-Nicin		
		Nia-Bid		
		Niaplus		
		Nicobid		
		Nicolar		
		Slo-Niacin		
		Enduracin		
Fibric acid derivatives	Clofibrate	Atromid S	2 g	2 g
	Gemfibrozil	Lopid	1200 mg	1200 mg
HMG CoA reductase	Lovastatin	Mevacor	20 mg hs	80 mg
inhibitors	Pravastatin	Pravachol	20 mg hs	40 mg
	Simvastatin	Zocor	10 mg hs	40 mg
Antioxidants	Probucol	Lorelco	1000 mg	1000 mg

HMG CoA = 3-hydroxy-3-methyl-glutaryl CoA; hs = at bedtime.
*With all the niacin agents, concomitant use of one aspirin daily may be indicated to prevent flushing.

continued to be used by many clinicians despite the frequent occurrence of the above side effects. In general, nicotinic acid is the most economical of all of the hypolipidemic drugs available, particularly in the immediate-acting form of nicotinic acid available without a prescription.[157,158] It should be pointed out that nicotinamide is frequently purchased by patients instead of nicotinic acid, and although it is well tolerated, nicotinamide has no lipid-lowering effect.[157]

In summary, nicotinic acid is effective in all forms of dyslipidemia as a result of its ability at maximal doses to lower triglyceride levels by 30 to 50%, to lower LDL-cholesterol levels by 20 to 30%, and to increase HDL-cholesterol levels by 10 to 35%[157,158] (Table 21–10). On first glance, nicotinic acid would appear to be the ideal drug for use in patients with diabetes. However, when nicotinic acid is used in clinically effective doses, the frequent side effect of increased insulin resistance, with a resultant worsening of hyperglycemia, significantly limits its usefulness in therapy for diabetic dyslipidemia.[36,108,161] In addition, the other side effects of nicotinic acid increase the difficulty associated with its use in patients with an underlying disease as complex as diabetes mellitus. It should be reserved for severe forms of hypertriglyceridemia such as the hyperchylomicronemia syndrome or the combined elevation of both VLDL and chylomicron triglyceride levels.[36] Whenever nicotinic acid is used to treat diabetic dyslipidemia, the effects on carbohydrate tolerance should be closely monitored.

Bile Acid Sequestrants

The bile acid sequestrants colestyramine (Questran or Cholybar) and colestipol (Colestid) are long-chain polymers containing strong, positively charged ionic groups.[156,157,162] These nonabsorbable anionic exchange resins are not absorbed and act primarily in the intestinal tract. By binding bile acids and interfering with their enterohepatic circulation, these agents force the liver to utilize cholesterol stores to synthesize additional bile acids. The resulting decrease in hepatic levels of intracellular free cholesterol results in an up-regulation of LDL receptors that increases LDL catabolism.[162] Again, the clinical usefulness of these agents is limited by a significant side-effect profile. Cholestyramine and colestipol administered at full dosage have been reported to result in constipation in 10 to 20% of patients, and gastric distress with bloating, nausea, vomiting, and increased flatulence has been noted in a significant number of patients.[156,157] Negatively charged drugs such as warfarin (Coumadin), digoxin, thyroxine, and thiazide diuretics will bind to these agents and thus should be taken at least 1 hour before or 4 hours after administration of the dose of the bile acid sequestrant. In addition, these agents are known to transiently increase the concentration of triglycerides and may result in a significant and prolonged elevation of triglyceride levels in individuals with pre-existing hypertriglyceridemia.[163]

The common side effects of these drugs can often be avoided by the use of an appropriate dosing schedule.[157] The starting dose of 4 g of cholestyramine or 5 g of colestipol once or twice daily should be given in a pleasant-tasting vehicle. These agents may be mixed in a variety of juices, water, or yogurt or added to oatmeal or other cereals. The fluid content of the diet should also be increased, and the incidence of constipation may be further reduced by adding to the diet a soluble-fiber preparation such as one of the psyllium-containing products. The dosage should be increased at 3- to 7-day intervals, with the minimal effective daily dose usually being 8 g of cholestyramine or 10 g of colestipol and the maximal dose being 24 g and 30 g, respectively.[156,157] Peak lipid effects are achieved within approximately 1 month. At maximal doses, the principal therapeutic effect of these agents is the lowering of LDL-cholesterol levels by 15 to 30% with little effect on HDL-cholesterol (Table

21–10). Concomitantly, as pointed out above, triglyceride levels may be increased by twofold or greater by the use of a bile acid sequestrant in patients with hypertriglyceridemia (i.e., >250 mg/dL).[126] For this reason, the bile acid sequestrants have significant limitations when applied to therapy for diabetic dyslipidemia.[108] The frequency of hypertriglyceridemia in diabetic patients and the propensity of this class of agents to further elevate triglyceride levels limit this drug as first-line therapy for many patients with diabetic dyslipidemia.[108] However, after triglyceride levels have been controlled, bile acid sequestrants may be used in combination with triglyceride-lowering drugs to bring levels of LDL-cholesterol within targeted levels.[157] Although few studies have been done with the bile acid resins specifically in diabetic patients, this class of hypolipidemic agents may be useful in those with isolated elevations in LDL levels.[108] However, the side effect of constipation, which may also be observed in patients with diabetes of long duration or with autonomic dysfunction, limits the use of bile acid resins in this group of patients.

Fibric Acid Derivatives

Clofibrate (Atromid-S) and gemfibrozil (Lopid) are presently the only fibric acid preparations available in the United States. Fenofibrate and bezafibrate are currently in clinical trials in the United States and have been used in Europe and other parts of the world for several years. All these drugs increase lipoprotein lipase activity, with a resulting increase in the clearance of VLDL triglycerides.[156,157,162] In patients with normal triglycerides and elevated levels of LDL-cholesterol, LDL clearance is also increased. Animal studies have suggested that this reduction in LDL-cholesterol may be the result of decreased hepatic cholesterol synthesis. There is an accompanying significant increase in HDL-cholesterol; however, the mechanism of this change is unknown.[93,156,157,162] Some patients with hypertriglyceridemia may experience a transient increase in LDL-cholesterol, and in some patients this increase may be sustained.[156,157] Both clofibrate and gemfibrozil are well tolerated, although they produce nausea and abdominal discomfort in 1 to 3% of patients. The usual dose of clofibrate is 1 g bid and that of gemfibrozil is 600 mg bid. Although gemfibrozil was not designated as a first-line drug in the initial report of the NCEP, with the release of the Helsinki Heart Study, most investigators now feel that gemfibrozil should also be considered a first-line drug for the treatment of hyperlipidemia.

The fibric acid derivatives comprise the class of hypolipidemic agent that has been studied most extensively in patients with diabetic dyslipidemia. Drugs in this group lower triglyceride levels by 20 to 50%, elevate HDL-cholesterol levels by 10 to 25%, and have variable effects on LDL-cholesterol levels[156,157] (Table 21–10). Similar effects on lipids have been documented in patients with diabetes.[164] Although the fibric acid derivatives are least effective in patients with isolated elevations of LDL-cholesterol, since the majority of patients with diabetic dyslipidemia have either hypertriglyceridemia or mixed hyperlipidemia, these drugs are of significant utility in many patients with diabetic dyslipidemia.[108]

Clofibrate was the first member of this class of agents used to treat hyperlipidemia. Although clofibrate has been used in diabetics with no evidence of adverse effects on glucose tolerance,[166] this drug has not been used extensively in the United States because of the results of the Coronary Drug Project study and the WHO study that indicated subjects treated with this agent experienced significant increases in cholelithiasis and other potentially deleterious side effects.[166–168]

Gemfibrozil is the other member of the fibric acid group available in the United States. Ever since the Helsinki Heart Study demonstrated a 34% reduction in cardiovascular mortality and morbidity in men with dyslipedia given this drug, it has been used extensively both in patients with and those without diabetes mellitus.[93] Although initial studies indicated that gemfibrozil might have a slight deleterious effect on carbohydrate tolerance, subsequent studies have indicated no significant change in blood sugar control in patients with diabetes treated with this drug.[164,169] Gemfibrozil is effective in diabetic patients with severe hypertriglyceridemia, including those with the hyperchylomicronemia syndrome.[70,171] It has also been useful in patients with mixed hyperlipidemia, although it may result in either a transient or a more prolonged increase in LDL-cholesterol levels.[164,172,173] In these situations, if the LDL-cholesterol level rises or is not sufficiently controlled to meet goal levels, a bile acid sequestrant can be added once the hypertriglyceridemia has been reduced.[162] A number of studies in patients with NIDDM have confirmed that gemfibrozil also increases levels of HDL-cholesterol in diabetic patients.[164,170–172] As stated previously, gemfibrozil is easily tolerated by most patients, producing minimal side effects. Because of the increased propensity for development of cholelithiasis in obese Type II diabetics, more studies are required to determine the safety of long-term therapy with gemfibrozil in these patients.

Bezafibrate and fenofibrate, the fibric acid derivatives not available in the United States, have also been used in patients with diabetes.[174–177] These agents appear to be similar to gemfibrozil in their effect on diabetic dyslipidemia and seem to be well tolerated and without deleterious effects on glucose control.

Probucol

Probucol (Lorelco), a lipophilic drug with modest cholesterol-lowering potential, has also been available for a number of years. The NCEP did not designate it as a first-line agent because it lowers LDL-cholesterol levels by only 10 to 20%, does not effect triglyceride levels, and decreases HDL-cholesterol levels by 15 to 30%[178] (Table 21–10).

The mechanism of action of probucol in lowering lipid levels is not fully explained; however, probucol has been shown to increase the fractional clearance rate of LDL and to increase the biliary excretion of cholesterol.[178] This increased removal of LDL may be due, at least in part, to a non-receptor-mediated pathway that is accelerated by the incorporation of probocol into the LDL particle. Its effect on HDL appears to be due primarily to a reduction in the cholesterol content of HDL particles, with less effect on the synthesis of HDL-specific apolipoproteins.[162,178] Side effects include mild diarrhea with accompanying flatulence, abdominal discomfort, and nausea in approximately 5% of patients.[155,178] The drug can also produce a prolongation of the Q-T interval, resulting in ventricular arrhythmias.[155,178]

Although probocol has not seen widespread use in the United States, there has been a recent resurgence of interest in this agent as a result of the demonstration that it is a potent anti-oxidant and that it may retard atherosclerosis at the cellular level within the arterial wall in addition to lowering cholesterol levels.[27] Few prospective clinical studies are available that demonstrate the efficacy of probucol to prevent coronary artery disease, either as a hypolipidemic agent or as an antioxidant/anti-atherosclerotic agent.

Although probucol has no significant effect on glucose tolerance, its limited efficacy in lowering LDL-cholesterol levels, its absence of effect on triglycerides, and its significant lowering of HDL-cholesterol levels make probucol a less than ideal agent for the treatment of diabetic dyslipidemia.[108] Although there is some evidence that diabetics may have an increased rate of LDL oxidation, the lack of proven clinical importance of probucol's antioxidant property in preventing atherosclerotic disease limits its usefulness in the prevention of the macrovascular complications of diabetes. However, if the studies currently being conducted demonstrate its efficacy as an anti-atherosclerotic agent, probucol may prove to be an important adjunct to hypolipidemic therapy in prevention of macrovascular disease in diabetics.

HMG CoA Reductase Inhibitors

Lovastatin (Mevacor) has been used extensively for the control of LDL-cholesterol since its release in 1988. Two additional drugs, pravastatin (Pravachol) and simvastatin (Zocor), have recently been released for clinical use, and several other derivatives are undergoing early clinical testing. These drugs competitively inhibit the rate-controlling enzyme of endogenous cholesterol biosynthesis, HMG CoA reductase, thus reducing cellular cholesterol production.[179] The resultant decrease in levels of intracellular free cholesterol increases the activity of LDL-receptor-mediated catabolism of LDL-cholesterol. In addition, conversion of VLDL remnants to LDL is significantly decreased in patients treated with an inhibitor of HMG CoA reductase. These drugs are the most effective single agents in reducing LDL-cholesterol levels and produce moderate decreases of triglyceride levels and increases in HDL levels.[157,162,179] At maximal doses, lovastatin consistently decreases LDL-cholesterol and triglyceride levels by 30 to 40% and 20 to 25%, respectively, and increases HDL-cholesterol levels by 5 to 15%[179-181] (Table 21-10). This class of drug seems extremely well tolerated, with liver dysfunction in the

form of elevations in levels of hepatic transaminases in fewer than 2% of lovastatin-treated patients.[180] Fewer than half of these patients will be forced to discontinue the medication because of a more significant elevation in transaminase levels (>3 times normal).[179,180] Approximately 0.1 to 0.5% of lovastatin-treated patients also have experienced myositis. The frequency of myositis is increased to approximately 5% when lovastatin is used in conjunction with gemfibrozil and to more than 30% when it is used with the immunosuppressant cyclosporin. Rhabdomyolysis and acute renal failure have been reported secondary to the combined use of lovastatin with cyclosporin or gemfibrozil.[162,182-184] Consequently, combination therapy with lovastatin and either gemfibrozil or cyclosporin should be undertaken with extreme caution in selected patients. Although there also appears to be an increased risk of myositis when lovastatin and nicotinic acid are used together, the lower frequency of myositis with this drug combination as compared with lovastatin and gemfibrozil allows combination therapy with lovastatin and nicotinic acid in patients who are at high risk for coronary artery disease because of significant hypercholesterolemia.[162] Recent reports also indicate that myositis has resulted from the concomitant use of lovastatin and erythromycin.[185] Although the possibility of cataract formation was initially of some concern, this has not proven to be a problem with wider use of lovastatin and the Food and Drug Administration has removed the requirement for a periodic slit-lamp examination for any of these HMG CoA reductase inhibitors.[179,180]

Lovastatin is given as initial therapy at a dosage of 20 mg daily.[179] This dose is most effective when taken at bedtime. The maximal total daily dose of 80 mg should be given as two doses. Although the data are still incomplete, there does not appear to be any significant difference between the other HMG CoA inhibitors and lovastatin with regard to the occurrence of side effects.[186] Both pravastatin and simvastatin are maximally effectve when given as a single dose at bedtime.

No adverse effects on glucose tolerance have been observed with lovastatin or with other drugs in this class during clinical trials.[108,164,173,181,187] Since these drugs are the agents most effective in lowering LDL-cholesterol levels, they are potentially useful in those diabetic patients with elevations in LDL cholesterol levels. Although lovastatin is not as effective as the fibric acid derivatives in lowering triglycerides, lovastatin has proven to be very effective in the treatment of the combined hyperlipidemia of diabetes.[108,164,173,182] Lovastatin is also not as effective as gemfibrozil in raising HDL-cholesterol levels; however, the observed moderate increase in HDL-cholesterol levels and the significant decline in LDL-cholesterol levels with lovastatin therapy has a very favorable effect on the ratio of LDL to HDL.[188] These drugs decrease the lithogenicity of the bile and theoretically should decrease the occurrence of cholelithiasis in obese patients.[179] Lovastatin is extremely well tolerated and has no apparent side effects of special concern for patients with diabetes.[180] However, the response of patients with diabetes to lovastatin and the other inhibitors of HMG CoA reductase needs to be studied more extensively.

Because of the effectiveness of lovastatin in reducing elevated lipid levels in patients with diabetes, lovastatin must be considered along with gemfibrozil as one of the drugs of choice for the treatment of diabetic dyslipidemia. The principal limitation of lovastatin for patients with diabetic dyslipidemia stems from its moderate ability to lower triglyceride levels. It is ineffective in patients with significant hypertriglyceridemia and of more limited effectiveness in patients with combined hyperlipidemia in which triglyceride elevation is the predominant disorder.[179]

Combination Drug Therapy

In patients with more severe elevations of triglyceride or cholesterol levels, the use of combinations of the above drugs is sometimes indicated. When patients who have been treated with gemfibrozil to control hypertriglyceridemia are noted to have an increase in LDL-cholesterol level or when the reduction of LDL does not reach goal levels, a bile acid sequestrant can be added to the treatment regimen once the triglycerides are under control. The combinations of gemfibrozil with a bile acid sequestrant and of nicotinic acid with a bile acid sequestrant have both been shown to be effective in the treatment of combined hyperlipidemia.[156,163,189] Probucol has also been used in conjunction with the bile acid resins, producing some increase in lipid-lowering efficacy.[162] Probucol, with its tendency to cause diarrhea, often will offset the constipation that commonly accompanies the use of a bile acid resin. The HMG CoA reductase inhibitors are also very effective in combination with bile acid sequestrants.[163,190] Triple drug therapy with nicotinic acid, a bile acid sequestrant, and lovastatin has been used in patients with severe hyperlipidemia.[191] This triple drug regimen is capable of lowering LDL-cholesterol levels by 70 to 80% and thereby of normalizing LDL levels even in patients with severe heterozygous familial forms of hypercholesterolemia or mixed hyperlipidemia. Although there is a slight increase in the incidence of myositis with the combination of nicotinic acid and lovastatin, this very effective combination can be used cautiously in individuals at high risk because of very elevated levels of LDL.[162] The observed increase in the incidence of myositis and the effects of nicotinic acid on glucose tolerance, as outlined previously, would limit this combination in the treatment of diabetic dyslipidemia. As discussed above, the combination of lovastatin and gemfibrozil should only be used in high-risk individuals, with caution, because of the significant increase in the rate of myositis to almost 5%.

OTHER CONSIDERATIONS

The Elderly Patient with Diabetes

Because the incidence of NIDDM and of hypercholesterolemia are observed to increase with age, diabetic dyslipidemia is a frequent finding in older individuals.

Although most of the major clinical trials have not studied elderly patients, the available data from a few studies and from epidemiologic studies such as the Framingham Study, indicate that lipid disorders continue to be of concern in the geriatric age group.[192,193] Since NIDDM frequently has its onset when individuals are older than 60 years of age, and since the presence of glucose intolerance increases the atherogenic potential of dyslipidemia and augments the natural tendency of cholesterol levels to increase with age, the elderly diabetic is of special concern to the clinician.[194] Studies from Framingham have suggested that the risk for coronary artery disease is significantly increased in elderly diabetic individuals; therefore, it seems appropriate to reduce cholesterol levels in this group.[195] Nonpharmacologic therapy should be effectively utilized before therapy with hypolipidemic drugs is considered. When drug therapy is necessary, both gemfibrozil and lovastatin are effective hypolipidemic agents and seem to have no age-specific side effects. However, as with all drug therapy for the elderly, special consideration should be given to the changes in metabolism that occur with aging, and dosage levels should be carefully titrated for older individuals.

Diabetic Nephropathy

Diabetic nephropathy is a frequent complication in both patients with IDDM and those with NIDDM. Diabetic renal disease usually presents with micro-albuminuria and hypertension and then progresses to nephrotic syndrome and/or chronic renal insufficiency.[196,197] A number of lipid abnormalities have been observed in patients with diabetic nephropathy, with hypertriglyceridemia and low levels of HDL-cholesterol being the most common. However, combined hyperlipidemia and the isolated elevation of LDL-cholesterol level also are seen in patients with diabetic renal disease.[198] The bile acid resins have been administered to patients with nephrotic syndrome secondary to diabetes, and since these agents are not absorbed through the gastrointestinal tract, they seem to result in no increases in side effects in patients with renal disease. However, because of their limited capacity to lower LDL-cholesterol levels and their propensity to elevate triglyceride levels, these agents are often not effective in controlling the lipid disorders of diabetic renal disease.[198]

More recently, lovastatin was used in patients with nephrotic syndrome, and it appears to be effective in lowering the LDL-cholesterol levels of patients with nephrotic syndrome who have no deterioration of renal function and is well tolerated by this group.[199] Because it is metabolized primarily by the liver, lovastatin should theoretically also be safe for patients with mild renal insufficiency. However, since lovastatin has not been studied in patients with more severe forms of diabetic nephropathy, it cannot be recommended for patients with significant deterioration of renal function.

For patients whose primary lipid problem secondary to diabetic nephropathy is hypertriglyceridemia, the fibric acid derivatives are of potential therapeutic benefit.[200]

Early studies with clofibrate in patients with renal insufficiency or nephrotic syndrome identified a significant problem with myositis, which in some cases was severe enough to produce rhabdomyolysis and worsening of renal failure. Although some studies have indicated that gemfibrozil and other fibric acid derivatives are beneficial in patients with nephrotic syndrome, fibric acid derivatives should be used with caution in patients with diabetic nephropathy because the predominant route of metabolism of these agents is renal excretion.[198]

CONCLUSION

Macrovascular disease is the number one cause of morbidity and mortality in NIDDM and is becoming increasingly important in IDDM. Although there has been an impressive decrease in mortality related to cardiovascular disease in the general population of the United States over the past 25 years,[201] patients with diabetes have not experienced this same decrease. Not only is diabetes an independent risk factor for arteriosclerosis, it is also frequently associated with other recognized risk factors such as obesity, hypertension, and dyslipidemia and with the recently proposed risk factors of insulin resistance and/or hyperinsulinemia. Hence, total risk factor management is mandatory in patients with diabetes mellitus. In addition, the therapeutic approach to any single risk factor must be designed so that it does not introduce or worsen other cardiovascular risk factors.

There is growing evidence that not only is dyslipidemia one of the most important contributors to arteriosclerosis but that with regard to coronary artery disease, the most frequent form of arteriosclerotic vascular disease, other risk factors may be lipid-dependent.[202] Hence, an understanding of the pathophysiology and treatment of diabetic dyslipidemia is essential for the successful management of patients with diabetes. Although many questions remain unanswered concerning the management of diabetic dyslipidemia, in this chapter we have attempted to summarize the current state of knowledge and to point out areas in which further basic and clinical research are indicated.

It seems particularly appropriate to end this discussion with an often quoted statement made by Dr. Elliot Joslin in 1927.

> I believe the chief cause of premature development of arteriosclerosis in diabetes, save for advancing age, is an excess of fat, an excess of fat in the body (obesity), an excess of fat in the diet, and an excess of fat in the blood. With an excess of fat diabetes begins and from an excess of fat diabetics die, formerly of coma, recently of arteriosclerosis.[203]

REFERENCES

1. Barrett-Connor E, Orchard T. Diabetes and heart disease. In: Diabetes in America. Diabetes data compiled 1984. National Diabetes Data Group. Washington, DC: US Dept of Health and Human Services, 1985;XVI 1–41: NIH publication no. 85–1468).
2. The Expert Panel. National Cholesterol Education Program. National Heart, Lung, and Blood Institute: report of the National Cholesterol Education Program Expert Panel on detection, evaluation, and treatment of high blood cholesterol in adults. Arch Intern Med 1988;148:36–69.
3. Gotto AM Jr, Pownall HJ, Havel RJ. Introduction to the plasma lipoproteins. Methods Enzymol 1986;128:3–4
4. Havel RJ. Origin, metabolic fate and metabolic function of plasma lipoproteins. In: Steinberg D, Olefsky JM, eds. Contemporary issues in endocrinology and metabolism. Hypercholesterolemia and atherosclerosis: pathogenesis and prevention. Vol 3. New York: Churchill Livingstone, 1987:117.
5. Assmann G, Lipid metabolism and atherosclerosis. Stuttgart: Schattauer, 1982.
6. Grundy SM. Cholesterol and atherosclerosis: diagnosis and treatment, Lippincott: Philadelphia, 1990.
7. Edelstein C, Kezdy FJ, Scanu AM, Shen BW. Apolipoproteins and the structural organization of plasma lipoproteins: human plasma high density lipoprotein-3. J Lipid Res 1979;20:143–53.
8. Havel RJ, Kane JP. Introduction: structure and metabolism of plasma lipoproteins. In: Scriver CR, Beaudet AL, Sly WS, Valle D, eds. The metabolic basis of inherited disease. 6th ed. New York: McGraw-Hill, 1989:1129–38.
9. Kane JP, Havel RJ. Disorders of the biogenesis and secretion of lipoproteins containing the B apolipoproteins. In: Scriver CR, Beaudet AL, Sly WS, Valle D, eds. The metabolic basis of inherited disease. 6th ed. New York, McGraw-Hill, 1989:1139–64.
10. Brown MS, Goldstein JL. The LDL receptor and HMG-CoA reductase—two membrane molecules that regulate cholesterol homeostasis. Curr Top Cell Regul 1985;26:3–15.
11. Havel RJ. Metabolism of triglyceride-rich lipoproteins. In: Schettler FD, ed. Atherosclerosis VI. Berlin-Heidelberg: Springer-Verlag, 1983:480.
12. Grundy SM. Cholesterol and coronary heart disease: a new era. JAMA 1986;256:2849–58.
13. Scanu AM, Fless GM. Lipoprotein (a): heterogeneity and biological relevance. J Clin Invest 1990;85:1709–15.
14. Castelli WP, Garrison RJ, Wilson PWF, et al. Incidence of coronary heart disease and lipoprotein cholesterol levels. The Framingham Study. JAMA 1986;256:2835–8.
15. Eisenberg S. High density lipoprotein metabolism. J Lipid Res 1984;25:1017–58.
16. Brewer HB Jr, Santamarina-Fojo S, Hoeg JM. Molecular biology of lipoproteins, their receptors, and lipoprotein lipase: primary hyperlipidemias. Vol 3, Chapter 3. In: Jeffers D, ed. Primary hyperlipidemias. New York: McGraw Hill, 1991:43–74.
17. Garfinkel AS, Schotz MC. Lipoprotein lipase. In: Gotto AM, ed. Plasma lipoproteins. Amsterdam: Elsevier, 1987:335.
18. Jackson RL. Lipoprotein lipase and hepatic lipase. In: Boyer PD, ed. The enzymes. Vol 16. New York: Academic Press, 1984:141.
19. Jauhiainen M, Dolphin PJ. Human plasma lecithin-cholesterol acyltransferase: an elucidation of the catalytic mechanism. J Biol Chem 1986;261:7032–43.
20. Fielding CJ, Fielding PE. Cholesterol transport between cells and body fluid: role of plasma lipoproteins and the plasma cholesterol esterification system. Med Clin North Am 1982;66:363–73.
21. Yki-Jarvinen H, Taskinen M-R, Koivisto VA, Nikkila EA. Response of adipose tissue lipoprotein lipase activity and serum lipoproteins to acute hyperinsulinemia in man. Diabetologia 1984;27:364–9.

22. Havel RJ, Hamilton RL. Hepatocytic lipoprotein receptors and intracellular lipoprotein catabolism. Hepatology 1988;8:1689–704.

23. Schonfeld G. Diabetes, lipoproteins, and atherosclerosis. Metabolism 1985;349(Suppl 1):45–50.

24. Sparks CE, Sparks JD, Bolognino M, et al. Insulin effects on apolipoprotein B lipoprotein synthesis and secretion by primary cultures of rat hepatocytes. Metabolism 1986;35:1128–36.

25. Goldberg IJ, Le NA, Paterniti JR Jr, et al. Lipoprotein metabolism during acute inhibition of hepatic triglyceride lipase in the cynomolgus monkey. J Clin Invest 1982;70:1184–92.

26. Packard CJ, Munro A, Lorimer AR, et al. Metabolism of apolipoprotein B in large triglyceride-rich very low density lipoproteins of normal and hypertriglyceridemic subjects. J Clin Invest 1984;74:2178–92.

27. Steinberg D, Parthasarathy S, Carew TE, et al. Beyond cholesterol: modifications of low-density lipoprotein that increase its atherogenicity. N Engl J Med 1989; 320:915–24.

28. Gwynne JT. High-density lipoprotein cholesterol levels as a marker of reverse cholesterol transport. Am J Cardiol 1989;64:10G–7.

29. Graham DL, Oram JF. Identification and characterization of a high density lipoprotein-binding protein in cell membranes by ligand blotting. J Biol Chem 1987;262:7439–42.

30. Howard BV. Lipoprotein metabolism in diabetes mellitus. J Lipid Res 1987;28:613–28.

31. Nikkila EA. Plasma lipid and lipoprotein abnormalities in diabetes. In: Jarrett RJ, ed. Diabetes and heart disease. New York: Elsevier, 1984:133–67.

32. Reaven GM. Non-insulin-dependent diabetes mellitus, abnormal lipoprotein metabolism, and atherosclerosis. Metabolism 1987;36(Suppl 1):1–8.

33. Goldberg RB. Lipid disorders in diabetes. Diabetes Care 1981;4:561–72.

34. Brunzell JD, Chait A, Bierman EL. Plasma lipoproteins in human diabetes mellitus. In: Alberti KGMM, Krall LD, eds. The diabetes annual. Amsterdam: Elsevier, 1985:463–79.

35. Ginsberg HN. Relationship between diabetes mellitus and coronary artery disease. Clin Diabetes 1988;6(Suppl 4):73–94.

36. Dunn FL. Treatment of lipid disorders in diabetes mellitus. Med Clin North Am 1988;72(6):1379–98.

37. Brunzell JD, Hazzard WR, Motulsky AG, Bierman EL. Evidence for diabetes mellitus and genetic forms of hypertriglyceridemia as independent entities. Metabolism 1975;24:1115–21.

38. Kissebah AH, Alfarsi S, Evans DJ, Adams PW. Integrated regulation of very low density lipoprotein triglyceride and apolipoprotein-B kinetics in non-insulin dependent diabetes mellitus. Diabetes 1982;31:903–10.

39. Abrams JJ, Ginsberg H, Grundy SM. Metabolism of cholesterol and plasma triglycerides in nonketotic diabetes mellitus. Diabetes 1982;31:903–10.

40. Ginsberg H, Grundy SM. Very low density lipoprotein metabolism in non-ketotic diabetes mellitus: effect of dietary restriction. Diabetologia 1982;23:421–5.

41. Dunn FL, Raskin P, Bilheimer DW, Grundy SM. The effect of diabetic control on very low-density lipoprotein-triglyceride metabolism in patients with Type II diabetes mellitus and marked hypertriglyceridemia. Metabolism 1984;33:117–23.

42. Howard BV, Abbott WGH, Beltz WF, et al. Integrated study

43. Taskinen MR. Lipoprotein lipase in diabetes. Diabetes Metab Rev 1987;3:551–70.

44. Streja DA, Marliss EB, Steiner G. The effects of prolonged fasting on plasma triglyceride kinetics in man. Metabolism 1976;36:505–6.

45. Tobey TA, Greenfield M, Kraemer F, Reaven GM. Relationship between insulin resistance, insulin secretion, very low density lipoprotein kinetics, and plasma triglyceride levels in normotriglyceridemic man. Metabolism 1981;30:165–71.

46. Howard BV, Abbott WG, Egusa G, Taskinen MR. Coordination of very low-density lipoprotein triglyceride and apolipoprotein B metabolism in humans: effects of obesity and non-insulin-dependent diabetes mellitus. Am Heart J 1987;113:522–6.

47. Patsch W, Franz S, Schonfeld G. Role of insulin in lipoprotein secretion by cultured rat hepatocytes. J Clin Invest 1983;71:1161–74.

48. Sparks CE, Sparks JD, Bolognino M, et al. Insulin effects on apolipoprotein B lipoprotein synthesis and secretion by primary cultures of rat hepatocytes. Metabolism 1986;35:1128–36.

49. Abbott WGH, Lillioja S, Young AA, et al. Relationship between plasma lipoprotein concentrations and insulin action in an obese hyperinsulinemic population. Diabetes 1987;36:897–904.

50. Garg A, Helderman JH, Koffler M, et al. Relationship between lipoprotein levels and in vivo insulin action in normal young white men. Metabolism 1988;37:982–7.

51. Schonfeld G, Birge C, Miller JP, et al. Apolipoprotein B levels and altered lipoprotein composition in diabetes. Diabetes 1974;23:827–34.

52. Patti L, Swinburn B, Riccardi G, et al. Alterations in very-low-density lipoprotein subfractions in normotriglyceridemic non-insulin-dependent diabetics. Atherosclerosis 1991;91:15–23.

53. Fielding CJ, Castro GR, Donner C, et al. Distribution of apolipoprotein E in the plasma of insulin-dependent and non-insulin-dependent diabetics and its relation to cholesterol net transport. J Lipid Res 1986;27:1052–61.

54. Eto M, Watanabe K, Iwashima Y, et al. Apolipoprotein E polymorphism and hyperlipemia in Type II diabetics. Diabetes 1986;35:1374–82.

55. Klein RL, Lyons TJ, Lopes-Virella MF. Metabolism of very low- and low-density lipoproteins isolated from normolipidaemic type 2 (non-insulin-dependent) diabetic patients by human monocyte-derived macrophages. Diabetologia 1990;33:299–305.

56. Steiner G, Vranic M. Hyperinsulinemia and hypertriglyceridemia, a vicious cycle with atherogenic potential. Int J Obesity 1982;6(Suppl 1):117–24.

57. Harris MI. Hypercholesterolemia in individuals with diabetes and glucose intolerance in the U.S. population. Diabetes Care 1991;14:366–74.

58. Gabor J, Spain M, Kalant N. Composition of serum very-low-density and high-density lipoproteins in diabetes. Clin Chem 1980;26:1261–5.

59. Kissebah AH, Alfarsi S, Evans DJ, Adams PW. Plasma low density lipoprotein transport kinetics in noninsulin-dependent diabetes mellitus. J Clin Invest 1983; 71:655–67.

60. Chait A, Bierman EL, Albers JJ. Low-density lipoprotein receptor activity in cultured human skin fibroblasts—

mechanism of insulin-induced stimulation. J Clin Invest 1979;64:1309–9.

61. Howard BV, Knowler WC, Vasquez B, et al. Plasma and lipoprotein cholesterol and triglyceride in the Pima Indian population: comparison of diabetics and nondiabetics. Arteriosclerosis 1984;4:462–71.

62. Fisher WR, Zech LA, Bardalaye P, et al. The metabolism of apolipoprotein B in subjects with hypertriglyceridemia and polydispense LDL. J Lipid Res 1980;21:760–74.

63. Hiramatsu K, Bierman EL, Chait A. Metabolism of low-density lipoprotein from patients with diabetic hypertriglyceridemia by cultured human skin fibroblasts. Diabetes 1985;34:8–14.

64. Kim HJ, Kurup IV. Nonenzymatic glycosylation of human plasma low density lipoprotein. Evidence for in vitro and in vivo glucosylation. Metabolism 1982;31:348–53.

65. Steinbrecher UP, Witztum JL. Glucosylation of low-density lipoproteins to an extent comparable to that seen in diabetes slows their catabolism. Diabetes 1984; 33:130–4.

66. Lorenzi M, Cagliero E, Markey B, et al. Interaction of human endothelial cells with elevated glucose concentrations and native and glycosylated low density lipoproteins. Diabetologia 1984;26:218–22.

67. Fielding CJ, Reaven GM, Fielding PE. Human noninsulin-dependent diabetes: identification of a defect in plasma cholesterol transport normalized in vivo by insulin and in vitro by selective immunoadsorption of apolipoprotein E. Proc Natl Acad Sci USA 1982;79:6365–9.

68. Golay A, Zech L, Shi M-Z, et al. High density lipoprotein (HDL) metabolism in noninsulin-dependent diabetes mellitus: measurement of HDL turnover using tritiated HDL. J Clin Endocrinol Metab 1987;65:512–8.

69. Harno K, Nikkila EA, Kuusi T. Plasma HDL cholesterol and postheparin plasma hepatic (HL) endothelial lipase activity: relationship to obesity and non-insulin dependent diabetes (NIDDM) [Abstract no. 165]. Diabetologia 1980;19:281.

70. Duell PB, Oram JF, Bierman EL. nonenzymatic glycosylation of HDL and impaired HDL-receptor-mediated cholesterol efflux. Diabetes 1991;40:377–84.

71. Bagdade JD, Buchanan WE, Kuusi T, Taskinen MR. Persistent abnormalities in lipoprotein composition in noninsulin-dependent diabetes after intensive insulin therapy. Arteriosclerosis 1990;10:232–9.

72. Bagdade JD, Porte D Jr, Bierman EL. Diabetic lipemia: a form of acquired fat-induced lipemia. N Engl J Med 1967;276:427–33.

73. Gonen B, White N, Schonfeld G, et al. Plasma levels of apoprotein B in patients with diabetes mellitus: the effect of glycemic control. Metabolism 1985;34:675–9.

74. Lopes-Virella MF, Wohltmann HJ, Loadholt CB, Buse MG. Plasma lipids and lipoproteins in young insulin-dependent diabetic patients: relationship with control. Diabetologia 1981;21:216–23.

75. Nikkila EA, Kekki M. Plasma triglyceride transport kinetics in diabetes mellitus. Metabolism 1973;22:1–22.

76. Lewis B, Mancini M, Mattock M, et al. Plasma triglyceride and fatty acid metabolism in diabetes mellitus. Eur J Clin Invest 1972;2:445–53.

77. Ginsberg H, Mok H, Grundy S, Zeck L. Increased production of very low density lipoprotein-triglyceride (VLDL-TG) in insulin-deficient diabetics [Abstract no. 182]. Diabetes 1977;26(Suppl 1):399.

78. Pietri AO, Dunn FL, Grundy SM, Raskin P. The effect of continuous subcutaneous insulin infusion on very-low-density lipoprotein triglyceride metabolism in Type I diabetes mellitus. Diabetes 1983;32:75–81.

79. Dunn FL, Carroll P, Vlachokosta F, Beltz B. Effect of treatment with the artificial beta-cell on triglyceride metabolism in Type I diabetes mellitus. Diabetes 1985;34(Suppl 1):86A.

80. Rosenstock J, Vega G-L, Raskin P. Improved diabetic control decreases LDL apoB synthesis in Type I diabetes mellitus [Abstract]. Arteriosclerosis 1985;5:513A.

81. Lopes-Virella MF, Sherer GK, Lees AM, et al. Surface binding, internalization and degradation by cultured human fibroblasts of low density lipoproteins isolated from Type I (insulin-dependent) diabetic patients: changes with metabolic control. Diabetologia 1982; 22:430–6.

82. Lopes-Virella MF, Sherer G, Wohltmann H, et al. Diabetic lipoprotein deficient serum: its effect in low density lipoprotein (LDL) uptake and degradation by fibroblasts. Metabolism 1985;34:1079–85.

83. Nikkila EA, Kuusi T, Taskinen MR. Role of lipoprotein lipase and hepatic endothelial lipase in the metabolism of high density lipoproteins: a novel concept on cholesterol transport in HDL cycle. In: Carlson LA, Personow B, eds. Metabolic risk factors in ischemic cardiovascular disease. New York: Raven Press, 1982:205–15.

84. Eckel RH, Albers JJ, Cheung MD, et al. High density lipoprotein composition in insulin dependent diabetes mellitus. Diabetes 1981;30:132–8.

85. Curtiss LK, Witztum JL. Plasma apolipoproteins AI, AII, B, CI, and E are glucosylated in hyperglycemic diabetic subjects. Diabetes 1985;34:452–61.

86. Gotto AM Jr, LaRosa JC, Hunninghake D, et al. The cholesterol facts: a summary of the evidence relating dietary fats, serum cholesterol, and coronary heart disease: a joint statement by the American Heart Association and the National Heart, Lung, and Blood Institute. Circulation 1988;81:1721–33.

87. Steiner G. From an excess of fat, diabetics die [Editorial]. JAMA 1989;262:398–9.

88. Sytkowski PA, Kannel WB, D'Agostino RB. Changes in risk factors and the decline in mortality from cardiovascular disease. The Framingham Heart Study. N Engl J Med 1990;322:1635–41.

89. Consensus Conference. Lowering blood cholesterol to prevent heart disease. JAMA 1985;253:2080–86.

90. Steinberg D. The cholesterol controversy is over. Why did it take so long? [Editorial] Circulation 1989;80:1070–8.

91. Lipid Research Clinics Program. The Lipid Research Clinics coronary primary prevention trial results. I. Reduction in incidence of coronary heart disease. JAMA 1984;251:351–64.

92. Canner PL, Berge KG, Wenger NK, et al. for the Coronary Drug Project Research Group. Fifteen year mortality in coronary drug project patients: Long-term benefit with niacin. J Am Coll Cardiol 1986;8:1245–55.

93. Frick MH, Elo O, Haapa K, et al. Helsinki Heart Study: primary-prevention trial with gemfibrozil in middle-aged men with dyslipidemia. Safety of treatment, changes in risk factors, and incidence of coronary heart disease. N Engl J Med 1987;317:1237–45.

94. Carlson LA, Rosenhamer G. Reduction of mortality in the Stockholm ischaemic heart disease secondary prevention study by combined treatment with clofibrate and nicotinic acid. Acta Med Scand 1988;223:405–18.

95. Blankenhorn DH, Nessim SA, Johnson RL, et al. Beneficial effects of combined colestipol-niacin therapy on coronary

atherosclerosis and coronary venous bypass grafts. JAMA 1987;257: 3233–40.

96. Brown G, Albers JJ, Fisher LD, et al. Regression of coronary artery disease as a result of intensive lipid-lowering therapy in men with high levels of apolipoprotein B. N Engl J Med 1990;323:1289–8.

97. Ornish D, Brown SE, Scherwitz LW, et al. Can lifestyle changes reverse coronary heart disease? The Lifestyle Heart Trial. Lancet 1990;336:129–33.

98. Buchwald H, Varco RL, Matts JP, et al. and the POSCH Group. Effect of partial ileal bypass surgery on mortality and morbidity from coronary heart disease in patients with hyper-cholesterolemia. Report of the program on the surgical control of the hyperlipidemias (POSCH). N Engl J Med 1990;323:946–55.

99. Kane JP, Malloy MJ, Ports TA, et al. Regression of coronary atherosclerosis during treatment of familial hypercholesterolemia with combined drug regimens. JAMA 1990; 264:3007–12.

100. Iwai M, Yoshino G, Matsushita M, et al. Abnormal lipoprotein composition in normolipidemic diabetic patients. Diabetes Care 1990;13:792–6.

101. American Diabetes Association. Role of cardiovascular risk factors in prevention and treatment of macrovascular disease in diabetes. Diabetes Care 1989;12:573–9.

102. West KM, Ahuja MMS, Bennett PH, et al. The role of circulating glucose and triglyceride concentrations and their interactions with other "risk factors" as determinants of arterial disease in nine diabetic population samples from the WHO multinational study. Diabetes Care 1983;6:361–9.

103. Fontbonne A, Eschwege E, Cambien F, et al. Hypertriglyceridemia as a risk factor of coronary heart disease mortality in subjects with impaired glucose tolerance or diabetes. Results from the 11-year follow-up of the Paris prospective study. Diabetologia 1989;32:300–4.

104. Abbott RD, Wilson PWF, Kannel WB, Castelli WP. High density lipoprotein cholesterol, total cholesterol screening, and myocardial infarction. The Framingham Study. Arteriosclerosis 1988;8:207–11.

105. Stern MP, Patterson JK, Haffner SM, et al. Lack of awareness and treatment of hyperlipidemia in Type II diabetes in a community survey. JAMA 1989; 262:360–4.

106. Kannel WB, McGee DL. Diabetes and cardiovascular disease. The Framingham Study. JAMA 1979;241:2035–8.

107. Walden CE, Knopp RH, Wahl PW, et al. Sex differences in the effect of diabetes mellitus on lipoprotein triglyceride and cholesterol concentrations. N Engl J Med 1984;311:953–9.

108. Garg A, Grundy SM. Management of dyslipidemia in NIDDM. Diabetes Care 1990;13:153–69.

109. NIH Consensus Development Conference Summary. Treatment of hypertriglyceridemia. Arteriosclerosis 1984;4:296–301.

110. Miller M, Mead LA, Kwiterovich PO Jr, Pearson TA. Dyslipidemias with desirable plasma total cholesterol levels and angiographically demonstrated coronary artery disease. Am J Cardiol 1990;65:1–5.

111. Technical Review. The American Diabetes Association Council on Exercise. Exercise and NIDDM. Diabetes Care 1990;13:785–9.

112. Position Statement. The American Diabetes Association Council on Exercise. Diabetes mellitus and exercise. Diabetes Care 1990;13:804–5.

113. National Institutes of Health. Consensus development

conference on diet and exercise in non-insulin-dependent diabetes mellitus. Diabetes Care 1987;10:639–44.

114. American Diabetes Association. Nutritional recommendations and principles for individuals with diabetes mellitus: 1986. Diabetes Care 1987;10:126–32.

115. Coulston AM, Hollenbeck CB, Swislocki ALM, Reaven GM. Persistence of hypertriglyceridemic effect of low-fat high-carbohydrate diets in NIDDM patients. Diabetes Care 1989;12:94–101.

116. Rivellese AA, Giacco R, Genovese S, et al. Effects of changing amount of carbohydrate in diet on plasma lipoproteins and apolipoproteins in Type II diabetic patients. Diabetes Care 1990;13:446–8.

117. Garg A, Bonanome A, Grundy SM, et al. Comparison of a high-carbohydrate diet with a high-monounsaturated-fat diet in patients with non-insulin-dependent diabetes mellitus. N Engl J Med 1989;319:829–34.

118. Abbott WGH, Swinburn B, Ruotolo G, et al. Effect of a high-carbohydrate, low-saturated-fat diet on apolipoprotein B and triglyceride metabolism in Pima Indians. J Clin Invest 1990;86:642–50.

119. Abbott WGH, Boyce VL, Grundy SM, Howard BV. Effects of replacing saturated fat with complex carbohydrate in diets of subjects with NIDDM. Diabetes Care 1989;12:102–7.

120. Simpson HCR, Carter RD, Lousley S, Mann JI. Digestible carbohydrate—an independent effect on diabetic control in type 2 (non-insulin-dependent) diabetic patients? Diabetologia 1982;23:235–9.

121. Hockaday TDR, Hockaday JM, Mann JI, Turner RC. Prospective comparison of modified-fat-high-carbohydrate with standard low-carbohydrate dietary advice in the treatment of diabetes: one year follow up study. Br J Nutr 1978;39:357–62.

122. Anderson JW, Chen W-JL, Sieling B. Hypolipidemic effects of high-carbohydrate, high-fiber diets. Metabolism 1980;29:551–8.

123. Stone DB, Connor WE. The prolonged effects of a low cholesterol, high carbohydrate diet upon the serum lipids in diabetic patients. Diabetes 1963;12:127–32.

124. Weinsier RL, Seeman A, Herrera MG, et al. High and low carbohydrate diets in diabetes mellitus. Study of effects on diabetic control, insulin secretion and blood lipids. Ann Intern Med 1974;80:332–41.

125. Simons LA, Ruys J, Chang S, Balasubramaniam S. Maintenance of plasma triglyceride-lowering through use of low-dose fish oils in the diet. Artery 1987;14:127–36.

126. Leaf A, Weber PC. Cardiovascular effects of n-3 fatty acids. N Engl J Med 1988;318:549–57.

127. Hendra TJ, Britton ME, Roper DR, et al. Effects of fish oil supplements in NIDDM subjects: controlled study. Diabetes Care 1990;13:821–9.

128. Friday KE, Childs MT, Tsunehara CH, et al. Elevated plasma glucose and lowered triglyceride levels from omega-3 fatty acid supplementation in Type II diabetes. Diabetes Care 1989;12:276–81.

129. Kasim S. Is there a role for fish oils in diabetes treatment? Clinical Diabetes 1989;7:93–100.

130. Mori TA, Vandongen R, Masarei JRL. Fish oil-induced changes in apolipoproteins in IDDM subjects. Diabetes Care 1990;13:725–32.

131. Sorisky A, Robbins DC. Fish oil and diabetes: the net effect [Editorial]. Diabetes Care 1989;12:302–4.

132. Lopes-Virella MF, Wohltmann HJ, Mayfield RK, et al. Effect of metabolic control on lipid, lipoprotein, and apolipoprotein levels in 55 insulin-dependent diabetic patients: a longitudinal study. Diabetes 1983;32:20–5.

133. Rosenstock J, Strowig S, Cercone S, Raskin P. Reduction in cardiovascular risk factors with intensive diabetes treatment in insulin-dependent diabetes mellitus. Diabetes Care 1987;10:729–34.

134. Dunn FL, Pietri A, Raskin P. Plasma lipid and lipoprotein levels with continuous subcutaneous insulin infusion in Type I diabetes mellitus. Ann Intern Med 1981; 95:426–31.

135. Ruotolo G, Micossi P, Galimberti G, et al. Effects of intraperitoneal versus subcutaneous insulin administration on lipoprotein metabolism in Type I diabetes. Metabolism 1990;39:598–604.

136. Stolar MW. Atherosclerosis in diabetes: the role of hyperinsulinemia. Metabolism 1988;37(Suppl 1):1–9.

137. Stout RW. Insulin and atheroma: 20-year perspective. Diabetes Care 1990;13:631–54.

138. Bierman E. Diabetes mellitus, hyperlipidemia and atherosclerosis. Lipid Rev 1989;3:17.

139. Gerich JE. Oral hypoglycemic agents. Medical Intelligence. N Engl J Med 1989;321:1231–45.

140. Melander A, Lebovitz HE, Faber OK. Sulfonylureas: why, which, and how? Diabetes Care 1990;13(Suppl 3):18–25.

141. Beck-Nielsen H, Hother-Nielsen O, Pedersen O. Mechanism of action of sulphonylureas with special reference to the extrapancreatic effect: an overview. Diabetic Med 1988;5:613–20.

142. Reaven GM. Abnormal lipoprotein metabolism in non-insulin-dependent diabetes mellitus: pathogenesis and treatment. Am J Med 1987;83(Suppl 3A):31–40.

143. Ronnemaa T, Laakso M, Puukka P, et al. Athero-sclerotic vascular disease in middle-aged, insulin-treated, diabetic patients: association with endogenous insulin secretion capacity. Arteriosclerosis 1988;8:237–44.

144. Janka HU, Ziegler AG, Standl E, Mehnert H. Daily insulin dose as a predictor of macrovascular disease in insulin treated non-insulin-dependent diabetics. Diabete Metab 1987;13:359–64.

145. Genuth S. Insulin use in NIDDM. Diabetes Care 1990; 13:1240–64.

146. Galloway JA. Treatment of NIDDM with insulin agonists or substitutes. Diabetes Care 1990;13:1209–39.

147. Turner RC, Holman RR. Insulin use in NIDDM: rationale based on pathophysiology of disease. Diabetes Care 1990;13:1011–20.

148. Taskinen MR, Kuusi T, Helve E, et al. Insulin therapy induces antiatherogenic changes of serum lipoproteins in noninsulin-dependent diabetes. Arteriosclerosis 1988; 8:168–77.

149. Hanefeld M, Schulze J, Fischer S, et al. The diabetes Intervention Study (DIS): a cooperative multi-intervention trial with newly manifested Type II diabetics: preliminary results. Monogr Atheroscler 1985;13:98–103.

150. Taskinen MR, Packard CJ, Shepherd J. Effect of insulin therapy on metabolic fate of apolipoprotein B-containing lipoproteins in NIDDM. Diabetes 1990;39:1017–27.

151. Lopes-Virella MF, Colwell JA. Pharmacological treatment of lipid disorders in diabetes mellitus. Diabetes Metab Rev 1987;3:691–722.

152. Bolinder J, Arner P. Antilipolytic effect of insulin in non-insulin-dependent diabetes mellitus after conventional treatment with diet and sulfonylurea. Acta Med Scand 1988;224:451–9.

153. Bailey TS, Mezitis NHE. Combination therapy with insulin and sulfonylureas for Type II diabetes. Diabetes Care 1990;13:687–95.

154. Lebovitz HE, Pasmantier RM. Combination insulin-sulfonylurea therapy. Diabetes Care 1990;13:667–75.

155. Christlieb AR. Treatment selection considerations for the hypertensive diabetic patient. Arch Intern Med 1990; 150:1167–74.

156. Illingworth DR. Lipid-lowering drugs: an overview of indications and optimum therapeutic use. Drugs 1987; 33:259–79.

157. Brown WV, Howard WJ. Treatment of lipoprotein disorders. Cardiovasc Clin 1990;20:157–76.

158. Brown WV, Field L, Howard WJ. Nicotinic acid and its derivatives. In: Rifkind B, ed. Drug treatment of hyperlipidemia. New York: Marcel Dekker, 1991.

159. Alderman JD, Pasternak RC, Sacks FM, et al. Effect of a modified, well-tolerated niacin regimen on serum total cholesterol, high density lipoprotein cholesterol and the cholesterol to high density lipoprotein ratio. Am J Cardiol 1989;64:725–9.

160. Henkin Y, Johnson KC, Segrest JP. Rechallenge with crystalline niacin after drug-induced hepatitis from sustained-release niacin. JAMA 1990;264:241–3.

161. Garg A, Grundy SM. Nicotinic acid as therapy for dyslipidemia in non-insulin-dependent diabetes mellitus. JAMA 1990;264:723–6.

162. Howard WJ, Brown WV. Pharmacologic therapy of hypercholesterolemia. Curr Opin Cardiol 1989;3:525–41.

163. Crouse JR III. Hypertriglyceridemia: a contraindication to the use of bile acid binding resins. Am J Med 1987; 83:243–8.

164. Garg A, Grundy SM. Gemfibrozil alone and in combination with lovastatin for treatment of hypertriglyceridemia in NIDDM. Diabetes 1989;38:364–72.

165. Kobayashi M, Shigeta Y, Hirata Y, et al. Improvement of glucose tolerance in NIDDM by clofibrate: randomized double-blind study. Diabetes Care 1988;11:495–9.

166. The Coronary Drug Project Research Group. Clofibrate and niacin in coronary heart disease. JAMA 1975; 231:360–81.

167. Report of the Committee of Principal Investigators. WHO cooperative trial on primary prevention of ischaemic heart disease using clofibrate to lower serum cholesterol: mortality follow-up. Lancet 1980;2:379–85.

168. Bateson MC, Maclean D, Ross PE, Bouchier IAD. Clofibrate therapy and gallstone induction. Am J Dig Dis 1978;23:623–8.

169. Pagani A, Dalmotto M, Pagano G, et al. Effect of short-term gemfibrozil administration on glucose metabolism and insulin secretion in non-insulin-dependent diabetics. Curr Ther Res 1989;45:14–20.

170. Bertolini S, Cordera R, Marcenaro A, et al. Metabolic effects of gemfibrozil in patients with primary hypertriglyceridemia. Diab Nutr Metab 1990;3:23–33.

171. Leaf DA, Connor WE, Illingworth DR, et al. The hypolipidemic effects of gemfibrozil in type V hyperlipidemia: a double-blind, crossover study. JAMA 1989;262:3154–60.

172. Marks J, Howard AN. A comparative study of gemfibrozil and clofibrate in the treatment of hyperlipidemia in patients with maturity-onset diabetes. Res Clin Forums 1982;4:97.

173. Vega GL, Grundy SM. Primary hypertriglyceridemia with borderline high cholesterol and elevated apolipoprotein B concentrations: comparison of gemfibrozil vs lovastatin therapy. JAMA 1990;264:2759–63.

174. Prager R, Schernthaner G, Kostner GM. Effect of bezafibrate on plasma lipids, lipoproteins, apolipoproteins AI, AII and B and LCAT activity in hyperlipidemic, non-

insulin-dependent diabetics. Atherosclerosis 1982; 2:321—7.

175. Jones IR, Swai A, Taylor R, et al. Lowering of plasma glucose concentrations with bezafibrate in patients with moderately controlled NIDDM. Diabetes Care 1990; 13:855—63.

176. Sommariva D, Branchi A, Tirrito M, et al. Differential effects of benfluorex and two fibrate derivatives on serum lipoprotein patterns in hypertriglyceridemic type 2 diabetic patients. Curr Ther Res 1986;40:859—70.

177. Smud R, Sermukslis B. Bezafibrate and fenofibrate in Type II diabetics with hyperlipoproteinemia. Curr Med Res Opin 1987;10:612—24.

178. Buckley MMT, Goa KL, Price AH, Brogden RN. Probucol: a reappraisal of its pharmacological properties and therapeutic use in hypercholesterolemia. Drugs 1989;37:761—800.

179. Grundy SM. HMG-CoA reductase inhibitors for treatment of hypercholesterolemia. N Engl J Med 1988;319:24—33.

180. Bradford RH, Shear CL, Chremos AN, et al. Expanded clinical evaluation of lovastatin (EXCEL) study results. I. Efficacy in modifying plasma lipoproteins and adverse event profile in 8245 patients with moderate hypercholesterolemia. Arch Intern Med 1991;151:43—9.

181. Garg A, Grundy SM. Treatment of dyslipidemia in non-insulin-dependent diabetes mellitus with lovastatin. Am J Cardiol 1988;62:44J-9.

182. Pierce LR, Wysowski DK, Gross TP. Myopathy and rhabdomyolysis associated with lovastatin-gemfibrozil combination therapy. JAMA 1990;264:71—5.

183. Scotto J, Hadchouel M, Hery C, et al. Detection of hepatitis B virus DNA in serum by a simple spot hybridization technique: comparison with results for other viral markers. Hepatology 1983;3:279—84.

184. Tobert JA. Rhabdomyolysis in patients receiving lovastatin after cardiac transplantation [Letter]. N Engl J Med 1988;318:48.

185. Spach DH, Bauwens JE, Clark CD, Burke WG. Rhabdomyolysis associated with lovastatin and erythromycin use. West Med J 1991;154(2):213—5.

186. Grundy SM, Vega GL, Garg A. Use of 3-hydroxy-3-methylglutaryl coenzyme A reductase inhibitors in various forms of dyslipidemia. Am J Cardiol 1990;18:31—8B.

187. Garg A, Grundy SM. Lovastatin for lowering cholesterol levels in non-insulin-dependent diabetes mellitus. N Engl J Med 1988;318:81—6.

188. Vega GL, Grundy SM. Comparison of lovastatin and gemfibrozil in normolipidemic patients with hypoalphalipoproteinemia. JAMA 1989;262:3148—53.

189. Witztum JL. Intensive drug therapy of hypercholesterolemia. Am Heart J 1987;113:603—9.

190. Vega GL, Grundy SM. Treatment of primary moderate hypercholesterolemia with lovastatin (mevinolin) and colestipol. JAMA 1987;257:33—8.

191. Malloy MJ, Kane JP, Kunitake ST, Tun P. Complementarity of colestipol, niacin and lovastatin in treatment of severe familial hyper-cholesterolemia. Ann Intern Med 1987; 107:616—22.

192. Denke MA, Grundy SM. Hypercholesterolemia in elderly persons: resolving the treatment dilemma. Ann Intern Med 1990;112:780—92.

193. Kafonek SD, Kwiterovich PO. Treatment of hypercholesterolemia in the elderly [Editorial]. Ann Intern Med 1990;112:723—5.

194. Stout RW. Diabetes and atheroma: 20-yr perspective. Diabetes Care 1990;13:631—54.

195. Castelli WP, Wilson PWF, Levy D, Anderson K. Cardiovascular risk factors in the elderly. Am J Cardiol 1989;63(16):12H—9.

196. Reddi AS, Camerini-Davalos RA. Diabetic nephropathy: an update. Arch Intern Med 1990;150:31—43.

197. Selby JV, FitzSimmons SC, Newman JM, et al. The natural history of epidemiology of diabetic nephropathy: implications for prevention and control. JAMA 1990; 263:1954—60.

198. Grundy SM. Management of hyperlipidemia of kidney disease [Editorial review]. Kidney Int 1990;37:847—53.

199. Vega GL, Grundy SM. Lovastatin therapy in nephrotic hyperlipidemia: effects on lipoprotein metabolism. Kidney Int 1988;33:1160—8.

200. Groggel GC, Cheung AK, Ellis-Benigni K, Wilson DE. Treatment of nephrotic hyperlipoproteinemia with gemfibrozil. Kidney Int 1989;36:266—71.

201. Levy RI. Causes of the decrease in cardiovascular mortality. Am J Cardiol 1984;54(5):7—13C.

202. Roberts WA. Atherosclerotic risk factors—are there ten or is there only one? [Editorial] Am J Cardiol 1989;64:552—4.

203. Joslin EP. Arteriosclerosis and diabetes. Ann Clin Med 1927;5:1061.

COLOR PLATES

ANIMAL MODELS OF DIABETES MELLITUS

Pancreatic islets from diabetic NOD (non-obese diabetic) mice and ICR (Institute for Cancer Research) mice. A. Islets from diabetic NOD mice (hematoxylin-eosin staining). Islets are infiltrated by immune cells (lymphocytes and macrophages). B. Islets from diabetic NOD mice (aldehyde-fuchsin-Masson staining). Note degranulation of insulin in the islet. C. Islets from control ICR mice (hematoxylin-eosin staining). D. Islets (blue) from control ICR mice (aldehyde-fuchsin-Masson staining). Note β-cells filled with insulin. Glomerulosclerosis of the kidneys. E. Glomerulus from a 6-month-old ICR mouse (periodic acid-Schiff staining). F. Glomerulus from a 6-month old diabetic mouse (periodic acid-Schiff staining). Note proliferation of the mesangium. Lipoprotein glomerulopathy of the kidney. G. Glomerulus from a 6-month old NON (non-obese nondiabetic) mouse (periodic acid-Schiff staining).

Plate I

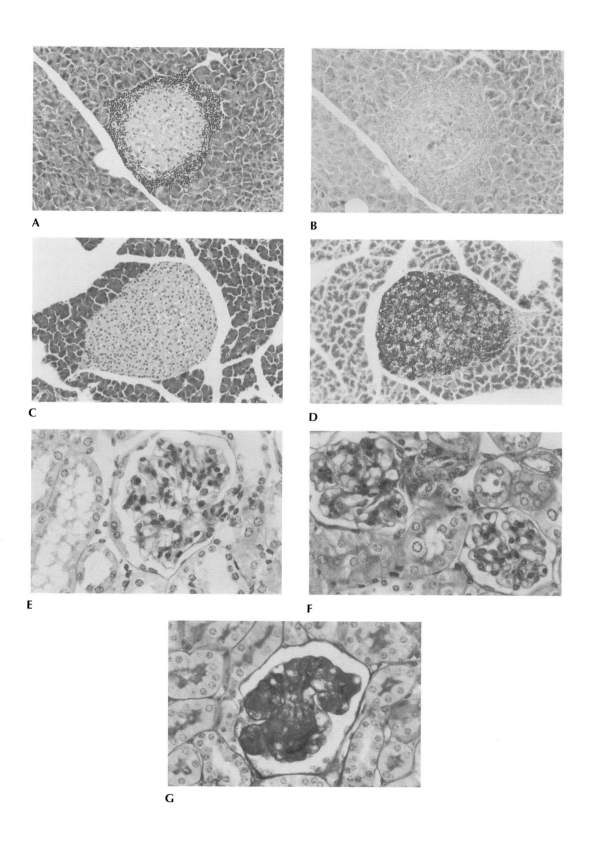

SKIN MANIFESTATIONS

A. Acute neuropathic ulcer in a 34-year-old man with diabetes who had previous amputations for osteomyelitis secondary to ulceration. B, C. Necrobiosis lipoidica in a 24-year-old with insulin-dependent diabetes. D. Disseminated granuloma annulare. E. Eruptive xanthomas on the abdomen of a 45-year-old with uncontrolled insulin-dependent diabetes. F, G. Perforating folliculitis in a 50-year-old with diabetes with retinopathy and nephropathy.

PLATE II

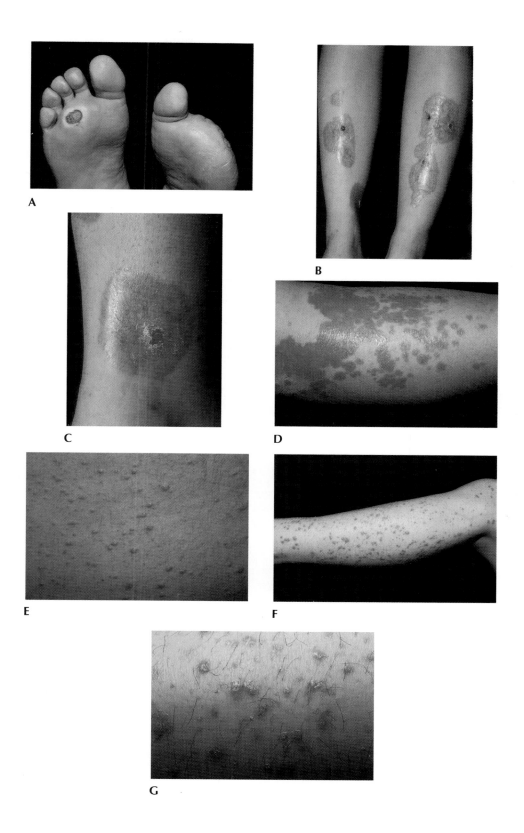

A

B

C

D

E

F

G

HYPOGLYCEMIA

A. Normal neonatal pancreas with insulin-secreting cells identified by immunoperoxidase labeling (brown). Note the presence of small aggregates and scattered single cells, some proximate to ductular epithelium, previously considered typical of "nesidioblastosis." B. The periphery of an islet in a child with intractable hyperinsulinemic hypoglycemia (double immunoperoxidase labeling: insulin, brown; somatostatin, blue). Note the irregular "ragged edge" of the islet and some prominent nuclei. There are ample numbers of somatostatin-secreting cells in close proximity to insulin-secreting cells. (The authors thank Dr. Victor E. Gould, Rush Medical College, for supplying these photomicrographs.)

PLATE III

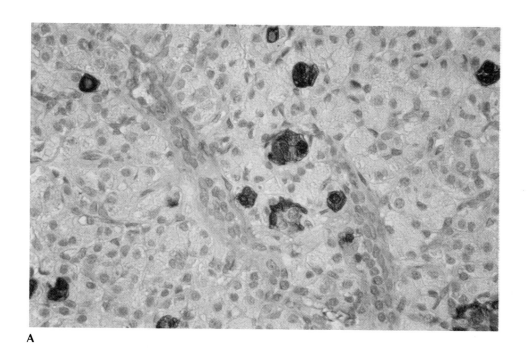

A

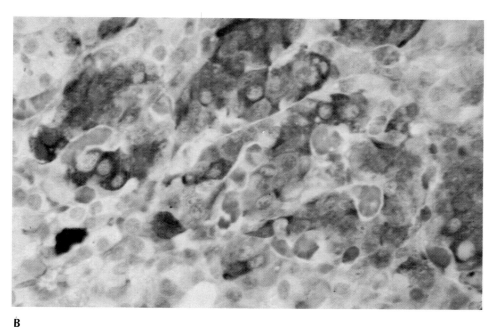

B

Chapter 22

GENERAL APPROACH TO THE TREATMENT OF DIABETES

RAMACHANDIRAN COOPPAN

Diabetes mellitus is a chronic disease affecting millions of people worldwide. In the last decade considerable progress has been made in understanding the pathophysiology of insulin-dependent (IDDM) and non-insulin-dependent diabetes (NIDDM). NIDDM is a syndrome that has heterogeneous manifestations and that is associated with a high risk for macrovascular complications.

At present, we cannot speak about a cure for diabetes. Cure is an appropriate future goal, especially for IDDM, for which progress in immunology, molecular biology, and immunotherapy has been dramatic.[1] In dealing with a chronic disease such as diabetes, our goals are maintenance of the well-being of the affected individual and minimization of long-term complications. The issue of the relationship of control to the development of long-term complications is the focus of much attention and has generated debate and controversy. With the use of self-monitoring of blood glucose (SMBG), the glycosylated hemoglobin assay, and intensive insulin treatment programs, we can now set goals for "tight control" and even achieve them for many of our patients. The larger question that faces us is whether this approach will prevent or even slow the progression of complications.[2] Furthermore, the risks of hypoglycemia associated with intensive therapy must be carefully assessed for each patient.[3] The Diabetes Control and Complications Trial (DCCT) is a multicenter study sponsored by the National Institutes of Health (NIH) designed to answer these questions.[4] The study concludes in 1993, and the results are eagerly awaited.

In patients with NIDDM, the risk for the development of macrovascular disease is greatly increased. The combinations of obesity, glucose intolerance, lipid abnormalities, hypertension, and cigarette smoking are major risk factors. Not only is glycemic control important in the approach to therapy for this type of diabetes, but care must also be taken to correct these other risk factors.

The treatment plan for patients with diabetes will also be affected by the prevalence of diabetes (especially NIDDM), which varies among different racial and ethnic groups. In minority groups such as Native Americans (especially the Pima Indians[5]), Hispanic Americans, and African-Americans,[6] the prevalence of NIDDM is higher than that in the white population. Furthermore, the prevalence of obesity is higher in all of these groups, and hypertension has been well documented to be more common in African-Americans.[7] For many in these groups, access to good medical care is affected by factors such as socioeconomic status, cultural background, language barriers, individual and group health beliefs, educational level, socioeconomic status, and peer behavior. These factors may present special problems in providing therapy.

The problem of diabetes in the older population is also a special issue—both for diagnosis and for setting goals of therapy. Although most elderly patients with diabetes have NIDDM, a significant proportion have IDDM. The elderly do not always present with the classical symptoms and signs of hyperglycemia, and the physician must always consider diabetes as a potential diagnosis,[8] even when patients are asymptomatic.

Although this chapter will focus on the general approach to the treatment of the patient with diabetes in the outpatient setting, the principles apply to inpatients as well. The material is presented as a general overview; other chapters in this text are devoted to specific issues.

AN INITIAL APPROACH

Once the diagnosis of diabetes has been made, the question of initiating therapy must be addressed. Those patients who present with diabetic ketoacidosis or who are markedly hyperglycemic and symptomatic will have to be admitted to a hospital. The need for hospitalization at diagnosis applies primarily to patients with IDDM; those with NIDDM can usually be treated in the outpatient setting.

At this initial stage of treatment, the physician should obtain a detailed history and perform a complete examination with appropriate laboratory testing. At this stage, the physician's treatment philosophy; the patient's competence at self-care; and the availability of a team consisting of a nutritionist, diabetes nurse educator, and physician are all extremely important in the development of the treatment plan, as they are for its future success.

The approach must consider the "whole person" with diabetes—not just the levels of glycemic control to be achieved or the therapy to be used to accomplish this (i.e., insulin or oral hypoglycemic agents). To this end a strong, integrated team approach is the one most likely to succeed. Although this complete team does not exist in most practitioners' offices, the physician and patient can make much progress together, and other components of the team—the nutritionist and diabetes nurse educator—are available in most community settings.

The Patient History

A detailed history is the foundation of good diabetes care. Knowledge about the age of the patient and the clinical presentation often can help the physician determine whether the patient has IDDM or NIDDM. A problem inherent to this determination is that of assigning a definite date to the onset of the disease—particularly for NIDDM. In the Joslin Diabetes Center, both patients with new-onset diabetes and those seeking consultation for existing disease are mailed a detailed metabolism questionnaire about symptoms, current therapy, family history, and other medical problems and therapy. Particular attention must be paid to histories of coronary artery disease, peripheral vascular disease, hypertension, and renal disease in the family. Patients are also asked to record on a dietary assessment sheet information on their diet for 2 days, including the times of their meals and the types and quantities of various foods eaten. This information helps the nutritionist design an appropriate meal plan based on the patient's food preferences.

Physical Examination

The physical examination is a fundamental part of the initial evaluation. Special attention should be paid to height and weight, blood pressure (lying and standing), and vascular status. The carotid and femoral vessels should be auscultated for bruits, especially in older patients with peripheral vascular disease. Neurologic examination of those with diabetes mellitus of 5 to 10 years' duration should include a careful assessment of reflexes and tests of sensation. Although these clinical methods of assessment lack sensitivity, they still permit the clinician to obtain a baseline picture and to carry out further investigations in appropriate patients. In a recent study of 189 patients with diabetes and 88 control subjects, Thivolet et al. used a graduated tuning fork to measure the sensitivity of the feet to vibratory sensations

and noted that 51% of patients with clinical symptoms of neuropathy in the extremities, 70% of those with absent tendon reflexes, and 75% of those with abnormal nerve conduction velocities had limited vibration sensation.[9]

The physician should pay special attention to the patient's feet, carefully palpating the dorsalis pedis and the posterior tibial, popliteal, and femoral pulses. Skeletal deformities such as hallux valgus, bunions, callouses, and hammer toes must be carefully documented. The combination of vascular disease and neuropathy is the major cause of diabetic foot infection and nontraumatic amputation.

Finally, a careful funduscopic examination is done, although this should not substitute for an evaluation by an ophthalmologist with experience in diabetes.

Laboratory Studies

At the patient's first visit, the minimum tests required are a complete urinalysis and determinations of blood glucose and glycosylated hemoglobin levels. It is now usual to add to these a chemistry panel that will measure lipids, liver and kidney function, electrolytes, a complete blood count. If possible, the lipid measurements should be done when the patient is in a fasting state in order to obtain an accurate determination of triglyceride levels. Total cholesterol and high-density lipoprotein (HDL) cholesterol also are measured. Lipid studies are an extremely important aspect of diabetes assessment because of the high risk of macrovascular disease.

A test for microalbuminuria may also be advisable, since the presence of early proteinuria heralds future renal disease[10] and may predict mortality in NIDDM.[11]

It is usually not necessary to measure islet cell antibodies or insulin autoantibodies in patients at the onset of diabetes. Tests for the presence of these antibodies, together with the intravenous glucose tolerance test, are used to determine those who are at high risk for developing IDDM.[12]

In the older patient or in patients with high blood pressure, a baseline electrocardiogram should be done. The physician can order a chest roentgenogram and other studies as needed.

Education

For the patient with a chronic disease, education is a life-long process. Access to printed educational materials and to the services of skilled diabetes nurse educators will help facilitate this process. Care must be taken not to overwhelm the patient with a surfeit of information. The onset of diabetes, either IDDM or NIDDM, is a difficult time emotionally for the patient, and the physician must be a source of encouragement as well as a provider of treatment. The family should also participate in the educational process.

The initial goals of education are that of helping the family understand the basic pathophysiology of diabetes and the differences between the insulin-dependent and non-insulin-dependent forms.

Patients with IDDM and their families learn basic skills necessary to the patient's survival. Such necessary skills include those of 1) insulin administration; 2) monitoring of blood and urinary glucose; 3) adjusting insulin dosage and food intake for exercise; and 4) sick-day care and prevention of ketoacidosis.

Patients with NIDDM are taught similar skills, although the emphasis is very much on the dietary program and weight control. It is important for patients to realize that the loss of even small amounts of weight (10 to 20 pounds) can be very beneficial. The ability to self-monitor blood glucose is also important. Exercise helps obese patients lose weight, and if they request more than a simple exercise prescription, it is appropriate for the physician to refer them to an exercise physiologist. Care should be taken in prescribing vigorous exercise programs to older patients, especially those with diabetic complications such as neuropathy or retinopathy. There is also the issue of coronary disease and silent ischemia. If a question arises about the presence of coronary artery disease and whether exercise can be undertaken with safety, the patient should be referred to a cardiologist for appropriate testing. Once the patient is cleared for an exercise program, he or she should exercise three to four times a week for the program to be of any benefit.

Those patients who will be receiving oral hypoglycemic therapy must become knowledgeable about the action of these medications and their adverse effects and understand that with time many patients will fail to respond to these agents and will need insulin therapy.

At the initial visit it is also appropriate to discuss briefly the rationale for glucose control and the potential for complications. At this time the physician's interpretation and understanding of the current literature on the relationship between the control of diabetes and complications will be extremely important. If the physician is vague and noncommittal in presenting this issue, the patient may assume that tight control is not necessary. By individualizing therapy and building on a solid foundation of basic skills acquired by the patient, the physician is in a unique position to guide the patient toward improved control.

CLINICAL GOALS

It is evident from the earlier discussion that the type of diabetes influences the form of therapy that is chosen. In the new-onset patient with acutely decompensated IDDM or in the previously diagnosed patient who is in poor control, goals will include the 1) elimination of ketosis; 2) elimination of symptoms of hyperglycemia such as polydipsia, polyuria, vaginitis, fatigue, or visual blurring; 3) restoration of normal blood chemistry values; 4) regaining of lost weight; and 5) restoration of sense of well-being.

Once the initial goals have been met, one can proceed to work on what will be necessary for long-term success. The general aim is the maintenance of health and well-being through control of the disease. It is important to not foster a life-style that is dominated by diabetes. Patients should control their diabetes and as much as possible follow their desired life-style. This is not always easy to accomplish, especially in patients with very

unstable or "brittle" IDDM. A minority of patients are severely incapacitated, and care must be taken to set realistic goals and to promote behavior that is not self-deprecating. For many patients, working with a psychologist or psychiatrist can help alleviate feelings of guilt and depression.

For young children the goals are the maintenance of normal growth and development. Again the life-style should be as close to normal as possible, without diabetes becoming the focal point of the entire family's existence. Children ideally should be comfortable at school, participate in sports, and socialize with their peers without being made to feel different.

Marrying and having a family is important for many women with diabetes. Helping them achieve a successful pregnancy is a very important aspect of their diabetes care. Unless the physician has considerable experience in this area, it is preferable for the patient to be referred to a multidisciplinary team skilled in managing these high-risk pregnancies.

Underlying all these goals is the desire to control the diabetes optimally so that long-term microvascular and macrovascular complications can be minimized. Since we cannot predict who will develop long-term complications, it seems prudent to try to control all patients optimally within the limits of safety.

Before proceeding with therapy, it is useful for the physician to discuss the different levels of success that may be achieved in the treatment of diabetes. In general, we now refer to minimal, average, and intensive goals of therapy. The American Diabetes Association[13] has defined these goals as follows:

Minimal goals

1. HbA_{1c}, 11 to 13%; or total glycosylated hemoglobin (HbA_1), 13.0 to 15.0%
2. Many SMBG values of >300 mg/dL
3. Tests for urinary glucose almost always positive
4. Intermittent, spontaneous ketonuria

Average goals

1. HbA_{1c}, 8 to 9.0%; or HbA_1, 10 to 11.0%
2. Pre-meal SMBG of 160 to 200 mg/dL
3. Tests for urinary glucose intermittently positive
4. Rare ketonuria

Intensive goals

1. HBA_{1c}, 6.0 to 7.0%; or HbA_1, 7 to 9%
2. Pre-meal SMBG of 70 to 120 mg/dL and post-meal SMBG of <180 mg/dL
3. Tests for urinary glucose essentially never positive
4. No ketonuria

Assessment of the level of diabetes control is best done by measurement of biochemical parameters. Reliance on clinical indexes such as body weight, frequency of polyuria, polydipsia, number of hypoglycemic reactions, fatigue, and sense of well-being is usually misleading. It is true that patients with very poor control can often be easily identified by their symptoms. But patients whose fasting glucose levels are 140 to 180 mg/dL and postprandial values are 180 to 240 mg/dL can feel quite well and present a false clinical picture of satisfactory diabetes control. In the past, daily urinary glucose measurements and random office glucose tests were relied upon. However, urine testing can prove less accurate in the presence of a high renal threshold, renal disease, or bladder neuropathy, and the use of a double-voided urine specimen does not remove these limitations.[14] Testing for the presence of ketones is still best accomplished with a urine sample.

During the last decade, two innovations revolutionized our approach to therapy. The first was self-monitoring of blood glucose (SMBG).[15] When first developed, the system used glucose oxidase reagent strips and a chart of colors corresponding to different glycemic ranges, which was compared visually with the reagent strips. The system has since developed into a sophisticated monitoring system. A variety of glucose monitoring devices are now available that give a digital readout of the blood glucose concentration. The devices employ a 120-, 60-, or 30-second time frame and may or may not require blotting. They are accurate enough for routine use by patients. For convenience, mechanical lancet devices are available for obtaining blood. Some of the newer glucose monitors include computerized memory to record the blood glucose levels, and some can be used in conjunction with more elaborate personal computers. Special machines are available for blind patients. One concern about SMBG is the accuracy of the recordings as compared with those obtained in the laboratories of large clinics or research settings that use more sophisticated instruments. In the patient's daily situation, many problems with SMBG may develop, even after careful instruction on the technique by a diabetes nurse educator. One such difficulty involves the patient's ability to obtain a drop of blood, place it accurately on the reagent strip, and time the monitor carefully. Newer monitors that do not require wiping or timing can help minimize these errors. A study performed by Jovanovic et al., in which four meter systems were compared, demonstrated the least variance from the control system (a glucose autoanalyzer) with a "no-wipe" system.[16] The use of this system, which eliminated the need for blood removal and timing, greatly decreased the variability in test results. Overall, SMBG must be considered one of the major advances in diabetes management in the last decade.

To be effective, the use of SMBG must be accompanied by an educational program that helps the patient understand the factors affecting any particular blood glucose level and provides appropriate options for corrections or adjustments. This knowledge is particularly necessary for patients involved in intensive insulin treatment programs.

There has been some discussion about the value of SMBG in patients with NIDDM or who are using diet or oral agents for control.[17] Although it is true that these patients will rarely make treatment changes on the basis of information from SMBG, it can reinforce dietary principles and reveal the benefits of exercise and medi-

cation. Patients with NIDDM who are receiving insulin should definitely use SMBG. Hypoglycemia occurs both in patients who are being treated with sulfonylurea drugs and those who are receiving insulin; in this setting SMBG can confirm a low glucose level. The frequency of monitoring can easily be adjusted to the individual patient's needs and circumstances. SMBG is therefore an extremely valuable tool for daily diabetes management.

The other important advance in diabetes management is the glycosylated hemoglobin assay. In normoglycemic subjects a small proportion of hemoglobin A is attached to a carbohydrate moiety, thus creating what is called *glycosylated* or *glycated* hemoglobin.[18] The glycosylated hemoglobin can be separated into three distinct fractions, which are designated A_{1a}, A_{1b}, and A_{1c}. Because of electrophoretic behavior of these minor hemoglobins, they are referred to as *fast hemoglobin*.

In conditions of sustained hyperglycemia, such as in diabetes mellitus, the proportion of hemoglobin that is glycosylated is increased substantially.[19,20] This glycosylation is the result of post-translational modification of hemoglobin A molecules; the binding of glucose is a nonenzymatic process that occurs continuously during the life of the red blood cell. Thus, the amount of glycosylated hemoglobin reflects the glycemic control of a patient during the 6- to 8-week period before the blood sample was obtained.[21]

Glycosylated hemoglobin can be measured by chromatographic, chemically based, or electrophoretic assays. The advantages and disadvantages of these assays will be reviewed briefly. Falsely high levels of glycohemoglobin can be produced in chromatographic assays by carbamylated hemoglobin (formed in uremia), acetaldehyde addition (in alcoholics), or increased fetal hemoglobin (elevated in thalassemia, aplastic anemia, myeloproliferative disorders, and pregnancy). Hemoglobin variants such as HbS or HbC also can cause falsely low results in these assays.

The labile fraction of glycohemoglobin (reflects reversibly bound component) is measured in ion-exchange assays but not in chemical assays employing affinity chromatography or calorimetry. Pretreatment of the sample in ion-exchange assays overcomes this problem.

The electrophoretic method that uses agar gel electrophoresis measures all of HbA_1, whereas isoelectric focusing on polyacrylamide gels gives wider separation of the different hemoglobin components and therefore can quantitate HbA_{1c}. In fact, while affinity chromatography measures all glycosylated hemoglobin, it is not affected by temperature or by the presence of hemoglobin variants or fetal hemoglobin. In general, ion-exchange columns (measure Hb_{A_1}) correlate quite well with affinity columns (measure all glycosylated hemoglobins) even though they measure two different substances. The glycosylated hemoglobin test gives an estimation of the average glycemic level during the 6 to 8 weeks preceding the test. It correlates well with fasting and postprandial blood glucose levels and 24-hour urinary glucose levels.[22–24] The glycosylated hemoglobin assay is presently one of the most widely applied tests in the management of diabetes. It is useful for the assessment of glycemic control in both patients with Type I and Type II diabetes.

Glycosylated hemoglobin values must be assessed with caution in patients with unstable diabetes. Levels of blood sugar in these patients fluctuate from very low to very high on an almost daily basis, a situation that can lead to unwanted symptoms of hyperglycemia and dangerous episodes of hypoglycemia.[25] The assay of glycosylated hemoglobin should be done every 3 to 4 months, with the goal of adjusting therapy to obtain the lowest value that does not place patients at undue risk for hypoglycemic reactions.

INITIATION OF THERAPY

For most adult patients, initiation of treatment is safely accomplished in the outpatient setting. Very young children and patients with diabetic ketoacidosis or severe, uncontrolled diabetes usually require hospitalization.

Although the decision to use insulin is usually made by the physician, it is extremely important to explain the rationale to patients and to include them in the decision process. Many have an understandable fear of injections and often regard this therapy as an indication of the presence of a more severe form of the disease. Insulin therapy needs to be presented as any other treatment option, and patients should be made to understand that one, two, or three injections per day may be needed, depending on their response. The physician should also review the issue of control and complications and develop initial goals with the patient.

At the Joslin Diabetes Center, the decision to start insulin therapy is followed by a referral to a diabetes nurse educator, who will instruct the patient or a family member on the techniques that will be required. Patients will administer their first injection at this time under supervision. This is also an opportunity to teach patients about the types of insulin available and their characteristic peaks and durations of activity, as well as to review strategies for dealing with hypoglycemia and hyperglycemia. The techniques for mixing regular with intermediate-acting insulins may be reviewed if the physician feels this is appropriate. Premixed insulin (70% NPH and 30% crystalline zinc insulin) can be used initially in patients who may not be able to master the mixing of insulins. This simplifies the treatment program, especially when patients have problems understanding and performing the mixing maneuvers. In many cases, the limitations are due to problems such as cataracts, degenerative joint disease, previous cerebrovascular accidents, or severe neuropathy.

The majority of new patients who require insulin will first be prescribed human insulin of recombinant DNA origin. Allergy and lipoatrophy are uncommon with the human insulins. Beef insulin and mixed beef-pork insulin should be avoided unless there are specific indications for their use. Patients also are instructed on SMBG at this time and are asked to keep in close contact with the nurse educator, who in turn reviews adjustments and the patient's progress with the physician. In most patients the diabetes can be expected to be brought under control over a 4- to 6-week period. The patient is often seen several times within this interval so that the physician can monitor progress, modify therapy, and review any interim problems or concerns.

Most patients are not started on an intensive management program at this time, as it is necessary to allow the patient to adjust to the emotional and life-style changes that follow a diagnosis of diabetes. Intensive therapy is used for patients who plan a pregnancy, those who cannot control their glucose levels by conventional therapies, or those whose life-styles demand the greater flexibility intensive programs offer.[26]

Patients with known diabetes that is in poor control or with diabetic complications will undergo a similar evaluation and physical examination. Attention is focused here on the patient's general approach to the disease, with particular attention being paid to the patient's acceptance of the disease and its treatment requirements. Many patients have an overwhelming fear of hypoglycemia. Some will deliberately avoid using rapid-acting insulin or will omit their evening injections, which predictably results in hyperglycemia. Others will overcompensate and treat any symptoms as a sign of potential hypoglycemia and some will start to monitor glucose levels with excessive frequency in an effort to discover lower values, in the hope of avoiding severe hypoglycemic reactions. For these patients, it is important to review their nutritional programs, exercise habits, alcohol intake, and psychosocial status. Even some patients with diabetes of long duration do not wait the required 30 minutes after injecting insulin before having their meals. Also some patients make the mistake of regularly injecting insulin at hypertrophied sites. In general, no acute changes in the insulin program are made, but frequently the patient is asked to monitor blood sugar three to four times a day for the next month, with the focus being on the nutritional program. Changes of insulin therapy are made by telephone or at future visits. Patients with major psychological problems are referred to a psychologist or psychiatrist. Unless these issues are addressed, diabetes control will continue to be a problem.

Some patients will require hospitalization. At the hospital, the focus of the treatment will be education and close monitoring to identify potential problems such as nocturnal hypoglycemia with rebound hyperglycemia, hypoglycemic unawareness, or inherently unstable diabetes. Even though the present economic climate is making it more difficult to hospitalize these patients, there is no way of satisfactorily addressing some of these problems in the outpatient setting. Complicated diabetes such as this requires individualized therapy that is both complex and time-consuming. However, if we are to provide proper care for our patients, we must address these issues carefully and sympathetically and offer solutions that will allow them to function optimally and to avoid some of the serious consequences of diabetes. Very often these individuals will need to have their glycemic goals changed to avoid dangerous hypoglycemia, despite earlier encouragement to maintain "tight control."

Patients with NIDDM may need insulin when they are first seen, particularly if they are very symptomatic and have lost weight. In some instances, the insulin can be discontinued when control is achieved and adherence to diet has taken effect.[28] However, many patients will require insulin indefinitely; this becomes obvious when they become ketonuric and hyperglycemic with a reduction in insulin dose.

The basis of therapy in NIDDM is nutritional, with a program designed to encourage weight loss. An exercise program is an essential part of any effort to lose weight. Glycemic control can often be improved by caloric restriction alone, even before significant weight loss occurs. Patients with NIDDM are also taught SMBG, and the frequency of testing is individualized. SMBG is always the preferred method of glucose monitoring, with urine testing being used only in special situations.

The decision to use oral sulfonylurea drugs generally is made after a trial of nutritional therapy. In general, a 4- to 12-week trial period is reasonable, and if the fasting glucose concentration remains above 140 mg/dL or postprandial values are above 200 mg/dL, treatment is started. A second-generation sulfonylurea usually is chosen. Patients must be aware that hypoglycemia can still occur with sulfonylureas, especially if meals are delayed.

Some patients who fail to obtain control with the maximal dose of sulfonylurea may benefit from the combined use of insulin and oral medication. Usually a bedtime dose of intermediate-acting insulin is given, with the oral drug being continued.[29] If the patient has high post-dinner blood glucose levels, a mixture of a regular and an intermediate-acting insulin can be given before supper. It is often useful to use a premixed insulin (70/30 mixture) in patients who have difficulty with mixing or adjusting insulin dose. Several studies of combination therapy have been done. Generally, patients who have residual endogenous insulin secretion respond best, although patients' responses vary greatly.[30]

For every patient, diabetes management must include a careful nutritional assessment and the implementation of a realistic dietary program. The goal of nutritional therapy in NIDDM is the control of blood glucose levels, normalization of lipid levels, and maintenance of ideal body weight. For young children with diabetes, the goal should be the maintenance of normal growth and development as well as of a reasonable body weight.

In general, the dietitian will prescribe a meal plan based on the individual patient's type of diabetes and mode of treatment. Patients receiving exogenous insulin must pay particular attention to the timing of meals and snacks to prevent undue fluctuation of the blood sugar levels. The meal plan is individualized with respect to weight goals, personal food preferences, and exercise habits. Many obese patients with diabetes may require special weight-loss programs and behavior modification therapy to maintain weight loss. Unfortunately, most patients do not succeed in their efforts to lose weight.

Diet therapy often is referred to as the cornerstone of treatment, particularly in NIDDM. For the patient to benefit maximally from this aspect of patient management, a team approach, which includes the services of a skilled registered dietitian, is recommended. Although these skills are not always available in physician's offices, they are offered in local community hospitals and by some dietitians in private practice. A detailed discussion on this component of treatment is presented in Chapter 24 on nutritional therapy.

Exercise plays an important role in diabetes management. In patients with IDDM, exercise should be thought of not as one of the major ways of improving glucose control but rather as part of the overall approach to maintaining a healthy life-style. Physical activity can benefit the patient by lowering the blood glucose level if overall control is good. However, care must be taken to instruct the patient on the possibility of physical exercise provoking hypoglycemic reactions or of worsening control when undertaken in the presence of higher blood glucose levels and ketonuria. Furthermore, patients with the complications of retinopathy and neuropathy can place themselves in jeopardy with excessive exercise.

In general, patients who are free of complications can engage in any type of exercise. They may often benefit from a consultation with an exercise physiologist. In patients with NIDDM, an exercise program should be part of the diet and medication therapy. Exercise helps promote weight loss, optimize glycemic control, and reduce cardiovascular risk factors. These patients need to be screened for early neuropathy or peripheral vascular disease before they start an exercise program. Silent ischemia is more common in patients with diabetes than in the general population, and patients over 35 years old should have a stress test before starting the exercise program. To be effective the program should be done three to four times a week with appropriate warm-ups, setting target exercise levels with monitoring of pulse rate and cooling-down time.

FOLLOW-UP

A critical part of diabetes management is regular follow-up of the patients. This is based on the initial management plan, which sets up goals with the patient. At each visit thereafter, the patient's progress is reviewed and ongoing problems are addressed.[31] The frequency of visits depends on the individual patient, type of diabetes, goals of control, and other medical conditions. Patients starting insulin therapy need close contact initially, but once their conditions have stabilized, they can be seen three to four times a year. In addition, patients are encouraged to keep in phone contact with the other team members. Some patients with NIDDM need to be seen only every 6 months.

As part of this follow-up process, an interim history is obtained, results of glucose monitoring are reviewed, and new problems or illnesses that affect diabetes control are addressed.

A comprehensive physical examination is done annually. At interim visits, previously abnormal findings are checked; height, weight, and blood pressure are determined; and previously abnormal findings are reevaluated.

For younger patients, an assessment of sexual maturation will be done. It is recommended that a complete eye examination be done annually in all patients over 30 years old and in younger patients 12 to 30 years old who have had diabetes for over 5 years.

A test for glycosylated hemoglobin should be done at least quarterly in patients with IDDM and semiannually in those with NIDDM. The patient with adult-onset diabetes also may benefit from having either a fasting or postprandial glucose level checked, as a means of judging overall glycemic control. A determination of fasting levels of triglycerides, cholesterol, and HDL cholesterol should be done annually and more often in patients with a dyslipidemia. Urinalysis done at least yearly is useful. After 5 years of diabetes, a test for microalbuminuria should be done yearly. If proteinuria is present, creatinine and blood urea nitrogen levels should be closely monitored; in addition, aggressive antihypertensive therapy and protein restriction should be considered.

At each visit the overall management plan, including the nutritional program and the exercise plan, is reviewed and modified as required. In addition, the overall emotional status of the patient is reviewed. This type of comprehensive care is extremely important for patients with a chronic, life-long disease such as diabetes.

This chapter has reviewed the general principles of management of diabetes. Many of the details will be found in other chapters in this textbook. To the practicing physician, diabetes offers the challenge of providing optimal patient care at every visit. It allows the physician the opportunity and privilege to practice not only the science but the art of medicine.

REFERENCES

1. Prevention of Type I diabetes mellitus. American Diabetes Association: position statement. Diabetes Care 1990;13:9:1026–7.
2. The DCCT Research Group. Diabetes control and complications trial (DCCT): results of feasibility study. Diabetes Care 1987;10:1–19.
3. Lager I, Attvall S, Blohme G, Smith U. Altered recognition of hypoglycaemic symptoms in type 1 diabetes during intensified control with continuous subcutaneous insulin infusion. Diabetic Med 1986;3:322–5.
4. DCCT Research Group. Diabetes control and complications trial (DCCT): update. Diabetes Care 1990;13:427–33.
5. Knowler WC, Pettit DJ, Savage PJ, Bennett PH. Diabetes incidence in Pima Indians: contributions of obesity and parental diabetes. Am J Epidemiol 1981;113:144–56.
6. Diehl AK, Stern MP. Special health problems of Mexican-Americans: obesity, gallbladder disease, diabetes mellitus and cardiovascular disease. Adv Intern Med 1989;34:73–96.
7. Douglas JG. Hypertension and diabetes in blacks. Diabetes Care 1990;13:4:1191–5.
8. Minaker KL. What diabetologists should know about elderly patients. Diabetes Care 1990;13(Suppl 2):34–46.
9. Thivolet C, El Farkh J, Petiot A, et al. Measuring vibration sensations with graduated tuning fork: simple and reliable means to detect diabetic patient at risk of neuropathic foot ulceration. Diabetes Care 1990;13:1077–80.
10. Mogensen CE. Prediction of clinical diabetic nephropathy in IDDM patients: alternatives to microalbuminuria? Diabetes 1990;39:761–7.
11. Mogensen CE. Microalbuminuria predicts clinical proteinuria and early mortality in maturity-onset diabetes. N Engl J Med 1984;310:6:356–60.
12. Ziegler AG, Ziegler R, Vardi P, et al. Life-table analysis of progression to diabetes of anti-insulin autoantibody-positive relatives of individuals with Type I diabetes. Diabetes 1989;38:1320–5.
13. Physician's guide to insulin-dependent (Type I) diabetes: diagnosis and treatment. Alexandria, VA: American Diabetes Association, 1988:18.
14. Feldman JM, Lebovitz FL. Tests for glucosuria: an analysis of factors that cause misleading results. Diabetes 1973;22:115–21.
15. Tattersall RB, Gale E. Patient self-monitoring of blood glucose and refinements of conventional insulin treatment. Am J Med 1981;70:177–82.
16. Jovanovic-Peterson L, Peterson CM, Dudley JD, et al. Identifying sources of error in self-monitoring of blood glucose. Diabetes Care 1988;11:10:791–4.
17. Allen BT, DeLong ER, Feussner JR. Impact of glucose self-monitoring on non-insulin-treated patients with Type II diabetes mellitus: randomized controlled trial comparing blood and urine testing. Diabetes Care 1990;13:1044–50.
18. Bunn HF, Haney DN, Gabbay KH, et al. Further identification of the nature and linkage of the carbohydrate in hemoglobin A_{1c}. Biochem Biophys Res Comm 1975;67:103–9.
19. Rahbar S. An abnormal hemoglobin in red cells of diabetics. Clin Chim Acta 1968;22:296–8.
20. Trivelli LA, Ranney HM, Lai H-T. Hemoglobin components in patients with diabetes mellitus. N Engl J Med 1971;284:353–7.
21. Koenig RJ, Peterson CM, Jones RL, et al. Correlation of glucose regulation and hemoglobin A_{1c} in diabetes mellitus. N Engl J Med 1976;295:417–20.
22. Paisey RB, Mcfarlane DG, Sherriff RJ, et al. The relationship between blood glycosylated haemoglobin and home capillary blood glucose levels in diabetics. Diabetologia 1980;19:31–4.
23. Gonen G, Rubenstein AH, Rochman H, et al. Haemoglobin A1: an indicator of the metabolic control of diabetic patients. Lancet 1977;2:734–7.
24. Gabbay KH, Hasty K, Breslow JL, et al. Glycosylated hemoglobins and long-term blood glucose control in diabetes mellitus. J Clin Endocrinol Metab 1977;44:859–64.
25. Schwartz JS, Clancy CM. Glycosylated hemoglobin assays in the management and diagnosis of diabetes mellitus. Ann Intern Med 1984;101:710–3.
26. Hirsch IB, Farkas-Hirsch R, Skyler JS. Intensive insulin therapy for treatment of Type I diabetes. Diabetes Care 1990;13:12:1265–83.
27. Cryer PE, Binder C, Bolli GB, et al. Hypoglycemia in IDDM. Diabetes 1989;38:1193–9.
28. Genuth S. Insulin use in NIDDM. Diabetes Care 1990;13:1240–64.
29. Riddle MC. Evening insulin therapy. Diabetes Care 1991;13:676–86.
30. Lebovitz HE, Pasmantier R. Combination insulin-sulfonylurea therapy. Diabetes Care 1990;13:667–75.
31. American Diabetes Association. Standards of medical care for patients with diabetes mellitus: position statement. Diabetes Care 1991;14:2:10–3.

Chapter 23

EDUCATION IN THE TREATMENT OF DIABETES

RICHARD S. BEASER
DONNA L. RICHARDSON
HUGO J. HOLLERORTH

This building given by thousands of patients and their friends provides an opportunity for many to control their diabetes by methods of teaching hitherto available to the privileged few

Chiseled in stone on the front of the Joslin Clinic Building, erected in 1955, the above inscription reflected Elliott P. Joslin's conviction that education was not just a part of diabetes treatment, it *was* the treatment. Dr. Joslin's concern about educating both patients with diabetes and their families began over 90 years ago, when such instruction was considered by many to be a luxury. Today, however, the importance of education is well recognized. As the World Health Organization has stated: "Education is a cornerstone of diabetic therapy and vital to the integration of the diabetic into society."[1]

The growing recognition of the vital role of education in the treatment of diabetes has led to the development of national standards for diabetes education by the National Diabetes Advisory Board in 1983.[2] This was followed by the development of a recognition program for diabetes education by the American Diabetes Association (ADA)[3] and of a certification program for diabetes educators by the American Association of Diabetes Educators.[4]

Unfortunately, progress in making educational programs available to everyone with diabetes has been slowed by the reluctance of third-party payers to reimburse for educational services, since actual financial benefits of such services have been difficult to demonstrate.[5] In spite of the obstacles, however, health-care professionals who care for people with diabetes continue their commitment to patient education through the development of new programs and research into more effective methods of teaching the principles and practice of diabetes self-care.

WHY IS EDUCATION IMPORTANT IN THE TREATMENT OF DIABETES?

For most medical conditions, the patient does not have to understand the condition in order to carry out the prescribed therapy properly. However, diabetes treatment requires careful balancing of various activities that are integral parts of the daily routine. Thus, treatment is a 24-hour-a-day activity and often includes important changes in life-style. It would seem that the more that people with diabetes understand how to make these required changes and the reasons for them, the more successful they will be in their diabetes treatment program.

With this as the assumption, many benefits have been ascribed to educating people with diabetes. Education allows people with diabetes to take control of their condition, integrating the daily routines of self-monitoring and discipline into their life-style rather than permitting this condition to overwhelm them and control their lives. It has been suggested, also, that education trains people to take the necessary actions to improve their metabolic control, which, it is postulated, may help maintain health and well-being and reduce the risk of diabetic complications. The well-educated person with diabetes may also decrease the costs related to the condition—both the direct cost of medical care and the indirect costs related to lost income or productivity. Finally, in this litigious age, provision by a health-care provider of proper education to people with diabetes may reduce the risk of malpractice suits. However, it is not unreasonable to question these assumptions about benefits and ask for proof, i.e., for scientific studies that demonstrate all of these benefits of education.

Herein lies the problem. Studies carried out so far have been difficult to design, perform, and evaluate, and when completed, their validity is often surrounded by controversy among health-care professionals. The results are questioned because of the many uncontrollable variables that affect both the ability to educate and the outcomes being measured. Nevertheless, since most diabetes health-care professionals still believe that education does provide many benefits and is therefore essential to the proper care of a person with diabetes, they continue to design studies that will prove the benefits of education.

Education Helps Patients Feel Better

People with diabetes must make life-style changes that may seem overwhelming, yet their failure to accept these changes may lead to inadequate diabetes control. Emotions related to nonacceptance, such as anxiety, depression, and poor self-confidence, have been shown to be associated with poor control.[6] Thus, a properly designed educational program should not only present facts but also address the emotional responses to diabetes.

Education may result in improved self-care practices,[7] but a mere increase in knowledge does not guarantee an improvement in metabolic parameters.[8] For individuals to be willing and able to make all the necessary life-style changes, they must have both knowledge and a positive emotional outlook about their diabetes and believe that the changes they make will lead to better health.

An educational program that demonstrably improves parameters of emotional well-being in addition to addressing self-care practices has been shown to lead to improved metabolic control that was sustained over 6 months.[9] The authors of the study suggested that emotional well-being itself may contribute to improved self-care.[9] Others contend that, for many patients, education about diabetes and self-care alone benefits emotional well-being,[10–12] which further boosts self-care ability. However, whether it is the emotional well-being that leads to improvement in self-care or vice versa has not been clearly determined nor has either factor alone, independent of the other, been proven to improve control.[13] Yet the impression stands that there are associations between education, improved self-care, and improved emotional outlook that are independent of improvements in metabolic control.

Education Improves Metabolic Control

A crucial question in diabetes management is how near to normal the metabolism of glucose needs to be to reduce the patient's risk of developing diabetes complications. This issue is currently under debate. Yet, regardless of the conclusion, many argue that no improvement in control can be achieved without proper patient education.

Although many people in the field of diabetes treatment have an intuitive belief that education will improve diabetes control, studies attempting to demonstrate this have produced variable results. For example, a trial comparing minimal vs. intensive education showed similar improvement in the two groups.[6] However, good control was related to the duration of school education, absence of anxiety, and quality of control and degree of self-confidence upon entry into the study. A similar study, with admitted socioeconomic bias affecting some of these factors, showed improvements in knowledge and behavior with education but not in metabolic control.[8]

Other studies also have underscored the importance of selecting the right outcome criteria for measurement. Education may not appear to be responsible for the desired improvements, both when looked at in relation to various outcomes other than metabolic control[14] and over extended periods,[7,15] if we examine the wrong outcomes. For example, the Diabetes Education Study[7] reported minimal differences between the education and control groups in measurements of their knowledge but found numerous, significant differences in their skills and self-care behaviors. Such studies also demonstrate the problems involved in measuring the effect of education on diabetes management. It is difficult to make comparisons with a true control group: How can one let someone with diabetes know nothing at all about self-management? Even if this were possible, it has been suggested that the placebo effect itself may be an educational experience[7] and that the comparison would be between two levels of education. These studies point out the difficulties of measuring the effects of education after a single educational intervention, focusing primarily on facts about diabetes rather than on behaviors, not including ongoing follow-up,[16] or measuring outcomes in terms of selected metabolic parameters only. Such limited studies often fail to detect all the potential long-term benefits of an ongoing educational experience.[17] Even if education does increase adherence, others have made the important point that improved glycemic control may not be apparent unless other treatment factors, such as the treatment regimen and individual metabolism, are taken into account.[18]

Therefore, although the studies cited may suggest that education does not improve metabolic control, another interpretation should also be considered—that education *alone* does not improve metabolic control, as has been demonstrated in studies that controlled for or randomized the other treatment factors.

For many patients, it is the use of a treatment program that matches normal physiology more accurately and is more responsive and flexible that improves diabetes control. However, for an individual both to agree to use such a program and to manage it correctly requires education, as is being demonstrated by the Diabetes Control and Complications Trial (DCCT),[19,20] which uses intensive education as a means of training patients to perform intensive insulin therapy. Furthermore, if the DCCT shows that intensified therapy does reduce the risk of developing complications, education would clearly be considered an important component, in addition to improved treatment design, in this multifactorial approach to diabetes management.

Education Decreases Costs of Care

"While it is generally agreed that education can be a major factor in decreasing costs of hospitalization, not until this fact can be proven conclusively regarding diabetic patients will ample money be made available for the needed education."[21]

So begins the section in the previous edition of this text that discusses how education can decrease the cost of diabetes care. Unfortunately, this paragraph is an apt beginning for this section of this edition as well. While medical professionals look to improvements in parameters such as levels of glycosylated hemoglobin (HbA_1) or complication rates, the people who pay the bills—the insurance companies and, ultimately, the consumers of health-care services—ask whether the benefits reaped by education warrant the expense.

Many people have tried to demonstrate that education saves money by using as an end point the reduction in costly hospitalizations. Geller and Butler[22] judged that 27% of the hospital admissions for diabetes complications over a 1-year period were the result of educational deficits and that an additional 20% were due to a combination of educational, psychological, and socioeconomic deficits. In the last edition of this text, Krall[21] recounted the classic, but not scientifically controlled, Joslin report of 100 patients surveyed who were admitted with foot infections. Only 38% of these patients had ever been exposed to diabetes education.

Experience reported by Scott et al. from New Zealand[23] suggested that education lowers admission rates among patients with diabetes. Seventy-nine of a group of 902 insulin-using patients required hospitalization, of whom 11% had received education previously and 89% had not. In a report from Maine,[24] a state that does provide some reimbursement for diabetes education, 38.5% fewer people were hospitalized and 28.3% fewer hospitalizations were necessary among patients who had participated in an educational program. The experience in Rhode Island reported by Fishbein[25] also demonstrated a reduction in the number of admissions after attendance in an outpatient education program.

However, these and various other studies that have appeared over the years have seemingly not been convincing enough to prove that education does save money. Criticisms of various studies, exemplified by a review by Kaplan and Davis,[26] typify the dilemma. They reviewed the studies used by the ADA to support third-party payment for outpatient education and nutritional counseling[27] and identified various defects in the design of these studies. They noted that studies often lacked control groups, random assignment, proper cost accounting, and clear demonstration of actual savings. They also pointed out that duration of hospital stay and rate of hospital admission can be affected by multiple factors influencing hospitalization practices that are unrelated to diabetes education or even to actual medical conditions.

The ultimate issue, pointed out by Anderson in a reply to the Kaplan and Davis article,[28] is that patients appear to need education to carry out their daily routine of diabetes self-care. Asking an educational program alone to result in cost reduction—or, for that matter, any particular medical goal—without considering the other variables that affect such outcome measures is ascribing more power to educational intervention than is warranted.

In summary, there is no evidence that education alone reduces health-care costs. To provide such evidence conclusively and convincingly would require studies that control for all the other factors that affect economic outcomes and that randomly assign patients to an education and a control group—studies that have significant ethical and practical obstacles.

Education does, however, seem to be an important component of a complete diabetes treatment program that also includes practitioners skilled at designing and carrying out diabetes management programs, at monitoring for complications, and at addressing psychosocial issues.

Thus, as the discussions about cost savings continue, most people who treat patients with diabetes still believe that education is cost-effective. However, since no one has been able to prove this convincingly, adequate financial support for diabetes education remains elusive. We hope that in the next edition of this textbook the report on the financing of diabetes education will be quite different!

Malpractice Protection

Sensitivity to the potential for malpractice lawsuits for alleged negligence has become part of the practice of medicine. This concern also extends to the act of conveying information about diabetes. Legal precedents in United States law exist that require health-care providers to be sure their patients receive adequate education and that outline the potential liability for either not educating or poorly educating their patients.[29]

The risk of potential lawsuits stemming from inadequate or improper education is likely to increase. Therefore, it is prudent for health-care professionals to ensure that their patients receive education of proper quality. Unless one is certain that a program meets established standards, programs that are recognized by the ADA or educators who are certified by the American Association of Diabetes Educators are the most reliable sources of proper education. It is strongly suggested that health-care professionals encourage patients to attend such programs.

THE DIABETES EDUCATION PROGRAM

The education of people with diabetes can be thought of as the process of providing them with experiences that favorably influence their understandings, attitudes, and practices related to living well with diabetes.[30] At its best, an educational program empowers those with diabetes to achieve optimal self-management of their condition.[31] Therefore, a successful educational program does not occur by accident. It is carefully planned by the health-care team and then executed by that team with the individual with diabetes, the student, targeting that person's specific needs.

The goal of any educational program is to help patients with diabetes gain the knowledge and skills that enable them to care for themselves and to develop the attitudes that will enable them to make behavioral changes. The ADA has set forth standards for diabetes education that include recommendations for the format of the program as well as a clear outline of the content areas that should be addressed.[3]

The Teachers

In the years after the discovery of insulin, Dr. Joslin was among the first to recognize that the responsibility of patient care lay mainly with the patients themselves. "The patient is his own nurse, doctor's assistant and chemist," he wrote in the first comprehensive guide to self-care, *A Diabetic Manual for the Mutual Use of Doctor and Patient,* in 1924,[32] shortly after the discovery of insulin. Recognizing the need for patient education, Dr. Joslin showed his nurses how to give insulin, calculate the diet, and balance insulin requirements with that diet. These nurses then visited patients throughout New England, sometimes staying with families for weeks, to teach patients to plan menus, prepare food, and administer several injections daily.

Since those days, the role of the "teaching nurse" has evolved and expanded and now includes other health-care providers with special diabetes-related skills. Diabetes educators, as they are now called, include nurses, nutritionists, social workers, exercise physiologists, psychologists, and physicians. Their expertise in diabetes care and education may qualify them to take an examination to become Certified Diabetes Educators. The person with diabetes, along with key family members, should be considered a part of the team and be involved in the educational program.[33]

These diabetes educators form the basis of the team approach to diabetes education.[34] Working together in both inpatient and outpatient settings, each member of the team provides the patient with specialized expert services. Nurses help patients master the skills necessary to inject insulin and monitor blood glucose levels, nutritionists work with patients to develop realistic meal plans, and social workers focus on coping mechanisms. It is such a team, working with the physician, that provides the most complete approach to diabetes education and care.

The Setting for Education

Education for diabetes care may be provided in a variety of settings, such as clinics, hospitals, education centers, or a physician's office. The program can be formalized and presented in a classroom setting or provided in a one-to-one fashion. It may be presented in a carefully planned educational session or may arise spontaneously from responses to questions asked during a routine office visit.

In educational sessions, the groups involved may be of various sizes and the forms of interaction used may include, but not be limited to, discussion, lecture, and interactive learning activities. Innovative educational techniques, such as programs incorporating computers and other audiovisual media, enhance the educational program.

Availability of staff, the needs of patients, the subject matter, and economics often dictate the choice of setting. For example, general information about the various kinds of insulin and their respective activity patterns might be presented in a group setting. However, the teaching of specific skills such as drawing insulin into the syringe is best carried out on an individual basis or in small groups no larger than six people. This small size provides the health professional with the opportunity to help each patient individually learn the necessary techniques for carrying out these essential skills. Similarly, general information about monitoring glucose levels might be presented in a group setting, but the actual learning of the skill should take place in a setting in which every patient can benefit from the individual attention of the health professional.

In addition, as with many other "school" settings, in which the educational experience is not limited to formalized instructional sessions, much of diabetes education occurs though the interactions among patients that occur in diabetes treatment units and camp-type settings. Information and understanding gained through the sharing of personal experiences can help patients improve both self-management and coping skills in ways that more formalized instruction cannot.

An example of such a program is that of the Diabetes Treatment Unit at the Joslin Diabetes Center. Patients who need inpatient medical treatment are admitted for an average of 5 days. The educational program includes classes run on a 3-day cycle from Monday through Wednesday and again from Wednesday through Friday (Fig. 23–1) as well as individual instruction. Free time also is available for social interaction among patients.

A similar program of education and patient care for people who do not need admission is offered in an outpatient setting for those who do not require hospital admission (Fig. 23–2) through the Diabetes Outpatient Intensive Treatment (DO-IT) program. Patients are evaluated medically and then enter the 3-day program of outpatient medical care and education. For most of these patients, periodic outpatient follow-up visits are necessary over the next few weeks or months to adjust treatment.

In addition, the educational program independent of coordinated medical care is available on selected weekends. Patients receiving routine office care may attend these programs to increase their knowledge about diabetes and their self-care skills and to benefit from interaction with other patients. Thus, similar educational pro-

TIMES	MONDAY	TUESDAY	WEDNESDAY	THURSDAY	FRIDAY
10:00 – 11:00			Meter Demo		
10:30 – 11:00		New Insulin	Self Blood Glucose Monitoring	New Insulin	Self Blood Glucose Monitoring
11:00 – 11:45	Factors Affecting Control	Treatment of High/Low Blood Sugar	Managing Sick Days	Treatment of High/Low Blood Sugar	Managing Sick Days
11:00 – 11:45			Factors Affecting Control		
1:00 – 2:00	Support Group Under age 40	Exercise Session	Exercise Session	Exercise Session	Relaxation
2:00 – 2:45	Meal Planning	Heart Healthy Meal Plan	Creative Meal Plan	Meal Planning	Heart Healthy Meal Plan
3:30 – 4:15	Relaxation		Exercise Lecture		Diabetes Discussion Group Over age 40
4:15 – 5:00	Research	Chronic Complications	Foot Care Lecture	Research	Chronic Complications
6:15 – 6:45			Insulin Information		

Fig. 23–1. Adult class schedule of the Diabetes Treatment Unit of the Joslin Diabetes Center/New England Deaconess Hospital.

grams are offered in different settings to meet various medical needs and patient preferences.

Who Should Be Educated

In its National Standards for Diabetes Education, the ADA recommends education for all people with diabetes at diagnosis and at regular intervals throughout life.[3] In these standards, the ADA recognizes the right of each person to understand the nature of his or her disease, to be given the tools to manage it, and to have this information updated routinely. The challenge for the team is to gain access to the patient at regular intervals and to meet the individual needs of every patient.

Patient Assessment

Assessment of the patient's and family's readiness to learn is the first step in the educational process. Concurrent illnesses, new diagnosis of diabetes, or psychosocial problems may affect a patient's willingness or ability to learn. A patient in whom pancreatic carcinoma has just been diagnosed may not be ready to discuss insulin administration. Similarly, a patient recovering from surgery may be more interested in starting on solid food than learning self-monitoring techniques. The key to assessment is communication with the patient. If education starts when the patient is emotionally and experientially ready, there is a better chance of engaging him or her in the entire educational process.[35]

The emotional response to diabetes can have an impact on the patient's ability to hear and absorb information. Denial may be the patient's first reaction to the diagnosis of diabetes and can impair his or her ability to learn.[36] The health-care provider can assist the patient by recognizing this response as denial, acknowledging that it may be a stage in the long process of adapting to a chronic

illness, and supporting the patient's effort to cope with the disease. Involvement in support groups and individual therapy may help the patient move from denial to successful adaptation.

Assessment of knowledge, skills, and attitudes about diabetes is an ongoing process that starts with the initial chart review and interview. Use of a conversational style, rather than a question-and-answer session, helps establish rapport and give the health-care professional some idea of the patient's life-style.[37] The health-care professional should learn to listen to the patient, to be sympathetic and understanding, and to accept that the patient's priorities may not be the same as the health-care team's. It is important to remember that diabetes is an intrusion into daily life, that most people will still have significant gaps in their knowledge about diabetes even after having the condition for 20 years, and that it is ultimately the patient who makes the final decisions about how he or she will approach the disease. Recognizing and accepting these realities will allow the health-care professional to set reasonable and achievable goals. The initial assessment should be documented in the chart and updated on a regular basis.

The assessment process provides an opportunity for the patient and family to express their health-care beliefs and their agenda for that visit and to voice particular needs or goals.[38] The information gained not only provides the health-care team with data about educational needs but also guides the team in management

TIMES	WEDNESDAY	THURSDAY	FRIDAY
7:30 – 7:45	Blood glucose measured	Blood glucose measured	Blood glucose measured
7:45 – 8:00	Insulin or Oral Agent taken	Insulin or Oral Agent taken	Insulin or Oral Agent taken
8:30 – 11:00	Individual Appointments with Physician, Nurse Educator, & Dietitian	Individual Appointments with Physician, Nurse Educator, & Dietitian	Individual Appointments with Physician, Nurse Educator, & Dietitian
11:00 – 11:45	Factors Affecting Control	Treatment of High/Low Blood Sugar	Managing Sick Days
11:45 – 12:00	Blood glucose measured	Blood glucose measured	Blood glucose measured
12:00 – 1:00	Lunch	Lunch	Lunch
1:00 – 2:00	Exercise Session	Exercise Session	Relaxation Class
2:00 – 2:45	Creative Meal Planning	Meal Planning	Heart Healthy Meal Plan
3:00 – 3:15	Blood Glucose Measured Snack	Blood Glucose Measured Snack	Blood Glucose Measured Snack
3:30 – 4:15	Exercise Lecture		Diabetes Support Group
4:15 – 5:00	Foot Care Lecture	Research	Chronic Complications
5:00 – 5:30			Post Test

Fig. 23–2. Schedule for 3-day program of the Diabetes Outpatient Intensive Treatment (DO-IT) program of the Joslin Diabetes Center/New England Deaconess Hospital.

issues. The team has the opportunity to answer questions, provide positive feedback, and encourage proper self-care behaviors.

In addition to assessing the patient's readiness to learn and stage of adaptation to diabetes, the health-care professional must obtain information on the patient's ethnic background, occupation, socioeconomic status, support systems, personality type, and health beliefs before looking at his or her knowledge of diabetes.[39] This information is invaluable in getting a sense of who the patient is and of what approach to education and treatment would be most helpful and reasonable.

An evaluation of functional ability aids the health-care provider in planning how to teach skills such as self-monitoring of blood glucose and insulin administration.[40] The patient's dexterity may be affected by arthritis or neuropathy. Vision changes due to retinopathy may be evident at a relatively young age. Some patients have a difficult time admitting to their vision deficit, so it is important to assess the patient's skill in these areas at the initial visit and again at regular intervals. Relatives or close friends should definitely be included in this part of the assessment process to determine whether they are willing and able to assume some responsibility for care of the patient.

Reported educational level appears to be a poor predictor of reading ability, since a person's actual reading level may be significantly lower. Nevertheless, it may be helpful to ask about educational experience.[41] In this context, a question concerning how the person learns best will provide some guidelines for deciding whether to use audio, video, or written materials or a one-on-one or a classroom setting.

What Is Taught

The educational plan is developed by the team, addressing educational needs and treatment goals identified by both the patient and the team. Education begins with "survival" knowledge, i.e., that information it is absolutely necessary for a person with diabetes to have to function independently and safely at home. For some, this may be as simple as identifying when to call the health-care provider. For others, self-monitoring of blood glucose and use of glucagon may be survival skills. Everyone with diabetes must also have some general knowledge about diabetes to understand when it is necessary to call the health-care provider for help.

The educational assessment provides the basis for the individualization of teaching. Having determined the patient's knowledge about diabetes, psychosocial history, and attitudes about diabetes, the educator can then formulate an educational plan that reflects the patient's specific needs.

As outlined by the ADA,[3] the content of the diabetes education program starts with an overview of the general facts. A definition of diabetes, information on its epidemiology and pathophysiology, and classification of diabetes should be included in this section. An explanation of treatment modalities, including the use of insulin, oral hypoglycemic agents, diet, and exercise, should follow. A description of hyper- and hypoglycemia, with explanations about prevention, recognition, and treatment, are also necessary and should be followed by a discussion of the adjustment of these forms of treatment on well days and sick days.

The effects of illness on diabetes are a critical part of any diabetes education. Guidelines for monitoring blood glucose and urine ketones and for modifying diet and about when to call the health-care team are essential skills for the patient.

The goals of monitoring; the kinds, descriptions, and limitations of monitoring devices; and instruction in the use and interpretation of test results are also necessary parts of initial and ongoing education.

The section on prevention, treatment, and rehabilitation of chronic complications should include strategies for coping with the physical changes and losses that complications bring. A discussion of personal adaptation to life with a chronic disease and the impact of diabetes on the family will also help patients understand some of their feelings.

Care of the skin, teeth, and feet are part of the hygiene segment of a diabetes education program. Self-care measures that help prevent complications, the need for regular checkups, and smoking, alcohol, and drug use are addressed in this section. The class on the benefits and responsibilities of care explores the patient-professional partnership in planning care and helps the patient develop short- and long-term goals. Exploration of the use of health-care systems and community resources can help the patient find support and services in the community.

Educational Methods

The use of some basic educational principles as guides can make a diabetes education program more successful, regardless of its setting. The active involvement of the patient in all aspects of the educational endeavor, including decisions about the treatment program, is one such principle.

Unfortunately, many diabetes education programs frequently foster a passive role for the patient.[42] However, it has been suggested that when patients participate in decisions about their care, improvements are seen in measures of both clinical condition and attitudes about health-related quality of life. In a controlled study, Greenfield and associates[43] met with patients before a scheduled office visit with their physicians to review past medical concerns and to focus and improve patients' information-seeking skills. Patients rehearsed negotiation skills, addressing obstacles that stood in the way of their gaining information from the physician, such as feelings of embarrassment or intimidation.

Patients so coached were twice as effective as those in the control group at eliciting information from the physician. Improvements in levels of HbA_1 were significantly greater in these individuals, as were reductions in factors such as days lost from work as a result of illness.

Others also have emphasized the relationship between compliance and the ways in which the physician and the patient reach treatment decisions.[44-47] Commenting on some of these studies, Sims and Sims concluded that patients will adhere to their treatment plans more consistently if they feel a sense of ownership of the plans.[48]

A study of adolescents[49] in a summer school program for young people with diabetes demonstrated another important principle: that education and learning are more effective when people have an opportunity to actively address the questions and problems that actually affect them. One group of participants was randomly assigned to a social learning intervention approach to identify situations in which social pressures made it difficult for them to maintain their treatment regimen, and they rehearsed appropriate responses to these situations. The second group of adolescents underwent a more didactic, fact-oriented diabetes education program.

Subsequent HbA_1 values were significantly lower among the adolescents in the social skills intervention group. Variables significantly correlated with good metabolic control included self-reported compliance with a diabetes regimen and attitudes toward self-care.

Of course, providing complete didactic information that is personally connected is also important and is associated with higher patient satisfaction. Ley et al.[50] provided patients with additional physician visits that were designed to assess previous patient education and understanding and to clarify areas of misunderstanding. These patients showed significantly more satisfaction with their care than did the control group. In a review of this subject, Tabak concurred that patients' satisfaction is clearly related to the amount of information available that contributes to their understanding of their condition and that they can use in caring for themselves.[51] It is also important that the provision and acquisition of information span a reasonable time period if it is to be remembered and utilized by patients. For example, a study of a diet education program given over either 3 days or 11 weeks showed that the longer program was associated with significantly greater improvements in dietary behaviors.[52] The need to pace both the provision and utilization of information has been demonstrated by others as well.[53]

Reinforcement and repetition are also important components of an educational program. Often, this is accomplished through the preparation of written materials for patients. Unfortunately, there is frequently a mismatch between a patient's reading skills and the level of comprehension required to understand the materials.

In one study,[54] only 28% of the patients had reading skills at or above the 9th-grade level. Fifty-nine percent read at the 5th- to 8th-grade level, while 13% had reading skills below the 5th-grade level. By contrast, an evaluation of the educational materials used with these patients showed that 87% were written at the 9th-grade level or above, 13% at the 5th- to 8th-grade level, and none below the 5th grade level. This means that 87% of the materials were comprehensible to only 28% of the patients, 13% were understood by 87%, and none of them were readable by 13%!

Formulas have been developed to determine the reading level of educational materials.[55–59] One of them, the Dale-Chall formula,[55] is particularly helpful. In addition to identifying the reading level of written material, it provides help for rewriting the material to make it simpler.

Finally, a successful education program provides an opportunity for patients to explore their attitudes toward the material being taught and to understand its implications for day-to-day living. Factors such as the patient's familial, social, and cultural environments; socioeconomic status; other health problems; and overall psychological and emotional well-being provide frames of reference from which patients approach diabetes care and their participation in it.[60] The goals for diabetes education developed by the ADA acknowledge the importance of these factors.[33] Anderson et al. suggest a means of adapting an educational program to the patient's frame of reference through activities that stimulate an exploration of the meaning of diabetes to the patient and of the psychological adaptations required for the patient to cope with his or her concept of the disease.[60]

Clearly, the effective implementation of the educational principles discussed above occurs most effectively when the health-care professional has been trained in teaching skills.[42,61–65] Unfortunately, many health professionals involved in diabetes education are not adequately trained in these skills. Their obtaining such skills is strongly encouraged.

When Education Should Take Place

Education for diabetes care is an ongoing, lifelong undertaking. However, there are identifiable stages in the progression of diabetes when educational interactions are particularly recommended.

Diagnosis Stage

Upon receiving a diagnosis of diabetes, many people are overwhelmed by the disease itself as well as by the idea of all the information they think they must absorb. Therefore, people with newly diagnosed diabetes should start by learning the minimum basic skills required for survival. They should learn to maintain reasonably satisfactory management of their diabetes while carrying out essential daily activities. They should become familiar with the dietary exchange system and be able to choose foods in the correct amounts to follow their meal plan. Patients should be taught how to self-monitor blood glucose, and some need to learn how to inject insulin. The ADA has prepared a booklet[33] identifying the educational requirements of this stage both for patients who require insulin and for those who do not.

This initial education provided at or around the time of diagnosis can occur over several days, particularly if the person is hospitalized, or in small increments over several days or weeks for those who are outpatients.

Ongoing Stage

Once patients have mastered the essential "survival skills" of diabetes management, they should progress to a more in-depth program of ongoing diabetes education to help them become even more sufficient at self-care. Such programs are available in many education centers, clinics, hospitals, and community public-health programs. For example, the Joslin Diabetes Center offers an intensive weekend program beginning on Friday evenings and continuing through Sunday afternoon. A similar intensive program is also offered in the Center's inpatient treatment unit. This in-depth experience provides the basis of knowledge and skills that permits people to live well with diabetes.

It is important that people also receive periodic educational updates after they complete this initial in-depth training to enable them to meet changing needs at different times of their lives. People can learn new ways of managing diabetes, develop skills that enable them to adapt their management program to changing needs, and familiarize themselves with new resources and advances available for diabetes care.

Major Points of Change

Times of major life and health changes can signal the need for revisions in diabetes management and often make supplementary educational exposure necessary. Throughout the course of a pregnancy, for example, nutritional needs will change and insulin treatment programs may become more intensified, and pregnant women must learn to make these changes properly.

Another milestone at which supplementary education is necessary is at the appearance of early symptoms or signs of a major complication. For example, patients can learn to make changes in their routine that, if instituted early enough, may slow down the progression of kidney dysfunction.

MAXIMIZING THE EFFICACY OF EDUCATION

As was pointed out previously, knowledge does not equal compliance. Noncompliance is not unique to diabetes. In fact, there are low rates of compliance with recommended treatment in a variety of chronic conditions. Studies show that only 50% of patients are compliant with long-term medication and that only 25% are compliant when the condition is asymptomatic.[66] In studies specific for diabetes, 80% of those studied administered insulin in an unacceptable manner, 58% gave the wrong dose, and 75% did not follow dietary recommendations.[67]

Noncompliance presents a substantial obstacle to the achievement of treatment goals, disrupts the potential benefits of the treatment regimen, and exposes the patient to otherwise unnecessary tests and therapies. It also interferes with the doctor/patient relationship and renders inaccurate any attempts to evaluate treatment efficacy.[68] There is no common profile of a noncompliant patient. Compliance cannot be predicted by age, sex, education, income, or personality type. Also, patients may be noncompliant in one area and not in others.[69]

Compliance and adherence are affected by a number of factors. The first is the treatment regimen. The greater the complexity and duration of the regimen, the more negative is its impact on compliance.[69] The more we ask patients to do and the longer we ask them to do it, the less likely they will be able to sustain compliance.

This compliance factor can be modified by the health-care team. A simplified and tailored regimen designed to meet individual life-style needs is more likely to gain compliance than is one that focuses on metabolic control alone. Clear, specific, simple, and concrete information and instructions in a diabetes education program will go far towards reducing the perceived complexity of treatment and improving the rate of compliance.[70]

Diabetes education can have an additional impact on the compliance rate by correcting misconceptions, teaching self-management, and encouraging changes in behavior by setting achievable and measurable goals. Acknowledgment of the imperfections and frustrations of the treatment plan helps to prepare the patient for the inevitable setbacks.[71]

The second factor that impacts on compliance is the patient's beliefs about health care. The health-belief model looks at whether the patient believes that he or she has diabetes, that it is serious, that the treatment is beneficial, and that the barriers to care are outweighed by its benefits.[72]

The characteristic coping styles of a patient may also be factors that determine adherence. Denial of diabetes will not allow the patient to enter into an aggressive treatment regimen. On the other hand, those patients who tend to be obsessive/compulsive may need to be given permission to do less rather than encouraged to do more. A compliance-oriented history will help identify barriers to care.

A third critical factor in compliance is the health-care provider, for he or she can influence the patient, modify the treatment regimen, and alter his or her relationship with the patient. In fact, the health-care provider is the key to adherence.

The health-care provider/patient relationship itself can have a positive or negative effect on compliance. Impersonality and lack of warmth in the relationship between the health-care provider and the patient can adversely affect patient compliance.[73] On the other hand, the health-care provider's use of self-disclosure and positive nonverbal communication, such as smile, touch, and eye contact, can have a positive impact on compliance.

In addition to working on a positive relationship with the patient, the health-care provider can simplify the form of treatment and support the patient's efforts to manage his or her care.

THE ECONOMICS OF DIABETES EDUCATION

Economic factors are exerting an increasing influence on the setting for and scope of diabetes patient education. Inpatient education programs are now restricted to people with medical conditions that cannot be adequately addressed in an outpatient setting, and shorter hospital stays limit what can be taught.[74] Increasingly, diabetes education must be delivered through outpatient programs.[75]

Ironically, economic factors also restrict the scope of outpatient programs as well. Inpatient education frequently was provided as part of the "overhead" service covered by the cost of hospitalization. However, because education is not adequately covered by insurance in any state, the cost of outpatient education is often borne directly by the patient. Thus, since inpatient education is restricted and outpatient education is unaffordable, *all* education may be unavailable for the vast majority.

In spite of continued recommendations to the contrary, many insurance programs still fail to cover outpatient education. The ADA stated that every patient has a right to accessible and affordable patient education services[76] and has issued a policy statement that "supports and encourages reimbursement for outpatient education and nutrition counseling that meet acceptable standards for persons with diabetes."[77] Yet Sinnock and Bauer, in 1984, noted great inconsistencies in the reimbursement policies of different states.[78] They recommended dissemination of Medicare policies on patient education, documentation of "successful" experiences, and the development of national education standards.[2-4]

Although some of these goals have since been met to various degrees, the situation has not improved substantially. Again, in 1990, the ADA issued a policy statement that noted "the omission of outpatient education as a benefit in many insurance and health-care financing plans constitutes a major barrier to the availability and accessibility of these services" and supported "adequate reimbursement and payment for outpatient diabetes education services that meet accepted standards."[79] Such lack of coverage may be the result either of the failure of insurance companies to include coverage in their policies or of a choice made by employers not to include such coverage in the insurance benefits they offer their employees when arranging insurance benefits.

Outpatient education does have advantages over inpatient education. There is flexibility of timing of the sessions, extension of the educational experience over weeks or months, ability to educate in a normal life-setting rather than in an artificial inpatient environment, and the opportunity for follow-up sessions. However, until the economics of outpatient education can be properly arranged, the full potential cannot be met.

ASSESSING OUTCOMES

"Outcome" refers to the hoped-for effect of an educational effort on diabetes management and overall quality of life for people with diabetes. Assessments of educational outcome have traditionally focused on physiologic improvements, which are the changes most easily measured. These assessments attempt to determine how changes in knowledge and skills contribute to better self-care behavior and improvements in blood glucose levels, decreased complications, reduced use of health-care services, and improved quality of life.[16,60,80]

However, as suggested earlier, health professionals are recognizing that assessing outcomes by examining only the knowledge acquired and the skills learned as the sole factors involved in effecting beneficial self-care practices and metabolic control is too narrow a focus.[18,28] There are many steps between an educational encounter and a medically or economically valuable outcome, with multiple factors influencing the process along the way. Knowledge and skills are only two factors that influence self-care behavior, and self-care behavior, while crucial for success, is only one component of a favorable outcome.

For example, improvements in self-care practices are unlikely to occur unless the patient is also helped to actively integrate his or her therapeutic regimen into the many facets of daily life. If the patient is expected to assume only a passive role in determining the regimen or in performing tasks and if his or her personal values and needs are ignored, no true progress is likely.[76]

The ultimate purpose of assessing outcomes of educational efforts is to justify the cost and to ensure that the desired goal of improved health is reached. However, measuring the efficacy of education has been limited by the difficulty or impracticality of demonstrating a direct link between educational interaction and desired outcome while controlling for the other variables.

Therefore, before beneficial outcomes can be measured, educational programs must be designed to address the multiple factors that encourage active patient participation in self-care that ultimately bring about an associated improvement in metabolic control and overall health. For example, one program made an effort to help patients develop a more accepting and positive personal response to having diabetes and to its treatment.[60] Another program successfully affected self-care patterns, levels of HbA$_1$, and emotional well-being by specifically addressing these issues.[9]

Currently, therefore, assessments of outcome look beyond knowledge and skills and focus on behaviors. Identification of about three specific, desired behavioral changes during the educational encounter permits subsequent evaluation based on whether these changes have occurred.

The challenge remains to design outcome assessments that trace the further progression from educational intervention, through behavioral changes, to desired outcome in terms of measurable medical or economic parameters. To determine the exact effect of education, however, one must control for the other variables that affect the outcome, a challenge that remains formidable.

CONCLUSION

It is hoped that the diabetes education programs that are evolving as part of multifaceted diabetes management efforts provided by skilled health-care teams will be able to help patients reach higher levels of adherence, metabolic control, and satisfaction by leading to their even more active participation in self-care. Perhaps, with such models of excellence, the economic costs of such educational programs will be recognized as the bargain they are rather than as an additional financial burden on society and that educational services will be accessible to all people with diabetes.

REFERENCES

1. WHO Expert Committee on Diabetes Mellitus. Education. Second report. Technical report series 646. Geneva: World Health Organization, 1980:58.
2. National Diabetes Advisory Board, November 1983. National standards for diabetes patient education programs. Diabetes Care 1984;7:XXXI–XXXV.
3. American Diabetes Association. Quality recognition for diabetes patient education programs. Review criteria for national standards from the American Diabetes Association. Diabetes Care 1986;9:XXXVI–XL.
4. National Certification Board for Diabetes Educators. Certification: progress and prospects for diabetes educators. Diabetes Educ 1987;13:206–8.
5. Sinnock P, Bauer DW. Reimbursement issues in diabetes. Diabetes Care 1984;7:291–6.
6. Korhonen T, Huttunen JK, Aro A, et al. A controlled trial on the effects of patient education in the treatment of insulin-dependent diabetes. Diabetes Care 1983;6:256–61.
7. Mazzuca SA, Moorman NH, Wheeler ML, et al. The diabetes education study: a controlled trial of the effects of diabetes patient education. Diabetes Care 1986;9:1–10.
8. Bloomgarden ZT, Karmally W, Metzger MJ, et al. Randomized controlled trial of diabetic patient education: improved knowledge without improved metabolic status. Diabetes Care 1987;10:263–72.
9. Rubin RR, Peyrot M, Saudek CD. Effect of diabetes education on self-care, metabolic control, and emotional well-being. Diabetes Care 1989;12:673–9.
10. Wilson W, Ary DV, Biglan A, et al. Psychosocial predictors of self-care behaviors (compliance) and glycemic control in non-insulin-dependent diabetes mellitus. Diabetes Care 1986;9:614–22.
11. Jacobson AM, Hauser ST, Wolfsdorf JI. Psychological predictors of compliance in children with insulin-dependent diabetes [Abstract no. 314]. Diabetes 1986;35(Suppl 1):79A.
12. Crabtree MK. Performance of diabetic self-care predicted by self-efficacy [Abstract no. 128]. Diabetes 1987;36(Suppl 1):32A.
13. Glasgow RE, McCaul KD, Schafer L, et al. Regimen adherence and glycemic control among persons with type I diabetes. Diabetes 1986;35(Suppl 1):20A.
14. Rettig BA, Shrauger DG, Recker RR, et al. A randomized study of the effects of a home diabetes education program. Diabetes Care 1986;9:173–8.
15. Mazzuca SA, Cohen SJ, Clark CM Jr, et al. The diabetes education study: two-year follow-up [Abstract no. 26]. Diabetes 1984;3(Suppl 1):7A.
16. Whitehouse FW, Whitehouse IJ, Smith J, Hohl RD. Teaching the person with diabetes: experience with a follow-up session. Diabetes Care 1979;2:35–8.
17. Anderson RM. Defining and evaluating diabetes patient education [Letter]. Diabetes Care 1983;6:619–20.
18. Glasgow RE, McCaul KD, Shafer LC. Self-care behaviors and glycemic control in type I diabetes. J Chronic Dis 1987;40:399–412.
19. Cahill GF. Diabetes control and complications [Editorial]. Diabetes Care 1983;6:310–1.
20. DCCT Research Group. Diabetes control and complications trial (DCCT): results of feasibility study. Diabetes Care 1987;10:1–19.
21. Krall LP. Education: a treatment for diabetes. In: Marble A, Krall LP, Bradley RF, et al. Joslin's diabetes mellitus. 12th ed. Philadelphia: Lea & Febiger, 1985:465–84.
22. Geller J, Butler K. Study of educational deficits as the cause of hospital admission for diabetes mellitus in a community hospital. Diabetes Care 1981;4:487–9.
23. Scott RS, Brown LJ, Clifford P. Use of health services by diabetic persons. II. Hospital admissions. Diabetes Care 1985;8:43–7.
24. Zaremba MM, Willhoite B, Ra K. Self-reported data: reliability and role in determining program effectiveness. Diabetes Care 1985;8:486–90.
25. Fishbein HA. Precipitants of hospitalization in insulin-dependent diabetes mellitus (IDDM): a statewide perspective. Diabetes Care 1985;8(Suppl 1):61–4.
26. Kaplan RM, Davis WK. Evaluating the costs and benefits of outpatient diabetes education and nutrition counseling. Diabetes Care 1986;9:81–6.
27. American Diabetes Association. Third-party reimbursement for outpatient education and nutrition counseling. Diabetes Care 1984;7:505–6.
28. Anderson RM. Assessing value of diabetes patient education [Letter]. Diabetes Care 1986;9:553.
29. McCaughrin WC. Legal precedents in American law for patient education. Patient Counsel Health Educ 1979;1:135–41.
30. Read DA, Greene WH. Creative teaching in health. New York: Macmillan, 1971:5.
31. Valentine V. Empowering patients for change. Practical Diabetol 1990;9:13.
32. Joslin EP. A diabetic manual for the mutual use of doctor and patient. 3rd ed. Philadelphia: Lea & Febiger, 1924:21.
33. Franz M, et al. Goals for diabetes education. American Diabetes Association Task Group on Goals for Diabetes Education. Alexandria, VA: American Diabetes Association, 1986.
34. Satterfield DW, Davidson JK. The team approach to evaluation, education, and treatment. In: Davidson JK, ed. Clinical diabetes mellitus: a problem-oriented approach. New York: Thieme, 1986:128–41.
35. Redman BK. The process of patient education. 6th ed. St. Louis: Mosby, 1988:21–48.
36. Hamburg BA, Inoff GE. Coping with predictable crises of diabetes. Diabetes Care 1983;6:409–16.
37. McLeod B. Program development for diabetes. Toronto: Canadian Diabetes Association, 1988.
38. Resler MM. Teaching strategies that promote adherence. Nurs Clin North Am 1983;18:799–811.
39. Rosenstock IM. Understanding and enhancing patient compliance with diabetic regimens. Diabetes Care 1985;8:610–6.
40. Alogna M. Assessment of patient knowledge and performance. In: Steiner G, Lawrence PA, eds. Educating diabetic patients. New York: Springer, 1981:146–53.
41. Barr P, Hess G, Frey ML. Relationship between reading levels and effective patient education [Abstract no. 192]. Diabetes 1986;35(Suppl 1):48A.
42. Lorenz RA. Teaching skills of health professionals. Diabetes Educ 1989;15:149–52.
43. Greenfield S, Kaplan SH, Ware JE Jr, et al. Patients' participation in medical care: effects on blood sugar control and quality of life in diabetes. J Gen Intern Med 1988;3:448–57.
44. Rost K. The influence of patient participation on satisfaction and compliance. Diabetes Educ 1989;15:140–3.
45. Roter DL. Patient participation in the patient-provider interaction: the effects of patient question asking on the quality of interaction, satisfaction and compliance. Health Educ Monographs 1977;5:281–315.

46. Rothert ML, Talarczyk GJ. Patient compliance and the decision-making process of clinicians and patients. J Compliance Health Care 1987;2:55–71.

47. Stewart MA. What is a successful doctor-patient interview? A study of interactions and outcomes. Soc Sci Med 1984;19:167–75.

48. Sims DF, Sims EAH. Commentary. Diabetes Spectrum 1990;3:227–8.

49. Kaplan RM, Chadwick MW, Schimmel LE. Social learning intervention to promote metabolic control in type I diabetes mellitus: pilot experiment results. Diabetes Care 1985;8:152–5.

50. Ley P, Bradshaw PW, Kincey JA, Atherton ST. Increasing patients' satisfaction with communications. Br J Soc Clin Psychol 1976;15:403–13.

51. Tabak ER. The relationship of information exchange during medical visits to patient satisfaction: a review. Diabetes Educ 1987;13:36–40.

52. Campbell LV, Barth R, Bosper JK, et al. Impact of intensive educational approach to dietary change in NIDDM. Diabetes Care 1990; 13:841–7.

53. Page P, Verstraete DG, Robb JR, Etzwiler DD. Patient recall of self-care recommendations in diabetes. Diabetes Care 1981;4:96–8.

54. McNeal B, Salisbury Z, Baumgardner P, Wheeler FC. Comprehension assessment of diabetes education program participants. Diabetes Care 1984;7:232–5.

55. Dale E, Chall JS. A formula for predicting readability. Columbus: Ohio State University Press, 1948.

56. Flesch RF. A new readability yardstick. J Appl Psychol 1948;32:221–33.

57. Fry E. A readability formula that saves time. J Reading 1958;11:513–78.

58. McLaughlin GH. SMOG grading—a new readability formula. J Reading 1969;12:639–46.

59. Doak CC, Doak LG, Root JH. Teaching patients with low literacy skills. Philadelphia: JB Lippincott, 1985.

60. Anderson RM, Nowacek G, Richards F. Influencing the personal meaning of diabetes: research and practice. Diabetes Educ 1988;14:297–302.

61. Boulton C, Garth RY. Students in learning groups: active learning through conversation. San Francisco: Jossey-Bass, June 1983:73–81. (Learning in groups: new directions for teaching and learning; no. 14).

62. Finkel DL, Monk GS. Teachers and learning groups: dissolution of the atlas complex. San Francisco: Jossey-Bass, June 1983:83–97. (Learning in groups: new directions for teaching and learning; no. 14).

63. Istre SM. The art and science of successful teaching. Diabetes Educ 1989;15:67–75.

64. Lorenz RA. Training health professionals to improve the effectiveness of patient education programs. Diabetes Educ 1986;12:204–9.

65. Sanson-Fisher RW, Campbell EM, Redman S, Hennrikus DJ. Patient-provider interactions and patient outcomes. Diabetes Educ 1989;15:134–8.

66. Sackett DL. The magnitude of compliance and non-compliance. In: Sackett DL, Haynes RB, eds. Compliance with therapeutic regimens. Baltimore: The Johns Hopkins University Press, 1976:9–25.

67. Watkins JD, Williams TF, Martin DA, et al. A study of diabetic patients at home. Am J Public Health 1967;57:452–9.

68. Speers MA, Turk DC. Diabetes self care: knowledge, beliefs, motivation and action. Patient Counseling Health Educ 1982;3:144–9.

69. Eraker SK, Becker MH. Improving compliance for the patient with diabetes. Practical Diabetol 1984;3:6–11.

70. Strowig S. Patient education: a model for autonomous decision-making and deliberate action in diabetes self-management. Med Clin North Am 1982;66:1293–307.

71. Westberg J, Jason H. Building a helpful relationship: the foundation of effective patient education. Diabetes Educ 1986;12:374–8.

72. Maiman LA, Becker MH. The clinician's role in patient compliance. Trends Pharmacol Sci 1980;1:457–9.

73. Harris G. Filling the gaps between patients and professionals. Diabetes Educ 1986;13:133–6.

74. Martinez NC, Deane DM. Impact of prospective payment on the role of the diabetes educator. Diabetes Educ 1989; 15:503–9.

75. Hiss RG, Frey ML, Davis WK. Diabetes patient education in the office setting. Diabetes Educ 1986;12:281–5.

76. American Diabetes Association. ADA patient bill of rights. Diabetes Forecast 1983;36.

77. American Diabetes Association. Third-party reimbursement for outpatient education and nutrition counseling. Diabetes Care 1984;7:505–6.

78. Sinnock P, Bauer DW. Reimbursement issues in diabetes. Diabetes Care 1984;7:291–6.

79. American Diabetes Association. Third-party reimbursement for outpatient diabetes education and counseling. Diabetes Care 1990;13(Suppl 1):36.

80. Graber AL, Christman BG, Alogna MT, Davidson JK. Evaluation of diabetes patient education programs. Diabetes 1977;26:61–4.

Chapter 24

DIETARY MANAGEMENT

PHYLLIS A. CRAPO

Dietary modification is the oldest of the three treatment modalities recommended for diabetes. As early as 1550 B.C., as described in the Ebers Papyrus, the use or avoidance of particular foods has been recommended for those with diabetes.[1] Through the years, however, no clear agreement has been reached about which foods should be used or avoided. At first, patients were treated empirically with carbohydrate-rich diets geared to match urinary glucose loss. In 1797, however, Rollo first reversed this tradition by advocating diets high in animal fat and protein and low in carbohydrate.[1] He felt that carbohydrate was at the root of the problems in diabetes and that restriction of carbohydrates would curtail glycemia. Even after the discovery of insulin in 1921, and a consequent reappraisal of the role of diet, differences in opinion about diet remained. The "Joslin" treatment at the beginning of the insulin era consisted of an initial period of fasting or severe caloric restriction, followed by a maintenance diet aimed at keeping the person in a subnutritional state without undergoing a progressive loss of weight.[2] But there was controversy about whether the diet should be high or low in carbohydrate. In the 1930s Rabinowitch and Himsworth advocated the use of high-carbohydrate, low-fat, and low-calorie diets for treatment of diabetes,[3,4] while others still recommended carbohydrate restriction. The significant use of high-carbohydrate diets did not occur until more than three decades later. As evidence of the changing views on dietary carbohydrate, Glick[5] reported that the "high-carbohydrate theory" covered 6½ pages in the fifth (1935) and sixth (1937) editions of *Joslin's Diabetes Mellitus* text but that the coverage fell to only three pages in the seventh edition (1940), to an italicized section in the eighth edition (1946), and to nothing at all in the ninth edition (1952).

In the 1970s the high-carbohydrate diet was rediscovered,[6,7] and today the "officially" recommended diet (Table 24–1)[8] is higher in complex carbohydrate and lower in fat and protein than most earlier diets and the attitude toward sucrose and other sugars is more liberal.

Table 24–1. American Diabetes Association Recommended Daily Intake (to Be Tailored to Individual Needs)

Carbohydrate (%)	Protein (g/mg)	Fat (%)[†]			Cholesterol (mg)	Fiber (g)
		PU	S	MS		
≤60	0.8*	6–8	<10	30 − (PU + S)	<300	40

*The recommended dietary allowance for protein is 0.8 g/kg body weight for adults. Patients with incipient renal failure may need to lower their protein intake.
†If the amount of total fat is reduced, all components, i.e., polyunsaturated (PU), saturated (S), and monounsaturated (MU) fat, should be reduced proportionally.
For people with low-calorie diets, fiber intake should be 25 g/1000 kcal.

These changes reflect a move from a sphere of concern about shielding patients from the lethal effects of ketoacidosis to a new sphere of concern about long-term complications. Of interest is the recognition by Dr. Elliott P. Joslin early in this century that complications would be reduced if blood glucose levels were kept as near normal as possible. But at that time, not everyone was in agreement about his aggressive therapeutic approach.[9]

Current nutritional recommendations for diabetes management are similar to those given in the *Surgeon's General Report on Nutrition and Health*,[10] by the American Heart Association (Table 24–2)[11] and by health organizations such as the National Cancer Institute (Table 24–3),[12] indicating that there is some uniformity of thought about what constitutes a healthy diet. But even this dietary approach to diabetes management has not received universal support in the diabetes health-care community, and although significant advances in dietary management have been made, much of our dietary advice is still without adequate research substantiation.

Yet the volume of research on issues of nutrition and diabetes and the number of changes made in the dietary management of diabetes as a consequence of research findings have never been greater. Newly evolving knowledge is rapidly affecting how the diet of the diabetic patient is managed. A greater variety in insulin regimens and the availability of technology for the self-monitoring of blood glucose, as well as other advances, have allowed increased flexibility in meal planning. A continued research focus on the glycemic response to different types of foods is gradually changing the way we think about diet in diabetes. We are now more aware of differences in metabolic responses to different types of carbohydrates and fats, and the impact of these differences when these foods are used in meals and over longer periods is becoming clearer.

The role of protein in attentuating the progressive loss of renal function that accompanies diabetes is now recognized. That the dietary management of non-insulin-dependent diabetes mellitus (NIDDM) is quite different from that of insulin-dependent diabetes mellitus (IDDM) has also been accepted. Our knowledge about the treatment of obesity in diabetes has also increased. In addition, new attention is being placed on the special considerations required among different subgroups of

Table 24-3. National Cancer Institute Dietary Guidelines

1. Reduce fat intake to ≤30% of calories
2. Increase fiber intake to 20–30 g daily, with an upper limit of 35 g
3. Include a variety of vegetables and fruits in daily diet
4. Avoid obesity
5. Consume alcoholic beverages in moderation, if at all
6. Minimize consumption of salt-cured, salt-pickled, and smoked foods

Table is adapted from Butrum et al.[12]

people with diabetes. The needs of ethnic minority groups with distinct dietary patterns, of pregnant women, of growing children, and of the elderly have been given increased recognition and attention. Emphasis is being placed on providing individualized, flexible diets that people can and will follow. Recent years have also seen dramatic changes in our methods of diabetes education. New strategies, knowledge, and techniques for teaching and obtaining compliance are improving the overall management of diabetes as well as dietary management. Teaching is often done in teams, and the patient and family often participate together in the process.

Despite the incomplete scientific underpinnings for some dietary approaches, the goals of dietary treatment can often be achieved through the use of individualized diets, self-monitoring of blood glucose, and the provision of pharmacotherapy on a more physiologic basis. Diet remains the cornerstone of management, but additional research is necessary to improve the contribution that diet can make to effective diabetes management.

MANAGEMENT GOALS

The goals of dietary management of diabetes are summarized in Table 24–4, which outlines the recommendations of the American Diabetes Association.[8]

Type I or Insulin-Dependent Diabetes Mellitus

The primary goals of therapy for persons with Type I diabetes are the maintenance of appropriate body weight and the prevention of hypoglycemia and hyperglycemia. The patient reaches these goals by consuming meals with an appropriate caloric content at regular intervals in coordination with the timing of insulin injections and the level of physical activity. Individuals with Type I diabetes are usually young and lean, and their caloric intake should be adequate to support normal growth and development.

Type II or Non-Insulin-Dependent Diabetes Mellitus

Eighty to ninety percent of individuals with Type II diabetes are overweight, and the first goal of dietary therapy is weight loss. For many of these persons, restriction of caloric intake and increased physical activity will produce a moderate weight loss that may be sufficient to control blood glucose levels and make insulin or oral medication unnecessary. Once they achieve a desirable weight, persons with Type II diabetes

Table 24-2. American Heart Association Low-Fat, Low-Cholesterol Diets

Dietary Factor	Percentage of Calories	
	Step 1	Step 2
Total fat	<30	<30
Saturated	<10	<7
Monounsaturated	10–15	10–15
Polyunsaturated	≤10	≤10
Carbohydrate	50–60	50–60
Protein	15–20	15–20
Cholesterol	<300 mg/d	<200 mg/d

Table is adapted from American Heart Association.[11]

Table 24-4. Goals for Diabetes Management

1. Restoration of normal blood glucose and optimal lipid levels. Maintenance of blood glucose levels as near to physiologic levels as possible to 1) prevent hyperglycemia and/or hypoglycemia; 2) prevent or delay the development of long-term cardiovascular renal, retinal, neurologic complications associated with diabetes mellitus; 3) contribute to a normal outcome of pregnancies for women with diabetes.
2. Maintenance of normal growth rate in children and adolescents as well as the attainment and maintenance of reasonable body weight in adolescents and adults. Any abnormal of unexplained deviation in growth rate or weight gain and/or loss as plotted or standard grids warrants an assessment of diabetes control, eating behavior, and caloric intake as well as consideration of alternative problems and/or diagnosis.
3. Provision of adequate nutrition for the pregnant woman, the fetus, and lactation.
4. Consistency in the timing of meals and snacks to prevent inordinate swings in blood glucose levels for people using exogenous insulin.
5. Determination of a meal plan appropriate for the individual's life-style and based on a diet history. Results of blood-glucose monitoring can then be used to integrate insulin therapy with the usual, as well as unanticipated eating and exercise patterns.
6. Management of weight for obese people with non-insulin-dependent diabetes mellitus. Weight management involves specific changes in food intake and eating behaviors as well as increased activity level. Continued support and follow-up by qualified health professionals are important if long-term changes in life-style are to be made.
7. Improvement in the overall health of people with diabetes through optimal nutrition.

Table is adapted from American Diabetes Association.[8]

must continue to adhere to dietary guidelines to maintain the reduction in weight and blood glucose control.

Both Type I and Type II Diabetes

For persons with either Type I or Type II diabetes, dietary therapy is concerned with 1) the maintenance of proper nutrition, 2) the total number of calories ingested, 3) the distribution of calories throughout the day, and 4) the individual food sources that contribute those calories. The American Diabetes Association has issued general dietary recommendations for persons with diabetes; these are summarized in Table 24-5 and discussed in more detail below.[8,10]

DIETARY RECOMMENDATIONS

Calories

The caloric intake prescribed should achieve and maintain a desirable weight in the person with diabetes. The caloric prescription is an important element of nutritional management and should be carefully considered. Caloric requirements for persons with diabetes are not different from those for persons without diabetes, if the person with diabetes is not losing calories through glycosuria. Caloric needs vary with the patient's age, sex, and activity level. The recommended caloric level is based on an individual's desired weight (whether the goal is weight loss, maintenance, or gain) and his or her activity patterns.

Table 24-5. American Diabetes Association Dietary Recommendations for Persons with Diabetes

Dietary Factor	Recommendations
Calories	Should be prescribed to achieve and maintain a desirable body weight
Carbohydrate	Ideally should comprise 55–60% of the calories, with the form and amount to be determined by individual eating patterns and blood glucose and lipid responses. Unrefined carbohydrates should be substituted for refined carbohydrates to the extent possible. Modest amounts of sugars may be acceptable as long as metabolic control and desirable body weight are maintained.
Protein	The recommended dietary allowance[69] of 0.85 g/kg body weight for adults is an appropriate guide for those with diabetes. Some reduction in protein intake from previously high consumption levels may help prevent or delay the onset of the renal complications of diabetes.
Fat/cholesterol	Should comprise ≤30% of total calories, and all components should be reduced proportionately. Replacement of saturated with polyunsaturated fat is desirable to reduce cardiovascular risk. Cholesterol should be restricted to ≤300/d to reduce cardiovascular risk.
Alternative sweeteners	Both nutritive and non-nutritive sweeteners are acceptable in diabetes management.
Sodium	Should be restricted to 1000 mg/1000 kcal, not to exceed 3000 mg/d, to minimize symptoms of hypertension. Severe sodium restriction may, however, be harmful for persons whose diabetes is poorly controlled and for those with postural hypotension (low blood pressure and consequent dizziness when first standing up) or fluid imbalance.
Alcohol	Should be used in moderation and may need to be restricted entirely by persons with diabetes and insulin-induced hypoglycemia, neuropathy, poor control of blood sugar or blood lipids, or obesity.
Vitamins and minerals	Should meet recommended levels for good health. Supplements are unnecessary for persons with diabetes except when caloric intake is exceptionally low or the variety of foods consumed is limited. Calcium supplements may be necessary under special circumstances.

Table is adapted with permission from reference 8 (American Diabetes Association. Nutritional recommendations and principles for individuals with diabetes mellitus: 1986. Diabetes Care 1987;10:126–32; copyright © of the American Diabetes Association).

Most people with IDDM are thin when first diagnosed with diabetes, and a caloric intake that ensures normal growth and development and is adequate to sustain the usual level of physical activity is necessary. For infants, children, and adolescents, the caloric needs associated with normal growth and sexual maturation must be carefully considered and growth rates should be vigilantly followed on standard growth charts at frequent intervals, with adjustments made in meal plans as necessary. If diabetes is not properly controlled during the growth years, growth may be retarded and the height potential not reached. Thus, any abnormal or unexplained deviation in growth rate or loss or gain in weight demands an assessment of the adequacy of diabetes control, including eating patterns and caloric intake, as well as consideration of any other potential problems. Failure of the person to develop normally indicates an inadequacy of caloric intake or insulin dosage or both. Activity levels and caloric requirements can vary considerably among children, and so the dietary prescription must be adjusted on a regular basis to accommodate the changes that occur in growth patterns, participation in sports, or in school or vacation schedules.

In contrast, most persons with NIDDM are overweight when first diagnosed and need to restrict their caloric intake. A reduction in caloric intake is perhaps the most important aspect of therapy and is associated with a reduction in hyperlipidemia as well as in hyperglycemia. Caloric restriction independent of weight loss can have a significant initial effect on glycemic control. Several days of fasting or severe caloric restriction have been found to produce significant reductions in levels of glucose and insulin even before a significant weight loss has occurred.[13,14] The rapid drop in blood glucose levels is a response to the abrupt decrease in calories and carbohydrate ingested. True weight loss, however, leads to a reduction in resistance to insulin and has a long-term effect on maintenance of the reduced blood glucose levels.

Overweight patients with NIDDM should be encouraged to establish their weight within a desirable range, but unrealistic targets, such as achievement of "ideal" weight, should not be insisted upon. Often, when large weight losses are necessary, setting intermediate goals may be useful and help the patient from becoming overwhelmed by the magnitude of the necessary weight loss. Weight management should include not only caloric control but behavioral modification (to encourage eating behaviors that will promote weight reduction) and increased physical activity. A reduction in caloric intake to approximately 500 kcal/day less than the requirements for weight maintenance can result in losses of 1 to 2 kg/month, a rate that should be considered satisfactory. Losses of 2 to 4 kg/month are excellent. Weight loss can be accelerated through the use of diets low or very low in calories, both of which have been quite effective in achieving weight loss and rapid glycemic control in obese NIDDM subjects.[15] The relatively rapid loss of weight can also motivate the patient to adhere to a longer-term weight management plan. However, the successful use of these diets in obese patients with NIDDM requires more intensive follow-up and monitoring by the physician. In lean patients with IDDM or NIDDM, appetite and hunger are usually reliable guides to caloric needs, although body weight is the definitive guide.

Several different means of estimating desirable body weight and caloric needs are available. Some examples are included in Table 24–6[16] and Figure 24–1.[17] Detailed information on diet, weight, and family histories;

Table 24-6. Estimating Caloric Intake and Desirable Body Weight for Adults

A. Estimating caloric intake
Basal calories: 10 kcal/lb desirable body weight
Add calories for activity
  If sedentary add 10% of estimated base calories
  If moderately active add 20% of estimated base calories
  If strenuously active add 40% of estimated base calories
Adjustments*
  Add calories for indicated weight gain, growth (pregnancy), or lactation
  Subtract calories for indicated weight loss
B. Estimating desirable body weight from frame size
Medium frame
  Women   100 lb for first 5 ft plus 5 lb for each additional inch
  Men   106 lb for first 5 ft plus 6 lb for each additional inch
Small frame   Subtract 10%
Large frame   Add 10%

Table is adapted from Vinik and Wing.[16]
*Adjustments are approximate; weight changes should be monitored and compared with caloric intake.

analysis of exercise routines; and a 24-hour dietary recall can all make important contributions to the process of establishing a recommended caloric level. Estimations of caloric needs and the recommended caloric level need not be absolutely precise but should be considered a starting point for fine-tuning during follow-up until a level is established that will help the patient achieve the desired weight and health goal.

Carbohydrate

Carbohydrates should comprise 55 to 60% of caloric intake of the diabetic patient, with the form and amount of carbohydrate determined by individual eating patterns and the levels of blood glucose and lipids achieved. Unrefined carbohydrates should be substituted for refined carbohydrates to the extent possible. Modest amounts of sugars may be acceptable as long as metabolic control and desirable body weight are maintained.

A diet in which approximately 60% of the total calories are from carbohydrate is now recommended for individuals with diabetes because it results in a reduction in dietary fat—particularly saturated fat—thought to be beneficial in reducing cardiovascular risk. Studies indicating that high-carbohydrate diets improve glucose tolerance and insulin sensitivity[6,18,19] support the advisability of this recommendation. Still, some disagreement remains about what constitutes the optimal percentage of carbohydrate for persons with diabetes.[20,21] The role of fiber has become the pivotal point of this issue. One concern about high-carbohydrate diets is their potential for increasing levels of very-low-density lipoprotein (VLDL). Several researchers have noted such an increase when dietary carbohydrate is increased,[22,23] but some also have demonstrated that the limited elevation in VLDL can be prevented if carbohydrate and fiber in the diet are increased in parallel.[24,25] Consequently, recommendations for increased carbohydrate consumption are now coupled with the recommendation that foods high in fiber, especially soluble fiber (e.g., legumes, lentils, some

NOMOGRAPH FOR BODY MASS INDEX (KG/M²)

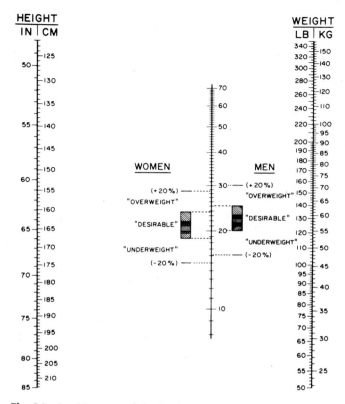

Fig. 24–1. Nomograph for body mass index (kg/m²) The ratio weight/height² is read from the central scale. The ranges suggested as "desirable" from life insurance data must be interpreted with clinical judgment regarding relative skeletal and muscle mass. Reprinted with permission from reference 17 (Thomas AE, McKay DA, Cutlip MB. A nomography for assessing body weight. Am J Clin Nutr 1973;29:302–4; © American Society for Clinical Nutrition).

fruits, oats, and barley), be encouraged. This caveat, however, raises perhaps the more controversial issue of what constitutes the optimal relative proportions of simple and complex carbohydrates for people with diabetes, i.e., the quality of carbohydrate consumed as distinct from the amount.

Traditionally, all complex carbohydrates were thought to generate equivalent blood glucose responses and all simple carbohydrates (or sugars) were thought to generate similar blood glucose responses. The responses to simple sugars were felt to be greater than those to complex carbohydrates. It is now known, however, that both blood glucose and insulin levels may respond differently to different types of simple and complex carbohydrates in the diet.[26–31] In 1981 Jenkins et al.[29] suggested that this response could be expressed as a "glycemic index," which is defined as the increase in the blood glucose level following ingestion of a food as a percentage of the increase that follows ingestion of a standard food (Table 24–7).[31] Glycemic responses to food have been shown to be affected by a variety of factors, including the form of the food, fiber type and

amount, nature and digestibility of the starch, cooking, preparation, and storage procedures, as well as a person's age, concomitant diseases, race, sex, and other individual factors (Table 24–8).

Some studies have found that the glycemic responses to meals can be predicted from the glycemic index of the carbohydrate components,[32–35] whereas others have failed to demonstrate the expected differences in glycemic responses.[36,37] Apart from this issue, several studies have suggested that positive clinical effects are produced when diets contain foods that have low glycemic indexes.[38–40] Some believe that differences are seen only with extreme variations in glycemic indexes (very high and very low) and consider that our understanding of this issue is still too preliminary for it to be considered a basis for therapy.[41] Of interest is a study by Gulliford and colleagues from the United Kingdom,[42] who measured the glucose and insulin responses of patients with NIDDM who were fed meals containing 25 g of carbohydrate as potato or spaghetti alone, with the addition of protein, and with the addition of both protein and fat. When eaten alone, potato elicited a higher glycemic and insulin response than did spaghetti. When protein was added, the insulin response to both meals was increased but the glycemic response to meals containing potato was reduced. With the addition of fat to the meal, the blood glucose response to meals containing potato dropped

Table 24-7. Glycemic Index

80–90%	50–59%	30–39%
Cornflakes	Buckwheat	Butter beans (lima)
Carrots*	Spaghetti (white)	Haricot beans
Parsnips*	Sweet corn	Blackeye peas
Potatoes (instant)	All-Bran	Chick peas
Maltose	Digestive biscuits	Apples (golden
Honey	Oatmeal biscuits	delicious)
	"Rich Tea" biscuits	Ice cream
70–79%	Peas (frozen)	Milk (skim)
Bread (whole meal)	Yam	Milk (whole)
Millet	Sucrose	Yogurt
Rice (white)	Potato chips	Tomato soup
Weetabix (a cereal)		
Broad beans (fresh)	40–49%	20–29%
Potato (new)	Spaghetti (whole	Kidney beans
Swede (a vegetable)*	meal)	Lentils
	Porridge oats	Fructose
60–69%	Potato (sweet)	
Bread (white)	Beans (canned	10–19%
Rice (brown)	navy)	Soya beans
Muesli (a cereal)	Peas (dried)	Soya beans (canned)
Shredded wheat	Oranges	Peanuts
"Ryvita" (a cracker)	Orange juice	
Water biscuits		
Beetroot*		
Bananas		
Raisins		
Mars bar		

Table is reprinted with permission from the American Diabetes Association, from reference 31 (Jenkins DJA. Lente carbohydrate: a newer approach to the dietary management of diabetes. Diabetes Care 1982;5:634–41). The glycemic index is defined as the area under the blood glucose response curve for each food expressed as a percentage of the area after taking the same amount of carbohydrate as glucose (glycemic index, 100%).
*Carbohydrate portions of 25 g were tested.

Table 24-8. Factors Affecting Glycemic Response

Food factors
  Nature of starch structure and physical form
  Cooking and processing procedures (e.g., particle size, blending, grinding)
  Storage procedures
  Ripeness or maturity
  Type and amount of fiber content
  Fat content
  Protein/starch interrelationships
Human factors
  Time of day
  Sex
  Age
  Ethnicity/race
  Medical condition (presence of diabetes)
  Preprandial blood glucose value
  Body mass/weight
  Prior meal and diet composition
  Gastric emptying
  Exercise/physical activity

further but the glycemic response to spaghetti did not change. The addition of other elements to a meal can variably affect the blood glucose response. Thus, while it is well accepted that the meal setting can result in a blunting of the glycemic response, the decrease may not be uniform. In addition, it has been pointed out that the glycemic response to meals or food may be related not only to the complexity and absorption of nutrients but also to the dynamics of insulin secretion in NIDDM.[35]

Because knowledge of food composition and physiology was not sufficient to permit a consistent prediction of glycemic responses, a National Institutes of Health (NIH) consensus development panel, when reviewing the use of glycemic index tables in 1986, did not recommend their use for people with diabetes.[43] However, the principle that food choices can be refined to obtain maximal control of blood glucose remains a possibility for motivated individuals who closely monitor their blood glucose levels. Awareness of differences in glycemic response to food has played an important role in expanding our thinking about how to improve dietary management and our understanding of what occurs in the daily management of individuals with diabetes.

Studies have now been reported that suggest the consumption of modest amounts of sucrose by persons with diabetes is acceptable as long as metabolic control is maintained.[8,44] For instance, several investigators found no significant difference between the blood sugar responses of persons with diabetes when they consumed sucrose and when they consumed only starch.[45-49] In an interesting study of the effect of sucrose that was conducted at Camp Granada in Illinois,[50] 16 staff members with IDDM were assigned to a sucrose or control group. Both groups ate the standard camp meals except for the morning and afternoon snacks, which were sweetened with sucrose for the sucrose group and with aspartame for the control group. The sucrose given comprised 7% of the total calories for the day. The researchers found that the addition of sucrose to snacks

for 5 days of camp did not affect blood glucose control. Another study in Italy of eight pairs of individuals with NIDDM found that a 10% substitution of sucrose for complex carbohydrate over a 6-month period did not worsen metabolic control.[51] Other studies around the world have had similar findings. For example, a study of the effects of sucrose, as compared with aspartame, in the diets of Australians with NIDDM[52] found no adverse effects of sucrose on blood glucose or lipid control when a total of 45 g, 9% of the day's calories, was ingested each day spread out in the day's meals and snacks, and no differences between the sucrose and aspartame diets.

In a recent study[53] children with IDDM in controlled settings had similar blood glucose responses to diets with and without added sucrose. The postprandial blood glucose values of patients with NIDDM fed meals in which potato was substituted for by a portion of chocolate cake of equal carbohydrate value were not significantly different from the values obtained from the same diet without the substitution. If chocolate cake was added rather than substituted into a meal, the blood glucose values rose.[54] It was suggested that children and young adults might feel less constrained by diabetes if they were allowed a diet more consistent with the sucrose-containing diets of their peers. Realistic guidelines for including sucrose-containing foods in the diet might improve patient cooperation with overall diet management. Of course, sucrose contains calories, encourages the development of dental caries, and in desserts is often associated with high amounts of fat, which may raise levels of serum lipids in some people. The recent NIH Consensus Development Conference[43] recommended that only persons who are lean and do not have carbohydrate-aggravated hyperlipidemia be permitted sucrose in their diet. In any case, the recommended sucrose content was not to exceed 5% of the dietary carbohydrate calories. Despite these concerns, the available studies show that sucrose is not as bad for blood glucose control as previously believed. These new findings are indications of how the idea of glycemic indexing is forcing us to reconsider strongly held doctrines. Since asking questions is the first step in discovery, application of the glycemic index is generating new studies of the diabetic diet that will allow us to develop improved dietary recommendations.

Fiber

Recent studies suggest that increased consumption of dietary fiber (Table 24-9)[55] might improve many clinical conditions, including diabetes. Some studies have demonstrated that diets containing higher amounts of fiber (particularly water-soluble fiber) and carbohydrates are associated with lower levels of blood glucose and serum lipids.[56-60] The results of studies of fiber in diabetes have been somewhat inconsistent—probably as a consequence of previously unrecognized differences in types and properties of fiber.

The water-insoluble fibers, such as cellulose, lignin, and most hemicelluloses found in whole grain breads, cereals,

Table 24-9. Fiber Content of Selected Foods

Food	Portion Size	Plant fiber
Breads, cereals and starchy vegetables (cooked/prepared)		
Beans, kidney	½ cup	4.5
Bran (100%), cereal	½ cup	10.0
Bread		
Rye	1 slice	2.7
White	1 slice	0.8
Whole-grain wheat	1 slice	2.7
Corn, kernels	⅓ cup	2.1
Parsnips	⅔ cup	5.9
Peas	½ cup	5.2
Potato, white	1 small	3.8
Rice, brown	½ cup	1.3
Rice, white	½ cup	0.5
Squash, winter	½ cup	3.6
Sweet potatoes	¼ cup	2.9
Fruit (uncooked)		
Apple	1 small	3.9
Banana	½ small	1.3
Blackberries	½ cup	3.6
Grapefruit	½	1.3
Orange	1 small	2.1
Peach	1 medium	1.0
Pineapple	¾ cup	1.3
Strawberries	¾ cup	2.4
Vegetables (cooked unless indicated by R)		
Asparagus	½ cup	1.2
Beans, string	½ cup	1.7
Beets	½ cup	1.5
Broccoli	½ cup	2.6
Carrots	½ cup	2.2
Cauliflower	½ cup	0.9
Cucumber (R)	½ cup	0.8
Lettuce (R)	½ cup	0.5
Squash, summer	½ cup	2.3
Turnips	½ cup	1.3

Reprinted with modifications with permission from the American Diabetes Association from reference 55 (Anderson JW, Ward K. Long-term effects of high-fiber diets on glucose and lipid metabolism: a preliminary report on patients with diabetes. Diabetes Care 1978;1:77-82; Copyright © American Diabetes Association).

and wheat bran, affect gastrointestinal transit time and fecal bulk but have little impact on plasma glucose, insulin, or cholesterol levels.[61,62] The effects of insoluble fibers on baseline blood glucose levels over the long-term need to be evaluated further. However, highly viscous water-soluble fibers, such as the pectins, gums, storage polysaccharides, and a few hemicelluloses found in fruits, legumes, lentils, roots, tubers, oats, and oat bran, have little influence on fecal bulk but, when eaten in purified form, reduce serum levels of glucose and insulin.[55-58] Recently, Wolever, considering whole foods, reported that the amount of soluble fiber in the food is not closely related to glucose response.[63] He reported a weak, but significant, correlation between the amount of total dietary fiber and the glycemic response to a food. The cellulose and uronic acid contents were the best predictors of glycemic response. Purified cellulose does not have a significant impact on blood glucose levels[64,65] but uronic acids are a part of the matrix of cell walls, Wolever postulated that the cell walls of foods that elicited a low

glycemic response were strong and high in cellulose and hemicellulose.[63] It should also be noted that differences in fiber components of foods did not explain all the variation in glycemic response.

Nevertheless, diets very high in carbohydrates and fiber, providing 70% of calories as carbohydrate and 35 g of plant fiber per 1000 calories, consistently improve glucose tolerance, decrease fasting levels of plasma glucose, lower insulin needs, and decrease serum cholesterol concentrations. These results have been confirmed in longer-term studies comparing a more moderate diet that provides 55 to 60% of calories as carbohydrate and 25 g of plant fiber per 1000 calories.[66,67]

These benefits may be related more to other factors than to dietary fiber content. For example, studies have suggested that fiber content is not the major determining factor in the serum glucose response to consumption of cereals.[59,68] In these studies, the form of the food (whole food vs. ground food; bread vs. pasta) affected the glycemic response more than did the fiber content. Nevertheless, increasing the level of fiber in the diet of a person with diabetes is recommended.[8] The amount and type of fiber that elicits the optimal improvement in diabetes symptoms are not well defined, however. A practical way of proceeding is to determine the current level of fiber in a patient's diet and to increase it gradually to a maximum of 35 to 40 g/day. Gradual introduction of the fiber minimizes gastrointestinal problems such as osmotic diarrhea and flatulence. Increased fiber intake should be accompanied by increased fluid intake and careful attention to self-monitoring of blood glucose levels. Intake of large quantities of fiber can delay or reduce peak glucose responses to carbohydrate and perhaps predispose an individual receiving antidiabetic medication to hypoglycemia if dosage of the medication is not adjusted to compensate for this effect. Use of commercial fiber supplements is generally not recommended.

Protein

The recommended dietary allowance (RDA) of protein of 0.85 g/kg of body weight for adults suggested by the National Research Council in 1980 and 1989[69] is an appropriate guide for those with diabetes. Some reduction in the consumption of protein from previously high levels may help prevent or delay the onset of the renal complications of diabetes.

Individuals whose diabetes is under good control appear to have the same protein requirements as nondiabetic individuals. Thus, when insulin levels are normal, protein is conserved in the body and the use of amino acids for glucose synthesis is limited.[70] However, individuals with poorly controlled diabetes may have increased needs for protein because it may be used by the liver to synthesize glucose.

There is now evidence that individuals with diabetes and renal insufficiency should avoid eating the excessive amounts of protein normal for many Americans. Glomerular hyperfiltration leads to impaired renal function, and increased protein intake can exacerbate the problem (see Chapter 40 on diabetic nephropathy). Limiting protein consumption can slow the rate of decline in renal function in individuals with diabetic nephropathy.[71] Because past dietary recommendations for persons with diabetes sometimes emphasized protein and because the average American eats more protein than is necessary to maintain health, current recommendations suggest that people with diabetes reduce protein intake to 0.85 g/kg body weight, a level below that consumed by most Americans.[8]

Fat

Consumption of total fat, saturated fat, and cholesterol by individuals with diabetes should be restricted. Total fat should comprise less than 30% of total calories, and the amount of cholesterol should be less than 300 mg/day.

People with diabetes have higher levels of plasma cholesterol and triglycerides and lower levels of high-density lipoproteins than do nondiabetic control populations. A diet low in total fat, saturated fat, and cholesterol consistent with that recommended by the American Heart Association[11] (see Chapter 21 on treatment of lipid disorders) has been recommended for individuals with diabetes to help decrease this risk for coronary heart disease.[8] Although the effectiveness of these recommendations in reducing the incidence and severity of cardiovascular complications in individuals with diabetes has not been established, they are felt to be appropriate.

In recent years, studies have demonstrated that some saturated fatty acids (stearic acid and medium-chain triglycerides) do not increase serum cholesterol levels[72,73] and that some unsaturated fatty acids ("trans" fatty acids found in hydrogenated products[74] do not help to lower them. As with carbohydrates, different types of fatty acids appear to exert variable effects. However, research has not yet evolved to the point that permits formulation of clear changes in dietary recommendations. Eventually we may be able to make such recommendations and reformulate products on the basis of an understanding of which fatty acids elevate serum cholesterol levels and which lower them. For the present, reducing total dietary fat is still of primary importance, with a particular emphasis being placed on reducing total saturated fats.

Alternative Sweeteners

Both nutritive and non-nutritive sweeteners are acceptable in diabetes management (Table 24–10).

Sucrose, glucose, and foods containing large amounts of the two refined sugars have been restricted in various dietary approaches as a means of limiting excursions of blood glucose and, more recently, of limiting calories in the overweight person. Consequently, alternative sweeteners, both caloric (fructose, sorbitol, mannitol, xylitol, hydrogenated starch hydrolysates) and noncaloric (saccharin, aspartame, and acesulfame K) (Table 24–10), play a dominant role in providing sweetness to the diabetic diet, much as they do for those without diabetes. Various surveys have shown that a high percentage of

Table 24-10. Available Alternative Sweeteners

Caloric	Non-caloric
Fructose	Saccharin
Sugar alcohols	Aspartame
Sorbitol*	Acesulfame K
Mannitol*	
Xylitol*	
Hydrogenated starch hydrolysates*	

*Used primarily in food production.

individuals desire sweetness in their diet, use alternative sweeteners, and feel that the sweeteners help them adhere to their diet.[75,76] But, there is little scientific evidence supporting these beliefs. It is not known whether alternative sweeteners contribute to better diabetes control and are beneficial for weight reduction in Type II diabetes. Because persons with diabetes may ingest larger amounts of alternative sweeteners than do the general public, issues of side effects, safety, and risk are extremely important. None of the available sweeteners is "ideal" in the sense of its not being associated with any disadvantages. The American Diabetes Association finds these sweeteners acceptable in treatment[8] but has recommended that the characteristics, advantages, and disadvantages of each be known and that their use be adjusted accordingly. For example, aspartame has no bitter aftertaste, which saccharin has for some, but cannot be heated without losing sweetness. Neither aspartame or saccharin provides the "bulk" needed in some products for proper texture. An alternative such as fructose provides bulk but also adds calories. Fortunately, consumers can pick and choose, obtaining the best compromise or fit for their own needs.

As has been discussed earlier, in recent years many have questioned whether the avoidance of sucrose really facilitates metabolic control. However, most clinicians and health professionals advocate some degree of limitation of sucrose, if only to decrease the incidence of dental caries, as is recommended for the population at large.

Caloric Sweeteners

The caloric sweeteners provide 4 calories/g. The alternatives to sucrose include fructose and the sugar alcohols.

Fructose. Fructose (levulose or fruit sugar) is a common monosaccharide in nature that is found in its free form in honey, fruits, and other plants and in a combined form as half of the disaccharide sucrose. It is one of the sweetest of the naturally occurring sugars, being 1.0 to 1.8 times sweeter than sucrose,[77] although the sweetness varies with the tasting medium. It tastes sweetest when in a cool, dilute, and slightly acidic medium. In some food applications caloric savings can be realized through the use of fructose but not on the order of the savings gained through the use of noncaloric sweeteners. There are no data supporting the use of fructose in weight reduction. Fructose leads to lower acute glycemic excursions than those produced by glucose, sucrose, high-fructose corn syrups, or even many complex carbohydrates.[45,78-80] However, in the setting of severe insulin deprivation and/or fasting levels of glucose lower than 200 mg/dL, fructose can produce a considerable increase in plasma glucose levels.

Recent longer-term studies of the effects of moderate intake of fructose have noted no adverse effects of such use on mean levels of glucose and insulin in patients with NIDDM or IDDM.[46,81-86] The main concern about fructose has been about its potential for increasing triglyceride levels.[82,83,87,88] In some susceptible NIDDM subjects, particularly those with increased hepatic synthesis and secretion of VLDL triglycerides, fructose can cause a dramatic increase in insulin levels and thus exacerbate the hypertriglyceridemia, indicating that fructose may be potentially harmful in the presence of pre-existing marked hypertriglyceridemia.[86,87]

Xylitol, Sorbitol, Mannitol, and Hydrogenated Starch Hydrolysates. Xylitol, sorbitol, mannitol, and hydrogenated starch hydrolysates are sugar alcohols, which like other sugars contain 4 calories/g but are absorbed more slowly and elicit less of a rise in blood glucose levels than sugars such as sucrose and glucose.[89,90] Slow absorption constitutes the main drawback to the use of sugar alcohols because it can cause osmotic diarrhea when these substances are ingested in larger quantities (>30 to 50 g).

Noncaloric Sweeteners

Saccharin. Saccharin is a synthetic sweetener some 300 to 400 times sweeter than sucrose and without caloric value. It is not metabolized or stored in humans. Concern about the carcinogenic potential of saccharin has lingered for years, although reviews of the literature have yielded little that can justify governmental restriction.[91] The issue hinges on the Delaney Clause of the Food and Drug Act, which does not allow assessment of quantitative risk. While those with diabetes could be at greater risk for any adverse effects because of their potentially larger intake, there appears to be little justification for restricting the reasonable use of saccharin.[92]

Acesulfame K. Acesulfame K (acesulfame potassium) is a white, odorless, crystalline sweetener approximately 200 times sweeter than sucrose. It is described as having a clean, fresh taste that does not linger, but some perceive a bitter taste when it is used at very high concentrations.[93] Acesulfame K is a derivative of acetoacetic acid and has a structure somewhat similar to that of saccharin. Approved for use by the Food and Drug Administration (FDA) in 1988, it is marketed in the United States under the brand name Sunette when used as an ingredient in foods and as Sweet One when sold as a table-top sweetener. Its advantages are its remarkable stability both in liquids and during baking or cooking. It is the only sweetener currently on the market that is not required to carry some type of health or safety warning.

Aspartame. Aspartame, a protein sweetener, is the methyl ester of L-phenylalanine and L-aspartic acid and is 180 to 200 times sweeter than sucrose.[94] It was first approved for use in 1981 and is marketed as NutraSweet both in food products and as a table-top sweetener. Although it is nutritive, containing 4 calories/g, so little is used to confer sweetness that it is effectively a noncaloric sweetener and is so classed. Aspartame does not alter glycemic control in individuals with diabetes.[95] The main concerns about its use have been those of safety, which is felt to be no different for individuals with and without diabetes. A variety of safety concerns about aspartame have been raised. For example, it has been suggested that mild nonspecific symptoms, such as headaches, dizziness or menstrual irregularities, are associated with its ingestion, that the byproducts of metabolism (methanol and diketopiperazine) are toxic, that it might alter brain neurotransmitter activity and thus result in functional or behavioral changes, that it might lead to brain tumors or neurotoxicity, or that prolonged heating would produce denatured molecular forms that might be harmful.[96] Despite these concerns, aspartame has repeatedly been determined to be safe for both the general public and people with diabetes.[97]

Sodium

Sodium intake should be restricted to 1000 mg/1000 kcal, not to exceed 3000 mg/day, to minimize symptoms of hypertension. Severe sodium restriction, however, may be harmful for persons whose diabetes is poorly controlled or have postural hypotension or fluid imbalance.

Concern about sodium intake is primarily directed at individuals with congestive heart failure or hypertension or who are susceptible to its development. Since people with diabetes are frequently hypertensive, it has been deemed prudent to make modest restrictions in their sodium intake. The degree of restriction is that recommended by the American Heart Association.[11] It should be cautioned, however, that salt can be beneficial, and thus its use should not be severely restricted in patients whose diabetes is severely out of control or who have problems with fluid balance or postural hypotension.

Alcohol

Alcohol use should be moderate and may need to be restricted entirely in persons with diabetes and insulin-induced hypoglycemia, neuropathy, poor control of blood sugar or blood lipids, or obesity.

Abstinence from alcohol is not required for adults with diabetes, but some issues regarding its use require attention. First, alcohol adds calories without nutritional benefit and has been shown to supplement rather than displace other calories.[98] In addition, restriction of calories provided by ethanol is one of the few dietary strategies positively correlated with success in weight reduction.[99] Consequently, the use of alcohol may need to be restricted in overweight persons. Second, excessive alcohol consumption by a person who is fasting or skipping meals can lead to hypoglycemia via inhibition of gluconeogenesis and may pose a serious risk for persons taking insulin or oral agents to control hyperglycemia. Intoxication can impair a person's ability to follow a prescribed management plan or to recognize symptoms of hypoglycemia and treat them appropriately.[100] Last, ingestion of alcohol may raise fasting and postprandial levels of triglycerides.[101,102] Since persons with diabetes are at increased risk for cardiovascular disease, ingestion of alcohol should be limited if the person is hypertriglyceridemic. Of course, it is also recommended that pregnant women avoid alcohol. Peripheral neuropathy is a frequent complication of diabetes, and the neuropathic effects of alcohol may be additive with those of diabetes. Therefore, on this basis as well, excessive use should be avoided in diabetic patients.

When alcohol is part of the meal plan of an individual on a weight loss regimen, fat intake should be reduced accordingly to account for the calories provided by the alcohol (7 kcal/g). In general, 2 ounces of alcohol may be consumed in addition to the meal plan if desired but should be consumed with other food.[8] The sugar content of sweetened alcoholic mixed drinks or liquors should be considered in the diabetic diet.

Vitamins and Minerals

Intake of vitamins and minerals should meet recommended levels for good health. There is no evidence that the requirements of vitamins and minerals is different in patients with and without diabetes, and supplements are unnecessary for persons with diabetes except those for whom caloric intake is exceptionally low or the variety of food intake is limited.

EDUCATIONAL STRATEGIES

Concern about diet should begin with the initial visit, when dietary habits, nutritional status, and weight history, as well as the growth and development of children, should be assessed.[103] The initial management plan should include individualized recommendations and instructions on nutrition, preferably given by a dietitian trained in diabetes care.[104] Diet education should be given continuously, and a nutritional evaluation should be made at each regular visit.

The American Association of Diabetes Educators (AADE) has provided rigid guidelines and a core curriculum for diabetes educators. Educators can now become certified by the National Certification Board for Diabetes Educators, which promotes formal recognition of health professionals who have met specific experiential and educational requirements. Those individuals are awarded certification and may add CDE (Certified Diabetes Educator) to their title.

A qualified dietitian is an important member of the health team, working with other team members to help the patient understand the relationships between nutrition, exercise, and therapy. A dietitian can gather a detailed nutritional history, including, for example, information on how often a person eats out, ethnic influences on food choices, favorite foods, diets followed in the past, and usual eating patterns. Nutritional status, energy expenditure, and dietary needs can be assessed. A dietitian can estimate caloric needs and develop an appropriate meal plan adjusted to an individual's lifestyle, activity level, food preferences, type of diabetes,

medicines, and other dietary restrictions. Consideration of these individual dietary, sociocultural, economic, and life-style characteristics and the involvement of the person with diabetes in devising the diet plan are considered critical to success.[104] The dietitian can also instruct and counsel the patient and family members about other aspects of nutritional care, such as sick-day food management, eating away from home, and strategies for coping with different eating situations for children, teenagers, or adults. Behavioral modification techniques often are used. Regrettably, a great disparity has been noted between knowledge about the benefits of some educational techniques, such as behavioral modification, and their actual application by dietitians.[105] It seems trite to say, but strategies felt to be important in diet education must be used as well as known and understood.

Because behavioral change is a slow process, dietary counseling may be more effective when it provides information in small, sequential steps[106] and presents nutrition information in stages. In the first stage, basic food selection skills ("survival skills") can be taught and simplified and individualized meal plans can be developed. In later stages, more detailed information can be provided that extends and reinforces existing knowledge and will help the individual change dietary behavior. Reinforcement is necessary through continuous reviews of dietary management, evaluation of adherence to the recommended diet, provision of motivations for improving dietary behavior, and incorporation of new information into the management plan.[107] In recent years, the importance of tailoring diet programs to suit the individual's cultural framework and include traditional foods has been emphasized. It is recognized that educators must use educational techniques that are appropriate to the cultural background and literacy of the individual. The need for a variety of tools and techniques suitable for various ethnic groups or learning styles has led to the development of a wide variety of teaching tools and educational materials.[108,109]

Videotaped instruction is an example of a technique that has been found effective in providing at least initial instruction in dietary principles to patients with diabetes.[110] The use of videotapes or other methods of self-instruction can free the dietitian for other types of counseling but, of even greater importance, can augment the resources available in institutions, particularly small ones.

MEAL PLANNING

Several meal planning alternatives are available for persons with diabetes. The following are some examples.

1) Exchange lists: Exchange lists group foods into categories containing similar amounts of calories, protein, carbohydrate, and fat. The foods within each group—starch/bread, meat and substitutes, vegetables, fruits, milk, and fat—can be substituted or exchanged for each other in the prescribed amounts. The "exchange" system is used extensively in diet counseling and meal planning. Instruc-

tion and assistance from a trained dietitian is necessary to tailor the diet to the individual's needs and to assess the individual's understanding of what constitutes a proper diet.[111]

2) Dietary guidelines, such as *Dietary Guidelines for Americans*.[112]

3) Counting systems that control caloric intake and/or glucose consumption.

4) Sample menus designed by a dietitian for the specific needs of individuals.[113]

Any of these methods can be appropriate for any given individual, but development of an individual meal plan requires that the patient be educated in both the principles of good nutrition and their effective implementation.

Improved overall management of diabetes reduces hospitalizations and other personal and economic costs. But for persons with diabetes to achieve these benefits, their self-care must be optimal. The quality of self-care will depend on their having the necessary knowledge and a supportive environment. Education of persons with diabetes often is associated with improvement in their self-care skills, dietary adherence, and control of blood glucose and blood lipid levels.[114–116] Such changes can result in cost savings greater than the costs of the educational program.[117] However, traditional educational approaches to effecting dietary change can often be ineffectual or achieve only temporary change.[118–120] The possible reasons for this failure are outlined in Table 24–11.[121] Intensive educational approaches can achieve better dietary compliance and improvements in total cholesterol levels but may not necessarily improve glycemic control.[114] Although intensive education helps, it does not need to be complex; simplified instruction can often be as effective as the more-complex traditional approaches.[114]

Table 24-11. Major Deterrents to Successful Diet Therapy

1. Failure to understand that elevated blood glucose levels are frequently associated with obesity and that attainment and maintenance of desirable body weight is one main and profoundly beneficial objective in treatment of Type II diabetes
2. Failure to determine appropriate diet prescription
3. Failure to use appropriately trained dietitians for counseling
4. Use of old, incomplete, or inappropriate diet materials for individual needs
5. Failure to adapt diet to individual's life-style and other needs
6. Failure to change patient's behavior because of inadequate education or follow-up care
7. Failure to understand magnitude and number of obstacles to be overcome in achieving results
8. Failure to adapt teaching techniques to individuals
9. Confusion about dietary goals, strategies, and priorities for individual patients
10. Uncertainty about influence of diet on blood glucose and lipid levels
11. Limited educational programs because of economic factors, including lack of third-party coverage for good counseling programs

Table is adapted from Davidson.[12]

The acknowledged problem with dietary noncompliance emphasizes the importance of an understanding of dietary management goals and methods by both the patient and the health-care team.[105] Although physicians may perceive dietary noncompliance as the patient's fault, persons with diabetes report that their compliance depends on environmental factors such as family, job, economic status, or physiologic factors such as visual and ambulation problems that interfere with food purchase and/or preparation.[16] An understanding of these different perceptions can help provide a broad basis of support for individuals with diabetes that enables them to assume greater responsibility for their own care.[122]

Because of the need for support and expertise on a variety of fronts, coordinated multidisciplinary programs of outpatient education that intimately involve the patient and his or her family are frequently the most effective setting for education.[123] The lack of third-party reimbursement for such programs, however, has hindered their development. While the availability of third-party reimbursement for comprehensive education and dietitian services is improving, the fit between the needs of people with diabetes and the provision and reimbursement of services is still not optimal. Health-care providers and patients must demand both quality care and third-party reimbursement for educational services.[122]

SPECIAL CONSIDERATIONS FOR DIETARY MANAGEMENT IN THE ELDERLY

As persons age, greater attention needs to be paid to their nutritional status and to dietary recommendations and advice. The provision of optimal nutrition for the elderly is a major concern,[124] even without the complicating presence of diabetes. Unfortunately, the nutritional needs of the elderly and particularly of the elderly with diabetes have not been well evaluated.[124] Only in recent years has this problem drawn the special attention it deserves. Nevertheless, the health-care provider who takes into consideration the changes occurring with age can vastly improve the care given to the elderly patient.

In general, the elderly have a higher percentage of body fat, a lower lean body mass, and a lower caloric requirement. The extent of the decrease in caloric needs is to some extent dependent on health status and continuance of activity levels. Currently, the nutrient requirements recommended for those over 51 years of age are extrapolated from the needs of younger individuals, but efforts are being made to correct this lack in specific data for the elderly.[69]

The eating patterns in the elderly can be significantly influenced by the many physical, mental, and emotional factors that affect them.[125] Impaired vision, smell, hearing, and/or taste, decreasing dexterity and memory, loneliness and depression, dental problems, illness and use of many medications, limited financial resources, and problems of mobility and transportation can all cause problems with eating. Poor teeth and gums or ill-fitting dentures are widespread problems in the elderly and commonly lead to their consumption of softer foods high in sugar and fat. Foods containing greater amounts of fiber, such as fresh fruits and vegetables or whole-grain cereals or breads, can be more difficult for them to chew. Depression and physical limitations can limit their access to food or ability to prepare it.

All of these factors contribute to the increased difficulties that the elderly person has in coping with the many demands imposed by diabetes and make the job of the health-care team even more challenging. Perhaps among no other patients is the consideration of the uniqueness of each individual more essential.

The important first step in nutritional management for the elderly patient is the thorough assessment of all factors that affect nutrition.[126] Obtaining necessary information from some elderly persons may be difficult because of their short attention spans or poor short-term memory. Older persons may not be able to recall their diet clearly enough to provide the educator with the information necessary for making appropriate dietary recommendations, and some elderly patients may present even more severe deficits in mental capacity.

Calories—both too many and too few—are of primary importance in the elderly. In the obese elderly, caloric restriction and weight reduction will usually help in diabetes management but can be more difficult to accomplish than in younger patients because of decreasing caloric needs. Desirable body weight, rather than ideal body weight, should usually be established as the goal. On the other hand, the elderly may have difficulty obtaining adequate calories. Decreased mobility and transportation complexities can limit the ability of elderly persons to shop for or transport food and may make it difficult for them to prepare it. Episodes of recurrent hypoglycemia in drug-treated elderly patients can be a result of their inability to get enough or appropriate food after injecting the day's insulin dose or ingesting oral medication.

Unfortunately, evaluation of both the optimal levels of macro- and micronutrients and the ideal body composition for elderly persons, particularly for the diabetic elderly, has been neglected, and their requirements remain uncertain. It does appear, however, that requirements for most nutrients either go up or stay stable but do not decrease. Thus, despite the decreasing energy needs (decreased activity, decreased metabolic rates, and thus decreased caloric needs), the elderly person must ingest the same or perhaps slightly more nutrients than may be necessary for younger individuals with higher caloric needs. This situation emphasizes the importance of foods of high nutrient density in the diets of the elderly. The potential for deficiencies means that the use of vitamin or mineral supplementation should be considered. Two micronutrients are often discussed in relationship to diabetes and aging. A role for chromium deficiency in the pathogenesis of diabetes in the elderly has been claimed, and zinc deficiency in a subset of Type II patients has been noted.[127,128] Evidence to support the use of chromium to treat established diabetes is weak, and zinc supplementation does not lower the blood glucose response to a glucose load.[129]

Once therapeutic decisions are made and the time comes for educating the patient, the educator may need extra time and patience because some patients may have difficulty remembering even simple verbal instructions. Educational sessions may need to be short and frequent, and all diet advice may need to be provided in simple written form in large print.[125] In addition, it is necessary to remember that visual acuity is highly involved in food selection and preparation. Elderly patients may have trouble reading labels on food or on grocery store shelves and may not be able to find the foods they are told to purchase. Thus, they may continue to buy foods they are familiar with or can locate easily.

In general, it is probably best to keep the diabetic diet regimen of the elderly simple. The maintenance of normoglycemia may not be realistic for some. Nutritional goals should aim at the provision of simple, balanced, consistent meals that fit long-standing eating habits, life-style, and the physical and psychological needs of the individual. Trying to change long-standing food habits by imposing new, rigid, and/or complicated meal plans may not be successful. On the other hand, many elderly have the time and interest to get highly involved in their diabetes management and will eagerly follow instructions when given the necessary support and information.

Last, financial difficulties and social isolation of the elderly and the dietary problems they create cannot be neglected. The counselor needs to be sensitive to these needs and be prepared with useful suggestions. Since many communities have a variety of support services for elderly citizens, all health professionals should be familiar with the resources and services available and assist elderly patients in utilizing these programs.

DIABETES AND PREGNANCY

In general, the basic dietary recommendations for a normal pregnancy are used as the foundation of guidelines for the management of diabetes in pregnancy. The nutritional requirements of a diabetic pregnancy are felt to be essentially the same as those of a nondiabetic pregnancy. In addition, pregnancy does not significantly change the basic tenets of dietary management of diabetes, although it does magnify the importance of adherence to management principles. The remarkable decreases in the morbidity and mortality rates among infants born to women with diabetes since the 1920s[130] are thought to be due, in large part, to the emphasis that has been placed on rigid control of maternal glucose levels throughout the course of pregnancy and on the avoidance of ketonuria.

Dietary deprivation—through either the skipping of meals or a substantial limitation in carbohydrate intake—in the later half of pregnancy can cause a more rapid and severe mobilization of fat and resultant increases in the formation of ketones,[131] a more rapid and greater decrease in levels of blood glucose and amino acids, and an increase in intrahepatic gluconeogenesis. The drop in blood glucose levels can progress to frank fasting hypoglycemia. Because of this risk, the use of an evening snack and the maintenance of carbohydrate intake at an adequate level must be carefully considered. However, many find that the higher carbohydrate levels recommended for nonpregnant diabetics may not be consistent with the requirements for the rigid control of blood glucose during pregnancy. Consequently, levels of carbohydrate of 30 to 40% of total caloric intake are often recommended.[132,133]

Whether obese, pregnant women should restrict caloric intake is controversial, and the use of such diets has been approached with caution. Both obesity and diabetes significantly increase the risk for perinatal complications. Caloric restriction in obese pregnant women has raised concern both because low weight gain during pregnancy is associated with poor pregnancy outcome and because the risk of ketonemia may be more exaggerated in these individuals. Nevertheless, some centers have used caloric restriction with no reported ill effects.[134,135] In general, however, obese, diabetic pregnant women should not be on weight-reduction diets unless they are managed by teams experienced in the careful monitoring and other procedures necessary to safety.

There is little, if any, evidence of any adverse effects of the use of the sweeteners saccharin[136] or aspartame[137] during pregnancy. However, since saccharin can cross the placental barrier in small concentrations and is cleared slowly from fetal circulation and because of concerns about the possible effects on pregnancy of altered amounts of the constituents of aspartame—aspartic acid, phenylalanine, and methanol—some clinicians have recommended that use of these sweeteners during pregnancy be curtailed. Since individuals with diabetes may ingest larger-than-average quantities of these sweeteners, this concern needs to be addressed carefully. Nutrition science as it relates to the diabetic diet is a rapidly growing and dynamic field, and what is considered sound practice today may not be so tomorrow.

CHILDREN AND ADOLESCENTS

Food and feeding issues are very important in the physical and psychological growth of children. Diet education must be approached differently and be responsive to each child, his or her developmental stage, and family dynamics. The child with diabetes is adding the complexities of balancing food, insulin, and activity to the already demanding needs of physical maturation and psychological, social, and cultural development. Dietary recommendations must be carefully adapted to these needs. Adolescents with diabetes likewise face unique challenges. At a time when they are attempting to separate from and become independent of parents and authority, they must follow management routines frequently in conflict with this need as well as their need to attain peer uniformity. Special attention must be paid to these needs in order to achieve the young person's maximal cooperation with dietary management.

For the child with diabetes, frequent assessment of diet and careful monitoring of growth are necessary. Nutritional assessment should include the regular plotting of height and weight measurement on standard growth grids in an effort to detect any shift in growth velocity.[138] Meal plans will need to be adjusted on a regular basis to account for changes in growth rate and activity. There can be wide seasonal variation in caloric needs as children change activity patterns from school to vacation and from periods of sports activity to lulls between seasons. The meal plan needs to be flexible enough to permit adjustment of calories on a daily basis as well as to changes in activities. The needs of the patient and family must be the guide for nutritional treatment.

Educators need to be especially attuned to parental concerns such as having their child eat appropriate foods at appropriate times and handling events such as parties and holidays. When the child reaches adolescence, special attention must be given to his or her need to not appear different from peers. At that time, the youth needs special attention and support to help adjust meal plans to changes in eating times and variety of foods. The educator can help adolescents with choices in these areas that will enable them to maintain control without appearing different from their peers. The use of self-monitoring of blood glucose fortunately provides a means by which greater flexibility in diet can be achieved.

The child and his or her parents must be able to integrate nutritional treatment into their lives and to manipulate it in response to rapidly changing developmental needs. Dietitians with advanced training in diabetes management are essential in promoting an educational process that will ensure this flexibility.

SUMMARY

Although a great deal of new information has been generated to improve our ability to manage diabetes more effectively through dietary means, we do not have final answers about what constitutes the "ultimate" dietary maneuvers. It is therefore important for the clinician to stay abreast of new knowledge and to be willing to try new approaches to dietary management of diabetes.

REFERENCES

1. Wood FC Jr, Bierman EL. New concepts in diabetic dietetics. Nutr Today 1972;7(3):4–12.
2. Mann JI. Diet and diabetes. Diabetologia 1980;18:89–95.
3. Rabinowitch IM. Effects of the high carbohydrate-low calorie diet upon carbohydrate tolerance in diabetes mellitus. Can Med Assoc J 1935;33:136–44.
4. Himsworth HP. The dietetic factor determining the glucose tolerance and sensitivity to insulin of healthy men. Clin Sci 1935;2:67–94.
5. Glick SM. Diet for diabetic patients [Letter]. N Engl J Med 1971;285;58.
6. Brunzell JD, Lerner RL, Hazzard WR, et al. Improved glucose tolerance with high carbohydrate feeding in mild diabetes. N Engl J Med 1971;284:521–4.
7. Anderson JW, Herman RH, Zakim D. Effect of high glucose and high sucrose diets on glucose tolerance of normal men. Am J Clin Nutr 1973;26:600–7.
8. American Diabetes Association. Nutritional recommendations and principles for individuals with diabetes mellitus: 1986. Diabetes Care 1987;10:126–32.
9. Joslin EP. The treatment of diabetes mellitus. 9th ed. Philadelphia: Lea & Febiger, 1952.

10. U.S. Department of Health and Human Services. The Surgeon General's report on nutrition and health. Washington, DC: U.S. Government Printing Office, 1988.

11. American Heart Association. The American Heart Association diet—an eating plan for healthy Americans [#51-018-B(SA)]. Dallas: American Heart Association, 1985.

12. Butrum RR, Clifford CK, Lanza E. NCI dietary guidelines: rationale. Am J Clin Nutr 1988;48(Suppl 3):888–95.

13. Henry RR, Schaeffer L, Olefsky JM. Glycemic effects of intensive caloric restriction and isocaloric refeeding in non-insulin-dependent diabetes mellitus. J Clin Endocrinol Metab 1985;61;917–25.

14. Hughes TA, Gwynne JT, Switzer BR, et al. Effects of caloric restriction and weight loss on glycemic control, insulin release and resistance, and atherosclerotic risk in obese patients with Type II diabetes mellitus. Am J Med 1984;77:7–17.

15. Henry RR, Wallace P, Olefsky JM. Effects of weight loss on mechanisms of hyperglycemia in obese non-insulin-dependent diabetes mellitus. Diabetes 1986;35:990–8.

16. Vinik A, Wing RR. Nutritional management of the person with diabetes. In: Rifkin H, Porte D Jr, eds. Diabetes mellitus. 4th ed. New York: Elsevier, 1990.

17. Thomas AE, McKay DA, Cutlip MB. A nomograph method for assessing body weight. Am J Clin Nutr 1976;29:302–4.

18. Brunzell JD, Lerner RL, Porte D Jr, Bierman EL. Effect of a fat free, high carbohydrate diet on diabetic subjects with fasting hyperglycemia. Diabetes 1974;23:138–42.

19. Thompson RG, Hayford JT, Danney MM. Glucose and insulin responses to diet. Effect of variations in source and amount of carbohydrate. Diabetes 1974;27:1020–6.

20. Reaven GM. How high the carbohydrate [Editorial]. Diabetologia 1980;18:409–13.

21. Jarrett RJ. More about carbohydrates [Letter]. Diabetologia 1981;21:427–8.

22. Rivellese AA, Giacco R, Genovese S, et al. Effects of changing amount of carbohydrate in diet on plasma lipoproteins and apolipoproteins in Type II diabetic patients. Diabetes Care 1990;13:446–8.

23. Coulston AM, Holenbeck CB Swislock ALM, et al. Deleterious metabolic effects of high-carbohydrate, sucrose-containing diets in patients with non-insulin-dependent diabetes mellitus. Am J Med 1987;82:213–20.

24. Rivellese A, Riccard G, Giacco A, et al. Effect of dietary fibre on glucose control and serum lipoproteins in diabetic patients. Lancet 1980;2:447–50.

25. O'Dea K, Traianedes K, Ireland P, et al. The effects of diet differing in fat, carbohydrate, and fiber on carbohydrate and lipid metabolism in Type II diabetes. J Am Diet Assoc 1989;89:1076–86.

26. Otto H, et al. In: Otto H, Spaethe R, eds. Diabetetik bei Diabetes Mellitus. Hamburg: Verlag Hans Huber, 1973:41.

27. Crapo PA, Reaven G, Olefsky J. Postprandial plasma-glucose and -insulin responses to different carbohydrates. Diabetes 1977;26:1178–83.

28. Crapo PA, Insel J, Sperling M, Kolterman OG. Comparison of serum glucose, insulin, and glucagon responses to different types of complex carbohydrate in noninsulin-dependent diabetic patients. Am J Clin Nutr 1981;34:184–90.

29. Jenkins DJA, Wolever TM, Taylor RH, et al. Glycemic index of foods: a physiological basis for carbohydrate exchange. Am J Clin Nutr 1981;34:362–6.

30. Jenkins DJA, Wolever TMS, Jenkins AL, et al. The glycemic index of foods tested in diabetic patients: a new basis for carbohydrate exchange favouring the use of legumes. Diabetologia 1983;24:257–64.

31. Jenkins DJA. Lente carbohydrate: a newer approach to the dietary management of diabetes. Diabetes Care 1982;5:634–41.

32. Collier GR, Wolever TMS, Wong GS, Josse RG. Prediction of glycemic response to mixed meals in noninsulin-dependent diabetic subjects. Am J Clin Nutr 1986;44:349–52.

33. Bornet FRJ, Costagliola D, Rizkalla SW, et al. Insulinemic and glycemic indexes of six starch rich foods taken alone and in a mixed meal by type 2 diabetics. Am J Clin Nutr 1987;45:588–95.

34. Wolever TMS, Nuttall FQ, Lee R, et al. Prediction of the relative blood glucose response of mixed meals using the white bread glycemic index. Diabetes Care 1985;8:418–28.

35. Cohen C, Wylie-Rosett J, Shamoon, H. Insulin response and glycemic effects of meals in non-insulin-dependent diabetes. Am J Clin Nutr 1990;52:519–23.

36. Coulston AM, Hollenbeck CB, Swislocki ALM, Reaven GM. Effect of source of dietary carbohydrate on plasma glucose and insulin responses to mixed meals in subjects with NIDDM. Diabetes Care 1987;10:395–400.

37. Laine DC, Thomas W, Levitt MD, Bantle JP. Comparison of predictive capabilities of diabetic exchange lists and glycemic index of foods. Diabetes Care 1987;10:38–94.

38. Kinmonth A-L, Angus RM, Jenkins PA, et al. Whole foods and increased dietary fibre improve blood glucose control in diabetic children. Arch Dis Child 1982;57:187–94.

39. Jenkins DJA, Woleer TMS, Collier GR, et al. Metabolic effects of a low-glycemic-index diet. Am J Clin Nutr 1987;46:968–75.

40. Jenkins DJA, Wolever TMS, Kalmusky J, et al. Low glycemic index carbohydrate foods in the management of hyperlipidemia. Am J Clin Nutr 1985;42:604–17.

41. Chiasson J-L, LaFrance L, Poisson D, Ducros F. The effect of the glycemic index of the diet on insulin requirement during intensive insulin therapy in IDDM [Abstract no. 187]. Diabetes 1990;39(Suppl 1):47A.

42. Gulliford MC, Bicknell EJ, Scarpello JH. Differential effect of protein and fat ingestion on blood glucose responses to high and low-glycemic-index carbohydrates in noninsulin-dependent diabetic subjects. Am J Clin Nutr 1989;50:773–7.

43. National Institutes of Health. Consensus development conference on diet and exercise in non-insulin-dependent diabetes mellitus. Diabetes Care 1987;10:639–44.

44. American Diabetes Association. Glycemic effects of carbohydrates. Diabetes Care 1984;7:607–8.

45. Lenner RA. Specially designed sweeteners and food for diabetics: a real need? Am J Clin Nutr 1976;29:726–33.

46. Bantle JP, Laine DC, Thomas JW. Metabolic effects of dietary fructose and sucrose in types I and II diabetic subjects. JAMA 1986;256:3241–6.

47. Jellish WS, Emanuele MA, Abraira C. Graded sucrose/carbohydrate diets in overtly hypertriglyceridemic diabetic patients. Am J Med 1984;77:1015–22.

48. Emanuele MA, Abraira C, Jellish WS, DeBartolo M. A cross-over trial of high and low sucrose-carbohydrate diets in Type II diabetics with hypertriglyceridemia. J Am Coll Nutr 1986;5:429–37.

49. Peterson DB, Lambert J, Gerring S, et al. Sucrose in the diet of diabetic patients—just another carbohydrate? Diabetologia 1986;29:216–20.

50. Wise JE, Keim KS, Huisinga JL, Willmann PA. Effect of sucrose-containing snacks on blood glucose control. Diabetes Care 1989;12:423–6.

51. Porta M, Pigino M, Minonne A, Guidetti LM. Moderate amounts of sucrose with mixed meals do not impair metabolic control in patients with Type II (non-insulin-dependent diabetes). Diabetes Nutr Metab 1989;2:133–7.

52. Colagiuri S, Miller JJ, Edwards RA. Metabolic effects of adding sucrose and aspartame to the diet of subjects with noninsulin-dependent diabetes mellitus. Am J Clin Nutr 1989;50:474–8.

53. Loghmani E, Rickard K, Washburne L, et al. Glycemic response to sucrose in the daily diets of children with IDDM [Abstract no. 184]. Diabetes 1990;39(Suppl 1):46A.

54. Peters AL, Davidson MB, Eisenberg K. Effect of isocaloric substitution of chocolate cake for potato in Type I diabetic patients. Diabetes Care 1990;13:888–92.

55. Anderson JW, Ward K. Long-term effects of high-carbohydrate, high-fiber diets on glucose and lipid metabolism: a preliminary report on patients with diabetes. Diabetes Care 1978;1:77–82.

56. Anderson JW. The role of dietary carbohydrate and fiber in the control of diabetes. Adv Intern Med 1980;26:67–96.

57. Anderson JW, Chen WL. Plant fiber: carbohydrate and lipid metabolism. Am J Clin Nutr 1979;32:346–63.

58. Wheeler ML, ed. Fiber and the patient with diabetes mellitus: a summary and annotated bibliography. Chicago: American Dietetic Association, 1983.

59. Vahouny GV. Conclusions and recommendations of the symposium "Dietary Fibers in Health and Disease," Washington, DC, 1981. Am J Clin Nutr 1982;35:152–6.

60. Jenkins DJA, Wolever TM, Jenkins AL, et al. Glycemic response to wheat products: reduced response to pasta but no effect of fiber. Diabetes Care 1983;6:155–9.

61. McMurry JF Jr, Baumgardner B. A high-wheat bran diet in insulin-treated diabetes mellitus: assessment with the artificial pancreas. Diabetes Care 1984;7:211–4.

62. Hall SEH, Bolton TM, Hetenyi G Jr. The effect of bran on glucose kinetics and plasma insulin in non-insulin-dependent diabetes mellitus. Diabetes Care 1980;3:520–5.

63. Wolever TMS. Relationship between dietary fiber content and composition in foods and the glycemic index. Am J Clin Nutr 1990;51:72–5.

64. Monnier L, Pham TC, Aguirre L, et al. Influence of indigestible fibers on glucose tolerance. Diabetes Care 1978;1:83–8.

65. Jefferys DB. The effect of dietary fibre on the response to orally administered glucose [Abstract]. Proc Nutr Soc 1974;33:11A–12.

66. Anderson JW, Tietyen-Clark J. Dietary fiber: hyperlipidemia, hypertension, and coronary heart disease. Am J Gastroenterol 1986;81:907–19.

67. Anderson JW, Gustafson NJ, Bryant CA, Tietyen-Clark J. Dietary fiber and diabetes: a comprehensive review and practical application. J Am Diet Assoc 1987;87:1189–97.

68. O'Dea K, Nestel PJ, Antonoff L. Physical factors influencing postprandial glucose and insulin responses to starch. Am J Clin Nutr 1980;33:760–5.

69. National Research Council. Recommended dietary allowance. 10th ed. Requirements established under the guidelines of 9th ed, 1980. Washington, DC: National Academic Press, 1989.

70. Cahill GF Jr. Starvation in man. N Engl J Med 1970;282:668–75.

71. Evanoff GV, Thompson CS, Brown J, Weinman EJ. The effect of dietary protein restriction on the progression of diabetic nephropathy: a 12-month follow-up. Arch Intern Med 1987;147:492–5.

72. Bonanome A, Grundy SM. Effect of dietary stearic acid on plasma cholesterol and lipoprotein levels. N Engl J Med 1988;318:1244–8.

73. Johnson RC, Cotter R. Metabolism of medium-chain triglyceride lipid emulsion. Nutr Int 1986;2:150.

74. Mensink RP, Katan MB. Effect of dietary trans fatty acids on high-density and low-density lipoprotein cholesterol levels in healthy subjects. N Engl J Med 1990;323:439–45.

75. Court JM. Diet in the management of diabetes; why have special diabetic foods? Med J Aust 1976;1:841–3.

76. Mehnert H. Zuckeraustauschstoffe in der Diabetesdiat. In: Ritzel G, Brubacher G, eds. Monosaccharides and polyalcohols in nutrition, therapy and dietetics. Bern: Huber, 1976.

77. Moskowitz HR. The psychology of sweetness. In: Sipple HL, McNutt KW, eds. Sugars in nutrition. New York: Academic Press, 1974:37–64.

78. Bohannon NV, Karam JH, Forsham PH. Advantages of fructose ingestion (FTT) over sucrose (STT) and glucose (GTT) in humans [Abstract no. 31]. Diabetes 1978;27(Suppl 2):438.

79. Lamar CP. Comparative oral glucose and fructose tolerance tests in normal subjects and in diabetic patients. J Fla Med Assoc 1959;46:180–6.

80. Crapo PA, Kolterman OG, Olefsky JM. Effects of oral fructose in normal, diabetic, and impaired glucose tolerance subjects. Diabetes Care 1980;3:575–82.

81. Anderson JW, Story LJ, Zettwoch NC, et al. Metabolic effects of fructose supplementation in diabetic individuals. Diabetes Care 1989;12:337–44.

82. Crapo PA, Kolterman OG, Henry RR. Metabolic consequence of two-week fructose feeding in diabetic subjects. Diabetes Care 1986;9:111–9.

83. Grigoresco C, Rizkalla SW, Halfon P, et al. Lack of detectable deleterious effects on metabolic control of daily fructose ingestion for 2 months in NIDDM patients. Diabetes Care 1988;11:546–50.

84. McPherson JD, Shilton BH, Walton DJ. Role of fructose in glycation and cross-linking of proteins. Biochemistry 1988;27:1901–7.

85. Osei K, Falko J, Bossetti BM, Holland GC. Metabolic effects of fructose as a natural sweetener in the physiologic meals of ambulatory obese patients with Type II diabetes. Am J Med 1987;83:249–55.

86. Thorburn AW, Crapo PA, Griver K, et al. Long-term effects of dietary fructose on carbohydrate metabolism in non-insulin-dependent diabetes mellitus. Metabolism 1990;39:58–63.

87. Thorburn AW, Crapo PA, Beltz WF, et al. Lipid metabolism in non-insulin-dependent diabetes: effects of long-term treatment with fructose-supplemented mixed meals. Am J Clin Nutr 1989;50:1015–22.

88. Hallfrisch J, Reiser S, Prather ES. Blood lipid distribution of hyperinsulinemic men consuming three levels of fructose. Am J Clin Nutr 1983;37:740–8.

89. Adcock LH, Gray CH. The metabolism of sorbitol in the human subject. Biochem J 1957;65:554–60.

90. Wheeler ML, Fineberg SE, Gibson R, Fineberg N. Metabolic response to oral challenge of hydrogenated starch hydrolysate versus glucose in diabetes. Diabetes Care 1990;13:733–40.

91. Food and Drug Administration. Cancer Assessment Committee Report. Washington, DC: U.S. Government Printing Office, FDA docket no. 82F–0320, 1984.

92. American Diabetes Association. Policy statement: saccharin. Diabetes Care 1978;1:209.

93. Lipinski GWV. The new intense sweetener acesulfame-K. Food Chemistry 1985;16:259–69.

94. Mazur RH. Aspartame—a sweet surprise. J Toxicol Environ Health 1976;2:243–9.

95. Nehrling JK, Kobe P, McLane MP, et al. Aspartame use by persons with diabetes. Diabetes Care 1985;8:415–7.

96. Crapo PA. Use of alternative sweeteners in diabetic diet. Diabetes Care 1988;11:174–82.

97. Council on Scientific Affairs. Aspartame: review of safety issues. JAMA 1985;254:400–2.

98. De Castro JM, Orozco S. Moderate alcohol intake and spontaneous eating patterns of humans: evidence of unregulated supplementation. Am J Clin Nutr 1990; 52:246–53.

99. Blair AJ, Booth DA, Lewis VJ, Wainwright CJ. The relative success of official and informal weight reduction techniques: retrospective correlational evidence. Psychol Health 1989;3(3):195–206.

100. American Diabetes Association. Physician's guide to insulin-dependent (Type I) diabetes: diagnosis and treatment. Alexandria, VA: American Diabetes Association, 1988.

101. Ginsberg H, Olefsky J, Farquhar JW, Reaven GM. Moderate ethanol ingestion and plasma triglyceride levels: a study in normal and hypertriglyceridemic persons. Ann Intern Med 1974;80:143–9.

102. Lieber CS. Hepatic and metabolic effects of alcohol. Gastroenterology 1966;50:119–33.

103. American Diabetes Association. Standards of medical care for patients with diabetes mellitus. Diabetes Care 1989;12:365–8.

104. Nuttall FQ, Maryniuk MD, Kaufman M. Individualized diets for diabetic patients. Ann Intern Med 1983;99:204–7.

105. Hauenstein DJ, Schiller MR, Hurley RS. Motivational techniques of dietitians counseling individuals with Type II diabetes. J Am Diet Assoc 1987;87:37–42.

106. Franz MJ, Holler H, Powers MA, et al. Exchange lists: revised 1986. J Am Diet Assoc 1987;87:28–34.

107. Franz MJ, et al, eds. Goals for diabetes education. Alexandria, VA: American Diabetes Association, 1986.

108. Diabetes Care and Education Practice Group. American Dietetic Association. Selected diabetes and nutrition education resources: for the person with diabetes. Chicago: American Dietetic Association, 1989.

109. American Dietetic Association/American Diabetes Association. Ethnic and regional food practices, A series (Mexican American, Jewish). Chicago: American Dietetic Association; Alexandria, VA: American Diabetes Association, 1989.

110. Bethea CD, Stallings SF, Wolman PG, Ingram RC. Comparison of conventional and videotaped diabetic exchange lists instruction. J Am Diet Assoc 1989;89:405–6.

111. Slowie LA. Using the new exchange lists for instructing patients with diabetes. J Am Diet Assoc 1977;70:59–61.

112. U.S. Department of Agriculture. Dietary guidelines for Americans. 3rd ed. Washington, DC: U.S. Department of Health and Human Services, Government Printing Office, 1990:273–93.

113. Green JA. Diabetes nutritional management: a need for meal planning alternatives. Diabetes Educ 1987;13:145.

114. Campbell LV, Barth R. Gosper JK, et al. Impact of intensive educational approach to dietary change in NIDDM. Diabetes Care 1990;13:841–7.

115. Mazzuca SA, Moorman NH, Wheeler ML, et al. The diabetes education study: a control trial of the effects of diabetes patient education. Diabetes Care 1986;9:1–10.

116. American Diabetes Association. Diabetes outpatient education: the evidence of cost savings. Alexandria, VA: American Diabetes Association, 1986.

117. Davidson JK, Delcher HK, Englund A. Spin-off cost benefits of expanded nutritional care. J Am Diet Assoc 1979;75:250–7.

118. Kaplan RM, Wilson DK, Hartwell SL, et al. Prospective evaluation of HDL cholesterol changes after diet and physical conditioning programs for patients with Type II diabetes mellitus. Diabetes Care 1985;8:344–8.

119. Bloomgarden ZT, Karmally W, Metzger MJ, et al. Randomized, controlled trial of diabetic patient education: improved knowledge without improved metabolic status. Diabetes Care 1987;10:263–72.

120. Scott RS, Reaven DW, Stafford JM. The effectiveness of diabetes education for non-insulin-dependent diabetic persons. Diabetes Educ 1984;1:36.

121. Davidson JK. A new look at diet therapy. Diabetes Forecast 1976;May/June:14.

122. House WC, Pendleton L, Parker L. Patients' versus physicians' attributions of reasons for diabetic patients' noncompliance with diet [Letter]. Diabetes Care 1986;9:434.

123. Conference Summary. Financing the care of diabetes mellitus in the 1990's. Diabetes Care 1990;13:1021–3.

124. Morely JE, Mooradian AD, Silver AJ, et al. Nutrition in the elderly. Ann Intern Med 1988;109:890–904.

125. Powers MA, Kohrs MB, Raimondi MP. Diabetes nutrition management for the elderly. Diabetes Educ 1983;9:26.

126. Templeton DL. Comment. Diabetes Spectrum 1989;2:179.

127. Schroeder HA, Balassa JJ, Tipton IH. Abnormal trace metals in man: chromium. J Chronic Dis 1962;15:941–64.

128. Niewoehner CB, Allen JI, Boosalis M, et al. Role of zinc supplementation in Type II diabetes mellitus. Am J Med 1986;81:63–8.

129. Greeley SJ, Taylor ML. Acute effects of a zinc supplement taken before a glucose load. J Am Coll Nutr 1988;7:137–40.

130. Freinkel N, Dooley SL, Metzger BE. Care of the pregnant woman with insulin-dependent diabetes mellitus. N Engl J Med 1985;313:96–101.

131. Metzger BE, Ravnikar V, Vileisis RA, et al. "Accelerated starvation" and the skipped breakfast in late normal pregnancy. Lancet 1982;1:588–92.

132. Pedersen J. Management of diabetic pregnancy and the newborn infant. In: Pedersen J. The pregnant diabetic and her newborn. 2nd ed. Baltimore: Williams & Wilkins, 1977:221–32.

133. Jovanovic-Peterson L, Peterson CM. Dietary manipulation as a primary treatment strategy for pregnancies complicated by diabetes. J Am Coll Nutr 1990;9:320–5.

134. Algert S, Schragg P, Hollingsworth DR. Moderate caloric restriction in obese women with gestational diabetes. Obstet Gynecol 1985;65:487–91.

135. Coetzee EJ, Jackson WPU, Berman PA. Ketonuria in pregnancy—with special reference to calorie-restricted food intake in obese diabetics. Diabetes 1980;29:177–81.

136. Pitkin RM, Reynolds WA, Filer LJ, et al. Placental transmission and fetal distribution of saccharin. Am J Obstet Gynecol 1971;111:280–6.

137. Sturtevant FM. Use of aspartame in pregnancy. Int J Fertil 1985;30(1):85–7.

138. Brink SJ. Pediatric and adolescent diabetes mellitus. Chicago: Year Book Medical Publishers, 1987.

Chapter 25

PSYCHOSOCIAL ASPECTS OF DIABETES

ALAN M. JACOBSON
STUART T. HAUSER
BARBARA J. ANDERSON
WILLIAM POLONSKY

"I'm just a normal kid who takes two shots a day."

"I worried and waited for the other shoe to fall. Once I got diabetes, I knew it would get me like it did my father."

"Diabetes has changed the way I live; I lost 30 pounds and now I eat healthy."

"My husband is so afraid of getting complications that he always keeps his sugars low so he has lots of reactions, some while he's driving. I'm afraid he'll have an unconscious reaction while he's driving with the kids."

"My daughter seems to deny the illness; she needs two shots daily but won't take them."

These comments touch on some of the varied experiences of patients and families with diabetes; no single description can summarize this diversity. Patients and families are affected by the timing and severity of the illness, its duration and complications, as well as by available social supports and methods of coping. However, whether the patient takes care of the diabetes and appears unworried or is clearly troubled and floundering, the requirements for conscientious daily self-care in regard to diet, insulin, and exercise; the need for learning detailed information critical to survival; and the threat or presence of physical complications raise a considerable

number of psychosocial issues. We will examine these issues in this chapter.

ADAPTATION TO ILLNESS

A growing number of studies[1-4] have examined psychosocial dimensions that are important determinants of health status and adaptation to illness. Three broad psychosocial factors have been identified by these studies: stressful life situations, coping ability, and social environment. Each contributes to problems and successes in the maintenance of health and the handling of chronic illness and consequently influence the adaptation to diabetes. These factors and health status interplay. For example, social environment can influence factors important to health outcome, such as adherence to the diabetic regimen. In turn, health outcomes themselves affect the patient's social supports and coping abilities. Although these factors interact, each can be considered separately for purposes of review.

Stress

Numerous reports have examined the influence of emotionally stressful experiences on health status. For example, Rahe et al.,[5] using scaled measures of life events, found that acute medical illnesses tend to occur at times of change. Other studies suggest that stressful experiences can be important etiologic factors in the pathophysiology of disabling chronic conditions, such as coronary vessel disease.[6] The course of a chronic illness such as diabetes can also be affected by stressful experiences.[7] Studies often emphasize the additive effects of multiple stressful life events. In addition to the number and intensity of these life events, their particular meaning to the individual also contributes to their ultimate influence on health status.[7-9]

Stress and Diabetes Onset

Interest in examining the role of psychological or environmental stressors in diabetes has a long history. Early reports[10] suggested that the onset of Type I diabetes may be triggered by psychological stress in a physiologically susceptible individual. Stein and Charles,[10] using retrospective documentation, found a higher prevalence of disturbances in infant feeding patterns in a small group of diabetic children than in their siblings. Since psychological stress can alter activity in the sympathetic nervous and adrenomedullary systems, elevate plasma cortisol levels, and possibly enhance the secretion of glucagon and growth hormone,[11] as well as affect immune functions,[12] a theoretically relevant set of biologic pathways are present that could mediate a relationship between psychosocial stressors and diabetes onset. Indeed, recent animal studies using the BB rat as a model of Type I diabetes indicate that an increase in environmental stress shortens the time to onset of overt diabetes mellitus.[13]

Another recent line of research has examined the role of stress as a trigger for Type II diabetes. Surwit and Feinglos[14] noted the "mounting experimental evidence of altered sympathetic nervous system activity in Type II diabetes" identified from several animal models. For example, Surwit and colleagues have demonstrated that *ob/ob* mice differ from their lean litter mates in having exaggerated blood glucose responses to environmental stressors and to the exogenous administration of epinephrine.[15-17] Other research suggests that *ob/ob* mice may have enhanced adrenergic responses to environmental stress.[18]

Research on obese but otherwise healthy men[19] shows that they exhibit an alteration in autonomic nervous system functioning, specifically a decrease in sympathetic and parasympathetic activity, associated with an increase in body fat. This finding indicates that a disordered homeostatic mechanism may exist that could promote excessive storage of energy by decreasing sympathetic activity but at the same time defend against weight gain by decreasing parasympathetic activity.

It is not clear whether these and other changes in neuroendocrine activity are causative, are related to the onset of hyperglycemia and/or hyperinsulinemia, or are simply chance findings without significance for the problem of Type II diabetes. However, this is an area in which further research may elaborate the role of stress and central nervous system control in the onset and course of Type II diabetes.

Stress and Metabolic Control

Research examining the role of psychological stress in metabolic control among patients with Type I diabetes has been extensive. These studies have suggested some interesting, albeit poorly documented, relationships between emotionally stressful experiences and the diabetic metabolic state. The earliest work of this type was performed by Hinkle and Wolf,[20] who demonstrated that stressful interviews—those that focused on personal problems and conflicts identified during prior psychotherapy sessions—usually led to decreases in blood glucose levels. The changes in blood glucose levels seemed to vary with the type of emotions elicited during these sessions. Experiences of anxiety and tension were associated with decreases in glucose levels, whereas experiences of anger and resentment were associated with increases in glucose levels. Because these authors used a case-study method, it is difficult to interpret the results of these first studies. Vandenbergh et al.,[21] using hypnotic suggestion to induce a stressful experience, also found that blood glucose levels usually dropped in response to stress. Weller et al.,[22] however, found no significant changes in glucose response to stress in patients under hypnosis. It is striking that the usual effect of these stress interviews has been a decrease in blood glucose levels, a response that contradicts the experimental effects of stress hormones on blood glucose.[23]

In the most sophisticated study of the role of short-term psychological stress on metabolic control among Type I diabetic patients, Kemmer et al.[11] found that short-term psychological stress, which was induced with mental arithmetic tasks and public-speaking experiences, did not lead to increases in blood glucose levels.

Research on the effect of psychosocial stress on levels of free fatty acids and ketone bodies has more consistently matched the hypothesized expectations. Both Vandenbergh et al.,[21] using hypnosis, and Baker et al.,[24,25] using stress from family interviews, demonstrated regular increases in fatty acids levels. Baker et al.[24,25] also reported that diabetic children with very "brittle" glycemic control and major family problems could be differentiated from both children with easily managed diabetes and children with known difficulties with regimen adherence. During stressful family interviews, plasma levels of free fatty acids in the children with extremely brittle control were more elevated and returned more slowly to a baseline level than did the levels in children from either comparison group. Baker et al. concluded that the children with brittle control experienced a direct effect of emotional state on level of free fatty acids that was not found in the other two groups. Thus, it appeared that family conflicts could induce emotional responses in a subset of diabetic children that could lead directly to recurrent ketoacidosis, regardless of regimen adherence. However, Coyne and Anderson[26,27] have pointed out that this research had methodologic problems and that nontraditional methods were used for data analysis. Furthermore, Kemmer et al.[11] failed to replicate the effect of stress on levels of ketone bodies and free fatty acids. The work of Kemmer et al., while the most experimentally sophisticated, used a random sample of Type I diabetic patients. In contrast, Baker et al.[24,25] studied specific, at-risk patients with a postulated sensitivity to stress. Further research might profitably apply more careful methods, such as those used by Kemmer et al.,[11] in special subgroups of patients who are at risk. The idea that individual differences in stress sensitivity may exist among children and adults with diabetes is further evidenced in a study by Stabler and colleagues,[28] who compared the responses of diabetic children with "Type A" behavior patterns with those of children with "Type B" behavior patterns to a psychosocial stressor. The investigators found that the Type A children had a greater blood glucose response to the psychosocial stressor than did the Type B children. In a series of studies, Type A personality has been associated with risk for cardiovascular disease. The study by Stabler et al. suggests that individuals with this behavioral pattern may also be at risk for exhibiting greater metabolic responses to psychosocial stress.

In summary, there are intriguing suggestions from initial studies of animal models of diabetes that psychosocial stress may play a role in the onset of both Type I and Type II diabetes. Laboratory research on the influence of stress on metabolic control in Type I diabetic patients has yielded mixed results when applied to random samples. The application of a research model from cardiovascular disease has provided a useful method for subtyping diabetic patients who may be at special risk for the direct psychological impact on metabolic control.[28] Although it is unclear whether psychosocial stress exerts a direct "psychosomatic" effect on the neuroendocrine regulatory mechanisms that influence metabolic control, it is quite clear that stress can influence patients' compliance behaviors in ways that lead to difficulties in metabolic control. Several studies (e.g., Peyrot and McMurray[29]) have identified such relationships. At the very least, stress has an important impact on glycemic control through its impact on patient behaviors.

Coping Ability

Individual differences in personality and coping skills influence health status and adaptation to diabetes. For example, longitudinal studies have evaluated personality traits as risk factors for later physical illness. Vaillant,[30] in a long-term follow-up study of physically healthy and successful college students, found that those students who coped best were the least likely to have major physical illnesses over a 40-year follow-up period. Thomas and McCabe[3] observed that levels of ability to cope with anxiety-producing situations predicted later development of coronary vascular disease among a group of medical students followed after 30 years. The nature of the specific influences of personality on development of disease is unclear from these reports. Personality may

influence health status by affecting health-related behaviors such as eating, smoking, and seeking health care; by predisposing to or protecting from psychiatric illness; or by affecting personal reactions to life stresses.

Bibring[8] has emphasized that patients with different personality types find different aspects of their illness upsetting and use different methods of coping with these difficulties. For example, overly dependent individuals with diabetes may find hospitalization comforting and even pleasant but may find the demands of managing their own insulin and diet problematic. Although more obsessional patients adapt to the rigors of self-management, they may be intolerant of the passivity of bed rest or bitterly frustrated when careful self-management does not prevent the development of later complications. Recognition of these traits by health-care providers may help them both to understand variations in the reactions of patients to their illness and to employ a variety of methods for helping patients adapt to their illness. For example, the obsessive person who is prescribed bed rest may find it helpful to be delegated appropriate tasks with detailed instructions for their implementation. The following vignette highlights the impact of individual personality differences on illness experience.

> The patient, a 45-year-old woman with a 35-year history of diabetes, developed retinopathy that caused major visual impairment such that she could no longer work. She was an extremely independent woman, who thrived in her work environment because she felt needed. She became depressed and suicidal when she was forced to stay at home. Her family, friends, and employer had all attempted to care for her, to the extent that she felt overprotected and unneeded. Her employer told her she could take a year's leave with pay, and her husband tried to take over all the chores of the household. She rebelled by slipping out of the house during the day to learn how to use public transportation. This frightened her family, who were concerned that she would be hurt. Together with her physician and a consulting psychiatrist, she planned a series of steps that would return her to work. Her family was consulted and shown that this could be done safely. Consequently, she felt more in control of her life and less depressed.[31]

Differences in coping styles and personality types influence the appraisal of stress[32] and therefore can affect the individual's experience of what constitutes a stressful life situation. Such individual differences may affect not only the emotional and behavioral consequences of stress, as noted earlier, but also the hormonal components of the stress response in cardiovascular illness[33] and perhaps in diabetes.[28] Similarly, Wolff et al.[34] found that variations in personal coping styles are associated with variations in corticosteroid levels of individuals under stress.

Clearly, individual differences color the meaning and experience of being ill as well as the specific problems posed by that illness. These differences influence the management of a complex chronic illness such as diabetes. Understanding such individual differences can contribute to the thoughtful design of treatment plans.

Coping and Course of Diabetes

An increasing number of systematic studies point to the influence of individual characteristics on the course of diabetes, with respect to management (adherence), metabolic control, and overall adjustment.[35,36] Self-esteem is one of the aspects of personality important in adaptation to diabetes. High or robust self-esteem may serve as a protective factor in a patient's adjustment to the vicissitudes of this complicated illness and to the potentially confusing, and at times inadvertently hurtful, responses of significant others such as family members, close friends, schoolmates, and colleagues. Along these lines, Jacobson et al. have found that preadolescents and adolescents with low self-esteem had lower levels of adherence at the time of diagnosis and over time than did those with better self-esteem.[37,38]

Several studies have found that other aspects of patient adjustment and coping ability are linked to adherence and glycemic control (e.g., Jacobson et al.[37,38]). For example, a number of investigators have considered how the patient's level of socioemotional (ego) development may bear upon his or her experience of and response to Type I diabetes. Ego development reflects the individual's maturation along the lines of impulse control, moral development, cognitive complexity, and interpersonal relationships.[39] Barglow and colleagues[40] found that ego development was the best predictor of an adolescent's responsiveness to a brief intervention designed to enhance adherence and glycemic control. In contrast, psychopathology was not associated with the response to the educative intervention. These findings and theoretical considerations suggest that the level of ego development a patient has achieved can affect the benefits of educational and medical interventions designed to improve metabolic control, adherence, or coping strategies. "A higher level of ego development may provide an individual with the cognitive and emotional maturity that is needed to deal effectively with the demands of having a chronic illness."[41] Further research is needed to develop interventions that are either tailored to individual differences in psychosocial functioning or designed to alleviate problems in psychosocial functioning that impede adherence among patients with diabetes.

Social Environment

Social environment is the third major psychosocial mediator of adaptation to chronic illness and maintenance of health.[42] Friends, family, and health-care providers may be important sources of support. Berkman and Syme[43] have shown, in studies of individuals matched for age, sex, and health status, that the availability of friends and close family for support has a long-term effect on mortality rates. Men and women rated lowest in the availability of friendships were more than twice as likely to suffer a fatal illness in the course of this 9-year study than were those rated highest in such friendships. Nuckolls et al.[44] showed that social supports moderated the problematic impact of life stress on pregnancy complications. Women with high levels of stress and few supports had a longer labor and more delivery complications than did women with high stress but many available supports. Social support made no difference in complication rates for women with low stress levels. Yet it is too simple to assume that important others are always positive influences. Disorganized and conflicted family relationships can negatively influence health status.[45]

A variety of studies have made several suggestions on the influence of social support on the ability of the child and the family to cope with diabetes.[36] Almost all of these studies address one aspect of social environment—the family context. While this consistent focus on the family with respect to social support does not exclude the possibility of peer and other forms of community support (e.g., religious and self-help groups), it is important to note that the most consistent evidence for social support factors in diabetes is based on family studies.

Family Context

Families of children and adolescents with newly diagnosed insulin-dependent diabetes are affected by this chronic illness in many ways.[46,47] Mealtime routines, adolescent bodily care, and adolescent yearnings for independence are all suddenly disrupted, and the longevity of the patient is threatened. Successful management of a child's diabetes may make it necessary for families to redistribute responsibilities, reorganize their daily routines, and renegotiate family roles.[48] Not surprisingly, there has been considerable interest in the ways that family forces influence patients' adaptation to diabetes.[49-59] Much of this research originally concentrated on the mother-child relationship and its effect on the young patient's adjustment.[49,60,61] Attention was then broadened to include the family unit and the ways it influences the youngster with diabetes, as investigations described the importance of maladaptive parenting styles,[62] parental self-esteem,[63] and marital satisfaction,[64] as well as specific family orientations and relationships.[55,57,65,66] Yet, as Schafer et al.[67] observe, it is only very recently that empiric studies have focused on the ways families influence diabetes, such as how they facilitate and impede adherence to treatment.

Significant family influences can contribute to the child's and adolescent's adherence, metabolic control, early complications, and overall adjustment. Although some studies that consider the family with respect to metabolic control[50] and the overall adjustment of the youngster with diabetes,[59] the largest corpus of work carefully examines contributions of family processes to the child or adolescent's adherence to the management program.[52,55,62,67-69] Variables described as associated with adherence include family support, cohesion, expressiveness, conflict, and organization. In a recent 4-year follow-up study, perceived family cohesiveness at onset was found to be associated with better short-term and long-term adherence.[70] In the same study, when parents and youngsters perceived more family conflict, levels of adherence in the first year were lower.[70] Over the 4 years, youngsters' perceptions of family conflict were associated with lower levels of adherence. These findings converge with previous cross-sectional studies describing a deleterious impact of family conflict on specific indicators of diabetes outcome.[52,58,62]

Another family dimension highlighted in these recent studies is organization, defined as clear coordination and structure in planning of family activities and responses to problem situations. Anticipation and coordination are required for successful adherence. These strengths probably are enhanced in families in which organization is valued and likely to be implemented in daily functioning. Parents' perceptions of family organization are associated with youngsters' higher self-esteem and more favorable adjustment to diabetes during their first year of illness.[57,65] Moreover, parents' perceptions of family organization during the months following their child's diagnosis are associated with higher levels of adherence during the first year as well as over several years of follow-up.

The next generation of family studies should take us one step further toward a more precise identification of risk (e.g., high conflict, low cohesion) and competence factors within the family that might then be applied to the design of family interventions, firmly grounded on the results of controlled studies, that could ensure the optimal adjustment, adherence, and metabolic control of youngsters with diabetes. As we locate the specific paths of action from family life to individual behaviors, we will be in a position to pinpoint specific family beliefs and interactions that may be the most amenable to change, instead of pursuing more global, and elusive, family factors.

Doctor-Patient Relationship

One important source of support that may be overlooked is the health-care provider. Laron and colleagues[71] have shown that an approach to health care that focuses on the psychosocial issues of diabetic children and their families, as compared with a strictly medical approach, has a beneficial effect in reducing the number of episodes of diabetic ketoacidosis and hypoglycemia. Anderson et al.[72] and Warren-Boulton et al.[73] similarly found that interdisciplinary and group approaches improve adherence and metabolic control in adolescents and young adults. Eisenberg[74] argues for the importance of social factors in medical care by suggesting that medical treatment is more helpful when therapeutic recommendations are directed at correcting the social determinants of the illness experience. Consequently, the physician's role includes the diagnosis of social components of disease and the encouragement of links between the patient and his or her family with culturally appropriate social and religious organizations, such as self-help groups and lay associations.

The physician is also in a position to help the patient set reasonable goals and to provide appropriate information for achieving these goals together with acceptance even if the patient does not achieve these goals because of physical, social, or psychological limitations. At times when the physician and patient seem to have reached their limits in treating the medical condition, the physician can be a strong source of support by listening to and acknowledging the patient's frame of reference.

One woman, writing a letter to the editor of the *Joslin Diabetes Center Newsletter*,[75] highlighted the importance of the physician in understanding her concerns as a patient. She found that her physician gave "medical" advice but failed to recognize the emotional consequences of her diabetes: "The point is that I will do anything to avoid the embarrassment of an insulin reaction in a public place. One doctor was amazed when I told him this. He seemed to think that knowing what measures to take was security enough." She wanted her physician to accept a compromise with ideal medical management that enabled her to feel more comfortable socially. Her quality-of-life goals and the medical-management goals did not match.[31]

The establishment of agreed-upon goals is an important aspect of success in the medical encounter. The physician can enhance the treatment process by seeking the underlying and often unstated requests and goals of the patient.[76] For example, the mother of an 11-year-old boy referred for regulation of newly diagnosed diabetes complained about the lack of proper care for her son. The reasons for these complaints were not readily apparent until she was asked to review her reasons for seeking specialty care. Although she wanted the education and training she and her son were receiving, she also believed that an undiagnosed cancer might be a cause of her son's diabetes. Consequently, she expected the specialists to test him extensively and thus diagnose his condition definitively. It was this worry and expectation that brought her for help. Once this less-visible agenda was elicited, the health-care team reviewed the methods of diagnosing diabetes with the child's mother. When this previously masked request was fully discussed with her, she was relieved of this anxiety.[31]

Recent studies have emphasized the importance of encouraging active patient participation in their medical appointments beyond asking questions. This research indicated that patients with diabetes who were already more active in setting the agenda of the appointment or who were trained to be more active through a single preparatory session were more likely to follow physicians' recommendations after the appointment and to have better glycemic control as a consequence.[77]

Diabetes as a chronic illness is a challenge to the coping skills of patients and their families. Since the course of diabetes is influenced by biologic and social-psychological forces, the physician who engages the patient and assesses both sets of factors will be in the strongest position to enhance medical outcome and personal adaptation.

DIABETES AND THE LIFE CYCLE

The stages of the human life cycle influence the adaptive consequences of diabetes. At each stage in the life cycle, the individual is confronted with a series of "developmental tasks" or goals in physical, psychological, and social domains. In addition, diabetes presents patients with the task of mastering the demands of diabetes self-care while they also are addressing the normal developmental tasks of a given age period. These demands of diabetes may exacerbate the pressures of normal development. At each stage of development, diabetes confronts family members with the task of being sensitive to the importance of establishing a balance between the patient's need for independence and his or her need for family support and involvement in self-care tasks. This dilemma raises different issues for families at different stages of child and adult development. The struggle to balance independence and dependence in the relationships between the person with diabetes and family members presents major coping tasks for families.

Childhood and Adolescence

A discussion of the interface between diabetes and the developmental tasks during infancy, childhood, and adolescence to young adulthood is presented in Chapter 30 by Wolfsdorf et al. and will not be repeated in this review.

Middle Adult Years

The developmental tasks of middle adulthood are complex and take a long time to master. These tasks include household and life-style management, child rearing, and career management. During the middle adult years, each of these tasks involves acceptance of the inevitable processes of aging as well as an investment in external social systems. During middle adulthood, the adult assesses self-worth in relation to physical functioning and contributions to other complex social units. "The tasks of middle adulthood demand an expanded conceptual analysis of social systems and a capacity to balance individual needs with system goals. The adult not only learns how to function effectively within larger groups, s/he comes to invest energy in those groups with which s/he can most readily identify."[78]

In contrast to the extensive empiric literature on development of the diabetic individual earlier in life, relatively little research has been carried out on adaptation to diabetes during middle adulthood. Diabetes constantly imposes conflicts between diabetic adults' responsibilities for maintaining their own health and blood sugar levels with their responsibilities for meeting the needs of other family members.[79] Few studies have been done on the impact of diabetes in a parent on the family environment of children.[80] When these middle years have been the focus of study, interest has centered on the influence of spouse support. Ahfield et al.[81] studied young adults with insulin-dependent diabetes with regard to the impact of the disease on their marriage and quality of daily life. The spouses of half of the sample also were studied. Although the adults comprising this sample had not yet reached the developmental period of middle adulthood we are discussing here, several findings from this research are relevant to issues facing adults with diabetes during middle adulthood. Ahfield and colleagues[81] found that diabetic patients perceived that the disease interfered with family activities and finances more

than did their nondiabetic spouses. Significantly more male than female patients found diabetes a source of friction in their marriage.

Given the importance of goals concerning family life during the middle adult years, it is appropriate that empiric studies of middle-aged adults with diabetes have focused primarily on spouse response and support. Katz[82] found that middle-aged women whose husbands had diabetes often reported that conflicts in the marriage were acted out through the medium of diabetes. A central source of marital conflict concerned the extent of the wife's involvement in the husband's treatment regimen. On the more positive side, Shenkel and colleagues[83] reported that the importance of the diabetic treatment regimen to the nondiabetic spouse was directly related to level of compliance in the diabetic spouse. A more complex set of findings concerning the attitudes of patient and spouse toward diabetes treatment was reported recently by Pieper et al.[84] These investigators reported that in a sample of patients 40 years or older who had Type II diabetes, the higher the nondiabetic spouses rated the benefits of diet, the lower they perceived their ability to help the diabetic partner. Dietary changes were most frequently rated as the most difficult part of the diabetic treatment regimen. Pieper et al.[84] concluded: "For the married person diagnosed as having diabetes in middle age or later life, life-style changes, especially in regard to diet and medications, may impact on marital adjustment. A lack of understanding of the impact of diabetes on the marital relationship may allow a couple to use diabetes to negatively influence their marriage and disease control."

Late Adulthood

In the later adult years, the primary developmental tasks concern the redirection of energy to new roles and activities, the acceptance of one's life and the physical and cognitive changes of the aging process, and the development of a point of view about death. Little has been written about diabetes in the later adult years (see Halter and Christensen[85] for an important exception and Chapter 31 by Morrow and Halter in this volume). Empiric data on coping issues facing the elderly patient with diabetes are not available. The period of "retirement" that faces many people who must retire in their later years means that elderly patients with diabetes must find new outlets for their intellectual capacities and social involvements. However, this is a period when the normal physical deterioration of the aging process in combination with the onset and progression of diabetes complications realistically limits the functioning of many elderly patients compared their functioning during their middle adult years. Moreover, elderly diabetic patients frequently cope with multiple medical conditions and medications. Thus, it may be difficult for family members and elderly patients to distinguish the deterioration related to the normal aging process from the progression of diabetes complications. Despair and alienation may result from the decline in level of functioning. Combined with society's typical devaluation of the disabled person, depression may become a threat to the elderly patient with diabetes. If the elderly patient's self-care abilities decline, stresses increase on family members for involvement in diabetes treatment and decision-making. Younger family members find that they must become educated in diabetes and make decisions concerning living arrangements for an elderly diabetic parent who is no longer able to inject insulin independently, to take medications, or to eat reliably.

In summary, across the life span—from infancy to the later adult years—the struggle to balance independence and dependence in the relationships between the person with diabetes and family members, especially with respect to self-care, presents chronic coping tasks for patients and families.

Pregnancy

The experience of pregnancy for a woman with diabetes is shaped by a number of forces: the development of her self-concept, sexuality, and body image during childhood and adolescence; information she has received about her ability to become pregnant and have a "normal, healthy" baby; the stability and level of her diabetes control before pregnancy; the level of her health and the presence of any diabetes complications before pregnancy; her access to the highly specialized high-risk prenatal care recommended for diabetic women during pregnancy; her resources for coping with both the physically demanding medical management necessary during pregnancy and with the emotional stress that must be endured as she faces uncertain health outcomes for herself and the baby; and, finally, the availability of involvement and support from a partner and from her extended family and peer group before, during, and immediately after the pregnancy.

Much new research documents the potential ability of diabetic women to give birth to "normal, healthy" infants if strict blood glucose control is in effect at conception and is maintained throughout the pregnancy (See Chapter 48 by Hare for additional information). More information is now available on the impact of pregnancy on the health of the diabetic woman. Women with more advanced ocular, vascular, and renal complications are frequently advised not to become pregnant because of the potential for the pregnancy to accelerate these physical complications and cause severe physical disability or even death in the diabetic woman. For patients who are involved in making decisions about risks to their own health as well as risks to the unborn child from a pregnancy, the decision about if and when to become pregnant is complex. The involvement of the partner is critical during this stressful decision-making period, especially if there are contraindications for a pregnancy such as adolescence, poor diabetes control, or the presence of serious diabetes complications.

There are three types of diabetic pregnancies: Type I, Type II, and gestational diabetes. (See Folkman and Hollerorth[86] and Chapter 48 for a more comprehensive discussion of pregnancy with these three types of diabetes.) For each of these types of diabetes, the medical management during pregnancy is intense, in terms of both the frequency of contact with specialists required and the daily treatment regimens recommended. Insulin needs often decrease during the first trimester of pregnancy but increase during the second and third trimesters. Throughout the pregnancy, most women must increase the frequency of blood sugar monitoring to at least four times a day because stabilization of blood sugar levels is more difficult during pregnancy and because hypoglycemia and hyperglycemia present risks to the developing fetus.

Despite the research advances and the realistic increases in the likelihood of the delivery of a "healthy, normal" baby, a great deal of apprehension accompanies a diabetic pregnancy. In addition to the normal changes that all pregnant women undergo, the pregnant diabetic woman must cope with concerns about the health of her baby and the impact of the pregnancy on her own health. Pregnant diabetic women must undergo multiple physiologic tests to assess the health and condition of the developing fetus throughout the pregnancy. The increased work involved in managing a diabetic pregnancy in conjunction with the intense emotional experience of the pregnancy make support from the husband or partner an extremely important factor in the pregnancy outcome. Support from extended family and friends is also critical in helping the pregnant woman maintain the discipline and emotional stability needed for the duration of the pregnancy.

DIABETES AND ITS COMPLICATIONS

The onset of complications is a critical point in the life of an individual with diabetes. For those patients who have struggled to ignore the disease or to mute its significance, the initial development of complications may point to the absolute and irrefutable "reality" of having diabetes. Even the most minor of long-term complications may challenge the previously successful denial of worries over the irreversible life-threatening and disabling effects of the illness. Acute episodes of depression or anxiety are not uncommon.

> [The patient was] 24 years old when she was told that the pains she was experiencing in her legs were due to neuropathy. A diabetic for 17 years, she had faithfully cared for her illness, always thinking that such care would protect her from complications. After the short bout of painful neuropathy, this patient developed what she thought were symptoms of recurrent hypoglycemia: nighttime sweating episodes, palpitations, and nervousness. During a hospital admission to sort out this problem, her blood sugars were found to be well maintained by her current regimen. Two episodes in the hospital were not accompanied by hypoglycemia. Reevaluation suggested that anxiety attacks caused her symptoms. Her anxiety stemmed from the unexpected onset of complications and the terror associated with future diabetic complications.[31]

For those patients who had anticipated this status, complications are a reaffirmation of their own worst fears.

Others, who believed that good care would decrease the likelihood of complications, may feel betrayed. When patients are faced with complications, their self-care behaviors often may change: 1) they may despair that good blood glucose control is of no further value and therefore relax or even quit their self-care regimen; 2) they may become mobilized by the onset of complications and become increasingly willing to care for themselves; or 3) they may become intensely fearful of hyperglycemic readings (reaffirming the possibility of further disability and/or impending death), which may promote an obsessive, overzealous approach to self-care.

Renal Disease

Several investigators have described the major psychosocial consequences of severe nondiabetic renal disease. However, few studies have examined the specific psychosocial consequences of renal disease in diabetic patients.[87-90] The ability of diabetic patients to adjust successfully to hemodialysis and subsequent transplantation varies considerably, and researchers have yet to pinpoint the best predictors of such adjustment. If the process of adjustment is congruent with that in patients with nondiabetic renal disease, factors such as social support, financial changes, ability to work, and the perceived "intrusiveness" of the illness may all contribute to the diabetic patient's adjustment.[91-94] In contrast to patients with nondiabetic renal disease, however, the diabetic patient—even after successful transplantation and a return to near-normal renal function—must still struggle to cope with a progressively disabling disease. In particular, coincident visual impairment appears to contribute to poor adjustment in the diabetic patient. The burden of vision loss and other diabetic complications also may impact strongly on the family's morale such that the institution of home dialysis may be particularly difficult among diabetic patients with renal disease. Also, the failure of renal transplantation may prove to be a critical setback leading to the decision to refuse further treatment. D'Elia et al.[88] state, "As these patients experience greater expectations and aspirations for an improved life-style following transplantation, they become more vulnerable to severe, and at times suicidal, depressions if there is subsequent failure of the allograft." The health-care team is a major source of support for the patient and family during the prolonged adaptation to the stresses of repeated treatment failure.

Erectile Dysfunction

There is little research and conflicting evidence on the existence of diabetes-associated sexual problems in women.[95,96] It is well established, however, that men commonly develop sexual difficulties (primarily erectile dysfunction) secondary to diabetes. The prevalence of erectile dysfunction in diabetic men has been estimated at 35 to 70%.[97] Retrograde ejaculation develops with far less frequency.

While the organic component has been widely recognized, psychosocial factors also may contribute to the development of erectile dysfunction in a significant subset of diabetic men. Indeed, some recent studies have suggested that in as many as 20% of diabetic men with reported impotence, the dysfunction may be primarily psychogenic in origin.[98,99] In addition, nocturnal penile tumescence, commonly monitored to assess organic pathology in erectile dysfunction, may be dramatically attenuated by major depressive episodes.[100,101] Any evaluation of erectile dysfunction must therefore include a sensitivity both to primary psychological factors and to secondary factors that may influence sexual functioning (A. Zeidler, D. A. Baron, J. Tang, and W. R. Procci, unpublished observations). For example, anxiety about performance may further exacerbate a partially dysfunctional episode in organically impaired individuals. Ignorance also may contribute to such problems. Many couples do not realize and are not informed that diabetes can promote erectile dysfunction, and they may misinterpret the source of the problem, believing that it is due to loss of love or an extramarital interest. Also, couples may not be aware and informed that orgasmic satisfaction can be achieved even if the penis is not tumescent. Most frequently, organic and psychological factors coexist so that behavioral and psychological interventions may be valuable in facilitating adjustment to the limitations posed by the organic impairment.

Surgical intervention, with the implantation of penile prostheses, appears to provide safe and satisfying results.[102] However, care must be taken to select couples with stable relationships, who are those most likely to experience a positive outcome.[102] Little research has been done on the impact of newer approaches, such as the use of vacuum devices and intracavernosal injection of vasodilators like papaverine, on quality of life and well-being. These procedures do provide alternatives to permanent surgical implants and therefore may be useful in the first phases of helping couples adjust to impotence.

Peripheral Neuropathy

Little has been written concerning the psychosocial consequences of painful peripheral neuropathy. Anecdotal evidence suggests that patients' responses to peripheral neuropathy vary significantly. When neuropathic pain becomes chronic, it is not uncommon for a self-reinforcing chronic-pain syndrome to develop, whereby the patient becomes increasingly depressed and the depression leads to an intensification of pain. Forced inactivity, muscle atrophy, social withdrawal, and dependence and/or addiction to pain medications all may contribute to further depression and pain.[103] Patients also may express fear, anger, and resentment and, it is important to note, frequently may manifest changes in personality secondary to the chronic pain. Pain reduction can lead to an improvement in apparent personality disturbances.

Given the strong association between depression and pain, antidepressants (e.g., amitriptyline, nortriptyline, or desipramine) are often helpful in conjunction with analgesics and analgesia-potentiating agents such as the phenothiazines in treating painful neuropathy.[104,105] When pain is more intractable, referral to a rehabilitation program specializing in pain may help the patient cope with this difficult experience. Such programs use group psychotherapy, stress management, and behavioral interventions to aid the patient in reducing dependence on medication, in changing pain-related behaviors, and in expressing feelings.[106]

Chronic pain often creates provocative interactions between patients and physicians, with cycles of requests for medication by the patient and frustration on the part of the physician. When the pain of neuropathy does not resolve, chronic treatment with synthetic narcotic agents may be needed as part of the treatment regimen for these patients. The administration of narcotic agents is best handled through selection of a stable dosage and frequent prescriptions (e.g., every other week for the same number of pills), with the clear understanding that these will be given in a stable, predictable manner. In resistant chronic-pain syndrome, this approach will help stabilize the patient's condition and decrease frustrating interchanges. Patients may test the limits of these prescriptions but usually settle into the ritual and may show an increase in their ability to function. When this testing occurs, time spent exploring the patient's concerns and worries may help decrease the fears frequently associated with pain and the escalating demands for medication. A consulting psychiatrist can be extremely helpful in establishing treatment goals and programs for such patients.

Vision Loss

Blindness is among the most feared complications of diabetes. The anticipation anxiety over this complication may become pronounced years before its onset, so that the identification of even early background retinopathy may represent a frightening event for the patient.[108] Actual threats to vision, such as fluctuating vision experienced throughout diabetic retinopathy, provoke a host of feelings, ranging from guilt and self-blame to anger for the presence of the complication. Although the prospect of blindness carries with it increased dependence on others, initial decreased mobility, decreased social interactions, and alterations in life-style and occupation, the actual onset of severe impairment may be perceived as a relief from the daily "changing realities" and "limbo" of fluctuating vision loss.[108,109] Once visual loss has stabilized, the process of grieving for the loss of vision can begin and successful adjustment to new realities can take place.

Psychological adjustment to blindness or severe visual impairment may be enhanced by social supports such as family and friends,[110] group support from other rehabilitated diabetics,[109] acquisition of orientation and mobilization skills (e.g., guide-dog training, cane use), introduction to visual aids, and occupational rehabilitation and placement, if necessary. These avenues provide the blind individual with the means and support necessary to his or her reclaiming at least some independence and overall reintegration of identity.

PSYCHOSOCIAL IMPACTS OF DIABETES

Effect on Neurobehavioral Functions

An increasing number of studies have examined neurobehavioral or cognitive functions in patients with Type I and Type II diabetes. Early studies found that diabetes mellitus may cause electroencephalographic (EEG) and neuropathologic changes to the central nervous system. More recent evidence has suggested that cognitive or neurobehavioral disorders may be a complication of diabetes mellitus.[111–114] A series of studies by Ryan and colleagues,[111–113] Rovet et al.,[114] Ack et al.,[115] and Holmes et al.[116] have indicated more clearly the nature of the problem found in patients with diabetes. The studies indicate that patients with Type I diabetes with onset prior to age 5 years are at particular risk for the development of neurobehavioral problems. These studies also show that mild cognitive impairments are found in greater numbers in these children than among comparable children or adolescents without diabetes or with diabetes onset at a later age. In most instances, these neurobehavioral problems are mild, leading to statistically significant but clinically subtle decreases in verbal intelligence quotients, fine motor coordination, memory, and learning. However, the research by Ryan et al.[111–113] also suggests that as many as one-fourth of adolescents with early onset of diabetes met criteria for serious neurobehavioral impairment, as compared with 6% of adolescents with later-onset diabetes and 6% of nondiabetic control adolescents. Research by Rovet et al.[117] confirms the general directions of these findings.

The mechanisms underlying the impact of Type I diabetes on cognitive impairment is suggested by this and other research. First, a number of studies have indicated that patients with early-onset Type I diabetes are subject to more serious hypoglycemic episodes. Second, neuropathologic and EEG studies show that serious hypoglycemic episodes involving seizures or unconscious reactions lead to EEG or neuropathologic impairments. Finally, several studies indicate that mild hypoglycemia impairs cognitive functions during the period of hypoglycemia.[116,118–124] In addition, previous research has suggested that poor metabolic control is associated with the increase in number and severity of neurobehavioral deficits.[125,126] Thus, it seems possible that severe hypoglycemia affects the young child's brain, causing neuropsychological impairment. It is not clear whether this effect is a function of host susceptibility or of the higher incidence of severe hypoglycemia in this age group.

The question of whether repeated episodes of hypoglycemia can affect adults has not yet been answered. Given the increasing use of methods to normalize blood glucose levels in an effort to retard microvascular complications and the recognition that such regimens lead to an increased frequency of severe hypoglycemic reactions, neurobehavioral deficits could be an unexpected and untoward outcome of more aggressive treatment.[127] This hypothesis is now subject to careful scrutiny as part of the Diabetes Control and Complications Trial.[127]

Other studies indicate that children and adolescents with diabetes demonstrate lower levels of school performance.[128,129] These decreased capacities on school achievement tests and in neuropsychological test batteries may reflect neurologic damage or the demonstrated effects of diabetes on school absence rates.[129] Thus, it is distinctly possible that those individuals with the worst diabetic control, including repeated episodes of severe hypoglycemia, may miss the most school and thereby demonstrate the most problems in tests of achievement and psychological functioning.

Research on Type II diabetic patients is more sparse. Perlmuter et al.[130] demonstrated patterns of cognitive deficits similar to those in children and adults in elderly patients with Type II diabetes. This research suggested that elderly diabetic patients had more difficulty with learning tasks and memory than did age-matched nondiabetic individuals. These cognitive problems of the elderly were associated with the degree of metabolic control as indexed by levels of glycosylated hemoglobin and extent of peripheral neuropathy as estimated from vibratory thresholds. The cognitive deficits found by Perlmuter et al.[131] could not be accounted for by the presence of peripheral neuropathy since these neurobehavioral deficits were not related to motor functions. It seems likely that among the elderly, cognitive dysfunction reflects the development of central complications parallel to those developing in the peripheral nervous system. It is not yet clear whether this dysfunction is related to macrovascular or to microvascular processes. Since Type II diabetic patients do not usually experience severe hypoglycemia, the pathophysiology of cognitive deficits in the elderly differs from such problems in young children.

In summary, it appears that cognitive functions may be impaired to a mild degree in Type I diabetic patients, especially those with a more serious history of metabolic control problems. In addition, for a small number of individuals, particularly those young children who have a history of repeated serious hypoglycemic episodes, there may be especially serious cognitive deficiencies. Furthermore, subtle problems in cognitive functioning could play a role in determining the capacity of patients to master and maintain the task of self-regulation implicit in the diabetic experience. Patients with subtle memory deficits may be less able to master the complex tasks of diabetes self-care. Therefore, when evaluating causes of adherence problems, one must evaluate cognitive functioning among other psychosocial factors known to affect diabetes adjustment.

Psychiatric Impacts

There has been long-standing awareness of the possibility that diabetes mellitus may place children and adults at greater risk for psychiatric disturbances. Early case reports[132–135] presented patients with extreme psychiatric disturbance and suggested that Type I diabetes in particular could have severe psychiatric consequences. Subsequent empiric investigations have led to more complex sets of findings. Simonds[136,137] assessed the degree of psychiatric disturbance, interpersonal conflict, and intrapsychic conflict among these children. He found that the number of psychiatric diagnoses and levels of conflict were equivalent in diabetic and nondiabetic children. Subsequent studies by Jacobson et al.[138] and Kovacs et al.[139] have shown that at diabetes onset children typically appear to experience, at most, mild transient situational disruptions without showing signs of early severe psychiatric pathology. In a similar vein, Sullivan[140] found mild increases in depression among adolescent campers but no differences in level of self-esteem in comparison to normative data. Ongoing longitudinal studies by Jacobson et al.[138] and Kovacs et al.[139] will provide data in the near future on the longer-term psychological effects of Type I diabetes in adolescents.

A few studies have suggested an increased risk of depression and anxiety disorders in patients with Type I and Type II diabetes. In particular, Lustman et al.[141] studied a randomly selected group of insulin-dependent and non-insulin-dependent diabetic adults. These patients were identified at the time they applied to a clinical research center for evaluation. Using the Diagnostic Interview Schedule (DIS), a structured psychiatric diagnostic interview designed to provide DSM-III diagnoses (American Psychiatric Association[142]), Lustman et al.[141] found that 71% of patients had a life-time history of at least one psychiatric diagnosis. A history of major depression was found in 33% of the patients, with 14% of the patients suffering from an episode at the time of study. No differences were found in the rates of depression in Type I and Type II diabetic patients. The patient sample consisted of individuals with long-standing diabetes and some clinical evidence of diabetic complications. Within this particular sample, an increasing number of complications was not associated with an increasing level of depression. In a similar study, Popkin et al.[143] evaluated insulin-dependent diabetic patients who were candidates for a pancreatic transplant. All patients had at least 10 years of illness and some degree of nephropathy. Using the DIS, Popkin et al. found that 59% of the candidates had a psychiatric diagnosis, with 23% of the women and 26% of the men having a life-time history of major depression. They also found unexpectedly high rates of phobic anxiety in this group of patients.

Other studies provide preliminary evidence for an increased prevalence of diabetes among patients with manic-depressive illness. Lilliker,[144] in a retrospective chart review of 203 manic-depressive patients admitted to a state hospital, found a higher prevalence of diabetes among the manic-depressive patients than among patients in other psychiatric diagnostic categories. Diabetes was present in 12.4% of the manic-depressive patients and in fewer than 4% of patients with personality disorders, schizophrenia, and transient situational disturbances. In one study of Type II diabetic patients, Wing et al.[145] compared 32 obese subjects with their obese nondiabetic spouses, all of whom were attending a weight-loss program. They found that the diabetic subjects reported significantly more symptoms than did their overweight nondiabetic spouses on the Beck Depression Inventory.

In summary, these studies suggest that insulin-dependent and non-insulin-dependent diabetic patients with long-standing illness and usually with some complications are at increased risk for affective and anxiety disorders. Clearly, further research is needed to examine whether adults who have a shorter duration of illness and fewer complications experience similar high rates of affective disorder. The work by Kovacs et al.[139,146–148] with adolescents suggests that the risk may be only slight among more-recently diagnosed adults.

Both psychological and humoral mechanisms could play a role in this apparent increased risk of depression among adult diabetic patients. The clear psychosocial demands and threats of this chronic illness are the most obvious likely precipitants of psychiatric illness.[149] The manifestations of altered function of the hypothalamic-pituitary-adrenocortical axis among depressed and diabetic patients are remarkably similar. In particular, abnormal cortisol production has been demonstrated among patients with major depression and insulin-dependent diabetes.[150,151] Other research has suggested that diabetics experience a range of mood shifts with hyperglycemic and hypoglycemic experience.[152] These can include periods of depression, euphoria, and irritability. It is possible that the presence of diabetes, particularly long-term poor glycemic control or extreme shifts in blood glucose levels, could place certain diabetic individuals at higher risk for subsequent affective disorder.

Eating Disorders

There has been considerable interest in examining the impact of Type I diabetes on the development of eating disorders. Although results conflict, most studies suggest an increase in rates of anorexia nervosa and bulimia among female patients with Type I diabetes. For example, Rosmark et al.[153] compared 86 patients with Type I diabetes with a normal control population. Using a standardized self-report questionnaire, these authors found that a greater proportion of diabetic patients than normal controls had clinical eating disorders. Steel et al.[154] found a higher rate of clinically apparent eating disorders among female adolescents than that expected from the rate in community populations. Finally, Rodin et al.[155] assessed 58 women with Type I diabetes for at least 1 year using standardized self-report interviews based on DSM-III criteria. They reported that 20.7% had a clinically significant eating disorder, among whom 6.9% experienced anorexia nervosa and 6.9% experienced bulimia. The rate of anorexia in this study was approximately seven times that expected in a general population. Nielsen et al.[156] also found an approximately sixfold increase in the prevalence of eating disorders at a tertiary-care center in Denmark. On the other hand, Birk and Spencer,[157] using standardized self-report surveys, studied 385 women 13 to 45 years old with Type I diabetes who were attending a large multispeciality group practice. The prevalence rates of anorexia (1%) were lower than those reported in other studies, and the

prevalence of current bulimia was 10%. The authors concluded that their data contradicted previous studies in that the prevalence of bulimia and anorexia nervosa in diabetes found in their study was within the range considered to exist in the general population. Since the rate of bulimia varies widely in general populations, it is clear that better controlled studies are needed to address this research issue.

Our current state of knowledge about the psychiatric impact of diabetes mellitus is at an early stage. Few studies have used standardized criteria. Most studies have failed to use control samples. Furthermore, investigations frequently depend on samples of convenience, and it is often not clear whether the control samples, when used, come from comparable populations. This is true of many studies done at tertiary-care centers, where patients may be preselected because of unusually severe problems with illness. Inclusion of such patients could easily lead to higher-than-expected rates of psychiatric disturbances such as anorexia, bulimia, and depression since all of these can lead to secondary problems of glycemic control that might trigger referral to the specialized center for care. There is a clear need for further studies of this complex problem in both Type I and Type II diabetes.

Impact on Development and Personality

A growing literature focuses on how diabetes may affect personality and development in children, adolescents, and adults. Studies disagree about whether diabetes has a distinct impact on aspects of personality and development.[158] Several studies report no significant differences in self-esteem between groups of children with and without diabetes.[36,159–161] On the other hand, some findings indicate that subtle developmental alterations may occur in adolescents with Type I diabetes.[39,162,163] These studies incorporate an approach that considers the influence of diabetes on the child or adolescent's psychological maturation, especially socio-emotional (ego) development. Two different, largely middle-class, samples of adolescents with diabetes were found to be functioning at significantly lower levels of ego development than the comparison population. In one instance diabetic patients were studied within 2 years of diagnosis and were compared with a sample of patients of similar age with a recent acute illness.[70] Similar observations have been reported in studies of adolescents with longer and more variable durations of diabetes.[39,163,164] However, Silver and colleagues,[41] comparing a smaller (eight patients) and more heterogeneous sample of chronically ill adolescents (with asthma, diabetes, and other chronic illnesses) with a comparable peer group, found no difference in ego development. The considerably lower socioeconomic class of their sample, together with the smaller number of diabetic patients included, make it difficult to determine how much their results differ from the results of previous studies.

One way to understand the reason for the lower ego development among the patients with diabetes is to consider that these young patients are responding to the introduction and accumulation of many new stressors (e.g., diet changes, daily insulin injections). Rather than continuing the normal inner psychological explorations of inner experiences, perceptions, and relationships (all of which would be consistent with progressive ego development among adolescents), the diabetic adolescent is involved in new conflicts and preoccupations (e.g., being "different" or getting complications) that may lead him or her to subtly withdraw from these developmentally appropriate tasks of adolescence to protect the newly more-vulnerable self.[162]

Impact on the Family

Certain aspects of diabetes make its impact on the family particularly powerful. Because dietary control is a basic feature of diabetes management, meal rituals are disrupted. Potential conflicts in parent/child relationships around such issues as independence and dependence in self-care tasks are magnified by the presence of diabetes. The administration of insulin by injection is taken on as an early task by the mother or the father of the diabetic child. In adolescence, this responsibility eventually shifts to the child. However, parental involvement in matters concerning their child's body, which ordinarily are diminishing in adolescence, often does not decrease from that during childhood. Parents also are continuously involved in other forms of increased attentiveness by monitoring the child's metabolic control. Moreover, the conscientious parent also may monitor the young child's physical activities outside the home, so as to be sure that the child is engaged in the proper amount of exercise.

When diabetes is first diagnosed in a child, families often are shocked and grieve deeply.[163,165,166] Other feelings frequently experienced and expressed by family members are anger, anxiety, and guilt. In addition to their receiving disturbing news, families must assimilate a vast amount of new information regarding management of the diabetes, master new medical skills, and make difficult medical decisions, such as the choice of a specific doctor and treatment site. Some families seem to accept the illness relatively easily, incorporating the new diabetic regimen into their daily life. Others adjust more slowly, continuing to deny the presence of the illness or maintaining a state of helplessness and sadness.[48,62,167]

Much of the empiric research about how the onset and continued presence of diabetes in the child or adolescent influences the family has focused on only one or two relationships in the family. Along these lines, studies report that parents of diabetic children reveal greater marital strain and greater disagreement over child-management issues than do parents of nondiabetic children.[53] Other studies consider the effect of the child's diabetes on the relationship between the parent and child. Parents may have difficulty dealing with their emotional reactions to the child, frequently responding with behaviors characterized as overprotective, overindulgent, or rejecting.[60,168] In addition, parents may have more difficulty disciplining a child with diabetes, leading in turn to additional anxiety and guilt about their child-rearing abilities.[62] On the other hand, it is important to note that some studies describe diabetic children as deriving much emotional support from their parents and as feeling closer to them through coping with their illness.[168]

Recent work in this area focuses on the impact of Type I diabetes on the family as a total system. Dimensions of the family that have been examined in relation to diabetes onset include strain on family roles,[53] family conflict,[169] activity orientation,[170] family cohesion,[57] and family enabling and constraining interactions.[56] For example, mothers of adolescents with recently diagnosed diabetes were found to be more accepting and supportive of their spouses and their diabetic child than were mothers of nondiabetic adolescents during research interviews designed to elicit family interactions.[171] In contrast, fathers of diabetic children appeared to be more judgmental and indifferent in these same research procedures. In addition, these families reported higher levels of organization and more shared activities than the comparison group.[48] Other studies describe an increase in conflict among families of diabetic children.[53]

Thus, studies show a complex set of effects of diabetes on the family, in which both an accentuation of closeness and an increase in tension are brought about by the new and strenuous demands of illness.

PSYCHOSOCIAL AND EDUCATIONAL INTERVENTIONS

An increasing number of studies have assessed various psychosocial and educational interventions among patients with Type I and Type II diabetes. These include information transfer in large-group, family, and individual settings; education enhanced by behavioral and counseling techniques; relaxation training; supportive counseling; treatment based on social learning theory; and behavior modification. The conclusions that can be drawn from these studies are complex. For example, a number of large and small educational studies have presented a wide variety of outcomes. Large, well-designed trials examining the impact of diabetes education performed by Rettig et al.,[172] Korhonen et al.,[173] and Mazucca et al.[174] reported rather mixed or weak effects of these interventions on self-care practices and metabolic control. Similarly, the study by Campbell et al.[175] of an intensive educational approach to dietary change for Type II diabetic patients showed improvements in dietary compliance without improvements in glycemic control. The only biologic variable shown to be affected was level of total cholesterol. Otherwise, the intensively treated group could not be differentiated from the conventionally treated group. Rubin et al.,[176] in a single uncontrolled group study, found distinct benefits of educational interventions for patients with Type I or Type II diabetes. Glycemic control and psychosocial variables such as emotional well-being and compliance were found to improve with educational interventions. However, this study did not use a randomized control design, making it difficult to draw conclusions about the actual benefits of treatment. The authors point out an important issue worthy of further consideration: the value of measuring quality-of-life as well as biologic end points. The authors note that studies have documented the importance of emotional status as a direct risk factor for development and progression of other medical illnesses, such as coronary heart disease.[177] Thus, improvement in quality-of-life outcomes through educational or psychological interventions could have indirect, longer-term benefits not evaluated in the assessment of biomedical end points immediately after intervention.

Other studies have described the value of psychological counseling programs used in combination with educational interventions. These studies (e.g., Anderson et al.[72]) suggest that small-group peer counseling for adolescents and children at the time of clinic visits enhances not only adherence outcomes but also glycemic control.[72] More recently, a study by Delamater et al.[179] suggested similar benefits of such a program for newly diagnosed adolescents.

In a comprehensive review and meta-analysis of the effects of educational and psychological interventions, Padgett et al.[178] presented a comprehensive view of 94 such studies. The author compared eight forms of intervention, including patient education with a didactic emphasis; patient education with both behavioral and educational techniques; diet instruction; exercise instruction; self-monitoring instructions; social learning and behavioral modification; relaxation training including biofeedback; and meditation and counseling. The studies reviewed were carried out in a variety of settings but were predominantly among outpatients. Patients in the study groups included an even mix of Type I and Type II of a wide range of ages and duration of illness. The sample size for the meta-analysis was maximized by including studies that used both single-group and control-group designs: 40% were single-group and 60% were control-group designs. Multiple outcomes were assessed, including biologic, psychological, information, and compliance. Biologic outcomes included glycemic control and weight loss. Because of the paucity of studies measuring psychological outcomes, none of the end points reached statistical significance. This finding underscores the point made by Rubin et al.[176] concerning the potential importance of including end points concerned with well-being in future studies to broaden the evaluation of these interventions.

For the 71 studies in which biologic effects were measured, diet instruction and social learning/behavioral modification had the greatest impact. Of interest, relaxation training had the least effect, such that benefits did not reach statistical significance. These findings confirm the overall clinical impression that educational and psychological interventions may influence important medical end points, but the effects remain modest. The strongest effects were found in dietary and psychological interventions that included a behavioral or social-learning component. The impact of interventions on Type I and Type II patients were similar. Study methodology was found to be associated with the level of effect, i.e., in weaker studies the size of the effect was greater than that in the better-designed studies. This underlines the critical importance in future research for the implementation of studies that are carefully controlled and designed. Con-

clusions are inflated by studies that appear to be poorly designed. This meta-analysis also examined longer-term vs. shorter-term effects on selected outcomes. Overall evidence confirms that the effectiveness of intervention decreases over time. The impact of intervention on levels of blood glucose, weight loss, and glycosylated hemoglobin and on the results of knowledge testing were much less impressive when there were 6- and 12-month follow-up points. This decrease in effect over time was especially notable in studies that evaluated weight loss.

In summary, some psychological and educational interventions hold promise for helping patients improve relevant medical outcomes. A variety of psychological and educational approaches, especially those that include psychological interventions based on social-learning approaches, may be valuable adjuncts for treatment. However, it is clear from this review that further study will be required to develop effective psychosocial interventions for diabetic patients.

CLINICAL DIABETES PROBLEMS

Assessing Adherence Difficulties

While faithful adherence to the self-care regimen is believed to be the most essential ingredient in preventing the development of complications, patients commonly have difficulty in adhering to the regimen required for maintenance of glycemic control.[180,181] To complicate the matter, recent evidence suggests that adherence is not a univariate phenomenon. One patient's adherence to his meal plan, for example, may be unrelated to his adherence to his prescribed regimen of blood glucose monitoring. In general, few significant correlations have been found between the different components of adherence to the self-care regimen.[182–185] It is therefore important that we do not assume that a patient's difficulty with adherence to one component of the regimen is necessarily an indication of a global disavowal of the regimen. Initial assessment must include a careful examination of patients' adherence to each aspect of the regimen.

Understanding and influencing the patient's difficulties with adherence may be one of the most challenging tasks in the treatment of diabetes. As discussed earlier, attitudinal and emotional factors are believed to play an important role in determining adherence to the self-care regimen.[31,186] Contributors to poor adherence include 1) psychiatric problems such as affective and eating disorders, 2) family conflict, 3) stressful life experiences, 4) cognitive deficits, and 5) coping ability. Therefore, evaluation of patients with suspected adherence problems requires a comprehensive review of their social and emotional lives.

In addition, specific elements of the diabetes experience may play an important role in a patient's self-care decisions and actions. These elements can include the patient's perceptions of hypoglycemia and hyperglycemia. Episodes of symptomatic hypoglycemia usually promote unpleasant physical symptoms as well as negative mood states[152] and lead to embarrassment. Always looming is the possibility that a hypoglycemic episode may become more severe, with serious cognitive and/or motor dysfunction, coma, or even death. Given the aversive nature of hypoglycemia, it is not surprising that some patients develop a fear of hypoglycemia. Such fear may lead to difficulties in adhering to the diabetic regimen[187] and may promote behaviors that result in the maintenance of elevated blood glucose levels.[188,189] Ironically, fears of hypoglycemia may be stronger deterrents to better glycemic control among patients with Type II diabetes[190] than among those with Type I diabetes (W. H. Polonsky, C. L. Davis, A. M. Jacobson, and B. J. Anderson, unpublished observations).

Recent research has suggested that Type I patients who have chronically poor control of blood glucose levels perceive hyperglycemia differently from patients who have good control.[191] Those in poor control reported feeling physically better at a blood glucose level higher than the level at which those with good control reported feeling their best. Also, those in poor control reported first perceiving hyperglycemic symptoms at a blood glucose level higher than that reported by those in good control. A subsequent study replicated and extended these findings, discovering that poor glycemic control was associated with the patient's initiation of treatment for hyperglycemia at a higher glucose level, the setting of higher minimal and maximal glucose levels as treatment goals, and reports of less-frequent testing for blood glucose.[192] Together, these data suggest that attempts to improve adherence to a self-care regimen may be thwarted in those patients for whom hyperglycemia is not negatively reinforced (i.e., who feel best when blood glucose levels are higher). In an initial assessment, patients should be questioned about the blood glucose level at which they feel best, the level at which they feel "too high," and their history of symptoms during previous attempts to improve adherence and reduce elevated blood glucose levels.

As discussed earlier, young women with Type I diabetes appear to be at high-risk for serious eating disorders.[193] Recent surveys[194,195] have reported a relationship between subclinical eating disorders and glycemic control in young women with Type I diabetes. Of particular concern, women with Type I diabetes may use insulin manipulation (i.e., omission) as a means of post-binge purging. Insulin omission is a particularly effective method of calorie purging and therefore has the potential for becoming psychologically addictive. Studies of eating disorders in women with diabetes have established that insulin manipulation is linked to poor glycemic control.[190]

Where weight is a concern, attitudes toward insulin management may be very influential in determining regimen adherence. In a recent study of adolescent and adult women with diabetes (all insulin-dependent), 42.5% feared that keeping their blood glucose in good control would cause weight gain, 44.3% believed that taking insulin would cause weight gain, and 35.9% believed that good control would cause them to become fat. These results suggest that it is common for women with Type I diabetes, especially those with poor diabetes control, to express a "fear of normoglycemia," which can translate into the avoidance of insulin to avoid weight gain (W. H. Polonsky, C. L. Davis, A. M. Jacobson, and B. J. Anderson, unpublished observations). Unfortunately, recent evidence has emerged that improved glycemic control often leads to weight gain.[127]

Disordered eating behaviors are often well hidden, but patients should be encouraged to bring up and discuss issues such as their current level of satisfaction with their weight, their weight goals, and—if willing—their experiences with binging.

Surreptitious Insulin Administration and/or Repeated Episodes of Hypoglycemia

Along the continuum of adherence difficulties and regimen manipulation in diabetes, the secretive use of insulin by patients with Type I diabetes represents one of the most frightening and potentially life-threatening examples of "noncompliance." When the patient administers insulin surreptitiously, the usual outcome is a recommendation by the health-care team (or parent) for the patient to decrease the usual insulin dose. Children have been known to inject insulin in secret to lower their level of blood sugar before undergoing a regular blood-sugar monitoring by their parents in an attempt to convince parents that diabetes is no longer present or that the insulin dose should be lowered, to avoid a feared weight gain if the dose had to be increased. Adolescent patients with Type I diabetes, desperate to escape from stressful living situations, have been known to surreptitiously take extra insulin to cause a predictable "medical emergency" and hospitalization for a severe hypoglycemic reaction. The documented[196] number of cases of surreptitious insulin administration among Type I patients thought to be "brittle" has forced some inpatient hospital units for diabetic patients to keep all insulin bottles and syringes away from the bedside and to insist that all insulin be administered to patients by the nursing staff. Unexplained "good" or "normal" blood sugar levels or unpredictable low blood sugar levels should be "red flags" for surreptitious insulin misuse.

Repeated Episodes of Diabetic Ketoacidosis

On the spectrum of adherence difficulties, repeated episodes of unexplained diabetic ketoacidosis (DKA) and unexplained hypoglycemia have a significant cost, both in terms of loss of human functioning and of hospitalization expenses. Shade et al.[196] reported, in one of the studies of so-called brittle diabetes or repeated DKA, that all cases in which patients were initially suspected of having brittle diabetes or so-called insulin resistance were, in fact, a consequence of insulin omission or manipulation by the patient. This form of self-destructive behavior frequently has a pragmatic basis, that is, repeated insulin omission, with consequent DKA and repeated hospitalization, is an effective strategy for removing the patient from a difficult, stressful, or abusive home or life situation. Less frequently, a severe personality disorder may trigger insulin omission and repeated DKA. Tattersall and Walford[197] describe several case studies of patients with severe personality disorders who skillfully deceived medical staff by repeatedly inducing DKA. These authors called this disorder "metabolic Munchausen." While many of these patients are diagnosed as having brittle diabetes, in fact, strategic, purposeful omission of insulin to escape an overwhelming home situation, a severe personality disorder, or to deal with fears of weight gain[198] is the most frequent cause of repeated DKA and repeated hospitalization.

Parent/Child Alienation

One of the "predictable crises of diabetes"[199] in families with children with Type I diabetes is diabetes-related conflict and possible alienation that can occur between parents and children. The origin of this deterioration in the relationship between parent and child is the erosion of self-esteem of both parent and child or adolescent in response to frustration over the child's inability to adhere "perfectly" to the diabetes treatment regimen and/or to consistently achieve blood sugar levels in an acceptable range. The child may be held responsible for having blood sugar levels deemed unacceptable or unsafe by the parent or health-care team. Although the developing youngster may be blamed for "cheating," it is important to keep in mind that high or fluctuating blood sugar levels may, in fact, be caused by a factor other than the child's eating behavior, such as an insufficient insulin dose in the context of recent physical growth, puberty, stress, or infectious illness. Anger and resentment toward diabetes as well as toward parents can build up in the child who is chronically accused. Such children or adolescents may begin to label themselves "bad diabetics" and experience a deteriorating sense of self-worth. Even when parents are not overly critical of the young diabetic patient, the child's obvious inability to meet treatment expectations can leave him or her with a profound sense of failure and hopelessness about the future. Moreover, when parents are trying everything within their power to help the child achieve blood sugar levels that are stable and acceptable and do not succeed, they may blame themselves for this failure. Parents may blame themselves for not having a more disciplined child or for not being able to provide the food or schedule necessary for the child to achieve more acceptable blood sugar readings. Parents with a diabetic child, who may have been blamed by health-care providers at one point in the course of diabetes, sometimes carry this sense of blame for years. They may also be particularly worried about their failures causing devastating complications of diabetes. Unfortunately, in some families, years of conflicts and accusations, along with the problems of self-esteem in the child and parents caused by difficulties in adhering to treatment requirements, can contribute to a profound alienation between parent and child.

Repeated family conflicts over nonadherence to treatment or severe parental or child distress or depression over blood sugar readings should be "red flags" for a referral to a child or family therapist for parent-child counseling that is focused on family communication about diabetes, and sharing of responsibility for regimen tasks.

CONCLUSION

Understanding psychosocial issues can help the health-care provider develop more effective treatment plans for patients with Type I and Type II diabetes. This chapter has focused on particular areas that should be of interest to the practitioner facing this task. It is especially important to realize that caring physicians and nurses are frequently their patients' best allies. Even if medical treatment does not appear to be most effectively used by the patient and family, the health-care provider can help the sick and worried patient by being supportive and approachable. By providing such an accepting atmosphere, health-care providers will, in the long run, help patients with this chronic illness do their best in caring for themselves.

REFERENCES

1. Dimsdale JE, Eckenrode J, Haggerty RJ, et al. The role of social supports in medical care. Soc Psychiatry 1979; 14:175–80.
2. Sosa R, Kennell J, Klaus M, et al. The effect of a supportive companion on perinatal problems, length of labor, and mother-infant interaction. N Engl J Med 1980;303:597–600.
3. Thomas CB, McCabe OL. Precursors of premature disease and death: habits of nervous tension. John Hopkins Med J 1980:147:137–45.
4. Turk D. Factors influencing the adaptive process with chronic illness. In: Sarason IG, Spielberger CD, eds. Stress and anxiety. New York: Wiley, 1979:291–312.
5. Rahe R, Meyer, M, Smith M, et al. Social stress and illness onset. J Psychosom Res 1964;8:35–44.
6. Goldband S, Katkin E, Morell M. Personality and cardiovascular disorder: steps toward demystification. In: Sarason IG, Spielberger CD, ed. Stress and anxiety. New York: Wiley, 1979:351–70.
7. Johnson JH, Sarason IG. Moderator variables in life stress research. In: Sarason IG, Spielberger CD, eds. Stress and anxiety. New York: Wiley, 1979:159–68.
8. Bibring GL. Psychiatry and medical practice in a general hospital. N Engl J Med 1956;254:366–72.
9. Klerman GL, Izen JE. The effects of bereavement and grief on physical health and general well-being. Adv Psychosom Med 1977;9:63–104.
10. Stein SP, Charles ES. Emotional factors in juvenile diabetes mellitus: a study of the early life experiences of eight diabetic children. Psychosom Med 1975;37:237–44.
11. Kemmer FW, Bisping R, Steingrüber HJ, et al. Psychological stress and metabolic control in patients with Type I diabetes mellitus. N Engl J Med 1986;314:1078–84.
12. Kiecolt-Glaser JK, Fisher LD, Ogrocki P, et al. Marital quality, marital disruption, and immune function. Psychosom Med 1987;49:13–34.
13. Carter WR, Herrman J, Stokes K, Cox DJ. Promotion of diabetes onset by stress in the BB rat. Diabetologia 1987;30:674–5.

14. Surwit RS, Feinglos MN. Stress and autonomic nervous system in Type II diabetes: a hypothesis. Diabetes Care 1988;11:83–5.

15. Surwit RS, Feinglos MN, Livingston EG, et al. Behavioral manipulation of the diabetic phenotype in *ob/ob* mice. Diabetes 1984;33:616–8.

16. Surwit RS, McCubbin JA, Kuhn CM, et al. Alprazolam reduces stress hyperglycemia in *ob/ob* mice. Psychosom Med 1986;48:278–82.

17. Surwit RS, McCubbin JA, Livingston EG, Feinglos MN, et al. Classically conditioned hyperglycemia in the obese mouse. Psychosom Med 1985;47:565–8.

18. Kuhn CM, Cochrane C, Feinglos MN, Surwit RS. Exaggerated peripheral responses to catecholamines contributes to stress-induced hypoglycemia in the *ob/ob* mouse. Pharmacol Biochem Behav 1987;26:491–5.

19. Peterson HR, Rothschild M, Weinberg CR, et al. Body fat and the activity of the autonomic nervous system. N Engl J Med 1988;318:1077–83.

20. Hinkle L, Wolf S. A summary of experimental evidence relating life stress to diabetes mellitus. J Mt Sinai Hosp 1952;19:567–70.

21. Vandenbergh RL, Sussman KE, Titus CC. Effects of hypnotically induced acute emotional stress on carbohydrate and lipid metabolism in patients with diabetes mellitus. Psychsom Med 1966;28:382–90.

22. Weller C, Linder M, Nuland W, Kline MV. The effects of hypnotically-induced emotions on continuous, uninterrupted blood glucose measurements: a preliminary evaluation. Psychosomatics 1961;2:375–8.

23. Eigler N, Saccà L, Sherwin RS. Synergistic interactions of physiologic increments of glucagon, epinephrine, and cortisol in the dog: a model for stress-induced hyperglycemia. J Clin Invest 1979;63:114–23.

24. Baker L, Barcai A, Kaye R, Haque N. Beta-adrenergic blockade and juvenile diabetes: acute studies and long-term therapeutic trial. Evidence for the role of catecholamines in mediating diabetic decompensation following emotional arousal. J Pediatr 1969;75:19–29.

25. Baker L, Minuchin S, Rosman B. Report of the National Commission on Diabetes. Appendix 33–43, Update. Washington, DC: US Public Health Service, 1976.

26. Coyne JC, Anderson BJ. The "psychosomatic family" reconsidered: diabetes in context. J Marital Family Ther 1988;14(2):113–23.

27. Coyne JC, Anderson BJ. The "psychosomatic family" reconsidered. II. Recalling a defective model and looking ahead. J Marital Family Ther 1989;15(2):139–48.

28. Stabler B, Surwit RS, Lane JD, et al. Type A behavior pattern and blood glucose control in diabetic children. Psychosom Med 1987;49:313–6.

29. Peyrot M, McMurray JF Jr. Psychosocial factors in diabetes control: adjustment of insulin-treated adults. Psychosom Med 1985;47:542–57.

30. Vaillant GE. Natural history of male psychologic health: effects of mental health on physical health. N Engl J Med 1979;301:1249–54.

31. Jacobson AM, Hauser ST. Behavioral and psychological aspects of diabetes. In: Ellenberg M, Rifkin H, eds. Diabetes mellitus: theory and practice. 3rd ed. New York: Medical Examination Publishing Co, 1983:1037–52.

32. Lazarus RS. Psychological stress and coping in adaptation and illness. Int J Psychiatry Med 1974;5:321–33.

33. Cohen F. Personality, stress, and the development of physical illness. In: Stone GC, Cohen F, Adler NE, eds. Health psychology. San Francisco: Jossey-Bass, 1979: 77–112.

34. Wolff CT, Friedman SB, Hofer MA, Mason JW. Relationship between psychological defenses and mean urinary 17-hydroxycorticosteroid excretion rates. I. A predictive study of parents of fatally ill children. Psychosom Med 1964;26:576–91.

35. Helz JW, Templeton B. Evidence of the role of psychosocial factors in diabetes mellitus: a review. Am J Psychiatry 1990;147:1275–82.

36. Wertlieb D, Jacobson AM, Hauser ST. The child with diabetes: a developmental stress and coping perspective. In: Costa PY Jr, Vanden Bos GR, eds. Psychological aspects of serious illness: chronic conditions, fatal diseases, and clinical care. Washington, DC: The American Psychological Association, 1990.

37. Jacobson AM, Hauser ST, Wolfsdorf JI, et al. Psychologic predictors of compliance in children with recent onset of diabetes mellitus. J Pediatr 1987;110:805–11.

38. Jacobson AM, Hauser ST, Lavori P, et al. Adherence among children and adolescents with insulin-dependent diabetes mellitus over a four-year longitudinal follow-up. I. The influence of patient coping and adjustment. J Pediatr Psychol 1990;15:511–26.

39. Hauser ST, Jacobson AM, Noam G, Powers S. Ego development and self-image complexity in early adolescence: longitudinal studies of psychiatric and diabetic patients. Arch Gen Psychiatry 1983;40:325–32.

40. Barglow P, Edidin DV, Budlong-Springer AS, et al. Diabetic control in children and adolescents: psychosocial factors and therapeutic efficacy. J Youth Adolesc 1983;12:77–94.

41. Silver EJ, Bauman LJ, Coupey SM, et al. Ego development and chronic illness in adolescents. J Pers Soc Psychol 1980;59:305–10.

42. House JS, Landis KR, Umberson D. Social relationships and health. Science 1988;241:540–5.

43. Berkman LF, Syme SL. Social networks, host resistance, and mortality: a nine-year follow-up study of Alameda County residents. Am J Epidemiol 1979;109:186–204.

44. Nuckolls KB, Cassel J, Kaplan BH. Psychosocial assets of life crisis and the prognosis of pregnancy. Am J Epidemiol 1972;95:431–41.

45. Minuchin S, Baker L, Rosman BL, et al. A conceptual model of psychosomatic illness in children: family organization and family therapy. Arch Gen Psychiatry 1975;32:1031–8.

46. Patterson J. Chronic illness in children and the impact on families. In: Chilmas C, Nunnaly E, Cox F, eds. Chronic illness and disability. Beverly Hills, CA: Sage, 1988.

47. Rolland JS. A conceptual model of chronic and life-threatening illness and its impact on the family. In: Chilmas C, Nunnaly E, Cox F, eds. Chronic illness and disability. Beverly Hills, CA: Sage, 1988.

48. Hauser S, Solomon ML. Coping with diabetes: views from the family. In: Ahmed PI, Ahmed N, eds. Coping with diabetes. Springfield, IL: Charles C Thomas: 1985:234–66.

49. Anderson BJ, Auslander WF. Research on diabetes management and the family: a critique. Diabetes Care 1980;3:696–702.

50. Anderson BJ, Miller JP, Auslander WF, Santiago JV. Family characteristics of diabetic adolescents: relationship to metabolic control. Diabetes Care 1981;4:586–94.

51. Benoliel JQ. Role of the family in managing young diabetics. Diabetes Educ 1977;5:8.

52. Bobrow ES, Asruskin TW, Siller J. Mother-daughter interaction and adherence to diabetes regimens. Diabetes Care 1985;8:146–51.

53. Crain AJ, Sussman MB, Weil WB Jr. Effects of a diabetic child on mental integration and related measures of family functioning. J Health Hum Behav 1966;7:122–7.

54. Baker L, Minuchin S, Milman L, et al. Psychosomatic aspects of juvenile diabetes mellitus: a progress report. Diabetes in juveniles. Mod Probl Pediatr 1975; 17:332–43.
55. Hanson CL, Henggeler SW, Burghen GA. Social competence and parental support as mediators of the link between stress and metabolic control in adolescents with insulin-dependent diabetes mellitus. J Consult Clin Psychol 1987;55:529–33.
56. Hauser ST, Jacobson AM, Wertlieb D, et al. Children with recently diagnosed diabetes: interactions within their families. Health Psychol 1986;5:273–96.
57. Hauser ST, Jacobson AM, Wertlieb, et al. The contribution of family environment to perceived competence and illness adjustment in diabetic and acutely ill adolescents. Family Relations 1985;34:99–108.
58. Koski M-L, Ahlas A, Kumeto A. A psychosomatic follow-up study of childhood diabetics. Acta Paedopsychiatrica 1976;42:12–26.
59. Wertlieb D, Hauser ST, Jacobson AM. Adaptation to diabetes: behavior symptoms and family context. J Pediatr Psychol 1986;11:463–79.
60. Pond H. Parental attitudes toward children with a chronic medical disorder: special reference to diabetes mellitus. Diabetes Care 1979;2:425–31.
61. Vandenbergh RL. Emotional aspects. In: Sussman KE, ed. Juvenile-type diabetes and its complications. Springfield, IL: Charles C Thomas, 1971:411–38.
62. Stein J. Family interaction and adjustment, adherence, and metabolic control in adolescents with insulin-dependent diabetes [Dissertation]. Boston: Boston University, 1989.
63. Grey MJ, Genel M, Tamborlane WV. Psychosocial adjustment of latency-aged diabetics: determinants and relationship to control. Pediatrics 1980;65:69–73.
64. Hanson CL, Jenggeler SW, Harris MA, et al. Family system variables and the health status of adolescents with insulin-dependent diabetes mellitus. Health Psychol 1989; 8:239–53.
65. Hauser ST, et al. Family contexts of self-esteem and illness adjustment in diabetic and acutely ill children. In: Ramsey C, ed. The science of family medicine. New York: Guilford Press, 1989.
66. Mendlowitz D. The relationship between level of metabolic control in children with juvenile onset diabetes and dimensions of family functioning. Dissertations Abstracts International 1983;44.
67. Schafer LC, Glasgow RE, McCaul KD, Dreher M. Adherence to IDDM regimens: relationship to psychosocial variables and metabolic control. Diabetes Care 1983;6:493–8.
68. Galatzer A, Amir S, Gil R, et al. Crisis intervention program in newly diagnosed diabetic children. Diabetes Care 1982;5:414–9.
69. Shouval R, Ber R, Galatzer A. Family social climate and the health status and social adaptation of diabetic youth. In: Laron Z, Galatzer A, Tikva P, eds. Psychological aspects of diabetes in children and adolescents. New York: Karger, 1982:89–93. (Pediatric and adolescent endocrinology; vol 10).
70. Hauser ST, Jacobson AM, Lavori P, et al. Adherence among children and adolescents with insulin-dependent diabetes mellitus over a four-year longitudinal follow-up. II. Immediate and long-term linkages with the family milieu. J Pediatr Psychol 1990;15:527–42.
71. Laron Z, Galatzer A, Amir S, et al. A multidisciplinary, comprehensive, ambulatory treatment scheme for diabetes mellitus in children. Diabetes Care 1979; 2:342–8.
72. Anderson BJ, Wolf FM, Burkhardt MT, et al. Effects of peer-group intervention on metabolic control of adolescents with IDDM: randomized outpatient study. Diabetes Care 1989;12:179–83.
73. Warren-Boulton E, Anderson BJ, Schwartz NL, Drexler AJ. A group approach to the management of diabetes in adolescents and young adults. Diabetes Care 1981; 4:620–3.
74. Eisenberg L. What makes persons "patients" and patients "well"? Am J Med 1980;69:277–86.
75. Joslin Diabetes Center Newsletter 1980;9(1):2.
76. Lazare A, Cohen F, Jacobson AM, et al. The walk-in patient as a 'customer': a key dimension in evaluation and treatment. Am J Orthopsychiatry 1972;42:872–83.
77. Kaplan SH, Greenfield S, Ware JE Jr. Assessing the effects of physician-patient interactions on the outcomes of chronic disease. Med Care 1989;27(Suppl):S110–27.
78. Newman BM, Newman PR. Development through life: a psychosocial approach. Homewood IL: Dorsey Press, 1975.
79. Anderson BJ. Diabetes and adaptations in family systems. In: Holmes CS, ed. Neuropsychological and behavioral aspects of diabetes. New York: Springer-Verlag, 1990:85–101.
80. Anderson BJ, Kornblum HK. What's with that kid? Diabetes Forecast 1984;37(5):39–43,74.
81. Ahlfield JE, Soler NG, Marcus SD. The young adult with diabetes: impact of the disease on marriage and having children. Diabetes Care 1985;8:52–6.
82. Katz AM. Wives of diabetic men. Bull Menninger Clin 1969;33:279–94.
83. Shenkel RJ, Rogers JP, Perfetto G, Levin RA. Importance of "significant others" in predicting cooperation with diabetic regimen. Int J Psychiatry Med 1985–86; 15:149–55.
84. Pieper B, Kushion W, Gaiuda S. The relationship between a couple's marital adjustment and beliefs about diabetes mellitus. Diabetes Educ 1990;16(2):108–12.
85. Halter JB, Christensen NJ. Diabetes mellitus in elderly people. Diabetes Care 1990;13(Suppl 2):1990.
86. Folkman J, Hollerorth HJ, eds. A guide for women with diabetes who are pregnant or plan to be. Boston: Joslin Diabetes Center, 1986.
87. Comty CM, Leonard A, Shapiro FL. Psychosocial problems in dialyzed diabetic patients. Kidney Int 1974;6(Suppl 1):144–51.
88. D'Elia JA, Piening S, Kaldany A, et al. Psychosocial crisis in diabetic renal failure. Diabetes Care 1981;4:99–103.
89. Simmons RG, Schilling KJ. Social and psychological rehabilitation of the diabetic transplant patient. Kidney Int 1974;6(Suppl 1):152–8.
90. Peterson LG, Perl M. Diabetic patients and the impact of renal transplantation. Psychosomatics 1982;23:173–85.
91. Malmquist A. A prospective study of patients in chronic hemodialysis. II. Predicting factors regarding rehabilitation. J Psychosom Res 1973;17:339–44.
92. Hagberg B, Malmquist A. A prospective study of patients in chronic hemodialysis. IV. Pretreatment psychiatric and psychological variables predicting outcome. J Psychosom Res 1974;18:315–9.
93. Hagberg B. A prospective study of patients in chronic hemodialysis. III. Predictive value of intelligence, cognitive deficit, and ego defence structures in rehabilitation. J Psychosom Res 1974;18:151–60.
94. Devins GM, et al. Illness intrusiveness and quality of life in end-stage renal disease: comparison and stability across treatment modalities. Health Psychol 1990;9:117–42.

95. Kolodny RC. Sexual dysfunction in diabetic females. Diabetes 1971;20:557–9.

96. Ellenberg M. Sexual aspects of the female diabetic. Mt Sinai J Med 1977;44:495–500.

97. Meisler AW, Carey MP, Lantinga LJ, Krauss DJ. Erectile dysfunction in diabetes mellitus: a biopsychosocial approach to etiology and assessment. Ann Behav Med 1989;11:18–27.

98. Karacan L, Salis PJ, Ware JC, et al. Nocturnal penile tumescence and diagnosis in diabetic impotence. Am J Psychiatry 1978;135:191–7.

99. Lehman TP, Jacobs JA. Etiology of diabetic impotence. J Urol 1983;129:291–94.

100. Roose SP, Glassman AH, Walsh BT, et al. Reversible loss of nocturnal penile tumescence during depression: a preliminary report. Neuropsychobiology 1982;8:284–8.

101. Thase ME, Reynolds CF III, Glanz LM, et al. Nocturnal penile tumescence in depressed men. Am J Psychiatry 1987;144:89–92.

102. Beaser RS, Van der Hoek C, Jacobson AM, et al. Experience with penile prostheses in the treatment of impotence in diabetic men. JAMA 1982;248:943–8.

103. Turk DC, Meichenbaum D, Gerest M. Pain and behavioral medicine. New York: Guilford Press, 1983.

104. Davis JL, Lewis SB, Gerich JE, et al. Peripheral diabetic neuropathy treated with amitriptyline and fluphenazine. JAMA 1977;238:2291–2.

105. Kvinesdal B, Molin J, Frøland A, Gram LF. Imipramine treatment of painful diabetic neuropathy. JAMA 1984;251:1727–30.

106. Sternbach RA. Mastering pain. New York: GP Putnam and Sons, 1987.

107. Jacobson AM, de Groot M. Psychology of visual loss. In: Albert DM, Jacobeic FA, eds. Principles and practices of ophthalmology: the Harvard system. Philadelphia: WB Saunders (in press).

108. Wulsin LR, Jacobson AM, Rand LI. Psychosocial aspects of diabetic retinopathy. Diabetic Care 1987;10:367–73.

109. Oehler-Giarrantana J, Fitzgerald RG. Group therapy with blind diabetics. Arch Gen Psychiatry 1980;37:463–67.

110. Perle T. A matter of adjustment: a personal reaction to visual loss. J Vis Impair Blind 1978;72:255–58.

111. Ryan C, Vega A, Drash A. Cognitive deficits in adolescents who developed diabetes early in life. Pediatrics 1985;75:921–7.

112. Ryan CM. Neurobehavioral complications of Type I diabetes: examination of possible risk factors. Diabetes Care 1988;11:86–93.

113. Ryan C, Vega A, Longstreet C, Drash A. Neuropsychological changes in adolescents with insulin-dependent diabetes. J Consult Clin Psychol 1984;52:335–42.

114. Rovet JF, Ehrlich RM, Hoppe M. Intellectual deficits associated with early onset of insulin-dependent diabetes mellitus in children. Diabetes Care 1987;10:510–5.

115. Ack M, Miller I, Weil WB Jr. Intelligence of children with diabetes mellitus. Pediatrics 1961;28:764–70.

116. Holmes CS, Hayford JT, Gonzalez JL, Weydert JA. A survey of cognitive functioning at different glucose levels in diabetic persons. Diabetic Care 1983;6:180–5.

117. Rovet JF, Ehrlich RM, Hoppe M. Specific intellectual deficits in children with early onset diabetes mellitus. Child Dev 1988;59:226–34.

118. Gilhaus KH, Daweke H, Lülsdorf HG, et al. EEG-Veränderungen bei diabetischen Kindern. Dtsch Med Wochenschr 1973;98:1449–54.

119. Haumont D, Dorchy H, Pelc S. EEG abnormalities in diabetic children: influence of hypoglycemia and vascular complications. Clin Pediatr 1979;18:750–3.

120. Hirabayashi S, Kitahara T, Hishida T. Computed tomography in perinatal hypoxic and hypoglycemic encephalopathy with emphasis on follow-up studies. J Comput Assist Tomogr 1980;4:451–6.

121. Ernhart CB, Graham FK, Eichman PL, et al. Brain injury in the preschool child: some developmental considerations. II. Comparison of brain injured and normal children. Psychol Monogr 1963;77(11):17–33.

122. Teuber H-L, Rudel RG. Behavior after cerebral lesions in children and adults. Dev Med Child Neurol 1962; 4:3–20.

123. Dikmen S, Matthews CG, Harley JP. The effect of early versus late onset of major motor epilepsy upon cognitive-intellectual performance. Epilepsia 1975;16:73–81.

124. Ingram TTS, Stark GD, Blackburn I. Ataxia and other neurological disorders as sequels of severe hypoglycaemia in childhood. Brain 1967;90:851–62.

125. Skenazy JA, Bigler ED. Neuropsychological findings in diabetes mellitus. J Clin Psychol 1985;40:246–58.

126. Holmes CS. Neuropsychological profiles in men with insulin-dependent diabetes. J Consult Clin Psychol 1986;54:386–9.

127. Ryan C, et al. Neurobehavioral assessment of medical patients in clinical trials: the DCCT experience. In: Mohr E, Brouwer P, eds. Handbook of clinical trials: The neurobehavioral approach. Swits Publishing (in press).

128. Gath A, Smith MA, Baum JD. Emotional, behavioral, and educational disorders in diabetic children. Arch Dis Child 1980;55:371–5.

129. Ryan C, Longstreet C, Morrow L. The effects of diabetes mellitus on the school attendance and school achievement of adolescents. Child Care Health Dev 1985; 11:229–40.

130. Perlmuter LC, Tun P, Sizer N, et al. Age and diabetes related changes in verbal fluency. Exp Aging Res 1987;13:9–14.

131. Perlmuter LC, Hakami MK, Hodgson-Harrington C, et al. Decreased cognitive function in aging non-insulin-dependent diabetic patients. Am J Med 1984;77:1043–8.

132. Swift CR, Seidman F, Stein H. Adjustment problems in juvenile diabetes. Psychosom Med 1967;29:555–71.

133. O'Leary DS, Lovel MR, Sackellares JC, et al. Effects of age of onset of partial and generalized seizures on neuropsychological performance in children. J Nerv Ment Dis 1983;171:624–9

134. Slawson PF, Flynn WR, Kollas EJ. Psychological factors associated with the onset and course of diabetes mellitus. JAMA 1963;185:166–70.

135. Sanders K, Mills J, Martin FIR, Del Horne DJ. Emotional attitudes in adult insulin-dependent diabetics. J Psychosom Res 1975;19:241–6.

136. Simonds JF. Psychiatric status of diabetic youth matched with a control group. Diabetes 1977;26:921–5.

137. Simonds JF. Psychiatric status of diabetic youth in good and poor control. Int J Psychiatry Med 1976–77; 7:133–51.

138. Jacobson AM, Hauser ST, Wertlieb D, et al. Psychological adjustment of children with recently diagnosed diabetes mellitus. Diabetes Care 1986;9:323–9.

139. Kovacs M, Brent D, Steinberg TF, et al. Children's self-reports of psychologic adjustment and coping strategies during first year of insulin-dependent diabetes mellitus. Diabetes Care 1986;9:472–9.

140. Sullivan BJ. Adjustment in diabetic adolescent girls: II.

Adjustment, self-esteem, and depression in diabetic adolescent girls. Psychosom Med 1979;41:127–38.

141. Lustman PJ, Griffith LS, Clouse RE, et al. Psychiatric illness in diabetes mellitus, relationship to symptoms and glucose control. J Nerv Ment Dis 1986;174:736–42.

142. American Psychiatric Association. Diagnostic and statistics manual. 3rd ed. Washington, DC: American Psychiatric Press, 1980.

143. Popkin MK, Callies AL, Lentz RD, et al. Prevalence of major depression, simple phobia, and other psychiatric disorders in patients with long-standing Type I diabetes mellitus. Arch Gen Psychiatry 1988;45:64–8.

144. Lilliker SL. Prevalence of diabetes in a manic-depressive population. Compr Psychiatry 1980;21:270–5.

145. Wing RR, Marcus MD, Blair EH, et al. Depressive symptomatology in obese adults with Type II diabetes. Diabetes Care 1990;13:170–2.

146. Kovacs M, Feinberg T. Coping with juvenile onset diabetes. In: Baum A, Singer J, eds. Handbook of health and psychology. Vol 2. Hillsdale, NJ: Lawrence Erlbaum Associates, 1982:165–212.

147. Kovacs M, Feinberg RE, Paulauskas S, et al. Initial coping responses and psychosocial characteristics of children with insulin-dependent diabetes mellitus. J Pediatr 1985;106:827–34.

148. Kovacs M, Kass RE, Schnell TM, et al. Family functioning and metabolic control of school-aged children with IDDM. Diabetes Care 1989;12:409–14.

149. Geringer ES. Affective disorders and diabetes mellitus. In: Holmes CS, ed. Neuropsychological and behavioral aspects of diabetes. New York: Springer-Verlag, 1990:239–72.

150. Ettigi PG, Brown GM. Psychoneuroendocrinology of affective disorders: an overview. Am J Psychiatry 1977;134:493–501.

151. Cameron OG, Kronfol Z, Greden JF, Carroll BJ. Hypothalmic-pituitary-adrenocortical activity in patients with diabetes mellitus. Arch Gen Psychiatry 1984;41:1090–5.

152. Gonder-Frederick LA, Cox DJ, Bobbitt SA, Pennebaker JW. Mood changes associated with blood glucose fluctuations in insulin-dependent diabetes mellitus. Health Psychol 1989;8:45–59.

153. Rosmark B, Berne C, Holmgren S, et al. Eating disorders in patients with insulin-dependent diabetes mellitus. J Clin Psychiatry 1986;47:547–50.

154. Steel JM, Young RJ, Lloyd GG, Clarke BF. Clinically apparent eating disorders in young diabetic women: associations with painful neuropathy and other complications. BMJ 1987;294:859–62.

155. Rodin GM, Johnson LE, Garfinkel PE, et al. Eating disorders in female adolescents with insulin dependent diabetes mellitus. Int J Psychiatry Med 1986–87;16:49–57.

156. Nielsen S, Borner H, Kabel M. Anorexia nervosa/bulimia in diabetes mellitus: a review and a presentation of five cases. Acta Psychiatr Scand 1987;75:464–73.

157. Birk R, Spencer ML. Prevalence of anorexia nervosa, bulimia, and induced glycosuria in IDDM females. Diabetes Educ 1989;15:336–41.

158. Dunn SM, Turtle JR. The myth of the diabetic personality. Diabetes Care 1981;4:640–6.

159. Jacobson AM, Hauser ST, Powers S, Noam G. The influences of chronic illness and ego development on self-esteem in diabetic and psychiatric adolescent patients. J Youth Adolesc 1985;13:489–507.

160. Jacobson AM. Current status of psychosocial research in diabetes [Editorial]. Diabetes Care 1986;9:546–8.

161. Ryan CM, Morrow LA. Self-esteem in diabetic adolescents: relationship between age at onset and gender. J Consult Clin Psychol 1986;54:730–1.

162. Hauser ST. The study of families and chronic illness: ways of coping and interacting. In: Brody G, Sigel I, eds. Methods of family research. New York: Plenum, 1990:59–86.

163. Jacobson AM, Hauser ST, Powers S, Noam G. Ego development in diabetics: a longitudinal study. Pediatr Adolesc Endocrinol 1982;10:1–8.

164. Hauser ST, Pollets D, Turner BL, et al. Ego development and self-esteem in diabetic adolescents. Diabetes Care 1979; 2:465–71.

165. Mattsson A. Juvenile diabetes: impacts on life stages and systems. In: Hamburg BA, Liset LF, Inoff GE, Drash AL, eds. Behavioral and psychosocial issues in diabetes. Washington, DC: Government Printing Office, 1979:43–55.

166. Wishner WJ, O'Brien MD. Diabetes and the family. Med Clin North Am 1978;62:849–56.

167. Sargent J. Juvenile diabetes mellitus and the family. In: Ahmed PI, Ahmed N, eds. Coping with juvenile diabetes. Springfield, IL: Charles C Thomas, 1985:205–33.

168. Farrell FZ, Hutter JJ Jr. The family of the adolescent: a time of challenge. In: Eisenberg MG, Sutkin LC, Jansen MA, eds. Chronic illness and disability through the life span: effects on self and family. New York: Springer, 1984:150–63.

169. McCubbin H, Patterson J. Family adaptation to crises. In: McCubbin H, Cauble A, Patterson J, eds. Family stress coping and social support. Springfield, IL: Charles C Thomas, 1982:169–88.

170. Powers S, et al. The coping strategies and psychological resources of seriously ill adolescents. Presented at Family Systems and Health Pre-Conference Workshop, National Council on Family Relations, San Francisco, CA, 1984.

171. Hauser ST, Jacobson AM, Wertlieb D, et al. Children with recently diagnosed diabetes: interactions within their families. Health Psychol 1986;5:273–96.

172. Rettig BA, Shrauger DG, Recker RR, et al. A randomized study of the effects of a home diabetes education program. Diabetes Care 1986;9:173–8.

173. Korhonen T, Huttunen JK, Aro A, et al. A controlled trial on the effects of patient education in the treatment of insulin-dependent diabetes. Diabetes Care 1983;6:256–61.

174. Mazucca S, Mazzuca SA, Moorman NH, et al. The diabetes education study: a controlled trial of the effects of diabetes patient education. Diabetes Care 1986;9:1–10.

175. Campbell LV, Barth R, Gosper JK, et al. Impact of intensive educational approach to dietary change in NIDDM. Diabetes Care 1990;13:841–7.

176. Rubin RR, Peyrot M, Saudek CD. Effect of diabetes education on self-care, metabolic control, and emotional well-being. Diabetes Care 1989;12:673–9.

177. Booth-Kewley S, Friedman HS. Psychological predictors of heart disease: a quantitative review. Psychol Bull 1987;101:343–65.

178. Padgett D, Mumford E, Hynes M, Carter. Meta-analysis of the effects of educational and psychosocial interventions on management of diabetes mellitus. J Clin Epidemiol 1988;41:1007–30.

179. Delamater AM, Smith JA, Kurtz SM, White NH. Dietary skills and adherence in children with Type I diabetes mellitus. Diabetes Educ 1988;14:33–6.

180. Bloom-Cerkoney KA, Hart LK. The relationship between the health belief model and compliance of persons with diabetes mellitus. Diabetes Care 1980;37:594–8.

181. Watkins JD, Williams TF, Martin DA, et al. A study of diabetic patients at home. Am J Public Health 1967;57:452–9.

182. Glasgow RE, McCaul KD, Schafer LC. Barriers to regimen adherence among persons with insulin-dependent diabetes. J Behav Med 1986;9:65–77.

183. Glasgow RE, McCaul KD, Schafer LC. Self-care behaviors and glycemic control in Type I diabetes. J Chronic Dis 1987;40:399–412.

184. Glasgow RE, Wilson W, McCaul KD. Regimen adherence: a problematic construct in diabetes research [Editorial]. Diabetes Care 1985;8:300–1.

185. Johnson SB, Silverstein J, Rosenbloom A, et al. Assessing daily management in childhood diabetes. Health Psychol 1986;5:545–64.

186. Surwit RS, Feinglos MN. The effects of relaxation on glucose tolerance in non-insulin-dependent diabetes. Diabetes Care 1983;6:176–9.

187. Weiner MF, Skipper FP Jr. Euglycemia: a psychological study. Int J Psychiatry Med 1978–79;9:281–8.

188. Cox DJ, Irvine A, Gonder-Frederick L, et al. Fear of hypoglycemia: quantification, validation, and utilization. Diabetes Care 1987;10:617–21.

189. Surwit RS, Feinglos MN, Scovern AW. Diabetes and behavior: a paradigm for health psychology. Am Psychol 1983;38:255–62.

190. Polonsky WH, Anderson BJ, Lohrer PA. Disordered eating and regimen manipulation in women with diabetes: relationships to glycemic control. Diabetes 1991;40(Suppl 1):540A.

191. Jacobson AM, Adler AG, Wolfsdorf JI, et al. Psychological characteristics of adults with IDDM: comparison of patients in poor and good glycemic control. Diabetes Care 1990;13:375–81.

192. Polonsky WH, Davis CL, Jacobson AM, Anderson BJ. Attitudes toward hyperglycemia and hypoglycemia in diabetes: associations with glycemic control [Abstract no. 651]. Diabetes 1990;39(Suppl 1):163A.

193. Marcus MD, Wing RR. Eating disorders and diabetes. In: Holmes CS, ed. Neuropsychological and behavioral aspects of Diabetes. New York: Springer-Verlag, 1990:102–21.

194. Wing RR, Nowalk MP, Marcus MD, et al. Subclinical eating disorders and glycemic control in adolescents with Type I diabetes. Diabetes Care 1986;9:162–7.

195. LaGreca AM, Schwartz LT, Satin W. Eating patterns in young women with IDDM: another look [Letter]. Diabetes Care 1987;10:659–60.

196. Schade DS, Drumm DA. Duckworth WC, Eaton RP. The etiology of incapacitating, brittle diabetes. Diabetes Care 1985;8:12–20.

197. Tattersall R, Walford S. Brittle diabetes in response to life stress: 'cheating and manipulation'. In: Pickup JC, ed. Brittle diabetes. London: Blackwell Scientific Publications, 1985:76–102.

198. Fairburn CG. The current status of the psychological treatments for bulimia nervosa. J Psychosom Res 1988;32:635–45.

199. Hamburg BA, Inoff GE. Coping with predictable crises of diabetes. Diabetes Care 1983;6:409–16.

Chapter 26

EXERCISE AND DIABETES

LAURIE J. GOODYEAR
ROBERT J. SMITH

Exercise tends to lower the blood sugar in the diabetic in whose body there is an adequate supply of insulin whether this be of endogenous or exogenous origin. This effect is so striking and so beneficial that exercise along with diet and insulin is now accorded a definite and prominent place in the everyday treatment of diabetes.

These words from the 1935 edition of *The Treatment of Diabetes Mellitus* by Joslin, Root, White, and Marble[1] reflect a recognition of the metabolic effects of exercise in patients with diabetes. As early as the eighteenth century, exercise was advocated as beneficial for patients with diabetes.[2] After insulin became available, exercise—together with insulin and diet—was considered one of the three central elements in the management of diabetes. Today, we have much better methods for administering insulin to patients with diabetes and for monitoring blood glucose control. We also have a greater understanding of the metabolic effects of exercise.

In this chapter, we will review current knowledge regarding the physiologic adaptations and hormonal responses to acute exercise and fitness training and will discuss the potential benefits and risks associated with exercise in the diabetic population. In addition, we will suggest guidelines for exercise prescription for patients with non-insulin-dependent diabetes mellitus (NIDDM) and insulin-dependent diabetes mellitus (IDDM).

METABOLIC AND HORMONAL CHANGES WITH EXERCISE

An acute bout of exercise can place enormous metabolic demands on the human organism. To maintain homeostasis during exercise, a person must meet increased requirements for oxygen and metabolic substrates through the precise functioning of several regulatory systems. These include cardiopulmonary responses that ensure delivery of oxygen and substrates to the working tissues and the removal of metabolic by-prod-

ucts, the regulation of insulin and counterregulatory hormone secretion by the neural and endocrine systems, and the regulation of metabolism in liver, muscle, and adipose tissue.

As illustrated in Table 26–1, only a small pool of circulating fuels—a total of about 100 kilocalories (kcal)—is available to meet increased metabolic demands during exercise. If used in its entirety, this fuel will permit a person to maintain a sitting posture for about 1 hour or to play tennis for 15 minutes. It is obvious, therefore, that metabolic homeostasis during exercise requires the mobilization of tissue substrate stores. These include muscle and hepatic glycogen—about 1500 and 350 kcal, respectively—and very large reserves of adipose tissue fat. Body protein represents a large potential caloric reserve, but protein breakdown does not ordinarily make a significant contribution to energy metabolism.

The changes in body fuel metabolism that occur during exercise are illustrated schematically in Figure 26–1. At rest, the major source of fuel for skeletal muscle is circulating free fatty acids, which provide approximately

Table 26–1. Postabsorptive Substrate Reserves in Normal Man (70 kg)

	Weight (kg)	Energy (kcal)
Circulating substrates		
Glucose	0.020	80
Free fatty acids	0.004	36
Total		116
Tissue depots		
Glycogen (muscle)	0.350	1,400
Glycogen (liver)	0.085	340
Adipose triglycerides	15	135,000
Protein (muscle)	6	24,000
Total		159,840

Recalculated from Wahren et al.[3]

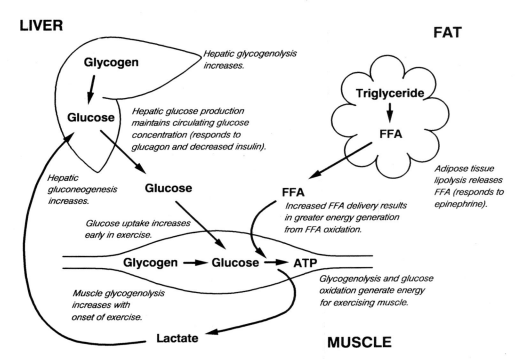

Fig. 26–1. Changes in body fuel metabolism with exercise. FFA = free fatty acids.

85 to 90% of the required fuel.[4] With the onset of exercise, the requirement for generation of high-energy phosphates by muscles to maintain levels of adenosine triphosphate (ATP) and replace phosphocreatine is met by a rapid increase in the oxidation of glucose. Initially, the oxidation of glucose occurs almost entirely through the breakdown of muscle glycogen (glycogenolysis). With physical exercise, there is also an increase in blood flow to the working muscle. This adaptation ensures delivery of glucose to the muscles and also provides additional fatty acids, which have been released by adrenergic stimulation of fat-cell lipolysis. Reliance on both circulating glucose and free fatty acids becomes more important during long-term exercise, as glycogen stores gradually become depleted.

Despite the tremendously increased rate of glucose uptake by muscle during exercise, which should exhaust blood glucose in minutes, the circulating level of glucose, at least in persons without diabetes, remains quite stable. This glucose homeostasis reflects a precise matching of glucose production by the liver with glucose uptake by muscle. During exercise, circulating insulin concentrations decrease as a result of an inhibition of insulin secretion in response to increased activity of the sympathetic nervous system.[5–7] At the same time, concentrations of glucagon and other counterregulatory hormones, such as epinephrine, norepinephrine, growth hormone, and cortisol, increase in the circulation.[8–11] Although the interaction of all these hormones contributes to glucose homeostasis, the balanced effects of insulin and glucagon on hepatic glucose production during exercise appear to be most important.[12] Epinephrine also plays a significant role by stimulating adipose tissue lipolysis. This results in the release of free fatty acids, which can be taken up and

oxidized by the muscle, and the production of glycerol, a gluconeogenic precursor for the liver.

The changes in concentrations of insulin and glucagon prevent a decrease in blood glucose levels during exercise initially by stimulating hepatic glycogenolysis and later by increasing hepatic gluconeogenesis.[4,13] Hepatic glycogen stores are readily mobilized but are limited in supply. As exercise progresses and the working muscles release gluconeogenic precursors (e.g., lactate, pyruvate, and alanine), the relative contribution of gluconeogenesis to hepatic glucose production increases. Hepatic gluconeogenesis is thus most important during long-term exercise, when muscle and hepatic glycogen stores become depleted.

Even though hepatic gluconeogenesis markedly increases with prolonged exercise, the amount of glucose produced by gluconeogenic pathways alone is not adequate to meet the energy requirements of exercising muscle. Hypoglycemia does not develop with continued exercise after glycogen pools have been depleted, however, because the importance of free fatty acids as a muscle fuel increases and the use of glucose by muscle decreases. Both the release of free fatty acids from adipose tissue and the oxidation of fatty acids in muscle increase progressively, such that after several hours of exercise of moderate intensity approximately twice as much energy is derived from free fatty acids as from glucose. Because of the precise regulation of hepatic glucose production and the increasing utilization of fat-derived fuels, hypoglycemia seldom occurs in nondiabetic individuals, even during very prolonged exercise.

The intensity of the exercise, as well as its duration, is an important determinant of the relative amounts of glucose and free fatty acids metabolized. Generally, as the intensity of exercise increases, so does the utilization of glucose. With very-high-intensity exercise (>90% of maximal oxygen consumption, Vo_{2max}), the substrate of choice is almost exclusively glucose, which results in very rapid depletion of glycogen stores and an early onset of fatigue. In this situation, even though rates of muscle glucose uptake are very high, plasma glucose concentrations may actually increase as hepatic production of glucose overshoots glucose utilization. With more moderate but still strenuous exercise (70 to 75% of Vo_{2max}), glucose is still the predominant fuel, but free fatty acids also play an important role. With lower-intensity exercise (50% of Vo_{2max}), fatty acids and glucose are used about equally. The contribution of amino acids to the fuel used during exercise appears to be limited under most conditions.

Since physical work results in increased glucose uptake by muscle, it is not unexpected that a single bout of exercise causes an increased rate of whole-body disposal of glucose.[14–16] Exercise increases sensitivity and responsiveness to insulin in skeletal muscle,[17] and evidence indicates that exercise and insulin can act synergistically to increase glucose uptake.[18,19] These effects of a single, acute bout of exercise on glucose uptake and the sensitivity and responsiveness of skeletal muscle to insulin can last for more than 12 hours, and perhaps for as long as 48 hours, after exercise ends.[16,20,21] This "persistent effect" of exercise on glucose uptake has important implications for individuals with diabetes.

The mechanism of increased glucose uptake during and after exercise is not well understood. Factors that may be involved include an increased rate of blood flow to the exercising muscle, a change in the energy status of the muscle, increases in insulin binding, and/or changes in cytoplasmic calcium concentrations. Since glucose transport in muscle is the major rate-limiting step in glucose utilization,[22–24] regulation of this system must play an important role with exercise. Recently, several studies have demonstrated that exercise can increase the number and intrinsic activity of glucose transporter proteins present in the plasma membrane of skeletal muscle.[25–28] However, the cellular signaling mechanism(s) that stimulates these glucose transporters is still not known.

METABOLIC EFFECTS OF ACUTE EXERCISE IN DIABETES

Non-Insulin-Dependent Diabetes

In individuals with NIDDM, the regulation of blood glucose during exercise is different from that in individuals without diabetes. Typically, circulating glucose concentrations fall modestly during exercise in persons with NIDDM because insulin secretion is not inhibited while the peripheral utilization of glucose is increased.[29] It is not known whether this lack of inhibition of insulin secretion reflects a primary abnormality of β-cell function or the prevention of adrenergic responses by hyperglycemia. Despite the fall in glucose concentrations, hypoglycemia usually does not occur in patients who are receiving only dietary therapy. However, patients treated with sulfonylureas or insulin are at risk of hypoglycemia during exercise as a result of insulin-induced depression of hepatic glucose production.[30,31]

As in persons without diabetes, in individuals with NIDDM peripheral glucose uptake is increased during and after exercise. Strenuous, glycogen-depleting exercise increases both peripheral insulin sensitivity and glucose disposal in patients with NIDDM, and, as in nondiabetic persons, these responses can persist for 12 hours or longer following exercise.[21] This raises the possibility that an exercise regimen that results in frequent episodes of glycogen depletion may be of benefit in the management of NIDDM.

Insulin-Dependent Diabetes

The blood glucose response to exercise in individuals with IDDM is influenced by multiple factors, including the state of metabolic control, the timing of insulin injections, and the type and intensity of exercise. As in patients with NIDDM, in patients with IDDM who have good metabolic control, exercise may result in a lowering of blood glucose concentrations (Fig. 26–2). This occurs

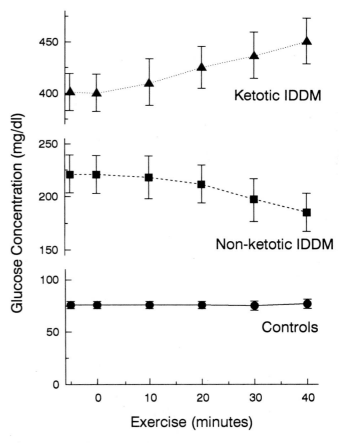

Fig. 26–2. Effects of moderate-intensity exercise (60% Vo_{2max}) on arterial glucose concentrations. In subjects with insulin-dependent diabetes (IDDM), insulin was withheld for 24 hours prior to study. Redrawn from Wahren et al.[3]

because the increase in peripheral glucose uptake with exercise is not accompanied by a coordinate increase in hepatic glucose production, since circulating insulin concentrations are not decreased. In addition, insulin entry into the circulation from exogenous injection sites continues during exercise, and in some cases, exercise can actually increase the rate of insulin absorption (Fig. 26–3). This may result from mechanical stimulation of the injection site during exercise or from exercise-induced hyperemia in the region of insulin injection. An increased rate of insulin absorption during exercise has the potential to cause hypoglycemia.[32] Furthermore, as in persons without diabetes, insulin sensitivity and glucose uptake by muscle may be increased for 12 hours or longer in persons with diabetes after glycogen-depleting exercise.[21] Thus, if additional calories are not provided or the insulin dosage is not reduced, severe hypoglycemia can develop lor.g after exercise stops, even if the exercise has been of relatively short duration (<1 hour).

A very different metabolic response can occur if exercise is performed during periods of poor control and severe insulin deficiency. In this situation, in which hyperglycemia and ketosis are present, exercise does not increase peripheral glucose utilization. Instead, rates of fat-cell lipolysis, hepatic glucose production, and keto-genesis outmatch utilization by the tissues. The inability

of exercise to increase glucose utilization under these conditions may be a function of the increased mobilization and oxidation of free fatty acids and ketones, inhibiting glucose oxidation by a feedback mechanism that involves an increase in cellular citrate concentration.[33] The net result is a worsening of hyperglycemia (Fig. 26–2), increased ketosis, and accompanying acidosis. For this reason, exercise by the poorly controlled, ketotic diabetic patient is contraindicated.

METABOLIC EFFECTS OF EXERCISE TRAINING

In recent years, a multitude of retrospective, cross-sectional, and prospective studies have suggested that physical exercise performed on a regular basis may be beneficial for health and longevity. The effects of exercise training may range from psychosocial factors (e.g., increased self-esteem), to favorable changes in whole-body physiology (e.g., enhanced aerobic capacity), to adaptive responses in cellular biochemistry. There is considerable evidence that the performance of regular physical exercise is associated with decreased risk of cardiovascular disease, possibly reflecting the combined effects of all of these factors. Since accelerated atherosclerotic cardiovascular disease represents one of the most significant complications of diabetes, it is important to consider the potential long-term benefits of exercise training in individuals with NIDDM and IDDM.

Endurance exercise training involves the performance of prolonged, intense physical activities such as running, swimming, or cycling at frequent intervals over a period of weeks, months, or years. An endurance training regimen can result in a remarkable increase in the capacity for performance of aerobic exercise as a result of numerous metabolic adaptations in the skeletal muscle, cardiovascular system, autonomic nervous system, and endocrine system. These adaptations include an increased maximal ability to consume oxygen (Vo_{2max}), increased endurance at submaximal workloads, increased cardiac output, decreased heart rate at submaximal workloads, and increased lean body mass along with decreased body fat.[34,35] Endurance training can also improve blood lipid profiles by increasing the high-density lipoprotein (HDL) subfraction of cholesterol, increasing the ratio of HDL to total cholesterol, and decreasing circulating triglyceride concentrations.[36–38] In skeletal muscle, exercise training can result in an increase in the number and size of mitochondria and in cellular respiratory capacity as evidenced by increased activity of citric acid cycle and other oxidative enzymes (e.g., succinic dehydrogenase, reduced nicotinamide adenine dinucleotide [NADH] dehydrogenase, and cytochrome oxidase).[34,35,39,40] In addition, skeletal muscle of trained individuals is characterized by an increased activity of enzymes for β oxidation, resulting in more effective utilization of free fatty acids for metabolic fuel and a sparing of muscle glycogen.[41]

One of the most important questions in regard to diabetes, and one that has not been resolved, is whether exercise training can improve glucose tolerance, glucose homeostasis, and the sensitivity of skeletal muscle to

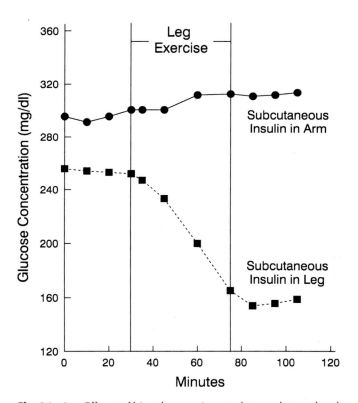

Fig. 26–3. Effects of bicycle exercise on plasma glucose levels in patients with insulin-dependent diabetes following insulin administration in the arm (immobilized, nonexercising limb) or in the thigh (exercising limb). Data are derived from the same subject on two different occasions. Data are from Zinman et al.[32]

insulin. Several studies in persons without diabetes have shown that trained individuals have a smaller increase in plasma insulin concentrations in response to a glucose load than do sedentary individuals but have unchanged or improved glucose tolerance despite the lower insulin levels.[42-47] Additional studies using the hyperinsulinemic euglycemic clamp procedure have demonstrated that exercise training results in a higher rate of insulin-stimulated glucose disposal at a defined insulin dose.[48-52] These results have been interpreted as evidence that exercise training increases tissue sensitivity to insulin. There is also evidence that a single bout of exercise can produce similar effects on glucose disposal and metabolism that can last for several hours after cessation of exercise.[14-17,20,21,53-57] It is likely that the effects of a regular exercise program on glucose tolerance and tissue insulin sensitivity reflect the combined influences of the metabolic adaptations of training plus acute metabolic responses to each bout of exercise.

METABOLIC EFFECTS OF ENDURANCE TRAINING IN DIABETES

An endurance exercise training program in individuals with diabetes results in changes in glucose metabolism similar to those that occur in individuals without diabetes. In one study, a vigorous exercise training program in patients with mild NIDDM was shown to normalize glucose tolerance.[58] Figure 26–4 describes the results of a study on the effects of a 6- to 10-week exercise training program on glucose tolerance in a group of patients with NIDDM.[59] Both the fasting plasma glucose level and the integrated rise in plasma glucose after administration of oral glucose are decreased in the trained subjects. Other investigators have confirmed increased insulin-stimulated

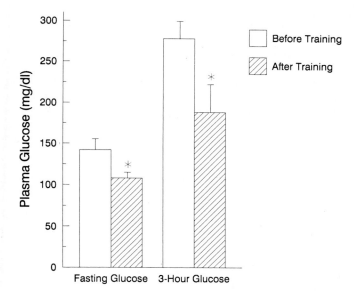

Fig. 26–4. Effects of a 6- to 10-week intensive exercise training program in obese patients with non-insulin-dependent diabetes on fasting plasma glucose concentrations and 3-hour integrated glucose response to ingestion of 75 g of glucose. Data are from Reitman et al.[59]

glucose disposal following exercise training in persons with NIDDM,[60,61] but beneficial effects on glucose tolerance have been variable.[48,62,63] It is probable that the effects of an exercise training program in persons with NIDDM are influenced by the degree of insulin resistance and insulin deficiency, the frequency and intensity of exercise, and multiple other factors, such as improved adherence to diet and loss of weight that often accompany a commitment to physical training. Under favorable circumstances, this can result in a modest improvement in long-term glucose control.[64]

In patients with IDDM, a program of exercise training can increase Vo_{2max} and the activities of mitochondrial enzymes that support glucose oxidation in muscle.[19,65] As in patients with NIDDM, regular physical exercise has been shown to improve insulin sensitivity.[19,66] Most studies, however, have not demonstrated an improvement in glucose control following an exercise program in patients with IDDM.[19,66,67-69] The available data thus would suggest only minor benefits for most patients if improved glucose control were the only objective of an exercise program in diabetes. However, since exercise training also can lead to improved cardiovascular fitness and blood lipid profiles, the potential effects on morbidity and mortality in IDDM as well as in NIDDM may be quite significant.

GENERAL GUIDELINES FOR EXERCISE PRESCRIPTION

Although the long-term benefits of regular exercise training on glucose tolerance and metabolic control have yet to be rigorously established, the current data suggest that an exercise program may be a valuable adjunct to diet, insulin, and oral agents in the management of diabetes.[70] In NIDDM, with the frequent occurrence of insulin resistance, obesity, blood lipid abnormalities, and cardiovascular disease, the potential benefits of exercise are obvious and the risk of serious hypoglycemia relatively low. Thus, a component of physical exercise should be considered in designing a management regimen for the majority of patients with NIDDM. In IDDM, the risk of serious hypoglycemia or worsened hyperglycemia and ketosis consequent to exercise merits a more cautious approach. A physical training program should be considered to be a potentially useful adjunct in management for many patients with IDDM, but appropriate care must be given to balancing insulin, diet, and exercise so that the consequences of hypoglycemia do not outweigh the benefits of exercise.

In all individuals with diabetes, once the decision to undertake an exercise program has been made, a careful and thorough medical examination should be performed. This should include a review of recent blood glucose control and an assessment of long-term complications of diabetes that may represent contraindications to exercise. If blood glucose control is poor, it should be regulated before the patient starts exercising. As a general rule, the blood glucose level should be less than 250 mg/dL, ketosis should be absent, and episodes of hypoglycemia should be infrequent. Severe or progressive retinopathy is a contraindication to intense exercise, since changes in blood pressure during exercise can increase the risk of vessel leakage and hemorrhage. This is an especially important consideration if patients are receiving laser therapy. Exercise involving the lower extremities in patients with peripheral neuropathy requires extremely close observation for foot injuries and may be totally contraindicated. For patients with neuropathy, it may be necessary to select activities, such as swimming, that do not carry significant risk of trauma to lower extremity soft tissue or to joints.

In addition to these considerations, before patients start an exercise program, it is advisable for them to undergo exercise stress testing if they are older than 30 years of age or have had diabetes for more than 20 years. Exercise stress testing should be considered mandatory in all patients with symptoms consistent with cardiovascular disease. For many individuals, it may be simplest and safest for them to enroll in a fitness program for cardiac patients. These programs provide supervised exercises of appropriate intensity and duration and also minimize the chance of injury by teaching proper techniques for stretching, warming-up, and cooling-down. Information about programs of this type can generally be obtained from a local cardiologist or cardiology department.

The goals and needs of each individual patient must be considered when prescribing exercise. Some patients may wish to undertake a less-intensive program, while others may want to participate in exercise of prolonged duration and intensity, such as marathon running and competitive sports. Some improvement in cardiovascular fitness in sedentary individuals can be expected to occur with almost any degree of increase in regular physical activity. However, according to the guidelines of the American College of Sports Medicine, the generation and maintenance of a good level of aerobic fitness probably requires three exercise sessions per week, performed on nonconsecutive days. The duration of each exercise session should be between 20 to 30 minutes at approximately 50 to 55% of maximal aerobic capacity or approximately 70% of age-adjusted maximal heart rate (maximal heart rate = 220 − age in years). Each exercise session should also include a 5- to 10-minute warm-up and cool-down component. The type of exercise performed should involve the use of a large muscle mass, such as that accomplished with brisk walking, aerobic dancing, running, swimming, cycling, rowing, or cross-country skiing. In addition to the goals or desires of the patient, the occurrence of complications of diabetes or other medical problems, such as cardiovascular disease, neuropathy, and retinopathy, should influence the choice of an appropriate exercise regimen.

When an exercise program is initiated in a patient with diabetes, it is very important to increase the intensity and duration of exercise gradually. In individuals with NIDDM, who may not have been physically active for a long period, a program of gradually increasing exercise will provide adequate time for the cardiovascular system to adapt and will allow for progressive development of flexibility and muscle strength. In patients with IDDM, a progressive exercise regimen will make it possible to adjust diet and insulin incrementally with minimal risk of hypoglycemia.

As mentioned above, 20 to 30 minutes of exercise three times per week will significantly improve cardiovascular fitness. It also will result in an increased caloric consumption of approximately 600 to 900 kcal per week. For patients with NIDDM on weight-reduction programs, if good adherence and tolerance of an exercise program is established, a greater frequency and duration of exercise may be indicated. Exercising at 70 to 85% of maximal heart rate for 30 to 60 minutes three to five times per week will result in a significantly greater caloric consumption (1000 to 3000 kcal per week). Furthermore, the post-exercise changes in glucose disposal and glucose tolerance discussed earlier in this chapter may also have a significant impact on overall glucose homeostasis when exercise is performed at this intensity, duration, and frequency.

Probably the most common risk for the exercising patient with diabetes is the development of hypoglycemia. Hypoglycemia can occur as a result of an acceleration of insulin absorption, an increase in whole-body glucose disposal, muscle glycogen depletion, an impairment in the response of counterregulatory hormones to exercise, and/or the interaction of glucose-lowering agents and exercise.

Several steps that patients with diabetes can take to reduce the risk of hypoglycemia are outlined in Table 26–2. The risk of hypoglycemia in patients taking insulin can be minimized if exercise is not undertaken immediately after insulin injection. In patients with tight control, additional calories in the form of readily absorbable carbohydrate should be taken before, during, and after exercise as needed. For this purpose, diluted fruit juice can be used to provide both calories and adequate amounts of water. An approximation of the calories expended by various forms of exercise is listed in Table 26–3. Blood glucose levels should be monitored frequently, and it should be recognized that hypoglycemia can develop as long as 24 hours after cessation of exercise as a result of increased caloric consumption during exercise and increased insulin responsiveness following

Table 26-2. Guidelines For Prevention of Hypoglycemia during and after Exercise

1. Monitoring blood glucose concentrations before, during, and after exercise. Frequent monitoring especially important when new exercise regimen or type of exercise initiated. Each person should learn how he or she responds to different types and intensities of exercise.
2. If blood glucose is <100 mg/dL, a carbohydrate snack should be eaten before exercise. For prolonged exercise, 15–30 g of carbohydrates may need to be eaten every 30 min during the exercise period and food intake may need to be increased for as long as 24 hours after exercise.
3. Avoid exercise at time of peak insulin action and exercise that involves muscles into which short-acting insulin has recently been injected.

Table 26-3. Caloric Expenditures of Physical Exercise

Activity	kcal/kg/hr	kcal/hr (in 68-kg human)
Light	0.73-2.93	50-200
Lying down	1.17	80
Sitting	1.47	100
Standing	2.05	140
Moderate	2.93-5.13	200-350
Walking (2.5 mph)	3.08	210
Golf	3.67	250
Swimming (0.25 mph)	4.40	300
Walking (3.75 mph)	4.40	300
Square dancing	5.13	350
Vigorous	>5.13	>350
Ice skating	5.87	400
Tennis	6.16	420
Skiing (10 mph)	8.80	600
Cycling (13 mph)	9.68	660
Running (10 mph)	13.20	900

Recalculated from reference 71 (Biermann J, Toohey B. Chart of calorie expenditures. Appendix E. In: The diabetic's sports and exercise book. Philadelphia: JB Lippincott, 1977:241-2).

exercise. In patients with NIDDM, hypoglycemia is much less likely to occur as a result of exercise. Patients with NIDDM will frequently not need to increase carbohydrate ingestion to prevent hypoglycemia and may have a tendency to overeat in anticipation of exercise. This obviously will offset the potential benefits of exercise on weight control.

In patients with IDDM who become involved in strenuous, prolonged sports activities, such as distance running and team sports, increased carbohydrate intake alone is unlikely to compensate adequately for the metabolic effects of exercise. Insulin dosage should be slowly decreased, typically in 10% increments, as exercise intensity is increased until an adequate prescription is developed for altered insulin dosage in anticipation of exercise. These patients should monitor glucose levels closely following exercise even after an effective program for insulin adjustment has been established.

With the availability of modern forms of insulin and glucose-monitoring methods, exercise is probably not as critical a component of the "everyday management of diabetes" as it was in Dr. Elliot Joslin's practice in 1935.[1] However, as an adjunct to other forms of therapy, regular physical exercise will play an important role in lowering the risk for cardiovascular disease and in reducing weight and may play a valuable supporting role in improving glucose control. With a carefully and sensibly designed exercise program, almost all individuals with IDDM or NIDDM can be encouraged to participate in their choices of recreational sports and activities, fitness programs, or even competitive athletics.

REFERENCES

1. Joslin EP, Root HF, White P, Marble A. The treatment of diabetes mellitus. 5th ed. Philadelphia: Lea & Febiger, 1935:299.
2. Rollo J. Cases of the diabetes mellitus; with the results of the trials of certain acids and other substances, in the cure of the lues venerea. 2nd ed. Dilly: London, 1798.
3. Wahren J, Felig P, Hagenfeldt L. Physical exercise and fuel homeostasis in diabetes mellitus. Diabetologia 1978; 14:213-22.
4. Ahlborg G, Felig P, Hagenfeldt L, et al. Substrate turnover during prolonged exercise in man: splanchnic and leg metabolism of glucose, free fatty acids, and amino acids. J Clin Invest 1974;53:1080-90.
5. Wahren J, Felig P, Ahlborg G, Jorfeldt L. Glucose metabolism during leg exercise in man. J Clin Invest 1971; 50:2715-25.
6. Hartley LH, Mason JW, Hogan RP, et al. Multiple hormonal responses to graded exercise in relation to physical training. J Appl Physiol 1972;33:602-6.
7. Hermansen L, Pruett EDR, Osnes JB, Giere FA. Blood glucose and plasma insulin in response to maximal exercise and glucose infusion. J Appl Physiol 1970;29:13-6.
8. Galbo H. Hormonal and metabolic adaptation to exercise. New York: Thieme Verlag, 1983.
9. Galbo H, Holst JJ, Christensen NJ. Glucagon and plasma catecholamine responses to graded and prolonged exercise in man. J Appl Physiol 1975;38:70-6.
10. Gray DE, Lickley HLA, Vranic M. Physiologic effects of epinephrine on glucose turnover and plasma free fatty acid concentrations mediated independently of glucagon. Diabetes 1980;29:600-8.
11. Vranic M, Berger M. Exercise and diabetes mellitus. Diabetes 1979;28:147-63.
12. Vranic M, Wasserman D, Bukowiecki L. Metabolic implications of exercise and physical fitness in physiology and diabetes. In: Rifkin H, Porte D. Diabetes mellitus: theory and practice. 4th ed. New York: Elsevier, 1990:198-219.
13. Felig P, Wahren J. Fuel homeostasis in exercise. N Engl J Med 1975;293:10'8-84.
14. Pruett EDR, Oseid S. Effect of exercise on glucose and insulin response to glucose infusion. Scand J Clin Lab Invest 1970;26:277-85.
15. Bogardus C, Thuillez P, Ravussin E, Vasquez B. Effect of muscle glycogen depletion on in vivo insulin action in man. J Clin Invest 1983;72:1605-10.
16. Mikines KJ, Sonne B, Farrell PA, et al. Effect of physical exercise on sensitivity and responsiveness to insulin in humans. Am J Physiol 1988;254:E248-59.
17. Richter EA, Mikines KJ, Galbo H, Kiens B. Effect of exercise on insulin action in human skeletal muscle. J Appl Physiol 1989;66:876-85.
18. Defronzo RA, Ferrannini E, Sato Y, Felig P. Synergistic interaction between exercise and insulin on peripheral glucose uptake. J Clin Invest 1981;68:1468-74.
19. Wallberg-Henriksson H, Gunnarsson R, Henriksson J, et al. Increased peripheral insulin sensitivity and muscle mitochondrial enzymes but unchanged blood glucose control in type I diabetics after physical training. Diabetes 1982; 31:1044-50.
20. Devlin JT, Horton ES. Effects of prior high-intensity exercise on glucose metabolism in normal and insulin-resistant men. Diabetes 1985;34:973-9.
21. Devlin JT, Hirshman M, Horton ED, Horton ES. Enhanced peripheral and splanchnic insulin sensitivity in NIDDM men after single bout of exercise. Diabetes 1987;36:434-9.
22. Berger M, Hagg S, Ruderman NB. Glucose metabolism in perfused skeletal muscle: interaction of insulin and exercise on glucose uptake. Biochem J 1975;146:231-8.

23. Elbrink J, Bihler I. Membrane transport: its relation to cellular metabolic rates. Science 1975;188:1177–84.

24. Richter EA, Garetto LP, Goodman MN, Ruderman NB. Muscle glucose metabolism following exercise in the rat: increased sensitivity to insulin. J Clin Invest 1982; 69:785–93.

25. Douen AG, Ramlal T, Klip A, et al. Exercise-induced increase in glucose transporters in plasma membranes of rat skeletal muscle. Endocrinology 1989;124:449–54.

26. Hirshman MF, Wallberg-Henriksson H, Wardzala LJ, et al. Acute exercise increases the number of plasma membrane glucose transporters in rat skeletal muscle. FEBS Lett 1988;238:235–9.

27. Goodyear LJ, Hirshman MF, King PA, et al. Skeletal muscle plasma membrane glucose transport and glucose transporters after exercise. J Appl Physiol 1990;68:193–8.

28. King PA, Hirshman MF, Horton ED, Horton ES. Glucose transport in skeletal muscle membrane vesicles from control and exercised rats. Am J Physiol 1989; 257:C1128–34.

29. Minuk HL, Vranic M, Marliss EB, et al. Glucoregulatory and metabolic response to exercise in obese noninsulin-dependent diabetes. Am J Physiol 1981;240:E458–64.

30. Kemmer FW, Tacken M, Berger M. Mechanism of exercise-induced hypoglycemia during sulfonylurea treatment. Diabetes 1987;36:1178–82.

31. Horton ES. Role and management of exercise in diabetes mellitus. Diabetes Care 1988;11:201–11.

32. Zinman B, Murray FT, Vranic M, et al. Glucoregulation during moderate exercise in insulin treated diabetics. J Clin Endocrinol Metab 1977;45:641–52.

33. Randle PJ, Garland PB, Hales CN, Newsholme EA. The glucose fatty-acid cycle its role in insulin sensitivity and the metabolic disturbances of diabetes mellitus. Lancet 1963;1:785–9.

34. Holloszy JO, Rennie MJ, Hickson RC, et al. Physiological consequences of the biochemical adaptations to endurance exercise. Ann NY Acad Sci 1977;301:440–50.

35. Holloszy, JO, Coyle EF. Adaptations of skeletal muscle to endurance exercise and their metabolic consequences. J Appl Physiol 1984;56:831–8.

36. Haskell WL, Taylor HL, Wood PD, et al. Strenuous physical activity, treadmill exercise test performance and plasma high-density lipoprotein cholesterol: the Lipid Research Clinics Program Prevalence Study. Circulation 1980; 62(Suppl 4):53–61.

37. Goodyear LJ, Fronsoe MS, Van Houten DR, et al. Increased HDL-cholesterol following eight weeks of progressive endurance training in female runners. Ann Sports Med 1986;3:33–8.

38. Haskell WL, Stefanick ML, Superko R. Influence of exercise on plasma lipids and lipoproteins. In: Horton ES, Terjung RL, eds. Exercise, nutrition, and energy metabolism. New York: Macmillan, 1988:213–27.

39. Holloszy JO. Biochemical adaptations in muscle: effects of exercise on mitochondrial oxygen uptake and respiratory enzyme activity in skeletal muscle. J Biol Chem 1967;242:2278–82.

40. Gollnick PD. Metabolism of substrates: energy substrate metabolism during exercise and as modified by training. Fed Proc 1985;44:353–7.

41. Holloszy JO. Metabolic consequences of endurance exercise training. In: Horton ES, Terjung RL. Exercise, nutrition, and energy metabolism. New York: Macmillan, 1988:116–31.

42. Björntorp P, Fahlén M, Grimby G, et al. Carbohydrate and lipid metabolism in middle-aged, physically well-trained men. Metabolism 1972;21:1037–44.

43. Lohmann D, Liebold F, Heilmann W, et al. Diminished insulin response in highly trained athletes. Metabolism 1978;27:521–4.

44. Johansen K, Munck O. The relationship between maximal oxygen uptake and glucose tolerance/insulin response ratio in normal young men. Horm Metab Res 1979;11:424–7.

45. Leblanc J, Nadeau A, Richard D, Tremblay A. Studies on the sparing effect of exercise on insulin requirements in human subjects. Metabolism 1981;30:1119–24.

46. Leblanc J, Nadeau A, Richard D, Tremblay A. Variations in plasma glucose, insulin, growth hormone and catecholamines in response to insulin in trained and non-trained subjects. Metabolism 1982;31:453–6.

47. Seals DR, Hagberg JM, Allen WK, et al. Glucose tolerance in young and older athletes and sedentary men. J Appl Physiol 1984;56:1521–5.

48. Saltin G, Lingärde F, Houston M, et al. Physical training and glucose tolerance in middle-aged men with chemical diabetes. Diabetes 1979;28(Suppl 1):30–2.

49. Rosenthal M, Haskell WL, Solomon R, et al. Demonstration of a relationship between level of physical training and insulin-stimulated glucose utilization in normal humans. Diabetes 1983;32:408–11.

50. Hollenbeck CB, Haskell W, Rosenthal M, Reaven GM. Effect of habitual physical activity on regulation of insulin-stimulated glucose disposal in older males. J Am Geriatr Soc 1985;33:273–7.

51. King DS, Dalsky GP, Staten MA, et al. Insulin action and secretion in endurance-trained and untrained humans. J Appl Physiol 1987;63:2247–52.

52. Mikines KJ, Sonne B, Tronier B, Galbo H. Effects of acute exercise and detraining on insulin action in trained men. J Appl Physiol 1989;66:704–11.

53. Holloszy JO, Narahara HT. Studies of tissue permeability. X. Changes in permeability to 3-methylglucose associated with contraction of isolated frog muscle. J Biol Chem 1965;240:3493–500.

54. Elbrink J, Phipps BA. Studies on the persistence of enhanced monosaccharide transport in rat skeletal muscle following the cessation of the initial stimulus. Cell Calcium 1980;1:349–58.

55. Fell RD, Terblanche SE, Ivy JL, et al. Effect of muscle glycogen content on glucose uptake following exercise. J Appl Physiol 1982;52:434–7.

56. Ivy JL, Young JC, McLane JA, et al. Exercise training and glucose uptake by skeletal muscle in rats. J Appl Physiol 1983;55:1393–6.

57. Mikines KJ, Sonne B, Farrell PA, et al. Effect of training on the dose-response relationship for insulin action in men. J Appl Physiol 1989;66:695–703.

58. Holloszy JO, Schultz J, Kusnierkiewicz J, et al. Effects of exercise on glucose tolerance and insulin resistance: brief review and some preliminary results. Acta Med Scand Suppl 1986;711:55–65.

59. Reitman JS, Vasquez B, Klimes I, Nagulesparan M. Improvement of glucose homeostasis after exercise training in non-insulin-dependent diabetes. Diabetes Care 1984; 7:434–41.

60. Trovati M, Carta Q, Cavalot F, et al. Influence of physical training on blood glucose control, glucose tolerance, insulin secretion, and insulin action in non-insulin-dependent diabetic patients. Diabetes Care 1984;7:416–20.

61. Yki-Järvinen H, Koivisto VA. Continuous subcutaneous

insulin infusion therapy decreases insulin resistance in type I diabetes. J Clin Endocrinol Metab 1984;58:659–66.

62. Ruderman NB, Ganda OP, Johansen K. The effect of physical training on glucose tolerance and plasma lipids in maturity-onset diabetes. Diabetes 1979;28(Suppl 1):89–92.

63. Rogers MA, Yamamoto C, King DS, et al. Improvement in glucose tolerance after 1 wk of exercise in patients with mild NIDDM. Diabetes Care 1988;11:613–8.

64. Schneider SH, Amorosa LF, Khachadurian AK, Ruderman NB. Studies on the mechanism of improved glucose control during regular exercise in type 2 (non-insulin-dependent) diabetes. Diabetologia 1984;26:355–60.

65. Costill DL, Cleary P, Fink WJ, et al. Training adaptations in skeletal muscle of juvenile diabetics. Diabetes 1979;28:818–22.

66. Koivisto VA, Yki-Jörvinen H, Defronzo RA. Physical training and insulin sensitivity. Diabetes Metab Rev 1986;1:445–81.

67. Zinman B, Zuniga-Guajardo S, Kelly D. Comparison of the acute and long-term effects of exercise on glucose control in type I diabetes. Diabetes Care 1984;7:515–9.

68. Wallberg-Henriksson H, Gunnarsson R, Henriksson J, et al. Influence of physical training on formation of muscle capillaries in type I diabetes. Diabetes 1984;33:851–7.

69. Landt KW, Campaigne BN, James FW, Sperling MA. Effects of exercise training on insulin sensitivity in adolescents with type I diabetes. Diabetes Care 1985;8:461–5.

70. National Institutes of Health. Consensus development conference on diet and exercise in non-insulin-dependent diabetes mellitus. Diabetes Care 1987;10:639–44.

71. Biermann J, Toohey B. Chart of calorie expenditures. Appendix E. In: The diabetic's sports and exercise book. Philadelphia: JB Lippincott, 1977:241–2.

Chapter 27

PRINCIPLES OF INSULIN THERAPY

JAMES L. ROSENZWEIG

A thorough knowledge and understanding of the use of insulin is essential to the proper treatment of diabetes. Currently, approximately one-third of all patients in the United States with diagnosed diabetes, including essentially all those with Type I diabetes, are being treated with insulin. It is thought that a significant proportion of the patients who are not now receiving insulin have suboptimal diabetes control and would benefit from the use of insulin. Those who do take insulin are often poorly managed, have inadequate or inappropriate insulin regimens, receive deficient education on the management of their disease, and are in poor communication with their physicians. Insulin is often viewed by both patient and physician as a treatment of last resort—a club or weapon to stave off disasters such as ketoacidosis and coma rather than a tool to correct or reverse the metabolic derangements that accompany diabetes.

Normally, the physiologic secretion of insulin into the portal circulation to control the concentration of glucose in the blood is timed precisely to meet the body's needs for glucose disposal and is regulated exquisitely by circulating body fuels and hormones. Once such control is lost, as in diabetes, it is extremely difficult to duplicate with subcutaneous injections of insulin released into the peripheral circulation.[1,2] Although it has been said that "the goal of physiologic replacement remains elusive,"[3] much can be done to approach that end, and our knowledge and abilities to achieve this goal have improved steadily. Because blood glucose levels can be so variable and are subject to changes in response to activity, diet, and numerous other factors, the establishment of good control is extremely labor-intensive, requiring vigilance by both patient and physician. Blood glucose levels must be monitored and evaluated continually, with adjustments in insulin dosage and regulation of activity and diet. Perhaps no area of therapy in internal medicine requires such close contact and communication between patient and physician.

Many developments have been made in insulin therapy since the publication of the previous edition of this text. Much has been learned about the chemistry and pharmacologic effects of insulin, as well as about the mechanisms of insulin action. The purity of commercially available insulins has improved, with a resultant decrease in their immunogenicity and related lipoatrophy, allergy, and immunologic insulin resistance. The use of human insulin as a therapeutic tool has continued to increase, now being dominant compared with animal insulins. Home blood glucose monitoring has become a routine component of diabetes management and has largely replaced urine testing. Periodic measurement of glycosylated hemoglobin levels is now a routine feature of diabetes care.

Debate continues about the indications for insulin treatment in many key situations, as well as about the role of insulin versus sulfonylureas in the early stages of diabetes. Debate has been resolved, however, on one other issue; it is clear that improved control of blood glucoses can decrease or prevent the microvascular complications of diabetes. New insulin regimens have been advocated, including "intensive" insulin treatment involving multiple daily injections, home blood glucose monitoring, and the adjustment of insulin dose on the basis of blood glucose measurements. There has been an increased use of long-acting ultralente insulins instead of the intermediate-acting insulins in certain situations. Alternative insulin injection systems, such as pen-type cartridge devices, are now widely used in some parts of the world. Open-loop, continuous, subcutaneous insulin-pump delivery systems continue as a mode of treatment for intensive diabetic control, but this form of therapy has been restricted to a relatively small subset of patients. Implantable insulin delivery systems are now in experimental use in patients with Type I and Type II diabetes.[4]

Further developments are anticipated in the near future. Monomeric insulin analogues have been developed that have more-rapid subcutaneous absorption profiles than regular insulin. These are expected to provide improved control of postprandial glucose levels.[5,6] Other insulin analogues with extremely long half-lives may prove superior to ultralente insulin for the delivery of basal insulin. The development of insulin preparations that will be absorbed nasally continues.[7] The creation of a reliable and accurate implantable glucose sensor remains the missing link in the development of a closed-loop insulin delivery system,[4] and islet cell transplantation is still in the experimental stage. Pending further developments in these areas, the mainstay of therapy for the near future will probably continue to be subcutaneous insulin injection.

HISTORICAL BACKGROUND

We now have 70 years of experience with the use of insulin. Insulin was first isolated by Banting and Best from dog pancreas in 1921,[8] and the first injection of insulin was given to a patient with diabetes at the Toronto General Hospital on January 12, 1922.[9] In the next few years, great strides were made in the extraction and purification of insulin, such that insulin became widely available for the treatment of patients with insulin-dependent diabetes mellitus (IDDM). At that time, because of the relatively short duration of action of soluble insulin, it was necessary to inject insulin subcutaneously three to four times a day to control blood glucose levels adequately.

In 1936, Hagedorn discovered that the activity of insulin after injection could be delayed or prolonged with the addition of various basic proteins, such as fish protamine, which kept the insulin in suspension so that it was absorbed more slowly from subcutaneous sites.[10] In the same year, Scott and Fisher showed that zinc and other heavy metals could extend the duration of action of protamine insulin even further, a finding that led to the development of protamine zinc insulin (PZI), the first really stable insulin preparation with prolonged action.[11] An injection of PZI could lower the blood glucose level for 48 to 72 hours and could be administered once a day by the patient for blood glucose control. The availability of protamine insulin and PZI ushered in the "Hagedorn Era," which revolutionized insulin therapy, leading to the predominance of once-a-day regimens of intermediate and long-acting insulins in the treatment of diabetes, as opposed to the multiple daily injections of soluble insulin used previously. In subsequent years, other insulins with prolonged action were developed. Isophane insulin, a more stable form of protamine insulin also known as NPH insulin (neutral protamine Hagedorn), was introduced in 1946[12] and has become the most widely used insulin in the United States. Insulin zinc suspensions that contain no added protamine or modifying proteins—referred to as the "lente" (slow-acting) series—were developed and introduced in the early 1950s.[13]

The past 20 years have seen a progressive improvement in the purity of commercially available insulins. This has resulted in a marked decrease in the medical problems attributed to immunogenicity of the insulin preparations. In 1980, human insulin was introduced, and its use has increased steadily.[15] The treatment of diabetes with insulin has been greatly influenced by the increased use of home blood glucose monitoring, which has allowed patients to adjust their insulin doses with algorithms based on their blood glucose levels. This has resulted in the development of a number of insulin regimens designed to accommodate physiologic needs for insulin, as will be discussed later in this chapter.

TYPES OF INSULIN

A list of the most commonly used insulins commercially available in the United States is given in Table 27–1. Similar preparations, often under different commercial names, are available throughout the world. Recent years have seen increasing standardization of the insulin preparations, as the production of insulin has become concentrated in the hands of fewer pharmaceutical companies as a result of mergers. Nevertheless, in recent years the number of different types of insulin available has increased because of the development of insulins from many species, of many degrees of purity, and of new insulin delivery systems such as pen-type devices.

Rapid-Acting Insulins

Regular insulin (also called crystalline zinc insulin, or CZI) is clear in solution to permit the most rapid

Table 27-1. Characteristics of Insulins Available in the United States

Types and Preparations	Composition	Action profile (hr)*			Insulin Species†
		Onset	Peak	Duration	
SHORT-ACTING					
Regular	Insulin solution, unbuffered	0.5	2-5	6-8	H,P,B/P
Buffered regular	Insulin solution, phosphate buffer	0.5	2-5	6-8	H,P
INTERMEDIATE-ACTING					
NPH	Protamine zinc suspension, phosphate buffer	1-2	4-12	18-26	H,P,B,B/P
Lente	Amorphous and crystalline suspension, acetate buffer	1-3	6-15	18-26	H,P,B,B/P
Isophane/regular	NPH 70%, regular 30%	0.5	2-12	24	H,P
U-500	Concentrated, unmodified insulin solution	1-3	6-12	12-18	P
LONG-ACTING					
Ultralente	Crystalline suspension, acetate buffer	4-6	8-30	24-36	H,B,B/P

*The times listed for onset, peak, and duration of action of the insulins listed are variable, with marked differences from one injection to another and variability due to location of injection, injection technique, insulin antibodies, insulin species, and other factors that affect insulin pharmacokinetics.
†H = human insulin; P = pork insulin; B = beef insulin; B/P = mixture of beef and pork insulins.
‡Production of PZI was recently discontinued in the United States.

absorption possible after injection, with peak activity usually 2 to 4 hours after subcutaneous injection. Its total duration of action after subcutaneous injection is generally considered to be approximately 6 hours, but a great degree of variability has been demonstrated both between subjects and at different times in the same individual. Daily insulin treatment programs most often use regular insulin to counteract the surge in blood glucose level that occurs after a meal. When regular insulin is given subcutaneously, onset of action is delayed, so it should be injected 30 to 45 minutes before a meal. In many treatment regimens, regular insulin is often mixed in the syringe with an intermediate- or long-acting insulin. Often the patient can adjust the dose of regular insulin according to blood glucose measurements determined by home monitoring and the application of pre-set algorithms. In addition, boluses of regular insulin can be given to supplement the usual insulin dose when there is hyperglycemia or ketosis in situations of acute illness. Regular insulin can also be injected from prefilled cartridges in pen devices for frequent before-meal administration.

Administration of insulin by continuous subcutaneous infusion (CSII) with insulin pumps is done exclusively with regular insulin. However, it has been found that the standard form of regular insulin, which is in an unbuffered solution, is subject to denaturation and aggregation in the tubing.[16] This problem is less common with phosphate-buffered forms of regular insulin, such as Velosulin (Novo Nordisk), which are now preferred for use in insulin pumps.[17]

Regular insulin is the only insulin that can be used intravenously. It is therefore used in infusions for treatment of diabetic ketoacidosis, hyperosmolar nonketotic coma, and the maintenance of blood glucose levels during surgery, trauma, and metabolic emergencies.

Semilente insulin has a longer duration of action than regular insulin, with a peak activity 2 to 8 hours after injection. It is now prescribed infrequently. It has some value as a substitute for intermediate-acting insulins in those patients for whom the action of these insulins tends to be delayed and may also be used in place of regular insulin in those patients with extremely rapid hypoglycemic responses to injected insulin.

Intermediate-Acting Insulins

All insulins other than regular insulin are modified into a suspension form to delay their absorption from subcutaneous sites, thereby prolonging their action. This modification can be accomplished by the addition of protamine, as in NPH insulin, or with zinc, as in the lente series of insulins. NPH and lente insulins are both commonly used, as their durations of action are similar and permit satisfactory glycemic control with one or two injections a day. Lente insulin is a stable mixture of 30% semilente insulin and 70% ultralente insulin. Although it is often said that these two insulins are interchangeable, lente insulin frequently has a more prolonged duration of action than NPH insulin. In theory, lente insulin may be preferable because it contains no additional protein that might serve as an allergen. However, this difference has not been found to be of clinical significance,[18] and NPH insulin is used widely. In addition, the use of NPH insulin in mixtures with regular insulin may offer some benefits, as will be discussed later in this chapter.

Long-Acting Insulins

In recent years, ultralente insulin has been used more frequently in a variety of regimens. Its slow onset of action, long duration, and relatively small peak of hypo-glycemic effect make it useful in regimens requiring a constant basal action of insulin. In many cases, beef ultralente insulin can be given once a day to provide a relatively "peakless" effect. In some individuals, however, this insulin has a more rapid effect, making two injections per day necessary for a "peakless" effect. Ultralente insulin has a very long half-life of activity after injection, and many days of treatment with this insulin may be necessary before a steady-state level of circulating insulin is achieved. Some advocate giving a large initial loading dose to a patient starting ultralente insulin.[19] Human ultralente insulin has a shorter duration of action than beef ultralente[20] and is therefore not "peakless" when given once a day. It is usually given twice a day to achieve a basal effect of insulin activity. Human ultralente insulin is also useful as a replacement for intermediate-acting insulins in those patients for whom these insulins have too rapid an effect. For example, some patients take NPH insulin along with regular insulin before supper to cover their needs until morning. Often, the action of NPH insulin will not last through the night. This may be remedied by delaying until bedtime the patient's night-time NPH injection; alternatively, ultralente can be used before supper to achieve the same effect. Similarly, human ultralente insulin can occasionally be used for the morning insulin injection when NPH or lente insulin have been found to have their peak hypoglycemic effect too early in the afternoon. PZI has a slow onset and long duration of action similar to ultralente insulin but is now rarely used in the United States.

INSULIN PURITY, SPECIES, AND CONCENTRATION

As mentioned earlier, the purity of insulin preparations available from pharmaceutical companies has increased during the past 20 years. Prior to 1970, the insulin formulations available for clinical use were purified by recrystallization and contained significant amounts of impurities, including proinsulin, insulin intermediates, and contaminating proteins from islet tissue or exocrine pancreas such as glucagon, somatostatin, and pancreatic polypeptide.[21] Standard insulin preparations contained proinsulin, a marker of impurities, in concentrations of 10,000 to 20,000 parts per million (ppm). Subsequently, insulin preparations have been routinely purified by gel filtration and, more recently, by ion-exchange chromatography and other molecular-sieving techniques. There has been a progressive improvement in the purity of commercially available insulins, such that "standard" insulins currently have only 10 to 20 ppm of proinsulin and "purified" monocomponent insulins have less than 1 ppm.[22] These improvements have resulted in a marked decrease in the medical problems attributed to immunogenicity of the insulin preparations, such as insulin allergy, insulin resistance, and localized lipoatrophy.[23]

Beef and Pork Insulins

Until recently, the most commonly used insulins were extracted from beef and pork pancreata. Beef insulin differs from human insulin by three amino acids, while pork insulin differs from human insulin by only one amino acid. Thus, the use of beef insulin has been associated with higher levels of circulating antibodies to insulin, as well as to an increased incidence of insulin allergy, insulin resistance, and other antibody-mediated complications of treatment. However, these problems related to immunogenicity have been relatively rare in comparison to the those seen when commercial insulins were less purified.[24] In a number of patients, the action of beef insulin preparations appears to have a slower onset, a later peak, and a longer duration than corresponding preparations of pork insulin.[25] The reasons for this are unclear but may be related to the insulin binding to circulating antibodies or possibly to differences in the properties of insulin binding to protamine and zinc.

"Standard" insulin in the United States manufactured by Eli Lilly (Iletin I) is a mixture of beef and pork insulin, in a ratio of approximately three to one. The "standard" insulin available from Novo Nordisk Pharmaceuticals consists of beef insulin in the intermediate- and long-acting forms and pork regular insulin. More-purified preparations of both pork and beef insulin are available for those patients with specific clinical needs—usually related to the immunogenicity of the insulins.

Human Insulin

Until 1982, human insulin for human use was unavailable commercially. It had been synthesized chemically by several groups in the early and mid-1960s, but total chemical synthesis was too technically difficult and expensive to apply to large-scale pharmaceutical production. Human insulin extracted from cadaveric pancreas was available in small quantities,[26] but the limited supply of specimens and the capacity of the pancreas to undergo autodigestion after death made this an impractical source. This was changed by the development of techniques to produce insulin by recombinant DNA technology. The DNA sequences encoding the A and B chains of insulin were synthesized and inserted into plasmids in *Escherichia coli*. The proteins encoded by these DNA inserts were synthesized in culture, harvested and purified, and reassembled with the appropriate disulfide linkages to form human insulin.[27] Human insulin can also been made by a single fermentation process to produce proinsulin, which can be converted to insulin by enzymatic cleavage.[28] Human insulin has been produced with these techniques for clinical use by Eli Lilly since 1981. Human insulin was also produced from pork insulin by enzymatically removing the amino acid alanine from the carboxy terminal position of the B-chain and replacing it with the amino acid threonine.[29] These substitutions resulted in the production of insulin with an amino acid sequence identical to that of insulin of human origin and was the method by which Novo Nordisk Pharmaceuticals produced insulin for clinical use. More recently, this company began producing human insulin by recombinant DNA technology in yeast (*Saccharomyces cerevisiae*).[30]

All of the preparations of human insulin that are currently available have few or no impurities and show no evidence of contamination with bacterial protein, pancreatic peptides, or insulin breakdown products.[31]

The biologic activity and pharmacokinetics of action of each of the types of human insulin are similar to those of purified pork insulin[32]; and human NPH, lente, and ultralente insulin were indeed formulated to have onset and duration of action similar to that of their corresponding animal insulins. Nevertheless, there is some evidence that human regular insulin is more rapidly absorbed from subcutaneous sites, with a more rapid onset of action after injection.[33] This may also be true of the longer-acting human insulins,[34] with human NPH insulin having a more rapid onset of activity than human lente insulin.[35] As mentioned earlier, human ultralente insulin acts more rapidly than beef ultralente insulin and must be administered twice a day in divided doses to achieve a basal "peakless" level in the circulation. Because of variations in the pharmacokinetics of different species of insulin and even of different brands of insulin of some species, it is inadvisable for patients to interchange insulin preparations indiscriminately without the supervision of a prescribing physician. Patients should be carefully instructed about the changes that might occur when a switch of insulin preparation is necessary.

Human insulin is less antigenic than beef insulin in most patients, a difference resulting in lower titers of antibodies to insulin and in a decrease in incidence of allergy and insulin resistance.[36] It is probably less antigenic than purified pork insulin as well, although in this case the difference between the insulins is small and rarely clinically significant.[37] Circulating antibodies to insulin are still generated even with the use of human insulin, albeit in lower titers than those reached with the use of animal insulins. Although there is no good evidence suggesting that human insulin is preferable to purified pork insulin for clinical use, human insulin has become much more widely used in North America because of its lower cost and increasing availability. Currently, human insulin represents 67% of the insulin sold in the United States and 74% of the all the insulin sold in the industrialized nations.[38] Because human insulin has become less and less expensive to produce, it is likely that it will continue to dominate the market and eventually to replace animal insulins except in isolated clinical circumstances.

There are some specific medical indications for switching a patient from animal insulin to human insulin: It is particularly helpful in eliminating medical problems caused by the antigenicity of animal insulins such as insulin allergy, insulin resistance, and localized lipoatrophy at injection sites.[39] Human insulin can also be used in patients treated with the animal regular insulins for whom the hypoglycemic effect is too delayed to counteract the rise in blood glucose level after meals. Currently, at the Joslin Diabetes Center, most patients beginning therapy with insulin are given human insulin. It would seem best, at least theoretically, to use human insulin in those patients who are being exposed to insulin for the first time or who may be receiving insulin temporarily, such as women with gestational diabetes. Stopping and starting the administration of insulin increases its antigenic potential.[40]

However, if a patient is using "standard" animal insulin and has good glycemic control with no adverse effects of therapy, there is no good reason to change to human insulin. Indeed, the more rapid onset and shorter duration of action of human insulin could present problems in some clinical situations. Patients who administer NPH or lente insulin before breakfast may sometimes find that the human insulin has an earlier peak of activity, causing hypoglycemia earlier in the afternoon, differences necessitating changes in diet, activity, or adjustments in the insulin regimen. Recently, there have been reports that the use of human insulin may be associated with a decrease in the development of warning symptoms of hypoglycemia in comparison to those noted with purified pork insulin.[41-44] The significance of these findings is unclear, and they will require further confirmation. Other studies show no difference in the effects of human and animal insulins on counterregulatory responses in normal patients[45] or in warning symptoms or incidence of hypoglycemia in diabetic patients.[46] It is possible that lack of awareness of hypoglycemia may be associated more with improved overall glycemic control than with the use of human insulin. Nevertheless, if a patient were to develop hypoglycemia unawareness while taking human insulin, a trial of purified pork insulin could be considered if other adjustments to minimize severe hypoglycemia were unsuccessful.

Insulin Concentrations

Almost all insulins now used in the United States are at a concentration of 100 units/mL (U-100). The syringes currently available are designed for this concentration. Some preparations of U-40 (40 units/mL) insulin are still available and may be used in infants and patients requiring very small doses of insulin more easily handled with dilution, but they are rarely used in this country. U-500 and U-5000 insulin are used in rare situations of insulin resistance when very high doses are required. These concentrated insulins are available only as regular (soluble) insulin, although their duration of action is more prolonged because of their higher concentration. Worldwide, insulin is available in a wider range of concentrations, including U-40, U-80, and U-100. Patients traveling outside the United States must be cautioned about this and instructed to use syringes appropriate to the concentration of insulin they are using to avoid dosage errors.

INITIATION OF INSULIN THERAPY

The decision to start insulin therapy may depend on a number of factors. Clearly, a patient with clinically evident Type I diabetes (IDDM) and hyperglycemia with glycosuria should be treated with insulin. Insulin acts directly to counteract the metabolic effects of insulin deficiency. In addition, there is some evidence that early, aggressive treatment with insulin may have a beneficial effect on progression to total insulin deficiency in Type I diabetes by decreasing islet cell antigenicity and autoimmune destruction of β-cells.[47] For this reason, temporary use of an oral hypoglycemic agent, rather than insulin, in the early stages of Type I diabetes is currently not advised because it may exacerbate progression to insulin deficiency later on. In a very young, thin patient with extreme hyperglycemia and ketosis, the decision to start insulin is straightforward. In patients for whom it is not clear clinically whether the diabetes is Type I or Type II, noting the presence of circulating islet cell antibodies or the relative absence of C-peptide after stimulation with glucagon can be helpful for diagnosis. In practice, however, these tests are rarely needed. Most pregnant patients with diabetes mellitus, whether Type I or Type II, will require treatment with insulin because oral hypoglycemic agents are contraindicated during pregnancy.[48]

Patients with Type I diabetes who initially receive insulin are at initial risk of hypoglycemia and require only small doses of insulin because of the induction of some recovery of residual insulin secretion and improvement in insulin sensitivity by insulin therapy. In the first few months of therapy, it is not uncommon to see a decline, to very low levels, of the daily dose of insulin necessary for glycemic control, and in many cases, use of insulin could potentially be stopped temporarily. This remission, often called the "honeymoon phase," may last a few weeks to several months. During this period it is advisable to continue therapy with insulin at a low dose rather than stopping it entirely, because intermittent use of insulin can increase its antigenicity.[23] As previously mentioned, insulin therapy to suppress islet cell secretion early in the course of IDDM may also have a beneficial effect in preserving residual β-cell function.[47]

GOALS OF THERAPY

The principal goal of the use of insulin for treatment of diabetes is elimination of the clinical symptoms of hyperglycemia and the prevention of diabetic ketoacidosis and hyperosmolar coma (Table 27–2). Secondary goals include the restoration of lean body mass and exercise capacity, decrease in the incidence and severity of infections, and improvement in the patient's sense of well-being. This can commonly be achieved with one or two injections of an intermediate-acting or long-acting insulin per day. The time and dose of insulin injections can be adjusted in coordination with meals and exercise to avoid hypoglycemic episodes and thus decrease the symptoms of polydipsia, polyuria, and weight loss. When necessary, regular insulin can be

Table 27–2. Goals of Insulin Therapy

1. Elimination of prime glycosuric symptoms
2. Prevention of diabetic ketoacidosis, hyperosmolar coma
3. Restoration of lost lean body mass
4. Improvement in exercise capability and work performance
5. Improvement in sense of well-being
6. Reduction of frequent infections
7. Decrease in fetal malformations, fetal and maternal morbidity, in pregnancy
8. Delay, arrest, or prevention of the microvascular and macrovascular complications of diabetes

added to the regimen to reduce postprandial hyperglycemia. These so-called standard regimens have been used by the majority of patients with diabetes and are not expected to achieve perfect control of blood glucose. Their main advantages are simplicity, safety, and ease of compliance for the patient.

There are other situations, however, when the goals of standard therapy are insufficient and insulin must be administered in a manner that will bring blood glucose levels to normal, nondiabetic values throughout the day. Regimens that achieve this are called "intensive" regimens because they require multiple injections or boluses of insulin during the day to mimic the physiologic needs of the patient for an insulin response to the increase in blood glucose level that follows meals.[49] These regimens are commonly used for the control of diabetes during pregnancy, when the achievement of near normoglycemia has been shown to decrease the incidence of fetal malformations and to reduce both fetal and maternal morbidity.[50]

Until recently, it was debated whether intensive regimens in the general diabetic population are safe and whether they can ameliorate or prevent the development of long-term microvascular and macrovascular changes of diabetes. Past studies of a large clinic population demonstrated a correlation between poor glycemic control and the occurrence of long-term complications of diabetes, but this did not indicate whether the initiation of intensive control could actually effect a change in the incidence or progression of complications.[51] Previously published prospective randomized studies comparing intensive and standard insulin therapy have been inconclusive[52] and involved relatively few subjects.[53,54] Most have shown that after switching to intensive control, retinopathy may worsen in the first 6 to 8 months.[55–57] This is probably a transient effect and may be followed by some amelioration of retinopathy.[58,59] Intensive control has also been shown to decrease proteinuria in patients with nephropathy[60] and lower GFR in patients with hyperfiltration related to diabetes.[61] All of these studies involved patients with some preexisting microvascular complications, and did not address the issue of whether intensive control can prevent the long-term complications of diabetes in patients who have not yet developed any microvascular and macrovascular changes.

Fortunately, these questions have been conclusively answered by the Diabetes Control and Complications Trial (DCCT).[186,187] This study, involving 1443 patients, was a prospective, randomized study comparing the effects of intensive with standard insulin treatment on both primary prevention and secondary intervention in the course of long-term diabetic complications.[62] One-half of the patients were in the primary prevention study; these patients had a duration of IDDM of 1 to 5 years, showed no evidence of diabetic retinopathy, and excreted less than 40 mg of albumin in the urine daily. The other one-half of the subjects were in the secondary intervention trial; these patients had diabetes for less than 15 years, with minimal nonproliferative retinopathy at the start of the study, and excreted less than 200 mg of albumin daily. All of the patients were randomized to either standard therapy (one or two injections of insulin a day), or intensive therapy (either three or more injections of insulin a day or continuous subcutaneous insulin infusion with insulin pumps, with frequent self blood glucose monitoring and adjustment of their insulin dose based upon the results of monitoring.) The results were conclusive, showing that intensive therapy reduced clinically important progression of retinopathy by 76% in primary prevention patients, and by 54% in secondary intervention patients. Intensive therapy also decreased the incidence of clinically significant proteinuria by about 56% and reduced microalbuminuria by about 46%. Clinically significant neuropathy was decreased by about 61%. A more comprehensive summary of the DCCT findings is presented in Appendix A.

The DCCT has already added to our understanding of the risks and complications of intensive therapy. The feasibility phase of the study determined that intensive therapy could indeed be accomplished in a large population group and result in significant declines in average blood glucose levels and in levels of hemoglobin A_{1c}, although not entirely to "normoglycemic" levels.[63] Intensive therapy resulted in an increased frequency of episodes of severe hypoglycemia, especially in a subgroup of patients with a previous history of hypoglycemic episodes.[64] Other studies have shown that intensive therapy decreases the threshold of responsiveness of epinephrine to hypoglycemia and enhances the suppression of glucose production in the liver by insulin, thereby increasing the risk of severe hypoglycemia.[65]

In the DCCT, intensive insulin therapy has been shown to be associated with a significantly greater weight gain than standard therapy.[66] Weight gain was greatest in those patients who started out with the highest levels of glycosylated hemoglobin and had the greatest declines in these levels with intensive therapy. This suggests that major improvements in glycemic control can put patients at risk for significant weight gain and development of obesity. Careful attention to diet and caloric restriction is extremely important in these patients. Also, certain complications have been reported specifically with the use of CSII, namely infections at the subcutaneous infusion sites and increased incidence of ketoacidosis with pump failures.[67]

To be successful, intensive insulin therapy also requires a great amount of time, effort, and motivation on the part of the patient. Although intensive therapy can now be recommended for most IDDM patients, care should be taken in the selection of appropriate patients for this form of therapy. Any decision to use a form of intensive therapy should take into account its possible risks and benefits, as outlined in Table 27–3.

TREATMENT STRATEGIES

If patients with IDDM of recent onset present to their physician with extreme hyperglycemia or diabetic ketoacidosis, they are initially treated with regular insulin infused intravenously. Once the blood glucose and electrolyte levels are stabilized and ketones are cleared

Table 27–3. Intensive Insulin Therapy

BENEFITS
1. More rational control of blood glucose with the ability to adjust insulin doses to changes in diet, activity, and illness
2. Improved sense of well-being
3. Delay in onset and progression of diabetic retinopathy
4. Decreases in microalbuminuria and clinical proteinuria
5. Decreased development of neuropathy
6. Reduced risk of hypercholesterolemia
7. Decreased fetal and maternal morbidity during pregnancy

DISADVANTAGES
1. Increased episodes of severe hypoglycemia
2. Hypoglycemia unawareness
3. Increased weight gain
4. In pump patients, increased ketoacidosis, infections, and inflammation of infusion sites
5. Early exacerbation (transiently) of preexisting retinopathy
6. Increased time, effort, and cost
7. Less suitable in patients with advanced complications and in small children

from the circulation, they can then be switched to a daily regimen of subcutaneous insulin injections. Patients who present with more stable hyperglycemia can initially be treated with insulin directly as outpatients. Care must be taken at this time to insure that patients receive a thorough education on the use of insulin, understand the rules for adjustment of insulin doses, learn to recognize and treat hypoglycemia, and understand the relation of insulin to the diet. Patients with acute illness and learning problems, as well as children, adolescents, and the elderly, often may benefit from hospitalization when insulin therapy is started, in an environment where intensive education can be carried out over several days and insulin adjustments can be made under the close supervision of a physician.

Single-Dose Regimens

Treatment with insulin usually is initiated with a single daily injection of intermediate-acting insulin, given before breakfast. The starting dose of insulin should be in the range of 0.2 to 0.3 U/kg per day. Most patients with IDDM who have no endogenous insulin secretion ultimately require higher daily doses, in the range of 0.5 to 1.0 U/kg per day, but it is prudent to start with a lower dose to avoid hypoglycemia and because the patient may have some endogenous insulin secretion. Patients should be instructed to monitor and record their blood glucose levels at least twice a day, especially before breakfast to obtain fasting glucose levels and in the late afternoon to note the peak effect of the intermediate-acting insulin. The insulin dose is increased gradually in small increments until the blood glucose values fall into an acceptable range or the patient starts to experience symptoms of hypoglycemia. Frequently, regular insulin can be added to the morning dose of intermediate-acting insulin to decrease the increase in glucose level that follows breakfast. If regular insulin is added, the insulin should be given 30 to 45 minutes before breakfast to synchronize the action of the insulin with the rise in blood glucose level after meals.

Twice-Daily Regimens

In patients with some endogenous insulin secretion, such as those with Type II diabetes, a single injection of intermediate-acting insulin may sometimes be sufficient to control blood glucose levels. Often this is the case during the first few months following initial treatment of Type I diabetes. However, endogenous secretion of insulin tends to decrease subsequently. Because the duration of action of NPH and lente insulin is usually much less than 24 hours, one can often see a pattern of high fasting blood glucose levels and low or normal glucose levels in the afternoon and evening. In this situation, it is necessary to add a second injection of intermediate-acting insulin, which can be given either before supper or at bedtime. Some diabetologists recommend that two injections of insulin be given per day at the start of insulin therapy in order to achieve more rapid control and because two injections will likely be needed eventually.[68] Although this regimen may speed the time to optimal control in some patients, it also may increase the risk of hypoglycemia, especially during the middle of the night in response to the action of the evening dose of intermediate-acting insulin.

When the second injection is given before supper, regular insulin can be added to the intermediate-acting insulin to cover the rise in blood glucose level that follows the evening meal. This commonly used regimen (often called a split-mix regimen) will often suffice for standard glucose control (Fig. 27−1A). Twice-daily insulin regimens are commonly used because of their convenience and simplicity for the patient. However, these advantages often are offset by their lack of flexibility. With two injections a day, adjustments to changes in diet and activity can sometimes be difficult; the hypoglycemic effect of the intermediate-acting insulin during the course of the day mandates scheduling lunch and supper at fairly precise times after breakfast and, in many patients, the addition of mid-morning and mid-afternoon snacks. The dietary content of each meal, especially of carbohydrate, must be kept fairly constant in order to avoid hypoglycemia. Increases or decreases in the amount or timing of exercise or physical activity can have adverse effects on glycemic control. The activity of both the short-acting and intermediate-acting components of the regimen also necessitate the administration of insulin at approximately the same time each day. Patients with erratic life-styles and changes in routine involving travel or variability in work hours may have problems with good glycemic control with this regimen.

In many cases, when NPH or lente insulin is given before supper, the peak action and duration are too short to last through the night, resulting in hypoglycemia in the middle of the night and hyperglycemia in the morning hours.[69] In addition, hepatic glucose output in the early morning hours increases in association with an increase in the basal insulin requirement, which is thought to be caused by pulses of growth hormone secretion during the middle of the night. This problem, often called the "dawn phenomenon," results in elevated fasting blood glucose values. This situation can be remedied by giving the intermediate-acting insulin at bedtime, rather than before supper, a regimen necessitating three injections per day if regular insulin is still given before supper (Fig. 27−1B). Alternatively, ultralente insulin can be given before supper for adequate duration of control of glucose overnight. This may, however, be more complicated for some patients, who will now have to use three different types of insulin during the course of the day.

Multiple Daily Injections

In most patients, the achievement of more tight control of blood glucose values requires the administration of at least three injections per day. The goal of intensive therapy is no longer merely the alleviation of symptoms of hyperglycemia but rather the maintenance of the average blood glucose level within a range as close as possible to that of a normal nondiabetic individual. For this to be achieved, insulin must be given in a manner that duplicates the normal diurnal patterns of insulin in the circulation as it is secreted from the islets in the postprandial and basal states. This can be achieved in a number of ways. Three injections can be given per day with use of a mixture of intermediate- and short-acting insulins in the morning before breakfast, with regular insulin before supper, and intermediate-acting insulin at bedtime (Fig. 27−1B). This regimen is commonly used because it is easily evolved from the split-mix regimen. It is especially useful in those diabetic patients who have frequent episodes of hypoglycemia in the middle of the night and subsequent hyperglycemia in the early morning before breakfast. Its major disadvantage is that the timing of meals and amounts of food have to be fixed fairly rigidly in sequence to the morning insulin dose and that little flexibility in diet and activity is allowed if good glycemic control is to be achieved.

Good glycemic control can also be achieved with four injections of insulin a day, using regular insulin before each meal and an intermediate-acting insulin at bedtime (Fig. 27−1C). This enables patients to vary their mealtimes a bit more; however, extremely long intervals between meals cannot be permitted because the relatively short duration of action of regular insulin would leave patients without insulin coverage for their basal needs during the day. In addition, patients can adjust their doses of regular insulin to cover variations in the carbohydrate content of individual meals. As with other intensive insulin regimens, the dose of regular insulin is determined according to an algorithm based on the blood glucose values before each meal (Table 27−4). Some patients prefer this regimen because they do not have to mix different types of insulin in the syringe. The preprandial doses of regular insulin can be easily administered using a pen-type insulin injection system.

Good glycemic control can also be achieved by using ultralente insulin instead of an intermediate-acting insulin to cover basal insulin needs, with regular insulin given before each meal as well (Fig. 27−1D). The ultralente insulin can be given as a single daily injection. If,

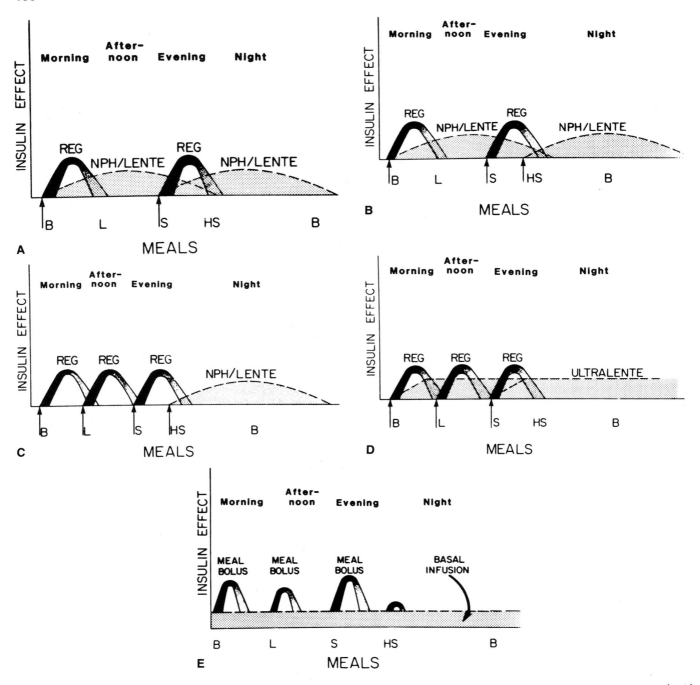

Fig. 27—1. Visualized representation of the peaks of action of insulin in various insulin injection regimens (A, B, C, D) and with continuous subcutaneous insulin infusion (E). The details of each regimen are discussed in the text. B = breakfast; L = lunch; S = supper; HS = bedtime snack; NPH = neutral protamine Hagedorn insulin. Arrows show the time of insulin injection or bolus 30 to 25 minutes before each meal. Reprinted with permission from reference 1 (Schade DS, Santiago JV, Skyler JS, Rizza RA. Insulin secretion in non-diabetics and insulin-dependent subjects. In: Schade DS, Santiago JV, Skyler JS, Rizza RA, eds. Intensive insulin therapy. Princeton, NJ: Excerpta Medica, 1983:23—35).

however, human ultralente insulin is used, it is best to split the dose into two injections a day, most often given before breakfast and before supper. This method is used to imitate the constant basal delivery of insulin that is best achieved with an insulin pump. Usually, approximately one-half of the total daily insulin dose will be given as ultralente insulin, but this proportion may vary from patient to patient. The regular insulin is taken by the patient before each meal, and occasionally before bedtime, with its dose adjusted according to the blood glucose values monitored by the patient (Table 27—5). This regimen offers the patient an increased degree of

Table 27–4. Intensive Insulin Therapy Algorithm: Example of a Four-Injection-a-Day Regimen*

Blood Glucose (mg/dL)	Breakfast	Lunch	Supper	Bedtime Snack
REGULAR INSULIN: Premeal regular insulin doses				
0–50	4U	3U	3U	0
51–100	6U	5U	5U	0
101–150	7U	6U	6U	0
151–200	8U	7U	7U	0
201–250	9U	8U	8U	2U
251–300	10U	9U	9U	3U
301–350	11U	10U	10U	4U
351–400	12U	11U	11U	5U
>400	13U	12U	12U	6U
INTERMEDIATE ACTING INSULIN (NPH or LENTE)			16U	
ADJUSTMENTS IN REGULAR INSULIN DOSE FOR EXERCISE	–2U	–2U	–2U	–2U

*The insulin doses listed here are representative samples of what may be used to treat an adult with IDDM. Actual insulin requirements, as well as the gradations of increase in the algorithm, may vary widely from patient to patient.

flexibility in the timing of meals and in adjusting insulin to changes in meal pattern that is not seen with the other regimens.

Goals of Intensive Therapy

In all of these regimens, the fasting blood glucose level is used as a guide for adjustment of the dose of the intermediate- or long-acting insulin to be used. Fasting blood glucose levels should ideally be kept within the range of 70 to 120 mg/dL for optimal control. To avoid nocturnal hypoglycemia, patients should check the blood glucose level at 3 a.m. once a week or so, maintaining this level above 70 mg/dL. Patients must be willing to check blood glucose levels a minimum of four times a day— before each meal and at bedtime. Glucose levels before meals should generally be within the same range as the fasting blood glucose levels. In addition, 2-hour postprandial blood glucose values should be monitored on a regular basis, with the goal of maintaining these levels between 70 and 140 mg/dL. The doses of regular insulin to be given before meals are usually determined from a sliding scale according to the patient's blood glucose levels, as previously illustrated in Tables 27–4 and 27–5, and the algorithms are adjusted up and down by trial and error. Careful adherence to the monitoring schedule with maintenance of blood glucose records, along with frequent communication with the physician and teaching nurse for review of the glucose results, is essential for success of intensive insulin therapy. It should be stressed that for this form of treatment the health-care providers must spend a great deal of effort and time with the patient in working out problems and adapting the insulin therapy to the patient's daily needs.

Continuous Subcutaneous Insulin Infusion

An alternative to multiple daily injections for intensive insulin therapy is continuous subcutaneous insulin infusion (CSII). For this form of treatment, regular insulin is contained in a syringe or reservoir of a pump that is worn externally and the insulin is delivered subcutaneously, usually to the abdomen, via a plastic catheter. The patient can program the pump to give insulin automatically in a basal mode, usually from 0.5 to 2.0 U/hour. With most currently available pumps, more than one basal rate can be selected over a 24-hour period to mimic the changes in basal insulin needs in some individuals. Such a change is seen most commonly in relation to the dawn phenomenon, in which higher basal rates are used in the early morning hours. Insulin can also be given before each meal or snack as a bolus to cover postprandial insulin requirements. The doses of these boluses can be adjusted to the preprandial blood value with use of sliding scales similar to those used in multiple daily injection regimens. In fact, CSII regimens (Fig. 27–1E) are similar in concept to ultralente-regular regimens, with the basal rate of insulin delivery substituting for the ultralente insulin dose. In general, however, the total daily dose of insulin needed with CSII is less than that necessary with the various multiple daily injection regimens, perhaps because of improved bioavailability of insulin with pump therapy.

When a patient starts CSII and is in reasonably good glycemic control, it is customary to begin with a daily insulin dose that is approximately 80% of his or her previous total insulin dose. Initially, approximately one-half of this dose is given at a single basal rate of infusion, with the rest of the insulin given as premeal boluses according to the relative carbohydrate content of the meals.[70] Patients will usually require a relatively larger bolus of insulin before breakfast than before other meals.

Table 27–5. Intensive Insulin Therapy Algorithm: Example of a Three-Injection-a-Day Regimen*

Blood Glucose (mg/dL)	Breakfast	Lunch	Supper	Bedtime Snack
REGULAR INSULIN: Premeal regular insulin doses				
0–50	3U	2U	2U	0
51–100	5U	4U	4U	0
101–150	6U	5U	5U	0
151–200	7U	6U	6U	0
201–250	8U	7U	7U	2U
251–300	9U	8U	8U	3U
301–350	10U	9U	9U	4U
351–400	11U	10U	10U	5U
>400	12U	11U	11U	6U
LONG-ACTING INSULIN (ULTRALENTE)	8U		8U	
ADJUSTMENTS IN REGULAR INSULIN DOSE FOR EXERCISE	–2U	–2U	–2U	–2U

*These are only representative insulin doses, as discussed in Table 27–4.

The basal insulin doses and boluses will then be adjusted according to the fasting, preprandial, postprandial, and 3 a.m. blood glucose levels. This is best achieved with an initial stay in the hospital of 3 to 5 days for adequate monitoring and insulin adjustment. After the patient is discharged from the hospital, close contact with the caregivers is essential, with frequent telephone contact and outpatient visits to review blood glucose results and to adjust insulin doses. A health-care provider must be available at all times to deal with any acute problems that may arise during the course of pump therapy.

Use of the insulin pump has several advantages over multiple daily injection regimens. Because regular insulin is the only insulin used, the absorption of insulin from subcutaneous tissues is more predictable than with intermediate- and long-acting insulin. Both the adjustment of bolus size before meals and the use of additional basal rates can help to achieve a pattern of circulating insulin levels closer to the physiologic range. Hypoglycemia may be easier to treat because no subcutaneous depot of long-acting insulin is present. There is evidence from some studies, but not all, that episodes of severe hypoglycemia can be reduced in some patients by switching from multiple daily injections to CSII.[71] Patients are spared the process of multiple injections and can be more flexible with their exercise patterns and eating habits. Patients with erratic schedules and those who cannot snack at fixed times benefit particularly by CSII. Nevertheless, although several studies have shown that CSII is at least as good as multiple daily injections in helping to achieve normoglycemia, it has been difficult to show that CSII is better.[72,73] CSII carries some risks and disadvantages to the patient that are not encountered with multiple daily injections (Table 27–6). Because regular insulin is the only insulin used, interruption of insulin delivery by pump malfunction, blocked catheter, leakage from the catheter connections, or displacement of the subcutaneous connection can result in a rapid rise in blood glucose levels with ketonuria in a matter of a few hours, and an increase in the incidence of diabetic ketoacidosis has been documented.[74] Patients are most often subject to these problems at night during sleep. Abscesses and cellulitis can occur at the sites of subcuta-neous needle insertion. Insulin can aggregate in the catheters, causing decreased bioavailability and catheter blockage, although this problem has been reduced with the use of buffered forms of regular insulin.[75] In addition, many patients find it cumbersome and difficult to adapt the pump to daily activities such as exercise and sports, swimming, showering, and sexual intercourse. The pump cannot always be concealed from others, which may present problems for those who do not wish to advertise that they have diabetes. These reasons, as well as the substantial cost of equipment and supplies, have limited pump use at present to a relatively small subgroup of patients with diabetes.

INSULIN TREATMENT OF NON-INSULIN-DEPENDENT DIABETES

The preceding sections of this chapter have focused on the role of different insulin treatment regimens in achieving good glycemic control by attempting to duplicate the physiologic response of the pancreas in supplying insulin for the body's normal needs. Although these approaches to treatment can be applied both to non-insulin-dependent diabetes (NIDDM) and IDDM, they tend to neglect the role of endogenous insulin secretion and insulin resistance, features unique to NIDDM. NIDDM is by far the most common of all the forms of diabetes. It affects from 3 to 6% of the general population, and an estimated 76% of all insulin-treated patients in the United States have NIDDM.[76]

A number of features of NIDDM make the approach to treatment with insulin substantially different from that to IDDM. Of particular importance are the dual abnormalities of insulin resistance and insulin deficiency that play such an important role in the pathogenesis of this disease (see Chapter 14 on pathogenesis of NIDDM). Much debate has been raised over the primacy of each of these processes in NIDDM, but it is clear that insulin resistance and insulin deficiency may each exacerbate the other.[77,78] The increased demands on the pancreas imposed by insulin resistance can lead to β-cell exhaustion, and the insulin secretory defect in NIDDM can lead to insulin resistance through atrophy of insulin-sensitive

Table 27–6. Comparison of Continuous Subcutaneous Insulin Injection (CSII) and Multiple Daily Injection (MDI) Regimens

CSII	MDI
ADVANTAGES	
1. Increased flexibility in adjustment of regimen to changes in diet, activity	1. Depot of insulin to prevent hyperglycemia
2. No need for injections	2. No need for catheter and external device
3. Improved control over MDI in some patients	3. Decreased cost
4. Possible decrease in risk of severe hypoglycemia	
5. Ease of treatment of hypoglycemic episodes	
DISADVANTAGES	
1. Cumbersome and inconvenient for some people	1. Variable absorption of longer-acting insulins
2. Catheter inflammation and infections	2. Need for three or four injections a day
3. Risk for mechanical malfunction	3. Decreased flexibility in dosage adjustments
4. Increased incidence of ketoacidosis	

metabolic pathways. These processes can work together to produce hyperglycemia, which has the secondary affect of worsening the situation through the proposed mechanism of glucose toxicity.[79] The functional capacity of the islets to secrete insulin is further impaired by prolonged elevations in plasma glucose levels, which also can exacerbate insulin resistance in insulin target tissues. The result is additional hyperglycemia caused by persistent excess hepatic production of glucose and poor utilization of glucose by the target tissues of insulin.

The hyperglycemia of NIDDM is manifested in two distinct, but interrelated, processes: the excess hepatic glucose production is found in the basal state, which results in elevated fasting plasma glucose levels. The defect in peripheral glucose utilization together with the insulin secretory defect result in elevated postprandial glucose excursions. Aggressive treatment with insulin can partially reverse these processes. In a significant proportion of patients with NIDDM—often those who are obese who have significant residual insulin secretion—lowering of fasting plasma glucose levels alone with the administration of long-acting basal insulin can counteract insulin resistance and glucose toxicity. This can result in recovery of insulin secretion and improvement of postprandial glucose excursions as well.[80] In many other patients with NIDDM, however, the addition of short-acting insulin before meals is necessary to return postprandial glucose levels to normal values.

The relative benefits of insulin and oral hypoglycemic agents in the treatment of NIDDM have been the subject of controversy and have been reviewed elsewhere.[81] In studies comparing the effectiveness of conventional insulin with sulfonylureas in the treatment of patients with NIDDM for whom dietary treatment has failed, the two forms of treatment were similarly effective in improving glycemic control, although insulin was slightly more effective in some studies. It should be noted, however, that the sulfonylureas were usually used at their maximal doses in these studies, while the insulin doses used appeared to be suboptimal for therapy. There was no difference in the safety of the two forms of therapy. Insulin treatment was associated with greater weight gain in most studies but also with an increase in levels of high-density lipoprotein. The findings of the University Group Diabetes Program study, which suggested that tolbutamide was associated with an increased risk of cardiovascular-related death,[82] have been questioned and debated because of problems with the study design, and have not been confirmed by subsequent studies.[83] A better understanding of the relative risks of insulin and oral agents and their effects on the microvascular complications of NIDDM will await the findings of the large multicenter study in the United Kingdom currently in progress that compares several treatment regimens in patients with more severe NIDDM.[84]

The decision to use insulin or sulfonylureas in an individual with NIDDM is influenced by a number of factors. An algorithm for the use of insulin based on these factors is illustrated in Figure 27–2. Clearly, insulin is more effective than sulfonylureas in those patients with NIDDM who have ketonuria, weight loss, and/or severe hyperglycemic symptoms. Patients in this category should be started on insulin without going through a trial of diet or oral agents. Some of these patients may, in fact, have "evolving IDDM." Those under age 40 years who are underweight are more likely to fit into this category, but many patients of this type could still be managed with oral agents. As mentioned earlier, measurement of stimulated C-peptide levels has been suggested as a screening test for candidates for insulin therapy, but its value in general clinical practice is limited by its expense and the time needed for results when clinical decisions have to be made. Older, obese patients with NIDDM do not need to be treated with insulin initially unless their blood glucose levels are extremely elevated or if they are in the midst of acute illness or undergoing surgery. In these situations, they can often be treated with insulin temporarily and switched to another form of therapy once their condition has stabilized.

Those patients who are not ketonuric and are without severe hyperglycemic symptoms or significant weight loss should be started on dietary therapy. If diet alone is unsuccessful in controlling blood glucose levels, sulfonylurea therapy should be started. If the patient's glucose levels cannot be controlled with maximal doses of a sulfonylurea agent, insulin treatment should be initiated. Metformin, another effective oral agent, is currently not available for use in the United States. Several different insulin treatment regimens, each with its relative advantages and disadvantages, have been advocated specifically for the treatment of NIDDM. At present, the data available are not sufficient to indicate which is the best form of therapy. The most widely advocated approaches are summarized below.

Intermediate-Acting Insulins

Patients are commonly started with a morning injection of NPH or lente insulin at a dosage of 0.2 to 0.5 U/kg of body weight. Significantly higher doses may ultimately be needed in obese individuals. Fasting blood glucose levels are followed sequentially, and the insulin dose is increased progressively until fasting glucose values are optimal or if presupper hypoglycemia supervenes. If the latter occurs, the morning insulin dose is decreased by 20% and a second injection of intermediate-acting insulin is given, usually before supper. This dose of the second injection is increased until the fasting blood glucose level is brought under control. If postprandial blood glucose values are still elevated with this regimen, regular insulin can be added before breakfast and supper to bring glucose values under control. This results in the standard split-mix regimen discussed previously. Premixed preparations of NPH and regular insulin have become more popular in the treatment of NIDDM. Such preparations may be useful for some patients who are elderly and have difficulty mixing insulins.

This regimen can be effective in many patients. Its principal disadvantage lies in the short duration of action of intermediate-acting insulins, which can be inadequate to control fasting blood glucose levels without producing hypoglycemia at other times. This problem is exacer-

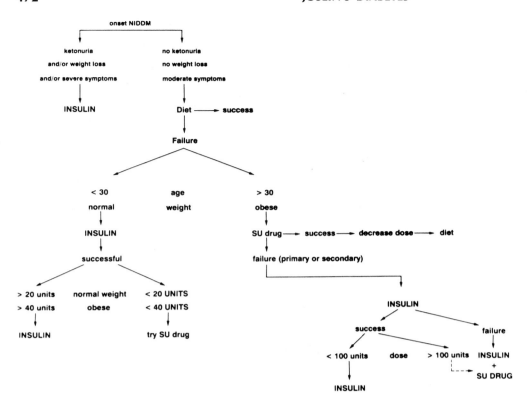

Fig. 27–2. Proposed decision flow diagram for treatment of non-insulin-dependent diabetes mellitus (NIDDM). Su = sulfonylurea. Reprinted with permission from reference 81 (Genuth S. Insulin use in NIDDM. Diabetes Care 1990;28:227–30; copyright © of the American Diabetes Association).

bated with the human insulins, whose duration of action is shorter than that of their beef and pork counterparts. For this reason, animal insulins may be preferable to human insulin as a single morning injection for some patients.

Ultralente Insulin

Since a principal goal of therapy for NIDDM is to provide basal insulin to normalize fasting glucose levels, ultralente insulin has been advocated and used effectively, especially in the United Kingdom.[19] This can be given as a single dose at bedtime or in two equal doses daily to avoid any peak hypoglycemic effect. Recommendations for the initial daily dose have been given based on the fasting plasma glucose level and patient's weight as a percentage of ideal body weight,[85] but it is prudent to start with a daily dose of 0.4 to 0.5 U/kg. Because of the long half-life of beef or beef/pork ultralente insulin, a loading dose that is two to four times the initial daily dose can be given on the first day without resulting in any complications from hypoglycemia.[19] When fasting blood glucose levels are optimized, postprandial glucose excursions often improve as well. If this does not occur, regular insulin can be administered before meals, with dosage adjustments as previously described for multiple-dose injection regimens. If regular insulin is to be mixed in the same syringe as the ultralente insulin, it should be injected immediately after mixing to avoid blunting the effect of the regular insulin (see section on mixing insulins).

Delivery of basal insulin with the use of CSII[86,87] as well as with implantable insulin delivery systems, is currently under experimental investigation as a treatment for NIDDM.[88] Very long acting analogues of insulin and proinsulin with no discernible peak of activity are currently being tested and may have a future therapeutic role in providing a more steady basal insulin level than that attained with ultralente insulin. Orally administered insulin preparations, which have a slow rate of release into the circulation, are also under investigation as a source of background insulin in mild NIDDM, in which variations in insulin delivery from day to day may be less of a problem.[89]

Bedtime Insulin

A single injection of NPH insulin can be given at bedtime to decrease the excess hepatic glucose production overnight and to normalize fasting plasma glucose levels. The rationale for this approach is similar to that for the above ultralente regimen. It assumes that postprandial endogenous insulin secretion will improve sufficiently to control glucose levels during the day once fasting glucose levels are controlled. In two studies, administration of NPH insulin at bedtime resulted in better parameters of glucose control than those attained with the same dose of insulin given in the morning.[90,91] This regimen has the benefit of simplicity for the patient and of protecting the patient from unnecessary exposure to hypoglycemia during the day. Unfortunately, many patients will develop hyperglycemia during the day and require the addition of either a sulfonylurea or morning insulin injections to control this problem.

Combined Insulin and Sulfonylurea

Regimens using the two forms of therapy for NIDDM have been studied for the past 10 years, with controversial results.[92] Initially, it was thought that oral agents could aid in glycemic control by improving tissue sensitivity to insulin. In fact, oral agents added to insulin therapy have been found to act by stimulating endogenous secretion of insulin.[93,94] Some reports of the effects of the addition of a sulfonylurea to an insulin regimen have indicated that glucose control may improve to a small degree and that insulin doses can be reduced.[95,96] In some cases, however, these benefits have been only transient, and the improvements in glucose control might have alternatively been accomplished by improving the insulin regimen alone. Concerns over the possibility that insulin therapy may increase atherogenesis have led some to advocate the addition of sulfonylureas as a means of decreasing episodes of hyperinsulinemia, but there is no evidence of clinical benefit for this at present.[81] A recent meta-analysis of 17 trials indicated that combined insulin-sulfonylurea therapy leads to modest improvements in fasting plasma glucose levels and hemoglobin A_1 over insulin therapy alone, especially in obese patients with high fasting C-peptide levels.[97] However, the routine use of combined therapy as an initial treatment for NIDDM is probably not advisable unless it can be proven to be clearly superior to insulin alone.[98,99]

Combined therapy may be indicated in certain special situations. If a patient is poorly controlled with large doses of insulin or requires more than 100 U/day for adequate control, the addition of a sulfonylurea may help make the insulin regimen more manageable. Sulfonylureas may also benefit those obese patients who continue to gain weight with insulin therapy, with spiraling increases in insulin requirements that result in further hyperglycemia and weight gain. It is also possible that the sequential use of bedtime insulin with a short-acting oral agent such as glipizide before meals will have a role in therapy, and further investigations of this approach are warranted. This form of therapy has appeal because of the ease with which small doses of evening insulin can be added to a pre-existing regimen with an oral agent.

PRACTICAL ASPECTS OF INSULIN USE

Storage

Commercially available insulin preparations are relatively stable at room temperature. Insulin in use can be kept at room temperature (68 to 75° F) for 6 to 8 weeks without loss in potency. Extremes in temperature should be avoided, especially during travel. Vials of insulin should not be frozen. Unopened vials or cartridges should be stored in the refrigerator at about 40° F. In situations when patients are unable to draw up insulin in their syringes, it is recommended that prefilled syringes be kept in the refrigerator and used within 3 weeks.

Insulin Injection Technique

Although pen-cartridge devices and prefilled disposable syringes have become popular in Europe, the vast majority of patients in the United States currently administer their insulin with disposable plastic syringes. If the insulin is in suspension, the vial should be rolled gently upside-down and sideways between the hands before the syringe is loaded to ensure that the suspension is uniform. The vial is turned upside-down and air is injected first from the syringe in an amount roughly equaling the space occupied by the amount of insulin to be withdrawn from the vial. The proper amount of insulin is then withdrawn downward into the syringe and the air bubbles are expelled. If two types of insulin are to be mixed in a single injection, the appropriate amount of air is first injected into the vial with insulin in suspension (e.g., NPH or lente) without withdrawing any insulin from the vial. Air is then injected into the vial of regular insulin, and the appropriate dose of regular insulin is then withdrawn into the syringe. One then returns to the vial of insulin in suspension to add the appropriate amount of insulin to the syringe. The insulin should be at room temperature at the time of injection.

Before the insulin is injected, an appropriate area of skin is selected and wiped with alcohol. The skin is gently pinched between the thumb and forefinger; the syringe is held as one would hold a pencil and the needle is pushed directly through the skin and into the subcutaneous tissue at a perpendicular angle. The plunger is pushed all the way down without drawing back, the pinch is released, and the needle is withdrawn. In extremely thin individuals and in some children, it may be necessary to inject at a 45° angle to avoid intramuscular injection.

Visually impaired individuals who have difficulty loading a syringe accurately may benefit from any of a variety of injection aids available, including magnifying glasses that fit around the syringe and guides for setting the proper depth of the plunger. Insulin may be prefilled in syringes by another individual and kept in the refrigerator for up to 3 weeks. Some visually impaired individuals who are unable to load syringes are able to use pen-type injection devices without difficulty. It is important to enable each patient to administer his or her own insulin whenever possible to foster self-reliance and decrease dependency on others. The age at which this can properly be initiated in children varies with the maturity and motivation of the individual child.

For those patients whose extreme fear of needles makes it difficult for them to penetrate the skin, spring-loaded injection aids can be attached to the syringe to facilitate injection. In practice, however, most patients overcome these fears with practice, repetition, and mental conditioning. In those situations when fear of needles impairs a patient's ability to take insulin, jet injectors can be used. These devices forcibly inject insulin under pressure through the skin and into the subcutaneous tissues without the use of needles. With these devices, however, the rate of insulin absorption often increases and the decline in blood glucose levels are more rapid than for an equal amount of insulin administered by syringe.[100] Duration of action of NPH and regular insulins can be reduced with jet injection, and insulin doses and times of injection may have to be adjusted to accommodate these changes. The shortened duration of action may make jet injection less feasible for patients receiving one or two injections a day. There is no conclusive evidence that jet injectors can be used to improve overall glycemic control over that accomplished with syringe injection. The increased cost of these devices is only partially offset by the savings incurred by not having to purchase syringes. In addition, their larger size and the difficulty of mixing insulins in them and verifying dosage have limited their acceptance.

Site of Injection

The best sites for routine insulin administration are the areas of the body with the most subcutaneous fat, which include the abdomen, buttock, anterior thigh, and dorsal area of the arm. Injection of insulin into areas with little subcutaneous fat may result in intramuscular administration, which is painful, associated with more rapid insulin absorption,[101] and can cause tissue scarring. Studies have shown that insulin is absorbed faster from the abdomen than from the leg or arm, resulting in a more rapid attainment of peak concentrations in the circulation.[14] However, insulin may be absorbed more rapidly from an extremity that is subsequently exercised because of increased local blood flow.[102] Thus, intermittent injection of an extremity that is sometimes exercised can result in erratic absorption of insulin and irregular glucose profiles. It is best, therefore, to avoid injecting extremities that undergo strenuous exercise; for example, long-distance runners might do better to restrict injections to their abdomen. Other factors also may influence the rate of insulin absorption[14] (Table 27–7). Massage of a local area that has been injected can increase the rate of insulin absorption, as can increased local skin temperature (in hot baths or very hot weather, for example). Maintaining an upright posture for a prolonged period has been shown to decrease subcutaneous blood flow to the legs and, to a lesser extent, to the abdominal wall, with a resulting slowing of insulin absorption from those areas. Smoking also is associated with reduced insulin absorption.

Table 27–7. Factors Affecting Insulin Bioavailability

1. Type of insulin
2. Insulin species
3. Insulin concentration and dose injected
4. Depth of injection and injection technique
5. Location of injection
6. Exercise
7. Ambient temperature
8. Local blood flow
9. Alterations in hepatic and renal function
10. Insulin antibodies
11. Insulin receptor defects
12. Subcutaneous insulin degradation (very rare, if it exists)
13. Unexplained daily variation in the same individual

Rotation of Injection

In the past, it has been customary to have patients routinely rotate the site of injection to minimize the formation of lipoatrophy and lipohypertrophy. The incidence of lipoatrophy has decreased, however, because of the improved purity of current insulin preparations. Because insulin absorption from different sites is so different and is so affected by exercise of the extremities, it is now recommended that patients rotate their injection sites within a particular anatomic region rather than between regions.[103] Patients should inject within the same general region at the same time each day but in different locations in that region (e.g., in the abdomen in the morning and in the thigh before bedtime). In many cases, the restriction of all injections to the abdomen may result in an improvement in the consistency of insulin and glucose profiles.

Adjustments to Exercise and Meals

Exercise is associated with an increase in the sensitivity of peripheral tissue to insulin and with a decrease in blood glucose levels in patients treated with insulin (see Chapter 26). The hypoglycemic effect can occur acutely during exercise and for as long as 12 to 24 hours afterwards (the so-called lag effect).[104] To avoid hypoglycemia, it is necessary to make adjustments to the insulin regimen or to the meal plan on days when patients exercise. Particular care is required when the exercise is of long duration (more than 2 hours), is of high intensity, and occurs during the peak of action of the insulin the patient is taking. The dose of the insulin that peaks in its activity during the exercise period can be decreased by as little as 5% for exercise of low intensity and intermediate to long duration and by as much as 30% for exercise of high intensity and long duration. Some practical guidelines for these adjustments are given in Table 27–8. In general, it is easier to make day-to-day changes in doses of regular insulin than in doses of intermediate- or long-acting insulin. It is helpful for patients to check blood glucose levels routinely before and after exercise to monitor the effectiveness of these dose adjustments. Patients also can add an additional carbohydrate snack before exercise to avoid hypoglycemia, while keeping their insulin dose the same. The amount of carbohydrate to be added can range between 10 g for exercise of short duration to as much as 50 g for high-intensity exercise of long duration, with addition of protein as well.

Although patients usually are taught to keep their intake of carbohydrate from meals relatively constant from day to day, with careful adherence to their meal plans, it is inevitable that the amount of food in meals occasionally will vary. Patients taking regular insulin before a meal can be taught to compensate for these changes by decreasing or increasing the dose. In general, most patients can add an additional unit of insulin before a meal for every additional 10 g of carbohydrate consumed. This amount may vary from patient to patient, however, and dose adjustments to meals often are decided by trial and error.

Table 27–8. Guidelines for Adjusting Insulin Dose to Exercise

Percentage to Decrease Peaking Insulin	Intensity of Exercise[†]	Duration of Exercise[‡]
0%	Low, moderate, or high intensity	Short duration
5%	Low intensity	Intermediate to long duration
10%	Moderate intensity	Intermediate duration
20%	Moderate intensity	Long duration
20%	High intensity	Intermediate duration
30%	High intensity	Long duration

*The specific insulin dose to be adjusted is that with its peak of action during the time of exercise.
[†]Low intensity = walking, golfing, or leisure cycling; moderate intensity = tennis, swimming, jogging, cycling, low-impact aerobics; high intensity = football, hockey, racquetball, basketball; strenuous running, cycling, or swimming; or intermediate or advanced aerobics.
[‡]Short duration = <30 minutes; intermediate duration = 30 to 60 minutes; long duration = ≥60 minutes.

Blood Glucose Monitoring

The ability of patients to monitor their own blood glucose levels has had a major impact on the therapy for diabetes. With self-monitoring, patients can evaluate their goals of therapy and change their regimens as their needs for insulin change. Written records of blood glucose results should be kept by the patient and brought in for evaluation by the physician. Records of self-monitoring, if they are done accurately, can be important aids for the physician in adjusting the insulin regimen to accommodate the fluctuation in blood glucose levels during the course of the day. Many of the currently available glucose meters have memories that allow the patient or health-care provider to recover individual glucose measurements, with the time and date of the reading. Because of the improved accuracy and reliability of meter readings, the patient should be encouraged to use a meter rather than to estimate visually the color on test strips. The use of meters that are simpler to use and include fewer steps, such as those that eliminate the need for wiping or blotting of the blood, reduces the introduction of patient-induced errors into the monitoring process and is thus preferable.

Having patients monitor blood glucose levels is of value only if the patients are motivated to perform the tests regularly and accurately. Poor training in glucose monitoring and lack of education can impair the usefulness of the testing, studies having shown that technical errors in testing can be responsible for a large variation in the accuracy of the results obtained. The competence of the patient in blood testing should be directly evaluated by the health-care provider. Glucose testing is of little use if the patient performs it only intermittently and does not make use of the results. In addition, insisting that the patient perform the test extremely frequently—beyond his or her ability to be motivated and to comply—is also futile. It is not uncommon for patients in this situation to consistently "forget" to bring in their test results to their physician or to produce neatly annotated monitoring sheets that turn out to be extensive fabrications that bear no relationship to the patients' glycohemoglobin levels. Studies have shown that the use of blood glucose monitoring alone does not bring about an improvement in blood glucose control in patients on standard treatment regimens.[105]

The frequency of glucose monitoring should be tailored to the individual patient's needs and level of education and motivation. Patients with standard insulin treatment regimens, (one or two injections per day) may do well monitoring once or twice a day, measuring the fasting blood glucose level as well as the glucose level at the time of peak effect of their dose of intermediate-acting insulin. More frequent glucose monitoring can be performed intermittently at scheduled intervals and before visits to the physician as a way of better defining daily blood glucose profiles. This is often called "block testing." In patients with intensive insulin regimens, self-monitoring of glucose is generally performed at least four times a day—before each meal and at bedtime, with additional testing done periodically at 3 a.m. to look for nighttime hypoglycemia and 2 hours postprandially at regular intervals to evaluate glucose excursions after meals.

Urine Testing

Testing urine for glucose has largely been supplanted by blood glucose monitoring in a significant proportion of patients with diabetes. Patients with elevated blood glucose levels and a high renal threshold for glucose will often have glucose in their urine in undetectable concentrations. Also, urine testing cannot detect or verify hypoglycemia. The principal advantages of urine testing are its simplicity and low cost. It is still useful for patients with limited goals for glycemic control and for those unwilling or unable to perform blood glucose monitoring. Urine testing done well is more valuable to the care of the patient than is blood testing done poorly. However, there is little need for patients who are performing blood glucose monitoring satisfactorily to check their urine for glucose as well.

Urine testing for ketones should continue to be performed in patients whose blood glucose levels are consistently above 240 mg/dL and in patients with acute illness and symptomatic hyperglycemia. It is important that such testing not be neglected in patients who no longer test their urine for the presence of glucose.

Use of Glycosylated Hemoglobin Measurements

Periodic measurement of glycosylated hemoglobin is an important aid to the physician in the care of insulin-treated patients with diabetes. Hemoglobin A is nonenzymatically glycosylated in the circulation, and the level of glycosylated hemoglobin in the blood has been shown to correlate directly with the mean blood glucose level over the 2 to 3 months preceding the measurement. The results are an accurate measure of overall blood glucose control[106]—more useful for this purpose than random or fasting blood glucose values. Levels of glycosylated hemoglobin can be used for assessing the accuracy of self-monitoring of blood glucose. Changes in levels of glycosylated hemoglobin, along with the health-care provider's assessment of the significance of the level, should be regularly reported to the patient. The sharing of such information is often a powerful behavioral tool for motivating patients to improve compliance and glycemic control.

Mixing Insulins

During the past few years, the increasing use of mixtures of regular insulin with longer-acting insulins in intensive therapy regimens has prompted investigations into the clinical effects of mixing different types of insulin. Some rules and guidelines for the mixing of insulins that have been established are summarized in Table 27–9. It should be noted that these rules may apply only to U-100 insulins and those types available in the United States. Studies have shown that different rules may apply to U-40 mixtures, and concentrations of protamine may be different in NPH preparations available in other countries.

Currently, in mixtures of NPH and regular insulin, the regular insulin retains its potency in a stable fashion for prolonged periods.[107] This is true for human insulins as well as for animal insulins. Unlike in the past, all the preparations of NPH insulin currently available from the major pharmaceutical companies have similar levels of protamine and do not contain excess protamine that might bind to the added regular insulin.[108] Mixtures of NPH and regular insulin at any of the ratios needed for clinical purposes can be used without resulting in any clinical difference in glycemic effect compared with that produced by separate injection of each of the insulins. Syringes can be prefilled with these mixtures and stored in the refrigerator for as long as 21 days for later use.[109] Commercially available mixtures of NPH and regular insulin in a 70 to 30% ratio, as well as in a 50 to 50% ratio, are currently available in the United States. Their clinical utility is best seen in patients with Type II diabetes who would benefit from simplified regimens that do not require them to mix insulins in the syringe. The ratios of NPH to regular insulin needed by most patients with Type I diabetes are too variable and subject to change to be accommodated by a single fixed ratio. In Europe, a wider variety of mixtures (NPH/regular) are currently available, including 90/10, 80/20, and 60/40, and these may be available for use in North America in the near future.

The clinical effects of using mixtures of regular insulin and lente are much more problematic. The lente series of insulins contain excess zinc, which tends to bind to added regular insulin and to cause it to precipitate out of solution. With beef-pork insulin, this process starts 15 minutes after mixing and progresses for up to 24 hours[108]; with human insulins, it occurs even more rapidly.[110] The effect is even more pronounced when the ratio of lente insulin to regular insulin is high. The binding of regular insulin by the zinc has been shown to be associated with a blunting of the increase in levels of circulating insulin after injection, but it is unclear whether this has any significance in the practical clinical situation. Given these findings, patients should be instructed to inject their insulin immediately after mixing the two types in the syringe and to keep their procedures for injection standardized. Similarly, mixing human regular and ultralente insulins is also associated with a blunting of the effect of the regular insulin.[111] Because of these problems, the mixing of lente series insulins with regular insulin is not generally recommended[103]; nevertheless, these insulins are commonly mixed together in intensive insulin regimens without undue effect in most patients.

Different insulins of the lente series can be mixed together without any problems. Phosphate-buffered insulins such as NPH and PZI, as well as buffered regular insulins (Humulin BR or Velosulin), are incompatible with lente series insulins because the phosphate precipitates the zinc from the suspension and allows more insulin to go into solution. The excess protamine in PZI insulin will bind added regular insulin in an unpredictable manner. Human insulin can be mixed with other species of insulins, but this rarely is necessary in clinical practice.

COMPLICATIONS OF INSULIN THERAPY

Hypoglycemia

By far the most frequently encountered problem in patients treated with insulin for diabetes is hypoglycemia. Virtually all insulin-treated patients develop hypoglycemia at one time or another and are constantly anticipating this problem and dealing with its consequences. Hypoglycemia is involved either primarily or secondarily as a

---

Table 27–9. Guidelines for Mixing Insulins

1. NPH insulin may be mixed with regular insulin without difficulty
2. Mixtures of NPH and regular insulin in prefilled syringes can be stored under refrigeration for up to 21 days
3. Lente series insulins may be mixed with each other
4. When lente series insulins are mixed with regular insulin, the insulin should be injected immediately after mixing in the syringe
5. Acetate-buffered insulins should not be mixed with phosphate-buffered insulins
6. PZI insulin should not be mixed with regular insulin
7. Insulins of different species can be mixed, but this is to be avoided if possible

NPH = neutral protamine Hagedorn insulin; PZI = protamine zinc insulin.

cause of death in 4 to 7% of patients with IDDM.[112] Severe hypoglycemia with loss of consciousness can have a profound effect on a patient, both physically and psychologically, and fear of developing hypoglycemia can play a great role in his or her behavior and approach to insulin administration. Severe hypoglycemia can cause brain damage and death, and the danger of hypoglycemia to the patient and others if it occurs during driving or the operation of machinery is considerable. A complete discussion of hypoglycemia can be found in Chapter 55. This chapter will focus on those aspects of hypoglycemia as they apply to insulin therapy.

Most patients experience some symptoms of hypoglycemia when their plasma glucose levels decrease to 50 mg/dL or less (blood glucose levels less than 45 mg/dL). As plasma glucose values decrease further, mentation may become impaired, although the degree to which this is clinically evident to others is quite variable.[113] Some individuals can be seemingly alert and conversant when their blood glucose levels are 20 mg/dL or less, although testing of cognitive function would show evidence of impairment. Others would be comatose if their blood glucose level was this low. As the blood glucose level falls, most patients experience adrenergic warning signs of hypoglycemia before they develop neuroglycopenic symptoms related to impairment of central nervous system functioning. The responses of the autonomic nervous system to a drop in blood glucose level result in anxiety, palpitations, diaphoresis, hunger, and tremulousness. Although it used to be thought that these symptoms were related to the rapidity of the fall of blood glucose level, this has since been found not to be true; the set point triggering adrenergic symptoms is usually that glucose level that triggers secretion of the counterregulatory hormones (60 to 65 mg/dL).[114] Nevertheless, these symptoms can be masked or unapparent when the blood glucose level decreases slowly and steadily, as can be seen in patients with insulinomas. Subsequently, the patient will develop clinical signs and symptoms of the effect of hypoglycemia on brain function[115]; these include headache, paresthesias of the tongue or lips, blurred vision, unsteady gait, impaired mentation, confusion, focal neurologic signs, seizures, and coma.

In most cases patients receiving insulin develop hypoglycemia because of a mismatch between the timing of insulin, meals, and exercise. Any of the insulin regimens previously discussed must take this into account. Increased intensity or frequency of exercise can cause hypoglycemia, as can omissions of meals or decreased daily caloric intake. Weight loss can cause hypoglycemia by increasing insulin sensitivity and lowering daily insulin requirements. Several clinical conditions can predispose a patient receiving insulin to hypoglycemia, including adrenal or pituitary deficiency, liver disease, renal insufficiency, use of alcohol, and drugs that cause β-adrenergic blockade. A careful history is important in assessing the possible causes of hypoglycemia in a patient with previously stable glycemic control with insulin.

The counterregulatory hormones glucagon and epinephrine have been shown to be of primary importance in the response to insulin-induced hypoglycemia.[116] If glucagon secretion is blocked, augmented epinephrine secretion can compensate to cause a rise in blood glucose level. Similarly, when epinephrine is blocked, glucagon release alone can provide for a recovery of blood glucose. When the response of both hormones is inadequate, however, hypoglycemia can become more severe and persist. This is of clinical importance because patients with diabetes progressively lose their counterregulatory hormone responses to hypoglycemia. The first hormone response that is lost is that of glucagon. After 5 years of IDDM, almost all patients have an impaired glucagon response to hypoglycemia. This is a selective deficiency, because glucagon secretion in response to amino acids and other secretogogues remains intact.[117] The problem is also seen in patients with NIDDM treated with insulin, but with decreased frequency. The cause of the deficient glucagon response is not known, and it is not reversible with improved glycemic control. The result of glucagon deficiency is to limit hepatic glucose production in response to hypoglycemia and to make the counterregulatory response of epinephrine more critical.

Hypoglycemia Unawareness

A common problem seen in patients with diabetes is the development of hypoglycemia unawareness or an inability to perceive the warning signs of hypoglycemia. This occurs more commonly in patients with diabetes of long duration and in patients with an increased frequency of hypoglycemic episodes. Counterregulatory responses of norepinephrine, epinephrine, and glucagon are impaired, resulting in hypoglycemic episodes that can be more severe and prolonged than they would be otherwise. Epinephrine secretion in response to hypoglycemia begins to be diminished after 5 to 10 years of IDDM, and this significantly impairs counterregulation in the absence of glucagon.[113] The prevalence of deficient epinephrine secretion in patients with long-standing diabetes may be as high as 40%. The deficiency can be attributed in large part to autonomic neuropathy and is often associated with other autonomic symptoms. Defects in glucose counterregulation can be diagnosed with insulin-infusion tests,[118] but these are rarely used in routine clinical practice.

As discussed earlier, hypoglycemia unawareness is seen with increased frequency in patients on intensive insulin therapy regimens,[65] and this unawareness is associated with an increased incidence of severe episodes of hypoglycemia.[64] This problem can be reversed, and counterregulatory responses often are regained when intensive therapy is discontinued. In those patients who develop this problem, it is best to avoid extremely tight glycemic control because of the risks of severe hypoglycemia.[119] This is best achieved by raising target blood glucose levels—e.g., from less than 120 mg/dL to less than 150 mg/dL.

Nocturnal Hypoglycemia: Somogyi Effect, Waning Insulin, and the Dawn Phenomenon

Frequently, hyperglycemia develops after an episode of insulin-induced hypoglycemia. Most commonly, this occurs overnight, when fasting blood glucose levels tend to be high, and worsen after the preceding nighttime insulin dose is increased. This problem was described by Somogyi in 1938, who hypothesized that hypoglycemia activates the process of glycogenolysis in the liver, leading to release of an excess of glucose into the circulation, resulting in hyperglycemia.[120] Blood glucose determinations were not done at that time. It was found that morning glycosuria with ketonuria could be successfully treated in some patients by decreasing, rather than increasing, the evening insulin dose. The existence of this phenomenon has been confirmed in a number of studies.[121,122] It is thought to be mediated by increases in the levels of circulating counterregulatory hormones in response to the transient hypoglycemia that may occur during sleep without the patient's experiencing any symptoms. This problem did not occur in patients with hypopituitarism.[123,124] β-Adrenergic blockade could ameliorate the hyperglycemic response but not the initial hypoglycemia.[125]

More recently, however, it has been recognized that counterregulatory hormone responses are not the only cause of hyperglycemia following hypoglycemia. The waning effect of the insulin dose given the previous evening can also be an important factor.[126] In patients given a dose of intermediate-acting insulin in the evening, the duration of effect of the insulin may result in a peak of hypoglycemic activity in the middle of the night and in a relative lack of circulating insulin in the early waking hours.[127,128] In this situation, insulin deficiency, rather than excessive counterregulatory responses, may be implicated in the resulting hyperglycemia. The relative importance of the waning effect of insulin and the Somogyi phenomenon in morning hyperglycemia has been a recurring subject of debate because of the different implications for therapy. In one case, the evening dose of insulin should be increased or delayed, and in the other, it should be decreased.

A third process, the so-called dawn phenomenon, is also involved in the pathogenesis of morning hyperglycemia.[129] In normal subjects, as well as in patients with diabetes, glucose production by the liver is increased and sensitivity to the action of insulin is decreased in the early morning hours from 4 a.m. to 8 a.m. Thus, higher levels of insulin are required to maintain euglycemia in the early morning hours, as seen in studies of intravenous insulin infusion.[123] The dawn phenomenon has been shown to be caused by nocturnal surges in secretion of growth hormone, which result in a subsequent, transient insulin resistance.[130] These surges are physiologic and are not caused by counterregulatory responses to hypoglycemia. In diabetic patients treated with insulin infusion pumps, the basal rate of infusion during the early morning hours is often increased by as much as one-third to deal with this problem. In patients treated with injections, the peak effect of the preceding insulin dose should be timed to coincide with this period of increased insulin requirement. In practical terms, it may often be necessary to use an intermediate-acting insulin late at bedtime rather than ultralente insulin in the evening, because the "peakless" absorption of ultralente insulin through the night may not fully coincide with the increased physiologic requirement for insulin in the early morning hours.

Treatment of Hypoglycemia

Hypoglycemic episodes can usually be treated successfully by ingestion of rapidly absorbed carbohydrate containing 20 g of glucose in the form of sugar, honey, candy, fruit juice, or a soft drink.[131] Remediation is best accomplished if the principal sugar is glucose—not fructose or sucrose. For this purpose, glucose tablets are particularly useful because of their portability and accuracy of dosage in acute conditions. Glucose gel preparations are also helpful and can be placed in the pouch between the cheek and gums to eliminate the danger of aspiration in patients who are stuporous or have difficulty swallowing. Glucagon, available in kits of 1-mg doses, should be given subcutaneously or intramuscularly by companions or family members when patients are comatose or unable to swallow. If these remedies are not immediately successful, intravenous administration of glucose is necessary.

Patients should be carefully instructed in how to recognize the warning signs and symptoms of hypoglycemia and should be well educated about the proper methods of treatment. They should always have the appropriate amount of oral carbohydrate available, wherever they are, especially in potentially dangerous situations such as while driving a car. Training of family members and companions in the recognition and treatment of hypoglycemia is important in dealing with situations involving changes in mental status. Patients should be instructed to carry identification in their wallets identifying them as insulin-dependent and should wear an identification tag or bracelet at all times.

After a severe hypoglycemic episode occurs, it is important for the patient and the physician to try to identify and analyze the principal factors responsible for the event. Commonly, a meal or snack was delayed, the exercise or activity pattern was changed, or the timing or dose of insulin was changed. If no obvious explanation can be identified, the daily dosage of the insulin active at the time of the event should be reduced by at least 2 units, and the patient should be followed-up closely and perform frequent glucose monitoring. Patients can be given dosage adjustment guidelines for these situations, but these guidelines should not be used as a substitute for communication between patient and physician.

Brittle Diabetes

For most patients with diabetes, an insulin treatment regimen can be devised that provides relatively stable control of blood glucose values. A small subgroup of patients, however, experience extremely erratic patterns of glycemic control, with large fluctuations in glucose levels for no obvious reason. These patients are usually said to have "brittle" diabetes, although the exact meaning of the term is frequently debated.[132,133] These patients either have marked and often incapacitating excursions of blood glucose levels on a daily basis or have frequent decompensations in their glycemic control, often with recurrent ketoacidosis or hypoglycemia that significantly interferes with their lifestyle. Of particular concern is the apparent randomness of the blood glucose excursions, which do not appear to show any obvious diurnal pattern or predictable response to changes in diet or exercise.

The problem is heterogenous, with a number of causes (Table 27–10). Some patients may have insulin resistance with high titers of circulating insulin antibodies, causing abnormalities in the kinetics of insulin action.[134] This, however, is relatively uncommon and has become increasingly rare with the introduction of human and purified insulins. An extremely rare syndrome of subcutaneous insulin resistance has been described that involves local degradation of injected insulin by proteases,[135] but it is not clear whether this syndrome has been adequately documented.[136] The genetic and acquired syndromes of insulin resistance and acanthosis nigricans, manifested by defects in insulin action at the cellular level or by the presence of circulating antibodies to the insulin receptor, can also be associated with erratic fluctuations in glucose levels.[137] The Somogyi phenomenon, as well as the defects in glucose counterregulation previously discussed, can often be overlooked as causes of erratic glycemic control. Gastroparesis diabeticorum can lead to erratic absorption of nutrients from the gastrointestinal tract, making it extremely difficult to coordinate insulin administration with meals. Chronic undiagnosed infections and underlying hormonal disorders such as adrenal insufficiency or pheochromocytoma can have adverse effects on glycemic control. Poor injection technique and/or confusion by the patient with regard to times and dosages of insulin often are implicated in patients diagnosed as "brittle." Of particular importance are psychosocial problems that lead to factitious disease (surreptitious administration of insulin by the patient, with no obvious motive or gain by the patient).[138] Manipulative behavior is also frequent, particularly in adolescents and young adults,[139] and poor glycemic control is often associated with eating disorders.[140,141] Patients concerned about weight gain in relation to insulin therapy discover they can use poor glycemic control as a means of losing weight or preventing weight gain. Alcohol and drug abuse also are causes of apparent "brittle" diabetes. In one recent study of 30 patients with this diagnosis, factitious disease and insulin manipulation were found to cause the problem in more than half the cases and cognitive and language deficits were present in another seven cases.[133]

Brittle diabetes is best managed with a sequential approach. A detailed, careful history and physical examination must be taken by a physician who is familiar with this problem so that complicating medical problems can be identified and screened. Prior hospitalizations should be carefully reviewed. It should be carefully determined that the apparent brittle control is not the result of an inappropriate treatment regimen or failure or inability of the patient to follow an appropriate regimen. Dietary issues must be carefully evaluated, and the patient should be taught home blood glucose monitoring and placed on a regimen that includes consistent exercise and a meal schedule the patient is judged to be capable of following. If these measures are unsuccessful for no apparent reason, the patient should be hospitalized for further evaluation. At that time, blood can be sampled frequently, with measurements of blood glucose levels before and after meals and through the night to look for nocturnal hypoglycemia or the dawn phenomenon. Inpatient education on insulin administration and diet can be instituted and the patient's activities evaluated and supervised. Insulin injections should be performed by the nursing staff, and access to insulin by the patient should be restricted. If metabolic control does not improve at this point, a detailed medical evaluation is initiated, with tests of adrenal, pituitary, thyroid, and renal function. A gastric-emptying scan and tests of autonomic neurologic functioning can be performed if deemed appropriate to the situation. When immunologic insulin resistance is suspected, circulating levels of free insulin and titers of antibodies to insulin can be measured. Some clinicians recommend testing with both an intravenous and a subcutaneous insulin challenge as an initial part of the evaluation,[133] but this has not been necessary at our institution. A search for occult infection, inflammatory disease, or surreptitious drug use may be initiated as well. Of prime importance is a careful psychological evaluation by a trained professional familiar with these problems to search for learning disorders, depression, eating disorders, or possible causes of manipulative behavior.

Once the underlying cause of the brittle diabetes is determined, steps can be taken to correct the problem. There is no single specific approach. Underlying hormonal and systemic disorders can be treated, and insulin

Table 27–10. Causes of Brittle Diabetes

1. Abnormalities in glucose counterregulation
   a. Somogyi effect
   b. Dawn phenomenon
   c. Hypoglycemia unawareness
2. Hormonal disorders
   a. Adrenal insufficiency
   b. Pituitary insufficiency
   c. Isolated growth hormone deficiency
   d. Acromegaly
   e. Glucocorticoid excess
   f. Thyroid hormone excess or deficiency
   g. Pheochromocytoma
3. Disorders of insulin pharmacokinetics
   a. Insulin antibodies
   b. Renal insufficiency
   c. Liver disease and cirrhosis
   d. Insulin-receptor disorders
   e. Subcutaneous insulin resistance
4. Gastrointestinal disease
   a. Gastroparesis diabeticorum
   b. Malabsorption syndromes
5. Systemic illness
6. Psychological disorders
   a. Factitious disease
   b. Insulin manipulation
   c. Bulemia and eating disorders
   d. Cognitive and language-processing disorders
   e. Depression
   f. Alcohol and drug abuse

and dietary regimens can be modified. Frequent blood glucose monitoring by the patient and food records may be helpful in understanding the problem. Regimens of multiple daily injections using primarily regular insulin have been advocated for some patients with unpredictable responses to intermediate and long-acting insulins. CSII has been reported to be of help to patients already receiving multiple daily infections who have severe hypoglycemic episodes,[142] but CSII also is subject to abuse by depressed or manipulative patients. Invasive procedures, such as intravenous and intraperitoneal delivery systems, are as of yet unproven treatments for this problem and should be used only on an experimental basis. Behavioral modification and psychotherapy may be of help in treating some of the underlying psychological disorders, and close follow-up and open communication are important for success.

Insulin Edema

Patients who have had poor glycemic control in the past sometimes develop peripheral edema when their blood glucose levels are rapidly brought under control.[143,144] This is most commonly seen in patients with newly diagnosed diabetes and extreme hyperglycemia when they start insulin therapy or in patients with long-standing chronic hyperglycemia who have started a more intensive insulin regimen. The edema may be present in local areas only, such as the feet and ankles, but also may be manifested as generalized anasarca with facial and periorbital swelling. Congestive heart failure has also been reported.[145] More commonly, a transient weight gain is seen that may be unaccompanied by any overt physical findings. Patients who have been treated for diabetic ketoacidosis and hyperosmolar coma often experience transient signs and symptoms of fluid overload. These are usually attributed to overly aggressive use of intravenous fluids but may be a manifestation of insulin edema. The edema and fluid retention are usually self-limited and will resolve after several days unless there is underlying cardiac or renal disease. In rare situations, a diuretic can be used temporarily to relieve the symptoms.

Several different mechanisms have been proposed to explain insulin-induced edema. Poorly controlled diabetes is associated with chronic volume depletion, which is corrected by the administration of insulin. Also, levels of circulating antidiuretic hormone are increased in situations of chronic hyperglycemia and poor control; this may lead to fluid retention and inability to excrete a water load during volume repletion. Insulin may act directly on the kidney to cause it to reduce excretion of sodium and to increase retention of free water.[146] Poor glycemic control also is associated with high levels of circulating glucagon, which inhibit the effect of circulating aldosterone. When glucagon levels decrease after correction of hyperglycemia, fluid retention can occur. This development is the mirror image of the effect of fasting and low-carbohydrate diets, which cause natriuresis and fluid loss. In addition, chronic hyperglycemia has been shown to be associated with an increase in capillary permeability, which may contribute to peripheral edema with volume repletion.[147]

Lipoatrophy

Injection of insulin can sometimes lead to a localized loss or to the absence of subcutaneous fat in the areas of chronic injection. This problem used be encountered frequently but has decreased in incidence with the advent of more purified insulins. Lipoatrophy is more common in young children and female patients and tends to occur in the first 6 months following the initiation of insulin therapy. The problem is primarily cosmetic and is not associated with systemic or metabolic problems other than insulin allergy. Most likely, the cause of lipoatrophy is a local immunologic reaction to impurities in the insulin.[148] Immune complexes have been found in biopsy specimens of lipoatrophic tissue.

At present, the principal treatment of lipoatrophy is to switch the patient to a more purified type of insulin and to change from beef insulin to human or pork insulin.[39] If the affected sites are left alone, adipose tissue tends to be restored gradually over a few years. It has been found that this process can be accelerated if purified insulin is chronically injected into the areas immediately surrounding the sites of lipoatrophy.

Lipohypertrophy

Increased swelling of the subcutaneous fat also can occur at a localized site of repeated insulin injections. These areas tend to be associated with decreased sensitivity to pain and are therefore overused for injection. Occasionally, masses of fibrous tissue develop at the sites. Absorption of insulin from areas of lipohypertrophy may be retarded, leading to erratic glycemic control. Lipohypertrophy probably is the direct effect of insulin on local tissue lipogenesis[149] and not related to immunogenicity. The problem is treated by the injection of insulin at alternative sites and regular rotation of the sites. With this approach, the areas of lipohypertrophy usually will regress gradually.

Insulin Antibodies

It has long been known that insulin acts as an antigen, and antibodies specifically directed to insulin appear in the circulation in all patients treated with insulin. Indeed, it was the characterization of these antibodies by Berson and Yalow in 1956 that led to the development of the radioimmunoassay for insulin and other hormones.[150] More recently, some patients with Type I diabetes were found to develop antibodies to insulin before being treated with insulin, and, indeed, before developing overt clinical diabetes.[151] Presumably, endogenous insulin may develop some antigenic properties as part of the autoimmune pathogenesis of Type I diabetes.

A number of factors can affect the development of antibodies to insulin. Insulin purity is one. The insulin preparations currently available are associated with lower titers of circulating antibodies than are insulin preparations that are not chromatographed in the preparatory process.[23] Insulin species may be a factor as well. Use of beef insulin is associated with higher antibody titers than is use of pork or human insulin.[36] Titers of antibody to human insulin tend to be lower than those to purified pork insulin.[37] Stopping and starting insulin therapy is associated with increased antibody formation through an anamnestic response. There is also one report claiming that intensive insulin regimens may be associated with increased immunogenicity.[152] Genetic factors also may play a role in the development of antibodies to insulin. Certain HLA phenotypes are associated with decreased antibody formation, while others are associated with increased levels.[23] Patients with Type II diabetes treated with insulin, who have some endogenous insulin secretion, have a decreased immune response to pork and human insulins (but not to mixed beef/pork insulin) compared with that of patients who are completely insulin-deficient.[39]

The presence of circulating antibodies to insulin can affect the absorption profile and bioavailability of injected insulin. IgG antibodies to insulin can bind to insulin after it enters the circulation following subcutaneous injection, thus decreasing the amount of free insulin available for binding to the insulin receptors of target tissues. This can cause a delay in the time to peak biologic activity of the insulin after injection and to a more prolonged duration of action. In patients with high antibody titers, less than 1% of circulating insulin remains unbound to antibodies. The bound insulin can provide a reservoir of circulating insulin with a prolonged capacity to lower blood glucose levels. In consequence, insulin that is not being absorbed subcutaneously can be released from circulating antibodies to produce hypoglycemia at inappropriate times.[153]

The specific clinical effects of the presence of antibodies to insulin on the control of blood glucose levels is a subject of controversy and in need of further study. It has been suggested that high levels of antibodies to insulin can adversely affect endogenous insulin secretion,[154] but this has not been proven.[39] The binding of endogenous insulin to antibodies may result in a worsening of overall glycemic control because of decreased bioavailability at appropriate times, as well as increased availability at inappropriate times, especially if the postprandial effect of secreted insulin is attenuated.[155,156] Alternatively, insulin antibodies may act as a buffer of levels of free insulin, preventing large variability and lability of the levels of insulin as it is released from the subcutaneous depot.[157] High titers of antibodies to insulin have been associated with insulin resistance, as is discussed later in this chapter.

It has been suggested that insulin antibodies might play a role in the pathogenesis of the long-term complications of diabetes because of the finding of insulin immune complexes in experimental models of nephropathy and retinopathy in animals.[158,159] High antibody titers have also been found to correlate with severe complications in patients with diabetes.[160] Insulin-antibody complexes have been shown to stimulate procoagulant activity, which may play a role in the pathogenesis of large-vessel disease.[161] However, a direct causal link between antibodies and complications has not yet been demonstrated. In pregnant women with diabetes, IgG antibodies to insulin can cross the placenta and enter the fetal circulation; they also may facilitate the transfer of insulin from the maternal to the fetal circulation.[162] A role of these antibodies on the development of fetal macrosomia has been postulated,[162] but any possible effects of insulin antibodies on fetal complications is as of yet speculative.[163]

Insulin Allergy

Allergic reactions to insulin, once extremely common,[164] are now seen relatively rarely because of the increased use of purified insulins.[165] These reactions occur either locally at the site of injection or as a generalized, systemic reaction. The symptoms of insulin allergy occur only after a patient has been treated with insulin for the first time for at least 7 days, and most episodes of insulin allergy have become manifest within 6 months after the start of treatment. People who develop insulin allergy, whether systemic or localized, have an increased incidence of allergies to penicillin and other drugs. In addition, they are more likely to have taken insulin intermittently, stopping and starting it several times. Patients with allergy to insulin also are more likely to develop insulin resistance, often subsequent to their allergic symptoms, and are more likely to have localized lipoatrophy.[166]

Localized Insulin Allergy

Localized reactions to insulin usually develop as patches of swelling and redness at the site of injection and are usually pruritic and often painful. They can also appear in milder forms as small subcutaneous nodules that can be palpated but not seen. The immunologic mechanisms that underlie local allergy are actually heterogeneous and can be differentiated clinically by their time of onset after injection of the insulin. Nevertheless, it is often difficult to distinguish the different types of local reactions without performing a skin biopsy. The most common type of local hypersensitivity is IgE-mediated and involves a biphasic response to insulin.[39] There is an immediate reaction after insulin injection involving urticaria at the injection site with induration and pruritus. This is followed by a late-phase response lasting 6 to 12 hours, with progressive swelling, redness, and pruritus at the site of injection. The swelling may last as long as 2 or 3 days. In some situations, the immediate-phase symptoms can predominate, while in others, the late-phase symptoms can occur without the early signs. Levels of IgE antibody to insulin in the circulation tend to be elevated in patients with these types of local hypersensitivity.[167] Dermal skin testing is associated with development of an immediate wheal-and-flare reaction in these individuals.

Less commonly seen is an intermediate hypersensitivity reaction of an Arthus type involving deposition of antigen-antibody complexes in dermal sites. This reaction has an onset 4 to 8 hours after injection, peaking at 12 hours. The lesions are pruritic and indurated, with pain at the injection site, but the patient does not have a wheal-and-flare reaction. Patients also can develop a classical cell-mediated delayed hypersensitivity reaction to insulin. In this situation, pruritus, induration, erythema, and burning appear 12 hours after injection and peak in intensity at 24 to 48 hours.[167]

The use of purified pork and human insulins has been associated with a decline in the incidence of these local reactions, which used to occur in as many as 50% of patients receiving unchromatographed insulins,[164] to 2% or less of patients started on purified pork insulin.[39] Similar results have been found with human insulin, although it is not clear that human insulin is any more beneficial than purified pork insulin in preventing local hypersensitivity. Local allergy is less common with the use of regular insulin alone than with the use of insulin in suspension, but it does occur in patients treated with regular insulin. It has also been reported in patients treated with CSII therapy.[74]

Hypersensitivity to the protamine and zinc in intermediate- and long-acting insulins has also been seen as a cause of local allergy, but its incidence is extremely low. Allergy to protamine can be identified with dermal skin testing and treated by switching the patient from NPH or PZI insulins to the lente series of insulins. Currently, all of the commercially available insulins contain zinc, although the concentration varies. A small number of patients with local reactions to purified insulins may benefit from treatment with zinc-free insulins, which are available on special request from the major pharmaceutical companies that produce insulin.[39]

Local reactions to insulin tend to be self-limited and generally resolve spontaneously within 1 to 2 months after onset of symptoms. Most patients with mild symptoms do not require treatment for this condition. If treatment is needed, patients can be switched to human insulin. If this is not successful after several injections, purified pork insulin or purified beef insulin can be tried. Oral antihistamines can be of help in decreasing local symptoms, especially those of IgE-mediated insulin allergy. However, antihistamines should not be injected locally in the syringe with the insulin because of their chemical incompatibility.[39] Local injection of glucocorticoids in low doses with the insulin has been used with some success in a small number of patients.

Generalized Insulin Allergy

Systemic allergy to insulin is uncommon, occurring in 0.05% of diabetic patients admitted to the hospital.[168] Patients with this condition may present with a number of clinical symptoms, including generalized urticaria, pruritus, angioedema, rash, flushing, palpitations, and bronchospasm. Acute anaphylaxis with respiratory and circulatory collapse can occur but is extremely rare. No deaths known to be due to generalized insulin allergy have been reported. These reactions are thought to be mediated by reaction of insulin with insulin-specific IgE that is bound to basophils and tissue mast cells.[169] These cells then release mediators of acute hypersensitivity, such as histamine and serotonin, which produce the symptoms. Patients with this condition generally have

high levels of circulating insulin-specific IgE,[168] but these antibody levels may also be elevated in patients without insulin allergy.[170]

Generalized insulin allergy can also be associated with symptoms similar to those of serum sickness, with arthralgias, myalgias, fever, headache, and gastrointestinal symptoms. Less commonly, autoimmune thrombocytic purpura and a Coombs-positive hemolytic anemia have been reported. Circulating insulin-specific IgG has been implicated in the pathogenesis of these symptoms. Similar symptoms have been reported in a few patients starting treatment with recombinant DNA human insulin and proinsulin, with the condition resolving after treatment with the insulin is stopped. No evidence was found of contamination of the insulin with bacterial proteins.[39]

Most systemic allergic reactions occur in patients who have stopped and then restarted insulin therapy. The insulin molecule itself is usually the offending antigen, but occasionally patients have specific reactivity to protamine. Patients may have severe allergy to a specific species of insulin, usually beef insulin, and tolerate other types. In these patients, however, there is frequently cross-reactivity between the offending insulin and other insulins, including human insulin.

A careful history and notation of the temporal relationship of the symptoms to insulin injections is necessary for the diagnosis of insulin allergy. Exposure to other offending antigens and other drug allergies should be ruled out. Intradermal skin testing with insulin is often of value. Patients can be given an initial dose of 0.001 U of purified beef insulin, purified pork insulin, and human insulin in 0.02-mL volumes injected intradermally into separate, clearly marked sites. Control injections containing saline and histamine can be given as well. If there is no response to the injected insulins, the doses of the insulins can be increased first to 0.1 U intradermally and then, if no response, to 1 U. If there is no response to 1 U intradermally in the presence of the appropriate positive control, it can be presumed that the patient does not have insulin allergy and that the symptoms are a response to some other antigen.

If generalized insulin allergy persists after the patient is switched to human insulin, desensitization should be initiated while the patient is hospitalized. Human insulin is used for this process unless it can be demonstrated that the patient has a milder allergic response to another species of insulin. If the patient is in stable metabolic control, an abbreviated desensitization schedule can be started with a dose of insulin equal to one-third of the dose that normally produces the reaction. The insulin dose can be increased by 5 U every 12 hours as tolerated until blood glucose levels are within a satisfactory range.[39] If the symptoms of systemic allergy are severe or if glycemic control is poor, rapid desensitization should be started. A syringe containing epinephrine diluted 1/100 should be available at the bedside and be given if a severe allergic response occurs. Antihistamines and glucocorticoids should be avoided because they could mask allergic symptoms. Desensitization kits can be obtained for the purpose (Eli Lilly), or serial dilutions of human insulin can be prepared such that the first injection delivers 0.001 U in 0.1 mL intradermally. Progressively larger doses of insulin can be given at 30-minute intervals in the following sequence: 0.002, 0.004, 0.01, 0.02, 0.04, 0.1, 0.2, 0.4, 1, 2, and 8 U. The first two doses can be given intradermally, and the subsequent doses, subcutaneously. If a local or systemic allergic reaction is seen (greater than 1 cm of wheal, flare, or induration), the sequence should be dropped back by two dilutions and then continued up the scale as before. If the patient reacts to the initial injection, desensitization should be started with 0.0001 U and increased at the same relative scale.

This procedure has be shown to be successful in about 94% of patients in a study performed with purified pork insulin,[39] and similar results should be expected with human insulin. Following desensitization, patients can be switched to intermediate-acting or long-acting insulin, alone or with regular insulin. It is important to have constant basal coverage with injected insulin; gaps in treatment or omission of doses can lead to the return of the systemic allergy, necessitating a repeat of the desensitization procedure. Patients who fail to become desensitized can be treated with oral antihistamines, low doses of systemic steroids, or a combination of the two.[171] Allergy to zinc should also be considered when desensitization is not successful; skin testing with zinc-free insulin can be performed to rule this out.

Although it is not fully clear how desensitization works, the process seems to involve depletion of the mediators of hypersensitivity from mast cells and basophils. In addition, IgG blocking antibodies are developed that prevent the binding of insulin to IgE on mast cells that triggers the immediate hypersensitivity response.[169] In addition, levels of circulating insulin-specific IgE fall during desensitization, so IgE production may be suppressed. The rise in levels of IgG blocking antibodies in this situation is occasionally associated with the development of insulin resistance.

Insulin Resistance

Insulin resistance refers to the clinical condition in which the biologic response to insulin is diminished to below normal levels.[172] Diabetic patients with insulin resistance require larger than normal daily doses of insulin. There is an intrinsic form of insulin resistance seen in patients with NIDDM that is involved in the pathogenesis of the disease and is separate from the insulin resistance of obesity, which may also be present.[79] Clinically significant insulin resistance is usually identified when an adult patient requires more than 200 U of insulin a day or when a child requires more than 2.5 U/kg of body weight.[173,174] In fact, patients who require smaller daily doses of insulin than those may still have some degree of insulin resistance, since the daily insulin output of the adult pancreas is only between 20 to 50 U.

Insulin resistance is associated with a number of clinical states. Acute illness, surgery, infection, and ketoacidosis can be accompanied by transient insulin resistance that increases the daily insulin requirements. Cushing disease, adrenal adenoma, ectopic adrenocorticotropic hormone syndrome, and exogenous steroid use can cause insulin resistance because of the metabolic effects of glucocorticoid excess. Similarly, insulin resistance caused by excess levels of growth hormone is seen in acromegaly. Insulin resistance is invariably seen in the later stages of pregnancy. A variety of syndromes with severe tissue resistance to the actions of insulin are encountered but are extremely uncommon (see Chapter 16).

Obesity and Weight Gain

The most common insulin-resistant state is obesity. Obesity is associated with decreased responsiveness to insulin in all of the major target tissues (muscle, liver, and fat) caused by a combination of defects in insulin receptor and post-receptor tissue.[175] Distribution of fat in the abdomen and upper body (as opposed to lower body or peripheral obesity) is especially associated with peripheral and hepatic resistance to insulin and a decrease in hepatic insulin extraction.[176,177] This is discussed in depth in Chapter 19. In practical terms, in patients treated with insulin, the magnitude of insulin resistance is proportional to the degree of excess weight. This can be a particularly difficult problem for obese patients treated with insulin because insulin treatment is associated with weight gain both in patients with IDDM and those with NIDDM. In a number of studies of patients treated with insulin for up to 12 months, weight gains of 2.0 to 4.5 kg were reported.[81] The problem of weight gain was well documented in IDDM patients in the DCCT, in which patients randomized to intensive insulin therapy gained a mean of 5.1 kg more then their counterparts receiving standard treatment during the first year of therapy. Weight gain was especially seen in those patients whose glycemic control improved the most and in those patients who had severe hypoglycemic episodes.[66] Most of the early weight gain following the initiation of insulin therapy is due to rehydration and correction of the catabolic state of poorly controlled diabetes, but subsequent chronic weight gain (in non-obese subjects) is two-thirds due to fat and one-third due to lean body mass.[178]

Probably several mechanisms are responsible for the weight gain associated with insulin use. Increasing insulin doses can cause recurrent hypoglycemia that can force intake of excess calories. The hypoglycemic episodes are frequently very mild, without adrenergic warning symptoms, and manifested only by hunger. Weight gain can also result from the direct lipogenic effects of insulin on adipose tissue, independent of food intake.[179]

The result of weight gain in insulin-treated patients is the often-cited vicious cycle of increased insulin resistance, leading to the need for more exogenous insulin, to further weight gain, which increases the insulin resistance even more. Diet therapy and weight loss are extremely important in reversing this process,[180] but the long-term results of these therapies have generally been disappointing, even in patients not receiving insulin.[181] More drastic measures, such as very-low-calorie diets, can be employed in patients with Type II diabetes who are receiving insulin, but such diets should be used with great caution in patients with Type I diabetes.[182] Insulin doses can be decreased dramatically in anticipation of weight loss and decreased carbohydrate intake during the fast, and in most cases, patients with Type II diabetes can discontinue taking insulin entirely. Unfortunately, patients subsequently gain back most or all of the weight lost during the fast if they do not continue afterward with a weight-maintenance behavior modification program.

Immunologic Insulin Resistance

The development of high titers of antibodies to insulin can be a rare cause of insulin resistance in patients with diabetes, occurring in fewer than 0.01% of patients treated with beef insulin.[168] This syndrome has not yet been reported in any patients who had not received beef insulin in the past, so it should cease to be a clinical consideration as the use of human insulin becomes more widespread. Immunologic insulin resistance is seen more commonly in patients with a history of insulin allergy or with interrupted or intermittent insulin therapy. The development of insulin resistance can occur when insulin allergy is resolving, as high titers of circulating IgG block IgE from causing cause allergic symptoms.[183] The exact mechanism by which the circulating antibodies cause insulin resistance is unclear, but it is thought that bound insulin may be sequestered from action at the insulin receptor. Furthermore, the kinetics of insulin turnover are markedly altered. Patients with this condition often have very high insulin requirements, with one-half requiring 1000 U or more of insulin per day.[23]

To make the diagnosis of immunologic insulin resistance, one should take a careful history to identify associated findings such as insulin allergy. Other causes of insulin resistance should be ruled out, such as glucocorticoid excess, acromegaly, the use of drugs that cause insulin resistance, occult lymphoma, and the rare forms of extreme insulin resistance and acanthosis nigricans. The concurrent presence of obesity can often confuse the picture and make the diagnosis more difficult. Confirmation of the diagnosis can be made by finding elevated titers of antibodies to insulin, as well as high levels of plasma free and total insulin, which are usually extremely high (greater than 20,000 U/mL).[184]

The first step in treatment is to switch the patient from beef-containing insulin to human or purified pork insulin. Divided doses of regular insulin per day are used, and their duration of action is sufficiently prolonged by the insulin antibody binding as to make the use of intermediate-acting insulins unnecessary. If extremely high doses of insulin are required, U-500 insulin can be used. After the titers of insulin antibody decrease, which usually takes 4 to 6 weeks, the use of intermediate or long-acting insulins can be resumed. If patients do not respond to human or pork insulin, they can be treated with glucocorticoids, usually starting with prednisone at a dosage of 20 mg/day or higher.[185] Daily insulin requirements usually decrease rapidly in the first 3 to 5 days. Sulfated insulin has also been used successfully in the past to treat this condition when other measures have failed,[23] but now that human insulin is available, this form of therapy is unlikely to be necessary.

REFERENCES

1. Schade DS, Santiago JV, Skyler JS, Rizza RA. Insulin secretion in non-diabetics and insulin dependent subjects. In: Schade DS, Santiago JV, Skyler JS, Rizza RA, eds. Intensive insulin therapy. Princeton, NJ: Excerpta Medica, 1983:23–35.
2. Marble A, Insulin in the treatment of diabetes. In: Marble A, Krall LP, Bradley RF, et al, eds. Joslin's diabetes mellitus. 12th ed. Philadelphia: Lea & Febiger, 1985:380–405.
3. Zinman B. The physiologic replacement of insulin: an elusive goal. N Engl J Med 1989;321:363–70.
4. Selam JL, Charles MA. Devices for insulin administration. Diabetes Care 1990;13:955–79.
5. Brange J, Owens DR, Kang S, Vølund A. Monomeric insulins and their experimental and clinical implications. Diabetes Care 1990;13:923–54.
6. Howey DC, Hooper SA, Bowsher RR. [Lys(B28), Pro(B29)]-human insulin: an equipotent analog of human insulin with rapid onset and short duration of action. Diabetes 1991;40(Suppl 1):423A.
7. Salzman R, Manson JE, Griffing GT, et al. Intranasal aerosolized insulin: mixed-meal studies and long-term use in Type I diabetes. N Engl J Med 1985;312:1078–84.
8. Banting FM, Best CH. The internal secretion of the pancreas. J Lab Clin Med 1922;7:256–71.
9. Best CH. The first clinical use of insulin. Diabetes 1956;5:65–7.
10. Hagedorn HC, Jensen BN, Krarup NB, Wodstrup I. Protamine insulinate. JAMA 1936;106:177–80.
11. Scott D, Fisher A. Studies on insulin with protamine. J Pharmacol Exp Ther 1936;58:78–92.
12. Krayenbuhl C, Rosenberg T. Crystalline protamine insulin. Rep Steno Mem Hosp 1946;1:60–73.
13. Hallas-Møllor K. The lente insulins. Diabetes 1956; 5:7–14.
14. Skyler JS. Insulin pharmacology. Med Clin North Am 1988;72:1337–54.
15. Riggs AD. Bacterial production of human insulin. Diabetes Care 1984;4:64–8.
16. Lougheed WD, Woulfe-Flanagan H, Clement JR, Albisser AM. Insulin aggregation in artificial delivery systems. Diabetologia 1980;19:1–9.
17. Mecklenburg RS, Guinn TS. Complication of insulin pump therapy: the effect of insulin preparation. Diabetes Care 1985;8:367–70.
18. Chance RE, Root MA, Galloway JA. The immunogenicity of insulin preparations. Acta Endocrinol 1976;83(Suppl 205):185–98.
19. Turner RC, Phillips MA, Ward EA. Ultralente based insulin regimens—clinical applications, advantages and disadvantages. Acta Med Scand Suppl 1983;671:75–86.
20. Reeves ML, Seigler DE, Goldberg RB, et al. Pharmacokinetics of ultralente (U) insulin preparations [Abstract no. 252]. Diabetes 1986;35(Suppl 1):63A.
21. Galloway JA, Root MA, Chance RE, et al. New forms of insulin. In: Kryston LJ, Shaw RA, eds. Endocrinology and diabetes. New York: Grune & Stratton, 1975:329–42.
22. Brange J. Galenics of insulin. Berlin: Springer-Verlag, 1987.
23. Kahn CR, Rosenthal AS. Immunologic reactions to insulin: insulin allergy, insulin resistance, and the autoimmune insulin syndrome. Diabetes Care 1979;2:283–95.
24. Yue DK, Turtle JR. New forms of insulin and their use in the treatment of diabetes. Diabetes 1977;26:341–7.
25. Nosadini R. Noy G, Kurtz AB, Alberti KGMM. Differential response to infusions of highly purified and conven-

tional bovine and porcine insulins. Diabetes 1981; 30:650–55.

26. Mirsky IA, Jinks R, Perisutti G. The isolation and crystallization of human insulin. J Clin Invest 1963;42:1869–72.

27. Chance RE, Kroeff EP, Hoffmann JA, Frank BH. Chemical, physical, and biologic properties of biosynthetic human insulin. Diabetes Care 1981;4:147–54.

28. Frank BH, Pettee JM, Zimmermann RE, et al. The production of human proinsulin and its transformation to human insulin and C-peptide. In: Rich DH, Gross E, eds. Peptides: synthesis-structure-function. Proceedings of the Seventh Peptide Symposium. Rockford, IL: Pierce Chemical, 1981:729–38.

29. Markussen J, Damgaard U, Pingel M et al. Human insulin (Novo): chemistry and characteristics. Diabetes Care 1983;6(Suppl 1):4–8.

30. Markussen J, Damgaard U, Diers I, et. al. Biosynthesis of human insulin in yeast via single chain precursors [Abstract no. 324]. Diabetologia 1986;29:568A–69.

31. Karam JH, Etzwiler DD, eds. International Symposium on Human Insulin. Diabetes Care 1983;6(Suppl 1):1–68.

32. Skyler JS. Human insulin of recombinant DNA origin: clinical potential. Diabetes Care 1982;5(Suppl 2):181–6.

33. Gulan M, Gottesman IS, Zinman B. Biosynthetic human insulin improves postprandial glucose excursions in Type I diabetes. Ann Intern Med 1987;107:506–9.

34. Galloway JA, Spradlin CT, Root MA, Fineberg SE. The plasma glucose response of normal fasting subjects to neutral regular and NPH biosynthetic human and purified pork insulins. Diabetes Care 1981;4:183–8.

35. Houtzagers CMGJ, Berntzen PA, van der Stap H, et al. Absorption kinetics of short- and intermediate-acting insulins after jet injection with Medi-Jector II. Diabetes Care 1988;11:739–42.

36. Fineberg SE, Galloway JA, Fineberg SN, Goldman J. Effects of species of origin, purification levels and formulation on insulin immunogenicity. Diabetes 1983;32:592–9.

37. Galloway J, Fireman P, Fineberg S. Complications of insulin therapy: a brief overview of four years experience with human insulin (rDNA) in diabetes mellitus: achievements and skepticisms. R Soc Med Int Cong Symp Ser 1984;77:55.

38. IMS Drug Store and Hospital Audits. New York: IMS International, 1991.

39. Galloway JA, deShazo RD. Insulin chemistry and pharmacology; insulin allergy, resistance, and lipodystrophy. In: Rifkin H, Porte D, eds. Ellenberg and Rifkin's diabetes mellitus: theory and practice. 4th ed. New York: Elsevier, 1990:497–513.

40. Federlin K, Kelcorsky H, Maser E. Clinical aspects of immunity to insulin. In: Keck K, Erb P, eds. Basic and clinical aspects of immunity to insulin. New York: Walter de Gruyter, 1981:250.

41. Teuscher A, Berger WG. Hypoglycaemia unawareness in diabetics transferred from beef/porcine insulin to human insulin. Lancet 1987;2:382–5.

42. Berger W, Keller U, Honegger B, Jaeggi E. Warning symptoms of Hypoglycaemia during treatment with human and porcine insulin in diabetes mellitus. Lancet 1989;1:1041–4.

43. Heine RJ, van der Heyden EAP, van der Veen EA. Responses to human and porcine insulin in healthy subjects. Lancet 1989;2:946–9.

44. Kern W, Lieb K, Kerner W, et al. Differential effects of human and pork insulin-induced hypoglycemia on neuronal functions in humans. Diabetes 1990;39:1091–8.

45. Jones TW, Caprio S, Diamond MP, et al. Does insulin

46. Mühlhauser I, Heinemann L, Fritsche E, et al. Hypoglycemic symptoms and frequency of severe hypoglycemia in patients treated with human and animal insulin preparations. Diabetes Care 1991;14:745–9.

47. Shah SC, Malone JI, Simpson NE. A randomized trial of intensive insulin therapy in newly diagnosed insulin-dependent diabetes mellitus. N Engl J Med 1989;320:4.

48. Jovanovic L, Peterson CM. Optimal insulin delivery for the pregnant diabetic patient. Diabetes Care 1982;5(Suppl 1):24–37.

49. Hirsch IB, Farkas-Hirsch R, Skyler JS. Intensive insulin therapy for treatment of Type I diabetes. Diabetes Care 1990;13:1265–83.

50. Skyler JS, O'Sullivan MJ. Diabetes and pregnancy. In: Kohler PO, ed. Clinical endocrinology. New York: Wiley, 1986:603–22.

51. Pirart J. Diabetes mellitus and its degenerative complications: a prospective study of 4,400 patients observed between 1947 and 1973. Diabetes Care 1978;1:168–88.

52. The DCCT Research Group. Are continuing studies of metabolic control and microvascular complications in insulin-dependent diabetes mellitus justified? The diabetes control and complications trial. N Engl J Med 1988; 318:246–50.

53. Beck-Nielsen H, Richelsen B, Mogensen CE, et. al. Effect of insulin pump treatment for one year on renal function and retinal morphology in patients with IDDM. Diabetes Care 1985;8:585–9.

54. Holman RR, Dornan TL, Mayon-White V, et al. Prevention of deterioration of renal and sensory-nerve function by more intensive management of insulin-dependent diabetic patients: a two-year randomised prospective study. Lancet 1983;1:204–8.

55. Lauritzen T, Frost-Larsen K, Larsen HW, et al. Effect of 1 year of near-normal blood glucose levels on retinopathy in insulin-dependent diabetics. Lancet 1983;1:200–4.

56. Kroc Collaborative Study Group. Blood glucose control and the evolution of diabetic retinopathy and albuminuria: a preliminary multicenter trial. N Engl J Med 1984; 311:365–72.

57. Dahl-Jørgensen K, Brinchmann-Hansen O, Hanssen KF, et al. Rapid tightening of blood glucose control leads to transient deterioration of retinopathy in insulin dependent diabetes mellitus: the Oslo Study. BMJ 1985; 290:811–5.

58. Dahl-Jørgensen K, Brinchmann-Hansen O, Hanssen KF, et al. Effect of near normoglycaemia for two years on progression of early diabetic retinopathy, nephropathy, and neuropathy: the Oslo study. BMJ 1986; 293:1195–9.

59. Lauritzen T, Frost-Larsen K, Larsen HW, Deckert T. Two-year experience with continuous subcutaneous insulin infusion in relation to retinopathy and neuropathy. Diabetes 1985;34(Suppl 3):74–9.

60. Dahl-Jørgensen K, Hanssen KF, Kierulf P, et al. Reduction of urinary albumin excretion after 4 years of continuous subcutaneous insulin infusion in insulin-dependent diabetes mellitus: the Oslo study. Acta Endocrinol 1988; 117:19–25.

61. Deckert T, Lauritzen T, Parving HH, et al. Diabetic Nephropathy 1983;2:6–12.

62. The DCCT Research Group. The Diabetes Control and Complications Trial (DCCT): design and methodologic considerations for the feasibility phase. Diabetes 1986; 35:530–45.

63. The DCCT Research Group. Diabetes Control and Complications Trial (DCCT): results of feasibility study. Diabetes Care 1987;10:1–19.

64. The DCCT Research Group. Epidemiology of severe hypoglycemia in the Diabetes Control and Complications Trial. Am J Med 1991;90:450–9.

65. Amiel SA, Tamborlane WV, Simonson DC, et al. Defective glucose counterregulation after strict glycemic control of insulin-dependent diabetes mellitus. N Engl J Med 1987;316:1376–83.

66. The DCCT Research Group. Weight gain associated with intensive therapy in the Diabetes Control and Complications Trial. Diabetes Care 1988;11:567–73.

67. Mecklenberg RS. Acute complications associated with the use of insulin infusion pumps. Endocrinologist 1991;1: 19–24.

68. Clements RS Jr, Bell DSH, Benbarka A, Capper SA. Rapid insulin initiation in non-insulin-dependent diabetes mellitus. Am J Med 1987;82:415–20.

69. Gale EAM, Tattersall RB. Unrecognised nocturnal hypoglycemia in insulin-treated diabetics. Lancet 1979;1: 1049–52.

70. Skyler JS, Seigler DE, Reeves ML. Optimizing pumped insulin delivery. Diabetes Care 1982;5:135–47.

71. Eichner HL, Selam JL, Holleman CB, et al. Reduction of severe hypoglycemic events in Type I (insulin-dependent) diabetic patients using continuous subcutaneous insulin infusion. Diabetes Res 1988;8:189–93.

72. Reeves ML, Seigler DE, Ryan EA, Skyler JS. Glycemic control in insulin-dependent diabetes mellitus: comparison of outpatient intensified conventional therapy with continuous subcutaneous insulin infusion. Am J Med 1982;72:673–80.

73. Schiffrin A, Belmonte MM. Comparison between continuous subcutaneous insulin infusion and multiple injections of insulin: a one-year prospective study. Diabetes 1982;31:255–64.

74. Mecklenburg RS, Benson EA, Benson JW Jr, et al. Acute complications associated with insulin infusion pump therapy: report of experience with 161 patients. JAMA 1984;252:3265–69.

75. Mecklenburg RS, Guinn TS. Complications of insulin pump therapy: the effect of insulin preparation. Diabetes Care 1985;8:367–70.

76. Galloway JA. Treatment of NIDDM with insulin agonists or substitutes. Diabetes Care 1990;13:1209–39.

77. Weir GC. Non-insulin-dependent diabetes mellitus: interplay between β-cell inadequacy and insulin resistance [Editorial]. Am J Med 1982;73:461–4.

78. Reaven GM, Chen YI, Coulston AM, et al. Insulin secretion and action in noninsulin-dependent diabetes mellitus: is insulin resistance secondary to hypoinsulinemia? Am J Med 1983;75(Suppl 5B):85–93.

79. DeFronzo RA. Lilly Lecture 1987. The triumvirate beta-cell, muscle, liver: a collusion responsible for NIDDM. Diabetes 1988;37:667–87.

80. Holman RR, Turner RC. Maintenance of basal plasma glucose and insulin concentrations in maturity-onset diabetes. Diabetes 1979;28:227–30.

81. Genuth S. Insulin use in NIDDM. Diabetes Care 1990; 13:1240–64.

82. University Group Diabetes Program. A study of the effects of hypoglycemic agents on vascular complications in patients with adult-onset diabetes. I. Design, methods, and baseline results. Diabetes 1970;19:747–83.

83. Sartor G, Scherstén B, Carlström S, et al. Ten-year follow-up of subjects with impaired glucose tolerance: prevention of diabetes by tolbutamide and diet regulation. Diabetes 1980;29:41–9.

84. Multi-Centre Study. UK prospective study of therapies of maturity-onset diabetes. I. Effect of diet, sulphonylurea, insulin or biguanide therapy on fasting plasma glucose and body weight over one year. Diabetologia 1983;24: 404–11.

85. Holman RR, Turner RC. A practical guide to basal and prandial insulin therapy. Diabetic Med 1985;2:45–53.

86. Garvey WT, Olefsky JM, Griffin J, et al. The effect of insulin treatment on insulin secretion and insulin action in Type II diabetes mellitus. Diabetes 1985;34:222–34.

87. Jennings AM, Lewis KS, Murdoch S, et al. Randomized trial comparing continuous subcutaneous insulin infusion and conventional insulin therapy in Type II diabetic patients poorly controlled with sulfonylureas. Diabetes Care 1991;14:738–44.

88. Blackshear PJ, Roussell AM, Cohen AM, Nathan DM. Basal-rate intravenous insulin infusion compared to conventional insulin treatment in patients with Type II diabetes: a prospective crossover trial. Diabetes Care 1989;12:455–63.

89. Turner RC, Holman RR. Insulin use in NIDDM: rationale based on pathophysiology of disease. Diabetes Care 1990;13:1011–20.

90. Riddle MC. Evening insulin strategy. Diabetes Care 1990;13:676–86.

91. Seigler DE, Olsson M, Skyler JS. Morning versus bedtime NPH insulin in Type II (non-insulin-dependent) diabetes mellitus [Abstract no. 504]. Diabetologia 1987;30:581A.

92. Lebovitz HE, Pasmantier R. Combination insulin-sulfonylurea therapy. Diabetes Care 1990;13:667–75.

93. Simonson DC, Delprato S, Castellino P, et al. Effect of glyburide on glycemic control, insulin requirement, and glucose metabolism in insulin-treated diabetic patients. Diabetes 1987;36:136–46.

94. Gutniak M, Karlander S-G, Efendić, S. Glyburide decreases insulin requirement, increases β-cell response to mixed meal, and does not affect insulin sensitivity: effects of short- and long-term combined treatment in secondary failure to sulfonylurea. Diabetes Care 1987;10:545–54.

95. Kabadi U, Birkenholz MR. Improved metabolic control in insulin-dependent diabetes mellitus with insulin and tolazamide. Arch Intern Med 1988;148:1745–9.

96. Burke BJ, Hartog M, Waterfield MR. Improved diabetic control in insulin-dependent diabetics treated with insulin and glibenclamide. Acta Endocrinol 1984;107:70–7.

97. Pugh JA, Wagner ML, Sawyer J, et al. Is combination sulfonylurea and insulin therapy useful in NIDDM patients? Metaanalysis. Diabetes Care 1992;15:953–9.

98. Genuth SM. Treating diabetes with both insulin and sulfonylurea drugs: what is the value? Clin Diabetes 1987;5:74–9.

99. Peters AL, Davidson MB. Insulin plus a sulfonylurea agent for treating Type 2 diabetes. Ann Intern Med 1991;115:45–53.

100. Task Force on Jet Injectors, Council on Youth. Position statement on jet injectors. Diabetes Care 1988; 11:600–1.

101. Vaag A, Handberg A, Lauritzen M, et al. Variation in absorption of NPH insulin due to intramuscular injection. Diabetes Care 1990;13:74–6.

102. Koivisto VA, Felig P. Effects of leg exercise on insulin absorption in diabetic patients. N Engl J Med 1978; 298:79–83.

103. American Diabetes Association. Position statement: insulin administration. Diabetes Care 1991;14(Suppl 2):30–3.

104. Koivisto VA, Vki-Järvinen H, DeFronzo RA. Physical training and insulin sensitivity. Diabetes Metab Rev 1986;1:445–81.

105. Worth R, Home PD, Johnston DG, et al. Intensive attention improves glycaemic control in insulin-dependent diabetes without further advantage from home blood glucose monitoring: results of a controlled trial. BMJ 1982; 285:1233–40.

106. Nathan DM, Singer DE, Hurxthal K, Goodson JD. The clinical information value of the glycosylated hemoglobin assay. N Engl J Med 1984;310:341–6.

107. Galloway JA, Root MA. Bergstrom R, et al. Clinical pharmacologic studies with human insulin (recombinant DNA). Diabetes Care 1982;5(Suppl 2):13–22.

108. Galloway JA, Spradlin CT, Jackson RL, et al. Mixtures of intermediate-acting insulin (NPH and lente) with regular insulin: an update. In: Skyler JS, ed. Insulin update: 1982. Amsterdam: Excerpta Medica, 1982:111–9.

109. Anderson JH, Campbell RK. Pharmacy update: mixing insulins in 1990. Diabetes Educ 1990;16:380–7.

110. Heine RJ, Bilo HJG, Fonk T, et al. Absorption kinetics and action profiles of mixtures of short- and intermediate-acting insulins. Diabetologia 1984;27:558–62.

111. Colagiuri S, Villalobos S. Assessing effect of mixing insulins by glucose-clamp technique in subjects with diabetes mellitus. Diabetes Care 1986;9:579–86.

112. Deckert T, Poulsen J, Larsen M. Prognosis of diabetics with diabetes onset before the age of thirty one. I. Survival, causes of death, and complications. Diabetologia 1978;14:363–70.

113. Gerich JE, Campbell PJ. Overview of counterregulation and its abnormalities in diabetes mellitus and other conditions. Diabetes Metab Rev 1988;4:93–111.

114. Cryer PE, Gerich JE. Glucose counterregulation, hypoglycemia, and intensive insulin therapy in diabetes mellitus. N Engl J Med 1985;313:232–41.

115. Herold KC, Polonsky KS, Cohen RM, et al. Variable deterioration in cortical function during insulin-induced hypoglycemia. Diabetes 1985;34:677–85.

116. Gerich J, Cryer P, Rizza R. Hormonal mechanisms in acute glucose counterregulation: the relative roles of glucagon, epinephrine, norepinephrine, growth hormone and cortisol. Metabolism 1980;29(Suppl 1):1164–75.

117. Gerich JE, Langlois M, Noacco C, et al. Lack of glucagon response to hypoglycemia in diabetes: evidence for an intrinsic pancreatic alpha cell defect. Science 1973; 182:171–3.

118. DeFronzo R, Hendler R, Christensen N. Stimulation of counterregulatory hormonal responses in diabetic man by a fall in glucose concentration. Diabetes 1980;29:125–31.

119. Amiel SA, Tamborlane WV, Saccà L, Sherwin RS. Hypoglycemia and glucose counterregulation in normal and insulin-dependent diabetic subjects. Diabetes Metab Rev 1988;4:71–89.

120. Somogyi M. Insulin as a cause of extreme hyperglycemia and instability. Bull St Louis Med Soc 1938;32:498–500.

121. Bolli GB, Gottesman IS, Campbell PJ, et al. Glucose counterregulation and waning of insulin in the Somogyi phenomenon (posthypoglycemic hyperglycemia). N Engl J Med 1984;311:1214–9.

122. De Feo P, Perriello G, Bolli GB. Somogyi and dawn phenomena: mechanisms. Diabetes Metab Rev 1988;4:31–49.

123. Mintz DH, Finster JL, Taylor AL, Fefer A. Hormonal genesis of glucose intolerance following hypoglycemia. Am J Med 1968;45:187.

124. Oakley NW, Jacobs HS, Turner RC, et al. The effect of hypoglycaemia on oral glucose tolerance in normal subjects and patients with pituitary and adrenal disorders. Clin Sci 1970;39:663–74.

125. Popp DA, Shah SD, Cryer PE. Role of epinephrine-mediated β-adrenergic mechanisms in hypoglycemic glucose counterregulation and posthypoglycemic hyperglycemia in insulin-dependent diabetes mellitus. J Clin Invest 1982;69:315–26.

126. Gale EAM, Kurtz AB, Tattersall RB. In search of the Somogyi effect. Lancet 1980;2:279–82.

127. Schmidt M, Hadji-Georgopoulos A, Rendell M, et al. Fasting hyperglycemia and associated free insulin and cortisol changes in "Somogyi-like" patients. Diabetes Care 1979;2:457–64.

128. Gale EAM, Pramming S, Lauritzen T, Binder C. Insulin escape curves—and the myth of rebound hyperglycemia [Abstract no. 102]. Diabetologia 1982;23:168.

129. Schmidt MI, Hadji-Georgopoulos A, Rendell M, et al. The dawn phenomenon, an early morning glucose rise: implications for diabetic intraday blood glucose variation. Diabetes Care 1981;4:579–85.

130. Campbell PJ, Bolli GB, Cryer PE, Gerich JE. Pathogenesis of the dawn phenomenon in patients with insulin-dependent diabetes mellitus: accelerated glucose production and impaired glucose utilization due to nocturnal surges in growth hormone secretion. N Engl J Med 1985;312:1473–9.

131. Brodows RG, Williams C, Amatruda JM. Treatment of insulin reactions in diabetics. JAMA 1984;252:3378–81.

132. Gill GV, Walford S, Alberti KGMM. Brittle diabetes: present concepts. Diabetologia 1985;28:579–89.

133. Schade DS. Brittle diabetes: strategies, diagnosis, and treatment. Diabetes Metab Rev 1988;4:371–90.

134. Renie A, Hamilton RG, Adkinson NF, Rendell MS Jr. Hyperlabile diabetes accompanied by insulin resistance. Clin Chem 1981;27:1463–4.

135. Paulsen EP, Courtney JW III, Duckworth WC. Insulin resistance caused by massive degradation of subcutaneous insulin. Diabetes 1979;28:640–5.

136. Schade DS, Duckworth WC. In search of the subcutaneous-insulin-resistance syndrome. N Engl J Med 1986;315:147–53.

137. Flier JS. Syndromes of insulin resistance. In: Becker KL, ed. Principles and practices of endocrinology and metabolism. Philadelphia: Lippincott, 1990:1118–27.

138. Schade DS, Drumm DA, Eaton RP, Sterling WA. Factitious brittle diabetes mellitus. Am J Med 1985;78:777–83.

139. Stearns S. Self-destructive behavior in young patients with diabetes mellitus. Diabetes 1959;8:379–82.

140. Wing RR, Nowalk MP, Marcus MD, et al. Subclinical eating disorders and glycemic control in adolescents with Type I diabetes. Diabetes Care 1986;9:162–7.

141. Rodin GM, Johnson LE, Garfinkel PE, et al. Eating disorders in female adolescents with insulin dependent diabetes mellitus. Int J Psychiatry Med 1986–87;16:49–57.

142. Nathan DM. Successful treatment of extremely brittle, insulin-dependent diabetes with a novel subcutaneous insulin pump regimen. Diabetes Care 1982;5:105–10.

143. Saudek C, Boulter PR, Knopp RH, Arky RA. Sodium retention accompanying insulin treatment of diabetes mellitus. Diabetes 1974;23:240–6.

144. Bleach NR, Dunn PJ, Khalafalla ME, McConkey B. Insulin oedema. BMJ 1979;2:177–8.

145. Sheehan JP, Sisam DA, Schumacher OP. Insulin-induced cardiac failure. Am J Med 1985;79:147–8.

146. Rabkin R, Ryan MP, Duckworth WC. The renal metabolism of insulin. Diabetologia 1984;27:351–3.

147. O'Hare JA, Ferriss JB, Twomey B, O'Sullivan DJ. Poor metabolic control, hypertension and microangiopathy independently increase the transcapillary escape rate of albumin in diabetes. Diabetologia 1983;25:260–3.

148. Reeves WG, Allen BR, Tattersall RB. Insulin-induced lipoatrophy: evidence for an immune pathogenesis. BMJ 1980;280:1500–3.

149. Renold AE, Marble A, Fawcett DW. Action of insulin on deposition of glycogen and storage of fat in adipose tissue. Endocrinology 1950;46:55–66.

150. Berson SA, Yalow RS. Studies with insulin-binding antibody. Diabetes 1957;6:402–7.

151. Palmer JP, Asplin CM, Clemons P, et al. Insulin antibodies in insulin-dependent diabetics before insulin treatment. Science 1983;222:1337–9.

152. Dahl-Jørgensen K, Torjesen P, Hanssen KF, et al. Increase in insulin antibodies during continuous subcutaneous insulin infusion and multiple-injection therapy in contrast to conventional treatment. Diabetes 1987;36:1–5.

153. Bolli GB, Dimitriadis GD, Pehling GB, et al. Abnormal glucose counterregulation after subcutaneous insulin in insulin-dependent diabetes mellitus. N Engl J Med 1984;310:1706–11.

154. Ludvigsson J. Insulin antibodies in diabetic children treated with monocomponent porcine insulin from the onset: relationship to B-cell function and partial remission. Diabetologia 1984;26:138–41.

155. Francis AJ, Hanning I, Alberti KGMM. The influence of insulin antibody levels on the plasma profiles and action of subcutaneously injected human and bovine short-acting insulins. Diabetologia 1985;28:330–4.

156. Frikke MJ, Gingerich RL, Stranahan PD, et al. Distribution of injected insulin and insulin-antibody complexes in normal and insulin-immunized animals. Diabetologia 1974;10:345–51.

157. Dixon K, Exon PD, Hughes H. Insulin antibodies in aetiology of labile diabetes. Lancet 1972;1:343–51.

158. Wehner H, Huber H, Kronenberg KH. The glomerular basement membrane of the rabbit kidney on long-term treatment with heterologous insulin preparations of different purity. Diabetologia 1973;9:255–63.

159. Wehner H. The influence of insulin and insulin antibodies on the glomerular structure. Acta Endocrinol 1976; 83(Suppl 205):241–50.

160. Andersen OO. Anti-insulin-antibodies and late diabetic complications. Acta Endocrinol 1976;83:329–40.

161. Uchman B, Bang NU, Rathbun MJ, et al. Effect of insulin immune complexes on human blood monocyte and endothelial cell procoagulant activity. J Lab Clin Med 1988;112:652–9.

162. Menon RK, Cohen RM, Sperling MA, et al. Transplacental passage of insulin in pregnant women with insulin-dependent diabetes mellitus: its role in fetal macrosomia. N Engl J Med 1990;323:309–15.

163. Schwartz R. Hyperinsulinema and macrosomia. N Engl J Med 1990;323:340–2.

164. Arkins JA, Engbring NH, Lennon EJ. The incidence of skin reactivity to insulin in diabetic patients. J Allergy 1962; 33:69–72.

165. Wright AD, Walsh CH, Fitzgerald MG, Malins JM. Very pure porcine insulin in clinical practice. BMJ 1979; 1:25–7.

166. Chance RE. Amino acid sequences of proinsulins and intermediates. Diabetes 1972;21(Suppl 2):461–7.

167. deShazo RD, Boehm TM, Kumar D, et al. Dermal hypersensitivity reactions to insulin: correlations of three patterns to their histopathology. J Allergy Clin Immunol 1982;69:229–37.

168. Granić M, Renar IP, Metelkož, Škrabalo Z. Insulin allergy [Letter]. Diabetes Care 1986;9:99–100.

169. Patterson R, Lucena G, Metz R, Roberts M. Reaginic antibody against insulin: demonstration of antigenic distinction between native and extracted insulin. J Immunol 1969;103:1061–71.

170. Grammer LC, Chen PY, Patterson R. Evaluation and management of insulin allergy. J Allergy Clin Immunol 1983;71:250–4.

171. Cockel R, Mann S. Insulin allergy treated by low-dosage hydrocortisone. BMJ 1967;3:722.

172. Kahn CR. Insulin resistance, insulin insensitivity, and insulin unresponsiveness: a necessary distinction. Metabolism 1978;27:1893–902.

173. Shipp JC, Cunningham RW, Russell RO, Marble A. Insulin resistance: clinical features, natural course and effects of adrenal steroid treatment. Medicine (Baltimore) 1965; 44:165–86.

174. Field JB. Chronic insulin resistance. Acta Diabetol Lat 1970;7:220–42.

175. Kolterman OG, Insel J, Saekow M, Olefsky JM. Mechanisms of insulin resistance in human obesity: evidence for receptor and postreceptor defects. J Clin Invest 1980; 65:1272–4.

176. Evans DJ, Murray R, Kissebah AH. Relationship between skeletal muscle insulin resistance, insulin-mediated glucose disposal, and insulin binding: effects of obesity and body fat topography. J Clin Invest 1984;74:1515–25.

177. Peiris AN, Struve MS, Mueller RA, et al. Glucose metabolism in obesity: influence of body fat distribution. J Clin Endocrinol Metab 1988;67:760–7.

178. Groop L, Widén E, Franssila-Kallunki A, et al. Different effects of insulin and oral antidiabetic agents on glucose and energy metabolism in Type 2 (non-insulin-dependent) diabetes mellitus. Diabetologia 1989;32:599–605.

179. Torbay N, Bracco E, Geliebter A, et al. Insulin increases body fat despite control of food intake and physical activity. Am J Physiol 1985;258:R2120–4.

180. Reaven GM. Beneficial effect of moderate weight loss in older patients with non-insulin-dependent diabetes mellitus poorly controlled with insulin. J Am Geriatr Soc 1985;33:93–5.

181. Wing RR, Koeske R, Epstein LH, et al. Long-term effects of modest weight loss in Type II diabetic patients. Arch Intern Med 1987;147:1749–53.

182. Genuth S. Supplemented fasting in the treatment of obesity and diabetes. Am J Clin Nutr 1979;32:2579–86.

183. Patterson R, Mellies CJ, Roberts M. Immunologic reactions against insulin. II. IgE anti-insulin, insulin allergy and combined IgE and IgG immunologic insulin resistance. J Immunol 1973;110:1135–45.

184. Davidson JK, DeBra DW. Immunologic insulin resistance. Diabetes 1978;27:307–18.

185. Oakley WG, Jones VE, Cunliffe AC. Insulin resistance. BMJ 1967;2:134–8.

186. The DCCT Research Group. Presented at the 53rd Annual Meeting of the American Diabetes Association, Las Vegas, Nevada, June 13, 1993.

187. The DCCT Research Group. N Engl J Med, *in press*.

Chapter 28

IATROGENIC HYPOGLYCEMIA

BARBARA WIDOM
DONALD C. SIMONSON

Diabetes and its treatment are the primary causes of episodes of hypoglycemia encountered clinically. Although there has been intense interest in the pathophysiology of iatrogenic hypoglycemia and glucose counterregulation during the past decade, it should be recognized that the signs, symptoms, and consequences of insulin-induced hypoglycemia were clearly described by Banting et al. within a year of the first therapeutic use of insulin.[1] Although our understanding of diabetes and its treatment has advanced remarkably during the twentieth century, hypoglycemia remains the most common and serious iatrogenic cause of morbidity in patients with diabetes.

DEFINITIONS OF HYPOGLYCEMIA

Traditionally, hypoglycemia has been defined operationally by Whipple's triad, that is, as a decrease in the plasma glucose concentration to a level sufficient to produce symptoms, with attenuation of symptoms upon restoration of a normal glucose concentration.[2,3] Unfortunately, this definition does not specify an absolute glucose level as representing "hypoglycemia." Such specification is rendered difficult by the wide differences in glucose levels required to stimulate hypoglycemic symptoms, which can differ depending on the age and sex of the patient, the presence of concomitant diseases, the duration and frequency of the hypoglycemic stimulus, and many other factors.

To circumvent the problems associated with the use of an operational definition of hypoglycemia, many investigators have used fixed (and somewhat arbitrary) biochemical criteria. Depending on the question under study, one may define hypoglycemia as a plasma glucose level that is 1) below the normal range for the laboratory (<65 to 70 mg/dL), 2) associated with the first detectable rise in counterregulatory hormones (<60 to 65 mg/dL), 3) accompanied by classic adrenergic symptoms (<50 to 60 mg/dL), or 4) associated with clinically meaningful impairment of cognitive function (<50 mg/dL). Thus, it is readily apparent that any study of hypoglycemia must carefully define the criteria (in operational or biochemical terms), the measurement technique, and the end point under investigation.

Patients with insulin-dependent diabetes mellitus (IDDM) are particularly susceptible to the adverse effects of hypoglycemia. Such patients often lack the classic symptoms of hypoglycemia as a result of autonomic dysfunction, intensive glucose control, or impaired sensitivity to adrenergic stimuli. In addition, defects in the production and action of key counterregulatory hormones may increase the time required to restore euglycemia. Thus, the group of patients for whom adequate glucose counterregulatory mechanisms are most critical are the same individuals who most frequently exhibit defects in this important homeostatic physiologic system.

EPIDEMIOLOGY

Although published estimates of rates of mild hypoglycemic episodes in patients with IDDM range from 40 to 70%,[4-9] it is likely that with careful questioning almost all patients will recall having experienced some symptom of hypoglycemia during the course of a year. Severe hypoglycemia (an episode for which the patient requires assistance from another person or that results in seizure or coma) is reported to occur at rates ranging from 4% to as high as 26% per patient-year.[4-9] In a survey of children with IDDM,[10] 16% experienced severe hypoglycemia with seizure or coma over a 1-year period. Severe recurrent hypoglycemia has been reported in approximately 3% of diabetic patients,[8] and hypoglycemia is thought to be the primary cause or a contributory cause of death in up to 4% of patients with diabetes.[11,12]

In a survey of 125 emergency room visits in which the patient's measured glucose level was less than 60 mg/dL,[13] 68 of the patients had diabetes. Similarly, a review of hospitalized patients[14] revealed that 45% of those whose measured glucose level was less than 50 mg/dL had diabetes mellitus, often with coexisting illnesses. Thus, as many as half of all cases of well-documented hypoglycemia in the hospital setting are in patients with diabetes and most likely have an iatrogenic cause.

Strict glycemic control in IDDM is associated with an increase in the frequency and severity of hypoglycemia. One study in which 24-hour glucose profiles were obtained for patients receiving insulin-pump therapy revealed that a measured glucose level of less than 50 mg/dL occurred in 9 of 10 subjects.[15] Results from the Diabetes Control and Complications Trial,[16,17] in which patients were randomized to receive conventional insulin therapy or intensified treatment via multiple injections or continuous insulin infusion, noted a two- to threefold increase in the incidence of severe hypoglycemia in the intensively treated group.

Neither multiple daily injections nor insulin-pump therapy per se appear to be associated with an increased risk of hypoglycemia. Rather it appears that the strict glycemic control generally sought with such regimens leaves little margin for error between euglycemia and hypoglycemia. In some patients with recurrent severe hypoglycemia, the initiation of insulin-pump therapy may actually reduce the frequency of hypoglycemic episodes.[8,18]

Hypoglycemia is also observed in patients with non-insulin-dependent diabetes (NIDDM). Postprandial hypoglycemia is found occasionally in patients with NIDDM before diagnosis or treatment. Estimates of rates of hypoglycemia in patients receiving sulfonylurea treatment vary widely but are reported to be as high as 20% over a 6-month treatment period.[19] Because of the older age of this patient population, the consequences of hypoglycemia can be severe. Although one study estimates that up to 10% of episodes of hypoglycemia related to sulfonylurea therapy are fatal, other studies report a rate closer to 4%.[20,21] The relatively high mortality rate may in part be due to a lack of adequate education about the symptoms and treatment of hypoglycemia among older and non-insulin-using patients.[22]

NORMAL GLUCOSE REGULATION

Under normal conditions, the central nervous system is dependent on glucose as its primary metabolic fuel. Since the brain is unable to synthesize or store significant amounts of glucose, a continuous supply from the systemic circulation is critical. Therefore, the body has a complex homeostatic system designed to maintain euglycemia.

In a healthy individual, after an overnight fast glucose is delivered into the circulation at a rate of 2.0 to 2.2 mg/kg body weight per minute.[23] Glucose is delivered primarily from the liver, with 75% of hepatic production of glucose from glycogenolysis and 25% from gluconeogenesis.[24] In the postabsorptive state, lactate, glycerol, and the gluconeogenic amino acids (particularly alanine) serve as the major substrates for de novo synthesis of glucose. Fifty to sixty percent of the glucose produced (approximately 1 mg/kg body weight per minute) is used by the brain, 20% is taken up by other insulin-insensitive tissues (intestines, renal medulla), and 20% is used by insulin-sensitive tissues such as muscle and adipose tissue.[23,25]

With a more prolonged fast, liver glycogen stores are depleted. Thus, gluconeogenesis becomes the primary process sustaining glucose production. Renal gluconeogenesis substantially supplements hepatic gluconeogenesis and may be responsible for as much as 45% of the body's total glucose production[26,27] during prolonged fasting. With an extended period of starvation, the brain begins to use ketone bodies as an alternate metabolic substrate, thus diminishing its absolute requirement for glucose. This utilization of ketone bodies may explain the substantial reduction in plasma glucose levels observed in healthy individuals following a 72-hour fast (mean nadir plasma glucose level 66 ± 3 mg/dL in men and 48 ± 3 mg/dL in women[28]) without the appearance of frankly hypoglycemic symptoms.

During the transition from the fasting (or postabsorptive) state to the postprandial state, the plasma glucose concentration increases as a result of absorption of the ingested carbohydrate. Subsequently, the plasma glucose concentration often falls to levels that are slightly lower than baseline values as a result of suppression of endogenous glucose production and increased glucose utilization by peripheral tissues. Finally, the glucose concentration returns to the baseline value following the resumption of endogenous glucose production.[29]

Changes in levels of insulin and glucagon are the most important hormonal factors in the control of this "normoglycemic counterregulation."[23] Insulin is secreted upon nutrient ingestion and inhibits hepatic glycogenolysis and gluconeogenesis, thus transforming the liver into an organ of net glucose uptake and storage. In addition, insulin stimulates glucose uptake, glycolysis, glucose oxidation, lipid synthesis, and glycogen formation by other insulin-sensitive tissues. The concentration of insulin required to stimulate glucose uptake in peripheral tissues is generally much greater than that required to inhibit hepatic glucose production.[30]

As the glucose level begins to decline, insulin secretion is suppressed and glucagon release is stimulated. Glucagon opposes the action of insulin on the liver, and hepatic production of glucose resumes. Deficiency of glucagon results in a 30% lower plasma glucose level following glucose ingestion, but the glucose level eventually does stabilize and begin to rise.[31] Levels of epinephrine also may rise 3 to 5 hours after ingestion of glucose[32];

however, epinephrine deficiency alone does not impair the restoration and maintenance of euglycemia.[31]

HYPOGLYCEMIC GLUCOSE COUNTERREGULATION

The mechanisms of recovery from insulin-induced hypoglycemia have been thoroughly studied during the intravenous administration of insulin by bolus or continuous infusion. After intravenous injection of crystalline insulin, the plasma glucose concentration in humans typically reaches a nadir at 25 to 30 minutes and returns to near basal levels at 120 minutes. Levels of counterregulatory hormones increase after the induction of hypoglycemia, with levels of epinephrine rising significantly approximately 20 minutes after insulin administration; of norepinephrine, at 25 minutes; of cortisol and glucagon, at approximately 30 minutes; and of growth hormone, at 40 minutes[33] (Fig. 28–1).

As a consequence of insulin administration, peripheral glucose utilization (predominantly by muscle) increases and hepatic glucose production declines. During recovery, glucose production increases and insulin-stimulated glucose uptake declines towards baseline levels.[33] This increase in glucose production is initially due to activation of glycogenolysis, but this wanes rapidly. Gluconeogenesis is activated more slowly but subsequently becomes the primary process that sustains glucose production.[34,35] During the recovery from short-term hypoglycemia, the primary means of recovery is an increase in the rate of glucose production, whereas with prolonged hypoglycemia, both an increase in glucose production and a decrease in glucose utilization are important.[36]

Since the onset of glucose counterregulation and the accompanying increase in the rate of glucose production can occur while insulin concentrations are elevated, it is clear that a waning of insulin levels is not the sole mechanism responsible for recovery from insulin-induced hypoglycemia.[37] Although endogenous insulin secretion is not completely suppressed until the arterial glucose concentration decreases to 50 mg/dL,[38] glucose counterregulation typically begins when glucose levels are at 60 to 65 mg/dL.

The rate of decline of plasma glucose levels does not appear to influence the magnitude of the counterregulatory hormone response to hypoglycemia.[36,39] In nondiabetic individuals a rapid drop from high to normal glucose levels does not stimulate the release of counterregulatory hormones.[40] The duration of hypoglycemia, however, may be an important determinant of levels of counterregulatory hormones,[41] with prolonged hypoglycemia producing a waning in the secretion of counterregulatory hormones and the intensity of symptoms.[38,42] Age may also be an important determinant of the counterregulatory hormone response. The epinephrine (but not the cortisol or growth hormone) response to hypoglycemia is approximately twofold greater in children than in adults.[43]

The relative importance of the individual counterregulatory hormones in the maintenance of glucose homeostasis has been studied by producing isolated pharmacologic deficiencies of each of the hormones and examining recovery from insulin-induced hypoglycemia. When α-adrenergic blockade with phentolamine or β-adrenergic blockade with propranolol is used, either alone or in combination, the alteration in the kinetic response to insulin-induced hypoglycemia is minimal.[44–46] From these studies, it has been concluded that adrenergic mechanisms do not normally play a critical role in glucose counterregulation (Fig. 28–2).

Subsequent studies using somatostatin to inhibit secretion of glucagon and growth hormone in nondiabetic subjects showed potentiation of insulin-induced hypoglycemia and attenuation of the recovery to euglycemia.[45–47] Replacement of glucagon, but not of growth hormone, restored the response to normal, thus establishing a primary role for glucagon in glucose counterregulation. With the inhibition of glucagon secretion, glucose recovery is impaired further during adrenergic blockade.[45,46] Under extreme circumstances, e.g., in adrenalectomized subjects in whom epinephrine is totally absent,

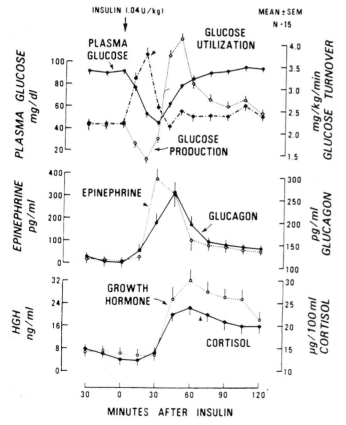

Fig. 28–1. Changes in plasma glucose kinetics and in concentrations of counterregulatory hormones during induction and reversal of short-term insulin-induced hypoglycemia in normal volunteers. HGH = human growth hormone. Reprinted with permission from reference 23 (Gerich JE, Campbell PJ. Overview of counterregulation and its abnormalities in diabetes mellitus and other conditions. Diabetes Metab Rev 1988;4:93–111; copyright © of John Wiley and Sons, Ltd.).

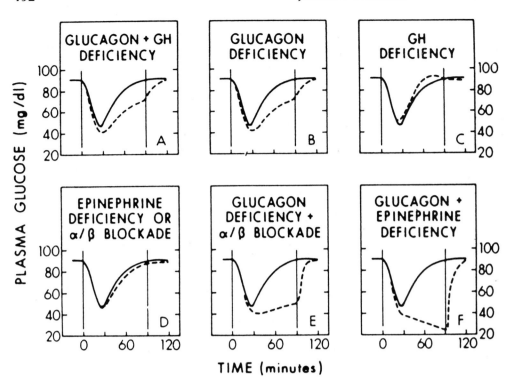

Fig. 28—2. Plasma glucose levels during insulin-induced hypoglycemia in normal subjects during control studies (solid lines) and as modified (dashed lines) by somatostatin infusion (A); somatostatin plus growth hormone infusion (B); somatostatin plus glucagon infusion (C); phentolamine plus propranolol infusion or studies in bilaterally adrenalectomized patients (D); somatostatin plus phentolamine and propranolol infusion (E); and somatostatin infusion in bilaterally adrenalectomized patients (F). Reprinted with permission from reference 44 (Cryer PE. Glucose counterregulation in man. Diabetes 1981; 30:261—4; copyright © of the American Diabetes Association).

euglycemia is not restored.[47] Thus, adrenergic mechanisms become critical for glucose recovery when glucagon secretion is impaired (Fig. 28—2). Epinephrine may also play a more important role during prolonged hypoglycemia, when the increase in the level of epinephrine outlasts that of glucagon,[38] and during severe hypoglycemia, when adrenergic blockade delays glucose recovery even when glucagon secretion is intact.[48,49]

Although studies of acute insulin-induced hypoglycemia have failed to demonstrate an important role for growth hormone or cortisol,[50] during prolonged insulin infusion, subjects with deficiencies of growth hormone or cortisol exhibit enhanced sensitivity to insulin and develop more profound hypoglycemia than control subjects.[51] Thus, these hormones may play an important permissive role during sustained hypoglycemia.

Glucagon exerts its hyperglycemic effect by stimulating hepatic glucose production. Glucagon transiently increases glycogenolysis but has a sustained stimulatory effect on gluconeogenesis via stimulation of hepatic gluconeogenic pathways and increased extraction of gluconeogenic precursors such as alanine.[34] Epinephrine acts in a variety of ways to restore euglycemia. First, it transiently increases hepatic production of glucose by stimulating glycogenolysis and gluconeogenesis via β-adrenergic mechanisms.[32,52] Second, epinephrine results in a sustained inhibition of glucose disposal in peripheral and splanchnic tissues.[32,53] Third, an important indirect hyperglycemic action of epinephrine is α-adrenergic-mediated inhibition of insulin secretion.[32] Fourth, epinephrine may increase glucagon secretion,

further contributing in an indirect manner to the restoration of euglycemia.[32] Finally, there appears to be a synergistic interaction of the counterregulatory hormones whereby infusion of glucagon and epinephrine in combination is more effective at reversing the hypoglycemic actions of insulin than is infusion of either hormone alone.[54]

Infusion of cortisol alone has only a minimal effect on hepatic glucose production. However, the addition of cortisol to epinephrine or glucagon markedly increases the glycemic response by prolonging the stimulatory effect on hepatic gluconeogenesis.[55] Thus, glucocorticoids generally are considered to have a permissive effect on the gluconeogenic actions of epinephrine and glucagon. Moreover, glucocorticoids also act peripherally to depress the oxidation of glucose by muscle and adipose tissue, thereby reducing insulin-mediated uptake of glucose. Although administration of growth hormone results in an initial transient decrease in plasma glucose levels (by enhancing utilization of glucose through its insulin-like effect), growth hormone plays an important role in counterregulation during prolonged hypoglycemia by increasing glucose production and limiting the transport of glucose into cells.[52,56,57]

The brain appears to play an important role in glucose recovery during insulin-induced hypoglycemia. This role was established through a canine model in which peripheral hypoglycemia was produced by insulin administration but brain hypoglycemia was prevented by the infusion of glucose into the carotid and vertebral arteries. With the maintenance of brain euglycemia, the glucagon level failed to increase, the normal increase in epinephrine and cortisol was blunted, and the production of glucose was attenuated by 75%.[58]

The hypothalamic region has traditionally been considered the counterregulatory center. However, a number of recent studies have demonstrated that the forebrain (including the hypothalamus) is not essential for glucose regulation. When the cerebral aqueduct is blocked in rats, infusion of the nonmetabolized glucose analogue 5-thioglucose into the fourth ventricle (but not infusion into the lateral ventricles) results in hyperglycemia, indicating that the receptors that mediate the hyperglycemic response to glucose deprivation are located caudal to the forebrain.[59] Likewise, when moderate or severe hypoglycemia is induced in dogs but forebrain euglycemia is maintained by infusion of glucose into the carotid artery, the counterregulatory hormone response is not altered.[60,61]

Hepatic autoregulation also may play an important role in the restoration and maintenance of euglycemia. Hepatic autoregulation is the term used to describe the process by which the liver can alter its output of glucose in response to changes in the circulating glucose level independent of neuronal or hormonal influences.[62] This process has been observed both in vivo and in vitro. The glucose output from the isolated perfused liver is increased when the glucose concentration in the perfusate is reduced.[63,64] Likewise, studies in dogs indicate that hypoglycemia stimulates hepatic glucose production by mechanisms in addition to hormone secretion.[34] The enzymatic basis for hepatic autoregulation appears to be modulation of hepatic glycogen synthetase and phosphorylase activities by the ambient glucose concentration. Studies in humans, however, have defined a role for hepatic autoregulation in the recovery from severe (30 mg/dL) but not from moderate (50 mg/dL) hypoglycemia.[62,65]

HYPOGLYCEMIC GLUCOSE COUNTERREGULATION IN DIABETES MELLITUS

Numerous studies have demonstrated delayed recovery from insulin-induced hypoglycemia in patients with IDDM.[49,66–68] This delayed restoration of normoglycemia in diabetes generally is due to a blunting or absence of the normal increase in hepatic glucose production during hypoglycemia.[66,67]

The most consistent abnormality in counterregulation in IDDM is an impairment or absence of the glucagon response to hypoglycemia.[49,66–70] This defect in glucagon secretion occurs in virtually all patients (children and adults) after 5 years of IDDM[71,72] but not in patients with newly diagnosed IDDM (less then 1 month).[71] The secretory defect is specific to the hypoglycemic stimulus, as the glucagon response to amino acid infusion or a protein meal may be exaggerated.[70,73] A number of hypotheses have been set forth to explain the loss of the glucagon response to hypoglycemia, including the presence of a defect in the "glucose sensor" of the α-cell,[74,75] a dependence on residual β-cell function acting in a paracrine fashion to regulate glucagon secretion,[76] or an

effect of endogenous prostaglandins.[77] However, no definitive cause has been established.

Normally, epinephrine compensates for the defective glucagon secretory response to hypoglycemia in patients with IDDM. When β-adrenergic blockade is established in these patients, glucose recovery is markedly impaired.[78] The incidence of defective epinephrine response to hypoglycemia in patients with long-standing IDDM is as high as 40%.[79,80] Impaired epinephrine secretion is a frequent finding in patients with autonomic neuropathy[71,81] but also is seen in patients without overt evidence of autonomic dysfunction.[66,67,80] As is the case with glucagon, the defective epinephrine response to hypoglycemia appears to be stimulus-specific, since the epinephrine response to exercise is normal or exaggerated.[82] The defects in glucagon and epinephrine responses to hypoglycemia are not restored by improved metabolic control.[83–85]

Pancreatic polypeptide also is secreted in response to hypoglycemia, and its release is mediated by the vagus nerve.[86] A reduction in the pancreatic polypeptide response to hypoglycemia is observed in some diabetic patients as well as in subjects with nondiabetic autonomic neuropathy.[87,88] In diabetic patients, a reduced epinephrine response to hypoglycemia is associated with a reduced pancreatic polypeptide response.[86,89] It has been suggested that an impaired pancreatic polypeptide response to hypoglycemia may be an earlier manifestation of diabetic autonomic neuropathy than abnormalities of the standard cardiovascular reflexes[89] and that the defective epinephrine response is due to autonomic neuropathy that is not clinically evident.

Other investigators have postulated that autoimmune adrenal disease may contribute to the defective epinephrine response to hypoglycemia, although this would not explain the stimulus specificity of the defect. One study in children with IDDM demonstrated a significant negative correlation between the titer of anti-adrenal medullary antibodies and the epinephrine response to insulin-induced hypoglycemia.[18]

The presence of antibodies to insulin may also delay recovery from hypoglycemia by prolonging the circulating half-life of injected insulin.[71] The recovery from hypoglycemia induced by a subcutaneous injection of insulin was found to be most impaired in patients with higher levels of free insulin after the induction of hypoglycemia, which was positively correlated with binding of antibody to insulin.[79] Glucagon replacement normalized recovery from insulin-induced hypoglycemia in a group of patients with IDDM and no antibodies to insulin but failed to normalize recovery in patients with significant titers of antibodies to insulin.[71]

Patients with NIDDM may also manifest defects in secretion of counterregulatory hormones, although this has been less thoroughly investigated in patients with NIDDM than in patients with IDDM. In patients with NIDDM, the glucagon response to hypoglycemia may be reduced but is seldom absent.[90] Lack of a glucagon response to hypoglycemia has been seen in patients with NIDDM complicated by autonomic neuropathy.[91] One study, in which insulin was administered subcutaneously to 13 non-obese patients with NIDDM and to control subjects, found similar nadir glucose levels in the two groups but a slower rate of recovery in the patients with NIDDM as a result of persistent suppression of glucose production. Overall, the plasma cortisol and growth hormone responses, as well as the glucagon response, were lower in the patients with NIDDM.[90] However, a second study[92] in patients with NIDDM controlled by oral hypoglycemic agents failed to find a significant difference in glucose recovery or counterregulatory hormone secretion as compared with matched controls.

Despite multiple defects in counterregulatory hormone production, patients with diabetes are capable of recovering spontaneously from most episodes of insulin-induced hypoglycemia. This ability may be related to an enhanced hyperglycemic response to epinephrine, which can be attributed in part to the inability of insulin levels to increase once the glucose level rises above basal levels.[93,94] In addition, patients with autonomic neuropathy exhibit a further enhancement in the hyperglycemic response to epinephrine,[95] possibly as a result of up-regulation of adrenergic receptors.

SYMPTOMS OF HYPOGLYCEMIA

The symptoms of hypoglycemia are commonly divided into "autonomic" (also called "adrenergic" or "neurogenic") and "neuroglycopenic" symptoms (Table 28–1). In healthy individuals, the glucose level at which a significant change in symptomatology is perceived appears to be significantly below the level required to stimulate the onset of counterregulatory hormone secretion[96] (Fig. 28–3). Autonomic symptoms are those resulting from an increase in activity of the autonomic nervous system and/or an increase in circulating epinephrine level. These include symptoms such as tremor and palpitations, which are primarily under adrenergic control, and sweating, which is regulated by the cholinergic system. Neuroglycopenic symptoms, such as confusion, blurred vision, and—under conditions of marked hypoglycemia—seizures and coma, result from a decrease in the delivery of glucose to the central nervous system. An unusual manifestation of hypoglycemia is hemiplegia. This may occur in patients with no other symptoms of hypoglycemia, can occur in young as well as older individuals, and is often confused with a cerebrovascular accident.[97]

Several unique responses to hypoglycemia are observed in patients with diabetes. For example, pallor is almost invariably found in hypoglycemic diabetic patients, whereas cutaneous hyperemia caused by vasodilation and increased cutaneous blood flow is seen in nondiabetic patients.[98] Patients with autonomic neuropathy may develop profound postural hypotension in association with hypoglycemia,[99] a condition that may be due to defective sympathetic outflow to the muscle bed.[100] Such an increase in sympathetic outflow normally counteracts the vasodilation and depletion in intravascular volume that occurs with insulin administration.[100,101] In these patients, the symptoms of hypotension may be difficult to distinguish from those of hypoglycemia.

The central nervous system, because of its inability to store significant amounts of glucose, requires a continuous glucose supply. Glucose transport across the blood-brain barrier is half-maximally saturated at a normal glucose concentration and becomes rate-limiting for glucose utilization as the plasma glucose level drops below the normal fasting level.[102] Thus, the utilization of glucose by the brain decreases linearly as the plasma concentration of glucose falls,[103] and when the plasma glucose level is 20 to 40 mg/dL, the metabolic rate of glucose in the brain is decreased to approximately one-half the normal rate.[104] Physiologic insulin concentrations do not appear to have an effect on cerebral glucose extraction in vivo.[105] However, marked hyperinsulinemia (1500 µU/mL) was found to increase glucose flux across the blood-brain barrier in one study.[106]

A number of investigators have examined the cognitive changes associated with insulin-induced hypoglycemia. Studies in healthy nondiabetic individuals have demonstrated alterations in fine motor skills and information processing at a glucose level of 61 mg/dL[107] and a decrease in reaction time at a glucose level of 45 mg/dL,[108] that persisted for as long as 40 minutes after recovery of normal glucose levels. Studies in subjects with IDDM have demonstrated 1) an increase in visual reaction time and a decline in simple mathematical skills but no change in short-term memory at a glucose level of 60 mg/dL,[109] 2) a decrease in verbal skills at a glucose level of 55 mg/dL,[110] and 3) a decrease in visual tracking, concentration, and planning ability at a glucose level of

Table 28–1. Symptoms of Hypoglycemia

Neuroglycopenic symptoms
Global
Difficulty thinking
Confusion
Poor coordination
Headache*
Hunger*
Weakness*
Dizziness
Faintness
Drowsiness
Irritability
Nightmares
Abnormal or belligerent behavior
Somnolence
Seizures
Coma
Focal
Blurred or double vision
Slurred speech
Paresthesias*
Tinnitus
Hemiplegia
Autonomic (adrenergic or neurogenic) symptoms
Tremor
Nervousness
Palpitations
Diaphoresis
Anxiety or apprehension
Pallor

*These symptoms are sometimes classified as autonomic.

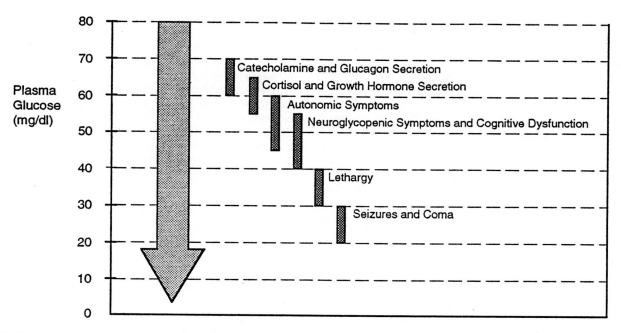

Fig. 28–3. Relationships among signs, symptoms, and counterregulatory hormone responses to progressive hypoglycemia.

50 mg/dL.[111] When assessed, the presence of symptoms of hypoglycemia did not correlate with cognitive performance,[108] and in one study in which diabetic patients were examined when their glucose level was 52 mg/dL,[112] 12 of 16 patients had subnormal scores on a battery of neuropsychological tests, while all failed to recognize any symptoms of hypoglycemia.

Electrophysiologic changes during hypoglycemia have been documented. The earliest electroencephalographic (EEG) change appears to be slowing of α-wave activity with a frontal preponderance, a pattern indicating that the frontal regions may be more sensitive than the occipital areas to hypoglycemia.[113] The auditory evoked potentials, recorded as the P300 wave latency, have been explored as a means of detecting subtle cerebral neuroglycopenia. One study[114] found an increase in the P300 wave latency at a glucose level as high as 72 mg/dL, with this change preceding any increase in levels of counterregulatory hormones.

Seizures and coma are manifestations of profound neuroglycopenia. Seizures occur in an estimated 22 to 37% of children with IDDM.[115] Recurrent, severe hypoglycemia can result in long-term developmental or cognitive deficits. In one study of 11 diabetic children with a history of seizure or coma associated with hypoglycemia, four had significant neurologic abnormalities, including ataxia, tremor, and severe developmental delay.[116] A comparison of 100 patients with long-term IDDM with matched controls revealed evidence of general cortical damage in 17 of the diabetic subjects and in none of the controls. Of these 17 subjects, only one had never required medical treatment for severe hypoglycemia.[117] One study[118] found that the frequency of asymptomatic hypoglycemia in children with IDDM correlated with lower scores on the abstract/visual reason-

ing subscale of the revised Stanford-Binet intelligence scale, suggesting that even mild hypoglycemia may produce permanent neuropsychological changes.

The mechanism of cortical damage from hypoglycemia does not appear to be completely analogous to that of anoxia or ischemia. Hypoglycemia affects the cerebral cortex and basal ganglia more diffusely than anoxia or ischemia and tends to spare the brain stem and cerebellum,[119] although the pathologic changes can be quite diverse.[120] Gross cerebral dysfunction with hypoglycemia can occur even when brain energy reserves are normal.[104] When nuclear magnetic resonance spectroscopy was used to determine the content of high-energy phosphate compounds such as adenosine triphosphate in the brain during insulin-induced hypoglycemia, no changes were found in any phosphate metabolite at a glucose level of 25 mg/dL.[121] It has been proposed that the distribution of neuronal necrosis with hypoglycemia suggests that the direct cause of brain-cell death is not lack of fuel but the release of excitatory toxins (including amino acids such as glutamate) that accelerate cell destruction.[104,122]

HYPOGLYCEMIC UNAWARENESS

Hypoglycemic unawareness is characterized by the absence of the classical autonomic warning symptoms of hypoglycemia, such that neuroglycopenia is the initial and only manifestation of hypoglycemia.[123] Frequently, the result of such a lack of premonitory symptoms is recurrent, severe hypoglycemic episodes requiring assistance.[81]

Since hypoglycemic unawareness is noted during insulin-induced hypoglycemia in nondiabetic patients with cervical spine transections,[124] it has been suggested that lack of neurally directed secretion of counterregulatory hormone secretions is the etiologic factor. When a group of patients with IDDM and hypoglycemic unawareness were studied during conditions of hypoglycemia, the patients failed to show any increase in epinephrine response at a glucose level of 58 mg/dL and showed a significant blunting of the epinephrine response at a glucose level of 45 mg/dL.[125] Similarly, when seven patients with recurrent severe hypoglycemia and hypoglycemic unawareness were compared with seven patients with enhanced perception of hypoglycemia (symptoms of hypoglycemia at a glucose level of 80 mg/dL), the patients with hypoglycemic unawareness showed a delayed increase in epinephrine response to hypoglycemia and a lower glucose threshold for stimulation of an increase in the levels of epinephrine, cortisol, and growth hormone.[9] However, a study of diabetic children younger than 5 years old who had severe recurrent hypoglycemia found normal increases in epinephrine, norepinephrine, and growth hormone.[18] An additional study in adults failed to find a difference in the epinephrine response to hypoglycemia in patients with severe recurrent hypoglycemia and a lack of adrenergic warning signs. However, the heart rate response of these patients to isoproterenol was significantly blunted, a finding that led the authors to suggest that a decrease in sensitivity to catecholamines may play a role in the absence of adrenergic symptoms with hypoglycemia.[126]

Recently, there has been concern that the use of human insulin may be associated with a reduced awareness of hypoglycemia. These concerns stemmed from a report that of 176 patients whose therapy was changed from beef/porcine insulin to human insulin, 66 (36%) reported that their early hypoglycemic warning symptoms had changed from sympathoadrenal to neuroglycopenic symptoms. When seven patients were changed back to animal insulin, the autonomic warning symptoms returned.[127] In a survey of patients changed from porcine to human insulin without a change in glycemic control, as assessed by levels of glycosylated hemoglobin, 64% noted that their recognition of hypoglycemia was increased when they were using porcine insulin and 50% noted that they perspired less when they used human insulin.[128] Finally, a double-blind randomized crossover trial comparing human and porcine insulin in 32 patients with IDDM over a 24-week period noted that during treatment with human insulin the awareness of hypoglycemia was significantly decreased and the incidence of neuroglycopenic warning symptoms in the absence of adrenergic symptoms during hypoglycemia was significantly higher.[129] However, a number of other investigators failed to find an increase in the incidence of severe hypoglycemia in patients treated with preparations of human insulin.[130-132] No increase in deaths attributed to diabetes were noted in Great Britain during 1985 to 1988, the period when most patients' therapy was changed from animal insulin to human insulin.[133]

Most attempts to delineate differences in counterregulatory hormone responses to hypoglycemia induced by different insulin species have failed. One study did demonstrate significantly greater norepinephrine and heart rate responses to hypoglycemia induced by porcine insulin than to hypoglycemia induced by semisynthetic human insulin.[134] A recent study[135] found greater changes in auditory evoked potentials during hypoglycemia induced by porcine insulin than during hypoglycemia induced by semisynthetic human insulin. However, a number of studies of symptomatic and hormonal responses to hypoglycemia induced by porcine and human insulin administered by a variety of routes have shown identical responses.[130,136-138] Thus, there is presently no convincing evidence supporting a variation in the hormonal or symptomatic response to hypoglycemia based on the porcine or human origin of the insulin.

GLYCEMIC CONTROL, HYPOGLYCEMIA, AND COUNTERREGULATION

As discussed above, strict glycemic control is generally associated with an increase in the frequency and severity of hypoglycemic episodes. Although a contributing factor to this phenomenon is clearly the goal of lower blood glucose levels sought with such regimens,[4] evidence is emerging that the glucose level at which symptoms and counterregulatory hormones are activated is related to the degree of glycemic control.

In diabetic subjects with fasting hyperglycemia, a fall in the glucose level from a supranormal level to one of 100 mg/dL can be associated with an increase in levels of catecholamines, growth hormone, and cortisol.[40,139] Such increases are not observed in healthy individuals. Furthermore, the glucose threshold at which an increase in the symptoms of hypoglycemia occurs is significantly greater in patients with IDDM with poor glycemic control than in normal individuals[140] or in patients with diabetes in good control.[98]

Further studies have examined the counterregulatory hormone response to insulin-induced hypoglycemia in patients with IDDM before and during intensive insulin therapy. These studies demonstrated a decrease in the epinephrine, growth hormone, and cortisol responses to a hypoglycemic stimulus of 50 mg/dL[141] as well as a decrease in the glucose level necessary to stimulate secretion of epinephrine, norepinephrine, growth hormone, and cortisol[142] when patients were receiving intensive insulin therapy (Fig. 28–4). Similarly, when a low-dose insulin infusion (0.3 mU/kg · min) was administered to normal volunteers, to patients with well-controlled IDDM, and to patients with poorly controlled IDDM, the patients with good glycemic control all had a glucose nadir lower than 45 mg/dL, whereas the patients in poor control and normal subjects showed glucose stabilization at a level higher than 55 mg/dL.[143] The attenuated counterregulatory hormone response to hypoglycemia in well-controlled diabetic subjects has not been shown to be associated with enhanced cognitive function under hypoglycemic conditions.[144]

Studies in rats suggest that cerebral glucose transport[145-147] and levels of transporters[147,148] are decreased in animals with poorly controlled diabetes. Conversely, glucose uptake is increased in the brains of rats made hypoglycemic by implantation of insulin-secreting tumors or by insulin administration.[149] Thus, enhanced cerebral glucose transport, and higher

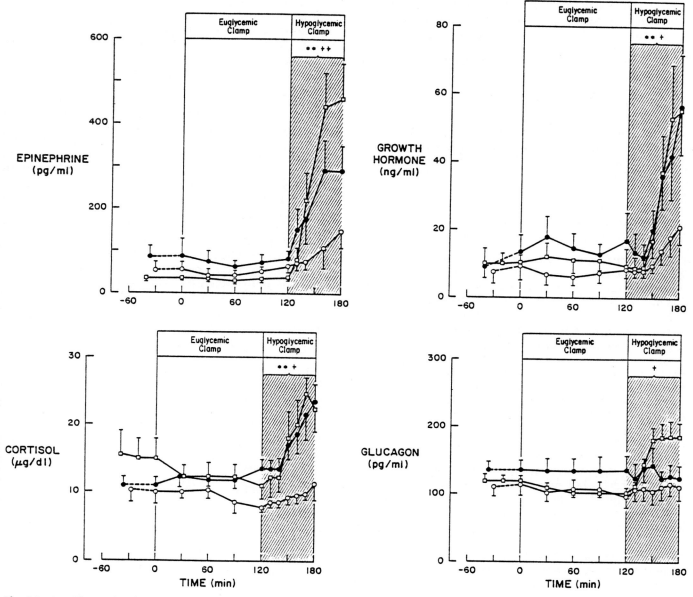

Fig. 28–4. Plasma levels of epinephrine, growth hormone, cortisol, and glucagon during the basal state, euglycemic clamp (90 mg/dL), and hypoglycemic clamp (50 mg/dL) in healthy controls (open squares) and in patients with insulin-dependent diabetes mellitus (IDDM) before (solid circles) and after (open circles) intensive insulin pump therapy. *P<.05 for patients with IDDM before vs. after pump treatment; **P<.01 for patients with IDDM before vs. after pump treatment; †P<.05 for healthy controls vs. patients with IDDM after pump treatment; ‡P<.01 for healthy controls vs. patients with IDDM after pump treatment. Reprinted with permission from reference 141 (Simonson DC, Tamborlane WV, DeFronzo RA, Sherwin RS. Intensive insulin therapy reduces counterregulatory hormone responses to hypoglycemia in patients with type I diabetes. Ann Intern Med 1985;103:184–90).

glucose levels in the brain during hypoglycemia, may underlie the observed defects in counterregulatory hormone production in diabetic patients who are maintaining strict glycemic control and experience frequent episodes of hypoglycemia.

HYPOGLYCEMIA IN PREGNANCY

Attempts at strict glycemic control in pregnant women with IDDM also lead to an increase in the incidence of hypoglycemia.[150–152] One prospective study[150] of pregnant women with IDDM found a 33% incidence in hypoglycemia of sufficient severity to produce an alteration in level of consciousness.

Although such efforts at strict glycemic control are undertaken in an attempt to improve fetal outcome, there is some evidence from in vitro and animal studies that exposure of the fetus to hypoglycemia may have deleterious effects.[153,154] There are periods during the embryonic development of the rat when an absolute dependence on glycolysis exists. In cultured rat embryos, prolonged hypoglycemia during this developmental period can have adverse effects on embryogenesis. Such effects are prevented by the addition of glucose even if insulin levels remain elevated.[155] One study of rat embryos exposed to hypoglycemic serum for 1 hour demonstrated major lesions in 7.1% of the embryos and minor lesions in 23.5%.[156] Finally, when pregnant rats were rendered hypoglycemic with a 1-hour insulin infusion, 3.6% of the embryos developed an open posterior neural pore.[157] Thus, frequent glucose monitoring during pregnancy is more critical than ever as a means of detecting and preventing episodes of severe hypoglycemia.

PREVENTION AND TREATMENT OF HYPOGLYCEMIA

A number of important measures can be taken to prevent severe hypoglycemia in diabetic patients, whether they are receiving insulin or oral hypoglycemic agents. These include home blood-glucose monitoring, careful attention to meal timing and content, appropriate reductions in insulin or supplementation of food intake with exercise, accuracy in the administration of medication, education regarding the symptoms of hypoglycemia, and prompt, appropriate treatment of hypoglycemia when it does occur. The simple addition of a bedtime snack if the blood glucose level at 10:30 p.m. was less than 120 mg/dL completely prevented nocturnal hypoglycemia in one group of patients receiving insulin-pump therapy.[158]

The Sleep Sentry (Teledyne Avionics, Charlottesville, VA), is a device designed to provide a signal to an individual who becomes hypoglycemic during sleep or who is otherwise unaware of hypoglycemia. The device monitors two cutaneous phenomena associated with hypoglycemia: diaphoresis and decreased skin temperature.[159,160] Initial studies showed that the monitors were capable of detecting the cutaneous changes associated with a glucose level lower than 50 mg/dL approximately 80% of the time.[159,160] However, in a test of the Sleep Sentry in 18 patients with IDDM during periods of hypoglycemia (mean nadir glucose level approximately 52 mg/dL) induced by a continuous insulin infusion, the alarm was triggered in only 10 (56%) of the subjects.[159] Metabolic and cutaneous parameters did not differ in the "alarmers" and the "non-alarmers." Thus, such devices may be of use only in a selected subset of patients.

Given that intensive insulin therapy can be associated with an increase in the incidence of severe hypoglycemia, it has been proposed that patients be screened for the adequacy of hypoglycemic counterregulation before they start intensive insulin therapy. Two similar insulin infusion tests have been devised for such use.[80,161] Following overnight administration of a low dose of insulin, insulin is infused intravenously at a rate of 30 mU/m^2 · min or 40 mU/kg · hr. Adequate counterregulation is defined by a nadir glucose level greater than 35[80] or 45[161] mg/dL and/or the absence of neurologic manifestations of

hypoglycemia. Both of these tests have been shown to be reproducible and have good predictive value in determining the frequency of severe hypoglycemia during intensive insulin therapy.[80,161,162] Conversely, in a study of 14 patients with severe recurrent hypoglycemia,[8] 12 patients developed neuroglycopenia during a similar insulin infusion test protocol. However, the practical use of these tests may be limited by the ultimate development of defective counterregulation in many, if not all, patients receiving intensive insulin therapy.[141–143]

The mainstay of treatment of hypoglycemia is the oral administration of carbohydrate-containing nutrients (Table 28–2). The suggested initial dose of carbohydrate is 15 g. The form of carbohydrate administered may be an important determinant of the glycemic response. One study compared various forms of oral carbohydrate for the treatment of hypoglycemia induced by intravenous insulin administration.[164] Fifteen grams of glucose or sucrose in tablet or liquid form were equally effective in increasing the blood glucose level and alleviating the symptoms of hypoglycemia. However, 15 g of glucose in gel form or 125 mL of orange juice (which according to the package information contained 15 g of carbohydrate but on analysis was found to contain 11.5 g) gave

Table 28–2. Treatment of Hypoglycemia

Oral
Juice
    4 ounces orange juice
    3 ounces cranberry juice
    3 ounces sweetened grape juice
Fruit drink
    4 ounces Tang or Hi-C
Soda (non-diet)
    6 ounces ginger ale
    5 ounces cola
Sugar
    4 teaspoons dissolved in water
Syrups
    1 tablespoon honey, maple syrup, or corn syrup
Dried fruit
    3 tablespoons raisins
    10 dried apricot halves
    4 prunes
Candy
    8 Lifesavers
    6 jelly beans
    9 small gumdrops
    3 large marshmallows
    25 miniature marshmallows
Cake icing
    1 small tube
Marshmallow cream
    1 tablespoon
Glucose tablets
    3 B-D Glucose Tablets (5 g each)
Glucose gel (40% dextrose)
    1½ tubes Glutose or Monojel (10 g dextrose per tube)
    1 tube Insta-Glucose (12 g dextrose per tube)
Parenteral
50% dextrose in water
    50 mL intravenously
Glucagon
    1 mg subcutaneously or intramuscularly

Adapted from Holleroth.[163]

consistently lower glycemic responses and resulted in alleviation of hypoglycemic symptoms in only 42% of patients at 20 minutes.

For more severe hypoglycemia in which the level of consciousness is depressed, treatment with parenteral glucose or glucagon is necessary. A randomized study compared 25 g of 50% dextrose with 1 mg of glucagon, each administered intravenously, in 52 consecutive insulin-treated outpatients with hypoglycemic coma (mean initial glucose level 18 mg/dL). The group treated with glucagon was slower to regain a normal level of consciousness (6.5 minutes vs. 4 minutes with dextrose treatment). All patients had a normal level of consciousness by 30 minutes.[165]

In the nonmedical setting, glucagon administration is the treatment of choice for severe hypoglycemia for which oral carbohydrate administration is not possible because of a depressed level of consciousness in the patient. Glucagon exerts its acute hyperglycemic effect via stimulation of hepatic glycogenolysis, but it also has a prolonged stimulatory effect on gluconeogenesis.[52] Thus, glucagon is less effective when liver function is impaired[166] or glycogen stores are depleted—as with starvation. Nausea and vomiting are the major side effects of parenteral administration of glucagon. Intramuscular, subcutaneous, and intravenous routes of administration appear to be equally effective.[167,168] Although the usual recommended initial dose is 1 mg, a study comparing doses of 10 and 20 μg/kg for treatment of hypoglycemia in diabetic children demonstrated that although recovery was slower with the lower dose, it was adequate. Only the 20-μg/kg dose produced nausea.[168]

Recently, there has been interest in the intranasal administration of glucagon. The bioavailability of intranasal glucagon is approximately 10%.[169] One study comparing 50 g of oral glucose to 1 mg of intranasal glucagon found a faster increase in glucose levels with glucagon.[170] Intranasal glucagon has been shown to produce a rapid increase in plasma glucose levels in diabetic patients with insulin-induced hypoglycemia. However, the glucose level falls 25 to 50 minutes after the administration of glucagon,[169,171] indicating the need for rapid supplementation with oral carbohydrate. Intramuscular glucagon has a more prolonged hyperglycemic effect.[170]

THE SOMOGYI EFFECT

In 1938, Somogyi and Kirstein suggested that insulin excess resulting in hypoglycemia could lead to activation of the glucose-raising systems and to subsequent hyperglycemia.[172,173] Recently, however, the clinical relevance of the Somogyi phenomenon (posthypoglycemic hyperglycemia) has been questioned.[31,174–176]

Clear theoretical grounds exist for the development of posthypoglycemic hyperglycemia. The key predisposing factor in patients with IDDM is the inability to increase insulin secretion in response to the hyperglycemia induced by prolonged elevation in levels of counterregulatory hormones. However, hyperglycemia in the morning following nocturnal hypoglycemia appears to be the result of both the dissipation of injected insulin and the

activation of glucose counterregulatory systems (particularly catecholamines and possibly growth hormone and cortisol[174,177]). One study demonstrated insulin resistance up to 12 hours after the induction of nocturnal hypoglycemia despite the return of levels of counterregulatory hormones to normal.[178]

Monitoring studies performed in hospitalized patients with IDDM indicate that nocturnal hypoglycemia occurs in up to 30% of patients.[73,179] However, in one overnight observational study of patients with IDDM or NIDDM, the average blood glucose level at 7:00 a.m. was 113 ± 10 mg/dL in the 15 patient profiles with a 3:00 a.m. glucose level measuring 50 mg/dL or less. Of the 80 patient profiles in which the glucose level at 3:00 a.m. was 100 mg/dL or less, the 7:00 a.m. glucose level was greater than 150 mg/dL in only 13 and greater than 200 mg/dL in only 6.[175] Similar findings were seen in children with IDDM observed overnight.[180] Two studies actually noted lower morning blood glucose values in patients with either naturally occurring[181] (Fig. 28–5) or induced[174] hypoglycemia, and a third study[182] found equal daytime plasma glucose levels following induction of hypoglycemia and following attempts at prevention of nocturnal hypoglycemia. The first study[181] showed that those patients with a glucose level greater than 180 mg/dL at 7:00 a.m. consumed greater amounts of carbohydrate in

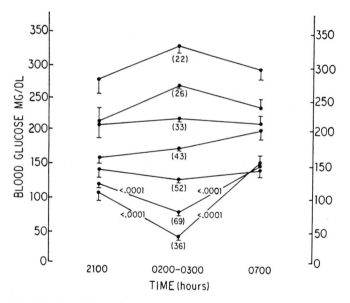

Fig. 28–5. Blood glucose concentrations (mean ± SE) at 2100 hr, 0200–0300 hr, and 0700 hr in 66 patients (281 profiles) with insulin-dependent diabetes mellitus (IDDM). Profiles are grouped by 50-mg/dL intervals on the basis of blood glucose level at 0200 to 0300 hr. Numbers in parentheses refer to number of profiles in each group. Patients with hypoglycemia at 0200 to 0300 hr had lower glucose values the preceding evening (2100 h) and the following morning (0700 h) than patients without nocturnal hypoglycemia. Reprinted with permission from reference 181 (Lerman IG, Wolfsdorf JI. Relationship of nocturnal hypoglycemia to daytime glycemia in IDDM. Diabetes Care 1988;11:636–42; copyright © of the American Diabetes Association).

response to the nocturnal hypoglycemia than did the patients with lower morning levels of blood glucose.

The Somogyi phenomenon may be more apparent in patients maintaining stricter glycemic control. One study[183] of patients with IDDM receiving insulin-pump therapy showed significantly higher 7:00 a.m. and 10:00 a.m. glucose values in patients who were given insulin to induce moderate (45 mg/dL) nocturnal hypoglycemia for 1½ hours, as compared with a group who received insulin similarly but in whom hypoglycemia was prevented by glucose infusion. The morning blood glucose levels correlated with peak levels of epinephrine, growth hormone, and cortisol and were associated with an increase in glucose production and a decrease in glucose clearance. Similarly, in nine patients with IDDM who were receiving multiple daily injections or insulin-pump therapy, hypoglycemia induced in the morning was found to be associated with increased glucose levels from 1 hour after lunch to 1 hour after dinner, whereas when hypoglycemia was prevented with intravenous glucose administration on a control study day, these postprandial glucose levels were not increased. The degree of hyperglycemia correlated with the peak growth hormone level attained during hypoglycemia.[184]

OTHER FACTORS CONTRIBUTING TO HYPOGLYCEMIA IN DIABETIC PATIENTS

Other Endocrine Diseases

A variety of autoimmune endocrinopathies associated with IDDM can increase the frequency of hypoglycemia. These conditions include glucocorticoid deficiency (due to Addison's disease, autoimmune hypophysitis resulting in generalized pituitary dysfunction, or isolated deficiency in adrenocorticotropic hormone)[185–187] and hypothyroidism (which prolongs the circulating half-life of insulin). A decrease in the insulin requirement following pregnancy may be a sign of postpartum hypopituitarism in women with IDDM.[188]

Antibodies to Insulin and the Insulin Receptor

Exogenous administration of insulin can result in the development of antibodies to insulin, which appear to be capable of binding and releasing large amounts of insulin. This results in the alternation of periods of relative insulin resistance and hyperglycemia with periods of apparently unexplained hypoglycemia.[189–191] The observed hypoglycemia may be due to release of the bound insulin from the antibodies, action of the antibody-insulin complex on the insulin receptor, and/or prolongation of the circulating half-life of injected insulin.[189,191] There are reports of fasting[191,192] and postprandial[189] hypoglycemia in both patients with IDDM and those with NIDDM[193] who have high titers of antibodies to insulin. Such antibodies can even be seen in patients treated exclusively with human insulin preparations. In addition, patients occasionally develop antibodies to insulin and associated hypoglyce-

mia without having been exposed to exogenous insulin.[194,195]

Hypoglycemia can also develop as a result of the development of antibodies directed at the insulin receptor.[196–198] The majority of patients with antibodies to the insulin receptor have diabetes mellitus associated with extreme insulin resistance and acanthosis nigricans.[196,198] Occasionally, however, antibodies are found in association with other autoimmune diseases that appear to be capable of causing hypoglycemia via exerting a stimulatory effect on the insulin receptor.[196] Hypoglycemia associated with antibodies to the insulin receptor may improve with glucocorticoid therapy.[196,197]

Exercise

During exercise, redundant glucoregulatory systems are involved in matching glucose production with the increase in glucose utilization.[199] Activation of the sympathochromaffin system plays a primary role in the maintenance of adequate plasma glucose levels.[124,199] Changes in the secretion of pancreatic islet hormones (i.e., glucagon and insulin) are not normally critical but become so when catecholamine action is deficient.[199] The activation of counterregulatory hormones during exercise appears to be regulated by glucose-independent mechanisms.[200]

Increases in peripheral insulin sensitivity may be seen after a single bout of exercise and more certainly after a few days of exercise.[201] Although patients are usually well informed regarding the need to increase carbohydrate intake or decrease the insulin dose prior to exercise, late-onset hypoglycemia following exercise can be significant. One prospective study of 300 patients with Type I diabetes over 2 years found that 48 patients had episodes of moderate or severe hypoglycemia (32 patients had a seizure or loss of consciousness) more than 4 hours after exercise.[202]

Renal Failure

Renal insufficiency is associated with hypoglycemia in both Type I and Type II diabetes mellitus. Hypoglycemia may also be observed in up to 3% of patients with renal failure who do not have diabetes.[203–205] In insulin-treated patients, a decline in renal function results in a decrease in insulin clearance, an increase in insulin half-life, and thus in a decrease in the insulin requirement. In patients with Type II diabetes who are receiving sulfonylureas that are partially dependent on kidney function for clearance, a decline in renal function may result in a similar prolongation of action, a decrease in dose requirement, and/or an increase in hypoglycemia. A decline in renal gluconeogenesis is also seen in patients with renal insufficiency. However, as discussed above, renal gluconeogenesis makes an important contribution to total glucose production only during a prolonged fast. One study[206] suggested that the response of counterregulatory hormones to hypoglycemia is blunted in patients receiving chronic hemodialysis, but this suggestion needs to be confirmed.

Medications

Nonselective β-adrenergic blockade impairs glucose recovery from hypoglycemia in most patients with IDDM since epinephrine plays a primary role in glucose recovery in the absence of glucagon.[78,207-209] Small doses of β_1-selective adrenergic blockers may be safer, but with larger doses the receptor selectivity is lost. Despite these theoretical concerns, one controlled trial of 50 insulin-treated diabetic patients[210] found no increase in the frequency or severity of hypoglycemia when β-adrenergic blockers were administered.

As discussed above, hypoglycemia is common in patients receiving sulfonylurea therapy. In a large review of drug-induced hypoglycemia,[211] more than 80% of deaths due to hypoglycemia were attributed to sulfonylureas or alcohol. However, metformin and other biguanides, even in great excess, generally do not cause clinical hypoglycemia.[20] A large number of drugs have been reported to potentiate the hypoglycemic effects of the sulfonylureas, including alcohol, sulfonamides, coumarin, clofibrate, monoamine oxidase inhibitors, tricyclic antidepressants, H_2-receptor blockers, phenylbutazone, chloramphenicol, and probenecid.[20,212-215]

A number of other medications have been reported to cause hypoglycemia in healthy individuals or in patients with diabetes. Aspirin and other salicylates most commonly result in hypoglycemia in children.[20,211] Recently, pentamidine was reported to cause both hypoglycemia and hyperglycemia, possibly as a result of its cytotoxic effects on β-cells, which result in early insulin release and subsequent insulin depletion.[216,217] Hypoglycemia has been seen in patients with malaria receiving quinine, although it is not clear whether the low circulating levels of glucose are secondary to quinine treatment or to the underlying infection.[218-221] Other rare reported causes of hypoglycemia include bordetella pertussis vaccine, haloperidol, propoxyphene, p-aminobenzoic acid, and chlorpromazine.[20,211]

Alcohol

Excessive alcohol consumption by insulin- or sulfonylurea-treated patients with diabetes may result in severe hypoglycemia.[222,223] Alcohol inhibits hepatic gluconeogenesis by increasing the ratio of reduced to oxidized nicotinamide adenine nucleotide (NAD), thus resulting in a depletion of NAD, which is required for the conversion of gluconeogenic precursors to glucose.[20,34] In nondiabetic individuals, alcohol-induced hypoglycemia occurs only when glycogen stores are depleted. However, gluconeogenesis does play an important role in the recovery from prolonged insulin-induced hypoglycemia.[34,35,224] Thus, alcohol may impair the ability of diabetic individuals to recover from hypoglycemia. This situation is particularly dangerous when the individual is intoxicated and is unable to recognize and appropriately treat the symptoms of hypoglycemia.

REFERENCES

1. Banting FG, Campbell WR, Fletcher AA. Further clinical experience with insulin (pancreatic extracts) in the treatment of diabetes mellitus. BMJ 1923;1:8–12.
2. Whipple AO. The surgical therapy of hyperinsulinism. J Int Chir 1938;3:237–76.
3. Whipple AO. Hyperinsulinism in relation to pancreatic tumors. Surgery 1944;16:289–305.
4. Goldstein DE, England JD, Hess R, et al. A prospective study of symptomatic hypoglycemia in young diabetic patients. Diabetes Care 1981;4:601–5.
5. Potter J, Clarke P, Gale EAM, et al. Insulin-induced hypoglycaemia in an accident and emergency department: the tip of an iceberg? BMJ 1982;285:1180–2.
6. Goldgewicht C, Slama G, Papoz L, Tchobroutsky G. Hypoglycaemic reactions in 172 type I (insulin-dependent) diabetic patients. Diabetologia 1983;24:95–9.
7. Casparie AF, Elving LD. Severe hypoglycemia in diabetic patients: frequency, causes, prevention. Diabetes Care 1985;8:141–5.
8. Sjöbom NC, Adamson U, Lins PE. The prevalence of impaired glucose counter-regulation during an insulin-infusion test in insulin-treated diabetic patients prone to severe hypoglycaemia. Diabetologia 1989;32:818–25.
9. Grimaldi A, Bosquet F, Davidoff P, et al. Unawareness of hypoglycemia by insulin-dependent diabetics. Horm Metab Res 1990;22:90–5.
10. Daneman D, Frank M, Perlman K, et al. Severe hypoglycemia in children with insulin-dependent diabetes mellitus: frequency and predisposing factors. J Pediatr 1989;115:681–5.
11. Deckert T, Poulsen JE, Larsen M. Prognosis of diabetics with diabetes onset before the age of thirty-one: survival, causes of death and complications. Diabetologia 1978;14:363–70.
12. Tunbridge WMG. Factors contributing to deaths of diabetics under fifty years of age. Lancet 1981;2:569–72.
13. Malouf R, Brust JCM. Hypoglycemia: causes, neurological manifestations, and outcome. Ann Neurol 1985;17:421–30.
14. Fischer KF, Lees JA, Newman JH. Hypoglycemia in hospitalized patients: causes and outcomes. N Engl J Med 1986;315:1245–50.
15. Arias P, Kerner W, Zier H, et al. Incidence of hypoglycemic episodes in diabetic patients under continuous insulin infusion and intensified conventional insulin treatment: assessment by means of semiambulatory 24-hour continuous blood glucose monitoring. Diabetes Care 1985;8:134–40.
16. DCCT Research Group. Diabetes Control and Complications Trial (DCCT): results of feasibility study. Diabetes Care 1987;10:1–19.
17. DCCT Research Group. Diabetes Control and Complications Trial (DCCT): update. Diabetes Care 1990;13:427–33.
18. Brambilla P, Bouneres PF, Santiago JV, et al. Glucose counterregulation in pre-school-age diabetic children with recurrent hypoglycemia during conventional treatment. Diabetes 1987;36:300–4.
19. Jennings AM, Wilson RM, Ward JD. Symptomatic hypoglycemia in NIDDM patients treated with oral hypoglycemic agents. Diabetes Care 1989;12:203–8.
20. Bailey CJ, Flatt PR, Marks V. Drugs inducing hypoglycemia. Pharmacol Ther 1989;42:361–84.
21. Berger W, Caduff F, Pasquel M, Rump A. Die relative

Häufigkeit dea schweren Sulfonylharnstoff-Hypoglykämie in den letzten 25 Jahren in der Schweiz. Schweiz Med Wochenschr 1986;116:145–51.

22. Mutch WJ, Dingwall-Fordyce I. Is it hypo? Knowledge of the symptoms of hypoglycaemia in elderly diabetic patients. Diabetic Med 1985;2:54–6.

23. Gerich JE, Campbell PJ. Overview of counterregulation and its abnormalities in diabetes mellitus and other conditions. Diabetes Metab Rev 1988;4:93–111.

24. Felig P. The glucose-alanine cycle. Metabolism 1973; 22:179–207.

25. Huang S-C, Phelps ME, Hoffman EJ, et al. Noninvasive determination of local cerebral metabolic rate of glucose in man. Am J Physiol 1980;238:E69–82.

26. Owen OE, Felig P, Morgan AP, et al. Liver and kidney metabolism during prolonged starvation. J Clin Invest 1969;48:574–83.

27. Cahill GF Jr. Starvation in man. N Engl J Med 1970; 282:668–75.

28. Merimee TJ, Tyson JE. Stabilization of plasma glucose during fasting. N Engl J Med 1974;291:1275–78.

29. Radziuk J, McDonald TJ, Rubenstein D, Dupre J. Initial splanchnic extraction of ingested glucose in normal man. Metabolism 1978;27:657–69.

30. Rizza RA, Mandarino LJ, Gerich JE. Dose-response characteristics for effects of insulin on production and utilization of glucose in man. Am J Physiol 1981;240:E630–9.

31. Tse TF, Clutter WE, Shah SD, Cryer PE. Mechanisms of postprandial glucose counterregulation in man: physiologic roles of glucagon and epinephrine vis-a-vis insulin in the prevention of hypoglycemia late after glucose ingestion. J Clin Invest 1983;72:278–86.

32. Clutter WE, Rizza RA, Gerich JE, Cryer PE. Regulation of glucose metabolism by sympathochromaffin catecholamines. Diabetes Metab Rev 1988;4:1–15.

33. Garber AJ, Cryer PE, Santiago JV, et al. The role of adrenergic mechanisms in the substrate and hormonal response to insulin-induced hypoglycemia in man. J Clin Invest 1976;58:7–15.

34. Frizzell RT, Campbell PJ, Cherrington AD. Gluconeogenesis and hypoglycemia. Diabetes Metab Rev 1988;4:51–70.

35. LeCavalier L, Bolli G, Cryer P, Gerich J. Contributions of gluconeogenesis and glycogenolysis during glucose counterregulation in normal humans. Am J Physiol 1989; 256:E844–51.

36. DeFeo P, Perriello G, De Cosmo S, et al. Comparison of glucose counterregulation during short-term and prolonged hypoglycemia in normal humans. Diabetes 1986;35:563–9.

37. Saccà L, Sherwin R, Hendler R, Felig P. Influence of continuous physiologic hyperinsulinemia on glucose kinetics and counterregulatory hormones in normal and diabetic humans. J Clin Invest 1979;63:849–57.

38. Bolli GB, Gottesman IS, Cryer PE, Gerich JE. Glucose counterregulation during prolonged hypoglycemia in normal humans. Am J Physiol 1984;247:E206–14.

39. Amiel SA, Simonson DC, Tamborlane WV, et al. Rate of glucose fall does not affect counterregulatory hormone responses to hypoglycemia in normal and diabetic humans. Diabetes 1987;36:518–22.

40. DeFronzo RA, Andres R, Bledsoe TA, et al. A test of the hypothesis that the rate of fall in glucose concentration triggers counterregulatory hormonal responses in man. Diabetes 1977;26:445–52.

41. Kerr D, MacDonald IA, Tattersall RB. Influence of duration of hypoglycemia on the hormonal counterregulatory response in normal subjects. J Clin Endocrinol Metab 1989;68:1118–22.

42. Kerr D, MacDonald IA, Tattersall RB. Adaptation to mild hypoglycaemia in normal subjects despite sustained increases in counter-regulatory hormones. Diabetologia 1989;32:249–54.

43. Amiel SA, Simonson DC, Sherwin RS, et al. Exaggerated epinephrine responses to hypoglycemia in normal and insulin-dependent diabetic children. J Pediatr 1987; 110:832–7.

44. Cryer PE. Glucose counterregulation in man. Diabetes 1981;30:261–4.

45. Clarke WL, Santiago JV, Thomas L, et al. Adrenergic mechanisms in recovery from hypoglycemia in man: adrenergic blockade. Am J Physiol 1979;236:E147–52.

46. Rizza RA, Cryer PE, Gerich JE. Role of glucagon, catecholamines, and growth hormone in human glucose counterregulation: effects of somatostatin and combined α- and β-adrenergic blockade on plasma glucose recovery and glucose flux rates after insulin-induced hypoglycemia. J Clin Invest 1979;64:62–71.

47. Gerich JE, Davis J, Lorenzi M, et al. Hormone mechanisms of recovery from insulin-induced hypoglycemia in man. Am J Physiol 1979;236:E380–5.

48. Abramson EA, Arky RA, Woeber KA. Effects of propranolol on the hormonal and metabolic responses to insulin-induced hypoglycaemia. Lancet 1966;2:1386–8.

49. Gelfand RA, DeFronzo RA. Hypoglycemic counterregulation in normal and diabetic man. Ann Clin Res 1984;16:84–93.

50. Amiel SA, Tamborlane WV, Saccà L, Sherwin RS. Hypoglycemia and glucose counterregulation in normal and insulin-dependent diabetic subjects. Diabetes Metab Rev 1988;4:71–89.

51. Boyle PJ, Cryer PE. Roles of growth hormone and cortisol in defense against prolonged hypoglycemia [Abstract]. Diabetes 1990;39:5A.

52. Cryer PE, Tse TF, Clutter WE, Shah SE. Roles of glucagon and epinephrine in hypoglycemic and nonhypoglycemic glucose counterregulation in humans. Am J Physiol 1984;247:E198–205.

53. Saccà L, Vigorto C, Cicala M, et al. Mechanisms of epinephrine-induced glucose intolerance in normal humans: role of the splanchnic bed. J Clin Invest 1982; 69:284–93.

54. Saccà L, Eigler N, Cryer PE, Sherwin RS. Insulin antagonistic effects of epinephrine and glucagon in the dog. Am J Physiol 1979;237:E487–92.

55. Eigler N, Saccà L, Sherwin RS. Synergistic interactions of physiologic increments of glucagon, epinephrine and cortisol in the dog: a model for stress-induced hyperglycemia. J Clin Invest 1979;63:114–23.

56. MacGorman LR, Rizza RA, Gerich JE. Physiological concentrations of growth hormone exert insulin-like and insulin antagonistic effects on both hepatic and extrahepatic tissues in man. J Clin Endocrinol Metab 1981;53:556–9.

57. DeFeo P, Perriello G, Torlone E, et al. Demonstration of a role for growth hormone in glucose counterregulation. Am J Physiol 1989;256:E835–43.

58. Biggers DW, Myers SR, Neal D, et al. Role of brain in counterregulation of insulin-induced hypoglycemia in dogs. Diabetes 1989;38:7–16.

59. Ritter RC, Slusser PG, Stone S. Glucoreceptors controlling feeding and blood glucose: location in the hindbrain. Science 1981;213:451–3.

60. Cane P, Artal R, Bergman RN. Putative hypothalamic

glucoreceptors play no essential role in the response to moderate hypoglycemia. Diabetes 1986;35:268–77.

61. Cane P, Haun CK, Evered J, et al. Response to deep hypoglycemia does not involve glucoreceptors in carotid perfused tissue. Am J Physiol 1988;255:E680–7.

62. Bolli GB, De Feo P, Perriello G, et al. Role of hepatic autoregulation in defense against hypoglycemia in humans. J Clin Invest 1985;75:1623–31.

63. McCraw EF, Peterson MJ, Ashmore J. Autoregulation of glucose metabolism in the isolated perfused rat liver. Proc Soc Exp Biol Med 1967;126:232–6.

64. Glinsmann WH, Hern EP, Lynch A. Intrinsic regulation of glucose output by rat liver. Am J Physiol 1969;216:698–703.

65. Hansen I, Firth R, Haymond M, et al. The role of autoregulation of the hepatic glucose production in man: response to a physiologic decrement in plasma glucose. Diabetes 1986;35:186–91.

66. Polonsky K, Bergenstal R, Pons G, et al. Relation of counterregulatory responses to hypoglycemia in type I diabetics. N Engl J Med 1982;307:1106–12.

67. Kleinbaum J, Shamoon H. Impaired counterregulation of hypoglycemia in insulin-dependent diabetes mellitus. Diabetes 1983;32:493–8.

68. Bolli GB, Calabrese G, De Feo P, et al. Lack of glucagon response in glucose counter-regulation in type I (insulin-dependent) diabetics: absence of recovery after prolonged optimal insulin therapy. Diabetologia 1982;22:100–5.

69. Boden G, Reichard GA Jr, Hoeldtke RD, et al. Severe insulin-induced hypoglycemia associated with deficiencies in the release of counterregulatory hormones. N Engl J Med 1981;305:1200–5.

70. Gerich JE, Langlis M, Noacco C, et al. Lack of glucagon response to hypoglycemia in diabetes: evidence for an intrinsic pancreatic alpha cell defect. Science 1973;182:171–3.

71. Bolli GB, De Feo P, Compagnucci P, et al. Abnormal glucose counterregulation in insulin-dependent diabetes mellitus: interaction of anti-insulin antibodies and impaired glucagon and epinephrine secretion. Diabetes 1983;32:134–41.

72. Singer-Granick C, Hoffman RP, Kerensky K, et al. Glucagon responses to hypoglycemia in children and adolescents with IDDM. Diabetes Care 1988;11:643–9.

73. Wise JK, Hendler R, Felig P. Evaluation of alpha-cell function by infusion of alanine in normal, diabetic and obese subjects. N Engl J Med 1973;288:487–90.

74. Unger RH, Aguilar-Parada E, Müller WA, Eisentraut AM. Studies of pancreatic alpha cell function in normal and diabetic subjects. J Clin Invest 1970;49:837–48.

75. Robertson RP, Porte DP. The glucose receptor: a defective mechanism in diabetes mellitus distinct from the beta adrenergic receptor. J Clin Invest 1973;52:870–76.

76. Fukuda M, Tanaka A, Tahara Y, et al. Correlation between minimal secretory capacity of pancreatic β-cells and stability of diabetic control. Diabetes 1988;37:81–8.

77. Giugliano D, Giannetti G, Di Pinto P, et al. Normalization by sodium salicylate of the impaired counterregulatory glucagon response to hypoglycemia in insulin-dependent diabetes: a possible role for endogenous prostaglandins. Diabetes 1985;34:521–5.

78. Popp DA, Tse TF, Shah SD, et al. Oral propranolol and metoprolol both impair glucose recovery from insulin-induced hypoglycemia in insulin-dependent diabetes mellitus. Diabetes Care 1984;7:243–7.

79. Bolli GB, Dimitriadis GD, Pehling GB, et al. Abnormal glucose counterregulation after subcutaneous insulin in insulin-dependent diabetes mellitus. N Engl J Med 1984;310:1706–11.

80. White NH, Skor DA, Cryer PE, et al. Identification of type I diabetic patients at increased risk for hypoglycemia during intensive therapy. N Engl J Med 1983;308:485–91.

81. Hoeldtke RD, Boden G, Shuman CR, Owen OE. Reduced epinephrine secretion and hypoglycemia unawareness in diabetic autonomic neuropathy. Ann Intern Med 1982;96:459–62.

82. Hirsch BR, Shamoon H. Defective epinephrine and growth hormone responses in type I diabetes are stimulus specific. Diabetes 1987;36:20–6.

83. Ensinck JW, Kanter RA. Glucagon responses to hypoglycemia in type I diabetic man after 24-hour glucoregulation by glucose-controlled insulin infusion. Diabetes Care 1980;3:285–9.

84. Bergenstal R, Polonsky KS, Pons G, et al. Lack of glucagon response to hypoglycemia in type I diabetics after long-term optimal therapy with a continuous subcutaneous insulin infusion pump. Diabetes 1983;32:398–402.

85. Bolli GB, De Feo P, De Cosmo S, et al. Effects of long-term optimization and short-term deterioration of glycemic control on glucose counterregulation in type I diabetes mellitus. Diabetes 1984;33:394–400.

86. White NH, Gingerich RL, Levandoski LA, et al. Plasma pancreatic polypeptide response to insulin-induced hypoglycemia as a marker for defective glucose counterregulation in insulin-dependent diabetes mellitus. Diabetes 1985;34:870–5.

87. Levitt NS, Vink AI, Sive AA, et al. Impaired pancreatic polypeptide responses to insulin-induced hypoglycemia in diabetic autonomic neuropathy. J Clin Endocrinol Metab 1980;50:445–9.

88. McGrath BP, Stern AI, Esler M, Hansky J. Impaired pancreatic polypeptide release to insulin hypoglycaemia in chronic autonomic failure with postural hypotension: evidence for parasympathetic dysfunction. Clin Sci 1982;63:321–3.

89. Kennedy FP, Bolli GB, Go VLW, et al. The significance of impaired pancreatic polypeptide and epinephrine responses to hypoglycemia in patients with insulin-dependent diabetes mellitus. J Clin Endocrinol Metab 1987;64:602–8.

90. Bolli GB, Tsalikian E, Haymond MW, et al. Defective glucose counterregulation after subcutaneous insulin in noninsulin-dependent diabetes mellitus. J Clin Invest 1984;73:1532–41.

91. Levitt NS, Vinik AI, Sive AA, et al. Studies on plasma glucagon concentration in maturity-onset diabetics with autonomic neuropathy. Diabetes 1979;28:1015–21.

92. Boden G, Soriano M, Hoeldtke RD, Owen OE. Counterregulatory hormone release and glucose recovery after hypoglycemia in non-insulin-dependent diabetic patients. Diabetes 1983;32:1055–9.

93. Berk MA, Clutter WE, Skor D, et al. Enhanced glycemic responsiveness to epinephrine in insulin-dependent diabetes mellitus is the result of the inability to secrete insulin. J Clin Invest 1985;75:1842–51.

94. Shamoon H, Hendler R, Sherwin RS. Altered responsiveness to cortisol, epinephrine, and glucagon in insulin-infused juvenile-onset diabetics. Diabetes 1980;29:284–91.

95. Hilsted J, Richter E, Madsbad S, et al. Metabolic and cardiovascular responses to epinephrine in diabetic autonomic neuropathy. N Engl J Med 1987;317:421–6.

96. Schwartz NS, Clutter WE, Shah SD, Cryer PE. Glycemic thresholds for activation of glucose counterregulatory systems are higher than the threshold for symptoms. J Clin Invest 1987;79:777–81.

97. Foster JW, Hart RG. Hypoglycemic hemiplegia: two cases and a clinical review. Stroke 1987;18:944–6.

98. Åman J, Berne C, Ewald U, Tuvemo T. Lack of cutaneous hyperemia in response to insulin-induced hypoglycemia in IDDM. Diabetes Care 1990;13:1029–33.

99. Page MM, Watkins PJ. Provocation of postural hypotension by insulin in diabetic autonomic neuropathy. Diabetes 1976;25:90–5.

100. Fagius J, Niklasson F, Berne C. Sympathetic outflow in human muscle nerves increased during hypoglycemia. Diabetes 1986;35:1124–9.

101. Fisher BM, Baylis PH, Frier BM. Plasma oxytocin, arginine vasopressin and atrial natriuretic peptide responses to insulin-induced hypoglycemia in man. Clin Endocrinol 1987;26:179–85.

102. Pardridge WM. Brain metabolism: a perspective from the blood-brain barrier. Physiol Rev 1983;63:1481–535.

103. Cryer PE, Gerich JE. Glucose counterregulation, hypoglycemia, and intensive insulin therapy in diabetes mellitus. N Engl J Med 1985;313:232–41.

104. Siesjo BK. Hypoglycemia, brain metabolism, and brain damage. Diabetes Metab Rev 1988;4:113–44.

105. Brooks DJ, Gibbs JSR, Sharp P, et al. Regional cerebral glucose transport in insulin-dependent diabetic patients studied using [^{11}C]3-O-methyl-D-glucose and positron emission tomography. J Cereb Blood Flow Metab 1986;6:240–4.

106. Hertz MM, Paulson OB, Barry DI, et al. Insulin increases glucose transfer across the blood-brain barrier in man. J Clin Invest 1981;67:597–604.

107. Stevens AB, McKane WR, Bell PM, et al. Psychomotor performance and counterregulatory responses during mild hypoglycemia in healthy volunteers. Diabetes Care 1989;12:12–7.

108. Herold KC, Polonsky KS, Cohen RM, et al. Variable deterioration in cortical function during insulin-induced hypoglycemia. Diabetes 1985;34:677–85.

109. Holmes CS, Hayford JT, Gonzalez JL, Weydert JA. A survey of cognitive functioning at different glucose levels in diabetic persons. Diabetes Care 1983;6:180–85.

110. Holmes CS, Koepke KM, Thompson RG, et al. Verbal fluency and naming performance in type I diabetes at different blood glucose concentrations. Diabetes Care 1984;7:454–9.

111. Hoffman RG, Speelman DJ, Hinnen DA, et al. Changes in cortical functioning with acute hypoglycemia and hyperglycemia in type I diabetes. Diabetes Care 1989; 12:193–7.

112. Pramming S, Thorsteinsson B, Theilgaard A, et al. Cognitive function during hypoglycaemia in type I diabetes mellitus. BMJ 1986;292:649–50.

113. Tamburrano G, Lala A, Locuratolo N, et al. Electroencephalography and visually evoked potentials during moderate hypoglycemia. J Clin Endocrinol Metab 1988;66:1301–6.

114. DeFeo P, Gallai V, Mazzotta G, et al. Modest decrements in plasma glucose concentration cause early impairment in cognitive function and later activation of glucose counterregulation in the absence of hypoglycemic symptoms in normal man. J Clin Invest 1988;82:436–44.

115. Eeg-Olofsson O. Hypoglycemia and neurological disturbances in children with diabetes mellitus. Acta Paediatr Scand Suppl 1977;270:91–5.

116. Ingram TTS, Stark GD, Blackburn I. Ataxia and other neurological disorders as sequels of severe hypoglycaemia in childhood. Brain 1967;90:851–62.

117. Bale RN. Brain damage in diabetes mellitus. Br J Psychiatry 1973;122:337–41.

118. Golden MP, Ingersoll GM, Brack CJ, et al. Longitudinal relationship of asymptomatic hypoglycemia to cognitive function in IDDM. Diabetes Care 1989;12:89–93.

119. Kalimo H, Olsson Y. Effects of severe hypoglycemia on the human brain: neuropathological case reports. Acta Neurol Scand 1980;62:345–56.

120. Patrick AW, Campbell IW. Fatal hypoglycemia in insulin-treated diabetes mellitus: clinical features and neuropathological changes. Diabetic Med 1990;7:349–54.

121. Hilsted J, et al. Maintenance of high-energy brain phosphorous compounds during insulin-induced hypoglycemia in men. Diabetes 1988;37:760–2.

122. Auer RN. Progress review: hypoglycemic brain damage. Stroke 1986;17:699–708.

123. Cryer PE. The metabolic impact of autonomic neuropathy in insulin-dependent diabetes mellitus. Arch Intern Med 1986;146:2127–9.

124. Cryer PE, White NH, Santiago JV. The relevance of glucose counterregulatory systems to patients with insulin-dependent diabetes mellitus. Endocrine Rev 1986;7:131–9.

125. Heller SR, MacDonald IA, Herbert M, Tattersall RA. Influence of sympathetic nervous system on hypoglycaemic warning symptoms. Lancet 1987;2:359–63.

126. Berlin I, Grimaldi A, Landault C, et al. Lack of hypoglycemic symptoms and decreased β-adrenergic sensitivity in insulin-dependent diabetic patients. J Clin Endocrinol Metab 1988;66:273–8.

127. Teuscher A, Berger WG. Hypoglycaemia unawareness in diabetics transferred from beef-porcine insulin to human insulin. Lancet 1987;2:382–5.

128. Berger WG, Althaus BU. Reduced awareness of hypoglycemia after changing from porcine to human insulin in IDDM. Diabetes Care 1987;10:260–1.

129. Berger W, Honegger B, Keller U, Jaeggi E. Warning symptoms of hypoglycaemia during treatment with human and porcine insulin in diabetes mellitus. Lancet 1989;1:1041–4.

130. Berger M. Human insulin: much ado about hypoglycemia (un)awareness. Diabetologia 1987;30:829–33.

131. Mühlhauser I, Berger M, Heinemann L, et al. Hypoglycemic warning symptoms and incidence of severe hypoglycaemia during treatment with human and animal insulin [Abstract]. Diabetologia 1990;33:A122.

132. Anderson JH, Holcombe JH, Grimes JA, Galloway JA. Hypoglycemia unawareness and human insulin [Abstract]. Diabetologia 1990;33:A122.

133. Stephenson J, Fuller J. Hypoglycaemia as cause of death in human insulin era. Lancet 1990;335:661.

134. Heine RJ, Van der Heyden EAP, Van der Veen EA. Responses to human and porcine insulin in healthy subjects. Lancet 2:946–9, 1989.

135. Kern W, Lieb K, Kerner W, et al. Differential effects of human and pork insulin-induced hypoglycemia on neuronal functions in humans. Diabetes 1990;39:1091–8.

136. Müller-Esch G, Ball P, Bekemeyer U, et al. Comparative study of hormonal counterregulation during GCIIS-guided insulin hypoglycemia tests using human insulin (recombinant DNA) and pork insulin. Diabetes Res 1985;2:121–5.

137. Leroith D, Leslie N, Pickens W, Sperling MA. Similar counterregulatory hormonal responses to hypoglycemia

induced by semisynthetic human and porcine insulin. Diabetes 1984;33:104A.

138. Perez Fernandez R, Casanueva FF, Devesa J, Cabezas-Cerrato J. Metabolic and hormonal parameters after insulin-induced hypoglycemia in man, comparison between biosynthetic human insulin and purified pork insulin. Horm Metabol Res 1985;17:351–4.

139. DeFronzo RA, Hendler R, Christensen N. Stimulation of counterregulatory hormonal responses in diabetic man by a fall in glucose concentration. Diabetes 1980;29:125–31.

140. Boyle PJ, Scwartz NS, Shah SD, et al. Plasma glucose concentrations at the onset of hypoglycemic symptoms in patients with poorly controlled diabetes and in nondiabetics. N Engl J Med 1988;318:1487–92.

141. Simonson DC, Tamborlane WV, DeFronzo RA, Sherwin RS. Intensive insulin therapy reduces counterregulatory hormone responses to hypoglycemia in patients with type I diabetes. Ann Intern Med 1985;103:184–90.

142. Amiel SA, Sherwin RS, Simonson DC, Tamborlane WV. Effect of intensive insulin therapy on glycemic thresholds for counterregulatory hormone release. Diabetes 1988;37:901–7.

143. Amiel SA, Tamborlane WV, Simonson DC, Sherwin RS. Defective glucose counterregulation after strict glycemic control of insulin-dependent diabetes mellitus. N Engl J Med 1987;316:1376–83.

144. Widom B, Simonson DC. Glycemic control and neuropsychologic function during hypoglycemia in patients with insulin-dependent diabetes mellitus. Ann Intern Med 1990;112:904–12.

145. McCall AL, Millington WR, Wurtman RJ. Metabolic fuel and amino acid transport into the brain in experimental diabetes mellitus. Proc Natl Acad Sci USA 1982;79:5406–10.

146. Gjedde A, Crone C. Blood-brain glucose transfer: repression in chronic hyperglycemia. Science 1981;214:456–7.

147. Pardridge WM, Triguero D, Farrell CR. Downregulation of blood-brain barrier glucose transporter in experimental diabetes. Diabetes 1990;39:1040–4.

148. Matthaei S, Horuk R, Olefsky JM. Blood-brain glucose transfer in diabetes mellitus. Diabetes 1986;35:1181–4.

149. McCall AL, Fixman LB, Fleming N, et al. Chronic hypoglycemia increases brain glucose transport. Am J Physiol 1986;251:E442–7.

150. Rayburn W, Piehl E, Jacober S, et al. Severe hypoglycemia during pregnancy: its frequency and predisposing factors in diabetic women. Int J Gynaecol Obstet 1986;24:263–8.

151. Bergman M, Seaton TB, Auerhahn CC, et al. The incidence of gestational hypoglycemia in insulin-dependent and non-insulin-dependent diabetic women. N Y State J Med 1986;86:174–7.

152. Bergman M, Newman SA. Hypoglycemia in pregnancy: unknown risks [Letter]. Diabetes Care 1987;10:380.

153. Buchanan T, Freinkel N, Schemmer JK. Maternal hypoglycemia impairs embryo development in the rat: implications for diabetic control in early pregnancy [Abstract]. Clin Res 1985;33:888A.

154. Bergman M, Frenz DA, McCreery LA, et al. Impaired chondrogenesis at abnormal glucose levels [Abstract]. Clin Res 1986;34:681A.

155. Akazawa S, Akazawa M, Hashimoto M, et al. Effects of hypoglycaemia on early embryogenesis in rat embryo organ culture. Diabetologia 1987;30:791–6.

156. Akazawa M, et al. Effects of brief exposure to insulin-induced hypoglycemic serum during organogenesis in rat embryo culture. Diabetes 1989;38:1573–8.

157. Buchanan TA, Schemmer JK, Freinkel N. Embryotoxic effects of brief maternal insulin-hypoglycemia during organogenesis in the rat. J Clin Invest 1986;78:643–9.

158. Schiffrin A, Suissa S. Predicting nocturnal hypoglycemia in patients with type I diabetes treated with continuous subcutaneous insulin infusion. Am J Med 1987;82:1127–32.

159. Clarke WL, Carter WR, Moll M, et al. Metabolic and cutaneous events associated with hypoglycemia detected by sleep sentry. Diabetes Care 1988;11:630–5.

160. Teledyne Avionics. Sleep Sentry: clinical testing summary. Charlottesville, VA: Teledyne, 1983.

161. Bolli GB, De Feo, De Cosmo S, et al. A reliable and reproducible test for adequate glucose counterregulation in type I diabetes mellitus. Diabetes 1984;33:732–7.

162. Santiago JV, White NH, Skor DA, et al. Defective glucose counterregulation limits intensive therapy of diabetes mellitus. Am J Physiol 1984;247:E215–20.

163. Holleroth HJ. Diabetes teaching guide for people who use insulin. Boston: Joslin Diabetes Center, 1988.

164. Slama G, Traynoar P-Y, Desplanque N, et al. The search for an optimized treatment of hypoglycemia: carbohydrates in tablets, solution, or gel for the correction of insulin reactions. Arch Intern Med 1990;150:589–93.

165. Collier A, Steedman DJ, Patrick AW, et al. Comparison of intravenous glucagon and dextrose in treatment of severe hypoglycemia in an accident and emergency department. Diabetes Care 1987;10:712–5.

166. Hall-Boyer K, Zaloga GP, Chernow B. Glucagon: hormone or therapeutic agent? Crit Care Med 1984;12:584–9.

167. Mühlhauser I, Koch J, Berger M. Pharmacokinetics and bioavailability of injected glucagon: differences between intramuscular, subcutaneous, and intravenous administration. Diabetes Care 1985;8:39–42.

168. Åman J, Wranne L. Hypoglycaemia in childhood diabetes. II. Effect of subcutaneous or intramuscular injection of different doses of glucagon. Acta Paediatr Scand 1988;77:548–53.

169. Freychet L, Rizkalla SW, Desplanque N, et al. Effect of intranasal glucagon on blood glucose levels in healthy subjects and hypoglycaemic patients with insulin-dependent diabetes. Lancet 1988;1:1364–6.

170. Pontiroli AE, Calderara A, Pajetta E, et al. Intranasal glucagon as remedy for hypoglycemia: studies in healthy subjects and type I diabetic patients. Diabetes Care 1989;12:604–8.

171. Pontiroli AE, Alberetto M, Pozza G. Metabolic effects of intranasally administered glucagon: comparison with intramuscular and intravenous injection. Acta Diabetol Lat 1985;22:103–10.

172. Somogyi M, Kirstein M. Insulin as a cause of extreme hyperglycemia and instability. Week Bull St Louis Med Soc 1938;32:498–500.

173. Somogyi M. Exacerbation of diabetes by excess insulin action. Am J Med 1959;26:169–91.

174. Tordjman KM, Havlin CE, Levandoski LA, et al. Failure of nocturnal hypoglycemia to cause fasting hyperglycemia in patients with insulin-dependent diabetes mellitus. N Engl J Med 1987;317:1552–9.

175. Havlin CE, Cryer PE. Nocturnal hypoglycemia does not commonly result in major morning hyperglycemia in patients with diabetes mellitus. Diabetes Care 1987;10:141–7.

176. Shamoon H, Hendler R, Sherwin RS. Synergistic interactions among antiinsulin hormones in the pathogenesis of

stress hyperglycemia in humans. J Clin Endocrinol Metab 1981;52:1235–41.

177. Bolli GB, Gottesman IS, Campbell PJ, et al. Glucose counterregulation and waning of insulin in the Somogyi phenomenon (posthypoglycemic hyperglycemia). N Engl J Med 1984;311:1214–9.

178. Kollind M, Adamson U, Lins PE. Insulin resistance following nocturnal hypoglycaemia in insulin-dependent diabetes mellitus. Acta Endocrinol (Copenh) 1987;116:314–20.

179. Pramming S, Thorsteinsson B, Bendtson I, et al. Nocturnal hypoglycaemia in patients receiving conventional treatment with insulin. BMJ 1985;291:376–9.

180. Shalwitz RA, Farkas-Hirsch R, White NH, Santiago JV. Prevalence and consequences of nocturnal hypoglycemia among conventionally treated children with diabetes mellitus. J Pediatr 1990;116:685–9.

181. Lerman IG, Wolfsdorf JI. Relationship of nocturnal hypoglycemia to daytime glycemia in IDDM. Diabetes Care 1988;11:636–42.

182. Hirsch IB, Smith LJ, Havlin CE, et al. Failure of nocturnal hypoglycemia to cause daytime hyperglycemia in patients with IDDM. Diabetes Care 1990;13:133–42.

183. Perriello G, De Feo P, Torlone E, et al. The effect of asymptomatic nocturnal hypoglycemia on glycemic control in diabetes mellitus. N Engl J Med 1988;319:1233–9.

184. Fowelin J, Attvall S, von Schenck H, et al. Postprandial hyperglycaemia following a morning hypoglycaemia in type I diabetes mellitus. Diabetic Med 1990;7:156–61.

185. Abramson EA, Arky RA. Coexistent diabetes mellitus and isolated ACTH deficiency. Metabolism 1968;17:492–5.

186. Kojima I, Nejima I, Ogata E. Isolated adrenocorticotropin deficiency associated with polyglandular failure. J Clin Endocrinol Metab 1982;54:182–6.

187. Sandler R, Proudfoot GR. Isolated ACTH deficiency contributing to frequent hypoglycemia in type I diabetes. Diabetes Care 1985;8:302–4.

188. Dorfman SG, Dillaplain RP, Gambrell RD. Antepartum pituitary infarction. Obstet Gynecol 1979;53:21S–4S.

189. Sklenar I, Wilkin TJ, Diaz J-L, et al. Spontaneous hypoglycemia associated with autoimmunity specific to human insulin. Diabetes Care 1987;10:152–9.

190. Berson SA, Yalow RS. Kinetics of reaction between insulin and insulin-binding antibody. J Clin Invest 1957;36:873–4.

191. Albert SG, Popp DA. Hypoglycemia due to serum-complexed insulin in a patient with diabetes mellitus. Diabetes Care 1984;7:285–90.

192. Harwood R. Insulin-binding antibodies and "spontaneous" hypoglycemia. N Engl J Med 1960;262:978–9.

193. Van Haeften TW, Krom BA, Gerich JE. Prolonged fasting hypoglycemia due to insulin antibodies in patients with non-insulin-dependent diabetes mellitus: effect of insulin withdrawal on insulin-antibody-binding kinetics. Diabetes Care 1987;10:160–3.

194. Ichihara K, Shima K, Saito Y, et al. Mechanism of hypoglycemia observed in a patient with insulin autoimmune syndrome. Diabetes 1977;26:500–6.

195. Benson EA, Ho P, Wang C, et al. Insulin autoimmunity as a cause of hypoglycemia. Arch Intern Med 1984;144:2351–4.

196. Moeller DE, Ratner RE, Borenstein DG, Taylor SI. Autoantibodies to the insulin receptor as a cause of autoimmune hypoglycemia in systemic lupus erythematosus. Am J Med 1988;84:334–8.

197. Taylor SI, Grunberger G, Marcus-Samuels B, et al. Hypo-

glycemia associated with antibodies to the insulin receptor. N Engl J Med 1982;307:1422–6.

198. Kahn CR, Flier JS, Bar RS, et al. The syndromes of insulin resistance and acanthosis nigricans: insulin-receptor disorders in man. N Engl J Med 1976;294:739–45.

199. Hoelzer DR, Dalsky GP, Clutter WE, et al. Glucoregulation during exercise: hypoglycemia is prevented by redundant glucoregulatory systems, sympathochromaffin activation, and changes in islet hormone secretion. J Clin Invest 1986;77:212–21.

200. Sotsky MJ, Shilo S, Shamoon H. Regulation of counterregulatory hormone secretion in man during exercise and hypoglycemia. J Clin Endocrinol Metab 1989;68:9–16.

201. Heath GW, Gavin JR III, Hinderliter JM, et al. Effects of exercise and lack of exercise on glucose tolerance and insulin sensitivity. J Appl Physiol 1983;55:512–7.

202. Macdonald MJ. Postexercise late-onset hypoglycemia in insulin-dependent diabetic patients. Diabetes Care 1987;10:584–8.

203. Block MB, Rubenstein AH. Spontaneous hypoglycemia in diabetic patients with renal insufficiency. JAMA 1970;13:1863–6.

204. Avram MM, Wolf RE, Gan A, et al. Uremic hypoglycemia: a preventable life-threatening complication. N Y State J Med 1984;84:593–6.

205. Rutsky EA, McDaniel HG, Tharpe DL, et al. Spontaneous hypoglycemia in chronic renal failure. Arch Intern Med 1977;138:1364–8.

206. Ramirez G, Brueggemeyer C, Ganguly A. Counterregulatory hormonal response to insulin-induced hypoglycemia in patients on chronic hemodialysis. Nephron 1988;49:231–6.

207. Lager I, Blohmé G, Smith U. Effect of cardioselective and non-selective β-blockade on the hypoglycaemic response in insulin-dependent diabetics. Lancet 1979;1:458–62.

208. Kleinbaum J, Shamoon H. Effect of propranolol on delayed glucose recovery after insulin-induced hypoglycemia in normal and diabetic subjects. Diabetes Care 1984;7:155–62.

209. Simonson DC, Koivisto V, Sherwin RS, et al. Adrenergic blockade alters glucose kinetics during exercise insulin-dependent diabetics. J Clin Invest 1984;73:1648–58.

210. Barnett AH, Leslie D, Watkins PJ. Can insulin-treated diabetics be given beta-adrenergic blocking drugs? BMJ 1980;280:976–8.

211. Seltzer HS. Drug-induced hypoglycemia: a review based on 473 cases. Diabetes 1972;21:955–66.

212. Cooper AJ. The action of mebanazine, a monoamine oxidase inhibitor antidepressant drug in diabetes. II. Int J Neuropsychiatry 1966;2:342–5.

213. True BL, Perry PJ, Burns EA. Profound hypoglycemia with the addition of a tricyclic antidepressant to maintenance sulfonylurea therapy. Am J Psychiatry 1987;44:1220–1.

214. Lee K, Mize R, Lowenstein SR. Glyburide-induced hypoglycemia and ranitidine [Letter]. Ann Intern Med 1987;107:261–2.

215. MacWalter RS, El Debani AH, Feely J, Stevenson IH. Potentiation by ranitidine of the hypoglycaemic response to glipizide in diabetic patients [Abstract]. Br J Clin Pharmacol 1985;19:121P-2P.

216. Waskin H, Stehr-Green JK, Helmick CG, Sattler FR. Risk factors for hypoglycemia associated with pentamidine therapy for pneumocystis pneumonia. JAMA 1988;260:345–7.

217. Karboski JS, Godley PJ. Inhaled pentamidine and hypoglycemia [Letter]. Ann Intern Med 1988;108:490.

218. Okitolonda W, Delacollette C, Malengreau M, Henquin JC. High incidence of hypoglycaemia in African patients treated with intravenous quinine for severe malaria. BMJ 1987;295:716–8.

219. Taylor TE, Molyneux ME, Wirima JJ, et al. Blood glucose levels in Malawian children before and during the administration of intravenous quinine for severe falciparum malaria. N Engl J Med 1988;319:1040–7.

220. Phillips RE, Looareesuwan S, White NJ, et al. Hypoglycaemia and antimalarial drugs: quinidine and release of insulin. BMJ 1986;292:1319–21.

221. White NJ, Warrell DA, Chanthavanich P, et al. Severe hypoglycemia and hyperinsulinemia in falciparum malaria. N Engl J Med 1983;309:61–6.

222. Arky RA, Veverbrants E, Abramson EA. Irreversible hypoglycemia: a complication of alcohol and insulin. JAMA 1968;206:575–8.

223. Melander A, Lebovitz HE, Faber OK. Sulfonylureas: why, which, and how? Diabetes Care 1990;13(Suppl 3):18–25.

224. Caprio S, Saccà L, Tamborlane WV, Sherwin RS. Relationship between changes in glucose production and gluconeogenesis during mild hypoglycemia in humans. Metabolism 1988;37:707–10.

Chapter 29

ORAL ANTIDIABETIC AGENTS

HAROLD E. LEBOVITZ

APPROACHES TO MANAGEMENT OF HYPERGLYCEMIA IN NON-INSULIN-DEPENDENT DIABETES MELLITUS

The treatment of hyperglycemia in patients with non-insulin-dependent diabetes (NIDDM) is directed toward achieving the following goals: 1) alleviating symptoms; 2) minimizing acute complications; 3) increasing the sense of well-being and the quality of life and; 4) eliminating or minimizing the chronic complications of microvascular, neuropathic, and accelerated macrovascular disease.[1] No controversy surrounds claims of the beneficial effects of reducing blood glucose values to levels defined as acceptable (Table 29–1) by the American Diabetes Association regarding the first three goals.[2] Whether the achievement of normal glycemic control in patients with NIDDM will markedly reduce or eliminate the chronic complications is still an unresolved

Table 29–1. Biochemical Indices of Glycemic Control in Type II Diabetes

Biochemical Index	Normal	Acceptable	Poor
Fasting plasma glucose (mmol/L)	6.4 (115)	7.8 (140)	>11.1 (>200)
Postprandial (2 hr) plasma glucose (mmol/L)	7.8 (140)	11.1 (200)	>13.1 (>235)
HbA$_{1c}$ (%)	6	8	>10

Values in parentheses in mg/dL.
Modified from Lebovitz.[2]

issue.[3–5] Many empiric observations suggest that chronic complications occur less frequently in patients with near-normoglycemic control.[6–10] However, to date, no large well-controlled study has demonstrated that near-normoglycemic regulation does indeed eliminate or markedly decrease the chronic complications of NIDDM. Therefore, it is reasonable to strive for acceptable glycemic control in all patients with NIDDM. Near-normoglycemic control should be the goal only for those patients who are likely to benefit from the prevention of chronic complications and are willing to put forth the effort necessary to achieve it in anticipation of findings in future controlled studies that such control will indeed significantly retard or prevent chronic complications.

Reducing hyperglycemia in patients with NIDDM involves using therapeutic procedures that ameliorate the underlying defects responsible for the hyperglycemia. Patients with NIDDM have been shown to have abnormalities in both insulin secretion and insulin action.[11–15] Some studies have suggested that insulin resistance is the underlying defect in NIDDM[16–18] and eventually causes a relative and, finally, an absolute deficiency in insulin secretion. Other studies show that the primary defect in NIDDM is a decrease in insulin secretion that ultimately leads to insulin resistance.[19–21] From a therapeutic viewpoint the following facts are germane. 1) All patients with NIDDM who are hyperglycemic have some deficiency in insulin secretion.[11–21] 2) The higher the fasting plasma glucose level the greater the degree of insulin deficiency.[12] 3) Insulin resistance is present in some but not all patients with NIDDM.[15,22,23] 4) The magnitude of insulin resistance varies considerably among patients with NIDDM and is significantly influenced by obesity.[23] An estimate of the relative roles played by insulin resistance and insulin deficiency in the pathogenesis of hyperglycemia in a particular patient may be useful in deciding which therapeutic modalities are likely to be most effective.

The mode by which the abnormalities of insulin secretion and action cause hyperglycemia can be traced to their effects on the liver and peripheral tissues.[12,15,23,24] The fasting levels of plasma glucose are regulated primarily by hepatic glucose production.[12,25,26] Levels of insulin and glucagon in the portal vein are major regulators of gluconeogenesis and glycogenolysis. Postprandial levels of plasma glucose are determined primarily by the nature of the diet and insulin-mediated peripheral glucose uptake.[27-29] Hepatic glucose production is regulated at insulin concentrations significantly lower than those regulating peripheral glucose uptake.[12,14,15] The sequence of abnormal glucose metabolism therefore goes from impaired glucose tolerance, to minimal fasting hyperglycemia with significant postprandial hyperglycemia, to fasting hyperglycemia with marked postprandial hyperglycemia as the deficiency in insulin secretion and action go from mild to moderate to severe.

Therapeutic approaches to treatment of hyperglycemia in patients with NIDDM can be constructed on this pathogenetic framework. Table 29–2 outlines such a conceptual approach and thoughts on how currently available agents exert their effects.[30] It is obvious that the various antidiabetic drugs available for treatment worldwide (sulfonylureas, metformin, acarbose) and in experimental trials (glucagon-like peptide 1, ciglitazone analogues) reduce hyperglycemia by different mechanisms. This implies not only that some agents may be better for

certain types of patients with NIDDM but also that combinations of agents that lower blood glucose by different mechanisms are likely to be more effective than any one agent alone.

Of the agents listed in Table 29–2, three are available (though unfortunately not everywhere) for the treatment of patients with NIDDM: sulfonylureas, metformin, and acarbose. This chapter focuses on the use of these three oral antidiabetic agents in the treatment of patients with NIDDM.

SULFONYLUREAS

Oral hypoglycemic sulfonylureas have been used in the treatment of NIDDM since 1955. Although a voluminous literature on both the pharmacology and clinical use of these drugs has been presented over the last 40 years, many clinical questions are still unresolved, and major new insights into the mechanism and significance of this class of drugs have occurred just recently. Unresolved clinical issues include questions such as, Why are sulfonylureas ineffective in about 20% of newly diagnosed patients with NIDDM? Why do some patients with NIDDM who initially show a good glycemic response to sulfonylureas lose this response after several years? What are the long-term results, benefits, and risks of sulfonylurea therapy in patients with NIDDM? Are extrapancreatic effects of sulfonylureas important in their antidiabetic actions? Will sulfonylurea therapy in patients with impaired glucose tolerance prevent or delay the progression to overt NIDDM? Are combinations of sulfonylureas with other antidiabetic agents useful and effective in the management of patients with NIDDM who are not achieving their desired glycemic goals with sulfonylureas alone?

New insights into the pharmacology of sulfonylureas include the identification and characterization of a plasma membrane sulfonylurea receptor and the discovery that sulfonylureas cause the closing of an adenosine triphosphate (ATP)-sensitive potassium channel, resulting in a change in the flux of K^+ and Ca^{++} across membranes. An update of sulfonylurea therapy in the 1990s therefore differs considerably from that of previous years.

Pharmacology

Sulfonylurea drugs are a class of compounds containing the sulfonylurea moiety that are related to the sulfonamide drugs. The discovery of the hypoglycemic action of sulfonylurea drugs was made inadvertently in 1942 when the original analogue (glyprothiazole) was used to treat patients with typhoid fever.[31,32] Subsequent modifications of the compound (elimination of an NH_2 moiety on the benzene ring and opening of the heterocyclic nitrogen ring) enhanced hypoglycemic activity and reduced toxicity.[33,34] This led to the development of the so-called first-generation sulfonylureas (Figure 29–1). The introduction of a cyclohexyl group to replace the aliphatic side chain and the addition, many years later, of another ring structure linked to glycine at the other end of the molecule created the so-called second-generation

Table 29–2. Sites for Intervention in Treatment of Hyperglycemia in Patients with Non-Insulin-Dependent Diabetes

I. Alter nutrient absorption
  A. Nonpharmacologic: dietary management
  B. Pharmacologic
    1. Gum guar
    2. α-Glucosidase inhibitors: acarbose
    3. Metformin?
II. Increase insulin secretion
  A. Sulfonylureas
  B. α-Adrenergic receptor antagonist
  C. Gastrointestinal hormones: GLP-1
III. Decrease hepatic glucose production
  A. Insulin and insulin analogues
  B. Inhibitors of lipolysis: acipimox
  C. Inhibitors of fatty acid oxidation
  D. Inhibitors of glucagon action
  E. Inhibitors of enzymes of gluconeogenesis
IV. Increase insulin action
  A. Sulfonylureas
  B. Metformin
  C. Ciglitazone analogues
V. Increase peripheral glucose metabolism independent of insulin inhibitors of fatty acid oxidation: methylpalmoxirate

GLP = glucagon-like peptide.

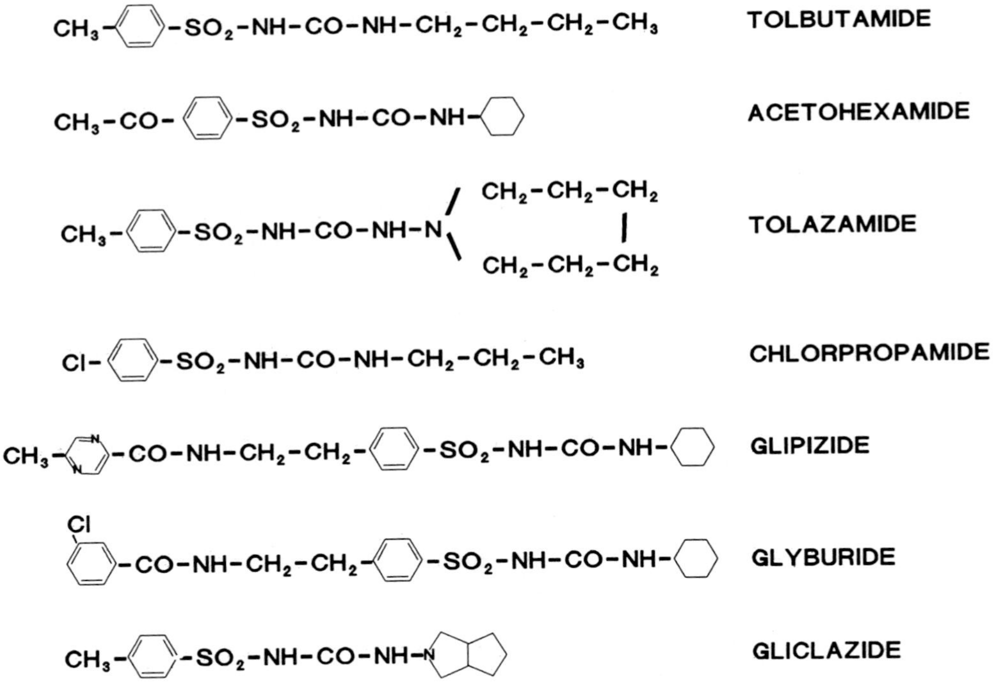

CH₃-⟨⟩-SO₂-NH-CO-NH-CH₂-CH₂-CH₂-CH₃ **TOLBUTAMIDE**

CH₃-CO-⟨⟩-SO₂-NH-CO-NH-⟨⟩ **ACETOHEXAMIDE**

CH₃-⟨⟩-SO₂-NH-CO-NH-N⟨ CH₂-CH₂-CH₂ / CH₂-CH₂-CH₂ ⟩ **TOLAZAMIDE**

Cl-⟨⟩-SO₂-NH-CO-NH-CH₂-CH₂-CH₃ **CHLORPROPAMIDE**

CH₃-⟨N⟩-CO-NH-CH₂-CH₂-⟨⟩-SO₂-NH-CO-NH-⟨⟩ **GLIPIZIDE**

Cl-⟨⟩-CO-NH-CH₂-CH₂-⟨⟩-SO₂-NH-CO-NH-⟨⟩ **GLYBURIDE**

CH₃-⟨⟩-SO₂-NH-CO-NH-N⟨⟩ **GLICLAZIDE**

Fig. 29–1. Commonly used sulfonylurea drugs. The "first-generation" sulfonylureas are tolbutamide, acetohexamide, tolazamide, and chlorpropamide. The "second-generation" sulfonylureas are glipizide, glyburide (glibenclamide), and gliclazide.

sulfonylureas (Figure 29–1). The antidiabetic mechanisms of all sulfonylureas are similar; however, the second-generation agents have much greater intrinsic activity.[33-38]

It was quickly recognized that the hypoglycemic activity of sulfonylureas was related, in large part, to their ability to stimulate insulin secretion. This action of sulfonylureas was demonstrated initially by showing that they did not lower the blood glucose of pancreatectomized humans or animals or patients with insulin-dependent diabetes (IDDM).[32,39-42] This effect on insulin secretion was demonstrated conclusively by showing increased plasma insulin levels in vivo following administration of sulfonylureas[43] or increased insulin secretion by pancreas pieces, isolated islets, or β-cells in culture incubated with sulfonylureas.[44,45]

For 30 years it was not clear why these drugs should stimulate the β-cell to secrete insulin. Equally confusing was the relationship, if any, between the numerous extrapancreatic effects of sulfonylureas described[46,47] and their pancreatic actions. Presently, it is recognized that sulfonylureas exert their pharmacologic actions by several different mechanisms.

Sulfonylurea Receptors and Ionic Fluxes

The presence of sulfonylurea binding sites on the surface of β-cells was initially suggested by studies indicating that all sulfonylureas but glyburide (glibenclamide) had a distribution volume in isolated islets similar to that for extracellular markers.[48] Glyburide, as an exception, enters the islet cells and is internalized.[49,50] Using ³H-labeled glyburide or glipizide, several investigators demonstrated and characterized sulfonylurea recep-

tors on the plasma membrane of β-cells derived from rat or hamster islet cell tumors.[51-56] The sulfonylurea receptor has a high affinity for second-generation sulfonylureas (K_d = 0.3 to 7.0 nM), and β-cell plasma membranes bind about 1 pmol of sulfonylurea per mg of protein.[56] The insulin-releasing potency of the various sulfonylureas is highly correlated with their affinity for the sulfonylurea receptor.[53,54,56]

The sulfonylurea receptor on the β-cell is coupled to an ATP-sensitive K⁺ channel in the plasma membrane (Figure 29–2).[53,57,58] The ATP-sensitive K⁺ channel in the basal state pumps K⁺ from the inside of the β-cell to the extracellular space and maintains the resting potential of the plasma membrane. When sulfonylureas bind to their plasma membrane receptors, K⁺ efflux through the ATP-sensitive K⁺ channel decreases and the membrane depolarizes. Depolarization of the membrane opens a voltage-dependent Ca⁺⁺ channel in the membrane that allows extracellular Ca⁺⁺ to enter the cell. The rise in Ca⁺⁺ in the cytosol of the β-cell triggers the movement of the insulin granule to the cell surface, where its contents of insulin and C-peptide are released into the circulation (see Chapter 4).[59,60]

Glucose and amino acid stimulation of insulin secretion by β-cells occurs by means of a similar mechanism (Figure 29–2).[45,61-63] The nutrients enter the β-cell and are metabolized. This metabolism leads to an increase in ATP and an increased ATP/ADP ratio. The increased ratio acts on the cytoplasmic side of the ATP-sensitive K⁺ channel to decrease K⁺ efflux from the cell, causing the cell membrane to depolarize and thus opening the voltage-sensitive Ca⁺⁺ channel. Nutrients and sulfonylureas act through the same ATP-sensitive K⁺ channel but by means of different interactions, as noted above. All

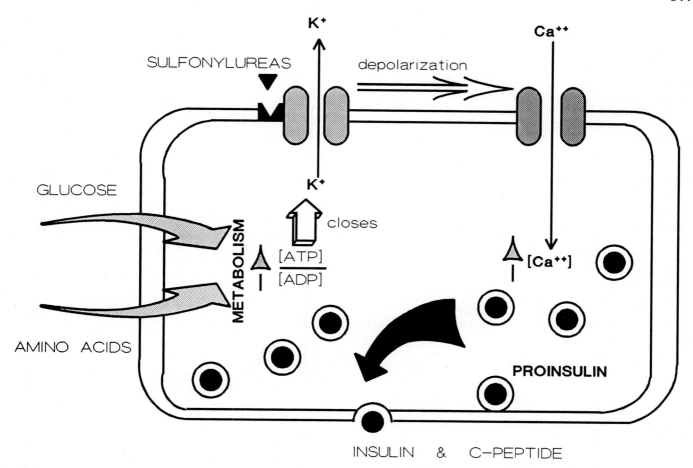

Fig. 29–2. Mechanism of insulin secretion. In the basal state, an ATP-modulated K^+ channel is open and maintains polarization of the plasma membrane. A voltage-dependent Ca^+ channel is closed. Metabolism of glucose and nutrients increases ATP production. An increase in the ATP/ADP ratio causes a closure of the K^+ channel. K^+ increases at the plasma membrane and causes its depolarization, which opens the voltage-dependent Ca^{++} channel and allows Ca^{++} to enter the cell. The increase in cytosolic Ca^{++} stimulates the secretion of insulin. Sulfonylureas bind to a receptor on the extracellular side of the ATP-modulated K^+ channel and cause its closure. The membrane is depolarized, the entry of Ca^{++} into the cell through the voltage-dependent Ca^{++} channel proceeds, and insulin secretion is stimulated. Sulfonylureas and metabolic products of nutrient metabolism affect the same ATP-modulated K^+ channel but by different mechanisms.

insulin secretogogues stimulate insulin secretion by increasing cytosolic Ca^{++}.

Although sulfonylureas and glucose stimulate insulin secretion through similar changes in ion fluxes, other actions of sulfonylureas on β-cells are markedly different from those of glucose.[44,45,62,63] Glucose stimulates proinsulin biosynthesis, and its insulin secretory responses consist of a rapid initial peak (first-phase insulin release) and a second, slower and more sustained, rise (second-phase insulin release). In contrast, sulfonylureas have either no effect or perhaps even an inhibitory effect on proinsulin biosynthesis. Sulfonylurea stimulation of insulin secretion consists primarily of the initial rapid peak (first-phase insulin release). Sulfonylureas and glucose effect the intermediary metabolism of the β-cell differently.

We therefore can summarize the major pharmacologic action of sulfonylureas on β-cells as that of changing ionic fluxes and membrane electrical activity. This effect

occurs within seconds of exposure of the β-cell to sulfonylureas.

Sulfonylureas receptors in many regions of the brain have also been identified and characterized.[51,64–66] The affinity constants of these receptors for sulfonylureas are similar to those noted for β-cells, but their concentration in plasma membranes is only about 10% that in β-cells. The highest concentration of sulfonylurea receptors in the brain is in the substantia nigra.[66] Sulfonylureas can block K^+ efflux from ATP-regulated K^+ channels in the substantia nigra. The significance of this effect is unclear, although the ATP-sensitive K^+ channel may be involved in the release of γ-aminobutyric acid from substantia nigra neuronal terminals.

ATP-sensitive K^+ channels that are responsive to sulfonylureas have also been described in cardiac muscle cells[66–70] and smooth muscle cells.[71] Mammalian heart cells contain high-affinity sulfonylurea receptors that have characteristics similar to those in pancreatic β-cells and also are associated with an ATP-sensitive K^+ channel. The duration of action potentials of cardiac cells in culture that have been drastically reduced by lowering concentrations of ATP are restored to near-normal values by the addition of a sulfonylurea to the medium.[69] Studies of diabetic cardiomyopathy in rats suggest that sulfonylureas increase cardiac function by improving Ca^{++} transport—independent of their effects on carbohydrate metabolism.[70]

Sulfonylurea Action on Liver, Muscle, and Adipose Tissue

Numerous in vitro actions of sulfonylurea drugs on liver, muscle, and adipose tissue have been demonstrated (Table 29–3). The relevance of these effects in vivo and their significance in the antidiabetic action of sulfonylureas continue to be debated. Although occasional reports suggest that these tissues may have specific sulfonylurea-binding sites, the data supporting the existence of such sites is equivocal and not consistent with that reported for pancreatic β-cell and neuronal sulfonylurea receptors. The characteristics of the actions of sulfonylureas on adipose tissue, muscle, and liver are inconsistent with an effect on ionic fluxes. The effects generally require an induction period of several hours or more and frequently require new protein synthesis.[79,88,90,94,95] In some in vitro studies, the concentrations of sulfonylureas required to demonstrate an effect are beyond the usual in vivo pharmacologic range. The effects described both have been independent of insulin action and have involved augmentation of insulin action. Augmentation of insulin action, when described, has not involved alterations in insulin binding.

The major question in evaluating these extrapancreatic actions of sulfonylureas is whether they occur in vivo in humans and, if they do, how relevant they are to the clinically observed actions of sulfonylureas. Since sulfonylureas have no effects on blood glucose levels in vivo in the absence of functioning β-cells, it seems unlikely that an in vitro effect that occurs in the absence of insulin can play a significant role in the antidiabetic action of these agents. Some clinical data do support the possibility that potentiation of insulin action on liver and muscle by sulfonylureas may contribute to their antidiabetic actions.[98–103]

Clinical Pharmacology

Clinical pharmacologic studies with sulfonylureas have provided considerable insight into how they reduce hyperglycemia in patients with diabetes mellitus. Acute treatment of hyperglycemic patients with NIDDM usually results in an increase in both fasting and postprandial plasma insulin levels.[25,99,104–108] As chronic management evolves and the fasting plasma glucose levels decrease toward normal values, plasma insulin levels readjust and stabilize, resulting in a decrease in fasting and postprandial insulin levels to pretreatment, or even lower, levels.[99,109–112] Thus, more-normal glucose metabolism is established at levels of insulin secretion that may be lower than those present initially. This type of data led to the hypothesis that the sulfonylureas exert a major antidiabetic action by increasing tissue (muscle and liver) responsiveness to insulin and that the sequence of events is an initial pancreatic effect (perhaps to as long as 1 year) and a later and more prolonged extrapancreatic action.

Several features of both sulfonylurea action and the pathophysiology of NIDDM exist that limit support for such a hypothesis. Though sulfonylurea drugs stimulate insulin secretion in vitro in the absence of glucose,[44] their effects are greatly enhanced by increasing glucose concentrations.[44,113] In humans, sulfonylureas and glucose potentiate one another's insulin secretory activity such that in patients with NIDDM treatment with a sulfonylurea partially restores the sensitivity of the β-cell to glucose as an insulin secretogogue.[21,106] At the same glucose concentration, the patient with NIDDM secretes more insulin with sulfonylurea treatment than without such treatment. Thus, the decrease in plasma insulin level during chronic sulfonylurea therapy occurs because the plasma glucose is lower but β-cell function is more efficient.[114]

Additionally, it is now known that hyperglycemia itself can decrease insulin sensitivity of liver and muscle.[115,116] Reduction of hyperglycemia by any mechanism may improve insulin sensitivity, and thus endogenous insulin can be more effective in lowering blood glucose levels.[116–120] Thus, the major antidiabetic action of sulfonylureas may be explained by their ability to increase insulin secretion. The clinical data that correlate successful sulfonylurea therapy with a significant β-cell insulin secretory reserve[121–127] and the numerous studies that show little or no effect of sulfonylurea therapy on insulin sensitivity in patients with IDDM[128–130] support the suggestion that increased endogenous insulin secretion is the major antidiabetic action of sulfonylureas.

Table 29–3. Extrapancreatic Actions of Sulfonylureas Proposed as Contributing to Their Antidiabetic Actions

I. Liver
   A. Direct effects
      1. Increase fructose-2, 6-biphosphate[72,73]
      2. Increase glycolysis[74,75]
      3. Decrease gluconeogenesis[73–75]
      4. Decrease oxidation of long-chain fatty acids[75,76]
   B. Potentiate insulin action
      1. Increase hepatic glycogen synthase and glycogen synthesis[77–80]
      2. Increase hepatic lipogenesis[81]
   C. Decrease hepatic extraction of insulin[82–85]
II. Skeletal muscle
   A. Direct effects
      1. Increase glucose transport[86]
      2. Increase fructose-2, 6-biphosphate[87]
   B. Potentiation of insulin stimulation of carbohydrate transport[88–90]
III. Adipose tissue
   A. Direct effects
      1. Increase of adenosine-3'5'-monophosphate diesterase and inhibition of lipolysis[91,92]
      2. Increase glycogen synthase[93]
   B. Potentiation of insulin-mediated glucose transport[94–96] and translocation of glucose transport molecules[97]

Although it is clear that increased insulin secretion is the major effect of sulfonylurea therapy, the possibility that some extrapancreatic effects contribute to antidiabetic actions cannot be ignored.[35,46,47,131,132] Several recent studies indicate that sulfonylureas alter the rate of hepatic extraction of insulin and may increase peripheral insulin levels through this mechanism.[83-85] Some studies suggest that sulfonylureas can potentiate insulin action on liver and muscle in both patients with NIDDM and those with IDDM.[98-103,131]

In evaluating the effects of sulfonylureas, it is important to compare the differences between administering exogenous insulin and increasing the endogenous secretion of insulin through administering sulfonylurea.[14,107,131-135] Exogenously administered insulin results in peripheral hyperinsulinemia. Sulfonylurea administration, although it increases β-cell sensitivity to glucose, results in little or no hyperinsulinemia in responsive patients since the lowered plasma glucose levels counteracts the increased responsiveness. In addition, endogenous insulin secretion is responsible for the normal gradient in plasma insulin levels from portal vein to peripheral vein whereas exogenous insulin administration abolishes this gradient.

A number of studies have evaluated the effects of sulfonylurea treatment on the abnormal levels of serum lipid and lipoprotein in patients with NIDDM. Poor glycemic control in patients with NIDDM is associated with elevations in serum levels of very-low-density lipoprotein (VLDL), total triglycerides, and low-density lipoprotein (LDL) cholesterol and with decreases in serum levels of high-density lipoprotein (HDL) cholesterol and lipoprotein lipase activity.[136-143] Improved glycemic control following sulfonylurea therapy decreases levels of serum VLDL, total triglycerides, and LDL-cholesterol[136-143] and increases serum lipoprotein lipase activity.[137,141] The effects of sulfonylurea therapy on serum HDL-cholesterol are inconsistent, with various studies showing increases,[136] decreases,[143] and no effect.[138,141] Comparison of the effects of sulfonylurea therapy with those of insulin on the serum lipid and lipoprotein levels of patients with NIDDM suggests that the effects of sulfonylurea therapy are due to the better glycemic control and not to specific effects of sulfonylureas on lipid or lipoprotein metabolism.[137,142]

Platelet and coagulation abnormalities are a consequence of poor metabolic regulation in patients with NIDDM. Improved glycemic control results in some improvement in these abnormalities. Although claims have been made that specific sulfonylureas have unique beneficial effects on some of these abnormalities, they have not been validated by conclusive, well-controlled studies.[34,144,145]

Pharmacokinetic and Pharmacologic Relationships

The underlying mechanisms of the antidiabetic actions of the different sulfonylureas are virtually identical. The differences noted in their clinical effects are a result of differences in their pharmacokinetic and pharmacodynamic actions. These differences are categorized in Table 29-4 and define the characteristics by which to select a sulfonylurea for clinical use.

Table 29-4. Characteristics by Which to Select Specific Sulfonylurea

Intrinsic antidiabetic activity
Rapidity of onset of action
Duration of action
Mode of metabolism and excretion
Beneficial and detrimental side effects

Table is modified from Lebovitz.[38]

Intrinsic Antidiabetic Potency

The intrinsic antidiabetic potency of a sulfonylurea is the effect of the drug per milligram in an in vitro system. The most reliable way of assessing this activity has been to quantitate the effect on insulin secretion. More recently, intrinsic activity has been assessed in terms of the binding constant with which the drug interacts with the sulfonylurea receptor of the β-cell.[51-54,56] As assessed by these techniques, the second-generation compounds glyburide and glipizide are about 1000 times more potent than the first-generation compounds tolbutamide and chlorpropamide.

While the intrinsic potency is an important characteristic of a sulfonylurea drug, a more important characteristic is the maximal therapeutic benefit that can be obtained from that drug and the dosage necessary for achievement of that effect (Table 29-5). From the few available well-controlled studies, it appears that, with the exception of tolbutamide (which is less effective[149,167]), the therapeutic benefit of all currently available sulfonylureas is approximately the same.[33,34,37,38,156,160,168-170] A sulfonylurea with a high intrinsic activity achieves this therapeutic benefit at a significantly lower dose than does one of low intrinsic activity. The use of a lower dose of a sulfonylurea has the advantage of being associated with a reduced likelihood of adverse reactions related to some component of the molecule other than the sulfonylurea moiety and of significant interactions with other drugs in terms of competition for binding sites or of common pathways of metabolism.

Rapidity of Onset of Action

Since the insulin secretory action of sulfonylureas is dependent on activation of the sulfonylurea receptor, the rapidity with which an orally administered dose achieves significant plasma levels can determine the rapidity with which insulin secretion is augmented in response to meals,[38,168] particularly for sulfonylurea drugs with a duration of action of 24 hours or less. For example, acute studies indicate that administration of glipizide 30 minutes before breakfast provides even better glycemic control than administration with the meal.[171] Glyburide, which is more slowly absorbed than glipizide, will have a slower but more prolonged effect on morning meal-induced glycemia.[172] Rapidity of action can be influenced by factors that alter the rate of absorption of sulfonylureas.[173-175] Distention of the stomach secondary to poor glycemic regulation and interference with absorption by meals can delay absorption.

Table 29–5. Characteristics of Commonly Used Sulfonylurea Drugs

	Dose (mg/day)		Peak Level (hr)	Half-life (hr)	Duration of Action (hr)	Metabolites	Excretion
	Average	Range					
Tolbutamide [146–150]	1500	500–3000	3–4	4.5–6.5	6–10	Inactive	Kidney
Chlorpropamide [151,152]	250	100–500	2–4	36	60	Active or unchanged	Kidney
Tolazamide [153]	250	100–1000	3–4	7	16–24	Weakly active	Kidney
Acetohexamide [154,155]	250	250–1500	4–6*	5†	12–18	More active than parent drug	Kidney
Glipizide [156–165]	10	2.5–40	1–3	2–4	15–24	Inactive	Kidney 80% Bile 20%
Glyburide [159–165]	7.5	1.25–20	4	10	24	Inactive and weakly active	Kidney 50% Bile 50%
Gliclazide [144,166]	160	40–320	?	6–12	16–24	Probably inactive	Kidney 70% Bile 30%

*Active metabolite (parent drug 0.8–2.4).
†Active metabolite.

A very-long-acting drug such as chlorpropamide maintains steady-state plasma levels, and rapidity of onset of action is not an issue although desensitization may be a consideration.

Duration of Action

The duration of action of a sulfonylurea (Table 29–5) is important for several reasons. Obviously, the dosage schedule will depend on the duration of action. A drug such as chlorpropamide with a very long half-life and duration of action needs to be given only once daily. Tolbutamide, which has a very short duration of action, needs to be administered two or three times daily. Drugs with a duration of action of 16 to 24 hours can be given once a day when an average dose is used but may need to be given twice a day when maximal doses are necessary because high dose requirements reflect either a need for higher plasma concentrations to elicit a therapeutic response or a more rapid rate of metabolism (genetically determined or drug-induced) of the sulfonylurea.

The extent and frequency of severe hypoglycemic reactions appear to be related to duration of action of the sulfonylurea drug used.[176] As noted in the section of this chapter on hypoglycemia, severe and sometimes intractable hypoglycemic reactions have been observed most often with patients receiving the longer-acting sulfonylureas chlorpropamide and glyburide.[177] In contrast, the lowest incidence of severe hypoglycemic reactions is observed in patients receiving short-acting agents such as tolbutamide and glipizide.

Another, possibly important, issue is raised by the question of whether desensitization to the insulin secretory effects of sulfonylureas occurs in vivo. Several years ago, Karam et al. showed that patients receiving oral sulfonylureas were unresponsive to an intravenous infusion of tolbutamide.[178] Responsiveness returned following discontinuation of therapy with the oral agent for 12 hours or longer. Several in vitro studies have demonstrated that continuous stimulation of islet cells with sulfonylureas for many hours leads to loss of stimulated

insulin secretion by several insulin secretogogues.[179,180] Some experimental details make it difficult to interpret these studies and to extrapolate the findings to the therapeutic use of sulfonylureas. If desensitization does occur in humans under clinical conditions, treatment with multiple doses of short-acting agents might be preferable to once-a-day administration of long-acting preparations. This area of sulfonylurea clinical pharmacology needs further study.

Mode of Metabolism and Excretion

Sulfonylurea drugs are bound extensively to serum protein (primarily albumin).[181–183] Binding, which ordinarily exceeds 95% of the plasma level of drug, is both ionic and non-ionic for first-generation sulfonylureas and only non-ionic for second-generation sulfonylureas.[183–185] Sulfonylureas and other drugs that bind to serum proteins compete for binding sites. Since plasma levels of second-generation sulfonylureas are quite low and they bind only non-ionic sites, the likelihood of interactions with other drugs is less than it is with the first-generation agents.

All sulfonylureas are metabolized by the liver. Some sulfonylureas are almost totally converted to inactive or weakly active metabolites, whereas others, such as chlorpropamide, are only partially metabolized. The metabolites of acetohexamide are more active than the native molecule. Excretion of the unchanged form or the metabolites of the first-generation sulfonylureas is accomplished exclusively by the kidney. The second-generation sulfonylurea drugs and their metabolites are excreted by the kidney or in the feces (Table 29–5) in differing proportions.

Since hepatic metabolism is the major mode of sulfonylurea inactivation, it is clear that these agents should not be used in individuals with significant hepatic dysfunction. The risk of serious hypoglycemia is markedly increased, and the ability to counterregulate is significantly impaired. In patients with decreased renal function, chlorpropamide is contraindicated. Sulfonylureas that are metabolized to inactive derivatives and excreted in part in the feces are least likely to cause serious hypoglycemia in patients with mild to moderate impairment of renal function.

Beneficial and Detrimental Side Effects

Certain side effects or complications of sulfonylurea therapy are unique to the specific agents because of the substituent groups rather than the sulfonylurea moiety. The antidiuretic property of chlorpropamide, which leads to water retention and hyponatremia, falls into this category.[186–188]

Other side effects, such as alcohol-induced flushing, may be related to properties of the sulfonylureas but are influenced by the absolute quantity of drug administered. Chlorpropamide frequently and tolbutamide occasionally cause alcohol-induced flushing.[36]

Sulfonylureas in the Treatment of Patients with NIDDM

Candidates for sulfonylurea therapy are patients with NIDDM who still have adequate β-cell function and have not achieved targeted glycemic regulation with dietary therapy and an exercise program.[2,3,34,35,37,38,168] With the exception of patients with maturity-onset diabetes of youth (MODY), the diagnosis of hyperglycemia will have been made after the age of 30 years in most patients.[189–191] Patients should be of normal weight or obese, since underweight diabetic patients are likely to be insulin-dependent.[189–191] Patients who have had diagnosed hyperglycemia for less than 5 years are more likely to show good glycemic responses to sulfonylureas than are those who have had a diagnosis for more than 5 years.[189–191]

About 15 to 20% of patients with newly diagnosed NIDDM have little or no glycemic response to sulfonylureas (primary failures).[4,189,191] Approximately 50% will achieve acceptable or normal glycemic control (Table 29–1), and the remainder will achieve between acceptable and poor glycemic control.[4,189–194] To achieve acceptable or normal glycemic control, the patient must follow some dietary program. Sulfonylurea drugs supplement dietary control and do not substitute for it. Each year of treatment, about 3 to 5% of patients with NIDDM who have achieved acceptable or better glycemic control are said to lose their responsiveness to sulfonylureas (secondary failure).[123,191,195]

Acceptable or normal glycemic control with sulfonylurea therapy is characterized by a reduction in fasting hyperglycemia and hepatic glucose production; a decrease in postprandial increases in blood glucose level; an initial increase in fasting- and nutrient-stimulated insulin secretion but, with chronic therapy, either a return to initial levels or a decrease but with improved β-cell responsiveness to glucose; and improvement in peripheral and hepatic sensitivity to insulin; and no consistent alterations in glucagon secretion.[25,98–100,104,105,196–199]

Sulfonylurea therapy can induce a near-normoglycemic remission in a small but significant percentage of patients with NIDDM.[174,200,201] This remission can last in excess of 12 months if therapy is discontinued. No data exist as to whether it is more efficacious to continue patients who are in a near-normoglycemic remission on low-dose sulfonylurea therapy or to discontinue the drug until a hyperglycemic relapse has occurred. Some investigators recommend the use of sulfonylureas in patients with NIDDM with minimal hyperglycemia,[4,5,202] while others prefer to use them only when glycemic control exceeds acceptable levels.

Most studies of sulfonylurea therapy of patients with NIDDM have involved small numbers of patients, have been relatively short in duration (<2 years), or have been uncontrolled. They usually show mean decreases in levels of plasma glucose of 25 to 30% and lowering of levels of glycosylated hemoglobin of 1 to 2%. Although data on sulfonylurea treatment are abundant in the literature, most do not give significant insights into the long-term effectiveness or value of sulfonylurea therapy. Only two long-term multicenter controlled trials of sulfonylurea therapy in NIDDM exist: the University Group Diabetes Program and the United Kingdom Prospective Diabetes Study.

The University Group Diabetes Program was a multicenter study designed to evaluate and compare the effectiveness of five therapeutic regimens in preventing the vascular complications of patients with adult-onset diabetes mellitus.[203,204] From 1961 to 1966, 1027 patients with newly diagnosed diabetes were entered into the study and randomized to one of five treatment programs (approximately 200 patients per regimen): placebo, tolbutamide 1.5 g/day, a standard daily dose of insulin based on the patient's body surface area, a variable dose of insulin to maintain "normal" blood glucose, and phenformin 100 mg/day. The study lasted for 9¾ years, when it was terminated because the investigators felt that their results indicated that tolbutamide treatment was associated with an increase in presumed cardiovascular mortality.[204,205] The validity of the study and its conclusions have been debated and analyzed extensively.[206–211] It is fair to say that this large multicenter study had many flaws that make it likely the conclusions are invalid. However, several points from the study are worth noting. The fixed dose of tolbutamide lowered the mean fasting blood glucose level by 25% for the first year and progressively lost its effectiveness over the ensuing 3 years, such that by 4½ years there was no difference between the fasting blood glucose levels of the group treated with placebo and those of the group treated with the fixed tolbutamide dose. The same type of glycemic responses were observed in the group treated with a standard insulin dose.[205] Persistent reductions in fasting blood glucose levels to near-normal values were seen only in the group treated with variable doses of insulin and required an increase of mean insulin dose from an initial dose of 10.5 U/day to one of 47.0 U/day at the end of the study.[5] The event rates for microvascular and macrovascular complications were low.[205] Maintaining near-normal glycemic control with insulin failed to result in a difference in vascular complication rates as compared with the rates in the placebo group or the tolbutamide group.[5]

The United Kingdom Prospective Diabetes Study is an ongoing study designed to answer the following two major questions: 1) whether improved glycemic control of maturity-onset diabetes diminishes the morbidity and mortality of the disease and 2) whether it is preferable to lower the blood glucose concentrations with insulin or with oral hypoglycemic agents.[4,194] Several thousand patients with newly diagnosed NIDDM are being randomized to treatment with diet, sulfonylurea (chlorpropamide or glyburide), metformin, or insulin. Preliminary results indicate that 83% of patients with dietary therapy fail within 1 year and need drug treatment.[4] Sulfonylurea therapy and insulin therapy are about equally effective in reducing the fasting levels of plasma glucose and glycosylated hemoglobin for the first year.[4,194] Follow-up at 3 and 6 years of 1503 patients with newly presenting NIDDM[212] revealed the following. At 3 years, 85% of the sulfonylurea-treated patients were still well controlled with sulfonylurea (median fasting plasma glucose level, 7.2 mmol/L), 10% needed the addition of metformin to the sulfonylurea regimen, and 5% had to be switched to insulin therapy. The insulin-treated group had a median fasting plasma glucose level of 7.2 mmol/L, and the placebo-treated group had a median level of 9.0 mmol/L. By 6 years, 20% of the sulfonylurea-treated patients required the addition of metformin and 12% had to be treated with insulin. The median fasting plasma glucose level for the sulfonylurea-treated group was 7.8 mmol/L as compared with a level of 6.7 mmol/L in the insulin-treated group. Sulfonylurea therapy became progressively more inadequate, with 50% of the patients having a fasting plasma glucose level >7.0 mmol/L at 3 years and 65%, at 6 years. Those conducting the study found that the higher the fasting plasma glucose level at initial randomization (after a trial of diet treatment) the greater the likelihood of failure of sulfonylurea therapy at 6 years (median fasting plasma glucose level: successful patients, 7.7 mmol/L; unsuccessful patients, 8.8 mmol/L). The preliminary results of the United Kingdom Prospective Diabetes Study help quantitate conclusions that have been noted qualitatively in many other studies.

Many investigators have tried to define the causes of both primary and secondary failure of sulfonylurea therapy. Little insight into the cause of primary failure has been obtained other than the observation that marked insulin deficiency is a potential, although not the only, cause.[121,195] Table 29–6 lists the potential causes of secondary failure. Some secondary failures, obviously, are reversible whereas others are not.[213,214] Some investigators have suggested that a course of intensive insulin treatment can restore sulfonylurea responsiveness; however, this reversal may be only temporary.

Sulfonylureas in the Management of Patients with Impaired Glucose Tolerance

Impaired glucose tolerance (IGT) is defined as a fasting plasma glucose level of <7.8 mmol/L and a 2-hour plasma glucose level after a 75-g oral glucose load of 7.8 to 11.2 mmol/L. The glycosylated hemoglobin level is usually

Table 29–6. Common Causes of Secondary Failure of Sulfonylureas

Patient-related factors
  Overeating and weight gain
  Poor patient compliances
  Lack of physical activity
  Stress
  Intercurrent illnesses
Disease-related factors
  Decreasing β-cell function
  Increasing insulin resistance
Therapy-related factors
  Inadequate drug dosage
  Desensitization to chronic sulfonylurea exposure
  Impaired absorption of drug because of hyperglycemia
  Concomitant therapy with diabetogenic drugs

Table is modified from Groop et al.[213]

normal. The significance of IGT is that approximately 30% of patients with IGT progress to NIDDM over a 10-year follow-up period and that it increases the risk of coronary artery disease (only slightly less than that in patients with NIDDM).[215–218]

Over the years many investigators have attempted to determine whether sulfonylurea treatment in individuals with IGT could prevent the progression to NIDDM and decrease the risk of cardiovascular disease. While most such studies failed to show any significant beneficial effects,[218–220] one study carried out in Sweden suggested that sulfonylurea treatment could prevent progression to NIDDM[221] and protect against the development of cardiovascular disease.[222–224] In this study, in which the number of subjects treated was small, by 12 years, 29% of subjects with IGT who received no treatment had progressed to NIDDM whereas 13% who received dietary instruction with or without placebo and 0% who received dietary instruction with tobutamide had progressed to NIDDM. Cardiovascular complications developed in 18% receiving no treatment, 10% of those with dietary restriction, and 0% of those with dietary restriction and tolbutamide. The tolbutamide-treated group, which was quite small (29 patients), showed improvement in diastolic blood pressure and serum triglyceride and cholesterol levels.

The relatively limited number of subjects with IGT who progress to NIDDM and the conflicting data on the benefits of sulfonylurea treatment presently preclude the advocation of such treatment of individuals with IGT. However, it would seem that studies of sulfonylurea treatment in appropriate populations with a high prevalence of IGT and NIDDM are justified and should be done.

Complications of Sulfonylurea Therapy

Hypoglycemia

The major complication of sulfonylurea therapy is hypoglycemia.[176] Estimates of the true frequency of hypoglycemic reactions in patients with NIDDM taking sulfonylureas are quite inaccurate. Many patients with

NIDDM are elderly, and hypoglycemic symptoms may be misinterpreted. The use of self-monitoring of blood glucose is infrequent in patients with NIDDM. One recent study of 40- to 65-year-old patients attending a diabetes clinic found that 20.2% of those receiving sulfonylureas experienced hypoglycemic symptoms during a 6-month period.[225] Approximately 6% had hypoglycemic symptoms monthly. The prevalence of hypoglycemic symptoms was significantly higher in patients treated with glyburide than in those treated with the other commonly used sulfonylureas, gliclazide and chlorpropamide. Hypoglycemic symptoms were observed most frequently in patients who had better glycemic control, had received sulfonylureas for less than 4 years, and were taking drugs that potentiate the hypoglycemic action of sulfonylureas.

Sulfonylurea drugs are the major cause of severe drug-induced hypoglycemia necessitating hospitalization. In his most recent review of 1418 reported cases of drug-induced hypoglycemia, Seltzer noted that 59% (842) were caused by sulfonylureas and that 9% of these patients died (63) or experienced permanent neurologic or cardiovascular sequelae (13).[177] The prevalence of sulfonylurea-associated hypoglycemia necessitating hospital treatment has been reported as 0.25 per 1000 treatment years in Switzerland,[226] 0.19 per 1000 treatment years in Sweden,[227] and 4.2 per 1000 treatment years in the Swedish island of Gotland.[227] Of considerable concern are the observations in the Swiss survey that the prevalence of and mortality due to sulfonylurea-associated hypoglycemia in the two 10-year periods 1960 through 1969 and 1975 through 1984 were essentially the same (respective prevalence, 0.22 vs. 0.24 per 1000 treatment years; mortality, 6.4% vs. 4.3% of the patients hospitalized for sulfonylurea-induced hypoglycemia).

Long-acting sulfonylureas such as glyburide and chlorpropamide are associated with severe and prolonged hypoglycemia much more frequently than are short-acting sulfonylureas such as tolbutamide and glipizide.[176,177,226,228] In the recent Swiss survey, the number of sulfonylurea-associated hypoglycemic episodes necessitating hospitalization was 0.38, 0.34, 0.15, and 0.07 per 1000 treatment years for glyburide, chlorpropamide, glipizide, and tolbutamide, respectively.[226] Data from the Swedish Board of Health and Welfare for 1975 through 1985 are similar; the number of long-lasting hypoglycemic episodes per 1,000,000 defined daily doses was 0.195 for glyburide, 0.184 for chlorpropamide, 0.004 for glipizide, and 0.072 for tolbutamide.[227]

The predisposing factors associated with severe sulfonylurea-associated hypoglycemia are age (>65 years); inadequate nutrition; intercurrent illness; chronic renal, hepatic, or cardiovascular disease; and concomitant administration of drugs that either potentiate sulfonylurea action or cause hypoglycemia themselves.[177,226,228]

While overdoses of sulfonylurea will cause hypoglycemia, many cases of severe and intractable hypoglycemia have been associated with relatively low doses of sulfonylureas. Therefore, when sulfonylurea therapy is initiated in individuals who are predisposed to hypoglycemia it is important to start with minimal doses and to increase the dose slowly. **Long-acting sulfonylureas** and drugs that have the potential to **interact with** sulfonylureas to increase hypoglycemia should be avoided or used with great caution.

The treatment of mild hypoglycemic symptoms usually involves a change in drug dosage or an adjustment in meal schedules. On occasion, change to a sulfonylurea with a shorter duration of action may be necessary. Management of severe hypoglycemic reactions requires hospitalization of the patient. Patients should be given a bolus of 50% glucose followed by a continuous infusion of 10 or 20% glucose. Blood glucose levels should be monitored for at least 3 days and maintained at 6 to 8 mmol/L. An occasional patient who does not respond adequately to glucose infusions may need treatment with glucocorticoids, glucagon, or agents that inhibit the release of insulin.

Since sulfonylureas cross the placenta, severe hypoglycemia can occur in newborn infants of mothers who may have been treated with sulfonylureas. However, this should not be a significant problem since sulfonylureas are contraindicated in **pregnancy**, although Seltzer, in his review, noted 14 such cases.[177] Sulfonylurea-induced hypoglycemia has been seen in persons with diabetes who have attempted suicide, with pharmacists' errors in dispensing prescriptions, and in patients with diabetes insipidus receiving chlorpropamide.

Drug Interactions

Patients who are treated with sulfonylureas generally are middle-aged or elderly, frequently have concomitant illnesses such as hypertension, arthritis, and cardiovascular disease; and usually are taking other medications or will need to take them during the course of their sulfonylurea treatment. Sulfonylurea drugs interact with many different drugs and either modify the effects of those drugs or are modified by them.[37,38,229] It is important for the physician to understand and plan appropriately for these drugs interactions. Table 29–7 list the major mechanisms by which drugs influence the action of sulfonylurea drugs to increase or decrease their effects on blood glucose regulation.

Toxicity

The most common adverse effects associated with sulfonylurea drug administration are gastrointestinal problems, i.e., nausea, vomiting, and nonspecific abdominal discomfort (1 to 3%), and skin rashes (0.5 to 1.5%).[144,150,156,193,196,229] Rare cases of hematologic disorders (hemolytic anemia, agranulocytosis), liver disease (cholestatic jaundice, granulomatous hepatitis), and immune disorders have been reported. Most cases of toxicity occur within the first several months of therapy.

Water retention and hyponatremia are relatively frequent side effects of chlorpropamide therapy,[186,188] which occur in perhaps as many as 7% of patients and is related to both increased secretion and activity of antidiuretic hormone.[187] Other sulfonylureas do not produce this effect.

Table 29–7. Major Drug Interactions with Sulfonylureas

A. Increase in hypoglycemia
  1. Drugs that displace sulfonylurea from albumin-binding sites: aspirin, fibrates, trimethoprim
  2. Competitive inhibitors of sulfonylurea metabolism: alcohol, H_2 blockers, anticoagulants
  3. Inhibitors of urinary excretion of sulfonylureas: probenecid, allopurinol
  4. Concomitant use of drugs with hypoglycemic activities: alcohol, aspirin
  5. Antagonists of counterregulatory hormones: β-adrenergic blockers, sympatholytic drugs
B. Worsening of glycemic control
  1. Drugs that increase sulfonylurea metabolism: barbiturates, rifampin
  2. Inhibitors of insulin secretion: thiazides and loop diuretics, β-adrenergic blockers, phenytoin
  3. Inhibitors of insulin action: corticosteroids, growth hormone, estrogens, catecholamines

Table is modified from Lebovitz and Melander.[227]

Alcohol-induced flushing reaction is common in patients taking chlorpropamide. The mechanism of this response has not been elucidated but may involve interactions among plasma acetaldehyde levels, opiate peptides, and prostaglandins.[36] This flushing reaction is rarely, if ever, seen during treatment with so-called second-generation sulfonylureas.

The most frequently discussed side effect of sulfonylureas is the increase in incidence of sudden death (presumed to be cardiovascular) in patients with NIDDM treated with tolbutamide, which was reported by the University Group Diabetes Program (UGDP).[204] As noted previously, the validity and significance of the UGDP study were debated for 10 years, and many arguments have been developed to show that the conclusions are probably invalid. The most compelling have been subsequent studies showing that, if anything, tolbutamide treatment improves survival from cardiovascular disease in patients with NIDDM.[222,230–232] The recent data showing that sulfonylureas improve myocardial function by inhibiting K^+ efflux and increasing Ca^{++} entry further argue against the sulfonylureas having any detrimental effects on the heart.[67–70]

Comparison of Sulfonylurea with Insulin Therapy in Patients with NIDDM

Since hyperglycemia develops in patients with NIDDM only when relative or absolute insulin deficiency occurs, the question arises whether insulin therapy should be the treatment of choice for all such patients. Clearly, the patient with NIDDM whose fasting plasma glucose level is greater than 15 mmol/L when managed by diet is best served by some form of insulin therapy, since an acceptable or normal glycemic response to sulfonylurea therapy is highly unlikely. For patients with lesser degrees of fasting hyperglycemia (on some dietary regimen), sulfonylurea therapy has a reasonable probability of providing acceptable or normal glycemic control for at least several years. Among patients who have had such glycemic responses to sulfonylureas, the clinical differences between the results of sulfonylurea and insulin therapy appear to be minimal.[4,107,133,134,212,233]

Several arguments can be posed for the preferential use of sulfonylureas over insulin in patients with NIDDM with mild to moderate fasting hyperglycemia. Table 29–8 lists the advantages and disadvantages of both forms of therapy. Insulin therapy is more difficult and time consuming for the patient. If hyperinsulinemia is a significant risk factor for macrovascular disease, insulin therapy would be less desirable than sulfonylurea therapy. Insulin therapy is frequently associated with excessive weight gain. On the other hand, sulfonylurea therapy is associated with primary failures, and the frequency of secondary failure increases as the duration of NIDDM increases. The selection of the type of therapy is therefore individualized by a consensus decision of the health-care team and each patient.[2,233–235]

Contraindications for Sulfonylurea Therapy

It is obvious from a review of the pharmacology, clinical effects, and complications of sulfonylurea therapy that the use of these agents is contraindicated in a

Table 29–8. Advantages and Disadvantages of Sulfonylurea Therapy and Insulin Therapy in Patients with Non-Insulin-Dependent Diabetes (NIDDM)

Advantages	Disadvantages
SULFONYLUREA	
Normal portal:peripheral vein gradient of plasma insulin (2:1 or 3:1)	Only about 50% of patients achieve acceptable or normal control
Relatively little or no hyperinsulinemia	Secondary failure occurs in many by 5 years
Extrapancreatic effects may exert some benefits (possible decrease in insulin resistance)	Ineffective during severe stress, surgery, or intercurrent illnesses
Administered orally	Contraindicated during pregnancy
INSULIN	
Can achieve acceptable or normal glycemic control in most patients	Abnormal portal:peripheral vein gradient of plasma insulin (1:1)
Effective throughout the clinical course of NIDDM	Hyperinsulinemia almost always present
Effective during stress, surgery, or intercurrent illnesses	Hypoglycemia more common than with sulfonylureas
	Excessive weight gain may be a problem
	Multiple injections frequently needed
	Doses >60 units/day frequently needed

number of clinical situations (Table 29–9). It is of particular importance to note that these agents are ineffective in the absence of functional β-cells (IDDM and pancreatic destruction or removal).

Combination with Other Antidiabetic Agents

In the event that therapy with sulfonylurea drugs does not achieve acceptable or normal glycemic control, the option for treatment is the use of a combination of antidiabetic agents or the abandonment of oral therapy and the institution of an insulin regimen that frequently requires the administration of multiple insulin injections per day.

The rationale behind combination therapy is based on multiple factors. Sulfonylureas achieve their effects primarily by increasing the endogenous secretion of insulin and, perhaps to a lesser degree, by potentiating insulin action. As the defect of endogenous insulin secretion becomes more extensive, the addition of insulin administered at an appropriate time might establish acceptable glycemic control with a simple regimen and a relatively low dose of insulin. The extrapancreatic actions of sulfonylureas might increase the efficacy of the exogenous insulin. The addition of metformin to a sulfonylurea regimen provides an agent with a different mode of antidiabetic action (see section on metformin) and thus compliments sulfonylurea therapy. Inhibitors of α-glucosidase lower postprandial plasma glucose levels by delaying absorption of glucose and would be expected to be additive to sulfonylurea therapy.

Combination insulin and sulfonylurea therapy has been studied extensively and reviewed even more extensively.[236–241] Unfortunately, the experimental designs have differed remarkably, the data are conflicting, and no clear conclusions are justified. Two types of combination insulin-sulfonylurea therapy have been used: concurrent administration and sequential administration (insulin in the evening and sulfonylureas during the day). The data from studies of both types indicate that insulin-sulfonylurea therapy is neither useful nor justified in patients with IDDM. The data regarding concurrent sulfonylurea-insulin therapy in patients with NIDDM that is poorly controlled with sulfonylurea or insulin therapy alone indicate that the exogenous insulin requirements are uniformly reduced and that some patients, although clearly not the majority, will show some improvement in glycemic control with insulin-sulfonylurea therapy as compared with that seen with insulin therapy alone. Any beneficial effects achieved from the addition of sulfonylureas to an insulin regimen are attributable to increased endogenous secretion of insulin and potentiation of its action.

A somewhat more rational approach to combining insulin and sulfonylurea therapy is that of administering intermediate or long-acting insulin in the evening and sulfonylureas during the day.[240,242–245] The insulin dose in the evening is adjusted to a level that will achieve near-normal fasting levels of plasma glucose and hepatic production of glucose. The usual dose needed (10 to 25U) is modest and is achieved by starting at a low dose (6 to 10U) and increasing by 2U every 2 to 3 days until the desired fasting plasma glucose level is achieved. The sulfonylurea dose should be maximal since the regimen is indicated only for patients with NIDDM whose glycemic control with previous maximal sulfonylurea therapy has been inadequate. The administration of insulin in the evening and the achievement of near-normal fasting plasma glucose levels allows the β-cell to respond maximally to the stimuli provided during the day by the sulfonylurea and meals. There are no large, well-controlled studies validating the effectiveness of this therapy. Del Prata and co-workers treated seven patients who experienced secondary failure to sulfonylurea therapy for 2 months with ultralente insulin, at supper plus glibenclamide before each meal and showed a reduction in fasting plasma glucose level and hepatic glucose production and an improvement in the concentration of hemoglobin A_{1c} (HbA_{1c}).[246] Pasmantier et al. found similar results in a double-blind, placebo-controlled study of the efficacy of therapy with human proinsulin at bedtime and glipizide before meals.[245] Sequential insulin sulfonylurea therapy needs to be evaluated more thoroughly before its long-term risks and benefits can be defined.

Combination sulfonylurea-metformin therapy has been used for many years. Several studies show that, in about 50% of patients for whom sulfonylurea therapy has failed, the addition of metformin to the regimen achieves adequate glycemic control.[247,248]

The addition of an inhibitor of α-glucosidase such as acarbose to the regimen of patients with inadequate control with sulfonylurea alone will lower postprandial levels of glucose about 3 mmol/L and HbA_{1c} about 0.6%.[249]

METFORMIN

Biguanides, which are guanidine derivatives, were introduced into clinical use for the treatment of hyperglycemia in patients with Type II diabetes mellitus in the 1950s. Three biguanides (phenformin, metformin, and butformin) were available initially. Phenformin, which was widely prescribed in the United States, and butformin have been banned for clinical use because of a significant incidence of associated lactic acidosis. Metformin, which was introduced in France in 1959, continues to be used worldwide and is undergoing clinical investigation in the United States.

Metformin is an oral antidiabetic agent with a structure (Figure 29–3) and mode of action different from sulfonylurea drugs.[250–252] It is effective and safe for the control of

Table 29–9. Contraindications for Sulfonylurea Therapy

Insulin-dependent diabetes
Diabetes secondary to destruction or removal of the pancreas
Pregnancy
Major surgery or trauma
Severe infections
History of sensitivity to sulfa drugs or another sulfonylurea
Patients predisposed to development of severe hypoglycemia

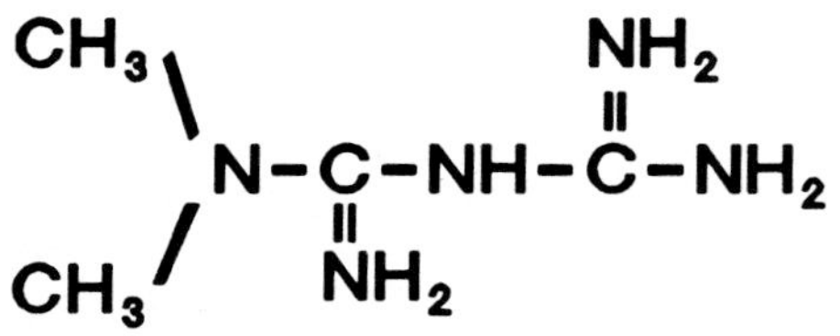

Fig. 29–3. The structure of metformin.

hyperglycemia in patients with Type II diabetes. Because of its different mechanism of action, it can be used instead of or in combination with sulfonylureas. The mechanisms of the antidiabetic action of metformin are still in question. Table 29–10 lists the various mechanisms that have been proposed. Several facts are clear. Metformin does not increase basal or meal-stimulated insulin secretion. It lowers blood glucose levels in hyperglycemic patients with Type II diabetes but has no effect on blood glucose levels in normal subjects. It does not cause hypoglycemia. Successful metformin therapy usually is associated with no weight gain or with some weight loss.[250–252]

Several studies have shown that phenformin decreases the intestinal absorption of glucose.[253,254] It is unclear whether this effect occurs at ordinary pharmacologic doses in humans or whether it occurs with metformin. Direct effects of biguanides in reducing hepatic glucose production[255–258] and in potentiating the action of insulin in decreasing hepatic glucose production[259] have been proposed by some as the primary antidiabetic actions of metformin but have been refuted by others.[270] Most studies, but not all, suggest that metformin increases insulin-mediated uptake of glucose by peripheral tissues.[261,263,266–270] Although a few in vitro and in vivo studies have demonstrated an effect of metformin on increasing the binding of insulin to the plasma membrane of insulin-sensitive cells,[260,262,264,265] most studies in patients with Type II diabetes show no effect on insulin binding,[266–269] results suggesting that metformin increases glucose uptake through post-binding mechanisms. Klip and Leiter recently suggested that metformin increases glucose transport by increasing the concentration of glucose transporter 4 (GLUT-4) in the plasma membrane of insulin-responsive cells.[271]

Table 29–10.   Proposed Mechanisms of Action of Metformin

I. Causes anorexia[250]
II. Decreases intestinal absorption of glucose[253,254]
III. Decreases hepatic glucose production
   A. Direct effect[33,255-258]
   B. Potentiates insulin action[259]
IV. Increases muscle and adipose tissue glucose uptake
   A. Direct effect[33,250]
   B. Potentiates insulin action
      1. By increasing insulin receptor binding[260–265]
      2. By postbinding mechanisms[263,266–270]
V. Increases GLUT-4 glucose transporters in insulin-sensitive cells[271]

Clinical studies have shown that metformin is as effective as chlorpropamide, tolbutamide, or gliclazide in lowering fasting and postprandial hyperglycemia in patients with newly diagnosed Type II diabetes.[272–276] However, metformin treatment produces a modest mean weight loss of 1 to 2 kg as compared with a mean weight gain of 1.5 to 5.0 kg produced by sulfonylurea therapy. Therapy with metformin results in what we would consider acceptable or better glycemic control in about 80% of patients with newly diagnosed Type II diabetes.[248,250] This response occurs in both[272] obese and non-obese patients. Reported rates of primary failure with metformin are about 12%, and those of secondary failure are about 5%.[272–275] The rate of secondary failure with metformin is said to be considerably lower than that with sulfonylureas.[250] Metformin therapy is initiated with 500 mg once or twice a day and is increased by 500 mg at weekly intervals until the target glycemic control is achieved or a maximal dose of 2.5 g/day is achieved.

Metformin used in combination with sulfonylureas has been extremely useful in the treatment of patients with Type II diabetes who have experienced secondary failure of sulfonylurea therapy. Table 29–11 presents the results of a 3-year study of 200 patients with failure of sulfonylurea therapy who were treated with a combination of metformin and a sulfonylurea.[277] The therapy is quite effective in achieving acceptable glycemic control in about 50% of patients 40 years or older. The results of most of the other reported studies of combined sulfonylurea-metformin treatment have been similar.[278–283]

Unique advantages of metformin therapy are its additional metabolic effects, some of which are useful in the management of patients with Type II diabetes. As noted previously, its use is frequently associated with a modest weight loss. Patients treated with metformin have either no increase in insulin secretion or a small decrease. Metformin treatment is associated with a decrease in plasma triglyceride levels and perhaps in a change in the composition of some lipoprotein particles.[284–286]

The most common side effects of metformin treatment are gastrointestinal problems, with anorexia, nausea, and diarrhea predominating.[250,287–289] These effects are present in 5 to 20% of patients, are usually transient, and rarely necessitate discontinuation of therapy. They are minimized by initiating therapy with low doses (500 mg/day) and by increasing the dose slowly.

The most serious side effect of biguanide therapy is associated lactic acidosis.[288,289] The reported incidence of lactic acidosis was greatest with phenformin therapy (0.6, 0.40, 0.31 and 0.23 cases per 1000 patient-years of therapy in Sweden, Switzerland, Finland, and France, respectively) and was responsible for the removal of the drug from clinical use. The mortality from phenformin-associated lactic acidosis was 67%. In contrast, the reported incidence of metformin-associated lactic acidosis ranges from 0.01 to 0.067 cases per 1000 patient-years of therapy, and the associated mortality is 33%.[288,289] Almost all cases of metformin-associated lactic acidosis were in patients with impaired renal function, which is a contraindication for biguanide therapy. Metformin-asso-

Table 29–11. Effect of Combined Sulfonylurea-Metformin Treatment in Patients with Failure of Sulfonylurea Treatment

Age at start of treatment (yr)	Outcome*	% of patients	Blood glucose (mmol/L)	
			Initial	3 yr
≤ 40	Complete success	11.5	14.5	7.8
	Partial success	. . .	. . .	. . .
	Failure	88.5	13.5–16.9	. . .
41–60	Complete success	47.4	15.1	7.2
	Partial success	. . .	. . .	. . .
	Failure	52.6	14.6	. . .
>60	Complete success	42.7	16.4	8.2
	Partial success	22.0	18.1	12.1
	Failure	35.4	17.2	. . .

Table is adapted from Clarke et al.[277]

*Complete success = blood glucose level 2 to 3 hours after meals is <11.1 mmol/L in patients >60 years old and <10 mmol/L in younger patients. Failure = blood glucose level 2 to 3 hours after meals is >13.9 mmol/L in patients <60 years old and >10 mmol in younger patients.

ciated lactic acidosis is quite rare when the drug is used appropriately. Since the introduction of metformin in Canada in 1972, not a single documented case of associated lactic acidosis has occurred in some 56,000 patient-years of treatment.[251] This safety record can be attributed to strict observance of contraindications (renal or hepatic impairment), limitation of the maximal dose to 2.5 g/day, and careful monitoring of patients with illnesses likely to cause hypoxia. The relative safety of metformin reflects its unique pharmacokinetic properties. It is not bound by serum proteins, has a mean plasma half-life of 1.5 to 2.8 hours, is not metabolized by the liver, and is excreted by the kidney.[33,250]

Malabsorption of vitamin B_{12} occurs in about 30% of metformin-treated patients, and pathologically low serum levels of B_{12} have been reported in 5.6 and 17.5% of metformin-treated patients in two series.[288] Pernicious anemia during metformin therapy is extremely rare.[288]

INHIBITORS OF α-GLUCOSIDASE

Clinical observations indicate that food intake plays a prominent role in regulating hyperglycemia in patients with Type II diabetes. Dietary management, although the cornerstone of treatment (see Chapter 24) is usually unable to achieve acceptable glycemic control in these patients. Experiments evaluating the ingestion of multiple small feedings as contrasted to one or more large meals show increased insulin sensitivity, decreased insulin secretion, decreased secretion of gastrointestinal hormone, improved lipid profiles, and frequently better glycemic control in patients.[29,290] The Bayer Pharmaceutical Company explored the concept that delayed digestion and absorption of carbohydrates would result in better glycemic regulation in patients with diabetes by developing drugs that block the α-glucosidase enzymes in the brush border of the intestinal enterocyte.[291,292] One such drug, acarbose, is in clinical use, and others (miglitol) are in clinical investigation.

Acarbose is a nonabsorbable α-glucosidase inhibitor.[249,293] It blocks the digestion of starch, sucrose, and maltose. The digestion of complex carbohydrates is delayed and occurs throughout the small intestine rather than in the upper part of the jejunum. Absorption of glucose and other monosaccharides are not affected.[294] The net result is a decrease in the postprandial increase in plasma glucose levels. Most carbohydrate is eventually absorbed; that which is not, is metabolized by the bacteria in the colon to short-chain fatty acids, which are absorbed in the colon. Additionally, acarbose decreases meal-stimulated secretion of gastric inhibitory polypeptide and other gastrointestinal peptide hormones.[295] The smaller increases in postprandial plasma glucose levels result in smaller postprandial rises in plasma insulin levels.[296,297] Acarbose does not cause weight loss, because no significant malabsorption occurs with appropriate pharmacologic doses.

Acarbose is administered orally three times a day and chewed with the first mouthful of food. The initial recommended dosage is 50 mg three times a day. The dose may be increased after 2 weeks to 100 mg three times a day. Thereafter, the dose may be increased in a stepwise fashion at 4-week intervals until the desired glycemic goal is achieved or the maximal drug dose (200 mg three times a day) is attained. The preferred method of titrating the dose is by the measurement of the 1-hour postprandial plasma glucose level. The dose of the drug should be increased for values ≥11.1 mmol/L.

In patients with Type II diabetes on a diet consisting of at least 50% carbohydrate, acarbose as primary therapy is likely to lower the mean fasting plasma glucose level by 1 mmol/L, the mean postprandial increase in level of plasma glucose by 3 mmol/L, and the level of glycosylated hemoglobin by 1%.[297–299] As an adjunct to sulfonylurea or insulin therapy, acarbose lowers postprandial glucose levels by 2.0 to 3.0 mmol/L and glycosylated hemoglobin levels by 0.5%.[299,300] This means that acarbose is useful as primary therapy in patients with Type II diabetes whose fasting plasma glucose level is ≤11.1 mmol/L and in whom use of sulfonylureas or metformin is likely to be associated with significant adverse effects. Because its mode of action is different from that of other agents, acarbose will have an additive glycemic effect when combined with sulfonylureas, metformin, or insulin in the treatment of patients with Type II diabetes patients. In insulin-treated patients, acarbose therapy results in a modest decrease in the insulin dose necessary (10 to 30%).

The major side effects of α-glucosidase inhibitors are gastrointestinal, i.e., abdominal fullness, borborygmus, increased intestinal flatulence, and diarrhea.[293,297] Side effects are reduced if acarbose therapy is initiated with low doses and the dose is increased slowly. Side effects abate significantly as the duration of treatment increases. Hypoglycemia does not occur with α-glucosidase inhibitors as primary therapy.

Concomitant use of antacids, bile acid resins, intestinal absorbents, or digestive enzyme preparations may interfere with the effectiveness of acarbose and should be used with care. Contraindications to acarbose use are primary therapy for Type I diabetes, significant gastrointestinal disorders, and pregnancy or lactation.

REFERENCES

1. Lebovitz HE. Goals of treatment. In: Lebovitz HE, ed. Therapy for diabetes mellitus and related disorders. Alexandria, VA: American Diabetes Association, 1991:1–2.
2. Lebovitz HE, ed. Physician's guide to non-insulin-dependent (type II) diabetes: diagnosis and treatment. 2nd ed. Alexandria, VA: American Diabetes Association, 1988.
3. Alberti KGMM, Gries FA. Management of non-insulin-dependent diabetes mellitus in Europe: a consensus view. Diabetic Med 1988;5:275–81.
4. Multi-centre study. UK prospective study of therapies of maturity-onset diabetes. I. Effect of diet, sulphonylurea, insulin or biguanide therapy on fasting plasma glucose and body weight over one year. Diabetologia 1983; 24:404–11.
5. University Group Diabetes Program. Effects of hypoglycemia agents on vascular complications in patients with adult-onset diabetes. VIII. Evaluation of insulin therapy: final report. Diabetes 1982;31(Suppl 5):1–26.
6. Mauer SM, Barbarosa J, Vernier RL, et al. Development of diabetic vascular lesions in normal kidneys transplanted into patients with diabetes mellitus. N Engl J Med 1976;295:916–20.
7. Pirart J. Diabetes mellitus and its degenerative complications: a prospective study of 4400 patients observed between 1947 and 1973. Diabetes Care 1978;1:168–88, 252–63.
8. Pettitt DJ, Knowler WC, Lisse JR, Bennett PH. Development of retinopathy and proteinuria in relation to plasma glucose concentrations in Pima Indians. Lancet 1980;2:1050–2.
9. Knuiman MW, Welborn TA, McCann VJ, et al. Prevalence of diabetic complications in relation to risk factors. Diabetes 1986;35:1332–9.
10. Klein R, Klein BEK, Moss SE, et al. Glycosylated hemoglobin predicts the incidence and progression of diabetic retinopathy. JAMA 1988;260:2864–71.
11. Reaven GM. Role of insulin resistance in human disease. Diabetes 1988;37:1595–607.
12. DeFronzo RA. The triumvirate: beta-cell, muscle, liver. A collusion responsible for NIDDM. Diabetes 1988; 37:667–87.
13. Unger RH, Grundy S. Hyperglycaemia as an inducer as well as a consequence of impaired islet cell function and insulin resistance: implications for the management of diabetes [Editorial]. Diabetologia 1985;28:119–21.
14. Firth R, Bell P, Rizza R. Insulin action in non-insulin-dependent diabetes mellitus: the relationship between hepatic and extrahepatic insulin resistance and obesity. Metabolism 1987;36:1091–5.
15. Banerji MA, Lebovitz HE. Insulin-sensitive and insulin-resistant variants of NIDDM. Diabetes 1989;38:784–92.
16. Lillioja S, Mott DM, Howard BV, et al. Impaired glucose tolerance as a disorder of insulin action: longitudinal and cross-sectional studies in Pima Indians. N Engl J Med 1988;318:1217–25.
17. Haffner SM, Stern MP, Hazuda HP, et al. Increased insulin concentrations in nondiabetic offspring of diabetic parents. N Engl J Med 1988;319:1297–301.
18. Eriksson J, Franssila-Kallunk A, Ekstrand A, et al. Early metabolic defects in persons at increased risk for non-insulin-dependent diabetes mellitus. N Engl J Med 1989;321:337–43.
19. O'Rahilly SP, Nugent Z, Rudenski AS, et al. Beta-cell dysfunction rather than insulin insensitivity is the primary defect in familial Type 2 diabetes. Lancet 1986;2:360–4.
20. Temple RC, Carrington CA, Luzio SD, et al. Insulin deficiency in non-insulin dependent diabetes. Lancet 1989;1:293–5.
21. Ward WK, Beard JC, Halter JB, et al. Pathophysiology of insulin secretion in non-insulin-dependent diabetes mellitus. Diabetes Care 1984;7:491–502.
22. Arner P, Pollare T, Lithell H. Different aetiologies of type 2 (non-insulin-dependent) diabetes mellitus in obese and non-obese subjects. Diabetologia 1991;34:483–7.
23. Banerji MA, Lebovitz HE. Insulin action in black Americans with non-insulin dependent diabetes mellitus. Diabetes Care 1992;15 (in press).
24. Campbell PJ, Mandarino LJ, Gerich JE. Quantification of the relative impairment in actions of insulin on hepatic glucose production and peripheral glucose uptake in non-insulin-dependent diabetes mellitus. Metabolism 1988;37:15–21.
25. Best JD, Judzewitsch RG, Pfeifer MA, et al. The effect of chronic sulfonylurea therapy on hepatic glucose production in non-insulin-dependent diabetes. Diabetes 1982; 31:333–8.
26. Glauber H, Wallace P, Brechtel G. Effects of fasting on plasma glucose and prolonged tracer measurement of hepatic glucose output in NIDDM. Diabetes 1987; 36:1187–94.
27. Hadden DR, Montgomery DAD, Skelly RJ, et al. Maturity-onset diabetes mellitus: response to intensive dietary management. BMJ 1975;3:276–8.
28. Firth RG, Bell PM, Marsh HM, et al. Postprandial hyperglycemia in patients with noninsulin-dependent diabetes mellitus: role of hepatic and extrahepatic tissues. J Clin Invest 1986;77:1525–32.
29. Jenkins DJA, Wolever TMS, Vuksan V, et al. Nibbling versus gorging: metabolic advantages of increased meal frequency. N Engl J Med 1989;321:929–34.
30. Lebovitz HE. New pharmacological approaches to the management of hyperglycemia in patients with NIDDM. In: Cameron S, Colagiuri S, Heding L, et al, eds. Non-insulin dependent diabetes mellitus. Amsterdam: Excerpta Medica, 1989:62–7.

31. Janbon M, Chaptal J, Vedel A, Schaap J. Accidents hypoglycemiques graves par un sulfamidothiadiazole. Montpellier Med 1942;441:21–2.

32. Loubatieres A. The hypoglycemic sulfonamides: history and development of the problem from 1942 to 1945. Ann NY Acad Sci 1957;71:4–11.

33. Marchetti P, Navalesi R. Pharmacokinetic-pharmacodynamic-relationships of oral hypoglycaemic agents: an update. Clin Pharmacokinet 1989;16:100–28.

34. Melander A, Bitzén P-O, Faber O, Groop L. Sulphonylurea antidiabetic drugs: an update of their clinical pharmacology and rational therapeutic use. Drugs 1989;37:58–72.

35. Lebovitz HE, Feinglos MN. Sulfonylurea drugs: mechanism of antidiabetic action and therapeutic usefulness. Diabetes Care 1978;1:189–8.

36. Lebovitz HE. Oral hypoglycemic agents. In: Alberti KGMM, Krall LP, eds. The diabetes annual/I. Amsterdam: Elsevier, 1985:93–110.

37. Gerich JE. Oral hypoglycemic agents. N Engl J Med 1989;321:1231–45.

38. Lebovitz HE. Sulfonylurea drugs. In: Lebovitz HE, ed. Therapy of diabetes mellitus and related disorders. American Diabetes Association: Alexandria, VA, 1991:112–9.

39. Houssay BA, Penhos JC. Action of the hypoglycemic sulfonyl compounds in hypophysectomized, adrenalectomized and depancreatized animals. Metabolism 1958; 5:727–32.

40. Mirsky IA, Perisutti G, Jinks R. Ineffectiveness of sulfonylureas in alloxan diabetic rats. Proc Soc Exp Biol Med 1956;91:475–7.

41. Parker ML, Pildes RS, Chao K-L, et al. Juvenile diabetes mellitus, a deficiency in insulin. Diabetes 1968;17:27–32.

42. Joffe BI, Jackson WPU, Bank S, Vinik AI. Effect of oral hypoglycemic agents on glucose tolerance in pancreatic diabetes. Gut 1972;13:285–8.

43. Yalow RS, Black H, Villazon M, Berson SA. Comparison of plasma insulin levels following administration of tolbutamide and glucose. Diabetes 1968;9:356–62.

44. Grodsky GM, Epstein GH, Fanska R, Karam JH. Pancreatic action of the sulfonylureas. Fed Proc 1977;36:2714–9.

45. Malaisse WJ, Lebrun P. Mechanisms of sulfonylurea-induced insulin release. Diabetes Care 1990;13(Suppl 3):9–17.

46. Feldman JW, Lebovitz HE. Appraisal of the extra-pancreatic actions of sulfonylureas. Arch Intern Med 1969; 123:314–22.

47. Beck-Nielsen H, Hother-Nielsen O, Pedersen O. Mechanism of action of sulphonylureas with special reference to the extrapancreatic effect: an overview. Diabetic Med 1988;5:613–20.

48. Hellman B, Sehlin J, Täljedal I-B. The pancreatic beta-cell recognition of insulin secretagogues. IV. Islet uptake of sulfonylureas. Diabetologia 1973;9:210–6.

49. Hellman B, Sehlin J, Täljedal I-B. Glibenclamide is exceptional among hypoglycaemic sulphonylureas in accumulating progressively in β-cell-rich pancreatic islets. Acta Endocrinol 1984;105:385–90.

50. Carpentier J-L, Sawano F, Ravazzola M, Malaisse WJ. Internalization of ^{3}H-glibenclamide in pancreatic islet cells. Diabetologia 1986;29:259–61.

51. Kaubisch N, Hammer R, Wollheim C, et al. Specific receptors for sulfonylureas in brain and in a β-cell tumor of the rat. Biochem Pharmac 1982;31:1171–4.

52. Geisen K, Hitzel V. Ökomonopoulos R, et al. Inhibition of ^{3}H-glibenclamide binding to sulfonylurea receptors by oral antidiabetics. Arzneim Forsch 1985;35:707–12.

53. Schmid-Antomarchi H, DeWeille J, Fosset M, Lazdunski M. The receptor for antidiabetic sulfonylureas controls the activity of the ATP-modulated K$^+$ channel in insulin-secreting cells. J Biol Chem 1987;262:15840–4.

54. Gaines KL, Hamilton S, Boyd AE III. Characterization of the sulfonylurea receptor on beta cell membranes. J Biol Chem 1988;263:2589–92.

55. Kramer W, Oekonomopulos R, Pünter J, Summ H-D. Direct photoaffinity labeling of the putative sulfonylurea receptor in rat beta-cell tumor membranes by [^{3}H]glibenclamide. FEBS Lett 1988;229:355–9.

56. Siconolfi-Baez L, Banerji MA, Lebovitz HE. Characterization and significance of sulfonylurea receptors. Diabetes Care 1990;13(Suppl 3):2–8.

57. Cook DL, Satin LS, Ashford MLJ, Hales CN. ATP-sensitive K$^+$ channels in pancreatic β-cells; spare channel hypothesis. Diabetes 1988;37:495–8.

58. Boyd AE III. Sulfonylurea receptors, ion channels, and fruit flies. Diabetes 1988;37:847–50.

59. Nelson TY, Gaines KL, Rajan AS, et al. Increased cytosolic calcium: a signal for sulfonylurea-stimulated insulin release from beta cells. J Biol Chem 1987;262:2608–12.

60. Prentki M, Wollheim CB. Cytosolic free Ca^{2+} in insulin secreting cells and its regulation by isolated organelles. Experientia 1984;40:1052–60.

61. Rorsman P, Trube G. Glucose dependent K$^+$-channels in pancreatic β-cells are regulated by intracellular ATP. Pflugers Arch 1985;405:305–9.

62. Panten U, Zünkler BJ, Scheit S, et al. Regulation of energy metabolism in pancreatic islets by glucose and tolbutamide. Diabetologia 1986;29:648–54.

63. Wollheim CB, Biden TJ. Signal transduction in insulin secretion: comparison between fuel stimuli and receptor agonists. Ann NY Acad Sci 1986;488:317–33.

64. Lupo B, Bataille D. A binding site for [^{3}H]glipizide in the rat cerebral cortex. Eur J Pharmacol 1987;140:157–69.

65. Bernardi H, Fosset M, Lazdunski M. Characterization, purification and affinity labeling of the brain [3H]glibenclamide-binding protein, a putative neuronal ATP regulated K$^+$ channel. Proc Natl Acad Sci USA 1988;85:9816–20.

66. Schmid-Antomarchi H, Amoroso S, Fosset M, Lazdunski M. K$^+$ channel openers activate brain sulfonylurea-sensitive K$^+$ channels and block neurosecretion. Proc Natl Acad Sci USA 1990;87:3489–92.

67. Belles B, Hescheler J, Trube G. Changes of membrane currents in cardiac cells induced by long whole-cell recordings and tolbutamide. Pflugers Arch 1987; 409:582–8.

68. Escande D, Thuringer D, Leguern S, Cavero I. The potassium channel opener cromakalim (BRL 34915) activates ATP-dependent K$^+$ channels in isolated cardiac myocytes. Biochem Biophys Res Commun 1988; 154:620–5.

69. Fosset M, De Weille JR, Green RD, et al. Antidiabetic sulfonylureas control action potential properties in heart cells via high affinity receptors that are linked to ATP-dependent K+ channels. J Biol Chem 1988;263:7933–6.

70. Mozaffari MS, Allo S, Schaffer SW. The effect of sulfonylurea therapy on defective calcium movement associated with diabetic cardiomyopathy. Can J Physiol Pharmacol 1989;67:1431–6.

71. Standen NB, Quale JM, Davies NW, et al. Hyperpolarizing vasodilators activate ATP-sensitive K+ channels in arterial smooth muscle. Science 1989;245:177–80.

72. Matsuda M, Kaku K, Hatao K, Kaneko T. Tolbutamide and insulin stimulation of fructose-2,6-bisphosphate formation

in hepatocytes differs. Diabetes Res Clin Pract 1986; 2:347–51.

73. Monge L, Mojena M, Ortega JL, et al. Chlorpropamide raises fructose-2,6-bisphosphate concentration and inhibits gluconeogenesis in isolated rat hepatocytes. Diabetes 1986;5:89–96.

74. Patel TB. Effects of tolbutamide on gluconeogenesis and glycolysis in isolated perfused rat liver. Am J Physiol 1986;250:E82–6.

75. McCormick K, Williams MC, Sicoli R, Chen L. Effect of tolazamide on basal ketogenesis, glycogenesis and gluconeogenesis in liver obtained from normal and diabetic rats. Endocrinology 1986;119:1268–73.

76. Patel TB. Effect of sulfonylureas on hepatic fatty acid oxidation. Am J Physiol 1986;251:E241–6.

77. Blumenthal SA. Potentiation of the hepatic action of insulin by chlorpropamide. Diabetes 1977;26:485–9.

78. Rinninger F, Kirsch D, Haring HU, Kemmler W. Extrapancreatic action of the sulphonylurea gliquidone: postreceptor effect on insulin-stimulated glycogen synthesis in rat hepatocytes in primary culture. Diabetologia 1984; 26:462–5.

79. Fleig WE, Noether-Fleig G, Fussgaenger R, Ditschuneit H. Modulation by a sulfonylurea of insulin-dependent glycogenesis, but not of insulin binding in cultured rat hepatocytes: evidence for a postreceptor mechanism of action. Diabetes 1984;33:285–90.

80. McGuinness OP, Green DR, Cherrington AD. Glyburide sensitizes perfused rat liver to insulin-induced suppression of glucose output. Diabetes 1987;36:472–6.

81. Salhanick AI, Konowitz P, Amatruda JM. Potentiation of insulin action by a sulfonylurea in primary cultures of hepatocytes from normal and diabetic rats. Diabetes 1983;32:206–12.

82. Mirsky IA, Perisutti G, Diengott D. The inhibition of insulinase by hypoglycemic sulfonamides. Metabolism 1956;5:156–61.

83. Almér L-O, Johansson E, Melander A, Wahlin-Boll E. Influence of sulfonylureas on the secretion, disposal and effect of insulin. Eur J Clin Pharmacol 1982;22:27–32.

84. Scheen AJ, Lefebvre PJ, Luyckx AS. Glipizide increases plasma insulin but not C-peptide level after a standardized breakfast in Type 2 diabetic patients. Eur J Clin Pharmacol 1984;26:471–4.

85. Groop LC, Groop P-H, Stenman S, et al. Do sulfonylureas influence hepatic insulin clearance? [Letter] Diabetes Care 1988;1:689–90.

86. Rogers BJ, Standaert ML, Pollet RJ. Direct effects of sulfonylurea agents on glucose transport in the BC 3H-1 myocyte. Diabetes 1987;36:1292–6.

87. Matsuda M, Kaku K, Kaneko T. Regulation of muscle fructose 2,6-bisphosphate levels by sulfonylureas. Endocrinol Japon 1986;33:913–7.

88. Feldman JM, Lebovitz HE. An insulin-dependent effect of chronic tolbutamide administration on the skeletal muscle carbohydrate transport system. Diabetes 1969;18:84–95.

89. Putnam WS, Andersen DK, Jones RS, Lebovitz HE. Selective potentiation of insulin-mediated glucose disposal in normal dogs by the sulfonylurea glipizide. J Clin Invest 1981;67:1016–23.

90. Wang PH, Beguinot F, Smith RJ. Augmentation of the effects of insulin and insulin-like growth factors I and II on glucose uptake in cultured rat skeletal muscle cells by sulfonylureas. Diabetologia 1987;30:797–803.

91. Solomon SS, Deaton J, Shankar TP, Palazzolo M. Cyclic AMP phosphodiesterase in Diabetes: effect of glyburide. Diabetes 1986;35:1233–6.

92. Okuno S, Inaba M, Nishizawa Y, et al. Effect of tolbutamide and glyburide on cAMP-dependent protein kinase activity in rat liver cytosol. Diabetes 1988;37:857–61.

93. Altan N, Altan VM, Mikolay L, et al. Insulin-like and insulin-enhancing effects of the sulfonylurea glyburide on rat adipose glycogen synthase. Diabetes 1985;34:281–6.

94. Maloff BL, Lockwood DH. In vitro effects of a sulfonylurea on insulin action in adipocytes: potentiation of insulin-stimulated hexose transport. J Clin Invest 1981;68:85–90.

95. Jacobs DB, Hayes GR, Lockwood DH. Effect of chlorpropamide on glucose transport in rat adipocytes in the absence of changes in insulin binding and receptor-associated tyrosine kinase activity. Metabolism 1987; 36:548–54.

96. Martz A, Jo I, Jung CY. Sulfonylurea binding to adipocyte membranes and potentiation of insulin-stimulated hexose transport. J Biol Chem 1989;264:13672–8.

97. Jacobs DB, Jung CY. Sulfonylurea potentiates insulin-induced recruitment of glucose transport carrier in rat adipocytes. J Biol Chem 1985;260:2593–6.

98. Lebovitz HE, Feinglos MN, Bucholtz HK, Lebovitz FL. Potentiation of insulin action: a probable mechanism for the anti-diabetic action of sulfonylurea drugs. J Clin Endocrinol Metab 1977;45:601–4.

99. Kolterman OG, Gray RX, Shapiro G, et al. The acute and chronic effects of sulfonylurea therapy in type II diabetic subjects. Diabetes 1984;33:346–54.

100. Ward G, Harrison LC, Proietto J, et al. Gliclazide therapy is associated with potentiation of postbinding insulin action in obese non-insulin-dependent diabetic subjects. Diabetes 1985;34:241–5.

101. Pontiroli AE, Alberetto M, Bertoletti A, et al. Sulfonylureas enhance in vivo the effectiveness of insulin in type 1 (insulin-dependent) diabetes mellitus. Horm Metab Res 1984;16(Suppl):167–70.

102. Pernet A, Trimble ER, Kuntschen F, et al. Sulfonylureas in insulin-dependent (type 1) diabetes: evidence for an extrapancreatic effect in vivo. J Clin Endocrinol Metab 1985;61:247–51.

103. Faber OK. Beck-Nielsen H, Binder C, et al. Acute actions of sulfonylurea drugs during long-term treatment of NIDDM. Diabetes Care 1990;13(Suppl 3):26–31.

104. Greenfield MS, Doberne L, Rosenthal M, et al. Effect of sulfonylurea treatment on in vivo insulin secretion and action in patients with non-insulin-dependent diabetes mellitus. Diabetes 1982;31:307–12.

105. Judzewitsch RG, Pfeifer MA, Best JD, et al. Chronic chlorpropamide therapy of non-insulin-dependent diabetes augments basal and stimulated insulin secretion by increasing islet sensitivity to glucose. J Clin Endocrinol Metab 1982;55:321–8.

106. Pfeifer MA, Halter JB, Judzewitsch RG, et al. Acute and chronic effects of sulfonylurea drugs on pancreatic islet function in man. Diabetes Care 1984;7(Suppl 1):25–34.

107. Firth R, Bell P, Marsh M, Rizza RA. Effects of tolazamide and exogenous insulin on pattern of postprandial carbohydrate metabolism in patients with non-insulin-dependent diabetes mellitus: results of a randomized crossover trial. Diabetes 1987;36:1130–8.

108. Groop L, Groop P-H, Stenman S, et al. Comparison of pharmacokinetics metabolic effects and mechanism of action of glyburide and glipizide during long-term treatment. Diabetes Care 1987;10:671–8.

109. Reaven G, Dray J. Effect of chlorpropamide on serum glucose and immunoreactive insulin concentrations in patients with maturity-onset diabetes mellitus. Diabetes 1967;16:487–92.

110. Feldman JM, Lebovitz HE. Endocrine and metabolic effects of glybenclamide: evidence for an extrapancreatic mechanism of action. Diabetes 1971;20:745–55.

111. Duckworth WC, Solomon SS, Kitabchi AE. Effect of chronic sulfonylurea therapy on plasma insulin and proinsulin levels. J Clin Endocrinol Metab 1972;35:585–91.

112. Elkeles RS, Heding LG, Paisey RB. The long-term effects of chlorpropamide on insulin C-peptide and proinsulin secretion. Diabetes Care 1982;5:427–9.

113. Kadowaki S, Taminato T, Chiba T, et al. Effect of tolbutamide on insulin glucagon and somatostatin release from the diabetic rat pancreas with special reference to glucose concentration. Endocrinology 1983; 112:2187–92.

114. Sumi S, Ichihara K, Nonaka K, Tarui S. Effect of the discontinuation of long-term sulfonylurea treatment on blood glucose and insulin secretion in non-insulin-dependent diabetes mellitus. Endocrinol Japon 1982;29:41–7.

115. Yki-Järvinen H, Helve E, Koivisto VA. Hyperglycemia decreases glucose uptake in Type I diabetes. Diabetes 1987;36:892–6.

116. Rossetti L, Smith D, Shulman GI, et al. Correction of hyperglycemia with phlorizin normalizes tissue sensitivity to insulin in diabetic rats. J Clin Invest 1987;79:1510–5.

117. Garvey WT, Olefsy JM, Griffin J, et al. The effect of insulin treatment on insulin secretion and insulin action in type II diabetes mellitus. Diabetes 1985;34:222–34.

118. Scarlett JA, Gray RS, Griffin J, et al. Insulin treatment reverses the insulin resistance of Type II diabetes mellitus. Diabetes Care 1982;5:353–3.

119. Scarlett JA, Kolterman OG, Ciaraldi TP, et al. Insulin treatment reverses the post-receptor defect in adipocyte 3-0-methylglucose transport in type II diabetes mellitus. J Clin Endocrinol Metab 1983;56:1195–201.

120. Ginsberg H, Rayfield EJ. Effect of insulin therapy on insulin resistance in type II diabetic subjects: evidence for heterogeneity. Diabetes 1981;30:739–45.

121. Sartor G. Ursing D, Nilsson-Ehle P, et al. Lack of primary effect of sulphonylurea (glipizide) on plasma lipoproteins and insulin action in former type 2 diabetics with attenuated insulin secretion. Eur J Clin Pharmacol 1987; 33:279–82.

122. Snehalatha C, Ramachandran A, Mohan V, et al. Beta cell function in long term NIDDM (type 2) patients and its relation to treatment. Horm Metab Res 1986;18:391–4.

123. Groop LC, Pelkonen R, Koskimies S, et al. Secondary failure to treatment with oral antidiabetic agents in non-insulin-dependent diabetes. Diabetes Care 1986; 9:129–33.

124. Gutniak M, Karlander S-G, Efendić S. Glyburide decreases insulin requirement increases β-cell response to mixed meal and does not affect insulin sensitivity: effects of short-and long-term combined treatment in secondary failure to sulfonylurea. Diabetes Care 1987;10:545–54.

125. Mauerhoff T, Ketelslegers JM, Lambert AE. Effect of glibenclamide in insulin-treated diabetic patients with a residual insulin secretion. Diabetes Metab 1986;12:34–7.

126. Stenman S, Groop P-H, Saloranta C, et al. Effects of the combination of insulin and glibenclamide in type 2 (non-insulin-dependent) diabetic patients with secondary failure to oral hypoglycemic agents. Diabetologia 1988;31:206–13.

127. Castillô M, Scheen AJ, Paolisso G, Lefebvre PJ. The addition of glipizide to insulin therapy in type-II diabetic patients with secondary failure to sulfonylureas is useful only in the presence of a significant residual insulin secretion. Acta Endocrinol 1987;116:364–72.

128. Grunberger G, Ryan J, Gorden P. Sulfonylureas do not affect insulin binding or glycemic control in insulin-dependent diabetics. Diabetes 1982;31:890–6.

129. Ratzmann KP, Schulz B, Heinke P, Besch W. Tolbutamide does not alter insulin requirement in type 1 (insulin-dependent) diabetes. Diabetologia 1984;27:8–12.

130. Simonson DC, Delprato S, Castellino P, et al. Effect of glyburide on glycemic control, insulin requirement, and glucose metabolism in insulin-treated diabetic patients. Diabetes 1987;36:136–46.

131. Nankervis A, Proietto J, Aitken P, et al. Differential effects of insulin therapy on hepatic and peripheral insulin sensitivity in type 2 (non-insulin-dependent) diabetes. Diabetologia 1982;23:320–5.

132. Lebovitz HE. Oral hypoglycemic sulfonylureas: pancreatic vs extrapancreatic effects. In: Shigeta Y, Lebovitz HE, Gerich JE, Malaisse WJ, eds. Best approach to the ideal therapy of diabetes mellitus. Amsterdam: Excerpta Medica, 1987:21–6.

133. Hidaka H, Nagulesparan M, Klimes I, et al. Improvement of insulin secretion but not insulin resistance after short term control of plasma glucose in obese type II diabetics. J Clin Endocrinol Metab 1982;54:217–22.

134. Firth RG, Bell PM, Rizza RA. Effects of tolazamide and exogenous insulin on insulin action in patients with non-insulin-dependent diabetes mellitus. N Engl J Med 1986;314:1280–6.

135. Firth RC. Insulin: either alone or combined with oral hypoglycemic agents. Primary Care 1988;15:665–83.

136. Greenfield MS, Doberne L, Rosenthal M, et al. Lipid metabolism in non-insulin-dependent diabetes mellitus: effect of glipizide therapy. Arch Intern Med 1982; 142:1498–500.

137. Pfeifer MA, Brunzell JD, best JD, et al. The response of plasma triglyceride cholesterol and lipoprotein lipase to treatment in non-insulin-dependent diabetic subjects without familial hypertriglyceridemia. Diabetes 1983; 32:525–31.

138. Huupponen RK, Viikari JS, Saarimaa H. Correlations of serum lipids with diabetes control in sulfonylurea-treated diabetic patients. Diabetes Care 1984;7:575–8.

139. Taskinen M-R, Bogardus C, Kennedy A, Howard BV. Multiple disturbances of free fatty acid metabolism in noninsulin-dependent diabetes: effect of oral hypoglycemic therapy. J Clin Invest 1985;76:637–44.

140. Hughes TA, Kramer JO, Segrest JP. Effects of glyburide therapy on lipoproteins in non-insulin-dependent diabetes mellitus. Am J Med 71985;9(Suppl 3B): 86–91.

141. Taskinen M-R, Beltz WF, Harper I, et al. Effects of NIDDM on very-low-density lipoprotein triglyceride and apolipoprotein B metabolism: studies before and after sulfonylurea therapy. Diabetes 1986;35:1268–77.

142. Kasim SE, LeBoeuf RC, Rockett MJ, et al. The effects of oral agent or insulin treatments on the plasma lipoproteins and the plasma lipoprotein lipase activator in diabetic patients. Horm Metab Res 1986;18:190–3.

143. Schmitt JK, Harriman K, Poole JR. Modification of therapy from insulin to chlorpropamide decreases HDL cholesterol in patients with non-insulin-dependent diabetes mellitus. Diabetes Care 1987;10:692–6.

144. Holmes B, Heel RC, Brogden RN, et al. Gliclazide: a preliminary review of its pharmacodynamic properties and therapeutic efficacy in diabetes mellitus. Drugs 1984;27:301–27.

145. Blumenthal SA. Sulfonylureas and platelet function [Letter]. Am J Med 1983;74:795.

146. Thomas RC, Ikeda GJ. The metabolic fate of tolbutamide in man and in the rat. J Med Chem 1966;9:507–10.

147. Melander A, Sartor G, Wåhlin E, et al. Serum tolbutamide and chlorpropamide concentrations in patients with diabetes mellitus. BMJ 1978;1:142–4.

148. Scott J, Poffenbarger PL. Pharmacogenetics of tolbutamide metabolism in humans. Diabetes 1979;28:41–51.

149. Fineberg SE, Schneider SH. Glipizide versus tolbutamide an open trial: effects on insulin secretory patterns and glucose concentrations. Diabetologia 1980;18:49–54.

150. O'Donovan CJ. Analysis of long-term experience with tolbutamide (orinase) in the management of diabetes. Curr Ther Res 1959;1:69–87.

151. Brotherton PM, Grieveson P, McMartin C. A study of the metabolic fate of chlorpropamide in man. Clin Pharmacol Ther 1969;10:505–14.

152. Taylor JA. Pharmacokinetics and biotransformation of chlorpropamide in man. Clin Pharmacol Ther 1972; 13:710–8.

153. Thomas RC, Duchamp DJ, Judy RW, Ikeda GJ. Metabolic fate of tolazamide in man and in the rat. J Med Chem 1978;21:725–32.

154. Smith DL, Vecchio TJ, Forist AA. Metabolism of antidiabetic sulfonylureas in man. I. Biological half-lives of the p-acetylbenzenesulfonylureas, U-18536 and acetohexamide, and their metabolites. Metabolism 1965;14:229–40.

155. Galloway JA, McMahon RE, Culp HW, et al. Metabolism, blood levels and rate of excretion of acetohexamide in human subjects. Diabetes 1967;16:118–27.

156. Lebovitz HE. Glipizide: a second-generation sulfonylurea hypoglycemic agent: pharmacology, pharmacokinetics and clinical use. Pharmacotherapy 1985;5:63–77.

157. Brogden RN, Heel RC, Pakes GE, et al. Glipizide: a review of its pharmacological properties and therapeutic use. Drugs 1979;18:329–53.

158. Wåhlin-Boll E, Almér L-O, Melander A. Bioavailability pharmacokinetics and effect of glipizide in type 2 diabetics. Clin Pharmacokinet 1982;7:363–72.

158a. Groop L, Luzi L, Melander A, et al. Different effects of glyburide and glipizide on insulin secretion and hepatic glucose production in normal and NIDDM subjects. Diabetes 1987;36:1320–8.

160. Groop L, Wåhlin-Boll E, Goop P-H, et al. Pharmacokinetics and metabolic effects of glibenclamide and glipizide in type 2 diabetics. Eur J Clin Pharmacol 1985;28:697–704.

161. Balant L, Fabre J, Zahnd GR. Comparison of the pharmacokinetics of glipizide and glibenclamide in man. Eur J Clin Pharmacol 1975;8:63–9.

162. Rogers HJ, Spector RG, Morrison PJ, Bradbrook ID. Pharmacokinetics of intravenous glibenclamide investigated by high performance liquid chromatographic assay. Diabetologia 1982;23:37–40.

163. Arnquist HJ, Karlberg BE, Melander A. Pharmacokinetics and effects of glibenclamide in two formulations, HB 419 and HB 420, in type 2 diabetes. Ann Clin Res 1983; 15(Suppl 37):21–5.

164. Matsuda A, Kuzuya T, Sugita Y, Kawashima K. Plasma levels of glibenclamide in diabetic patients during its routine clinical administration determined by a specific radioimmunoassay. Horm Metab Res 1983;15:425–8.

165. Ikegawi H, Shima K, Tanaka A, et al. Interindividual variation in the absorption of glibenclamide in man. Acta Endocrinol 1986;111:528–32.

166. Campbell DB, Adriaenssens P, Hopkins YW, et al. Pharmacokinetics and metabolism of gliclazide: a review. In: Keen H, Caldwell ADS, Murphy M, Bowker C, eds. Gliclazide and the treatment of diabetes. International Congress and Symposium Series no. 20. London: Academic Press, 1980:71–82.

167. Singer DL, Hurwitz D. Long-term experience with sulfonylureas and placebo. N Engl J Med 1967;277:450–6.

168. Melander A, Lebovitz HE, Faber OK. Sulfonylureas: why, which, and how? Diabetes Care 1990;13(Suppl 3):18–25.

169. Ferner RE, Chaplin S. The relationship between the pharmacokinetics and pharmacodynamic effects of oral hypoglycemic drugs. Clin Pharmacokinet 1987; 12:379–401.

170. Clarke BF, Campbell IW. Long term comparative trial of glibenclamide and chlorpropamide in diet-failed, maturity-onset diabetics. Lancet 1975;1:246–8.

171. Wåhlin-Boll E, Melander A, Sartor G, Scherstén B. Influence of food intake on the absorption and effect of glipizide in diabetics and healthy subjects. Eur J Clin Pharmacol 1980;18:279–83.

172. Sartor G, Lundquist I, Melander A, et al. Improved effect of glibenclamide on administration before breakfast. Eur J Clin Pharmacol 1982;21:403–8.

173. Sartor G, Melander A, Scherstén B, Wåhlin-Boll E. Influence of food and age on the single dose kinetics and effects of tolbutamide and chlorpropamide. Eur J Clin Pharmacol 1980;17:285–93.

174. Antal EJ, Gillespie WR, Phillips JP, Albert KS. The effect of food on the bioavailability and pharmacodynamics of tolbutamide in diabetic patients. Eur J Clin Pharmacol 1982;22:459–62.

175. Samanta A, Jones GR, Burden AC, Shakir I. Improved effect of tolbutamide when given before food in patients on long-term therapy [Letter]. Br J Clin Pharmacol 1984; 18:647–8.

176. Ferner RE, Neil HAW. Sulphonylureas and hypoglycaemia. BMJ 1988;296:949–50.

177. Seltzer H.S. Drug-induced hypoglycemia: a review of 1418 cases. Endocrinol Metab Clin North Am 1989;18:163–83.

178. Karam JH, Sanz N, Salamon E, Nolte MS. Selective unresponsiveness of pancreatic β-cells to acute sulfonylurea stimulation during sulfonylurea therapy in NIDDM. Diabetes 1986;35:1314–20.

179. Grodsky GM. A new phase of insulin secretion. How will it contribute to our understanding of β-cell function? Diabetes 1989;38:673–8.

180. Bailey TS, Lebovitz HE. Continuous sulfonylurea exposure desensitizes beta cell insulin secretion at a distal site [Abstract no. 548]. Diabetes 1990;39(Suppl 1):137A.

181. Judis J. Binding of sulfonylureas to serum proteins. J Pharm Sci 1972;61:89–93.

182. Hsu P-L, Ma JKH, Luzzi LA. Interactions of sulfonylureas with plasma proteins. J Pharm Sci 1974;63:570–3.

183. Crooks MJ, Brown KF. The binding of sulphonylureas to serum albumin. J Pharm Pharmacol 1974;26:304–11.

184. Crooks MJ, Brown KF. Interaction of glipizide with human serum albumin. Biochem Pharmacol 1975;24:298–9.

185. Brown KF, Crooks MJ. Displacement of tolbutamide, glibenclamide and chlorpropamide from serum albumin by anionic drugs. Biochem Pharmacol 1976;25:1175–8.

186. Weissman PN, Shenkman L, Gregerman RI. Chlorpropamide hyponatremia: drug-induced inappropriate antidiuretic hormone activity. N Engl J Med 1971;284:65–71.

187. Moses AM, Numann P, Miller M. Mechanism of chlorpropamide-induced antidiuresis in man: evidence for release of ADH and enhancement of peripheral action. Metabolism 1973;22:59–66.

188. Kadowaki T, Hagura R, Kajinuma H, et al. Chlorpropamide-

induced hyponatremia: incidence and risk factors. Diabetes Care 1983;6:468–71.

189. Berhhard H. Long-term observations of oral hypoglycemic agents in diabetes: the effect of carbutamide and tolbutamide. Diabetes 1965;14:59–70.

190. Cervantes-Amezcua A, Naldjian S, Camerini-Dávalos R, Marbel A. Long-term use of chlorpropamide in diabetes. JAMA 1965;193:759–62.

191. Balodimos MC, Camerini-Dávalos RA, Marble A. Nine years experience with tolbutamide in the treatment of diabetes. Metabolism 1966;15:957–70.

192. Powell T, Howells L. Diabetes mellitus treated with chlorpropamide and tolbutamide: a four-year clinical study. Diabetes 1966;15:269–75.

193. Muller R, Bauer G, Schroder R, Saito S. Summary report of clinical investigation of the oral antidiabetic drug HB 419 (glibenclamide). Horm Metab Res 1969;1(Suppl):88–92.

194. Multicenter Study: UK Prospective Diabetes Study. II. Reduction in HbA_{1c} with basal insulin supplement sulfonylurea or biguanidine therapy in maturity-onset diabetes. Diabetes 1985;34:793–8.

195. Turner RC, Holman RR, Matthews DR. Sulfonylurea failure and inadequacy. In: Cameron D, Colagiuri S, Heding L, et al, eds. Non-insulin-dependent diabetes mellitus. Hong Kong: Excerpta Medica, 1989:52–6.

196. Sachs R, Frank M, Fishman SK. Overview of clinical experience with glipizide. In: Glipizide: a worldwide review. Amsterdam: Excerpta Medica, 1984:163–72.

197. Beck-Nielsen H, Pedersen O, Lindskov HO. Increased insulin sensitivity and cellular insulin binding in obese diabetics following treatment with glibenclamide. Acta Endocrinol 1979;90:451–62.

198. Lebovitz HE, Feinglos MN. Mechanism of action of the second-generation sulfonylurea glipizide. Am J Med 1983;75(Suppl 5B):46–54.

199. Simonson DC, Ferrannini E, Bevilacqua S, et al. Mechanism of improvement in glucose metabolism after chronic glyburide therapy. Diabetes 1984;33:838–45.

200. Lev-Ran A. Trial of placebo in long-term chlorpropamide-treated diabetics. Diabetologia 1974;10:197–200.

201. Banerji MA, Lebovitz HE. Remission in non-insulin-dependent diabetes mellitus: clinical characteristics of remission and relapse in black patients. Medicine (Baltimore) 1990;69:176–85.

202. Bitzén P-O, Melander A, Schersten B, Wåhlin-Boll E. The influence of glipizide on early insulin release and glucose disposal before and after dietary regulation in diabetic patients with different degrees of hyperglycaemia. Eur J Clin Pharmacol 1988;35:31–7.

203. University Group Diabetes Program. A study of the effects of hypoglycemic agents on vascular complications in patients with adult-onset diabetes. I. Design, methods and baseline results. Diabetes 1970;19(Suppl 2):747–83.

204. University Group Diabetes Program. A study of the effects of hypoglycemic agents on vascular complications in patients with adult-onset diabetes. II. Mortality results. Diabetes 1970;19(Suppl 2):789–830.

205. University Group Diabetes Program. Means and standard errors for selected response variables for specified cohorts of patients. Diabetes 1982;31(Suppl 5):32–71.

206. Schor S. The University Group Diabetes Program: a statistician looks at the mortality results. JAMA 1971;217:1671–5.

207. Leibel B. An analysis of the University Group Diabetes Study Program: data results and conclusions. Can Med Assoc J 1971;105:292–4.

208. Seltzer HS. A summary of criticisms of the findings and conclusions of the University Group Diabetes Program (UGDP). Diabetes 1972;21:976–9.

209. Kolata GB. Controversy over study of diabetes drugs continues for nearly a decade. Science 1979;203:986–9.

210. American Diabetes Association. The UGDP controversy (policy statement). Diabetes Care 1979;2:1–3.

211. Kilo C, Miller JP, Williamson JR. The crux of the UGDP: spurious results and biologically inappropriate data analysis. Diabetologia 1980;18:179–85.

212. Matthews DR, Cull CA, Holman RR, Turner RC. Sulphonylurea and insulin therapy: the 3 and 6 year glycaemic outcome in the United Kindgom Prospective Diabetes Study [Abstract no. 1222]. Diabetes 1991;40(Suppl 1):306A.

213. Groop L, Eriksson J, Schalin C, Ahola A. Does secondary oral failure represent slowly evolving type 1 diabetes. In: Cameron D, Colagiuri S, Heding L, et al., eds. Non-insulin-dependent diabetes mellitus. Hong Kong: Excerpta Medica, 1989:48–51.

214. Groop LC, Bottazzo GF, Doniach D. Islet cell antibodies identify latent type 1 diabetes in patients aged 35–75 years at diagnosis. Diabetes 1986;35:237–41.

215. Kadowaki T, Miyake Y, Hagura R, et al. Risk factors for worsening to diabetes in subjects with impaired glucose tolerance. Diabetologia 1984;26:44–9.

216. Saad MF, Knowler WC, Pettitt DJ, et al. The natural history of impaired glucose tolerance in Pima Indians. N Engl J Med 1988;319:1500–6.

217. Jarrett RJ, Keen H, Fuller JH, McCartney M. Worsening to diabetes in men with impaired glucose tolerance ("borderline diabetes"). Diabetologia 1979;16:25–30.

218. Jarrett RJ, Keen H, McCartney P. The Whitehall Study: ten-year follow up report on men with impaired glucose tolerance with reference to worsening to diabetes and predictors of death. Diabetic Med 1984;1:279–83.

219. Stowers JM. Treatment of chemical diabetes with chlorpropamide and the associated mortality. Adv Metab Disorders 1973;2(Suppl 2):549–55.

220. Keen H, Jarrett RJ, McCartney P. The ten-year follow-up of the Bedford survey (1962–1972): glucose tolerance and diabetes. Diabetologia 1982;22:73–8.

221. Sartor G, Scherstén B, Carlström S, et al. Ten year follow-up of subjects with impaired glucose tolerance: prevention of diabetes by tolbutamide and diet regulation. Diabetes 1980;29:41–9.

222. Persson G. Cardiovascular complications in diabetics and subjects with reduced glucose tolerance. Acta Med Scand Suppl 1977;605:7–48.

223. Knowler WC, Sartor G, Scherstén B. Effects of glucose tolerance and treatment of abnormal tolerance on mortality in Malmöhus County Sweden [Abstract no. 280]. Diabetologia 1987;30:541A.

224. Melander A, Bitzén P-O, Sartor G, et al. Will sulfonylurea treatment of impaired glucose tolerance delay development and complications of NIDDM? Diabetes Care 1990;13(Suppl 3):53–8.

225. Jennings AM, Wilson RM, Ward JD. Symptomatic hypoglycemia in NIDDM patients treated with oral hypoglycemic agents. Diabetes Care 1989;12:203–8.

226. Berger W, Caduff F, Pasquel M, Rump A. Die relativ Häufigkeit der schweren Sulfonylharnstoff—Hypoglykämie in den letzten 25 Jahren in der Schweiz. Schweiz Med Wochenschr 1986;116:145–51.

227. Lebovitz HE, Melander A. Sulfonylureas: basic and clinical aspects. In: Alberti KGMM, DeFronzo R, Keen H, Zimmet

P, eds. International textbook of diabetes mellitus. London: Wiley, 1992:745–72.

228. Asplund K, Wiholm B-E, Lithner F. Glibenclamide-associated hyperglycaemia: a report on 57 cases. Diabetologia 1983;24:412–7.

229. Jackson JE, Bressler R. Clinical pharmacology of sulphonylurea hypoglycaemic agents. Drugs 1981;22:211–45, 295–320.

230. Paasikivi J, Wahlberg F. Preventive tolbutamide treatment and arterial disease in mild hyperglycaemia. Diabetologia 1971;7:323–7.

231. Keen H, Jarrett RJ, Fuller JH. Tolbutamide and arterial disease in borderline diabetics. In: Mailaisse WJ, Pirat J, eds. Diabetes: Proceedings of the 8th Congress of the International Diabetes Federation. Amsterdam: Excerpta Medica, 1973:588–602.

232. Ohneda A, Maruhama Y, Itabashi H, et al. Vascular complications and long-term administration of oral hypoglycemic agents in patients with diabetes mellitus. Tohoku J Exp Med 1978;124:205–22.

233. Nathan DM, Roussell A, Godine JE. Glyburide or insulin for metabolic control in non-insulin-dependent diabetes mellitus: a randomized double-blind study. Ann Intern Med 1988;108:334–40.

234. Frazier LM, Mulrow CD, Alexander LT Jr, et al. Need for insulin therapy in type II diabetes mellitus: a randomized trial. Arch Intern Med 1987;147:1085–89.

235. Martin DB. Type II diabetes: insulin versus oral agents [Editorial]. N Engl J Med 1986;314:1314–5.

236. Scheen AJ, Lefèbvre PJ. Insulin versus insulin plus sulfonylureas in type 2 diabetic patients with secondary failure to sulfonylureas. Diabetes Res Clin Practice 1989;6(4):S33–43.

237. Groop LC, Groop P-H, Stenman S. Combined insulin-sulfonylurea therapy in treatment of NIDDM. Diabetes Care 1990;13(Suppl 3):47–52.

238. Lebovitz HE, Pasmantier RM. Combination insulin-sulfonylurea therapy. Diabetes Care 1990;13:667–75.

239. Bailey TS and Mezitis NHE. Combination therapy with insulin and sulfonylureas for type II diabetes. Diabetes Care 1990;13:687–95.

240. Riddle MC. Evening insulin strategy. Diabetes Care 1990;13:676–86.

241. Peters AL, Davidson MB. Insulin plus a sulfonylurea agent for treating type 2 diabetes. Ann Intern Med 1991;115:45–53.

242. Riddle MC, Hart JS, Bouma DJ, et al. Efficacy of bedtime NPH insulin with daytime sulfonylurea for subpopulation of Type II diabetic subjects. Diabetes Care 1989;12:623–9.

243. Taskinen M-R, Sane T, Helve E, et al. Bedtime insulin for suppression of overnight free-fatty acid blood glucose and glucose production in NIDDM. Diabetes 1989;38:580–8.

244. Trischitta V, Italia S, Borzi V, et al. Low-dose bedtime NPH insulin in treatment of secondary failure to glyburide. Diabetes Care 1989;12:582–5.

245. Pasmantier R, Chaiken RL, Hirsch SR, Lebovitz HE. Metabolic effects of combination glipizide and human proinsulin treatment in NIDDM. Diabetes Care 1990; 13(Suppl 3):42–6.

246. Del Prato S, Vigili de Kreutzenberg S, Riccio A, et al. Partial recovery of insulin secretion and action after combined insulin-sulfonylurea treatment in type 2 (non-insulin-dependent) diabetic patients with secondary failure to oral agents. Diabetologia 1990;33:688–95.

247. Clarke BF, Duncan LJP. Combined metformin-chlorpro-

248. Hermann LS. Biguanides and sulfonylureas as combination therapy in NIDDM. Diabetes Care 1990;13(Suppl 3):37–41.

249. Lebovitz HE. Oral antidiabetic agents: the emergence of alpha-glucosidase inhibitors. Drugs 1992 (in press).

250. Vigneri R, Goldfine ID. Role of metformin in treatment of diabetes mellitus. Diabetes Care 1987;10:118–22.

251. Lucis OJ. The status of metformin in Canada. Can Med Assoc J 1983;128:24–6.

252. Lebovitz HE. Metformin. In: Lebovitz HE, ed. Therapy of diabetes mellitus and related disorders. Alexandria, VA: American Diabetes Association, 1991:120–3.

253. Czyzyk A, Tawecki J, Sadowski J, et al. Effect of biguanides on intestinal absorption of glucose. Diabetes 1969; 17:492–8.

254. Caspary WF. Biguanides and intestinal absorptive function. Acta Hepato-Gastroenterol 1977;24:473–80.

255. Dietze G, Wicklmayr M, Mehnert H, et al. Effect of phenformin on hepatic balances of gluconeogenic substrates in man. Diabetologia 1978;14:243–8.

256. Meyer F, Ipaktchi M, Clauser H. Specific inhibition of gluconeogenesis by biguanides. Nature 1967;213:203–4.

257. Searle GL, Gulli R. The mechanism of the acute hypoglycemic action of phenformin (DBI). Metabolism 1980; 29:630–5.

258. Bratusch-Marrain PR, Korn A, Waldhäusl WK, et al. Effect of butformin on splanchnic carbohydrate and substrate metabolism in healthy man. Metabolism 1981;30:946–52.

259. Jackson RA, Hawi MI, Jaspan JB, et al. Mechanism of metformin action in non-insulin-dependent diabetes. Diabetes 1987;36:632–40.

260. Vigneri R, Pezzino V, Wong KY, Goldfine ID. Comparison of the in vitro effect of biguanides and sulfonylureas on insulin binding to its receptors in target cells. J Clin Endocrinol Metab 1982;54:95–100.

261. Pagano G, Tagliaferro V, Carta Q, et al. Metformin reduces insulin requirements in type 1 (insulin-dependent) diabetes. Diabetologia 1983;24:351–4.

262. Trischitta V, Gullo D, Pezzino V, Vigneri R. Metformin normalizes insulin binding to monocytes from obese nondiabetic subjects and obese type II patients. J Clin Endocrinol Metab 1983;57:713–8.

263. Lord JM, White SI, Bailey CJ, et al. Effect of metformin on insulin receptor binding and glycaemic control in type II diabetes. BMJ 1983;286:830–31.

264. Goldfine ID, Iwamoto Y, Pezzino V, et al. Effects of biguanides and sulfonylureas on insulin receptors in cultured cells. Diabetes Care 1984;7(Suppl 1):54–8.

265. Benzi L, Trischitta V, Ciccarone A, et al. Improvement with metformin in insulin internalization and processing in monocytes from NIDDM patients. Diabetes 1990; 39:844–9.

266. Prager R, Schernthaner G. Insulin receptor binding to monocytes insulin secretion and glucose tolerance following metformin treatment: results of a double-blind crossover study in Type II diabetics. Diabetes 1983;32:1083–6.

267. Gin H, Messerchmitt C, Brottier E, Aubertin J. Metformin improved insulin resistance in type 1 insulin-dependent diabetic patients. Metabolism 1985;34:923–5.

268. Schernthaner G. Improvement in insulin action is an important part of the antidiabetic effect of metformin. Horm Metab Res Suppl 1985;15:116–20.

269. Nosadini R, Avogaro A, Trevisan R, et al. Effect of metformin on insulin-stimulated glucose turnover and

insulin binding to receptors in type II diabetes. Diabetes Care 1987;10:62–7.

270. Hother-Nielsen O, Schmitz O, Andersen PH, et al. Metformin improves peripheral but not hepatic insulin action in obese patients with type II diabetes. Acta Endocrinol (Copenh) 1990;120:257–65.

271. Klip A, Leiter LA. Cellular mechanisms of action of metformin. Diabetes Care 1990;13:696–704.

272. Clarke BF, Duncan LJP. Comparison of chlorpropamide and metformin treatment on weight and blood-glucose response of uncontrolled obese diabetics. Lancet 1968; 1:123–6.

273. Lim P, Khoo O.T. Metformin compared with tolbutamide in the treatment of maturity-onset diabetes mellitus. Med J Aust 1970;1:271–3.

274. Clarke BF, Campbell IW. Comparison of metformin and chlorpropamide in non-obese maturity-onset diabetics uncontrolled by diet. BMJ 1977;2:1576–8.

275. Collier A, Watson HH, Patrick AW, et al. Effect of glycaemic control metformin and gliclazide on platelet density and aggregabilty in recently diagnosed Type 2 (non-insulin-dependent) diabetic patients. Diabetes Metab 1989;15:420–5.

276. Josephkutty S, Potter JM. Comparison of tolbutamide and metformin in elderly diabetic patients. Diabetic Med 1990; 7:510–4.

277. Clarke BF, Marshall A, McGill RC, et al. A 3-year evaluation of combined sulphonylurea-metformin treatment in 200 diabetic ketoacidosis resistant sulfphonylurea failures. In: Butterfield WJH, Van Westering, eds. Tolbutamide . . . . after ten years. New York: Excerpta Medica, 1967:312–20.

278. Krall LP, Balodimos MC. Combined sulfonylurea-biguanide therapy of diabetes mellitus. In: Butterfield WJH, Van Westering, eds. Tolbutamide . . . . after ten years. New York: Excerpta Medica, 1967:303–11.

279. Nattrass M, Hinks L, Smythe P, et al. Metabolic effects of combined sulphonylurea and metformin therapy in maturity-onset diabetics. Horm Metab Res 1979;11:332–7.

280. Higginbotham L, Martin FIR. Double-blind trial of metformin in the therapy of non-ketotic diabetics. Med J Aust 1979;2:154–6.

281. Capretti L, Bonora E, Coscelli C, Butturini U. Combined sulphonylurea-biguanide therapy for non-insulin-dependent diabetics. Metabolic effects of glibenclamide and metformin or phenformin in newly diagnosed obese patients. Curr Med Res Opin 1982;7:677–83.

282. Groop L, Widén E, Franssila-Kallunki A, et al. Different effects of insulin and oral antidiabetic agents on glucose and energy metabolism in type 2 (non-insulin-dependent) diabetes mellitus. Diabetologia 1989;32:599–605.

283. Gregorioa F, Ambrosi F, Marchetti P, et al. Low dose metformin in the treatment of type II non-insulin-dependent diabetes: clinical and metabolic evaluations. Acta Diabetol Lat 1990;27:139–55.

284. Wu M-S, Johnston P, Sheu WH-H, et al. Effect of metformin on carbohydrate and lipoprotein metabolism in NIDDM patients. Diabetes Care 1990;13:1–8.

285. Schneider J, Erren T, Zöfel P, Kaffarnik H. Metformin-induced changes in serum lipids lipoproteins, and apoproteins in non-insulin-dependent diabetes mellitus. Atherosclerosis 1990;82:97–103.

286. Lalor BC, Bhatnagar D, Winocour PH, et al. Placebo-controlled trial effects of guar gum and metformin on fasting blood glucose and serum lipids in obese type 2 diabetic patients. Diabetic Med 1990;7:242–5.

287. Dandona P, Fonseca V, Mier A, Beckett AG. Diarrhea and metformin in a diabetic clinic. Diabetes Care 1983; 6:472–4.

288. Berger W. Incidence of severe side effects during therapy with sulfonylureas and biguanides. Horm Metab Res Suppl 1985;15:111–5.

289. Campbell IW. Metformin and the sulphonylureas: the comparative risk. Horm Metab Res Suppl 1985; 15:105–11.

290. Jenkins DJA, Wolever TMS, Ocana AM, et al. Metabolic effects of reducing rate of glucose ingestion by single bolus versus continuous sipping. Diabetes 1990; 39:775–81.

291. Puls W, Keup U. Influence of an α-amylase inhibitor (Bay d 7791) on blood glucose serum insulin and NEFA in starch loading tests in rats dogs and man. Diabetologia 1973;9:97–101.

292. Puls W, Bischoff H. The pharmacological rationale of diabetes mellitus therapy with acarbose. In: Creutzfeldt W, ed. Acarbose for the treatment of diabetes mellitus: 2nd International Symposium on Acarbose. Berlin: Springer-Verlag, 1988:29–38.

293. Clissold SP, Edwards C. Acarbose: a preliminary review of its pharmacodynamic and pharmacokinetic properties, and therapeutic potential. Drugs 1988;35:214–43.

294. Joubert PH, Venter HL, Foukaridis GN. The effect of miglitol and acarbose after an oral glucose load: a novel hypoglycaemic mechanism? Br J Clin Pharmacol 1990;30:391–6.

295. Requejo F, Uttenthal LO, Bloom SR. Effects of alpha-glucosidase inhibition and viscous fibre on diabetic control and postprandial gut hormone responses. Diabetic Med 1990;7:515–20.

296. Schnack C, Prager RJF, Winkler J, et al. Effects of 8-week α-glucosidase inhibition on metabolic control C-peptide secretion hepatic glucose output and peripheral insulin sensitivity in poorly controlled type II diabetic patients. Diabetes Care 1989;12:537–43.

297. Hanefeld M, Fischer S, Schulze J, et al. Therapeutic potentials of acarbose as first-line drug in NIDDM insufficiently treated with diet alone. Diabetes Care 1991; 14:732–7.

298. Tuomilehto J. Acarbose monotherapy in the treatment of non-insulin dependent diabetes mellitus: a review. In: Creutzfeldt W, ed. Acarbose for the treatment of diabetes mellitus: 2nd International Symposium on Acarbose. Berlin: Springer-Verlag, 1988:104–18.

299. Coniff R. Results of U.S. trials with acarbose in the treatment of NIDDM. FDA Application, 1991.

300. Sachse G. Acarbose in non-insulin-dependent diabetes—long-term studies in combination with oral agents. In: Creutzfeldt W, ed. Acarbose for the treatment of diabetes mellitus: 2nd International Symposium on Acarbose. Berlin: Springer-Verlag, 1988:92–103.

Chapter 30

TREATMENT OF THE CHILD WITH DIABETES

JOSEPH I. WOLFSDORF
BARBARA J. ANDERSON
CYNTHIA PASQUARELLO

THE DIABETES TEAM

Optimal care of children and adolescents with insulin-dependent diabetes mellitus (IDDM) is complex and time-consuming and requires the coordinated efforts of several disciplines. Because few general practitioners or pediatricians have the expertise or can devote the time required to provide all of the various components of an optimal treatment program, we believe that the goals of treatment are best accomplished by a diabetes treatment team that works with the child's primary care physician.[1] The members of the pediatric diabetes team should be trained in pediatric diabetes management, and the team should include a physician, a diabetes nurse specialist/educator, a dietitian, and a mental health professional—either a social worker or a clinical psychologist. All should understand the intricacies of diabetes care, the complications of diabetes, and the impact of the disease on child and adolescent development and family interaction. The most important members of the team, however, are the patient and his or her family, whose goals and concerns should receive priority in planning and implementing the treatment program.

PATIENT EDUCATION

All members of the diabetes team participate in the educational process. The diabetes management of children and adolescents is based on a structured diabetes education curriculum adapted to the individual child and family.[2] The process of educating parents and children in diabetes care should begin at the time of diagnosis. Initially, most parents and children are too upset and anxious to assimilate an extensive body of largely abstract information. Therefore, the education program is staged[3]; initial goals are limited to imparting an understanding of the fundamental nature of the disease and how it is treated and to ensuring that the essential survival skills are acquired to enable the child to be cared for safely at home and reintegrated into his or her daily routine. During the next several weeks, the basic aspects of diabetes care are consolidated by practical experience at home and by frequent contact with the diabetes educator and physician. As the grief reaction subsides, most families are more ready to learn the intricate details of diabetes management necessary for maintaining optimal glycemic control while coping with the challenges imposed by exercise, fickle appetite, and varying food intake, intercurrent illnesses, and other normal variations in a child's daily routine.

In addition to imparting facts and teaching practical skills, the education program should attempt to promote desirable health beliefs and attitudes in the young person who has to live with a chronic and as yet incurable disease.[4] For the child, this is often accomplished best in a nontraditional educational setting such as a summer camp for children with diabetes and/or other age-specific peer support groups. The educational curriculum must be concordant with the child's level of cognitive development and adapted to the learning style and intellectual ability of the individual child and family.[5,6] We urge that parents be fully involved and encourage the diabetes team to supervise a gradual and flexible transfer of responsibility from parents to the adolescent child such that the normal process of separation and attainment of independence that occurs during the teenage years is not impeded.[7] Periods of intensive re-education are often necessary during developmental transitions, such as that between childhood and adolescence and when the adolescent leaves home.

GOALS OF THERAPY

In 1976, the American Diabetes Association issued a policy statement to publicize the belief that the weight of evidence strongly supports the concept that the microvascular complications of diabetes are decreased by a reduction in blood glucose concentrations: "The goal of appropriate therapy for those with diabetes should thus include a serious effort to achieve levels of blood glucose as close to those in the nondiabetic as feasible. Obviously, patients' needs and resources must be carefully assessed and the goals individualized accordingly. This concept is particularly applicable to the diabetics at greatest risk of developing the microvascular complications—the young and the middle-aged."[8] The theoretical goal of treatment, therefore, is to restore metabolic function to as near normal as possible while avoiding serious complications of therapy, especially episodes of severe hypoglycemia. This goal is based on the belief that achievement and long-term maintenance of nearly normal glycemia will reduce the risk of development of microvascular and macrovascular complications of diabetes.[9–13]

Although accumulating evidence indicates that glycemic control is an important factor in the genesis of diabetic complications, the relation between long-term control and the development of complications remains incompletely defined. The data currently available do not provide a clear answer to the vexing question: What level of glycemic control will prevent tissue damage and diabetic complications? Studies such as the Diabetes Control and Complications Trial (DCCT) are attempting to answer this crucial question.[14] The attempt to define therapeutic goals for children is further complicated by clinical and epidemiologic data that suggest the prepubertal years of diabetes may contribute minimally to long-term prognosis.[15] Several studies indicate that chil-

dren who develop diabetes before their fifth birthday may be at increased risk for the subsequent development of cognitive impairment.[16–19] Such impairment is presumed to be the result of multiple episodes of severe hypoglycemia, which may be more frequent in the very young child.[20–23] Therefore, maintaining very tight control of glucose levels in children with very early onset diabetes may be harmful, given the risk of causing recurrent, severe, and potentially debilitating episodes of hypoglycemia.

The prepubertal child may be relatively protected from diabetic nephropathy; for example, microalbuminuria, an index of renal glomerular damage, is less prevalent in children younger than 12 years old than in those older than 12 years old matched for duration of diabetes.[24] Despite these considerations, the importance of glycemic control is evident from the findings of a recent study of a large cohort of youths followed longitudinally. No subject whose mean level of glycosylated hemoglobin (HbA_1) was within 1.1 times the upper limit of the normal range had either retinopathy or increased albuminuria.[25] In contrast, among subjects whose mean HbA_1 was consistently greater than 1.5 times the upper limit of normal, 29% had increased albuminuria and 37% had evidence of diabetic retinopathy. While evidence relating quality of glycemic control to late microvascular complications continues to accumulate,[9–13] a survey of glycemic control of patients attending diabetes clinics serving large numbers of children and adolescents indicates that the majority of children and adolescents with diabetes are not achieving desired targets of glycemic control (Table 30–1).[26–37] In the absence of definitive answers to these important questions, we aim for the best control that the child, family circumstances, and available treatment permit. However, those who take care of children and adolescents with diabetes are faced with the problem that the techniques of diabetes management currently available cannot be applied to the majority of children with an intensity sufficient to achieve nearly normal glycemia within the constraints of an acceptable life-style that permits normal emotional development without the hazard of frequent and severe hypoglycemia.

Therefore, "good control" must be defined in a broader context of achievable goals.[38,39] These goals are the prevention of diabetic ketoacidosis and severe hypoglycemia; sustained elimination of the symptoms of uncontrolled diabetes such as polydipsia, polyuria, and hunger; promotion of a sense of physical and emotional well-being; and maintenance of normal physical growth, sexual development, and ideal body weight. Patients and parents are expected to perform self-monitoring of blood glucose (SMBG) regularly and should be able to adjust insulin dose(s) and diet guided by the results of SMBG. In biochemical terms, we aim to achieve a level of glycemic control, while avoiding episodes of severe hypoglycemia, such that most measurements of blood glucose levels before meals and before the bedtime snack are in the range 70 to 180 mg/dL. Patients are expected to test their urine for ketones whenever blood glucose levels exceed 250 mg/dL and/or when they are ill. Ketones should be

Table 30–1. Average Levels of Glycosylated Hemoglobin (HbA$_1$) for Children and Adolescents Attending Diabetes Clinics at Referral Center

Center	No. of Patients	Mean HbA$_1$ Levels*		
		Controls	Patients	C†
Glostrup Hospital, Denmark[26]	92	6.5	11.0	1.7
Children's Hospital, Vancouver, Canada[27]	91	4.3	8.3	1.9
University Hospital, Nottingham, England[28]	148	6.5	13.1	2.0
University of Missouri-Columbia Medical Center, USA[29]	180	5.3	10.0	1.9
University of Oulu Hospital, Finland[30]	177	8.6	14.0	1.6
Children's Hospital, Pittsburgh, USA[31]	477	6.1	11.8	1.9
Hospital for Sick Children, Bristol, UK[32]	94	8.9	14.7	1.7
Hospital for Sick Children, Toronto, Canada[33]	311	5.0	8.7	1.7
Karolinska Hospital, Stockholm, Sweden[34]	131	7.3	11.7	1.6
Children's Hospital, Pittsburgh, USA[35]	340	6.1	10.2	1.7
Montreal Children's Hospital, Canada[36]	219	6.8	11.8	1.7
Joslin Clinic, Boston, USA[37]	198	6.4	11.4	1.8

*HbA$_1$ levels are expressed as the percentage of total hemoglobin.
†C = control factor (the mean HbA$_1$ value expressed as a multiple of the mean value for nondiabetic controls).

consistently absent from the urine. Blood lipid levels should be in the normal range for age,[40–42] and associated disease, e.g., autoimmune thyroiditis, should be detected and, if necessary, treated before it becomes clinically significant.[43–45]

Coping with the unrelenting demands of this chronic incurable disease, for which treatment is complex, difficult, and impacts on the patient's life-style, is stressful. It is not surprising, therefore, that emotional problems are common. Consequently, an important goal of therapy is the prevention, as well as the identification and treatment, of emotional problems and the provision of continuous psychosocial support and encouragement to patients and their families. Despite the above general description of the goals of therapy, it is critically important to tailor the goals of treatment to the capabilities of the individual patient and family.

INSULIN THERAPY

Insulin regimens used to treat IDDM in children and adolescents range from a single daily injection of intermediate-acting insulin (NPH [neutral protamine Hagedorn]/isophane or lente) to intensive regimens of three or four injections each day (multiple daily injections) or continuous subcutaneous insulin infusion.

Conventional Insulin Therapy

Patients with newly diagnosed IDDM usually require a total daily insulin dose of 0.5 to 0.75 U/kg per day. However, initial insulin requirements of patients diagnosed early—before the onset of ketonuria—may be even lower (0.25 to 0.5 U/kg per day). Patients who are less sensitive to insulin, e.g., adolescents, obese patients, patients recovering from diabetic ketoacidosis, or patients with an infection, often require more than 1.0 U/kg per day initially to establish satisfactory glycemic control. Doses of insulin are adjusted according to the results of blood glucose measurements performed before meals

and the bedtime snack and at 2 to 3 a.m. The goal is the attainment of preprandial blood glucose levels between 80 and 120 mg/dL with the maintenance of blood glucose levels at or above 70 mg/dL at 2 to 3 a.m. Adjustments in insulin dose(s) are based on the observation of patterns of hypoglycemia or hyperglycemia over a period of 2 to 3 days that cannot be explained by alterations in the level of physical activity, amount and timing of meals and snacks, or other factors that affect blood glucose levels. When the dose(s) of insulin is adjusted, the dose most likely to be responsible for the high or low blood glucose level at a particular time of the day should be increased or decreased, as appropriate, by approximately 10% of the current dose. A period of 2 to 3 days should be allowed to elapse to permit an evaluation of the effect of the altered insulin dose before further adjustments are made. Within a few weeks of starting insulin therapy, approximately two-thirds of children enter a remission ("honeymoon") period[46–51] and require considerably less insulin (<0.5 U/kg per day) to maintain normal or nearly normal glycemic control. During this period, many children require only a single daily dose of intermediate-acting insulin given in the morning, possibly combined with a small amount of regular insulin if levels of blood glucose before lunch exceed the target range. When the honeymoon period comes to an end as a result of progressive loss of β-cell function,[52] insulin requirements increase steadily over several weeks to months. Most prepubertal children ultimately require 0.6 to 1.0 U/kg per day, whereas pubertal patients usually need 1.0 to 1.5 U/kg per day[53] as a result of physiologic resistance to insulin.[54–58] Caloric requirements decrease and insulin resistance is less pronounced when the pubertal growth spurt ends, and the average insulin requirement drops to 0.8 to 1.0 U/kg per day.

A single daily injection of intermediate-acting insulin, with or without the addition of rapid-acting insulin, does not mimic the normal pattern of insulin release[59–61]; nevertheless, while substantial endogenous insulin secretion persists in patients diagnosed very early and during the honeymoon or remission period, normal or nearly normal glycemic control can be achieved with a single daily injection of insulin.[62] When insulin deficiency is more severe, e.g., in patients who present with severe metabolic derangements or with diabetic ketoacidosis or when the honeymoon period ends, optimal 24-hour glycemic control cannot be achieved with a single daily injection of intermediate-acting insulin even with the addition of rapid-acting insulin. Inadequate blood levels of insulin during the night result in unrestrained hepatic glucose production and fasting hyperglycemia, whereas the delayed absorption of the morning injection of intermediate-acting insulin results in marked postprandial hyperglycemia. Consequently, most children with severe insulin deficiency require a mixture of rapid- and intermediate-acting insulins (NPH/isophane or lente) twice daily, before breakfast and before the evening meal or at bedtime (a so-called split-mixed regimen), to remain free of symptoms and to achieve acceptable levels of glycemic control throughout the day and night.[63-67] The two types of insulin are mixed together in the same syringe and given as a single injection. Because independent adjustment in the dose(s) of the rapid- and intermediate-acting insulins is often necessary and desirable, the use of premixed insulins is not recommended unless indicated by special circumstances. Nevertheless, premixed insulins are useful for patients who have difficulty mixing insulins; e.g., patients with a learning disability who may have difficulty executing the complex series of steps necessary to prepare and inject a mixed insulin dose.

A mixed injection of rapid- and intermediate-acting insulins given before breakfast provides both a rapidly developing peak level of plasma insulin to match nutrient absorption after breakfast and a more slowly developing peak that occurs at the time of the midday meal. The mixed injection of insulin before the evening meal should be adjusted to provide sufficient rapid-acting insulin to dispose of the meal itself and intermediate-acting insulin to provide the basal insulin required to suppress hepatic glucose production overnight. The peak action of the second dose of intermediate-acting insulin administered before the evening meal, however, tends to occur from midnight to 4 a.m., the time when normal insulin requirements are at their lowest. Subsequently, plasma levels of insulin tend to decrease when basal insulin requirements normally increase between 6 a.m. and 9 a.m.[68] This mismatch between insulin delivery and insulin requirement frequently causes nocturnal and/or early morning hypoglycemia[69-75] followed by pre-breakfast or "dawn" hyperglycemia.[76-80] Despite these limitations, most children with "total diabetes" i.e., those without significant residual insulin secretion, can achieve satisfactory glycemic control with a twice-daily insulin regimen consisting of a mixture of rapid- and intermediate-acting insulins given before breakfast and supper. Of the total daily dose, usually 60 to 75% is given before breakfast and 25 to 40% is given before the evening meal. Regular insulin usually comprises 25 to 35% of the morning dose and 30 to 50% of the pre-supper dose; however, the optimal ratio of rapid- to intermediate-acting insulins required for each patient is influenced by the relative size and composition of his or her meals and must be based on results of SMBG and determined by trial and error.

Rapid-acting insulin should be taken at least 30 minutes before meals so that plasma levels of insulin coincide more closely with insulin needs during the postprandial period.[81-84] If the patient performs accurate and reliable SMBG, the timing of the insulin injection can be varied according to the results.[84] Thus, if the blood glucose level is greater than 180 mg/dL, the interval between the injection and the meal can be extended to 45 to 60 minutes. In contrast, if the blood glucose level is less than 70 mg/dL, rapidly absorbed carbohydrate should be consumed immediately and the meal should be started within 15 minutes. Patients should be taught to adjust their insulin doses in response to blood glucose measurements and to circumstances in which insulin needs are different from the usual. For example, they should increase or decrease doses when the blood glucose concentration is high or low before a meal (compensatory adjustment) or in anticipation of exercise or a larger-than-usual meal (anticipatory adjustments). Also, highly motivated and intelligent patients can be taught to use an algorithm or "sliding scale" to select the dose of rapid-acting insulin before meals when the blood glucose level deviates from the target range.[85]

Using a split-mixed regimen, many children experience either nocturnal hypoglycemia,[69-75] rising levels of blood glucose between 3 a.m. and 8 a.m. (the "dawn phenomenon"),[76-79] or both.[74,80] Therefore, adjustments in insulin doses should be based on the results of blood glucose measurements performed both at 2 to 4 a.m. and at 6 to 8 a.m. For patients in whom nocturnal hypoglycemia and/or fasting hyperglycemia cannot be eliminated by adjustments in the dose of intermediate-acting insulin administered before the evening meal, a three-injection regimen consisting of a mixed dose before breakfast, rapid-acting insulin before the evening meal, and intermediate-acting insulin at bedtime is particularly useful because the peak of insulin action occurs when insulin requirements rise the following morning.[86] Before resorting to three injections each day (a bedtime injection of intermediate-acting insulin), we would consider a trial of a twice-daily regimen in which human ultralente insulin replaces NPH before the evening meal.[87] We have found this regimen to be quite successful in many young children who have supper early, and it improves overnight glycemic control in a substantial number of children unwilling or unable to take three injections of insulin each day.

Human insulin is prescribed for newly diagnosed children. However, some children may have difficulty with control that is attributable to the more-rapidly developing peak effect and the shorter duration of action of human intermediate-acting insulin,[88-90] and this may warrant a change to animal-source insulin. Patients already using animal insulins need not change to human insulin unless a specific indication exists, such as insulin allergy, lipoatrophy, or poor metabolic control attributable to the development of antibodies to insulin. The pharmacokinetics of insulin from different species varies.

Therefore, patients should be cautioned not to change to an insulin from another species without careful professional supervision.

Intensive Insulin Therapy (Basal-Bolus Method)

Normoglycemia is rarely achieved in patients with severe insulin deficiency whose insulin regimens involve one or two injections daily. Therefore, if the therapeutic goal is the achievement of blood glucose levels within or close to the normal range (70 to 120 mg/dL before meals and <160 to 180 mg/dL 90 minutes after meals) insulin must be delivered in a manner that simulates normal insulin secretion more closely.[91,92] Endogenous glucose production by the liver is suppressed during the night by a variable basal rate of insulin secretion,[93] which reaches a nadir at 3 a.m. before it rises gradually from 4 to 8 a.m.[68,76–78] In individuals without diabetes, during meals the abrupt increase in insulin levels in portal vein plasma further reduces hepatic glucose production and stimulates hepatic glucose uptake. The increase in insulin levels in peripheral plasma promotes glucose uptake in muscle and fat. Thus, normoglycemia is maintained by the dual effects of insulin on the liver and on insulin-sensitive peripheral tissues. During the past decade, there has been renewed emphasis on the development of treatment regimens that attempt to make insulin available in a manner that mimics the normal pattern of insulin secretion. All these approaches to insulin replacement therapy attempt to provide a basal level of insulin upon which boluses of rapid-acting insulin administered before meals are superimposed. The mimicking of physiologic insulin delivery requires either multiple daily injections of insulin (MDI) or continuous subcutaneous insulin infusion (CSII) by means of a portable insulin pump.[94] The dose of regular insulin given before each meal is selected on the basis of the pre-meal blood glucose level, the size of the meal, and the anticipated exercise.[85] The basal insulin requirement is provided by either a constant slow infusion of regular insulin (using CSII) or a subcutaneous injection of either a long-acting insulin (ultralente) or an intermediate-acting insulin.[95] The basal component of the insulin regimen usually provides 40 to 60% of the total daily insulin dose, and prandial insulin, supplied by injections of rapid-acting insulin before meals, provides the remaining 40 to 60%. However, the insulin regimen, per se, provided that it simulates physiologic insulin availability, is not the major determinant of improved glycemic control. Increased attention to all the elements of the treatment program is essential to the achievement of sustained improvement in glycemic control.[96]

CSII and MDI regimens have been used successfully to improve glycemic control in selected young adults,[96,97] adolescents,[98–100] and young children[101–103] with IDDM in the context of clinical research programs involving intensive patient instruction and supervision by a research team. In the usual diabetes clinic, however, consistent and long-term sustained improvement in glycemic control through the use of CSII has not been observed in children and adolescents.[104–107] CSII is clearly not a therapeutic solution for adolescents with management difficulties stemming from psychosocial problems and poor adherence to prescribed treatment. Successful application of intensive insulin therapy toward the achievement of normoglycemia requires intensification of all aspects of diabetes management: i.e., more frequent SMBG, detailed record keeping, meticulous attention to meal planning, and more frequent contact with the diabetes team. Therefore, pediatric diabetologists have generally been reluctant to use pumps or MDI to treat children because of concerns about patient acceptance, safety, and efficacy.[108] Because CSII and MDI regimens are more complex and demanding to use than a split-mixed insulin regimen, they should be reserved for exceptionally motivated patients committed to the goal of maintaining long-term normoglycemia and capable of achieving it. Therefore, considerable care should be exercised in the selection of pediatric patients for MDI or CSII regimens, and the clinic must be able to provide the intensive instruction and supervision required to achieve sustained benefit from this form of therapy and to monitor its safe implementation.

In addition to psychosocial considerations, a persuasive argument against striving for normoglycemia in children with diabetes is the concern that this would be accompanied by more frequent and more severe hypoglycemia.[109,110] For example, if a child's blood glucose level is 60 to 80 mg/dL, unexpected exercise or a missed meal or snack could quickly lead to serious hypoglycemia. The most important safeguard against hypoglycemia is frequent SMBG, and many children are reluctant or unable to perform such intensive monitoring. Because most children and adolescents are unable or unwilling to sustain the considerable commitment necessary to maintaining near-normal metabolic control safely, we generally do not encourage either CSII or MDI regimens for diabetic children or teenagers. Under special circumstances (such as when diabetes is unusually difficult to control and manipulation and psychosocial factors do not appear to explain the diabetic instability), a more intensive regimen, i.e., more than two injections each day, is offered to patients who cannot achieve optimal control with a split-mixed regimen and who are intelligent, highly motivated, and receive the support and encouragement of their families to achieve ideal goals for blood glucose control. A "basal-bolus" regimen has the advantage of allowing greater flexibility in timing of meals, a feature that may have considerable attraction to some adolescents, especially college students, whose patterns of sleeping and eating are notoriously irregular.

DIET THERAPY

Principles

The nutritional needs of children with diabetes do not differ from those of children who do not have diabetes, nor do they require special foods or different amounts of vitamins or minerals. The total intake of energy (calories) and nutrients must balance the daily expenditure of energy and satisfy the requirements for normal growth. The energy content of the meal plan is based on the child's age, sex, current height, weight, stage of sexual development, and level of physical activity and on the dietitian's nutritional assessment, which may include use of 24-hour dietary recall, a food-frequency table, dietary food records, and food models. The dietary prescription is based on the nutritional assessment and on one of the methods of estimating energy and protein allowances. A method commonly used to estimate energy requirements is based on age and can be used as a crude approximation for children up to 12 years old: basal needs for all children = 1000 kilocalories (kcal); for boys add to the basal needs 125 kcal × age in years, and for girls add 100 kcal × age in years. For very active children, add up to 20% more kcal. Table 30–2 serves as a guide to recommended daily energy allowances for protein and energy for children and adolescents.[111]

The American Diabetes Association currently recommends that carbohydrates provide 50 to 60% of the total calories and that protein and fat provide no more than 15 to 20% and 30%, respectively.[112] Because the requirements change with growth and physical development, the diet prescription has to be reviewed and adjusted, if necessary, at least every 6 months to ensure maintenance of a normal rate of physical growth and maturation.[113]

When insulin is given subcutaneously, it is absorbed from the injection site in a more or less predictable fashion, depending on the type of insulin or combination of insulins used, and exhibits a characteristic time of onset, peak effect, and total duration of action. Therefore, meals and snacks must be consumed at times that match the anticipated time-course of action of injected insulin. Meals and snacks have to be eaten at the same times each day, and the total consumption of calories and the proportions of carbohydrate, protein, and fat in each meal and snack should be consistent from day to day. Because insulin is released continuously from the injection site, hypoglycemia may occur if snacks are not eaten between the main meals. Hence, most children receiving twice-

daily injections of a mixture of rapid- and intermediate-acting insulins have a snack between each meal and at bedtime. An additional snack containing carbohydrate should always precede strenuous exercise unless the blood glucose level is known to be very high.

The clinical nutritionist or dietitian has the important task of educating the patient and family in the basic principles of nutrition and the application of these principles to the formulation of an individualized meal plan. The aim is to lay a foundation for lifelong healthy eating habits for the child and family. Even the most intensive regimens of insulin administration are not successful without careful attention to dietary management.[114] A single instructional session is totally inadequate. Nutrition education, like all aspects of diabetes education, must be an ongoing process, with periodic review and revision of the meal plan and assessment of the child's and parents' levels of comprehension and adherence. Teaching should be followed by systematic assessment of the patients' ability to perform. The assessment should approximate as closely as possible the behaviors expected in the natural environment.[115]

Exchange System

A meal plan based on the system of food exchanges is formulated in consultation with a clinical nutritionist and is individualized to meet the ethnic, religious, and economic circumstances of each family and the food preferences of the individual child. The exchange system is based on six food groups: milk, fruit, vegetable, bread (starch), meat (protein), and fat.[116] Individual food choices (exchanges) included in the list of foods in a particular category contain approximately the same amount of carbohydrate, fat, and protein. The portion size of each exchange is given either by weight or volume. Thus, the meal plan is prescribed in terms of the number of exchanges from each food group that should be

Table 30–2. National Research Council Recommended Daily Allowances (RDAs), 1989: Median Heights and Weights and Recommended Energy and Protein Intakes

	Age in Years	Weight		Height		Calories		Protein (g)
		kg	lb	cm	in	/kg	/day	
Infants	0–0.5	6	13	60	24	108	650	13
	0.5–1.0	9	20	71	28	98	850	14
Children	1–3	13	29	90	35	102	1300	16
	4–6	20	44	112	44	90	1800	24
	7–10	28	62	132	52	70	2000	28
Males	11–14	45	99	157	62	55	2500	45
	15–18	66	145	176	69	45	3000	59
	19–24	72	160	177	70	40	2900	58
Females	11–14	46	101	157	62	47	2200	46
	15–18	55	120	163	64	40	2200	44
	19–24	58	128	164	65	38	2200	46

Table is adapted from Recommended Dietary Allowances.[111] From birth to age 10 years, no distinction between sexes is made regarding energy requirement. Separate allowances are recommended for boys and girls older than 10 years because of differences in the age of onset of puberty and patterns of physical activity. Considerable variability is seen in the timing and magnitude of the adolescent growth spurt and in activity patterns. Consequently, the range of the recommendation for children older than 10 years is wider, and energy allowances should be adjusted individually to take into account body weight, physical activity, and rate of growth.

included in each meal and snack. This method provides a means of ensuring day-to-day consistency of total calories, carbohydrate, protein, and fat while permitting the patient a wide selection of foods. The food choice or exchange system may also be used to instruct patients in other healthy eating practices, such as low-fat, low-cholesterol, and high-fiber meal planning.

Prudent Fat

Because individuals with diabetes are predisposed to atherosclerosis, the amount of fat should not exceed 30% of the total daily calories, and dietary cholesterol should not exceed 300 mg/day. Saturated fat, monounsaturated fat, and polyunsaturated fat should constitute less than 10%, 10 to 15%, and up to 10%, respectively, of the total calories. Fat intake is reduced by the consumption of lean cuts of red meat, more chicken and turkey without skin, fish and seafood, skim and low-fat milk and milk products, and vegetable proteins (legumes).

Fiber

Dietary fiber may benefit the diabetic patient by blunting the rise in blood glucose after meals. Soluble fiber also can reduce levels of serum cholesterol and triglycerides. Unrefined or minimally processed foods such as grains, legumes, whole fruits, nuts, and vegetables should replace highly refined carbohydrates. To avoid abrupt increases in blood glucose, children should eat fruit whole and avoid fruit juices, which should be reserved for treating episodes of hypoglycemia.

Adherence

Adherence to a planned diet is one of the behaviors patients must maintain for optimal management of IDDM. However, diet is the most difficult part of diabetes management for many patients, especially adolescents.[117,118] Patients frequently do not adhere to their prescribed meal plan,[119] and many children (and their parents) do not possess the knowledge and skill required for good dietary adherence regardless of motivation.[115,120] Despite its paramount importance in diabetes management, the successful implementation of nutritional management is achieved in a minority of patients, and, in general, dietary compliance is notoriously poor. There are many barriers to adherence,[121] but these should not discourage health-care professionals involved in the care of children with diabetes from helping their patients overcome these difficulties and enjoy the benefits of good diabetes control. SMBG makes a greater degree of dietary flexibility possible and can enable adolescents to take a more active and informed role in their nutritional management.[122,123]

EXERCISE

The effects of exercise on fuel metabolism in patients with diabetes are complex[124-126] and have not been studied extensively in children.[127-130] Exercise lowers the blood glucose concentration acutely to an extent that depends on the intensity and duration of the exercise and the concurrent level of insulinemia. In part, this effect of exercise is the result of accelerated insulin absorption from the injection site in response to increased regional blood flow and to the massaging effect of contracting limb musculature.[131,132] If exercise is planned, the preceding insulin injection should be given in a site least likely to be affected by exercise. For example, insulin might be injected into the anterior abdominal wall on the morning preceding a sports event. Because children's activities tend to be spontaneous, this advice is difficult, if not impossible, to implement consistently. Consequently, bursts of increased energy expenditure should be "covered" by consumption of an extra snack before and, if the exercise is prolonged, during the activity. A rule of thumb is to provide one bread or fruit exchange (15 g of carbohydrate) for each 30 minutes of vigorous physical activity. Also, rapidly absorbed carbohydrate should be available during and after exercise. The optimal amount of additional carbohydrate must be individually determined guided by SMBG before, during, and after exercise.

Acute vigorous exercise in a patient whose diabetes is poorly controlled can aggravate hyperglycemia and stimulate ketoacid production.[133] Therefore, the child whose diabetes is out of control (pronounced hyperglycemia with ketonuria) should be discouraged from exercising until satisfactory control has been restored.

Physical training increases tissue sensitivity to insulin.[129,134] Consequently, when the frequency and duration of physical activity increases consistently, as occurs when a child attends a summer camp or plays on a competitive school team, the total daily insulin dose should be reduced by 10 to 20% to avoid the occurrence of severe hypoglycemia. Youths who participate in organized competitive sports should be advised to adjust their insulin dose in anticipation of sustained physical activity during a specific period of the day, e.g., reduction in the morning dose of intermediate-acting insulin on those days when the athlete participates in an after-school sports program. The precise amount of such adjustments of insulin dose must be determined empirically. Guidelines for avoiding hypoglycemia or hyperglycemia with exercise are outlined in Table 30–3.

Post-exercise hypoglycemia is a common problem for the child with diabetes.[135] Episodes of hypoglycemia that occur 6 to 15 hours after unusually strenuous exercise or play are thought to be the result of increased insulin sensitivity coupled with increased glucose uptake and glycogen synthesis in previously exercised muscle groups.[136] Hepatic glycogen stores also are rebuilt after exercise but at a slower rate than in muscle, so that increased requirements for dietary carbohydrate may persist for up to 24 hours after prolonged glycogen-depleting exercise.

Some studies have indicated that physical training in children with diabetes improves glycemic control as measured by glycosylated hemoglobin levels,[127,128] whereas others have not demonstrated any beneficial effects of similar exercise programs on metabolic control.[129,130] Exercise helps to maintain ideal body weight

Table 30–3. Strategies for Avoiding Hypoglycemia or Hyperglycemia with Exercise

Food
  Eat 1–3 hours before exercise
  If exercise is vigorous and prolonged, consume supplemental carbohydrate every 30 min during exercise
  Increase food intake after strenuous and prolonged exercise
Insulin
  Avoid exercising immediately after taking insulin
  Decrease insulin dose before exercise
  Consider reducing doses of insulin taken after exercise
Blood glucose monitoring
  Monitor blood glucose before, during, and after exercise and especially at bedtime
  Delay exercise if blood glucose is ≥250 mg/dL and ketonuria is present
  Learn individual glucose responses to different types of exercise

Table is adapted from Horton.[126]

and increases insulin sensitivity. Thus, in combination with appropriate adjustments in the insulin regimen and meal plan, exercise may be a useful adjunct to efforts at achieving optimal glycemic control. Although some studies fail to demonstrate improved glycemic control resulting from physical training programs that improve cardiovascular fitness, other benefits of regular exercise continue to make this an important component of a comprehensive program of diabetes management in children.[137] Exercise plays an important role in the amelioration of risk factors for coronary artery disease (obesity, hypertension, and hyperlipidemia). Of equal importance, children with diabetes are likely to benefit from the enjoyment and enhanced feeling of self-worth derived from participation in physical activities.

MONITORING

Blood Glucose

Since its introduction into clinical practice more than a decade ago,[138,139] self-monitoring of blood glucose (SMBG) has been widely accepted as an important tool in the management of diabetes.[140] It serves four principal functions: to guide physicians in long-term treatment planning; to guide patients in short-term adjustments; to signal possible emergency situations; and to enhance patients' education.[140] Early studies showed that 67 to 95% of children accepted SMBG[72,141–143] and that a majority of children prefer SMBG to urine testing.[143] SMBG has gained widespread acceptance and is now the preferred method of metabolic monitoring. Most children and adolescents can be trained to obtain results that are sufficiently accurate to guide routine clinical decision-making. For example, in one study 68% of tests done by visual reading of the reagent strip were within 20% of the correct figure.[144] The technique should be taught to all patients with IDDM, and their ability to obtain accurate results must be confirmed. Inaccurate test results are common and are usually the result of poor technique. Frequent problems include the patient's failing to obtain

an adequate drop of blood to cover the reagent strip, failing to time carefully the chemical reaction, and wiping or blotting the reagent strip too vigorously. Some of these technical problems have been eliminated by newer glucose meters that are less dependent on meticulous technique and enable the user to obtain measurements of glucose concentration from a single drop of capillary blood that are within 10% of the value obtained in a clinical chemistry laboratory. Nevertheless, studies that use meters equipped with an electronic memory have shown that compliance may be poor and that many children (and adults) fabricate and/or do not consistently record results in a logbook.[145,146] Results may be fabricated to please parents or physicians and to avoid allegations of cheating and/or harsh criticism for "bad blood sugars."

Monitoring schedules vary depending on the intensity of control. The frequency and timing of glucose monitoring should be dictated by the particular needs and goals of the patient. Testing should be performed consistently in relation to injections, meals, and exercise. A minimum of two tests each day usually provides sufficient information to confirm that the current insulin dose and diet are achieving satisfactory control. Additional tests before, during, and after exercise are an invaluable guide to maintaining optimal control in association with exercise and avoiding severe hypoglycemia or excessive hyperglycemia. Patients who monitor infrequently should be encouraged to vary the times of their tests to obtain data about their blood glucose patterns over the entire day. However, at the initiation of therapy, during periods of unstable control that necessitate adjustments of the insulin dose, and for patients using intensive insulin therapy regimens (CSII or MDI) aimed at achieving near normoglycemia, SMBG should be performed before each meal and at bedtime. For most children, this frequency of testing is impractical or intolerable. A satisfactory compromise is for the patient to perform SMBG before each dose of insulin, with additional tests before lunch and at bedtime twice each week (once during the school week and once on the weekend) and at 2 to 3 a.m. once or twice each month. Bedtime tests are especially important for children who have had strenuous or increased exercise during the day because it serves as a basis for judging the size of the bedtime snack necessary to avert delayed or late hypoglycemia.[70,147] For patients using fixed insulin doses who are reluctant or unable to monitor two or three times each day or who cannot afford the reagent strips, a period of intensive monitoring before each meal, at bedtime, and between 2 and 3 a.m. for several consecutive days before an office visit can provide sufficient information to confirm acceptable glycemic control or indicate a trend such that rational adjustments to the insulin regimen can be made.

Frequent SMBG (every 3 to 4 hours throughout the day and night) in conjunction with urine tests for ketones is essential to the management of intercurrent illnesses and the prevention of ketoacidosis. SMBG is of great value to parents uncertain of the cause of their young child's crankiness or unusual behavior when the question of possible hypoglycemia frequently arises. SMBG is also valuable in helping patients to distinguish symptoms of hypoglycemia from symptoms of anxiety and in training individuals to recognize their unique responses to high and low blood glucose levels.[148]

Early studies showed no significant statistical or clinical difference in glycemic control between patients who performed SMBG and those who performed urine tests.[143,149] Presumably, no difference was seen because the data from SMBG were underutilized by patients and their parents. Few patients make active use of their SMBG data for making either compensatory or anticipatory changes in insulin dose.[7] Consequently, SMBG, per se, may not improve glycemic control. The therapeutic benefits are indirect and are mediated by a number of compliance and utilization factors.[150] Teaching patients how and when to monitor their blood glucose levels and a physician's recommending use of SMBG are not in themselves sufficient to improve glycemic control.[36,151,152] Furthermore, failure to improve control often is the result of the patient's not actually performing SMBG in addition to not using the information to make appropriate adjustments.[36,153,154] However, when used in selected patients and in conjunction with intensified insulin regimens and educational programs that teach patients how to use the data to select appropriate insulin doses and adjust their diet, SMBG is an invaluable tool that enables children and adolescents with diabetes to improve their glycemic control and to have greater flexibility in their lives.[100,149,154–156]

Urine Testing

The concentration of glucose in urine correlates poorly with the concentration of glucose in blood,[157–159] and urine glucose testing has many limitations as a means of optimally monitoring control of diabetes. In patients with a normal renal threshold, a negative urine test cannot be used to distinguish between a blood glucose level in the hypoglycemic range from one that is normal or even slightly or moderately increased. Therefore, parents fearful of a hypoglycemic reaction when their young child's urine contains no sugar often deliberately undertreat the child with insulin to ensure that "there is always a little sugar in the urine."

The urine should always be tested for the presence of ketones whenever the child is sick or when the blood glucose level exceeds 250 mg/dL. First morning specimens should be tested for ketones when the possibility of nocturnal hypoglycemia is suspected.

Glycosylated Hemoglobin

Blood glucose levels of patients with IDDM characteristically fluctuate during the course of a single day as well as from day to day.[160,161] Assessment of glycemic control based on symptoms, urinary glucose excretion, or measurements of blood glucose performed infrequently at home or in the office is unreliable and does not accurately reflect the level of long-term glycemia.[162,163] The level of glycosylated hemoglobin (HbA$_1$ or HbA$_{1C}$) formed when glucose is bound non-enzymatically to the N-terminal valine of the β chain of the hemoglobin molecule[164] is directly proportional to the integrated blood glucose concentration over the preceding 2 to 3 months.[165–167] The percentage of glycosylated hemoglobin, after the removal of the labile fraction, provides a reliable index of average glycemia during the preceding 6 to 10 weeks.[165–168] Therefore, determinations at 3-month intervals should be used to provide an objective measure of average glycemia in the intervals between measurements. This test is objective, being independent of both the patient's cooperation and the time elapsed since the last meal. There are several different methods of measuring glycosylated hemoglobin[169,170]; therefore, to allow meaningful comparisons of results from one evaluation to the next, it is advisable to perform all the assays in the same laboratory.

Discrepancies between the determinations of glycosylated hemoglobin level and the results of SMBG or urine glucose testing usually indicate that the latter was inaccurately performed or the results were fabricated.[26,171,172] Factors other than the average blood glucose concentration may affect the test.[169,170] Hemoglobin F spuriously elevates the glycosylated hemoglobin value in most assays,[173] whereas hemoglobins S, C, and G lower the values.[174,175] In patients whose glycosylated hemoglobin value is unexpectedly high or low, it is prudent to perform hemoglobin electrophoresis to rule out any hemoglobinopathy before confronting patients with any allegations of their having fabricated monitoring data.[176] The variant hemoglobin, hemoglobin South Florida, increases the HbA$_{1c}$ value as measured by ion-exchange chromatography but gives normal levels by the thiobarbituric acid (TBA) and affinity-chromatography methods. Hemoglobin electrophoresis does not identify this abnormal variant, which co-elutes with HbA$_{1c}$. Therefore, when no explanation for a patient's elevated HbA$_{1c}$ is apparent, the measurement should be made by the TBA or affinity-chromatography method.[177] If any hemoglobinopathy is identified, an assay method unaffected by the specific hemoglobinopathy should be used to monitor that individual's long-term glycemic control.[169,170]

Levels of glycosylated hemoglobin that are high at the time of diagnosis fall abruptly after insulin therapy is started, reaching a nadir 3 weeks to 6 months after diagnosis and correlating with a decrease in insulin dosage and rising again as the remission wanes.[178] On the basis of measurements of glycosylated hemoglobin reported from children's diabetes clinics in Europe and North America, it is evident that very few children with IDDM in the post-remission phase of the disease achieve normal or even nearly normal glycemic levels. Mean HbA$_1$ levels in children and adolescents with IDDM treated with conventional methods are 1.5 to 2 times the mean for the nondiabetic population, and after the remission, fewer than 5% of these children treated with either one or two doses of insulin each day have HbA$_1$ levels within the normal range (Table 30–1).[26–37]

ACUTE COMPLICATIONS

Diabetic Ketoacidosis

Diabetic ketoacidosis is discussed in Chapter 41.

Prevention of Diabetic Ketoacidosis

Management of Sick Days in Children with Diabetes. Relatively minor illness, such as an upper respiratory tract infection, can destabilize the metabolic state of a child with diabetes and lead to the development of diabetic ketoacidosis (DKA). The stress of infection, surgery, injury, or severe emotional disturbances is associated with increased secretion of the stress or counterregulatory hormones: glucagon, epinephrine, growth hormone, and cortisol. Acting in synergy, these hormones produce a state of insulin resistance and cause increased hepatic glucose production and reduced glucose utilization,[179,180] Thus, despite a reduced intake of carbohydrate associated with the underlying illness, levels of blood glucose usually increase, and enhanced production of ketoacids results in ketonuria. Unchecked, these metabolic disturbances may rapidly progress to full-blown DKA. The objective of sick-day management is to minimize deterioration of metabolic control and to prevent the development of DKA.[181]

The major principles of treatment are 1) to never omit administration of insulin, 2) to prevent dehydration, 3) to monitor levels of blood glucose and urine ketones frequently, 4) to give supplemental insulin according to the accompanying guidelines, and 5) to monitor the child's condition for signs and symptoms that demand immediate attention of a physician. These principles should be an integral component of the educational program provided to patients with IDDM and the family members who provide the child's care.

Never Omit Insulin Injections. Patients with IDDM always need insulin and the child's schedule of insulin injections should not be changed. If the child's level of blood glucose is low, the dose of insulin is reduced (see Table 30–4); however, supplemental injections of regular insulin are usually required because blood glucose levels tend to be high and ketonuria is frequently present.

Treat the Underlying Illness. The underlying illness should be treated appropriately on its own merits with antibiotics, if necessary; with antipyretics for fever; and with bed rest and other necessary therapy.

Prevent Dehydration. It is important to ensure a high fluid intake to prevent dehydration. The child should be encouraged to drink at least 2 mL of liquids/lb of body weight per hour, or 3 L/M^2 per 24 hours. The fluids chosen should contain salt and potassium to replace those electrolytes lost with metabolic decompensation. A combination of different types of fluids is recommended, thereby ensuring that the child receives salt, glucose, and potassium in addition to fluid. Suitable fluids for sick days are broth or bouillon, water, carbonated beverages, and fruit juices. Sugar-free fluids are recommended if, despite the illness, the child is able to follow his or her meal plan and thereby obtain an adequate amount of carbohydrate. However, if the child is unable to eat solid foods, the liquids chosen should contain a source of glucose: e.g., fruit juices, popsicles, regular fruit gelatin, or sweetened carbonated beverages (e.g., cola, lemonade, ginger ale).

Monitor Every 4 Hours. Weight loss is a reliable sign of dehydration; therefore, the child should be carefully weighed several times each day. SMBG and urine tests for ketones should be done every 3 to 4 hours around the clock.

Give Supplemental Insulin. Depending on the results of SMBG and urine ketone tests, it may be necessary to administer additional regular insulin every 3 to 4 hours until the blood glucose level is reduced to less than 250 mg/dL. As a general guideline, an additional 10 to 20% of the child's usual total daily dose of insulin may be given safely. Table 30–4 is an empiric guide to supplementation of regular insulin.

Signs and Symptoms that Demand Medical Attention. Parents should be taught to look out for signs that indicate the child needs to be examined by a physician. If any of the following circumstances pertain, the child must be seen immediately by a physician because continued self-management at home without the child's being seen by a physician may not be safe.

Table 30–4. A Guide to Supplementation of Regular Insulin When Diabetic Children Are Sick

Blood Glucose Level (mg/dL)	Urinary Ketones More Than Trace Positive	Amount of **Extra** Insulin Needed*
<80	Yes or no	Omit regular insulin; decrease NPH/lente insulin by 20%; contact physician; test again in 3–4 hr
80–250	Yes or no	No extra insulin; test again in 3–4 hr
250–400	No	Give 10% of usual total daily dose; test again in 3–4 hr and repeat if no improvement
	Yes	Give 20% of usual total daily dose; test again in 3–4 hr and repeat if no improvement
>400	Yes or no	Give 20% of usual total daily dose; test again in 3–4 hr and repeat if no improvement

*Supplemental insulin is given exclusively as regular (soluble) insulin. The dose of supplemental insulin, however, is calculated as a percentage of the usual total daily dose of insulin (regular and intermediate-acting insulin, NPH or lente). For example, for a patient whose usual total daily dose is 50 units, a 10% supplemental booster dose would be 5 units and a 20% supplemental dose would be 10 units.

1. If the child exhibits any signs of dehydration, such as dry mouth or tongue, cracked lips, sunken eyes, dry flushed skin, or weight loss.
2. If the child is unable to consume the recommended amount of fluid or carbohydrate or if vomiting persists for more than an hour or two.
3. If the child develops symptoms of DKA, such as nausea, abdominal pain, vomiting, hyperventilation, or drowsiness.
4. If high levels of blood glucose (>250 mg/dL) and ketonuria persist for more than 12 hours.

Extensive experience has shown that by assiduously following the guidelines outlined in this protocol, families can successfully manage most intercurrent illnesses in children at home without recourse to a hospital emergency room.

Hypoglycemia

Hypoglycemia is the most frequent acute complication of IDDM.[182] Its clinical manifestations range from minor annoyances (tremors, hunger, weakness) to catastrophic events such as coma and seizures. Occasional, mild hypoglycemia may be one of the prices to be paid for the achievement of good metabolic control.[75,183,184] Although infrequent, mild, and brief symptomatic hypoglycemia is perhaps an inevitable consequence of good diabetic control, there is evidence that cognitive function deteriorates when blood glucose levels are low, even in the absence of typical symptoms.[185] Moderate and severe hypoglycemia, however, is disabling, and considerable effort should be made to avoid such events, which affect school performance and make operating a car or dangerous machinery extremely hazardous.[186-188] Repeated or prolonged severe hypoglycemia can cause permanent damage to the central nervous system,[189] especially in very young children.[190] The confidence of the patient and members of the patient's family is often shaken after experiencing an episode of severe hypoglycemia, and some patients develop a pathologic fear of hypoglycemia that leads them to chronically overeat or to select inadequate doses of insulin in an effort to maintain the high blood glucose levels they perceive as being safe.[191] The fear of hypoglycemia may become a barrier to the patient's attaining and maintaining optimal glycemic control and, not infrequently, causes more anxiety for parents than any other aspect of diabetes, including the fear of long-term complications.

Frequency

A prospective study over a 14-week period found that the average incidence of symptomatic hypoglycemia among a random sample of 47 children attending a diabetes clinic was once every 33 days (range, 0–5.2 times/month). Hypoglycemia occurred more frequently in children with the lowest levels of HbA$_1$, and was more frequent in the evening, in the early morning, and around midday.[75] A recent survey of children attending the diabetes clinic at The Hospital for Sick Children in Toronto found that 31% reported having had an episode of severe hypoglycemia, 22% had more than one episode, and 16% had an episode in a single year.[33] Our experience with a sample of 198 children attending the Joslin Clinic is similar. In a 2-year period, 14.8% had at least one episode of severe hypoglycemia, and 12.2 episodes of severe hypoglycemia occurred per 100 patient-years. All patients reported having experienced mild or moderate hypoglycemia at least once.[37] The incidence of severe hypoglycemia was 6.8% in a 1-year prospective study of 350 children receiving conventional insulin therapy at the diabetes clinic at Montreal Children's Hospital.[192] A similar average yearly incidence, 6.5 per 100 person-years, occurred in an 8-year longitudinal study (from 1981 to 1988) of 155 children with IDDM. The average yearly incidence was 4.4 per 100 person-years over the first 4 years and increased significantly to 7.4 per 100 person-years during the second 4 years.[193] In a population-based study conducted over a 12-month period that involved 92 children 7 to 18 years old who had IDDM for more than 1 year, severe hypoglycemia (defined as an event that required the child to be assisted by an adult to relieve the hypoglycemia) occurred in 44%, and 17% experienced either unconsciousness or convulsions.[194] Mild episodes (managed by the child without assistance) occurred in 97% of children and at least once a week in 53%. Among 684 children aged 7 to 17 years attending, for the first time, a summer camp for children with diabetes, 123 (18%) reported one or more episodes of severe hypoglycemia. This figure may be an underestimate of the actual incidence because some parents may not send a child who has had seizures to camp.[195]

Predisposing Factors

Patient errors relating to insulin dosage, decreased food intake, or unplanned exercise could be implicated in 64 to 85% of the episodes.[33,37,192] It appears that many patients or their families become careless and conduct the daily diabetes routine by rote, without thinking about the intricate interplay of insulin, food intake, and exercise. Recent evidence indicates that the frequency of hypoglycemic coma in children increases with intensification of insulin treatment (an increase in the number of daily injections) and a decrease in HbA$_1$.[193] Table 30–5 lists the common causes of hypoglycemia in children and adolescents.

Presentation and Treatment of Mild, Moderate, and Severe Reactions

Symptoms of clinical hypoglycemia result from adrenergic and/or neuroglycopenic responses to low levels of blood glucose, and insulin reactions or hypoglycemia can be classified as mild, moderate, or severe.

Mild Reactions. The most common early symptoms are tremor (shakiness), tiredness, weakness, faintness, dizziness, or hunger.[7,19] Parents are most often alerted to the presence of hypoglycemia in a very young child by noting pallor, drowsiness, unexplained irritability, or behavioral change. Cognitive deficits usually do not accompany mild reactions, and older children are able to treat themselves. Mild symptoms abate within 10 to 15

Table 30–5. Common Causes of Hypoglycemia

Insulin errors (deliberate or inadvertent)
Reversal of morning and evening dose
Reversal of short- and intermediate-acting insulin
Improper timing of insulin in relation to food
Excessive insulin dosage
Surreptitious insulin administration, suicide gesture or attempt
Erratic or altered absorption
Inadvertent intramuscular injection
More rapid absorption from exercising limbs
Unpredictable absorption from lipohypertrophy at injection sites
Use of more purified insulin preparations
Changes from mixed species to pure pork or human insulin
Diet
Omission or inadequate amounts of food
Timing errors: late snacks or meals
Exercise
Unplanned activity
Prolonged duration or increased intensity of physical activity
Alcohol and/or drugs
Impaired hepatic gluconeogenesis resulting from excessive alcohol consumption
Impaired thinking associated with use of alcohol, marijuana, cocaine, and other recreational drugs

minutes after oral administration of 5 to 15 g of simple carbohydrate. Carbohydrate-containing liquids (fruit juices, carbonated drinks), Lifesavers, corn syrup, packets of granulated sugar, or sugar cubes all provide rapidly absorbed carbohydrate suitable for terminating mild reactions. Glucose tablets (5 g/tablet) raise blood glucose levels more rapidly than does orange juice or milk, and the dosage is easily calibrated. Therefore, glucose tablets are considered the treatment of choice.[197] Patients who use glucose tablets may be less likely to overtreat their insulin reactions. Glucose gels and cake frosting are especially useful for treating infants or toddlers who refuse to drink. Chocolate and ice cream are not recommended because their high fat content slows gastric emptying and retards the absorption of available sugar.

Moderate Reactions. Moderate reactions have neuroglycopenic as well as adrenergic symptoms, e.g., headache, mood changes, irritability, decreased attentiveness, and drowsiness. Patients may require assistance with treatment because they are often confused and have impaired judgment, and weakness and poor coordination may make self-treatment difficult. Moderate reactions produce longer-lasting and more severe symptoms and may make a second dose of simple carbohydrate necessary.

Severe Reactions. Severe reactions are characterized by unresponsiveness, unconsciousness, or convulsions and require emergency treatment with parenteral glucagon administered by a family member or intravenous glucose given by an emergency medical technician or by hospital personnel. Buccal and rectal administration of glucose is useless.[198,199] Glucagon is as effective in treating severe hypoglycemia in children[200] as it is in adults.[201,202] Most studies in adults have found that glucagon rapidly raises blood glucose levels and relieves symptoms of hypoglycemia.[203–204] If the period of

hypoglycemia was prolonged or extremely severe and the patient had a seizure, complete recovery of normal mental function may take several hours despite restoration of blood glucose to a normal level. The postictal period may be complicated by headache, lethargy, nausea, vomiting, and aching muscles.

Symptoms of experimentally induced hypoglycemia in diabetic children are relieved within 10 minutes of administration of glucagon by either subcutaneous (SC) or intramuscular (IM) injection, although mean levels of blood glucose and plasma glucagon are slightly but not significantly higher after IM than SC injection.[200] Both 10-μg/kg and 20-μg/kg doses of glucagon relieve clinical signs and symptoms, but the increment in blood glucose concentration after 10 minutes is less after the 10-μg/kg dose (1.1 $\pm$ 0.3 vs. 1.7 $\pm$ 0.7 mmol/L); however, the differences after 20 and 30 minutes are not significant. Nausea and/or vomiting can be expected to occur 1 to 3 hours after the injection in a minority of children who receive a dose of 20 μg/kg but usually do not occur after a dose of 10 μg/kg. In diabetic children[200] and in healthy adults,[206] there appears to be no important difference between the effects of glucagon injected SC and that injected IM. The levels of plasma glucagon attained are higher than those seen in peripheral venous or portal blood of healthy adults during insulin-induced hypoglycemia and are probably higher than those necessary for maximal effect. Excessively high levels of plasma glucagon seem more likely to cause nausea and/or vomiting. The increase in blood glucose concentration after glucagon administration is sustained for at least 30 minutes. Therefore, it is not necessary to repeat the dose or force the child to eat or drink for at least 30 minutes.

Although glucagon was available in 82% of patients' homes and all caregivers had been instructed in its use, Daneman et al.[33] found that it was actually administered in only 37% of cases. Similarly, Aman et al.[194] found that glucagon was administered in only 15% of cases, while 12% required intravenous glucose and 16% were admitted to the hospital.

PSYCHOSOCIAL ISSUES

What distinguishes diabetes from most other chronic diseases of childhood is the incessant demands it makes on patients and families for self-care and the clinical decision-making responsibilities it gives patients almost immediately after diagnosis.[207] To meet these demands requires major adjustments of life-style. As is clear from the preceding discussion in this chapter, diabetes management affects many components of family life—eating, physical activity, finances, and time. The daily treatment required of children with diabetes impacts and intrudes on expectations for everyday behavior in the family, alters family routines, and affects relationships among family members. How the family handles these intrusions determines the effectiveness with which diabetes is managed at home.[208] The single most important psychosocial issue concerning families with diabetic youngsters is how responsibilities for diabetes management are defined and supported within the family, how these treatment responsibilities are shared among family members, and how and when responsibilities are transferred from parent(s) to child as the child develops.[209] Moreover, over the past decade, recommendations about appropriate ages at which responsibilities should be transferred to children with diabetes have shifted significantly.[5,7]

With the current emphasis on prevention in the treatment of childhood diabetes, we want to emphasize that the negative effects of two specific psychosocial or emotional complications of IDDM in young children—the premature assumption of independent responsibility for diabetes care tasks by children and the sole assumption of diabetes responsibilities by one parent (usually the mother)—can be prevented by a thoughtful team approach from the time of diagnosis. In this section, we address these two specific problems, both of which concern the family's division of responsibility for the tasks of managing IDDM.

The Crisis at Diagnosis

The diagnosis of diabetes in a child or adolescent hurls the parent from a secure and known reality into a frightening and foreign world. At points of crisis such as the diagnosis of IDDM, parents face competing stresses. They must begin the process of grieving the loss of their healthy child and cope with normal distress reactions such as shock, disbelief and denial, fear, anxiety, anger, and rage, as well as with extreme feelings of blame or guilt that follow the diagnosis of any serious, chronic childhood disorder.[210] Despite grieving and coping with emotional distress, parents must acquire sufficient cognitive understanding and behavioral skills to manage the illness at home and achieve acceptable blood glucose control in their child soon after diagnosis. Moreover, parents must continue to meet the normal developmental needs of their newly diagnosed child as well as attend to the needs of other family members. In addition, at diagnosis many parents have other ongoing stresses that consume time and energy, such as financial problems, conflicts with extended family, another ill family member, or marital difficulties. A common problem for parents at the time of diagnosis is the introduction of entirely too many facts and guidelines during a time when they are still in shock, which only compounds their emotional upheaval. Guidelines and the number of different medical staff should be kept to a minimum during the early days following diagnosis, and the program of diabetes education must be addressed to both parents or, if this is a single-parent family, to another adult—a grandparent, neighbor, or babysitter—who should be encouraged to participate as a support for the primary parent.

As was emphasized earlier in this chapter, diabetes education is an ongoing process, and it is vital that parents receive the emotional support necessary for them to begin to cope with the emotional distress caused by the discovery of this serious illness and not to be overwhelmed by unrealistic cognitive or behavioral expectations from a well-meaning diabetes treatment team. Pacing the introduction of new medical concepts, technologies, and personnel to the learning "readiness" of the parents of a newly diagnosed child is critically important for launching the family toward successful mastery of the very difficult task that lies ahead. Parents must find their own sense of balance in the crisis that follows the diagnosis and should be encouraged to progress at their own pace, with a staff member or another parent offering emotional support.

Diabetes and Child Development

Across all developmental stages, diabetes presents family members with the task of being sensitive to the balance between the child's simultaneous needs for independence and mastery in terms of self-care and for family support and involvement in carrying out self-care tasks. The struggle to balance independence and dependence in relationships between the child with diabetes and family members presents a chronic coping task for families and raises different issues for families at different stages of child and adolescent development. The most effective means of assessing how families can best share treatment tasks is to focus on the normal developmental tasks at each stage of the child's growth and development and to consider how diabetes impacts on normal childhood tasks as well as how normal childhood tasks impact on diabetes and its management.[211]

The Infant and Toddler (0 to 3 Years)

At this earliest stage of child development, the parent(s) is the only appropriate patient with respect to learning about and taking responsibility for diabetes management. Leaverton[212] reported that management problems facing parents with diabetic infants and toddlers included monitoring diabetic control, establishing a meal schedule despite the child's "normally" irregular eating patterns, coping with the very young child's inability to understand the need for injections, and managing the conflicts with older siblings that result from unequal sharing of parental attention brought about by the requirements of caring for the very young diabetic child. Children diagnosed before the age of 5 years may be at greater risk for severe hypoglycemic episodes[19] because of the inherent difficulties in administering and adjusting the very small insulin doses needed by most babies and toddlers as well as the inability of the preverbal child to recognize and communicate symptoms of hypoglycemia.[20] At this stage of development, two important and interrelated aspects of clinical treatment concern the sharing of treatment responsibilities between parents and the prevention of severe hypoglycemic episodes.

The primary developmental task during infancy is the achievement of a stable, reciprocal relationship of trust between the infant and primary caregiver. With the potential for frightening episodes of hypoglycemia, diabetes in a baby especially exaggerates the parent's sense of responsibility or vigilance and the baby's helplessness. Many parents with diabetic babies and toddlers have considerable difficulty finding child care to relieve the relentless 24-hour-a-day burden of diabetes management.

It is critical at this stage of development that a single parent does not have full responsibility for diabetes care at home; if no spouse or partner is available, we strongly recommend that a grandparent, neighbor, or adult friend be educated in diabetes care so as to be able to provide support for the mother. Very frequently in two-parent families the mother carries a disproportionate share of the burden of diabetes care, an unbalance that may be reinforced during the hospitalization at diagnosis and at follow-up medical appointments that do not require the father's participation. Not infrequently, if fathers do not participate in the initial diabetes education at diagnosis, they continue to feel out of touch with the complexities of diabetes management in a baby or toddler. Moreover, some mothers may need a "push" from the health-care team to begin to let go of some aspect of the responsibilities for diabetes care at home.

The central task of the child from 1 year to 3 years old is to establish a sense of autonomy and mastery over his or her world. Toddlers do not have the cognitive skills to permit them to understand why their cooperation with the intrusive, sometimes painful procedures of the diabetic treatment regimen is necessary. Thus, injections or finger sticks for blood glucose monitoring may become battlegrounds when the toddler resists with all his or her strength. Parenting a toddler with IDDM who resists and rejects the regimen requires a great deal of emotional stamina. Because of the emotional drain on parents and the potential for undetected hypoglycemia in very young children, Golden and colleagues have emphasized the critical importance of ongoing psychosocial support in addition to medical guidance for families with babies or toddlers.[20]

The Preschool and Early Elementary School Child (4 to 7 Years)

During the preschool and early school years, the child's primary developmental task is to put his or her newly established sense of autonomy to work by actively investigating the environment outside the home. The child is involved in gaining a sense of gender identity, joining with peers for group play, and in using newly developed cognitive skills called "concrete operations," which permit the child to use more cause-and-effect thinking strategies. With the child's entrance into school, he or she also must master separation from the family, adapt to the expectations of teachers, and learn to feel safe away from home. It has been suggested that school entrance by diabetic children may represent the first public context in which both parents and children must cope with the social meaning of diabetes, including the tasks of educating others about the disease.[211,213] Thus, school entry makes it necessary for both the child with diabetes and the parent to trust individuals outside the family and to talk about the disease and its treatment with them. The separation problems that often appear in children at this age may be heightened in the child with IDDM. The 4- to 7-year-old child with IDDM often applies cause-and-effect thinking to diabetes and may blame himself or herself for having the disease or may see

injections and restrictions as punishments. It is important for diabetic youngsters at this age to begin to relate to other children with IDDM and their families. At this critical period, many families will benefit from informal contact and group interactions (diabetes camps, support groups) with other families with diabetic children who are beginning school and broadening their base of diabetes "supervisors." Many families will need assistance from their health-care team to educate school personnel, coaches, and scout leaders about diabetes.

At this stage of development, the parent(s) continues to be the primary recipient of diabetes education and to interact with the health-care team. However, the child's increasing motor coordination and cognitive skills enable him or her to become a more involved partner in diabetes self-care tasks at home. Children at this age can select from among several appropriate choices for snacks, select and clean the site for injections, and begin to identify symptoms of low blood sugar. The goal is for elementary school-aged children to be drawn into their own care in a positive way without their being pressured with premature and unrealistic expectations for independence or autonomy while parental control and supervision continue.

Later Elementary School Years (8 to 11 Years)

The later elementary school years are characterized by the rapid growth of intellectual, athletic, and artistic skills. The preadolescent child forms close friendships with children of the same sex, strives to gain approval from this peer group, and begins to evaluate himself or herself seriously by comparing abilities with those of peers. It is important that diabetic youngsters in the process of making these social comparisons develop a strong, positive self-image.[214,215] Grey et al.[216] have pointed out that preadolescent diabetic children with adjustment problems often are overlooked because they are not overtly rebellious and hostile but instead are often overdependent on family members and withdrawn from peers. "Participation" and "positive self-image" are key concepts at this stage of development, and health-care providers may need to emphasize to parents the importance of the child's engaging in a wide range of activities with peers. One way to help parents feel comfortable in trusting their diabetic child in wider and wider circles outside the home is to focus diabetes education on realistic goals for blood sugar levels and safety guidelines for prevention of hypoglycemia. This usually means a willingness of parent and child to increase the frequency of SMBG and to plan ahead to provide additional snacks when the child's activity increases.

It is important to continue to emphasize the long-term benefits of continued parental involvement, even during this "skill-building" phase of the later elementary school years. Although some children at this age may demand to take over primary responsibility for diabetes management tasks, research has shown that youngsters at this age are not capable of sustained independence in carrying out diabetes tasks.[7] While it is important at this age for parents to retain their primary role in diabetes care, youngsters at this age can begin to test blood sugar levels and give injections on occasion without supervision, such as at a slumber party or when visiting grandparents for the weekend. As a shift in responsibility for diabetes care occurs in families during the later elementary school years, it is important for members of the health-care team to begin to negotiate more directly with the child concerning issues and problems with diabetes, rather than talking solely to the parents.[217]

Early Adolescence (12 to 15 Years)

During early adolescence, the conflict intensifies in the changing balance of responsibility between the diabetic child and the family for diabetes management tasks. The early adolescent years are confusing for teenagers and parents alike. On both sides, there is pushing toward independence and pulling back toward the familiar comforts of childhood. Dramatic changes occur in five areas: physical development, family dynamics, school experiences, cognitive development, and social networks.[218] Pubertal changes start during the early adolescent years, and adjusting to dramatic changes in height, weight, complexion, and size of body parts is a critical coping task for young teenagers. Young adolescents and their parents must begin to integrate these physical changes into their image of who the teenager is and must collectively acknowledge that the young teenager is no longer a child but is on the threshold of becoming an adult. It is common at this time for families to change their expectations of the young adolescent for a broad range of responsibilities (e.g., selecting clothes and friends, doing homework).[209] Therefore, parents frequently "turn over" responsibility for diabetes management to the young teenager along with other responsibilities.[219] However, a factor that complicates an abrupt transition of responsibility for diabetes management within families is the new physiologic difficulty of controlling blood glucose concentrations during puberty. Recently, investigators have demonstrated that the physiologic changes of puberty are associated with insulin resistance in both nondiabetic and diabetic adolescents, and reduced sensitivity to insulin probably contributes significantly to the difficulty experienced by many young diabetic adolescents in achieving optimal glycemic control.[54,55]

As teenagers become aware that they are no longer children, they begin to search for a new role in the family and to test the limits of family rules. The work of defining a new role in the family is often done indirectly. For example, a conflict over diabetes self-care or over friends or clothes may often be a fight over who holds the power in the family. Changes in the school environment are also confusing at this age. Entering junior high school or middle school means the introduction to more teachers, choices, rules, freedoms, and friends. These many different changes leave the young teenager very vulnerable and with few coping skills necessary to confront these new challenges. Friends assume a new importance, and building new loyalties outside the family is a natural stepping stone on the way to mature independence. However,

classmates may be at considerably different stages of their physical maturity and emotional growth, and their interests may differ enormously, making for an unstable group. Fitting in with the peer group is perhaps the biggest task of young teens. It usually takes a while for the young adolescent to figure out how diabetes fits in with this task. At this vulnerable stage, if the diabetes care regimen makes a teenager stand out from the peer group, conflicts will arise. Some teenagers may stop their self-care and try to prove they are "normal." Others may use diabetes as an excuse to withdraw. Many youngsters who never before "hid" their diabetes may now refuse to talk about it with friends.

Young teenagers have an increasing cognitive ability and are able to analyze themselves and the world around them and do not accept authority but examine, criticize, and question. This growing ability to analyze the "bigger picture" leads many diabetic teenagers to a new sensitivity about their disease. For the first time, they may vent their anger about having diabetes. At the same time, however, the behavior of younger teenagers is not future oriented. They make decisions based on the present and concrete. It has been suggested that parents and healthcare professionals frequently overestimate teenagers' conceptual understanding of diabetes,[219] and parents likewise often overestimate adolescents abilities to follow through with diabetes care tasks without their receiving immediate positive reinforcements and support, mistakenly assuming that "long-term good health" will provide motivation for adherence to the diabetes treatment plan. This is the root of many conflicts about diabetes in families, with parents focused on, and fearful of, the future and young teenagers able to cooperate only in relation to the here and now.

Diabetes can further threaten young teenagers' self-confidence. It makes their bodies seem even more different. Fluctuating blood sugar levels that defy control contribute to younger teenagers' uneasy feelings about their bodies. Insulin reactions, injections, and blood sugar monitoring can further undermine the younger teenagers' ability to feel attractive—or simply "normal."[220] Concerns about body image need to be taken seriously by parents and health-care providers. For example, a frequent problem in young adolescent girls distressed about weight gain is a dramatic increase in blood sugar levels. When young adolescent girls are worried about their weight and parents and the health care team focus exclusively on "good control," many patients secretly begin to reduce their insulin and thereby "purge" calories and lose weight. This self-destructive cycle of behavior is similar to bulimia nervosa, and this type of diabetes-specific "eating disorder" often results in repeated hospitalizations for diabetic ketoacidosis in adolescent girls.[221] The adolescent girl concerned about her weight or the shape of her body needs to work more closely with different members of the diabetes-care team to gradually lower the calorie level of her meal plan and reduce the insulin dose as guided by the results of more frequent SMBG, while increasing her level of physical activity.

When serious personal problems or family conflicts over diabetes care develop at this age, a referral for problem-focused family counseling should be made to help parents and teenagers who are having difficulty negotiating responsibilities. Because of the physiologic barriers to the control of blood sugar levels caused by puberty and the psychological and social vulnerabilities of this age period, it is generally recommended that parents continue their involvement in and supervision of the administration of insulin and testing of blood sugars through the early adolescent years. This is definitely the wrong developmental period during which to expect adequate self-care by diabetic youths. For some 12- to 15-year-old youngsters, it may work best for the parent to give almost all of the injections, while in other families, young teenagers may need the support of a parent-observer only during injection times. It is critical to negotiate continued support and supervision, even if the young adolescent initially rejects it. Likewise, it is critical to recruit some participation from the young adolescent, even if the notion is rejected initially. The key is to negotiate and not to force diabetes care on the young, vulnerable adolescent. It is well documented that negative family interactions surrounding diabetes management contribute to problems of compliance and control in adolescents with diabetes.[222]

At this stage, families should also be encouraged to begin to change their pattern of relationships with diabetes health-care providers.[223] Young teenagers often have issues that they do not feel comfortable discussing in the presence of their parents, such as concerns about sexuality, depression, complications of diabetes, and communication problems at home. For this reason, it is important for diabetes health-care providers to begin seeing parents and young teenagers individually and sequentially so that the needs of each for information, support, and confidentiality are respected. Both young adolescents and their parents may benefit from contact with other youngsters and families coping with the same struggles over diabetes care during this extremely complex and difficult developmental period. Diabetes camps often provide an important forum for peer identification for youth at this age, and peer group educational and support programs have been reported to be helpful for both young teenagers with diabetes and their parents.[224]

Later Adolescence (16 to 19 Years)

The intensity of the changes that occur during the early adolescent years decreases somewhat during later adolescence, and as growth decreases and changes stabilize, frequently so do conflicts over diabetes self-care. The central developmental tasks of older adolescents include making decisions regarding their plans after high school, living more independently of parents, strengthening relationships with a smaller number of friends, and assuming more independent responsibility for health, including health care. Some older diabetic teenagers who feel overwhelmed with the pressures of high school and the need to plan for the future ignore all but the most essential requirements of their self-care. When peer relationships are insecure or school work seems beyond their abilities, some teenagers may use their diabetes to

avoid the conflicts at school. This sets up a vicious cycle in which they get further behind in school, with chronic school absences and re-entries increasing problems with their peers at high school. The very poor metabolic control of some older teenagers reflects a chronic, unmet need for more family support for self-care tasks. Sometimes poor control in a teenager is a reflection of chaos and dysfunction at home. Nothing alienates parents and teenagers at this stage of development more than do conflicts over friendships. This is especially true when issues of safety (driving) and sexual activity are raised. Many parents feel that their youngsters are unprepared to handle the pressures on adolescents in the 1990s, especially sexuality. Health-care professionals can initiate an offer to assist parents with this dilemma. Older teenage patients have a need for and a right to honest discussion and facts about recreational drugs and alcohol, contraception, sexually transmitted diseases, and the stresses associated with being an adolescent parent. Many older teenage girls (and their parents) have not been educated about the importance of maintaining good metabolic control before conception or about the difficulties of managing a diabetic pregnancy.

During this stage of development, the growth and dramatic changes of puberty have slowed down and insulin needs stabilize. Many older adolescent females continue to be concerned about a weight gain that may have occurred when the insulin dose increased and the meal plan provided significantly more calories to meet the requirements of accelerated growth. An evaluation for insulin manipulation should be done whenever poor metabolic control remains unexplained in an adolescent female concerned about her weight. Because of the emerging independent status of the older teenager, a strong relationship between at least one member of the health-care team and the older adolescent is very important. Expectations are that older adolescents can manage diabetes independently; however, each family situation must be assessed individually. The presence of a personality disorder or learning disability, extreme poverty, or family dysfunction may necessitate the continued involvement of another person in the adolescent's self-care tasks.

Young Adult Years (19 to 24 Years)

Except when a college education or job shortages prolong economic dependency, the primary developmental task facing the young adult is the completion of the process of establishing his or her independence; the assumption of control over many aspects of daily life, including health care; and the consolidation of decisions about a career and life-style. The first "real" job is often the first experience in learning to cope with an authority system more rigid than either the home or school environment. For many young adults with diabetes, their first job is also their first experience in implementing a diabetes management plan within an environment in which no one else is motivated to ensure adherence to the regimen. Learning to be assertive about one's needs as a person with diabetes can be very stressful, especially for young adults who are insecure about their employability. Health-care providers should anticipate patients' fears of having hypoglycemic episodes on the job.

A team approach to diabetes care continues to be critical during the young adult years. As young adults, patients may experience their first diabetes-related physical complications, and the discovery of retinopathy or the diagnosis of neuropathy or nephropathy may lead to depression and hopelessness or to an increase in risk-taking behavior. It is important to refer young adults for psychological therapy when they are frightened or depressed about complications of diabetes. Some young adult patients choose to maintain their relationships with their pediatric caregivers. Others may choose to transfer to adult clinics or college health services. Even though providers of adult health care have not known their young adult patients for long, it is important for the health-care provider to initiate discussions about intimate relationships and to offer to discuss the stresses of diabetes with a fiancé(e) or spouse. Developing mature intimate relationships is another important task of the young adult. Discussions on family planning should also be initiated by health-care providers, and genetic counseling can help young adults address their concerns about having children. Young adults are for the first time independent consumers of health care. It is well known that interventions to assist older adolescents and medical caregivers with this transition from pediatric to adult medical delivery systems are vitally needed.[225] If older adolescents are more comfortable maintaining connections with their pediatric providers, this should be accepted as an appropriate and reasonable option for care. The goal is to not lose young adult patients in the cracks between our pediatric and adult medical delivery systems.[226]

In summary, at every stage of child development, the tasks and demands of normal development interface with the coping tasks confronted by children and families managing diabetes. Furthermore, the tasks of normal child development have repercussions for the structure of the continuously evolving triangle of parent, patient, and health-care provider. From the crisis of diagnosis of IDDM in a child, the primary challenge is to manage the "burden of care"—the unending and arduous work of controlling blood sugar in a developing child—so that neither child nor parent feels frustrated and discouraged but rather that they both feel the goals of diabetes management can be achieved. Responsibilities must not be transferred unevenly to the parent(s) or abruptly and prematurely to the child or adolescent but instead should be assumed and mastered by the older adolescent and young adult who is cognitively and emotionally prepared to handle the burden of care and to ask for the support necessary to living with IDDM. At all stages in this journey, the resources of a multidisciplinary health-care team—physician, educator, nurse, social worker, nutritionist, psychologist, exercise physiologist, and ophthalmologist—are essential for the successful management of IDDM by the child or adolescent and family.

REFERENCES

1. Laron Z, Galatzer A, et al. A multidisciplinary, comprehensive, ambulatory treatment scheme for diabetes mellitus in children. Diabetes Care 1979;2:342–8.
2. Committee on Youth Education American Diabetes Association. Curriculum for youth education. Alexandria, VA: American Diabetes Association, 1983.
3. Etzwiler DD. Education of the patient with diabetes. Med Clin North Am 1978;62:857–66.
4. Rosenstock IM. Understanding and enhancing patient compliance with diabetic regimens. Diabetes Care 1985; 8:610–6.
5. Kohler E, Hurwitz LS, Milan D. A developmentally staged curriculum for teaching self-care to the child with insulin-dependent diabetes mellitus. Diabetes Care 1980; 5:300–4.
6. Johnson SB, Pollak T, Silverstein JH, Rosenbloom AL, et al. Cognitive and behavioral knowledge about insulin-dependent diabetes among children and parents. Pediatrics 1982;69:708–13.
7. Ingersoll GM, Orr DP, Herrold AJ, Golden MP. Cognitive maturity and self-management among adolescents with insulin-dependent diabetes mellitus. J Pediatr 1986; 108:620–3.
8. Cahill GF Jr, Etzwiler DD, Freinkel N. "Control" and diabetes [Editorial]. N Engl J Med 1976;294:1004–5.
9. Skyler JS. Complications of diabetes mellitus: relationship to metabolic dysfunction. Diabetes Care 1979;2:499–509.
10. Tchobroutsky G. Relation of diabetic control to development of microvascular complications. Diabetologia 1978; 15:143–52.
11. Tamborlane WV, Sherwin RS. Diabetes control and complications: new strategies and insights. J Pediatr 1983; 102:805–13.
12. Leslie ND, Sperling MA. Relation of metabolic control to complications of diabetes mellitus. J Pediatr 1986; 108:491–7.
13. Raskin P, Rosenstock J. Blood glucose control and diabetic complications. Ann Intern Med 1986;105:254–63.
14. The DCCT Research Group. Are continuing studies of metabolic control and microvascular complications in insulin-dependent diabetes mellitus justified? The Diabetes Control and Complications Trial. N Engl J Med 1988;318:246–50.
15. Kostraba JN, Dorman JS, Orchard TJ, et al. Contribution of diabetes duration before puberty to development of microvascular complications in IDDM subjects. Diabetes Care 1989;12:686–93.
16. Ack M, Miller I, Weil WB Jr. Intelligence of children with diabetes mellitus. Pediatrics 1961;28:764–70.
17. Ryan C, Vega A, Drash A. Cognitive deficits in adolescents who developed diabetes early in life. Pediatrics 1985; 75:921–7.
18. Holmes CS, Richman LC. Cognitive profiles of children with insulin-dependent diabetes. J Dev Behav Pediatr 1985;6:323–6.
19. Rovet JF, Ehrlich RM, Hoppe M. Intellectual deficits associated with early onset of insulin-dependent diabetes mellitus in children. Diabetes Care 1987;10:510–5.
20. Golden MP, Russell BP, Ingersoll GM, Gray DL, et al. Management of diabetes mellitus in children younger than 5 years of age. Am J Dis Child 1985;139:448–52.
21. Francois R, Hermier M, Jurlot JC, et al. Occurrence of diabetes in infants less than one year old. Mod Prob Paediatr 1975;12:60–6.

22. Grunt JA, Banion CM, Ling L, et al. Problems in the care of the infant diabetic patient. Clin Pediatr 1978;17:772–7.

23. Ternand C, Go VLW, Gerich JE, Haymond MW. Endocrine pancreatic response of children with onset of insulin-requiring diabetes before age 3 and after age 5. J Pediatr 1982;101:36–9.

24. Dahlquist G, Rudberg S. The prevalence of microalbuminuria in diabetic children and adolescents and its relation to puberty. Acta Paediatr Scand 1987;76:795–800.

25. Chase HP, Jackson WE, Hoops SL, et al. Glucose control and the renal and retinal complications of insulin-dependent diabetes. JAMA 1989;261:1155–60.

26. Mortensen HB, Vestermark S, Kastrup KW. Metabolic control in children with insulin dependent diabetes mellitus assessed by hemoglobin A_{1c}. Acta Paediatr Scand 1982;71:217–22.

27. Tze WJ, Thompson KH, Leichter J: HbA_1—an indicator of diabetic control. J Pediatr 1978;93:13–6.

28. Mann NP, Johnston DI. Total glycosylated haemoglobin (HbA_1) levels in diabetic children. Arch Dis Child 1982;57:434–7.

29. Goldstein DE, Walker B, Rawlings SS. Hemoglobin A_{1c} levels in children and adolescents with diabetes mellitus. Diabetes Care 1980;3:503–7.

30. Kaar M-L, Åkerblom HK, Huttunen N-P, et al. Metabolic control in children and adolescents with insulin-dependent diabetes mellitus. Acta Paediatr Scand 1984; 73:102–8.

31. Daneman D, Wolfson DH, Becker DJ, Drash AL. Factors affecting glycosylated hemoglobin values in children with insulin-dependent diabetes. J Pediatr 1981; 99:847–53.

32. Williams ML, Savage DCL. Glycosylated hemoglobin levels in children with diabetes mellitus. Arch Dis Child 1979;54:295–8.

33. Daneman D, Frank M, Perlman K, et al. Severe hypoglycemia in children with insulin-dependent diabetes mellitus: frequency and predisposing factors. J Pediatr 1989; 115:681–5.

34. Dahlquist G, Blom L, Bolme P, et al. Metabolic control in 131 juvenile-onset diabetic patients as measured by HbA_{1c}: relation to age, duration, insulin dose, and one or two injections. Diabetes Care 1982;5:399–403.

35. Drash AL, Kingsley LA, Doft B, et al. Observations on the effects of changing therapeutic strategies on metabolic status and microvascular complications in IDDM. Pediatr Adolesc Endocrinol 1988;17:206–14.

36. Belmonte MM, Schiffrin A, Dufresne J, et al. Impact of SMBG on control of diabetes as measured by HbA_1: 3-year survey of a juvenile IDDM clinic. Diabetes Care 1988;11:484–8.

37. Bhatia V, Wolfsdorf JI. Severe hypoglycemia in youth with insulin-dependent diabetes mellitus: frequency and causative factors. Pediatrics 1991;88:1187–93.

38. Drash A. The control of diabetes mellitus. Is it achievable? Is it desirable? [Editorial] J Pediatr 1976;88:1074–6.

39. Copeland KC. Too uptight about tight control? [Editorial]. Diabetes Care 1990;13:1089–91.

40. The Lipid Research Clinics Population Studies Data Book. Vol 1. The prevalence study. US Department of Health and Human Services. Publication no. 80–1527. Washington, DC: Goverment Printing Office, July 1980.

41. American Academy of Pediatrics Committee on Nutrition. Indications for cholesterol testing in children. Pediatrics 1989;83:141–2.

42. American Heart Association. Diagnosis and treatment of primary hyperlipidemia in childhood. Circulation 1986; 74:1181A–8.

43. Riley J, MacLaren NK, Lezotte DC, et al. Thyroid autoimmunity in insulin-dependent diabetes mellitus: the case for routine screening. J Pediatr 1981;98:350–4.

44. Gilani BB, MacGillivray MH, Voorhess ML, et al. Thyroid hormone abnormalities at diagnosis of insulin-dependent diabetes mellitus in children. J Pediatr 1984;105:218–22.

45. McKenna MJ, Herskowitz R, Wolfsdorf JI. Screening for thyroid disease in children with IDDM. Diabetes Care 1990;13:801–3.

46. Brush JM. Initial stabilization of the diabetic child. Am J Dis Child 1944;67:429–44.

47. Baker L, Kaye R, Root AW. The early partial remission of juvenile diabetes mellitus. The roles of insulin and growth hormone. J Pediatr 1967;71:825–31.

48. Grajwer LA, Pildes RS, Horwitz DL, Rubenstein AH. Control of juvenile diabetes and its relationship to endogenous insulin secretion as measured by C-peptide immunoreactivity. J Pediatr 1977;90:42–8.

49. Cahill GF Jr, McDevitt HO. Insulin-dependent diabetes mellitus: the initial lesion. N Engl J Med 1981; 304:1454–65.

50. Madsbad S. Prevalence of residual B cell function and its metabolic consequences in type 1 (insulin-dependent) diabetes. Diabetologia 1983;24:141–7.

51. Sochett EB, Daneman D, Clarson C, Ehrlich RM. Factors affecting and patterns of residual insulin secretion during the first year of type 1 (insulin-dependent diabetes mellitus in children. Diabetologia 30:453,1987.

52. Ferner RE. The natural history of insulin secretion in type 1 diabetes. Diabetic Med 1989;6:299–302.

53. Mann NP, Johnston DI. Improvement in metabolic control in diabetic adolescents by the use of increased insulin dose. Diabetes Care 1984;7:460–4.

54. Amiel SA, Sherwin RS, Simonson DC, et al. Impaired insulin action in puberty: a contributing factor to poor glycemic control in adolescents with diabetes. N Engl J Med 1986;315:215–9.

55. Bloch CA, Clemons P, Sperling MA. Puberty reduces insulin sensitivity. J Pediatr 1987;110:481–7.

56. Rosenbloom AL, Wheeler L, Bianchi R, et al. Age-adjusted analysis of insulin responses during normal and abnormal oral glucose tolerance tests in normal children and adolescents. Diabetes 1975;24:280–8.

57. Hindmarsh P, Di Silvio L, Pringle PJ, et al. Changes in serum insulin concentration during puberty and their relationship to growth hormone. Clin Endocrinol 1988;28:381–8.

58. Caprio S, Plewe G, Diamond MP, et al. Increased insulin secretion in puberty: a compensatory response to reductions in insulin sensitivity. J Pediatr 1989;114:963–7.

59. Ginsberg S, Block MB, Mako ME, Rubenstein AH. Serum insulin levels following administration of exogenous insulin. J Clin Endocrinol Metab 1973;36:1175–9.

60. Rasmussen SM, Heding LG, Parbst E, Vølund AV. Serum IRI in insulin-treated diabetics during a 24-hour period. Diabetologia 1975;11:151–8.

61. Gokal R, Harding P, Turner RC. Comparison between the plasma insulin and glucose reponses to five different insulin regimens in diabetic patients. Clin Endocrinol 1977;7:301–5.

62. Werther GA, Turner RC, Jenkins PA, Baum JD. Twenty-four-hour profiles of plasma C-peptide in type 1 (insulin-dependent) diabetic children. Diabetologia 1982; 22:245–9.

63. Sterky GCG, Persson BEH, Larsson YAA. Dietary fats, the diurnal blood lipids and ketones in juvenile diabetes. Diabetologia 1966;2:14−9.

64. Åkerblom HK, Hiekkala H. Diurnal blood and urine glucose and acetone bodies in labile juvenile diabetics on one- and two-injection insulin therapy. Diabetologia 1970;6:130−4.

65. Åkerblom H, Hiekkala H, Salmenperä L, Koivukanges T. One or two daily injections of insulin? Mod Probl Paediatr 1975;12:320−4.

66. Werther GA, Jenkins PA, Turner RC, Baum JD. Twenty-four-hour metabolic profiles in diabetic children receiving insulin injections once or twice daily. BMJ 1980; 281:414−8.

67. Langdon DR, James FD, Sperling MA. Comparison of single- and split-dose insulin regimens with 24-hour monitoring. J Pediatr 1981;99:854−61.

68. Clarke WL, Haymond MW, Santiago JV. Overnight basal insulin requirements in fasting insulin-dependent diabetics. Diabetes 1980;9:78−80.

69. Winter RJ. Profiles of metabolic control in diabetic children: frequency of asymptomatic nocturnal hypoglycemia. Metabolism 1981;30:666−72.

70. Whincup G, Milner RDG. Prediction and management of nocturnal hypoglycaemia in diabetes. Arch Dis Child 1987;62:333−7.

71. Annotation. Nocturnal hypoglycaemia in childhood diabetes. Lancet 1987;2:253−4.

72. Baumer JH, Edelstein AD, Howlett BC, et al. Impact of home blood glucose monitoring on childhood diabetes. Arch Dis Child 1982;57;195−9.

73. Shalwitz RA, Farkas-Hirsch R, White NH, Santiago JV. Prevalence and consequences of nocturnal hypoglycemia among conventionally treated children with diabetes mellitus. J Pediatr 1990;116:685−9.

74. Lerman IG, Wolfsdorf JI. Relationship of nocturnal hypoglycemia to daytime glycemia in IDDM. Diabetes Care 1988;11:636−42.

75. Macfarlane PI, Walters M, Stutchfield P, Smith CS. A prospective study of symptomatic hypoglycaemia in childhood diabetes. Diabetic Med 1989;6:627−30.

76. Schmidt MI, Hadji-Georgopoulous A, Rendell M, et al. Fasting hyperglycemia and associated free insulin and cortisol changes in "somogyi-like" patients. Diabetes Care 1979;2:457−64.

77. Bolli GB, Gerich JE. The "dawn phenomenon"—a common occurrence in both non-insulin-dependent and insulin-dependent diabetes mellitus. N Engl J Med 1984; 310:746−50.

78. Campbell PJ, Bolli GB, Cryer PE, Gerich JE. Pathogenesis of the dawn phenomenon in patients with insulin-dependent diabetes mellitus. Accelerated glucose production and impaired glucose utilization due to nocturnal surges in growth hormone secretion. N Engl J Med 1985; 312:1473−21.

79. Perriello G, De Feo P, Bolli GB. The dawn phenomenon: nocturnal blood glucose homeostasis in insulin-dependent diabetes mellitus. Diabetic Med 1988;5:13−21.

80. Duncan BB, Schmidt MI, Ellis GJ III, et al. Frequency of early-morning rise in blood glucose in children with diabetes at camp. Diabetes Care 1988;11:574−8.

81. Kinmonth AL, Baum JD. Timing of pre-breakfast insulin injection and postprandial metabolic control in diabetic children. BMJ 1980;280:604−6.

82. Kraegen EW, Chisholm DJ, McNamara ME. Timing of insulin delivery with meals. Horm Metab Res 1981; 13:365−7.

83. Dimitriadis GD, Gerich JE. Importance of timing of preprandial subcutaneous insulin administration in the management of diabetes mellitus. Diabetes Care 1983;6:374−7.

84. Witt MF, White NH, Santiago JV. Roles of site and timing of the morning insulin injection in type 1 diabetes. J Pediatr 1983;103:528−33.

85. Skyler JS, Skyler DL, Seigler DE, O'Sullivan MJ. Algorithms for adjustment of insulin dosage by patients who monitor blood glucose. Diabetes Care 1981;4:311−8.

86. Francis AJ, Home PD, Hanning I, et al. Intermediate acting insulin given at bedtime: effect on blood glucose concentrations before and after breakfast. BMJ 1983;286:1173−6.

87. Wolfsdorf JI, Laffel LMB, Pasquarello C, et al. Split-mixed insulin regimen with human ultralente before supper and NPH (isophane) before breakfast in children and adolescents with IDDM. Diabetes Care 1991;14:1100−6.

88. Galloway JA, Root MA, Bergstrom R, et al. Clinical pharmacologic studies with human insulin (recombinant DNA). Diabetes Care 1982;5(Suppl 2):13−22.

89. Ebihara A, Kondo K, Ohashi K, et al. Comparative clinical pharmacology of human insulin (Novo) and porcine insulin in normal subjects. Diabetes Care 1983;6(Suppl 1):17−22.

90. Starke AAR, Heinemann L, Hohmann A, Berger M. The action profiles of human NPH insulin preparations. Diabetic Med 1989;6:239−44.

91. Schade DS, Santiago JV, Skyler JS, Rizza RA. Intensive insulin therapy. Amsterdam: Excerpta Medica, 1983.

92. Holman RR, Turner RC. A practical guide to basal and prandial insulin therapy. Diabetic Med 1985;2:45−53.

93. Sherwin RS. Role of the liver in glucose homeostasis. Diabetes Care 1980;3:261−5.

94. Rizza RA, Gerich JE, Haymond MW, et al. Control of blood sugar in insulin-dependent diabetes: comparison of an artificial endocrine pancreas, continuous subcutaneous insulin infusion and intensified conventional insulin therapy. N Engl J Med 1980;303:1313−8.

95. Deckert T. Intermediate-acting insulin preparations, NPH and lente. Diabetes Care 1980;3:623−6.

96. Skyler JS, Seigler DE, Reeves ML. A comparison of insulin regimens in insulin-dependent diabetes mellitus. Diabetes Care 1982;5(Suppl 1):11−8.

97. Tamborlane WV, Sherwin RS, Genel M, Felig P. Outpatient treatment of juvenile-onset diabetes with a preprogrammed portable subcutaneous insulin infusion system. Am J Med 1980;68:190−6.

98. Rudolf MC, Ahern JA, Genel M, et al. Optimal insulin delivery in adolescents with diabetes: impact of intensive treatment on psychosocial adjustment. Diabetes Care 1982;5(Suppl 1):53−7.

99. Schiffrin A, Desrosiers M, Moffat M, Belmonte MM. Feasibility of strict diabetes control in insulin-dependent diabetic adolescents. J Pediatr 1983;103:522−7.

100. Schiffrin A, Desrosiers M, Aleyassine H, Belmonte MM. Intensified insulin therapy in the type 1 diabetic adolescent: a controlled trial. Diabetes Care 1984;7:107−13.

101. Bougneres PF, Landier F, Lemmel C, et al. Insulin pump therapy in young children with type 1 diabetes. J Pediatr 1984;105:212−7.

102. de Beaufort CE, Houtzagers CMGT, Bruining GJ, et al. Continuous subcutaneous insulin infusion (CSII) versus conventional injection therapy in newly diagnosed diabetic children: two year follow-up of a randomized, prospective trial. Diabetic Med 1989;6:766−71.

103. de Beaufort CE, Bruining GJ. Continuous subcutaneous insulin infusion in children. Diabetic Med 1987;4:103−8.

104. Brink SJ, Stewart C. Insulin pump treatment in insulin-dependent diabetes mellitus: children, adolescents, and young adults. JAMA 1986;255:617–21.

105. Knight G, Boulton AJM, Ward JD. Experience of continuous subcutaneous insulin infusion in the outpatient management of diabetic teenagers. Diabetic Med 1986; 3:82–4.

106. Greene SA, Smith MA, Baum JD. Clinical application of insulin pumps in the management of insulin dependent diabetes. Arch Dis Child 1983;58:578–81.

107. Becker DJ, Kerensky KM, Transue D, et al. Current status of pump therapy in childhood. Acta Paediatr Jpn 1984; 26:347–8.

108. Kaye R. Research and practice in the treatment of insulin-dependent diabetes: a survey of 53 pediatric diabetologists. Pediatrics 1984;74:1079–85.

109. Unger RH. Meticulous control of diabetes: benefits, risks and precautions. Diabetes 1982;31:479–85.

110. The DCCT Research Group. Diabetes Control and Complications Trial (DCCT): results of feasibility study. Diabetes Care 1987;10:1–19.

111. Recommended Dietary Allowances. 10th ed. National Research Council, National Academy of Science. Washington, DC: National Academy Press, 1989.

112. American Diabetes Association. Nutritional recommendations and principles for individuals with diabetes mellitus: 1986. Diabetes Care 1987;10:126–32.

113. National Diabetes Advisory Board. National standards and review criteria for diabetes patient education programs. Diabetes Educ 1986;12:286–91.

114. Grinvalsky M, Nathan DM. Diets for insulin pump and multiple daily injection therapy. Diabetes Care 1983; 6:241–4.

115. Lorenz RA, Christensen NK, Pichert JW. Diet-related knowledge, skill, and adherence among children with insulin-dependent diabetes mellitus. Pediatrics 1985; 75:872–6.

116. American Diabetes Association, American Dietetic Association. Exchange lists for meal planning. Alexandria, VA: American Diabetes Association; Chicago, IL: American Dietetic Association, 1986.

117. Anderson BJ, Miller JP, Auslander WF, Santiago JV. Family characteristics of diabetic adolescents: relationship to metabolic control. Diabetes Care 1981;4:586–94.

118. Lockwood D, Frey ML, Gladish NA, Hiss RG. The biggest problem in diabetes. Diabetes Educ 1986;12:30–33.

119. Christensen NK, Terry RD, Wyatt S, et al. Quantitative assessment of dietary adherence in patients with insulin-dependent diabetes mellitus. Diabetes Care 1983; 6:245–50.

120. Delameter AM, Smith JA, Kurtz SM, White NH. Dietary skills and adherence in children with type 1 diabetes mellitus. Diabetes Educ 1988;14:33–6.

121. Sims DF. Barriers to adherence. Diabetes Care 1979; 2:524–5.

122. Daneman D, Siminerio L, Transui D, et al. The role of self-monitoring of blood glucose in the routine management of children with insulin-dependent diabetes mellitus. Diabetes Care 1985;8:1–4.

123. Templeton CL, Burkhart MT, Anderson BJ, Bacon GE. A group aproach to nutritional problem solving using self-monitoring of blood glucose with diabetic adolescents. Diabetes Educ 1988;14:189–91.

124. Wahren J, Felig P, Hagenfeldt L. Physical exercise and fuel homeostasis in diabetes mellitus. Diabetologia 1978; 14:213–22.

125. Zinman B, Murray FT, Vranic M, et al. Glucoregulation during moderate exercise in insulin treated diabetics. J Clin Endocrinol Metab 1977;45:641–52.

126. Horton ES. Role and management of exercise in diabetes mellitus. Diabetes Care 1988;1:201–11.

127. Dahl-Jørgensen K, Meen HD, Hanssen KF, Aagenaes Ø. The effect of exercise on diabetic control and hemoglobin $A_1(HbA_1)$ in children. Acta Paediatr Scand Suppl 1980;283:53–6.

128. Campaigne BN, Gilliam TB, Spencer ML, et al. Effects of a physical activity program on metabolic control and cardiovascular fitness in children with insulin-dependent diabetes mellitus. Diabetes Care 1984;7:57–62.

129. Landt K, Campaigne BN, James FW, Sperling MA. Effects of exercise training on insulin sensitivity in adolescents with type 1 diabetes. Diabetes Care 1985;8:461–5.

130. Rowland TW, Swadba LA, Biggs DE, et al. Glycemic control with physical training in insulin-dependent diabetes mellitus. Am J Dis Child 1985;139:307–10.

131. Koivisto VA, Felig P. Effects of leg exercise on insulin absorption in diabetic patients. N Engl J Med 1978; 298:79–83.

132. Berger M, Halban PA, Assal JP, et al. Pharmacokinetics of subcutaneously injected tritiated insulin: effects of exercise. Diabetes 1979;28(Suppl 1):53–7.

133. Berger M, Berchtold P, Cüppers HJ, et al. Metabolic and hormonal effects of muscular exercise in juvenile type diabetics. Diabetologia 1977;13:355–65.

134. Wallberg-Henriksson H, Gunnarsson R, Henriksson J, et al. Increased peripheral insulin sensitivity and muscle mitochondrial enzymes but unchanged blood glucose control in type 1 diabetics after physical training. Diabetes 1982;31:1044–50.

135. MacDonald MJ. Postexercise late-onset hypoglycemia in insulin-dependent diabetic patients. Diabetes Care 1987;10:584–8.

136. Bogardus C, Thuillez P, Ravussin E, Vasquez B. Effect of muscle glycogen depletion on in vivo insulin action in man. J Clin Invest 1983;72:1605–10.

137. Rowland TW. Physical fitness in children: implications for the prevention of coronary artery disease. Curr Probl Pediatr 1981;11:1–54.

138. Sönksen PH, Judd SL, Lowy C. Home monitoring of blood glucose: method for improving diabetic control. Lancet 1978;1:729–32.

139. Walford S, Gale EAM, Allison SP, Tattersall RB. Self-monitoring of blood glucose: improvement of diabetic control. Lancet 1978;1:732–5.

140. American Diabetes Association. Consensus statement on self-monitoring of blood glucose. Diabetes Care 1987; 10:95–9.

141. Geffner ME, Kaplan SA, Lippe BM, Scott ML. Self-monitoring of blood glucose levels and intensified insulin therapy: acceptability and efficacy in childhood diabetes. JAMA 1983;249:2913–6.

142. Burghen GA. Therapy in childhood diabetes [Editorial]. JAMA 1983;490:2938–9.

143. Daneman D, Siminerio L, Transue D, et al. The role of self-monitoring of blood glucose in the routine management of children with insulin-dependent diabetes mellitus. Diabetes Care 1985;8:1–4.

144. Clarson C, Daneman D, Frank M, et al. Self-monitoring of blood glucose: how accurate are children with diabetes at reading Chemstrip bG? Diabetes Care 1985; 8:354–8.

145. Wilson DP, Endres RK. Compliance with blood glucose monitoring in children with type 1 diabetes mellitus. J Pediatr 1986;108:1022–4.

146. Mazze RS, Shamoon H, Pasmantier R, et al. Reliability of blood glucose monitoring by patients with diabetes mellitus. Am J Med 1984;77:211–7.

147. Schiffrin A, Suissa S. Predicting nocturnal hypoglycemia in patients with type 1 diabetes treated with continuous subcutaneous insulin infusion. Am J Med 1987; 82:1127–32.

148. Freund A, Johnson SB, Rosenbloom A, et al. Subjective symptoms, blood glucose estimation, and blood glucose concentrations in adolescents with diabetes. Diabetes Care 1986;9:236–43.

149. Carney RM, Schechter K, Homa M, et al. The effects of blood glucose testing versus urine sugar testing on the metabolic control of insulin-dependent diabetic children. Diabetes Care 1983;6:378–80.

150. Wysocki T. SMBG: has the promise been fulfilled? Diabetes Spectrum 1988;1:83–7.

151. Hermansson G, Ludvigsson J, Larsson Y. Home blood glucose monitoring in diabetic children and adolescents: a 3-year feasibility study. Acta Paediatr Scand 1986; 75:98–105.

152. Mann NP, Noronha JL, Johnston DI. A prospective study to evaluate the benefits of long-term self-monitoring of blood glucose in diabetic children. Diabetes Care 1984; 7:322–6.

153. Wing RR, Lamparski DM, Zaslow S, et al. Frequency and accuracy of self-monitoring of blood glucose in children: relationship to glycemic control. Diabetes Care 1985; 8:214–8.

154. Delamater AM, Davis SG, Bubb J, et al. Self-monitoring of blood glucose by adolescents with diabetes: technical skills and utilization of data. Diabetes Educ 1989; 15:56–61.

155. Delamater AM, Bubb J, Davis SG. et al. Randomized prospective study of self-management training with newly diagnosed diabetic children. Diabetes Care 1990; 13:492–8.

156. Schiffrin A, Belmonte M. Multiple daily self-glucose monitoring: its essential role in long-term glucose control in insulin-dependent diabetic patients treated with pump and multiple subcutaneous injections. Diabetes Care 1982;5:479–84.

157. Malone JI, Rosenbloom AL, Grgic A, Weber FT. The role of urine sugar in diabetic management. Am J Dis Child 1976;130:1324–7.

158. Ohlsen P, Danowski TS, Rosenblum DH, et al. Discrepancies between glycosuria and home estimates of blood glucose in insulin-treated diabetes mellitus. Diabetes Care 1980;3:178–83.

159. Tattersall R, Gale E. Patient self-monitoring of blood glucose and refinements of conventional insulin treatment. Am J Med 1981;70:177–82.

160. Alberti KGMM, Dornhorst A, Rowe AS. Metabolic rhythms in normal and diabetic man: studies in insulin-treated diabetes. In: Shafrir E, ed. Contemporary topics in the study of diabetes and metabolic endocrinology. New York: Academic Press, 1975:45–54.

161. MacGillivray MH, Voorhess ML, Putnam TI, et al. Hormone and metabolic profiles in children and adolescents with type 1 diabetes mellitus. Diabetes Care 1982;5(Suppl 1):38–47.

162. Malone JI, Hellrung JM, Malphus EW, et al. Good diabetic control—a study in mass delusion. J Pediatr 1976; 88:943–7.

163. Nathan DM, Singer DE, Hurxthal K, Goodson JD. The clinical information value of the glycosylated hemoglobin assay. N Engl J Med 1984;310:341–6.

164. Bunn HF, Haney DN, Kamin S, et al. The biosynthesis of human hemoglobin A_{1c}: slow glycosylation of hemoglobin in vivo. J Clin Invest 1976;57:1652–9.

165. Koenig RJ, Peterson CM, Jones RL, et al. Correlation of glucose regulation and hemoglobin A_{1c} in diabetes mellitus. N Engl J Med 1976;295:417–20.

166. Gabbay KH, Hasty K, Breshlow JL, et al. Glycosylated hemoglobins and long-term blood glucose control in diabetes mellitus. J Clin Endocrinol Metab 1977;44:859–64.

167. Gonen B, Rubenstein AH. Haemoglobin A_1 and diabetes mellitus. Diabetologia 1978;15:1–8.

168. Svendsen PA, Lauritzen T, Segaard U, Nerup J. Glycosylated haemoglobin and steady-state mean blood glucose concentration in type 1 (insulin-dependent) diabetes. Diabetologia 1982;23:403–5.

169. Goldstein DE, Little RR, Wiedmeyer HM, et al. Glycated hemoglobin: methodologies and clinical applications. Clin Chem 1986;32(Suppl 10):B64–70.

170. Health and Public Policy Committee, American College of Physicians. Glycosylated hemoglobin assays in the management and diagnosis of diabetes mellitus. Ann Intern Med 1984;101:710–3.

171. Belmonte MM, Gunn T, Gonthier M. The problem of "cheating" in the diabetic child and adolescent. Diabetes Care 1981;4:116–20.

172. Citrin W, Ellis GJ III, Skyler JS. Glycosylated hemoglobin: a tool in identifying psychological problems [Editorial]. Diabetes Care 1980;3:563–4.

173. Krause JR, Stolc V, Campbell E. The effect of hemoglobin F upon glycosylated hemoglobin determinations. Am J Clin Pathol 1982;78:767–9.

174. Aleyassine H. Low proportions of glycosylated hemoglobin associated with hemoglobin S and hemoglobin C. Clin Chem 1978;25:1484–6.

175. Sosenko JM, Flückiger R, Platt OS, Gabbay KH. Glycosylation of variant hemoglobins in normal and diabetic subjects. Diabetes Care 1980;3:590–3.

176. Allen DB, MacDonald MJ. Artifacts in glycosylated hemoglobin values in pediatric patients. J Pediatr 1986; 109:655–7.

177. Shah SC, Malone JI, Boissell J-P, Kasper TJ. Hemoglobin South Florida: new variant with normal electrophoretic pattern mistaken for glycosylated hemoglobin. Diabetes 1986;35:1073–6.

178. Daneman D, Tsalikian E, Hengstenberg F, et al. Glycosylated haemoglobin in children with insulin-dependent diabetes mellitus. Diabetologia 1980;19:423–6.

179. Schade DS, Eaton RP. Pathogenesis of diabetic ketoacidosis: a reappraisal. Diabetes Care 1979;2:296–306.

180. Schade DS, Eaton RP. The temporal relationship between endogenously secreted stress hormones and metabolic decompensation in diabetic man. J Clin Endocrinol Metab 1980;50:131–6.

181. Schade DS, Eaton RP. Prevention of diabetic ketoacidosis. JAMA 1979;242:2455–8.

182. Frier BM. Hypoglycaemia and diabetes. Diabetic Med 1986;3:513–25.

183. Goldstein DE, England JD, Hess R, et al. A prospective study of symptomatic hypoglycemia in young diabetic patients. Diabetes Care 1981;4:601–5.

184. Daneman D, Ehrlich RM. Children with insulin-dependent diabetes mellitus. Med North Am 1987;15:2926–34.

185. Pramming S, Thorsteinsson B, Theilgaard A, et al. Cognitive function during hypoglycaemia in type 1 diabetes mellitus. BMJ 1986;292:647–506.

186. Frier BM, Matthews DM, Steel JM, Duncan LJP. Driving and insulin-dependent diabetes. Lancet 1980;1:1232–7.

187. Songer TJ, La Porte RE, Dorman JS, et al. Motor vehicle accidents and IDDM. Diabetes Care 1988;11:701–7.

188. Ratner RE, Whitehouse FW. Motor vehicles, hypoglycemia, and diabetic drivers. Diabetes Care 1989; 12:217–22.

189. Brierley JB. Brain damage due to hypoglycaemia. In: Marks V, Rose FC, eds. Hypoglycemia. 2nd ed. Oxford: Blackwell, 1981:488–94.

190. Aynsley-Green A, Soltesz G. Hypoglycaemia in infancy and childhood. New York: Churchill Livingstone, 1985:29–31.

191. Cox DJ, Irvine A, Gonder-Frederick L, et al. Fear of hypoglycemia: quantification, validation, and utilization. Diabetes Care 1987;10:617–21.

192. Bergada I, Suissa S, Dufresne J, Schiffrin A. Severe hypoglycemia in IDDM children. Diabetes Care 1989; 12:239–44.

193. Egger M, Gschwend S, Davey Smith G, Zuppinger K. Increasing incidence of hypoglycemic coma in children with IDDM. Diabetes Care 1991;14:1001–5.

194. Aman J, Karlsson I, Wranne L. Symptomatic hypoglycemia in childhood diabetes: a population-based questionnaire study. Diabetic Med 1989;6:257–61.

195. Travis LB. Hypoglycemia in insulin-dependent diabetes mellitus [Editorial]. J Pediatr 1989;115:740–2.

196. Eastman BG, Johnson SB, Silvestein J, et al. Understanding of hypo- and hyperglycemia by youngsters with diabetes and their parents. J Pediatr Psychol 1983;8:229–43.

197. Brodows RG, Williams C, Amatruda JM. Treatment of insulin reactions in diabetics. JAMA 1984;252:3378–81.

198. Gunning RR, Garber AJ. Bioactivity of instant glucose— failure of absorption through the oral mucosa. JAMA 1978;240:1611–2.

199. Åman J, Wranne L. Treatment of hypoglycemia in diabetes: failure of absorption of glucose through rectal mucosa. Acta Paediatr Scand 1984;73:560–1.

200. Åman J, Wranne L. Hypoglycemia in childhood diabetes. II. Effect of subcutaneous or intramuscular injection of different doses of glucagon. Acta Paediatr Scand 1988; 77:548–53.

201. Muhlhauser I, Berger M, Sonnenberg G, et al. Incidence and management of severe hypoglycemia in 434 adults with insulin-dependent diabetes mellitus. Diabetes Care 1985;8:268–73.

202. Matthews DM, Patrick AW, Collier DA, et al. Awareness and use of glucagon in diabetics treated with insulin. BMJ 1986;293:367–8.

203. Shipp JC, Delcher HK, Munroe JF. Treatment of insulin hypoglycemia in diabetic campers: comparison of glucagon (1 and 2 mg) and glucose. Diabetes 1964;13:645–8.

204. Elrick H, Witten TA, Arai Y. Glucagon treatment of insulin reactions. N Engl J Med 1958;258:476–86.

205. Schulman JL, Greben SE. The effect of glucagon on the blood glucose level and the clinical state in the presence of marked insulin hypoglycemia. J Clin Invest 1957; 36:74–80.

206. Mühlhauser I, Koch J, Berger M. Pharmacokinetics and bioavailability of injected glucagon: differences between intramuscular, subcutaneous and intravenous administration. Diabetes Care 1985;8:39–42.

207. Drash AL, Becker D. Diabetes mellitus in the child: course, special problems, and related disorders. In: Katzen HM, Mahler RJ, eds. Diabetes, obesity, and vascular disease. Advances in modern nutrition. Vol 2. New York: Wiley, 1978:615–43.

208. Hauser S, Solomon ML. Coping with diabetes: views from the family. In: Ahmed R, Ahmed N, eds. Coping with juvenile diabetes. Springfield, IL: Charles C Thomas, 1985:234–66.

209. Anderson BJ. Diabetes and adaptations in family systems. In: Holmes C, ed. Neuropsychological and behavioral aspects of diabetes. New York: Springer-Verlag, 1990:85–101.

210. Sabbeth B. Understanding the impact of chronic childhood illness on families. Pediatr Clin North Am 1984; 31:47–57.

211. Anderson BJ. The impact of diabetes on the developmental tasks of childhood and adolescence: a research perspective. In: Natrass M, Santiago JV, eds. Recent advances in diabetes. New York: Churchill Livingstone, 1984:165–71.

212. Leaverton DR. The child with diabetes mellitus. In: Call JD, et al, eds. Basic handbook of child psychiatry. Vol 1. New York: Basic Books, 1979:452–8.

213. Hagen JW, Anderson BJ, Barclay CR. Issues in research on the young chronically ill child. Top Early Childhood Spec Ed 1986;5:49–57.

214. Bregani P, Della Porta V, Carbone A, et al. Attitudes of juvenile diabetics and their families towards dietetic regimen. Pediatr Adolesc Endocrinol 1979;7:159–63.

215. Zuppinger K, Schmid E, Schutz B. Attitude of the juvenile diabetic, his family and peers toward a restricted dietetic regimen. Pediatr Adolesc Endocrinol 1979;7:153–8.

216. Grey MJ, Genel M, Tamborlane WV. Psychosocial adjustment of latency-age diabetics: determinants and relationship to control. Pediatrics 1980;65:69–73.

217. Anderson BJ, White NW. A comprehensive approach to the management of insulin-dependent diabetes mellitus (IDDM) in children, adolescents, and families. Part 1. Pediatric Rounds C.S. Mott Children's Hospital 1988; 8(3):1–5.

218. Hamburg BA. Early adolescence: a specific and stressful stage of the life cycle. In: Coelho GV, Hamburg DA, Adams JE, eds. Coping and adaptation. New York: Basic Books, 1974:110–24.

219. Cerreto MC, Travis LB. Implications of psychological and family factors in the treatment of diabetes. Pediatr Clin North Am 1984;31:689–710.

220. Anderson BJ, White NH. A comprehensive approach to the management of insulin-dependent diabetes mellitus (IDDM) in children, adolescents, and families. Part 2. Pediatric Rounds C.S. Mott Children's Hospital 1988; 8(4):1–8.

221. La Greca AM, Schwarz LT, Satin W. Eating patterns in young women with IDDM: another look [Letter]. Diabetes Care 1987;10:659–60.

222. Anderson BJ, Auslander WF. Research on diabetes management and the family: a critique. Diabetes Care 1980;3:696–702.

223. Green LW, Horton D. Adolescent health: issues and challenges. In: Coates T, Peterson A, Perry P, eds. Promoting adolescent health. New York: Academic Press, 1982:23–43.

224. Citrin WS, La Greca AM, Skyler JS. Group interventions in type I diabetes mellitus. In: Ahmed PI, Ahmed N, eds. Coping with juvenile diabetes. Springfield, IL: Charles C Thomas, 1985:184–204.

225. Gortmaker SL, Sappenfield W. Chronic childhood disorders: prevalence and impact. Pediatr Clin North Am 1984;31:3–18.

226. Barbero GJ. Leaving the pediatrician for the internist [Editorial]. Ann Intern Med 1982;96:673–4.

Chapter 31

TREATMENT OF THE ELDERLY WITH DIABETES

LINDA A. MORROW
JEFFREY B. HALTER

Men and women 65 years and older currently make up more than 12% of the United States population. This number is expected to increase to 22% by the year 2040.[1] At present, included in this population are almost 3 million of the "oldest old"—those individuals 85 years and older. This number is expected to grow to 13 million by the year 2040.[2] These demographic changes will have profound effects on health care and its delivery in the United States. Because diabetes mellitus may affect up to 20% of individuals over the age of 65 years, treatment of older patients with diabetes mellitus demands careful consideration.

Diabetes mellitus is a disease associated with aging. Uncommon in children and younger adults, its prevalence increases with age. The National Health and Nutrition Examination Survey (NHANES II), conducted by the National Center for Health Statistics from 1976 through 1980, provided estimates of diagnosed and undiagnosed diabetes mellitus in the United States for individuals aged 19 to 74 years.[3] Among those 65 to 74 years old, almost 10% had previously diagnosed diabetes and an equal number were found to have undiagnosed diabetes mellitus by the criteria used in this study (oral glucose tolerance testing). Other abnormalities in carbohydrate metabolism were found to be present in this age group as well, with an additional 22.7% meeting the criteria for impaired glucose tolerance.

The incidence of diabetes mellitus also increases with age. The incidence rate is approximately 2 per 1000 among those individuals aged 25 to 44, increasing to approximately 5 per 1000 among individuals older than 45. This high incidence rate is maintained even for those individuals greater than 75 years old.[4]

Although the classification of diabetes mellitus in older adults is difficult, the majority of individuals with diabetes mellitus who are older than 65 have non-insulin-dependent diabetes (NIDDM). Insulin-dependent diabetes mel-litus (IDDM) occurs in this age group as well; perhaps 5 to 10% of older individuals with newly diagnosed diabetes mellitus have IDDM.[5] In addition, a small proportion of older individuals who initially have NIDDM appear to become insulin-dependent over time. The relation between the clinical syndromes of NIDDM and IDDM and the etiologic categories of Type I and Type II diabetes mellitus is not well-defined for older adults. The presence of ketosis at the time of diagnosis in older adults with diabetes mellitus suggests that insulin therapy will be necessary. However, some elderly individuals with diabetes and ketosis can subsequently be treated with oral agents. While HLA-DR3 is more common in older adults who require insulin treatment, the frequency of antibodies to islet cells in this group is not increased.[5]

CHANGES IN CARBOHYDRATE METABOLISM IN AGING

The prevalence of both diabetes mellitus and glucose intolerance increases with advancing age. These abnormalities in carbohydrate metabolism have features in common, and the glucose intolerance associated with aging may predispose to the development of overt diabetes mellitus. There is no evidence to suggest that the pathophysiology of NIDDM is any different in older adults than in younger adults. However, physiologic changes that appear to accompany the aging process produce glucose intolerance even in very healthy older individuals. These changes are manifested primarily as an elevation in postprandial blood glucose levels, which may increase by as much as 15 mg/dL (0.8 mM) per decade after the age of 30.[6,7] Age-related changes in fasting blood glucose levels are small, perhaps 1 to 2 mg/dL (0.05 to 0.09 mM) per decade after age 30. Figure 31–1 illustrates these changes with data from oral glucose tolerance testing for three different age groups.[8]

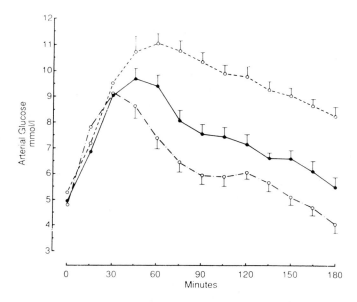

Fig. 31–1. Influence of age on oral glucose tolerance (100 g) in non-obese healthy men. Dashed line: 70–83 years old (*n* = 9); Solid line: 30–45 years old (*n* = 12); Stippled line: 19–24 years old (*n* = 11). Reprinted with permission from reference 8 (Jackson RA, Blix PM, Matthews JA, et al. Influence of ageing on glucose homeostasis. J Clin Endocrinol Metab 1982;55:840–8; © The Endocrine Society).

The pathophysiology of the change in glucose tolerance associated with aging is not yet completely defined. Glucose absorption following oral glucose ingestion may be slowed with increasing age, and hepatic glucose production is delayed (most likely as a result of delayed insulin secretion).[9] Subtle age-related changes in regulation of insulin secretion[10] have been described but have not been demonstrated in all studies. There is general agreement about the presence of insulin resistance in the elderly.[11,12] Such resistance is a result of post-receptor events, but the identification of the specific site or sites of such age-related changes is still being investigated.[13–15]

In addition to intrinsic changes of aging, extrinsic factors may contribute to glucose intolerance. Both the decline in lean body mass and the increase in body fat that accompany aging[16] may contribute to insulin resistance. Levels of physical activity also may decline with aging,[17] and such changes may precipitate or accelerate changes in body composition. Studies of both master athletes and older non-athletes suggest that some of these changes can be either prevented or modified with exercise.[18] Diet also can have adverse effects on carbohydrate metabolism, and a high-carbohydrate diet has been shown to improve insulin sensitivity in older individuals.[19] Drugs commonly used by older individuals, including diuretics, estrogen, sympathomimetics, glucocorticoids, niacin, phenytoin, and tricyclic antidepressants, can adversely affect glucose metabolism, exacerbating glucose intolerance. Stress states such as myocardial infarction, infection, burns, and surgery can worsen glucose tolerance and precipitate fasting hyperglycemia.

The clinical significance of glucose intolerance has been demonstrated in several studies. Glucose intolerance is a risk factor for the development of cardiovascular disease. The Honolulu Heart Study, a 12-year prospective study, found that the risk for fatal myocardial events among older nondiabetic men was 2.4 times higher in those in the highest quintile for post-challenge glucose levels than in those in the lowest quintile.[20] In addition, glucose intolerance in the elderly, as in younger adults, increases the risk for the development of overt diabetes mellitus. The risk for the development of diabetes mellitus among those over age 70 who are glucose intolerant is 2% per year, as compared with a risk of 0.04% per year for those older individuals with normal glucose tolerance.[21]

DIAGNOSIS OF DIABETES MELLITUS IN THE ELDERLY

The diagnostic criteria for diabetes mellitus and glucose intolerance are not adjusted for age and may be found in Chapter 11. In fact the criteria proposed by the National Diabetes Data Group (NDDG) in 1979 and currently in use were relaxed from previous criteria. This change was made, in part, to account for the high prevalence of diabetes mellitus in older adults that would be found if the earlier criteria were used. However, in spite of these changes, the testing situation should be carefully controlled to reduce the roles of factors such as drugs and intercurrent illness. In addition, the recommendations made for the preparations used for oral glucose tolerance testing should be followed carefully to avoid false-positive results in older adults. The best screening test for diabetes mellitus in older adults is a determination of fasting serum glucose levels. Oral glucose tolerance testing may be considered for individuals with fasting serum glucose levels between 115 and 140 mg/dL (6.4 to 7.8 mM) and for whom a definite diagnosis of diabetes mellitus or glucose intolerance is necessary (e.g., for experimental protocols, insurance requirements). For most elderly individuals, the decision about instituting treatment if fasting glucose levels are lower than 140 mg/dL (7.8 mM) will not be changed by the results of the two oral glucose tolerance tests necessary to establish the diagnosis of diabetes mellitus. Therefore, the indications for oral glucose testing should be carefully considered.

TREATMENT OF THE OLDER ADULT WITH DIABETES MELLITUS

For younger patients, aggressive management with the goal of achieving euglycemia is considered by many to be standard therapy, and little, if any, consideration is given to any other treatment goal. For the chronically ill patient in nursing home, rigorous glycemic control is probably not indicated. However, few of the approximately 6 million individuals older than 65 who have diabetes mellitus are chronically ill and residing in nursing homes. Therefore, an aggressive approach to therapy should at least be considered for these individuals.

The initial approach to the older adult with diabetes mellitus should include a careful assessment of the patient's current medical status and consideration of remaining life expectancy. Motivation and commitment of the patient and family also play large roles in determining what level of treatment is appropriate. Other issues that may be important are the support services available in the community and economic considerations.

Care for older adults with diabetes mellitus may be divided into two levels: basic care and aggressive care. Basic care is indicated for those individuals for whom the primary goal of treatment is the prevention of symptomatic hyperglycemia. The average glucose levels necessary for achievement of this goal are approximately 200 mg/dL (11 mM) or the glucose level at which glycosuria is minimal. The elimination of glycosuria is an important therapeutic threshold, as glycosuria predisposes older individuals with diabetes to volume depletion and risks of secondary problems related to hypotension and poor tissue perfusion. The most severe complication of diabetes in older individuals is hyperglycemic hyperosmolar nonketotic coma. Glycosuria also is associated with weight loss caused by the loss of calories in the urine. This associated catabolic state, one that results in excess protein metabolism and the loss of lean body tissue, may predispose to infections and other complications of malnutrition.

Aggressive care is appropriate when the goals of treatment include the prevention of long-term complications of diabetes. Euglycemia, with a fasting glucose level lower than 115 mg/dL (6.4 mM) is optimal, with a mean glucose level between 110 and 140 mg/dL (6 to 8 mM) and normal levels of glycosylated hemoglobin. These treatment goals are similar to those for younger patients with diabetes. Appropriate modifications should be made in these goals as new information becomes available regarding optimal levels of blood glucose for prevention of long-term complications.

The decision regarding treatment goals may be the single most important one in diabetes management, as this drives the remainder of the evaluation and treatment program. Usually this decision is made jointly by the patient (or the responsible party) and the primary care giver. Additional input from family members and consultants such as geriatricians, diabetologists, cardiologists, and nephrologists may be helpful in individual cases to provide a clearer picture of the current medical condition and estimates of life expectancy. The patient may also be aided in decision-making by information obtained from a diabetes educator, dietician, and/or nurse.

Several arguments can be made against the choice of an aggressive management program for older adults with diabetes. One is that some elderly patients may be less capable than younger patients of carrying out activities requiring the high levels of skill, commitment, and diabetes education necessary to their achieving an aggressive treatment goal. However, while methods of learning and memory do change with age, most older individuals are fully able to learn complicated concepts and tasks.[22-24] To the extent that older adults lead a less

hectic, more ordered life than younger adults, it may actually be easier for them to make the type of adjustments in life-style necessary for adherence to a good diabetes treatment program.

A common argument against aggressive diabetes management in older adults is based on inaccurate estimates of life expectancy (i.e., why try to prevent complications in someone who is likely to die soon?). Recent data reveal that the mean remaining life expectancy for individuals aged 65 is more than 17 years, for those aged 75 is 10 years, and for those aged 85 is 6 years. Furthermore, these are mean estimates, which will be exceeded by approximately 50% of the people in a given age cohort. While the presence of diabetes may reduce these figures for any given patient, age alone should not be a significant contributor to the decision process for the "young old"—those individuals aged 65 to 85 years who are otherwise in reasonably good health. Examination of the life expectancy data reveals that there is substantial time for the development of diabetes complications in a patient for whom the diagnosis is made during their sixties or seventies. It is also clear that elderly individuals are susceptible to virtually all of the chronic complications of diabetes mellitus. Age and diabetes frequently interact to worsen the risk for many of these complications. For example, creatinine clearance declines with normal aging,[25] and age is an independent risk factor for the development of peripheral neuropathy.[26,27] Until studies are available demonstrating that the risks of tight glycemic control outweigh the benefits in older adults or that glycemic control does not prevent the development of complications, many elderly patients deserve the same consideration as younger adults regarding aggressive management of their disease.

All older adults with diabetes mellitus should receive a care program that meets minimum standards, regardless of treatment goals. These standards, shown in Table 31–1, include a complete history and physical examination at the time of diagnosis that is directed toward the complications of diabetes mellitus and the presence of risk factors for diabetic complications. A geriatric assessment, sometimes also referred to as a functional assessment, should be performed at the time of diagnosis. This

Table 31–1. Minimum Standards of Care for Older Adults with Diabetes Mellitus

Initial evaluation
Complete history and physical examination
Geriatric assessment
Laboratory examination: fasting blood glucose, glycosylated hemoglobin, fasting lipid profile, creatinine, urinalysis, electrocardiogram
Ophthalmologic examination
Dietary assessment
Continuing care
Use of treatment as needed to meet target glucose levels: diet, oral agents, or insulin
Assessment of blood glucose levels as frequently as needed to assure that treatment goals are being met
Annual assessment for diabetes complications
Annual review of geriatric assessment

is an assessment of the patient's capabilities for self-care, both for the basic activities involved in daily life (bathing, grooming, dressing, feeding, toileting, and transferring) and the instrumental activities of daily life (e.g., shopping, telephoning, finances, and housework), and indicates what amount of assistance, if any, the patient needs. Geriatric assessment also includes an evaluation of the patient's social support systems and frequently includes assessment of financial and insurance status. Nursing and social-work assistance are invaluable for the geriatric assessment. At the minimum, the initial laboratory evaluation for older patients with diabetes should include determinations of fasting serum glucose level, glycosylated hemoglobin (to assess previous level of control and to be used as a baseline), fasting lipid profile, and serum creatinine; urinalysis with examination for proteinuria; and an electrocardiogram. Ophthalmologic evaluation at the time of diagnosis is recommended by the American Diabetes Association for all patients with NIDDM.[28] This recommendation applies to elderly patients as well, who are at high risk for ocular diseases other than retinopathy. Dietary assessment is also indicated to provide the background for an initial dietary therapeutic intervention for a patient with newly diagnosed NIDDM.

Once the level of care is decided, subsequent management of older adults becomes clearer. In short, the treatment regimen chosen is the one necessary to achieve treatment goals. The four standard modalities of diabetes therapy—diet, exercise, use of oral hypoglycemic agents, and administration of insulin—all merit consideration for older adults.

DIET

Many older adults with diabetes mellitus are managed with diet alone with various degrees of success. There is no evidence to suggest that dietary therapy is any more or less effective in older patients than in younger patients. One study has shown that elderly patients with diabetes are able to improve diabetes control with diet and weight loss.[29] However, as with younger patients with diabetes, older adults may find it difficult to adhere to a strict dietary regimen and maintain weight loss. In older adults with mobility problems, for whom exercise to increase caloric expenditure is not possible, the amount of caloric restriction necessary to achieve weight loss may be substantial. These individuals are at risk for the development of nutrient and vitamin deficiencies, and aggressive dietary management cannot be recommended under these circumstances. Other considerations specific to older adults may limit the effectiveness of dietary therapy (Table 31–2).

No specific modifications in the diet currently recommended by the American Diabetes Association have been recommended for older adults. A diet relatively high in carbohydrate (50 to 60% of total calories), low in fat (<30% of total calories from fat, with 10% saturated fat, 10% polyunsaturated fat, and 10% monosaturated fat), and moderate in protein (~20% of total calories) appears at this time to be appropriate for the elderly in general,

Table 31–2. Dietary Therapy: Special Considerations for Older Adults with Diabetes

Financial difficulty
Difficulty with shopping because of transportation or mobility problems
Poor food-preparation skills (particularly elderly widowed men)
Ingrained dietary habits
Difficulty following dietary instruction because of impaired cognitive function
Decreased taste
Increased frequency of constipation

although data are lacking. These restrictions should be liberalized for the malnourished or chronically ill elderly patient, whose protein and energy intake should be increased. Vitamin and mineral supplements are indicated when caloric intake falls below 1000 kilocalories per day to prevent deficiency syndromes.

EXERCISE

The role of exercise in the management of diabetes mellitus is controversial. Although the beneficial effect of exercise on glucose tolerance has been well-documented for both individuals with and without diabetes,[30] its effectiveness in lowering plasma glucose levels is unclear. In addition, the effects of exercise on glucose tolerance are transient, disappearing within several days of discontinuance of an exercise program.[31] The use of exercise as a treatment modality for older adults with diabetes may pose additional problems. One study found that 81% of older men with newly diagnosed mild diabetes were unable to participate in a regular training program because of other diseases or medical treatment. For those who ultimately participated in the study, no differences in glucose control, glucose tolerance, or lipoprotein levels were found when they were compared with a control group of diabetic men not participating in the training program.[32] This study suggests that exercise, as a significant therapy for control of hyperglycemia, may not be feasible for many older adults. Nonetheless, substantial benefits of exercise apart from its effect on glucose metabolism make it worth recommending to older adults. Most of these benefits relate to improvements in the risk factors for cardiovascular disease, a significant complication of diabetes mellitus in the elderly. These benefits and the risks of exercise in older adults are outlined in Table 31–3. Because of the prevalence of silent coronary artery disease in this population, older adults with diabetes should be given an exercise tolerance test before they begin any exercise program.

SULFONYLUREAS

Although one-third of all patients with NIDDM are being treated with sulfonylureas, approximately 70% of the prescriptions for these drugs from office-based physicians are for individuals over the age of 60.[33] In spite of widespread use of these drugs in older adults, few studies have assessed the risks and benefits in this population.

Table 31–3. Potential Benefits and Risks of Exercise for Older Adults with Diabetes

Benefits	Risks
Improved exercise tolerance	Sudden cardiac death
Improved glucose tolerance	Foot and joint injuries
Improved maximal oxygen consumption	Hypoglycemia
Increased muscle strength	
Decreased blood pressure	
Decreased body fat and increased muscle mass	
Improved lipid profile	
Improved sense of well-being.	

The mechanism of action and efficacy of sulfonylureas have been discussed extensively in Chapter 29. There is no evidence to suggest that these drugs act any differently in older adults. The safety profile and easy dosing schedule make sulfonylureas an attractive family of drugs for the management of elderly diabetic patients for whom treatment beyond diet and exercise is indicated. Because IDDM is uncommon in older adults, most are eligible for a trial of oral agents when dietary management fails.

The major risk for older adults treated with sulfonylureas is hypoglycemia. Several papers have identified age alone as a major risk factor for hypoglycemia in those patients treated with oral agents.[34–36] There are multiple factors associated with aging that might increase the risk for hypoglycemia. These include age-associated impairments in hepatic and renal function that alter drug metabolism and excretion. The impairment of hepatic oxidative pathways associated with aging may increase the half-lives of sulfonylureas, which are metabolized extensively by the liver. Renal function, as measured by creatinine clearance, declines with age,[25] and insulin clearance has been shown to be reduced.[37] Aging also is associated with impairments in the autonomic nervous system[38,39] and reductions in β-adrenergic receptor function,[40] suggesting that the sensation of glycemia may not be as acute in older adults as in younger adults. The elderly are frequent users of drugs that are known to increase the risk for hypoglycemia, including β-adrenergic blockers, salicylates, warfarin, sulfonamides, and alcohol. Because of the physiologic changes associated with aging, the longer-acting drugs have been postulated to cause more episodes of hypoglycemia. In fact, several studies do report this,[34–36] although the longer-acting drugs are used by more patients than are the shorter-acting ones, and this factor has not been taken into account. Direct comparisons with controlled studies have not been done in elderly patients with diabetes.

Another important risk associated with the use of oral hypoglycemic agents in older adults is hyponatremia. The risk appears to be greatest with chlorpropamide, although both first- and second-generation sulfonylureas have been implicated. The addition of a thiazide diuretic to an oral hypoglycemic agent appears to increase both the risk and the severity of hyponatremia.[41] Intrinsic changes in water metabolism with aging may present a particular risk to older adults.

INSULIN

Although the initiation of insulin therapy is sometimes considered to be a difficult and momentous step for elderly patients, insulin is indicated for any patient when treatment goals are not being met without it. No studies have demonstrated that elderly patients cannot use insulin effectively and safely. Insulin therapy should be instituted when necessary. Insulin therapy can result in euglycemia (while oral hypoglycemic agents may not) in those patients for whom this is the goal. Insulin should also be used for elderly patients with symptomatic hyperglycemia whose glucose levels cannot be controlled with diet and oral agents.

No special insulin regimens have been identified as being more or less efficacious in older patients. As in younger adults, it is probably difficult to obtain normoglycemia with a single dose of intermediate-acting insulin. Therefore, when aggressive management is indicated, a split-mixed regimen is usually necessary. A single dose of insulin may be appropriate, however, to prevent symptomatic hyperglycemia when this is the treatment goal. The addition of insulin to a regimen including an oral hypoglycemic agent has not been studied in older adults and should be considered very cautiously.

Insulin therapy does require some special considerations when used in older adults (Table 31–4). Aging alone, or complications secondary to diabetes, may impair vision and the fine motor skills necessary for insulin administration. Blood glucose monitoring, indicated for patients treated with insulin, requires additional skills that may also be impaired with aging or disease processes. Hyperglycemia and poor diabetes control may be associated with subtle impairments of cognitive function in older adults.[42,43] Such impairments, combined with the high prevalence of cognitive disorders in older populations, may adversely affect the ability of an older individual to adhere to a complicated insulin regimen. Elderly individuals who live alone without adequate family or support services may be at increased risk for serious sequelae of insulin administration, i.e, hypoglycemia. However, none of these considerations are absolute contraindications to insulin therapy. If problems are recognized before or at the time of institution of insulin therapy, solutions can usually be found for each.

Table 31–4. Insulin Therapy in Older Adults: Special Considerations

Vision
Manual dexterity
Sensation in hands
Access to injection sites
Cost
Ability to do blood glucose monitoring
Cognitive function
Family support

Family members are frequently the most valuable resource. Community support services such as Meals on Wheels, Visiting Nurse Services, and Home Health Aides or Homemaker Services are able to provide primary assistance or fill in the gaps.

Hypoglycemia is a major potential complication for elderly patients treated with insulin. While little is known about counter-regulatory mechanisms in older adults with diabetes mellitus, the key to successful management of this complication is prevention. The strategies for prevention of hypoglycemia include frequent monitoring of blood glucose levels; adequate diabetes education, with special emphasis on the recognition and treatment of hypoglycemia; dietary assessment and instruction; and the intervention of family, friends, or support services to provide frequent (at least daily) contact for the older adult with diabetes.

MANAGEMENT OF THE ELDERLY PATIENT WITH DIABETES IN SPECIAL SITUATIONS

The Nursing-Home Patient

Approximately 3 to 5% of the population over the age of 65 are residing in nursing homes at any given time,[44] and at least 20% of elderly individuals will ultimately be cared for in a nursing home.[45] The prevalence of diabetes in the nursing-home population is about twice that in the general population.[46] The 1977 Nursing Home Survey found that diabetic patients in nursing homes had a high prevalence of diseases associated with diabetes, such as heart disease, and a high prevalence of amputations and immobility.[47] In contrast, the prevalence of chronic brain syndrome was low in the nursing-home patients with diabetes. A more recent study by Mooradian et al. of patients in a nursing home found that chronic renal failure, retinopathy, and neuropathy were more common among the patients with diabetes than among a similarly aged group of patients without diabetes.[48] Urinary tract infections and skin infections were also more common in the patients with diabetes.

The approach to most nursing-home patients with diabetes should be that of providing basic care with control of hyperglycemia and prevention of acute complications. Tight glycemic control for the prevention of chronic complications may not be appropriate, as life expectancy is markedly reduced for most individuals admitted to nursing homes. A recent study of 563 patients discharged from 24 nursing homes revealed that 30% were dead at discharge and 75.8% of the original group were dead within 2 years of discharge.[49] While diabetes was not identified as a predictor for outcome, functional status was. Patients with diabetes, who have been shown to be less mobile than their counterparts, may be more likely to have poorer survival rates as well.

Control of hyperglycemia in patients in nursing homes is achieved primarily through the use of diet and medications. Exercise will probably not play a major role in the management of diabetes in these patients. However, patients who are capable of an exercise program

should be encouraged to participate to enhance mobility and functional status. Diet is an important therapeutic option, but weight maintenance may be as important as weight loss for many elderly patients with diabetes in nursing homes. One study found that over 20% of patients with diabetes in nursing homes were more than 20% underweight,[48] a finding that raises the concern about malnutrition in this population. Thus, all patients with diabetes should be evaluated by a dietitian at the time of admission to the nursing home. Adjustments in recommended caloric intake should be made for wounds, infections, and level of activity. Patients should be weighed monthly, and further dietary adjustments should be made as needed.

As in other situations, the decision regarding use of sulfonylureas or insulin should be based on the level of glycemic control desired. Often an oral agent is preferable both to the patient and to the nursing home staff, but insulin is needed for those patients for whom glycemic goals cannot be achieved with a sulfonylurea. Glucose control may be more easily obtained in the patient with diabetes who is in a nursing home because medications and meals are delivered on a regular schedule. In the nursing-home setting, glucose monitoring may be done more frequently and the response of the physician may be more immediate than in the outpatient setting. In fact, Mooradian et al. found that patients with diabetes in the nursing home had lower levels of glycosylated hemoglobin, fewer episodes of hypoglycemia, and were thinner than a younger group of outpatients with diabetes.[48]

In addition to glycemic control, particular attention should be paid to the prevention of conditions that may be related to, or are exacerbated by, diabetes mellitus. Infections, particularly skin and urinary tract infections, are more common in nursing-home patients with diabetes. The incidence of urinary tract infections may be reduced by limiting the use of indwelling bladder catheters and by ensuring good urinary output through adequate hydration. Skin infections may be prevented by strict decubitus precautions, such as frequent turning of immobilized patients, the use of adequate bed and wheelchair cushioning, and the use of heel protectors. The prevalence of all infections is reduced with good staff hygiene, particularly by the enforcement of strict hand-washing regimens. The use of annual influenza vaccination and one-time pneumococcal vaccination for all nursing-home patients will provide herd immunity and protect against epidemics of these illnesses in the nursing home. Immunization and PPD (purified protein derivative) status should be verified and documented for all new admissions to the nursing home. Patients with diabetes who have a positive PPD reaction should be considered for prophylaxis with isoniazid if they have not been treated previously for tuberculosis.

Routine preventive medicine should continue for nursing-home patients with diabetes, including regular ophthalmologic, dental, and foot care. Many institutions offer these services in the nursing home itself. These interventions will maintain quality of life and, in some circumstances, may serve to detect and ameliorate potentially life-threatening events.

The Hospitalized Elderly Patient with Diabetes

The rate of hospitalization among elderly patients with diabetes is 1.7 times the rate among elderly people without diabetes. In the NHANES II conducted from 1976 through 1980, only 16.5% of individuals without diabetes 65 to 74 years old reported having been hospitalized once or more within the previous year, whereas 29.8% of those older individuals with known diabetes reported having been hospitalized. These include hospitalizations both for diabetes and for other reasons.

Regardless of the reason for hospitalization, an appropriate goal for glycemic management should be established for each patient. In general, efforts should emphasize minimization of the likelihood of insulin deficiency, which can contribute to a catabolic state. If this is the primary goal, tight control is not necessary. Reasonable goals would be a mean plasma glucose level of less than 250 mg/dL (14 mM) and minimal glycosuria. Stressful illnesses such as myocardial infarction, pneumonia, influenza, and stroke can exacerbate hyperglycemia and may even precipitate hyperosmolar hyperglycemic nonketotic coma in a patient who is already hospitalized. Thus, elderly patients with these conditions (including patients previously managed with oral agents or diet alone or even patients not previously recognized as having diabetes) may need to be treated temporarily with insulin. Attention must also be given to fluid status, with the use of appropriate intravenous fluid therapy to prevent dehydration and worsening of hyperglycemia. Frequent glucose monitoring is recommended to prevent wide perturbations in glycemia. Sliding scales of regular insulin can be useful for the acutely ill patient or postoperative patient who is unable to eat. However, once their oral intake is adequate, most hospitalized patients are better managed with split-mixed dosing of insulin with adjustments made as needed on the basis of the results of frequent glucose monitoring.

An important risk for the hospitalized older adult with diabetes mellitus is hypoglycemia. Although there are no specific studies that apply only to elderly patients, hypoglycemia is a significant problem for all hospitalized patients with diabetes. In general, hypoglycemia in the hospital results from decreased caloric intake or inappropriate changes in insulin dosage.[50] Hypoglycemia may be prevented by frequent glucose monitoring, with adjustments being made in the insulin dose as the patient's medical condition changes and with the establishment of appropriate in-hospital goals for glycemic control.

The basic principles of geriatric medicine apply to the management of hospitalized elderly patients with diabetes. Some general recommendations include strict decubitus precautions, restriction of the use of indwelling catheters, and judicious use of psychoactive drugs (their administration should not be on a "prn" [as required] basis). Mobility should be encouraged, and physical therapy should begin early in the hospital course, as indicated. Planning for discharge should begin at the time of admission, with input from the social-work service. Involvement of a consultant in geriatric medicine should be considered, particularly if the patient has multiple medical problems and is taking multiple medications, is functionally impaired, and requires or may require home care or nursing-home placement at the time of discharge.

REFERENCES

1. Siegel JS. Recent and prospective trends for the elderly population and some implications for health care. In: Haynes S, Feinleib M. Second conference on the epidemiology of aging. DHHS (NIH) publication no. 80–969. Washington, DC: US Government Printing Office, 1980.
2. Guralnik JM, Fitzsimmons SC. Aging in America: a demographic perspective. Cardiol Clin 1986;4:175–83.
3. Harris MI, Hadden WC, Knowler WC, et al. Prevalence of diabetes and impaired glucose tolerance and plasma glucose levels in U.S. population aged 20–74 years. Diabetes 1987;36:523–34.
4. Harris MI. Epidemiology of diabetes mellitus among the elderly in the United States. Clin Geriatr Med 1990; 6:703–19.
5. Kilvert A, Fitzgerald MG, Wright AD, et al. Clinical characteristics and aetiological classification of insulin-dependent diabetes in the elderly. Q J Med 1986;60:865–72.
6. Andres R. Aging and diabetes. Med Clin North Am 1971; 55:835–46.
7. Davidson MB. The effect of aging on carbohydrate metabolism: a review of the English literature and a practical approach to the diagnosis of diabetes mellitus in the elderly. Metabolism 1979;28:688–705.
8. Jackson RA, Blix PM, Matthews JA, et al. Influence of ageing on glucose homeostasis. J Clin Endocrinol Metab 1982; 55:840–8.
9. Jackson RA, Hawa MI, Roshania RD, et al. Influence of aging on hepatic and peripheral glucose metabolism in humans. Diabetes 1988;37:119–29.
10. Chen M, Bergman RN, Pacini G, et al. Pathogenesis of age-related glucose intolerance in man: insulin resistance and decreased beta-cell function. J Clin Endocrinol Metab 1985;60:13–20.
11. DeFronzo RA. Glucose intolerance and aging. Diabetes Care 1981;4:493–501.
12. Lipson LG. Diabetes in the elderly: diagnosis, pathogenesis, and therapy. Am J Med 1986;80(Suppl 5A):10–21.
13. Fink RI, Kolterman OG, Kao M, et al. The role of the glucose transport system in the postreceptor defect in insulin action associated with human aging. J Clin Endocrinol Metab 1984;58:721–5.
14. Belfiore F, Vagnoni G, Napoli E, Rabuazzo M. Effect of ageing on key enzymes of glucose metabolism in human adipose tissue. J Mol Med 1977;2:89–95.
15. Trischitta V, Reaven GM. Evidence of a defect in insulin-receptor recycling in adipocytes from older rats. Am J Physiol 1988;254:E39–44.
16. Forbes Gβ, Reina JC. Adult lean body mass declines with age: some longitudinal observations. Metabolism 1977; 19:653–63.
17. Sallis JF, Haskell WL, Wood PD, et al. Physical activity assessment methodology in the Five-City Project. Am J Epidemiol 1985;121:91–106.
18. Seals DR, Hagberg JM, Allen WK, et al. Glucose tolerance in

young and older athletes and sedentary men. J Appl Physiol 1984;56:1521–5.

19. Chen M, Bergman RN, Porte D Jr. Insulin resistance and beta-cell dysfunction in aging: the importance of dietary carbohydrate. J Clin Endocrinol Metab 1988;67:951–7.

20. Donahue RP, Abbott RD, Reed DM, et al. Postchallenge glucose concentration and coronary heart disease in men of Japanese ancestry: Honolulu Heart Program. Diabetes 1987;36:689–92.

21. Agner E, Thorsteinsson B, Eriksen M. Impaired glucose tolerance and diabetes mellitus in elderly subjects. Diabetes Care 1982;5:600–4.

22. Albert MS. Cognitive function. In: Albert MS, Moss MB, eds. Geriatric neuropsychology. New York: The Guilford Press, 1988:33–53.

23. Ciocon JO, Potter JF. Age-related changes in human memory: normal and abnormal. Geriatrics 1988; 43(10):43–8.

24. Einstein GO, McDaniel MA. Normal aging and prospective memory. J Exp Psychol Learn Mem Cogn 1990;16 :717–26.

25. Rowe JW, Andres R, Tobin JD, et al. The effect of age on creatinine clearance in man: a cross-sectional and longitudinal study. J Gerontol 1976;31:513–63.

26. Mackenzie RA, Phillips LH II. Changes in peripheral and central nerve conduction with aging. Clin Exp Neurol 1981;18:109–16.

27. Naliboff BD, Rosenthal M. Effects of age on complications in adult onset diabetes. J Am Geriatr Soc 1989;37:838–42.

28. American Diabetes Association. Standards of medical care for patients with diabetes mellitus. Diabetes Care 1989; 12:365–8.

29. Reaven GM. Beneficial effect of moderate weight loss in older patients with non-insulin-dependent diabetes mellitus poorly controlled with insulin. J Am Geriatr Soc 1985; 33:93–5.

30. Holloszy JO, Schultz J, Kursnierkiewicz J, et al. Effects of exercise on glucose tolerance and insulin resistance. Brief review and some preliminary results. Acta Med Scand Suppl 1986;711:55–65.

31. Schneider SH, Amorosa LF, Khachadurian AK, et al. Studies on the mechanism of improved glucose control during regular exercise in type 2 (non-insulin-dependent) diabetes. Diabetologia 1984;26:355–60.

32. Skarfors ET, Wegener TA, Lithell H, et al. Physical training as treatment for type 2 (non-insulin-dependent) diabetes in elderly men. A feasibility study over 2 years. Diabetologia 1987;30:930–3.

33. Kennedy DL, Piper JM, Baum C. Trends in the use of oral hypoglycemic agents: 1964–1986. Diabetes Care 1988; 11:558–62.

34. Asplund K, Wiholm BE, Lithner F. Glibenclamide-associated hypoglycaemia: a report on 57 cases. Diabetologia 1983; 24:412–7.

35. Seltzer HS. Severe drug-induced hypoglycemia: a review. Compr Ther 1979;5(4):21–9.

36. Sonnenblick M, Shilo S. Glibenclamide induced prolonged hypoglycaemia. Age Ageing 1986;15:185–9.

37. Minaker KL, Rowe JW, Tonino R, Pallota JA. Influence of age on clearance of insulin in man. Diabetes 1982;31: 851–5.

38. Dorfman LJ, Bosley TM. Age-related changes in peripheral and central nerve conduction in man. Neurology 1979; 29:38–44.

39. O'Brien IA, O'Hare P, Corrall RJM. Heart rate variability in healthy subjects: effect of age and the derivation of normal ranges for tests of autonomic function. Br Heart J 1986; 5:348–54.

40. Heinsimer JA, Lefkowitz RJ. The impact of aging on adrenergic receptor function: clinical and biochemical aspects. J Am Geriatr Soc 1985;33:184–8.

41. Kadowaki T, Hagura R, Kajinuma H, et al. Chlorpropamide-induced hyponatremia: incidence and risk factors. Diabetes Care 1983;6:468–71.

42. U'Ren RC, Riddle MC, Lezak MD, et al. The mental efficiency of the elderly person with Type II diabetes mellitus. J Am Geriatr Soc 1990;38:505–10.

43. Reaven GM, Thompson LW, Nahum D, et al. Relationship between hyperglycemia and cognitive function in older NIDDM patients. Diabetes Care 1990;13:16–21.

44. Ouslander JG, Martin S. Assessment in the nursing home. Clin Geriatr Med 1987;3:155–74.

45. Brock DB, Brody JA. Statistical and epidemiological characteristics. In: Andres R, Bierman EL, Hazzard WR, eds. Principles of geriatric medicine. New York: McGraw-Hill, 1985:53–71

46. Tonino RP. Diabetes education. What should health care providers in long-term nursing care facilities know about diabetes? Diabetes Care 1990;13(Suppl 2):55.

47. Van Nostrand JF. Nursing home care for diabetics. In: Diabetes in America: diabetes data compiled in 1984. DHHS publication no. 85–1468. Washington, DC: US Government Printing Office, 1985.

48. Mooradian AD, Osterweil D, Petrasek D, et al. Diabetes mellitus in elderly nursing home patients. A survey of clinical characteristics and management. J Am Geriatr Soc 1988;36:391–6.

49. Lewis M, Kane RL, Cretin S, et al. The immediate and subsequent outcomes of nursing home care. Am J Public Health 1985;75:758–62.

50. Fischer KF, Lees JA, Newman JH. Hypoglycemia in hospitalized patients. Causes and outcomes. N Engl J Med 1986;315:1245–50.

Chapter 32

WHOLE-PANCREAS AND ISLET-CELL TRANSPLANTATION

DAVID SHAFFER
ANTHONY P. MONACO

Since publication of the last edition of *Joslin's Diabetes Mellitus,* significant advances have been made in both whole-pancreas and islet-cell transplantation. With improvements in surgical technique and immunosuppressive therapy, the results of simultaneous pancreas-kidney transplantation have become comparable to the results of other solid-organ transplantation,[1] and this has become established therapy for uremic diabetic patients. Improvements in graft survival and reduction in surgical morbidity following the combined procedure have prompted proposals of criteria for the use of pancreas transplantation alone before the onset of end-stage diabetic nephropathy.[2] While transplantation of pancreatic islet cells is still in the experimental stage, important advances are being made both in the laboratory and clinically. This chapter will review the current status of both whole-pancreas and islet-cell transplantation. For additional information and detailed bibliographies, the reader is referred to several recent comprehensive reviews.[3-7]

HISTORY

The concept of pancreas transplantation long preceded the discovery of insulin. In 1890, von Mering and Minkowski[8] reported that removal of the pancreas caused diabetes, and 2 years later, Minkowski[9] and Hédon[10] transplanted portions of a whole pancreas to reverse diabetes in animals. In 1894, Williams attempted both the first xenograft and the first islet-cell transplant by transplanting fragments of the pancreas of a sheep into a child with diabetes.[11] Following Carrel's pioneering studies of vascular anastomoses,[12] others reported successful grafts of vascularized whole pancreas and several investigators refined surgical techniques in large animals.[13-15]

Kelly et al.[16] performed the first transplant of human pancreas in 1966, a simultaneous segmental pancreas and kidney transplant in a young woman with diabetes and end-stage renal disease who was given prednisone and azathioprine for immunosuppression. Although both allografts functioned immediately and the patient became insulin-independent, both grafts were removed because of rejection and development of pancreatic fistula, and the patient died of a pulmonary embolism 2 months after transplantation. Between 1966 and 1973, Lillehei and associates performed 13 pancreatic transplants, only one of which functioned for more than a year.[17] Through 1977, 15 institutions throughout the world reported 64 pancreas transplants to the International Pancreas Transplant Registry (IPTR). The overall rate of 1-year graft survival was only 5%.[3]

Improvements in the results of heart, liver, and kidney transplantation following the introduction of cyclosporine in 1978 launched a resurgence of interest in pancreas transplantation. Thus, while 15 whole-pancreas transplants were reported to the IPTR in 1978, 419 were reported 10 years later. From October 1, 1987, when the United Network for Organ Sharing (UNOS) Registry was established to collect data on pancreas transplants in the United States, through December 31, 1990, 1197 pancreas transplants were reported by 60 centers in the United States (Fig. 32–1), with an overall 1-year patient survival rate of 92% and 1-year graft survival rate of 72%.[18] This dramatic improvement over the rates during the previous decade can be attributed to better immunosuppressive therapy, improved organ preservation with

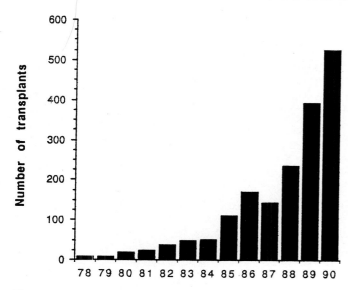

Fig. 32—1. Number of pancreas transplants performed in the United States by year from 1978 through 1990 (data are from reference 18).

UW-Belzer solution, adoption of the bladder-drainage technique for pancreatic exocrine secretions, and the use of simultaneous transplantation of the pancreas and kidney.

WHOLE-PANCREAS TRANSPLANTATION

Recipient Categories and Selection

The goals of pancreatic transplantation are the eradication of the morbidity associated with labile blood glucose, stabilization or improvement of secondary diabetic complications, and improvement in the quality of life of patients with insulin-dependent diabetes mellitus (IDDM) by the establishment of normal glucose metabolism. Recipients of pancreas transplants can be divided into three categories: 1) patients who are pre-uremic who receive a pancreas transplant alone (PTA); 2) patients who receive a pancreas transplant after undergoing a successful cadaver or living-related kidney transplantation (PAK); and 3) uremic patients who simultaneously receive a pancreas and kidney transplant from the same cadaver donor (SPK). Simultaneous pancreas-kidney transplants are the most common, comprising 82% of all pancreas transplants in the current UNOS Registry, with PAK and PTA accounting for 11% and 7% of the total, respectively.[18] The morbidity of surgery and chronic immunosuppression following pancreatic transplantation must be weighed against the potential benefit of improved or normal glucose metabolism in diabetic recipients. Thus, until more long-term data are available showing that the benefits of transplantation in pre-uremic diabetic patients in terms of quality of life and effects on secondary diabetic complications outweigh the risks of surgery and chronic immunosuppression, patients receiving SPK will remain the largest group undergoing pancreas transplantation, since they are already obligated to surgery and immunosuppression for the treatment for chronic renal failure. In addition, the ability to use the simultaneously transplanted kidney as a marker for pancreas rejection contributes to improved graft survival rates in the SPK group. However, as better methods of diagnosing early rejection of pancreas grafts are developed, such as the monitoring of urinary amylase[19] or serum anodal trypsinogen[20] levels, PAK and PTA should become more widely applicable.

Actual patient selection criteria vary from center to center, but in general, patients with IDDM who have end-stage renal disease without significant cardiovascular disease are ideal candidates for SPK. Table 32—1 outlines the specific selection criteria for SPK that are followed at the authors' institution, the New England Deaconess Hospital. Advanced retinopathy per se is not a contraindication for pancreatic transplantation, and the presence of a functioning graft may significantly improve the quality of life for these patients. The timing of SPK relative to the course of nephropathy is somewhat controversial, although most centers recommend that transplantation be done before dialysis, if possible, both to reduce perioperative morbidity and to potentially halt or improve secondary neurovascular complications at an earlier stage. However, until more data on long-term survival and secondary complications with SPK are available and because of the excellent long-term results of living-related donor (LRD) kidney transplantation in patients with diabetes,[21] the policy at the authors' institution and elsewhere[4] is to recommend LRD kidney transplantation alone if there is a suitable family donor. Recipients of LRD kidney transplants also become candidates for a subsequent cadaver-pancreas transplant (PAK).

Surgical Technique

Although the University of Minnesota has performed a series of LRD pancreas transplants,[22] virtually all other centers have used only cadaver donors. The whole pancreas is procured with an 8- to 10-cm segment of

Table 32—1. Criteria for Simultaneous Pancreas-Kidney Transplantation

CRITERIA FOR INCLUSION
1. Insulin-dependent diabetes mellitus
2. Age 18-55 years
3. Established diabetic nephropathy (serum creatinine ≥2 mg/dL)

CRITERIA FOR EXCLUSION
1. Insufficient cardiac reserve
   a. Stress thallium or dipyridamole thallium test demonstrating significant uncorrectable coronary heart disease
   b. Inadequate myocardial function demonstrated by echocardiogram
2. Evidence of severe peripheral vascular disease (ischemic ulcers, dependent rubor, rest pain, or amputation of major limb)
3. Major psychiatric illness/refractory noncompliance
4. Ongoing substance abuse (alcohol or drug)
5. Cancer (except non-melanoma skin cancer) unless free of disease without recurrence for >5 years
6. Active infection

duodenum at the head of the pancreas and with the spleen in continuity with the tail of the pancreas. The arterial blood supply consists of the splenic artery and superior mesenteric artery, and the venous outflow consists of a short segment of portal vein at the superior border of the pancreas. Most grafts obtained in the United States are preserved by cold storage in UW-Belzer solution. Although at the authors' institution, the average preservation time is less than 12 hours, pancreas grafts stored for up to 30 hours before transplantation have had good functional outcome.[18,23]

Over the past 25 years, numerous surgical techniques have been used in pancreatic transplantation: either the whole organ (pancreaticoduodenal) or a segment (body and tail) can be used[24,25]; the allograft can be placed retroperitoneally or intraperitoneally[26]; the graft can be drained into the portal or systemic venous circulation[27]; and pancreatic exocrine secretions can be drained into the bladder,[28-30] into a loop of recipient intestine,[31] directly into the peritoneal cavity,[32] or the pancreatic duct can be ligated[16] or obliterated with an inert polymer such as neoprene[33] or prolamine.[34] Although enteric drainage of exocrine secretions is used in Europe,[31] most centers in the United States use bladder-drained, whole-organ pancreaticoduodenal grafts because of the decrease in incidence of perioperative complications and the ability to monitor graft function by measuring serial urinary amylase levels.[19] From October 1967 to 1990, 96% of pancreas transplants reported in the UNOS registry were bladder-drained.[18]

In the operation in the recipient, the pancreas graft is revascularized with anastomoses between the donor splenic artery and superior mesenteric artery (either on an intact patch of donor aorta or after reconstruction with a bifurcation graft using donor iliac artery) and the recipient external iliac artery and donor portal vein and recipient external iliac vein (Fig. 32-2). The proximal and distal ends of the donor duodenum are oversewn, and a duodenocystostomy is performed between the recipient bladder and the midportion of the duodenal segment. This is essentially the mirror image of the procedure used in a standard kidney transplant, which is implanted to the contralateral iliac vessels in the usual fashion. The donor spleen, which is left in continuity during the procurement procedure to reduce handling and trauma to the pancreas, is removed.

Postoperative Management

Cyclosporine and prednisone form the cornerstone of immunosuppressive therapy after pancreas transplantation. At the authors' institution, the postoperative immunosuppressive protocol is the same as that for kidney transplantation alone and consists of triple therapy with cyclosporine, prednisone, and azathioprine.[21] Other centers routinely employ quadruple immunosuppressive therapy, with the addition of a 7- to 14-day course of induction therapy with antilymphocyte globulin or the anti-T cell monoclonal antibody OKT3.[36,37] Rejection episodes are treated initially with a pulse of intravenous methylprednisolone, 250 to 500 mg daily for 3 to 5 days.

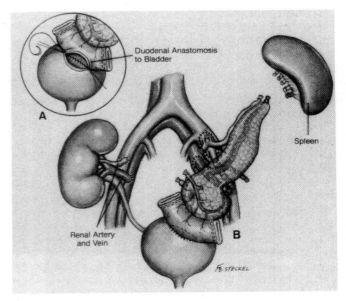

Fig. 32-2. Simultaneous kidney-pancreas transplantation using systemic venous drainage to the iliac vessels and bladder drainage of exocrine secretions via a duodenocystostomy. Reprinted with permission from reference 35 (Warren KW, Jenkins RL, Steele GD. Atlas of surgery of the liver, pancreas and biliary tract. Norwalk, CT: Appleton & Lange, 1991).

Rejection episodes unresponsive to steroids are treated with a 10- to 14-day course of OKT3. While the new immunosuppressive agent FK 506 appears to be extremely effective following liver transplantation,[38,39] the clinical data regarding its use in whole-pancreas transplantation are limited. Unfortunately, a common side effect of FK 506 administration appears to be impaired glucose metabolism, and initial reports of the use of FK 506 in liver or kidney transplantation document a 14 to 22% incidence of de novo development of IDDM.[39,40] However, data on the use of FK 506 in rats suggest that the deterioration in glucose metabolism may be reversible[41] and that islet allograft survival may be prolonged.[42] At the time of this writing, the potential role of newer immunosuppressive agents such as RS-61443, rapamycin, and 15-deoxyspergualin in whole-pancreas transplants is unknown.

Rejection remains the most common cause of failure of pancreas grafts. The pancreas is highly immunogenic, and rejection episodes occur in almost 90% of SPK recipients, roughly twice the frequency following kidney transplantation alone.[26,37,43] By the time plasma glucose levels rise, which is a relatively late sign of pancreas rejection, a significant portion of β-cells may have already been destroyed. In SPK recipients, an elevated creatinine level usually precedes by several days an elevated plasma glucose level, and thus renal allograft function becomes the major guide to postoperative immunosuppressive therapy. This early marker of rejection may account for the better graft survival rates with SPK compared with rates with PAK or PTA. In addition, in patients with bladder-drained pancreas grafts, pancreatic exocrine function serves as a marker for rejection.[19] Thus a 50% drop in level of urinary amylase from the baseline value is indicative of rejection. Transcystoscopic transduodenal biopsy of the pancreas, originally reported by Perkins et al.,[44] can provide a histologic diagnosis of rejection and is used routinely in some centers. Finally, newer serum markers of pancreas allograft rejection have been developed, notably pancreatic-specific protein[45] and serum anodal trypsinogen,[20] which may permit earlier, noninvasive diagnosis of rejection of a pancreas transplanted without a simultaneous kidney transplant.

The most common postoperative complications following pancreas transplantation are rejection and infection, particularly cytomegalovirus infection. Wound infections are a frequent complication of retroperitoneally placed grafts but can be prevented by placing the graft intraperitoneally through a standard midline incision.[26,46] Because of its susceptibility to postoperative edema and pancreatitis, graft thrombosis was a major cause of graft loss in early series[5] and led many centers to administer anticoagulants to pancreas recipients during the early postoperative period. Bleeding complications and improvements in organ preservation that reduced postoperative swelling of the graft prompted discontinuation of this protocol, and recipients are now usually given one aspirin a day to prevent thrombosis.[37] Urine leaks from the duodenocystostomy of the oversewn duodenum segment, which are reported in 13 to 15% of pancreas transplant recipients,[37,46] usually require operative closure. Late graft pancreatitis secondary to reflux of urine into the pancreatic duct is an uncommon but increasingly recognized problem in bladder-drained grafts. A neurogenic bladder may predispose to reflux; symptoms resolve quickly following placement of a Foley catheter. Recurrent cases have been treated with somatostatin,[4] with oral pancreatic enzymes,[47] and by conversion from bladder to enteric drainage.[48]

Results of Pancreas Transplantation

Rates of patient and graft survival comparable to those seen with other solid-organ allografts have been reported by single centers in the United States with large series of SPK transplants.[36,37,49-51] In the initial series of 27 pancreas transplants by Shaffer et al., actuarial rates of 1-year patient, kidney, and pancreas graft survival were 96%, 88%, and 85%, respectively, and were not significantly different from rates for a concurrent control group of diabetic patients receiving cadaver kidney transplants alone.[46]

Fewer centers have a large experience with either PTA or PAK. Sutherland et al. reported rates of 1-year patient and pancreas graft survival of 97% and 53% for PTA and 91% and 48% for PAK, respectively.[36] In a smaller series, Sollinger et al. reported rates of 1-year pancreas graft survival of 50% for pancreas grafts after living-related donor kidney transplants and 100% with pancreas grafts after cadaver kidney transplants (PAK).[52]

For all cases reported to the UNOS Registry for the period October 1987 through October 1990, the overall rates of 1-year of patient and pancreas graft survival were 92% and 72%, respectively.[18] The rates of 1-year graft survival for SPK, PAK, and PTA recipients were 77%,

52%, and 54%, respectively, and the rate of 1-year kidney graft survival in SPK recipients was 86% in the UNOS Registry, indicating that the addition of the pancreas graft does not jeopardize the outcome of a cadaver kidney transplant with regard to either patient or graft survival.

Effect of Pancreas Transplantation on Glucose Metabolism and Secondary Complications

Glucose Metabolism

Available data suggest an important relationship between long-term glycemic control and the progression or prevention of neurovascular complications of Type I diabetes mellitus.[53,54] Early studies from the University of Minnesota showed that a successful pancreas transplant results in the attainment of normal fasting blood glucose levels and 24-hour metabolic profiles, with most patients showing normal results in oral and intravenous glucose tolerance tests.[55,56] More recently, the same group reported normalization of glycosylated hemoglobin (HbA_1) levels, with mean values of 6.7% and 6.5% 1 and 2 years after transplantation. These values were significantly lower than preoperative levels (10.8%) and levels in diabetic patients receiving conventional insulin therapy but were not different from values in nondiabetic kidney-transplant recipients.[57] Similar results were reported by Nathan et al.[51] In our own series, we observed normalization of glycosylated hemoglobin values in SPK recipients, with mean values significantly lower than preoperative levels or levels in a concurrent group of diabetic patients receiving kidney transplants alone and the same immunosuppressive regimen[46] (Fig. 32-3).

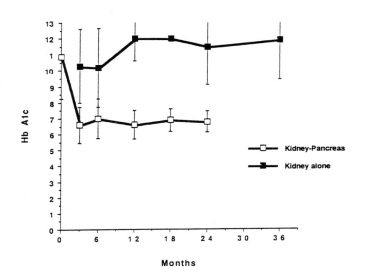

Fig. 32-3. Serial levels of glycosylated hemoglobic HbA_{1c} in diabetic recipients of simultaneous pancreas-kidney transplants vs. levels in recipients of kidney transplants alone at the New England Deaconess Hospital, 1988 through 1991. Reprinted with permission from reference 46 (Shaffer D, Madras PN, Sahyoun AI, et al. Kidney-pancreas transplantation: a 3-year experience. Arch Surg 1992;127:574-8; copyright of the American Medical Association).

Other studies have shown improved counterregulation of hypoglycemia, as manifested by increased glucagon secretion, following pancreas transplantation.[58]

Because of technical factors, virtually all transplantation groups place the pancreas allograft in the pelvis with systemic (i.e., iliac vein) drainage as opposed to portal venous drainage. This placement, because it produces changes in hepatic insulin clearance, results in elevated basal levels of insulin and C-peptide and in elevated insulin responses to glucose and arginine.[59] Katz et al. also found systemic hyperinsulinemia in patients with systemic drainage of pancreas transplants but no differences in postprandial glucose metabolism as compared with that in nondiabetic kidney-transplant recipients receiving the same immunosuppressive regimen.[60] Because hyperinsulinemia may be a risk factor for hypertension and macrovascular disease,[61,62] portal venous drainage of pancreatic allografts may be preferable to systemic drainage.[59]

Nephropathy

Diabetic nephropathy occurs in normal kidneys transplanted into diabetic recipients,[63] although it is not an issue of major clinical significance because of the long period required for the development of important functional changes. Simultaneous transplantation of a pancreas with the kidney prevents recurrent diabetic nephropathy, with the Stockholm group reporting normal glomerular basement membrane thickness and mesangial volume on serial biopsy specimens after transplantation.[64]

Studies in rats with streptozotocin-induced diabetes suggest that normalization of blood glucose levels can reverse the morphologic features of diabetic nephropathy.[65] Clinically, Bilous et al. reported that successful pancreas transplantation may halt the progression of diabetic nephropathy in previously transplanted kidneys.[66] Glomerular volumes were also smaller in PAK recipients than in a group of matched diabetic recipients of kidney transplants alone.[66]

Finally, Bilous et al. also found that morphologic parameters of diabetic nephropathy improved in the native kidneys of non-uremic recipients of PTA, although creatinine clearance was reduced, perhaps in response to the nephrotoxic effects of cyclosporine.[67]

Neuropathy

The natural history of diabetic polyneuropathy is one of progression, which is not halted by the presence of a functioning kidney transplant alone in uremic diabetic patients.[68] Symptomatic autonomic neuropathy is also a marker for significant morbidity and mortality in patients with Type I diabetes.[69] Several studies have reported improvement in indexes of diabetic polyneuropathy after pancreatic transplantation.[70–73] In a prospective study, Kennedy et al. reported significant improvement in both motor and sensory indexes of diabetic neuropathy 12 months after transplantation and in a sensory index 24 months after transplantation in comparison with values in a control group of patients with IDDM who did not receive transplants.[70] In a previous study, the same group

reported improvement in neurophysiologic scores in pre-uremic diabetic recipients of pancreatic transplants alone, a finding that suggests the improvement was due to restoration of normoglycemia as opposed to elimination of uremia.[71] The latter was suggested by Wilczek et al. in a study of SPK recipients.[74] Other groups have also shown that successful pancreas transplantation may slow the progression of peripheral[72] and autonomic neuropathy.[73] In these studies, the degree of improvement noted was small, a finding that reflects either the relatively late stage in progression of the disease at which the patients undergo transplantation or the relatively short follow-up.

Retinopathy

In contrast to the encouraging reports of improvement in diabetic nephropathy and neuropathy, reports from the University of Minnesota indicate that successful pancreas transplantation fails to reverse or slow the progression of diabetic retinopathy.[75] The probability of progression of retinopathy within 3 years following transplantation was the same in patients with a successful pancreas transplant as in those with a transplant that failed within 3 months. The effects of either a longer period of euglycemia on the progression of retinopathy or a reversal of hyperglycemia earlier in the course of retinopathy remain unknown.

ISLET-CELL TRANSPLANTATION

Clearly the major disadvantage of whole-pancreas transplantation limiting its wider application to both uremic and non-uremic diabetic patients is the morbidity associated with the surgical procedure and concomitant immunosuppression. For non-uremic diabetic patients in particular, the risks of long-term immunosuppression must be weighed against the risks of development of secondary neurovascular complications. From a theoretical standpoint, transplantation of pancreatic islet cells has potential advantages over transplantation of the whole pancreas: minimal surgical morbidity, since islets may be infused via simple intravenous injection; lack of problems associated with exocrine function; and the possibility of modulating or manipulating islets in vitro to reduce their immunogenicity and the concurrent requirements for immunosuppressive therapy. Islet transplantation has been shown to reverse diabetes both in streptozotocin-induced diabetic rats[76,77] and, more recently, in spontaneously diabetic BB rats[78,79] and NOD (non-obese diabetic) mice.[80–82] Studies in animal models have shown that functioning islet-cell transplants can reverse or prevent secondary diabetic complications.[65] From a practical standpoint, two major problems, islet isolation and rejection, have prevented successful clinical application of islet-cell transplantation until quite recently.

Islet Isolation

Early attempts at islet isolation consisted of various methods of simple mechanical disruption or fragmentation. The use of enzymatic digestion with collagenase, initially described by Moskalewski[83] and perfected by Lacy and Kostianovsky,[84] allowed better separation of islets from surrounding acinar tissue. Simple enzymatic digestion and Ficoll density-gradient separation, however, still gave relatively poor yields of islets, particularly in larger animals with more-fibrous pancreatic tissue. The introduction of intraductal perfusion of collagenase in the dog permitted better dispersion of pancreatic tissue with the preservation of islet viability.[85] Subsequently, this technique was applied to rodent models, with significant improvements in islet yields.[86]

Several modifications of these basic techniques have been applied to the isolation of human islets. Gray et al. reported that prewarming the collagenase to 39° C facilitated digestion of acinar tissue and, when mesh filtration was used, reduced loss of islets from Ficoll density-gradient separation alone.[87] Others reported improvements in islet yield with the use of constant intraductal perfusion.[6] Ricordi et al., using the pig, injected collagenase prewarmed to 24° C, dispersed pancreatic cells with a mechanical macerator, and purified with mesh filtration and Ficoll density-gradient centrifugation.[88] Subsequently, Ricordi et al. modified this procedure for human islet isolation.[89,90]

Rejection

Rejection is currently the major problem limiting the clinical application of islet-cell transplantation. Early experience with islet allografting suggested that islets are rejected more rapidly than primarily vascularized solid-organ allografts, including whole-pancreas allografts.[91] In addition, by the time islet-cell rejection becomes evident by the development of elevated blood glucose levels, it is too late to reverse the rejection process. Approaches to the prevention of rejection of pancreatic islets fall into three general categories: immunosuppression; immunomodulation; and immunoisolation.

Immunosuppression

Conventional nonspecific immunosuppressive agents are relatively ineffective in preventing rejection of islet allografts. Corticosteroids are not effective,[92] and azathioprine prolongs graft survival to only about 25 days in the rat.[93] Cyclosporine, which has led to significantly improved graft survival of other solid-organ allografts, including the whole pancreas, has also been disappointing in regard to allografts with islets alone.[94] In addition, high doses of cyclosporine may impair glucose metabolism.[95] Antilymphocyte serum (ALS) has been the most effective conventional agent in rodent models, resulting in prolonged survival[96] and, in some strain combinations, in donor-specific unresponsiveness.[97,98] Although newer immunosuppressive agents such as FK 506[42] and RS-61443[99] appear promising, the relative resistance of islet allografts to nonspecific immunosuppression has led numerous investigators to pursue ways of decreasing the immunogenicity of islet tissue.

Immunomodulation

A major advantage of cellular transplantation is the potential for manipulating tissue in vitro to alter or decrease its immunogenicity.[7] Several methods have proved effective with islet allografts. Lacy et al. found that islet immunogenicity could be reduced by 7-day culture at 24° C, with all of the rat-islet allografts surviving longer than 100 days in recipients given a single dose of ALS.[100] Others have shown that islet immunogenicity could be reduced and allograft survival prolonged by culture of islets in 95% O_2 and 5% CO_2,[101] islet cryopreservation[102] or use of cultured fetal islet tissue.[103]

Passenger leukocytes or dendritic cells that express class II histocompatibility antigens appear to play a major role in allograft rejection, a concept first introduced by Snell.[104] Using a mouse model, Faustman et al. obtained prolonged survival of islet allografts by pretreating the islets with monoclonal antibody to class II antigen and complement[105] or with monoclonal antibody to dendritic cells and complement.[106] Lau et al., using the rat, successfully used ultraviolet (UV) irradiation to inactivate class II-bearing passenger leukocytes and obtained prolonged survival of islet-cell grafts in animals given a short course of cyclosporine.[107] Whether these methods can be effectively applied to humans, who also express class II antigens on vascular endothelium, remains to be seen.

Another approach to the reduction of immunogenicity that has direct clinical applicability is the transplantation of small numbers of islets from multiple donors. Gotoh and associates[108] found that 50 mouse islets transplanted under the kidney capsule, although they did not restore normoglycemia, did not provide a potent enough stimulus to cause rejection. However, transplantation of 50 islets each from four different donors restored euglycemia without being rejected.

Immunoisolation

A third approach to the problem of islet immunogenicity is immunoisolation. In animal models, certain anatomic sites have been found to be immunologically privileged, presumably because of the presence of a natural barrier to immunoreactive cells or immunoglobulins. Thus, prolonged survival of allografts placed into the cerebral cortex[109] or testicle[110] has been obtained without immunosuppression. Although these findings are not applicable clinically, they form the conceptual basis for immunoisolation techniques, in which islets are placed in a membrane permitting diffusion of insulin and glucose but not lymphocytes or antibodies. This may take the form of "microencapsulation," in which donor islets are encapsulated in biocompatible, porous microspheres and injected into the free peritoneal cavity[111,112] or subcutaneous tissue[113] or as a biohybrid artificial pancreas that is placed in continuity with the recipient's bloodstream via vascular grafts.[114,115] Encapsulating islets in biocompatible, selective membranes may be particularly useful in protecting islet xenografts from rejection.[116] Although some encouraging results with these immunoisolation techniques have been reported, problems include the maintenance of islet viability in solution, the development of a fibroproliferative response limiting diffusion with capsules placed in nonvascularized sites, and thrombosis or fibrin deposition with intravascular devices.

58. Diem P, Redmon JB, Abid M, et al. Glucagon, catecholamine and pancreatic polypeptide secretion in type I diabetic recipients of pancreas allografts. J Clin Invest 1990;86:2008–13.

59. Diem PD, Abid A, Redmon JB, et al. Systemic venous drainage of pancreas allografts as independent cause of hyperinsulinemia in type I diabetic recipients. Diabetes 1990;39:534–40.

60. Katz H, Homan M, Velosa J, et al. Effects of pancreas transplantation on postprandial glucose metabolism. N Engl J Med 1991;325:1278–83.

61. Welborn TA, Breckenridge A, Rubinstein AH, et al. Serum-insulin in essential hypertension and in peripheral vascular disease. Lancet 1966;1:1336–7.

62. Zavaroni I, Bonora E, Pagliara M, et al. Risk factors for coronary artery disease in healthy persons with hyperinsulinemia and normal glucose tolerance. N Engl J Med 1989;320:702–6.

63. Mauer SM, Steffes MW, Connett J, et al. The development of lesions in the glomerular basement membrane and mesangium after transplantation of normal kidneys to diabetic patients. Diabetes 1983;32:948–52.

64. Bohman S-O, Wilczek H, Tydén G, et al. Recurrent diabetic nephropathy in renal allografts placed in diabetic patients and protective effect of simultaneous pancreatic transplantation. Transplant Proc 1987;19:2290–3.

65. Steffes MW, Brown DM, Basgen JM, Mauer SM. Amelioration of mesangial volume and surface alterations following islet transplantation in diabetic rats. Diabetes 1980;29:509–15.

66. Bilous RW, Mauer SM, Sutherland DER, et al. The effects of pancreas transplantation on the glomerular structure of renal allografts in patients with insulin-dependent diabetes. N Engl J Med 1989;321:80–5.

67. Bilous RW, Mauer SM, Sutherland DER, Steffes MW. Glomerular structure and function following successful pancreas transplantation (PTx) for insulin-dependent diabetes mellitus (IDDM) [Abstract no. 171]. Diabetes 1987;36(Suppl 1):43A.

68. Van der Vliet JA, Navarro X, Kennedy WR, et al. Long-term follow-up of polyneuropathy in diabetic kidney transplant recipients. Diabetes 1988;37:1247–52.

69. Navarro X, Kennedy WR, Loewenson RB, Sutherland DER. Influence of pancreas transplantation on cardiorespiratory reflexes, nerve conduction, and mortality in diabetes mellitus. Diabetes 1990;39:802–6.

70. Kennedy WR, Navarro X, Goetz FC, et al. Effects of pancreatic transplantation on diabetic neuropathy. N Engl J Med 1990;322:1031–7.

71. Sutherland DER, Kendall DM, Moudry KC, et al. Pancreas transplantation in nonuremic, Type I diabetic recipients. Surgery 1988;104:453–64.

72. Secchi A, Martinenghi S, Galardi G, et al. Effects of pancreatic transplantation on diabetic polyneuropathy. Transplant Proc 1991;23:1658–9.

73. Gaber AO, Cardoso S, Pearson S, et al. Improvement in autonomic function following combined pancreas-kidney transplantation. Transplant Proc 1991;23:1660–2.

74. Wilczek H, Solders G, Gunnarsson R, et al. Effects of successful combined pancreatic and renal transplantation on advanced diabetic neuropathy: a one-year follow-up study. Transplant Proc 1987;19:2327–8.

75. Ramsay RC, Goetz FC, Sutherland DER, et al. Progression of diabetic retinopathy after pancreas transplantation for insulin-dependent diabetes mellitus. N Engl J Med 1988;318:208–14.

76. Ballinger WF, Lacy PE. Transplantation of intact pancreatic islets in rats. Surgery 1972;72:175–86.

77. Reckard CR, Barker CF. Transplantation of isolated pancreatic islets across strong and weak histocompatibility barriers. Transplant Proc 1973;5:761–3.

78. Naji A, Silvers WK, Plotkin SA, et al. Successful islet transplantation in spontaneous diabetes. Surgery 1979;86:218–26.

79. Hegre OD, Enriquez AJ, Ketchum RJ, et al. Islet transplantation in spontaneously diabetic BB/Wor rats. Diabetes 1989;38:1148–54.

80. Nomikos IN, Prowse SJ, Carotenuto P, Lafferty KJ. Combined treatment with nicotinamide and desferrioxamine prevents islet allograft destruction in NOD mice. Diabetes 1986;35:1302–4.

81. Maki T, Ichikawa T, Blanco R, Porter J. Long-term abrogation of autoimmunity in spontaneously diabetic NOD mice by immunotherapy with anti-lymphocyte serum. Proc Natl Acad Sci USA 1992;89:3434–8.

82. Weber C, Krekun S, Koschitzky T, et al. Prolonged functional survival of rat-to-NOD mouse islet xenografts by ultraviolet-B (UV-B) irradiation plus microencapsulation of donor islets. Transplant Proc 1991;23(1 Pt 1):764–6.

83. Moskalewski S. Isolation and culture of the islets of Langerhans of the guinea pig. Gen Comp Endocrinol 1965;5:342–53.

84. Lacy PE, Kostianovsky M. Method for the isolation of intact islets of Langerhans from the rat pancreas. Diabetes 1967;16:35–9.

85. Horaguchi A, Merrell RC. Preparation of viable islet cells from dogs by a new method. Diabetes 1981;30:455–8.

86. Gotoh M, Maki T, Kiyoizumi T, et al. An improved method for isolation of mouse pancreatic islets. Transplantation 1985;40:437–8.

87. Gray DWR, McShane P, Grant A, Morris PJ. A method for isolation of islets of Langerhans from the human pancreas. Diabetes 1984;33:1055–61.

88. Ricordi C, Finke E, Lacy PE. A method for the mass isolation of islets from the adult pig pancreas. Diabetes 1986;35:649–53.

89. Ricordi C, Lacy PE, Finke EH, et al. Automated method for isolation of human pancreatic islets. Diabetes 1988;37:413–20.

90. Ricordi C, Socci C, Davalli AM, et al. Isolation of the elusive pig islet. Surgery 1990;107:688–94.

91. Perloff LJ, Naji A, Silvers WK, et al. Vascularized pancreas versus isolated islet allografts: an immunological comparison. Surgery 1990;88:222–30.

92. Schulak JA, Franklin W, Reckard CR. Morphological and functional changes following intraportal islet allograft rejection: irreversibility with steroid pulse therapy. Surg Forum 1977;28:296–9.

93. Marquet RL, Heystek GA. The effect of immunosuppressive treatment on the survival of allogeneic islets of Langerhans in rats. Transplantation 1975;20:428–31.

94. Gray DWR, Morris PJ. Cyclosporine and pancreas transplantation. World J Surg 1984;8:230–5.

95. Hahn HJ, Laube F, Lucke S, et al. Toxic effects of cyclosporine on the endocrine pancreas of Wistar rats. Transplantation 1986;41:44–7.

96. Gray BN, Watkins E Jr. Prolonged relief from diabetes after syngeneic or allogeneic transplantation of isolated pancreatic islets in rats. Surg Forum 1974;25:382–4.

97. Ziegler MM, Reckard CR, Naji A, Barker CF. Extended

function of isolated pancreatic islet isografts and allografts. Transplant Proc 1975;7(Suppl 1):743–5.

98. Zitron IM, Ono J, Lacy PE, Davie JM. Active suppression in the maintenance of pancreatic islet allografts. Transplantation 1981;32:156–8.

99. Hao L, Lafferty KJ, Allison AC, Eugui EM. RS-61443 allows islet allografting and specific tolerance induction in adult mice. Transplant Proc 1990;22:876–9.

100. Lacy PE, Davie JM, Finke EH. Prolongation of islet allograft survival following in vitro culture (24° C) and a single injection of ALS. Science 1979;204:312–3.

101. Simeonovic CJ, Bowen KM, Kotlarski I, Lafferty KJ. Modulation of tissue immunogenicity by organ culture: comparison of adult islets and fetal pancreas. Transplantation 1980;30:174–9.

102. Coulombe MG, Warnock GL, Rajotte RV. Prolongation of islet xenograft survival by cryopreservation. Diabetes 1987;36:1086–8.

103. Mandel TE, Transplantation of organ-cultured fetal pancreas: experimental studies and potential clinical application in diabetes mellitus. World J Surg 1984;8:158–8.

104. Snell GD. The homograft reaction. Annu Rev Microbiol 1957;11:439–58.

105. Faustman D, Hauptfeld V, Lacy P, Davie J. Prolongation of murine islet allograft survival by pretreatment of islets with antibody directed to Ia determinants. Proc Natl Acad Sci USA 1981;78:5156–9.

106. Faustman DL, Steinman RM, Gebel HM, et al. Prevention of rejection of murine islet allografts by pretreatment with anti-dendritic cell antibody. Proc Natl Acad Sci USA 1984;81:3864–8.

107. Lau H, Reemtsma K, Hardy MA. The use of direct ultraviolet irradiation and cyclosporine in facilitating indefinite pancreatic islet allograft acceptance. Transplantation 1984;38:566–9.

108. Gotoh M, Porter J, Kanai T, et al. T. Multiple donor allotransplantation: a new approach to pancreatic islet transplantation. Transplantation 1988;45:1008–12.

109. Tze WJ, Tai J. Successful intracerebral allotransplantation of purified pancreatic endocrine cells in diabetic rats. Diabetes 1983;32:1185–7.

110. Selawry HP, Whittington K. Extended allograft survival of islets grafted into intra-abdominally placed testis. Diabetes 1984;33:405–6, 1984.

111. Weber CJ, Zabinski S, Koschitzky T, et al. The role of CD4+ helper T cells in the destruction of microencapsulated islet xenografts in NOD mice, Transplantation 1990;49:396–404.

112. O'Shea MG, Sun AM. Encapsulation of rat islets of Langerhans prolongs xenograft survival in diabetic mice. Diabetes 1986;35:943–6.

113. Lacy PE, Hegre OD, Gerasimidi-Vazeou A, et al. Maintenance of normoglycemia in diabetic mice by subcutaneous xenografts of encapsulated islets. Science 1991;254:1782–4.

114. Maki T, Ubhi CS, Sanchez-Farpon H, et al. Successful treatment of diabetes with the biohybrid artificial pancreas in dogs. Transplantation 1991;51:43–51.

115. Sullivan SJ, Maki T, Borland KM, et al. Biohybrid artificial pancreas: long-term implantation studies in diabetic, pancreatectomized dogs. Science 1991;252:718–21.

116. Lanza RP, Butler DH, Borland KM, et al. Xenotransplantation of canine, bovine, and porcine islets in diabetic rats without immunosuppression. Proc Natl Acad Sci USA 1991;88:11100–4.

117. Sutherland DER, Kendall D. Clinical pancreas and islet transplant registry report. Transplant Proc 1985;17:307–11.

118. Scharp DW, Lacy PE, Santiago JV, et al. Insulin independence after islet transplantation into type I diabetic patient. Diabetes 1990;39:515–8.

119. Scharp DW, Lacy PE, Santiago JV, et al. Results of our first nine intraportal islet allografts in type 1, insulin-dependent diabetic patients. Transplantation 1991;51:76–85.

120. Warnock GL, Kneteman NM, Ryan E, et al. Normoglycaemia after transplantation of freshly isolated and cryopreserved pancreatic islets in type I (insulin-dependent) diabetes mellitus. Diabetologia 1991;34:55–8.

121. Kneteman NM, Warnock GL, Ryan E, et al. Prolonged insulin independence after clinical pancreatic islet transplantation. Transplantation 1992 (in press).

122. Ricordi C, Tzakis A, Carroll P, et al. Human islet allotransplantation under FK 506. Transplant Proc 1991;23:3207.

123. Ricordi C, Tzakis A, Alejandro R, et al. Detection of pancreatic islet tissue following islet allotransplantation in man. Transplantation 1991;52:1079–80.

124. Calne RY, Sells RA, Pena JR, et al. Induction of immunological tolerance by porcine liver allografts. Nature 1969;223:472–6.

Chapter 33

ALTERNATIVE APPROACHES TO INSULIN THERAPY AND RECENT ADVANCES IN IMPLANTABLE GLUCOSE SENSORS

ALAN C. MOSES
DAVID GOUGH

In this chapter we will consider a variety of new approaches to insulin therapy and new methods of monitoring ambient glucose concentrations with implantable glucose sensors. These areas of insulin therapeutics and glucose monitoring are evolving rapidly. It is anticipated that some changes in therapy based on these approaches will have occurred between the time of submission of this chapter and the time of its publication.

Recently, clinical investigators and practitioners have placed an increasing emphasis on the concept of basal-bolus insulin therapy.[1] There is a widely held assumption, which still awaits definitive proof, that the achievement of a level of glycemic control in subjects with diabetes that is similar to the level in the nondiabetic population will reduce the risk of long-term complications of diabetes.[2-4] These issues are discussed in greater detail elsewhere in this volume. The belief that complications of diabetes are correlated with the level of glycemic control[2,3,5] and the attempts that have been made to reduce the increased risks of hypoglycemia associated with intensified insulin therapy regimens[4] have led to a variety of innovative routes of insulin administration. Recent efforts also have been directed toward modification of the structure of insulin itself as a means of altering the rate and predictability of its absorption.[6]

New approaches to insulin therapy differ according to whether the goal is the achievement of a steady-state insulin level in the postabsorptive or fasting state (basal therapy) or of a rapid increment in insulin concentration at mealtime to simulate postprandial release of insulin from the normal pancreatic β-cell (bolus therapy). In this chapter the discussion of insulin therapies is divided arbitrarily into those that provide basal insulin and those that provide bolus insulin. Some of the technologies discussed are applicable to both types of insulin administration. Segmental, whole, and islet cell pancreatic transplantation is not discussed in this chapter since this area of therapy is covered in detail elsewhere (Chapter 32).

BASAL INSULIN THERAPY

General Considerations

The goal of basal insulin administration is the maintenance of a blood glucose level during the postabsorptive state that is within the narrow range found in persons without diabetes.[7-10] Basal insulin therapy, by definition, requires the maintenance of blood insulin levels within a narrow range, but a range that is effective and safe both during times of physiologic insulin resistance and during times of insulin sensitivity.[11,12] Increased serum levels of insulin appear to be required in the early morning hours to "overcome" mild, physiologic insulin resistance induced by nocturnal increases in secretion of growth hormone and cortisol.[11,12] Thus, one goal of basal insulin administration is the provision of "precise" serum insulin levels. Unfortunately, currently available repository forms of insulin cannot provide the narrow range of serum insulin levels required for optimal therapy. In large part this inability is due to variation in the rates of insulin absorption from the subcutaneous repository.[13-17] In addition, it recently has been recognized that the very long-acting forms of insulin such as human ultralente are absorbed more rapidly than similarly formulated animal insulins.[18] Further, the problems involved in the administration of basal insulin by subcutaneous injection are intensified by the need to mix short-acting with long-acting insulins.[19-21] Mixing the various formulations of insulin can alter the relative proportion of these forms in the subcutaneous space and can result in different and unpredictable rates of insulin absorption.[19] As suggested above, even if insulin were absorbed at a constant rate, variation in insulin requirements in the "basal state" at different times of day or from day to day probably would result in a level of glycemic control that was not acceptable or safe for all subjects with diabetes.[9,22]

A variety of approaches have been used to overcome problems associated with basal insulin administration (Table 33-1). Chief among these approaches is the use of mechanical insulin pumps that can either be implanted with catheter insertion into the systemic venous circulation or the peritoneum[23-26] or be used externally in conjunction with a subcutaneously placed catheter.[27-29] Insulin pumps are discussed in greater detail elsewhere in this volume (Chapter 27). However, a major limitation of any mechanical insulin pump is the lack of a reliable, long-lived, internally implanted glucose sensor (see below). Novel means of basal insulin delivery that are discussed in greater detail in this chapter include 1) the use of polymeric, subcutaneous insulin-containing pellets; 2) iontophoresis; and 3) the development of modified insulins with "designed" aggregation or solubility properties.

Subcutaneous Insulin-Impregnated Polymeric Pellets

One novel approach to the provision of a constant rate of insulin administration has been the development of polymers that are impregnated with insulin and implanted subcutaneously. Langer[30] and his associates have developed a number of polymers that are well-tolerated in the subcutaneous space and that provide stable rates of insulin release over long periods in animals[31] (Fig. 33-1). The biocompatible polymers originally used by this group were stable compounds such as ethylene-vinyl acetate copolymers that released insulin and were inert in the presence of biologic fluids. Later, this group turned to biodegradable polymers made of polyanhydrides that

Table 33-1. New Approaches to Basal Insulin Therapy

Insulin infusion pumps
    External pump with subcutaneous catheter
    Implantable pump with intravenous or peritoneal catheter
Subcutaneous, insulin-impregnated polymeric capsules
Iontophoresis
Insulin analogues with slow-absorption characteristics.

All of these approaches, except the use of insulin infusion pumps, are experimental, with little or no data on long-term efficacy in humans with diabetes. Significant impediments to these methods remain. See Chapter 27 for additional discussion of the data on insulin infusion pumps.

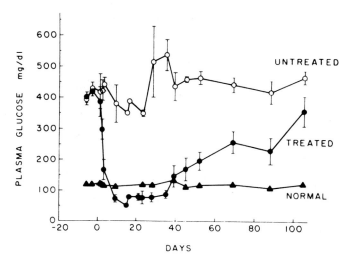

Fig. 33-1. Effects of subcutaneous implantation of insulin-containing polymeric pellets on blood glucose concentrations in diabetic rats. Ethylene-vinyl acetate copolymers containing sodium insulin were implanted subcutaneously in rats made diabetic by the intravenous administration of streptozotocin at day 0. Plasma glucose concentration was monitored for 100 days in these animals and compared with concentrations in untreated diabetic control animals and normal littermates. Implantation of the insulin-containing copolymers reduced plasma glucose concentration in the treated animals and had a sustained effect that lasted more than 2 months. Reprinted with permission from reference 31 (Creque HM, Langer R, Folkman J. One month of sustained release of insulin from polymer implant. Diabetes 1980;29:37-40; copyright © of the American Diabetes Association).

would both release insulin at a fixed and predictable rate and "dissolve" in the subcutaneous space.[30,32]

By incorporating magnetic particles into the insulin-containing polymers and by exposing these particles to a magnetic field, Langer et al.[33] and Kost et al.[34] demonstrated a reduction in blood glucose concentration in diabetic rats.

The geometry of the pellets can be altered to provide the desired rate of insulin release both in vitro and in vivo.[35,36] By modifying insulin itself and by incorporating glucose oxidase into the polymer, Fischel-Ghodsian et al. developed a glucose-sensitive insulin pellet.[37] Unfortunately, the bioactivity of the modified insulin is considerably less, on a weight basis, than that of native insulin.[37] No data are yet available that suggest such a system would be feasible in humans. Nonetheless, this approach offers a number of alternatives for new insulin delivery systems that could offer both basal and bolus insulin release. Moreover, the direct coupling of glucose "sensing" to insulin release through chemical means establishes a prototype of a nonmechanical "artificial" pancreas.

Iontophoresis

Iontophoresis refers to the process of "forcing" molecules across a barrier through the use of an electrical charge. The rate of absorption of a molecule across a barrier (skin or mucosal surface) depends on the size of the molecule, its charge, and the composition of the barrier itself.[38] In the case of the human skin, the stratum corneum and epidermis themselves produce significant barriers to drug absorption. Iontophoresis of small molecules has been accomplished in a number of animal and human models.[38,39] However, there have been major limitations to the successful transcutaneous passage of insulin and other large peptides or small proteins.[38,39]

Therapeutically relevant amounts of insulin can be delivered to alloxan-diabetic rabbits[40] and to pigs[41] with an iontophoretic device. However, even in these models, the concentrations of insulin used were high and abrasion of the cutaneous surface to remove the keratinized epidermal layer was necessary before physiologically relevant amounts of insulin could be absorbed. More recently, investigators have begun to explore the role of the pretreatment of the skin with surface-active agents before the iontophoretic administration of insulin.[39,42,43] It is not yet certain whether the rate of insulin absorption across the cutaneous barrier with iontophoretic devices is predictable and constant enough to be of therapeutic value in humans.

Insulin Analogues with Delayed Absorption Characteristics

Much has been learned about the crystal structure and aggregation properties of insulin.[7] Major changes in insulin therapy accompanied the development of crystalline insulin suspensions containing both protamine and zinc (NPH series) or excess zinc alone. Long-acting forms of insulin provided a major advance in the days when large volumes of nonhomogeneous insulin were administered three to four times daily in that they permitted the patient with diabetes to reduce the number of injections to one or two daily. Unfortunately, these long-acting forms of insulin did not and do not provide stable basal insulin levels and still leave the patient susceptible to unacceptable hypoglycemia or excessive postprandial glucose excursions.[1]

As the crystal structure of insulin was defined and the structure-function relationships were elucidated, it became clear that substitutions of specific amino acids within the primary structure of insulin could alter both the biologic activity of insulin and its aggregation and solubility properties[7] (Fig. 33–2). In the development of a form of insulin suitable for basal therapy, the goal has been to engineer the solubility characteristics of insulin crystals in the environment of the subcutaneous space. One such approach has been to develop an insulin molecule that remains in solution at acid pH but that forms uniform crystals in the subcutaneous space.[44,45] These crystals would "dissolve" at a fixed, slow rate at neutral pH. Information on the utility of this form of insulin is preliminary and concerns only one analogue— insulin substituted with arginine for threonine at B27, with threonine amide for threonine at B30 (COOH-terminus), and with glycine for asparagine at A21.[46,47] It is of interest that although the time required for 50% absorption of this analogue is longer than that for human ultralente insulin (35 vs. 25 hours) the reproducibility of the kinetics of absorption is better than that for human ultralente insulin.[47] Although this analogue may offer some advantages over currently available long-acting insulin formulations, it is unlikely to resolve the problems related to having a fixed, although steady, rate of insulin absorption in the face of variations in insulin sensitivity at various times of the day. In other words, although the rate of insulin absorption might be more predictable than that of currently available insulin formulations, this insulin

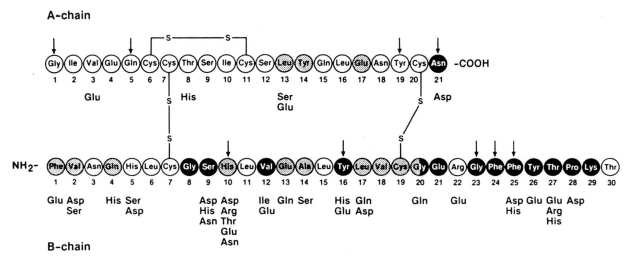

Fig. 33–2. Potential insulin analogues: sites of amino acid substitutions in human insulin. The primary amino acid sequence of human insulin is shown, with emphasis placed on residues involved in dimer (black residues) and hexamer formation (gray residues). Residues reported to be involved in high-affinity receptor binding are identified with arrows. Various amino acid substitutions for these residues that have been constructed are shown beneath each residue. Reprinted with permission from reference 7 (Brange J, Owens DR, Kang S, Vølund A. Monomeric insulins and their experimental and clinical applications. Diabetes Care 1990;13:923–54; copyright © of the American Diabetes Association).

delivery system would still not be dependent on the ambient glucose concentration.

Another approach to the development of a stable, slow-release form of insulin has been the incorporation of insulin into liposomes prior to subcutaneous injection.[48] The data available are insufficient to permit a determination of whether this approach will be useful in therapy for insulin-dependent diabetes (IDDM).

BOLUS INSULIN THERAPY

General Considerations

The goal of bolus insulin therapy is the provision of a reproducible and rapid increment in serum insulin levels at the time of meals to blunt postprandial glycemic excursion.[1] Ideal bolus insulin therapy would reproduce the secretion of insulin from the pancreatic β-cell and would result in high levels of insulin in the portal and peripheral circulations within minutes. An equally important attribute of successful bolus insulin therapy is a decline in serum insulin levels after absorption of the substrate is complete. In this regard, new approaches to bolus insulin therapy seek both to increase the rate of insulin absorption initially and to ensure complete insulin absorption or insulin inactivation in the postabsorptive state. Current formulations of short-acting insulin are not absorbed rapidly enough to provide predictable control of postprandial glucose excursion.[7,13,14,49] Moreover, these formulations are characterized by marked variability in the rate and extent of absorption and by a half-life that is much longer than ideal for the control of postprandial glucose excursion.[7,13]

Many approaches to bolus insulin therapy have been tested (Table 33–2). These involve devices that increase the rate of absorption of conventional short-acting insulins, the synthesis of insulin analogues absorbed rapidly from the subcutaneous space, and the development of new routes of insulin administration that circumvent current problems encountered with subcutaneous injection.

Table 33–2. New Approaches to Bolus Insulin Therapy

Jet injectors and sprinkler needles
  Enzyme-linked
  Magnetic particles
Insulin analogues with rapid absorption characteristics
New routes of insulin administration
  Pulmonary aerosols
  Vaginal insulin
  Ophthalmic insulin
  Oral insulin
  Rectal insulin
  Nasal insulin

None of these approaches except jet injection have been proven safe and effective in long-term clinical trials. Major emphasis is currently on the development of short-acting insulin analogues and alternative routes of insulin administration, of which nasal insulin holds the most promise.

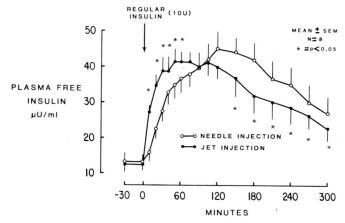

Fig. 33–3. Concentrations of plasma-free insulin in subjects with Type I diabetes mellitus following the administration of identical 10U doses of insulin subcutaneously by standard needle injection and by jet injection. Peak concentrations of plasma-free insulin are reached more rapidly after jet injection than after subcutaneous needle injection. Reprinted with permission from reference 50 (Pehling GB, Gerich JE. Comparison of plasma insulin profiles after subcutaneous administration of insulin by jet spray and conventional needle injection in patients with insulin-diabetes mellitus. Mayo Clin Proc 1984; 59:751–4).

In this section these new approaches to bolus therapy will be categorized as follows: artificial injectors; subcutaneous insulin-containing pellets linked to enzymes or imbedded with magnetic particles; insulin analogues; and "new" routes of insulin administration, including oral, buccal, rectal, vaginal, ophthalmic, and nasal application.

Jet Injectors

The rate of absorption of short-acting insulin from the subcutaneous space depends in part on the ratio of surface area to volume of the injected insulin. The mechanics of insulin administration as a subcutaneous "bolus" injection result in a spherical deposit of highly concentrated insulin in the subcutaneous space.[7] The ratio of surface area to volume decreases as the volume of injected insulin increases, and thus the rate of insulin absorption is inversely proportional to the volume of injected material. A number of jet injectors have been developed that force a stream of insulin across the cutaneous barrier with compressed air instead of with a needle.[50–55] Insulin administered as a jet spray theoretically is dispersed more widely in the subcutaneous space than is insulin administered via injection. It might be predicted—and has been proven—that regular insulin administered via a jet spray is absorbed more rapidly than conventionally administered insulin.[50,51,53,54] (Fig. 33–3). This more rapid absorption might provide some advantage at mealtimes to blunt postprandial glycemic excursion. This approach has not completely resolved the problems associated with the long absorption profile (i.e., continued insulin absorption for hours after administration) of subcutaneous regular insulin[50,51,53,54] (Fig. 33–3). There are no data to demonstrate that this route of insulin administration decreases the incidence of late postprandial hypoglycemia.

Another approach to the dispersion of insulin in the subcutaneous space has been the development of the "sprinkler" needle,[56] which is a conventional needle with multiple holes on the sides rather than a hole at the end. While this needle has not been widely tested, preliminary results demonstrate that the rate of insulin absorption is more rapid than that with conventional insulin injection.[56]

Subcutaneous Insulin Pellets

The potential role of subcutaneous insulin pellets was described in greater detail in the section on basal insulin therapy. When the subcutaneous pellets are modified to include small magnetic particles, the rate of insulin absorption can be increased on demand by placing a small electromagnet over the particles.[33,34] The magnet increases the motion of the particles and increases the rate of insulin release. This system has been demonstrated to increase insulin release from the subcutaneous pellets in diabetic rats.[34] It has not yet been tested in humans. With modifications in the solubility characteristics of insulin and the coupling of glucose oxidase to the insulin-containing polymer, the rate of insulin release can be increased as a function of ambient glucose concentration.[37] It is not yet clear whether the kinetics of this process are appropriate for basal/bolus insulin therapy in humans. Moreover, this system currently is limited by the significantly lower biologic activity of the modified insulin than the native porcine or human insulin.[37] Nonetheless, these approaches offer some interesting possibilities for mechanically simple, feed-back loop, systems of insulin delivery.

Insulin Analogues with Rapid Absorption Characteristics

As the structure-function relationships of insulin have been elucidated, it has become apparent that the residues involved in insulin dimer and hexamer formation are not the same as those involved in interaction of insulin with the insulin receptor.[7] The majority of residues involved in dimer formation are in the COOH-terminus of the B chain of insulin; residues involved in hexamer formation are more widely distributed[7] (see Fig. 33–2). Thus, on the basis of this information, it has become possible to design insulin analogues that have altered solubility characteristics but retain potent biologic activity. Several different approaches have been used to create monomeric or dimeric ("designer") insulins: i.e., insulins that do not form macromolecular complexes. These include the removal of metal-binding sites (Zn binding), which decreases the hydrophobicity of certain portions of the insulin molecule and thus produces steric hindrance that interferes with the association of insulin monomers into larger complexes, and the use of charge repulsion to inhibit insulin association into multimeric forms.[7] A

whole series of insulin analogues has been designed and expressed with the use of recombinant vectors.[6] These insulin analogues display a range of association characteristics and biologic potencies in vitro and in vivo.[6,57,58] It should be noted that pioneering work on the development of insulin analogues began with the tedious procedure of solid-phase synthesis in the laboratory of Katsoyannis.[59] However, only with the efficiency and ease of manipulation of recombinant DNA technology has it been possible to develop a whole series of insulin analogues for clinical testing.

The majority of clinical studies of insulin analogues have been accomplished with three analogues developed at Novo Nordisk.[7] These include analogues with the following substitutions: 1) aspartic acid for histidine at position 10 of the B chain (AspB10); 2) aspartic acid for proline at position 28 of the B chain (AspB28); and 3) a double substitution of aspartic acid for serine at position B8 and glutamic acid for serine at position B27 (AspB9, GluB27)(see Fig. 33–2). Each of these analogues is characterized by absorption from the subcutaneous space that is more rapid than that of U100 regular human insulin[7,58,60,61] (Fig. 33–4). There is an excellent correlation between the disappearance of insulin from the subcutaneous injection site and the appearance of insulin in the systemic circulation.[7,61] It is interesting that for some of these analogues the glucose-lowering effect in vivo is not directly correlated with biologic activity in vitro.[7,57,61] The clearance of the analogue and the internalization of the activated insulin receptor appear to be major determinants of biologic effects in vivo.[7]

Whereas only 50% of soluble human insulin is absorbed during the first 3 hours after injection, more than 75% of each of the analogues is absorbed during this interval[7] (Fig. 33–5). It is important to note that this means that 25% or less of each of these analogues is absorbed during the interval 3 to 8 hours after subcutaneous administration whereas almost 50% of native human insulin is absorbed during this time.[7] Although the metabolic clearance rates of these three insulin analogues differ, each is more effective than soluble human insulin in blunting postprandial glycemic excursion.[7] This is true even when the analogues are administered immediately before a meal and when soluble human insulin is administered 30 minutes before the meal[7] (Fig. 33–6). The area under the plasma insulin concentration curve is greater and the area under the plasma glucose concentration curve is smaller with the AspB10, GluB28 analogue than those achieved with the soluble human insulin[7] (Fig. 33–7).

Relatively little information is available about the effectiveness of these analogues in the long-term treatment of diabetes. These analogues appear to be no more immunogenic than recombinant regular human insulin.[7] However, on the basis of kinetic considerations, one can predict that the analogues tested to date would reduce both postprandial glycemic excursion and the risk of postabsorptive hypoglycemia. One practical advantage of the analogues tested to date is that, unlike native human insulin, short-acting insulin analogues can be adminis-

MONOMERIC INSULINS

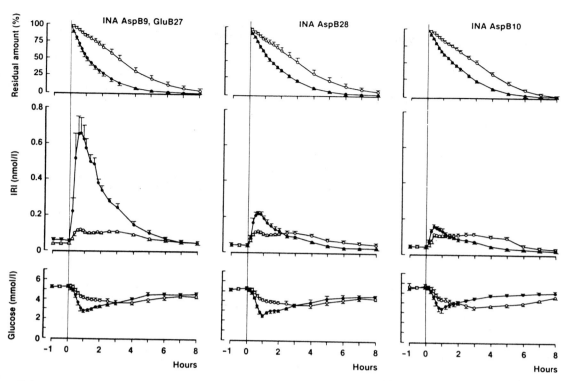

Fig. 33–4. Relative rates of absorption of three short-acting insulin analogues (INA) in comparison with regular human insulin. The absorption of each of three insulin analogues (closed circles) was compared with that of an identical dose of regular human insulin (open circles) following subcutaneous administration to healthy human volunteers. The upper panel shows the disappearance of ^{125}I from the subcutaneous space, the middle panel shows changes in plasma immunoreactive insulin (IRI) concentrations, and the lower panel shows changes in blood glucose concentration. Each of the insulin analogues was absorbed more rapidly than regular human insulin, as assessed both by disappearance of ^{125}I-insulin from the subcutaneous space and by its appearance in the circulation. Reprinted with permission from reference 7 (Brange J, Owens DR, Kang S, Vølund A. Monomeric insulins and their experimental and clinical applications. Diabetes Care 1990;13:923–54; copyright © of the American Diabetes Association).

tered subcutaneously immediately before a meal and be absorbed rapidly enough to reduce postprandial glucose levels.[7] Work continues on development of additional insulin analogues that are nonimmunogenic, have a long shelf-life, provide reproducible kinetics with high biologic potency, and have some degree of tissue specificity with regard to their biologic effects.

Alternate Routes of Insulin Administration

Shortly after Banting, Best, and Collip isolated insulin and administered it by subcutaneous injection to patients with Type I diabetes, investigators began to seek different routes of insulin administration. A wide variety of published reports have documented the administration of insulin as rectal suppositories,[62] oral suspensions,[63] vaginal douches or suppositories,[64] pulmonary aerosols,[65] and nasal sprays.[66,67] Each of these routes of insulin administration offers specific advantages and disadvantages. All have been developed in an attempt to alter the rate of insulin absorption and to avoid insulin injection.

Pulmonary Aerosols

Pulmonary aerosols have received relatively little attention to date. The advantage of pulmonary aerosols is the apparent occurrence of significant insulin absorption by formulations that do not contain absorption-enhancing agents. Unfortunately, the methods developed so far have required the use of cumbersome devices that preclude portability and ease of use.[65,68] No data have been published regarding the efficacy of this approach for the chronic treatment of diabetes. The kinetics of absorption of insulin administered as a pulmonary inhalant suggest that such a route of administration might have beneficial effects on postprandial glycemic control.[65] Clearly, more efforts are needed to determine if this route of administration is safe, tolerable, and efficacious.

Vaginal Administration

Insulin can be absorbed across the vaginal mucosa when administered as a suppository.[64] Unfortunately, no recent studies on this route of administration have been

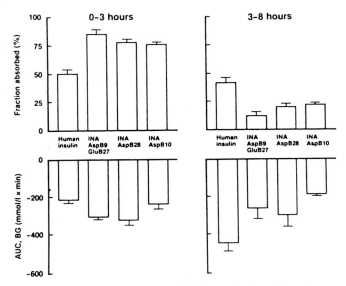

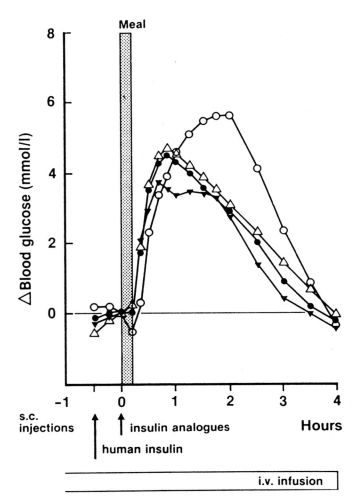

Fig. 33–5. Rate of absorption of short-acting insulin analogues (INA) vs. regular human insulin. The rates of absorption 0 to 3 hours and 3 to 8 hours following subcutaneous injection were determined for the three listed analogues and for regular human insulin. The upper panel shows the percentage of insulin absorbed over time, and the lower panel shows the area under the plasma glucose concentration curve (AUC,BG). A greater percentage of each of the analogues than of regular human insulin was absorbed between 0 and 3 hours after injection, and a smaller percentage of each of the analogues than of regular insulin was absorbed from 3 to 8 hours after injection. Reprinted with permission from reference 7 (Brange J, Owens DR, Kang S, Vølund A. Monomeric insulins and their experimental and clinical applications. Diabetes Care 1990;13:923–54; copyright © of the American Diabetes Association).

can be timed to food ingestion; and 3) it potentially delivers insulin to the portal circulation in a manner that mimics the secretion of insulin from the pancreatic β-cell. Unfortunately, insulin by itself is degraded by intestinal enzymes and is not absorbed intact across the gastrointestinal mucosa.[63,70,71] In an effort to circumvent this problem, investigators have taken a number of different approaches. The first approach was the encapsulation of insulin in liposomes that would protect it from degrada-

Fig. 33–6. Effect of insulin analogues on postprandial glycemic excursion in subjects with Type I diabetes mellitus. Subjects were administered intravenous insulin by constant infusion to maintain a steady concentration of blood glucose in the fasting state. At time 0, subjects ate a 500-kcal test meal. They received either regular human insulin subcutaneously in the anterior abdominal wall 30 minutes before the test meal (open circles) or an equivalent dose of one of the three analogues in the same location immediately before the meal. The analogues studied were AspB9 (closed triangles), AspB10 (open triangles), and AspB9,GluB27 (closed circles). Each of the analogues reduced postprandial glycemic excursion more effectively than did the regular human insulin. Reprinted with permission from reference 7 (Brange J, Owens DR, Kang S, Vølund A. Monomeric insulins and their experimental and clinical applications. Diabetes Care 1990;13:923–54; copyright © of the American Diabetes Association).

published and no direct comparisons have been made of the kinetics, efficiency of absorption, and tolerability of this route and other routes of insulin administration. On the basis of cultural considerations and ease of use, it is unlikely that this route of insulin administration will ever achieve widespread use.

Ophthalmic Insulin

Preliminary studies have demonstrated that insulin mixed with surface-active agents can be absorbed into the systemic circulation after administration on the conjunctivae.[69] The time course of insulin absorption suggests that some, if not the majority, of the absorption occurs across the nasal mucosa after transport of the solution down the lacrimal duct into the nasal cavity.[69] Few data are available concerning the clinical efficacy of this route of insulin administration, and more work needs to be completed before this becomes a viable delivery route for insulin.

Oral Insulin

The appeal of oral insulin has prompted numerous investigators to pursue this route of administration. The theoretical advantages of oral insulin administration are that 1) it obviates the need for injectable therapy; 2) it

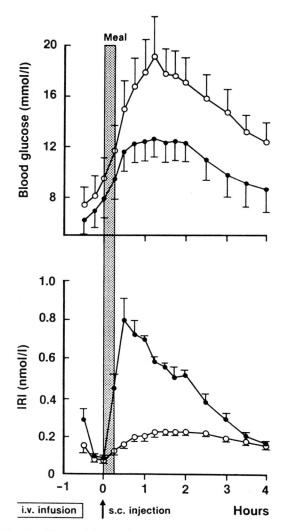

Fig. 33–7. Effect of the analogue AspB9,GluB27 on postprandial glycemic excursion and plasma insulin levels in patients with Type I diabetes mellitus. Six subjects ate a 500-kcal test meal immediately after the injection of equivalent doses (10U) of regular human insulin (open circles) or the AspB9, GluB27 insulin analogue (closed circles). The blood glucose concentration is shown in the upper panel, and plasma-free immunoreactive insulin concentration (IRI) is shown in the lower panel. The insulin analogue produced a more rapid and greater increment in levels of plasma-free insulin than that produced by the regular human insulin. This resulted in a blunting of postprandial glycemic excursion in those who received the analogue. Reprinted with permission from reference 7 (Brange J, Owens DR, Kang S, Vølund A. Monomeric insulins and their experimental and clinical applications. Diabetes Care 1990;13:923–54; copyright © of the American Diabetes Association).

tion and facilitate its uptake by the intestinal mucosal cells. Patel and colleagues clearly demonstrated that insulin incorporated into liposomes can be absorbed across the intestinal mucosa of animals and humans.[72,73] However, to date, it has been necessary to administer the insulin directly into the duodenal lumen via direct enteral

infusion.[70,73] Saffran et al. have taken a different approach by incorporating insulin into microspheres protected from digestion in the upper gastrointestinal tract by azoaromatic cross-linked polymers.[74] After the azo bonds of the polymer are degraded by colonic bacteria, insulin is released and can be absorbed directly across the colonic mucosa.[74] Administration of insulin encapsulated in this way can lower blood glucose concentration in diabetic rats.[74] So far, there are no reports of efficacy of such encapsulated insulin in humans.

More recently, Gwinup et al. encapsulated insulin with a methacrylic acid copolymer and demonstrated a decrease in endogenous C-peptide secretion that begins 2 to 3 hours after peroral insulin ingestion and is followed by an increase in immunoreactive insulin at 4 to 5 hours.[75] This time course of insulin absorption supports the dissolution of the microcapsules in the distal small bowel or proximal colon. Results of administration of these preparations in patients with diabetes have not yet been reported. Moreover, the long "lag-phase" from ingestion to substantial insulin absorption might present some therapeutic difficulties with regard to the timing of insulin administration and the desired biologic effects. Damgé et al. have reported that polyalkylcyanoacrylate nanocapsules (nanometer-size capsules) loaded with insulin produce physiologically relevant insulin absorption both in normal and in diabetic rats.[76] It is interesting that these nanocapsules appear to have a long duration of action in rats, lasting up to 20 days in a dose-dependent fashion. The role of this formulation of insulin in therapy for human diabetes is only in the early stages of testing.

The constancy of bioavailability, kinetics, and reproducibility of oral insulin all must meet the same criteria developed for parenteral insulin formulations. Unfortunately, few or no data addressing these issues have yet been published.

Rectal Insulin

A large number of studies have been performed in animals and humans that demonstrate sufficient amounts of insulin can be absorbed across the rectal mucosa to lower blood glucose concentrations.[62,77–83] Whether the use of rectal insulin will ever be a practical approach to insulin therapy has not been resolved. Nonetheless, major advances in our understanding of the process of transmucosal transport have been made on the basis of mechanistic studies in which insulin was used as a therapeutic agent.[80,84,85] There is precedence from findings about the rectal administration of a large number of therapeutically important agents to suggest that insulin absorption might occur via this route.[86] In fact, insulin by itself is not absorbed to an appreciable degree across the rectal or any other mucosal surface[62,81] (except for the pulmonary mucosa, as described above). For this reason, most studies have been directed toward the identification of safe agents that will enhance the rate and efficiency of insulin absorption.

Yamasaki et al. brought attention to the therapeutic possibilities of rectal insulin administration with their studies in dogs.[81] Later, many groups explored the mechanism of action of a wide variety of diverse adjuvant molecules that promote insulin absorption across the rectal mucosa and other mucosal surfaces.[62,78,80,84,85,87] These agents range from salicylic acid to bile acid salts.[62] Most are characterized by having lipophilic or amphiphilic properties.[85] Some agents, such as EDTA, uniquely enhance rectal insulin absorption without altering the absorption of insulin across the nasal or buccal mucosal membrane.[85] The effects of EDTA suggest some intrinsic differences between the ciliated epithelial cells lining the colon/rectum or some differences in intercellular connections of the rectal mucosa as compared with those of other mucosal surfaces.[85,87] Insulin can be administered either in suppository form or as a rectal gel or solution.[79,82,84,88] The pharmaceutical form appears to be a less important determinant of insulin absorption than the adjuvant molecule used.

These adjuvant molecules increase both the rate and efficiency of insulin absorption across the rectal mucosa.[62,83,85] Serum insulin levels peak within 30 minutes of rectal administration of insulin, producing a serum insulin profile reminiscent of insulin release by pancreatic β-cells following a meal.[8] Insulin absorption occurs over a relatively short period, thereby lessening the potential for postabsorptive hypoglycemia. Some of the biologic effects of rectally administered insulin may result from direct transport across the rectal mucosa into the portal venous system through the superior rectal vein. However, most of the venous drainage of the lower rectum empties into the systemic rather than the portal circulation.

Although research focused at defining formulations of rectal insulin that are more effective and well tolerated continues, the practical problems involved in administering a drug via the rectal route multiple times per day suggest that this approach will not meet with widespread enthusiasm in the United States. Despite these limitations, however, the kinetics of insulin absorption across the rectal mucosa and studies on the mechanisms by which adjuvant molecules promote absorption have provided important information applicable to the development of other routes of insulin administration.

Nasal Insulin

Physicians had attempted to administer insulin as a nasal spray as early as 1923. These initial attempts were unsuccessful because insulin by itself does not cross the nasal mucosa.[66,89] However, Collens and Goldzieher demonstrated in 1932 that when insulin is mixed with a detergent such as the tree-bark extract saponin, pharmacologically relevant amounts of insulin can be absorbed across the nasal mucosa.[67] These early attempts to promote insulin absorption were met with poor reproducibility and significant limitations in the amount of insulin that could be administered and/or absorbed. For this reason and because long-acting forms of parenteral insulin were being developed, attempts to perfect alternative routes of insulin administration waned.

Interest in the potential for intranasal administration of insulin was reawakened in the late 1970s and early 1980s with some important observations by Hirai and colleagues at Takeda Pharmaceuticals.[90,91] These investigators demonstrated that although neutral insulin was not absorbed across the dog's nasal mucosa, lowering the pH of the insulin solution or mixing bile acid salts with the insulin promoted the absorption of enough to lower blood glucose concentration.[91] These investigators then proceeded to carry out structure-function studies on a variety of potential adjuvant molecules, including polyoxyethylene ethers and bile acid salts.[90] A major advance was their development of a rat model for the study of insulin absorption across the nasal mucosa.[90] Among the various agents found to promote insulin absorption, two were studied in depth in animals and in humans.

Pontiroli et al. demonstrated that a mixture of sodium glycocholate and insulin permitted the absorption of enough insulin to lower blood glucose concentrations to hypoglycemic levels in normal human volunteers.[66] Moses and colleagues extended these observations by demonstrating that another bile acid salt, sodium deoxycholate, was more potent than sodium glycocholate[89,92] (Fig. 33–8). It is important to note that both glycocholate and deoxycholate mixed with insulin and administered as a nasal spray produced peak serum insulin levels in 10 to 15 minutes.[89,92] These adjuvant effects are not limited to bile acid salts. Investigators have used adjuvant molecules ranging from bile acid salts, polyoxyethylene ethers such as laureth 9,[93] derivatives of the antibiotic fusidic acid (sodium taurodihydrofusidate),[94] to lecithin.[95] A number of studies were directed at defining the structure-function relationship of adjuvant molecules.[92] To date, the mechanisms of action of the various absorption-enhancing agents have not been defined completely. It is likely that by defining these mechanisms, modifications of the structure of the adjuvant molecules may be made that may lead to the formulation of more effective and better tolerated formulations for nasal administration.

Long-term clinical trials of nasally administered insulin are just beginning. Several important conclusions can be drawn from the preliminary studies completed to date.[93,96,97] First, the kinetics of insulin absorption across the nasal mucosa in the presence of an absorption-enhancing agent are rapid and predictable.[89,93,96] Depending on the adjuvant molecule used, peak blood concentrations of insulin are achieved within 8 to 20 minutes after application of a nasal spray.[89,93,95,96] The kinetics and bioavailability of absorption appear to depend on the absorption-enhancing agent and not on the concentration of insulin in the solution[89,92] (Fig. 33–9). Of importance, the intrasubject and intersubject variations in the kinetics of nasal insulin absorption are small.[98] This method of administration provides a highly predictable pattern of insulin absorption and one that is most suitable for preprandial administration. Insulin administered as a nasal spray in the presence of an adjuvant molecule that enhances absorption blunts glucose excursion in subjects with either Type I or Type II

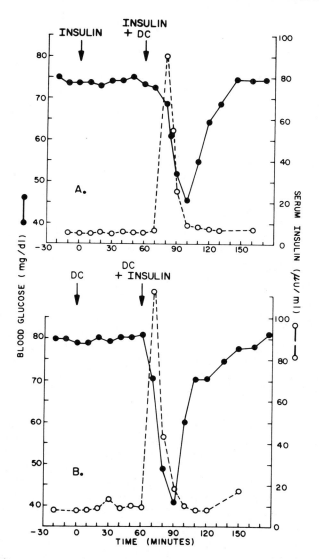

Fig. 33–8. Biologic effects of nasal insulin in normal human volunteers. Regular human insulin was mixed with sodium deoxycholate (DC; final concentration, 1%) and administered as a metered-dose nasal spray to 29 normal human volunteers. Upper panel shows serum insulin levels as an increment over basal levels; lower panel shows blood glucose concentration as a percentage of the value at time 0. Plasma insulin levels peaked rapidly (10 min) and produced a decrease in blood glucose concentration. Reprinted with permission from reference 89 (Moses AC, Gordon GS, Carey MC, Flier JS. Insulin administered intranasally as an insulin-bile salt aerosol: effectiveness and reproducibility in normal and diabetic subjects. Diabetes 1983;1040–7; copyright © of the American Diabetes Association).

diabetes [93,96,97] (Fig. 33–10). Theoretically, nasal insulin meets many of the criteria required for a reproducible, predictable bolus form of insulin administration. The therapeutic value of this route of insulin administration, however, still awaits clinical trials of long-term use to establish efficacy and safety in subjects with Type I or Type II diabetes.

It is obvious from the discussion above that a major limitation of insulin therapy, regardless of the route of administration, is the lack of feedback-controlled insulin delivery. The development of mechanical insulin delivery systems that are safe as well as efficacious will depend on the development of long-lived, biocompatible, implantable glucose sensors. Major advances in the development of such devices have taken place relatively recently.

IMPLANTABLE GLUCOSE SENSORS

General Considerations

The concept of employing implantable glucose sensors in the management of diabetes has been of interest for many years. The attraction of this idea is the potential for truly continuous glucose monitoring, rather than the discrete sampling possible at present. Continuous glucose monitoring with an implanted sensor would make possible a quantitative warning of hypoglycemia, earlier detection of hyperglycemia, and more aggressive approaches to therapy. An implanted sensor that is acceptable to the patient would also result in a greater degree of compliance with glucose monitoring because sample collection by the patient would be minimized.

There are many possible clinical applications for an implantable glucose sensor once one becomes available. There are several sensor configurations, various modes of sensor operation, and distinct options for the use of the resulting information. Some configurations under development are 1) a catheter-like sensor for acute intravenous blood glucose monitoring in hospitalized patients; 2) a needle-like sensor, or a sensor introduced through a removable needle, that would be implanted in subcutaneous tissues for acute monitoring of glucose concentrations in tissue fluids and that would be used in conjunction with a small, external instrumentation unit incorporating an algorithm for estimation of blood glucose concentration from tissue fluid glucose concentration; 3) a catheter-like sensor that would be chronically implanted in the vena cava, coupled to an implanted telemeter that would transmit the glucose concentration signal to a small, external receiver; 4) a sensor that would be chronically implanted in tissues and coupled to an implanted telemeter and that employs an algorithm that correlates tissue fluid glucose concentrations with blood glucose concentration.

Each of these sensors also could be used with an external or implantable insulin infusion pump and the appropriate control algorithms as an "artificial mechanical β-cell."

The feasibility of these glucose sensor configurations and various sensing principles is being explored. The excitement and expectations created by the introduction of the concept of the glucose sensor decades ago have been tempered by slow progress in their development, but their potential remains good. Recently, some encouraging advances have been made that may lead to clinical applications in the near future, but significant challenges

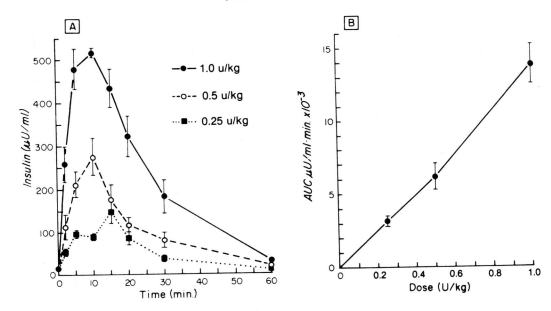

Fig. 33–9. Dose-dependent absorption of insulin from an insulin nasal spray in sheep. Insulin at various concentrations was mixed with sodium taurodihydrofusidate and administered as a nasal spray to fasting sheep. Plasma insulin levels (Fig. A) and the area under the plasma insulin concentration curve (AUC; Fig. B) were determined. Both peak plasma insulin concentrations and the AUC were a function of the dose of insulin administered. Similar data have been obtained for healthy human volunteers.[98] Reprinted with permission of the American Pharmaceutical Association from reference 94 (Longenecker JP, Moses AC, Flier JS, et al. Effects of sodium taurodihydrofusidate on nasal absorption of insulin in sheep. J Pharm Sci 1987;76:351–5).

must be addressed before the sensor becomes widely available.

Physical Principles of Glucose Sensors

Several principles of glucose sensors are based on the following reaction catalyzed by glucose oxidase:

glucose + ½ O_2 + H_2O ↔ gluconic acid + H_2O_2 + H_2O

Glucose oxidase can be immobilized in a gel that contacts an electrochemical sensor that detects either the consumption of oxygen[99,100] or the production of hydrogen peroxide,[101–104] thereby providing an indirect measurement of glucose concentration. In either case, concentration of ambient oxygen must be accounted for by a combination of a reference oxygen sensor and an appropriate sensor design, since availability of oxygen may limit the enzymatic reaction.[105] Alternatively, an electrochemically active redox agent such as ferrocene can be incorporated into the gel to take the place of oxygen and hydrogen peroxide.[106] The potential advantage of the enzyme electrode approach is the specificity of the enzyme for glucose, which permits the sensor, if properly designed, to also be specific. The technical problems are interference by other electrochemically active molecules, limited stability of the electrochemical process, the supply of oxygen or the redox agent, and the catalytic lifetime of the enzyme. These problems range from relatively insignificant to severe, depending on the enzyme electrode principle and sensor design.[107]

An alternative to this approach is direct electrochemical oxidation of glucose at a membrane-covered, catalytic metal electrode.[108,109] In sensors based on this principle, the oxidation of glucose produces a concentration-dependent current that is dependent on the electrochemical potential, electrode surface conditions, and membrane characteristics. The potential advantage of this system is the possibility of long life of the metal catalyst. The major problems with this system are difficulties in achieving acceptable selectivity for glucose in the presence of many other electrochemically active biochemicals, the design and fabrication of the sensor, and the possibility of generation of toxic electrochemical byproducts.

Many other sensing approaches have been proposed, including, for example, approaches based on other electrochemical principles,[110,111] on various optical principles,[112–115] or on thermal effects.[116] In general, these approaches are less well developed than those discussed above and present additional disadvantages.

In Vivo Applications

Use of implantable glucose sensors has been limited to research applications. Of the many reports of implant studies, only a few have appeared in the peer-reviewed literature. Some of the most promising studies are summarized here.

Short-Term Subcutaneous Implants

The development of a short-term sensor that can be placed percutaneously in the subcutaneous tissues and operated for several days has been the goal of several research groups. A variety of potential difficulties are associated with both the sensor design and its operation

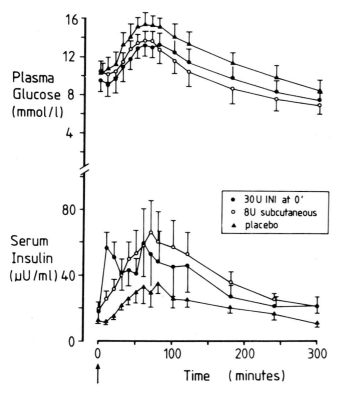

Fig. 33–10. Plasma glucose and serum insulin levels in subjects with Type II diabetes mellitus. Six subjects received a standard mixed meal on separate occasions. In addition, they received 30U of regular insulin administered intranasally (INI) mixed with sodium glycocholate (1% w/v final concentration; closed circles), 8U of regular insulin injected subcutaneously (open circles), or placebo (adjuvant alone) (closed triangles). Plasma glucose concentrations are shown in the upper panel, and serum insulin concentrations are shown in the lower panel. Intranasal insulin produced a more rapid increment in serum insulin concentrations than subcutaneously administered insulin. Both intranasal and subcutaneous insulin blunted postprandial glycemic excursion relative to placebo administration. Reprinted with permission from reference 97 (Frauman AG, Jerums GJ, Louis WJ. Effects of intranasal insulin in non-obese Type II diabetics. Diabetes Res Clin Pract 1987;3:197–202).

in subcutaneous tissues. The sensor would have to be small enough to not cause significant tissue injury, edema, or inflammation. The glucose determination must not be affected by variations in local skin temperature, tissue composition, microvascular perfusion, tissue oxygenation, or movement at the implant site. At present, the relative importance of these effects on the glucose assay is unknown.

Short-term subcutaneous sensors have been used on an experimental basis in humans. A needle-shaped, hydrogen peroxide-based enzyme electrode was implanted in the subcutaneous tissues of diabetic volunteers.[102] Initially, a linear correlation between blood glucose concentration and sensor signal was claimed, but a 43% decay in sensitivity to glucose was seen over 4 days of continuous use. In another study,[117] a needle-like, redox agent-based enzyme electrode was implanted on a short-term basis in

the subcutaneous tissues of the forehead of diabetic subjects. The decay in sensitivity was 50% over the 2-day period of use.

Other short-term subcutaneous implantation studies have been carried out in anesthetized animals for periods of several hours. A needle-like, redox agent-based enzyme electrode has been implanted in pigs,[118] and a similar hydrogen peroxide-based sensor has been implanted in rats[119] and dogs.[103] In each case, some response was obtained to blood glucose excursions caused by glucose infusions, but actual values of glucose concentration were difficult to ascertain. The relationship between tissue fluid glucose concentration and blood glucose concentration was assumed to be linear, but conflicting values of glucose partitioning from blood to tissue were reported.

An oxygen-based enzyme electrode has been implanted in a rat skin chamber developed for study of the response of chronically implanted sensors in nonanesthetized animals.[120] The chamber, permanently mounted on the animal's back, supports the growth of vascularized subcutaneous tissues around the sensor. A total of 12 glucose sensors and 14 oxygen reference sensors were implanted in 9 rats for 10 days. A detailed histologic analysis at termination of the experiment revealed an increase in microvascular density in the immediate vicinity of the sensor and no collagenous encapsulation of the sensors. The sensor response in the unanesthetized rats showed sensitivity to glucose and exhibited fluctuations that may be attributable to vasomotion.

The results of these studies are encouraging but point to a need for further investigation. In some cases, the sensitivity to glucose before implantation and the absolute current were substantially and unpredictably reduced by implantation, as judged by the response to blood glucose perturbations. Certain investigators[117] reported that the sensor signal followed rapid changes in blood glucose concentration but were not able to indicate absolute concentration values. In addition, a decay in sensitivity to glucose with duration of implant was reported in most studies. The reasons for these phenomena are unclear, but may be related to electrochemical interference, tissue oxygen limitations, tissue structure, local physiologic processes such as wound healing, or other factors. If the understanding of these issues remains incomplete, at best this sensor would have to be used in conjunction with frequent blood sampling, which would counter some of the advantages of the sensor.

Intravascular Implants

A catalytic metal electrode sensor has been fabricated at the tip of a catheter and implanted intravenously in the dog for several hours.[121] The sensor signal correlated with changes in blood glucose concentration during certain parts of the experiment but not during other parts. Recalibration of the sensor was necessary after implantation because of a substantial change in sensitivity that was due primarily to electrochemical interference. The formation of a fibrous deposit over the electrochemically active region of the sensor may have been a result of the sensor design, in which electric current passed through the blood/sensor interface. Clearly, a more basic understanding of this sensor is required.

An oxygen-based enzyme electrode was implanted intravenously in six dogs for 1 to 15 weeks.[122] The catheter-like glucose sensor and a similar reference oxygen sensor were implanted in the superior vena cava near the entrance of the right atrium. The sensor response was transmitted externally by a telemetry system[123] implanted nearby, by surgically accessed subcutaneous leads, or by chronically maintained percutaneous leads. The longest single implant was for 108 days, during which time the sensor response showed quantitative agreement with blood glucose concentration based on preimplantation calibration.[122] In each case, the sensor signal closely followed blood glucose concentration based on the in vitro calibration before implantation and the glucose sensitivity from preimplantation to postexplantation changed only minimally. In this sensor design, the current is totally confined within the sensor, eliminating the possibility of current-induced thrombosis. Systemic anticoagulants were not used. Although no adherent thrombi or evidence of emboli was found, one of six sensors was totally encapsulated by a thin layer of tissue, which lengthened the time necessary for response to glucose but had a minimal effect on sensitivity. These experiments were limited by electrical and mechanical failures of the telemetry and by other components rather than by biocompatibility, enzyme lifetime, biochemical interference, oxygen availability, or other effects related directly to the sensor. This suggests that long-term operation of a chronically implanted intravenous sensor is feasible but still unproven.

Conclusions

Implantable glucose sensors are not yet ready to be used with confidence in humans, but significant progress in their development has been made. After many years of research, it is clear that a systematic scientific approach must be employed to obtain more information about the sensor and its interaction with the biologic environment. With improvements in the understanding of the sensor system and its application in the body, a variety of novel clinical applications can be foreseen.

REFERENCES

1. Hirsch IB, Farkas-Hirsch R, Skyler JS. Intensive insulin therapy for treatment of Type 1 diabetes. Diabetes Care 1990;13:1265–83.
2. DCCT Research Group. Are continuing studies of metabolic control and microvascular complications in insulin-dependent diabetes mellitus justified? The Diabetes Control and Complications Trial. N Engl J Med 1988;318:246–50.
3. Hanssen KF, Dahl-Jørgensen K, Lauritzen T, et al. Diabetic control and microvascular complications: the near-normalglycaemic experience. Diabetologia 1986;29:677–84.
4. DCCT Research Group Diabetes Control and Complications Trial (DCCT): results of feasibility study. Diabetes Care 1987;10:1–19.

5. Dahl-Jørgensen K, Brinchmann-Hansen O, Hanssen KF, et al. Rapid tightening of blood glucose control leads to transient deterioration of retinopathy in insulin dependent diabetes mellitus: the Oslo Study. BMJ 1985;290:811–15.
6. Brange J, Ribel U, Hansen JF, et al. Monomeric insulins obtained by protein engineering and their medical implications [Letter]. Nature 1988;333:679–82.
7. Brange J, Owens DR, Kang S, Vølund A. Monomeric insulins and their experimental and clinical implications. Diabetes Care 1990;13:923–54.
8. Rizza RA, Gerich JE, Haymond MW, et al. Control of blood sugar in insulin-dependent diabetes: comparison of an artificial endocrine pancreas, continuous subcutaneous insulin infusion, and intensified conventional insulin therapy. N Engl J Med 1980;303:1313–8.
9. Cahill GF Jr, Herrera MG, Morgan AP, et al. Hormone-fuel interrelationships during fasting. J Clin Invest 1966;45:1751–69.
10. Ferrannini E, Bjorkman O, Reichard GA Jr, et al. The disposal of an oral glucose load in healthy subjects. A quantitative study. Diabetes 1985;34:580–8.
11. Schmidt MI, Hadji-Georgopoulos A, Rendell M, et al. The dawn phenomenon, an early morning glucose rise: implications for diabetic intraday blood glucose variation. Diabetes Care 1981;4:579–85.
12. Bolli GB, Gerich JE. The "dawn phenomenon"—a common occurrence in both non-insulin-dependent and insulin-dependent diabetes mellitus. N Engl J Med 1984;310:746–50.
13. Galloway JA, Spradlin CT, Nelson RL, et al. Factors influencing the absorption, serum insulin concentration, and blood glucose responses after injections of regular insulin and various insulin mixtures. Diabetes Care 1981;4:366–76.
14. Gardner DF, Arakaki RF, Podet EJ, et al. The pharmacokinetics of subcutaneous regular insulin in Type I diabetic patients: assessment using a glucose clamp technique. J Clin Endocrinol Metab 1986;63:689–94.
15. Moore EW, Mitchell ML, Chalmers TC. Variability in absorption of insulin-I[31] in normal and diabetic subjects after subcutaneous and intramuscular injection. J Clin Invest 1959;38:1222–7.
16. Chap Z, Ishida T, Chou J, et al. First-pass hepatic extraction and metabolic effects of insulin and insulin analogues. Am J Physiol 1987;252:E209–17.
17. Lauritzen T, Pramming S, Deckert T, Binder C. Pharmacokinetics of continuous subcutaneous insulin infusion. Diabetologia 1983;24:326–9.
18. Hildebrandt P, Berger A, Vølund A, Kuhl C. The subcutaneous absorption of human and bovine ultralente insulin formulations. Diabetic Med 1985;2:355–9.
19. Heine RJ, Sikkenk AC, Eizenga WH, van der Veen EA. Delayed onset of action of soluble insulin after premixing with U100 lente insulin. Diabetes Res Clin Pract 1986;2:353–8.
20. Heine RJ, Bilo HJG, Fonk T, et al. Absorption kinetics and action profiles of mixtures of short- and intermediate-acting insulins. Diabetologia 1984;27:558–62.
21. Nolte MS, Poon V, Grodsky GM, et al. Reduced solubility of short-acting soluble insulins when mixed with longer-acting insulins. Diabetes 1983;32:1177–81.
22. Perlman K, Ehrlich RM, Filler RM, Albisser AM. Waveform requirements for metabolic normalization with continuous intravenous insulin delivery in man. Diabetes 1981;30:710–7.

23. Blackshear PJ, Shulman GI, Roussell AM, et al. Metabolic response to three years of continuous, basal rate intravenous insulin infusion in Type II diabetic patients. J Clin Endocrinol Metab 1985;61:753–60.

24. Saudek CD, Selam J-L, Pitt HA, et al. A preliminary trial of the programmable implantable medication system for insulin delivery. N Engl J Med 1989;321:574–9.

25. Blackshear PJ, Roussell AM, Cohen AM, Nathan DM. Basal-rate intravenous insulin infusion compared to conventional insulin treatment in patients with Type II diabetes: a prospective crossover trial. Diabetes Care 1989;12:455–63.

26. Saudek CD, Fischell RE, Swindle MM. The programmable implantable medication system (PIMS): design features and pre-clinical trials. Horm Metab Res 22:201–206, 1990.

27. Birch K, Hildebrandt P, Jensen BM, et al. Insulin appearance of subcutaneously infused insulin: influence of the basal rate pulse interval of the infusion pump. Diabetes Res 1985;2:141–3.

28. Tamborlane WV, Sherwin RS, Genel M, Felig P. Reduction to normal of plasma glucose in juvenile diabetes by subcutaneous administration of insulin with a portable infusion pump. N Engl J Med 1989;300:573–8.

29. Nathan DM, Lou P, Avruch J. Intensive conventional and insulin pump therapies in adult Type I diabetes: a cross-over study. Ann Intern Med 1982;27:31–6.

30. Langer R. New methods of drug delivery. Science 1990;249:1527–33.

31. Creque HM, Langer R, Folkman J. One month of sustained release of insulin from a polymer implant. Diabetes 1980;29:37–40.

32. Mathiowitz E, Kline D, Langer R. Morphology of polyanhydride microsphere delivery systems. Scanning Microsc 1990;4:329–40.

33. Langer R, Siegel R, Brown L, et al. Controlled release and magnetically modulated systems for macromolecular drugs. Ann N Y Acad Sci 1985;446:1–13.

34. Kost J, Wolfrum J, Langer R. Magnetically enhanced insulin release in diabetic rats. J Biomed Mater Res 1987;21:1367–73.

35. Brown L, Munoz C, Siemer L, et al. Controlled release of insulin from polymer matrices: control of diabetes in rats. Diabetes 1986;35:692–7.

36. Brown L, Siemer L, Munoz C, Langer R. Controlled release of insulin from polymer matrices: in vitro kinetics. Diabetes 1986;35:684–91.

37. Fischel-Ghodsian F, Brown L, Mathiowitz E, et al. Enzymatically controlled drug delivery. Proc Natl Acad Sci USA 1988;85:2403–6.

38. Chien YW, Siddiqui O, Sun Y, et al. Transdermal iontophoretic delivery of therapeutic peptides/proteins. I. insulin. Ann N Y Acad Sci 1987;507:32–51.

39. Srinivasan V, Higuchi WI, Sims SM, et al. Transdermal iontophoretic drug delivery: mechanistic analysis and application to polypeptide delivery. J Pharm Sci 1989;78:370–5.

40. Kari B. Control of blood glucose levels in alloxan-diabetic rabbits by iontophoresis of insulin. Diabetes 1986;35:217–21.

41. Stephen RL, Petelenz TJ, Jacobsen SC. Potential novel methods for insulin administration. I. Iontophoresis. Biomed Biochim Acta 43:553–558, 1984.

42. Piborský J, Takayama K, Nagai T, et al. Combination effect of penetration enhancers and propylene glycol on in vitro transdermal absorption of insulin. Drug Des Deliv 1987;2:91–7.

43. Liedtke RK, Sorger M, Merk F, Vetter H. Transdermale Applikation von Insulin bei Typ-II-Diabetikern: Ergebnisse einer klinischen Pilotstudie. Arzneimittelforschung 1990;40:884–6.

44. Markussen J, Diers I, Hougaard P, et al. Soluble, prolonged-acting insulin derivatives. III. Degree of protraction, crystallizability and chemical stability of insulins substituted in positions A21, B13, B23, B27 and B30. Protein Eng 1988;2:157–66.

45. Markussen J, Diers I, Engesgaard A, et al. Soluble, prolonged-acting insulin derivatives. II. Degree of protraction and crystallizability of insulins substituted in positions A17, B8, B13, B27 and B30. Protein Eng 1987;1:215–23.

46. Vølund A, Meador M, Watanabe R, Bergman RN. Insulin analogs with altered absorption kinetics exhibit metabolic effects similar to native insulin [Abstract]. Diabetes Res Clin Pract 1988;5:59.

47. Jørgensen S, Vaag A, Langkjaer L, et al. NovoSol Basal: pharmacokinetics of a novel soluble long acting insulin analogue. BMJ 1989;299:415–9.

48. Stevenson RW, Patel HM, Parsons JA, Ryman BE. Prolonged hypoglycemic effect in diabetic dogs due to subcutaneous administration of insulin in liposomes. Diabetes 1982;31:506–11.

49. Galloway JA, Root MA, Bergstrom R, et al. Clinical pharmacologic studies with human insulin (recombinant DNA). Diabetes Care 1982;5(Suppl 2):13–22.

50. Pehling GB, Gerich JE. Comparison of plasma insulin profiles after subcutaneous administration of insulin by jet spray and conventional needle injection in patients with insulin-dependent diabetes mellitus. Mayo Clin Proc 1984;59:751–4.

51. Worth R, Anderson J, Taylor R, Alberti KGMM. Jet injection of insulin: comparison with conventional injection by syringe and needle. BMJ 1980;281:713–4.

52. Cohn L, Chez RA, Hingson RA, et al. Use of jet insulin injection in diabetes mellitus therapy. Diabetes 1972;21:39–44.

53. Malone JI, Lowitt S, Grove NP, Shah SC. Comparison of insulin levels after injection by jet stream and disposable insulin syringe. Diabetes Care 1986;9:637–40.

54. Hallé JP, Lambert J, Lindmayer I, et al. Twice-daily mixed regular and NPH insulin injections with new jet injector versus conventional syringes: pharmacokinetics of insulin absorption. Diabetes Care 1986;9:279–82.

55. Houtzagers CM, Visser AP, Berntzen PA, et al. The Medi-Jector II: efficacy and acceptability in insulin-dependent diabetic patients with and without needle phobia. Diabetic Med 1988;5:135–8.

56. Edsberg B, Herly D, Hildebrandt P, Kuhl C. Insulin bolus given by sprinkler needle: effect on absorption and glycaemic response to a meal. BMJ 1987;294:1373–6.

57. Vora JP, Owens DR, Atiea JA, et al. Recombinant DNA derived monomeric insulin analogue: comparison with soluble human insulin in normal subjects. BMJ 1988;297:1236–9.

58. Ribel U, Hougaard P, Drejer K, Sørensen AR. Equivalent in vivo biological activity of insulin analogues and human insulin despite different in vitro potencies. Diabetes 1990;39:1033–9.

59. Cosmatos A, Okada Y, Katsoyannis PG. Synthesis of two biologically active insulin analogues with modifications at the N-terminal and N- and C-terminal amino acid residues. Biochemistry 1976;15:4076–82.

60. Heinemann L, Starke AAR, Heding L, et al. Action profiles of fast onset insulin analogues. Diabetologia 1990;33:384–6.

61. Kang S, Owens DR, Vora JP, Brange J. Comparison of insulin analogue B9AspB27Glu and soluble human insulin in insulin-treated diabetes. Lancet 1990;335:303–6.

62. Nishihata T, Rytting JH, Kamada A, et al. Enhancement of rectal absorption of insulin using salicylates in dogs. J Pharm Pharmacol 1983;35:148–51.

63. Murlin JR, Gibbs CBF, Romansky MJ, et al. Effectiveness of per-oral insulin in human diabetes. J Clin Invest 1940;19:709–22.

64. Fisher NF. The absorption of insulin from the intestine, vagina and scrotal sac. Am J Physiol 1923;67:65–71.

65. Wigley FM, Londono JH, Wood SH, et al. Insulin across a respiratory mucosae by aerosol delivery. Diabetes 1971;20:552–6.

66. Pontiroli AE, Alberetto M, Secchi A, et al. Insulin given intranasally induces hypoglycaemia in normal and diabetic subjects. BMJ 1982;284:303–6.

67. Collens WS, Goldzieher MA. Absorption of insulin by nasal mucous membrane. Proc Soc Exp Biol Med 1932;29:756–9.

68. Elliott RB, Edgar BW, Pilcher CC, et al. Parenteral absorption of insulin from the lung in diabetic children. Aust Paediatr J 1987;23:293–7.

69. Chiou GCY, Chuang CY, Chang MS. Reduction of blood glucose concentration with insulin eye drops [Letter]. Diabetes Care 1988;11:750–1.

70. Dapergolas G, Gregoriadis G. Hypoglycaemic effect of liposome-entrapped insulin administered intragastrically into rats. Lancet 1976;2:824–7.

71. Earle MP. Experimental use of oral insulin. Israel J Med Sci 1992;8:899–900.

72. Patel HM, Ryman BE. The gastrointestinal absorption of liposomally entrapped insulin in normal rats. Biochem Soc Trans 1977;5:1054–5.

73. Patel HM, Harding NGL, Logue F, et al. Intrajejunal absorption of liposomally entrapped insulin in normal man. Biochem Soc Trans 1978;6:784–5.

74. Saffran M, Kumar GS, Savariar C, et al. A new approach to the oral administration of insulin and other peptide drugs. Science 1986;233:1081–4.

75. Gwinup G, Elias AN, Domurat ES. Insulin and C-peptide levels following oral administration of insulin in intestinal-enzyme protected capsules. Gen Pharmacol 1991;22:243–6.

76. Damgé C, Michel C, Aprahamian M, Couvreur P. New approach for oral administration of insulin with polyalkylcyanoacrylate nanocapsules as drug carrier. Diabetes 1988;37:246–51.

77. Yamasaki Y, Shichiri M, Kawamori R, et al. The effectiveness of rectal administration of insulin suppository on normal and diabetic subjects. Diabetes Care 1981;4:454–8.

78. Kim S, Kamada A, Higuchi, Nishihata T. Effect of enamine derivatives on the rectal absorption of insulin in dogs and rabbits. J Pharm Pharmacol 1983;35:100–3.

79. Ichikawa K, Ohata I, Mitomi M, et al. Rectal absorption of insulin suppositories in rabbits. J Pharm Pharmacol 1980;32:314–8.

80. Hauss DJ, Ando HY. The influence of concentration of two salicylate derivatives on rectal insulin absorption enhancement. J Pharm Pharmacol 1988;40:659–61.

81. Yamasaki Y, Shichiri M, Kawamori R, et al. The effect of rectal administration of insulin on the short-term treatment of alloxan-diabetic dogs. Can J Physiol Pharmacol 1981;59:1–6.

82. Ritschel WA, Ritschel GB, Ritschel BEC, Lücker PW. Rectal delivery system for insulin. Methods Find Exp Clin Pharmacol 1988;10:645–56.

83. Strazzulla G, Cotrozzi G, Guazzelli R, et al. L'administration d'insuline par voie rectale. Ann Med Interne (Paris) 1988;139:148–9.

84. van Hoogdalem EJ, Heijligers-Feijen CD, Verhoef JC, et al. Absorption enhancement of rectally infused insulin by sodium tauro-24,25-dihydrofusidate (STDHF) in rats. Pharm Res 1990;7:180–3.

85. Aungst BJ, Rogers NJ. Site dependence of absorption-promoting actions of laureth-9, Na salicylate, Na2EDTA, and aprotinin on rectal, nasal, and buccal insulin delivery. Pharm Res 1988;5:305–8.

86. Sekine M, Sasahara K, Okada R, Awazu S. Improvement of bioavailability of poorly absorbed drugs. IV. Mechanism of the promoting effect of medium chain glyceride on the rectal absorption of water soluble drugs. J Pharmacobiodyn 1995;8:645–52.

87. Aungst BJ, Rogers NJ, Shefter E. Comparison of nasal, rectal, buccal, sublingual and intramuscular insulin efficacy and the effects of a bile salt absorption promoter. J Pharmacol Exp Ther 1988;244:23–7.

88. Ritschel WA, Ritschel GB, Sathyan G. Insulin drug delivery systems: rectal gels. Res Commun Chem Pathol Pharmacol 1988;62:103–12.

89. Moses AC, Gordon GS, Carey MC, Flier JS. Insulin administered intranasally as an insulin-bile salt aerosol effectiveness and reproducibility in normal and diabetic subjects. Diabetes 1983;32:1040–7.

90. Hirai S, Yashiki T, Mima H. Effect of surfactants on the nasal absorption of insulin in rats. Int J Pharm 1981;9:165–72.

91. Hirai S, Ikenaga T, Matsuzawa T. Nasal absorption of insulin in dogs. Diabetes 1978;27:296–9.

92. Gordon GS, Moses AC, Silver RD, et al. Nasal absorption of insulin: enhancement by hydrophobic bile salts. Proc Natl Acad Sci USA 1985;82:7419–23.

93. Salzman R, Manson JE, Griffing GT, et al. Intranasal aerosolized insulin: mixed-meal studies and long-term use in Type I diabetes. N Engl J Med 1985;312:1078–84.

94. Longenecker JP, Moses AC, Flier JS, et al. Effects of sodium taurodihydrofusidate on nasal absorption of insulin in sheep. J Pharm Sci 1987;76:351–5.

95. Drejer K, Vaag A, Bech K, et al. Pharmacokinetics of intranasally administered insulin with phospholipid as absorption enhancer [Abstract no. 198]. Diabetologia 1990;33(Suppl):A61.

96. Frauman AG, Cooper ME, Parsons BJ, et al. Long-term use of intranasal insulin in insulin-dependent diabetic patients. Diabetes Care 1987;10:573–8.

97. Frauman AG, Jerums GJ, Louis WJ. Effects of intranasal insulin in non-obese Type II diabetics. Diabetes Res Clin Pract 1987;3:197–202.

98. Nolte MS, Taboga C, Salamon E, et al. Biological activity of nasally administered insulin in normal subjects. Horm Metab Res 1990;22:170–4.

99. Updike SJ, Hicks GP. The enzyme electrode. Nature 1967;214:986–8.

100. Gough DA, Leypoldt JK, Armour JC. Progress toward a potentially implantable enzyme-based glucose sensor. Diabetes Care 1982;5:190–8.

101. Clark LC Jr. The hydrogen peroxide sensing platinum anode as an analytical enzyme electrode. Methods Enzymol 1979;56:448–79.

102. Shichiri M, Kawamori R, Yamasaki Y, et al. Wearable artificial endocrine pancreas with needle-type glucose sensor. Lancet 1982;2:1129–31.

103. Abel P, Müller A, Fischer U. Experience with an implantable glucose sensor as a prerequisite of an artificial beta cell. Biomed Biochim Acta 1984;43:577–84.

104. Kerner W, Zier H, Steinbach G, et al. A potentially implantable enzyme electrode for amperometric measurement of glucose. Horm Metab Res Suppl 1988;20:8–13.

105. Gough DA, Lucisano JY, Tse PHS. A two-dimensional enzyme electrode for glucose. Anal Chem 1985;57:2351–7.

106. Cass AEG, Davis G, Francis GD, et al. Ferrocene-mediated enzyme electrode for amperometric determination of glucose. Anal Chem 56:667–71.

107. Gough DA. Issues related to in vitro operation of potentially implantable enzyme electrode glucose sensors. Horm Metab Res Suppl 1988;20:30–3.

108. Lerner H, Soeldner JS, Colton CK, Giner J. Measurement of glucose concentration in the presence of coreactants with a platinum electrode. Diabetes Care 1982;5:229–37.

109. Preidel W, Saeger S. In vitro measurements with electrocatalytic glucose sensor in blood. Biomed Biochim Acta 1989;48:897–903.

110. Degani Y, Heller A. Direct electrical communication between chemically modified enzymes and metal electrodes. I. Electron transfer from glucose oxidase to metal electrodes via electron relays, bound covalently to the enzyme. J Physical Chem 1987;91:1285–9.

111. Wilkins ES, Wilkins MG. The coated wire electrode glucose sensor. Horm Metab Res Suppl 1988;20:50–5.

112. Rabinovitch B, March WF, Adams RL. Noninvasive glucose monitoring of the aqueous humor of the eye. I. Measurement of very small optical rotations. Diabetes Care 1982;5:254–8.

113. Gough DA. The composition and optical rotary dispersion of bovine aqueous humor. Diabetes Care 1982;5:266–70.

114. Janatsch G, Kruse-Jarres JD, Marbach R, Heise HM. Multivariate calibration for assays in clinical chemistry using attenuated total reflection infrared spectra of human blood plasma. Anal Chem 1989;61:2016–23.

115. Schultz JS, Mansouri S, Goldstein I. Affinity sensor: a new technique for developing implantable sensors for glucose and other metabolites. Diabetes Care 1982;5:245–53.

116. Muehlbauer MJ, Guilbeau EJ, Towe BC. Model for a thermoelectric enzyme glucose sensor. Anal Chem 1989;61:77–83.

117. Pickup JC, Shaw GW, Claremont DJ. In vivo molecular sensing in diabetes mellitus: an implantable glucose sensor with direct electron transfer. Diabetologia 1989;32:213–7.

118. Claremont DJ, Sambrook IE, Penton C, Pickup JC. Subcutaneous implantation of a ferrocene-mediated glucose sensor in pigs. Diabetology 1986;29:817–21.

119. Velho G, Froguel P, Sternberg R, et al. In vitro and in vivo stability of electrode potentials in needle-type glucose sensors: influence of needle material. Diabetes 1989;38:164–71.

120. Ertefai S, Gough DA. Physiological preparation for studying the response of subcutaneously implanted glucose and oxygen sensors. Biomed Eng 1989;11:362–8.

121. Sarangapani S, Giner J, Soeldner JS, et al. Electrocatalytic glucose sensor. Horm Metab Res Suppl 1988;20:43–7.

122. Armour JC, Lucisano JY, McKean BD, Gough DA. Application of chronic intravascular blood glucose sensor in dogs. Diabetes 1990;39:1519–26.

123. McKean BD, Gough DA. A telemetry-instrumentation system for chronically implanted glucose and oxygen sensors. IEEE Trans Biomed Eng 1988;35:526–32.

Chapter 34

ECONOMIC AND SOCIAL COSTS OF DIABETES

KENNETH E. QUICKEL, JR.

Diabetes is the prototype chronic disease. In 1991, there were about 14 million people with diabetes in the United States, representing 5 to 6% of the population, about half of whom were aware of the diagnosis.[1] Diabetes is a leading cause of death and disability and imposes large economic and social costs. These not only affect individuals with diabetes and their families but have a major impact on the entire society.

Diabetes is nearly ubiquitous, occurring in all age and racial groups but affecting certain minority and economically disadvantaged segments of the population disproportionately. Diabetes is commonly listed among the leading causes of death, especially in assessments that include deaths due to diabetes-related conditions. In 1991, more than 150,000 people in the United States died as a result of diabetes and its complications, and the mortality rate for people with diabetes was 20 times that for the general population. Diabetes is the leading cause of blindness in Americans of working age, of end-stage renal disease, and of nontraumatic amputations, and it is a major risk factor for coronary artery disease and adverse outcomes of pregnancy. It is more prevalent among black and Hispanic populations and is especially common among the Pima Indians of Arizona and several other native American groups (Table 34–1).

The financial costs of diabetes are very high, for both society as a whole and individuals with diabetes. For each of the 6,800,000 persons known to have diabetes, this cost amounted to about $3000 in 1987.[2] Even at this level of expenditure, many essential services required by people with diabetes are not covered by their insurance

Table 34–1. Prevalence off Diabetes by Race or Ethnic Group

Race/Ethnic Group	Prevalence
White	6.2
Black	10.2
Cuban	9.3
Mexican	13.0
Puerto Rican	13.4
Japanese-American	13.9
Pima Indian	27.5

Data are from the American Diabetes Association.[1]

plans and must be paid out of pocket or simply be foregone. Society pays a high price for diabetes, but the individual with diabetes encounters many additional economic and social costs. Persons with diabetes frequently experience employment limitations and even job discrimination.[3–7] They often have difficulty obtaining health or life insurance and often must pay significantly more than nondiabetic persons for coverage.[8,9]

At a national level, the economic impact of diabetes is significant. In 1987, the cost of diabetes in the United States, including the direct cost of care and indirect costs associated with loss of productivity and other factors, was an estimated $20.4 billion.[2] According to the United States Department of Health and Human Services, health-care expenditures in 1990 amounted to $666.2 billion, or 12.2% of the gross national product (GNP).[10] For these statistics, the United States led the industrialized nations

(Fig. 34–1). In the United States (Fig. 34–2) and all other nations, expenditures for health care are increasing rapidly, and some authorities project that by the year 2000 the United States will expend nearly 17% of its GNP on health care.[11] This increase imposes major economic burdens, and nations have developed health-care payment policies designed to balance the growth of health-care expenditures against other national priorities. Often these policies further limit the services that are paid for. In many cases the emphasis is on providing acute and short-term care rather than on providing longer-term care and preventive medical services. Thus, national priorities for the distribution of limited funds for health care often make it more difficult for individuals with diabetes to receive services.

In addition to the expense of providing diabetes services, research expenditures constitute part of the cost of diabetes in those nations with major medical research commitments. In the United States, the 1991 budget of the National Institutes of Health (NIH) was $8.3 billion.[12] Research on diabetes is focused in several of the individual institutes of the NIH, the primary one being the National Institute of Diabetes, Digestive and Kidney Diseases, which had a budget of $615 million in 1991.[12] In 1991, $261 million was expended for diabetes research in the various institutes of the NIH. Significant additional research funding in the United States is provided by national organizations such as the Juvenile Diabetes Foundation, the American Diabetes Association, a variety of other foundations and philanthropies, and the pharmaceutical and medical-device industries.

The economic burdens of diabetes are only part of the story, however. The person with diabetes and his or her family face important social issues. Children with diabetes deal with the special challenge of growing up in a society in which few others have physical constraints. Going to school, staying overnight at a friend's house, dating, and getting married are but a few of the major personal issues that young people with diabetes and their parents must resolve. Driving a motor vehicle, drinking alcoholic beverages, and smoking are other issues affecting people with diabetes in special ways. Eligibility for various forms of employment, job discrimination, and participation in leisure activities such as scuba diving, hiking, and mountain climbing are considerations that patients with diabetes must address. People with diabetes and their families worry about these matters, and the professionals who advise them must recognize the nature of their concerns and be prepared to counsel them wisely.

This chapter presents a review of the economic and social costs of diabetes from the perspective of both the individual with diabetes and the nation. Many of the same factors of individual economic and social cost apply to both developed and emerging nations, although less-developed nations have more limited health-care services and lower overall economic resources. For instance, payment for outpatient diabetes education and special shoes might be major issues in an affluent nation, but availability of insulin itself may be a primary issue in another. In most countries, individual and national economic constraints commonly affect those with chronic diseases such as diabetes to a greater extent than they affect the general population.

ECONOMICS OF DIABETES

Use of Health Care in Diabetes

People with diabetes require more than the average amount of health care. Diabetes is the fourth leading reason for physician contacts in the United States among every age group, exceeded only by hypertension, acute

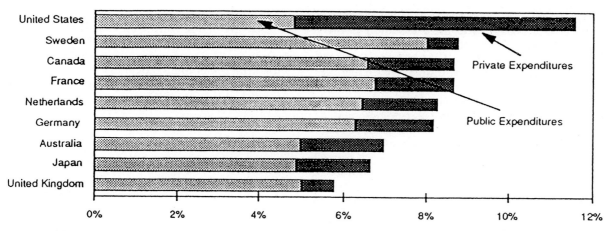

Fig. 34–1. Total health expenditures, public and private, as a percentage of gross domestic product (GDP), 1989. The most recent data for public and private health expenditures are for 1987. Figure is from the Employee Benefits and Research Institute (EBRI)[36] (from data from the U.S. Department of Health and Human Services, Health Care Financing Administration. Health Care Financing Review Annual Statistical Supplement, 1989. Washington, DC: US Government Printing Office, 1990; Organization for Economic Cooperation and Development. News From OECD. Washington, DC: Organization for Economic Cooperation and Development, 1991). EBRI assumes that, because no major changes have occurred in these countries' health-care systems, the division of private and public expenditures in 1989 will be similar to that in 1987.

Percentage

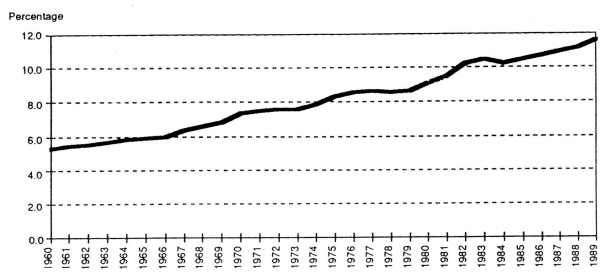

Fig. 34—2. National health expenditures as a percentage of gross national product, 1961—1989. Data are from Lazenby and Letsch.[70]

respiratory infections, and otitis media.[1] Among individuals under age 20, 78.4% of those with diabetes see a physician each year vs. 67.4% of those without diabetes. Among those over age 65, the corresponding numbers are 81.1% and 69.1%.

Hospital use is also higher among patients with diabetes. Approximately 7.2% of hospitalizations in the United States have diabetes listed as either a primary or secondary diagnosis. Individuals with diabetes not only are more likely to be hospitalized than are those without diabetes but when admitted then stay in the hospital longer. In one study performed by the National Insurance Association of America[13,14] people with diabetes were hospitalized 2.4 times more frequently than people without diabetes and stayed in the hospital 30% longer. The duration of a hospital stay by persons with diabetes exceeded that of non-diabetics by 1.7 days. The most common primary discharge diagnosis for patients with diabetes was diseases of the circulatory system. According to the 1987 National Hospital Discharge Survey, people with diabetes are hospitalized 10 times more often for cerebrovascular accidents, 10 times more often for atherosclerosis, 15 times more often for peripheral vascular disease, and 22 times more often for skin ulcers and/or gangrene than are people without diabetes.[16] While most of the excess hospital use among people with diabetes is related directly to the disease and its complications, the rate of hospitalizations for conditions unrelated to diabetes or its complications is also about 10% higher among patients with diabetes.[2] Presumably, this excess occurs because the threshold for admitting people with diabetes who have unrelated conditions is lower than that for other patients, and those with diabetes tend to be kept in the hospital longer once they are admitted.

In the United States, there are significant regional and racial differences affecting hospitalization of persons with diabetes (Table 34—2). Black women have the highest age-adjusted rate of hospitalizations related to diabetes.[15] In 1987, this rate was 183 per 10,000 — 36% higher than the rate for black men, 95% higher than the rate for white women, and 109% higher than the rate for white men. The rate of hospital discharges listing diabetes as the primary diagnosis was lowest in western states and highest in southern states. Diabetes-related hospital discharges tended to increase during the early 1980s, reaching a peak in 1984 and stabilizing thereafter. In light of the general increase in prevalence of diabetes, this stabilization probably was the result of the national implementation of Medicare regulations in 1983 that encouraged the use of outpatient services for the care of less-acute problems.[17]

The use of other health-related services is also consistently higher among individuals with diabetes (Table 34—3), including short-stay hospitalizations and telephone contacts and use of podiatrists and physical therapists.[1] The total impact of these statistics on persons with diabetes is higher personal cost, higher insurance rates, greater loss of productive work time, and significant personal and family disruption.

Table 34—2. Hospital Discharges of Patients with Diabetes, by Race and Sex

Group	Discharge Rate*	Ratio†
White males	87.5	1.00
White females	93.6	1.07
Black males	135.1	1.54
Black females	183.2	2.09

Data are from the Centers for Disease Control.[15]
*Age-adjusted rate per 10,000 discharges.
†Ratio of the adjusted rate to the rate for white males.

Table 34–3. Health-Care Use for Individuals with Diabetes Over Age 20

Source of Care	Percentage Using Service During Previous 12 Months	
	Diabetes	General Population
Physician's office	78.4	67.4
Hospital outpatient	30.9	19.0
Short-stay hospital	22.9	12.8
Clinic	6.7	7.1
Telephone contact	17.5	13.6
Home visit	2.9	1.6
Dentist	38.3	48.8
Podiatrist	6.4	3.2
Chiropractor	5.7	5.0
Physical therapist	3.9	2.0

Data are from the American Diabetes Association.[1]

Cost of Having Diabetes

Each patient with diabetes is different, and individual costs related to diabetes vary widely. For the patient with uncomplicated Type II diabetes controlled with diet alone, the costs may be limited to periodic physician visits, laboratory work, periodic home glucose testing, periodic eye screening, and modest additional costs for diet. Increments in health-care insurance and life insurance can also be included as related costs. As the years pass, several events will frequently intervene to increase costs. The progression of diabetes may necessitate the use of oral hypoglycemic agents or insulin, which add to the cost of medications and create the need for closer self-monitoring and more frequent physician visits. Should complications of diabetes develop, major increases in costs are incurred for laser therapy, renal dialysis, transplantation, vascular surgery, and many other events.

Among an unselected group of 205 residents of Ottawa, Canada, who had diabetes, the total annual costs of care in 1986 averaged $2944 in Canadian dollars, 64% of which was for hospital services, 14% for treatment needs, 10% for physician services, and 8% for supplies.[18] Costs of routine outpatient care averaged $962 annually, of which 45% was for treatment supplies, 21% for physician services, and 10% for miscellaneous items. These routine outpatient costs were determined in large measure by the nature of the patient's treatment regimen. The average annual cost for routine outpatient care was $236 for those requiring oral hypoglycemic agents, $362 for those who injected insulin, and $1603 for those who used insulin pumps.

Among individuals receiving medical care for any reason, in every age group the average out-of-pocket cost per person with diabetes is higher than that for people without diabetes.[9,19,20] In the United States in 1977, expenditures for direct medical care among patients with diabetes of all ages averaged $1514, vs. $548 for patients without diabetes.[9] Despite significant inflation since 1977, the general trend should be relatively constant over time. However, the greatest increase in out-of-

pocket expenses for patients with diabetes was for prescribed medicines, for which patients over 20 years old spent 2.5 times more than patients without diabetes. Other significantly higher costs included expenditures for health insurance (1.7-fold), physician services (1.6-fold), hospital care (1.3-fold), and dental care (1.3-fold). The differences were greatest among younger patients with diabetes, but significant differences were apparent even among patients over 65. Although expenditures were higher for whites than nonwhites with diabetes, there were no significant racial differences in the expenditure ratios for persons with diabetes vs. the ratios for the general population within each racial group. These data included only those individuals who had medical expenses in the year they were surveyed. Since a higher proportion of diabetic than nondiabetic individuals incur direct medical-care expenses each year (99% vs. 87%), the impact of diabetes on average medical-care expenses is even greater across the entire population.

National Costs of Diabetes in the United States

Diabetes has many implications for public health on a national basis, and cost of care is among the most obvious of these. Estimates of the economic impact of diabetes are important for planning allocation of health-care resources and for evaluating the cost benefit of health-care initiatives. In recent years, several important studies and reviews have estimated the national cost of diabetes in the United States using one or more established methods of estimating the economic impact of diseases.[2,21–24] Other studies have presented data from Minnesota,[25] Kentucky,[26] France,[27,28] Great Britain,[29,30] and Sweden.[31] The national cost of diabetes changes each year in response to a number of factors. The costs of health-care services evolve continuously in response to general economic factors. Like death and taxes, inflation and rising health-care costs are a certainty. Both the increasing prevalence of diabetes and the implementation of new technologies will continue to increase the national economic burden of diabetes.[32]

Among the methods used for estimating the economic impact of a disease, the "human capital approach" of Rice et al. has been the one most widely used.[24] With this method, two categories of cost are evaluated: direct medical costs of providing services, and indirect costs resulting from productivity losses due to disability and premature death. Using this methodology, Entmacher et al. estimated the total cost of diabetes in the United States for selected years from 1969 to 1984.[23] During this period, the United States spent a rather constant 3.9 to 4.0% of health-care expenditures on diabetes care, despite the increasing prevalence of diabetes. In 1975, the total cost of diabetes in the United States was $5.3 billion; by 1984, the total cost had risen to $13.8 billion. Over the entire period from 1969 through 1984, the proportion of the total cost categorized as direct cost increased from 38 to 54%, undoubtedly reflecting the more rapid increase in health-care costs than of general inflation. However, these earlier studies underestimate the impact of diabetes, since they do not account for all of the costs related to diabetes.

The total economic cost of diabetes care includes, in addition to the categories of costs included in earlier studies, the impact of diabetes as a secondary condition on the complexity of concurrent diseases. For instance, a patient with diabetes who develops pneumonia is more likely to be hospitalized and might be expected to have a longer and more costly hospitalization than a patient without diabetes. A patient with diabetes who is undergoing surgery might need to be admitted for additional evaluation and stabilization both before and after the surgery. To include estimates of the effects of diabetes on the intensity of other health-care services received, the Center for Health Economic Studies in Medicine modified the human-capital approach.[2] They estimated that in 1987 the direct cost of diabetes was $9.6 billion, the indirect cost was $10.8 billion, and the total cost was $20.4 billion (Table 34–4) and that 6.51 million people in the United States had known diabetes, making the average cost per individual with diabetes $3130. This amount is the total average per-case impact of diabetes on society, not the out-of-pocket expenses paid by an individual with diabetes. Although it is certainly not valid to extrapolate endlessly, it is tempting to point out that this amounts to over $60,000 (in 1987 dollars) over a 20-year duration of diabetes. This study is being updated as this chapter is being prepared. By applying an inflation rate of 5.75% to the 1987 data (half of the actual health-care inflation rate in 1991) and ignoring any changes in the prevalence of diabetes, one can estimate that diabetes will cost the United States about $32 billion in 1992, or $4915 per year for each individual with known diabetes.

The economic costs of diabetes to society as a whole and to affected individuals and their families are great. Having outlined the cumulative costs of diabetes from the broad societal perspective, it is now appropriate to consider how these costs are paid, since the specific financial impact of diabetes is determined by the manner in which the health-care system pays for services.

Table 34–4. Total Cost of Diabetes, 1987

Cost Category	Total Cost ($ Millions)	Percentage of Total Costs
Direct costs		
Institutional (hospitals, nursing homes)	7,871.4	38.6
Outpatient	1,727.8	8.5
Total direct costs	9,599.2	47.1
Indirect costs		
Short-term morbidity	141.9	0.7
Long-term disability	3,143.2	15.4
Mortality	7,488.8	36.8
Total indirect costs	10,773.9	52.9
Total costs	20,373.1	100.0

Data are from the American Diabetes Association.[2]

Health-Care Reimbursement Systems and Diabetes

Health-care reimbursement systems control how the services are provided and paid for, affecting the availability of services for the people who use them and even influencing the career choices of young physicians and other health-care providers.[33] These payment systems have different impacts on different diseases. The general trend is for urgent and acute care to be paid for, while chronic and preventive care often are deferred. As a result, the reimbursement system has special impact on diabetes, whose chronic nature imposes a compelling need for preventive care. Most medical schools and other training programs for health-care personnel provide little information about how the health-care reimbursement system works. Health professionals must have a clear knowledge of the reimbursement system in order to understand the economic factors that control the services available to their patients with diabetes.

Evolution of the Health-Care System

Before 1900, few effective medical therapies existed. Health care was both relatively ineffective and quite inexpensive. However, the rise of scientific medicine in the first half of the twentieth century brought many effective diagnostic and therapeutic advances, such as anesthetics, radiography, and antibiotics. The discovery of insulin in 1921 was just one of these many advances. As new and effective medical methods became available, the cost of providing them increased. Not only were the new technologies themselves expensive, but patients who otherwise would have died were surviving and requiring continuing care. Nowhere was this more obvious than in diabetes, which was converted by the advent of insulin from an acute and generally fatal disease into a chronic disease that included risks of long-term complications. By the Great Depression in 1929, the demand for effective care had increased and the cost of care had risen, yet financial collapse made health care inaccessible to many people. During the 1930s, new methods of financing health care developed, including private insurance plans for those who could afford them, and employers and governments began to assume more responsibility for paying for health care. This emphasis on improving access to care continued after World War II. In 1946 the Hill-Burton Act provided low-cost federal loans to encourage hospitals to build new facilities. During the 1960s and 1970s, federal programs were developed to encourage the expansion of medical schools and medical training programs in an effort to increase the supply of physicians, and the funding for NIH increased rapidly to promote advancements in medical science and technology. All of these programs improved access to scientific and effective medical care, but by the 1960s it had become apparent that the costs of health care would have to be constrained. In about 1970, the emphasis shifted from increasing access to care to developing tactics to restrain the escalating costs of medical progress. Many innovative policies and programs to reduce costs began to be developed, and much of the reduction required putting restraints on people's access to care. These

Table 34–5. National Health Expenditures According to Source of Funds: Selected Years, 1965–1988

Year	All Health Expenditures ($ Billions)	Private Funds Amount ($ Billions)	Private Funds Percentage of Total	Public Funds Amount ($ Billions)	Public Funds Percentage of Total
1965	41.6	31.3	75.3	10.3	24.7
1970	74.4	46.7	62.8	27.7	37.2
1975	132.9	77.8	58.5	55.1	41.5
1980	241.1	143.9	57.8	105.2	42.2
1985	420.1	245.2	58.4	174.9	41.6
1988	539.9	312.4	57.9	227.5	42.1

Data are from the Office of National Cost Estimates.[35]

cost-containment policies have had particular impact on diabetes care.

Diabetes and the Health-Care System

People with diabetes must depend on a wide variety of reimbursement options to pay for necessary health care. Each reimbursement mechanism operates by somewhat different principles and differs in the diabetes services it will pay for. Significant economic barriers block patients with diabetes from receiving the care they need.[34] Although many of these barriers exist because patients simply cannot afford care, others are incorporated into the health-care reimbursement system, and it is important to understand how this system operates.

As health-care costs rise, society as a whole is forced to make decisions about the allocation of resources among a variety of compelling national priorities. In the United States, the proportion of the health-care expenditure burden paid by the government increased rapidly after the implementation of Medicare in 1965 and has remained around 42% since 1974 (Table 34–5). At the national level, the old "guns or butter" conflict has taken on the flavor of a "butter or Band-Aids" discussion, as the issues of access vs. cost are weighed. Generally, the decision-making process does not simply involve decisions on how much the nation should spend on health care and allocation of this amount for specific services. Instead, the allocation systems are hidden in the complex laws, rules, and regulations determining how reimbursement systems work. These policies, by establishing incentives, determining payment levels, and controlling eligibility for payment, determine how health-care services are allocated. Because diabetes is the prototype chronic disease, diabetes services are especially at risk in such an environment.

In the United States in 1991, $800 billion was spent on health care, representing 14% of the GNP. Both the total amount spent on health care and the proportion of the GNP expended for this purpose have increased dramatically and consistently in recent decades, with health-care costs rising faster than the general rate of inflation[36] (Fig. 34–2). The average annual increase in health-care expenditures between 1980 and 1988 was 10.6%. The distribution of national health-care expenditures in 1989 is summarized in Table 34–6; hospital care accounted for 38.5% and physician services for 19.5%. In the United

States, the payment for health-care services comes from a wide variety of sources, including government programs such as Medicare and Medicaid, individually purchased insurance, employer-purchased insurance, and out-of-pocket. Table 34–7 presents a breakdown of this health coverage in the United States in 1989.[37] It is important to note that in 1991 an estimated 34 million Americans had no health insurance coverage whatsoever and that only about 17% of those individuals were unemployed (Fig. 34–3).

Medicare

Medicare is the dominant health-care reimbursement system in the United States. In 1989, it covered 17% of medical-care costs in the United States.[37] Medicare policies have an impact on all health-care reimbursement, since health-care insurance programs throughout the country have a strong tendency to follow Medicare's lead when implementing new policies. Medicare was established by the federal government in 1965 to provide health-care coverage for the elderly as part of the social-security system. It has subsequently been expanded to cover certain other groups, including the disabled and those with end-stage renal disease.[38] For those who are eligible, Medicare provides payment for hospital services through the Part A program and for physician and certain outpatient services through the Part

Table 34–6. National Health Expenditures by Type of Expenditure, 1989

Type of Expenditure	Expenditure ($ Billions)	Percentage of Total
Hospital care	232.8	38.5
Physician services	117.6	19.5
Other personal health care*	87.8	14.5
Other spending†	73.4	12.2
Nursing-home care	47.8	7.9
Total	559.5	100.0

Data are from Lazenby and Letsch.[70]
*Includes dental services, home health care, medical durables, and other professional services.
†Includes program administration, insurance premiums in excess of claims, government public health program, and research and construction.

Table 34–7. Health-Care Insurance Coverage in the United States, 1989

Insurance Coverage	Percentage of U.S. Population
Employer insurance	58
Medicare	17
Medicaid	9
Individual insurance	6
Uninsured	13

Adapted from the Source Book of Health Insurance Data.[37]

B program. Federal legislation passed by Congress directs overall Medicare policy, and the Health Care Finance Administration (HCFA) establishes and oversees the policies by which Medicare operates. Throughout the nation, day-to-day operation of Medicare reimbursement is managed by regional Medicare intermediaries—usually the local Blue Cross-Blue Shield organizations. This results in considerable local variation in payment policies, since the intermediaries in each region often interpret the nationally established rules differently. A primer on Medicare for people with diabetes is available.[39]

Until 1983, Medicare Part A provided payment for hospital care on a per diem basis, calculating an allowable cost per day of hospital care for each hospital and paying retrospectively for each day of a patient's hospitalization. Under this system, the longer the patient remained in the hospital, the more the hospital was paid. In 1983, Medicare shifted to a prospective payment system based on 467 diagnosis-related groups (DRGs), each of which was assigned a reimbursement level reflecting its average cost. Each patient admitted to the hospital was assigned to a DRG, and the hospital was paid the set amount established for that group. Simultaneously, to prevent overutilization of hospitals, review organizations called "Professional Review Organizations" were established throughout the country to determine the appropriateness of each hospitalization. Since hospitals were now penalized by long hospital stays and patients were precluded from more frequent hospitalizations, there were major reductions in expenditures for hospital care. In 1990, expenditures for hospital care were estimated to be $18 billion less than expected as a result of this change.[17] Of importance is the adoption of the DRG system by many other health-care insurance plans.

These changes in Medicare's hospital payment system have had a significant effect on hospitalization for diabetes care.[40] The major effect has been to shift patient care from the inpatient setting to the outpatient setting, especially for patients with less-intensive health-care needs. Hospital admissions for initiation or adjustment of insulin regimens and for comprehensive diabetes education have decreased significantly. At Joslin Diabetes Center, outpatient visits have increased steadily each year, while inpatient admissions to the Diabetes Treatment Unit have fallen. Admissions to hospitals for diabetic complications and other more-acute needs initially de-

creased under the DRG system, then stabilized, and began to move upward in parallel with the increasing prevalence of diabetes.

Medicare Part B pays for physician services on a fee-for-service basis. Traditionally, payment levels for individual services have been set according to the usual customary and reasonable charges of physicians in each region. During the 1980s, there was a growing concern that these payment levels had become distorted, overpaying for many surgical services and procedures and underpaying for so-called cognitive services. In 1992, Medicare implemented a new system of payment that was based on a resource-based relative value system (RB-RVS) developed by Hsiao et al.[41] Under this system, each service is assigned a relative value that relates to the amount of effort and cost required to deliver the service. The impact of this change on the availability of various services needed by people with diabetes is likely to be mixed, although it is hoped that the RB-RVS will attract more physicians to the specialties of endocrinology and diabetology and will encourage the office consultations that persons with diabetes use so heavily.

Medicaid

Medicaid, another important government program, is designed to provide health-care coverage for the indigent of all ages.[38] Medicare and Medicaid were created by the same federal legislation in 1965, and HCFA oversees both. Unlike Medicare, however, Medicaid is jointly funded by the federal and state governments and administered by 53 individual states and territories. Although a state must follow broad federal guidelines to be eligible for federal funds, each jurisdiction establishes its own rules for determining who is eligible for benefits, what services are covered, and what payment levels and methods are used. Because of funding constraints, some services required by people with diabetes may not be covered. In view of the higher prevalence of diabetes in minority groups, Medicaid's inadequacies have special effects on diabetes care.

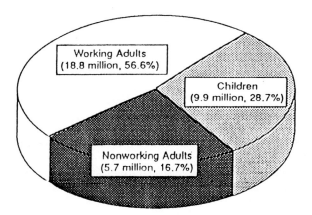

Fig. 34–3. Civilian population under age 65 without health insurance, by own work status, 1989. Data are from Foley.[71]

Private Health Insurance

In addition to government programs such as Medicare and Medicaid, as many as 700 private insurance companies provide health insurance throughout the United States. Traditional private health insurance is purchased by an individual or his or her employer to cover services described by a contract between the insurance company and the individual who is covered.[38] Because of the abundance of private health insurance plans in the United States, this is the most variable form of health insurance. Private insurance can be divided into two categories: Blue Cross/Blue Shield plans and commercial insurance programs.

Collectively, the largest private insurers are the Blue Cross and Blue Shield plans. These plans grew out of health-care trust funds established by hospitals in the 1930s to ensure that their patients could purchase health-care insurance that would enable them to afford care. These funds were later authorized by state legislation that charged them with responsibility to provide broad coverage and offered the protection of tax exemption. The Blues are fundamentally local insurance companies, but they are rather loosely linked into a national confederation. Blue Cross provides insurance for hospital care, and Blue Shield covers physician services. The commercial health-insurance companies differ from the Blues, in that they are for-profit companies that design and sell health-insurance policies, generally without the legal requirement for providing broad coverage to the community. Over the years, extensive competition between the Blues and the commercial insurers has diluted the public-welfare mission of the Blues, such that the distinction between them has become increasingly blurred.

The policies available from each private insurance company are different, ranging from very comprehensive policies covering almost any health-care service to very restrictive policies covering only a limited range of services. The prices of private insurance vary widely, depending on the extent of services covered and the health risks of the individuals permitted to purchase each plan. An important feature of traditional forms of private insurance is that the patient chooses the physician, hospital, or other provider and the insurance company pays for the services it has agreed to cover on a fee-for-service basis. Of particular importance to individuals with diabetes, premium payments may be significantly increased for the person who has an underlying health condition, and many private insurance policies may either delay or exclude coverage for persons with certain conditions preexisting before purchase of insurance.[8] It is important for people with diabetes to understand their own health-insurance policies and to choose insurance that will pay for the services they need. Several articles have been published that provide guidance for the patient with diabetes looking for health insurance.[42,43]

Alternative Delivery Systems

Alternative delivery systems refer to a variety health-care programs in which the providers work in some arrangement other than the traditional fee-for-service mode. By far the most rapidly growing health-care payment systems in the United States are the prepaid-care programs. In their classical form, they are called health maintenance organizations (HMOs). In an HMO, the patient pays a set monthly price for health-care services and the HMO provides the services, determining which physicians, hospitals, or other providers will render the services. Sometimes the HMO pays a set amount, called a capitated payment, to the provider, who is then responsible for rendering a broad range of services. In other instances, the HMO pays the provider a discounted fee, withholding a percentage, and pays the provider a portion of the withheld amount at the end of the year if there has been a cost savings. These mechanisms place the provider "at risk" and are intended to create an incentive for the provider to reduce the unnecessary use of services and to maintain the good health of patients through the use of good preventive medicine practices. HMOs endeavor to control the costs of health care by selecting efficient, effective, low-cost providers of care. In group- or staff-model HMOs, groups of salaried physicians provide the care. A common form of HMO is the independent practice association (IPA), in which independently practicing physicians in a community contract with the HMO to provide care. It is common for HMOs to assign each patient to a primary care physician, referred to as a "gatekeeper," who is the point of first contact for care, referring patients only when special needs arise. For the individual with diabetes, HMOs generally are capable of providing excellent care,[44,45] but there are several potential pitfalls. It is important to evaluate whether the specific specialty physicians, hospitals, and other services needed for competent diabetes care are available and used appropriately by the HMO. Like many other forms of health-care coverage, some HMOs offer only limited diabetes-specific and preventive services and may restrict their patients' access to specialty referrals. Like all health-insurance companies, HMOs are most profitable when their clients are healthy, so patients with preexisting conditions such as diabetes are sometimes excluded from coverage.

Employer-Based Health-Care Coverage

While many Americans buy their own health insurance or are eligible for various government-sponsored programs such as Medicare or Medicaid, the Employee Benefit Research Institute has reported that 66% of Americans receive employer-sponsored health care as an employment benefit. Employers utilize many kinds of insurance programs to provide health-care coverage for their employees. Some of them purchase group plans from private insurance companies, including Blue Cross and Blue Shield. Others purchase HMO coverage for their employees, and a few even have their own health-care arrangements with providers. Many employers offer a range of options to their employees, and the employer and employees generally share in the costs of the insurance. The proportion of an employee's health care that is paid by the employer varies widely and has tended to increase as the costs of health care have increased. Many small employers provide no health insurance at all. In general, because employers can purchase group health insurance for their employees, the risk is spread across a larger population and the premiums are lower than if the individual purchases insurance on his or her own. This is a special advantage for people with diabetes, whose individual insurance premiums might otherwise be very high. However, a special problem arises for employees with diabetes who leave their jobs, since a new employer's health insurance may regard the diabetes as a preexisting condition. With the Consolidated Omnibus Budget Reconciliation Act of 1986, also known as COBRA, the federal government required larger employers to continue to offer the same group-rate health insurance coverage to former employees and their families for a period of up to 3 years, although the responsibility for paying the entire premium shifted to the former employee. The problem arises when an individual with diabetes seeks new health-care insurance thereafter. They then not only must deal with higher premiums because of their diabetes but are required by many insurance programs to forego coverage for diabetes-related needs for some interval because diabetes is a preexisting condition. One important effect of these rules and programs is that people with diabetes are more tightly locked into their jobs than is the general population.

Cost-Containment Methods

All health-insurance plans attempt to reduce unnecessary use of health-care services among the people holding policies. As a means of accomplishing this, the plan may simply not cover some necessary services or decline to provide some forms of specialty care. Many insurance plans require the individual to pay deductibles and co-payments. Deductibles are amounts the patient must pay for services before the insurance provides payment. For example, a plan may cover all services over $500 in a given year, with the patient paying the first $500. Co-payments are payments the patient must make for a given service covered by the insurance company. For instance, the patient may be required to make a small payment for each visit to a physician. These co-payments are referred to as point-of-service payments.

Another currently popular concept in health-care payment is managed care, which is defined by Slee and Slee[46] as an arrangement by which an authority interposed between the patient and physician can place restraints on how and from whom the patient may obtain medical and health services. Managed care is a technique for controlling costs by directing care, not a specific payment mechanism or form of insurance. This system is used in some form by virtually every organization that pays for health care and contrasts with a system in which the patient may select any providers of services that he or she wishes and use them anytime. In such managed care, various techniques are commonly used to control costs and to identify the most appropriate care for each patient, including the use of gatekeepers to control specialty

referrals, a requirement for second opinions before elective surgery, the placement of restrictions on hospitalization, and arrangements that permit the performance of very expensive procedures such as transplants in only selected institutions. These techniques are used in some form by nearly every payer and are thus widespread. More recently, managed-care firms have emerged to provide these services to employers, smaller insurance companies, and other payers who do not operate their own managed-care organizations. For the individual with diabetes, the specific managed-care policies applied by each insurance company, HMO, government program, or employer are of major significance in determining what economic barriers are interposed between the patient and required services.

An additional factor in health-insurance coverage for people with diabetes involves how insurance companies calculate the premiums paid. Premiums may be "community rated" or "experience rated." Under the community-rating mechanism, the premium is calculated for all insured individuals in the community, regardless of individual health risk. This spreads the economic risk across the entire community, tending to protect the higher-risk individuals from higher premium payments. Experience rating, on the other hand, calculates the insurance premium separately for each group of individuals. Under experience rating, employers who have a disproportionate number of higher-risk employees will find their insurance premiums are higher than those of other employers. Many insurance companies like to use experience rating, since it permits them to target lower-risk segments of the population, leaving the higher-risk individuals for somebody else to insure. For people with diabetes, whose health-care expenditures are relatively high, experience rating has several adverse effects. Their employers are placed at a disadvantage, and it is almost certain that this factor leads to some of the employment discrimination to which people with diabetes are subjected.[3] In addition, small employers are especially at risk in an experience-rated system, and many small employers elect not to provide any health insurance at all. In the United States there are at least 34 million people without health insurance, of whom 57% are employed, 17% are nonworking adults, and 28% are children. It is interesting that among people with diabetes, the proportion without health insurance is about the same as that of the general population.[9] Individuals with diabetes who have no insurance tend to be younger, members of minority groups, in good health, and to reside outside metropolitan areas.

In some states, risk pools have been established to assist individuals who cannot obtain affordable health insurance because of the existence of a condition such as diabetes that increases the risk. In 1991, 22 states had established such pools.[42] While the individual state programs differ, they all follow the general concept that the insurance companies in the state form an association to offer health insurance to individuals regardless of their health status, thereby spreading the risk by creating a kind of group plan for high-risk people. Co-payments, deductibles, waiting periods for coverage of preexisting conditions, and other mechanisms to control costs are commonly used in these risk pools. The premiums are often quite high, and many states require that they be capped—usually at 150% of standard individual premiums in the state.

Implications of Reimbursement on Diabetes Care

Health-care reimbursement systems have a wide variety of potential implications for people with diabetes. The most obvious of them result from the payment policies of the particular reimbursement system in relation to the needs of persons with diabetes. The American Diabetes Association has established standards of care for people with diabetes[47,48] that describe the best professional consensus concerning what constitutes the acceptable quality of care for people with diabetes. Ideally, a reimbursement system should provide payment for the services necessary to meet these standards. In actual practice, however, cost constraints and the cost-containment tactics outlined above have restricted coverage of many necessary forms of care for people with diabetes. Table 34–8 provides a compilation of the some of the services, equipment, and supplies that are essential to the provision of care meeting the standards of the American Diabetes Association. Since there is great variability among reimbursement mechanisms, health professionals must counsel their patients with diabetes to shop carefully for their health insurance.

There have been a few studies of the impact of various reimbursement mechanisms on the quality of care provided to individuals with diabetes. In a chart-review study of elderly Medicare patients with diabetes, patients in HMOs and patients in a fee-for-service system were judged to be receiving comparable care.[45] Songer et al. compared mortality rates among patients with insulin-dependent diabetes (IDDM) in Allegheny County with those in Finland.[34] The mortality rate in the United States group was higher, and it was suggested that this might be due to the greater health-system barriers that exist in the United States.

Life Insurance

Improvements in the life expectancy of people with diabetes have made life insurance more available to them,
although they may be required to pay higher premiums. Life-insurance companies use data from the medical literature to guide them concerning what factors constitute risks for people with diabetes, then examine their own data to determine mortality and calculate premiums for individuals in various risk groups.[49] The data are always retrospective and often based on outdated studies, so for a disease for which mortality is improving, such as diabetes, premiums tend to be higher than actual future experience would justify. An example of the kind of mortality data upon which such calculations are based is presented in Table 34–9, which depicts mortality ratios for groups of individuals insured between 1955 and 1959 and followed through 1974. From these kinds of data, standard tables can be developed to guide the establishment of premiums. Table 34–10 shows a typical rating table, in which the basic rating is the percent increase in recommended premiums over and above standard premiums for healthy individuals. For instance, an individual with IDDM in the 36- to 45-year age group would have a basic rating of +125 and pay a life-insurance premium 225% of the standard premium. Tables such as this are available to outline the ratings for a wide range of variables that life-insurance companies use to determine premiums for people with diabetes. Life-insurance companies commonly require the following kinds of information to determine the premiums for people with diabetes: 1) present age and age at onset of diabetes; 2) method of control; 3) adequacy of control; 4) history of diabetic coma or hypoglycemic episodes; 5) frequency of medical supervision; 6) complications.

Life-insurance companies also take into account whether the individual has gestational diabetes or mild abnormalities of glucose tolerance tests. Although the methods life-insurance companies use to calculate the ratings vary considerably, the resulting ratings established by the companies for each class of individuals with diabetes are often quite similar. Some companies are unwilling to provide life insurance for individuals in the higher risk categories. Like health insurance, group life insurance—such as that available through employment—is often less expensive than individually purchased life insurance for people with diabetes.

Table 34–8. Coverage of Services, Equipment, and Supplies for Diabetes Care

	Medicare	Medicaid	Blue Cross/ Blue Shield	Commercial Insurance
Outpatient visits to physician	Yes	Yes	Most	Most
Annual eye examination	Yes	Yes	Most	Some
Treatment of retinopathy	Yes	Yes	Yes	Most
Routine foot care	Yes	A few	Most	Some
Outpatient education	Yes	A few	A few	Some
Self-monitoring of glucose	Yes	A few	Most	Most
Insulin and supplies	No	Most	A few	Yes
Prescription drugs	No	Yes	A few	Yes
Insulin pumps	No	A few	A few	Most
Therapeutic shoes	No	A few	A few	A few

Data are from Bransome.[22]

Table 34–9. Mortality Ratios of Individuals with Diabetes by Type of Treatment

	Actual Deaths*	Expected Deaths†	Mortality Ratio
Males			
Diet	125	119	105
Oral drugs	60	40	151
Insulin	85	47	183
Females			
Diet	200	151	133
Oral drugs	56	49	117
Insulin	117	71	165

Adapted from the Birmingham Actuarial Society's Continuing Investigation into the Mortality of Diabetics, 1974.[72]
*Deaths among 3673 males and 2237 females identified with diabetes in 1955–1959 and followed up in 1964, rounded off to the nearest whole number.
†Deaths in the general population insured in 1955–1959 and followed up in 1974, rounded off to the nearest whole number.

SOCIAL ISSUES IN DIABETES

Despite enormous strides in our knowledge of diabetes and its management, people with diabetes continue to face an endless array of day-to-day issues that affect nearly every aspect of their lives. For instance, each child with diabetes must deal with special challenges in the school setting, where he or she may be the only person receiving insulin, requiring a special diet, and possibly having insulin reactions. Teachers and school nurses are understandably insecure and fearful, and the children themselves can feel very different from their peers. Leisure activities, too, are affected by diabetes. Should children with diabetes be permitted on overnight outings with their friends? What about activities like driving a car, scuba diving, mountain climbing, and going to summer camp? People with diabetes face questions about future employment, wondering what kinds of jobs they should avoid and what types of employment are available to them, knowing that they will have to contend with employment discrimination. Travel raises issues relating not only to the management of the diabetes itself during travel but also to transport of medications and supplies, finding physicians far from home, and adjusting to unaccustomed diets.

The decision about how to advise patients with diabetes concerning employment and participation in various leisure activities that involve some degree of risk is a serious responsibility of health professionals. The health professional not only has an obligation to advise the patient wisely but also has a responsibility to protect society. When obvious disabilities, such as visual impairment, amputations, end-stage renal failure, and severe diabetic neuropathy are present, the health professional can evaluate the risks and give advice with relative confidence. The health professional must understand not only the patient's health status but also the nature of the activity that the patient is seeking to participate in. When the risks of activities derive from the possibility of the patient's having a hypoglycemic episode, however, the circumstance can be considerably more difficult to judge.

Current standards of care for people with diabetes call for tighter control of blood sugar levels. Innovations in self-monitoring of blood glucose and improvements in insulin-delivery systems now permit tighter glycemic control—but at the price of effecting some increase in the frequency of hypoglycemia. Early information from the Diabetes Control and Complications Trial indicated that the frequency of severe hypoglycemic reactions was increased threefold among the groups with tight control of glucose levels.[50] While severe hypoglycemia presents a clear risk, there is evidence that even modest reductions in plasma glucose levels may also be associated with alterations in reaction times and in neuropsychological skills.[51,52] An additional complexity is presented by the occasional patient who manifests hypoglycemic unresponsiveness, in which the usual early hypoglycemic warning symptoms resulting from the secretion of counter-regulatory hormones are not experienced before neuroglycopenic manifestations develop.

Patients who are prone to hypoglycemic episodes can usually be identified by the health professional. Such individuals can be counseled to avoid risky activities or to maintain their blood glucose level a bit higher than usual when they prepare to undertake such activities. Self-monitoring of blood glucose levels before undertaking certain activities can afford significant protection. Some individuals whose occupations are intrinsically risky might even elect to maintain less stringent glycemic control over longer periods, although this choice must be balanced against the increased health risks incurred. In the sections that follow, we discuss many of these issues of life-style, occupation, and social life.

School

Children attending school must balance the medical need to maintain good glycemic control, the developmental need not to be unnecessarily restricted from normal activities, and the social desire not to be regarded as "different." At the beginning of the school year, the parents should meet with the child's teacher and school nurse to discuss the child's needs, including the requirement for snacks and timely meals, and any restrictions on physical activity and its timing. The school nurse should instruct the teacher about the management of insulin reactions, and the child must be made comfortable in

Table 34–10. Life Insurance Rating Table for Individuals with Diabetes

Age at Application (yr)	Basic Rating	
	IDDM	NIDDM
Under 16	+350	+250
16–25	+200	+150
26–35	+150	+100
36–45	+125	+ 50
46–54	+100	Standard
55 and older	+ 50	Standard

Data are from Brackenridge.[49] IDDM = insulin-dependent diabetes; NIDDM = non-insulin-dependent diabetes.

notifying the teacher when he or she has special needs during the school day. The teacher should be careful not to be overprotective and to avoid making obvious special allowances for the child.

Boarding-school circumstances impose additional challenges. Colleges do not place admission restrictions on students with diabetes, expecting that students of college age will be proficient in the techniques of self-care. However, younger students may require more support, and some secondary boarding schools may not be prepared to deal with diabetes. Parents of college and secondary boarding-school students should consider the individual student's degree of self-reliance and investigate the health-care support available at the school. The social pressures and irregular schedule of a boarding school or college environment place considerable responsibility in the hands of the student, and these years are frequently a time of major personal growth for adolescents with diabetes. There must be clear understanding on the part of the school health officials about the student's medical condition and diabetic regimen, with assurance that these needs will be met. In addition, any roommates must be aware of the student's diabetes and should be instructed on how to help with insulin reactions.

Marriage

Most young people with diabetes and their parents worry about how diabetes will affect their ability to marry and have families. In general, for the person with diabetes, there are significant benefits to having a partner in life who is understanding, supportive, and knowledgeable about diabetes. However, marriage in the face of diabetes does pose special problems, and the spouse should be as well-informed as the partner with diabetes about the disease, its management, and implications. The couple must candidly discuss and understand several important matters before marriage.

1) Diabetes is associated with long-term complications that sometimes, but not always, cause disability or premature death. Among the complications are an increased frequency of impotence in males.

2) Women with diabetes face increased risk in pregnancy and childbearing. Although the current outcomes of diabetic pregnancies are excellent, diabetic control before and during pregnancy requires special attention, and the genetic implications of diabetes must be understood. Adoption or artificial insemination are possibilities if the genetic consequences seem overwhelming to the couple.

3) Employment, health-care insurance, and life insurance may present special financial challenges for both partners in a marriage including a partner with diabetes.

4) The nondiabetic spouse must become fully educated about diabetes and its management and must be willing to provide the necessary support.

For most people with diabetes, once having openly considered these issues and having made the necessary decisions relating to them, there is no reason why they cannot marry and have families. In fact, Dr. Elliott P. Joslin wrote many years ago that "It is a great advantage for a diabetic to be married because of the intimate protection and care thereby attained." In advising those who are considering marriage in the face of diabetes, the happiness of the two partners will always outweigh any other factors. It is the responsibility of those providing advice to offer factual information in a supportive manner that encourages the clear understanding the couple needs to make good decisions.

Smoking

There is an increasing trend toward less use of tobacco products, especially in the United States. The health-care industry has taken a strong and effective stand against smoking. Increasingly, public gathering places and places of work are banning smoking, as national attention is paid to both the personal risks of smoking and the added risks of secondary smoke inhalation. Nationally, it is recognized that tobacco use is associated with increases in the incidence of cancer, chronic pulmonary disease, cardiovascular disease, and even motor-vehicle accidents. As important as it is for the general population to avoid tobacco, it is even more so for individuals with diabetes. The increase in risk of cardiovascular diseases makes smoking especially dangerous for persons with diabetes. The vasoconstrictive effects of tobacco, especially on smaller blood vessels, impose the risk of impeding the already endangered peripheral circulation in patients with diabetes. Simply stated, people with diabetes should not smoke.

Alcohol

In the early years of the Joslin Clinic, Dr. Joslin took a notoriously firm stand against alcohol use by individuals with diabetes. Not only did he admonish his patients about this, but there are sad memories among the more senior members of the Joslin staff of Dr. Joslin intercepting holiday presents of liquor and wine from thankful patients and dramatically pouring them down the nearest sink. In recent years the use of alcoholic beverages in the United States has decreased significantly in parallel with the greater attention to the adoption of healthier lifestyles, the recognition of the major risk of motor-vehicle accidents related to alcohol, and a broad public awareness of the ravages of alcoholism. Nevertheless, the use of alcohol continues to be a widespread social and business custom to which nearly everybody is exposed at some time.

Today, there is a trend toward slightly greater flexibility in our advice to people with diabetes about alcohol consumption, although special care and great moderation are still strongly recommended. Alcohol affects the control of diabetes in several important ways. It is a source of calories and can elevate the blood sugar level. It impairs gluconeogenesis by the liver and can thereby blunt the response to hypoglycemia. This latter effect can set up a circumstance in which oral hypoglycemic agents can cause hypoglycemia—a particular risk with the longer-acting sulfonylureas. As a central nervous system depressant, alcohol can impair the recognition of the symptoms of hypoglycemia and can lead to a reduction in the self-control necessary to avoid the dietary indiscretions often associated with the situations in which alcohol is used. Alcoholic neuropathy can provide an added risk in diabetes, particularly when superimposed on diabetic neuropathy and impaired peripheral circulation.

Most physicians now permit their patients to consume modest amounts of alcohol if they desire, and diabetic exchange lists have been developed to reflect the dietary impacts of various alcoholic beverages. In general, 1 g of alcohol supplies 7 calories. Beer, wine, and mixed drinks include components that provide additional calories as well. For this reason, hard liquor is a less-complex form of alcohol to consume and less variable in caloric content. Some details about the management of alcohol use in diabetes are presented in Chapter 24.

Alcohol use and driving is a most dangerous mix for anyone, but the risk is increased for the individual with diabetes. The symptoms of hypoglycemia often mimic the symptoms of alcohol intoxication. Many law enforcement officers are not familiar with the symptoms of hypoglycemia, and there are numerous instances of patients with diabetes being mistakenly arrested for driving under the influence of alcohol when they are actually experiencing an insulin reaction. It is not uncommon for a patient with diabetes to attend a party, consume a modest amount of alcohol, delay eating, and then experience an insulin reaction while driving home. It requires a very broad-minded police officer to accept the explanation that a patient with alcohol on his breath who exhibits symptoms of intoxication is having an insulin reaction. In addition to taking care to avoid such circumstances, the person with diabetes should be advised to carry some form of clear identification of his or her diabetes status.

Driving

Driving a motor vehicle has become a necessity of modern life for many people and a rite of passage for many teenagers. Every state in the nation permits individuals with diabetes to hold licenses for driving noncommercial motor vehicles, although the requirements vary considerably from state to state and some states require medical certification. More stringent limitations are placed on commercial vehicle licenses for individuals with diabetes who require insulin, as noted later in this chapter.

Concerns about the safety of operating a motor vehicle arise when there are severe complications of the diabetes or when insulin therapy imposes a risk of hypoglycemia.[53] A number of studies have attempted to ascertain the risk among insulin-taking individuals.[54-62] From a selection of these studies (Table 34–11), the results can be seen to be highly variable. Drivers with diabetes have been reported to have both increased and decreased rates of traffic violations and accidents. The traffic violation rates reported range from a 44% increase to a 24% decrease in drivers with diabetes, and the accident rates, from a 78% increase to a 35% decrease. One defect of

Table 34–11. Summary of Studies of Driving Experience of Drivers with Diabetes

Study	No. of Diabetics	Ratio of Diabetics to Controls	
		Traffic Violations	Accidents
Ysander[54]	256	0.76	0.65
Waller[55]	257	1.39	1.78
Davis et al.[56]	108	1.44	1.04
Crancer and McMurray[57]	7646	0.90	1.14
Hansotia and Broste[59]	484	1.14	1.32
Stevens et al.[60]	354	...	1.09

many of these studies is that they include both individuals with insulin-dependent diabetes (IDDM) and those with non-insulin-dependent diabetes (NIDDM) and another is that they do not take into account the effects of age. The risk of hypoglycemia among persons with NIDDM should be low, which should decrease risk, but they are older than the general population used as controls in some studies, which may increase the risk in this group. Two studies not included in Table 34–11 have focused on drivers who take insulin. Frier et al. noted that 13% of drivers taking insulin had experienced accidents, but this study did not include a control group.[61] Only 5.2% of the accidents among these persons with IDDM were due to hypoglycemia. Songer examined the driving experiences of 158 sibling pairs with and without diabetes.[62] There were more accidents among the siblings with diabetes, but the difference was not statistically significant. One intriguing finding of the sibling study was that of an unexplained significant increase in accidents among young, unmarried women with diabetes. A significant number of individuals with diabetes voluntarily elect not to drive because of visual and other disabilities.

When counseling an individual with IDDM about operating a motor vehicle, one must take into account the frequency, timing, and predictability of hypoglycemic episodes. Those who are unreliable in self-monitoring blood glucose or who are otherwise incapable of predicting, detecting, and avoiding hypoglycemia should be advised not to operate motor vehicles. However, by monitoring blood glucose levels appropriately and taking proper action in assuring that levels do not fall to hypoglycemic levels during driving, most individuals who require insulin can operate motor vehicles safely.

Travel

Almost everybody travels for pleasure or business. Modern travel often involves traveling during mealtimes, crossing time zones, waiting in unfamiliar places, and passing through foreign customs. For the patient whose diabetes does not require insulin, shifting the timing of medications and meals is a relatively simple matter, since hypoglycemia is not a major concern. There is little reason why most individuals with diabetes, even those with IDDM, cannot—with careful planning—manage extensive travel. The individual with IDDM should be advised about several issues when preparing to travel:

1) The patient and his or her physician should carefully review the travel plans and adjust the timing of meals and insulin dosages accordingly. How this is done will depend on the individual regimen, as outlined in Chapter 27.

2) The patient should be supplied with a note from the physician outlining the diagnosis, listing the generic and proprietary names of medications, giving the physician's name and telephone number, and listing physicians at the destination who can be consulted in an emergency. Most foreign countries have diabetes associations that can assist international visitors.

3) The patient should carry adequate supplies of medications and materials to treat hypoglycemia. These should never be checked in baggage that is inaccessible or that might reach a different destination. On some trips, it may be advisable to carry extra prescriptions for insulin, syringes, and other essential supplies in case of loss or theft.

4) The patient should conduct frequent glucose monitoring throughout the trip, especially when the travel involves changes in time zones and meal schedules.

5) The patient should take special precautions to avoid motion sickness or travelers' diarrhea, both of which may contribute to hypoglycemia, dehydration, or ketoacidosis, and must be especially careful to have the proper immunizations when traveling abroad.

Employment and Diabetes

Both patients and employers must deal with challenging issues relating to the employability of individuals with diabetes, including issues of job safety, absenteeism, health and disability insurance costs, and employment discrimination. There is a considerable body of data about the employment experience of workers who have diabetes and an extensive and constantly evolving body of federal and state law relating to employment discrimination.

For many years, efforts were made to define what occupations could be safely engaged in by people with diabetes. Employment standards for persons with diabetes were first recommended by the American Diabetes Association in 1972 and were intended to guide physicians in advising their patients about what jobs were safe for them.[63] However, in 1982 the Board of Directors of the American Diabetes Association shifted gears and issued this statement about employment policy: "Any diabetic, whether insulin-dependent or non-insulin-dependent, should be able to accept any employment for which he or she is individually qualified." The significance of this policy is that it calls for individualization of the decision about employment. It does not state that all people with diabetes should be eligible for all jobs but

rather that each person's qualifications should be evaluated individually, taking into account the nature of the job and the patient's ability to perform it safely and effectively.

In most industries few formal restrictions have been placed on the employment of people with well-controlled diabetes. Nevertheless, employment discrimination and job refusal have been documented for workers with diabetes. Songer et al. studied the employment experiences of 158 sibling pairs, one with IDDM and the other without diabetes.[3] The siblings with IDDM were significantly more likely than those without it to have been refused a job at some point in their lives (56% vs. 42%). Among the siblings with diabetes, those who revealed their diabetes during job interviews were much more likely to report job refusal (64%) than were those who did not mention their diabetes (44%). Job refusal of the siblings with diabetes did not appear to be fully explained by their higher rate of disability, since job refusal was also more likely to have been experienced by the able-bodied siblings with diabetes than among their nondiabetic siblings. Klesges et al. asked 295 business students to rate job applications and videotaped interviews of individuals with diabetes and obesity and interviews of normal controls with comparable qualifications and to recommend whether they should be hired.[4] Applicants with diabetes were less likely than controls to be rated as qualified, although they were rated similarly on personal appearance, attitude, and communication skills. The applicants with diabetes were viewed as having poorer work habits and being more likely to have medically related job absences. Robinson et al. found that 13% of individuals with diabetes in Great Britain had experienced difficulties in obtaining employment because of their diabetes.[5] These data appear to substantiate the existence of rather widespread, yet subtle, employment discrimination against persons with diabetes.

In addition to the safety risks some employers fear in employing people with diabetes, employers are also apprehensive about the productivity and job performance of workers with diabetes. Unemployment is higher among people with diabetes,[6] and much of this is due to medical disability among a subgroup of individuals with diabetes. Although increased frequencies of disability and/or absenteeism have been reported in several studies of employment of workers with diabetes, other studies have actually reported lower absenteeism.[3,61,64] In a study of employment experience among siblings with and without IDDM, Songer et al. found that work disability was significantly more frequent among the siblings with diabetes than among siblings without diabetes (32% vs. 5%).[3] This disability was related primarily to diabetic complications. Among the siblings with diabetes reporting severe disabilities that prevented them from working, the causes cited were kidney disease (55%), blindness (40%), severe retinopathy (20%), heart disease (15%), less severe forms of retinopathy (10%), and amputations (10%). Largely as a result of this higher rate of disability, a lower proportion of the IDDM siblings were participants in the work force (67% vs. 85%). The siblings with IDDM were less likely than their nondiabetic siblings to be employed full-time (55% vs. 73%), and 13% of the diabetic siblings had not worked at all during the preceding year. The 1978 Survey of Work and Disability, which grouped persons with IDDM and NIDDM together, reported a threefold increase in work disability among those with diabetes. Despite these problems, individuals with diabetes do not appear to experience greater problems in the workplace than do individuals without diabetes.[65]

It is not surprising that workers with diabetes have a higher rate of unemployment and disability than workers without diabetes, in view of the well-known complications of diabetes. A number of studies have dealt with absenteeism among workers with diabetes.[66-69] In the sibling study,[3] the rate of absenteeism among those siblings with diabetes who were employed was nearly identical to that of their nondiabetic siblings. Other studies have actually reported lower absenteeism rates among employed persons with diabetes, suggesting that some people with diabetes may be especially highly motivated to perform their jobs reliably. Even the studies that have reported higher absenteeism among workers with diabetes strongly suggest that the excess absenteeism is confined to a cluster representing only about 30% of the diabetic population. For instance, studies conducted by the Ford Motor Company and the DuPont Company revealed that over 70% of those with diabetes had entirely satisfactory records of absenteeism related to illness.[66-68] It has been pointed out that in those studies that reported higher absenteeism rates among workers with diabetes, the average age of these workers was higher than that of nondiabetic workers.[69] The consensus of studies suggest that people with diabetes are absent more frequently than persons without diabetes, that this excess is limited primarily to a minority of about 30% of the workers with diabetes, and that the remaining 70% have at least as good work records as the general population.

Several special types of employment controlled largely by government regulations have been of considerable recent interest, including the employment of drivers in interstate commerce, airline pilots, and air traffic controllers. Individuals with IDDM as a group have been excluded from employment in these professions. Commercial drivers with diabetes are permitted to drive vehicles in interstate commerce only if they do not require insulin. Airline pilots and, until recently, air traffic controllers have faced similar restrictions.

As recently as 1977, the American Diabetes Association supported the Federal Highway Administration's policy of not permitting individuals with diabetes who required insulin to drive in interstate commerce. The obvious concern was that drivers would develop hypoglycemia while transporting passengers or dangerous freight. Commercial driving differs from the operation of private motor vehicles in several respects that may be important for individuals with IDDM. Professional drivers spend longer periods behind the wheel as they press to keep schedules, and they may have less choice about when to stop for meals. They are often required to load and unload their vehicles and to make deliveries. Despite these theoretical concerns, there are no good studies on the safety of interstate commercial driving for persons with IDDM, largely because most have been disqualified from driving. While many states do permit intrastate commercial driving among individuals with IDDM, record-keeping is inadequate to determine their accident experience.

Several events caused the American Diabetes Association to request that the Federal Highway Administration reevaluate this policy. The development and widespread use of home glucose monitoring, along with more flexible insulin regimens, has permitted many individuals with diabetes to achieve more precise glucose control and to detect and avoid hypoglycemia more reliably. In many cases it was apparent that drivers were refusing to initiate insulin treatment because of this regulation, and many drivers who were taking insulin were not reporting it to their employers. This situation resulted in the potentially dangerous circumstance of drivers who should not be driving continuing to do so and the absence of standards to assure that they monitor their blood sugar levels carefully while driving. New national legislation prohibiting blanket employment discrimination has stimulated interest in establishing criteria to identify drivers with well-controlled IDDM who might safely be permitted to drive commercially. Regulations are currently being studied by the Federal Highway Administration that would allow drivers with diabetes to seek individual exemptions from the rule preventing them from driving commercially. If a qualified physician certifies that a diabetic individual has been free of severe hypoglycemia and if the person follows strict rules about glucose monitoring and record-keeping while driving and is reexamined and recertified annually, he or she would be granted the right to employment as an interstate commercial driver even if taking insulin for control of diabetes.

Similar issues have arisen concerning air-traffic controllers and airline pilots and crews. In 1990, an air-traffic controller was reported to have had a severe hypoglycemic reaction while on duty, and the Federal Aviation Administration (FAA) immediately took all controllers who were taking insulin off the job. After considerable discussions between the union representing the controllers and the FAA, in 1992 the air-traffic controllers who required insulin were permitted to return to their duties under increased medical supervision.

A somewhat more problematic issue has been whether insulin-dependent airline pilots should be permitted to fly. In this instance, there has been a widespread feeling that the risks of piloting aircraft are greater than those of driving commercial ground vehicles or serving as air-traffic controllers. The existing regulations regarding airline pilots are more restrictive than those applying to the other groups, since even pilots who require oral hypoglycemic agents are not permitted to fly. Earlier editions of this text have referred to a Joslin Clinic series in which early diagnosis and vigorous dietary treatment of pilots resulted in a number of cases in which individuals were able to maintain sufficient control with diet alone to continue to fly for a number of years. The exceptional motivation of some of these individuals to salvage their careers was unquestionably the key to their success. Nevertheless, there is now growing interest in extending the right to continue flying to carefully screened and selected pilots, although there is considerable opposition from the FAA and the airline companies and their insurers.

With regard to flight attendants and other nonoperating members of air crews, each airline has established its own sets of rules. Some have prohibited all individuals with diabetes who require antidiabetic medications from flying, operating on the theory that in the event of an accident these individuals might be unable to function effectively.

Antidiscrimination Laws

The attitudes of society about employment discrimination have advanced in recent decades, and federal laws relating to discrimination have evolved that seek to prevent blanket employment discrimination against groups of individuals. These laws have potential significance for people with diabetes. In 1973, Congress passed the Rehabilitation Act, Public Law 93–112, which went into effect in 1979. This law was designed to prevent discrimination in the employment of handicapped persons in the federal government and in organizations supported by federal funds. This law did not address people with diabetes directly except with regard to the disabilities falling within the general definition of the law, such as amputations or blindness, and those who were federally employed. A more recent law has been passed that will have a broader impact on employment of people with diabetes. Under the newer Rehabilitation Act of 1991—the Americans with Disabilities Act—the provisions of the previous act were expanded to apply to all employers with at least 15 employees and diabetes itself was added as a defined disability. While there was concern about the implications of defining diabetes as a "disability," the possibility of reducing employment discrimination for people with diabetes seemed attractive. This law makes it illegal to discriminate against anyone just because he or she has diabetes, thereby providing a legal basis supporting the policy of the American Diabetes Association on employment of people with diabetes. The full impact of this legislation on employment of people with diabetes will only be apparent after several years. In coming years, considerable activity will be expended to define the conditions under which people with diabetes can safely be employed in specific occupations, and the demand for research into the effect of the new policies will increase.

DIABETES ORGANIZATIONS

Various government and nongovernment organizations have been established throughout the world that serve the needs of both those with diabetes and the professionals who give them care or conduct diabetes research. While all national and local government health departments and many national and international health-care organizations are involved in diabetes in some way, a number of important organizations are specifically dedicated to diabetes. Some are international in scope, others are essentially national, and still others are local. The missions, goals, organizational structures, and services of each organization differ; these often include setting and administering national policy, advocating on behalf of the needs and rights of individuals with diabetes, raising funds for diabetes research, providing publications and other services for people with diabetes, and conducting professional education and scientific seminars.

International Diabetes Federation

With headquarters in Brussels, Belgium, the International Diabetes Federation (IDF) is composed of over 100 member associations in more than 80 countries and includes a total membership of over 950,000 individuals. With a close working relationship with the World Health Organization and in collaboration with its member associations throughout the world, the IDF is engaged in a worldwide effort to ensure the availability of quality care, essential drugs, education, and appropriate modes of treatment for people with diabetes. For instance, the IDF surveyed its member organizations in 1991 and found that some 19 countries reported that diabetes was not incorporated into the national health plan. The IDF has since encouraged universal inclusion of diabetes in these nations' plans. In the event of wars and national emergencies, when distribution of diabetes supplies has been hampered, the IDF has mobilized activities to address the shortages throughout the world. In nations in which inflation and fragile economies have threatened even the most basic diabetes services, the IDF has sought to provide support. Every 3 years, the IDF, under the aegis of one of its member organizations, conducts an international meeting of both professionals and volunteers from around the world. These conventions are the largest diabetes-related meetings in the world.

The IDF periodically publishes a directory of its affiliated organizations. This directory provides considerable information about the state of diabetes in each nation represented, as well as the names and addresses of the affiliated organizations in each country. The address of IDF is Fédération Internationale du Diabète, 40 rue Washington, 1050 Brussels, Belgium (telephone 32–2/647–4414).

American Diabetes Association

The mission of the American Diabetes Association (ADA) is "to prevent and cure diabetes and to improve the lives of all people affected by diabetes." Based in Alexandria, VA, and with 270,000 members (including over 10,000 professional members), the ADA is the largest single volunteer health organization dedicated to diabetes in any nation. Founded primarily as a professional organization, the ADA initially focused on providing forums, conferences, and professional publications to serve the needs of health-care professionals in diabetes. Among its early publications was the journal *Diabetes*, which now has a circulation of over 10,000. Today, the ADA has expanded to become a comprehensive volunteer health organization providing a wide range of services to patients and health-care professionals. It is organized into state affiliates and local chapters in many communities throughout the nation. Its publications include *Diabetes, Diabetes Care, Clinical Diabetes,* and *Diabetes Forecast,* as well as a broad array of patient and professional education materials and cookbooks. Through its Government Relations Committee, the ADA engages in extensive advocacy activities to influence public policy concerning diabetes, continuously monitoring legislation, seeking new legislation, and providing expert testimony before congressional committees. Through its Professional Practice Committee, the ADA has developed standards of care for people with diabetes, defining and describing what constitutes the highest quality of care. The ADA sponsors a major annual conference of professionals and volunteers on the national level, as well as hundreds of courses and meetings at a local level.

Supported by membership fees, sale of publications, philanthropy, and proceeds from professional meetings, the ADA has had a major influence on diabetes in the United States. The address of the ADA is 1660 Duke Street, Alexandria, VA 22314 (telephone 800–232–3472).

Many other countries have national diabetes associations resembling the ADA. The most comprehensive listing is found in the IDF directory mentioned above.

Juvenile Diabetes Foundation

The Juvenile Diabetes Foundation (JDF) was founded in 1970 by a group of parents and friends of children with diabetes who wanted a more aggressive volunteer commitment to finding a cure for diabetes through raising funds for research. At that time, the ADA was primarily a professional organization focusing on the needs of health professionals in diabetes, with a relatively small national organization of volunteers. Over its first 20 years of existence, JDF volunteers raised over $100 million to support diabetes research. Funds are allocated to support individual research projects and fellowships to train diabetes researchers. The preponderant focus of research supported by JDF has traditionally been Type I diabetes, and the stated mission has been to seek a cure for this disease.

The JDF is an international organization. Its world headquarters are at 432 Park Avenue South, New York, NY 10016–8013 (telephone 212–889–7575). Other national JDF offices are located in Chatswood, Australia; Willowdale, Ontario, Canada; London, England; Athens, Greece; Tel Aviv, Israel; São Paulo, Brazil; Santiago, Chile; Paris, France; Calcutta, India; and Rome, Italy.

Joslin Diabetes Center

In 1898, Elliott P. Joslin, M.D., opened a practice of medicine in his family home in the Back Bay section of Boston. More than 23 years later, the discovery of insulin changed diabetes from a largely acute and almost routinely fatal disease to the chronic disease we know today. Dr. Joslin's practice grew into the major group practice of diabetes as he added other physicians to his staff. The discovery of insulin and its first use in New England under the direction of Dr. Joslin and his associate, Dr. Howard Root, propelled the Joslin Clinic to international prominence. In addition to the commitment to patient care, Dr. Joslin and his staff dedicated themselves to expanding the knowledge of diabetes and to teaching clinicians and researchers. Over 600 physicians have been trained at Joslin, and today many of them are caring for patients, conducting research, and providing leadership in diabetes throughout the world.

The Joslin Diabetes Center is located on the Longwood Medical Campus of Boston, in affiliation with the Harvard Medical School, New England Deaconess Hospital, Brigham and Women's Hospital, Boston Children's Hospital, Beth Israel Hospital, and the Massachusetts Eye and Ear Infirmary. The Center includes the Joslin Clinic, a multispecialty group practice of about 50 physicians dedicated to providing comprehensive patient care to meet the full range of needs of patients with diabetes, and the Elliott P. Joslin Research Laboratories, where an extremely wide spectrum of basic and clinical research is conducted under the direction of 40 senior researchers. Additionally, Joslin conducts a summer camp for boys with diabetes and supports a sister camp for girls. By 1992, there were eight Joslin-affiliated diabetes clinics conducted in cooperation with major hospitals and medical groups in Jacksonville, FL; Indianapolis, IN; Livingston, NJ; Pittsburgh, PA; Clearwater, FL; Miami, FL; Charlotte, NC; and Berwyn, IL.

In addition to publishing the Joslin text, the Joslin Diabetes Center publishes a broad range of teaching manuals for professionals and patients and conducts numerous professional and patient education courses and conferences. The Joslin Diabetes Center is located at One Joslin Place, Boston, MA 02215 (telephone 617–732–2400).

REFERENCES

1. Diabetes. 1991 vital statistics. Alexandria, VA: American Diabetes Association, 1991.
2. American Diabetes Association. Direct and indirect costs of diabetes in the United States in 1987. Reston, VA: Center for Economic Studies in Medicine, Pracon, 1988.
3. Songer TJ, LaPorte RE, Dorman JS, et al. Employment spectrum of IDDM. Diabetes Care 1989;12:615–22.
4. Klesges RC, Klem ML, Hanson CL, et al. The effects of applicant's health status and qualifications on simulated hiring decisions. Int J Obesity 1990;14:527–35.
5. Robinson N, Yateman, NA, Protopapa LE, Bush L. Employment problems and diabetes. Diabetic Med 1990;7:16–22.
6. Robinson N, Yateman NA, Protopapa LE, Bush L. Unemployment and diabetes. Diabetic Med 1989;6;797–803.
7. Robinson N, Bush L, Yateman NA, Protopapa LE, Yateman NA. Employers attitudes to diabetes. Diabetic Med 1989; 6:692–7.
8. Frier BM, Sullivan FM, Stewart JC. Diabetes and insurance: a survey of patient experience. In: Living with diabetes. John Wiley and Sons, 1984:127–30.
9. Taylor AK. Medical expenditures and insurance coverage for people with diabetes: estimates from the National Medical Care Expenditure Survey. Diabetes Care 1987; 10:8794.
10. United States Department of Health and Human Services. Wall Street Journal, Oct. 13, 1991.

11. Sullivan LW. Healthy people 2000. N Engl J Med 1990; 323:1065–7.

12. United States House of Representatives, Committee on Appropriations. Report no. 102–121, June 20, 1991, Departments of Labor, Health and and Human Services, Education, and Related Agencies Appropriation Bill, 1992.

13. Peck SB, Musco TD, Jejich C. Diabetes coverage by commercial insurers in the U.S.A. Washington, DC: Health Insurance Association of America, 1986.

14. Bransome ED. Access to coverage: health insurance for people with diabetes. Diabetes Spectrum 1988;1:59–62.

15. Centers for Disease Control. Diabetes surveillance: annual report 1990. Atlanta GA: US Department of Health and Human Services, Centers for Disease Control, April 1990.

16. Jacobs J, Sena M, Fox N. The cost of hospitalization for the late complications of diabetes in the United States. Diabetic Med 1991;8:S23–29.

17. Russell LB, Manning CL. The effect of prospective payment on Medicare expenditures. N Engl J Med 1989; 320:439–44.

18. McKendry JBR. Direct costs of diabetes care: a survey in Ottawa, Ontario 1986. Can J Public Health 1989;80:124–8.

19. Bonham GS, Corder LS. National Healthcare Expenditure Study: instruments and procedures. 1. NMCS household interview instruments. DHHS publication no. PHS 81–3280. Washington, DC: US Government Printing Office, 1981.

20. Cohen SB, Farley PJ. National Healthcare Expenditure Study: instruments and procedures. 3. Estimation and procedures in the NMCS insurance surveys. DHHS publication no. PHS 84–3369. Washington, DC: US Government Printing Office, 1984.

21. Huse DM, Oster G, Killen AR, et al. The economic costs of non-insulin-dependent diabetes mellitus. JAMA 1989; 262:2708–13.

22. Bransome ED Jr. Financing the care of diabetes mellitus in the U.S.: Background, problems and challenges. Diabetes Care 1992;15(Suppl 1):1–5.

23. Entmacher PS, Sinnock P, Bostic E, Harris MI. Economic impact of diabetes. In: National Diabetes Data Group. Diabetes in America: diabetes data compiled 1984. Washington, DC: US Department of Health and Human Services, August 1985:XXXII-1–XXXII-13.

24. Rice DP, Hodgson TA, Kopstein AN. The economic costs of illness: a replication and update. Health Care Financing Rev 1985;7(1):61–80.

25. Centers for Disease Control. Economic cost of diabetes mellitus—Minnesota, 1988. MMWR 1991;40:229–31.

26. Leichter SB, Hernandex C, Fisher A, et al. Diabetes in Kentucky. Diabetes Care 1982;5:126–34.

27. Triomphe A. The socio-economic cost of diabetic complications in France. Diabetic Med 1991;8:S30–2.

28. Triomphe A, Flori YA, Costagliola D, Eschwege E. The cost of diabetes in France. Health Policy 1988;9:39–48.

29. Alexander WD. Diabetes care in a U.K. health region: acitivity, facilities and costs. Diabetic Med 1988;5:577–81.

30. Gerard K, Donaldson C, Maynard AK. The cost of diabetes. Diabetic Med 1989;6:164–70.

31. Jönsson B. Diabetes—the cost of illness and the cost of control: an estimate for Sweden 1978. Acta Medica Scand Suppl 1983;671:19–27.

32. Helms RB. Implications of population growth on prevalence of diabetes: look at the future. Diabetes Care 1992; 15(Suppl 1):6–9.

33. Prashker MJ, Meenan RF. Subspecialty training: is it financially worthwhile? Ann Intern Med 1991;115:715–9.

34. Songer TJ, DeBerry K, LaPorte RE, Tuomilehto J. International comparisons of IDDM mortality: clues to prevention and the role of diabetes care. Diabetes Care 1992;15(Suppl 1):15–21.

35. Office of National Cost Estimates, Office of Actuary. National Health expenditures, 1988. Health Care Financing Rev 1990;2(4).

36. Challenges and opportunities: issues facing the U.S. health care system: special report. Washington, DC: Employee Benefits and Research Institute, September 1991.

37. Source book of health insurance data. Washington, DC: Health Insurance Association of America, 1990.

38. Fein R. Medical care, medical costs: the search for a health insurance policy. Cambridge, MA: Harvard University Press, 1989.

39. Jewler D. A primer on Medicare for people with diabetes. Diabetes Forecast 1987;Sept:17–20.

40. Bransome ED Jr. Assessment of impact of Medicare prospective payment system of care of persons with diabetes mellitus. Diabetes Care 1986;9:415–9.

41. Hsiao WC, Braun P, Dunn D, et al. Results and policy implications of the resource-based relative-value study. N Engl J Med 1988;319:8818.

42. Horseman RE. Insiders guide to health insurance. Diabetes Self-Management 1991;Jan/Feb:1991:6–13.

43. Your insurance benefits checklist. Diabetes Forecast 1987; Oct:55–61.

44. Geffner DL. Diabetes care in health maintenance organizations. Diabetes Care 1992;15(Suppl 1):44–50.

45. Retchin SM, Preston J. Effects of cost containment on the care of elderly diabetics. Arch Intern Med 1991; 151:2244–8.

46. Slee VN, Slee DA. Health care terms. 2nd ed. St Paul, MN: Tringa Press, 1991.

47. American Diabetes Association. Clinical practice recommendations, 1991–1992. Diabetes Care 1992;15(Suppl 2):1–80.

48. Clark CM Jr, Kinney ED. Standards for the care of diabetes: origins, uses and implications for third-party payment. Diabetes Care 1992;15(Suppl 1):10–4.

49. Brackenridge RDC. Medical selection of life risks. 2nd ed. New York: The Nature Press, 1985.

50. The DCCT Research Group. Diabetes control and complications trial (DCCT): results of feasibility study. Diabetes Care 1987;10:1–19.

51. Harrad RA, Cockram CS, Plumb AP, et al. The effect of hypoglycaemia on visual function: a clinical and electrophysiological study. Clin Sci 1985;69:673–9.

52. Herold KC, Polonsky KS, Cohen RM, et al. Variable deterioration in cortical function during insulin-induced hypoglycemia. Diabetes 1985;34:677–85.

53. Ratner RE, Whitehouse FW. Motor vehicles, hypoglycemia and diabetic drivers. Diabetes Care 1989;12:217–22.

54. Ysander L. Sick and handicapped drivers. Acta Chir Scand Suppl 1970;409:1–82.

55. Waller JA. Chronic medical conditions and traffic safety: review of the California experience. N Engl J Med 1965; 273:1413–20.

56. Davis TG. Wehling EH, Carpenter RL. Oklahoma's medically restricted drivers: a study of selected medical conditions. J Okla State Med Assoc 1973;66:322–7.

57. Crancer A Jr, McMurray L. Accident and violation rates of Washington's medically restricted drivers. JAMA 1968; 205:272–6.

58. Eadington DW, Frier BM. Type I diabetes and driving experience: an eight-year cohort study. Diabetic Med 1989;6:137–41.

59. Hansotia P, Broste SK. The effect of epilepsy or diabetes mellitus on the risk of automobile accidents. N Engl J Med 1991;324:22–6.

60. Stevens AB, Roberts M, McKane R, et al. Motor vehicle driving among diabetics taking insulin and non-diabetics. BMJ 1989;299:591–5.

61. Frier BM, Matthews DM, Steel JM, Duncan LJP. Driving and insulin-dependent diabetes. Lancet 1980;1:1232–4.

62. Songer TJ, LaPort RE, Dorman JS, et al. Motor vehicle accidents and IDDM. Diabetes Care 1988;11:701–7.

63. American Diabetes Association. Employment of diabetics: a statement of the Committee on Employment and Insurance, American Diabetes Association. Diabetes 1972;21:834–5.

64. Robinson N. Disability and diabetes. Int Disabil Stud 1990;12:28–31.

65. Ardron M, MacFarlane I, Robinson C. Educational achievements, employment and social class of insulin-dependent diabetics: a survey of a young adult clinic in Liverpool. Diabetic Med 1987;4:546–8.

66. Pell S, D'Alonzo CA. Diabetes mellitus in an employed population. JAMA 1960;172:1000–6.

67. Pell S, D'Alonzo CA. Sickness absenteeism in employed diabetics. Am J Public Health 1967;57:253–60.

68. Nasr ANM, Block DL, Magnuson HJ. Absenteeism experience in a group of employed diabetics. J Occup Med 1966;8:621–5.

69. Moore RH, Buschbom RL. Work absenteeism in diabetics. Diabetes 1974;23:957–61.

70. Lazenby HC, Letsch SW. National health expenditures, 1989. Health Care Financing Rev 1990;12(2):1–26.

71. Foley JD. Uninsured in the United States: the nonelderly population without health insurance. Analysis of the March 1990 current population survey. EBRI special report SR-10. Washington, DC: Employee Benefit Research Institute, 1991.

72. Shaw BH. Mortality of diabetes. J Inst Act 1974;405–13.

Chapter 35

EPIDEMIOLOGY OF LATE COMPLICATIONS OF DIABETES

ANDRZEJ S. KROLEWSKI
JAMES H. WARRAM

This chapter reviews the descriptive epidemiology of the late complications of insulin-dependent (IDDM) and non-insulin-dependent diabetes mellitus (NIDDM), selectively emphasizing the findings with implications for the etiology of these problems. We use the same indices of frequency to describe the occurrence of various outcomes of diabetes as were defined in Chapter 12 of this volume. In illustrating the natural history of late diabetic complications, we frequently use data from cohort studies carried out in the patient population and the Joslin Diabetes Center. A less selective review of the epidemiology of late diabetic complications can be found in Chapter 2 of the previous edition of *Joslin's Diabetes Mellitus.*[1]

NATURAL HISTORY OF LATE COMPLICATIONS IN INSULIN-DEPENDENT DIABETES MELLITUS (IDDM)

Impact of Insulin Treatment on Survival

The natural history of IDDM has changed dramatically since the introduction of insulin into clinical practice in 1921. Survival rates among patients with juvenile-onset IDDM seen by Dr. Elliot P. Joslin between 1898 and 1919 have been calculated according to elapsed time after the diagnosis of diabetes.[1] One-half of these patients died in the first 20 months (Fig. 35–1)and fewer than 10% survived for 5 years. Deaths were due mainly to diabetic ketoacidosis.

The survival rates for a similar group of patients with juvenile-onset IDDM who came to the Joslin Diabetes Center with newly diagnosed diabetes between 1939 and

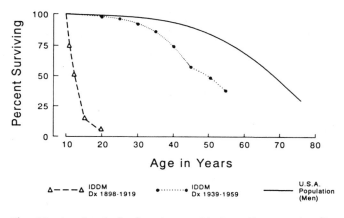

Fig. 35–1. Survival of patients with juvenile-onset insulin-dependent diabetes mellitus (IDDM) according to the availability of insulin for treatment (no insulin treatment: 1898–1919) compared with survival of the white juvenile population of the United States (figure is adapted from data in references 1–4).

1959 and were followed up until 1981 are also shown in Figure 35–1.[2,3] During that time, these patients received insulin therapy in an effort to achieve the best possible glycemic control as well as the benefits of modern medical technology such as hemodialysis and renal transplantation. Regardless of age at diagnosis, almost all of these patients survived to age 30 years, although one-half of them died before age 55. Thus, while insulin treatment had dramatically improved the survival of patients with juvenile-onset IDDM, their median survival was still lower, by 20 years, than that of the general population. In the absence of IDDM, one-half of these individuals would have survived to age 75 (if men) or age 80 (if women).

Diabetes Exposure and Its Consequences

Although insulin replacement therapy prevents diabetic ketoacidosis and death due to coma, it does not completely restore metabolic homeostasis. The result of this imperfect treatment is a novel condition that includes combinations of various metabolic and hormonal alterations such as hyperinsulinemia, hyperglycemia, ketonemia, hyperlipidemia, and many other abnormalities.[5,6] Each of these alterations, referred to as components of *diabetes exposure*, can be characterized by intensity, duration, and cumulative dose (intensity × duration). Although individual components of diabetes exposure may vary independently, many are correlated, and in practice their intensity is thought to be reflected in large measure by the level of blood glucose or glycosylated hemoglobin.

The distribution of intensity of diabetes exposure as estimated from glycosylated hemoglobin levels ranges widely. In the population of patients who visited the Joslin Diabetes Center in 1990, levels of glycosylated hemoglobin ranged from 7 to 20%, whereas 7.5% is the upper limit of normal in the nondiabetic population (Fig. 35–2). When these patients were stratified according to age, those 1 to 9 years old had the lowest glycosylated hemoglobin values: 11.1%, 9.7%, and 8.5% for 75th, 50th, and 25th percentiles, respectively. Patients 10 to 19 years old had the highest levels, while those 20 to 39

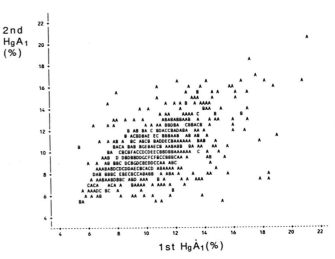

Fig. 35–3. Distribution of patients according to the HgA₁ value obtained in 1990 (1st HgA1) and a second measurement of HgA₁ obtained 6 to 18 months later (2nd HgA1). The patients are the same as those 20–29 years old in Fig. 35–2. A similar pattern was obtained for the other age groups. Spearman correlation coefficients were .58, .51, .57, and .67 for age categories 0–9, 10–19, 20–29, and 30–39, respectively. An "A" represents one patient, "B" represents two patients, and so forth (L.M.B. Laffel, M. Quinn, J.H. Warram, and A.S. Krolewski, unpublished data).

years old had values slightly below that peak. A similar distribution of glycosylated hemoglobin values was observed in a population-based study of patients with IDDM.[7] In the Joslin population, the medians of measurements repeated approximately a year later remained unchanged, and patients tended to maintain their position within the distribution (Fig. 35–3). Those who had a high glycosylated hemoglobin level at the first visit in 1990 had a similar value at the second visit 6 to 18 months later. This "tracking" of level of control is a notable feature and has been observed by others.[8,9]

As a consequence of diabetes exposure, diverse functional and morphologic alterations develop that lead to severe complications affecting the eyes, kidneys, and heart. Despite intensive research, it is unknown which components of diabetes exposure are responsible for particular complications. Various hypotheses have been proposed, ranging from global hypotheses that invoke a single mechanism and a single component of diabetes exposure as responsible for all complications[10–14] to separate hypotheses for each complication that invoke interactions among tissue-specific genetic factors, environment, and diabetes exposure.[15]

In the following sections, the development of each late complication is examined according to duration of IDDM, level of glycemic control, and to other, nondiabetic, factors. The respective patterns of occurrence are contrasted so conclusions can be drawn regarding the extent of commonality in their pathogenic mechanisms. Because of a sparsity of data on the occurrence of late complications in adult-onset IDDM, this review presents data on IDDM diagnosed before age 20 almost exclusively.

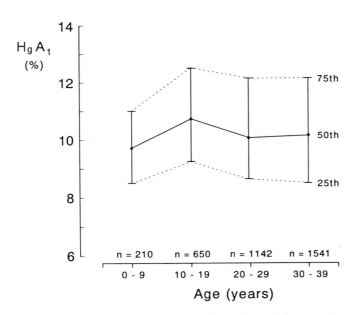

Fig. 35–2. Distribution of glycosylated hemoglobin (HgA₁) according to age in patients who visited the Joslin Diabetes Center in 1990. The 75th, 50th and 25th percentiles of the distribution are presented (L.M.B. Laffel, M. Quinn, J.H. Warram, and A.S. Krolewski, unpublished data).

Inevitability of Proliferative Diabetic Retinopathy

The most frequent complication of IDDM is retinopathy. After a lag period of about 4 years following diagnosis, the incidence rate of background retinopathy, manifested as microaneurysms and hemorrhages in the retina, increases rapidly with the duration of diabetes.[16,17] During the 5th year of IDDM, background retinopathy develops in only 1 of 100 patients, whereas in the 14th year, it develops in 11 of the 100 patients who had escaped it up to that time (Fig. 35–4A). After 14 years, almost all patients with IDDM have developed retinopathic lesions, with a cumulative incidence of 90% (Fig. 35–4B).

Since retinopathy is extremely rare in persons without diabetes, one can infer that it is a consequence of exposure to IDDM. However, the specific relation between exposure and development of early retinopathy is unclear. One possibility is that these retinal lesions occur after a sufficient accumulation (intensity × duration) of IDDM exposure. However, the duration of exposure may be more important than its intensity, provided that the intensity exceeds some relatively low threshold, a factor that could explain the 4-year delay before the appearance of retinal lesions and their almost ubiquitous occurrence within the first 15 years of IDDM.

With longer duration of disease, patients with IDDM are vulnerable to the development of proliferative retinopathy, which can lead to blindness. The emergence of this vulnerability is reflected in the incidence of proliferative retinopathy (Fig. 35–4A), which increases rapidly between the 10th and the 15th year of IDDM.[18] It should be noted that after this increase, the incidence rate remains at a constant level; proliferative retinopathy develops in about 3 of 100 previously unaffected patients each year, regardless of whether they have had diabetes for 20 or 40 years. This constant incidence rate yields a cumulative incidence of 62% after 40 years (Fig.

35–4B). The fact that the incidence rate of proliferative retinopathy does not decline even after most of the population has been affected suggests that almost all patients with Type I diabetes are susceptible to proliferative retinopathy.

A question remains, however, as to why some patients with IDDM develop proliferative diabetic retinopathy within the second decade of diabetes whereas others are spared for several decades. In studies conducted at the Joslin Diabetes Center, the level of glycemic control appears to be the major predictor of the early development of proliferative retinopathy. Those with the poorest glycemic control during the first 15 years of diabetes had the highest risk of developing proliferative retinopathy during the second decade of IDDM.[18,19] A strong relationship between the development of proliferative retinopathy and the level of glycemic control also was found in the Wisconsin Study.[20] While these studies demonstrate the validity of glycosylated hemoglobin and other indices of hyperglycemia as predictors of proliferative retinopathy, the indices must be viewed only as markers of risk, since the actual component of diabetes exposure that contributes to the development of proliferative diabetic nephropathy remains unknown.

Another factor found to be closely associated with the development of early-onset proliferative diabetic retinopathy is the presence of cardiovascular autonomic neuropathy.[19] All patients with early-onset proliferative nephropathy had some degree of cardiovascular autonomic neuropathy, whereas only 50% of those who had nonproliferative retinopathy had these abnormalities. The two most probable explanations for this patterns of association are 1) that autonomic neuropathy contributes to the development of retinal neovascularization or 2) that autonomic neuropathy is a risk indicator, i.e., a marker of a process that underlies the development of both autonomic neuropathy and early proliferative diabetic nephropathy.[19]

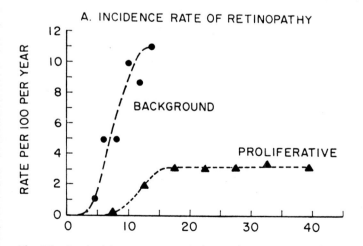

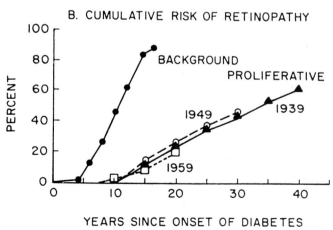

Fig. 35–4. Incidence rates (A) and cumulative risks (B) of background and of proliferative retinopathy according to the duration of insulin-dependent diabetes (IDDM). Cumulative risk of proliferative retinopathy is shown according to year of diagnosis of IDDM. Reprinted with permission from reference 15 (Krolewski AS, Warram JH, Rand LI, Kahn CR. Epidemiologic approach to the etiology of Type I diabetes mellitus and its complications. N Engl J Med 1987;317:1390–8).

While the proliferation of new vessels in proliferative retinopathy is the major factor responsible for blindness in patients with IDDM, it appears that visual loss is related primarily to neovascularization on the optic disc (NVD).[21,22] Whereas neovascularization elsewhere in the retina (NVE) develops in most patients with IDDM, NVD develops in only a subset.[23] In an analysis of data from a clinical trial of laser therapy for diabetic retinopathy, we found different patterns for the development of NVD and NVE.[23] While the risk of NVE appears to be determined by retinal lesions, a high risk of NVD might be determined by systemic factors that are related to the presence of NVD in the contralateral eye, young age, or the presence of renal complications. The possibility that there are different determinants of neovascularization on the optic disc and in the retina requires further investigation since their identification may provide a clue regarding the systemic factor(s) leading to subsequent blindness.

Susceptibility to Diabetic Nephropathy

Nephropathy is manifested initially as a persistent elevation in urinary excretion of albumin and subsequently as an increase in excretion of protein.[24-26] The incidence rate of proteinuria according to the duration of IDDM is shown in Figure 35–5A. After a lag of 5 years following diabetes onset, risk of nephropathy rises rapidly, peaks during the second decade, and then declines.[27] Other studies have reported similar findings.[28] Although nephropathy often is considered together with retinopathy as a "microangiopathic" complication, the pattern of risk is quite different from that for eye lesions (Fig. 35–4A) and suggests that only a subset of patients are susceptible to renal complications. The rarity of new cases of nephropathy among patients who have had IDDM for many years suggests that this complication had already affected almost all susceptible patients.[15]

The concept of susceptibility to diabetic nephropathy has also been supported by family studies. Seaquist et al. found an 83% prevalence of nephropathy among the diabetic siblings of IDDM probands selected because they had diabetic nephropathy but a prevalence of only 17% in diabetic siblings of IDDM probands selected because they did not have nephropathy.[29] The sibling concordance in families of probands with diabetic nephropathy was too high to be consistent with Mendelian genetic models.[30] Perhaps there was some bias toward ascertainment of concordant pairs. In a study conducted at the Joslin Diabetes Center that was designed to avoid ascertainment bias, we found prevalences of 53% and 18% in IDDM siblings of probands with and without nephropathy, respectively.[31] These family data are consistent with a hypothesis that genetic factors determine predisposition to diabetic nephropathy and that this predisposition may be caused by a major gene effect.[30,32]

Susceptibility to renal complications in IDDM could arise through several mechanisms, one being a genetic predisposition to hypertension. Patients who develop nephropathy within the first 20 years of diabetes frequently have parents with hypertension and also have higher sodium-lithium countertransport activity in their red cells (a presumed marker of hypertension risk) than a matched group of patients with IDDM without microalbuminuria.[33-36]

A feature diabetic nephropathy has in common with proliferative diabetic retinopathy is the relation of risk to the level of glycemic control. Several studies conducted at the Joslin Diabetes Center found a dose-dependent relationship between the index of hyperglycemia and the development of persistent proteinuria during the first 20 years of IDDM.[27,34,36] Of interest is the apparent interaction between predisposition to essential hypertension and poor glycemic control in the production of diabetic nephropathy.[34]

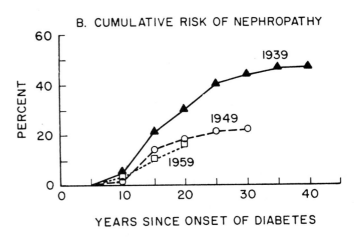

Fig. 35–5. Incidence rate (A) and cumulative risk (B) of nephropathy according to duration of insulin-dependent diabetes (IDDM). Cumulative risk is shown according to year of diagnosis of IDDM. Reprinted with permission from reference 15 (Krolewski AS, Warram JH, Rand LI, Kahn CR. Epidemiologic approach to the etiology of Type I diabetes mellitus and its complications. N Engl J Med 1987;317:1390–8).

In addition to the interaction between poor glycemic control and genetically determined susceptibility factors, some environmental exposures also influence the risk of diabetic nephropathy. The cumulative risk of persistent proteinuria in patients with IDDM diagnosed in 1949 and 1959 was only one-half that in patients with disease diagnosed in 1939[27] (Fig. 35–5B). A similar observation was made in Denmark.[37] One difference between patients who became diabetic in 1939 and those who became diabetic in 1949 or 1959 may have been the frequency of clinical and subclinical infections possibly damaging glomeruli.[27] If residual damage from infections adds to the injury caused by the intrarenal hemodynamic alterations in diabetes, such effects could explain the higher risk of diabetes-associated nephropathy in the 1939 cohort. Another factor that has changed over time is the recommended diet for diabetic patients. According to one hypothesis, a decrease in protein intake could contribute to the decline in the risk of nephropathy.[38] However, the main change in the recommended diet seems to have been a substitution of carbohydrates for excess fat rather than a reduction in protein.[39]

Once patients have persistent proteinuria, their prognosis is poor. Their median duration of survival is about 10 years, and most patients are dead within 20 years.[27,28] The duration of this stage is determined by two pathologic processes that progress simultaneously: a decline in renal function that leads to renal failure and an acceleration of atherosclerosis that leads to coronary artery disease.[40]

Promotion of Atherosclerosis

An excess of coronary artery disease (CAD) in patients with IDDM can only be observed in patients older than 30 years of age.[3,41] In a cohort of patients with juvenile-onset IDDM who were followed for 20 to 40 years, 33% had died of CAD between the age of 30 and 55 years (Fig. 35–6A), whereas in the nondiabetic participants in the Framingham Heart Study the comparable proportions were much lower: about 8% for men and 4% for women.[3] Not only was there excess mortality in the diabetic cohort, there was excess symptomatic and asymptomatic CAD among survivors. If all three levels of manifestation of CAD are combined, the cumulative risk by age 55 years is 50%.[3] It is important to note that the risks of CAD in men and women with IDDM are similar and increase after age 30 at the same rate, regardless of whether the onset of diabetes was in early childhood or in late adolescence (Fig. 35–6B).[3]

One possible hypothesis about why excess risk of CAD is absent in patients with IDDM until they reach age 30 is that diabetes cannot initiate atherosclerosis but can accelerate progression of early atherosclerotic lesions, which commonly appear, even in the absence of diabetes, during the third and fourth decades of life.[3,42] In the absence of these initial lesions, patients might endure the presence of diabetes for 40 years without showing any clinical evidence of CAD. At present it is unclear which components of diabetes exposure are responsible for accelerating the progression of atherosclerosis in coronary arteries. It has been established, however, that patients with diabetic nephropathy have the highest risk of death from CAD.[3,40,43,44]

Relationships among Late Complications in IDDM

A schematic summary can be made of the overlap of the late complications occurring in patients with a diagnosis of IDDM before age 21 on the basis of studies conducted at the Joslin Diabetes Center (Fig. 35–7).[3,18,27] During a 40-year observation period, about one-third of these patients developed overt proteinuria, most of whom developed proliferative retinopathy as

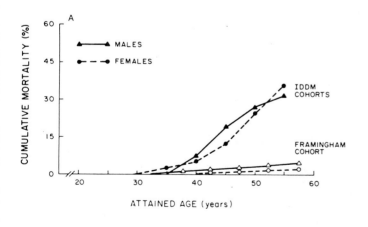

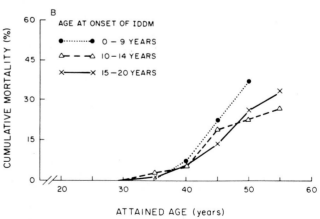

Fig. 35–6. A: Cumulative mortality from coronary artery disease according to attained age in patients with juvenile-onset insulin-dependent diabetes (IDDM) followed for 20 to 40 years and in the population of the Framingham Heart Study. B: Cumulative mortality from coronary artery disease according to attained age and according to age at onset of diabetes in patients with juvenile-onset IDDM followed for 20 to 40 years. Reprinted with permission from reference 3 (Krolewski AS, Kosinski EJ, Warram JH, et al. Magnitude and determinants of coronary artery disease in juvenile-onset, insulin-dependent diabetes mellitus. Am J Cardiol 1987;59:750–5).

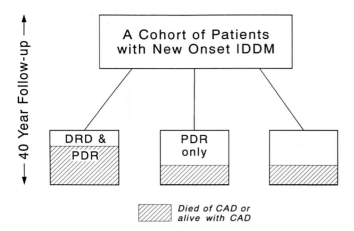

Fig. 35–7. Natural history of late complications of insulin-dependent diabetes (IDDM) during 40-year follow-up of a cohort of patients diagnosed before age 21 years and followed up from within 1 year of the diagnosis of IDDM. The category of diabetic renal disease (DRD) includes patients with persistent proteinuria as well as those who had progressed to renal failure.[27] Proliferative diabetic retinopathy (PDR) includes neovascularization on the optic disc or in the retina.[18] Coronary artery disease (CAD) includes the cases of symptomatic CAD among surviving patients as well as fatal CAD.[3]

well. An additional one-third developed proliferative retinopathy but not proteinuria, and the remaining one-third developed neither proliferative retinopathy nor nephropathy. It is interesting that during the last 40 years the risk of nephropathy has declined (Fig. 35–5B) but not the risk of proliferative retinopathy (Fig. 35–4B). Of the total cohort, about 50% died of or have symptoms of CAD. Among those with nephropathy, hypertension is almost universally present, and the majority have CAD.

It is important to note that some patients developed one complication but not another, the implication being all these complications cannot be caused by a single determinant or even by a single set of determinants and that each complication must have at least some distinctive etiologic feature. For example, the risks of proliferative retinopathy and nephropathy are each closely related to the level of glycemic control but diverge with respect to their occurrence in time after the onset of IDDM. Furthermore, while proliferative retinopathy is related to the presence of cardiovascular autonomic neuropathy,[19] nephropathy is related instead to predisposition to essential hypertension.[33–36] The risk of CAD is affected profoundly by many factors. In addition to its dependence on attained age (not duration of diabetes), CAD risk is strongly related to abnormalities involved in predisposition to hypertension (which precede the appearance of proteinuria) as well as to other abnormalities that accompany persistent proteinuria. A single pathogenic mechanism, fueled by the cumulative exposure to diabetes (i.e., level of hyperglycemia × duration), seems to be insufficient to explain these diverse relationships. One must postulate the existence of various modifiers (genetic or environmental) of the effects of diabetes exposure and, perhaps, different roles for the compo-

nents of exposure to account for the distinctiveness of the patterns of occurrence of specific complications.[15]

NATURAL HISTORY OF LATE COMPLICATIONS IN NON-INSULIN-DEPENDENT DIABETES MELLITUS (NIDDM)

In the following sections, salient characteristics of the occurrence of retinopathy, nephropathy, and CAD in patients with NIDDM are reviewed and contrasted with those in IDDM. Diabetes diagnosed after age 30 years is considered to be NIDDM. Because the occurrence of IDDM after this age is relatively rare in comparison with that of NIDDM (see Chapter 12), this operational definition of NIDDM introduces a negligible bias.

Metabolic Abnormalities

Late complications of NIDDM are determined by combinations of metabolic abnormalities present before as well as after the clinical onset of diabetes. Regarding the antecedent abnormalities, several studies have shown that hyperinsulinemia is a major feature.[45–47] The earliest documentation of this abnormality came from a follow-up study conducted at the Joslin Diabetes Center.[47] A large group of normoglycemic young adult offspring of two parents with NIDDM were recruited for a longitudinal study and followed for up to 25 years. During the first 8 years of follow-up, there was only the occasional case of NIDDM, but during the subsequent decade, one of six offspring developed NIDDM. Baseline characteristics of the group that developed NIDDM and the group that remained normoglycemic are compared in Table 35–1. Fasting and postchallenge (oral glucose tolerance test [OGTT]) blood glucose levels were similar in the two groups, but the groups differed significantly with regard to insulin levels. Fasting and postchallenge insulin levels of the offspring destined to develop NIDDM were almost twice those of the offspring who remained normoglyce-

Table 35–1. Baseline Characteristics of Prediabetic Individuals 15 to 25 Years before They Developed Diabetes Compared with Those of Individuals Followed Concurrently Who Did Not Develop Diabetes

Characteristic	Nondiabetic (n = 130)	Prediabetic (n = 25)
Men (%)	43	60
Age at baseline studies (yr)	32 ± 10	33 ± 8
Ideal body weight (%)	116 ± 20	146 ± 35
Results of OGTT		
Blood glucose (mg/dL)		
Fasting	77 ± 8	79 ± 8
2-hr	89 ± 18	102 ± 14
Plasma insulin (μU/mL)		
Fasting	17 ± 10	32 ± 23
Sum of all values*	594 ± 322	1029 ± 658

Reanalysis of data in reference 47. See text for description of study group. OGTT = oral glucose tolerance test.
*Sum of all insulin values during an OGTT with sampling times at 0, 15, 30, 45, 60, 90 and 120 minutes.

mic during 15 to 25 years of follow-up. The relative hyperinsulinemia of the prediabetic offspring persisted after the data were adjusted for the significant differences between the distributions of body weight in the two groups.

Thus, during the "prediabetic" period, one to two decades before the diagnosis of NIDDM, these offspring were insulin-resistant and were exposed to hyperinsulinemia—not hypoinsulinemia. Hyperglycemia emerged very slowly after many years of hyperinsulinemia. Longitudinal data on one of the offspring who developed NIDDM are summarized in Figure 35–8. This individual was followed for 17 years and subjected every other year to an OGTT, with measurements of glucose and insulin levels. Hyperglycemia, which was evident only after glucose challenge, was first detected at age 62, when postchallenge hyperinsulinemia was still clearly evident. Then, as postchallenge insulin levels declined, fasting hyperglycemia developed. Note that fasting hyperinsulinemia persisted through this stage of the process. A similar pattern for the emergence of hyperglycemia was seen in most offspring who developed NIDDM.

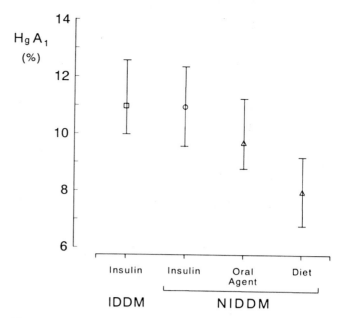

Fig. 35–9. Distribution of glycosylated hemoglobin (HgA$_1$) according to type of diabetes and treatment for hyperglycemia in a random sample of diabetic patients who visited the Joslin Diabetes Center in 1990. All patients had diabetes diagnosed after the age of 30 and were 45 to 59 years old in 1990 (L.M.B. Laffel, M. Quinn, J.H. Warram, and A.S. Krolewski, unpublished data).

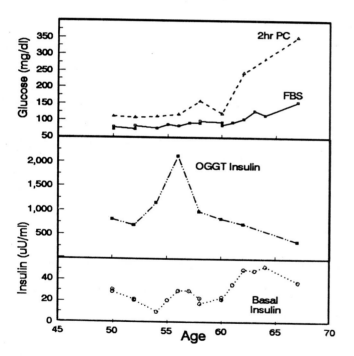

Fig. 35–8. Gradual emergence of non-insulin-dependent diabetes mellitus (NIDDM) in an offspring of two parents with NIDDM during 17 years of follow-up. The offspring's weight ranged from 135 to 140% of ideal for the first 5 years of follow-up and remained in the range 120 to 125% thereafter. The top panel shows the fasting (FBS) and 2-hour (PC) blood glucose levels during repeated oral glucose tolerance tests (OGTT). OGTT insulin is the sum of plasma insulin levels at 0, 15, 30, 45, 60, 90, and 120 minutes during the OGTT. The 90th percentile for OGTT insulin in a control group of individuals with no family history of diabetes was 875 μU/mL. For basal insulin, the 90th percentile in the control group was 22 μU/mL (J.H. Warram, B.C. Martin, A.S. Krolewski, J.S. Soeldner, and C.R. Kahn, unpublished data).

Of the metabolic abnormalities present after the onset of NIDDM, hyperglycemia is the most prominent. There is no evidence that conventional methods of treatment for hyperglycemia achieve normoglycemia in a majority of patients with NIDDM. Among a sample of patients with NIDDM aged 45 to 59 years who visited the Joslin Diabetes Center in 1990, the distribution of glycohemoglobin values among those treated with insulin was similar to that among patients with adult-onset IDDM (Fig. 35–9). The levels of glycosylated hemoglobin in patients with NIDDM treated with oral agents, and particularly in those treated with diet, were significantly below those in patients treated with insulin. Still, the non-insulin-treated groups had values far above the normal range (5 to 7.4%). Similar distributions of glycosylated hemoglobin values were observed in patients with NIDDM in a population-based study.[7]

In summary, patients with NIDDM have been exposed to hyperinsulinemia for decades before the emergence of hyperglycemia, a feature that contrasts sharply with the prediabetic phase of IDDM. Subsequently, in many of these patients, the hyperglycemia is as severe as in patients with IDDM. As a consequence of the metabolic abnormalities that exist before and after the onset of NIDDM, these patients are at high risk of developing some of the late diabetic complications.

Low Risk of Proliferative Retinopathy

Many cross-sectional surveys have been conducted to assess the prevalence of diabetic retinopathy in NIDDM.

The most informative was carried out among participants of the Framingham Heart Study.[48] The prevalence of nonproliferative retinopathy (determined by fundus photography) in diabetic patients in the Framingham cohort rose from 5% among those with a duration of diabetes of less than 5 years to 30%, 45%, and 62% among those with a duration of diabetes of 5 to 9 years, 10 to 14 years, and 15 or more years, respectively. It is noteworthy that changes in the retina characteristic of those in diabetes were found in 0.8% of persons without diabetes in that population. Proliferative retinopathy was detected in only a few individuals with NIDDM in the Framingham Study population.

Another population-based cross-sectional study that provided detailed data on the prevalence of eye complications in NIDDM was conducted in Wisconsin.[49] The prevalence of retinopathy was slightly higher in this population than in the Framingham Heart Study population (Fig. 35–10), but as before, not many patients had proliferative retinopathy despite a long duration of NIDDM. Patients treated with insulin had a higher prevalence of retinopathy than did patients treated with oral agents or diet.

There have been few prospective observations of the development of diabetic retinopathy in patients with NIDDM. In a study of the inception cohort of patients with NIDDM in the population studied in Rochester, Minnesota, nonproliferative retinopathy developed in 35% over a period of 20 years of follow-up, whereas the cumulative incidence of proliferative retinopathy was less than 4%.[50] The level of hyperglycemia at the baseline examination appeared to have a significant impact on the development of retinal changes.[51] During the follow-up

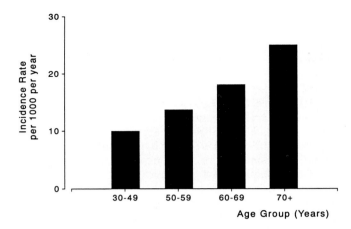

Fig. 35–11. Age-specific incidence rate of persistent proteinuria during the first 5 years after the diagnosis of non-insulin-dependent diabetes mellitus in the population of Rochester, Minnesota (adapted from reference 52).

component of the Wisconsin study, similar observations were made, i.e., the level of glycohemoglobin A_1 was the major predictor of the development of nonproliferative and proliferative retinopathy.[20]

In summary, nonproliferative retinopathy appears to be a frequent complication of NIDDM and is related to the severity of diabetes (level of glycemic control). Proliferative retinopathy, however, appears to be less frequent in NIDDM than in IDDM. There has been little investigation into factors that could account for the lower risk of proliferative retinopathy in NIDDM than in IDDM, although some of the difference may be due to a decreasing susceptibility with age.[23]

Difference in Natural History of Nephropathy from That in IDDM

Unlike young patients with IDDM, who rarely develop persistent proteinuria during the first 5 years of diabetes, patients with NIDDM frequently have proteinuria at diagnosis. Moreover, the prevalence of persistent proteinuria in patients with newly diagnosed NIDDM increases with age. For example in the Rochester study population, the prevalence of proteinuria increased from 2.7% in the group 30 to 49 years old at diagnosis to 12.4% in the group over 70 years old at diagnosis.[52] A strong effect of age on the risk of development of persistent proteinuria also was observed during follow-up.[52] In the first 5 years after the diagnosis of NIDDM, the incidence rate of persistent proteinuria rose from 10/1000 per year in the age group 30 to 49 to 25/1000 per year in those over age 70 (Fig. 35–11). In striking contrast to IDDM (see Fig. 35–5A), in NIDDM the incidence rate of persistent proteinuria did not vary with duration of diabetes. The incidence rate of persistent proteinuria during the first 5 years after diagnosis of NIDDM was 17/1000 per year and was similar during all subsequent intervals of observation.[52]

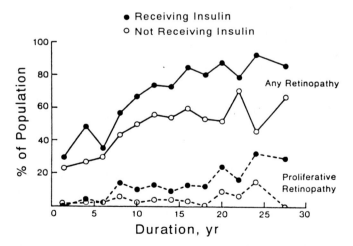

Fig. 35–10. Prevalence of retinopathy according to duration of diabetes and type of treatment for hyperglycemia. All patients had diabetes diagnosed after the age of 30 and presumably had non-insulin-dependent diabetes. Reprinted with permission from reference 49 (Klein R, Klein BEK, Moss SE, et al. The Wisconsin Epidemiologic Study of Diabetic Retinopathy. III. Prevalence and risk of diabetic retinopathy when age at diagnosis is 30 or more years. Arch Ophthalmol 1984; 102:527–32).

The risk of development of persistent proteinuria in NIDDM also was examined in the University Group Diabetes Program (UGDP). The cumulative incidence of persistent proteinuria was 9.2% in patients included in that study and followed for 10 years.[53] This corresponds roughly to an incidence rate of 9/1000 per year, a rate lower than that in the Rochester population. Since the UGDP participants included a substantial number with impaired glucose tolerance, the cumulative incidence of proteinuria would have been higher if the analysis had been limited to patients with NIDDM.

The relationship between severity of diabetes (or level of glycemic control) and the development of persistent proteinuria can be seen clearly in Figure 35–12, which shows the cumulative incidence of persistent proteinuria in the Rochester diabetic population computed according to duration of NIDDM and fasting glucose level at the diagnosis of diabetes.[52] Patients with NIDDM whose fasting blood glucose levels were lower than 205 mg/dL at diagnosis had a cumulative incidence of persistent proteinuria of about 15% after 25 years of diabetes, whereas in those whose fasting blood glucose at diagnosis was 205 mg/dL or greater had a cumulative incidence of almost 40%. The latter risk figure approaches that observed in IDDM.[27]

Other measures of the magnitude of renal complications in NIDDM include the incidence rate of end-stage renal disease (ESRD) and the mortality rate due to renal failure. Mortality data are available from a study conducted at the Joslin Diabetes Center (J. E. Manson, B. C. Martin, J. H. Warram, and A. S. Krolewski, unpublished data). A random sample of patients with recently diagnosed NIDDM who came to the Joslin Diabetes Center in 1923 and 1960 were traced until their death or until 1983. For deceased patients, all available information

Table 35–2. Distribution of the Joslin Cohort of Diabetic Patients, Age 35 to 62 Years at First Clinic Visit, According to Status at End of 24-Year Follow-up

Status at End of 24-yr Follow-up	Percentage With Status	
	Men (n = 407)	women (n = 470)
Death according to cause		
Coronary artery disease	38	39
Other cardiovascular diseases	11	18
Renal failure	4	3
Cancer	11	9
Other	15	11
Survival	13	12
Untraced	8	9

J.E. Manson, B.C. Martin, J.H. Warram, and A.S. Krolewski, unpublished data.

regarding causes of death were collected and classified according to the primary cause. In patients aged 35 to 62 at their first visit to the clinic, renal failure was the cause of only a small proportion of the deaths (Table 35–2). During a 24-year follow-up interval, the majority of patients died of CAD, and only 4% of the men and 3% of the women died of renal failure. The cumulative mortality due to renal failure among those with diabetes diagnosed between 1945 and 1960 was about the same as that among patients with a diagnosis between 1922 and 1944.

The incidence rate of ESRD was determined in the diabetic population of Rochester, Minnesota.[54] All patients who developed NIDDM between 1949 and 1979 were followed until 1984, and development of ESRD was recorded. The cumulative risk of ESRD in this population was 0.8% and 6.2% after 10 and 25 years of diabetes, respectively. This risk is very similar to the risk of death due to renal failure in the Joslin population (Table 35–2). Overall, the risk of ESRD in patients with NIDDM is about one-fourth that in patients with juvenile-onset IDDM.[27] However, since NIDDM is more common than IDDM in the U.S. population, NIDDM contributes almost as many individuals to the ESRD program as does IDDM. The age distribution of diabetic patients residing in Massachusetts who had a transplanted kidney or were in a dialysis program as of December 31, 1988, is shown in Table 35–3. Of 459 patients, 264 were 15 to 54 years old, and presumably the majority of them had IDDM. The remaining 195 patients were 55 or older, and presumably most of them had NIDDM.

In summary, persistent proteinuria is frequent in patients with NIDDM, but the risk of its progressing to renal failure is lower than in patients with IDDM. The mechanisms that would explain this are not clear. Two possibilities can be considered: first, that persistent proteinuria in many patients with NIDDM is caused by factors other than diabetes and that the rate of progression of proteinuria to renal failure might be minimal in such cases; second, that progression is interrupted by a competing cause of death such as CAD before ESRD is reached. The latter possibility is supported by several

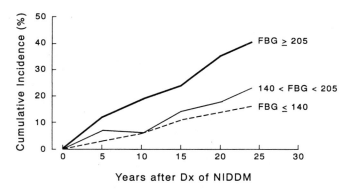

Fig. 35–12. Cumulative incidence of persistent proteinuria according to level of fasting blood glucose (FBG) at the time of diagnosis of non-insulin-dependent diabetes mellitus (NIDDM). The patients under observation had NIDDM diagnosed between 1949 and 1969 and were followed until 1985. Reprinted with permission from reference 52 (Ballard DJ, Humphrey LL, Melton LJ III, et al. Epidemiology of persistent proteinuria in type II diabetes mellitus. Population-based study in Rochester, Minnesota. Diabetes 1988;37:405–12; copyright © American Diabetes Association).

Table 35–3. Age distribution of Diabetic Massachusetts Residents, Alive as of December 31, 1988, Who Were Receiving Dialysis or Had Received a Renal Transplant

Age Category (yr)	No. of Diabetic Patients With ESRD
15–24	14
25–34	103
35–44	78
45–54	69
55–64	103
65–74	82
75+	10
Total	459*

Unpublished data from the U.S. Renal Data System, National Institute of Diabetes and Digestive and Kidney Diseases, National Institutes of Health, Bethesda, MD, supplied by Donna Zobel. ESRD = end-stage renal disease.
*Of these patients, 384 (84%) were white.

studies showing an excess mortality due to CAD in patients with NIDDM who have microalbuminuria or proteinuria.[55–57]

Coronary Artery Disease as the Major Health Problem

CAD and other cardiovascular diseases occur earlier and with greater frequency in patients with NIDDM than in the general population. Several mechanisms contribute to this excess. First, CAD and NIDDM frequently occur together (cluster) in families. For example, patients with NIDDM are more likely to have a parent with CAD or hypertension than are patients with IDDM or controls without diabetes.[58] The mechanisms responsible for these associations are unclear. They may reflect a shared etiologic factor—with a significant genetic determinant—shared by CAD and NIDDM.[59] Second, hyperinsulinemia and insulin resistance, which precede by many years the development of NIDDM (see Table 35–1), also are predictors of the development of elevated blood pressure and lipid abnormalities.[60,61] Several studies have demonstrated that an elevated serum insulin level in the fasting or postprandial state is an independent predictor of the development of CAD.[62–64] Thus, the hyperinsulinemia/insulin resistance that occurs during the prediabetic period together with elevated blood pressure and lipid abnormalities may accelerate atherosclerosis to advanced stages of CAD in many patients by the time a diagnosis of NIDDM is made.[65–67]

After NIDDM (hyperglycemia) develops, risk factors for CAD become more prevalent and more intense. It has been shown that a large proportion of patients with NIDDM are obese and have hypertension as well as changes in lipid profiles.[65–70] However, the long-term impact of exposure to hyperglycemia (overt NIDDM) on the risk of CAD is not clear. Certain authors have argued that only exposure before diabetes onset is important, but the studies that failed to demonstrate an increasing risk of

CAD with increasing duration of NIDDM had little statistical power to detect such an increase.[59,71]

The long-term effects of diabetes exposure on the development of CAD in patients with NIDDM was assessed in a 24-year follow-up study of patients with NIDDM who came to the Joslin Diabetes Center between 1922 and 1960.[58] The study group was a random sample of patients with NIDDM who resided in Massachusetts and came to the clinic soon after the diagnosis of diabetes. Patients were traced until death or until 1983, and all available information about the circumstances of each death was collected so that an assignment of the primary cause of death could be made according to criteria similar to those used in the Framingham Heart Study. Among patients 35 to 62 years old at the beginning of the 24-year follow-up, the cause of death was CAD in 38% of the men and in 39% of the women (Table 35–2). Other cardiovascular diseases contributed another 11% and 18% of the deaths among men and women, respectively.

Cumulative mortality due to CAD was computed separately for patients who came to the Joslin Diabetes Center between 1923 and 1944 and those who came between 1945 and 1960. The cumulative mortality due to CAD was slightly lower in the group with more recently diagnosed diabetes, but the decline in the CAD mortality rate was more evident among men than women. Whether the rate of decline of CAD mortality among men with diabetes is different from that among men in the general population cannot be assessed because of the small sample size. However, the lack of a distinct trend among diabetic women is not in agreement with the trend for women in the general population, among whom CAD mortality has declined as it has in men.[72]

The long-term effect of diabetes exposure on the mortality due to CAD was further examined by comparing the CAD mortality rates in the Joslin cohort with those from the Framingham Heart Study according to duration of follow-up (Fig. 35–13). CAD mortality is shown according to 4-year intervals of duration of follow-up. In the Framingham sample, the increasing risk of CAD with duration of follow-up reflects the effect of the aging process, whereas in patients with diabetes, the increased risk reflects the combined effect of aging together with accumulating diabetes exposure. Diabetic patients had higher CAD-related mortality than did the nondiabetic patients during the first 4 years of follow-up. During subsequent intervals of observation, the magnitude of this excess mortality increased, indicating the existence of a cumulative effect of exposure to diabetes that is independent of aging processes. The effect of diabetes exposure on CAD risk is much larger in women that in men.

It should be noted that whereas the difference in CAD mortality grew in each successive duration group the increase did not occur as a constant multiple of the rate in the Framingham population. The biologic implications of this are uncertain, but such a pattern would occur if the cumulative effect of diabetes accelerates the development of CAD in only a subset of patients.[3]

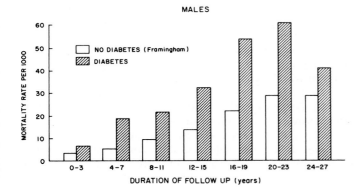

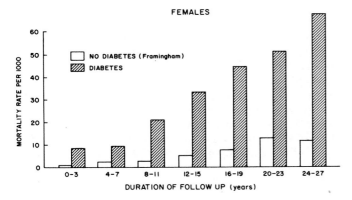

Fig. 35–13. Age-adjusted mortality rate from coronary artery disease during 24 years of follow-up of the Joslin Diabetes Center cohort of diabetic patients whose diabetes was diagnosed between ages 35 and 62 and who came to the center soon after diagnosis, compared with that in the Framingham cohort, according to sex and duration of follow-up. Diabetic patients are the same as those in Table 35–2 (unpublished data).

The determinants of CAD mortality in patients with NIDDM were studied further in another cohort of patients aged 40 to 62 years who came to the Joslin Diabetes Center between 1957 and 1963 with newly diagnosed diabetes and were followed until the end of 1971 (P.

Valsania, B.C. Martin, J.H. Warram, A.S. Krolewski, unpublished data). Cause-specific mortality in this cohort was compared with that in nondiabetic individuals participating in the Framingham Heart Study. Among patients in the Joslin cohort, the total mortality was approximately twofold higher than that among nondiabetic individuals in the Framingham cohort (Table 35–4), and the excess mortality was due primarily to CAD.

Determinants of the CAD excess mortality in the diabetic cohort are presented in Figure 35–14. Among patients with NIDDM treated with diet or oral agents at the beginning of the observation period, CAD mortality during the first 8 years of follow-up was similar to that for men and women in the Framingham cohort. Among those patients treated with insulin, however, CAD mortality was twofold higher in men and fivefold higher in women than in the nondiabetic cohort. After a longer duration of diabetes, i.e., 8 to 14 years after diagnosis, the difference between the CAD mortality the diabetic and nondiabetic populations was magnified. Patients treated at the beginning of the observation period with diet or oral agents alone had a risk of death due to CAD twofold or threefold higher than that for nondiabetic men and women, respectively. Patients treated from the beginning of follow-up with insulin now had respective risks of death due to CAD that were fourfold and sixfold higher than those in the nondiabetic cohort for men and women, respectively.

A high risk of CAD in insulin-treated patients with NIDDM has been demonstrated in several other studies. In cross-sectional studies in Finland, NIDDM patients with CAD had higher levels of endogenous insulin than did NIDDM patients without CAD.[69,70] In a cross-sectional study conducted in Germany, NIDDM patients with macrovascular disease had higher fasting levels of C-peptide and free plasma insulin than did similar patients who were free of macrovascular complications.[73] In the follow-up component of this study, patients treated with the highest daily insulin dose were found to have the highest risk of developing large-vessel complications.[74] Among a large cohort study in Poland, it was found, after adjustment for other known CAD risk factors, that patients with NIDDM treated with insulin had a significantly higher CAD mortality than did those treated with

Table 35–4. Age-Adjusted, Cause-Specific Rates in the Framingham Heart Study and in the 1958–1963 Joslin Diabetes Center Cohort Followed until 1972

	Mortality Rates (/1000 per yr)			
	Men		Women	
Cause of Death	Framingham (n = 1886)	Joslin (n = 1126)	Framingham (n = 2439)	Joslin (n = 1103)
CAD	8.2	16.5	3.5	12.0
Other CVD	3.0	4.5	2.2	4.0
Other	7.1	10.0	5.0	6.5
Total	18.3	31.0	10.5	22.5

P. Valsania, B.C Martin, J.H. Warram, and A.S. Krolewski, unpublished data. CAD = coronary artery disease; CVD = cardiovascular disease.

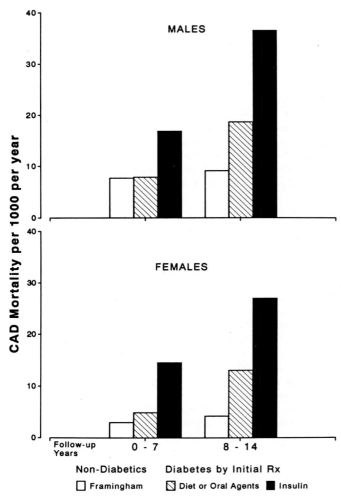

Fig. 35–14. Mortality rate from coronary artery disease (CAD) in a cohort of Joslin Diabetes Center patients compared with that in the Framingham cohort, according to sex, type of treatment for hyperglycemia, and duration of diabetes (P. Valsania, B.C. Martin, J.H. Warram, and A.S. Krolewski, unpublished data).

oral agents or diet (J. Kopczynski, D. Janeczko, A. Czyzyk, et al., unpublished data).

At present the interpretation of the high CAD mortality among patients with adult-onset diabetes (mostly NIDDM) treated with insulin is not clear. At least two possibilities can be considered. First, one can hypothesize that these patients have the poorest glycemic control and that it is hyperglycemia that accelerates atherosclerosis and leads to death due to CAD. Second, perhaps high plasma insulin levels, which are common in NIDDM, are increased even further by insulin treatment and that it is the hyperinsulinemia that accelerates the formation of atherosclerotic lesions.

In summary, premature mortality due to CAD emerges as the major health problem in NIDDM. Three factors contribute to this problem: 1) CAD is present in excess at the time of diagnosis of NIDDM[65–67]; 2) the incidence rate of CAD in patients with diagnosed NIDDM is several times that in nondiabetic populations[75–77]; and 3) the probability of surviving a heart attack is lower for persons with diabetes than for those without diabetes.[78,79] In terms of mechanisms, a high prevalence and aggregation of several risk factors for CAD is already evident in patients with NIDDM even at the time of diagnosis of diabetes. Once NIDDM is clinically manifested, the levels of risk factors increase and perhaps interact with some unknown components of diabetes exposure to augment their effect in ways as yet unknown, particularly in individuals treated with insulin. Finally, the unknown factors that protect nondiabetic women from CAD are lost in diabetic women so that their risk of CAD equals or exceeds that in diabetic men.

Difference in Risk of Coronary Artery Disease in Different NIDDM Populations

Data consistent with the observation made in the Joslin Diabetes Center population that CAD is the major health problem for patients with NIDDM have been obtained in other populations studied in the United States.[75,77,80] However, in some populations with NIDDM, CAD is an infrequent outcome.

The WHO Multinational Study of Vascular Disease in Diabetics has documented marked variation in the occurrence of CAD among 14 samples of middle-age diabetic patients throughout the world.[81,82] In the cross-sectional part of this study conducted in the 1970s, high prevalence rates of indicators of cardiovascular disease, such as electrocardiographic abnormalities and chest pain symptoms, were found in diabetic patients from Switzerland, Berlin, and London. Very low prevalence rates were found in diabetic patients from Tokyo and Hong Kong and in native Americans (Pima) from Arizona.[81] Similar findings were obtained during the 7-year follow-up study. The CAD mortality rate was highest in the samples of diabetic patients from Berlin, Switzerland, and London, whereas it was lowest in patients from Tokyo and Hong Kong and in the Pima.[82]

The low risk of CAD in the Pima with NIDDM is particularly curious.[81–83] This population has the highest incidence of NIDDM in the world, and most of these patients are insulin-resistant and hyperinsulinemic for most of their lives. In addition, the prevalence rates of hypertension and lipid abnormalities in patient with NIDDM in this population are similar to those in populations with a high CAD risk.[81] Furthermore, renal complications develop as frequently in the Pima with diabetes as in the white population with IDDM.[82]

In summary, the wide variation in the occurrence of CAD among different diabetic populations is consistent with the hypothesis that certain components of prediabetic exposures (e.g., hyperinsulinemia), as well as exposures during diabetes, have an impact only on progression of atherosclerotic lesions. However, these exposures have no impact on the frequency of atherosclerosis in diabetic patients from populations among which the initiation of atherosclerosis is infrequent, such as the Pima, Tokyo Japanese, and Hong Kong Chinese.[3,27]

REFERENCES

1. Krolewski AS, Warram JH, Christlieb AR. Onset, course, complications, and prognosis of diabetes mellitus. In: Marble A, Krall LP, Bradley RF, et al., eds. Joslin's diabetes mellitus. 12th ed. Philadelphia: Lea & Febiger, 1985:251–77.

2. Christlieb AR, Warram JH, Krolewski AS, et al. Hypertension: the major risk factor in juvenile-onset insulin-dependent diabetics. Diabetes 1981;30(Suppl 2):90–6.

3. Krolewski AS, Kosinski EJ, Warram JH, et al. Magnitude and determinants of coronary artery disease in juvenile-onset, insulin-dependent diabetes mellitus. Am J Cardiol 1987;59:750–5.

4. United States Life Tables for 1949–51. Vital statistics—special reports. Vol 41, no. 1. Washington, DC: US Public Health Service. National Office of Vital Statistics, 1954:28–9.

5. MacGillivray MH, Voorhess ML, Putnam TI, et al. Hormone and metabolic profiles in children and adolescents with Type I diabetes mellitus. Diabetes Care 1982;5(Suppl 1):38–47.

6. Waldhäusl WK. The physiological basis of insulin treatment—clinical aspects. Diabetologia 1986;29:837–49.

7. Klein R, Klein BEK, Moss SE, et al. Glycosylated hemoglobin in a population-based study of diabetes. Am J Epidemiol 1987;126:415–28.

8. Daneman D, Wolfson DH, Becker DJ, Drash AL. Factors affecting glycosylated hemoglobin values in children with insulin-dependent diabetes. J Pediatr 1981;99:847–53.

9. Janka HU, Warram JH, Rand LI, Krolewski AS. Risk factors for progression of background retinopathy in long-standing IDDM. Diabetes 1989;38:460–4.

10. Fagerberg S-E. Diabetic neuropathy: a clinical and histological study on the significance of vascular affections. Acta Med Scand 1959;164(Suppl 345):1–80.

11. Parving H-H, Viberti GC, Keen H, et al. Hemodynamic factors in the genesis of diabetic microangiopathy. Metabolism 1983;32:943–9.

12. Brownlee M, Cerami A, Vlassara H. Advanced glycosylation end products in tissue and the biochemical basis of diabetic complications. N Engl J Med 1988;318:1315–21.

13. Lee T-S, Saltsman KA, Ohashi H, King GL. Activation of protein kinase C by elevation of glucose concentration: proposal for a mechanism in the development of diabetic vascular complications. Proc Natl Acad Sci USA 1989;86:5141–5.

14. Baynes JW. Role of oxidative stress in development of complications in diabetes. Diabetes 1991;40:405–12.

15. Krolewski AS, Warram JH, Rand LI, Kahn CR. Epidemiologic approach to the etiology of Type I diabetes mellitus and its complications. N Engl J Med 1987;317:1390–8.

16. Palmberg P, Smith M, Waltman S, et al. The natural history of retinopathy in insulin-dependent juvenile-onset diabetes. Ophthalmology 1981;88:613–8.

17. Klein R, Klein BEK, Moss SE, et al. The Wisconsin Epidemiologic Study of Diabetic Retinopathy. II. Prevalence and risk of diabetic retinopathy when age at diagnosis is less than 30 years. Arch Ophthalmol 1984;102:520–6.

18. Krolewski AS, Warram JH, Rand LI, et al. Risk of proliferative diabetic retinopathy in juvenile-onset Type I diabetes: a 40-yr follow-up study. Diabetes Care 1986;9:443–52.

19. Krolewski AS, Barzilay J, Warram JH, et al. Risk of early-onset proliferative retinopathy in IDDM is closely related to cardiovascular autonomic neuropathy. Diabetes 1992;41:430–7.

20. Klein R, Klein BEK, Moss SE, et al. Glycosylated hemoglobin predicts the incidence and progression of diabetic retinopathy. JAMA 1988;260:2864–71.

21. Deckert T, Simonsen SE, Poulsen JE. Prognosis of proliferative retinopathy in juvenile diabetics. Diabetes 1967;16:728–33.

22. Rand LI, Prud'homme GJ, Ederer F, Canner PL. Diabetic Retinopathy Study Research Group. Factors influencing the development of visual loss in advanced diabetic retinopathy. Diabetic Retinopathy Study (DRS): report no. 10. Invest Ophthalmol Vis Sci 1985;26:983–91.

23. Valsania P, Warram JH, Rand IL, Krolewski AS. Different determinants of neovascularization on the optic disc and in the retina in patients with nonproliferative diabetic retinopathy. Arch Ophthalmol 1993;111:202–6.

24. Viberti GC, Hill RD, Jarrett RJ, et al. Microalbuminuria as a predictor of clinical nephropathy in insulin-dependent diabetes mellitus. Lancet 1982;1:1430–2.

25. Mathiesen ER, Oxenbll B, Johansen K, et al. Incipient nephropathy in type 1 (insulin-dependent) diabetes. Diabetologia 1984;26:406–10.

26. Mogensen CE, Christensen CK. Predicting diabetic nephropathy in insulin-dependent patients. N Engl J Med 1984;311:89–93.

27. Krolewski AS, Warram JH, Christlieb AR, et al. The changing natural history of nephropathy in Type I diabetes. Am J Med 1985;78:785–94.

28. Andersen AR, Christiansen JS, Andersen JK, et al. Diabetic nephropathy in type 1 (insulin-dependent) diabetes: an epidemiological study. Diabetologia 1983;25:496–501.

29. Seaquist ER, Goetz FC, Rich S, Barbosa J. Familial clustering of diabetic kidney disease: evidence for genetic susceptibility to diabetic nephropathy. N Engl J Med 1989;320:1161–5.

30. Reeders ST. Genetic factors in diabetic nephropathy [Letter]. N Engl J Med 1989;321:905.

31. Quinn M, Angelico MC, Cross A, et al. Concordance for kidney complications in siblings with IDDM [Abstract no. 433]. Diabetes 1992;41(Suppl 1):121A.

32. Krolewski AS, Doria A, Magre J, et al. Molecular genetic approaches to the identification of genes involved in the development of nephropathy in insulin-dependent diabetes mellitus. J Am Soc Nephrol 1992;3(Suppl 1):S9–17.

33. Viberti GC, Keen H, Wiseman MJ. Raised arterial pressure in parents of proteinuric insulin dependent diabetics. BMJ 1987;295:515–7.

34. Krolewski AS, Canessa M, Warram JH, et al. Predisposition to hypertension and susceptibility to renal disease in insulin-dependent diabetes mellitus. N Engl J Med 1988;318:140–5.

35. Mangili R, Bending JJ, Scott G, et al. Increased sodium-lithium countertransport activity in red cells of patients with insulin-dependent diabetes and nephropathy. N Engl J Med 1988;318:146–50.

36. Barzilay J, Warram JH, Bak M, et al. Predisposition to hypertension: risk factor for nephropathy and hypertension in IDDM. Kidney Int 1992;41:723–30.

37. Kofoed-Enevoldsen A, Borch-Johnsen K, Kreiner S, et al. Declining incidence of persistent proteinuria in Type I (insulin-dependent) diabetic patients in Denmark. Diabetes 1987;36:205–9.

38. Brenner BM. Hemodynamically mediated glomerular injury and the progressive nature of kidney disease. Kidney Int 1983;23:647–55.

39. Krall LP, Joslin AP. General plan of treatment and of diet regulation. In: Marble A, White P, Bradley RF, Krall LP, eds. Joslin's diabetes mellitus. 11th ed. Philadelphia: Lea & Febiger, 1971:255–86.

40. Warram JH, Laffel LMB, Ganda OP, Christlieb AR. Coronary artery disease is the major determinant of excess mortality in patients with insulin-dependent diabetes mellitus and persistent proteinuria. J Am Soc Nephrol 1992;3(Suppl 1):S104–10.

41. Valsania P, Zarich SW, Kowalchuk GJ, et al. Severity of coronary artery disease in young patients with insulin-dependent diabetes mellitus. Am Heart J 1991;122:695–700.

42. Krolewski AS, Warram JH, Valsania P, et al. Evolving natural history of coronary artery disease in diabetes mellitus. Am J Med 1991;90(Suppl 2A):56S–60S.

43. Borch-Johnsen K, Andersen PK, Deckert T. The effect of proteinuria on relative mortality in type 1 (insulin-dependent) diabetes mellitus. Diabetologia 1985;28:590–6.

44. Warram JH, Laffel LMB, Valsania P, et al. Excess mortality associated with diuretic therapy in diabetes mellitus. Arch Intern Med 1991;151:1350–6.

45. Savage PJ, Bennett PH, Gorden P, Miller M. Insulin responses to oral carbohydrate in true prediabetics and matched controls. Lancet 1975;1:300–2.

46. Haffner SM, Stern MP, Hazuda HP, et al. Increased insulin concentrations in nondiabetic offspring of diabetic parents. N Engl J Med 1988;319:1297–301.

47. Warram JH, Martin BC, Krolewski AS, et al. Slow glucose removal rate and hyperinsulinemia precede the development of Type II diabetes in the offspring of diabetic parents. Ann Intern Med 1990;113:909–15.

48. Leibowitz HM, Kreuger DE, Maunder LR, et al. The Framingham Eye Study monograph. V. Diabetic retinopathy. Surv Ophthalmol 1980;24(Suppl):401–59.

49. Klein R, Klein BEK, Moss SE, et al. The Wisconsin Epidemiologic Study of Diabetic Retinopathy. III. Prevalence and risk of diabetic retinopathy when age at diagnosis is 30 or more years. Arch Ophthalmol 1984;102:527–32.

50. Dwyer MS, Melton LJ III, Ballard DJ, et al. Incidence of diabetic retinopathy and blindness: a population-based study in Rochester, Minnesota. Diabetes Care 1985;8:316–22.

51. Ballard DJ, Melton LJ III, Dwyer MS, et al. Risk factors for diabetic retinopathy: a population-based study in Rochester, Minnesota. Diabetes Care 1986;9:334–42.

52. Ballard DJ, Humphrey LL, Melton LJ III, et al. Epidemiology of persistent proteinuria in Type II diabetes mellitus. Population-based study in Rochester, Minnesota. Diabetes 1988;37:405–12.

53. Knatterud GL, Klimt CR, Goldner MG, et al. The University Group Diabetes Program. Effects of hypoglycemic agents on vascular complications in patients with adult-onset diabetes. VIII. Evaluation of insulin therapy: final report. Diabetes 1982;31(Suppl 5):1–81.

54. Humphrey LL, Ballard DJ, Frohnert PP, et al. Chronic renal failure in non-insulin-dependent diabetes mellitus. A population-based study in Rochester, Minnesota. Ann Intern Med 1989;111:788–96.

55. Mogensen CE. Microalbuminuria predicts clinical proteinuria and early mortality in maturity-onset diabetes. N Engl J Med 1984;310:356–60.

56. Schmitz A, Vaeth M. Microalbuminuria: a major risk factor in non-insulin-dependent diabetes. A 10-year follow-up study of 503 patients. Diabetic Med 1988;5:126–34.

57. Mattock MB, Keen H, Viberti GC et al. Coronary heart disease and urinary albumin excretion rate in type 2 (non-insulin-dependent) diabetic patients. Diabetologia 1988;31:82–7.

58. Krolewski AS, Czyzyk A, Kopczynski J, Rywik S. Prevalence of diabetes mellitus, coronary heart disease and hypertension in the families of insulin dependent and insulin independent diabetics. Diabetologia 1981;21:520–4.

59. Jarrett RJ, Shipley MJ. Type 2 (non-insulin-dependent) diabetes mellitus and cardiovascular disease—putative association via common antecedents: further evidence from the Whitehall Study. Diabetologia 1988;31:737–40.

60. Reaven GM. Role of insulin resistance in human disease. Diabetes 1988;37:1595–607.

61. DeFronzo RA, Ferrannini E. Insulin resistance: a multifaceted syndrome responsible for NIDDM, obesity, hypertension, dyslipidemia, and atherosclerotic cardiovascular disease. Diabetes Care 1991;14:173–94.

62. Welborn TA, Wearne K. Coronary heart disease incidence and cardiovascular mortality in Busselton with reference to glucose and insulin concentrations. Diabetes Care 1979;2:154–60.

63. Pyörälä K, Savolainen E, Kaukola S, Haapakoski J. Plasma insulin as coronary heart disease risk factor: relationship to other risk factors and predictive value during 9½-year follow-up of the Helsinki Policemen Study Population. Acta Med Scand Suppl 1985;701:38–52.

64. Fontbonne A, Charles MA, Thibult N, et al. Hyperinsulinaemia as a predictor of coronary heart disease mortality in a healthy population: the Paris prospective study, 15-year follow-up. Diabetologia 1991;34:356–61.

65. Jarrett RJ, McCartney P, Keen H. The Bedford survey: ten year mortality rates in newly diagnosed diabetics, borderline diabetics and normoglycaemic controls and risk indices for coronary heart disease in borderline diabetics. Diabetologia 1982;22:79–84.

66. Uusitupa M, Siitonen O, Aro A, Pyörälä K. Prevalence of coronary heart disease, left ventricular failure and hypertension in middle-aged, newly diagnosed type 2 (non-insulin-dependent) diabetic subjects. Diabetologia 1985;28:22–7.

67. Laakso M, Rönnemaa T, Pyörälä K, et al. Atherosclerotic vascular disease and its risk factors in non-insulin-dependent diabetic and nondiabetic subjects in Finland. Diabetes Care 1988;11:449–63.

68. Assmann G, Schulte H. The prospective cardiovascular Munster (PROCAM) study: prevalence of hyperlipidemia in persons with hypertension and/or diabetes mellitus and the relationship to coronary heart disease. Am Heart J 1988;116:1713–24.

69. Rönnemaa T, Laakso M, Puukka P, et al. Atherosclerotic vascular disease in middle-aged, insulin-treated, diabetic patients: association with endogenous insulin secretion capacity. Arteriosclerosis 1988;8:237–44.

70. Rönnemaa T, Laakso M, Pyörälä K, et al. High fasting plasma insulin is an indicator of coronary heart disease in non-insulin-dependent diabetic patients and nondiabetic subjects. Arterioscler Thromb 1991;11:80–90.

71. Jarrett RJ. Type 2 (non-insulin-dependent) diabetes mellitus and coronary heart disease—chicken, egg or neither? Diabetologia 1984;26:99–102.

72. Patrick CH, Palesch YY, Feinleib M, et al. Sex differences in declining cohort death rates from heart disease. Am J Public Health 1982;72:161–6.

73. Standl E, Janka HU. High serum insulin concentrations in relation to other cardiovascular risk factors in macrovascular disease of type 2 diabetes. Horm Metab Res Suppl 1985;15:46–51.

74. Janka HU, Ziegler AG, Standl E, Mehnert H. Daily insulin dose as a predictor of macrovascular disease in insulin treated non-insulin-dependent diabetics. Diabete Metab (Paris) 1987;13:359–64.

75. Kannel WB, McGee DL. Diabetes and cardiovascular disease: The Framingham Study. JAMA 1979;241:2035–8.

76. Rosengren A, Welin L, Tsipogianna A, Wilhelmsen L. Impact of cardiovascular risk factors on coronary heart disease and mortality among middle aged diabetic men: a general population study. BMJ 1989;299:1127–31.

77. Manson JE, Colditz GA, Stampfer MJ, et al. A prospective study of maturity-onset diabetes mellitus and risk of coronary heart disease and stroke in women. Arch Intern Med 1991;151:1141–7.

78. Czyzyk A, Krolewski AS, Szablowska S, et al. Clinical course of myocardial infarction among diabetic patients. Diabetes Care 1980;3:526–9.

79. Savage MP, Krolewski AS, Kenien GG, et al. Acute myocardial infarction in diabetes mellitus and significance of congestive heart failure as a prognostic factor. Am J Cardiol 1988;62:665–9.

80. Kleinman JC, Donahue RP, Harris MI, et al. Mortality among diabetics in a national sample. Am J Epidemiol 1988;128:389–401.

81. West KM, Ahuja MMS, Bennett PH, et al. The role of circulating glucose and triglyceride concentrations and their interactions with other "risk factors" as determinants of arterial disease in nine diabetic population samples from the WHO Multinational Study. Diabetes Care 1983;6:361–9.

82. Head J, Fuller JH. International variations in mortality among diabetic patients: the WHO Multinational Study of Vascular Disease in Diabetics. Diabetologia 1990;33:477–81.

83. Nelson RG, Sievers ML, Knowler WC, et al. Low incidence of fatal coronary heart disease in Pima Indians despite high prevalence of non-insulin-dependent diabetes. Circulation 1990;81:987–95.

Chapter 36

RELATIONSHIP BETWEEN METABOLIC CONTROL AND LONG-TERM COMPLICATIONS OF DIABETES

DAVID M. NATHAN

For what a man had rather were true, he more readily believes.

—Roger Bacon, 1450

The relationship between metabolic control and development of long-term complications of diabetes mellitus remains one of the most contentious issues in medicine.[1-5] Whether intensive forms of diabetes therapy that have as their goal the achievement of near-normal glycemia will prevent the development or ameliorate the progression of diabetes-associated complications (the only testable question in humans) remains unanswered. In this chapter, the history of the debate and the human studies that shed light on this relationship are reviewed. Where relevant, studies in animal models of diabetes also are discussed. The resolution of this debate will determine future goals for the treatment of both insulin-dependent (Type I) and non-insulin-dependent (Type II) diabetes.

HISTORY

Although the recognition of diabetes mellitus itself has a venerable history,[6] the recognition and description of diabetic complications is relatively new. The first description of retinopathy in diabetes was recorded only 100 years ago,[7] and both the occurrence and character of retinal lesions in relation to diabetes were the subject of active debate as recently as 50 years ago.[8] The classic lesions of diabetic glomerulosclerosis were described less than 60 years ago.[9]

The major reason for the lack of clinical appreciation of diabetic complications is related to their dependence on duration of diabetes, the most potent known risk factor for complications.[10-16] In the pre-insulin era, the limited life-span of patients after their development of Type I diabetes precluded the development of long-term complications. Eight years after the introduction of insulin, diabetic children were described as having "invulnerable" eyes and a future of "limitless hope."[17] Twenty years after insulin became available, however, the results of long-term survival with insulin therapy were noted to include retinopathy, nephropathy, and peripheral and cardiovascular disease.[18-20] In a prescient set of observations made more than 30 years ago, Dolger noted that duration of diabetes appeared to be more important than age at onset or type of therapy, that all patients whose diabetes was of sufficient duration developed retinal lesions, that approximately 50% developed proteinuria, and that complications developed in patients whose long-term metabolic control was judged to be good as well as in those whose metabolic control was poor.[20] On the other hand, several retrospective studies suggested that children with "adequately" controlled diabetes were not vulnerable to growth retardation, cataracts, or retinal hemorrhages.[21] Thus, the debate on the effects of metabolic control on long-term complications was born.

The history of Type II diabetes and long-term complications is even more murky. Until the recent extension of the human life-span and accompanying increase in the prevalence of obesity led to a dramatic increase in the prevalence of Type II diabetes,[22] it was a relatively rare disease. More important, elderly patients with Type II diabetes rarely survived the 10 to 20 years after onset of diabetes that are necessary for the development of clinically significant complications. Major advances in general medical care, and especially in cardiac care, now have allowed older patients with Type II diabetes to live longer. This increased life expectancy has unmasked the risks of long-term complications in Type II diabetes, much as insulin therapy did for Type I diabetes. Type II diabetes is now widely recognized as a cause of duration-dependent complications similar to those in Type I diabetes.[12,14,23–25] Although the frequency of retinopathy and nephropathy is relatively lower in Type II than in Type I diabetes, the tenfold greater prevalence of Type II diabetes makes it the major contributor to visual loss and renal failure secondary to diabetes in the United States.[24,26] The association of Type II diabetes and elevated levels of blood glucose with microvascular complications has been recognized implicitly in the definition of blood glucose criteria for the diagnosis of Type II diabetes. The diagnostic blood glucose criteria for Type II diabetes are predicated on those glucose levels that are accompanied by microvascular complications.[27]

MAJOR ISSUES

Several major questions should be framed before a critical examination of the data is undertaken. The occurrence of retinopathy, nephropathy, and neuropathy as long-term, diabetes-specific complications of all types of diabetes is clear. As noted above, the diagnostic criteria for Type II diabetes include glucose levels selected specifically because of the risk they impart for development of long-term complications, specifically retinopathy. (The profound hyperglycemia and absolute requirement for insulin in Type I diabetes make diagnostic glucose criteria unnecessary.) Persons whose glucose levels are elevated but who are not vulnerable to diabetes-specific complications are not considered diabetic but are described nosologically as having impaired glucose tolerance.[27] Thus, the association of hyperglycemia with certain long-term complications is incorporated into the clinical definition of diabetes, and a glucose threshold for the development of specific complications is implicit in the accepted definition of Type II diabetes.

The glucose hypothesis, i.e., that the long-term complications of diabetes are a consequence of hyperglycemia, is a natural, although fallacious, outgrowth of these observations. Although diabetes of diverse etiologies is defined as being related to both hyperglycemia and long-term complications, the conclusion that one leads to the other, while attractive, is not necessarily true. A primary question, therefore, is what relationship exists between the level of hyperglycemia and the occurrence or development of complications.

Even if the relationship between different levels of hyperglycemia and complications is established and delineated, association does not necessarily impute causation. More important, even if hyperglycemia results in the development or progression of complications, the practical questions of whether control of glucose levels will prevent or reverse complications and what the costs are of such control must be answered.

Important subsidiary questions include the following: 1) Will all diabetes-specific complications respond similarly to changes in glucose level? 2) Is the timing of intervention important, i.e., whether treatment is instituted before the development of any complications (primary prevention) or after the development of complications (secondary intervention)? 3) Does maintenance of a specific glucose level prevent or ameliorate any or all complications? 4) Will different methods (e.g., exogenous administration of insulin vs. pancreatic transplantation) of achieving more normal glycemia have similar effects on complications? 5) Will long-term complications in Type I and Type II diabetes respond similarly to therapy? 6) Will nonspecific macrovascular complications, the severity and frequency of which are increased in diabetes, be affected by therapies directed at achieving glucose levels closer to physiologic values?

RETINOPATHY

Animal Studies

Although none of the animal models of diabetes and its complications are sufficiently similar to human diabetes to provide more than suggestive evidence, they overwhelmingly support the premise that therapies that normalize blood glucose levels can prevent and/or ameliorate retinopathy, nephropathy, and neuropathy. The animal models fall into three different groups. In one model, animals with chemically induced (with alloxan or streptozotocin) diabetes are treated with insulin with the goal of achieving either tight or loose control of blood glucose levels.[28,29] In another model, animals are pancreatectomized and treated with pancreatic or isolated islet cell transplantation.[30,31] Finally, animals with genetic diabetes and various degrees of glycemia have been studied.[32] Most studies have demonstrated efficacy of intensive therapy aimed at maintaining glucose levels close to the physiologic range in preventing primary complications. The ability of intensive diabetes therapy to affect complications once they have been initiated is arguable.

Studies by Engerman et al. of dogs with alloxan-induced diabetes are the most compelling of the animal studies.[28,29] The diabetic dogs developed microaneurysms and pericyte loss similar to those seen in diabetic humans, changes not generally found in nondiabetic dogs. In an early study, therapy with two daily injections of isophane insulin (NPH insulin) with the goal of aglycosuria ("good control") was initiated soon after the dogs were made diabetic.[28] Good control was shown to be associated with fewer microaneurysms than was therapy with one daily injection of isophane insulin ("poor control") over a 5-year period. A later study demonstrated that if dogs with alloxan-induced diabetes were treated with the poor-control regimen for 2.5 years followed by the good-control regimen for 2.5 years, they developed an intermediate number of microaneurysms, suggesting that secondary intervention was not as effective as primary prevention.[29] Of note, severe hypoglycemia resulted in the deaths of several dogs in "good control," presaging the results of human trials.

Human Studies

Type I Diabetes

Early studies that examined the relationship of retinopathy to glucose control used relatively insensitive measures of retinopathy and nonquantitative, imprecise measures of chronic glycemia. Knowles reviewed 47 studies of glucose control and development of complications conducted before 1964 and concluded that the studies were hampered by the absence of quantitative methods of evaluating long-term glucose control and complications and by a poor appreciation of clinical-trial methodology.[33] In the modern era, nondilated ophthalmoscopy has given way to seven-field stereoscopic fundus photography and fluorescein angiography, and sporadic blood glucose measurements and semiquantitative measures of glycosuria have been supplanted by assays for glycosylated hemoglobin (HbA_1 or HbA_{1c}).

Although lacking in these modern innovations, the noninterventional, longitudinal study of Pirart deserves mention, if only for its magnitude.[34] Pirart followed a large (4398) cohort of patients with early- and late-onset diabetes for as long as 25 years. He noted that retinopathy, nephropathy, and neuropathy were more common in patients with a higher glycemic index, a value derived from intermittent measurements of blood and urine glucose levels and other factors. The high attrition rate over time, the lack of objective measures of complications and glycemia, and the possibility that complications led to worsened glucose control—rather than vice versa—detract from this study.

In the modern era, the population-based, observational Wisconsin Epidemiologic Study of Diabetic Retinopathy (WESDR) examined an unselected population of diabetic residents of Wisconsin over time using measurements of glycosylated hemoglobin and seven-field stereoscopic fundus photography. Follow-up over 4 years included more than 90% of the original subjects and revealed a striking association between the incidence of any retinopathy, progression of retinopathy, progression to proliferative retinopathy,[35] macular edema,[36] and vision loss[37] and the level of glycosylated hemoglobin at baseline. The relationship between levels of glycosylated hemoglobin and retinopathy was continuous; no threshold for glycosylated hemoglobin with regard to risk of retinopathy was noted. The observed associations remained after the comparisons were controlled for duration of diabetes, age, and baseline retinopathy. Although WESDR subjects were not strictly categorized as Type I and Type II diabetics, the separation by age of onset (<30 years vs. ≥30 years) effectively provided Type I and Type II populations. Other observational studies have confirmed these findings in more-selected Type I populations[38–41] and have suggested that higher glycemic levels are a risk factor for the development of proliferative retinopathy.[16,39,41]

Although of interest, cross-sectional and longitudinal observational studies can only indicate associations between glycemic control (and other confounders) and complications. Randomized, controlled interventional clinical trials are required to document the effects of treatments designed to achieve near-normal glucose control on the development and progression of complications. The introduction and refinement of methods for self-monitoring of blood glucose levels and of intensive therapies, such as continuous subcutaneous insulin infusion (CSII) with pumps and multiple daily injection (MDI) regimens,[42] provided the opportunity to test whether such therapies would have salutary effects. Four well-designed randomized studies have been completed,[43–46] and the Diabetes Control and Complications Trial (DCCT), the most comprehensive of the clinical trials, is ongoing.[47–49]

The first four clinical trials included the multicenter study by the Kroc Collaborative Study Group,[43] and studies by the Steno Study Group,[44] the Oslo group,[45] and the Stockholm Diabetes Intervention Study group[46] (Table 36–1). All of these trials were secondary intervention studies, including only subjects with retinal lesions at baseline. In all of these studies, the mean duration of diabetes was relatively long. The duration of the trials ranged from 8 to 60 months and included 30 to 100 subjects. (By contrast, the DCCT is studying 1441 subjects with a mean follow-up of 7 years.) The total number of patient-years of study was less than 800 in the four previous secondary intervention trials combined. The total number of patient-years for the secondary-intervention component of the DCCT will be 5000 at the end of the study in 1993. Except for the Oslo study,

Table 36–1. Clinical Trials of Glycemic Control and Retinopathy in Type I Diabetes

Study	No. of Subjects	Range (mean) Duration[†] (yr)	Study Duration (mo)	Therapy[‡]
Kroc[43]	68	<30 (17)	8	Std vs. CSII
Steno[44]	30	9–33 (19)	24	Std vs. CSII
Oslo[45]	45	6–30 (13)	41	Std vs. MDI vs. CSII
Stockholm[46]	100	(17)	60	Std vs. MDI
DCCT*[49]				
Primary prevention	726	1–5 (2.6)	60–120	Std vs. CSII or MDI
Secondary intervention	715	1–15 (8.7)	60–120	Std vs. CSII or MDI

*DCCT = Diabetes Control and Complications Trial.
†Duration of diabetes at baseline.
‡Std = standard, conventional; CSII = continuous subcutaneous insulin infusion (external pump); MDI = multiple (≥3) daily injections of insulin.

which included two intensive-treatment groups, the studies compared Type I diabetic patients randomly assigned to conventional treatment with patients randomly assigned to CSII (Kroc and Steno) or MDI (Stockholm). The results of the Kroc,[43] Steno,[44,50] Oslo,[45,51] and Stockholm[46] studies were similar with regard to retinopathy. (End results of the Stockholm study have yet to be published; only interim results are available.) In the first 6 to 12 months, the Kroc, Steno, and Oslo studies demonstrated a transient worsening of retinopathy in the patients receiving intensive treatment (Table 36–2). By the end of the study, no significant differences were seen between treatment groups in any of the published studies, although the groups receiving intensive treatment maintained significantly lower levels of glycosylated hemoglobin than did those receiving standard treatment (Fig. 36–1). The Steno and Oslo study groups performed a meta-analysis of their combined results, after eliminating the MDI treatment group of the Oslo study, and concluded that intensive treatment decreases retinopathy risk.[52] The validity of this analysis has been questioned; when the Oslo results for MDI are included in the analysis, the difference between the retinopathy risks of the standard- and intensive-treatment groups evaporates.[53]

The DCCT, initiated in 1982, includes both a secondary intervention study, as did the previous clinical trials, and a primary prevention cohort, composed of 13- to 39-year-old volunteers with 1 to 5 years of Type I diabetes and no retinopathy, as based on the findings from seven-field stereoscopic fundus photography at baseline.[47] The more than 700 subjects in each of the primary prevention and secondary intervention cohorts will be studied for 5 to 10 years. The probability is greater than 90% of the study detecting a change as small as 33% in the hazard rate for either the appearance of retinopathy or the progression of retinopathy in the primary prevention and secondary intervention studies, respectively. Although the study can be terminated before its full term if the external monitoring group discovers a statistically and clinically significant difference between the two treatment groups, the DCCT continues in its eighth year. The investigators remain masked to the study outcomes until study

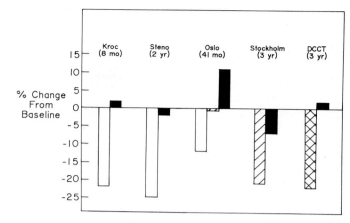

Fig. 36–1. Change of glycosylated hemoglobin level from baseline in five controlled clinical trials. Solid box: Conventional treatment. Open box: Continuous subcutaneous insulin infusion (CSII). Diagonal: Multiple daily injections of insulin (MDI). Hatched: CSII or MDI.

completion, so all of the interim publications have described only design, methods, and baseline analyses.

Type II Diabetes

An association between retinopathy and glycemia similar to that for Type I diabetes has recently been demonstrated for Type II diabetes. Both the WESDR[12] and a study of Type II diabetes in an aging population (55 to 75 years old)[14] showed that the relative risk of developing retinopathy increases as the level of HbA_{1c} increases (Fig. 36–2). The only clinical trial that examined the impact of glycemic control on retinopathy in Type II diabetes was that of the University Group Diabetes Program (UGDP).[54] This multicenter trial compared the effects of five different treatment modalities

Table 36–2. Results of Controlled Clinical Trials of Intensive Diabetes Therapy: Effects on Progression of Retinopathy

Study	Intensive vs. Conventional Therapy*
Kroc[43]	Intensive worse at 8 mo
Steno[44,50]	Intensive worse at 1 yr, NS at 24 mo
Oslo[45,51]	Intensive worse at 6 mo, NS at 41 mo
Stockholm[46]	NS at 36 mo†
DCCT‡	Pending

*NS = no significant difference between intensive therapy group and conventional therapy group.
†Five-year results pending.
‡DCCT = Diabetes Control and Complications Trial.

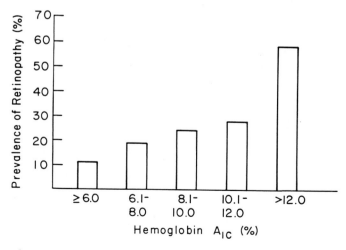

Fig. 36–2. Association between mean glucose level as measured by level of glycosylated hemoglobin (HbA_{1c}) and presence of retinopathy in older patients (55 to 75 years) with Type II diabetes.[14]

(diet, diet plus tolbutamide, diet plus phenformin, diet plus standard insulin dose, and diet plus variable-dose insulin) on long-term outcome in patients with newly diagnosed Type II diabetes. Although the variable-dose insulin regimen maintained mean fasting levels of blood glucose approximately 20% lower than baseline levels, compared with no significant changes from baseline glucose values over time with the other treatment regimens, no significant differences between any of the groups were noted in the degree of retinopathy as measured by fundus photography. Although far from definitive, the UGDP trial is the longest-duration and largest-scale controlled clinical trial of diabetes therapy and complications in Type II diabetes. The ongoing U.K. Prospective study[55] and a recently initiated multicenter Veterans Administration study may provide more satisfactory data.

In summary, an association between glycemia and retinopathy in Type I and Type II diabetes has been established in studies using accurate measures of retinopathy and chronic glycemia. The putative salutary effect of intensive treatment regimens directed at achieving near-normal glucose levels on established retinopathy, however, has not been demonstrated in the four clinical trials completed to date. Whether the inability of these trials to demonstrate efficacy is secondary to an incorrect hypothesis, inadequate power (type II error), inadequate glucose control, lengthy duration of diabetes before intervention, or other factors is unknown. The DCCT has sufficient power to detect even a relatively small difference between treatment groups and also will examine the effects of intensive therapy in the prevention of retinopathy.

Putative risk factors for diabetic retinopathy, other than the level of glycemia, include hypertension,[56] pregnancy,[57] and a family history of diabetic retinopathy.[58]

NEPHROPATHY

Animal Studies

Although glomerular lesions in several animal models of diabetes are similar to those seen in diabetic nephropathy in humans, the time course of the development of the lesions is different from that in human diabetes. In addition, the contribution of other factors that play important roles in the genesis of human diabetic nephropathy, cannot be evaluated in these models. As with retinopathy, studies of nephropathy in animal models can lend support to, but cannot prove, the glucose hypothesis.

Studies in animal models appear to demonstrate that nephropathy can be prevented or even reversed when diabetic animals are treated with pancreatic transplantation or with intensive insulin therapy. Rats with streptozotocin-induced diabetes develop mesangial thickening with immunoglobulin deposition within 6 to 9 months of diabetes onset.[30] Successful islet transplantation can prevent the development of such lesions or lead to stabilization and some improvement in established lesions concurrent with normalization of glucose levels.[30]

Several fundamental problems apply to this model. First, diabetic rats develop a renal lesion (mesangial expansion) that is distinctly different from the early lesion of human nephropathy (glomerular basement membrane expansion) and do not develop end-stage renal failure. Second, other potentially important variables that might predict or influence development of nephropathy in humans (e.g., hypertension) cannot be studied in animal models. Third, rats in which transplants of pancreatic islet cells do not succeed in correcting glucose levels also show improvements in renal results.[30] Despite these objections, studies in other animal models such as the BB/W rat (spontaneously diabetic)[59] and uninephrectomized, alloxan-treated dog[60] tend to support the role of glucose control in the genesis of nephropathy.

Human Studies

Diabetic nephropathy poses several different problems, when compared with retinopathy, regarding the analysis of its association with glucose levels and of the effects of intensive therapy on its development and course. The natural history of diabetic nephropathy, although duration-dependent, extends over many more years than retinopathy before clinical expression becomes evident.[61,62] Generally, a minimum of 12 years and usually 15 to 18 years of Type I diabetes is required before the development of clinical-grade (dipstick-positive, i.e., ≥500 mg/24 hours) proteinuria, the first incontrovertible sign of developing end-stage renal disease. After the development of clinical-grade proteinuria, a mean of 5 years is required for the decline in creatinine clearance that terminates in end-stage renal disease.[63] Thus, compared with the time course of diabetic retinopathy, for which signs will appear in 50% of individuals within 5 to 7 years of diabetes onset, the time course for the development of clinical nephropathy (dipstick-positive proteinuria), when it occurs, is much prolonged, requiring a duration of diabetes of approximately 15 years.

With the reluctance to perform kidney biopsies early in the course of diabetes for documentation of microscopic changes in the glomerulus and the less than perfect correlation between microscopic changes and clinical course, surrogate markers of evolving nephropathy have tentatively been identified. "Incipient" nephropathy, as demonstrated by microalbuminuria (generally >20−30 mg and <300 mg of urinary albumin/24 hours), has been identified as a predictor or marker for the development of end-stage renal disease in retrospective studies of Type I[64−67] (Table 36−3) and Type II diabetes.[68] Unfortunately, microalbuminuria can vary considerably in individuals over time, with levels fluctuating from abnormal to normal values. Therefore, a urinary albumin excretion rate of >20 μg/minute (>28 mg/24 hours) but <200 μg/minute (<288 mg/24 hours) in at least two of three urine collections within a 6-month period has been suggested as a definition of "persistent" microalbuminuria.[69] In addition, microalbuminuria may not be a predictor of nephropathy unless hypertension and a decreasing glomerular filtration rate (GFR) also are

Table 36–3. Longitudinal Studies of Microalbuminuria as a Risk Factor for Development of Clinical Proteinuria in Type I Diabetes Mellitus

Study	No. of Subjects	Diabetes Duration* (yr)	Study Duration (yr)	Baseline UAER† (mg/24 hr)	Progression to Dipstick-Positive Proteinuria (%)	RR‡
Viberti et al.[64]	55	7	14	<43	4	
	8	14		43–202	88	24
Parving et al.[65]	15	15	6	<35	13	
	8	19		80–153	50	3.8
Mathiessen et al.[66]	64	13	6	<100	5	
	7	19		>100	100	21
Mogensen and Christensen[67]	29	13	10	<22	0	
	14	13		>22	86	...

*At baseline.
†UAER = urinary albumin excretion rate.
‡Relative risk for development of clinical proteinuria for subjects with higher baseline UAER.

present.[70] Finally, all the data indicating an association between microalbuminuria and nephropathy are retrospective in nature. Whether any intervention that affects this presumed marker for nephropathy also will affect the course of nephropathy has yet to be demonstrated. Despite these limitations, changes in microalbuminuria have been used as renal end points in many controlled trials.

There are several reasons to suspect that the association between glucose control and nephropathy may be more complex than that with retinopathy. The occurrence of nephropathy in no more than 40% of patients with Type I diabetes and 25% of patients with Type II diabetes suggests that variables other than glycemia are operant. Hypertension and family history of hypertension have been suggested as possible mediators of nephropathy.[71,72]

Type I Diabetes

The association between levels of glycemia and nephropathy has not been as clearly delineated as that for retinopathy. Although the Pirart study[34] demonstrated an association between the derived glycemic index and an increase in creatinine level over time, cross-sectional or longitudinal studies using objective measurements of glycemia and proteinuria are rare and have not consistently revealed such an association. Only one longitudinal study has demonstrated an association between mean levels of glycosylated hemoglobin, measured over 7 years, and risk of microalbuminuria in Type I diabetes.[73] Although this association persisted when age and duration of diabetes were taken into account, measurements of microalbuminuria at baseline, blood pressure, and other possible confounders were not considered in the analysis.

Potential reasons for the difficulty in establishing a relationship between glycemia and nephropathy, if such a relationship exists, are numerous. First, the development of renal failure may influence glycemic control in a number of ways (e.g., alterations in sensitivity to insulin and development of hypertension and effects of antihypertensive medications on glycemia). Second, uremia,

anemia, and transfusions may interfere with or influence the accuracy of measurements of glycosylated hemoglobin. Finally, and most importantly, given the long duration of diabetes necessary before the development of renal failure, it is unlikely that infrequent measurements of glycosylated hemoglobin, representing a relatively brief period of exposure, would be predictive of the development of nephropathy.

Although the association between glucose control and nephropathy is not well established, studies in animal models have encouraged investigators to pursue this topic. Interventional studies are required to examine whether intensive treatment of diabetes will influence the development or progression of nephropathy. Early uncontrolled studies suggested that intensive diabetes therapy with CSII for periods as brief as 24 to 72 hours could decrease mean rates of urinary albumin excretion from 38 to 18 mg/24 hours[74] (Table 36–4). On the other hand, intensive therapy implemented at later stages of nephropathy, i.e., after clinical grade proteinuria had developed, were not effective.[75,79] The Kroc study was the first randomized, controlled trial to note an effect of intensive therapy on the progression of proteinuria when subjects were stratified according to retrospectively chosen cut-off levels of baseline albuminuria.[43] Other controlled trials have demonstrated insignificant[80,81] or only modest and questionably meaningful[77] differences in relatively low levels of baseline albuminuria when intensive treatment was compared with conventional treatment. Examination of the progression to clinical proteinuria (>500 mg/24 hours) has been more revealing. Although the Steno study of incipient nephropathy did not demonstrate any effects of intensive therapy, as compared with the effects of standard therapy, on GFR or albuminuria after 12 months,[82] after 24 months significantly fewer intensively treated than conventionally treated subjects progressed to clinical-grade (>300 mg of urinary albumin/24 hours) proteinuria[76] (Table 36–5). Three-year results from the Stockholm Diabetes Study have confirmed a reduction in progression to clinical-grade proteinuria with intensive therapy, although the number of subjects at risk (with microalbuminuria) was greater in the conventional treatment group at baseline.[78]

Table 36–4. Clinical Trials of Intensive Treatment and Nephropathy

Study	No. of Subjects	Diabetes Duration (yr)	Study Duration	UAER Therapy	Pre	Post	Significance (P*) Pre vs. Post	Intergroup
Viberti et al.[74]	7	15	3 d	CSII	55	25	<.02	...
Kroc[43]	20[†]		8 mo	Conv	9.6	9.8	NS	...
	19[†]			CSII	7.9	9.8	NS	...
	10[‡]			Conv			NS	...
	10[‡]			CSII	70	23	<.02	...
Steno[76]	18	15	12 mo	Conv	62	68	NS	NS
	18	15		CSII	63	60	NS	NS
			24 mo	Conv	160	360[§]	NS	
				CSII	170	160[§]	NS	<.05
Oslo[77]	15	13	48 mo	Conv	21	22	NS	
	15	13		MDI	17	14	NS	
	15	13		CSII	26	16	<.01	<.03
Stockholm[78]	51	18	36 mo	Conv	1.4	1.6[¶]	<.05	
	44	16		MDI	1.3	1.3	NS	<.05

Abbreviations: UAER = urinary albumi excretion rate (expressed as mg/24 hr unless noted); CSII = continuous subcutaneous insulin infusion; Conv = conventional therapy; MDI = multiple daily injections; Pre and Post = before and after therapy, respectively.
*Pre vs. Post = comparison within group; Intergroup = comparison between intensive therapy group and conventional therapy group from baseline to end of study.
[†]Stratified by baseline UAER <17 mg/24 hr.
[‡]Stratified by baseline UAER ≥17 mg/24 hr.
[§]Expressed as median fractional UAER.
[¶]Expressed as albuminuria index (/24 hr): 1 = <29 mg; 2 = 29 to 287 mg; 3 = >288 mg.

Although retinopathy is the primary study end point in the DCCT, microalbuminuria and glomerular filtration (creatinine clearance and iothalamate clearance) are being carefully studied. Eligibility criteria for the primary prevention and secondary intervention cohorts include a urinary albumin excretion rate (UAER) of <40 mg/24 hours and <200 mg/24 hours, respectively. The mean UAER at baseline is 11.8 mg/24 hours in the primary prevention group and 20 mg/24 hours in the secondary intervention group.[49] The large number of subjects and relatively long follow-up should provide more useful data regarding the ability of intensive therapy to prevent development and affect progression of diabetic nephropathy.

Type II Diabetes

An association between glycemia and renal disease (persistent proteinuria) has been demonstrated in one study of Type II diabetes,[83] and only one study has examined the effect of diabetes therapy on microalbuminuria in Type II diabetes.[84] Hypocaloric dietary treatment of obese, glucose-intolerant Pima Indians resulted in improved glycemia with weight loss and a significant decrease in microalbuminuria. Whether the change in blood glucose levels or the decrease in protein intake and/or blood pressure that accompanied the diet and weight loss was responsible for the decreased proteinuria is unknown. In the UGDP study, measurements of renal function through analyses of serum creatinine, creatinine clearance, and urinary protein did not reveal significant differences between therapy groups over time.[54]

In summary, the results of intensive treatment on nephropathy are somewhat more encouraging than those for retinopathy. Although data regarding primary prevention of nephropathy (prevention of development of renal lesions or microalbuminuria) with intensive diabetes therapy are not convincing, the apparent slowing of progression of microalbuminuria to clinical-grade proteinuria is an important finding. The duration of the

Table 36–5. Effect of Intensive Therapy on Progression to Clinical Proteinuria

Study	Duration of Therapy (mo)	Therapy	End-Point UAER (/24 hr)	No. With Progression/No. Treated
Steno[76]	24	Conv	>300 mg	5/18
		CSII		0/18
Stockholm[78]	36	Conv	>288 mg	5/13*
		MDI		1/8*

Abbreviations: UAER = urinary albumin excretion rate; Conv = conventional therapy; CSII = continuous subcutaneous insulin infusion; MDI = multiple daily injections.
*Baseline UAER = 29 to 288 mg/24 hr.

secondary-intervention effect, noted in the Steno[76] and Stockholm[78] studies, has not been studied. Whether intensive treatment merely delays progression to end-stage renal disease or actually halts the progression is unknown. Variables that may confound results in these studies include treatment of hypertension[85] and dietary protein content.[86]

NEUROPATHY

Diabetic neuropathy is composed of several protean elements, including distal, symmetrical, somatosensory neuropathy and autonomic neuropathy, both of presumed metabolic origin, and mononeuropathies, presumably of vascular origin. Although electrophysiologic measures of nerve conduction have been available for more than 30 years, their questionable relevance to symptomatic clinical diabetic neuropathy has made the study of glucose control and neuropathy problematic. For example, the early observation that insulin treatment of new-onset Type I diabetes increased slowed motor nerve conduction within 6 weeks in asymptomatic patients supported an acute effect of hyperglycemia on nerve conduction and cast doubt on the role of electrophysiologic testing.[87] The absence of histologic (sural nerve biopsy) has been a major impediment to our understanding of diabetic neuropathy. A weak association between glycemia and motor and sensory nerve conduction has been documented in Type I[88] and Type II[89] diabetes. Although uncontrolled[90] and controlled, randomized trials[91–93] have demonstrated improvements in motor nerve conduction,[92,93] sensory nerve conduction,[92] and sensory function[91,92] with intensive treatment, the changes have invariably been modest and of questionable clinical significance. In the DCCT, newly introduced quantitative measures of autonomic nerve function are being used in addition to measures of motor and sensory nerve function.

MACROVASCULAR DISEASE

The multifactorial etiology of cardiovascular disease (CVD) makes it unlikely that the association established between levels of glycemia and complications specific to diabetes such as retinopathy also will pertain to CVD. Almost all studies have been in populations with Type II diabetes or impaired glucose tolerance (IGT). Although the presence of diabetes (or IGT) increases the prevalence of CVD,[94–97] an association between the level of glycemia and the occurrence of CVD has not been easy to demonstrate.[98] Recently, however, studies that used more accurate measures of long-term glycemia found a correlation between glycemic levels and prevalence of CVD.[99,100] In the Framingham Study, level of HbA_{1c} correlated with prevalence of CVD, but only in women.[100] Whether diabetes affects CVD directly or through the established risk factors that accompany it, such as hypertension, hyperlipidemia, and obesity (in Type II diabetes), or through putative risk factors, such as hyperinsulinemia, is not known. The only randomized trial of diabetes intervention and CVD has been the UGDP trial, which did not demonstrate any impact of glucose control on CVD outcome.[54] The DCCT will examine macrovascular disease as an outcome, but its relatively young Type I population is unlikely to experience enough CVD events during the 10-year course of the study to provide any definitive answers.

CONCLUSIONS

Although several important issues in the study of metabolic control and diabetic complications have been settled, many important questions remain unanswered. With the use of objective measures that reflect long-term glycemia, epidemiologic studies have established a clear association between level of glycemia and occurrence of retinopathy but not nephropathy. The more relevant clinical question of whether intensive treatment aimed at achieving near-normal glucose levels will prevent or affect the progression of complications has been addressed in controlled clinical trials. To date, evidence has not emerged to support a salutary effect on retinopathy of intensive therapy as primary prevention or secondary intervention. Whether this lack of evidence is due to inadequate power, inadequate study duration, or imperfect glucose control in previous trials; to the inability to affect the course of retinopathy once lesions are established (in all completed trials, intervention has been secondary in nature); or to other factors is unknown. The DCCT, which includes both primary prevention and secondary intervention cohorts, has sufficient power to answer these questions.

With regard to nephropathy, no uniform effect of intensive therapy on relatively low-grade microalbuminuria has been demonstrated. Moreover, the relevance of any changes in such modest microalbuminuria with regard to development of end-stage renal disease needs to be established. On the other hand, two relatively small studies have demonstrated that intensive therapy can diminish the fraction of patients who progress from microalbuminuria to clinical-grade (dipstick-positive) proteinuria. This finding represents the strongest support for the glucose hypothesis in human diabetes. Whether the effect will be sustained or whether progression towards end-stage renal disease will continue, albeit at a slower rate, must be investigated. The DCCT will provide more detailed information on the long-term effects of intensive therapy on nephropathy.

Finally, for any benefits that accrue with intensive therapy, the costs of the therapy, both in terms of complications of therapy and financial cost, must be balanced against the benefits. The major complications of currently available intensive therapies have been described by the DCCT and include a two- to threefold increase in minor and severe hypoglycemia,[101] catheter-related problems such as infections and lipodystrophy for patients treated with external pumps, and weight gain.[102] The only currently established indication for intensive therapy in IDDM for which the benefits outweigh the risks is during pregnancy, or preferably in women planning pregnancy.[103] The benefit that accrues is for the neonate, rather than for the mother.[104]

Should the DCCT demonstrate an effect of intensive therapy on complications, critical questions will remain. Whether any results can be extrapolated to Type II diabetes will be of major interest, given the importance of this highly prevalent form of diabetes as a cause of morbidity and mortality. In addition, whether cardiovascular disease can be ameliorated will be another crucial issue for investigation. With the prospect of the emergence of scientifically satisfying, clinically relevant information during the next 1 to 2 years that will validate or disprove the glucose hypothesis, clinicians and patients need to postpone, or at least temper, their enthusiasm regarding intensive therapy. Currently, the risks of such therapy outweigh the documented benefits in nonpregnant diabetic patients. Answers that will guide rational therapy of diabetes mellitus are on the horizon.

REFERENCES

1. Cahill GF Jr, Etzwiler DD, Freinkel N. "Control" and diabetes [Editorial]. N Engl J Med 1976;294:1004–5.
2. Siperstein MD, Foster DW, Knowles HC Jr, et al. Control of blood glucose and diabetic vascular disease [Editorial]. N Engl J Med 1977;296:1060–3.
3. Ingelfinger FJ. Debates on diabetes. N Engl J Med 1977;296:1228–30.
4. Siperstein MD. Diabetic microangiopathy and the control of blood glucose. N Engl J Med 1983;309:1577–9.
5. Stern MP, Haffner SM. Prospective assessment of metabolic control in diabetes mellitus: the complications question. JAMA 1988;260:2896–7.
6. Von Engelhardt D, et al, eds. Diabetes: its medical and cultural history. New York: Springer-Verlag, 1989.
7. Nettleship E. Chronic retinitis, with formation of bloodvessels in the vitreous in a patient with diabetes; one eye lost by results of chronic iritis, accompanied by the formation of large vessels in the iris. Trans Ophthalmol Soc UK 1888;8:159–61.
8. Ballantyne AJ, Loewenstein A. The pathology of diabetic retinopathy. Trans Ophthalmol UK 1943;63:95–115.
9. Kimmelstiel P, Wilson C. Intercapillary lesions in the glomeruli of the kidney. Am J Pathol 1936;12:83–97.
10. Palmberg P, Smith M, Waltman S, et al. The natural history of retinopathy in insulin-dependent juvenile-onset diabetes. Ophthalmology 1981;88:613–8.
11. Frank RN, Hoffman WH, Podgor MJ, et al. Retinopathy in juvenile-onset Type I diabetes of short duration. Diabetes 1982;31:874–84.
12. Klein R, Klein BEK, Moss SE, et al. The Wisconsin epidemiologic study of diabetic retinopathy. III. Prevalence and risk of diabetic retinopathy when age at diagnosis is 30 or more years. Arch Ophthalmol 1984;102:527–32.
13. Klein R, Klein BEK, Moss SE, et al. The Wisconsin epidemiologic study of diabetic retinopathy. II. Prevalence and risk of diabetic retinopathy when age at diagnosis is less than 30 years. Arch Ophthalmol 1984;102:520–6.
14. Nathan DM, Singer DE, Godine JE, et al. Retinopathy in older Type II diabetics: association with glucose control. Diabetes 1986;35:797–801.
15. Ballard DJ, Melton LJ III, Dwyer MS, et al. Risk factors for diabetic retinopathy: a population-based study in Rochester, Minnesota. Diabetes Care 1986;334–42.
16. Krolewski AS, Warram JH, Rand LI, et al. Risk of proliferative diabetic retinopathy in juvenile-onset Type I diabetes: a-40 year follow-up study. Diabetes Care 1986;9:443–52.
17. White P. The future of the diabetic child. JAMA 1930;95:1160–2.
18. Joslin EP. Insulin's twenty-fifth anniversary. Diabetes Abstracts 1945;5:37.
19. Wagener HP. Retinopathy in diabetes mellitus. Proc Am Diabetes Assoc 1943;5:201–16.
20. Dolger H. Clinical evaluation of vascular damage in diabetes mellitus. JAMA 1947;134:1289–91.
21. Boyd JD, Jackson RL, Allen JH. Avoidance of degenerative lesions in diabetes mellitus. JAMA 1942;118:694–6.
22. Harris MI, Hadden WC, Knowler WC, Bennett PH. Prevalence of diabetes and impaired glucose tolerance and plasma glucose levels in U.S. population aged 20–74 yr. Diabetes 1987;36:523–4.
23. Nathan DM, Singer DE, Godine JE, Perlmuter LC. Non-insulin-dependent diabetes in older patients. Am J Med 1986;81:837–42.
24. Humphrey LL, Ballard DJ, Frohnert PP, et al. Chronic renal failure in non-insulin-dependent diabetes mellitus: a population based study in Rochester, Minnesota. Ann Intern Med 1989;111:788–96.
25. Cowie CC, Port FK, Wolfe RA, et al. Disparities in incidence of diabetic end-stage renal disease according to race and type of diabetes. N Engl J Med 1989;321:1074–9.
26. Dwyer MS, Melton LJ III, Ballard DJ, et al. Incidence of diabetic retinopathy and blindness: a population based study in Rochester Minnesota. Diabetes Care 1985;8:316–22.
27. National Diabetes Data Group. Classification and diagnosis of diabetes mellitus and other categories of glucose intolerance. Diabetes 1979;28:1039–57.
28. Engerman R, Bloodworth JMB Jr, Nelson, S. Relationship of microvascular disease in diabetes to metabolic control. Diabetes 1977;26:760–9.
29. Engerman RL, Kern TS. Progression of incipient diabetic retinopathy during good glycemic control. Diabetes 1987;36:808–12.
30. Mauer SM, Steffes MW, Sutherland DER, et al. Studies of the rate of regression of the glomerular lesions in diabetic rats treated with pancreatic islet transplantation. Diabetes 1975;24:280–5.
31. Gray BN, Watkins E Jr. Prevention of vascular complications of diabetes by pancreatic islet transplantation. Arch Surg 1976;254–7.
32. Cohen AJ, McGill PD, Rossetti RG, et al. Glomerulopathy in spontaneously diabetic rat. Diabetes 1977;36:944–51.
33. Knowles HC Jr. The problem of the relation of the control of diabetes to the development of vascular disease. Trans Am Clin Climatol Assoc 1964;76:142–47.
34. Pirart J. Diabetes mellitus and its degenerative complications: a prospective study of 4,400 patients observed between 1947 and 1973. Diabetes Care 1978;1:168–88, 252–66.
35. Klein R, Klein BEK, Moss SE, et al. Glycosylated hemoglobin predicts the incidence and progression of diabetic retinopathy. JAMA 1988;260:2864–71.
36. Klein R, Moss SE, Klein BEK, et al. The Wisconsin epidemiologic study of diabetic retinopathy. XI. The incidence of macular edema. Ophthalmology 1989;96:1501–10.
37. Moss SE, Klein R, Klein BEK. The incidence of vision loss

in a diabetic population. Ophthalmology 1989; 95:1340−8.

38. Doft BH, Kingsley LA, Orchard TJ, et al. The association between long-term diabetic control and early retinopathy. Ophthalmology 1984;91:763−9.

39. McCance DR, Atkinson AB, Hadden DR, et al. Long-term glycaemic control and diabetic retinopathy. Lancet 1989; 2:824−8.

40. Weber B, Burger W, Hartmann R, et al. Risk factors for the development of retinopathy in children and adolescents with Type I (insulin-dependent) diabetes mellitus. Diabetologia 1986;29:23−9.

41. Groop LC, Teir H, Koskimies S, et al. Risk factors and markers associated with proliferative retinopathy in patients with insulin-dependent diabetes. Diabetes 1986; 35:1397−1403.

42. Nathan DM. Modern management of insulin-dependent diabetes mellitus. Med Clin North Am 1988;72:1365−78.

43. The Kroc Collaborative Study Group. Blood glucose control and the evolution of diabetic retinopathy and albuminuria: a preliminary multicenter trial. N Engl J Med 1984;6:365−72.

44. Lauritzen T, Frost-Larsen K, Larsen H-W, Deckert T. The Steno Study Group: two-year experience with continuous subcutaneous insulin infusion in relation to retinopathy and neuropathy. Diabetes 1985;34(Suppl 3):74−9.

45. Brinchmann-Hansen O, Dahl-Jorgensen K, Hanssen KF-,Sandvik L. The response of diabetic retinopathy to 41 months of multiple insulin injections, insulin pumps, and conventional insulin therapy. Arch Ophthalmol 1988; 106:1242−6.

46. Reichard P, Britz A, Carlsson I, et al. Metabolic control and complications over 3 years in patients with IDDM: the Stockholm Diabetes Intervention Study (SDIS). J Intern Med 1990;228:511−7.

47. DCCT Research Group. The Diabetes Control and Complications Trial (DCCT): design and methodologic considerations for the feasibility phase. Diabetes 1986; 35:530−45.

48. DCCT Research Group. Diabetes Control and Complications Trial (DCCT): results of the feasibility study. Diabetes Care 1987;10:1−19.

49. DCCT Research Group. Diabetes Control and Complications Trial (DCCT): update. Diabetes Care 1990; 13:427−33.

50. Lauritzen T, Larsen H-W, Larsen K-F, Deckert T, and the Steno Study Group. Effect of 1 year of near-normal blood glucose levels on retinopathy in insulin-dependent diabetics. Lancet 1983;1:200−4.

51. Dahl-Jorgensen K, Brinchmann-Hansen O, Hanssen KF, et al. Rapid tightening of blood glucose control leads to transient deterioration of retinopathy in insulin dependent diabetes mellitus: the Oslo study. BMJ 1985; 290:811−5.

52. Hanssen KF, Dahl-Jorgensen K, Lauritzen T, et al. Diabetic control and microvascular complications: the near-normoglycaemic experience. Diabetologia 1986; 29:677−84.

53. DCCT Research Group. Are continuing studies of metabolic control and microvascular complications in insulin-dependent diabetes mellitus justified? The Diabetes Control and Complications Trial. N Engl J Med 1988; 318:246−50.

54. University Group Diabetes Program. A study of the effects of hypoglycemic agents on vascular complications in patients with adult-onset diabetes. VI. Supplementary report on nonfatal events in patients treated with tolbutamide. Diabetes 1976;25:1129−53.

55. Turner RC, Mann JI, Iceton S, et al. Multi-centre study: UK prospective study of therapies of maturity-onset diabetes. I. Effect of diet, sulphonylurea, insulin or biguanide therapy on fasting plasma glucose and body weight over one year. Diabetologia 1983;24:404−11.

56. Knowler WC, Bennett PH, Ballintine EJ. Increased incidence of retinopathy in diabetics with elevated blood pressure: a six-year follow-up study in Pima Indians. N Engl J Med 1980;302:645−50.

57. Klein BEK, Moss SE, Klein R. Effect of pregnancy on progression of diabetic retinopathy. Diabetes Care 1990; 13:34−40.

58. Leslie RDG, Pyke DA. Diabetic retinopathy in identical twins. Diabetes 1982;31:19−21.

59. Cohen AJ, McGill PD, Rossetti RG, et al. Glomerulopathy in spontaneously diabetic rat: impact of glycemic control. Diabetes 1987;36:944−51.

60. Steffes MW, Buchwald H, Wigness BD, et al. Diabetic nephropathy in the uninephrectomized dog: microscopic lesions after one year. Kidney Int 1982;21:721−4.

61. Andersen AR, Christiansen JS, Andersen JK, et al. Diabetic nephropathy in Type I (insulin-dependent) diabetes: an epidemiological study. Diabetologia 1983;25:496−501.

62. Rosenstock J, Raskin P. Early diabetic nephropathy: assessment and potential therapeutic interventions. Diabetes Care 1986;9:529−45.

63. Kussman MJ, Goldstein HH, Gleason RE. The clinical course of diabetic nephropathy. JAMA 1976;236:1861−3.

64. Viberti GC, Jarrett RJ, Mahmud U, et al. Microalbuminuria as a predictor of clinical nephropathy in insulin-dependent diabetes mellitus. Lancet 1982;1:1430−2.

65. Parving H-H, Oxenboll B, Svendsen PA, et al. Early detection of patients at risk of developing diabetic nephropathy. A longitudinal study of urinary albumin excretion. Acta Endocrinol 1982;100:550−5.

66. Mathiesen ER, Oxenboll B, Johansen K, et al. Incipient nephropathy in Type I (insulin-dependent) diabetes. Diabetologia 1984;26:406−10.

67. Mogensen CE, Christensen CK. Predicting diabetic nephropathy in insulin-dependent patients. N Engl J Med 1984;311:89−93.

68. Mogensen CE. Microalbuminuria predicts clinical proteinuria and early mortality in maturity-onset diabetes. N Engl J Med 1984;310:356−60.

69. Feldt-Rasmussen B, Mathieson ER. Validity of urinary albumin excretion in incipient diabetic nephropathy. Diabetic Nephrol 1984;3:101−4.

70. Chavers BM, Bilous RW, Ellis EN, et al. Glomerular lesions and urinary albumin excretion in Type I diabetes without overt proteinuria. N Engl J Med 189;320:966−70.

71. Viberti GC, Keen H, Wiseman MJ. Raised arterial pressure in parents of proteinuric insulin dependent diabetics. BMJ 1987;295:515−7.

72. Krolewski AS, Canessa M, Warram JH, et al. Predisposition to hypertension and susceptibility to renal disease in insulin-dependent diabetes mellitus. N Engl J Med 1988; 318:140−5.

73. Chase HP, Jackson WE, Hoops, SL, et al. Glucose control and the renal and retinal complications of insulin-dependent diabetes. JAMA 1989;261:1155−60.

74. Viberti GC, Pickup JC, Jarrett JR, et al. Effect of control of blood glucose on urinary excretion of albumin and beta-2 microglobulin in insulin-dependent diabetes. N Engl J Med 1979;300:638−41.

75. Viberti GC, Bilous RW, Mackintosh B, et al. Long term correction of hyperglycaemia and progression of renal failure in insulin dependent diabetes. BMJ 1983;286:598–602.

76. Feldt-Rasmussen B, Mathiesen ER, Deckert T. Effect of two years of strict metabolic control on progression of incipient nephropathy in insulin-dependent diabetes. Lancet 1986;2:1300–4.

77. Dahl-Jorgensen K, Hanssen KF, Kierulf P, et al. Reduction of urinary albumin excretion after 4 years of continuous subcutaneous insulin infusion in insulin-dependent diabetes mellitus: the Oslo Study. Acta Endocrinol 1988; 117:19–24.

78. Reichard P, Rosenqvist U. Nephropathy is delayed by intensified insulin treatment in patients with insulin-dependent diabetes mellitus and retinopathy. J Intern Med 1989;226:81–7.

79. Tamborlane WV, Puklin JE, Bergman M, et al. Long-term improvement of metabolic control with the insulin pump does not reverse diabetic microangiopathy. Diabetes Care 1982;5(Suppl 1):58–64.

80. Steno Study Group. Effect of 6 months of strict metabolic control on eye and kidney function in insulin-dependent diabetics with background retinopathy. Lancet 1982; 1:121–3.

81. Bending JJ, Viberti GC, Watkins PJ, Keen H. Intermittent clinical proteinuria and renal function in diabetes: evolution and the effect of glycaemic control. BMJ 1986; 292:83–6.

82. Feldt-Rasmussen B, Mathiesen ER, Hegedus L, et al. Kidney function during 12 months of strict metabolic control in insulin-dependent diabetic patients with incipient nephropathy. N Engl J Med 1986;314:665–70.

83. Ballard DJ, Humphrey LL, Melton LJ, et al. Epidemiology of persistent proteinuria in Type II diabetes mellitus. Diabetes 1988;37:405–12.

84. Vasquez B, Flock EV, Savage PJ, et al. Sustained reduction of proteinuria in type 2 (non-insulin-dependent) diabetes following diet-induced reduction of hyperglycaemia. Diabetologia 1984;26:127–33.

85. Mogensen CE. Long-term antihypertensive treatment inhibits progression of diabetic nephropathy. BMJ 1982; 285:685–88.

86. Cohen D, Dodds R, Viberti G. Effect of protein restriction in insulin dependent diabetics at risk of nephropathy. BMJ 1987;294:295–8.

87. Ward JD, Fisher DJ, Barnes CG, et al. Improvement in nerve conduction following treatment in newly diagnosed diabetics. Lancet 1971;1:428–30.

88. The DCCT Research Group. Factors in development of diabetic neuropathy. Diabetes 1988;37:476.

89. Porte D Jr, Graf RJ, Halter JB, et al. Diabetic neuropathy and plasma glucose control. Am J Med 1981;70:195–200.

90. Boulton AJM, Drury J, Clarke B, Ward JD. Continuous subcutaneous insulin infusion in the management of painful diabetic neuropathy. Diabetes Care 1982; 5:386–90.

91. Holman RR, Mayon-White V, Orde-Peckar C, et al. Prevention of deterioration of renal and sensory-nerve function by more intensive management of insulin-dependent diabetic patients: a two-year randomised prospective study. Lancet 1983;1:204–8.

92. Service FJ, Rizza RA, Daube JR, et al. Near normoglycaemia improved nerve conduction and vibration sensation in diabetic neuropathy. Diabetologia 1985;28:722–7.

93. Pietri A, Ehle AL, Raskin P. Changes in nerve conduction velocity after six weeks of glucoregulation with portable insulin infusion pumps. Diabetes 1980;29:668–71.

94. Kannel WB, McGee DL. Diabetes and cardiovascular disease. The Framingham Study. JAMA 1979;241:2036–8.

95. Gordon T, Castelli WP, Hjortland MC, et al. Diabetes, blood lipids, and the role of obesity in coronary heart disease risk for women. The Framingham Study. Ann Intern Med 1977; 87:393–7.

96. Jarrett RJ, McCartney P, Keen H. The Bedford Survey: ten year mortality rates in newly diagnosed diabetics, borderline diabetics and normoglycaemic controls and risk indices for coronary heart disease in borderline diabetics. Diabetologia 1982;22:79–84.

97. Wingard DL, Barrett-Connor E, Criqui MH, Suarez L. Clustering of heart disease risk factors in diabetic compared to nondiabetic adults. Am J Epidemiol 1983; 117:19–26.

98. The International Collaborative Group. Joint discussion. J Chronic Dis 1979;32:829–37.

99. Knuiman MW, Welborn TA, McCann VJ, et al. Prevalence of diabetic complications in relation to risk factors. Diabetes 1986;35:1332–9.

100. Singer DE, Nathan DM, Wilson PWF, et al. HbA1c as a risk factor for cardiovascular disease in the Framingham study. Diabetes 1992;41:202–8.

101. DCCT Research Group. Epidemiology of severe hypoglycemia in the DCCT. Am J Med 1991;90:450–9.

102. DCCT Research Group. Weight gain associated with intensive therapy in the Diabetes Control and Complications Trial. Diabetes Care 1988;11:567–73.

103. American College of Obstetrics and Gynecology. Management of diabetes in pregnancy. Am Coll Gynecol Tech Bull 1986;10:1–2.

104. Jovanovic L, Druzin M, Peterson CM. Effect of euglycemia on the outcome of pregnancy in IDDM as compared to normal controls. Am J Med 1981;71:921–6.

Chapter 37

MECHANISMS OF DIABETIC MICROVASCULAR COMPLICATIONS

GEORGE L. KING
NIRMAL K. BANSKOTA

Microvascular complications of diabetes represent one of the most serious consequences of the disease. It is likely that all blood vessels, both large and small, are abnormal in patients with diabetes of long duration. The changes involve both the vascular cells making up the capillaries and arterioles and their basement membranes. Although all microvascular blood vessels are involved clinically, only those in the retina, renal glomeruli, and possibly the large nerves exhibit significant pathology. It is not clear why these sites are particularly affected. No single hypothesis can provide a satisfactory explanation for all the pathologic abnormalities observed in the microvasculature in diabetes or the differences in morphologic changes in the vascular cells of different tissues. The specific clinical syndromes involving these sites are covered in other chapters and therefore will not be described here in detail. This chapter will review both the morphologic and biochemical features of the microangiopathy, focusing particularly on the renal and retinal vessels because most existing information on mechanisms has been derived from studies of these two microvascular beds.

The main function of the vasculature is to provide a conduit for the delivery of nutrients required by the individual tissues and for the removal of materials from specific tissues. To achieve this important goal, the cells of the vasculature need to monitor the needs of the tissue continuously and either increase or decrease functional capacity appropriately. To accomplish this, the vasculature must possess mechanisms for regulating coagulation, monitoring flow and contractility, establishing a level of permeability, and regenerating after injury. Not surprisingly, a wide range of the vascular abnormalities that have been described in diabetic patients and animals can be placed in one of these four categories.

MORPHOLOGIC FEATURES

The classic morphologic finding in diabetic microangiopathy is the thickening of basement membranes in capillaries.[1-3] This is a generalized phenomenon that affects basement membranes of both vascular and nonvascular tissues. The basement membranes of mammary ducts, testes, and sweat glands also are thickened, as are sarcoplasmic and perineural basement membranes and alveolar epithelium.[4-8] However, because of the relative clinical insignificance of basement membrane thickening in nonvascular tissues, these have been studied less extensively than vascular tissues. In general, thickening of the basement membrane is defined by light microscopy, but ultrastructural studies also confirm the increase. Because of their clinical significance, lesions of the retinal and renal basement membranes have received the most intensive study. What constitutes the basement membrane is defined slightly differently in light microscopic vs. electron microscopic reports. Basement membranes may be further characterized with the use of biochemical and immunocytochemical techniques. In most tissues, the basement membrane separates cells from the interstitial space. The exceptions are the glomerulus of kidney, in which the basement membrane is between endothelial cells of the capillary and epithelial cells of the Bowman's capsule, and in the central nervous system, in which the basement membrane is between the endothelial cell and the glial cell.[9] The glomerular basement membrane is continuous with the tubular basement membrane via the Bowman's capsule. In the retina, thickening of the basement membrane also is found between endothelial cells and pericytes (mural cells).[3,10-12] Ultrastructurally, the capillary basement membrane is composed of fine filaments embedded in a homogeneous matrix, with two clear zones (inner and outer) that are separated from a dense middle zone (the lamina internal).[13] The morphologic traits of the capillary basement membrane vary in different tissues, and its thickness often correlates with the intracapillary pressures.[14]

The chemical components of the basement membrane are now well recognized and include collagens (mainly type IV), chondroitin, heparan sulfate proteoglycans, and various glycoproteins such as laminin.[15-18] Basement membranes in normal tissues form boundaries between cells and different cell types. They provide structural support, maintain architecture, modify cellular functions such as proliferation, and provide a filtration barrier. Thus, these alterations in basement membrane morphology can easily be envisaged as having functional consequences.

The capillary basement membranes in the retina thicken with age. Basement membrane thickening is also a consistent feature in both diabetic patients and animal models of diabetes[19-21] (Fig. 37-1). In the retina of diabetic rats, capillary thickening is more prominent in the inner capillary bed (nerve and ganglion layer) than in the inner and outer plexiform layers.[22] Experimentally, thickening of the basement membrane of retinal capillaries similar to that in patients with diabetes is observed in galactose-fed rats and dogs.[10,23]

Since the initial description of diabetic renal glomeruli by Kimmelstiel and Wilson,[24] thickening of the glomerular basement membrane has been recognized as a prominent morphologic feature of diabetic nephropathy. This thickening of the basement membrane in diabetes has classically been described as a slow process that occurs over many years. Acute glomerular hypertrophy also occurs early in the course of diabetes mellitus, but it is uncertain whether this is a precursor of the classical

renal lesions of diabetes.[25-27] Similar structural changes have been described in rats with streptozotocin-induced diabetes. The expansion of the mesangium is the other major lesion observed in diabetic glomerulopathy. This expansion is thought to be the main factor leading to decreased renal function.[28] With the progressive increase in the mesangial matrix, there is a loss in capillary surface area (filtration area). Increase in mesangial volume fraction (mesangial volume/glomerular volume) also has a strong clinical correlation with declining glomerular filtration rate (GFR) and albuminuria. Such a functional correlation is not exhibited for increases in the thickness of the glomerular basement membrane.[29] Along with changes in the composition of the basement membrane, changes in the mesangium lead to altered permeability and eventually to glomerular occlusion, fibrosis, and decreased filtering capacity.

Functional changes also occur in early diabetes. The GFR and filtration fraction (GFR/renal plasma flow) increase early in the course of diabetes and can be corrected by intensive insulin treatment.[30-32] Permeability of the capillaries is altered such that the excretion of proteins with molecular weights of 44,000 to 150,000 is increased.[33] Albumin excretion is increased early in diabetes and, like an elevated GFR, can be normalized by intensive insulin treatment or islet-cell transplantation.[30-32] Similar changes are seen in diabetic rats. This initial alteration in permeability seems to be due primarily to increased filtration pressures across the glomerulus. Altered charge selectivity of the permeability barrier—changes that permit an increase in the leakage of plasma proteins—may also be involved. Fibrin accumulation, possibly related to decreases in fibrolysis, may contribute to the precapillary occlusion seen in diabetes.[34-37]

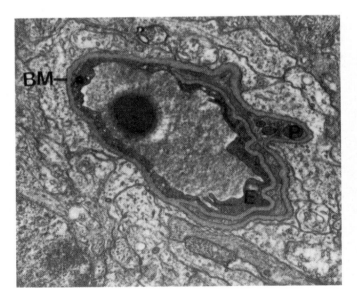
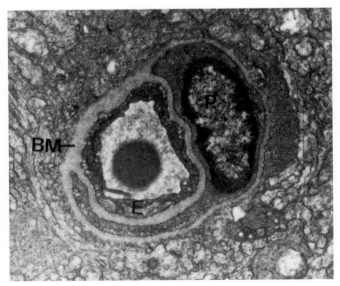

Fig. 37-1.   Retinal capillaries from control (left) and diabetic (right) rats. The basement membrane (BM) is thickened in the diabetic rat. E = endothelial cells; P = pericytes (courtesy of Dr. J. W. Williamson and Dr. R. Tilton, Washington University, St. Louis, MO).

CHEMISTRY AND METABOLISM OF BASEMENT MEMBRANES

The basement membrane is composed of collagen, glycoprotein such as fibronectin, laminin, entactin, proteoglycans, heparan, chondroitin, and dermatan. The collagenous proteins are rich in the amino acids glycine, hydroxyproline, and hydroxylysine, whereas the noncollagenous proteins are high in the amino acids hydroxyglycine and cysteine and in carbohydrates. The carbohydrates in basement membranes are of two distinct types: a complex asparagine-like heteropolysaccharide containing galactose, mannose, fructose, sialic acid, and glucosamine on more polar, less collagen-like parts of the peptide; and a glucose-galactose disaccharide attached to hydroxylysine.[13,16-18,38]

The composition of basement membrane has been analyzed in diabetic and normal tissues. The total amount of basement membrane protein is increased in the glomeruli of patients with chronic diabetes.[39-42] The basement membrane of diabetic patients also has an increase in hydroxylysine and a decrease in lysine content. The amount of carbohydrate, especially the glucose-galactose disaccharide units, also is increased. The levels of heparan sulfate proteoglycans and laminin are decreased while those of fibronectin are unchanged.[15,38-42]

The compositional changes observed in components of the basement membrane in diabetes may result from altered rates of synthesis, degradation, or both. The enzymatic activity of lysylhydroxylase, which hydroxylates lysine residues of newly synthesized peptide chains, is increased in homogenates of diabetic kidney, an increase that can be corrected by insulin treatment.[43-47] The addition of the galactose-glucose disaccharide units to the hydroxylysine is a two-step process catalyzed by two specific enzymes, galactosyltransferase and glucosyltransferase.[47,48] The levels of these enzymes have been reported by some to be increased in diabetic renal cortex.[45] Again, insulin treatment normalizes the activity of these enzymes but only if it is instituted early in the course of diabetes.[45]

Incorporation of amino acids into basement membrane proteins in diabetes has been analyzed directly, but the experimental methods are of questionable specificity. However, the results do suggest that basement membrane synthesis is accelerated.[49-55] Recent studies using cultured endothelial cells from human umbilicus also have noted an increase in the synthesis of type IV collagen and an increase in levels of mRNA for type IV collagen in cells incubated in media containing elevated levels of glucose.[56] However, these changes were rather small. Furthermore, direct extrapolation of these findings to the retina and renal glomeruli is very speculative.

CHANGES IN VASCULAR CELLS

Beside the generalized changes in the basement membrane, specific changes in vascular cells have been documented. These changes in vascular cells vary depending on the tissue. A schematic drawing of the histologic changes in the retina in diabetic patients and diabetic dogs is shown in Figure 37-2.[57-63]

The earliest histologic change in diabetic retinopathy is the loss of retinal pericytes.[57-61] Normally, the ratio of endothelial cells to pericytes in the retinal capillaries is 1:1.[57,58] This ratio is very different in peripheral capillaries, which have more endothelial cells than pericytes. For example, the ratio of endothelial cells to pericytes in the capillaries from muscle is 20:1.[62] The similarity in the numbers of pericytes and endothelial cells is found only in the retinal and central nervous system microvessels, suggesting that the relationship between pericytes and endothelial cells may be important in the function of microvessels—perhaps in the formation of a tight barrier in these microvessels. As initially shown by Cogan and co-workers, the ratio of pericytes to endothelial cells in trypsin digests of retinal vessels from diabetic patients is decreased to 1:4 after only several years of disease and decreased to 1:10 with even longer duration of disease.[59,60] In parallel with loss of pericytes, several other histologic changes are observed, including increased capillary diameter, thickening of the basement membrane, changes in retinal blood flow, increased vascular permeability, and formation of microaneurysms. It has been postulated that many of these changes are the consequence of the loss of pericytes. The existence of a closely regulated relationship between pericytes and endothelial cells is supported by the finding of gap junctions between these cells.[64]

Progress in cell culture technique has permitted the isolation and propagation of large quantities of retinal capillaries and pericytes.[65,66] In addition, specific markers for pericytes have been reported.[67] The discovery of a

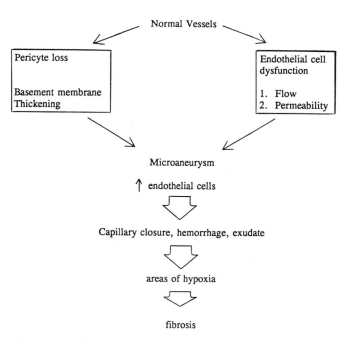

Fig. 37-2. Schematic drawing of the progression of diabetic retinopathy.

vital stain that allows pericytes to be separated from other cells has facilitated biochemical and molecular studies on the direct effects of hyperglycemia and growth factors on these cells. In culture, the endothelial cells retain their monolayer distribution and cuboidal shape whereas pericytes grow in a multilayered configuration with many pseudopods (Fig. 37–3). More recent studies have shown that the contact between pericytes and endothelial cells is quite important in the regulation of cytokines produced by the endothelial cells, which in turn can regulate the function and growth of endothelial cells.[68,69]

Once the early changes described above have occurred in nonproliferative diabetic retinopathy, the blood vessels lose their ability to regulate blood flow, and the capillaries in turn lose their ability to receive blood, a deficit that leads to the formation of ghost capillaries.[57–61] With an increase in the amount of hemorrhage and exudate and the formation of ghost vessels, areas of anoxia are formed. In addition, hemorrhage provides serum growth factors that, in combination with anoxia-induced local growth factors or the loss of inhibitors of vascular growth, lead to the more serious stage of diabetic retinopathy called proliferative retinopathy. Proliferative retinopathy is characterized by neovascularization of retinal capillaries both intraretinally and within the vitreous. These new vessels contain very few pericytes and do not form the usual retinal blood barrier. These properties increase the risk of bleeding, which in turn leads to fibrosis in the retina and, as a consequence, to an enhancement in the potential for retinal detachment and blindness. The development of proliferative and fibrotic changes in the later stages of diabetic retinopathy probably is due to factors not too different from those responsible for other proliferative diseases of the retina, since the pathologic changes observed are similar to those in other such retinal diseases.[70,71]

In the glomeruli, at least three different types of vascular cells are involved in microvascular changes[72–74]: glomerular endothelial cells, mesangial cells, and epithelial cells. The basement membrane of the glomeruli is formed primarily from products of the glomerular endothelial cells and epithelial cells, whereas nodules probably are formed from products of the mesangial cells in the glomerular tuft. Mesangial cells, like pericytes, have contractile properties but react differently to diabetes, increasing their size and possibly their number as well.[1,2,9,72–74] The loss of glomerular filtration function is directly related to the expansion of the mesangium and the loss of the filtration surface formed by the endothelial and epithelial cells. In early stages of diabetes, there appears to be an expansion of the mesangium and mesangial cells. The basement membrane is also thickened, and the combination of this thickening and the expansion of the mesangium results in a gradual loss of the endothelial and epithelial cells. At the later stage of nephropathy, general fibrosis of the glomeruli leads to end-stage kidney disease similar to other glomerulosclerotic diseases[1,2,9,24–28] (Fig. 37–4).

VASCULAR ABNORMALITIES

In general, the endothelial cells of the microvessel appear to retain their ability to proliferate in the diabetic milieu. For example, the formation of microaneurysms due to aggregation of endothelial cells consequent to either migration or proliferation has been reported in brain, heart, adipose tissue, and retina. In addition, neovascularization is observed in the retina and possibly in the glomeruli. This progression is different from that in macrovessels, in which endothelial cell injury may result in cell loss. Specific changes in various aspects of endothelial cell functions will be described in the following section.

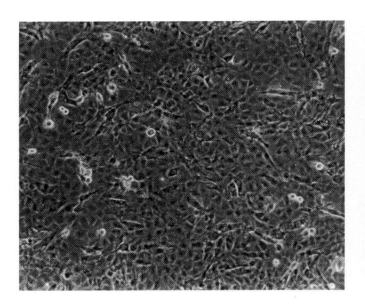
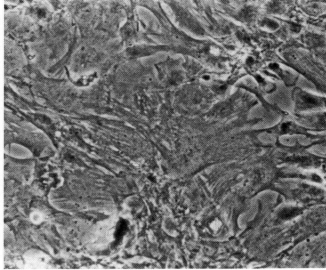

Fig. 37–3. Phase-contrast photography of cultured bovine retinal endothelial cells (left) and pericytes (right).

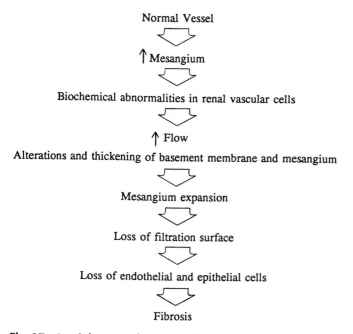

Normal Vessel

↑ Mesangium

Biochemical abnormalities in renal vascular cells

↑ Flow

Alterations and thickening of basement membrane and mesangium

Mesangium expansion

Loss of filtration surface

Loss of endothelial and epithelial cells

Fibrosis

Fig. 37–4. Schematic drawing of the pathway in the development of diabetic nephropathy.

Coagulation

The abnormalities found in the endothelial and vascular supporting cells from diabetic patients or animals can be separated into four general categories: 1) coagulation, 2) flow and contractility, 3) permeability, and 4) regeneration. Multiple alterations in coagulation have been reported. In the endothelium, abnormalities have been found in the levels of activity of factor VIII, prostaglandins, fibrinolysis, and other functions.[75,76] The levels of tissue plasminogen activator (TPA) and tissue plasminogen activator inhibitor (PAI) have been evaluated in several studies.[77–79] Some studies have found that TPA activity is decreased or absent in response to stimulation by desmopressin, although this correlated with obesity rather than with diabetes.[77] However, other studies have reported no change or an increase in TPA levels. A decrease in TPA activity would support the finding of diminished fibrinolysis activity in diabetic patients, since plasminogen, which is secreted by the endothelial cells, converts plasminogen to plasmin, which is involved in fibrinolysis. The activities of TPA can be inhibited by PAI.[78] Thus, it is possible that the decrease in TPA activities is due to an increase in PAI.[79]

Another parameter used in assessing the coagulation state is von Willebrand factor antigen (vWF), which complexes with factor VIII to form factor VIII Ag:vWF.[80–88] This complex is produced by endothelial cells and is involved in formation of thrombi and in adhesion of platelets to the subendothelium.[82,83] Most studies have reported that levels of vWF are increased in both insulin-dependent and non-insulin-dependent diabetic patients. Most studies have indicated that glycemic control, whether achieved by diet, sulfonylureas, or insulin, normalizes vWF levels in patients.[87,89] The

duration of the diabetic state seems to correlate with the level of vWF,[90,91] although vWF may be elevated in young diabetic patients without vascular disease as well as early in the diabetic state in streptozotocin diabetic rats.[91–93] This may simply reflect early endothelial cell injury or dysfunction secondary to hyperglycemia.[94]

Diabetes and hyperglycemia have been reported to affect the metabolism of prostaglandins, which are potent metabolites of endothelial cells that affect platelet aggregation and vascular thrombosis.[95,96] Prostaglandin I_2 (PGI_2) production in endothelial cells has been evaluated extensively because it is an inhibitor of platelet aggregation and adhesion and a strong vasodilator.[96] These properties suggest that a reduction in the level of PGI_2 may lead to an increase in thrombosis and contractility. PGI_2 levels are reduced in the sera of diabetic animals and patients, probably because of a decrease in its production. Exposure of endothelial cells to sera from diabetic patients and animals inhibits PGI_2 production. Treatment of diabetic rats with insulin reverses the inhibitory effect of the sera.[95,96] It is of interest that vitamin E treatment also reverses the inhibitory effect of sera from diabetic patients and animals, a finding that suggests a possible role for antioxidant in the treatment of vascular complications.

Permeability

Increase in vascular permeability is another hallmark of diabetic vascular disease. This is most obvious in the retina and renal glomeruli. In the retina, fluorescein leakage can easily be detected in areas of clinical pathology such as microaneurysms and exudates. Since fluorescein is a very small molecule, fluorescein leakage may be observed before clinical pathology is evident.[97–103] In animals, an increase in the permeability of microvessels to labeled albumin after 4 to 6 weeks of chemically induced diabetes has been reported.[101] This increase in permeability has been noted in many tissues, including nonvascular tissues such as the skin. Since peripheral microvessels contain endothelial cells with few vascular supporting cells such as pericytes, the effect of diabetes is likely a reflection of dysfunction in the endothelial cells.

In retinal vessels, the vascular barrier is formed by tight junctions between capillary endothelial cells. Increases in permeability are probably due to abnormalities in the endothelial cells. The pericytes also may play a major role, since the normal ratio of pericytes to endothelial cells is one. Recent studies in which retinal pericytes and endothelial cells have been co-cultured demonstrate that pericytes can regulate the endothelial cell barrier even if the cells are not in direct contact. If they are in contact, pericytes can regulate the growth of endothelial cells by altering the expression of stimulatory and inhibitory growth factors such as transforming growth factor β (TGF-β).[68,69]

Contractility and Flow

The third general area of vascular abnormality in diabetes is contractility and flow.[103–113] Some of the vasoactive substances that have been evaluated in diabetic patients and animals are listed in Table 37–1. Increase in blood flow in the renal glomeruli has been documented in diabetic patients and animals.[103,104] This increase appears to precede any pathologic changes. The mechanisms responsible for the increase in blood flow are not known. However, one report has suggested that vasoactive substance may be involved. Atrial natriuretic peptide (ANP) has been shown to increase renal blood flow and filtration rate.[104] Infusion of antibodies to ANP normalizes renal blood flow, suggesting that ANP may have a role in increasing renal blood flow in the diabetic state.[104] Other growth factors, such as growth hormone and insulin-like growth factor I (IGF-I), have been implicated, since they can cause renal enlargement and increase the GFR.[114–116] However, the expression of nephropathy that develops in transgenic mice with increased expression of either IGF-I or growth hormone is not exactly like that found in diabetes, although these animals do develop glomerular sclerosis.[115]

Not all vascular beds show increased flow. During the first 2 to 5 years of diabetes, retinal blood flow appears to be decreased.[117] Blood flow has been reported to be increased when background retinopathy is present.[57,101] However, with advanced proliferative retinopathy, retinal blood flow appears to decrease again.[118–122] This decrease could increase hypoxia and further induce neovascularization. Thus, the effect of diabetes on vascular flow varies according to the tissue and the duration of disease.

Reports regarding large-vessel contractility in animals are conflicting. In general, a delay in the relaxation phase, usually mediated by the release of endothelium-dependent releasing factor (EDRF), has been noted.[105–113] In the aorta, the endothelium-dependent relaxing phase in response to acetylcholine and Ca++ ionophore is decreased. This attenuated response is observed in the presence of endothelium but is not seen when nitroprusside or adenosine is added, suggesting that secretion of EDRF may be reduced or quenched by glycosylated proteins[123] or that the level of some vasoconstrictor may be increased.[124] Evidence in support of each possibility is available. In vitro, glycosylated proteins have been shown to reduce the effectiveness of nitric oxide, a major component of EDRF. However, Tesfamariam et al. reported that the hyperglycemia-induced lack of relaxation can be reversed by inhibitors of protein kinase C (PKC)

or prostaglandin inhibitors. A role for PKC is further supported by the observation that activators of PKC can mimic the effect of diabetes.[125]

The attenuated response of acetylcholine-induced vasodilation also is observed in microvascular circulation in the small mesenteric arteries[109] and in the microvessels of the penile corpora cavernosa.[112] In tissue from diabetic men with impotence, the endothelium-dependent relaxation response to acetylcholine is reported to be decreased, although the responses to sodium nitroprusside and papaverine are not diminished.

Abnormalities in vascular contractility could also be due to changes in the levels or actions of vasoactive hormones. Increased sensitivity to renin and angiotensin has been postulated, although little supporting evidence is available. Recent results have shown a possible relationship between diabetes and endothelin-1 (ET-1), a potent vasoconstrictor that can cause prolonged hypertension in vivo.[126–135] In diabetic patients receiving insulin therapy, the plasma level of ET-1 has been reported to be higher than that in nondiabetic patients controls.[131] One possible reason for this elevation is a stimulatory effect of glucose on ET-1 production in endothelial cells.[132] Another reason is the enhancement by insulin of the rate of transcription of ET-1 RNA by endothelial cells.[135] Alterations in vasoactive hormones could account for the abnormality in contractility and the high incidence of hypertension in the diabetic population.[136–138]

Cellular Regeneration

Both proliferation and loss of cells are prominent features of diabetic vascular disease. The appearance of capillary microaneurysms has been attributed to a loss of pericytes. The growth of retinal endothelial cells is inhibited by their co-culture with pericytes.[68,69] The inhibitory effect can be observed only if the two types of cells are in physical contact. Further studies have suggested that while endothelial cells and pericytes are in contact, the endothelial cells release active forms of TGF-β, which proceeds to inhibit the growth of endothelial cells.[68,69] Therefore, in the retinas of diabetic patients, the loss of pericytes caused by hyperglycemia may prevent the expression of active TGF-β by the endothelial cells, allowing the endothelial cells to proliferate and thus resulting in the formation of microaneurysms.[59–61]

Hyperglycemia can enhance proliferation of retinal endothelial cells directly as well as indirectly through its contribution to the loss of pericytes. Recent studies have shown that the exposure of cultured retinal endothelial cells to elevated levels of glucose (400 mg/dL) results in an increase in membrane-associated PKC activity, which represents the active pool of enzyme.[139] This activation of the PKC is probably due to an increase in the level of diacylglycerol (DAG), which is, along with Ca++ and phospholipids, a physiologic activator of PKC.[140,141] Such PKC activation could be important in the enhancement of cellular proliferation, since activation of PKC has been implicated in cellular regulation by many growth factors, including platelet-derived growth factor (PDGF).[142–146]

Table 37–1. Some Vasoactive Hormones That Have Been Evaluated in Diabetic Patients or Animals

Hormone	Relation to Levels in Controls*
Renin + angiotensin	↓ ↔
Vasopressin	↑ (when stimulated)
Histamine	↑
Endothelin	↑
Atrial natriuretic peptide	↑ ↔
Aldosterone	↑ ↔
Catecholamines	↑ (poorly controlled) ↔

*Arrows indicate whether levels are increased, decreased, or the same as those in controls.

In addition, a regulatory role for PKC in basement membrane synthesis, vascular contractility, and permeability has been suggested.[142-151]

Not much about the role of growth inhibitors in microangiopathy is known except that vitreous from normal eyes inhibits angiogenesis in various in vivo assays.[152-154] Taylor and Weiss have partially purified a 5700-dalton glycoprotein inhibitor of angiogenesis from the vitreous.[153] Both TGF-β and tumor necrosis factor-α (TNF-α) have the paradoxical effects of inhibiting proliferation of endothelial cells in vitro but appearing to be angiogenic in vivo.[155,156]

The exact identity of the growth factor or factors responsible for the development of neovascularization and fibrosis in the diabetic retina has not be determined. However, numerous types of growth factors have been identified in the retina (Table 37-2). In general, these factors can be classified as local or systemic growth factors. The systemic factors act primarily as enhancing factors, whereas the local factors probably play a major role in the initiation of proliferative changes.

The fibroblast-derived growth factor (FGF) family of polypeptides have been shown to be responsible for much of the mitogenic activity isolated from the retina and vitreous fluid in proliferative retinopathy.[157,158] Two types of FGF have been found in the retinal tissues, acidic FGF (aFGF) and basic FGF (bFGF). Both are 17-kilodalton proteins that can be isolated by their binding to heparin. The FGFs are not secreted from the cells but can be released by cell disruption. Once released, the FGFs are found bound to basement matrix and are presumed to be activated by turnover or degradation of the basement membrane.[159] The FGFs are angiogenic but can stimulate the growth of many types of cells in addition to endothelial cells.[160] The role of FGFs in proliferative diabetic retinopathy is not clear. Several studies involving a small number of patients and controls have had conflicting results.[161,162] Using an immunoassay for bFGF, Sivalingam et al. reported that patients with proliferative

diabetic retinopathy tend to have higher levels of bFGF than patients without diabetes or proliferative disease.[161]

TGF-β has also been found in the retina and can also be synthesized by retinal pigmented epithelial cells.[163,164] TGF-β has an inhibitory effect on endothelial cell proliferation but can be angiogenic in vivo, probably by the recruitment of monocytes through its chemotactic properties. Total TGF-β levels in the vitreous as measured by a radioreceptor assay are three times greater in patients with proliferative vitreoretinopathy (PVR) than in patients who have retinal detachment without PVR.[165] Since PVR occurs in a significant percentage of patients with late-stage diabetic proliferative disease, TGF-β may play a role both during early stages, with the formation of microaneurysms, and during late stages, with the formation of fibrosis.

Another growth factor that has been studied specifically with respect to retinal proliferative disease is endothelial cell-stimulating angiogenesis factor (ESAF). This is a low-molecular-weight (400) factor isolated from the retina and vitreous that is angiogenic and can activate procollagenase activities.[166,167] It is different from other growth factors; it is not a protein and may be specific for microvascular endothelial cells. Bioassays have suggested that ESAF levels may be increased in retinas and vitreous from kittens with oxygen-induced retrolental fibroplasia, a condition that also includes neovascularization among its pathologic features.[167] In a preliminary report, ESAF activity from vitreous aspirates from patients with neovascularization appeared to be higher than that in normal eyes. These findings are intriguing, especially since the biologic activities of ESAF and FGF are additive.

The last group of growth factors that need discussion are the factors first identified and include growth hormone and the insulin-like growth factors (IGF-I and IGF-II). Growth hormone (GH) was postulated to play a significant role in diabetic proliferative retinopathy when it was reported that diabetic patients who were GH-deficient showed an amelioration of their proliferative retinopathy.[63,168] However, levels of GH in serum are not predictive of the development or severity of diabetic retinopathy. Since GH mediates most of its growth effects by increasing the levels of IGF-I, Grant et al. measured IGF-I levels in the serum and vitreous.[169] This group found that IGF-I levels were increased in only a small group of patients who had particularly aggressive diabetic proliferative retinopathy. In vitro studies have demonstrated that retinal endothelial cells have receptors for IGF-I and respond to IGF-I by increased growth.[66] IGF-I has been demonstrated to have chemotactic and angiogenic activities as well.[66,169] Unfortunately, a study with a larger number of patients found no correlation between plasma IGF-I levels and the presence of proliferative retinopathy.[170]

Studies of insulin and IGF-I receptors and actions on vascular cells in culture have stimulated a great deal of interest because of the possible involvement of insulin and IGF-I in the development of hypertension, atherosclerosis, and other vascular complications prevalent in the diabetic population. Numerous publications have suggested that hyperinsulinemia or insulin resistance may be

Table 37-2. Growth Modulators Identified in Retina

Factors Identified in Retina	Relation of Levels in Diabetes to Those in Controls*
Fibroblast growth factors	↑ ↔†
Epidermal growth factor	↔
Transforming growth factor-β	↑
Platelet-derived growth factor	?
Insulin	↔
Insulin-like growth factor I	↑ ↔
Insulin-like growth factor II	↑ ↔
Growth hormone	↑
Endothelial cell-stimulating angiogenesis factor	?
Tumor necrosis factor	↔
Vascular endothelial cell growth factor	?

*Levels were determined in diabetic animals or patients. Arrows indicate whether levels are increased or the same as those in controls. A question mark indicates that factor has not been measured in diabetic patients or animals.
†Acidic or basic fibroblast growth factors.

a risk factor for the development of hypertension and acceleration of atherosclerosis that clearly occur in diabetic patients.[171-173] Insulin and IGF-I receptors have been noted on all vascular cells,[145,172,174-177] including cells from different vascular sites, such as retina, aorta, fat, renal glomeruli, brain, and umbilical vein.[72,145,172] In addition, insulin receptors have also been detected on vascular cells from different species. In general, insulin receptors on the vascular cells are structurally similar to those expressed on the "classical" insulin-sensitive tissues such as fat and liver (see Chapter 8 on insulin action). These receptors have a high affinity and specificity for their respective ligands, although IGF-I and IGF-II also can bind to insulin receptors, although with affinities 50 to 100 times lower than that of insulin (Fig. 37–5). As with other cell types, when insulin is added to vascular cells, phosphorylation of these receptors occurs immediately on both tyrosine and serine residues. However, there are major differences between endothelial cells and peripheral tissues with regard to location, processing, and actions of these receptors.

Endothelial cells, unlike muscle and fat cells, are polarized, with an apical surface that faces the intraluminal side of the blood vessel and a basolateral surface that is attached to the basement membrane. Most, if not all, of the insulin receptors are located on the apical surface.[178] This apical location is important for the function of insulin receptors on endothelial cells. Thus, the insulin receptors on the apical surface of the cell will bind and internalize insulin and transport it across the endothelial cell without significant degradation.[179] This process, called *receptor-mediated transcytosis*, probably also applies to the transport of IGF-I.[180]

Direct measurement of the transport of ^{125}I-insulin by aortic endothelial cells in vitro using a two-compartment system confirms that insulin can be rapidly and unidirectionally transported by receptor-mediated transcytosis. The transport is inhibited by an excess of unlabeled insulin and by specific antibodies to the insulin receptor but not by an excess of an unrelated polypeptide such as nerve growth factor.[181]

Thus, the insulin receptors on endothelial cells function as transporters of insulin across the vascular barrier. In the continuously lined capillaries of muscle and adipose tissue, where endothelial cells are the principal obstacles to the free diffusion of insulin from blood to tissue, receptor-mediated transcytosis most likely provides an efficient and highly regulated system of insulin delivery. An example of a physiologic role for receptor-mediated transcytosis is the special case of insulin transport across the blood-brain barrier. This scheme has been convincingly demonstrated in vivo.[179] The insulin receptors in both brain and retinal microvessel endothelial cells have the same structural and functional properties as those in non-neuronal tissues.[66] Wallum et al. found that peripheral intravenous infusion of insulin in human subjects raised insulin levels in plasma from 12 ± 1.2 to 268 ± 35 μU/mL and concomitantly raised insulin levels in cerebrospinal fluid from 0.9 ± 0.1 to 2.8 ± 0.4 μU/mL.[179] They interpreted these data as suggesting a mechanism by which peripheral insulin might provide a feedback signal to the central nervous system to regulate food intake.

In addition to their ability to transport insulin in a receptor-mediated pathway, insulin receptors on endothelial cells also can mediate "classical" effects of insulin. It is of interest that the endothelial cells of macro- and microvessels respond differently to insulin even though no differences have been found in their receptor binding affinity or number (Fig. 37–5). Capillary endothelial cells isolated from normal rats are responsive to both the metabolic and growth effects of insulin.[66] In contrast, the same cells isolated from capillaries of diabetic rats have been reported to have a decreased number of insulin receptors and actions as measured by receptor autophosphorylation and glucose incorporation into glycogen. The mRNA and the protein structure of the insulin receptors from the endothelial cells, as determined by northern

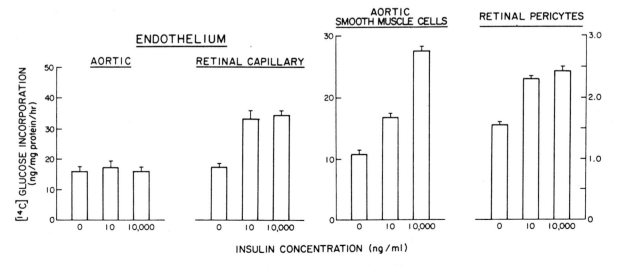

Fig. 37–5. Characteristics of the action of insulin in various vascular cells.

blot and trypsin-digest analysis, respectively, do not reveal any differences.[177] It is possible that the decreased number of insulin receptors in cells from diabetic rats may be due to alterations in receptor processing or degradation. We believe that such alterations in processing could be due to PKC activation, having shown that increased serine phosphorylation of the insulin receptor can enhance the rate of its internalization in the endothelial cell.[147,178]

Although macrovascular endothelial cells are rather insensitive to the classical actions of insulin, it has recently been reported that these cells are sensitive to the effect of insulin on the expression of the mRNA of ET-1, a potent vasoconstrictor synthesized in large quantity by the endothelial cells.[132-135] The rate of transcription of ET-1 can be enhanced three- to fourfold within 30 minutes by physiologic concentrations of insulin.[135]

MOLECULAR MECHANISMS OF HYPERGLYCEMIC DAMAGE

One of the major causes of vascular dysfunction is hyperglycemia, but the exact mechanism of its detrimental effect is not clear. Quite possibly, hyperglycemia mediates its adverse effects via multiple mechanisms, since glucose and its metabolites are utilized by numerous pathways. Over the last several years, several theories have been proposed to explain the adverse effects of hyperglycemia (Table 37–3).

The Sorbitol Pathway

The sorbitol theory of hyperglycemic damage has been the theory studied most intensively.[182-195] This postulate is based on the finding that glucose can be converted to sorbitol in most cells by the enzyme aldose reductase.[182,188,189,193] In situations in which the glucose level is not elevated, the intracellular concentration of sorbitol is very low because of the high K_m of aldose reductase for glucose. However, when the intracellular glucose level is increased in response to an elevation in glucose levels in either the plasma or media, the intracellular level of sorbitol will increase. Once formed, sorbitol can be metabolized by sorbitol dehydrogenase into fructose, with the production of reduced nicotinamide adenine dinucleotide (NADH) (Fig. 37–6). However, this degradation of sorbitol proceeds at a relatively slow rate, permitting sorbitol to accumulate in the vascular neuronal cells and other tissues.[182-195]

Since sorbitol does not diffuse across cell membranes easily, it may accumulate and cause osmotic changes that damage the cell. This mechanism is plausible for those

Table 37–3. Possible Mechanisms by Which Hyperglycemia Produces Vascular Complications

1. Aldose reductase, polyol pathway
2. Nonenzymatic glycosylation
3. Alteration of redox potential
4. Diacylglycerol–protein kinase C pathway

tissues in which sorbitol accumulates to a relatively high level, such as in the lens of the eye. In this setting, the osmotic changes lead to the development of cataracts. Aldose reductase inhibitors (ARIs) have been shown to prevent cataracts in animals with chemically induced diabetes.[182,186,193]

However, the extent of sorbitol accumulation in response to hyperglycemia differs greatly from tissue to tissue. Increases in sorbitol concentrations in neuronal and vascular tissues may not be high enough to cause significant osmotic changes, and thus other mechanisms of damage have been proposed. One possibility is that the elevated levels of both glucose and sorbitol compete for the uptake of myoinositol in the tissues and cells.[182,188] Myoinositol levels are decreased in neuronal tissues of diabetic animals,[182] and it has been postulated that this decrease may result in alterations in the level of the important phospholipids involved in signal transduction, which in turn could lead to damage or alteration in neuronal cell functions. However, myoinositol levels are not increased in the aorta of diabetic animals.[194,195] Perhaps one difference between nervous and vascular tissue is that increases in the sorbitol levels in vascular cells are minor relative to those in neuronal cells. In fact, myoinositol replacement or treatment with an ARI has been shown to normalize myoinositol levels in neuronal tissues of diabetic animals.[182] In addition, treatment with an ARI can improve nerve conduction velocity in diabetic animals. The activities of many other key enzymes are altered in neural or vascular tissue of diabetic animals. Na^+/K^+-ATPase activity also has been shown to be decreased in the vascular and neuronal tissues of diabetic animals.[182,195] This effect can be simulated in cultured vascular cells by exposing them to elevated levels of glucose. The changes in Na^+/K^+-ATPase activity have been linked to elevations in sorbitol level, since the addition of ARI will partially normalize the decrease of Na^+/K^+-ATPase activity.[182,195]

Increases in sorbitol levels have been documented in all vascular and neuronal tissues. The vascular tissues include retina, aorta, and renal glomeruli. However, the role of the sorbitol and polyol pathway in the pathogenesis of diabetic vascular complications is not clear. In trials of ARIs in diabetic rats, some results have been promising with respect to the neurologic dysfunction and possibly the increased renal GFR. However, clinical studies have not demonstrated a clear efficacy of ARI in neuropathy or retinopathy.[196,197] In addition, studies of ARI administration in diabetic dogs have not shown a significant reduction in the level of retinopathy.[198]

To determine whether polyol or aldose reductase might play a role in the development of diabetic complications, some investigators have studied dogs or rats fed a diet high in galactose.[10,20,23,198] Galactose will be converted into galactitol by aldose reductase. However, galactose, because of its inability to bind to sorbitol dehydrogenase, is not further converted to fructose. The elevation in galactitol level is thought to mimic the effect of sorbitol and to cause vascular dysfunction in the absence of the other metabolic changes found in diabetes. In fact dogs, and possibly rats, receiving a diet containing

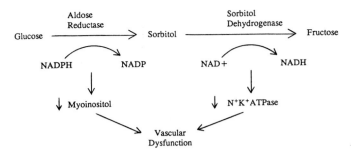

Fig. 37−6. Possible mechanisms of the polyol effect on cellular function and redox potential.

elevated levels of galactose develop cataracts and early changes in the retinal microvessels similar to those found in diabetic patients.[10,20,23,198] Again, ARI treatment does not appear to prevent the effects of galactose completely.[198] Of interest, dogs fed a high-galactose diet did not develop neuropathy or the classic changes of diabetic nephropathy.

One possible problem involved in using the galactose-fed dog model is that galactose might be metabolized by pathways beside the one converting it to galactitol. Preliminary studies have shown that galactose may increase the level of DAG, possibly via the glycolysis and de novo synthesis pathways. The limited effect of ARI in these studies might be due to the inability of ARI to reach the targeted tissue or to completely inhibit the increased flux in the sorbitol pathway.

Alteration in Redox Potential

Another possible effect of hyperglycemia involves the possible changes in redox potential caused by elevations in glucose level. Multiple pathways of glucose utilization could affect the redox potential and the production of NADH/NAD. The postulate is that glucose metabolism via glycolysis or through the polyol production pathway will increase the ratio of NADH to NAD. Specifically, increases in NADH can be derived from the metabolism of sorbitol (Fig. 37−6). The increased NADH/NAD ratio can affect the flux in many other pathways, such as the synthesis of DAG, DNA repair, and fatty acid oxidation. In support of this postulate, some groups have reported that the addition of pyruvate both in vivo and in cell culture models of diabetes complications improves the function of vascular cells that had been exposed either to diabetes or to elevated levels of glucose. The basis of the effect of pyruvate is its conversion to lactate, which in turn requires the conversion of NADH to NAD, thereby normalizing the redox potential.[199]

Activation of Protein Kinase C and the Diacylglycerol Pathway

Possible changes in phospholipid levels and in the activity of PKC in diabetes have interested many groups, since this enzyme system and phospholipids have been

shown to regulate a diverse range of vascular functions, including permeability, contractility, coagulation, flow, hormone action, growth factor effects, and ultimately the synthesis and turnover of basement membrane.[142−151] All of these parameters have been found to be abnormal in diabetes, as described above. In animals with chemically or genetically induced diabetes, the PKC activity in the membrane pool, which is the active fraction, is elevated in a variety of vascular tissues, including the retina, aorta, heart, and renal glomeruli.[139,140,200] Occurring in parallel with the changes in PKC activity in these tissues is an increase in total DAG level. The finding of such parallel changes suggests that diabetes enhances the PKC activity by increasing the total DAG content of the tissue. This suggestion is consistent with one known function of DAG—that of activating PKC by causing a translocation from the cytosolic pool to the membranous fraction. This effect of diabetes, however, is not observed in all tissues. For example, no changes in PKC or DAG are found in the brain, suggesting that the effect of elevated glucose levels or possibly diabetes is quite specific.

The reason for the specificity of the PKC and DAG response of the vasculature to diabetes is not known. However, this response may be related to the metabolism of glucose and its effect on the production of DAG. Elevated glucose levels appear to be able to increase the de novo synthesis of DAG in vascular cells in vitro, whereas in many other cells, the active pool of DAG is derived from the turnover of phosphoinositides. In cultured vascular cells such as smooth muscle and endothelial cells of the aorta and endothelial cells of the retina, an elevated glucose level leads to increases in total DAG and in the activity of the membranous pool of PKC (Fig. 37−7). Furthermore, fractionation of the various isoforms of PKC by immunoblotting has shown only α and βII isoforms of PKC in the vascular cells. Elevation of glucose level, or diabetes, appears to preferentially activate the βII form rather than the α form.[141] Further studies using radiolabeled free fatty acid have documented that the increase in DAG comes directly from the glucose. The changes in the PKC and DAG cannot be mimicked by osmotic changes and also appear not to be altered by ARI, suggesting that these effects of glucose are not due to osmotic effects or changes in the sorbitol pathway.

These effects on PKC and DAG normally represent acute changes. It is interesting to note, however, that the effect of elevated glucose levels in diabetes is not rapid but is delayed 3 to 5 days both in cultured cells and in intact animals. In diabetic rats, once the PKC and DAG changes have been established, the institution of euglycemia in the diabetic animal does not immediately reverse all of the biochemical manifestations.[141] These findings suggest that these changes in PKC and DAG are secondary to some other biochemical steps that precede the formation of DAG and the activation of PKC and result in structural changes that may not be easily reversible. In both diabetic animals and humans, many established vascular changes are difficult to reverse even by several months or years of euglycemic control.[141,200]

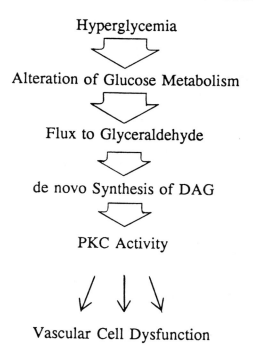

Hyperglycemia

⇓

Alteration of Glucose Metabolism

⇓

Flux to Glyceraldehyde

⇓

de novo Synthesis of DAG

⇓

PKC Activity

↙ ↓ ↘

Vascular Cell Dysfunction

Fig. 37–7. Schematic drawing on the effect of hyperglycemia on diacylglycerol (DAG) synthesis and protein kinase C (PKC) activation.

The consequences of changes in DAG and PKC activities are not yet clear. In studies using cultured vascular cells, the activation of PKC has been shown to affect a wide range of cellular substrates, including growth factors, hormones, cytokines, cytoskeletal proteins, and many signal transduction systems. Elevation of glucose levels and activation of PKC have been shown to cause increased phosphorylation of PKC substrates and regulation of growth factor receptors. In preliminary studies measuring physiologic parameters in diabetic rats, some reported results indicate that the increases in PKC and DAG parallel the changes in retinal blood flow. A decrease in retinal blood flow is observed in the initial few weeks after the onset of diabetes in both animals and humans with diabetes. Injection of an agonist of PKC into the vitreous will result in a mimicking of the decreased flow found in diabetic rats, whereas injection of PKC inhibitors actually can normalize the abnormality in retinal blood flow in diabetic rats. Thus, these data suggest that the changes in DAG and PKC can be chronic in nature and difficult to reverse even by euglycemia and can have pathophysiologic implications.

Nonenzymatic Glycosylation Pathway

The last theory for the mechanism of the effect of elevated glucose levels on cellular functions relates to the ability of glucose to form covalent products by nonenzymatic processes.[201–205] Glucose can form nonenzymatic glycosylation products such as glycosylated hemoglobin via a nucleophilic addition of glucose to the amino groups of proteins and possibly DNA. This reaction is slow and, depending on the half-life of the protein, can reach an apparent equilibrium over several weeks. The production of these intermediate glycosylated compounds eventually can lead to the formation of advanced glycosylation end-products (AGE) in a chemical reaction that is irreversible. These glycosylated proteins can cause changes in cellular functions or generate free radicals that may contribute to further cross-linking and alterations in cellular functions. The major factors that govern formation of these glycosylated products are the level of glucose and the duration of exposure to glucose. Therefore, the AGE products will form and accumulate primarily in those macromolecules with a prolonged half-life. For example, collagen, other proteins found in the basement membrane, and perhaps DNA are particularly disposed to the formation of AGE products because of their slow turnover rates. Vascular and neural tissues also may be particularly susceptible to the accumulation of nonenzymatic glycosylation products because of their slow turnover.

The consequences of nonenzymatic glycosylation can be separated into three different types. In the extracellular pool, glycosylated products can be formed with plasma proteins such as low-density lipopolysaccharide (LDL), albumin, and hemoglobin.[200–206] Glycosylated LDL could be cross-linked to collagen or other components of the basement membrane. In addition, glycosylation of LDL has been reported to change the binding of LDL to its receptor. All these changes might alter the metabolism of this important atherogenic substance. The complexing of glucose to the basement membrane is another way that elevated glucose can enhance the thickening of basement membrane. In vitro studies have shown that components of the basement membrane such as collagen that have been glycosylated or are cross-linked by glucose to each other are resistant to degradation. These alterations in the basement membrane could alter protein and affect the metabolism, function, and growth of vascular cells. Therefore, the accumulation of AGE products within collagen and basement membrane components may lead to a thickening of basement membrane and to alterations in the content of proteoglycans and may even affect the function of vascular cells by altering their signal transduction through receptors such as the integrin receptors.

AGE products that are released into the circulation can alter vascular function by binding to macrophages, which contain specific receptors to AGE. AGE products, once bound, have been shown to elicit several responses, such as an increase in the release of tumor necrosis factor (TNF), interleukin-1 (IL-1), and other cytokines.[201–210] Since TNF and IL-1 have receptors on endothelial cells that are known to increase vascular permeability and to affect the coagulation status of the endothelium, they may cause vascular dysfunction such as that described in diabetic patients.

Recent studies show that the infusion of AGE compounds can mimic some of the vascular abnormalities of diabetes such as thickened basement membrane and altered vascular contractility. AGE products also have been shown to quench the effect of nitric oxide, which is known to cause vasodilatation, or relaxation, of contractile vessels. Therefore, it is possible that an increase in glycosylated products can result in a loss of the relaxation phase in the vasculature, such as that described in the large arteries of diabetic animals. Studies have been done using inhibitors of nonenzymatic glycosylation such as aminoguanidine hydrochloride, which selectively blocks the reactive carbonyl group on early glycosylation products and prevents the formation of AGE products. In vitro, aminoguanidine will inhibit the formation of AGE and other proteins. In vivo, aminoguanidine can increase the accumulation of AGE-related products in the basement membrane and the plasma protein. Preliminary studies appear to show that chronic treatment with aminoguanidine may reduce basement membrane thickening and prevent some of the early changes in the retinal vasculature of diabetic rats.[203,210]

Besides resulting in cross-linking of protein, receptors, and other plasma factors, elevation of glucose levels has been shown in some recent in vitro studies to result in cross-linking of primary amine groups of nucleotides such as in DNA. If such changes occur in vivo they could have long-lasting effects.[212,213]

The effect of glycosylation on DNA is not known. However, it is associated with an increase in the frequency of mutations of either the deletion or insertion type and in alterations in gene expression. These changes can be measured by determining the fluorescent properties of the DNA in prokaryotic cells. In eukaryotic cells, elevated levels of glucose have been shown to affect DNA. Human endothelial cells cultured in 30 mM glucose appear to have an increase in single-strand breaks in DNA and a decrease in the DNA repair process.[214] However, this effect of glucose was not found in another study.[215]

In summary, elevations in glucose level can affect many important metabolic pathways in vascular cells. These changes can easily alter vascular cell functions and lead to the complications that have been described in diabetic patients and animals. It is not clear, however, which mechanism of injury plays the primary role in producing these alterations in cell function. Probably no one pathway is predominant, and any predominance may not apply to all vascular tissues. Indeed, it is likely that more than one of these pathways is responsible for the vascular changes observed in diabetes.

REFERENCES

1. Bergstrand A, Bucht H. The glomerular lesions of diabetes mellitus and their electron-microscope appearances. J Pathol Bacteriol 1959;77:231–42.
2. Mogensen CE, Østerby R, Gundersen HJG. Early functional and morphologic vascular renal consequences of the diabetic state. Diabetologia 1979;17:71–6.
3. Williamson JR, Kilo C. Extracellular matrix changes in diabetes mellitus. In: Scarpelli DG, Migaki G, eds, Comparative pathobiology of major age-related diseases. Modern aging research. Vol 4. New York: Alan R Liss, 1984:269–88.
4. Merriam JC Jr, Sommers SC. Mammary periductal hyalin in diabetic women: report of 20 cases. Lab Invest 1957; 6:412–20.
5. Schffling K, Federlin K, Ditschuneit H, et al. Disorders of sexual function in male diabetic. Diabetes 1963; 12:519–27.
6. Durand M, Durand A. Les altérations vasculaires dermo-hypodermiques des diabétiques: étude aux microscopes optique et électronique. Pathol Biol 1966;14:1005–19.
7. Johnson PC. Non-vascular basement membrane thickening in diabetes mellitus [Letter]. Lancet 1981;2:932–3.
8. Vracko R, Thorning D, Huang TW. Basal lamina of alveolar epithelium and capillaries: quantitative changes with aging and in diabetes mellitus. Am Rev Respir Dis 1979; 120:973–83.
9. Tisher CC. Anatomy of the kidney. In: Brenner BM, Rector FC Jr, eds. The kidney. Vol 2. 2nd ed. Philadelphia: WB Saunders, 1981:3–75.
10. Robison WG Jr, Kador PF, Kinoshita JH. Retinal capillaries: basement membrane thickening by galactosemia prevented with aldose reductase inhibitor. Science 1983; 221:1177–9.
11. Kelley C, D'Amore P, Hechtman HB, Shepro D. Microvascular pericyte contractility in vitro: comparison with other cells of the vascular wall. J Cell Biol 1987; 104:483–90.
12. Herman IM, D'Amore PA. Microvascular pericytes contain muscle and nonmuscle actins. J Cell Biol 1985; 101:43–52.
13. Farquhar MG. The glomerular basement membrane: a selective macromolecular filter. In: Hay ED, ed. Cell biology of extracellular matrix. New York: Plenum, 1981:335–78.
14. Simionescu M, Simionescu N. Ultrastructure of the microvascular wall: functional correlations. In: Renkin EM, Michel CC, eds. Handbook of physiology. Section 2. The cardiovascular system. Vol IV. Microcirculation. Part 1. Bethesda: American Physiological Society, Waverly Press, 1984:41–101.
15. Shimomura H, Spiro RG. Studies on macromolecular components of human glomerular basement membrane and alterations in diabetes: decreased levels of heparan sulfate proteoglycan and laminin. Diabetes 1987; 36:374–81.
16. Beisswenger PJ, Spiro RG. Studies on the human glomerular basement membrane: composition, nature of the carbohydrate units and chemical changes in diabetes mellitus. Diabetes 1973;22:180–93.
17. Grant ME, Heathcote JG, Orkin RW. Current concepts of basement-membrane structure and function. Biosci Rep 1981;1:819–42.
18. Sage H. Collagens of basement membranes. J Invest Dermatol 1982;79(Suppl 1):51S–59S.
19. Nagata M, Katz ML, Robison WG Jr. Age-related thickening of retinal capillary basement membranes. Invest Ophthalmol Vis Sci 1986 27:437–40.
20. Robison WG Jr, Kador PF, Akagi Y, et al. Prevention of basement membrane thickening in retinal capillaries by a novel inhibitor of aldose reductase, tolrestat. Diabetes 1986;35:295–9.
21. Waber S, Meister V, Rossi GL, et al. Studies on retinal microangiopathy and coronary macroangiopathy in rats with streptozotocin-induced diabetes. Virchows Arch [B] 1981;37:1–10.
22. Fischer F, Gärtner J. Morphometric analysis of basal laminae in rats with long-term streptozotocin diabetes. II. Retinal capillaries. Exp Eye Res 1983;37:55–64.

23. Robison WG Jr, Nagata M, Kinoshita JH. Aldose reductase and retinal capillary basement membrane thickening. Exp Eye Res 1988;46:343–8.

24. Kimmelstiel P, Wilson C. Intercapillary lesions in the glomeruli of the kidney. Am J Pathol 1936;12:83–98.

25. Østerby R, Gundersen HJG. Glomerular size and structure in diabetes mellitus. I. Early abnormalities. Diabetologia 1975;11:225–9.

26. Østerby R, Gundersen HJG. Fast accumulation of basement membrane material and the rate of morphological changes in acute experimental diabetic glomerular hypertrophy. Diabetologia 1980;18:493–500.

27. Østerby R. Early phases in the development of diabetic glomerulopathy. Acta Med Scand Suppl 1975;574:1–80.

28. Mauer SM, Steffes MW, Ellis EN, et al. Structural-functional relationships in diabetic nephropathy. J Clin Invest 1984;74:1143–55.

29. Steffes MW, Mauer SM. Diabetic glomerulopathy: a morphological approach to monitoring development, progression and reversibility. Diabetic Nephropathy 1985;4:114–7.

30. Wiseman MJ, Saunders AJ, Keen H, Viberti G. Effect of blood glucose control on increased glomerular filtration rate and kidney size in insulin-dependent diabetes. N Engl J Med 1985;312:617–21.

31. Rasch R. Prevention of diabetic glomerulopathy in streptozotocin diabetic rats by insulin treatment: albumin excretion. Diabetologia 1980;18:413–6.

32. Steffes MW, Brown DM, Basgen JM, Mauer SM. Amelioration of mesangial volume and surface alterations following islet transplantation in diabetic rats. Diabetes 1980;29:509–15.

33. Schnider S, Aronoff SL, Tchou P, et al. Urinary protein excretion in prediabetic (PD), normal (N), and diabetic (D) Pima Indians and normal caucasians (NC) [Abstract no. 37]. Diabetes 1977;26(Suppl 1):362.

34. Myers BD, Winetz, JA, Chui F, Michaels AS. Mechanisms of proteinuria in diabetic nephropathy: a study of glomerular barrier function. Kidney Int 1982;21:633–41.

35. Wahl P, Deppermann D, Hasslacher C. Biochemistry of glomerular basement membrane of the normal and diabetic human. Kidney Int 1982;21:744–9.

36. Parthasarathy N, Spiro RG. Effect of diabetes on the glycosaminoglycan component of the human glomerular basement membrane. Diabetes 1982;31:738–41.

37. Nakamura Y, Myers BD. Charge selectivity of proteinuria in diabetic glomerulopathy. Diabetes 1988;37:1202–11.

38. Spiro RG. Biochemistry of the renal glomerular basement membrane and its alterations in diabetes mellitus. N Engl J Med 1973;288:1337–42.

39. Spiro RG. Nature of the glycoprotein components of basement membranes. Ann NY Acad Sci 1978;312:106–21.

40. Beisswenger PJ, Spiro RG. Human glomerular basement membrane: chemical alteration in diabetes mellitus. Science 1970;168:596–8.

41. Kefalides NA. Biochemical properties of human glomerular basement membrane in normal and diabetic kidneys. J Clin Invest 1974;53:403–7.

42. Westberg NG, Michael AF. Human glomerular basement membrane: chemical composition in diabetes mellitus. Acta Med Scand 1973;194:39–47.

43. Peterson DT, Greene WC, Reaven GM. Effect of experimental diabetes mellitus on kidney ribosomal protein synthesis. Diabetes 1971;20:649–54.

44. Khalifa A, Cohen MP. Glomerular protocollagen lysylhydroxylase activity in streptozotocin diabetes. Biochim Biophys Acta 1975;386:332–9.

45. Cohen MP, Khalifa A. Effect of diabetes and insulin on rat renal glomerular protocollagen hydroxylase activities. Biochim Biophys Acta 1977;496:88–94.

46. Spiro MJ, Spiro RG. Studies on the biosynthesis of the hydroxylysine-linked disaccharide unit of basement membranes and collagens. II. Kidney galactosyltransferase. J Biol Chem 1971;246:4910–8.

47. Spiro RG, Spiro MJ. Studies on the biosynthesis of the hydroxylysine-linked disaccharide unit of basement membranes and collagens. I. Kidney glucosyltransferase. J Biol Chem 1971;246:4899–909.

48. Spiro RG, Spiro MJ. Effect of diabetes on the biosynthesis of the renal glomerular basement membrane: studies on the glucosyltransferase. Diabetes 1971;20:641–8.

49. Risteli J, Koivisto VA, Akerblom HK, Kivirikko KI, et al. Intracellular enzymes of collagen biosynthesis in rat kidney in streptozotocin diabetes. Diabetes 1976;25:1066–70.

50. Guzdek A, Sarnecka-Keller M, Dubin A. The activities of perfused livers of control and streptozotocin diabetic rats in the synthesis of some plasma proteins and peptides. Horm Metab Res 1979;11:107–11.

51. Beisswenger PJ. Glomerular basement membrane: biosynthesis and chemical composition in the streptozotocin diabetic rat. J Clin Invest 1976;58:844–52.

52. Cohen MP, Vogt CA. Collagen synthesis and secretion by isolated rat renal glomeruli. Biochim Biophys Acta 1975;393:78–87.

53. Grant ME, Harwood R, Williams IF. The biosynthesis of basement membrane collagen by isolated rat glomeruli. Eur J Biochem 1975;54:531–40.

54. Grant ME, Harwood R, Williams IF. Increased synthesis of glomerular basement membrane collagen in streptozotocin diabetes. J Physiol (Lond) 1976;257(1):1–56P–57P.

55. Brownlee M, Spiro RG. Glomerular basement membrane metabolism in the diabetic rat: in vivo studies. Diabetes 1979;28:121–5.

56. Cagliero E, Maiello M, Boeri D, et al. Increased expression of basement membrane components in human endothelial cells cultured in high glucose. J Clin Invest 1988;82:735–8.

57. Tilton RG, Miller EJ, Kilo C, Williamson JR. Pericyte form and distribution in rat retinal and uveal capillaries. Invest Ophthalmol Vis Sci 1985;26:68–73.

58. Petty RG, Pearson JD. Endothelium—the axis of vascular health and disease. J R Coll Physicians Lond 1989;23:92–102.

59. Cogan DG, Toussaint D, Kuwabara T. Retinal vascular patterns. IV. Diabetic retinopathy. Arch Ophthalmol 1961;66:366–78.

60. Kuwabara T, Cogan DG. Retinal vascular patterns. VI. Mural cells of the retinal capillaries. Arch Ophthalmol 1963;69:492–502.

61. Ashton N. Injection of the retinal vascular system in enucleated eyes in diabetic retinopathy. Br J Ophthalmol 1950;34:38–41.

62. Shepro D, D'Amore PA. Physiology and biochemistry of the vascular wall endothelium. In: Renkin EM, Michel CC, eds. Handbook of physiology. Section 2. The cardiovascular system. Vol IV. Microcirculation. Part I. Bethesda: American Physiological Society, Waverly Press, 1984:103–64.

63. Merimee TJ. Diabetic retinopathy: a synthesis of perspectives. N Engl J Med 1990;322:978–83.

64. Larson DM, Carson MP, Haudenschild CC. Junctional transfer of small molecules in cultured bovine brain

microvascular endothelial cells and pericytes. Microvasc Res 1987;34:184–99.

65. Buzney SM, Frank RN, Varma SD, et al. Aldose reductase in retinal mural cells. Invest Ophthalmol Vis Sci 1977; 16:392–6.

66. King GL, Goodman AD, Buzney S, et al. Receptors and growth-promoting effects of insulin and insulinlike growth factors on cells from bovine retinal capillaries and aorta. J Clin Invest 1985;75:1028–36.

67. Nayak RC, Berman AB, George KL, et al. A monoclonal antibody (3G5)-defined ganglioside antigen is expressed on the cell surface of microvascular pericytes. J Exp Med 1988;167:1003–15.

68. Antonelli-Orlidge A, Saunders KB, Smith SR, D'Amore PA. An activated form of transforming growth factor β is produced by cocultures of endothelial cells and pericytes. Proc Natl Acad Sci USA 1989;86:4544–8.

69. Sato Y, Rifkin DB. Inhibition of endothelial cell movement by pericytes and smooth muscle cells: activation of a latent transforming growth factor β1-like molecule by plasmin during co-culture. J Cell Biol 1989;109:309–15.

70. Burditt AF, Caird FI, Draper GJ. The natural history of diabetic retinopathy. Q J Med 1968;37:303–17.

71. Caird FI, Burditt AF, Draper GJ. Diabetic retinopathy: a further study of prognosis for vision. Diabetes 1968; 17:121–3.

72. Arnqvist HJ, Ballerman BJ, King GL. Receptors for and effects of insulin and IGF-1 in rat glomerular mesangial cells. Am J Physiol 1988;254:C411–6.

73. Striker GE, Killen PD, Farin FM. Human glomerular cells in vitro: isolation and characterization. Transplant Proc 1980;12(Suppl 1):88–99.

74. Kreisberg JI, Karnovsky MJ. Glomerular cells in culture. Kidney Int 1983;23:439–47.

75. Ishii H, Umeda F, Nawata H. Platelet function in diabetes. Diabetes Metab Rev 1992;8:53–66.

76. Ostermann H, van de Loo J. Factors of the haemostatic system in diabetic patients: a survey of controlled studies. Haemostasis 1986;16:386–416.

77. Grant MB, Fitzgerald C, Guay C, Lottenberg R. Fibrinolytic capacity following stimulation with desmopressin acetate in patients with diabetes mellitus. Metabolism 1989; 38:901–7.

78. Kruithof EKO. Plasminogen activator inhibitor type 1: biochemical, biological and clinical aspects. Fibrinolysis 1988;2:59–70.

79. Small M, Kluft C, MacCuish AC, Lowe GDO. Tissue plasminogen activator inhibition in diabetes mellitus. Diabetes Care 1989;12:655–8.

80. Moroose R, Hoyer LW. Von Willebrand factor and platelet function. Annu Rev Med 1986;37:157–63.

81. Banga JD, Sixma JJ. Diabetes mellitus, vascular disease and thrombosis. Clin Haematol 1986;15:465–92.

82. Jaffe EA, Hoyer LW, Nachman RL. Synthesis of von Willebrand factor by cultured human endothelial cells. Proc Natl Acad Sci USA 1974;71:1906–9.

83. Bloom AL. The biosynthesis of factor VIII. Clin Haematol 1979;8:53–77.

84. Colwell JA, Lopes-Virella M, Winocour PD, et al. New concepts about the pathogenesis of atherosclerosis in diabetes mellitus. In: Levin ME, O'Neal LW, eds. The diabetic foot. St Louis: CV Mosby, 1988:51–70.

85. Colwell JA, Lopes-Virella M, Halushka PV. Pathogenesis of atherosclerosis in diabetes mellitus. Diabetes Care 1981;4:121–33.

86. Porta M, Ricchetti I, La Selva M, et al. Quantitative and qualitative assessment of plasma von Willebrand fact-

or variations, as induced by forearm venous stasis in patients with diabetic microangiopathy. Diabetes Res 1984;1:219–21.

87. Gonzalez J, Colwell JA, Sarji KE, et al. Effect of metabolic control with insulin on plasma von Willebrand factor activity (VIIIR:WF) in diabetes mellitus. Thromb Res 1980;17:261–6.

88. Winocour PD, Lopes-Virella M, Laimins M, Colwell JA. Time course of changes in in vitro platelet function and plasma von Willebrand factor activity (VIIIR:WF) and factor VIII-related antigen (VIIIR:Ag) in the diabetic rat. J Lab Clin Med 1983;102:795–804.

89. Paton RC, Kernoff PBA, Wales JK, McNicol GP. Effects of diet and gliclazide on the haemostatic system of non-insulin-dependent diabetics. BMJ 1981; 283:1018–20.

90. Porta M, Maneschi F, White MC, Kohner EM. Twenty-four hour variations of von Willebrand factor and factor VIII-related antigen in diabetic retinopathy. Metabolism 1981;30:695–9.

91. Muntean WE, Borkenstein MH, Haas J. Elevation of factor VIII coagulant activity over factor VIII coagulant antigen in diabetic children without vascular disease: a sign of activation of the factor VIII coagulant moiety during poor diabetes control. Diabetes 1985;34:140–4.

92. Coller BS, Frank RN, Milton RC, Gralnick HR. Plasma cofactors of platelet function: correlation with diabetic retinopathy and hemoglobin A_{1a-c}: studies in diabetic patients and normal persons. Ann Intern Med 1978; 88:311–6.

93. Winocour PD, Lopes-Virella M, Laimins M, Colwell JA. Effect of insulin treatment in streptozotocin-induced diabetic rats on in vitro platelet function and plasma von Willebrand factor activity and factor VIII-related antigen. J Lab Clin Med 1985;106:319–25.

94. Stehouwer CDA, Stroes ESG, Hackeng WHL, et al. Von Willebrand factor and development of diabetic nephropathy in IDDM. Diabetes 1991;40:971–6.

95. Aanderud S, Krane H, Nordy A. Influence of glucose, insulin and sera from diabetic patients on the prostacyclin synthesis in vitro in cultured human endothelial cells. Diabetologia 1985;28:641–4.

96. Umeda F, Inoguchi T, Nawata H. Reduced stimulatory activity on prostacyclin production by cultured endothelial cells in serum from aged and diabetic patients. Atherosclerosis 1989;75:61–6.

97. Oosterhuis JA, Vink R. Fluorescein photography in diabetic retinopathy. In: Henkes HE, ed. Perspectives in ophthalmology. New York: Excerpta Medica, 1968:115–32.

98. Sosula L, Beaumont P, Hollows FC, Jonson KM. Dilatation and endothelial proliferation of retinal capillaries in streptozotocin-diabetic rats: quantitative electron microscopy. Invest Ophthalmol 1972;11:926–35.

99. Parving H-H, Larsen M, Hommel E, Lund-Andersen H. Effect of antihypertensive treatment on blood-retinal barrier permeability to fluorescein in hypertensive type I (insulin-dependent) diabetic patients with background retinopathy. Diabetologia 1989;32:440–4.

100. Wallow IHL, Engerman RL. Permeability and patency of retinal blood vessels in experimental diabetes. Invest Ophthalmol Vis Sci 1977;16:447–61.

101. Williamson JR, Chang K, Rowold E, et al. Sorbinil prevents diabetes-induced increases in vascular permeability but does not alter collagen cross-linking. Diabetes 1985; 34:703–5.

102. Llorach MAS, Böhm GM, Leme JG. Decreased vascular

reactions to permeability factors in experimental diabetes. Br J Exp Pathol 1976;57:747–54.

103. Cunha-Vaz J, De Abreu JRF, Campos AJ, Figo GM. Early breakdown of the blood-retinal barrier in diabetes. Br J Ophthalmol 1975;59:649–56.

104. Ortola FV, Ballermann BJ, Anderson S, et al. Elevated plasma atrial natriuretic peptide levels in diabetic rats: potential mediator of hyperfiltration. J Clin Invest 1987;80:670–4.

105. Kamata K, Miyata N, Kasuya Y. Involvement of endothelial cells in relaxation and contraction responses of the aorta to isoproterenol in naive and streptozotocin-induced diabetic rats. J Pharmacol Exp Ther 1989;249:890–4.

106. Pieper GM, Gross GJ. Oxygen free radicals abolish endothelium-dependent relaxation in diabetic rat aorta. Am J Physiol 1988;255:H825–33.

107. Mayhan WG. Impairment of endothelium-dependent dilatation of cerebral arterioles during diabetes mellitus. Am J Physiol 1989;256:H621–5.

108. Gebremedhin D, Koltai MZ, Pog tsa G et al. Differential contractile responsiveness of femoral arteries from healthy and diabetic dogs: role of endothelium. Arch Int Pharmacodyn Ther 1987;288:100–8.

109. Fortes ZB, Leme JG, Scivoletto R. Vascular reactivity in diabetes mellitus: possible role of insulin on the endothelial cell. Br J Pharmacol 1984;83:635–43.

110. Durante W, Sen AK, Sunahara FA. Impairment of endothelium-dependent relaxation in aortae from spontaneously diabetic rats. Br J Pharmacol 1988;94:463–8.

111. Gebremedhin D, Koltai MZ, Pog tsa G, et al. Influence of experimental diabetes on the mechanical responses of canine coronary arteries: role of endothelium. Cardiovasc Res 1988;22:537–44.

112. de Tejada IS, Goldstein I, Azadzoi K, et al. Impaired neurogenic and endothelium-mediated relaxation of penile smooth muscle from diabetic men with impotence. N Engl J Med 1989;320:1025–30.

113. Tanz RD, Chang KSK, Weller TS. Histamine relaxation of aortic rings from diabetic rats. Agents Actions 1989; 28:1–8.

114. Doi T, Striker LJ, Quaife C, et al. Progressive glomerulosclerosis develops in transgenic mice chronically expressing growth hormone and growth hormone releasing factor but not in those expressing insulinlike growth factor-I. Am J Pathol 1988;131:398–403.

115. Hirschberg R, Kopple JD. Evidence that insulin-like growth factor I increases renal plasma flow and glomerular filtration rate in fasted rats. J Clin Invest 1989; 83:326–30.

116. Fagin JA, Melmed S. Relative increase in insulin-like growth factor I messenger ribonucleic acid levels in compensatory renal hypertrophy. Endocrinology 1987; 120:718–24.

117. Clermont A, Bursell S-E, King GL, et al. Indication of retinal circulation changes in early stage diabetic patients. Invest Ophthalmol Vis Sci 1992;33:1366.

118. Grunwald JE, Riva CE, Martin DB, et al. Effect of an insulin-induced decrease in blood glucose on the human diabetic retinal circulation. Ophthalmology 1987; 94:1614–20.

119. Ditzel J, Standl E. The problem of tissue oxygenation in diabetes mellitus. I. Its relation to the early functional changes in the microcirculation of diabetic subjects. Acta Med Scand Suppl 1975;578:49–58.

120. Yoshida A, Feke GT, Morales-Stoppello J, et al. Retinal blood flow alterations during progression of diabetic retinopathy. Arch Ophthalmol 1983;101:225–7.

121. Hickam JB, Frayser R. A photographic method for measuring the mean retinal circulation time using fluorescein. Invest Ophthalmol 1965;4:876–84.

122. Kohner EM, Hamilton AM, Saunders SJ, et al. The retinal blood flow in diabetes. Diabetologia 1975;11:27–33.

123. Bucala R, Tracey KJ, Cerami A. Advanced glycosylation products quench nitric oxide and mediate defective endothelium-dependent vasodilatation in experimental diabetes. J Clin Invest 1991; 87:432–8.

124. Tesfamariam B, Jakubowski JA, Cohen RA. Contraction of diabetic rabbit aorta caused by endothelium-derived PGH_2-TXA_2. Am J Physiol 1989;257:H1327–33.

125. Tesfamariam B, Brown ML, Cohen RA. Elevated glucose impairs endothelium-dependent relaxation by activating protein kinase C. J Clin Invest 1991;87:1643–8.

126. Nyborg NCB, Prieto D, Benedito S, Nielson PJ. Endothelin-1-induced contraction of bovine retinal small arteries is reversible and abolished by nitrendipine. Invest Ophthal Vis Sci 1991; 32:27–31.

127. Arai H, Hori S, Aramori I, et al. Cloning and expression of a cDNA encoding an endothelin receptor. Nature 1990;348:730–2.

128. Van Renterghem C, Vigne P, Barhanin J, et al. Molecular mechanism of action of the vasoconstrictor peptide endothelin. Biochem Biophys Res Comm 1988; 157:977–85.

129. Marsden PA, Danthuluri NR, Brenner BM, et al. Endothelin action on vascular smooth muscle involves inositol triphosphate and calcium mobilization. Biochem Biophys Res Commun 1989;158:86–93.

130. Sugiura M, Inagami T, Hare GMT, Johns JA. Endothelin action: inhibition by a protein kinase inhibitor and involvement of phosphoinositols. Biochem Biophys Res Commun 1989;158:170–6.

131. Takahashi K, Ghatei MA, Lam H-C, et al. Elevated plasma endothelin in patients with diabetes mellitus. Diabetologia 1990;33:306–10.

132. Yamauchi T, Ohnaka K, Takayanagi R, et al. Enhanced secretion of endothelin-1 by elevated glucose levels from cultured bovine aortic endothelial cells. FEBS Lett 1990;267:16–8.

133. Yanagisawa M, Kurihara H, Kimura S, et al. A novel potent vasoconstrictor peptide produced by vascular endothelial cells. Nature 1988;332:411–5.

134. Takahashi K, Brooks RA, Kanse SM, et al. Production of endothelin-1 by cultured bovine retinal endothelial cells and presence of endothelin receptors on associated pericytes. Diabetes 1989;38:1200–2.

135. Oliver FJ, de la Rubia G, Feener EP, et al. Stimulation of endothelin-1 gene expression by insulin in endothelial cells. J Biol Chem 1991;266:23251–6.

136. World Health Organisation Multinational Study of Vascular Disease in Diabetics. Prevalence of small vessel and large vessel disease in diabetic patients from 14 centres. Diabetologia 1985;28(Suppl):615–40.

137. Drury PL. Hypertension. Baillieres Clin Endocrinol Metab 1988;2:375–89.

138. Simonson DC. Etiology and prevalence of hypertension in diabetic patients. Diabetes Care 1988;11:821–7.

139. King GL, Johnson S, Wu G. Possible growth modulators involved in the pathogenesis of diabetic proliferative retinopathy. In: Westermark B, Betsholtz C, Hkfelt B, eds. Growth factors in health and disease. International Congress Series 925. Amsterdam: Excerpta Medica, 1990; 303–7.

140. Craven PA, Davidson CM, DeRubertis FR. Increase in diacylglycerol mass in isolated glomeruli by glucose

from de novo synthesis of glycerolipids. Diabetes 1990; 39:667−74.

141. Inoguchi T, Battan R, Handler E, et al. Preferential activation of protein kinase C isoform βII and diacylglycerol levels in the aorta and heart of diabetic rats. Proc Natl Acad Sci USA 1992;89:11059−63.

142. Kikkawa U, Nishizuka Y. The role of protein kinase C in transmembrane signalling. Annu Rev Cell Biol 1986; 2:149−78.

143. Schlessinger J. Allosteric regulation of the epidermal growth factor receptor kinase. J Cell Biol 1986; 103:2067−72.

144. Backer JM, King GL. Regulation of receptor-mediated endocytosis by phorbol esters. Biochem Pharmacol 1991;41:1267−77.

145. Banskota NK, Carpentier J-L, King GL. Processing and release of insulin and insulin-like growth factor I by macro- and microvascular endothelial cells. Endocrinology 1986;119:1904−13.

146. Kariya K, Kawahara Y, Tsuda T, et al. Possible involvement of protein kinase C in platelet-derived growth factor-stimulated DNA synthesis in vascular smooth muscle cells. Atherosclerosis 1987;63:251−55.

147. Hachiya HL, Takayama S, White MF, King GL. Regulation of insulin receptor internalization in vascular endothelial cells by insulin and phorbol ester. J Biol Chem 1987; 262:6417−24.

148. Jiang MJ, Morgan KG. Intracellular calcium levels in phorbol ester-induced contractions of vascular muscle. Am J Physiol 1987;253:H1365−71.

149. Baraban JM, Gould RJ, Peroutka SJ, Snyder SH. Phorbol ester effects on neurotransmission: interaction with neurotransmitters and calcium in smooth muscle. Proc Natl Acad Sci USA 1985;82:604−7.

150. Forder J, Scriabine A, Rasmussen H. Plasma membrane calcium flux, protein kinase C activation and smooth muscle contraction. J Pharmacol Exp Ther 1985; 235:267−73.

151. Limas CJ, Limas C. Phorbol ester- and diacylglycerol-mediated desensitization of cardiac β-adrenergic receptors. Circ Res 1985;57:443−9.

152. Raymond L, Jacobson B. Isolation and identification of stimulatory and inhibitory cell growth factors in bovine vitreous. Exp Eye Res 1982;34:267−86.

153. Taylor CM, Weiss JB. Partial purification of a 5.7 k glycoprotein from bovine vitreous which inhibits both angiogenesis and collagenase activity. Biochem Biophys Res Comm 1985;133:911−6.

154. Lutty GA, Thompson DC, Gallup JY, et al. Vitreous: an inhibitor of retinal extract-induced neovascularization. Invest Ophthalmol Vis Sci 1983;24:52−6.

155. Schweigerer L, Malerstein B, Gospodarowicz D. Tumor necrosis factor inhibits the proliferation of cultured capillary endothelial cells. Biochem Biophys Res Commun 1987;143:997−1004.

156. Fràter-Schröder M, Risau W, Hallmann R, et al. Tumor necrosis factor type α a potent inhibitor of endothelial cell growth in vitro, is angiogenic in vivo. Proc Natl Acad Sci USA 1987;84:5277−81.

157. Schweigerer L, Neufeld G, Friedman J, et al. Capillary endothelial cells express basic fibroblast growth factor, a mitogen that promotes their own growth. Nature 1987;325:257−9.

158. Jaye M, Howk R, Burgess W, et al. Human endothelial cell growth factor: cloning, nucleotide sequence, and chromosome localization. Science 1986;233:541−5.

159. Klagsbrun M, Baird A. A dual receptor system is required for basic fibroblast growth factor activity. Cell 1991; 67:229−31.

160. Sprugel KH, McPherson JM, Clowes AW, Ross R. Effects of growth factors in vivo. I. Cell ingrowth into porous subcutaneous chambers. Am J Pathol 1987;129:601−13.

161. Sivalingham A, Kenny J, Brown GC, et al. In: Second International Symposium on Ocular Circulation and Neovascularization, Bethesda, MD: National Institutes of Health, 1989.

162. Lutty G, Chandler C, Bennett A, et al. Presence of endothelial cell growth factor in normal and diabetic eyes. Curr Eye Res 1986;5:9−17.

163. Glaser BM. Extracellular modulating factors and the control of intraocular neovascularization: an overview. Arch Ophthalmol 1988;106:603−7.

164. Glaser BM, Campochiaro PA, Davis JL Jr, Jerden JA. Retinal pigment epithelial cells release inhibitors of neovascularization. Ophthalmology 1987;94:780−4.

165. Connor TB Jr, Roberts AB, Sporn MB, et al. Correlation of fibrosis and transforming growth factor-β type 2 levels in the eye. J Clin Invest 1989;83:1661−6.

166. Taylor CM, Kissun RD, Schor AN, et al. Endothelial cell-stimulating angiogenesis factor in vitreous from extraretinal neovascularizations. Invest Ophthalmol Vis Sci 1989;30:2174−8.

167. Taylor CM, Weiss JB, McLaughlin B, et al. Increased procollagenase activating angiogenic factor in the vitreous humour of oxygen treated kittens. Br J Ophthalmol 1988;72:2−4.

168. Balodimos MC, Rees SB, Aiello LM, et al. Fluorescein photography in proliferative diabetic retinopathy treated by pituitary ablation. In: Goldberg MF, Fine SL, eds. Symposium on the treatment of diabetic retinopathy. Diabetes and Arthritis Control Program, US Department of Health, Education and Welfare. Washington, DC: US Government Printing Office, 1969:153−69.

169. Grant M, Russell B, Fitzgerald C, Merimee TJ. Insulin-like growth factors in vitreous: studies in control and diabetic subjects with neovascularization. Diabetes 1986; 35:416−20.

170. Lamberton RP, Goodman AD, Kassoff A et al. Von Willebrand factor (VIII R: Ag), fibronectin, and insulin-like growth factors I and II in diabetic retinopathy and nephropathy. Diabetes 1984;33:125−9.

171. Pyörälä K, Laakso M, Uusitupa M. Diabetes and atherosclerosis: an epidemiologic view. Diabetes Metab Rev 1987;3:463−524.

172. King GL, Buzney S, Kahn CR, et al. Differential responsiveness to insulin of endothelial and support cells from micro- and macrovessels. J Clin Invest 1983;71:974−79.

173. Stout RW. Insulin and atheroma—an update. Lancet 1987;1:1077−9.

174. Jialal I, King GL, Buchwald S, et al. Processing of insulin by bovine endothelial cells in culture: internalization without degradation. Diabetes 1984;33:794−800.

175. Jialal I, Crettaz M, Hachiya HL, et al. Characterization of the receptors for insulin and the insulin-like growth factors on micro- and macrovascular tissues. Endocrinology 1985;117:1222−9.

176. Bar RS, Boes M. Distinct receptors for IGF-I, IGF-II, and insulin are present on bovine capillary endothelial cells and large vessel endothelial cells. Biochem Biophys Res Commun 1984;124:203−9.

177. Kwok CF, Goldstein BJ, Muller-Wieland D, et al. Identification of persistent defects in insulin receptor structure

and function in capillary endothelial cells from diabetic rats. J Clin Invest 1989;83:127–36.

178. Bottaro DP, Bonner-Weir S, King GL. Insulin receptor recycling in vascular endothelial cells: regulation by insulin and phorbol ester. J Biol Chem 1989; 264:5916–23.

179. Wallum BJ, Taborsky GJ Jr, Porte D Jr,, et al. Cerebrospinal fluid insulin levels increase during intravenous insulin infusions in man. J Clin Endocrinol Metab 1987;64:190–4.

180. Bar RS, Boes M, Sandra A. IGF receptors in myocardial capillary endothelium: potential regulation of IGF-I transport to cardiac muscle. Biochem Biophys Res Commun 1988;152:93–8.

181. King GL, Johnson SM. Receptor-mediated transport of insulin across endothelial cells. Science 1985; 227:1583–6.

182. Greene DA, Lattimer SA, Sima AAF, et al. Sorbitol, phosphoinositides, and sodium-potassium-ATPase in the pathogenesis of diabetic complications. N Engl J Med 1987;316:599–606.

183. MacGregor LC, Matschinsky FM. Treatment with aldose reductase inhibitor or with myo-inositol arrests deterioration of the electroretinogram of diabetic rats. J Clin Invest 1985;76:887–9.

184. Hawthorne GC, Bartlett K, Hetherington CS, Alberti KGMM. The effect of high glucose on polyol pathway activity and myoinositol mechanism in cultured human endothelial cells. Diabetologia 1989;32:163–6.

185. Lightman S, Rechthand E, Terubayashi H, et al. Permeability changes in blood-retinal barrier of galactosemic rats are prevented by aldose reductase inhibitors. Diabetes 1987;36:1271–5.

186. Akagi Y, Yajima Y, Kador PF, et al. Localization of aldose reductase in the human eye. Diabetes 1984;33:562–6.

187. Chakrabarti S, Sima AAF, Nakajima T, et al. Aldose reductase in the BB rat: isolation, immunological identification and localization in the retina and peripheral nerve. Diabetologia 1987;30:244–57.

188. Winegrad AI. Does a common mechanism induce the diverse complications of diabetes? Diabetes 1987; 36:396–406.

189. Gabbay KH. The sorbitol pathway and the complications of diabetes. N Engl J Med 1973;288:831–6.

190. Kennedy A, Frank RN, Varma SD. Aldose reductase activity in retinal and cerebral microvessels and cultured vascular cells. Invest Ophthalmol Vis Sci 1983;24:1250–8.

191. Ludvigson MA, Sorenson RL. Immunohistochemical localization of aldose reductase. II. Rat eye and kidney. Diabetes 1980;29:450–9.

192. Lorenzi M, Toledo S, Boss GR, et al. The polyol pathway and glucose 6-phosphate in human endothelial cells cultured in high glucose concentrations. Diabetologia 1987;30:222–7.

193. Kador PF, Robison WG Jr, Kinoshita JH. The pharmacology of aldose reductase inhibitors. Annu Rev Pharmacol Toxicol 1985;25:691–714.

194. Sussman I, Carson MP, Schultz V, et al. Chronic exposure to high glucose decreases myo-inositol in cultured cerebral microvascular pericytes but not in endothelium. Diabetologia 1988;31:771–5.

195. Loy A, Lurie KG, Ghosh A, et al. Diabetes and the myo-inositol paradox. Diabetes 1990;39:1305–12.

196. Frank RN. Aldose reductase inhibition. The chemical key to the control of diabetic retinopathy? [Editorial] Arch Ophthalmol 1990;108:1229–31.

197. Judzewitsch RG, Jaspan JB, Polonsky KS, et al. Aldose reductase inhibition improves nerve conduction velocity in diabetic patients. N Engl J Med 1983;308:119–25.

198. Kern TS, Engerman RL. Development of complications in diabetic dogs and galactosemic dogs: effect of aldose reductase inhibitor. In: Proceedings of a workshop on aldose reductase inhibitors. NIH publication no. 91–3114. Bethesda, MD: National Institutes of Health, 1991.

199. Pugliese G, Tilton RG, Williamson JR. Glucose-induced metabolic imbalances in the pathogenesis of diabetic vascular disease. Diabetes Metab Rev 1991;7:35–59.

200. Wolf BA, Williamson JR, Easom RA, et al. Diacylglycerol accumulation and microvascular abnormalities induced by elevated glucose levels. J Clin Invest 1991;87:31–8.

201. Brownlee M, Cerami A, Vlassara H. Advanced glycosylation end products in tissue and the biochemical basis of diabetic complications. N Engl J Med 1988;318:1315–21.

202. Brownlee M, Vlassara H, Cerami A. Nonenzymatic glycosylation and the pathogenesis of diabetic complications. Ann Intern Med 1984;101:527–37.

203. Brownlee M, Vlassara H, Kooney A, et al. Aminoguanidine prevents diabetes-induced arterial wall protein cross-linking. Science 1986;232:1629–32.

204. Edelstein D, Brownlee M. Mechanistic studies of advanced glycosylation end product inhibition by aminoguanidine. Diabetes 1992;41:26–9.

205. Brownlee M. Glycosylation products as toxic mediators of diabetic complications. Annu Rev Med 1991; 42:159–66.

206. Gupta S, Rifici V, Crowley S, et al. Interactions of LDL and modified LDL with mesangial cells and matrix. Kidney Int 1992;41:1161–9.

207. Haitoglou CS, Tsilibary EC, Brownlee M, Charonis AS. Altered cellular interactions between endothelial cells and nonenzymatically glucosylated laminin/type IV collagen. J Biol Chem 1992;267:12404–7.

208. Makita Z, Vlassara H, Cerami A, Bucala R. Immunochemical detection of advanced glycosylation end products in vivo. J Biol Chem 1992;267:5133–8.

209. Makita Z, Radoff S, Rayfield EJ, et al. Advanced glycosylation end products in patients with diabetic nephropathy. N Engl J Med 1991;325:836–42.

210. Hammes HP, Martin S, Federlin K, et al. Aminoguanidine treatment inhibits the development of experimental diabetic retinopathy. Proc Natl Acad Sci USA 1991; 88:11555–8.

211. Vlassara H, Esposito C, Gerlach H, Stern. Receptor-mediated binding of glycosylated albumin to endothelium induces tissue necrosis factor and acts synergistically with TNF procoagulant activity [Abstract no. 329]. Diabetes 1989;38(Suppl 2):83A.

212. Bucala R, Model P, Cerami A. Modification of DNA by reducing sugars: a possible mechanism for nucleic acid aging and age-related dysfunction in gene expression. Proc Natl Acad Sci USA 1984;81:105–9.

213. De Bellis D, Horowitz MI. In vitro studies of histone glycation. Biochim Biophys Acta 1987;926:365–8.

214. Lorenzi M, Montisano DF, Toledo S, Barrieux A. High glucose induces DNA damage in cultured human endothelial cells. J Clin Invest 1986;77:322–5.

215. Weimann BJ, Lorch E, Baumgartner HR. High glucose concentrations do not influence replication and prostacyclin release of human endothelial cells [Letter]. Diabetologia 1984;27:62–3.

Chapter 38

PATHOGENESIS OF MACROVASCULAR DISEASE IN DIABETES

ALAN CHAIT
EDWIN L. BIERMAN

The prevalence of macrovascular disease is markedly increased among individuals with diabetes mellitus. Its major clinical manifestations are consequences of atherosclerosis of coronary arteries, cerebral arteries, and large arteries of the lower extremities. This atherosclerotic vascular disease is the major cause of mortality and significant morbidity in diabetes in Westernized populations.[1] Although other causes of large-vessel disease such as calcific medial sclerosis[2] or microvascular disease may play a role, the great excess of deaths attributable to coronary heart disease (CHD) in populations with both major types of diabetes compared with populations without the disorder is undoubtedly due to atherosclerosis. North American data suggest that about 75% of patients with diabetes ultimately die of CHD.[3]

ATHEROSCLEROSIS IN INDIVIDUALS WITH AND WITHOUT DIABETES

Autopsy studies have repeatedly demonstrated that atherosclerosis in diabetic individuals is more extensive and accelerated than atherosclerosis in individuals without diabetes. In a large multinational study in which 23,000 sets of coronary arteries from autopsies from 14 countries were examined, diabetes was associated with an increase in the extent of raised lesions in the arteries from all countries, whether the prevalence of CHD in the country was high or low.[4] Further, from other studies (reviewed in Pyörälä et al.[1]), patients with diabetes appear to have a greater narrowing of the left main coronary artery, a greater number of major coronary arteries involved, and a greater diffuseness of the distribution of atherosclerotic lesions. Younger individuals with insulin-dependent diabetes mellitus (IDDM) are not spared; severe and extensive luminal narrowing of major coronary arteries was found in subjects with onset of IDDM before age 15 years who died before the age of 40.[5] Coronary angiographic studies of patients with symptomatic CHD have generally confirmed these autopsy findings. The extent and severity of atherosclerosis in the aorta and in cerebral and peripheral arteries of the lower extremities are also increased in diabetes. In amputated legs, occlusive atherosclerotic lesions in arteries below the knee are more common among patients with diabetes than among individuals without diabetes.[1]

Clinical studies of morbidity and mortality from atherosclerotic macrovascular disease in diabetes serve to underscore the magnitude of the problem. While older data from the Joslin Clinic emphasize the progressive increase in deaths from CHD among all persons with diabetes from the start of the insulin era until the 1960s (when it reached the 75% mark), more recent data, focused specifically on IDDM, indicate that about one-third of individuals with this disorder die of CHD by the age of 55.[6] In persons with IDDM, CHD becomes the leading cause of death with longer duration of diabetes, while in non-insulin-dependent diabetes (NIDDM), CHD is the leading cause of death regardless of duration of diabetes. Persons with diabetes in the Framingham study population,[7] most of whom presumably have NIDDM, had a relative risk (diabetic vs. nondiabetic) of death due to cardiovascular disease of 2.1 for men and 4.9 for women. A two- to fourfold excess in deaths due to CHD among persons with diabetes of either sex has been found in prospective population studies, consisting of a variety of ethnic and racial groups, in Israel, Evans County (Georgia), Rancho Bernardo (California), Tecumseh (Michigan), Chicago, Puerto Rico, London, Paris, and Finland.[1] Even among some populations of individuals with impaired glucose tolerance (IGT) (not all of whom go on to develop clinical diabetes), there appears to be an excess mortality from CHD.[8]

Mortality from CHD in persons with diabetes is increased even in populations in which the incidence of CHD is low, such as in Asia. Men of Japanese ancestry with diabetes who live in Hawaii and have adopted a Western diet (and other aspects of Western life-style) show a threefold increase in the rate of death from CHD compared with the rate among Japanese men with diabetes who live in Japan,[9] a difference that stresses the important interactions of potentially reversible environmental factors in the pathogenesis of atherosclerosis in diabetes.

The incidence of all major clinical forms of macrovascular disease is increased in both main types of diabetes. For example, in the Framingham study, among diabetics the 20-year incidence of new CHD events was 1.7 times higher in men and 2.7 times higher in women than among nondiabetics.[7] Comparable incidences of "atherothrombotic brain infarctions" are 2.7-fold higher for men with diabetes and 3.8 times higher in women with diabetes, and those of peripheral vascular disease (intermittent claudication) are 4.0 times higher in men with diabetes and 6.4 times higher in women with diabetes. In most, but not all, studies, the relative excess of clinical atherosclerotic disease in patients with diabetes appears to be more marked in women than in men, effectively eliminating the relative "protection" from atherosclerosis in nondiabetic women in the middle years. Recent data suggest that this phenomenon may be more apparent in IDDM than in NIDDM.[10]

RISK FACTORS FOR ATHEROSCLEROSIS IN DIABETES

In general the prevalence of the known major risk factors for CHD in the general population is amplified in diabetes (Table 38–1). The major risk factors for CHD that are of particular importance in diabetes include alterations in lipoprotein concentration and composition (dyslipidemia), hyperinsulinemia, hypertension, and central obesity, some of which may have a genetic component.

Dyslipidemia

The dyslipidemia of diabetes includes hypertriglyceridemia, low levels of high-density lipoprotein (HDL) cholesterol, alterations in the composition of low-density lipoprotein (LDL; predominance of triglyceride-rich small, dense LDL particles), and an increase in apolipoproteins (apo) B and E.[11–13] The potential for glycation and oxidation of all lipoprotein classes is enhanced (see later), and alterations of lipid composition are manifold (Table 38–2). These changes may occur in both IDDM and NIDDM and are exaggerated by poor metabolic control but may be only partly reversible.

Hypertriglyceridemia, reflecting increased plasma levels of very-low-density lipoproteins (VLDL) and remnants of VLDL and chylomicron catabolism, is very common in both IDDM and NIDDM. Its presence is accentuated when nephropathy supervenes. The role of triglyceride as a cardiovascular risk factor in nondiabetic populations is debatable. Most studies demonstrate an increased risk of CHD with high triglyceride levels in univariate analyses, while others, taking into account other risk factors in multivariate analyses, do not.[14] However, multivariate analysis with closely linked risk factors may not be appropriate.[15] Further, population studies of diabetics consistently and strongly suggest that hypertriglyceridemia is a significant risk factor for CHD among both those with IDDM and those with NIDDM.[15–18] For

Table 38–1. Cardiovascular Risk Factors in Diabetes Mellitus

Risk Factor	IDDM	NIDDM
Dyslipidemia		
Hypertriglyceridemia	++	++
Low HDL	+/−	++
Small, dense LDL	+	++
Increased apoB	+	++
Hypertension	+	++
Hyperinsulinemia/insulin resistance	+	++
Central obesity	−	++
Family history of atherosclerosis	−	+
Cigarette smoking	−	−

IDDM = insulin-dependent diabetes mellitus; NIDDM = non-insulin-dependent diabetes mellitus; HDL and LDL = high-density and low-density lipoproteins; apoB = apolipoprotein B; + = moderately increased compared with nondiabetic populations; ++ = markedly increased compared with nondiabetic populations.

Table 38–2. Alterations of Lipoproteins in Diabetes

CONCENTRATION
Hypertriglyceridemia due to increased VLDL levels
Increased levels of remnants of triglyceride-rich lipoproteins
Low levels of HDL (normal in treated IDDM)
Decreased HDL$_{2b}$
LDL levels +/− normal (improve with glycemic control)
? increased levels of Lp(a)
Hyper-apoB

COMPOSITION
Cholesterol enrichment of VLDL (due to remnant accumulation)
Small, dense VLDL
Small, dense triglyceride-enriched LDL
Triglyceride-enriched HDL
Increased cholesterol/lecithin ratio in all lipoprotein classes
Glycation
Oxidation

VLDL, LDL, and HDL = very-low-density, low-density, and high-density lipoproteins; IDDM = insulin-dependent diabetes mellitus; Lp(a) = lipoprotein a; hyper-apoB = hyperapobetalipoproteinemia.

example, in the World Health Organization's cross-sectional multinational study of more than 1900 persons with diabetes, plasma triglyceride levels were significantly related to CHD, independent of other risk factors.[17] In the Paris prospective study, triglyceride levels predicted CHD both in persons with diabetes and in those with IGT, independent of plasma cholesterol levels.[19]

Hypertriglyceridemia is related in part to the degree of diabetic control[20] and is characteristic of the untreated diabetic state.[11] Triglyceride levels tend to slowly return toward normal levels after the institution of therapy appropriate to the individual patient.[11] Further improvement in triglyceride levels can sometimes be achieved by paying close attention to glycemic control.[21,22] Recent studies have shown that hypertriglyceridemia in the diabetic patient is associated with an increase in concentrations of chylomicron remnants[23] and that the size distribution of VLDL particles is shifted towards smaller, denser particles in the VLDL density range.[24] The reason hypertriglyceridemia predisposes the diabetic individual in particular to atherosclerosis is unknown, but it may be related to these small VLDL particles. Accelerated atherosclerosis also is a hallmark of familial combined hyperlipidemia, in which VLDL particles also are small and dense.[25] Further, an increase in levels of the remnants of catabolism of triglyceride-rich lipoproteins, which is seen in both these disorders, also appears to impart an increased risk of atherosclerosis. The mechanisms by which the triglyceride-rich lipoproteins interact with cells of the arterial wall and the extracellular matrix to form atheromata are unknown, although remnant lipoproteins resemble β-VLDL, i.e., atherogenic lipoproteins formed in response to consumption of diets rich in fat and cholesterol, and could potentially be taken up by macrophages, leading to lipid accumulation. Although the lipid that accumulates in atherosclerotic plaques is cholesterol rather than triglyceride, these remnant lipoproteins contain more molecules of cholesterol per particle than does LDL. Further, it is conceivable that the triglyceride component of internalized triglyceride-rich lipoproteins is removed preferentially, leaving the cholesterol behind.[26] It also is possible that the hypertriglyceridemia in diabetes is merely a marker of some other underlying abnormality of lipoproteins or risk factor that plays a more direct role in atherogenesis.

The impact of plasma cholesterol levels on CHD appears to be similar in diabetic and nondiabetic individuals.[27] However, elevated levels of total cholesterol in persons with diabetes need not be an index of increased levels of LDL-cholesterol, since VLDL and remnant cholesterol can disproportionately elevate the plasma total cholesterol level in diabetic patients. LDL has long been regarded as the most atherogenic of the circulating lipoproteins in nondiabetic individuals. Further, considerable evidence indicates that reduction of LDL levels leads to a reduction in cardiovascular risk[28] and slows or even reverses the atherosclerosis as evaluated by quantitative coronary angiography.[29] However, the role of LDL in atherogenesis in diabetes is less clear. Most studies that have evaluated LDL have shown either normal or only

mildly elevated levels in both types of diabetes.[12] Evaluation of LDL levels in diabetes is complicated because virtually all studies have used techniques for measuring LDL that included the remnant-enriched intermediate-density lipoprotein (IDL), which frequently is increased in diabetes (see earlier). Thus, little is known about the "true" LDL levels in diabetes. Despite the lack of evidence for marked elevations of LDL in diabetes, several studies have shown that improved glycemic control can further reduce LDL levels,[21,22] presumably because, at least in part, of improved LDL receptor-mediated clearance of this lipoprotein.[30] It is conceivable that the levels of LDL that adversely affect the arterial wall in diabetic persons are lower than those that affect the artery wall in nondiabetic persons. Preliminary analysis of the diabetes subgroup studied in the Multiple Risk Factor Intervention trial (MRFIT) provides some evidence in support of this view. Although the full details of that study have yet to be published, it appears that in the group with diabetes, as in the group without diabetes, cardiovascular risk was related to serum cholesterol but that the risk of cardiovascular events was much higher in those with diabetes than in those without diabetes at all levels of cholesterol, which to a large extent reflects LDL-cholesterol levels[31] (Fig. 38–1). The reason for the LDL-independent difference in cardiovascular risk remains unknown, however. Further, although levels of true LDL-cholesterol may not be increased in treated diabetic patients, the composition of the LDL particles is altered, resulting in a preponderance of small, dense particles. Although such particles have been associated with CHD in the general population,[32] no studies of this association in diabetes have been reported. The presence of such particles is linked to hypertriglyceridemia and to low levels of HDL-cholesterol. A lower threshold for concern about LDL levels and

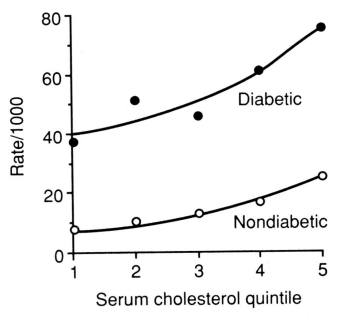

Fig. 38–1. Coronary artery disease events in diabetic subjects from the Multiple Risk Factor Intervention Trial (MRFIT).[31]

intervention to lower them may therefore be prudent in diabetes. An additional alteration in lipoprotein composition that is a good index of atherosclerosis risk, i.e., the cholesterol/lecithin ratio,[33] is increased in LDL[34] and other lipoproteins in subjects with diabetes.

Levels of HDL-cholesterol are uniformly low in untreated patients with IDDM and NIDDM. In patients with NIDDM, these low levels persist after treatment, perhaps in association with persisting obesity and insulin resistance. In patients with IDDM, low HDL levels may become normalized or even high following insulin treatment[35,36] but will remain low in the presence of nephropathy. The circulating level of HDL is widely recognized as one of the risk factors most predictive for coronary artery disease, with levels related inversely to cardiovascular disease risk in the nondiabetic population. Most studies show an association between low levels of HDL-cholesterol and CHD in both NIDDM and IDDM.[18,37] In the prospective data from the Framingham study, the HDL-cholesterol level was inversely related to CHD in the diabetic population, as in the general population.[38]

HDL particles are very heterogeneous and exist in several subclasses. There are two major classes of HDL particles: those that contain apoA$_I$ without apoA$_{II}$ and those that contain both apoA$_I$ and apoA$_{II}$.[39] Several subclasses with respect to size and density exist within both major classes of HDL.[40] Further, a very small HDL subclass with pre-β electrophoretic mobility appears to be important in promoting cholesterol efflux from cells.[41] However, the precise functions of these various HDL subclasses is unknown. Some studies have suggested that distribution of HDL particles in diabetes may be abnormal,[42] differences that might result in functional abnormalities facilitating atherosclerosis.

Thus, CHD in diabetes appears to be strongly associated with the dyslipidemia of diabetes, i.e., high triglyceride levels (VLDL and remnants); low HDL-cholesterol levels; and small, dense LDL particles. This dyslipidemia is accentuated in nephropathy. It is of interest that among Asian diabetic patients whose triglyceride and HDL levels are comparable to those of Western nondiabetics, these levels are still abnormal compared with those in the Asian nondiabetic population.[43] Migration and adoption of a Western life-style leads to an exaggeration of these lipid abnormalities,[9] and, as noted earlier, to higher rates of CHD.

Other lipoprotein-related risk factors for CHD include lipoprotein a [Lp(a)] and apoB. Lp(a) is a lipoprotein in which a unique apolipoprotein, apo(a), is present in disulfide linkage with the major apolipoprotein of LDL, apoB. Lp(a) has long been known to be a risk factor for CHD.[44] Recently, interest in this lipoprotein revived considerably since it was found to share considerable sequence homology with plasminogen,[45] which plays a role in clot lysis. Lp(a) thus may provide an important link between lipoprotein and thrombogenic cardiovascular risk factors. Lp(a) competes with plasminogen for binding to the plasminogen receptor and stimulates gene expression of an inhibitor to plasminogen activation.[46] Since Lp(a) does not have the thrombolytic effect of

plasminogen, it blocks the thrombolysis-stimulating action of plasminogen. Lp(a) may interact with other risk factors, since the level of Lp(a) is a powerful predictor of which individuals with familial hypercholesterolemia will develop early-onset atherosclerotic complications.[47] Little is known about the regulation of Lp(a) by dietary, hormonal, or other factors. Lp(a) levels are not readily lowered by lipid-lowering drugs. The potential role of Lp(a) in predisposing the diabetic patient to atherosclerotic disease is unknown. However, a spate of recent preliminary reports suggest that Lp(a) levels may be altered by glycemic control in diabetic subjects[48] and that Lp(a) levels are increased in diabetic patients with either micro- or macroalbuminuria,[49] alterations that may in part explain the increased CHD risk associated with the presence of proteinuria.[50] With assays for Lp(a) becoming more readily available, the information available concerning the role of Lp(a) in atherogenesis in diabetes should increase in the near future.

Apolipoprotein B$_{100}$ (apoB) is the major structural apolipoprotein of the atherogenic lipoproteins VLDL, its remnants, and LDL. Circulating levels of apoB increase when the concentration of these particles are increased in plasma. Since most of the cholesterol in plasma is present in LDL, concentrations of apoB are especially increased in the presence of high levels of this lipoprotein. However, levels of apoB can be increased in the presence of normal or only mildly elevated levels of LDL. This situation has been termed hyperapobetalipoproteinemia (hyper-apoB) and is associated with a markedly increased predisposition to early-onset cardiovascular disease.[51] Hyper-apoB without concomitant elevations of LDL-cholesterol levels is seen in some subjects with familial combined hyperlipidemia. Familial combined hyperlipidemia is characterized by the presence of small, dense, lipid-poor LDL particles,[25] a feature that accounts for the increase in apoB values relative to cholesterol levels. As indicated earlier, the presence of these small, dense LDL particles appears to be an inherited trait that predisposes individuals to cardiovascular disease.[32] Hypertriglyceridemia also is commonly associated with the presence of these small, dense LDL particles.[32] Diabetes, especially NIDDM, also is characterized by LDL particles with a smaller mean diameter and of higher density than those from nondiabetic subjects,[13] differences that may be another factor predisposing diabetics to increased CHD risk.

Hypertension

Hypertension is more prevalent both among persons with IDDM and those with NIDDM than in the general population. The role of hypertension as a risk factor for atherosclerosis is at least as strong for diabetic as for nondiabetic persons. Hypertension can be the result of diabetic nephropathy, although the frequency of hypertension also appears to be higher in the diabetic population without renal complications than in the general population.[52] In NIDDM, hypertension occurs as part of a syndrome in which it can coexist with central obesity, insulin resistance, and dyslipidemia (see next section).

Family studies have shown that there is a major genetic component to this syndrome.

Hyperinsulinemia, Insulin Resistance, and Central Obesity

In prospective studies of populations around the world, high plasma levels of insulin predict the development of CHD, independent of other risk factors.[53-55] Cross-sectional studies of subjects with NIDDM have also linked levels of insulin, free insulin, or C peptide with the prevalence of CHD.[56-58] Since patients with IDDM treated with exogenous insulin have increased circulating levels of free insulin much of the day and patients with NIDDM commonly have endogenous hyperinsulinemia in association with the insulin resistance, high plasma insulin levels must be considered in the pathogenesis of atherosclerosis in diabetes. Plausible pathobiologic mechanisms are discussed later. Of note, insulin treatment by subcutaneous injection delivers insulin first to the periphery rather than to the liver, where arteries are exposed to abnormally high concentrations of insulin.

Impaired insulin action (insulin resistance) in NIDDM frequently is associated with central (intra-abdominal) adiposity, leading to hyperinsulinemia.[59] Hyperinsulinemia has, in turn, been linked to hypertension and the dyslipidemia of diabetes, each of which can enhance the risk of atherosclerosis. A scheme depicting the key role of hyperinsulinemia can be proposed (Fig. 38-2).

The importance of central rather than peripheral obesity as a risk factor for CHD has long been appreciated. Recent studies have clarified the risk of abdominal obesity,[60] which can be semiquantified by the waist/hip ratio. In particular, visceral abdominal adiposity (which may not be so simple to detect clinically, although it can be detected by abdominal computed tomographic scan) confers more of a risk than does subcutaneous abdominal adiposity. This is the form of fat deposition that is associated with insulin resistance and compensatory

hyperinsulinemia.[61] When pancreatic reserve is surpassed, NIDDM ensues.[62] The major lipid abnormalities that occur in this situation are hypertriglyceridemia, low levels of HDL, and the presence of small, dense LDL particles,[63] all of which appear to signify increased cardiovascular risk when associated with central obesity or insulin resistance. When insulin resistance and glucose intolerance predominate, affected individuals tend to be classified as having NIDDM. When hypertension is the predominant feature and the disorder can be shown to be familial, patients are classified as having familial dyslipidemic hypertension. When lipid abnormalities are the major feature, affected individuals may be diagnosed as having familial combined hyperlipidemia or hyperapobetalipoproteinemia. All of them may have variants of the same disorder, the common features of which are a markedly increased risk of accelerated atherosclerosis, insulin resistance, and hyperinsulinemia.

Smoking

There is no good evidence that cigarette smoking is more common among persons with diabetes than among the population at large. However, there is strong evidence that smoking markedly increases the risk of both myocardial infarction[64] and complications of peripheral vascular disease[65] in those with diabetes, especially women.[66] Smoking is believed to be associated with adverse changes in plasma lipids and lipoproteins, especially with low levels of HDL-cholesterol.[67]

PATHOGENIC FACTORS UNIQUE TO THE DIABETIC STATE

Multivariate analysis of several prospective population studies has suggested that a large proportion of excess CHD among persons with diabetes cannot be explained by increases in the known risk factors for CHD that affect the general population.[1] Since risk factors cluster among diabetic individuals, multivariate analysis, which is appropriately applied only to a group of independent risk factors, would underestimate the contribution of known CHD risk factors. Also, some of the more recently appreciated risk factors, e.g., HDL-cholesterol and Lp(a), were not measured in earlier studies. Nevertheless, it appears that a large proportion of the excess CHD risk is not explained by the major CHD risk factors but can be attributed to the diabetic state itself.

Three recent prospective studies of diabetic individuals support this view. In the MRFIT studies of more than 350,000 men followed prospectively for 6 years, 5245 men had known diabetes. At every level of each major risk factor analyzed (serum cholesterol, blood pressure, cigarette smoking), the diabetic men had a three- to sixfold increase in CHD risk. Further, after segregation of individuals on the basis of the presence of one, two, or three risk factors, those with diabetes had a marked increase in CHD risk at every level of risk.

In another study, a population of approximately 7000 men in Göteborg was followed for 7 years.[68] The 232

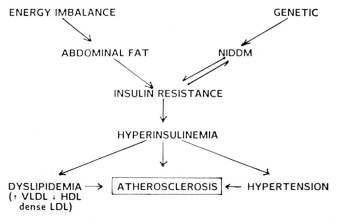

Fig. 38-2. Scheme depicting postulated role of hyperinsulinemia in atherosclerosis. NIDDM = non-insulin-dependent diabetes; mellitus; VLDL, HDL, and LDL = very-low-density, high-density, and low-density lipoproteins.

men with known diabetes had a two- to threefold increased incidence of CHD at both high and low cholesterol levels and regardless of smoking history. These observations in middle-aged diabetic men have now been noted in diabetic women. In the Nurses Health Study, which includes almost 1500 diabetic women among approximately 115,000 women, the incidence rate of CHD was fivefold higher in diabetic women whether their cholesterol levels were high or low.[69]

Thus, the diabetic state appears to have an independent influence on the incidence of CHD. The possible direct consequences of the diabetic state per se on the atherogenic process will be discussed in a later section.

ATHEROSCLEROSIS RISK IN THE PREDIABETIC STATE

Impaired glucose tolerance (IGT), defined arbitrarily by cut points in serum glucose levels after an oral glucose load, is a heterogeneous state.[70] Only a small proportion of individuals with IGT develop NIDDM, with the IGT thus representing a prediabetic state in these individuals. Nevertheless, several general population studies[1,8,53,71,72] have shown a nonlinear increase in CHD with increasing serum glucose levels following oral glucose loading, with a distinct rise at the high end of the glucose distribution. This threshold effect suggests that IGT, particularly the prediabetic state, may predispose to CHD.

Two recent studies have shown that CHD risk factors are increased in prediabetic individuals. In the San Antonio heart study of Mexican Americans,[73] individuals who were not diabetic at initial examination but who subsequently developed diabetes during an 8-year period had higher levels of total serum cholesterol, triglycerides, fasting glucose, and insulin; higher body mass index and blood pressure; and lower levels of HDL-cholesterol than individuals who remained nondiabetic. Exclusion of subjects with IGT did not influence this finding. Thus, individuals with confirmed pre-NIDDM have an atherogenic pattern of risk factors, perhaps linked to obesity and hyperinsulinemia, that may be present for many years before the onset of clinical diabetes. Similar findings consistent with this "ticking clock" hypothesis emerged from the Rancho Bernardo study of upper middle class men and women age 40 years or older.[74] Those individuals who went on to develop NIDDM after 10 to 15 years initially had a higher blood pressure, fasting plasma glucose level, triglyceride level, and body mass index than those whose glucose tolerance remained normal. (Fasting insulin and lipoprotein levels were not analyzed.) These trends were stronger among women than among men. Individuals who developed IGT had intermediate levels of these risk factors.

These findings have implications for the prevention or interruption of the progression of atherosclerosis in NIDDM, since modification of risk factors across the general adult population should reduce CHD morbidity and mortality among those who eventually develop NIDDM. No comparable findings have been reported for pre-IDDM.

BASIC MECHANISMS OF ATHEROGENESIS

During the past several years, considerable knowledge has accrued concerning basic mechanisms of atherogenesis (Fig. 38–3). The development of atherosclerotic lesions progresses over many years, starting as a fatty streak—the earliest lesion of atherosclerosis—and progressing to a fibro-fatty plaque and finally to a complicated lesion with fibrosis, plaque fissuring, hemorrhage, and thrombosis. Restriction of blood supply in the coronary arteries, cerebral arteries, or peripheral vasculature can result in angina, stroke, and intermittent claudication, respectively. Occlusion of the coronary arteries by thrombi leads to myocardial infarction and sudden death. As discussed earlier, all of these complications of atherosclerosis are more common in diabetes than in the nondiabetic state.

Monocyte-Endothelial Interaction

The earliest event that occurs during atherogenesis is adhesion of monocytes to an intact endothelial layer.[75] A family of leukocyte adhesion molecules have been discovered that are expressed after activation of endothelial cells by a variety of stimuli. A superfamily of molecules, integrins, also are expressed on the surface of circulating leukocytes, which adhere to specific receptors on endothelial cells.[76] Changes in both monocyte and endothelial adhesion molecules, e.g., those induced by hypercholesterolemia, may be required to trigger adhesion of circulating monocytes to arterial endothelial cells.[77] Other factors that affect expression of either monocyte or endothelial adhesion molecules may thereby initiate fatty-streak formation. Monocyte adherence to endothelial cells can be induced by exposure to LDLs that have been minimally or mildly oxidized.[78] This is but one potential mechanism by which lipoproteins modified by oxidation could promote atherogenesis (see later).

Monocyte Recruitment and Maturation to Macrophages

Adherent monocytes next penetrate between endothelial cells to enter the subendothelial space, where they mature into intimal macrophages. Monocytes are believed to infiltrate the endothelial layer at gap junctions in response to chemotactic stimuli. Monocyte chemotactic protein-1 (MCP-1), a chemotactic factor produced by macrophages and arterial smooth muscle cells, appears to specifically attract monocytes.[79] Its production also is increased by minimally oxidized LDL.[80] More extensively oxidized LDL is itself chemotactic for monocytes.[81] Thus, oxidative modification of LDL by endothelial cells may be another factor that triggers recruitment of monocytes into the arterial intima.

The factors that induce macrophage differentiation are unknown, but the appearance of T lymphocytes, some of which are activated, in close proximity to subendothelial macrophages[82] suggests a role for cytokines of T-cell origin. These cytokines might also lead to macrophage

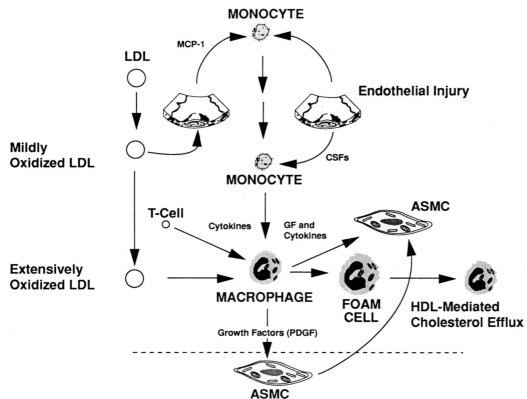

Fig. 38–3. Scheme for postulated sequence of events in atherogenesis. LDL and HDL = low-density and high-density lipoproteins; MCP-1 = monocyte chemotactic protein-1; CSFs = colony-stimulating factors; GF = growth factor; ASMC = arterial smooth muscle cell; PDGF = platelet-derived growth factor.

activation, which is associated with modulation of expression of several macrophage-derived genes.[83]

Macrophage Foam-Cell Formation

Subendothelial macrophages accumulate lipids, predominantly cholesteryl esters, to become arterial wall foam cells. These lipids are derived from lipoproteins that enter the subendothelial space, presumably after endothelial transcytosis. The mechanism by which macrophages take up lipoproteins has been studied extensively in vitro. Although LDL receptors are present on macrophages, uptake of unmodified LDL by this route does not lead to significant accumulation of lipid. Macrophages also possess scavenger receptors that bind several modified lipoproteins, the uptake of which leads to accumulation of cholesteryl esters and formation of foam cells.[84,85] A likely ligand for the scavenger receptor in vivo is oxidatively modified LDL (see later). Malondialdehyde-modified LDL, which also is a ligand for this receptor,[86] could potentially be formed in vivo as a by-product of lipid peroxidation or during prostaglandin synthesis. The consumption of diets high in fat and cholesterol results in the formation of cholesterol-enriched VLDL particles with unusual electrophoretic mobility, termed β-VLDL. Although these particles were initially believed to be taken up by a distinct class of receptors on macrophages,[87] it is now known that these particles are taken up by the LDL receptor[89] and that their uptake can lead to cholesterol accumulation and foam-cell formation.[89] Recently, another macrophage lipoprotein receptor was

described that binds VLDL from hypertriglyceridemic individuals.[90] These in vitro observations suggest that lipoproteins may need to be modified in vivo, possibly in the milieu of the artery wall, before they can lead to macrophage foam-cell formation.

Macrophages also can take up large amounts of lipid by phagocytosis of lipoprotein aggregates[91,92] or lipoprotein-immune complexes.[93] It is conceivable that lipoproteins aggregate in the artery wall following binding to extracellular matrix components. Lipoprotein-glycosaminoglycen (GAG) complexes can be taken up by macrophages. Lipoproteins that have been modified by glycation[94] or oxidative modification[95] can stimulate antibody production, which presumably could lead to the formation of lipoprotein-immune complexes in the vicinity of macrophages in the arterial wall that can also be taken up by these cells.

Macrophages contain a cell-surface binding site, the HDL receptor, that facilitates the translocation of cholesterol from intracellular pools to the cell membrane,[96] from where it can be picked up by cholesterol acceptors in the extracellular space.[97] Cholesterol accumulates when its net uptake exceeds efflux. Lipid-laden macrophages are the predominant cells in fatty streaks, but they also are common in more advanced lesions.

Smooth Muscle Cell Proliferation and Foam-Cell Formation

While it is believed that most fatty streaks do not progress to complicated lesions in humans, all complicated lesions are thought to start as fatty streaks. Thus, strategies aimed at the prevention of atherosclerosis ideally should attempt to inhibit fatty-streak formation. Lesions that are going to progress to fibro-fatty plaques are characterized by the migration of smooth muscle cells from the media to the intima and by subsequent proliferation of smooth muscle cells.[75] Mitogens for smooth muscle cells usually are both chemotactic and mitogenic. Several such mitogens can be produced by the cells in the developing plaque. One such growth factor that has received considerable attention is platelet-derived growth factor (PDGF). So-named because it was first isolated from platelets, it has since been found to be a ubiquitous growth factor produced by several cells of the arterial wall. For example, PDGF is secreted by macrophages, especially following activation.[98] It also is produced by endothelial cells[99] and even by smooth muscle cells themselves under certain conditions.[100] These cells, especially endothelial cells and macrophages, are likely to be more important sources of PDGF than are platelets in the early stages of lesion formation, when the endothelial layer is still intact. Breaks occur in the endothelial layer later during lesion formation, after which platelets adhere to subendothelial matrix components and macrophages and release PDGF.

Smooth muscle cells also accumulate lipid, although presumably by mechanisms different from those of macrophages. Smooth muscle cells were thought not to have scavenger receptors, although a recent study suggests that such receptors may be present in this type of cell type under certain conditions.[101] Alternate mechanisms for accumulation of lipids by arterial smooth muscle cells are by the LDL receptor, which may not be tightly regulated in this cell type,[102] or via net transfer of free cholesterol or cholesteryl ester from lipoproteins to cells.[103] Since cholesterol accumulates in smooth muscle cells without functional LDL receptors in both patients and animals, such mechanisms of uptake not mediated by the LDL receptor must occur.

Role of Cytokines and Growth Factors

Several cytokines and other growth factors have been implicated in the process of atherogenesis.[104] Interest in these molecules was stimulated by the observation that T lymphocytes, a well-known source of cytokines such as interferon-γ, are present at all stages of lesion development.[82] Other cytokines that may be involved include interleukins 1, 2, and 6 (IL-1, 2, and 6), tumor necrosis factor (TNF), the colony-stimulating factors (CSFs), and growth factors in addition to PDGF such as insulin-like growth factor 1 (IGF-1), fibroblast growth factor, vascular endothelial cell growth factor, platelet-derived endothelial growth factor, and transforming growth factors α and β that are produced in a variety of cells present in the arterial wall (Table 38–3). These molecules have a vast array of immunoregulatory and growth regulatory functions (including chemotaxis, regulation of cell proliferation, modulation of expression of cell surface receptors, antigen presentation, and formation of cell secretory products and extracellular matrix) believed to play a role

Table 38–3. Cytokines and Growth Factors Related to Atherogenesis

Molecule	Major Arterial Cell(s) of Origin
Colony-stimulating factors	Macrophage, EC, T-lymph
Fibroblast growth factor	EC, macrophage, SMC
Insulin-like growth factor	Macrophage, EC, SMC, platelet
Interferon-γ	T-lymph
Interleukins 1, 2, and 6	T-lymph, macrophage, SMC, EC
Platelet-derived endothelial growth factor	Platelet
Platelet-derived growth factor	Macrophage, EC, SMC, platelet
Transforming growth factor α	Macrophages
Transforming growth factor β	T-lymph, EC, macrophage, platelet
Tumor necrosis factor	T-lymph, macrophage, SMC, EC
Vascular endothelial growth factor	Macrophage, SMC

EC = endothelial cells; SMC = smooth muscle cells; T-lymph = T lymphocytes.

in atherogenesis,[105] although the exact mechanisms by which many of these growth factors and cytokines participate in this process are not known. The factors that regulate the expression of these cytokines and growth factors in arterial cells during atherogenesis also are largely unknown, although several of these molecules are secreted only by activated or injured cells. Further, several of these molecules appear to be modulated by oxidatively modified LDL. LDL that has been insufficiently oxidized (termed minimally modified LDL) to trigger its uptake by the macrophage scavenger receptor stimulates the expression of several CSFs by endothelial cells.[107] This might be important in the recruitment, differentiation, and activation of arterial wall macrophages. More extensively oxidized LDL inhibits the expression of PDGF by macrophages[107] and endothelial cells[99] and of TNF-α by macrophages.[108] Scavenger and LDL receptors are suppressed by macrophage activation,[109] which also modulates the expression of several macrophage secretory products that may be involved in atherogenesis, such as apoE[110] and lipoprotein lipase.[111]

Matrix Involvement

Another important component of the complicated lesion is deposition of connective tissue, which is newly synthesized by cells of the artery wall, especially smooth muscle cells. This leads to fibrosis and can result in platelet adhesion. Extracellular matrix components also can bind lipoproteins in a fairly specific manner,[112] thereby trapping them in the extracellular space, where they can be modified, stimulate the formation of antibodies, and lead to uptake of lipoprotein-immune complexes and lipoprotein-GAG complexes by macrophages.

EFFECT OF DIABETES MELLITUS ON ATHEROGENESIS

The reason for the marked acceleration of atherosclerosis seen in diabetes is unknown. However, accelerated atherosclerosis is a feature of both IDDM and NIDDM, suggesting common pathogenetic mechanisms in these two different diseases (see earlier). Features common to IDDM and NIDDM are an excess of several cardiovascular risk factors and prolonged hyperglycemia, which could lead to nonenzymatic glycation of long-lived proteins that may be involved in the atherogenic process. As noted, the increased atherosclerosis seen in diabetes might in part relate to an excess of several well characterized cardiovascular risk factors, such as dyslipidemia, hypertension, and central obesity. However, as discussed earlier, excesses of the conventional cardiovascular risk factors are insufficient to explain the tremendous increase in cardiovascular disease in diabetes, raising the likelihood that mechanisms unique to diabetes need to be invoked in addition. These mechanisms are likely to be operative in the arterial wall and may not be amenable to easy detection. Since prolonged hyperglycemia is characteristic of both IDDM and NIDDM, mechanisms of atherogenesis that occur as a result of excessive nonenzymatic glycation of proteins and from the formation of advanced glycation end-products need to be considered. Mechanisms of atherogenesis related to increased lipid peroxidation may be another explanation for the increased atherosclerosis seen in diabetes, since evidence suggests that the process of lipid peroxidation occurs to a greater extent in diabetic animals and humans than in nondiabetic controls. Other subtle alterations of lipoprotein structure and function consequent to the diabetic state also might render lipoprotein particles more atherogenic, thereby contributing to the increased cardiovascular risk that typifies diabetes. Figure 38–4 depicts the sites at which diabetes might influence the process of atherogenesis.

Prolonged Hyperglycemia and Protein Glycation

Both IDDM and NIDDM are characterized by periods of hyperglycemia, even under conditions of good control. Therefore, proteins with long half-lives are likely to undergo more extensive nonenzymatic glycation in those with diabetes than in those without diabetes. Since protein glycation has been linked to the aging process,[113] the diabetic state might be considered a state of accelerated aging, also characterized by progressive atherosclerosis. The mechanism by which protein glycation leads to atherosclerotic changes remains uncertain, however. Recent studies have shed new light on how protein glycation might be atherogenic. For example, increased glycation of circulating lipoproteins has been observed in diabetes,[114] even of lipoproteins with relatively short half-lives, presumably because some apolipoproteins, e.g., apoE and apoC, shuttle between lipoproteins and actually reside for a fairly long time in plasma. The effect of glycated lipoproteins on cellular lipoprotein metabolism is not entirely clear. While glycation of lipoproteins clearly reduces their binding to the LDL receptor,[115] thereby reducing their rate of catabolism, results have conflicted regarding the uptake of glycated lipoproteins by macrophages. Thus, some studies have demonstrated increased uptake of glycated LDL by macrophages,[116] whereas others have not.[117] Glycated HDL is cleared from plasma at an enhanced rate,[118] and its ability to stimulate cholesterol efflux from arterial cells is dimin-

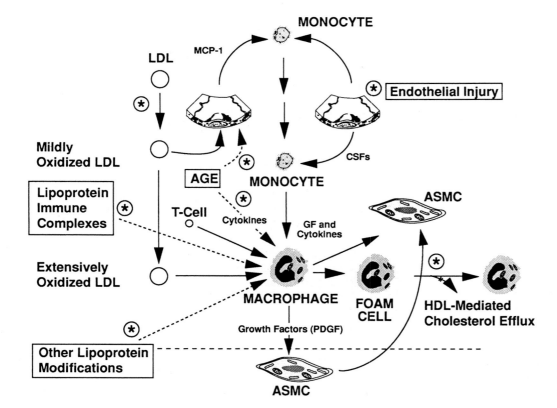

Fig. 38–4. Sites at which diabetes might influence the atherogenic process. See Figure 38–3 legend for abbreviations.

ished in comparison to that of native HDL.[119,120] Glycated lipoproteins also are likely to be immunogenic, since autoantibodies to them have been detected.[94] The potential importance of such autoantibodies is discussed later.

Longer-lived proteins are even more likely to undergo excessive nonenzymatic glycation in diabetic individuals. Increased glycation of collagen is well described in diabetes[121]; whether this increase plays a role in atherogenesis in diabetes is unclear. One potential mechanism by which glycated collagen might facilitate atherogenesis is by trapping lipoproteins in the extracellular matrix,[122] which would render them more susceptible to oxidative modification. Glycated collagen also stimulates platelet aggregation to a greater extent than does nonglycated collagen[123] and might thereby also facilitate the later stages of the atherosclerotic process.

Some of the early glycation products on collagen and other long-lived proteins undergo slow chemical changes leading to the formation of advanced glycation end-products (AGE).[124] These AGE proteins may have different biologic effects than the early glycation products. Thus, the recent finding that AGE proteins induce the transendothelial migration of monocytes and the subsequent expression of PDGF by macrophages[125] provides a potentially important mechanism whereby these modified proteins may be involved in the early stages of atherogenesis. Advanced glycation of LDL renders the modified lipoprotein as effective as other AGE proteins in the chemoattraction of monocytes.[125] AGE proteins can also be taken up by specific receptors on macrophages, which stimulate the expression of several cytokines[126] that may modulate the atherosclerotic process. Whether LDL that has been trapped on extracellular matrix components can undergo these advanced glycation changes and thereafter be taken up by these specific AGE-protein receptors on macrophages remains to be determined.

Other Lipoprotein Modifications and Diabetes

Diabetes might be associated with several lipoprotein modifications other than glycation that may increase their atherogenicity by altering their interaction with cells of the arterial wall. Additional lipoprotein modifications that potentially contribute to atherogenesis in diabetes include oxidative modification, formation of lipoprotein immune complexes, lipoprotein aggregation, and modification of the lipoprotein surface composition.

Oxidative Modification of Lipoproteins

Oxidatively modified lipoproteins are believed to play an important role in atherogenesis since, in vitro, oxidized LDL can induce adhesion of monocytes to endothelium,[78] stimulate monocyte chemotaxis by inducing the expression of MCP-1,[80] and is cytotoxic[127] to cells such as endothelial cells. Thus, this modified form of LDL could play a role in the earliest events in atherogenesis, i.e., monocyte adherence, monocyte chemoattraction, and endothelial cell damage.[75] Oxidized LDL also may facilitate the differentiation of monocytes to macrophages[128] and lead to macrophage activation, possibly by stimula-

tion of the expression of CSFs by cells such as endothelial cells.[106] Oxidized LDL also can deliver lipid via scavenger receptor pathways and lead to foam-cell formation.[85] Expression of growth factor and cytokine genes that may be involved in atherogenesis may also be modulated by exposure of macrophages or endothelial cells to oxidatively modified lipoproteins,[107,108] which also may affect vasoreactivity by inhibiting endothelium-derived relaxing factor.[129] Thus, oxidized lipoproteins could theoretically be atherogenic by a variety of mechanisms. The immunocytochemical demonstration of oxidatively modified lipoproteins in vivo in atherosclerotic lesions, but not in areas of artery without lesions, from experimental animals and humans[95,130,131] strongly supports their role in atherogenesis. Further, use of the antioxidants probucol and butylated hydroxytoluene is associated with reduction in lesion formation in atherosclerosis-prone hypercholesterolemic rabbits.[132,133]

In vitro, LDL can be oxidatively modified by endothelial cells,[85] arterial smooth muscle cells,[134,135] monocyte-macrophages,[136,137] and by cell-free systems in which redox-active transition metals are present.[138,139] Superoxide appears to play an important initiating role in arterial smooth muscle cells[134] and activated macrophages,[136] whereas lipoxygenase appears to be important in endothelial cells and unstimulated monocyte-macrophages.[140,141] Susceptibility of lipoproteins to oxidative modification is increased in cigarette smokers,[142,143] presumably because of the many free radicals in cigarette smoke. Although there is considerable evidence for the existence of oxidatively modified lipoproteins in atherosclerotic lesions from rabbits and humans,[130,131] little is known about the mechanisms of lipoprotein oxidation in vivo.

There are several reasons why lipoprotein oxidation might be accelerated in diabetes. First, the process of protein glycation has been shown to lead to the generation of reactive oxygen species such as superoxide,[144] the one-electron-reduced form of oxygen, which can initiate the oxidative modification of lipoproteins.[134,136] Thus, increased nonenzymatic glycation of proteins in the extracellular space could increase superoxide production, thereby facilitating the oxidative modification of adjacent lipoprotein particles. It also is conceivable that glycation of LDL itself might favor its oxidative modification. Indeed, a recent study suggests that LDL can become oxidatively modified during its nonenzymatic glycation.[145] This modification is most likely to occur with LDL that is bound to extracellular matrix components such as proteoglycans, glycosaminoglycans, and collagen. The production of superoxide by monocytes also has been shown to be increased in diabetes,[146] an increase possibly related to the hypertriglyceridemia that accompanies diabetes rather than to diabetes per se.[147] Most studies have suggested that oxidation stress is increased in diabetes,[113] although some studies have failed to confirm this finding, possibly, in part, because of the difficulty in measuring oxidation stress in vivo.

Second, the process of monosaccharide auto-oxidation also can generate reactive oxygen species[148] that could lead to oxidative modification of lipoproteins. When monosaccharides auto-oxidize, the predominant reactive oxygen species generated are hydrogen peroxide and the highly reactive hydroxyl radical. These species also could result in oxidative modification of lipoproteins in the microenvironment of the arterial wall. The ketoaldehydes generated during the process of monosaccharide auto-oxidation might lead to additional lipoprotein modification that might influence the interaction of lipoproteins with cells of the arterial wall. Although considerably larger quantities of reactive oxygen species are generated during the auto-oxidation of monosaccharides such as mannose, dihydroxyacetone, or even fructose than of glucose, auto-oxidation of glucose nonetheless could lead to significant generation of reactive oxygen species and modification of lipoproteins.

Third, the LDL heterogeneity that is characteristic of both types of diabetes may favor lipoprotein oxidation. As discussed earlier, both NIDDM and treated IDDM are characterized by the presence of an increased number of small, dense lipoprotein particles.[13] Since small, dense LDL particles have been shown to be more susceptible than larger particles to oxidative modification,[149] the lipoproteins present in diabetes are likely to be more susceptible to oxidative modification than are those present in the nondiabetic state.

Formation of Lipoprotein Immune Complexes

The demonstration of circulating antibodies to glycated[94] and oxidized LDL[95] suggests that these modified lipoprotein species can be immunogenic. The presence of circulating lipoprotein immune complexes has been associated with accelerated atherosclerosis,[150,151] presumably as a result either of macrophage foam-cell formation in response to the uptake of these immune complexes or of stimulation of atherogenic immune mechanisms in cells of the arterial wall. Immune complexes can be phagocytosed by macrophages after they bind to Fc receptors. If these complexes contain glycated or oxidized lipoproteins, they are likely to deliver large quantities of lipid, the presence of which would result in the formation of foam cells.

Lipoprotein Aggregation

The phagocytic uptake of lipoprotein aggregates by mechanisms mediated by LDL receptors also can lead to marked accumulation of lipids and formation of foam cells.[91,93] Aggregation of lipoproteins to extracellular matrix components has been demonstrated in vivo.[152] Since glycated matrix proteins, such as those likely to be found with increased frequency in diabetes, avidly bind LDL,[122] excess trapping and aggregation of lipoproteins that might occur in diabetes could lead to phagocytic uptake of these aggregated lipoproteins. Further, the small, dense LDL particles characteristic of diabetes preferentially bind to proteoglycans,[153] leading to further potentiation of cellular uptake of these particles by this mechanism.

Alteration in Lipoprotein Surface Composition

Qualitative abnormalities of lipoprotein surface and core composition occur frequently in diabetes and are independent of lipoprotein levels (Table 38–2). The free cholesterol/lecithin ratio in plasma, a striking index of cardiovascular disease risk,[33] is typically increased in both IDDM and NIDDM,[34,154] as a result of changes in this ratio for all lipoprotein classes. These compositional changes might affect the interaction of these lipoproteins with cells of the arterial wall by either facilitating the delivery of free cholesterol to cells[103] or altering the process of reverse cholesterol transport.[155] Reverse cholesterol transport could also be influenced by the increase in the ratio of sphingomyelin to lecithin in HDL in diabetes.[34,156] It is of interest that all these compositional changes tend to revert towards normal values with tight metabolic control in patients with IDDM.

Disturbances of Cell Replication and Growth Factors

Mitogens produced locally by arterial wall cells or derived from circulating blood cells such as platelets have been postulated to play important roles in the chemotaxis and proliferation of cells of the arterial wall, especially smooth muscle cells. However, there is little information concerning disturbances of any of these mitogens in diabetes. A low-molecular-weight growth factor was found in the plasma from subjects with NIDDM[157]; however, the nature of this growth factor has not been established. The expression of IGF-1, which is localized to the smooth muscle cell layer of rat aorta, is reduced in the diabetic state and can be regulated by insulin.[158] Although these findings are consistent with the hypothesis that increased expression of IGF-1, a potent mitogen for arterial smooth muscle cells, might be increased in the presence of hyperinsulinemia, much more needs to be learned concerning the role of mitogens in atherogenesis and their regulation by factors relevant to diabetes.

Propensity to Thrombosis

Clinical complications of atherosclerotic lesions often are precipitated by thrombosis at the site of the atheromatous lesion. There is an extensive and well-reviewed literature that amply demonstrates the association of diabetes with an increased propensity to thrombosis, as detected by many different in vitro measures.[159] Abnormalities of platelet adherence and aggregation have been observed in all forms of human and experimental diabetes. In addition, levels of several clotting factors and of the inhibitor to the anticoagulant tissue plasminogen activator (TPA) are increased in diabetes, thus potentially entering a procoagulant state in diabetes[42] (Table 38–4). Levels of fibrinogen are also increased.[160] However, more

Table 38–4. Procoagulant State in Diabetes

Related to hypertriglyceridemia
Increased factor VII clotting activity
Increased factor X clotting activity
Increased TPA inhibitor
Other
Increased platelet aggregatability
Increased Lp(a)

TPA = tissue plasminogen activator; Lp(a) = lipoprotein (a).

Table 38–5. Features of Diabetes Other than Lipoprotein Alterations that May Influence Atherogenesis

---

Disturbances of cellular function
    Reactive oxygen species
    Cytokines
    Phagocytosis
Disturbances of cell replication and growth factors
Modification of extracellular matrix
Propensity to thrombosis

---

evidence that the propensity to thrombosis is increased in vivo in diabetes is necessary. This obviously is of considerable practical importance, since dietary and pharmacologic measures that reduce intravascular coagulation could play an important role in the prevention of clinical events in patients with diabetes. Thus, it is apparent that a variety of features of diabetes unrelated to lipids and lipoproteins may influence atherogenesis (Table 38–5).

THERAPEUTIC IMPLICATIONS FOR THE PREVENTION OF ATHEROSCLEROSIS IN DIABETES

While our knowledge of the epidemiology and pathogenesis of macrovascular disease in diabetes is far from complete, strategies aimed at prevention of atherosclerosis in diabetes can be developed on the basis of currently available information. One approach would be to attempt to reduce all the traditional cardiovascular risk factors in individuals with diabetes. Thus, cigarette smoking should be discouraged in the strongest possible terms, hypertension should be treated with antihypertensive agents that are lipid-neutral or lipid-beneficial, and hyperlipidemia should be treated aggressively. In view of the dramatic increase in atherosclerotic complications in diabetes, an aggressive approach to the management of hypertension and the use of lower thresholds for initiating treatment of hyperlipidemia in diabetic patients than in nondiabetic subjects may be warranted. It seems reasonable to recommend a low-fat, low-cholesterol diet and participation in an exercise program as part of the general hygienic measures aimed at reducing cardiovascular disease. However, no information is currently available demonstrating that any of these strategies work in the prevention of cardiovascular complications in diabetes.

There also is little information about whether attention to the more recently appreciated risk factors will benefit patients with diabetes. Several approaches based on these pathophysiologic considerations may be considered, and even applied, before information regarding their value becomes available. For example, lipid-lowering agents that increase the size of lipoprotein particles and reduce levels of apoB might be worthy of consideration. With time, antihypertensive agents that improve the dyslipidemia of diabetes (e.g., the α-adrenergic blocking agents) or reduce microalbuminuria (e.g., the angiotensin-converting enzyme inhibitors) might prove to be of value in the prevention of atherosclerotic disease in diabetes. As drugs are discovered that are able to effectively lower

Lp(a) levels, their use in diabetic subjects with high Lp(a) levels should be entertained. The use of antioxidants for the prevention of atherosclerosis is controversial. Although some evidence from epidemiologic, experimental, basic, and clinical trial studies of the use of antioxidants for this purpose suggests a likely beneficial effect, the information available is insufficient to permit a recommendation for their widespread use in this context. Nonetheless, it has been suggested that both diabetic patients and smokers should consume more than the recommended daily allowance of vitamin C as a possible means of reducing damage done by the increased oxidant stress attributed to these conditions. While consumption of the dietary antioxidants vitamins C and E and β-carotene, even in fairly large doses, appears to be relatively safe, trials are necessary to test whether these agents, in either physiologic or pharmacologic doses, can reduce lipid peroxidation and atherosclerotic complications. The use of antioxidant drugs such as probucol also needs to be evaluated in diabetic subjects, and antioxidant drugs that do not lower HDL levels need to be developed.

The effect of long-term tight glycemic control might reduce the glycation of key proteins involved in the atherosclerotic process and thereby delay the onset of cardiovascular complications. The University Group Diabetes Project (UGDP) study of several years ago[161] did not achieve sufficiently good glycemic control over a long period to test this hypothesis adequately and paid little attention to other cardiovascular risk factors. Although evaluation of cardiovascular end points is not the primary intent of the ongoing DCCT trial, useful information concerning the effect of tight glycemic control on cardiovascular complications might be forthcoming.

Even less is known concerning management of the diabetic patient with established atherosclerotic complications. Because of the known existence of atherosclerotic disease in these subjects, an even stronger argument could be made for the application of safe strategies based on strong theoretical grounds. Of course, in the long run, studies will need to be performed to determine the efficacy of these various approaches in the prevention and management of atherosclerosis in diabetes. Further knowledge concerning the mechanisms of atherosclerosis in general, and in diabetes in particular, will no doubt ultimately lead to additional approaches to atherosclerosis prevention and, it is hoped, to a reduction in the alarming rate of cardiovascular complications in diabetes.

REFERENCES

1. Pyörälä K, Laakso M, Uusitupa M. Diabetes and atherosclerosis: an epidemiologic view. Diabetes Metab Rev 1987;3:463–524.
2. Everhart JE, Pettitt DJ, Knowler WC, et al. Medial arterial calcification and its association with mortality and complications of diabetes. Diabetologia 1988;31:16–23.
3. Steiner G. Atherosclerosis, the major complication of diabetes. Adv Exp Med Biol 1985;189:277–97.
4. Robertson WB, Strong JP. Atherosclerosis in persons with hypertension and diabetes mellitus. Lab Invest 1968; 18:538–51.
5. Crall FV Jr, Roberts WC. The extramural and intramural coronary arteries in juvenile diabetes mellitus: Analysis of

nine necropsy patients aged 19 to 38 years with onset of diabetes before age 15 years. Am J Med 1978;64:221–30.

6. Krolewski AS, Kosinski EJ, Warram JH, et al. Magnitude and determinants of coronary artery disease in juvenile-onset, insulin-dependent diabetes mellitus. Am J Cardiol 1987;59:750–5.

7. Kannel WB, McGee DL. Diabetes and cardiovascular disease: the Framingham study. JAMA 1979;241:2035–8.

8. Fuller JH, Shipley MJ, Rose G, et al. Coronary-heart-disease risk and impaired glucose tolerance: the Whitehall study. Lancet 1980;1:1373–6.

9. Kawate R, Yamakido M, Nishimoto Y, et al. Diabetes mellitus and its vascular complications in Japanese migrants on the island of Hawaii. Diabetes Care 1979; 2:161–70.

10. Morrish NJ, Stevens LK, Head J, et al. A prospective study of mortality among middle-aged diabetic patients (the London cohort of the WHO multinational study of vascular disease in diabetics). I. Causes and death rates. Diabetologia 1990;33:538–41.

11. Brunzell JD, Chait A, Bierman EL. Plasma lipoproteins in human diabetes mellitus. In: Alberti KG, Krall LP, eds. The diabetes annual. Vol 1. Amsterdam: Elsevier Medical Publishers, 1985:463–79.

12. Howard BV. Lipoprotein metabolism in diabetes mellitus. J Lipid Res 1987;28:613–28.

13. Barakat HA, Carpenter JW, McLendon VD, et al. Influence of obesity, impaired glucose tolerance, and NIDDM on LDL structure and composition: possible link between hyperinsulinemia and atherosclerosis. Diabetes 1990; 39:1527–33.

14. Hulley SB, Rosenman RH, Bawol RD, Brand RJ. Epidemiology as a guide to clinical decisions: the association between triglyceride and coronary heart disease. N Engl J Med 1980;302:1383–9.

15. Austin MA. Plasma triglyceride and coronary heart disease. Arter Thromb 1991;11:2–14.

16. Santen RJ, Willis PW III, Fajans SS. Atherosclerosis in diabetes mellitus: correlations with serum lipid levels, adiposity, and serum insulin levels. Arch Intern Med 1972;130:833–43.

17. West KM, Ahuja MMS, Bennett PH, et al. The role of circulating glucose and triglyceride concentrations and their interactions with other "risk factors" as determinants of arterial disease in nine diabetic population samples from the WHO multinational study. Diabetes Care 1983;6:361–9.

18. Laakso M, Pyörälä K, Sarlund H, Voutilainen E. Lipid and lipoprotein abnormalities associated with coronary heart disease in patients with insulin-dependent diabetes mellitus. Arteriosclerosis 1986;6:679–84.

19. Fontbonne A, Eschwège E, Cambien F, et al. Hypertriglyceridaemia as a risk factor of coronary heart disease mortality in subjects with impaired glucose tolerance or diabetes: results from the 11-year follow-up of the Paris prospective study. Diabetologia 1989;32:300–4.

20. Eckel RH, McLean EB, Albers JJ, et al. Plasma lipids and microangiopathy in insulin-dependent diabetes mellitus. Diabetes Care 1981;4:447–53.

21. Pietri AO, Dunn FL, Grundy SM, Raskin P. The effect of continuous subcutaneous insulin infusion on very-low-density lipoprotein triglyceride metabolism in type I diabetes mellitus. Diabetes 1983;32:75–81.

22. Taskinen M-R, Kuusi T, Helve E, et al. Insulin therapy induces antiatherogenic changes of serum lipoproteins in noninsulin-dependent diabetes. Arteriosclerosis 1988; 8:168–77.

23. Ochiai S, Onuma T, Boku A, et al. Change of chylomicron remnant in non-insulin-dependent diabetes mellitus [Abstract]. In: Eighth International Symposium on Atherosclerosis. Amsterdam: Excerpta Medica, 1989:677.

24. Rivellese A, Riccardi G, Romano G, et al. Presence of very low density lipoprotein compositional abnormalities in type 1 (insulin-dependent) diabetic patients: effects of blood glucose optimisation. Diabetologia 1988; 31:884–8.

25. Grundy SM, Chait A, Brunzell JD. Familial combined hyperlipidemia workshop. Arteriosclerosis 1987;7:203–7.

26. Parker F, Bagdade JD, Odland GF, et al. Evidence for the chylomicron origin of lipids accumulating in diabetic eruptive xanthomas: a correlative lipid biochemical, histochemical and electron microscopic study. J Clin Invest 1970;49:2172–87.

27. Kannel WB, McGee DL. Diabetes and cardiovascular risk factors: the Framingham study. Circulation 1979;59:8–13.

28. Report of the National Cholesterol Education Program expert panel on detection, evaluation, and treatment of high blood cholesterol in adults. Arch Intern Med 1988;148:36–69.

29. Brown G, Albers JJ, Fisher LD, et al. Regression of coronary artery disease as a result of intensive lipid-lowering therapy in men with high levels of apolipoprotein B. N Engl J Med 1990;323:1289–98.

30. Chait A, Bierman EL, Albers JJ. Regulatory role of insulin in the degradation of low density lipoprotein by cultured human skin fibroblasts. Biochim Biophys Acta 1978; 1529:292–9.

31. Stamler J. Epidemiology, established major risk factors, and the primary prevention of coronary heart disease. In: Parmley WW, Chatterjee K, eds. Cardiology. Vol 2. Philadelphia: JB Lippincott, 1989:1–41.

32. Austin MA, Breslow JA, Hennekens CH, et al. Low-density lipoprotein subclass patterns and risk of myocardial infarction. JAMA 1988;260:1917–21.

33. Kuksis A, Myher JJ, Geher K, et al. Decreased plasma phosphatidylcholine/free cholesterol ratio as an indicator of risk for ischemic vascular disease. Arteriosclerosis 1982;2:296–302.

34. Bagdade JD, Buchanan WE, Kuusi T, Taskinen M-R. Persistent abnormalities in lipoprotein composition in noninsulin-dependent diabetes after intensive insulin therapy. Arteriosclerosis 1990;10:232–9.

35. Nikkilä EA, Hormila P. Serum lipids and lipoproteins in insulin-treated diabetes: demonstration of increased high-density lipoprotein concentrations. Diabetes 1978; 27:1078–86.

36. Eckel RH, Albers JJ, Cheung MC, et al. High density lipoprotein composition in insulin-dependent diabetes mellitus. Diabetes 1981;30:132–6.

37. Laakso M, Voutilainen E, Pyörälä K, Sarlund H. Association of low HDL and HDL$_2$ cholesterol with coronary heart disease in noninsulin-dependent diabetics. Arteriosclerosis 1985;5:653–8.

38. Gordon T, Castelli WP, Hjortland MC, et al. Diabetes blood lipids and the role of obesity in coronary heart disease risk for women: The Framingham Study. Ann Intern Med 1977;87:393–7.

39. Cheung MC, Albers JJ. Characterization of lipoprotein particles isolated by immunoaffinity chromatography: particles containing A-I and A-II and particles containing A-I but no A-II. J Biol Chem 1984;259:12201–9.

40. Cheung MC, Wolf AC. Differential effect of ultracentrifugation on apolipoprotein A-I-containing lipoprotein subpopulations. J Lipid Res 1988;29:15–25.

41. Castro GR, Fielding CJ. Early incorporation of cell-derived cholesterol into pre-beta-migrating high-density lipoprotein. Biochemistry 1988;27:25–9.

42. Bierman EL. Atherogenesis in diabetes. Arter Thromb 1992;12 (in press).

43. Pan X-R, Walden CE, Warnick GR, et al. A comparison of plasma lipoproteins and apoproteins in Chinese and American non-insulin-dependent diabetic subjects and controls. Diabetes Care 1986;9:395–400.

44. Scanu AM, Lawn RM, Berg K. Lipoprotein (a) and atherosclerosis. Ann Intern Med 1981;115:209–18.

45. McLean JW, Tomlinson JE, Kuang W-J, et al. cDNA sequence of human apolipoprotein(a) is homologous to plasminogen. Nature 1987;330:132–7.

46. Etingin OR, Hajjar DP, Hajjar KA, et al. Lipoprotein(a) regulates plasminogen activator inhibitor-1 expression in endothelial cells: a potential mechanism in thrombogenesis. J Biol Chem 1991;266:2459–65.

47. Seed M, Hoppichler F, Reaveley D, et al. Relation of serum lipoprotein(a) concentration and apolipoprotein(a) phenotype to coronary heart disease in patients with familial hypercholesterolemia. N Engl J Med 1990;322:1494–9.

48. Stern MP, Haffner SM. Dyslipidemia in type II diabetes. Diabetes Care 1991;14:1144–59.

49. Takegoshi T, Haba T, Hirai J, et al. Alterations of lipoprotein(a) in patients with diabetic nephropathy [Letter]. Atherosclerosis 1990;83:99–100.

50. Morrish NJ, Stevens LK, Head J, et al. A prospective study of mortality among middle-aged diabetic patients (the London cohort of the WHO Multinational Study of Vascular Disease in Diabetics). II. Associated risk factors. Diabetologia 1990;33:542–8.

51. Brunzell JD, Sniderman AD, Albers JJ, Kwiterovich PO Jr. Apoproteins B and A-1 and coronary artery disease in humans. Arteriosclerosis 1984;4:79–83.

52. Wingard DL, Barrett-Connor E, Criqui MH, Suarez L. Clustering of heart disease risk factors in diabetic compared to nondiabetic adults. Am J Epidemiol 1983;117:19–26.

53. Pyörälä K, Savolainen E, Kaukola S, Haapakoski J. Plasma insulin as coronary heart disease risk factor: relationship to other risk factors and predictive value during 9½-year follow-up of the Helsinki Policemen Study Population. Acta Med Scand Suppl 1985;701:38–52.

54. Welborn TA, Wearne K. Coronary heart disease incidence and cardiovascular mortality in Busselton with reference to glucose and insulin concentrations. Diabetes Care 1979;2:154–60.

55. Fontbonne A, Charles MA, Thibult N, et a. Hyperinsulinaemia as a predictor of coronary heart disease mortality in a healthy population: The Paris Prospective Study, 15-year follow-up. Diabetologia 1991;34:356–61.

56. Standl E, Janka HU. High serum insulin concentrations in relation to other cardiovascular risk factors in macrovascular disease of type 2 diabetes. Horm Metab Res 1985 (Suppl 15);15:46–51.

57. Bergstrom RW, Leonetti DL, Newell-Morris LL, et al: Association of plasma triglyceride and C-peptide with coronary heart disease in Japanese-American men with a high prevalence of glucose intolerance. Diabetologia 1990;33:489–96.

58. Ronnemaa T, Laakso M, Pyörälä K, et al. High fasting plasma insulin is an indicator of coronary heart disease in non-insulin-dependent diabetic patients and nondiabetic subjects. Arter Thromb 1991;11:80–90.

59. DeFronzo RA, Ferrannini E. Insulin resistance: a multifaceted syndrome responsible for NIDDM, obesity, hypertension, dyslipidemia, and atherosclerotic cardiovascular disease. Diabetes Care 1991;14:173–94.

60. Després J-P, Moorjani S, Lupien PJ, et al. Regional distribution of body fat, plasma lipoproteins, and cardiovascular disease. Arteriosclerosis 1990;10:497–511.

61. Fujioka S, Matsuzawa Y, Tokunaga K, Tarui S. Contribution of intra-abdominal fat accumulation to the impairment of glucose and lipid metabolism in human obesity. Metabolism 1987;36:54–9.

62. Bierman EL, Bagdade JD, Porte D Jr. Obesity and diabetes: the odd couple. Am J Clin Nutr 1968;21:1434–7.

63. Terry RB, Wood PD, Haskell WL, et al. Regional adiposity patterns in relation to lipids, lipoprotein cholesterol, and lipoprotein subfraction mass in men. J Clin Endocrinol Metab 1989;68:191–9.

64. LaCroix AZ, Lang J, Scherr P, et al. Smoking and mortality among older men and women in three communities. N Engl J Med 1991;324:1619–25.

65. Palumbo PJ, O'Fallon WM, Osmundson PJ, et al. Progression of peripheral occlusive arterial disease in diabetes mellitus. What factors are predictive? Arch Intern Med 1991;151:717–21.

66. Freedman DS, Gruchow HW, Walker JA, et al. Cigarette-smoking and non-fatal myocardial infarction in women: is the relation independent of coronary artery disease? Br Heart J 1989;62:273–80.

67. Stamford BA, Matter S, Fell RD, Papanek P. Effects of smoking cessation on weight gain, metabolic rate, caloric consumption, and blood lipids. Am J Clin Nutr 1986;43:486–94.

68. Rosengren A, Welin L, Tsipogianni A, Wilhelmsen L. Impact of cardiovascular risk factors on coronary heart disease and mortality among middle aged diabetic men: a general population study. BMJ 1989;299:1127–31.

69. Manson JE, Colditz GA, Stampfer MJ, et al. A prospective study of maturity-onset diabetes mellitus and risk of coronary heart disease and stroke in women. Arch Intern Med 1991;151:1141–7.

70. Stern MP, Rosenthal M, Haffner SM. A new concept of impaired glucose tolerance: relation to cardiovascular risk [Editorial]. Arteriosclerosis 1985;5:311–4.

71. Jarrett RJ, Keen H, McCartney P. The Whitehall Study: ten year followup report on men with impaired glucose tolerance with reference to worsening of diabetes and predictors of death. Diabetic Med 1984;1:279–83.

72. Eschwege E, Richard JL, Thibult N, et al. Coronary heart disease mortality in relation with diabetes, blood glucose and plasma insulin levels: The Paris prospective study, ten years later. Horm Metab Res 1985 (Suppl 15);15:41–6.

73. Haffner SM, Stern MP, Hazuda HP, et al. Cardiovascular risk factors in confirmed prediabetic individuals: does the clock for coronary heart disease start ticking before the onset of clinical diabetes? JAMA 1990;263:2893–8.

74. Brown-McPhillips J, Barrett-Connor E, Wingard DL. Cardiovascular disease risk factors prior to the diagnosis of impaired glucose tolerance and non-insulin-dependent diabetes mellitus in a community of older adults. Am J Epidemiol 1990;131:443–53.

75. Ross R. The pathogenesis of atherosclerosis—an update. N Engl J Med 1986;314:488–500.

76. Ruoslahti E. Integrins. J Clin Invest 1991;87:1–5.

77. Gerrity RG, Goss JA, Soby L. Control of monocyte recruitment by chemotactic factor(s) in lesion prone areas of swine aorta. Arteriosclerosis 5:55–66.

78. Berliner JA, Territo MC, Sevanian A, et al. Minimally modified low density lipoprotein stimulates monocyte endothelial interactions. J Clin Invest 1990;85:1260–6.

79. Valente AJ, Rozek MM, Schwartz CJ, Graves DT. Characterization of monocyte chemotactic protein-I binding to human monocytes. Biochem Biophys Res Commun 1991;176:309–14.

80. Cushing SD, Berliner JA, Valente AJ, et al. Minimally modified low density lipoprotein induces monocyte chemotactic protein 1 in human endothelial cells and smooth muscle cells. Proc Natl Acad Sci USA 1990;87:5134–8.

81. Quinn MT, Parthasarathy S, Fong LG, Steinberg D. Oxidatively modified low density lipoproteins: a potential role in recruitment and retention of monocyte/macrophages during atherogenesis. Proc Natl Acad Sci USA 1987; 84:2995–8.

82. Hansson GK, Jonasson L, Seifert PS, Stemme S. Immune mechanisms in atherosclerosis. Arteriosclerosis 1989; 9:567–78.

83. Hamilton TA, Adams DO. Molecular mechanisms of signal transduction in macrophages. Immunol Today 1987; 8:151–8.

84. Goldstein JL, Ho YK, Basu SK, Brown MS. Binding site on macrophages that mediates uptake and degradation of acetylated low density lipoprotein, producing massive cholesterol deposition. Proc Natl Acad Sci USA 1979; 76:333–7.

85. Henriksen T, Mahoney EM, Steinberg D. Enhanced macrophage degradation of biologically modified low density lipoprotein. Arteriosclerosis 1983;3:149–59.

86. Fogelman AM, Shechter I, Seager J, et al. Malondialdehyde alteration of low density lipoproteins leads to cholesteryl ester accumulation in human monocyte-macrophages. Proc Natl Acad Sci USA 1980;77:2214–8.

87. Mahley RW, Innerarity TL, Brown MS, et al. Cholesteryl ester synthesis in macrophages: stimulation of β-very low density lipoproteins from cholesterol-fed animals of several species. J Lipid Res 1980;21:970–80.

88. Ellsworth JL, Cooper AD, Kraemer FB. Evidence that chylomicron remnants and β-VLDL are transported by the same receptor pathway in J774 murine macrophage-derived cells. J Lipid Res 1986;27:1062–72.

89. Brown MS, Goldstein JL. Lipoprotein metabolism in the macrophage: implications for cholesterol deposition in atherosclerosis. Annu Rev Biochem 1983;52:223–61.

90. Gianturco SH, Lin AH-Y, Hwang S-LC, et al. Distinct murine macrophage receptor pathway for human triglyceride-rich lipoproteins. J Clin Invest 1988;82:1633–43.

91. Suits AG, Chait A, Aviram M, Heinecke JW. Phagocytosis of aggregated lipoprotein by macrophages: low density lipoprotein receptor-dependent foam-cell formation. Proc Natl Acad Sci USA 1989;86:2713–7.

92. Khoo JC, Miller E, McLoughlin P, Steinberg D. Enhanced macrophage uptake of low density lipoprotein after self-aggregation. Arteriosclerosis 1988;8:348–58.

93. Lopes-Virella MF, Griffith RL, Shunk KA, Virella GT. Enhanced uptake and impaired intracellular metabolism of low density lipoproteins complexed with anti-low density lipoprotein antibodies. Arter Thromb 1991;11:1356–67.

94. Witztum JL, Koschinsky T. Metabolic and immunological consequences of glycation of low density lipoproteins. Prog Clin Biol Res 1989;304:219–34.

95. Palinski W, Rosenfeld ME, Ylä-Herttuala S, et al. Low density lipoprotein undergoes oxidative modification in vivo. Proc Natl Acad Sci USA 1989;86:1372–6.

96. Oram JF, Brinton EA, Bierman EL. Regulation of high density lipoprotein receptor activity in cultured human skin fibroblasts and human arterial smooth muscle cells. J Clin Invest 1983;72:1611–21.

97. Rothblat GH, Phillips MC. Cholesterol efflux from arterial wall cells. Curr Opin Lipids 1991;2:288–94.

98. Glenn KC, Ross R. Human monocyte-derived growth factor(s) for mesenchymal cells: activation of secretion by endotoxin and concanavalin A. Cell 1981;25:603–15.

99. Fox PL, Chisolm GM, DiCorleto PE. Lipoprotein-mediated inhibition of endothelial cell production of platelet-derived growth factor-like protein depends on free radical lipid peroxidation. J Biol Chem 1987;262:6046–54.

100. Majesky MW, Schwartz SM. Smooth muscle cell diversity in wound repair. Toxicol Pathol 1990;18:554–9.

101. Pitas RE. Expression of the acetyl low density lipoprotein receptor by rabbit fibroblasts and smooth muscle cells: up-regulation by phorbol esters. J Biol Chem 1990; 265:12722–7.

102. Bierman EL, Albers J. Regulation of low density lipoprotein receptor activity by cultured human arterial smooth muscle cells. Biochim Biophys Acta 1977;488:152–60.

103. Slotte JP, Chait A, Bierman EL. Cholesterol accumulation in aortic smooth muscle cells exposed to low density lipoproteins: contribution of free cholesterol transfer. Arteriosclerosis 1988;8:750–8.

104. Libby P, Hansson GK. Involvement of the immune system in human atherogenesis: current knowledge and unanswered questions. Lab Invest 1991;64:5–15.

105. Raines EW, Ross R. Mechanisms of plaque formation: cellular changes and the possibility of growth-regulatory molecules. Atherosclerosis Rev 1991;23:143–52.

106. Rajavashisth TB, Andalibi A, Territo MC, et al. Induction of endothelial cell expression of granulocyte and macrophage colon-stimulating factors by modified low-density lipoproteins. Nature 1990;344:254–7.

107. Malden LT, Chait A, Raines EW, Ross R. The influence of oxidatively modified low density lipoproteins on expression of platelet-derived growth factor by human monocyte-derived macrophages. J Biol Chem 1991; 25:13901–7.

108. Hamilton TA, Ma G, Chisolm GM. Oxidized low density lipoprotein suppresses the expression of tumor necrosis factor-' mRNA in stimulated murine peritoneal macrophages. J Immunol 1990;144:2343–50.

109. Fong LG, Fong AT, Cooper AD. Inhibition of mouse macrophage degradation of acetyl-low density lipoprotein by interferon-γ. J Biol Chem 1990;265:11751–60.

110. Werb Z, Chin JR, Takemura RL, et al. The cell and molecular biology of apolipoprotein E synthesis by macrophages. Ciba Found Symp 1986;118:155–71.

111. Mori N, Gotoda T, Ishibashi S, et al. Effects of human recombinant macrophage colony-stimulating factor on the secretion of lipoprotein lipase from macrophages. Arter Thromb 1991;11:1315–21.

112. Wiklund O, Camejo G, Mattsson L, et al. Cationic polypeptides modulate in vitro association of low density lipoprotein with arterial proteoglycans, fibroblasts, and arterial tissue. Arteriosclerosis 1990;10:695–702.

113. Wolff SP, Jiang ZY, Hunt JV. Protein glycation and oxidative stress in diabetes mellitus and ageing. Free Radic Biol Med 1991;10:339–52.

114. Curtiss LK, Witztum JL. Plasma apolipoproteins A-I, A-II, B, C-I and E are glycosylated in hyperglycemic diabetic subjects. Diabetes 1985;34:452–61.

115. Witztum JL, Mahoney EM, Branks MJ, et al. Nonenzymatic glucosylation of low-density lipoprotein alters its biologic activity. Diabetes 1982;31:283–91.

116. Lopes-Virella MF, Klein RL, Lyons TJ, et al. Glycosylation of low-density lipoprotein enhances cholesteryl ester syn-

thesis in human monocyte-derived macrophages. Diabetes 1988;37:550−7.

117. Gonen B, Baenziger J, Schonfeld G, et al. Nonenzymatic glycosylation of low density lipoproteins in vitro: effects on cell-interactive properties. Diabetes 1981;30:875−8.

118. Witztum JL, Fisher M, Pietro T, et al. Nonenzymatic glucosylation of high-density lipoproteins accelerates its catabolism in guinea pigs. Diabetes 1982;31:1029−32.

119. Duell PB, Oram JF, Bierman EL. Nonenzymatic glycosylation of HDL resulting in inhibition of high-affinity binding to cultured human fibroblasts. Diabetes 1990; 39:1257−63.

120. Duell PB, Bierman EL. Nonenzymatic glycosylation of HDL inhibits HDL receptor-mediated cholesterol efflux [Abstract]. Arteriosclerosis 1989;9(5):716a.

121. Monnier VM, Kohn RR, Cerami A. Accelerated age-related browning of human collagen in diabetes mellitus. Proc Natl Acad Sci USA 1984;81:583−7.

122. Brownlee M, Vlassara H, Cerami A. Nonenzymatic glycosylation products on collagen covalently trap low-density lipoprotein. Diabetes 1985;34:938−41.

123. LePape A, Guitton JD, Gutman N, et al. Nonenzymatic glycosylation of collagen in diabetes: incidence on increased normal platelet aggregation. Haemostasis 1983; 13:36−41.

124. Brownlee M, Cerami A, Vlassara H. Advanced glycosylation end products in tissue and the biochemical basis of diabetic complications. N Engl J Med 1988;318:1315−21.

125. Kirstein M, Brett J, Radoff S, et al. Advanced protein glycosylation induces transendothelial human monocyte chemotaxis and secretion of platelet-derived growth factor: role in vascular disease of diabetes and aging. Proc Natl Acad Sci USA 1990;87:9010−4.

126. Vlassara H, Brownlee M, Manogue KR, et al. Cachectin/ TNF and IL-1 induced by glucose-modified proteins: role in normal tissue remodeling. Science 1988; 240:1546−8.

127. Morel DW, Hessler JR, Chisolm GM. Low density lipoprotein cytotoxicity induced by free radical peroxidation of lipid. J Lipid Res 1983;24:1070−6.

128. Frostegård J, Nilsson J, Haegerstrand A, et al. Oxidized low density lipoprotein induces differentiation and adhesion of human monocytes and the monocytic cell line U937. Proc Natl Acad Sci USA 1990;87:904−8.

129. Henry PD, Bucay M. Effects of low-density lipoproteins and hypercholesterolemia on endothelium-dependent vasodilatation. Curr Opin Lipids 1991;2:306−10.

130. Boyd HC, Gown AM, Wolfbauer G, Chait A. Direct evidence for a protein recognized by a monoclonal antibody against oxidatively-modified LDL in atherosclerotic lesions from a Watanabe heritable hyperlipidemic rabbit. Am J Pathol 1989;135:815−25.

131. Ylä-Herttuala S, Palinski W, Rosenfeld ME, et al. Evidence for the presence of oxidatively modified low density lipoprotein in atherosclerotic lesions of rabbit and man. J Clin Invest 1989;84:1086−95.

132. Kita T, Nagano Y, Yokode M, et al. Probucol prevents the progression of atherosclerosis in Watanabe heritable hyperlipidemic rabbit, an animal model for familial hypercholesterolemia. Proc Natl Acad Sci USA 1987; 84:5928−31.

133. Carew TE, Schwenke DC, Steinberg D. Antiatherogenic effect of probucol unrelated to its hypocholesterolemic effect: evidence that the antioxidants in vivo can selectively inhibit low density lipoprotein degradation in macrophage-rich fatty streaks and slow the progression of

atherosclerosis in the Watanabe heritable hyperlipidemic rabbit. Proc Natl Acad Sci USA 1987;84:7725−9.

134. Heinecke JW, Baker L, Rosen H, Chait A. Superoxide-mediated modification of low density lipoprotein by arterial smooth muscle cells. J Clin Invest 1986; 77:757−61.

135. Morel DW, DiCorleto PE, Chisolm GM. Endothelial and smooth muscle cells alter low density lipoprotein in vitro by free radical oxidation. Arteriosclerosis 1984;4:357−64.

136. Hiramatsu K, Rosen H, Heinecke JW, et al. Superoxide initiates oxidation of low density lipoprotein by human monocytes. Arteriosclerosis 1987;7:55−60.

137. Parthasarathy S, Printz DJ, Boyd D, et al. Macrophage oxidation of low density lipoprotein generates a modified form recognized by the scavenger receptor. Arteriosclerosis 1986;6:505−10.

138. Heinecke JW, Rosen H, Chait A. Iron and copper promote modification of low density lipoprotein by human arterial smooth muscle cells in culture. J Clin Invest 1984; 74:1890−4.

139. Steinbrecher UP, Parthasarathy S, Leake DS, et al. Modification of low density lipoprotein by endothelial cells involves lipid peroxidation and degradation of low density lipoprotein phospholipids. Proc Natl Acad Sci USA 1984;81:3883−7.

140. Cathcart MK, McNally AK, Chisolm GM. Lipoxygenase-mediated transformation of human low density lipoprotein to an oxidized and cytotoxic complex. J Lipid Res 1991;32:63−70.

141. Parthasarathy S, Fong LG, Quinn MT, Steinberg D. Oxidative modification of LDL: comparison between cell-mediated and copper-mediated modification. Eur Heart J 1980;11(Suppl E):83−7.

142. Scheffler E, Huber L, Frühbis J, et al. Alteration of plasma low density lipoprotein from smokers. Atherosclerosis 1990;82:261−5.

143. Harats D, Ben-Naim M, Dabach Y, et al. Effect of vitamin C and E supplementation on susceptibility of plasma lipoproteins to peroxidation induced by acute smoking. Atherosclerosis 1990;85:47−54.

144. Gillery P, Monboisse JC, Maquart FX, Borel JP. Glycation of proteins as a source of superoxide. Diabetes Metab 1988;14:25−30.

145. Hunt JV, Smith CCT, Wolff SP. Autoxidative glycosylation and possible involvement of peroxides and free radicals in LDL modification by glucose. Diabetes 1990;39:1420−4.

146. Kitahara M, Eyre HJ, Lynch RE, et al. Metabolic activity of diabetic monocytes. Diabetes 1980;29:251−6.

147. Hiramatsu K, Arimori S. Increased superoxide production by mononuclear cells of patients with hypertriglyceridemia and diabetes. Diabetes 1988;37:832−7.

148. Thornalley PJ. Monosaccharide auto-oxidation in health and disease. Environ Health Perspect 1985;64:297−307.

149. Chait A, Brazg RL, Tribble DL, Krauss RM. Susceptibility of small, dense, low-density lipoproteins to oxidative modification in subjects with the atherogenic lipoprotein phenotype, pattern B. AM J Med 1993;94:350−6.

150. Wissler RW. Update on the pathogenesis of atherosclerosis. Am J Med 1991;91(Suppl):35−95.

151. Orekhov AN. Lipoprotein immune complexes and their role in atherogenesis. Curr Opin Lipids 1991;2:329−33.

152. Vijayogopal P, Srinivasan SR, Jones KM, et al. Complexes of low-density lipoproteins and arterial proteoglycan aggregates promote cholesteryl ester accumulation in mouse macrophages. Biochim Biophys Acta 837:251−61.

153. Hurt-Camejo E, Camejo G, Rosengren B, et al. Differential

uptake of proteoglycan-selected subfractions of low density lipoprotein by human macrophages. J Lipid Res 31:1387–98.

154. Bagdade JD, Subbaiah PV. Whole-plasma and high-density lipoprotein subfraction surface lipid composition in IDDM men. Diabetes 1989;38:1226–30.

155. Fielding CJ, Reaven GM, Fielding PE. Human noninsulin-dependent diabetes: identification of a defect in plasma cholesterol transport normalized in vivo by insulin and in vitro by selective immunoadsorption of apolipoprotein E. Proc Natl Acad Sci USA 1982;79:6365–9.

156. Bagdade JD, Ritter MC, Subbaiah PV. Accelerated cholesteryl ester transfer in patients with insulin-dependent diabetes mellitus. Eur J Clin Invest 1991;21:161–7.

157. Koschinsky T, Bünting CE, Rütter R, Gries FA. Vascular growth factors and the development of macrovascular disease in diabetes mellitus. Diabetes Metab 1987; 13:318–25.

158. Bornfeldt KE, Arnqvist HJ, Enberg B, et al. Regulation of insulin-like growth factor-I and growth hormone receptor gene expression by diabetes and nutritional state in rat tissues. J Endocrinol 1989;122:651–6.

159. Banga JD, Sixma JJ. Diabetes mellitus, vascular disease and thrombosis. Clin Haematol 1986;15:465–92.

160. Jones RL, Peterson CM. Hematologic alterations in diabetes mellitus. Am J Med 1981;70:339–52.

161. University Group Diabetes Program. Effects of hypoglycemic agents on vascular complications in patients with adult-onset diabetes. VIII. Evaluation of insulin therapy: final report. Diabetes 1982;31(Suppl 5):1–81.

Chapter 39

PATHOGENESIS OF DIABETIC NEUROPATHY

DAVID A. SIMMONS

In the absence of any universally accepted hypothesis to explain the relationship between the diverse clinical states referred to as diabetes mellitus and the wide variety of disorders of the peripheral nervous system with which diabetes is associated, these neuropathic syndromes have been divided empirically into two broad categories, the symmetrical neuropathies and the focal and multifocal neuropathies. It is generally agreed that these two broad groups of syndromes have distinct pathogenetic bases. A discussion of the efforts to explain the etiology of the distal, symmetrical, sensorimotor (predominantly sensory) polyneuropathy most frequently referred to as diabetic neuropathy is the topic of the bulk of this chapter. The limited information regarding the etiology of the focal neuropathies will be discussed separately.

PERIPHERAL NERVE BIOLOGY

Aspects of the structure and function of normal peripheral nerves relevant to an understanding of the information available regarding the pathogenesis of diabetic neuropathy will be discussed.

Histology

Peripheral nerves are composed of single or multiple bundles of nerve fibers, called *fascicles*. The fiber bundles are immediately enveloped in endoneurial connective tissue, enclosed in a perineurial membrane, and surrounded by epineurium.[1] The epineurium consists of areolar connective tissue, which contains fat, fibroblasts, mast cells, the vaso nervorum, and lymphatics.[1] The perineurium is a lamellated cellular membranous covering for the fascicle that serves as a perifascicular diffusion barrier.[1] The endoneurium consists of the nerve fibers per se and the endoneurial connective tissue. The perineurium is traversed by blood vessels that link the anastomotic vascular network in the epineurium with the intrafascicular capillary network in the endoneurium.[1] The endothelial barrier of these endoneurial capillaries contains tight junctions that also serve as a diffusion barrier.[2] As a result, the neuronal tissue of the peripheral nervous system appears to be protected by a blood-nerve barrier,[2] which is analogous in structure and function to the blood-brain barrier. The anastomotic nature of both the epineurial and endoneurial vascular networks creates a situation of redundant vascular supply, and experimental evidence suggests that it is difficult to restrict blood supply to the point of producing ischemia.[3] To produce ischemia, vascular occlusion must occur at multiple sites, whether the occlusion is in the small arteries,[4] the epineurial arterioles,[5] or in the microcirculation.[6,7] Although acute occlusion of large arteries resulting in limb gangrene is known to cause nerve degeneration, asymptomatic atherosclerosis of the large arteries has not been shown to cause fiber degeneration.[8]

Nerve axons are surrounded by specialized satellite cells called Schwann cells—probably of neuroectodermal origin.[1] The larger, myelinated nerve fibers (2 to 22

665

mm in diameter) are wrapped in a tube of myelin that consists of a succession of cylindrical segments called internodes. The myelin is derived from a chain of Schwann cells lying end to end, whose junctions form the nodes of Ranvier.[9] The myelin sheath consists of a concentric array of lamellae derived from the plasma membrane of Schwann cells and is therefore rich in phospholipids.[9] Unmyelinated nerves are those nerves invested by Schwann cells that have not produced a myelin sheath. In addition to including the large population of small nerve fibers that are normally not myelinated, unmyelinated fibers include developing fibers, regenerating fibers, and demyelinated nerves.[10]

Nerve Metabolism and Physiology

Under most physiologic conditions, mammalian cells maintain a precise dynamic balance between their rate of utilization and their rate of production of adenosine triphosphate (ATP) so that fluctuations in the ratio [ATP]/[adenosine diphosphate (ADP)]×[P_i] can be restricted.[11] This ratio determines the energy provided by the hydrolysis of a molecule of ATP and must be maintained within a restricted range to ensure that the free energy of hydrolysis is sufficient to determine the direction of the innumerable reactions that it controls. Mammalian cells are designed to function such that the rate of ATP utilization determines the rate at which substrates are used for ATP production,[11] i.e., the utilization and production of energy are in balance. This design permits rapid alterations in cellular activity without marked alterations in energy balance, a requirement for normal function and cell survival.[12] A significant imbalance between the utilization and production of ATP that results in a significant decrease in the [ATP]/[ADP]×[P_i] ratio rapidly leads to cell death.[11] Cells can adapt to transient restrictions on ATP production by 1) using their phosphocreatine (PCr) stores for ATP production (which results in a reduction in the ratio [PCr]/[Cr], a sensitive measure of the tissue's energy state); 2) decreasing energy-requiring biologic activities to reduce ATP utilization; 3) or increasing glycolysis for the production of ATP (when ATP production by oxidative phosphorylation is restricted by limitations on the availability of O_2).[13]

Regional blood flow is normally regulated in a manner that is coupled to the local rate of energy utilization to prevent restrictions on availability of ATP, a process termed *vascular autoregulation*. Autoregulation has been demonstrated in brain[14] and in virtually every mammalian tissue in which it has been critically examined. Cells cannot survive a prolonged restriction on ATP production,[11] particularly if it is the result of ischemia. Ischemia differs from hypoxia in that there is a restriction not only on the availability of O_2 but also on the provision of the greatly increased amounts of glucose required for glycolysis (16 molecules of glucose are required for the same level of ATP production via glycolysis vs. oxidative phosphorylation) and results in the rapid accumulation of lactate and development of acidosis. The relative rapidity

with which hypoxia or ischemia leads to cell damage is well documented for the heart.[15,16]

Although many neuronal energy-requiring processes are segregated in the nerve cell bodies and nerve termini, the energy requirements of the long axonal segments are subject to wide fluctuations under physiologic conditions. Because of the astronomic distances (in cellular dimensions) between cell bodies and their terminations, neither diffusion nor axoplasmic flow (see the discussion of axonal transport below) could conceivably provide ATP produced in the bodies or termini to the axonal segments with a rapidity sufficient to maintain dynamic energy balance. These nerve segments should be considered as a tissue, whose function is impulse conduction and whose energy metabolism merits consideration as a distinct problem,[13] as evidenced by their distinct vascular supply. The total capacity for glycolysis and oxidative phosphorylation in an axonal segment at any given time will depend on prior synthesis and transport of organelles and enzymes from the cell body,[17,18] but regional control of axonal ATP production is clearly required. The Schwann cells are an integral part of this impulse conduction tissue, but their relationship to axonal energy balance remains unknown. Current information on axonal energy balance is largely restricted to data on the composite energy metabolism of peripheral nerve axons and Schwann cells, the cell types comprising the peripheral nerve endoneurium.

Under most physiologic conditions, glucose is the major substrate for energy production in peripheral nerve endoneurium.[19,20] The diffusion barriers noted above protect peripheral nerve endoneurium from exposure to free fatty acids found in the plasma or epineurial extracellular fluid bound to albumin. Furthermore, the isolated tissue exhibits no capacity to derive energy from albumin-bound palmitate.[19] Insulin does not regulate energy metabolism in this tissue.[19,21] Alterations in energy metabolism induced by impulse conduction result from utilization of energy for the active transport of cations required to maintain ionic gradients.[14] In resting peripheral nerve, 30 to 40% of energy utilized is for the Na^+/K^+-ATPase activity that maintains the unequal distributions of Na^+ and K^+ across the cell membrane.[22,23] The relative contributions of axons and Schwann cells in these processes remain to be clarified. Impulse conduction per se is not an energy-requiring process, since the electrochemical gradients of Na^+ and K^+ across the axoplasmic membrane provide the driving force for the generation of the action potential by Na^+ influx through voltage-gated Na^+ channels and repolarization by K^+ efflux through voltage-gated K^+ channels.[24] The ionic flux associated with a single impulse is relatively small.[24] However, repetitive impulse conduction requires increased electrogenic axonal Na^+/K^+-ATPase activity for cation transport during the recovery period[23] (if active transport of K^+ into Schwann cells plays a role in buffering local changes in extracellular K^+ in some nerves, an increase in Na^+/K^+-ATPase activity in Schwann cells in response to impulse conduction would also be expected). This increased Na^+/K^+-ATPase activity induces an increase in glucose utilization,[23] which is required to prevent a rapidly developing restriction on the availability of ATP for this Na^+/K^+-ATPase activity. Under physiologic conditions, this restriction on the availability of ATP is prevented by the mechanisms that couple the rate of energy utilization to control of glucose oxidation and oxidative phosphorylation in functioning axons.[14]

Organization of the Peripheral Nervous System

Myelinated fibers include motor, proprioceptive, vibratory, and stretch afferent fibers. Unmyelinated and small myelinated fibers generally carry autonomic, pain, and temperature senses. Somatic afferent nerves transmit sensory impulses from the periphery to their nerve cell bodies in the dorsal root ganglion. Somatic efferent fibers have their cell bodies in the anterior horn and exit through the ventral root. Sympathetic autonomic fibers emerge from the thoracolumbar spinal cord as preganglionic fibers and terminate in ganglia located near the target organ. Parasympathetic fibers originate in the brain stem and sacral spinal cord as preganglionic fibers and also terminate in ganglia near the target organs.[25]

Nerve conduction velocity of unmyelinated nerves is on the order of 1 m/second and can be increased only with substantial increases in nerve diameter.[10] Myelinization results in substantial increases in conduction velocity to as high as 100 m/second without such large increases in diameter.[9] It should also be noted that the axons function as a chemical transport system for various axoplasmic constituents in the form of axonal transport (see below).[9]

HISTOPATHOLOGY OF DIABETIC NEUROPATHY

Diabetic neuropathy results from chronic, widely distributed lesions in the peripheral nerves. The most common form of diabetic neuropathy is a distal sensory polyneuropathy, with or without motor involvement, affecting fibers in a length-related pattern, with longer fibers being more vulnerable.[26] Histopathologic studies of autopsy and biopsy materials from patients with diabetic neuropathy have revealed lesions affecting nearly every component of peripheral nerves.[26] Attempts to deduce the pathogenesis of these lesions or the clinical syndromes that they accompany solely on the basis of the late-stage pathologic condition must be viewed with caution because the natural history of the lesions remains largely unknown and the biochemical basis for the individual aspects of the pathologic features remains conjectural. Furthermore, in large-scale studies assessing clinical findings (signs and symptoms), nerve conduction studies, and quantitative morphometric evaluations of nerve biopsy specimens, the correlation between clinical and electrophysiologic parameters and pathologic changes was imprecise.[27]

Pathologic studies of nerves from patients with clinically established polyneuropathy demonstrate a loss of axons in the peripheral nerve trunks, which is generally considered to be the characteristic lesion of this neuro-

pathy.[1] Myelinated and unmyelinated axons are affected,[1] and losses are greater distally than proximally.[1] Cases of "small fiber neuropathy" have been demonstrated, with selective loss of small myelinated and unmyelinated fibers.[28] On this basis, it was suggested that there is a spectrum of cases ranging from those with predominant loss of small unmyelinated and myelinated fibers to those with predominant loss of large myelinated fibers, corresponding to the anticipated spectrum of clinical deficits,[28] although cases of the latter have not yet been demonstrated.[26] In fact, in studies of both acute[29] and chronic[30] painful diabetic neuropathy, degeneration of fibers of all diameters, myelinated and unmyelinated, was found.

Some aspects of axonal loss remain controversial. Loss of cells in the dorsal root ganglion and the anterior horn has been reported but is not considered an important cause of axonal loss.[26] Focal intraneural lesions with a presumed vascular basis have been reported,[31,32] but not uniformly and usually in studies involving older patients. The suggestion has been made that this represents a distal axonopathy of the "dying-back" type,[33] but studies of the more rostral elements of the posterior columns that would be required to evaluate this hypothesis are not yet available, and the consistency of this interpretation with the available findings has been questioned.[34] (These observations are discussed in greater detail below.)

Evidence of axonal degeneration short of complete breakdown does exist[26] in the form of abnormal intra-axonal inclusions. Axonal atrophy occurs in animal models of diabetes[35] but has not yet been established in human neuropathy. Axonal regeneration occurs, which is seen as "regenerative clusters" of myelinated and unmyelinated axons or groups of small caliber unmyelinated axons.[26] (It has been proposed that ectopic impulses arising in regenerating sprouts from pain fibers provide an explanation for the occurrence of pain in painful neuropathy.[36])

There is significant disagreement over the basis of segmental demyelination and remyelination, which are generally agreed to be prominent features of diabetic neuropathy. The controversy centers on whether demyelination may exist as a primary lesion or whether it is secondary to axonal degeneration. (This issue has been considered by some authors as a critical issue in distinguishing between a metabolic and vascular pathogenesis for neuropathy, based on assumptions regarding the relative sensitivities of axons and Schwann cells to ischemia.) In one study, untreated diabetic patients without symptomatic neuropathy had as the predominant abnormality demyelination and remyelination; untreated diabetic patients with symptoms of neuropathy had the additional finding of degenerating axons; and treated diabetic patients had as the predominant abnormality axonal degeneration.[37] The same group subsequently reported the results of sural nerve biopsies in diabetic patients with and without neuropathy in which they concluded that demyelination and remyelination are secondary to nerve fiber loss.[38] Some authors have suggested that there is evidence of demyelination as both a primary and secondary process,[33] whereas others have reported no correlation between axonal loss and demyelination.[30,39] There is evidence of abnormalities in myelin at the node of Ranvier early in the course of neuropathy in experimental diabetes. Months after the onset of spontaneous diabetes in the BB rat, the terminal myelin loops detach from the plasma membrane of the axon,[40] a process termed *axoglial dysjunction.*[41] Axoglial dysjunction has recently been reported in patients with insulin-dependent diabetes mellitus (IDDM) with neuropathy.[42]

Abnormalities in the vascular and connective tissue components of peripheral nerve have also been reported in histologic studies of biopsy and autopsy material from patients with diabetic neuropathy. Endothelial cell proliferation and hypertrophy and thickening and reduplication of the capillary basal lamina have been reported,[43–45] as well as luminal narrowing.[44] Some authors have demonstrated an increase in capillary closure and platelet aggregations,[46] and others have noted a decrease in endoneurial capillary density.[44] Increased intrafascicular area and collagen deposition have been reported.[47] Fenestrations in the normally tightly junctioned capillary endothelial wall were also mentioned in a detailed analysis of these abnormalities.[26] A detailed discussion of these findings can be found in the section discussing evidence of a vascular basis for diabetic neuropathy.

A brief mention should be made regarding autonomic neuropathies. It has been suggested on the basis of their clinical epidemiology that the pathogenetic basis of these syndromes is similar to that of symmetrical polyneuropathy.[26] Pathologic studies of autonomic nerves are rare in comparison to those of peripheral nerves. Degenerative changes are reported in sympathetic ganglion cells,[48,49] and demyelination and axonal loss have been reported in the white rami communicantes of the vagus and splanchnic nerves.[50] Axonal loss has been demonstrated in the vagus in cases of gastroparesis diabeticorum[26] and diabetic diarrhea.[51] Degeneration of fibers and fiber loss have been demonstrated in the bladder wall,[52] the corpora cavernosa,[53] and the innervation of the vessels of the lower limb.[54] Finally, in an autopsy study of five patients with autonomic and sensorimotor neuropathy, inflammatory infiltrates were noted in autonomic ganglia and axons in visceral walls but not in nerve trunks, spinal cord, brain, or muscle.[55]

PATHOGENESIS OF FOCAL NEUROPATHIES ASSOCIATED WITH DIABETES

The clinical picture of focal nerve palsies is suggestive of a vascular etiology. They tend to be sudden in onset with spontaneous resolution and occur in older patients. The direct evidence for this etiology is extremely limited. Serial sections of the oculomotor nerve in two diabetic patients who died shortly after the onset of oculomotor palsy demonstrated intracavernous, noninflammatory, focal demyelinating lesions, which were interpreted as having an ischemic basis.[56] Microinfarcts were described in obturator, femoral, sciatic, and posterior tibial nerves

of a 73-year-old man with diabetes who died shortly after the onset of a focal limb neuropathy.[57] The authors have been criticized for interpreting Renaut's bodies as infarcts, although they are now known to be structures found in normal nerves.[58] Nonetheless, most investigators agree that these processes have a vascular basis.

MECHANISMS OF PATHOGENESIS OF DIABETIC NEUROPATHY

The risk for the complications of diabetes, including neuropathy, increases with increasing duration and severity of hyperglycemia.[59] Furthermore, all forms of diabetes mellitus convey risks for progressive structural alterations and eventual clinical manifestations in the same restricted group of tissues. This is true whether the hyperglycemia is related to an inherited or to an acquired syndrome[60–62] and regardless of the degree of insulin deficiency or the form of currently available therapy used.[63] It is therefore now generally accepted that hyperglycemia is what conveys the risk for the association between diabetes and its late complications.[64] The concept that the complications result from an inherited vascular abnormality, such as thickening of the basement membrane, independent of hyperglycemia and the metabolic consequences of diabetes, is no longer tenable and has been abandoned by its original proponents.[65]

Hypotheses regarding the pathophysiology of nerve dysfunction have generally fallen into two broad categories, the metabolic and the vascular. Since most of the available information has evolved in this context, the two categories will be discussed separately and in detail below. Current information would suggest that this is an artificial distinction, since the relationship between hyperglycemia and diabetic neuropathy noted above would suggest that if the basis for the pathogenesis of diabetic neuropathy is vascular (ischemic or hypoxic), the underlying vascular disease must also result from hyperglycemia or the metabolic abnormalities induced by the diabetic state. Therefore, current information on pathogenesis of diabetic neuropathy is best understood in the context of current information on the pathogenesis of the complications of diabetes in general.

Complications of Diabetes

The late clinical complications of diabetes are manifested in tissues by marked pathologic alterations. The pathogenesis of these complications should not be considered as a condition, but as a process that occurs in stages over years and even decades (Fig. 39–1). Early in the course of diabetes, functional alterations are known to occur in the tissues that are the targets of the late complications. These functional alterations are reversible by the correction of hyperglycemia and are detectable long before the appearance of the characteristic structural alterations.[66–70] The functional alterations are often followed by and accompany the appearance of early, initial structural modifications of these tissues that are distinct from the pathologic modifications seen in end-stage disease.[40,71,72] The evolving information regarding the natural history of nephropathy and retinopathy

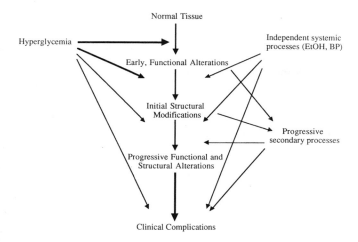

Fig. 39–1. The complications of diabetes as a process.

indicates that links connect hyperglycemia, the early functional alterations in those organs, and the initial patterns of structural changes.[71,73] The evidence further indicates that the progression of the initial structural and functional alterations creates conditions under which independent, superimposed pathologic processes develop whose progression is governed by factors other than hyperglycemia.[72,74] Each complication appears to result from a complex sequence of structural alterations unique to the tissue and usually not to the diabetic state[71,75] and therefore probably reflecting the biology of that tissue's response to injury. Furthermore, at various stages in the development of a complication, independent systemic processes (i.e., those related to hypertension, alcohol use, toxins, cigarette smoking, or dietary excesses or deficiencies) may become a primary determining factor in the progression of that complication. The natural history of diabetic neuropathy appears to be equally complex. The evidence regarding the various mechanisms by which hyperglycemia affects peripheral nerve must be seen in this light. Caution is required in the assumption that the nature of the early events can be extrapolated from the pathologic or metabolic alterations seen late in the disease process.

Vascular, Ischemic, and Hypoxic Hypotheses

The evidence upon which these hypotheses are based can be roughly divided into two sections. The first will deal with the morphologic evidence for vascular lesions that might be pathogenetic for diabetic neuropathy and the second with the evidence for nerve hypoxia as the pathogenetic basis for diabetic neuropathy.

Evidence for a Vascular Basis

The suggestion that diabetic neuropathy has a primarily vascular basis is nearly a century old.[76] It was initially supported predominantly by observations in amputated limbs or made at autopsy[77] and therefore of patients for whom occlusive atherosclerotic vascular disease of the affected limb could be clearly documented or seriously

suspected. Furthermore, in these studies Renaut's bodies were interpreted as nerve infarcts. Since diabetic neuropathy clearly occurs in the absence of clinically significant atherosclerotic disease of the peripheral arterial tree, it is now virtually uniformly agreed that such disease does not represent the pathogenetic basis of diabetic neuropathy.

The hypothesis that neuropathy results from pathologic developments in the small vessels in diabetes was initially suggested by the observation of a thickening of the walls of endoneurial capillaries in the nerves of diabetic patients as a result of an accumulation of periodic acid-Schiff (PAS)-positive material[78] subsequently identified as thickened basement membrane.[79] The pathogenetic significance of these observations was called into serious question by the observations that these changes were not found consistently in the peripheral nerves of patients with diabetic neuropathy[80,81] and that thickened basement membranes have been found in diverse acquired neuropathies other than those in diabetes.[30,82] Furthermore, basement membrane thickening has been shown to occur, on an age- and sex-related basis, in muscle biopsy specimens from subjects without diabetes,[83,84] as well as in the capillary beds of diabetic tissues that are not the targets of late complications.[85,86] For these reasons, the hypothesis that diabetic neuropathy has a primarily vascular basis had fallen into disfavor.

There has been a recent resurgence of support for vascular hypotheses regarding the pathogenesis of diabetic neuropathy. In a study of peripheral nerve tissue taken at autopsy from diabetic patients with neuropathy and from nondiabetic controls, multifocal loss of proximal fibers and diffuse loss of distal fibers were reported; the authors explained the distal losses on the basis of the summation of the proximal process.[34] In a series of sural nerve biopsies comparing diabetic patients with neuropathy with diabetic patients without neuropathy and with nondiabetic controls, the same authors reported a patchy and multifocal pattern of loss of myelinated fibers.[38] On the basis of a comparison of these findings with the morphology of nerve damage found in experimental models of peripheral nerve ischemia, it was suggested that this pattern of fiber loss provides direct evidence for an ischemic pathogenetic basis for diabetic neuropathy.[34,38] These studies have been criticized both because of the advanced age of the patient population and because of the younger comparative age of the controls.[58,87]

Evidence for the existence of focal lesions was presented in another study, in which autopsy specimens of lumbosacral trunk, posterior tibial nerve, and sural nerve from diabetic patients and nondiabetic controls were compared with sural nerve biopsy specimens from selected patients with vasculitis.[32] In the comparison of autopsy specimens, significant decreases in fiber number were found only in the sural nerves, whereas patchy lesions were found more commonly at all anatomic levels in the nerves of diabetic patients (although these lesion were apparently seen in the nerves of nondiabetic patients as well), and rare, focal proximal lesions predominantly affecting the perineurium were reported in the samples from the diabetic patients. The authors suggested that these rare, focal lesions have a vascular origin on the basis of the morphologic similarity of the lesions to those seen in sural nerve biopsy specimens from patients with vasculitis, although there was no apparent relationship to any discernible vascular abnormality in either circumstance.

In summary, several authors have concluded that a patchy, multifocal distribution of fiber loss reflects a vascular etiology for diabetic neuropathy, although the exact nature of the vascular lesion remains undefined.

This issue was addressed by comparing sural nerve biopsy specimens from a group of younger patients with diabetic neuropathy with those from a group of patients with type 1 hereditary motor and sensory neuropathy (HMSN).[88] These investigators found that although the patchy pattern of fiber loss in the diabetic patients was similar to that reported in those studies concluding that these findings had a vascular basis, this pattern was also identical to that found in the age-matched control group with type 1 HMSN. The authors concluded that since it is highly unlikely that HMSN has a primarily vascular basis, the occurrence of patchy, multifocal fiber loss in generalized polyneuropathies cannot be interpreted as an indication of a vascular etiology.[88] The pathogenetic basis for this pattern of fiber loss remains unclear.

Most of the more recent morphologic evidence provided in support of a vascular etiology for diabetic neuropathy has focused on the microcirculation. The most convincing evidence was provided in a study of the capillaries in sural nerve biopsy specimens from 36 diabetic patients and 45 age-matched controls.[46] The patients included 10 insulin-dependent (IDDM) and 26 non-insulin-dependent (NIDDM) diabetic patients; 32 had clinical evidence of neuropathy. The ages of these populations were not provided. The most striking feature reported was that the percentage of "closed" capillaries, i.e., those capillaries in which no lumen could be detected at high magnification, was significantly greater in the diabetic than in the control population and that the percentage of closed capillaries correlated with an "index of pathology" used to grade the severity of neuropathologic changes in the biopsy specimens.[46] The study was interpreted as providing direct evidence that capillary abnormalities play a role in the development of diabetic neuropathy. A subsequent study from the same laboratory[89] confirmed an excess of closed capillaries in diabetic patients with neuropathy. "Plugging" of capillaries with cellular debris was also reported in sural nerve biopsy material from a group of elderly diabetic patients who had predominantly motor neuropathy.[45]

Quantitative morphometric studies of the endoneurial capillaries of a group of relatively young diabetic patients have recently been reported.[90] Sural nerve biopsy specimens from 27 diabetic patients (25 with IDDM) were studied; all showed clinical and electrophysiologic evidence of distal symmetrical, predominantly sensory, polyneuropathy with or without clinical evidence of autonomic neuropathy. These were compared with biopsy specimens taken from nine patients with type 1 HMSN and from specimens obtained antemortem from nine organ donors. No occluded endoneurial capillaries were observed in this study (no focal lesions of the perineurium were encountered as well). These findings suggest that although evidence of vascular disease in the form of capillary closure may be superimposed in many cases of diabetic neuropathy, full-blown diabetic neuropathy frequently will develop in the absence of morphologic evidence for a vascular basis. In support of this conclusion is the observation from the original report of capillary closure that some of the severely affected nerves showed normal percentages of closed capillaries.[46] The authors suggested that this phenomenon could be explained by sampling error, more-proximal vascular abnormalities leading to loss of more-distal fibers, and the possibility that closure represents only the most severe lesion in a spectrum of capillary abnormalities. It should be noted that in that study, capillary closure was observed in the control nerves on an age-related basis.[46]

Capillary abnormalities in the absence of complete closure have been evaluated in a number of studies, including those already cited. The early suggestion that there is thickening of the basement membranes of endoneurial capillaries in diabetic individuals as compared with age-matched controls has been substantiated by numerous investigators.[30,43-45] The arguments discussed above, which strongly suggest that these changes do not reflect a primary pathogenetic process for diabetic neuropathy, are further substantiated by the report that basement membrane thickening was also observed in patients with type 1 HMSN.[90] Although the basis for thickening of the basement membrane is unknown, these authors suggest that increased turnover of endothelial cells, resistance to proteolytic degradation, or layering of basement membrane as a consequence of repeated alterations in vessel size may contribute to this abnormality.[91] It is generally accepted, even among investigators who support a vascular or hypoxic explanation for diabetic neuropathy,[8] that basement membrane thickening is not likely to limit the diffusion of oxygen, glucose, or small organic molecules. In fact, direct observations suggest an increase in the permeability of endoneurial capillaries to small molecules.[92]

Evidence that might suggest an abnormality in capillary luminal size is contradictory. In the study reporting capillary closure cited above, it was also reported that endoneurial luminal area in diabetic patients without neuropathy was greater than that in controls or diabetic patients with neuropathy, for whom no difference in luminal area was found.[89] In a study comparing sural nerve biopsy specimens from diabetic patients without neuropathy, or with mild or severe neuropathy, with specimens from age-matched controls, endoneurial capillary luminal size was evaluated as luminal perimeter but not as area or diameter.[44] The luminal perimeter was significantly greater in the diabetic patients without neuropathy and in those with severe neuropathy but not in those with mild neuropathy than in the controls. Other investigators have failed to confirm these findings. In one study endoneurial luminal size was determined as luminal diameter, which did not differ between diabetic patients with neuropathologic changes and control subjects.[43] The quantitative morphometric evaluation of endoneurial capillaries cited above revealed no significant difference between the mean luminal area or the distribution of capillary luminal size in diabetic patients with neuropathy and that in controls.[90] The bulk of the evidence suggests that there is no decrease in the size of the endoneurial capillary lumen in patients with diabetic neuropathy.

A number of other abnormalities have been reported in endoneurial capillaries in diabetic patients with neuropathy. The same investigators who found alterations in luminal perimeter reported a decrease in capillary density (expressed as the number of capillaries per square millimeter) in their severely neuropathic patients.[44] However, capillary density and minimum intercapillary distance were unaltered in diabetic patients with neuropathy both in the original study reporting capillary closure[46] and in the more recent report in which that finding could not be confirmed.[90] Endoneurial endothelial hyperplasia, expressed as both an increase in endothelial cell number and an increase in cross-sectional area, has been reported by several groups.[43,45] This observation was confirmed in the previously cited quantitative morphometric analysis but was found in type 1 HMSN as well, calling any causal relationship between endoneurial endothelial hyperplasia and diabetic neuropathy into question.[90]

Significantly less attention has been paid to the epineurial arteriolar circulation in diabetic neuropathy. In most studies it has not been evaluated. In one study, epineurial arteriolar intimal thickening as a result of endothelial cell proliferation was reported in diabetic patients with neuropathy, but no correlation was found between the degree of thickening and the degree of fiber loss.[93] Currently, there is no significant evidence to implicate arteriolar disease in the pathogenesis of diabetic neuropathy.

Finally, the pattern of peripheral nerve disturbance in diabetes is predominantly sensory and autonomic. This is not the pattern observed in those neuropathies with a known vascular basis.[58] Rather, motor involvement predominates and the onset is usually multifocal.[90] This discrepancy remains to be explained.

Evidence for a Hypoxic Basis

The chief proponents of a vascular or hypoxic etiology for diabetic neuropathy have contended that chronic nerve hypoxia could explain the pathogenesis outside of the evidence for structural vascular lesions.[8,94] Evidence to support this hypothesis has been generated from studies both of humans with diabetes and of animals with experimental diabetes. Two general lines of evidence have been pursued: 1) direct attempts to evaluate the energy status of peripheral nerves and 2) comparisons between the electrophysiologic data for models of neuropathy assumed to have an hypoxic basis and the data for diabetic neuropathies. A pathogenetic scheme based on the hypoxic hypothesis, postulated by one of its leading proponents, is provided in Figure 39–2.[95]

Direct Evidence for an Ischemic/Hypoxic Basis.
In the streptozotocin rat model, it has been reported that after 4 months of diabetes the endoneurial blood flow decreases by 30%, with an accompanying decrease in vascular resistance and a reduction in endoneurial O_2 tension.[96] The investigators have interpreted this evidence as suggesting that decreased endoneurial blood flow results in hypoxia sufficient to produce nerve dysfunction. There is disagreement over this interpretation. In vitro studies of intact preparations of peripheral nerve axons and Schwann cells have demonstrated that energy utilization in diabetic endoneurium is reduced by approximately 30%,[21] a change that reflects a decrease in Na^+/K^+-ATPase activity[97] (see below). It has been suggested that this decrease would provoke an anticipated decrease in tissue blood flow as a result of autoregulation of regional blood flow.[13] The proponents of a hypoxic model have suggested that mammalian peripheral nerve does not autoregulate (vascular autoregulation is discussed above) on the basis of the observation that sciatic nerve blood flow decreased by more than half when rats were supplied with 10% O_2 and became hypoxic.[98] Because these observations were made in regard to blood flow in the whole nerve of animals that were significantly hypotensive (circumstances in which the regulation of regional blood flow would be expected to be compromised for the preservation of cerebral and cardiac perfusion), the data permit no conclusion regarding vascular autoregulation in the neural components of peripheral nerve. The mechanism of the reported decreases in endoneurial blood flow remains controversial.

Decreased phosphocreatine (PCr) concentrations and increased lactate concentration also were reported in the sciatic nerves of rats with streptozotocin-induced diabetes.[99] This, in combination with the reduced endoneurial po_2, has been considered as direct evidence of hypoxic restrictions on nerve metabolism.[94] A number of objections to this interpretation have been raised. Previous studies reported decreased PCr and increased lactate concentrations in rabbit sciatic nerves 2 weeks after the induction of diabetes with alloxan.[21] In this model, it was demonstrated that the decrease in PCr is the result of a decrease in the total creatine (Cr) pool [Cr + PCr], which would be expected in a tissue in which decreased Na^+/K^+-ATPase activity resulted in a loss of the ionic gradients normally required to maintain their intracellular concentration (see below). No reduction was seen in the ratio of [PCr]/[Cr], a much more sensitive marker for limitations on the availability of ATP as a result of alterations in the energy charge than is the concentration of PCr alone.[19] The alterations in PCr and lactate and the decreased rate of energy utilization were not corrected during in vitro incubations in 95% O_2.[19] These observations are interpreted as being inconsistent with a hypoxic restriction on provision of energy to tissues and would suggest that the reported abnormalities are the result of metabolic alterations more directly associated with diabetes and hyperglycemia.

Endoneurial O_2 tension was measured in vivo in human diabetic patients with neuropathy, and the values were compared with those of a control group, which included the nondiabetic investigators and a diabetic patient without neuropathy.[101] In the neuropathic group, endoneurial O_2 tension was decreased and the normal gradi-

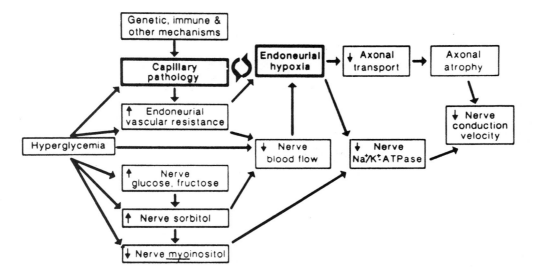

Fig. 39—2. A proposed hypoxic mechanism for the pathogenesis of diabetic neuropathy. Reprinted with permission from reference 95 (Low PA, Tuck RR, Takguchi M. Nerve microenvironment in diabetic neuropathy. In: Dyck PJ, Thomas PK, Asbury AK, et al., eds. Diabetic neuropathy. Philadelphia: WB Saunders, 1987:266—78).

ent of O_2 tension between the tissue and venous blood was reversed. The conclusion drawn, that these finding imply a hypoxic basis for neuropathy, has been disputed on a number of grounds. The mean age of the patient population was 70 years, whereas that of the controls was 38.8 years, a difference that restricts the ability to make conclusions from this data regarding the etiology of either the decreased O_2 tension or the neuropathology.

Direct observations of capillary blood flow in the nail fold of the toes in diabetic patients with and without neuropathy and in nondiabetic controls have been compared.[101] Capillary flow was increased threefold in the diabetic neuropathic subjects, and no capillary closure was evident,[101] although the report that in diabetes the endoneurial capillary morphologic abnormalities are more significant than those in skin capillaries[44] might restrict the significance of these findings. However, tissue O_2 tension, as measured by a transcutaneous oxygen electrode, in the legs and feet of diabetic patients with neuropathy was actually increased when compared with that in normal controls.[102] Finally, as discussed above in the section on metabolism, the expected effect of hypoxia sufficient in duration to restrict tissue energy balance is acute necrosis,[103] which is not a recognized feature of pathologic alterations of diabetic neuropathy in animals or humans. It has been asserted that chronic endoneurial hypoxia is associated with axonal pathology,[104] but this assertion is based on observations made of galactose neuropathy in rats.[105] The assertion that galactose neuropathy has a hypoxic basis is as controversial as that for diabetic neuropathy. Direct measurements of endoneurial O_2 tension and parameters of the tissue energy charge (such as the ratio of [PCr]/[Cr]) in diabetic patients with and without neuropathy and age-matched controls would be helpful in direct evaluations of this issue.

Electrophysiologic Evidence for an Ischemic/ Hypoxic Basis. Ischemia induced by the application of a pressure cuff to an extremity ultimately results in a failure in conduction of impulses in the nerves to that

extremity.[106,107] In the rat caudal nerve, which is a specialized trunk that innervates the tail, a delay in the time required before this phenomenon is observed in animals with streptozotocin-induced diabetes has been observed and termed *resistance to ischemic conduction block* (RICB).[99] The observation that RICB was significantly corrected by rearing rats with streptozotocin-induced diabetes in hyperbaric oxygen[108] led to the speculation that the phenomenon had its origin in hypoxia. This contention was supported by the observation that rats exposed to 4 weeks of chronic hypoxia (breathing 10% O_2) developed both RICB and decreased nerve conduction velocity (NCV),[109] a characteristic electrophysiologic abnormality in both human and experimental diabetic neuropathy (see below). Although it has been widely cited that O_2 supplementation partially prevented decreased NCV in rats with streptozotocin-induced diabetes,[110] the same investigators noted no improvement in NCV in streptozotocin-diabetic rats treated with hyperbaric oxygen.[109] The observation that human patients with arterial po_2 values lower than 60 mm Hg demonstrated RICB similar to that seen in 20 age-matched diabetic patients has been taken as further evidence for a hypoxic basis for both RICB and diabetic neuropathy.[111] However, the metabolic mechanism of RICB remains unknown,[111] and the previously cited reduction in energy utilization in peripheral nerves in diabetes as well as an increased availability of glucose substrate have been suggested as contributing factors.[99] Further, caution must be exercised in inferring a causal basis to observations made by correlation, the necessity of which is emphasized by the observation of RICB in rats 2 hours after the injection of streptozotocin and 95 minutes after the induction of hyperglycemia with glucose infusions.[112] These observations cast serious doubt on the hypothesis that RICB in diabetes is the result of chronic hypoxia.

Another piece of evidence that has been proposed as suggesting a hypoxic basis for diabetic neuropathy is the presence of peripheral neuropathy in some patients with chronic obstructive pulmonary disease (COPD).[113,114] Neuropathologic studies of a group of 47 patients with COPD revealed symptomatic neuropathy in 13%; segmental demyelination and unmyelinated fiber degeneration were the prominent pathologic features.[115] Although some of these studies have emphasized the role of hypoxia,[111,115] others have emphasized the role of a concomitant history of cigarette smoking.[113] Since the role of hypoxia has not been established as the etiologic basis for this neuropathy of COPD, an interpretation for these observations remains obscure. Furthermore, diabetic neuropathy is clinically indistinguishable from a number of neuropathies[59,116] for which the pathogenesis cannot be assumed to be identical. The observation that in a heterogeneous group of clinical disorders of various etiology (COPD) a neuropathic syndrome exists that is as yet poorly characterized but appears similar clinically to that seen in diabetes provides little insight into the pathogenesis of either disorder.

Summary

The clinical presentation of diabetic neuropathy, as discussed in the chapter detailing these syndromes, is frequently complex. Particularly in older patients, features will coexist that may suggest the superimposition of focal peripheral nerve lesions onto a picture of a symmetric, distal sensory polyneuropathy.[26] The evidence presented above suggests that the symmetric neuropathy can develop in the absence of a clear-cut vascular or hypoxic basis and that it likely results from a metabolic defect whereas the focal lesions may have a vascular basis.[90] The observation that focal nerve fiber loss is a prominent pathologic feature noted in sural nerve biopsy specimens from older patients with NIDDM but not in the group of younger patients with IDDM[42] would seem to support this analysis. However, the nature of the putative vascular lesions remains obscure.

Metabolic Hypotheses for the Pathogenesis of Diabetic Neuropathy

The diffuse and symmetric nature of the process and the peculiar vulnerability of sensory and autonomic fibers in diabetic neuropathy suggest but do not prove a metabolic basis for its pathogenesis.[58] The previously cited relationship between the severity and duration of hyperglycemia and the risk for neuropathy[59] and the clinical and pathologic similarity of diabetic neuropathy to other metabolic neuropathies[59] suggest that diabetic neuropathy is the result of the metabolic consequences of diabetes and hyperglycemia. In elucidating the mechanism by which hyperglycemia might *initiate* the risk for polyneuropathy, it is important to focus on early events. In attempting to understand the process by which these early events *progress* to clinical neuropathy, one must remember that the response of tissues to perturbations in structure and function, as well as general systemic processes, may become the primary factors governing the progression to clinical disease.

Evidence that Hyperglycemia Acts through a Common Mechanism in Initiation and Progression

Experimental Evidence that Hyperglycemia Acts through a Common Mechanism in Initiation. Evidence that a common biochemical mechanism initiates the processes that eventuate in the late clinical complications of diabetes has primarily been developed from observations of the functional alterations that occur within weeks after onset of hyperglycemia in the tissues that are the targets of the late complications of diabetes—including peripheral nerves, kidney, and retina—in humans[66–70] and experimental animals.[117–121] In each instance, both in diabetic patients and animals with experimental diabetes, the functional alterations are preventable or reversible with tight glycemic control and occur in the absence of the histopathologic features characteristic of the clinical complications. Direct observations of tissue homogenates from each of the animal models have related the functional alteration to decreased tissue Na^+/K^+-ATPase activity.[122–124] The most striking shared feature linking these functional alterations to a common pathogenetic mechanism is the ability of a distinctive panel of therapeutic interventions to prevent (and reverse, within a given time frame) the functional abnormalities.[64] In addition to rigorous glycemic control, treatment with aldose reductase inhibitors (ARIs) or dietary supplementation with pharmacologic levels of myoinositol designed to increase the normal plasma levels severalfold has each been shown to prevent or reverse decreases in NCV,[118,125,126] glomerular hyperfiltration,[127,128] and alterations in retinal function[124] in experimental animals.

Much of the information relating to a common initiating mechanism for the complications of diabetes was originally derived from studies involving peripheral nerve. Decreased NCV develops within weeks of the onset of hyperglycemia in rats with streptozotocin-induced diabetes[118] and in spontaneously diabetic BB rats[40] in the absence of the characteristic histopathologic features of chronic disease and is felt to be a model[35] for the decreased NCV seen shortly after the onset of Type I diabetes in humans.[66,67] The decreased NCV results from the effects of an abnormally high (increased approximately fourfold) intra-axonal $[Na^+]$ on Na^+ conductance and the function of the voltage-gated Na^+ channels at the nodes of Ranvier in large myelinated axons,[129] which appears to be the result of the decreased Na^+/K^+-ATPase activity that has been demonstrated in tissue homogenates[122,130] and intact tissue[21,130] in nerves from diabetic animals. The information regarding the mechanism by which hyperglycemia results in decreased Na^+/K^+-ATPase activity will be discussed below.

Hyperglycemia causes increased activity of the polyol pathway in nerves that fluctuates with the level of plasma glucose, as evidenced by the observation that hyperglycemia causes increased levels of glucose, sorbitol, and fructose[118,131] in nerve, and that these levels rapidly fall to normal levels when hyperglycemia is abruptly corrected with insulin.[132] The polyol pathway (Fig. 39–3) is

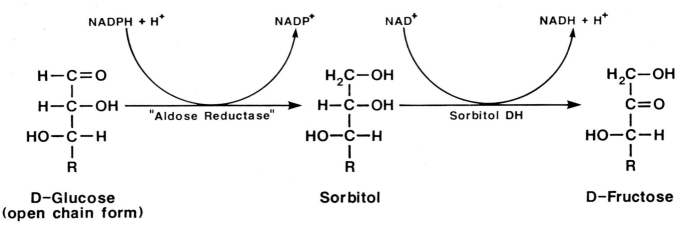

Fig. 39–3. The polyol pathway.

an alternate pathway for glucose metabolism with a ubiquitous distribution in mammalian tissues[64] but with a yet unknown function (except in seminal vesicles, where it provides a source of fructose for the metabolism of spermatozoa[133]). Normal concentrations of intracellular glucose are well below the apparent K_m of glucose for aldose reductase, the initial enzyme in the pathway (whose actual substrate may be the open-chain form of glucose). Activity through this pathway in most tissues, including nerve, is low but present under normal circumstances, as evidenced by the presence of detectable quantities of free sorbitol and fructose.[132,133] In the diabetic individual, increased concentrations of free intracellular glucose, which are the consequence of its unrestricted entry into nerves under hyperglycemic conditions,[19,21] results in increased activity of the polyol pathway.[132,133] However, it must be remembered that flux through the polyol pathway is difficult to measure and cannot be accurately assessed by measurements of the static concentrations of either sorbitol, which reflects a dynamic balance between its production and its oxidation, or fructose, which may be released into the extracellular fluid.[134,135]

The changes observed in activity of the polyol pathway in nerves of animals with diabetes of specific duration are associated with small (approximately 25%) decreases in the myoinositol content of composite tissue, although normal levels of plasma myoinositol are found in diabetic patients and animals.[118,126,136] Myoinositol is a cyclic hexitol found in abundance in mammalian tissues (1 to 50 mmoles/kg; approximately 4 mmoles/kg in nerve)[137–140] and plasma (10 to 50 μM, depending on the species).[118,137] When the rate of dietary intake is normal, plasma levels of myoinositol are tightly regulated by the kidney by oxidation to glucuronic acid.[141] Dietary intake of myoinositol is not required to maintain plasma levels[118,137] or the large gradients between the concentrations in plasma and tissue.[132] Tissue levels appear to be maintained primarily by synthesis (from glucose-6-phosphate[142,143]) and recovery of free myoinositol from inositol phosphates liberated by phosphoinositide hydrolysis.[144] Although active transport of myoinositol is known

to occur in a number of tissues,[145–147] including nerve,[148] the contribution of transport to the maintenance of normal tissue levels is unknown.[13,149]

The major metabolic fate of cellular myoinositol is its incorporation into phosphatidylinositol (PI), an integral membrane glycerophospholipid, which is the parent phosphoinositide for phosphatidylinositol-4-phosphate (PIP) and phosphatidylinositol-4,5-bisphosphate (PIP$_2$), which are formed by progressive phosphorylation of free hydroxyl groups on the inositol ring and are called polyphosphinositides. Receptor-mediated hydrolysis of PIP$_2$ by phospholipase C is now known to be the signal transduction mechanism for numerous hormones and neurotransmitters. Such hydrolysis stimulates a bifurcating signal pathway by liberating polyphosphorylated myoinositols (inositol phosphates [IPs]), which raise cytosolic [Ca^{++}] by releasing intracellular stores; and by generating sn-1,2-diacylglycerols (DAGs), which modulates the activity of protein kinases of the C type.[150,151] Phospholipase C hydrolysis of PI per se can also serve as a regulatory mechanism by releasing DAGs at specific membrane sites, but the IPs released from PI do not increase cytosolic [Ca^{++}].[150,151] Synthesis of a specific phosphoinositide pool utilized for metabolic regulation is usually independently regulated.[151]

The capacity of a distinctive panel of therapeutic interventions—tight glycemic control, aldose reductase inhibition, and dietary myoinositol supplementation—to prevent the alterations in tissue Na$^+$/K$^+$-ATPase activity[41,152] and NCV[117,131] led to the postulation of an initiating mechanism for diabetic neuropathy[153,154] (Fig. 39–4). Rigorous glycemic control prevents hyperglycemia, increased activity of the polyol pathway activity, and decreased tissue concentrations of myoinositol.[118,132] Treatment with an aldose reductase inhibitor prevents the increases in nerve sorbitol and fructose levels and the decreases in myoinositol levels without affecting plasma or nerve glucose levels.[126,136,155] Dietary myoinositol supplementation that raises plasma concentrations of myoinositol severalfold prevents the decrease in tissue concentrations of myoinositol but has no effect on plasma levels of glucose or tissue concentrations of glucose,

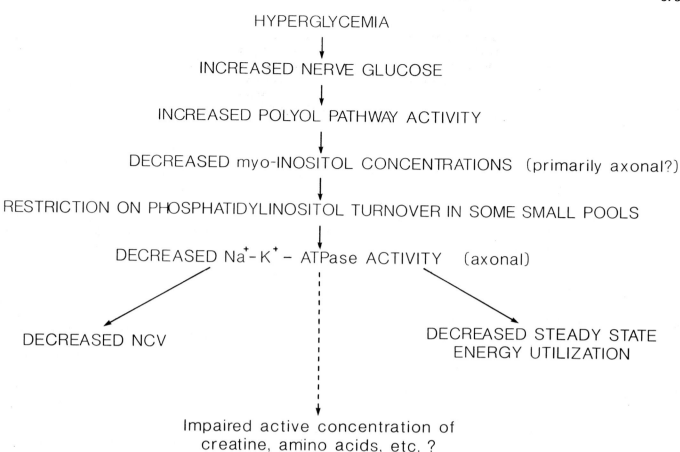

Fig. 39—4. The myoinositol depletion hypothesis: an early formulation of a mechanism for the pathogenesis of diabetic neuropathy.

sorbitol, or fructose.[118] These observations suggested (Fig. 39—4) that hyperglycemia causes increased intracellular concentrations of glucose in nerve (a tissue that does not require insulin for glucose uptake), a change resulting in increased activity of the polyol pathway. This increased activity of the polyol pathway acts through a mechanism, as yet unknown, to alter tissue metabolism of myoinositol, which in turn results in an inhibition of tissue Na^+/K^+-ATPase activity.[153,154]

The exact nature of this initiating mechanism has been elusive. Because consistently detectable decreases in NCV require weeks to develop in these animal models, the implicit assumption has been made that similar periods of hyperglycemia are required to express the underlying defect in Na^+/K^+-ATPase activity. Consequently, most of the available information has been derived from studies that compare levels of metabolite and Na^+/K^+-ATPase activity in tissues from normal animals and from treated and untreated animals with diabetes of several weeks' duration. On the basis of these observations, it was initially postulated that "myoinositol depletion" was a prerequisite for the effect on Na^+/K^+-ATPase activity in nerve and other tissues.[153,154] Numerous observations have proven to be inconsistent with this view. In isolated renal glomeruli from rats with strepto-

zotocin-induced diabetes, Na^+/K^+-ATPase activity is reduced before decreases are seen in myoinositol content,[156] even though the resultant alteration in glomerular filtration is preventable by dietary supplementation with myoinositol and therapy with an aldose reductase inhibitor.[127] One group of investigators has reported a decrease in myoinositol content and Na^+/K^+-ATPase activity in superior cervical ganglia from rats 8 weeks after the induction of diabetes with streptozotocin that could be prevented by an aldose reductase inhibitor (ARI).[157] Another group detected decreases in the myoinositol content—they did not measure Na^+/K^+-ATPase activity—of rat dorsal root ganglia after 2 weeks of streptozotocin diabetes that disappeared after 8 weeks of diabetes in untreated rats.[158] Another study found that the decrease in tibial nerve myoinositol content seen after 3 months of streptozotocin diabetes was preventable by therapy with an aldose reductase inhibitor but found a normal nerve myoinositol content after 6 months of diabetes in untreated animals, despite persistent decreases in NCV.[159] In a detailed analysis of specific cell types of various non-neural tissues from normal rabbits and rabbits with alloxan-induced diabetes after 19 days or 2 months of diabetes, the investigators detected numerous changes but no consistent pattern of change in the total myoinositol content in these tissues; they did not attempt to measure Na^+/K^+-ATPase activity or any functional parameters or the effect of any therapeutic intervention.[160]

One group of investigators has reported direct observations on the operation of a putatively common initiating mechanism in tissue from normal animals that provides a potential resolution for these apparently paradoxical observations.[22,161,162] These authors reported that approximately half of the normal resting Na^+/K^+-ATPase activity of tibial nerve endoneurium from normal rabbits incubated in glucose at normal extracellular fluid (ECF) concentrations could be inhibited by inhibiting transport of ECF myoinositol by deletion of myoinositol from the incubation medium,[22] despite the lack of a decrease in the composite myoinositol content of tissue beyond that attributable to a washout of the ECF myoinositol initially present in the tissue.[22,103] These observations were confirmed and clarified in studies of normal rabbit aortic intima-media (AIM), a preparation of intact arterial wall, which represents another excitable tissue susceptible to the effects of hyperglycemia.[161,162] On the basis of their further observations, these investigators concluded that in normal endoneurium and arterial wall a distinct fraction of normal resting Na^+/K^+-ATPase activity is controlled by a regulatory system in which PI turnover in a discrete pool serves as the transducing arm.[22,161] (This is unusual, in that the transducing system involves hydrolysis of PI per se and not polyphosphoinositides.) Direct observations in AIM suggest that endogenously released adenosine, acting through a novel adenosine receptor, acts as the stimulus for this system in that resting tissue.[163] The discrete, rapidly turning over PI pool is replenished by a distinct fraction of PI synthesis that is selectively inhibited when myoinositol uptake is prevented by deleting myoinositol from the ECF, without detectable decreases in total tissue myoinositol content.[22,161] (PI synthetases have been isolated from two cellular sites, endoplasmic reticulum, in which the reported K_m values for myoinositol are in the millimolar range; and plasma membrane, in which the reported K_m is 67 micromolar.[164]) These observations have been interpreted as suggesting that the presence of this regulatory system in a tissue should make it susceptible to a derangement in Na^+/K^+-ATPase activity, if hyperglycemia induced an increase in polyol pathway activity that impaired active transport of ECF myoinositol at normal ECF concentrations,[64] as was previously demonstrated in nerve.[126,131]

A glucose-induced inhibition of Na^+/K^+-ATPase activity with the identifying characteristics of the common initiating mechanism was reproduced and studied in vitro in normal AIM and was shown to result from inhibition of this normal regulatory system (Fig. 39–5).[162] At normal ECF levels of myoinositol (70 μM), raising the concentration of glucose from 5 mM (90 mg/dL) to 30 mM completely and specifically inhibited the component of Na^+/K^+-ATPase activity that requires ECF myoinositol, as well as the fraction of PI synthesis required to maintain the regulatory system in AIM.[162] ECF glucose concentrations of 10 mM and 20 mM had an identical effect on

Na^+/K^+-ATPase activity.[162] These effects occurred during incubation times totaling only 60 minutes[161] and under conditions demonstrated to have no effect on the normal total tissue myoinositol content (5.8 mmoles/kg).[161,165] These effects of an elevated ECF glucose level were completely prevented by raising the ECF myoinositol concentration severalfold (from 70 μM to 500 μM) or by adding one of two structurally distinct aldose reductase inhibitors at standard pharmacologic concentrations (10 μM sorbinil or 1 μM tolrestat).[162] The authors suggest that these observations demonstrate that the effects of hyperglycemia on Na^+/K^+-ATPase activity occur acutely and in the absence of "myoinositol depletion" and that alterations in composite tissue myoinositol content likely reflect delayed, secondary effects of hyperglycemia.[103,162]

The evidence regarding the content and turnover of phosphoinositides in nerve is complex, but no uniformly demonstrable global deficits in the nerve content of PI, PIP, or PIP_2 are apparent.[103] Several studies have demonstrated decreased amounts of inositol-containing lipids in the nerves of diabetic mice[130] and in biopsy[166] and autopsy[167] specimens of nerves from diabetic patients. Whereas one study of sciatic nerve endoneurium from rats with streptozotocin-induced diabetes revealed no global deficit in phosphoinositide content[168] and another revealed deficits only in polyphosphoinositide content after 6 and 9 weeks of diabetes,[169] another investigator reported decreased PI content in rat sciatic nerves after 20 weeks of streptozotocin-induced diabetes.[170] Several authors have reported diminished incorporation of [^{3}H]inositol into the sciatic nerves of diabetic rats[171,172] but normal incorporation of [^{32}P]phosphates into PI and increased incorporation into PIP_2,[169,173,174] which was corrected by insulin treatment.[174] Taken together, these findings would suggest that the abnormality in myoinositol and PI metabolism associated with increased activity of the polyol pathway activity is restricted to a selective inhibition of a specific fraction of the synthesis of PI per se in nerve.[103] This analysis is supported by the observation that the concentration of DAG in sciatic nerves from streptozotocin-diabetic rats was significantly reduced; analysis of the molecular species suggested that the bulk of this reduction was a consequence of decreased phosphoinositide hydrolysis.[175] Furthermore, the exposure of tibial nerve endoneurium from alloxan-diabetic rabbits to specific DAG analogues and other protein kinase C agonists acutely corrected the 40% reduction observed in their resting Na^+/K^+-ATPase activity without affecting the activity in normal controls.[176] These findings are in accord with the view that hyperglycemia initially decreases nerve Na^+/K^+-ATPase activity by inhibiting the PI turnover that normally maintains a distinct fraction of this activity.

It has been suggested that a defect in the regulation of Na^+/K^+-ATPase activity related to hyperglycemia and the polyol pathway could account for some of the early abnormalities noted in peripheral nerve in addition to decreased NCV.[64,154] In mammalian tissues, the Na^+ gradient is normally used for active concentration of numerous metabolites.[177] The decrease in the total creatine pool of diabetic peripheral nerve, discussed in

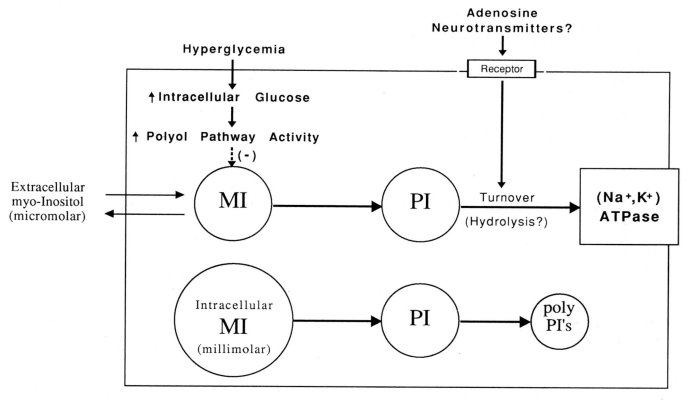

Fig. 39–5. A "common mechanism" for the pathogenesis of diabetic complications. Hyperglycemia inhibits a normal regulatory system that requires extracellular fluid myoinositol (MI) for the maintenance of a discrete pool of phosphatidylinositol (PI), whose turnover regulates a component of (Na+,K+)-ATPase activity (see text for details).

the sections of this chapter related to metabolism and hypoxia, has been ascribed to a reduction in Na+-dependent uptake of creatine.[21] A reported defect in the Na+-dependent uptake of amino acids in the nerve of rabbits after 2 weeks of alloxan diabetes was prevented by ARIs and dietary myoinositol supplementation.[178] Since a Na+-dependent myoinositol transport mechanism in nerve has been reported,[148] alterations in the components of myoinositol transport maintained by that mechanism may explain the delayed, secondary effects of hyperglycemia on total tissue myoinositol content discussed above. Furthermore, the Na+ gradient is used in nerve to maintain intracellular Ca++ homeostasis[179]; dysregulation of intracellular [Na+] would be expected to affect this function and potentially could account for altered responsiveness to neurotransmitters and hormones whose signals are transduced through effects on intracellular Ca++.

In summary, evidence from animal models suggests that hyperglycemia inhibits a distinct component of resting Na+/K+-ATPase activity in nerve that results in a reversible reduction in NCV (Fig. 39–5). Hyperglycemia appears to act through a mechanism involving increased activity of the polyol pathway to inhibit the uptake of ECF myoinositol, which is required to maintain the synthesis of a discrete pool of PI whose turnover represents the transducing arm of a regulatory system that normally maintains a distinct component of Na+/K+-ATPase activ-

ity. Inhibition of this myoinositol uptake inhibits the discrete pool of PI turnover and the Na+/K+-ATPase activity that it controls. This inhibition of Na+/K+-ATPase activity has been shown to induce a decrease in NCV and a decrease in uptake of amino acids and creatine. The impact of the other potential acute manifestations of this inhibition remains to be evaluated.

Experimental Evidence that the Common Mechanism Is Involved in Progression. The early, reversible functional abnormalities in diabetic nerve are soon accompanied by identifiable structural abnormalities demonstrated in experimental models, although the relationship of these early changes to the characteristic pathologic features of the late clinical complications remains unknown. The earliest reported structural abnormality in the nerves of diabetic animals is demonstrable in sciatic nerves within 14 days of the injection of streptozotocin into rats.[180] In these studies, the authors demonstrated a significant decrease in the number of electron-dense intramembranous particles on both the P-face (inner leaflet) and E-face (outer leaflet) of the freeze-fractured surfaces of the internodal myelin[180] in sciatic nerves from diabetic animals as compared with the number in normal control rats. These particles are felt to represent integral membrane proteins[180] that may be important in the maintenance of the integrity of the myelin sheath.[180,181] The decreases in the number of intramembranous particles were prevented in diabetic rats kept euglycemic with insulin therapy and in those diabetic rats that received diets supplemented with 1% myoinositol,[180] suggesting that the common mechanism described above is responsible for the development of this early abnormality in the myelin of peripheral nerves of diabetic animals.

Within 3 weeks of the onset of hyperglycemia in the spontaneously diabetic BB rat[40,41] and 4 weeks following hyperglycemia in the streptozotocin-diabetic rat,[182] histologic examination of the peripheral nerves reveals a characteristic swelling, referred to as paranodal swelling, in the area immediately surrounding the nodes of Ranvier. These changes can be directly related to the common mechanism, because in the BB rat paranodal swelling can be reversed with insulin therapy,[40] ARI therapy, and dietary supplementation with myoinositol[41] and in the streptozotocin-diabetic rat the swelling can be prevented by successful islet cell transplantation.[182] Paranodal swelling is presumed to result from the effects of increased intra-axonal Na$^+$ concentration[40] and therefore may represent a structural correlate to the decrease in NCV induced by impaired Na$^+$/K$^+$-ATPase activity. It had been postulated that "osmotic swelling" induced by accumulation of intermediates of the polyol pathway contributes to the pathogenesis of diabetic complications,[183,184] including neuropathy.[155] The role of osmotic swelling early in neuropathy can virtually be excluded by the observation that supplementation with myoinositol prevents or reverses paranodal swelling, decreased NCV, and reduced Na$^+$/K$^+$-ATPase activity without producing any effect on the concentration of glucose or intermediates of the polyol pathway. For this and numerous other reasons, most authors have rejected a role for osmotic swelling in the pathogenesis of neuropathy.[153,154]

Whereas the metabolic and functional alterations and the accompanying structural modifications observed in nerves of acutely diabetic animals are completely reversible, more prolonged hyperglycemia accompanying more chronic diabetes in these animal models is accompanied by the development of changes that are only partially reversible with strict glycemic control with insulin. As discussed above, the institution of rigorous glycemic control after 6 weeks of diabetes in BB rats normalizes NCV, Na$^+$/K$^+$-ATPase activity, Na$^+$ equilibrium and permeability, nerve glucose, polyol pathway intermediates, and myoinositol content, and paranodal swelling. However, if diabetes is allowed to persist untreated for 12 or 24 weeks in the BB rat, motor NCV continues to decline, and although the institution of rigorous glycemic control at these time points permits significant improvement in motor NCV, nerve conduction is no longer normalized.[185,186] In one study, motor NCV in animals after 6 weeks of rigorous insulin treatment following 12 weeks of diabetes was 118% of that in untreated diabetic animals but 90% of that in nondiabetic controls.[186] In another study, however, 3 weeks of rigorous insulin therapy after 24 weeks of hyperglycemia resulted in motor NCV that was 124% of that in the untreated diabetic control group but corresponded to only 80% of the value in age-matched nondiabetic animals.[185] The improvements in motor NCV following normalization of

blood glucose levels in the 12-week model were accompanied by normalization of the ouabain-inhibitable ATPase activity and nerve myoinositol content; levels of nerve glucose, sorbitol, and fructose were not reported.[186] In the 24-week model, electrophysiologic parameters were evaluated by voltage-clamp studies and revealed that the persistent decline in NCV was attributable to irreversible alterations in the Na$^+$ permeability and the Na$^+$ equilibrium potential, parameters that were completely normalized by euglycemia after 3 weeks of diabetes, when the motor NCV was also completely correctable (the degree to which the metabolic parameters in nerve were corrected by the period of euglycemia in the 24-week model was not assessed).[185]

The development of a component of decreased NCV after 12 weeks of diabetes that cannot be reversed with 6 weeks of tight glycemic control is associated with the development of irreversible structural abnormalities of the axons (maloriented neurofilaments) and the nodes of Ranvier (axoglial dysjunction, a detachment of the terminal myelin loops from the plasma membrane of the axon).[186] (Other structural abnormalities, including axonal glycogenosomes, honeycombing of the Schwann cell axon interface, and acute axonal degeneration, were reported but remained predominantly reversible.) There was no detectable decrease in mean fiber size, distribution of fiber-size frequency, or axon-myelin ratio that might account for decreased NCV, and the authors suggest that maloriented neurofilaments are unlikely to produce decreases in NCV. They concluded that axoglial dysjunction is the likely cause of the observed irreversible impairment in NCV.[186] These investigators suggest that a normal function of the axoglial junction is the limitation of the lateral migration of voltage-sensitive Na$^+$ channels away from the node and that loss of these junctional complexes leads to this migration, producing the electrophysiologic abnormalities cited above that result in nodal conduction delay and the resultant irreversible decreases in NCV.[35,185,186]

The pathogenetic basis of axoglial dysjunction is not yet understood. On the basis of sequential morphologic observations in the BB rat,[40] the streptozotocin-diabetic rat,[182] and human diabetic neuropathy,[42,187] it has been suggested that axoglial dysjunction may represent a progression from paranodal swelling[35] and that it likely constitutes the initial stage in the progression of structural changes to paranodal demyelination and remyelination.[35] The observations that axoglial dysjunction is prevented in the streptozotocin-diabetic rat by successful islet cell transplantation[182] and partially reversed in the human by long-term treatment with an ARI[187] link its development to hyperglycemia and the common mechanism.

In summary, evidence exists in animal models of a direct relationship between the common mechanism and the early, definable, predominantly reversible structural abnormalities in peripheral nerve. Further evidence has suggested a structural basis—axoglial dysjunction—for the appearance of irreversible decreases in NCV before the appearance of axonal atrophy characteristic of chronic diabetic neuropathy in animals and clinical neuropathy in humans and suggests a relationship of these lesions to the common mechanism. The pathogenetic basis for axonal loss remains undefined.

Evidence for Metabolic Abnormalities Related to Neurotrophism and Maintenance of Cellular Integrity

Numerous observations support the concept that there is an impairment in the capacity of the peripheral nervous system of diabetic animals to carry out the normal functions required for maintenance, repair, and regeneration. Since the exact mechanism underlying the axonal loss characteristic of diabetic neuropathy remains to be explained, it is tempting to speculate on the role of such abnormalities in its pathogenesis. However, these observations have not, in general, been organized under the rubric of any unifying hypothesis as to their etiology. Therefore, each must be discussed in the context in which it has been reported.

Evidence for Abnormalities in Axonal Transport and Protein Synthesis.
The role of the cell body in providing essential trophic functions for the nerve fibers has been recognized for nearly 150 years.[188] The synthesis of proteins, macromolecules, and organelles by the neuron occurs predominantly in the cell body (perikaryon), and the axon is dependent for its supply of these constituents on a process called axonal transport.[17,18] Three components of anterograde (central to peripheral, also called orthograde) axonal transport have been identified. The anterograde fast component (aFC; approximately 400 mm/day) involves predominantly endoplasmic reticulum and vesicles and the glycoproteins and enzymes associated with these organelles.[18] The slow component of anterograde transport has been divided into slow component a (SCa), consisting primarily of neurofilament polypeptides and the slowly moving component of tubulin (approximately 1 mm/day)[18]; and slow component b (SCb), which includes the rapidly moving component of tubulin as well as aldolase, pyruvate kinase, neuron-specific enolase, and creatine phosphokinase (approximately 4 mm/day).[18,189] Furthermore, a component of transport in the retrograde direction (retrograde fast component [rFC]; approximately 250 mm/day) has been identified, with molecular constituents similar to those of aFC, felt to represent secondary lysosomes.[18]

Conflicting results have been reported regarding the effect of diabetes on nearly every component of axonal transport. To a great degree, these contradictions can be accounted for by differences in experimental technique. Axonal transport is generally measured by following the movement of radioactive endogenous proteins labeled with pulses of radioactive precursors or by measuring the accumulation of specific endogenous enzyme activities (frequently choline acetyltransferase [CAT] or acetylcholinesterase [AcChE]) at the site of ligature or cold block. Retrograde transport may also be followed by labeling exogenous proteins. Difficulties with the enzyme technique noted include the observation that different isoforms of the same enzyme may be transported by different components and that the activity of a given enzyme, i.e., Na$^+$/K$^+$-ATPase, may be markedly different under different circumstances.[189] The estimation by isotopic techniques of amount of transport is complicated by the possibly differential effect of diabetes on rates of protein synthesis[190] and on the transport and therefore pool size of various amino acids,[191,192] as well as on the number and caliber of axons in a nerve fiber. In addition, delayed transport of individual molecular species within a given component might not be detected by this method.[193]

Observations have been made of defects in aFC related to diabetes.[194,195] Because aFC is extremely temperature sensitive,[196] these findings are probably the result of an artefact induced by inadvertent hypothermia of the nerve.[189] It is now generally agreed that diabetes is not associated with an abnormality in aFC.[189]

Abnormalities in the slow axonal transport have been consistently reported in experimental models of diabetes. Decreased velocity and quantity of SCa have been demonstrated in sensory and motor nerves of streptozotocin-diabetic rats[190,191,197,198] and in the motor nerves of db/db diabetic mice.[199] Slowing of specific components of SCb have been demonstrated in sciatic nerves of streptozotocin-diabetic rats[197,198] and in spontaneously diabetic BB rats.[193] Abnormalities in retrograde transport in streptozotocin-diabetic rats include a delay in turnaround from fast anterograde to retrograde transport[200] and in the retrograde transport of exogenous nerve growth factor (NGF).[201,202]

The significance of alterations in axonal transport for the pathogenesis of diabetic neuropathy remains unclarified. Several investigators have suggested that the decrease in transport of structural proteins associated with SCa, including neurofilaments and microtubular components, is responsible for the axonal atrophy characteristic of streptozotocin-induced diabetes.[189,191,193] (It should be remembered that streptozotocin-diabetic rats do not develop the fiber loss seen in diabetic neuropathy in BB rats and in humans.[35]) One group of investigators has specifically correlated changes in axonal caliber with retardation of slow axonal transport,[193] despite their observation that the retardation of transport of glycolytic enzymes associated with SCb is more impressive than the changes in SCa both in streptozotocin-diabetic[198] and in spontaneously diabetic BB rats,[193] and suggest that the decrease in axonal caliber is a direct consequence of the impaired transport of neurofilaments and microtubules.[203]

The metabolic basis of these alterations in axonal transport remains unknown. All of the defects are preventable or reversible with tight glycemic control with insulin.[194,200,201,204] The common mechanism (see Fig. 39–5) discussed above can be implicated by the observation that ARI therapy and dietary myoinositol supplementation can prevent or reverse the abnormality in CAT transport;[204] however, abnormalities in SCa were not prevented by these therapies.[205] Abnormalities in perikaryal protein synthesis have been reported in the retinas of diabetic rabbits[206] and in the dorsal root ganglia of streptozotocin-diabetic rats.[207] However, abnormalities in SCa and SCb in streptozotocin-diabetic and BB diabetic rats have been demonstrated in the absence of any defect in protein synthesis; it was therefore suggested that such a defect could not be the basis for these findings.[193,198] The same investigators found no evidence of nerve infarcts in their system,[193] and others have found that acute and chronic hypoxia did not induce abnormalities in the slow components of axonal transport.[208] It has been suggested that a selective impairment in transport might best be explained by the differential effects of nonenzymatic glycosylation on different proteins, but in the same report it was noted that there was no change in molecular weight or isoelectric point of the proteins involved in the abnormal transport,[193] although abnormalities have been reported in the polymerization of tubulin presumed to be related to glycosylation (see below).[209] Finally, it has been suggested that the abnormality in SCa is secondary to the loss of trophic function resulting from impaired retrograde transport of NGF and other neurotrophic factors,[189] although an explanation would still be required for the abnormality in retrograde transport.

Evidence for a Deficiency of Insulin or Other Neurotrophic Factors.

It has been suggested that decreased nerve-fiber size and a resultant decrease in NCV might be a consequence of insulin deficiency leading to growth retardation and thus to impaired nerve fiber maturation.[210,211] There are at least two lines of evidence suggesting that this is not the case. The first is the large body of evidence, discussed in detail above, that dietary myoinositol supplementation and ARI therapy can correct the abnormality in NCV without affecting insulin levels or body weight.[118,125,126] The second relates to the observation that when calorie-restricted rats, a situation in which plasma insulin levels are decreased, were compared with streptozotocin-diabetic rats, no comparable reduction in the size of myelinated fibers was noted.[212] It is therefore unlikely that alterations in growth related to insulin deficiency are the basis for alterations in NCV or size of myelinated fibers.

A key observation suggesting diminished neurotrophic function in experimental diabetes is that of the inhibition of fiber regeneration after nerve section in streptozotocin-diabetic rats.[213] A similar observation in galactose-fed rats[214] would suggest that this inhibition is not related to insulin deficiency and may be related to the polyol pathway. This contention is further supported by the observation of blunted regeneration in human diabetic patients that is corrected with 1 year of ARI therapy (see below).[187] The possibility that this effect is mediated through neurotrophic factors cannot be excluded. In one study, the serum of streptozotocin-diabetic rats was found to contain circulating inhibitors of somatomedin activity that were eliminated by continuous infusion of insulin.[215]

Evidence for a Role for Nonenzymatic Glycosylation.

Nonenzymatic glycosylation of proteins has been implicated as a potential pathogenetic mechanism in the vascular complications of diabetes.[216] Advanced glycosylation end-products (AGEs) have been identified in peripheral nerve myelin from diabetic patients.[217] Purified tubulin from rat brain, glycosylated nonenzymatically in vitro, forms insoluble aggregates that prevent normal polymerization, and tubulin monomers isolated from the brains of streptozotocin-diabetic rats form fewer polymers than those from control animals,[47] but the link between the two observations remains speculative. To date, there is no evidence of a deleterious effect of nonenzymatic glycosylation on neural function, and its role in the pathogenesis of neuropathy remains undefined.

Evidence for a Role for Gangliosides.

Gangliosides are a heterogeneous family of sphingolipid molecules found in most mammalian membranes and in particular abundance in neural tissue, where they are thought to be an important component of neurotransmitter receptors.[218] Defects in the catabolism of gangliosides are the basis for Tay-Sachs disease. There is no direct evidence for any alteration in ganglioside metabolism in diabetes. Despite this, experiments whose rationale is based on the apparent neurotrophic activity of gangliosides in a number of nondiabetic experimental systems[219,220] have shown that parenteral application of partially purified bovine brain gangliosides improve the defects in Na^+/K^+-ATPase activity,[221] NCV,[222] the axonal transport of 6-phosphofructokinase,[223] and nerve fiber diameter[224] in diabetic animals, although the group that reported the effects on Na^+/K^+-ATPase activity could show no effect on NCV[221] or the CAT component of axonal transport.[225] In some human trials, a small but significant improvement in NCV and a slight improvement in symptom scores have been found,[226-230] but in some others no improvement could be demonstrated.[231,232] The rational basis for any beneficial effect that might accrue remains to be elucidated.

Evidence for Involvement of Metabolic Mechanisms in the Pathogenesis of Human Diabetic Neuropathy

The plethora of information generated in experimental models regarding the adverse consequences of diabetes on peripheral nerve structure and function has produced insights into the pathogenesis of diabetic neuropathy that are relevant to human neuropathy. While it is true that rodents with short legs and that "do not smoke, drink beer, or develop atheroma" may not constitute a precise model for human diabetic neuropathy,[233] it is almost certainly equally true, as stated about experimental diabetic glomerulopathy, "If any therapeutic manoeuvre inhibits the initial stages in the development this is sufficient to warrant optimism about its long-term effect."[234] Nonetheless, a detailed understanding of the pathogenesis of axonal loss and segmental demyelination—the characteristic lesions of human diabetic neuropathy—has been elusive even with the diverse approaches available in the experimental models. Direct evaluations of human neuropathy are of necessity significantly more restricted. As a result, conclusions must be inferential and somewhat guarded.

Studies related to the pathogenesis of nephropathy in human diabetes have the decided advantage of numerous readily measured functional parameters that can be directly related to the natural history of the process as it is understood.[71,73] The same cannot be said of diabetic neuropathy, for which the accessibility of tissue is extremely limited and clinical parameters are indirect and the significance of each is controversial. Within the framework presented in Figure 39–1, by the time diabetic neuropathy has progressed to the point of clinical detectability, it is in some ways an end-stage process, representing a manifestation of widely distributed, presumably irreversible, axonal loss accompanied by segmental demyelination and remyelination.[26] Thus, improvements in clinical and physiologic measures of neuropathy must be based on reversal of functional impairments in the remaining nerve fibers in acute studies, as well as on the contribution to improved function made by regenerative fibers in chronic studies. It is not surprising that a variable but significant portion of this dysfunction is apparently irreversible with the therapies available to date. At the other end of the spectrum, although alterations in NCV and other electrophysiologic parameters represent a quantifiable measure of nerve dysfunction that may be related to a specific pathogenetic mechanism, decreased NCV is not equivalent to clinical neuropathy. No universally accepted parameters exist for the quantitative evaluation of the status of the peripheral nerve over the years and even decades during which the transition occurs from completely reversible nerve dysfunction to clinical neuropathy with axonal loss. As a result, our knowledge of the pathogenesis is indirect and must rely to a great degree on the evidence from experimental models discussed above.

Human studies concerned with the pathogenesis of diabetic neuropathy have generally addressed a few central issues. The evidence from human studies relating to vascular and hypoxic mechanisms in the pathogenesis of diabetic neuropathy has been discussed in detail above. The remaining literature can be divided into those studies that address the role of hyperglycemia and diabetic control in the pathogenesis of neuropathy, those studies concerned with the role of the polyol pathway and myoinositol metabolism in the pathogenesis of neuropathy, and those studies that have evaluated the efficacy of a number of agents for which the specific basis of their effects in the diabetic individual is less clearly defined. In the last case, clinical studies have addressed the efficacy of gangliosides (discussed in detail above), thiamine,[235] pyridoxine,[236] vitamin B_{12},[237] and isaxonine.[238] In each instance, the reported beneficial effects are limited or controversial,[238] and they do not provide insight into the specific mechanisms by which diabetes results in peripheral neuropathy.

Two major questions are addressed in human studies on the relationship between hyperglycemia and neuropathy. The first bears on the relationship between hyperglycemia and the development of neuropathy, addressed above in this chapter. The hypothesis that hyperglycemia is the etiologic agent in the pathogenesis of diabetic neuropathy[64] is supported by the following: 1) the information available from experimental diabetes; 2) the information regarding the risks for other complications; 3) the direct relationship between the duration and severity of hyperglycemia and the development of neuropathy in several large, retrospective studies[59,67,78]; and 4) the persistence of this relationship regardless of the diverse etiologies and treatments of hyperglycemia.[60,63] Although insulin deficiency or another metabolic derangement related to diabetes may contribute significantly to the pathogenesis or modify its course, no direct evidence suggests that any of these abnormalities is the primary pathogenetic factor.

The second question regards the relationship between improved glycemic control and neuropathy. In young, asymptomatic patients with Type I diabetes, progression of abnormalities in peripheral nerve electrophysiology and autonomic function tests has been related to poor glycemic control,[239] and, as noted above, the decreased NCV seen shortly after the onset of Type I diabetes in humans is reversible with tight glycemic control.[66,67] In untreated patients with Type II diabetes, NCV is inversely related to HbA_{1c} levels[240] and improves in proportion to improvement in this measure of control.[242] Numerous investigators have demonstrated improvements in NCV[241,243] and other electrophysiologic parameters[244] related to improved glycemic control in patients with Type I diabetes. The significance of these improvements in electrophysiologic parameters has been further substantiated by reports of symptomatic relief[245] and improvement in vibratory sense[246,247] related to improved glycemic control. Finally, improved glycemic control was reported to result in recovery from neuropathy and in weight gain in acute painful neuropathy with weight loss[29] and improvement in symptoms and NCV in chronic painful neuropathy.[248] Taken together, this information suggests that there are reversible components of peripheral nerve dysfunction related to hyperglycemia at nearly every stage in the development of clinical diabetic neuropathy and that progression of neuropathy can be prevented or retarded by tight glycemic control.

Although substantial evidence from clinical studies in humans relates diabetic neuropathy to the polyol pathway (through ARI therapy) and myoinositol metabolism, this topic still provokes considerable controversy. Most of the reports consist of short-term studies with small numbers of patients and incomplete outcome parameters. Large, multicenter, long-term, controlled trials of a number of ARIs are in progress but have not yet been reported. The earliest studies of ARI therapy in diabetic patients reported symptomatic improvement (but no objective response) in nine patients[249] and minor improvements in clinical and electrophysiologic parameters in 30 asymptomatic patients[250] treated with alrestatin; however, use of this drug has been discontinued because of its excess toxicity. Double-blind, placebo-controlled crossover studies of the drug sorbinil produced improvements in NCV in 39 patients after 2 months[251] that were similar in magnitude to those obtained with tight glycemic control[244]; improvement in pain, tendon reflexes, and nerve action potential amplitude, but not in NCV, in 15 patients after 1 month[252]; and improvements in autonomic function and electrophysiologic parameters after 6 months in 55 patients.[253] Some studies that reported a lack of efficacy of sorbinil have been criticized in regard to the advanced degree of neuropathy[254] or the advanced age of the patient population.[255] However, other, longer-term, studies have reported negative responses to this drug.[256,257] Preliminary reports on placebo-controlled trials with two newer drugs have demonstrated early (8 weeks)[258] and sustained (1 year)[259] improvement in subjective and objective parameters with tolrestat and long-term (2 years) improvement in subjective and objective parameters with the drug ONO-2235.[260] These studies suggest that at certain stages in the development of diabetic neuropathy, some components of peripheral nerve dysfunction can be related to increased activity of the polyol pathway.

Data from human therapeutic trials of dietary myoinositol supplementation, unlike that from trials of ARIs, are meager. The results have been disappointing as compared with those from animal trials, but a number of beneficial effects have been reported. A 2-week double-blind trial of myoinositol supplementation in seven patients showed improvements in nerve action potential but not in NCV.[261] A 4-month trial involving 20 patients showed clinical improvement and increased sensory NCV, but not motor NCV.[262] A double-blind, placebo-controlled study of four patients with painful neuropathy demonstrated improvements in clinical but not in electrophysiologic parameters.[263] However, a 6-month trial involving 30 patients and a 2-month trial with 14 patients revealed no effect on clinical or electrophysiologic parameters.[264,265] Levels of plasma myoinositol attained in all of these studies were significantly lower than the levels demonstrated to be effective in animal studies.[266] Appropriate doses have not been established, partly because of concerns raised from studies in diabetic rats[118] and uremic humans[267,268] that excessive levels of plasma myoinositol may be neurotoxic, and appropriate treatment intervals in established neuropathy are unknown.

Morphologic evidence of the effectiveness of ARIs in established diabetic neuropathy has been reported in one recent study.[187] In a placebo-controlled, double-blind, prospective clinical trial, data from quantitative morphometric and biochemical analysis of sural nerve biopsy specimens and selected clinical and electrophysiologic parameters were compared for 10 patients treated with sorbinil and 6 placebo-treated controls. Sorbinil treatment resulted in a fourfold increase in regenerating fibers, a 33% increase in fiber density, and a significant reduction in paranodal and segmental demyelination that was accompanied by modest but significant improvement in clinical and electrophysiologic parameters.[187] The changes were attributed to inhibition of the polyol pathway because a significant decrease in nerve sorbitol content was seen without any change being observed in nerve glucose or HbA$_{1c}$ levels.[187] Nerve myoinositol levels, which were initially decreased in diabetic patients as compared with levels in controls, returned toward normal levels in the treated group but continued to decline in the placebo group.[269] The study has been criticized because the repeat biopsy specimens were taken from the same side as the original specimens and because the significance of regeneration for clinical

improvement remains unknown.[270] However, these criticisms do not address the clinical improvements, the electrophysiologic improvements that were measured contralaterally, or the effects on demyelination.

The role of myoinositol metabolism in the pathogenesis of human diabetic neuropathy was challenged in the report of a study on human nerve biopsy specimens issued concurrently with the study discussed above. In this report, sural nerve biopsy specimens from diabetic patients with and without neuropathy (mean duration of diabetes, 14 years) and nondiabetic controls were evaluated for levels of glucose, fructose, sorbitol, and myoinositol, as well as for selected morphologic criteria.[271] The investigators found increased levels of endoneurial glucose and fructose in diabetic nerves and an inverse correlation between sorbitol levels and myelinated fiber density. They found no alteration in endoneurial myoinositol content in any of the groups analyzed.[271] The authors of the article and of an accompanying editorial conclude that myoinositol deficiency does not play a role in the pathogenesis of diabetic neuropathy.[270,271] This conclusion has been disputed on a number of grounds.[272,273] The decreases in nerve myoinositol content have been reported in acutely diabetic animals that did not have the characteristic neuropathology of chronic disease, and the significance of composite tissue content becomes obscured in a heterogeneous tissue as advancing pathologic developments alter the relative contributions of the individual cell types. This is particularly relevant in human neuropathy, where axonal loss is often accompanied by proliferation of Schwann cells and increased tissue levels of myoinositol.[274] Furthermore, the two studies have produced contradictory results regarding decrease in nerve myoinositol content,[269,271] although the latter has been criticized for its use of cadaveric organ donors as controls.[271] Finally, data regarding tissue myoinositol levels permit no conclusion about whether an alteration in myoinositol metabolism contributes to the pathogenesis of diabetic neuropathy.[273] As discussed in detail above, depletion of composite tissue myoinositol is not a part of the common mechanism by which hyperglycemia alters myoinositol metabolism and the regulation of Na$^+$/K$^+$-ATPase activity in the tissues that are the targets of the complications of diabetes (see Fig. 39–5).

The evidence from experimental models suggests that tight glycemic control, ARI therapy, and dietary myoinositol supplementation would all be most effective as primary prophylaxis rather than as secondary interventions. Long-term, prospective clinical trials of their prophylactic efficacy in new-onset, Type I diabetes are not likely to be undertaken. The available information does not permit the unqualified recommendation of any of these specific agents or therapies for clinical use. These studies do provide a body of evidence, when evaluated with the information available from experimental models, suggesting that hyperglycemia acting through increased activity of the polyol pathway and its effects on myoinositol metabolism is likely to be a primary mechanism in the pathogenesis of human diabetic neuropathy. The contribution of other metabolic mechanisms—impaired axonal transport, insulin and growth factor deficiency, nonenzymatic glycosylation, and altered ganglioside metabolism—to human neuropathy has been less extensively studied and remains to be defined.

SUMMARY

The details of the pathogenesis of the axonal loss and segmental demyelination and remyelination characteristic of clinically apparent human diabetic neuropathy are still unexplained. The morphologic evidence discussed would suggest that full-blown neuropathy can occur in the absence of any definable vascular lesion but that neuropathic lesions with a vascular basis are a frequent concomitant of diabetic neuropathy, especially in the older population. The information suggesting that diabetic neuropathy is predominantly a manifestation of chronic endoneurial hypoxia has been reviewed in detail, but most investigators now agree that diabetic neuropathy is most likely the prolonged consequence of metabolic derangements. Evidence that favors a common mechanism linking hyperglycemia, the polyol pathway, and alterations in myoinositol metabolism to the pathogenesis of neuropathy and the other complications of diabetes has been discussed in detail, and information regarding other potential metabolic mechanisms has also been presented.

REFERENCES

1. Thomas PK, Ochoa J. Microscopic anatomy of peripheral nerve fibers. In: Dyck PJ, Thomas PK, Lambert EH, Bunge R, eds. Peripheral neuropathy. 2nd ed. Vol 1. Philadelphia: WB Saunders, 1984:39–96.
2. Olsson Y. Vascular permeability in the peripheral nervous system. In: Dyck PJ, Thomas PK, Lambert EH, Bunge R, eds. Peripheral neuropathy. 2nd ed. Vol 1. Philadelphia: WB Saunders, 1984:579–97.
3. Stewart MA, Passonneau JV, Lowry OH. Substrate changes in peripheral nerve during ischaemia and Wallerian degeneration. J Neurochem 1965;12:719–27.
4. Korthals JK, Wisnieski HM. Peripheral nerve ischemia. I. Experimental model. J Neurol Sci 1975;24:65–76.
5. Dyck PJ, Conn DL, Okazaki H. Necrotizing angiopathic neuropathy: three-dimensional morphology of fiber degeneration related to sites of occluded vessels. Mayo Clin Proc 1972;47:472–5.
6. Nukada H, Dyck PJ. Acute ischemic injury causes axonal stasis swelling attenuation and secondary demyelination. Ann Neurol 1987;22:311–8.
7. Nukada H, Dyck PJ. Microsphere embolization of nerve capillaries and fiber degeneration. Am J Pathol 1984;115:275–87.
8. Dyck PJ. Hypoxic neuropathy: does hypoxia play a role in diabetic neuropathy? Neurology 1989;39:111–8.
9. Bischoff A, Thomas PK. Microscopic anatomy of myelinated nerve fibers. In: Dyck PJ, Thomas PK, Lambert EH, eds. Peripheral neuropathy. Vol 1. Philadelphia: WB Saunders, 1975:104.
10. Ochoa J. Microscopic anatomy of unmyelinated nerve fibers. In: Dyck PJ, Thomas PK, Lambert EH, eds. Peripheral neuropathy. Vol 1. Philadelphia: WB Saunders, 1975:131.
11. Alberts B, Bray D, Lewis J, et al. Molecular biology of the cell. New York: Garland Publishing Co, 1983.
12. Erecínska M, Wilson DF. Regulation of cellular energy metabolism. J Membr Biol 1982;70:1–14.
13. Winegrad AI, Simmons DA. Energy metabolism in peripheral nerve. In: Dyck PJ, Thomas PK, Asbury AK, et al. Diabetic neuropathy. Philadelphia: WB Saunders, 1987:279.
14. Yarowsky PJ Ingvar DH. Neuronal activity and energy metabolism. Fed Proc 1981;40:2353–62.
15. Jennings RB, Steenbergen C Jr. Nucleotide metabolism and cellular damage in myocardial ischemia. Annu Rev Physiol 1985;47:727–49.
16. Vary TC, Reibel DK, Neely JR. Control of energy metabolism of heart muscle. Annu Rev Physiol 1981;43;41–30.
17. Grafstein B, Forman DS. Intracellular transport in neurons. Physiol Rev 1980;60:1167–283.
18. Lasek RJ, Garner JA, Brady SI. Axonal transport of the cytoplasmic matrix. J Cell Biol 1984;99(1 pt 2):212S–21.
19. Greene DA, Winegrad AI. In vitro studies of the substrates for energy production and the effects of insulin on glucose utilization in the neural components of peripheral nerve. Diabetes 1979;28:878–87.
20. den Hertog A, Greengard P, Ritchie JM. On the metabolic basis of nervous activity. J Physiol (Lond) 1969;204:511–21.
21. Greene DA, Winegrad AI. Effects of acute experimental diabetes on composite energy metabolism in peripheral nerve axons and Schwann cells. Diabetes 1981;30:967–74.
22. Simmons DA, Winegrad AI, Martin DB. Significance of tissue *myo*-inositol concentrations in metabolic regulation in nerve. Science 1982;217:848–51.
23. Rang HP, Ritchie JM. On the electrogenic sodium pump in mammalian non-myelinated fibres and its activation by various external cations. J Physiol (Lond) 1968;1:183–221.
24. Hille B. Ionic channels of excitable membranes. Sunderland MA: Sinauer Associates, 1984.
25. Gardner E. Gross anatomy of the peripheral nervous system. In: Dyck PJ, Thomas PK, Lambert EH, eds. Peripheral neuropathy. Vol 1. Philadelphia: WB Saunders, 1975:9.
26. Thomas PK, Eliasson SG. Diabetic neuropathy. In: Dyck PJ, Thomas PK, Lambert EH, Bunger R, eds. Peripheral neuropathy. 2nd ed. Vol 2. Philadelphia: WB Saunders, 1984:1773–810.
27. Dyck PJ, Karnes JL, Daube J, et al. Clinical and neuropathological criteria for the diagnosis and staging of diabetic polyneuropathy. Brain 1985;108:861–80.
28. Brown MJ, Martin JR, Asbury AK. Painful diabetic neuropathy a morphometric study. Arch Neurol 1976;33:164–71.
29. Archer AG, Watkins PJ, Thomas PK, et al. The natural history of acute painful neuropathy in diabetes mellitus. J Neurol Neurosurg Psychiatry 1983;46:491–9.
30. Behse F, Buchthal F, Carlsen F. Nerve biopsy and conduction studies in diabetic neuropathy. J Neurol Neurosurg Psychiatry 1977;40:1072–82.
31. Sugimura K, Dyck PJ. Multifocal fiber loss in proximal sciatic nerve in symmetric distal diabetic neuropathy. J Neurol Sci 1982;53:501–9.
32. Johnson PC, Doll SC, Cromey DW. Pathogenesis of diabetic neuropathy. Ann Neurol 1987;19:450–7.
33. Said G, Slama G, Selva J. Progressive centripetal degeneration of axons in small fibre diabetic polyneuropathy: a clinical and pathological study. Brain 1983;106:791–807.

34. Dyck PJ, Karnes JL, O'Brien P, et al. The spatial distribution of fiber loss in diabetic polyneuropathy suggests ischemia. Ann Neurol 1986;19:440–9.

35. Sima AAF, Yagihashi S, Greene DA. Morphological features of human and animal diabetic nerve. In: Ward J, Goto Y, eds. Diabetic neuropathy. Chichester: John Wiley & Sons, 1990:17.

36. Asbury AK, Fields HL. Pain due to peripheral nerve damage a hypothesis. Neurology 1984;34:1587–90.

37. Dyck PJ, Sherman WR, Hallcher LM, et al. Human diabetic endoneurial sorbitol fructose and myo-inositol related to sural nerve morphometry. Ann Neurol 1980;85:90–6.

38. Dyck PJ, Lais A, Karnes JL, et al. Fiber loss is primary and multifocal in sural nerves in diabetic polyneuropathy. Ann Neurol 1986;19:425–39.

39. Yagihashi S, Matsunaga M. Ultrastructural pathology of peripheral nerves in patients with diabetic neuropathy. Tohoku J Exp Med 1979;129:357–66.

40. Sima AAF, Brismar T. Reversible diabetic nerve dysfunction structural correlates to electrophysiologic abnormalities. Ann Neurol 1985;18:21–9.

41. Greene DA, Chakrabarti S, Lattimer SA, Sima AAF. Role of sorbitol accumulation and myo-inositol depletion in paranodal swelling of large myelinated nerve fibers in the insulin deficient spontaneously diabetic Bio-breeding rat reversal by insulin replacement an aldose reductase inhibitor and myo-inositol. J Clin Invest 1987;79:1479–85.

42. Sima AAF, Nathaniel V, Bril V, et al. Histopathological heterogeneity of neuropathy in insulin-dependent and non-insulin-dependent diabetes and demonstration of axo-glial dysjunction in human diabetic neuropathy. J Clin Invest 1988;81:349–64.

43. Powell HC, Rosoff J, Myers RR. Microangiopathy in human diabetic neuropathy. Acta Neuropathol (Berl) 1985;68:295–305.

44. Malik RA, Newrick PG, Sharma AK, et al. Microangiopathy in human diabetic neuropathy: relationship between capillary abnormalities and the severity of neuropathy. Diabetologia 1989;32:92–102.

45. Timperley WR, Boulton AJM, Davies-Jones GAB, et al. Small vessel disease in progressive diabetic neuropathy associated with good metabolic control. J Clin Pathol 1985;38:1030–8.

46. Dyck PJ, Hansen S, Karnes J, et al. Capillary number and percentage closed in human diabetic sural nerve. Proc Natl Acad Sci USA 1985;82:2513–7.

47. Williams E, Timperly WR, Ward JD, Duckworth T. Electron microscopical studies of vessels in diabetic peripheral neuropathy. J Clin Pathol 1980;33:462–70.

48. Hensley GT, Soergel KH. Neuropathologic findings in diabetic diarrhea. Arch Pathol 1968;85:587–97.

49. Appenzeller O, Richardson EP Jr. The sympathetic chain in patients with diabetic and alcoholic and polyneuropathy. Neurology 1966;16:1205–9.

50. Appenzeller O, Ogin G. Myelinated fibres in human paravertebral sympathetic chain: white rami communicantes in alcoholic and diabetic patients. J Neurol Neurosurg Psychiatry 1974;37:1155–51.

51. Kristensson K, Nordborg C, Olsson Y, Sourander P. Changes in the vagus nerve in diabetes mellitus. Acta Pathol Microbiol Scand 1971;79A:684–5.

52. Faerman I, Glocer L, Celener D, et al. Autonomic nervous system and diabetes: histological and histochemical study of the autonomic nerve fibers of the urinary bladder in diabetic patients. Diabetes 1973;22:225–37.

53. Faerman I, Glocer L, Fox D, et al. Impotence and diabetes: histological studies of the autonomic nervous fibers of the corpora cavernosa in impotent diabetic males. Diabetes 1974;23:971–6.

54. Grover-Johnson NM, Baumann FG, et al. Abnormal innervation of lower limb epineurial arterioles in human diabetes. Diabetologia 1981;20:31–8.

55. Duchen LW, Anjorin A, Watkins PJ, Mackay JD. Pathology of autonomic neuropathy in diabetes mellitus. Ann Intern Med 1980;92:301–3.

56. Asbury AK, Aldredge H, Hershberg R, Fisher CM. Oculomotor palsy in diabetes mellitus a clinico-pathological study. Brain 1970;93:555–66.

57. Raff MC, Sangalang V, Asbury AK. Ischemic mononeuropathy multiplex associated with diabetes mellitus. Arch Neurol 1968;18:487–99.

58. Thomas PK. The pathogenesis of diabetic neuropathy: current problems and prospects. In: Ward J, Goto Y, eds. Diabetic neuropathy. Chichester: John Wiley & Sons, 1990:3.

59. Pirart J. Diabetes mellitus and its degenerative complications: a prospective study of 4400 patients observed between 1947 and 1973. Diabetes Care 1978;1:168.

60. Dymock IW, Cassar J, Pyke DA, et al. Observations on the pathogenesis complications and treatment of diabetes in 115 cases of haemochromatosis. Am J Med 1972;52:203–9.

61. Duncan LJP, Macfarlane A, Robson JS. Diabetic retinopathy and nephropathy in pancreatic diabetes. Lancet 1958;1:822–6.

62. Lukens FDW. Experimental diabetes and its relation to diabetes mellitus. Am J Med 1955;19:790–7.

63. Barbosa J, Saner B. Do genetic factors play a role in the pathogenesis of diabetic microangiopathy. Diabetologia 1984;27:487–92.

64. Winegrad AI. Does a common mechanism induce the diverse complications of diabetes? Diabetes 1987;36:396–406.

65. Feingold KR, Lee TH, Chung MY, Siperstein MD. Muscle capillary basement membrane width in patients with Vacor-induced diabetes mellitus. J Clin Invest 1986;78:102–7.

66. Ward JD, Barnes CG, Fisher DJ, Jessop JD. Improvement in nerve conduction following treatment in newly diagnosed diabetics. Lancet 1971;1:428–30.

67. Gregersen G. Diabetic neuropathy: influence of agesex metabolic control and duration of diabetes on motor conduction velocity. Neurology 1967;17:972–80.

68. Mogensen CE, Andersen MJF. Increased kidney size and glomerular filtration rate in untreated juvenile diabetes normalization by insulin treatment. Diabetologia 1975;11:221–4.

69. Krupin T, Waltman SR. Fluorophotometry in juvenile-onset diabetes long-term follow-up. Jpn J Ophthalmol 1985;29:139–45.

70. Cunha-Vaz J, Faria De Abreu JR, Campos AJ, Figo GM. Early breakdown of the blood-retinal barrier in diabetes. Br J Ophthalmol 1975;59:649–56.

71. Østerby R, Gundersen HJG, Hørlyck A, et al. Diabetic glomerulopathy: structural characteristics of the early and advanced stages. Diabetes 1983;32:79.

72. Kohner EM. Microangiopathy diabetic retinopathy. In: Crabbe MJC, ed. Diabetic complications. Edinburgh: Churchill Livingstone, 1987:41–65.

73. Mogensen CE. Management of diabetic renal involvement and disease. Lancet 1988;1:867–70.

74. Hørlyck A, Gundersen HJG, Østerby R. The cortical distribution pattern of diabetic glomerulopathy. Diabetologia 1986;29:146-50.

75. Kohner EM, McLeod D, Marshall J. Diabetic eye disease. In: Keen H, Jarrett, eds. Complications of diabetes. London: Edward Arnold,1982:19.

76. Pryce TD. On diabetic neuritis with a clinical and pathological description of three cases of diabetic pseudotabes. Brain 1893;16:416–24.

77. Woltman HW, Wilder RM. Diabetes mellitus: pathologic changes in the spinal cord and peripheral nerves. Arch Intern Med 1929;44:576–603.

78. Fagerberg SE. Diabetic neuropathy a clinical histological study on the significance of vascular affections. Acta Med Scand Suppl 1959;345:1–81.

79. Bischoff A. Die Ultrastruktur peripherer Nerven bei der diabetischen Neuropathie. Verh Dtsch Ges Inn Med 1967;72:1138–41.

80. Harriman D. Ischemic factor in diabetic neuropathy. In: Proceedings of the 4th International Congress on Neuropathology. Stuttgart: Theime, 1962;3:164.

81. Dolman CL. The morbid anatomy of diabetic neuropathy. Neurology 1963;13:135–42.

82. Vital C, Le Blanc M, Vallat JM, et al. Etude ultrastructurale du nerf périphérique chez 16 diabétiques sans neuropathie clinique: comparaisons avec 16 neuropathies diabétiques et 16 neuropathies non diabétiques. Acta Neuropathol (Berl) 1974;30:63–72.

83. Kilo C, Vogler N, Williamson JR. Muscle capillary basement membrane changes related to aging and to diabetes mellitus. Diabetes 1972;21:881–905.

84. Dunn PJ, Donald RA, Day T, et al. The association between diabetic retinopathy and skeletal muscle capillary basal lamina thickening corrected for the influence of age and duration of diabetes. Diabetes 2979;28:858–64.

85. Friederici HR, Tucker WR, Schwartz TB. Observations on small blood vessels of skin in the normal and in diabetic patients. Diabetes 1966;15:233–50.

86. Sosenko JM, Miettinen OS, Williamson JR, Gabbay KH. Muscle capillary basement-membrane thickness and long-term glycemia in type 1 diabetes mellitus. N Engl J Med 1984;311:694–8.

87. Greene DA, Sima AAF, Albers JW, Pfeifer MA. Diabetic Neuropathy. In: Rifkin H, Porte D Jr, eds. Ellenberg and Rifkin's diabetes mellitus: theory and practice. New York: Elsevier, 1990:710.

88. Llewelyn JG, Thomas PK, Gilbey SG, et al. Pattern of myelinated fibre loss in the sural nerve in neuropathy related to type 1 (insulin-dependent) diabetes. Diabetologia 1988;31:162–7.

89. Yasuda H, Dyck P. Abnormalities of endoneurial microvessels and sural nerve pathology in diabetic neuropathy. Neurology 1987;37:20–8.

90. Bradley J, Thomas PK, King RHM, et al. Morphometry of endoneurial capillaries in diabetic sensory and autonomic neuropathy. Diabetologia 1990;33:611–8.

91. King RHM, Llewelyn JG, Thomas PK, et al. Diabetic neuropathy abnormalities of Schwann cell and perineurial basal laminae. Implications for diabetic vasculopathy. Neuropathol Appl Neurobiol 1989;15:339–55.

92. Rechtland E, Smith QR, Latker CH, Rapoport SI. Altered blood-nerve barrier permeability to small molecules in experimental diabetes mellitus. J Neuropathol Exp Neurol 1987;46:302–14.

93. Korthals JK, Gieron MA, Dyck PJ. Intima of epineurial arterioles is increased in diabetic polyneuropathy. Neurology 1988;38:1582–6.

94. Low PA. Recent advances in the pathogenesis of diabetic neuropathy. Muscle Nerve 1987;10:121–8.

95. Low PA, Tuck RR, Takguchi M. Nerve microenvironment in diabetic neuropathy. In: Dyck PJ, Thomas PK, Asbury AK, et al. Diabetic neuropathy. Philadelphia: WB Saunders, 1987:266–78.

96. Tuck RR, Schmelzer JD, Low PA. Endoneurial blood flow and oxygen tension in the sciatic nerves of rats with experimental diabetic neuropathy. Brain 1984;107:935–50.

97. Greene DA, Lattimer SA. Impaired energy utilization and Na-K-ATPase in diabetic peripheral nerve. Am J Physiol 1984;246:E311–8.

98. Low PA, Tuck RR. Effects of changes of blood pressure respiratory acidosis and hypoxia on blood flow in the sciatic nerve of the rat. J Physiol (Lond) 1984;347:513–24.

99. Low PA, Ward K, Schmelzer JD, Brimijoin S. Ischemic conduction failure and energy metabolism in experimental diabetic neuropathy. Am J Physiol 1985;248:E457–62.

100. Newrick PG, Wilson AJ, Jakubowski J, et al. Sural nerve oxygen tension in diabetes. BMJ 1986;293:1053–4.

101. Flynn MD, Edmonds ME, Tooke JE, Watkins PJ. Direct measurement of capillary blood flow in the diabetic neuropathic foot. Diabetologia 1988;31:652–6.

102. Gaylarde PM, Fonseca VA, Llewellyn G. et al. Transcutaneous oxygen tension in legs and feet of diabetic patients. Diabetes 1988;37:714–6.

103. Winegrad AI, Simmons DA. Biochemical mechanisms for peripheral nerve disease in diabetics. In: Ward J, Goto Y, eds. Diabetic neuropathy. Chichester: John Wiley & Sons, 1990:123.

104. Low PA. Vascular and hypoxic factors in chronic experimental and human diabetic neuropathy. In: Ward J, Goto Y, eds. Diabetic neuropathy. Chichester: John Wiley & Sons, 1990:199.

105. Nukada H, Dyck PJ, Low PA, et al. Axonal caliber and neurofilaments are proportionally decreased in galactose neuropathy. J Neuropath Exp Neurol 1986;45:140–50.

106. Seneviratne KN, Peiris OA. The effect of ischaemia on the excitability of human sensory nerve. J Neurol Neurosurg Psychiatry 1968;31:338–47.

107. Caruso G, Labianca O, Ferrannini E. Effect of ischaemia on sensory potentials of normal subjects of different ages. J Neurol Neurosurg Psychiatry 1973;36:455–66.

108. Low PA, Schmelzer JD, Ward KK, et al. Effects of hyperbaric oxygenation on normal and chronic streptozotocin diabetic peripheral nerves. Exp Neurol 1988; 99:201–12.

109. Low PA, Schmelzer JD, Ward KK, Yao JK. Experimental chronic hypoxic neuropathy relevance to diabetic neuropathy. Am J Physiol 1986;250:E94–9.

110. Low PA, Tuck RR, Dyck PJ, et al. Prevention of some electrophysiologic and biochemical abnormalities with oxygen supplementation in experimental diabetic neuropathy. Proc Natl Acad Sci USA 1984;81:6894–8.

111. Masson EA, Church SE, Woodcock AA, et al. Is resistance to ischaemic conduction failure induced by hypoxia? Diabetologia 1988;31:762–5.

112. Shirabe S, Kinoshita I, Matsuo H, et al. Resistance to ischemic conduction block of the peripheral nerve in hyperglycemic rats: an electrophysiological study. Muscle Nerve 1988;11:582–7.

113. Faden A, Mendoza E, Flynn F. Subclinical neuropathy associated with chronic obstructive pulmonary disease: possible pathophysiologic role of smoking. Arch Neurol 1981;38:639–42.

114. Appenzeller O, Parks RD, MacGee J. Peripheral neuropathy in chronic disease of the respiratory tract. Am J Med 1968;44:873–80.

115. Malik RA, Masson EA, Sharma AK, et al. Hypoxic neuropathy: relevance to human diabetic neuropathy. Diabetologia 1990;33:311–8.

116. Thomas PK. Symptomatology and differential diagnosis of peripheral neuropathy: clinical features and diagnosis. In: Dyck PJ, Thomas PK, Lambert EH, eds. Peripheral neuropathy. Vol 1. Philadelphia: WB Saunders, 1975:39.

117. Sima AAF. The development and structural characterization of the neuropathies in the spontaneously diabetic BB Wistar rat. Metabolism 1983;32(Suppl 1):106–11.

118. Greene DA, De Jesus PV, Winegrad AI. Effects of insulin and dietary myoinositol on impaired peripheral motor nerve conduction velocity in acute streptozotocin diabetes. J Clin Invest 1975;55:1326–36.

119. Kaufmann F, Lacoste C. Vitreous fluorescein accumulation determined by in vivo fluorophotometry and by vitreous extraction in normal and diabetic rats. Diabetologia 1986;29:175–80.

120. Krupin T, Waltman SR, Scharp DW, et al. Ocular fluorophotometry in streptozotocin diabetes mellitus in the rat: effect of pancreatic islet isografts. Invest Ophthalmol Vis Sci 1979;18:1185–90.

121. Seyer-Hansen K. Renal hypertrophy in experimental diabetes mellitus. Kidney Int 1983;23:643–6.

122. Das PK, Bray GM, Aguayo AJ, Rasminsky M. Diminished ouabain sensitive sodium-potassium ATPase activity in sciatic nerves of rats with streptozotocin-induced diabetes. Exp Neurol 1976;53:285–8.

123. Cohen MP. Aldose reductase glomerular metabolism and diabetic nephropathy. Metabolism 1986;35(Suppl 1):55–9.

124. MacGregor LC, Matschinsky FM. Experimental diabetes mellitus impairs the function of the retinal pigmented epithelium. Metabolism 1986;34(Suppl 1):28–34.

125. Yue DK, Hanwell MA, Satchell PM, Turtle JR. The effect of aldose reductase inhibition on motor nerve conduction velocity in diabetic rats. Diabetes 1982;31:789–94.

126. Gillon KRW, Hawthorne JN, Tomlinson DR. myo-Inositol and sorbitol metabolism in relation to peripheral nerve function in experimental diabetes in the rat: the effect of aldose reductase inhibition. Diabetologia 1983;25:365–71.

127. Goldfarb S, Ziyadeh FN, Kern EFO, Simmons DA. The effects of polyol pathway inhibition and dietary myo-inositol on glomerular hemodynamic function in experimental diabetes mellitus in the rat. Diabetes 1991;40:465–71.

128. Pugliese G, Tilton RG, Speedy A, et al. Modulation of hemodynamic and vascular filtration changes in diabetic rats by dietary myo-inositol. Diabetes 1990;39:312–22.

129. Brismar T, Sima AAF. Changes in nodal function in nerve fibers of the spontaneously diabetic BB-Wistar rat: potential clamp analysis. Acta Physiol Scand 1981;113:499–506.

130. Greene DA, Lattimer SA. Impaired rat sciatic nerve sodium potassium adenosine triphosphatase in acute streptozocin diabetes and its correction by dietary myo-inositol supplementation. J Clin Invest 1983;72:1058–63.

131. Gillon KRW, Hawthorne JN. Sorbitol inositol and nerve conduction in diabetes. Life Sci 1983;32:1943–7.

132. Stewart MA, Sherman WR, Kurien MM, et al. Polyol accumulations in nervous tissue of rats with experimental diabetes and galactosaemia. J Neurochem 1967;14:1057–66.

133. Winegrad AI, Clements RS, Morrison AD. Insulin-independent pathways of carbohydrate metabolism. In: Steiner DF, Freinkel N, eds. Handbook of physiology. Section 7.

Endocrinology. Vol 1. Washington, DC: American Physiological Society, 1972:457–71.

134. Morrison AD, Clements RS Jr, Travis SB, et al. Glucose utilization by the polyol pathway in human erythrocytes. Biochem Biophys Res Commun 1970;40:199–205.

135. González RG, Barnett P, Aguayo J, et al. Direct measurement of polyol pathway activity in the ocular lens. Diabetes 1984;33:196–9.

136. Mayer JH, Tomlinson DR. The influence of aldose reductase inhibition and nerve myo-inositol on axonal transport and nerve conduction velocity in rats with experimental diabetes. J Physiol 1983;340:25p–6p.

137. Clements RS Jr, Reynertson R. Myoinositol metabolism in diabetes mellitus: effect of insulin treatment. Diabetes 1977;26:215–21.

138. Dawson RMC, Freinkel N. The distribution of free meso-inositol in mammalian tissues, including some observations of the lactating rat. Biochem J 1961;78:606–10.

139. Sherman WR, Stewart MA, Kurien MM, Goodwin SL. The measurement of myo-inositol, myo-inosose-2, and scyllo-inositol in mammalian tissues. Biochim Biophys Acta 1968;158:197–205.

140. Sherman WR, Packman PM, Laird MH, Boshans RL. Measurement of myo-inositol in single cells and defined areas of the nervous system by selected ion monitoring. Anal Biochem 1977;78:119–31.

141. Clements RS Jr, Diethelm AG. The metabolism of myo-inositol by the human kidney. J Lab Clin Med 1979;93:210–9.

142. Burton LE, Wells WW. Studies on the developmental pattern of the enzymes converting glucose-6-phosphate to myo-inositol in the rat. Dev Biol 1974;37:35–42.

143. Chen CH-J, Eisenberg F Jr. Myoinosose-2-1-phosphate an intermediate in the myoinositol-1-phosphate synthase reaction. J Biol Chem 1975;250:2963–7.

144. Sherman WR, Munsell LY, Gish BG, Honchar MP. Effects of systemically administered lithium on phosphoinositide metabolism in rat brain kidney and testes. J Neurochem 1985;44:798–807.

145. Caspary WF, Crane RK. Active transport of myo-inositol and its relation to the sugar transport system in hamster small intestine. Biochim Biophys Acta 1970;203:308–16.

146. Takenawa T, Tsumita T. myo-inositol transport in plasma membrane of rat kidney. Biochim Biophys Acta 1974;373:106–14.

147. Spector R. Cyclohexitol transport in the central nervous system. In: Wells WW, Eisenberg F Jr, eds. Cyclitols and phosphoinositides. New York: Academic Press, 1978:499–506.

148. Greene DA, Lattimer SA. Sodium- and energy-dependent uptake of myo-inositol by rabbit peripheral nerve: competitive inhibition by glucose and lack of insulin effect. J Clin Invest 1982:70:1009–18.

149. Greene DA, Lattimer SA. Altered myo-inositol metabolism in diabetic nerve. In: Dyck PJ, Thomas PK, Asbury AI, et al. eds. Diabetic neuropathy. Philadelphia: WB Saunders, 1987:289.

150. Berridge MJ. Inositol trisphosphate and diacylglycerol two interacting second messengers. Annu Rev Biochem 1987;56:159–93.

151. Hokin LE. Receptors and phosphoinositide-generated second messengers. Annu Rev Biochem 1985;54:205–35.

152. Greene DA, Lattimer SA. Action of sorbinil in diabetic peripheral nerve: relationship of polyol (sorbitol) pathway inhibition to a myo-inositol mediated defect in sodium- potassium ATPase activity. Diabetes 1984;33:712–6.

153. Winegrad AI, Simmons DA, Martin DB. Has one diabetic complication been explained? [Editorial]. N Engl J Med 1983;308:152–4.

154. Greene DA, Lattimer SA, Sima AAF. Sorbitol phosphoinositides and sodium-potassium-ATPase in the pathogenesis of diabetic complications. N Engl J Med 1987;316:599–606.

155. Finegold D, Lattimer S, Nolle S, et al. Polyol pathway activity and *myo*-inositol metabolism: a suggested relationship in the pathogenesis of diabetic neuropathy. Diabetes 1983;32:988–92.

156. Cohen MP. Effects of experimental diabetes and aldose reductase inhibitors on glomerular phosphoinositide metabolism. In: Proceedings of the 3rd International Symposium on Diabetes Mellitus. Amsterdam: Elsevier, 1989.

157. Greene DA, Mackaway AM. Decreased *myo*-inositol content and Na$^+$-K$^+$-ATPase activity in superior cervical ganglion of STZ-diabetic rat and prevention by aldose reductase inhibition. Diabetes 1986;35:1106–8.

158. Llewelyn JG, Simpson CM, Thomas PK, et al. Changes in sorbitol *myo*-inositol and lipid inositol in dorsal root sympathetic ganglia from streptozotocin-diabetic rats. Diabetologia 1986;29:876–81.

159. Cameron NE, Leonard MB, Ross IS, Whiting PH. The effects of sorbinil on peripheral nerve conduction velocity polyol concentrations and morphology in the streptozotocin-diabetic rat. Diabetologia 1986;29:168–74.

160. Loy A, Lurie KG, Ghosh A, et al. Diabetes and the *myo*-inositol paradox. Diabetes 1990;39:1305–12.

161. Simmons DA, Kern EFO, Winegrad AI, Martin DB. Basal phosphatidylinositol turnover controls aortic Na$^+$/K$^+$ ATPase activity. J Clin Invest 1986;77:503–13.

162. Simmons DA, Winegrad AI. Mechanism of glucose-induced (Na$^+$K$^+$)-ATPase inhibition in aortic wall of rabbits. Diabetologia 1989;32:402–8.

163. Simmons DA, Winegrad AI. Elevated extracellular fluid glucose inhibits an adenosine-(Na$^+$K$^+$)-ATPase regulatory system in rabbit aortic wall. Diabetologia 1991;34:157–63.

164. Imai A, Gershengorn MC. Independent phosphatidylinositol synthesis in pituitary plasma membrane and endoplasmic reticulum. Nature 1987;325:726–8.

165. Morrison AD, Orci L, Perrelet A, Winegrad AI. Studies of the effects of an elevated glucose concentration on the ultrastructure and composite metabolism of the intact rabbit aortic intima-media preparation. Diabetes 1979;28:720–3.

166. Brown MJ, Iwamori M, Kishimoto Y, et al. Nerve lipid abnormalities in human diabetic neuropathy: a correlative study. Ann Neurol 1979;5:245–52.

167. Mayhew JA, Gillon KRW, Hawthorne JN. Free and lipid inositol sorbitol and sugars in sciatic nerve obtained post-mortem from diabetic patients and control subjects. Diabetologia 1983;24:13–5.

168. Palmano KP, Whiting PH, Hawthorne JN. Free and lipid *myo*-inositol in tissues from rats with acute and less severe streptozotocin-induced diabetes. Biochem J 1977;167:229–35.

169. Hawthorne JN, Smith EM, Gillon KRW, Millar FA. Inositol sorbitol and diabetic neuropathy. In: Bleasedale JE, Eichberg J, Hauser G, eds. Inositol and phosphoinositides metabolism and regulation. Clifton, NJ: Humana Press, 1985:551.

170. Natarajan V, Dyck PJ, Schmid HHO. Alterations of inositol lipid metabolism of rat sciatic nerve in streptozotocin induced diabetes. J Neurochem 1981;36:413–9.

171. Hothersall JS, McLean P. Effects of experimental diabetes and insulin on phosphatidylinositol synthesis in rat sciatic nerve. Biochem Biophys Res Commun 1979;88:477–84.

172. Bell ME, Eichberg J. Decreased incorporation of [^{3}H]inositol and [^{3}H]glycerol into glycerolipids of sciatic nerve from the streptozotocin-diabetic rat. J Neurochem 1985;45:465–9.

173. Bell ME, Peterson RG, Eichberg J. Metabolism of phospholipids in peripheral nerve from rats with chronic streptozotocin-induced diabetes: increased turnover of phosphatidylinositol-45-bisphosphate. J Neurochem 1982;39:192–200.

174. Berti-Mattera L, Peterson R, Bell M, Eichberg J. The effects of hyperglycemia and its prevention by insulin treatment on the incorporation of ^{32}P into polyphosphoinositides and other phospholipids in peripheral nerve of the streptozotocin diabetic rat. J Neurochem 1985;45:1692–8.

175. Zhu X, Eichberg J. 12-diacylglycerol content and its arachidonyl-containing molecular species are reduced in sciatic nerve from streptozotocin-induced diabetic rats. J Neurochem 1990;55:1087–90.

176. Lattimer SA, Sima AAF, Greene DA. In vitro correction of impaired (Na$^+$K$^+$)-ATPase in diabetic nerve by protein kinase C agonists. Am J Physiol 1989;256:E264–9.

177. Kyte J. Molecular considerations relevant to the mechanism of active transport. Nature 1981;292:201–4.

178. Greene DA, Lattimer SA, Carroll PB, et al. A defect in sodium-dependent amino acid uptake in diabetic rabbit peripheral nerve: correction by an aldose reductase inhibitor or *myo*-inositol administration. J Clin Invest 1990;85:1657–65.

179. Carafoli E. Intracellular calcium homeostasis. Annu Rev Biochem 1987;56:395–434.

180. Fukuma M, Carpentier J-L, Orci L, et al. An alteration in internodal myelin membrane structure in large sciatic nerve fibres in rats with acute streptozotocin diabetes and impaired nerve conduction velocity. Diabetologia 1978;15:65–72.

181. Pinto da Silva P, Miller RG. Membrane particles on fracture faces of frozen myelin. Proc Natl Acad Sci USA 1975;72:4046–50.

182. Sima AAF, Zhang W-X, Tze WJ, et al. Diabetic neuropathy in STZ-induced diabetic rat and effect of allogenic islet cell transplantation: morphometric analysis. Diabetes 1988;37:1129–36.

183. Gabbay KH. The sorbitol pathway and the complications of diabetes. N Engl J Med 1973;288:831–6.

184. Cogan DG (moderator), Kinoshita JH, et al. (discussants). Aldose reductase and complications of diabetes. Ann Intern Med 1984;101:82–91.

185. Brismar T, Sima AAF, Greene DA. Reversible and irreversible nodal dysfunction in diabetic neuropathy. Ann Neurol 1987;21:504–7.

186. Sima AAF, Lattimer SA, Yagihashi S, Greene DA. Axo-glial dysjunction: a novel structural lesion that accounts for poorly reversible slowing of nerve conduction in the spontaneously diabetic bio-breeding rat. J Clin Invest 1986;77:474–84.

187. Sima AAF, Bril V, Nathaniel V, et al. Regeneration and repair of myelinated fibers in sural-nerve biopsy specimens from patients with diabetic neuropathy treated with sorbinil. N Engl J Med 1988;319:548–55.

188. Waller AV. Sur la reproduction des nerfs et sur la structure et les fonctions des ganglions spinaux. Arch Anat Physiol Wissench Med (Berl) 1852;392–401.

189. Sidenius P, Jakobsen J. Axonal transport in human and experimental diabetes. In: Dyck PJ, Thomas PK, Asbury AK, et al, eds. Diabetic neuropathy. Philadelphia: WB Saunders, 1987:260.

190. Sidenius P, Jakobsen J. Reversibility and preventability of the decrease in slow axonal transport velocity in experimental diabetes. Diabetes 1982;31:689–93.

191. Jakobsen J, Sidenius P. Decreased axonal transport of structural proteins in streptozotocin diabetic rats. J Clin Invest 1980;66:292–7.

192. Sidenius P, Jakobsen J. Axonal transport in early experimental diabetes. Brain Res 1979;173:315–30.

193. Medori R, Jenich H, Autilio-Gambetti L, Gambetti P. Experimental diabetic neuropathy: similar changes of slow axonal transport and axonal size in different animal models. J Neurosci 1988;8:1814–21.

194. Mendell JR, Sahenk Z, Warmolts JR, et al. The spontaneously diabetic BB Wistar rat: morphologic and physiologic studies of peripheral nerve. J Neurol Sci 1981;52:103–15.

195. Meiri KF, McLean WG. Axonal transport of protein in motor fibres of experimentally diabetic rats—fast anterograde transport. Brain Res 1982:238:77–88.

196. Whiteley SJ, Townsend J, Tomlinson DR, Brown AM. Fast orthograde axonal transport in sciatic motoneurones and nerve temperature in streptozotocin-diabetic rats. Diabetologia 1985;28:847–51.

197. Mayer JH, Tomlinson DR, McLean WG. Slow orthograde axonal transport of radiolabelled protein in sciatic motoneurones of rats with short-term experimental diabetes: effects of treatment with an aldose reductase inhibitor or myo-inositol. J Neurochem 1984;43:1265–70.

198. Medori R, Autilio-Gambetti L, Monaco S, Gambetti P. Experimental diabetic neuropathy: impairment of slow transport with changes in axon cross-sectional area. Proc Natl Acad Sci USA 1985;82:7716–20.

199. Vitadello M, Filliatreau G, Dupont JL, et al. Altered axonal transport of cytoskeletal proteins in the mutant diabetic mouse. J Neurochem 1985;45:860–8.

200. Sidenius P, Jakobsen J. Impaired retrograde axonal transport from a nerve crush in streptozotocin-diabetic rats. Diabetologia 1980;19:222–8.

201. Jakobsen J, Brimijoin S, Skau K, et al. Retrograde axonal transport of transmitter enzymes fucose-labeled protein and nerve growth factor in streptozotocin-diabetic rats. Diabetes 1981;30:797–803.

202. Schmidt RE, Modert CW, Yip HK, Johnson EM. Retrograde axonal transport in intravenously administered ^{125}I-nerve growth factor in rats with streptozotocin-induced diabetes. Diabetes 1983;32:654–63.

203. Medori R, Autilio-Gambetti L, Jenich H, Gambetti P. Changes in axon size and slow axonal transport are related in experimental diabetic neuropathy. Neurology 1988;38:597–601.

204. Mayer JH, Tomlinson DR. Prevention of defects of axonal transport and nerve conduction velocity by oral administration of myo-inositol or an aldose reductase inhibitor in streptozotocin diabetic rats. Diabetologia 1983;25:433–8.

205. Tomlinson DR, Sidenius P, Larsen JR. Slow component a of axonal transport nerve myo-inositol and aldose reductase inhibition in streptozocin-diabetic rats. Diabetes 1986;35:398–402.

206. Chihara E, Sakugawa M, Entani S. Reduced protein synthesis in diabetic retina and secondary reduction of slow axonal transport. Brain Res 1982;250:363–6.

207. Thomas PK, Wright DW, Tzebelikos E. Amino acid uptake by dorsal root ganglia from streptozotocin-diabetic rats. J Neurol Neurosurg Psychiatry 1984;47:912–6.

208. Nagata H, Brimijoin S, Low P, Schmelzer JD. Slow axonal transport in experimental hypoxia and in neuropathy induced by p-bromophenylacetylurea. Brain Res 1987;422:319–26.

209. Williams SK, Howarth NL, Devenny JJ, Bitensky MW. Structural and functional consequences of increased tubulin glycosylation in diabetes mellitus. Proc Natl Acad Sci USA 1982;79:6546–50.

210. Sharma AK, Thomas PK, DeMolina AF. Peripheral nerve fiber size in experimental diabetes. Diabetes 1977;26:689–92.

211. Sharma AK, Bajada S, Thomas PK. Influence of streptozotocin-induced diabetes on myelinated nerve fiber maturation and on body growth in the rat. Acta Neuropathol (Berl) 1981;53:257–65.

212. Jakobsen J. Axonal dwindling in early experimental diabetes. I. A study of cross-sectioned nerves. Diabetologia 1976;12:539–46.

213. Longo FM, Powell HC, Lebeau J, et al. Delayed nerve regeneration in streptozotocin diabetic rats. Muscle Nerve 1986;9:385–93.

214. Powell HC, Longo FM, LeBeau JM, Myers RR. Abnormal nerve regeneration in galactose neuropathy. J Neuropathol Exp Neurol 1986;45:151–60.

215. Taylor AM, Sharma AK, Avasthy N, et al. Inhibition of somatomedin-like activity by serum from streptozotocin-diabetic rats prevention by insulin treatment and correlation with skeletal growth. Endocrinology 1987;121:1360–5.

216. Brownlee M, Cerami A, Vlassara H. Advanced products of non-enzymatic glycosylation and the pathogenesis of diabetic vascular disease. Diabetes Metab Rev 1988;4:437–51.

217. Vlassara H, Brownlee M, Cerami A. Nonenzymatic glycosylation of peripheral nerve protein in diabetes mellitus. Proc Natl Acad Sci USA 1981;78:5190–2.

218. Lehninger AI. Lipids and membranes. In: Principles of Biochemistry. New York: Worth Publishers, 1982:303–30.

219. Gorio A, Aporti F, Norido F. Axon sprouting stimulated by gangliosides A new model for elongation and sprouting. In: Rappoport MM, Gorio A, eds. Gangliosides in neurological and neuromuscular function development and repair. New York: Raven Press, 1981.

220. Dimpfel W, Moller W, Mengs U. Ganglioside-induced neurite formation in cultured neuroblastoma cells. In: Rappoport MM, Gorio A, eds. Gangliosides in neurological and neuromuscular function development and repair. New York: Raven Press, 1981.

221. Calcutt NA, Tomlinson DR, Willars GB. Ganglioside treatment of diabetic rats; effects on nerve adenosine triphosphatase activity and motor nerve conduction velocity. Life Sci 1988;42:1515–20.

222. Spuler M, Dimpfel W, Tullner H-U. Effects of gangliosides on nerve conduction velocity during diabetic neuropathy in the rat. Arch Int Pharmacodynam Ther 1987;287:211–26.

223. Calcutt NA, Tomlinson DR, Willars GB. Ganglioside treatment of streptozotocin-diabetic rats prevents defective axonal transport of 6-phosphofructokinase activity. J Neurochem 1988;50:1478–83.

224. Norido F, Canella R, Gorio A. Ganglioside treatment of neuropathy in diabetic mice. Muscle Nerve 1982;5:107–10.

225. Tomlinson DR, Calcutt N, Robinson JP, Willars GB. Axonal transport and nerve conduction in experimental diabetes. In: Shafrir E, Reynold AE, eds. Frontiers in diabetes

research: lessons from animal diabetes II. London: John Libbey, 1988:482–7.

226. Pozza G, Saibene V, Comi G, et al. The effect of ganglioside administration in human diabetic peripheral neuropathy. In: Rappoport MM, Gorio A, eds. Gangliosides in neurological and neuromuscular function: development and repair. New York: Raven Press, 1981.

227. Bassi S, Albizzatti E, Calloni E, Frattola L. Electromyographic study of diabetic and alcoholic polyneuropathic patients treated with gangliosides. Muscle Nerve 1982; 5:351–6.

228. Fedele D, Crepaldi G, Battistin L. Multicentre trial on gangliosides in diabetic peripheral neuropathy. Adv Exp Med Biol 1984;174:601–6.

229. Horowitz SH. Ganglioside (Cronassial) therapy in diabetic neuropathy. Adv Exp Med Biol 1984;174:593–600.

230. Naarden A, Davidson J, Harris L, et al. Treatment of painful diabetic polyneuropathy with mixed gangliosides. Adv Exp Med Biol 1984;174:581–92.

231. Hallett M, Flood T, Slater N, Dambrosia J. Trial of ganglioside therapy for diabetic neuropathy. Muscle Nerve 1987;10:822–5.

232. Abraham RR, Abraham RM, Wynn V. A double-blind placebo controlled trial of mixed gangliosides in diabetic peripheral and autonomic neuropathy. Adv Exp Med Biol 1984; 174:60–24.

233. Tomlinson DR. General discussion (Chapter VIII). In: Sharir E, Reynold, eds. Frontiers in diabetes research: lessons from animal diabetes II. London: John Libbey, 1988: 549.

234. Østerby R. Glomerular structural abnormalities in early and late stages of experimental diabetes models for diabetic nephropathy? In: Shafrir E, Reynold AE, eds. Frontiers in diabetes research: lessons from animal diabetes II. London: John Libbey, 1988:522–7.

235. Thompson RHS. Biochemical aspects of diabetic neuropathy. In: Cummings JN, Kremer M, eds. Biochemical aspects of neurological disorders. 2nd Series. Oxford: Blackwell, 1965.

236. McCann VJ, Davis RE. Pyridoxine and diabetic neuropathy a double-blind controlled study [Letter]. Diabetes Care 1983;6:102–3.

237. Yamada K, Goto Y, Takebe K. Treatment of diabetic peripheral neuropathy with methylcobalamin. In: Goto Y, Horiuchi A, Kogure K, eds. Diabetic neuropathy. Amsterdam: Excerpta Medica, 1982:336–40.

238. Le Quesne PM. Trophic factors and vitamin therapy. In: Dyck PJ, Thomas PK, Asbury AK, et al. Diabetic neuropathy. Philadelphia: WB Saunders, 1987:194.

239. Young RJ, Macintyre CCA, Martyn CN, et al. Progression of subclinical polyneuropathy in young patients with Type 1 (insulin-dependent) diabetes: associations with glycaemic control and microangiopathy (microvascular complications). Diabetologia 1986;29:156–61.

240. Graf RJ, Halter JB, Halar E, Porte D Jr. Nerve conduction abnormalities in untreated maturity-onset diabetes: relation to levels of fasting plasma glucose and glycosylated hemoglobin. Ann Intern Med 1979;90:298–303.

241. Graf RJ, Halter JB, Pfeifer MA, et al. Glycemic control and nerve conduction abnormalities in noninsulin-dependent diabetic subjects. Ann Intern Med 1981;94:307–11.

242. Pietri A, Ehle AL, Raskin P. Changes in nerve conduction velocity after six weeks of glycoregulation with portable insulin infusion pumps. Diabetes 1980;29:668–71.

243. Service FJ, Daube JR, O'Brien PC, Dyck PJ. Effect of artificial pancreas treatment on peripheral nerve function in diabetes. Neurology 1981;31:1375–80.

244. Troni W, Carta QC. Cantello R, et al. Peripheral nerve function and metabolic control in diabetes mellitus. Ann Neurol 1984;16:178–83.

245. Boulton AJM, Clarke B, Drury J, Ward JD. Comparison of symptomatic relief with biothesiometer measurements in diabetic neuropathy treated with continuous subcutaneous insulin infusion [Abstract]. Diabetologia 1981; 21:505.

246. Holman RR, Dornan TL, Mayon-White V, et al. Prevention of deterioration of renal and sensory-nerve function by more intensive management of insulin-dependent diabetic patients: a two-year randomised prospective study. Lancet 1983;1:204–8.

247. Service FJ, Rizza RA, Daube JR, et al. Near normoglycaemia, improved nerve conduction and vibration sensation in diabetic neuropathy. Diabetologia 1985;28:722–5.

248. Bertelsmann FW, Heimans JJ, Van Rooy JCGM, et al. Peripheral nerve function in patients with painful diabetic neuropathy treated with continuous subcutaneous insulin infusion. J Neurol Neurosurg Psychiatry 1987;50:1337–41.

249. Handelsman DJ, Turtle JR. Clinical trial of an aldose reductase inhibitor in diabetic neuropathy. Diabetes 1981;30:459–64.

250. Fagius J, Jameson S. Effects of aldose reductase inhibitor treatment in diabetic polyneuropathy—a clinical and neurophysiological study. J Neurol Neurosurg Psychiatry 1981;44:991–1001.

251. Judzewitsch RG, Jaspan JB, Polonsky KS, et al. Aldose reductase inhibition improves nerve conduction velocity in diabetic patients. N Engl J Med 1983;308:119–25.

252. Young RJ, Ewing DJ, Clarke BF. A controlled trial of sorbinil an aldose reductase inhibitor in chronic painful diabetic neuropathy. Diabetes 1983;32:938–42.

253. Fagius J, Brattberg A, Jameson S, Berne C. Limited benefit of treatment of diabetic polyneuropathy with an aldose reductase inhibitor a 24-week controlled trial. Diabetologia 1985;28:323–9.

254. Guy RJC, Gilbey SG, Sheehy M, et al. Diabetic neuropathy in the upper limb and the effect of twelve months of sorbinil treatment. Diabetologia 1988;31:214–20.

255. Lewin IG, O'Brien IAD, Morgan MH, Corrall RJM. Clinical and neurophysiological studies with the aldose reductase inhibitor, sorbinil, in symptomatic diabetic neuropathy. Diabetologia 1984;26:445–8.

256. Christensen JE, Varnek L, Gregersen G. The effect of an aldose reductase inhibitor (sorbinil) on diabetic neuropathy and neural function of the retina a double-blind study. Acta Neurol Scand 1985;71:164–7.

257. O'Hare JP, Morgan MH, Alden P et al. Aldose reductase inhibition in diabetic neuropathy; clinical and neurophysiological studies of one year's treatment with sorbinil. Diabetic Med 1988;5:537–42.

258. The Tolrestat in Painful Neuropathy Study Group. Objective (nerve con:duction) and subjective (painful symptom) improvement in diabetic neuropathy following administration of tolrestat a new aldose reductase inhibitor [Abstract no. 436]. Diabetologia 1986;29:588A.

259. Boulton AJM, Atiea J, De Leeuw IH, et al. The efficacy and safety of the aldose-reductase inhibitor tolrestat in the treatment of chronic sensorimotor diabetic neuropathy [Abstract no. 57]. Diabetologia 1989;32:469A.

260. Hotta N, Kakauta H, Fukasawa H, et al. A long-term experimental and clinical study of an aldose reductase inhibitor ONO-2235 on diabetic neuropathy. In: Ward J, Goto Y, eds. Diabetic neuropathy. Chichester: John Wiley & Sons, 1990:149.

261. Salway JG, Whitehead L, Finnegan JA, et al. Effect of *myo*-inositol on peripheral nerve function in diabetes. Lancet 1978;2:1282–4.

262. Clements RS Jr, Vourganti B, Kuba T, et al. Dietary *myo*-inositol intake and peripheral nerve function in diabetic neuropathy. Metabolism 1979;28(Suppl 1):477–83.

263. Greene DA, Brown MJ, Braunstein SN, et al. Comparison of clinical course and sequential electrophysiological tests in diabetics with symptomatic polyneuropathy and its implications for clinical trials. Diabetes 1981;30:139–47.

264. Gregersen G, Børsting H, Theil P, Servo C. Myoinositol and function of peripheral nerves in human diabetics: a controlled clinical trial. Acta Neurol Scand 1978;58:241–8.

265. Gregersen G, Bertelsen B, Harbo H, et al. Oral supplementation of myoinositol: effects on peripheral nerve function in human diabetics and on the concentration in plasma, erythrocytes, urine and muscle tissue in human diabetics and normals. Acta Neurol Scand 1983;67:164–72.

266. Gregersen G. *Myo*-inositol supplementation. In: Dyck PJ, Thomas PK, Asbury AK, et al, eds. Diabetic neuropathy. Philadelphia: WB Saunders, 1987:188.

267. Clements RS Jr, DeJesus PV Jr, Winegrad AI. Raised plasma myoinositol levels in uraemia and experimental neuropathy. Lancet 1973;1:1137–41.

268. Servo C, Palo J, Pitkanen E. Polyols in the cerebrospinal fluid and plasma of neurological diabetic and uraemic patients. Acta Neurol Scand 1977;56:111–6.

269. Greene DA, Bril V, Lattimer SA, Sima AAF. Correction of *myo*-inositol depletion in diabetic human sural nerve by treatment with an aldose reductase inhibitor [Abstract no. 343]. Diabetes 1987;36(Suppl 1):86A.

270. Asbury AK. Understanding diabetic neuropathy. N Engl J Med 1988;319:577–8.

271. Dyck PJ, Zimmerman BR, Vilen TH, et al. Nerve glucose, fructose, sorbitol, *myo*-inositol, and fiber degeneration and regeneration in diabetic neuropathy. N Engl J Med 1988;319:542–8.

272. Sima AAF, Greene DA. Pathogenesis of diabetic neuropathy [Letter]. N Engl J Med 1989;320:58–9.

273. Winegrad AI, Simmons DA, Martin DB. Pathogenesis of diabetic neuropathy [Letter]. N Engl J Med 1989;320:57–8.

274. Kusuma H, Stewart MA. Levels of *myo*-inositol in normal and degenerating peripheral nerve. J Neurochem 1970;17:317.

Chapter 40

DIABETIC NEPHROPATHY

GIANCARLO VIBERTI
MARTIN J. WISEMAN
JOSÉ R. PINTO
JEANNIE MESSENT

Diabetic nephropathy is a relatively common microvascular complication of both insulin-dependent (IDDM) and non-insulin-dependent (NIDDM) diabetes mellitus. It is clinically defined by the presence of persistent proteinuria (>0.5 g/24 hour) in a patient with diabetes with concomitant retinopathy and elevated blood pressure, but without urinary tract infection, other renal disease, or heart failure.

Though proteinuria had been noted in patients with diabetes since the eighteenth century,[1,2] it was not until the late 1830s that it was postulated that albuminuria could reflect a serious renal disease specific to diabetes.[3,4] In 1936, Kimmelstiel and Wilson described the nodular glomerular intercapillary lesions in the diabetic kidney and related them to the clinical syndrome of profuse proteinuria and renal failure accompanied by arterial hypertension.[5]

The size of the problem of diabetic kidney disease became clear in the 1950s, with the longer survival afforded patients with IDDM after the discovery of insulin in 1921. Recent studies indicate that approximately 600 cases of end-stage diabetic renal failure occur every year in the United Kingdom (about 10 cases per million population).[6] About one-third of all patients beginning renal replacement therapy in the United States in 1985 were diabetic; the cost for caring for these patients with diabetes with renal failure approached $1 billion in 1985.[7]

EPIDEMIOLOGY

The epidemiology of diabetic nephropathy has been studied primarily, although not exclusively, in patients with IDDM. The largest studies are from Denmark and the Joslin Clinic. Although patients with NIDDM have not been investigated as thoroughly, major differences between ethnic groups have been found to exist. At present, it is prudent to treat the epidemiology of nephropathy for the two types of diabetes separately.

Insulin-Dependent Diabetes

Two major cohort studies have described the prevalence and incidence of diabetic nephropathy, as defined by persistent clinical proteinuria, in patients with IDDM who developed diabetes before the age of 31 years.[8–10] The prevalence (the number of cases at a given time) of nephropathy increases with duration of diabetes to a peak of 21% after 20 to 25 years, after which it declines to about 10% in those who have had diabetes for 40 years or more. After 5 years of diabetes, the annual incidence (the number of cases per given time) of nephropathy rises rapidly over the next 10 years to a peak after 15 to 17 years of about 3% per year. It then declines to around 1% per year in those with 40 years or more of diabetes.[11]

This pattern of risk indicates that accumulation of exposure to diabetes (i.e., intensity times duration) is not sufficient to explain the development of clinically manifest kidney disease and suggests that only a subset of patients are susceptible to renal complications. The paucity of new cases of nephropathy among patients with long-standing diabetes supports the view that this complication occurs in most of the susceptible individuals earlier in the course of diabetes. During the first 10 years of diabetes, only about 4% of patients develop nephropathy. The cumulative incidence increases thereafter to a plateau after about 25 years. Nephropathy develops in only 4% of patients with more than 35 years of diabetes. This indicates that only a proportion of patients with juvenile diabetes ever develop nephropathy. This proportion has changed over the years.[9,10] In cohorts of patients diagnosed before 1942, the cumulative risk up to 25 to 30 years of duration of diabetes was approximately 41%, but in patients diagnosed after 1949, it declined to around 25%. The reason(s) for the lower frequency of diabetic nephropathy in recent decades is not entirely clear. Cohort differences may be related to changes in diabetes care and control, to more intensive and early treatment of concomitant conditions such as hypertension, or, less likely, to dietary changes. An alternative explanation is that before 1942 in a proportion of patients with diabetes persistent proteinuria may have been the manifestation of some other form of renal disease, particularly glomerulonephritis, the incidence of which has declined during this century.[12] This interpretation would explain why a sharp decrease in incidence was seen in patients diagnosed in the late 1940s, but not since.

There is a male preponderance in the development of proteinuria, with the ratio of males to females of around 1.7. The cumulative incidence is 46% in male diabetics but only 32% in female diabetics in those cohort studies that have followed patients for 40 years or more. This difference in the incidence of renal disease in males and females is also found in subjects without diabetes.[13,14] It is of interest that some authors have also reported a male preponderance in the development of proliferative diabetic retinopathy.[15,16] It has been suggested that sex steroids may be of importance, since castrated diabetic rats seem less prone than non-castrated control animals to late diabetic complications.[17]

Age at diagnosis significantly influences the risk of nephropathy. The time to development of microvascular complications is not influenced by prepubertal duration of the disease,[18] and nephropathy develops more slowly in individuals with onset of diabetes before the age of 10 years than in those with diagnosis after puberty.[9] The highest cumulative incidence of 44% is seen in subjects who developed diabetes between 11 and 20 years of age,[10] while in those with a diagnosis after the age of 20, the cumulative incidence of nephropathy is about 35%. Current age has been found by some authors[9] but not by others[10] to influence the incidence of proteinuria, with a maximal risk in the age interval 18 to 35 years and a rapid decline in incidence after age 35 years regardless of duration of diabetes.[19] This discrepancy in findings may be related in part to the different age groups of the cohorts studied.

In one study the level of hyperglycemia during the first 15 years of diabetes was found to be positively related to the risk of persistent proteinuria.[9] However, the incidence of nephropathy rapidly declined after 15 years' duration of diabetes, even though there was no improvement in the control of glycemia, a finding suggesting that susceptibility to this condition is related to nonmetabolic factors, most probably genetic. The complex metabolic disturbances of diabetes thus appear necessary, but not sufficient, for the clinical manifestation of nephropathy.

The development of end-stage renal failure and its associated mortality closely conform to the occurrence of persistent proteinuria[9]; 25% develop end-stage renal failure within 6 years, and 75% within 15 years of onset of proteinuria. Progression to end-stage renal failure seems to take longer in patients diagnosed with diabetes before puberty. The median time between onset of persistent proteinuria and the development of end-stage renal failure was 14 years in the group of subjects with onset of diabetes before age 12 years and was 8 years in those with onset of diabetes between the ages of 12 and 20 years.[9] The range of survival after the onset of persistent proteinuria is wide—between 1 and 24 years. Median survival has been reported to be around 7 to 10 years.[8,9]

The ominous significance of renal involvement in IDDM is clearly shown by the comparison of long-term outcome in patients with and without nephropathy. After

40 years of diabetes, only 10% of patients with proteinuria are alive, in contrast to more than 70% of those without proteinuria.[8] Almost all of the latter have normal renal function, and up to about 70% are clinically well in all respects, only about 10% being seriously disabled by virtue of amputation or visual or cardiovascular complications.[20]

When renal replacement therapy was not widely available, the primary cause of death (~60%) in patients with IDDM with diabetic nephropathy was uremia, but a substantial proportion died before terminal renal failure from ischemic heart disease (19%) or stroke (5%). The proportion of cardiovascular deaths increases significantly to around 40% in those patients who develop proteinuria after more than 20 years of diabetes.[8] The advent of renal replacement therapy, which has postponed death due to uremia, has by the same token increased the pool of cardiovascular deaths, which usually now occur after institution of treatment for end-stage renal disease. The development of persistent proteinuria in patients with IDDM increases early mortality caused by cardiovascular disease by approximately ninefold.[21,22] The risk of developing coronary artery disease is estimated to be 15 times higher in those with proteinuria than in those without proteinuria,[23] and its cumulative incidence 6 years after onset of proteinuria is eight times higher than in matched controls without renal involvement[22] (Table 40–1). Whatever the cause, mortality from all causes by age 45 years in IDDM patients with proteinuria has been reported to be 20 to 40 times higher than that in patients without proteinuria, who experience a relative mortality only double that of the nondiabetic population.[11] Recent studies suggest that more effective antihypertensive treatment during the past decade has significantly improved the prognosis in patients with diabetic nephropathy. The 10-year survival rate after onset of persistent proteinuria has risen from 30 to 50%[8,9] to about 80%[24,25] (Fig. 40–1).

Non-Insulin-Dependent Diabetes

Data on the prevalence and incidence of nephropathy in patients with NIDDM, as indicated by persistent proteinuria, have been relatively scarce until recent years.

Table 40–1. Cumulative Incidence of Coronary Heart Disease in Patients with Insulin-Dependent Diabetes with and without Proteinuria

Group	Cumulative Incidence (%) at Indicated Year After Proteinuria		
	2	4	6
Patients with proteinuria	10	25	40*
Patients without proteinuria	2	5	5*

Table is adapted from Jensen et al.[22]
*P <.001: patients with proteinuria at 6 years vs. patients without proteinuria at 6 years.

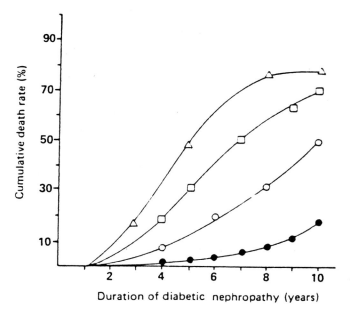

Fig. 40–1. Cumulative death rates from diabetic nephropathy in patients with insulin-dependent diabetes with (solid circle, n = 45) and without (open triangle, n = 45, Knowles et al.[26]; open square, n = 360, Anderson et al.[8]; open circle, n = 67, Krolewski et al.[9]) effective antihypertensive treatment. Reprinted with permission from reference 24 (Parving H-H, Hommel E. Prognosis in diabetic nephropathy. BMJ 1989;29:230–3).

The overall prevalence of proteinuria (>500 mg/24 hour) has been reported to be approximately 16% in one study of European patients with diabetes diagnosed after the age of 40 years.[27] Other studies in slightly differently selected populations have reported lower prevalences of 12 to 14%, with a higher prevalence in men (19%) than in women (4%).[28,30] The prevalence of proteinuria increases steadily with duration of diabetes—from 7 to 10% in patients with diabetes diagnosed less than 5 years previously to 20 to 35% in patients with diabetes diagnosed more than 20 to 25 years earlier.[27,28]

In non-European patients with NIDDM, the lowest prevalence of proteinuria (2.4%) has been reported in patients in Hong Kong,[30] but prevalences higher than in European patients have been found in American Indians,[30–32] Mexican-Americans,[33] African-Americans,[34] Japanese,[30] Nauruan from central Pacific islands,[35] and Asian Indians in the United Kingdom,[36] in whom an increased prevalence of microalbuminuria has also been described.[37] In some non-European ethnic groups, there also is a tendency for the prevalence to increase with duration of diabetes.

A male preponderance in the prevalence of proteinuria has been reported by some authors.[38] Both blood glucose control and level of arterial pressure have been related to prevalence of proteinuria in a number of ethnic groups. Sixty-two percent of European patients with NIDDM maintain normal protein excretion after 16 years of diabetes. Those who develop proteinuria have a higher prevalence of hypertension before onset of persistent

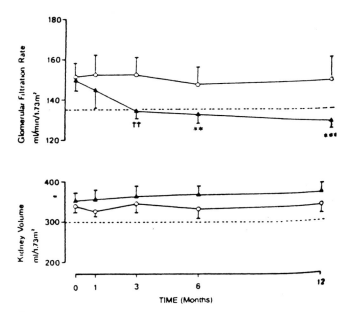

Fig. 40–4. Changes in glomerular filtration rate (GFR) and kidney volume in 12 patients with insulin-dependent diabetes with increased GFR, randomized to receive either continuous subcutaneous insulin infusion (CSII; solid triangle) or conventional insulin therapy (open circle). The reduction in GFR from baseline in the patients who received CSII was highly significant (††$P < .025$, ** $P < .005$, ***$P < .001$).

was described in two retrospective studies,[88,89] but these findings were not confirmed by a more recent study spanning an observation period of 18 years.[90] In all these reports, a number of potentially important confounding variables, such as albumin excretion rate, blood pressure, or protein intake, all of which can affect outcome, were not controlled for. The 5-year results of an ongoing prospective case-control study of patients with IDDM with and without hyperfiltration[91] suggest that diabetics with hyperfiltration, although showing a faster rate of GFR decline do not show an increased frequency of rising albuminuria or blood pressure.

Although in this silent phase, patients do not, by definition, demonstrate clinically detectable proteinuria, the use of a sensitive radioimmunoassay for urinary albumin has shown that in several circumstances a proportion of patients with relatively early diabetes have elevated, supranormal rates of albumin excretion. A significant increase in albumin excretion rate (AER) to three to four times above the normal level was first demonstrated in patients with NIDDM that was newly detected in a population survey.[92] Young subjects with newly diagnosed IDDM or subjects with short-term diabetes in poor control often demonstrate an elevated AER.[93–95] Subclinical elevations in rates of both albumin and IgG excretion also are found in patients with longer-term IDDM.[96] These abnormal, although subclinical, increases in AER have been termed *microalbuminuria.* Albumin excretion in healthy individuals ranges between 1.5 and 20 µg/min, with a geometric mean around 6.5 µg/min. These levels have been termed

normoalbuminuria. The wide use of chemical reagent "dipstix" has led to the definition of *persistent* or *clinical proteinuria* in patients whose urine is positive in these tests. Such patients generally have AERs in excess of 200 µg/min. Microalbuminuria thus defines the wide subclinical range of albumin hyperexcretion ranging between 20 and 200 µg/min.[97]

AER in both normal individuals and patients with diabetes tends to be about 25% higher during the day than during the night and exhibits an average day-to-day variation of about 40%.[93,98–102] Similar coefficients of variation are found for albumin/creatinine ratios, suggesting that this variability is a true biologic phenomenon and not due to inadequate urine collection.[93,100,101] An important practical implication of this variability is that the accurate classification of AERs should depend on measurements for at least three collections over a 6-month period. The prevalence of microalbuminuria in IDDM has been reported to range from 5 to 37% in different population-based and diabetes clinic-based studies.[103–107] These rather large differences in prevalence are most likely ascribable to patient selection. No correlation is found between AER and age, but there is a male preponderance among microalbuminuric patients with IDDM, who also tend to have an earlier onset and longer duration of diabetes than normoalbuminuric patients.[107,108] Persistent elevations in AER are exceptional in the first 5 years of diabetes,[104,108] and microalbuminuria has not been detected in children younger than 15 years of age.[103] The phase of persistent microalbuminuria has been termed *incipient nephropathy* by some authors.[109] AER is influenced by glycemic control, and correction of hyperglycemia can reduce microalbuminuria, in long-term as well as short-term IDDM.[94–96,110] Moderately strenuous exercise is also capable of provoking an exaggerated rise in AER in patients with diabetes whose resting values are normal.[111,112] The severity of the exercise-induced albuminuria seems related to duration of diabetes and is modulated by the level of blood glucose control.[113–115]

In NIDDM, prevalences of microalbuminuria have been reported of between 8% and 46% in Europeans[27,48,106,108,116] and of 47% in Pima Indians.[32] Microalbuminuria is found not only in patients with diabetes but also in patients with impaired glucose tolerance.[32,92,116] No correlation is found between microalbuminuria and sex, but significant positive associations are found between microalbuminuria and diastolic blood pressure and resting heart rate.[117]

The prognostic significance of microalbuminuria for development of persistent proteinuria and overt nephropathy has been demonstrated by five longitudinal studies of cohorts of IDDM patients.[88,99,118–120] These investigations have all suggested the existence of a threshold of AER above which the risk of progression to clinical nephropathy increases by about twentyfold. The overall findings of these studies are remarkably similar, the differences in methods of urine collection and length of follow-up probably being responsible for the different risk levels of AER (Table 40–2). Microalbuminuria is unlikely to be a marker of susceptibility to the develop-

Table 40–2. Predictive Value of Albumin Excretion Rate (AER) for Persistent Clinical Proteinuria in Patients with Insulin-Dependent Diabetes in Five Different Studies.

	No. of Subjects	Baseline AER (μg/min)	Follow-up (yr)	Type of Collection	Predictive Value
Viberti et al.[118]	63	>30	14	Overnight	88% (7/8)
Parving et al.[119]	23	>28	6	24 hr	63% (5/8)
Mathiesen et al.[99]	71	>70	6	24 hr	100% (7/7)
Mogensen and Christensen[88]	43	>15	10	Short-term	86% (12/14)
Jerums et al.[120]	53	>30	8	24 hr	25% (1/4)

ment of clinical nephropathy, as it is undetectable in the first 5 years of diabetes,[104] but is more likely a sign of early disease. This interpretation has recently been corroborated by the finding that patients with persistent microalbuminuria have more severe renal histologic lesions than do patients with normal AERs.[121] At present, there is no evidence that exercise-induced microalbuminuria improves the predictive power of resting microalbuminuria. A good correlation has been found between AER and albumin/creatinine ratios, particularly in first morning urine samples, and AER >30 μg/min correspond to albumin/creatinine ratios >2.5.[101]

Three retrospective studies also have examined the prognostic value of microalbuminuria in cohorts of patients with NIDDM.[48,50,51] Over an interval of 10 to 14 years, they have all shown an increased risk of cardiovascular death in these patients. A recent prospective study of 3 years' duration has confirmed the greater incidence of cardiovascular events in patients with NIDDM with microalbuminuria.[122] Moreover, microalbuminuria has been found to be predictive of risk of cardiovascular events in the nondiabetic population.[123]

Late Phase: Clinical Nephropathy

The onset of the clinical phase of diabetic nephropathy is signaled, by convention, by the appearance of persistent proteinuria (total protein excretion of ≥0.5 g/day), which corresponds to an AER greater than ~200 μg/min (i.e., ~300 mg/day). A phase of intermittent dipstick-positivity of urine for protein precedes persistent proteinuria,[124] but most likely this corresponds to the late phases of high microalbuminuria, with values intermittently breaking through the clinical threshold.[120,125] The value of the term and concept of intermittent proteinuria is limited to its being an indication for quantitative measurements of urinary albumin. Its use as a description of a specific phase of disease should be abandoned. In those patients in whom persistent proteinuria develops, there is a progressive decline of the GFR to end-stage renal failure.[126–129] Whether the fall in GFR starts at the time of or after the appearance of the microalbuminuric phase is a matter for debate.[125,130] The fall in GFR appears to be linear with time in all patients, but the rate of decline varies over an approximately fourfold range among individual patients.

The reasons for these different rates of progression are not entirely clear and do not seem to be related to age,

sex, duration of diabetes, or degree of proteinuria at onset. Adequacy of blood glucose control has only a limited impact on progression,[131,132] even though some, but not all, authors have reported a correlation between levels of glycosylated hemoglobin and rate of fall of GFR.[133,134] The level of diastolic blood pressure has been found to be correlated with the rate of progression of established diabetic nephropathy, and serum creatinine concentrations have been reported to rise sooner in those proteinuric patients with the higher blood pressure levels.[126,132,135] The failure by other authors[127–129] to confirm the relationship with blood pressure may result from the current more widespread treatment of mild hypertension in these patients. In evaluations of the rate and magnitude of fall of GFR, caution must be applied when serum creatinine or creatinine clearance is used as an index of glomerular function.[136] Because of the asymptotic relationship between serum creatinine and GFR, there may be no rise in serum creatinine level until more than 50% of the GFR has been lost. A linear decline in inverse creatinine is not seen for serum creatinine concentrations below 200 μmol/L.[127] Moreover, the use of creatinine clearance tends to overestimate GFR because of the enhanced tubular secretion of creatinine that takes place in advanced renal failure.[137]

In the past, end-stage renal failure occurred on average 7 years after the onset of persistent proteinuria. In recent years, this interval has probably more than doubled with early, more intensive treatment of hypertension,[24,25] and early restriction of dietary protein.[138,139]

Arterial pressure is almost invariably elevated in diabetic patients with established nephropathy. A small proportion (~25%) of patients may still have blood pressures within the so-called normal range at the onset of persistent proteinuria, although it may have risen within the normal range from previous lower levels before the onset of proteinuria.[99,140,141] With progression to renal insufficiency, virtually all patients become hypertensive.[24,124,132] Several studies suggest that the excess of arterial hypertension described in IDDM patients is almost entirely accounted for by patients with persistent proteinuria.[132,142,143] Patients with long-term IDDM without proteinuria have blood pressures that are indeed lower than those of age-matched controls.[144] The degree of proteinuria in patients with diabetes is usually in the subnephrotic range, but heavy protein excretion and nephrotic syndrome may occur, and this has been related to a poorer renal outcome.[145] The level of proteinuria is roughly related to the degree of severity of the glomerular lesions, but glomerular histologic damage has been reported in patients without proteinuria.[145,146] The clinical significance of this finding remains unclear. In our own experience of follow-up of more than 90 patients with IDDM and diabetic nephropathy, we have not encountered a single case of progressive renal failure in the absence of some degree of proteinuria.

Nonrenal Complications

Diabetic retinopathy is present in virtually all patients with IDDM with nephropathy.[107,146–148] In advanced renal disease retinopathy is usually severe with new vessel formation. Indeed, the absence of retinopathy should lead to more than usually careful consideration of other nondiabetic causes for proteinuria and renal disease (see below). Whereas all patients with nephropathy have retinopathy, the reverse is not true. Retinopathy, even of the proliferative kind, may occur in the absence of proteinuria and renal disease.[149] Up to one-third of patients with proliferative retinopathy may be free of proteinuria.[150,151] The exact reasons for this discrepancy in manifestations of microvascular disease are not clear, but epidemiologic evidence suggests that retinopathy and nephropathy are associated with different environmental determinants. The cumulative risk of retinopathy approaches 100% after 15 years of diabetes,[152] demonstrating a close relationship to a history of poor control of blood glucose. In contrast, levels of blood pressure are stronger determinants of the development of nephropathy. In patients with NIDDM with persistent proteinuria, retinopathy is present in 47 to 63%,[29,48,153] a finding consistent with the observation that in about 30% of patients with NIDDM with proteinuria it is of nondiabetic origin.

In a substantial number of proteinuric patients with diabetes, urinalysis shows the presence of microhematuria. A recent study has demonstrated that proteinuric diabetic patients with microhematuria exhibit a higher prevalence of concomitant nondiabetic renal disease.[154] However, microhematuria can occur in proteinuric patients with diabetes in the absence of other renal conditions as part of the diabetic nephropathy syndrome. It has been reported in 66% of all cases in a large series in which 136 consecutive renal biopsies were performed in patients with IDDM or NIDDM, and it has been claimed that the presence of microhematuria is of little use in distinguishing nondiabetic renal disease.[155] Red cell casts are unusual in diabetic nephropathy and their presence calls for further evaluation. Although the diagnostic significance is still controversial, the presence of red cells in the urinary sediment must alert the physician to the possibility of another renal disease.

End-Stage Renal Failure

The development of uremia in patients with diabetes is compounded by a number of other complications. Fluid retention and edema occur relatively early in the development of renal failure, in the absence of hypoalbuminemia.[156] The variable contributions, particularly in older patients, of cardiac insufficiency and of vasomotor defects secondary to neuropathy and peripheral vascular disease were recognized long ago.[157–159] Depressed renal function further compromises disposal of water and solutes and impairs osmotic diuresis, especially in the face of rapid compartmental shifts of fluid secondary to variations in glycemia.[160] Pulmonary edema may follow, and the prognosis at this stage is poor. Hyperkalemia may develop, partly as a result of the hyporeninemic hypoaldosteronism common in patients with advanced diabetic nephropathy,[161] which may itself aggravate the metabolic acidosis of chronic renal failure.

Peripheral neuropathy affects the majority of diabetic patients with renal failure. Uremia, itself a cause of neuropathy, is likely to contribute to the severity of symptoms in a number of cases. Foot sepsis leading to amputation may occur, a development that is probably due to a combination of neural and arterial disease. Foot sepsis can be a major cause of incapacity and morbidity in these patients, but it can often be prevented by good patient education and active involvement of the chiropodist. Autonomic neuropathy, notably postural hypotension, can make treatment of arterial hypertension particularly troublesome. Good control of blood pressure in the supine position is often accompanied by an unacceptable drop in standing blood pressures. Diabetic diarrhea[147] and gastroparesis[162] causing nausea and vomiting are sometimes hard to distinguish from the gastrointestinal symptoms of uremia. Impotence and profuse sweating are also common manifestations of autonomic neuropathy in uremic patients.[163] Neurogenic bladder, a particularly serious problem, will be discussed separately (see below). Arterial disease and medial calcification of larger arteries (Monckeberg's sclerosis) are present in almost all diabetic patients with advanced renal disease.[164] Disturbances of lipid metabolism of diabetes and uremia combined with arterial hypertension all contribute to the development of severe sclerotic damage. Coronary artery disease is the major cause of death in these patients, and peripheral artery disease may contribute to gangrene and amputation both before and particularly after renal replacement therapy.

PATHOPHYSIOLOGY

Early Functional Changes

Glomerular Hyperfiltration

Several studies that used accurate techniques for estimating GFR have confirmed that in patients with IDDM the GFR is 20 to 40% above normal. The investigation of the intrarenal hemodynamic basis for hyperfiltration is easier in animal models of IDDM than in humans because of the ability to make direct measurements in single nephrons of the major determinants of GFR: renal plasma flow, transglomerular hydraulic pressure gradient with a filtration coefficient, and oncotic pressure. Data from both human and animal studies are used in this chapter.

Renal Plasma Flow. Renal plasma flow (RPF), one of the major determinants of GFR, has been reported as elevated, normal, or reduced in patients with IDDM.[62,71,73] However, most recent work shows an elevation of renal plasma flow of 9 to 14%,[74] an elevation less than that of the GFR. Several studies have demonstrated a good correlation between the increases in RPF and GFR in patients with diabetes.[72,75,76] These findings suggest that at least some of the increase in GFR is accounted for by elevation of RPF.

Increased RPF, however, cannot account for the entire rise in GFR. In human studies in which GFR and RPF were measured simultaneously, RPF accounted for about 50 to 60% of the increase in GFR.[72,75] Increased filtration fraction, sometimes associated with elevated urinary albumin excretion, in patients with short-term IDDM is compatible with a suggested possible elevation in intraglomerular pressure under these circumstances.[95]

Hydraulic Filtration Pressure. Direct measurements of hydraulic filtration pressure cannot be obtained in humans, but micropuncture studies in moderately hyperglycemic rats have shown a significant increase in the transglomerular pressure gradient,[165,166] although this elevation has not always been confirmed.[167,168] Severely hyperglycemic rats show no elevation in intraglomerular pressure.[165,168,169] In the rat model, analysis of the arteriolar vasculature has shown that increases in both flow and pressure are achieved by a reduction of total arteriolar vascular resistance, which is more marked at the afferent than at the efferent end of the arteriole.[165] These findings have a counterpart in diabetic patients with glomerular hyperfiltration, whose calculated renal vascular resistance is reduced.[170] However, the renal lesion in the rat model is that of focal segmental glomerular sclerosis, not that of diabetic nephropathy, and not all strains of rats develop hyperfiltration and increased glomerular pressure (see Pathogenesis). The elevation in the glomerular transcapillary hydraulic pressure difference appears, therefore, to account for a further proportion of the rise in GFR, which is estimated at approximately 25%.

Glomerular Ultrafiltration Coefficient. A third determinant of GFR is the glomerular ultrafiltration coefficient, the product of the capillary hydraulic conductivity and the capillary surface area available for filtration. Although in animal studies the calculated glomerular ultrafiltration coefficient did not account for the increased filtration rate,[165,167,168] filtration surface area has been found to be increased in patients with IDDM[171] as well as in diabetic rats,[172] and a significant correlation has been described between GFR and filtration surface area in young patients with IDDM.[173] Thus, an increase in the surface area available for filtration (a component of the ultrafiltration coefficient) may be a determinant of the elevation in the GFR. Changes in GFR can occur with changes in metabolic control[68,94,170,174] within a time period that might not appear sufficient to alter the filtration surface area as assessed by conventional morphologic techniques.[171] However, filtration surface area may be affected dynamically by mesangial contraction in response to vasoactive stimuli such as angiotensin II. A reduction in the density of glomerular angiotensin II has been demonstrated in diabetic rats.[175] A close correlation has been found between GFR and kidney size. Kidney size, which is enlarged in 40% of patients with IDDM, has been found to be related to changes in the transglomerular pressure gradient and filtration surface area.[176]

Systemic Oncotic Pressure. A fourth determinant of GFR is systemic oncotic pressure, which has been reported to be normal in both diabetic humans[177] and animals.[168]

Metabolic and Hormonal Mediators of Elevation in Glomerular Filtration Rate

The cause of elevation of GFR appears to be multifactorial. Hyperfiltration is a phenomenon that occurs under conditions of moderate hyperglycemia, since severe hyperglycemia (>14 to 16 mmol/L) is associated not with an elevated GFR but with a normal or reduced GFR.[67,165,178] In unselected groups of patients with IDDM whose baseline GFRs range from normal to high, increasing the concentration of blood glucose to an average of 16 mmol/L by intravenous glucose infusion leads to an average rise in GFR of approximately 5%.[177] Other studies show that only those diabetic patients with glomerular hyperfiltration at baseline experience a significant increase in GFR (on average by 12%) in response to intravenous glucose infusion.[170] In normal individuals, elevations in blood glucose levels are associated either with an increase[177,179,180] or with no change in the GFR.[170] These differences may depend, at least in part, on the level of glycemia achieved. High blood glucose levels may induce vasodilation, which has been shown to occur in the retinal circulation.[181] A similar mechanism might apply to the glomerular arterioles. In rats, hyperglycemia and glycosuria, both separately and additively, affect the tubuloglomerular feedback mechanism by blunting the reduction in GFR in response to increased proximal tubular flow through a reduced sodium flux across the macula densa, thus producing relative hyperfiltration.[182] An increase in glucose-coupled reabsorption of sodium and water in the proximal tubule also may cause an increase in GFR.[183] Recently, infusion of ketone bodies in supraphysiologic doses in patients with diabetes has been shown to cause an increase of GFR of about 33%, the single most powerful effect so far described. This effect was accompanied by a concomitant rise of about 16% in RPF and a 14% increase in the filtration fraction.[184]

In addition to the altered level of glucose and other metabolites found in diabetes, a number of changes in circulating levels of, as well as in vascular responsiveness to, metabolic fuel-related and vasoactive hormones may be seen in diabetes. Acute reduction in blood glucose levels in patients with diabetes by insulin infusion reduces the GFR within 30 to 60 minutes, but the effect is small (~6%).[185] This reduction of the elevated GFR and RPF by insulin infusion does not occur if the blood glucose is maintained at euglycemic levels by concomitant glucose infusion.[186] Euglycemic insulin infusion in normal humans is not associated with changes in either GFR or RPF.[187,188] These findings have been interpreted as indicating that insulin per se has no effect on GFR and RPF. Daily administration of growth hormone for some days, although not by acute infusion,[189] increases GFR and RPF in normal subjects[190,191] and in patients with IDDM[192] by 7% and 6%, respectively, in the face of unchanged glycemic control. However, a correlation between plasma concentration of growth hormone and GFR has not been found in unselected patients with diabetes,[193] and diabetic patients with hyperfiltration have diurnal profiles of growth hormone levels not dissimilar to those of patients with diabetes with a normal GFR.[194] Intravenous infusion of glucagon to achieve plasma levels found in patients with poorly controlled diabetes raises the GFR in both normal[195] and diabetic[196] subjects. In patients with diabetes, this increase is accompanied by an equivalent increase in RPF, with a significant relationship between RPF and GFR. However, circulating levels of glucagon were found to be no higher throughout the day in diabetic patients with an increased GFR than in those patients with a normal GFR.[194] It is controversial whether infusion of glucagon into the renal artery causes consistent modification of GFR, but intra-portal infusion of the hormone induces a significant rise.[197,198] Recent evidence suggests that the glucagon effect on renal hemodynamics may be mediated through renal prostaglandin (PG) production.[199]

Small elevations of plasma renin activity, coupled with increased urinary excretion of 6-keto-PGF$_{1\alpha}$, have recently been described in patients with IDDM with glomerular hyperfiltration.[200] Other authors, however, studying similar patients, have found significantly lower levels of plasma renin activity and normal levels of urinary prostaglandin excretion.[201] In streptozotocin-diabetic rats, both the circulating levels of renin and the density of glomeruli angiotensin II receptor were found to be reduced,[175] a finding suggesting that the expected up-regulation of receptors with suppression of renin did not occur. Other workers have provided evidence in the animal model that renal prostaglandin production may be important in the genesis of glomerular hyperfiltration. In the isolated perfused kidney, the increased GFR and the vasodilation in response to hyperglycemia have been found to be blocked by indomethacin infusion, a finding that implicates renal prostanoids as possible mediators of this effect.[202] Administration of indomethacin to diabetic animals has been found to cause a significant reduction in GFR and RPF,[203] and an increased synthesis of prostaglandins in isolated glomeruli from diabetic rats has been described.[204] Administration of aspirin to streptozotocin-diabetic rats prevented early hyperfiltration as well as the decrease in GFR and accompanying increase in thickness of the glomerular basement membrane at 16 weeks in the control animals.[205]

The predominance of the prostaglandin system is further supported by the finding that inhibition of prostaglandin production by acetylsalicylate reduces GFR in patients with IDDM with hyperfiltration.[201] However, short-term administration of indomethacin to patients with newly diagnosed IDDM has been reported not to affect GFR.[206] However, a reduction in GFR in response to indomethacin administration was found in patients with IDDM with persistent proteinuria,[207] as has been reported for patients with other, nondiabetic, renal disease.

Some authors have postulated that a hepatic product could be responsible for the increased GFR. This substance, which has been named *glomerulopressin*, is thought to be a glucuronic acid conjugate[208] and has been reported to be increased in dogs with diabetes.[198] In diabetic rats, raised levels of atrial natriuretic peptide (ANP) have been found to be associated with glomerular hyperfiltration and intraglomerular hypertension. Reduction of plasma ANP levels by antibody blockade led to a parallel fall in GFR. It has been postulated that diabetes-induced volume expansion (as seen on average in these animals) may mediate the rise in ANP levels, which in turn could elevate the GFR.[209] ANP levels have been reported to be higher in diabetic patients with hyperfiltration,[210-212] but these findings were not confirmed by other authors.[213] The results in patients with microalbuminuria and persistent proteinuria have also been conflicting.[211,212,214] Similarly, different authors have found the volume of extracellular fluid to be normal or expanded.[213-216]

In conclusion, metabolic and hormonal mechanisms acting both systemically and locally are likely to be involved in the alteration of GFR in diabetes. The effects of a number of mediators, themselves small, may combine to induce the observed GFR elevations. These disturbances not only are related to the diabetic state but seem specifically to affect the function of susceptible kidneys in diabetes.

Renal Hypertrophy

The kidneys of patients with IDDM are, on average, larger than those of control subjects, and the kidneys of animals made diabetic enlarge within days of the induction of diabetes. The weight of the entire kidney increases by an average of 15% within the first 3 days of diabetes, and parallel increases in the protein and RNA content of the kidney are observed. DNA synthesis remains stable for the first 3 days but increases thereafter.[83,217] Treatment with insulin that is initiated soon after the induction of diabetes is capable of preventing the incremental increase in kidney weight,[82] but if insulin treatment is started after 28 days, the enlargement of the kidney is not reversed.[83] When near-normal glycemia is achieved by islet transplantation 4 weeks after induction of diabetes, a partial reduction in kidney size and normalization of RNA/DNA ratio, which is elevated in untreated diabetes, is obtained.[172] This situation resembles the findings in humans with diabetes, in whom good metabolic control at onset of diabetes appears capable of reversing kidney enlargement,[75] whereas chronic strict metabolic control in patients with longer-term diabetes with established kidney enlargement has been shown to have no effect or to produce only a partial reduction in kidney volume.[68,69,80,81] In the animal model, glomerular growth is prominent during the first 4 days following induction of diabetes. Tubular growth then catches up and eventually exceeds the glomerular growth over the first 6 weeks after onset of diabetes.[218] Glomerular capillary length appears to be the earliest change and is followed in the succeeding weeks by increases in the radial cross-sectional area of the capillary loop, which eventually becomes the dominant change responsible for the increased glomerular size.[219] The length of both the proximal and distal tubules increases by approximately 20%, but whereas proximal tubular cells retain their normal appearance, the distal cells in the cortex and outer medullary stripe appear laden with glycogen-like granules and show a marked reduction in the number of organelles and basal infoldings.[220] Some authors believe that these morphologic changes precede the early hemodynamic alterations and that they may, in fact, contribute to them.[217,221]

Microalbuminuria

In a percentage of patients with IDDM, the urinary AER is increased above the upper limit of normal but is still undetectable by current routine clinical tests. Exaggerated excretion of albumin can also be induced by periods of poor metabolic control[94] or moderately strenuous exercise.[111,112] In these situations microalbuminuria is not accompanied by an increase in the excretion rate of β_2-microglobulin, a protein that is freely filtered across the glomerular capillary barrier and almost entirely reabsorbed by proximal tubular cells, thus reflecting proximal tubular function.[222,223] The consistency of normal β_2-microglobulin excretion rate in the face of an augmented AER suggests that the excess albuminuria is not the result of a change in tubular reabsorption of the protein but more likely derives from increased glomerular leakage.

The glomerular capillary blood-urine barrier can be regarded functionally as a membrane perforated by pores of an average size of 5.5 nm and uniformly coated by a negative electrical charge.[224-228] Therefore, both the size and charge of the circulating molecule, as well as the set of hemodynamic forces operating across the capillary wall, determine the passage of proteins and other molecules across the glomerular membrane. In microalbuminuric patients with diabetes, the fractional clearances of albumin, a polyanion with a molecular radius of about 3.6 nm; and of IgG, a larger but electrically neutral molecule with radius of around 5.5 nm, are both increased.[229,230] These early increases are likely to be the consequence of alterations in glomerular hemodynamics and, in particular, of transglomerular pressure gradient, which is elevated in moderately hyperglycemic diabetic rats.[165;166,203] This is consistent with the findings of an increased filtration fraction in patients with poorly controlled diabetes[71,79,94] and of a raised absolute urinary clearance of neutral dextran over a wide range of molecular weights in parallel with the elevated glomerular filtration rate.[174]

As microalbuminuria becomes persistent and increases in degree, the selectivity index—the clearance of IgG as a proportion of the clearance of albumin—starts to fall, reaching its lowest values when albumin excretion is around 90 μg/min or higher. The decrease in this index is due to a disproportionate increase in the filtration of albumin as compared with that of IgG, and it marks a new selective stage of glomerular leakage of anionic albumin.[229,230] Experiments measuring the clearance of neutral dextrans have shown that medium-size pores are unchanged at this stage.[71,228] A likely reason for the increased glomerular filtration of albumin is a loss of the fixed negative electrical charge on the membrane.[231-234] This would permit increased permeation of anionic albumin, with its smaller molecular weight, but would have little influence on IgG, a larger neutral molecule, the filtration of which is regulated by pore radius or number and by glomerular pressures and flows. The mechanism of this transition from low to high levels of microalbuminuria is unknown but may be the result of a combination of hemodynamic abnormalities with the cumulative derangement of synthesis of the electronegative membrane glycosialoproteins and proteoglycans.[230,235-237] Recent studies suggest, however, that preferential filtration on the basis of charge discrimination resulting from loss of glomerular polyanion does not entirely explain the facilitated clearance of anionic proteins. Permeation of both large- and medium-sized molecules through a non-size-discriminatory shunt pathway could account for the observed renal clearances of albumin, IgG, and dextrans.[238] An alternative suggestion is that the facilitated clearance of anionic proteins, including IgG4,[239] may reflect, rather than a loss of glomerular polyanion, an increased expression of cationic sites on the glomerular filter.[240] This would be compatible with the consistent finding of a linear deposition of anionic albumin and IgG4 in the diabetic glomerular basement membrane.[241]

Exposure of structural and circulating proteins to high glucose concentrations increases the rate of their nonenzymatic glycosylation.[242,243] Recent studies indicate that microvessels isolated from rat epididymal fat pads preferentially take up glycosylated rat albumin by endocytosis; glycosylation of endothelial membrane components seems to enhance this process of pinocytosis even further.[244] Two recent reports seem to indicate that glycosylated proteins (including albumin) may undergo preferential transport across the glomerular barrier.[245,246] The reason for this facilitated flux of glycosylated macromolecules through the glomerular membrane barrier remains unknown, but it is possible that conformational changes such as those induced by glycosylation are important.[247]

The transition to high selectivity proteinuria signals the advent of heavier proteinuria. This may indicate the critical importance of the loss of the charge barrier in the unfolding sequence of pathogenic events.

Concomitants of Microalbuminuria

The positive association between urine flow and albumin excretion[248,249] has led to the suggestion that glucose-induced diuresis could impair proximal tubular reabsorption of albumin, as it does for several other solutes. However, in the rat, albumin excretion by the kidney is unaffected by osmotic diuresis, whereas it is increased after volume expansion, probably through a change in the GFR.[250] In the diabetic human, there is no correlation between glycosuria and urinary albumin excretion.[93,251] The transient microalbuminuria seen in normal subjects after water loading is likely to be mediated, as in the volume-expanded rat, by transient changes in glomerular filtration rate.[252] Whether acute worsening of glycemia by glucose ingestion or infusion increases AER remains somewhat controversial. Glucose ingestion has been reported to increase albuminuria in normal subjects but not in diabetic patients.[251] A number of other studies have failed to show any acute effect of either oral or intravenous glucose on urinary albumin excretion.[177,253] Mild metabolic acidosis has no effect on urinary albumin excretion but increases the excretion of β_2-microglobulin.[184]

Although a bolus intravenous injection of insulin was reported to increase urinary albumin excretion,[185] these findings have not been reproduced.[186,254] Neither glucagon nor growth hormone affect urinary albumin excretion in normal or in diabetic subjects.[191,192,195,196]

A consistent association of microalbuminuria is found with higher levels of arterial pressure (Fig. 40–5). A positive, linear and independent correlation between arterial pressure and AER has been confirmed by several investigators.[99,140] Furthermore, changes in blood pressure have been shown to be positively correlated to changes in AER in a prospective study.[131] This association is much closer than that between AER and blood glucose level and is independent of a number of other variables, including age, duration of diabetes, body mass index, sex, and blood glucose level itself. The observation of higher arterial pressures in microalbuminuric patients without reduced GFR speaks against the assumption that the higher blood pressure is a consequence of renal dysfunction and argues in favor of a more complex relationship. This raises the possibility either that the rise in blood pressure could be contributory to the renal disease or, alternatively, that microalbuminuria and high blood pressure may be related to a common determinant. It is of interest that microalbuminuric patients with elevation of arterial pressure show significantly more marked mesangial expansion than do patients with a similar duration of diabetes but with a lower AER and arterial pressure.[121]

Tubular Function

Changes in tubular function take place early in the course of IDDM, and all are related to the degree of metabolic control. Both the maximal rates of glucose reabsorption and the absolute rates of sodium reabsorption are elevated in these patients.[178] The increase in sodium reabsorption is probably due, at least in part, to its proximal tubular cotransport with glucose.[255] It has been suggested that enhanced proximal tubular reabsorption could diminish distal sodium delivery and thereby trigger tubulo-glomerular feedback mechanisms that would lead to an increase in glomerular filtration rate.[256] A direct effect of insulin—that of increasing distal sodium reabsorption—has been shown in both normal[187] and diabetic patients.[188] A number of tubular proteins, such as N-acetyl-β-D-glucosaminidase (NAG), have also been found to be increased in patients with IDDM, the elevation being related to the degree of glycemic control.[257,258] On the other hand, tubular phosphate absorption is diminished in patients with IDDM. The defect in phosphate reabsorption also appears to be related to blood glucose concentration. It has been proposed that there is a competition between these two solutes for tubular reabsorption.[259] Insulin has been shown to reduce the renal clearance of phosphate by stimulating its proximal reabsorption.[187,188] These abnormalities are rapidly corrected by improvement of blood glucose control, and their prospective significance for renal function outcome is largely unknown.

Late Functional Changes

Glomerular Filtration Rate

In established diabetic nephropathy, GFR declines relentlessly towards end-stage renal failure. The reduction in GFR is accompanied by a reduction in renal plasma flow, the filtration fraction remaining relatively constant.[232] Advancing renal disease is associated with progressive mesangial expansion and capillary occlusion. This process, by reducing filtering surface area, would be compatible with the suggestion that a reduction in the ultrafiltration coefficient contributes to the decline in GFR.[260] Although direct measurements of these variables are not possible in humans, indirect calculations, using neutral dextran sieving curves, support this view.[232,261] It is believed that in established renal disease the surviving glomeruli filter at or near their maximal capacity. This assumption is consistent with findings that administration of an oral protein load did not induce a further expansion of GFR over baseline values in diabetic patients with impaired renal function.[264] This loss of "renal functional reserve" has been suggested as one of the possible deleterious mechanisms that would lead to further renal damage. However, it seems more likely that this is a result not of a general loss of renal reserve but rather of a more

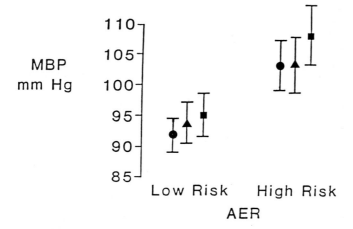

Fig. 40–5. Mean blood pressure (MBP) in patients with insulin-dependent diabetes with albumin excretion rate (AER) in the normal range (low-risk) and in the microalbuminuric range (high-risk). Data are from Wiseman et al.[140] (solid circle); Mathiesen et al.[99] (solid triangle); and Mogensen and Christensen[88] (solid square).

specific defect in the renal response to protein loading, as other stimuli have been shown to have profound effects on the GFR in patients with diabetic renal failure. Hyperglycemia, for instance, has been shown to induce a GFR rise of about 50% in these patients.[263] This glucose-induced effect seems to be mediated by changes in renal prostaglandin production, as it can be significantly blunted by cyclo-oxygenase inhibition.[246] Whether in the setting of renal failure the higher GFR that accompanies hyperglycemia represents an advantage or a disadvantage in the long-term remains an open question. It is worth noting that correction of hyperglycemia at this advanced stage of renal disease has no significant impact on the progression of renal failure.[125,131]

Clinical Proteinuria

As the degree of proteinuria progresses, a change from high- to low-selectivity proteinuria takes place. As the degree of proteinuria progresses and the GFR falls, more IgG relative to albumin is filtered, inducing a change from high- to low-selectivity proteinuria.[229] Studies of neutral dextran sieving curves have demonstrated that the proteinuria of the late stages of overt nephropathy is most likely the result of a defect in size selectivity of the glomerular membrane. The fractional clearance of neutral molecules with radii >4.6 nm is elevated, and mathematical analysis indicates that this increase is consistent with the appearance of a "shunt pathway" within the glomerular capillary wall. The development of a small population of unselective pores would allow the unrestricted movement of very large plasma proteins into the urine. Whether the defect in size selectivity completely explains the proteinuria of advanced nephropathy remains to be established.[228,238,261] It is likely that charge selectivity de-

fects as well as abnormal renal hemodynamics persist at this stage of advanced nephropathy. It is of interest that the sialic acid component of the glomerular barrier has been found to be reduced in patients with long-standing diabetes.[231,265,266] Moreover, a reduction in the synthesis of heparan sulfate within the glomerular basement membrane has been described in diabetic animals,[233,236,267–269] and a loss of heparan sulfate has been demonstrated in the glomerular basement membrane of IDDM patients with nephropathy.[270] This glycosaminoglycan is a major contributor of the fixed negative charge of the glomerular capillary wall.

Hyperlipidemia

With advancing renal disease, clear disturbances of plasma lipoproteins take place. Increases in cholesterol, low-density lipoprotein (LDL)-cholesterol, total triglycerides, very low-density lipoprotein (VLDL)-triglyceride and apolipoprotein-B1 have been described, and high-density lipoprotein 2 (HDL_2)-cholesterol has been found to be decreased.[271–274] The pathogenic role of these lipid disturbances in the progression of renal failure in human diabetes remain uncertain. However, studies in the Zucker rats (diabetic animal model) suggest that hyperlipidemia may contribute to late glomerular sclerotic changes.[275] Recent findings suggest that these lipid changes may not entirely be secondary to heavy proteinuria and advancing renal disease. Microalbuminuric patients with either IDDM[276,277] or NIDDM[278] with normal renal function have also been found to have a similar pattern of lipid abnormalities, though of a lesser degree (Fig. 40–6). It is clearly important now to establish the potential of early correction of the lipid disturbances for prevention of the deterioration of renal function as well as of histologic damage.

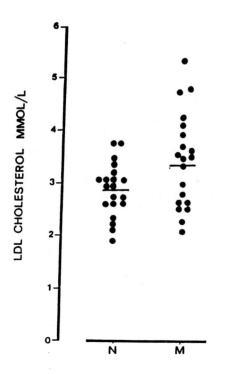

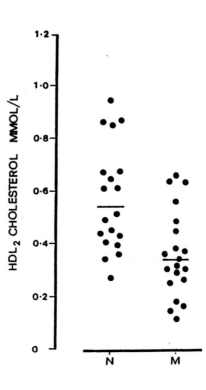

Fig. 40–6. Serum concentration of low-density lipoprotein (LDL) and high-density lipoprotein (HDL) cholesterol in 20 patients with insulin-dependent diabetes with microalbuminuria (M) and 20 matched patients with insulin-dependent diabetes with normoalbuminuria (N). Horizontal bars indicate geometric means.

PATHOGENESIS

Metabolic Pathways

Hyperglycemia

There is no doubt that a positive relationship between the abnormal glycemic milieu of diabetes and microvascular complications does exist. The view that small vessel disease, and particularly abnormalities in capillary basement membrane thickness, are primarily an inherited phenomenon[279] has been negated by an overwhelming body of evidence linking hyperglycemia to diabetic complications.[280,281] Small vessel complications can be found in secondary diabetes in humans[282,283] and in a variety of types of chemically induced and genetic diabetes in the animal model.[284] In the kidney, histologic lesions such as mesangial expansion may be reversed by the transplantation of a diabetic kidney into a normal animal[285] or by correcting diabetes with islet cell transplantation.[172,286,287] Moreover, in the rat model, renal histologic lesions[82,288] and albuminuria[289] can be prevented by near-normalization of blood glucose with intensified insulin treatment from the time of induction of diabetes.

There are, however, two important aspects to consider. The animal model most frequently used for the study of diabetic nephropathy is the rat. This animal does not develop advanced renal failure and severe histologic lesions such as those seen in the human with diabetes, and there are considerable species differences in the glomerular hemodynamic responses to different glycemic levels, making extrapolation of data to humans difficult.[284,290] In addition, the strains of rats used as models of chemically induced or genetic diabetes are highly inbred, a condition that is unrepresentative of the genetic heterogeneity encountered in human diabetes.

Indeed, in humans the evidence of a straightforward causal relationship between hyperglycemia and renal disease is less compelling than it is in the animal model. The development of clinically overt renal disease is not linearly related to the duration of diabetes and affects only between 35 and 50% of patients. The majority of patients with diabetes escape renal failure, and although some histologic damage occurs in their kidneys, their renal function remains essentially normal until death. Kidneys from nondiabetic human donors develop typical lesions of diabetic glomerulopathy when they are transplanted into a diabetic recipient,[291] but the rate of development of the lesions varies greatly in a manner independent of the blood glucose control over the years.[292] It therefore appears that in humans hyperglycemia is necessary but not sufficient to cause the renal damage that leads to kidney failure, and that other, possibly nonenvironmental, factors are needed for the manifestation of the clinical syndrome.

Nonenzymatic Glycosylation

The reaction between glucose and the lysine aminoterminal of circulating and structural proteins gives rise to glycosylation products by a nonenzymatic process.[293]

Two major classes of glycosylated products have been identified according to the half-life of the protein involved. Relatively short-lived proteins form a Schiff base, which undergoes an Amadori rearrangement, with the formation of a stable, but still chemically reversible, sugar-protein adduct. Structural proteins with a slower turnover, such as collagen, myelin, crystallins, and elastin, accumulate different products derived from slow reactions of dehydration, degradation, and rearrangement of the Amadori adducts to form chemically irreversible advanced glycosylation end-products.[293,294] Nonenzymatic glycosylation is thus likely to affect the glomerular basement membrane and other matrix components in the glomerulus.

The pathophysiologic consequences of this process are unsettled, but several possibilities have been suggested. Excess glomerular basement membrane glycosylation, as seen in diabetes, may lead to an increase in the degree of cross-linking of disulfide bridges between collagen components via increased oxidation of sulfhydryl groups. This process may induce molecular rearrangement and has been implicated in cataract formation in the lens.[295] Similar cross-linking by disulfide bonds might affect the assembly and architecture of the glomerular basement membrane and mesangial matrix. It has also been shown that advanced glycosylation end-products are capable of extensive cross-linking throughout the collagen molecule. Rotary shadowing electron microscopy of glycosylated basement membrane components has revealed increased collagen IV cross-linking and altered molecular morphology.[294] It is noteworthy that the compound aminoguanidine, which blocks the formation of advanced glycosylation end-products, has been shown to prevent, in Lewis alloxan-diabetic rats, both the increased aortic collagen cross-linking and the cross-linking of collagen to lipoproteins, as well as the thickening of glomerular basement membrane and the glomerular trapping of IgG molecules.[294]

However, the pathogenic consequences of enhanced cross-linking in the kidney remain obscure. The reaction of glycosylation may theoretically enhance the binding of circulating plasma proteins to structural components in the glomerular basement membrane and mesangial matrix by the presence of the reactive carbonyl group on the glucose attached to these structures. It has been suggested that this increased binding may account for the linear deposition of albumin and IgG observed along glomerular and tubular basement membranes in diabetes.[296] Glycosylation of structural proteins or of circulating proteins trapped in the glomerular structures may interfere with their degradation. Degradation of fibrin by plasmin has been found to be reduced by glycosylation.[297] Reduced degradation of glomerular components may result in accumulation and expansion of mesangial matrix and glomerular basement membrane. Other glycoproteins, such as fibronectin, which are found in the mesangial matrix and are involved in the control of cell growth, replication, and adhesion, are also susceptible to nonenzymatic glycosylation. This process has been shown to interfere in vitro with the binding characteristics of fibronectin, inhibiting its adhesion to matrix components[298] and enhancing its binding to glomerular basement membrane.[299] In vivo this phenomenon may result in alterations in the integrity and adhesive properties of the matrix and promote the development of defects in the selectivity properties of the capillary barrier. It has been claimed that an alteration of the charge distribution of glycosylated albumin could provide a mechanism for the abnormal flux of modified albumin across the glomerular membrane.[245] However, these results have not been confirmed by Nakamura and Myers,[238] who were unable to show differences in the isoelectric point distribution of glycosylated and nonglycosylated albumin. Recently, a membrane-associated macrophage receptor that specifically recognizes advanced glycosylation end-products in proteins has been identified.[300] This receptor enables the selective removal of senescent cross-linked denatured proteins. The binding of this receptor to protein with advanced glycosylation end-products induces synthesis by macrophages of monokines (interleukin-1 and tumor necrosis factor), which in turn stimulate nearby mesenchymal cells to synthesize extracellular proteases. These monokines also initiate a cascade of stimuli and interactions whose end-result is increased protein synthesis and cell proliferation and, in the endothelium, an increased vascular permeability.[294]

In conclusion, excessive formation of glycosylation products in the glomerulus may lead to enhancement in deposition of basement membrane-like material and circulating proteins in the mesangium, interference with mesangial clearance mechanisms, and alterations in the macrophage removal system and so contribute to mesangial expansion and glomerular occlusion.

The Polyol Pathway

Sorbitol is produced in cells from glucose by a reaction catalyzed by aldose reductase. In the normal kidney, aldose reductase is present in the papilla, glomerular epithelial cells, distal tubular cells, and probably mesangial cells.[301,302] In many tissues, the physiologic significance of aldose reductase is difficult to define, but in the renal medullary cells of the kidney, its primary role seems to be in the generation of sorbitol, an organic osmolyte, in response to the high salinity in the medullary interstitium. Sorbitol would aid in preventing osmotic stress.[303] It has been argued that, in tissues in which glucose entry into cells is insulin-independent, more glucose becomes available for reduction by aldose reductase, resulting in an increased concentration of sorbitol and/or a reduced intracellular concentration of myoinositol. These changes might contribute to diabetic complications, via an upset of cellular osmoregulation.[304,305] Depletion of tissue myoinositol has been observed in association with enhanced activity of the polyol pathway in sciatic nerve, lens, retina, and glomeruli of humans and animals.[306]

A series of trials has been carried out with various aldose reductase inhibitors, with the aim of blocking the intracellular conversion of glucose to sorbitol and thus of preventing some complications of diabetes. In glomeruli obtained from diabetic rats, the increased flux through the polyol pathway, with accumulation of sorbitol, depletion of myoinositol, and reduced Na^+/K^+-ATPase activity, has been shown to be preventable by the administration of the aldose reductase inhibitor sorbinil. The increased GFR and proteinuria in rats with streptozocin-induced diabetes have also been reported to be reduced by inhibitors of aldose reductase or by supplementation of myoinositol.[307-309] These studies, however, were not confirmed by a more recent report and have been criticized because large volumes of saline were infused during clearance studies, kidney hemodynamics were factored for body-weight, diabetes was of short-duration, and total urinary protein rather than albumin was measured.[310] There is some evidence that renal clearance of low-molecular-weight proteins may be affected to a greater degree by sorbinil than is the clearance of proteins the size of albumin or larger, which more directly reflect the glomerular barrier permeability function.[309] It has also been suggested that sorbinil may act as a vasoconstrictor[311,312] and lower renal prostaglandin synthesis,[313] thereby modifying renal hemodynamics independently of the aldose reductase pathway. It is of interest that sulindac, a potent inhibitor of prostanoid synthesis, also blocks aldose reductase, suggesting that the action of certain aldose-reductase inhibitors may be similar to that of nonsteroidal anti-inflammatory drugs.[314] Although sorbinil has been shown to prevent renal hypertrophy in galactose-fed rats,[315] all authors concur that aldose reductase inhibitors have no effect on the increased kidney weight in animals with streptozotocin-induced diabetes. Moreover, in the rat, the histologic lesions of glomerular disease after 6 months of diabetes were unaffected by the administration of statil, another aldose reductase inhibitor.[316]

In contrast with these data showing the relative inefficacy of statil on renal function and structure is the report of Tilton et al.,[317] who found, using three different aldose reductase inhibitors, a reduction in the clearance of ^{51}Cr-ethylenediamine tetraacetic acid (EDTA), in albuminuria, and in the permeation of ^{125}I-bovine serum albumin into the vascular wall in the streptozotocin-diabetic Sprague-Dawley rat. These authors concluded that "virtually all of the early functional and structural renal and vascular changes associated with diabetes in animals are aldose reductase-linked phenomena." The same group has also shown that myoinositol-supplemented diets that raise plasma myoinositol levels by fivefold reduce or normalize GFR, renal blood flow, urinary protein excretion, and serum albumin permeation of blood vessels.[306]

This diversity of effects of aldose-reductase inhibitors persists in the few studies carried out in humans. Reductions of GFR[318] and AER[319] in patients with IDDM have been claimed, but no effects have been reported in a controlled study of microalbuminuric patients with NIDDM.[320]

Biochemical Abnormalities of Extracellular Matrix

Diabetic glomerulopathy is characterized by an excessive accumulation of glomerular basement membrane and mesangial matrix. Studies in diabetic animals suggest that the rates of synthesis of matrix and glomerular basement membrane are significantly accelerated. Collagen represents a major component of extracellular membranes, and its biosynthesis, measured by the incorporation of radiolabeled amino acids, has been shown to be increased in diabetic rats.[321] The activity of lysylhydroxylase, an enzyme involved in the hydroxylation of peptide-bound lysine during collagen biosynthesis,[322] has been found to be increased in the glomeruli of diabetic rats. These abnormalities can be prevented by insulin therapy initiated at the time of induction of diabetes.

Synthesis of the non-collagenous moieties of the glomerular basement membrane and glomerular basement membrane-like material can be measured by the rates of incorporation of glucosamine, galactose, and sulfates into glomerular basement membrane sialoglycoproteins and glycosaminoglycans, its two major carbohydrate constituents. Glycosaminoglycan (GAG) polysaccharides account for approximately 90% of the total carbohydrate component of the glomerular basement membrane, with sialoproteins constituting the remainder. The principal GAG in the glomerular basement membrane is heparan sulfate, which, together with sialic acid, contributes to the negative charge of the glomerular capillary wall and thereby to the charge selectivity properties of the filtration barrier.[225,323] In diabetes there is reduced de novo synthesis of glomerular heparan sulfate, and the total GAG content in the glomerulus and glomerular basement membrane is reduced.[233,236,267–269] The heparan sulfate content of the glomerular basement membrane has been found to be decreased in patients with IDDM with nephropathy.[270] Moreover, findings in studies of both diabetic humans and experimental diabetic animals have also consistently reported a reduction in sialic acid components.[231,265,266] Sialoglycoproteins are highly negatively charged and coat glomerular epithelial cells, their foot processes, and the epithelial slit diaphragm. A loss of negative charge of the glomerular membrane may be responsible for foot process fusion, with consequent obliteration of the slit diaphragm, and could partly explain the albuminuria of diabetic nephropathy (see Pathology section).

Abnormalities in carbohydrate components of the glomerular basement membrane in diabetes remain more controversial. An increase in the hydroxylysine content of the glomerular basement membrane, as well as in the glucose and galactose disaccharide units attached to hydroxylysine residues, has been described. Elevated activity of the enzyme glycosyltransferase, responsible for the attachment of glucose to the glycoprotein, has also been reported. A number of other studies, however, have failed to confirm these findings.[231,265,266,324–326]

Glucotoxicity

Direct pathogenetic effects of glucose itself have only recently been described. Lorenzi et al.[327,328] have demonstrated convincingly that cultured human endothelial cells, after prolonged, although not acute, exposure to high ambient glucose concentrations, display consistent alterations in cell replication and maturation, which cannot be ascribed to abnormalities of the polyol pathway.[329] These abnormalities in cultured endothelial cells are associated with evidence of damage to DNA,[330] which has also been demonstrated in peripheral blood lymphocytes from patients with poorly controlled diabetes but not from those with better control.[331] Furthermore, high glucose concentrations can be shown to enhance the expression in cultured endothelial cells of those glycoproteins characteristically increased in diabetic basement membrane.[332] Similarly, cultured human endothelial cells show abnormal expression of tissue factor mRNA in response to thrombin and interleukin-1 after prolonged exposure to high glucose concentrations.[333]

Whether glucose exerts a direct toxic effect on human endothelial cells in vivo is currently unknown, but it is of interest that abnormalities of endothelial cell function have been implicated in the increased frequency of cardiovascular disease that is a feature of diabetic nephropathy. It has been shown that such abnormalities, evidenced by raised plasma levels of von Willebrand factor[334] and decreased release of tissue plasminogen activator in response to exercise,[335] are present even before overt nephropathy develops.

Hemodynamic and Hypertrophic Pathways

Glomerular hemodynamic disturbances with elevations of flows and pressures occur early in the course of diabetes. These alterations have been suggested to be directly responsible for the development of glomerulosclerosis and its attendant proteinuria.[235] The notion that increments in GFR, renal plasma flow, and glomerular capillary hydraulic pressure produce diabetic glomerular injury is based on several observations. Mesangial expansion and mesangial accumulation of circulating plasma proteins were found to be greater in uninephrectomized diabetic rats, in whom abnormalities of renal hemodynamics are known to occur, than in control animals without unilateral nephrectomy,[336] suggesting that altered microcirculatory dynamics may affect the rate of development of glomerular lesions. The induction of systemic hypertension in the diabetic rat, by the two-kidney one-clip Goldblatt hypertension model, resulted in the development of much more severe glomerular lesions in the unclipped kidney than in the kidneys of normotensive diabetic control animals.[337] The clipped kidney showed lesser degrees of glomerular damage than the kidney of diabetic control rats. Autopsy findings for two diabetic men with hypertension and unilateral renal artery stenosis showed that nodular glomerulosclerotic lesions were confined to the kidney with the patent renal artery, while the contralateral kidney was spared.[338,339] Finally, in the diabetic animal model, maneuvers that lessen disturbed renal hemodynamics, such as low protein diet or inhibition of converting enzyme, have been shown to prevent the increase in urinary albumin excretion and the glomerular histologic lesions that occur in the untreated diabetic control animal.[166,340,343]

How alterations in the set of glomerular hemodynamic forces lead to mesangial expansion, glomerular basement membrane thickening, and eventual sclerosis is uncertain, but several suggestions have been made. Elevated intraglomerular pressure may lead to an increase in the number of mesangial cells and in matrix production and to thickening of the glomerular basement membrane via an increase in arteriolar or capillary wall tension, as noted in smooth muscle cells exposed to higher pressures.[235,342,343] Physical stress and shear forces may damage endothelial and epithelial surfaces and disrupt the normal glomerular barrier, again by analogy to what is believed to occur at sites of turbulence in larger arteries in systemic hypertension.[344-346] The proteinuria associated with disruption of the normal glomerular barrier would lead to accumulation and deposition of plasma proteins and lipoproteins in the mesangial area. Their persistence because of reduced mesangial clearance of protein in diabetes[347] might act as a local stimulus for more mesangial matrix production and accumulation.[348-350]

The evidence that alterations in local physical forces within the glomerulus lead to later sclerotic changes in diabetes is, however, debatable and has recently been questioned.[351] A dissociation between the hemodynamic changes and the subsequent sclerosis has been reported in a number of studies. Severely hyperglycemic rats develop renal sclerotic changes[352] even though they have no evidence of raised pressures and flows early in the course of diabetes.[165] Bank et al.,[353] in a study of two strains of diabetic rats, found no relationship between levels of glomerular hyperfiltration and pressure and subsequent degree of glomerular sclerosis. The lowering of high lipid levels in the Zucker rat model has been reported to protect against renal sclerosis without affecting hemodynamics.[275] Moreover, maneuvers that affect renal hemodynamics also have marked effects on other cell functions. Unilateral nephrectomy, for instance, is a potent stimulus for glomerular hypertrophy and hyperplasia,[354] and Goldblatt hypertension leads to (compensatory) hypertrophy in the unclipped kidney.[355] Hypertrophic changes in the glomerulus have been shown to be invariably related to subsequent glomerular sclerosis.[351] It is of interest that marked renal hypertrophy is a very early event in diabetes. Treatments that modify renal hemodynamics and the degree of glomerular sclerosis also affect the accompanying glomerular hypertrophy. Low-protein diets and inhibitors of angiotensin-converting enzyme significantly attenuate the renal hypertrophy associated with nephrectomy or streptozotocin-induced diabetes.[356] In certain animal models of renal disease, reduction of hypertrophic and sclerotic changes has been obtained independently of modification of renal hemodynamics, and agents that affect glomerular and mesangial cell proliferation but are not known to have hemodynamic effects have been shown to ameliorate glomerular sclerosis.[357-364] It has been argued that hyperplastic and hypertrophic changes in the diabetic kidney precede the hemodynamic abnormalities.[217] Hypertrophic factors in diabetes may activate mesangial cell proliferation and augment mesangial matrix formation or suppress matrix degradation, giving rise to the histologic alterations that are pathognomonic of diabetic glomerulopathy. Perhaps

one of the clearest demonstrations linking glomerular hypertrophy to subsequent sclerosis has been obtained with the use of transgenic mice with chronic overexpression of growth hormone and growth hormone-releasing factor. These animals develop early enlargement of the glomerulus, which is followed by glomerulosclerosis.[365]

Familial/Genetic Pathways

In human diabetic renal disease, however, a central question remains to be answered. Why do only a proportion of diabetic patients develop renal failure? If a diabetes-induced abnormality in systemic or local growth promoters or in hemodynamic forces were sufficient to cause renal damage, all patients would develop overt renal disease given time. But this is not the case.

Diabetes induces important metabolic, hormonal, and growth factor changes. These changes, which are related in part to the degree of glycemic control, occur in virtually all patients, but, to date, it has been impossible to isolate a subset of individuals in whom the severity of these environmental perturbations is convincingly linked to the development of renal complications. On the contrary, there is ever-growing evidence that the degree of diabetic control is only a necessary component but is not linearly related to the development of renal failure. Moreover, there is the consistent observation in humans that early renal hypertrophic and hemodynamic changes occur only in a subgroup of subjects. To explain the susceptibility to renal failure in this subgroup, it is therefore necessary to formulate an alternative hypothesis that takes into account the host response to diabetes-induced environmental disturbances.

Familial clustering of diabetic kidney disease has been reported. In IDDM 83% of diabetic siblings of probands with diabetic nephropathy have evidence of nephropathy, compared with only 17% of diabetic siblings of probands without nephropathy, a significant fivefold difference.[366] (Table 40-3). A familial influence on development of nephropathy has also been described in

Table 40-3. Prevalence of Diabetic Kidney Disease (End-Stage Renal Failure and Elevated Albumin Excretion Rate) in Diabetic Siblings of Patients with Insulin-Dependent Diabetes with and without Nephropathy

	No. (%) of Siblings	
Kidney Function	Patients With Nephropathy	Patients Without Nephropathy
End-stage renal failure	12 (41.4)	0 (0)*
Raised albumin excretion rate (≥45 mg/24 hr)	12 (41.4)	2 (17)*
Normal albumin excretion rate (<45 mg/24 hr)	5 (17.2)	10 (83)*

Table is adapted from Seaquist et al.[366]
*P <.01.

Pima Indians with NIDDM.[44] The findings of these studies are consistent with the postulate that inherited factors play an important role in determining susceptibility to diabetic nephropathy but do not provide insight into the nature of these factors. A familial predisposition to raised arterial pressure has been suggested, by some—though not all—reports, as a possible contributing factor to the susceptibility to nephropathy in diabetes.[367-369] Parents of patients with IDDM who have proteinuria were found to have significantly higher arterial pressure or a higher prevalence of hypertension than matched parents of nonproteinuric patients with IDDM (Table 40–4). More recently, familial clustering of cardiovascular disease has been found in patients with IDDM and nephropathy, and a parental history of cardiovascular disease has been shown to increase significantly the risk of kidney disease in the diabetic offspring.[370]

Further insight into the predisposition to and mechanisms of diabetic renal disease, and possibly the attendant cardiovascular disease, has come from studies of red cell sodium-lithium countertransport, a cell membrane cation transport system whose activity is determined largely genetically and whose elevated rates are associated with essential hypertension.[371,372] The rates of sodium-lithium countertransport have been found to be higher in proteinuric patients with diabetes and their parents than in matched long-term normoalbuminuric controls[368,369,373,374] (Fig. 40–7). The risk of nephropathy seems to be magnified by the combination of a history of poor glycemic control and the possession of high sodium-lithium countertransport activity[368] (Fig. 40–8). Microalbuminuric diabetic patients, a group at increased risk of overt nephropathy, have also been found to have higher rates of sodium-lithium countertransport.[375] Moreover, an association has been described between plasma lipoprotein levels and sodium-lithium countertransport activity in patients with IDDM without persistent clinical proteinuria. Higher rates of countertransport were associated with elevated LDL cholesterol, total and VLDL triglycerides, and reduced HDL_2 cholesterol concentrations.[376] The mechanisms of the association between sodium-lithium countertransport activity, hypertension, and lipid abnormalities in the context of

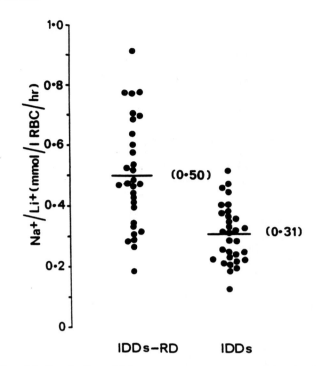

Fig. 40–7. Sodium-lithium countertransport activity in 31 (18M, 13F) patients with insulin-dependent diabetes with diabetic renal disease (IDDs-RD) and in 31 (16M,15F) age-matched (36 ± 10 vs. 35 ± 11 years) and diabetes duration-matched (23 ± 9 vs. 20 ± 7 years) patients with insulin-dependent diabetes without renal disease (IDDs) ($P < .001$).

susceptibility to diabetic renal and vascular disease are unclear, but they could be related to factors involved in the control of insulin sensitivity.[376] In a study of short-term, nonclinically proteinuric diabetic patients with arterial hypertension (blood pressure >140/90 mm Hg), the hypertensive patients with higher rates of sodium-lithium countertransport were more insulin-resistant and in addition had higher rates of albumin excretion, increased total body exchangeable sodium, enlarged kidneys, and left ventricular hypertrophy.[377] These associations were independent of the actual level of blood pressure or the duration of arterial hypertension. These findings suggest that it is the diabetic hypertensive patient with high sodium-lithium countertransport who displays those features (i.e., albuminuria, left ventricular and renal hypertrophy, and insulin resistance) that have been related to renal and vascular injury.[121,378-380] This combination of risk factors may not be confined to the diabetic population but may be a manifestation of a syndrome also described in the general population.[381]

Sodium-lithium countertransport shares certain similarities with the physiologic sodium-hydrogen antiport, a system crucial in the control of intracellular pH, cell growth, and the renal reabsorption of sodium and thus in the regulation of blood pressure.[382] Recently, leukocytes and cultured skin fibroblasts from IDDM patients with albuminuria have been reported to have elevated sodium-hydrogen antiport activity.[383,384] Moreover, an increased [³H]thymidine incorporation into DNA of skin fibroblasts

Table 40–4. Blood Pressure (BP) and Frequency of Hypertension in Parents of Patients with Insulin-Dependent Diabetes with and without Nephropathy (DN)

	Parents of Patients With DN	Parents of Patients Without DN
Systolic BP (mm Hg; mean ± SD)	161 ± 27	146 ± 21*
Diastolic BP (mm Hg; mean ± SD)	94 ± 14	86 ± 11†
Frequency of hypertension (%)	77	45†

Table is adapted from Viberti et al.[367] and Krolewski et al.[368]
*$P < .02$.
†$P < .05$.

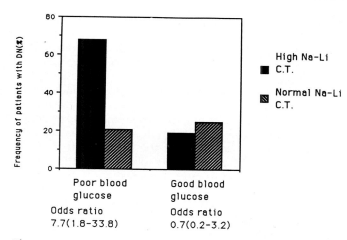

Fig. 40−8. Frequency of the development of nephropathy with high (≥0.35 mmol/L of red blood cells per hour) or normal Na⁺-Li⁺ countertransport activity in patients with good or poor blood glucose control. Adapted from Krolewski et al.[368]

of diabetic patients with nephropathy has been documented.[383] These findings are consistent with the view that cells of diabetic patients who develop nephropathy have an intrinsic enhanced capacity to proliferate and that this phenomenon is associated with high rates of sodium-hydrogen exchanger activity. Of note is the association of phases of growth of the entire body, such as puberty in humans, with insulin resistance.[385] Thus, the activity of the sodium-hydrogen antiport seems to act as an indicator of some mechanism, possibly genetically determined, controlling cell growth and hypertrophy on the one hand and intracellular sodium homeostasis on the other. The environmental changes brought about by diabetes could lead to dysregulation of these mechanisms in susceptible individuals and induce cell hypertrophy and hyperplasia contributing to glomerular hypertrophy and mesangial expansion in the kidney, as well as tubular hypertrophy and hyperplasia. Increased renal sodium reabsorption would augment systemic and renal perfusion pressure to maintain sodium balance. The increased perfusion pressure would be readily transmitted to the glomerular capillaries because of the general vasodilation present in diabetes.[386] This would lead to increased intraglomerular pressure, which determines, at least in part, the increase in GFR and may be responsible for the disruption of glomerular membrane permeability properties generating proteinuria. On the other hand, progressive mesangial expansion would lead to glomerulosclerosis and further disruption of glomerular basement membrane permeability selective properties. The insulin resistance associated with excessive growth and the consequent hyperinsulinemia may cause lipid abnormalities that, in the setting of the vascular hyperpermeability characteristic of diabetic microvascular disease,[387] would further aggravate the renal histologic damage[388] and contribute, in combination with hypertension, to the accelerated atherosclerosis of diabetic renal failure. That insulin resistance is associated with increased cardiovascular events has been reported with regard to the general

population.[389] The sequence of phenomena just described could trigger a vicious cycle of events producing reduction in renal function, more hypertension, more proteinuria, more severe glomerulosclerosis, more hyperlipidemia, and eventually renal failure and cardiovascular death (Fig. 40−9).

PATHOLOGY

The renal morphologic changes associated with diabetes mellitus were first described in 1936 by Kimmelstiel and Wilson.[5] In the early 1940s these findings were confirmed and extended by other workers.[390,391] Both the early autopsy and biopsy series and later studies[155,392] have shown that the histologic findings in kidneys of patients with IDDM and NIDDM are similar.

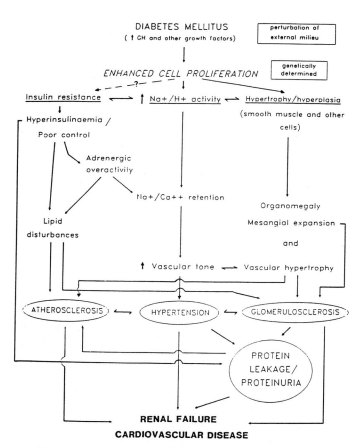

Fig 40−9. Hypothetical diagrammatic representation of a sequence of events leading to the development of renal and cardiovascular disease in a subset of susceptible patients with insulin-dependent diabetes (IDDM). It is speculative at present whether insulin resistance follows from an enhanced cell proliferation (thus the broken line and question mark). A primary role for insulin resistance has been advocated by other authors. Insulin resistance in these patients with IDDM would lead to an increased requirement for exogenous insulin and thus to hyperinsulinemia. Whether this sequence of events would apply to patients with non-insulin-dependent diabetes is presently unknown. In the latter situation, insulin resistance would lead to hyperinsulinemia from an endogenous source.

Light Microscopy

The nodular lesion described by Kimmelstiel and Wilson in 1936[5] has for a long time been considered virtually specific for diabetes.[158,159] Reports that it could be found in the absence of diabetes have not withstood critical review,[393] and some patients may have had the nodular form of light-chain nephropathy.

The nodules are well-demarcated hard masses, eosinophilic and periodic acid-Schiff (PAS)-positive, located in the central regions of peripheral glomerular lobules (Fig. 40–10). When not acellular they contain pyknotic nuclei, and not infrequently foam cells can be seen surrounding them. Relatively homogeneous when stained with hematoxylin, their structure is laminated when viewed in preparations with PAS or reticulin stains. They are characteristically irregular in size and distribution, both within and between glomerular loops, and located away from the hilus. A rim of mesangial cells can sometimes be seen between them and the adjoining capillary, which is often distended. The location and the morphogenesis of the nodules have been the subject of long dispute, as reflected by the use of both terms "intracapillary" and "intercapillary" to describe them. Recent evidence[394] seems to establish the mesangium as their site of origin and extends the original suggestion that mesangial disruption and lysis of the lobule center was related to prior microaneurysmal dilatation of the associated capillary, followed by a laminar reorganization of the mesangial debris.[395]

Although, when present, this lesion is pathognomonic for diabetes, it is a far from universal finding. Its incidence varies considerably from 12 to 46% in different series, which included both IDDM and NIDDM cases, probably because of differences in selection.[396] Nodules have been found in 55% of an autopsy series of Pima Indian patients with NIDDM.[392] Nodules are not seen in the absence of the diffuse lesion, and this reflects their appearance only after a long period of disease (14 years in the series of Gellman et al.[160]).

The diffuse glomerular lesion comprises an increase of the mesangial area and capillary wall thickening, with the mesangial matrix extending to involve the capillary loops (Fig. 40–11). The accumulated material has staining properties similar to those of the nodules. In its early stages it may be difficult to distinguish the minor mesangial expansion from changes present with aging or from other glomerular pathology.[145] In more severe cases, the capillary wall thickening and the mesangial expansion lead to capillary narrowing and eventually to complete hyalinization. In this advanced state, periglomerular fibrosis is often present. As with the nodules, the distribution of the diffuse lesion is non-uniform, both among lobules of the same glomerulus and between different glomeruli, leading to appearances suggestive of transition to nodule formation. The thickening of the capillary walls tends also to be non-uniform, and this is particularly evident when the histologic changes are not very severe. This lesion is more frequent than the nodular one, but again its incidence varies in different series.[396] In a large autopsy study, however, changes compatible with diabetic glomerulosclerosis were found in as many as 90% of patients with IDDM with disease duration of more than 10 years.[146] In patients with NIDDM, the reported prevalences of these changes ranges between 25 and 51%.[78,158,396]

The exudative lesions are highly eosinophilic, rounded homogeneous structures seen in the capsular space, overlying a capillary loop (fibrin cap) or lying on the inside of Bowman's capsule (capsular drop). They are

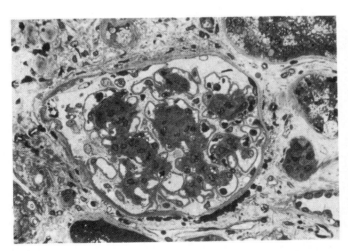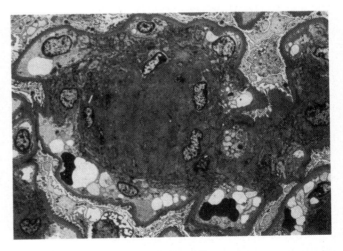

Fig. 40–10. Left: A nodular lesion in a 54-year-old with insulin-dependent diabetes. The mesangium shows enormous expansion with relatively acellular masses of material, with preservation of the patency of surrounding capillary loops and of the glomerular capillary walls (toluidine blue; original magnification ×400). Right: Electron microscopy shows again the complex texture of the mesangial nodule and its relative acellularity. Only three nuclei are clearly seen; as usual, these are around the periphery of the mass. A developing foam cell can be seen on the left (impregnated with osmium tetroxide and uranyl acetate; original magnification ×8950). Courtesy of Dr. Barrie Hartley, Department of Pathology, Guy's Campus, UMDS, London.

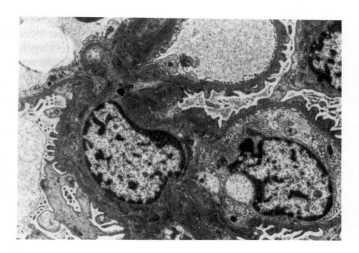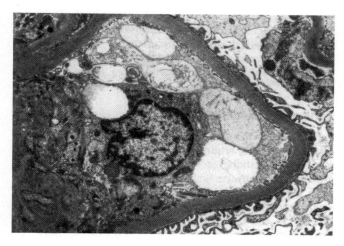

Fig. 40–11.   The diffuse capillary membrane lesion of diabetic nephropathy. Left: A capillary wall of normal thickness (250 to 350 nm) is shown. Right: A capillary loop from a diabetic patient with severe thickening of the capillary basement membrane; the basement membrane is at least twice as thick as normal, with a homogenous texture. Despite proteinuria, the architecture of the podocytes outside the capillary wall is relatively well preserved (impregnated with osmium tetroxide and uranyl acetate; original magnification ×850). Courtesy of Dr. Barrie Hartley, Department of Pathology, Guy's Campus, UMDS, London.

nonspecific, containing various proteins and sometimes lipid material, and similar lesions are seen in a variety of other renal conditions.

In patients with IDDM, an increase in glomerular volume and in luminal volume are noted 1 to 6 years after diagnosis.[397] Whereas the initial glomerular enlargement is not accompanied by hyperplasia, the number of nuclei in patients with 16 or more years of disease is increased and the volume of the patent glomeruli becomes even larger. This late hypertrophy has been considered distinct from the early hypertrophy and may be an expression of compensatory growth in the face of progressive glomerular loss.[398,399] Although atrophic ischemic glomeruli are present, some of the nonfunctioning obsolete glomeruli seem filled up with solid PAS-positive material and preserve their increased dimension. This hypertrophy has not been found in subjects with NIDDM,[400] although hyalinized non-atrophic glomeruli can be seen in these patients.[146]

Arteriolar lesions are prominent in diabetes, with hyaline material progressively replacing the entire wall structure. Bell[158] first underlined that both afferent and efferent arterioles could be affected (Fig. 40–12). He also pointed out that these lesions were often present in the absence of hypertension and that involvement of the efferent vessel was highly specific for diabetes. These arteriolar changes may be the first change detectible by light microscopy in the diabetic kidney, as judged by their recurrence at 2 years in nondiabetic kidneys transplanted into diabetic patients.[401]

The tubules and interstitium may show a variety of changes that are nonspecific and similar to those seen in other forms of progressive renal disease. The Armanni-Ebstein lesion is the result of accumulation of glycogen in tubular cells of the corticomedullary region in patients with profound glycosuria and was common in patients

with IDDM before the advent of insulin. More subtle tubular changes, consisting of vacuolization, a decrease in the intercellular spaces normally present between the macula densa cells, and a significant increase in the contact area between them and the extraglomerular

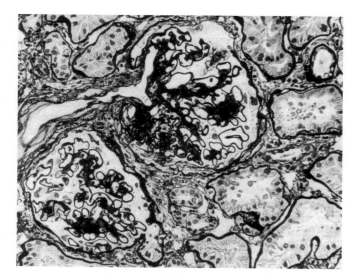

Fig. 40–12.   Cross-section of a glomerulus from a patient with diabetes showing the hilar region. Two arterioles are shown here with hyaline masses within their walls, seen as clear non-argyrophilic spaces. This lesion affecting also the efferent arteriole is believed to be relatively specific for diabetes and may be present in the absence of proteinuria and/or obvious glomerular changes (silver-methenamine/hematoxylin and eosin; original magnification ×250). Courtesy of Dr. Barrie Hartley, Department of Pathology, Guy's Campus, UMDS, London.

mesangial cells of Goormatigh, have been described at the ultrastructural level in the streptozotocin-diabetic rat. It was suggested that these changes may represent a morphologic counterpart to disturbed tubuloglomerular feedback, which might contribute to hyperfiltration in diabetes.[402]

Differential Diagnosis

The histologic changes described, although individually nonspecific, when present simultaneously are highly suggestive of diabetes. The degree of arteriolar hyalinization seen in diabetes is uncommon outside this condition, and its presence in the efferent arteriole has been suggested to be unique to diabetes.[158] Nodular masses similar to the diabetic nodule may be present in other conditions. In mesangiocapillary glomerulonephritis, the nodules tend to be much more evenly distributed, with characteristic loop changes and hypercellularity. In this and in light-chain nephropathy, in which similar nodular masses can be seen, the immunofluorescent findings should establish the diagnosis. In amyloid nephropathy the nodules may be unevenly distributed and the use of specific stains may be necessary to establish the distinction. When nodules are not present, the glomerular changes may have to be distinguished from those present in a number of other renal diseases. Specific stains for amyloid may again be of help. In membranous nephropathy, the thickening of the capillary loops and the degree of glomerular involvement are even, whereas this is rarely the case in diabetes. The differential diagnosis with nonspecific arteriolosclerosis and with the changes of aging may be difficult. In both these conditions, obsolete glomeruli tend to be reduced in size, whereas in diabetes large hyalinized glomeruli often are seen.

Immunopathology

Westberg and Michael[403] confirmed previous observations of thin linear staining of the glomerular basement membrane for IgG, IgM, albumin, and fibrinogen in kidneys of patients with IDDM and concluded that it represented a nonspecific consequence of increased permeability rather than an expression of immunologic binding. Their findings were later extended, and the presence of this linear positivity for IgG and albumin, along not only the glomerular basement membrane but also the Bowman's capsule and especially the outer aspect of the tubular basement membrane, was considered specific for diabetes.[404] This assertion has been supported by the demonstration of similar staining in kidneys from nondiabetic donors transplanted into patients with IDDM.[401]

Immunofluorescence techniques have shown increased mesangial amounts of types IV and V collagen, laminin, and fibronectin and the presence of antigens normally expressed in fetal glomeruli only.[405] Immunochemical analysis has confirmed the increase in type IV collagen but showed reduced levels of laminin and markedly decreased amounts of the heparan sulfate proteoglycan, whereas levels of fibronectin were not different from those in normal controls.[270] Collagens of type I[406] and type VI, but not of type III,[407] have also been described in the diabetic mesangium. Type VI collagen, which is probably synthesized only by mesangial cells and therefore absent from the basement membrane, has been found to be increased about threefold in the kidneys of those with long-standing diabetes as compared with the kidneys of nondiabetic controls.[408] The possibility of anomalies in the contractile properties of the mesangium has been considered following the demonstration of increased amounts of actomyosin.[409] Fibrin products as well as IgG and complement components have been found in the exudative lesions of the glomerulus and of the arterioles,[396] suggesting a role for coagulation processes in the genesis of glomerulosclerosis.[403,410]

Electron Microscopy

Thickening of the glomerular basement membrane is a prominent finding in the kidneys of patients with diabetes. It has been studied particularly in IDDM subjects, in whom it is absent at diagnosis,[411] becoming detectable after 2 to 5 years of disease.[412] The increased synthesis taking place during this period is reflected in the 80% increase in the area of the peripheral capillary wall found in young subjects with IDDM within months of diagnosis.[171] In advanced stages of the disease, the basement membrane can become very thick, and particularly so in association with nodular lesions[413] Whereas in early disease the increase in thickness is even, a marked irregularity in its width appears later.[414] Localized areas of electron-lucent material can make up to 10% of total volume of the basement membrane, and between 1 and 6% of the capillary length is lined by abnormally thin membrane.[399] Throughout all the stages up to sclerosis, features suggestive of immune deposits are absent, although subendothelial fibrillar electron-dense material interpreted as fibrin-fibrinogen products has been described.[410]

The foot processes of the epithelial cells in diabetes remain discrete soon after proteinuria has become persistent[415] and until renal function has declined to 20% of normal.[399] At this stage, epithelial cell cytoplasm preserves a healthy appearance and prominent organelles (rough endoplasmic reticulum, mitochondria, Golgi vesicles) that may be the expression of continued basement membrane synthesis. However, with further progression of disease, the foot processes appear wider in cross-section and the length of the filtration slits tends to decrease.[416] Aspects suggestive of degenerative changes have also been noted, accompanied by detachment from the underlying basement membrane that is left exposed.[417] Eventually, podocyte effacement and fusion are noted.[413]

Although normal at diagnosis of IDDM,[418] an increase of the fractional volume of the mesangium, initially involving an expansion of the matrix component, follows the thickening of the glomerular basement membrane.[419] Its delicate strands anastomose and widen, and collagen fibrils become detectable with progression of the disease.

The core of the typical nodules seems to correspond to local accumulation of these components,[420,421] while their laminated periphery may derive from expanded and folded basement membrane.[407] In more advanced stages of the disease, the number of mesangial nuclei is sometimes increased and the fractional volume of the mesangium can become more than double the value found in normal controls.[260]

The exudative lesions appear on electron microscopy as finely granular electron-dense material. In the arterioles, this material spreads from an initial subintimal location towards the media, sometimes to its near replacement. The "capsular drop" corresponds to accumulation of this material between the epithelial cells and Bowman's capsule basement membrane, whereas the "fibrin cap" represents its presence along the endothelial side of the glomerular basement membrane.[396]

Endothelial cell changes are not prominent in diabetes.

Structure-Function Relationship

Understanding the relationship between abnormal morphologic appearances and altered function may help clarify the pathogenesis of diabetic kidney disease. Information concerning this important issue is almost totally restricted to patients with IDDM.

Increased glomerular volume is a salient feature in the kidneys of patients with IDDM and is part of a generalized hypertrophic process that also involves the tubules and results in increased kidney volume. Larger glomeruli are probably a necessary condition for the early hyperfiltration of IDDM. Unlike most other renal diseases, in diabetes mellitus relatively large kidneys persist with advancing renal failure.

More than 30 years ago, Gellman et al.[159] were the first to show that the nodular lesions are of little functional significance and that it is the degree of diffuse glomerulosclerosis, encompassing changes in the glomerular capillary and the mesangial region, that correlates with the clinical manifestations of worsening renal function. In the early phases of IDDM, the increase in luminal volume and filtering surface area shown by light and electron microscopic studies offers a structural counterpart to the higher GFR.[171] With advancing renal disease, no correlation is seen between the width of the thickened basement membrane and any of the parameters of renal function, but a close association has been reported between these changes in function and mesangial expansion.[422] A fractional mesangial volume in excess of 37% has been claimed to characterize patients with clinical proteinuria.[260] Mesangial expansion also correlates inversely with the capillary filtering area, a variable closely associated with glomerular filtration rate, from levels of hyperfiltration to markedly reduced renal function.[423,424] It has therefore been suggested that it is the expansion of the mesangium, with the attendant reduction in glomerular filtration surface area, that is responsible for the progressive loss of renal function in IDDM. However, it should be remembered that there is overlap between the fractional mesangial volume of patients with and those

without proteinuria,[425,426] making the prognostic significance of this variable open to question.

In patients with IDDM, morphometric parameters did not correlate with albumin excretion rate up to 40 mg/day (~30 μg/min). In patients with higher albumin excretion rates, however, the fractional volume of mesangium was, on average, significantly increased and a minor reduction in creatinine clearance and an elevation in blood pressure were observed.[121] Similar findings in patients with NIDDM have recently been reported.[427] These data confirm the reliability of persistent microalbuminuria and the attendant blood pressure elevation as clinical markers of significant renal damage.[140]

Indications for Renal Biopsy in Patients with Diabetes

It can be argued that if a patient has diabetes and also shows urinary abnormalities there is no need to do a renal biopsy, which will almost certainly show changes consistent with diabetic nephropathy. While it is true that in the great majority of patients with clinical diabetes proteinuria with or without hematuria is the result of diabetic nephropathy, this is, however, far from always the case.

The first step in the investigation of a proteinuric patient with diabetes is to obtain information on the number, size, and position of the kidneys by ultrasonography. Should there be a suspicion of papillary necrosis or tuberculosis of the renal tract, conditions that have an increased incidence in diabetic patients and that may be associated with modest proteinuria, a full radiologic assessment of the urinary tract should be performed.

Several clues may suggest that the patient may have disease other than diabetic nephropathy. Retinopathy is almost invariably present in patients with diabetic nephropathy. A concordance rate ranging from 63% in NIDDM[29] and up to 85 to 99% in IDDM[107,146-148] makes the absence of retinopathy a strong argument for performing a biopsy.

The frequency of hematuria has been variably reported depending on the type of diabetes studied and on the definition of hematuria. In a large series of 136 consecutive biopsies in patients with IDDM and NIDDM, Taft et al.[155] found hematuria in excess of 10,000 cells/mL to be present in 66% of patients and to be of little help in distinguishing diabetic and nondiabetic renal disease. In a smaller biopsy series, Hommel et al.[154] reported that of 13 patients with IDDM with proteinuria and hematuria, 69% had a concomitant nondiabetic renal disease. Red cell casts have been noted in 4% of cases of biopsy-proven diabetic disease.[428] Although still controversial, the presence of hematuria, especially when accompanied by red cell casts, should alert to the possibility of other renal disease.

In IDDM proteinuria develops in only 4% of patients within 10 years of onset of diabetes. Thus, early onset of proteinuria is likely to indicate a disease other than diabetic nephropathy.[429] Conversely, the likelihood that a patient with diabetes with onset in childhood who develops proteinuria 20 years later has diabetic nephropathy approaches 100%.

In NIDDM, proteinuria can be present at diagnosis in as many as 8% of patients,[108] and the number presenting with proteinuria increases with increasing age at presentation.[147] Moreover, in these older patients the duration of diabetes is uncertain, and the presence of other renal disease is more likely.[429] Thus, early proteinuria is of lesser value in differentiating between renal injury of diabetic origin and that of nondiabetic origin.

The diagnosis of a coincident glomerular disease by renal biopsy may be helpful from both a therapeutic and a prognostic standpoint. Besides detecting a potentially treatable nondiabetic renal disease, renal biopsy may be useful in the future for monitoring the effect of treatment of the early potentially reversible phases of diabetic nephropathy.

Other Glomerular Diseases in Patients with Diabetes

Almost every form of glomerular disease has been shown to occur in patients with diabetes; this is not surprising considering that approximately 3% of the general population is diabetic.

IgA nephropathy and other forms of mesangial glomerulonephritis, acute glomerulonephritis, lupus, amyloidosis, mesangiocapillary glomerulonephritis types I and II, crescentic glomerulonephritis, and steroid responsive minimal-change disease in both children and adults[155,430–432] have all been reported in patients with diabetes. In a few patients, two additional glomerulopathies have been noted, as well as diabetic nephropathy.[433]

The overall incidence of nondiabetic glomerular disease in diabetic patients who underwent biopsies in various studies was 8% of 50,[434] 9% of 122,[430] 22% of 164,[432] and 10% of 136.[155] When only patients with NIDDM were examined, 27% of 33 were found to have nondiabetic renal disease.[29] In a retrospective study of renal biopsies in patients with diabetes, 12% of 49 of those with IDDM and 28% of 60 of those with NIDDM were found to have another disease.[429] These figures will undoubtedly be an overestimate of the true rate, since in most units routine renal biopsy of proteinuric diabetic patients is not practiced, and those submitted to biopsy will, because of selection bias, include a greater proportion of patients with nondiabetic glomerulopathies.

Membranous nephropathy is the glomerular disease most often been reported in association with diabetes. Since the first description by Churg's group,[421] at least 60 cases have been reported; many similar patients seen more recently have not been reported since the association is now well recognized (see Rao and Crosson,[434] Kobayashi et al.,[435] Kasinath et al.,[430] and Silva et al.[431] for reviews of published cases). The most common age at presentation was 40 to 60 years, a range similar to that of membranous nephropathy without diabetes as well as of NIDDM itself. However, patients as young as 13 years and several in their 20s have been reported. In most cases duration of diabetes was 10 years or more, and two-thirds of the patients were using insulin. Only 25% of the patients had retinopathy, although not all had undergone fluorescein angiography. Most of the patients were nephrotic, with urinary protein levels reaching as high as 35 g/24 hour. Histologic appearances ranged from typical membranous nephropathy to an almost typical diabetic glomerulosclerosis complicated by mild or occasional membranous changes.

It is difficult to be sure if this association is simply the coincidental appearance of one of the commoner glomerulopathies in middle age with diabetes of either type or whether it represents a specific association. Certainly the excess of cases of membranous nephropathy over cases of other glomerular pathologic disease noted in nephrotic patients aged 30 to 60 years is striking.

Although the superimposition of Heymann membranous nephropathy on streptozotocin-induced diabetes in rats has been found to lead to a more severe nephrotic syndrome and a higher mortality than that produced by either disease alone,[436] Chihara et al.[432] reported that coincidence of membranous nephropathy and diabetes did not affect the prognosis for kidney function in humans.

TREATMENT OF DIABETIC NEPHROPATHY

Blood Pressure Control

Up to 10 years ago, hypertension was viewed as a late phenomenon of diabetic nephropathy in IDDM and was thought to be a consequence of diabetes.[124] For NIDDM no consensus was achieved regarding the frequency or pathogenic importance of hypertension.[437]

It has, however, become apparent that rises in blood pressure take place in proteinuric patients with IDDM even in the face of normal, although declining, GFR.[128] Moreover, microalbuminuric patients with IDDM have also been shown to have higher arterial pressures than matched normoalbuminuric patients.[99,140] These observations, coupled with evidence for a central role of blood pressure level in the progression of diabetic renal disease,[132] have led to a different perception of the importance of arterial hypertension.

Mogensen[126] was the first to show, in a small number of patients with IDDM with established nephropathy, that reduction in blood pressure slowed the rate of loss of GFR and checked the increasing albuminuria. A prospective self-controlled study of 6 years' duration[438] demonstrated that effective blood pressure treatment reduced the rate of decline of GFR from 0.94 mL/min per month before therapy to 0.29 mL/min per month during the first 3 years and to 0.1 mL/min per month by 6 years of effective blood pressure treatment. This change was attended by a 50% reduction in albuminuria from 1038 μg/min to 504 μg/min. Despite the small number of patients and the lack of a randomized controlled design, these results were taken as evidence of the significant impact of antihypertensive treatment on the progression of diabetic kidney disease. The authors speculated that, should the slowing of progression be maintained, the survival of the kidneys of these patients might be extended from the current 7 to 10 years to more than 20 years. Recent longitudinal cohort studies seem to support this prediction, with a remarkable reduction in cumulative mortality—from over 50% at 10 years to only 18%—noted in patients receiving antihypertensive treatment[24,25] (Fig. 40–1).

In the earlier studies, multiple drug therapy for hypertension was used, including a β-blocker, a diuretic, and a vasodilator. During the last few years, great interest has surrounded the use of angiotensin-converting enzyme (ACE) inhibitors, not only in established diabetic nephropathy but also in nonhypertensive patients with microalbuminuria. Studies in experimentally diabetic animals,[340,341] by implicating glomerular hypertension as a determinant of glomerular damage, have led to the suggestion that ACE inhibitors may be specifically protective of renal function because of their ability to reduce efferent arteriolar vasoconstriction and thus to reduce intraglomerular hypertension. This "specific" effect has been claimed to be separate from any effect on systemic blood pressure, although this remains debatable.[439]

A reduction in proteinuria and in the rate of fall of GFR was shown to occur independently of significant changes in blood pressure in two uncontrolled studies by Taguma et al.[440] and Bjørck et al.[441] In more recent controlled trials, however, the effects on proteinuria lowering and on the rate of GFR decline were found to be associated with a reduction of systemic blood pressure, even when nonhypertensive proteinuric patients were investigated.[24,442,443] The decrease in the rate of fall of GFR obtained with treatment with ACE inhibitors does not appear to be of greater magnitude than that achieved with conventional antihypertensive therapy. A physiologic approach to the study of the antiproteinuric effect of converting-enzyme inhibitors has employed the fractional clearance of graded-size neutral dextrans. Three studies using different designs[444–446] have demonstrated that treatment of proteinuric diabetic patients with ACE inhibitors significantly reduces the augmented clearance of large-sized dextrans (molecular radii 5.6 to 7.4 nm) and of large, essentially neutral, plasma proteins such as IgG. This improvement in glomerular membrane size-selective properties seems to be unique to ACE inhibitors

and independent of changes in systemic blood pressure, since administration of other antihypertensive drugs (such as diuretics or clonidine) are not followed by the same effect in spite of similar reductions in systemic arterial pressure. However, the prognostic significance of these membrane changes on selectivity remains unknown.

The effect of ACE inhibition has also been studied prospectively in nonhypertensive patients with IDDM with microalbuminuria. In a randomized study, Marre et al.[447] showed a reduction in albumin excretion rate, with normalization in 50% of cases, after 1 year of treatment with enalapril. Mean blood pressure was reduced by about 10 mm Hg throughout the study and the GFR remained unchanged. By contrast, in the placebo group the mean blood pressure rose and GFR decreased significantly, with 30% of the patients becoming persistently proteinuric by 1 year. A decrease in the fractional clearance of albumin, in the absence of changes in GFR or RPF, was also found in a short-term cross-over study of the effects of enalapril on patients with normal albumin excretion rates.[448]

Antihypertensive treatment appears, therefore, to delay the progression of established diabetic nephropathy and, if started at the stage of microalbuminuria, even may prevent or at least retard the onset of clinically overt renal disease. Caution must be applied in the extrapolation of data based primarily on reduction of urinary protein excretion, and long-term trials are needed to establish a definite effect on the rate of deterioration of glomerular function. Table 40–5 summarizes some of the studies on the effect of antihypertensive treatment on the progression of kidney disease in patients with IDDM with persistent proteinuria or microalbuminuria.

Dietary Treatment

A reduction of protein intake has long been advocated for the treatment of chronic renal failure,[450] and diabetic nephropathy is no exception. Early studies by Attman et al.[451] provided no evidence of a beneficial effect of

Table 40–5. Effect of Antihypertensive Treatment on the Progression of Renal Disease in Four Studies of Patients with Insulin-Dependent Diabetes with Either Persistent Proteinuria or Microalbuminuria

Study*	Subject (n)	Duration (mo)	BP (mm Hg)		GFR decline (mL/min/mo)		AER (mg/min)	
			Control	Treatment	Control	Treatment	Control	Treatment
1. Parving et al.[438]	11	72	143/96	129/84	0.89	0.22†	1038	504‡
2. Bjørck et al.[441]	14	24	163/97	155/94	0.85	0.45†	2014	1944
3. Marre et al.[447]	10	12	137/82	124/72	1.67	0.58†	127.1	25.7
4. Parving[449]	15	12	128/78	122/77	6.4	3.1	378	336†

Parving et al. and Bjørck et al. studied patients with persistent proteinuria, and Marre et al. studied patients with microalbuminuria. BP = blood pressure; GFR = glomerular filtration rate; AER = albumin excretion rate.
*In studies 2, 3, and 4, patients were treated with angiotensin-converting enzyme inhibitor (ACEI), and in study 1, with metoprolol, hydralazine, and furosemide.
†P <.05.
‡P <.01.

protein restriction (as low as 0.3 g/kg per day) on the progression of renal disease in patients with IDDM, but the lack of a therapeutic effect in this study may have been due to the advanced stage of the disease, as indicated by serum creatinine levels at entry of about 800 μmol/L. Recent data on diabetic patients with less severe impairment of renal function seem more encouraging. Barsotti et al.[452] and Evanoff et al.[453] have claimed that a diet reduced in protein retards the progression of diabetic nephropathy in patients with IDDM. These studies have, however, been criticized because renal function was assessed by measurements of creatinine clearance or the reciprocal of serum creatinine levels, two indices that are unreliable markers of renal function in advanced renal disease and especially in patients fed a low-protein diet.[129,136,137] Other important potentially confounding variables, such as blood pressure, also were not controlled for.

Two long-term longitudinal studies have used reliable markers of glomerular function. Walker et al.,[138] in a 5-year self-controlled study of 19 patients with IDDM with moderate renal failure at entry (mean GFR about 60 mL/min), showed that the mean rate of decline of GFR, measured as plasma clearance of ^{51}Cr-EDTA, was reduced from 0.61 mL/min per month with a diet of 1.13 g/kg body weight of protein per day to 0.14 mL/min per month with a diet of 0.67 g/kg body weight of protein per day. The individual response to the low-protein diet was, however, heterogeneous, with four patients failing to respond and seven showing a nonsignificant reduction in the rate of GFR decline. The low-protein diet reduced the AER from 467 to 340 mg per 24 hours and checked the progressive rise in the fractional clearance of albumin. The effects of the diet seemed to be independent of changes in blood pressure, which contributed only 11% to the decreased rate of loss of GFR.

Zeller et al.[139] in a controlled 5-year prospective study of 35 patients with IDDM with nephropathy in whom GFR was assessed by iothalamate clearance, found that the rate of decline of GFR in the group receiving a protein- and phosphorus-restricted diet was 0.26 mL/min per month. By contrast, in the control group with a normal protein intake, the rate of decline of GFR was significantly faster, at 1.01 mL/min per month. A remarkable finding in this study was that 50% of the patients receiving dietary therapy showed no decline in GFR during a 31-month follow-up period. Blood pressure was similarly controlled in both groups. Table 40–6 illustrates the effect of protein restriction on the fall of GFR and AER in these two studies.

Diets restricted to 0.5 to 0.6 g of protein/kg body weight per day seem to have no long-term detrimental effects on nutritional status. Anthropometric measurements such as the mid-arm muscle circumference were not affected by such diets, and several authors noted an increase in serum albumin during protein restriction.[138,452,453]

Short-term studies of the physiologic mechanisms of action of low-protein diets in diabetic patients with nephropathy indicate that such diets lead to a reduction in the fractional clearance of albumin, IgG, and broad-sized neutral dextrans and thus to an improvement of the permeability selectivity of the glomerular membrane without affecting GFR or RPF.[454,455] Micropuncture studies in the streptozotocin-diabetic Munich-Wistar rat suggest that the antiproteinuric effect of a diet severely restricted in protein may be modulated by changes in intraglomerular pressure.[166] However, the mode of action of a low-protein diet is complex, unlikely to be mediated simply by hemodynamic changes[262,351] and probably involving the effects of changes in other nutritional components such as phosphorus and lipids.[138]

Reduction of dietary protein by approximately 50% has also been shown to reduce the fractional clearance of albumin in patients with microalbuminuria[457] and to lower GFR in patients with hyperfiltration,[457] independently of changes in glucose control and blood pressure.

The prognostic significance of these changes remains at present obscure, as no long-term studies of patients with early renal involvement are available. It also remains to be determined if the contributions of good blood pressure control and a low-protein diet may have an additive sparing effect on renal function. It is of interest that renal functional changes similar to those obtained by a low-protein diet can be induced in normal individuals by the administration of a vegetarian diet with normal protein content. The mediators of this effect are not entirely understood but may involve changes in glucagon secretion and the production of renal prostaglandins.[458]

Table 40–6. Effect of Low-Protein Diet (LPD), Compared with Normal Protein Diet (NPD) on Albumin Excretion Rate (AER) and the Decline in Glomerular Filtration Rate (GFR) in Two Studies of Patients with Insulin-Dependent Diabetes and Nephropathy

Study	Subjects (n)	Duration (mo)	Change in GFR (mL/min/mo)		Change in AER (mg/24 hr)	
			NPD	LPD	NPD	LPD
Walker et al.[138]	19	61	−0.61	−0.14*	...	−127†
Zeller et al.[139]	35	35	−1.01	−0.26*	+1024*	−196*

*P <.05.
†P <.01.

Glycemic Control

Blood glucose control appears to have only limited impact on the progression of diabetic renal failure. A positive correlation between levels of HbA_{1C} and rate of decline of GFR reported by some authors[133] has not been confirmed subsequently by others.[134] In a study of strict blood glucose control by continuous subcutaneous insulin infusion (CSII), long-term correction of hyperglycemia for nearly 2 years did not affect the rate of decline of GFR or the increasing rates of albumin and IgG fractional clearances in patients with IDDM with persistent proteinuria.[131] Similarly poor results of intensified insulin treatment have been obtained in a controlled study of patients with intermittent proteinuria.[125] It would appear that there is a point beyond which the diabetic metabolic abnormality is no longer necessary for progression of disease.

More encouraging are the effects of reducing elevated blood glucose levels at earlier stages of renal disease. The exaggerated albuminuric response to exercise in patients with IDDM is corrected by a relatively short period of better diabetic control.[113–115] Several authors have reported a significant correlation between indices of blood glucose control and albumin excretion rate in patients with IDDM without persistent proteinuria.[96,130,140] In patients with microalbuminuria, strict metabolic control by CSII has been effective in reducing the AER,[110,459,460] and in preventing the progressive increase in the fractional clearance of albumin in the long-term.[257] In the Steno study, over a 2-year period, 28% of conventionally treated patients progressed to clinical nephropathy, whereas no progression was seen in the patients who received intensified insulin treatment.[130] Similar reductions in AER can be obtained by multiple-injection therapy, provided that similar levels of blood glucose control are achieved, a finding suggesting that it is the attained blood glucose concentration rather than the modality of treatment that matters.[461] Improvement of blood glucose control by diet or oral therapy also reduced microalbuminuria in patients with NIDDM.[70,462]

The results of these studies are consistent with the epidemiologic observation of a fourfold increase in the risk of developing nephropathy in patients with IDDM with a record of poor glycemic control[9,368,463] and suggest a beneficial effect of tight glucose control on progression of microalbuminuria. Whether this effect may be translated to prevention of end-stage renal disease remains to be established.

Correction of hyperglycemia shortly after diagnosis of IDDM induces a decrease in GFR, which in some[79] but not all[68] studies was accompanied by a reduction in the increased kidney size. Recent evidence suggests that the increased kidney size is associated with an exaggerated renal hemodynamics to amino acid infusion and that both can be corrected by 3 weeks of intensified insulin therapy.[464] With more long-standing disease, however, near-normal glycemia lowers GFR while not affecting kidney hypertrophy. Cessation of strict glycemic control in these patients with large hyperfiltering kidneys leads to a prompt return of GFR to previous levels.[69] It has been suggested that the establishment of the irreversibility of kidney enlargement signals the onset of a phase of progressive renal disease in which overproduction of intrarenal growth factors perpetuates renal damage.[86]

Other Treatment Modalities

Although the amount of experimental data on the renal effect of aldose reductase inhibitors in rats is substantial (see Pathogenesis section), the number of studies in humans is limited. Whereas a reduction of GFR[318] and a decrease in AER[319] were noted in patients with IDDM who had either a normal AER or microalbuminuria, a controlled study on subjects with NIDDM with microalbuminuria failed to show any effects on renal function, blood pressure, or glucose control after a short period of treatment.[320] Longer-term studies will probably be needed to clarify the role of this class of compounds in human disease.

It has been claimed that a therapeutic regimen with aspirin and dipyridamole may delay the progression of chronic renal failure in some patients with diabetic nephropathy.[465] However, this study was uncontrolled and did not allow for the confounding effect of other variables.

OTHER MANIFESTATIONS OF DIABETIC RENAL DISEASE

Renal Papillary Necrosis

Diabetes has long been associated with renal papillary necrosis (RPN), whose prevalence in autopsy cases averages 4.4%.[466] This figure may be an underestimation, since diabetes has been found in up to 50% of cases of RPN.[467–469]

In a recent prospective series of 76 consecutive patients with IDDM with normal serum creatinine levels who underwent urography, RPN was diagnosed in 24%.[470] It tends to occur in patients with long-standing disease and affects both kidneys in up to 65% of cases.[466] When unilateral, it has been shown to involve the contralateral kidney in the ensuing years. It is more frequent in women, particularly those with recurrent urinary tract infection.

Viewed in the past as an acute devastating condition often leading to sepsis and death, it has become clear that RPN can be nearly asymptomatic and follow a more indolent course, with bouts of urinary infection and/or renal colic. Microscopic hematuria has been reported to be more frequent when this condition is present, and pyuria will often be present even in the absence of documented infection, a finding that should alert to the possibility of underlying silent papillary necrosis.[469,470] Proteinuria is often present but usually modest (<2 g/24 hours), and patients with persistent proteinuria do not seem to experience RPN at a prevalence in excess of that in patients without persistent proteinuria.[470] The urographic appearances of "moth-eaten" calyxes and the "ring-shadow" image of the necrotic papilla are highly suggestive of this condition.

The management of the acute form of RPN in the patient with diabetes is compounded by the need to maintain adequate metabolic control. If obstruction is present, its relief is urgent and will often condition the success of associated antibiotic therapy. In the chronic, indolent form of RPN, the use of nonsteroidal anti-inflammatory agents may further compromise medullary circulation and should therefore be avoided.

Autonomic Neuropathy of the Bladder

It is difficult to ascertain the true prevalence of autonomic neuropathy of the bladder in patients with diabetes because of the insidious onset of the condition. In the older literature, this uncertainty is reflected by prevalence figures that range from 1 to 26%,[471,472] whereas more recent studies, which based diagnosis on urodynamic criteria, report prevalence of bladder autonomic dysfunction in long-standing diabetes of ~40%.[473]

The first abnormality, usually detected in asymptomatic patients, is impairment of sensation with decreased awareness of bladder distention caused by involvement of proprioceptive afferent fibers. As a result, micturition occurs at progressively larger bladder volumes, and this, together with progressive damage of the parasympathetic innervation of the detrusor, leads to weaker bladder contraction, incomplete emptying, and increasing residual volume. Involvement of the efferent sympathetic innervation to the trigone may lead to functional incompetence of the vesicoureteric junction and to incomplete relaxation of the internal sphincter during micturition.[474,475]

Patients are often unaware of the extent of their bladder abnormality. Symptoms are scarce and at the initial stages may be confined to disappearance of previous nocturia, with less frequent daytime voiding of large volumes of urine. These changes may go unnoticed for a long time. Later, a weaker stream produced only on straining, terminal dribbling, and involuntary stream interruption or overflow incontinence due to detrusor-urethral sphincter dyssynergy, may become apparent. From the early stages, recurrent and/or persistent urinary tract infections may set in as a consequence of incomplete emptying and/or reflux.[476,477]

Recognition of the insidious course assists early diagnosis. Proper consideration given to recurring urinary infections in a patient with long-standing diabetes may lead to detection of an unsuspected enlarged bladder by physical examination or, alternatively, to disclosure of residue or residual volume by ultrasound scanning. Patients with diabetes are capable of developing other conditions (i.e., prostatic hypertrophy, asymptomatic stone) that may interfere with bladder function, and overt symptoms may occur in response to associated treatment with anticholinergic drugs.[478,479] Urodynamic studies with uroflowmetry (mictiography)[480] and cystometrogram study[481] can characterize the bladder dysfunction and may be invaluable for accurate prognosis and decisions about treatment.

Detection of autonomic bladder involvement in a patient with diabetes should lead to adoption of a policy of voluntary, regular voiding performed by the patient even in the absence of subjective urge. Suprapubic manual pressure will help complete emptying. Intermittent or temporary catheterization, and its association with parasympathomimetic drug treatment with betanechol chloride, may lead to reduction of bladder distention and recovery of detrusor function.[482] The effect of this drug seems unpredictable, however, and may be limited by adverse effects.[483] In the presence of detrusor-urethral dyssynergy, centrally acting muscle relaxants or an α-adrenergic blocking agent, depending on whether dysfunction involves the external or the internal sphincter, respectively, may be of help. Bladder neck resection is sometimes successful. More complex operations to reduce bladder capacity are sometimes performed. Long-term catheterization may be the only solution in severely disabled patients. The most serious complication of neurogenic bladder is an intractable urinary infection, which may render the patient unsuitable for renal transplantation.

Pregnancy in Diabetic Nephropathy

Up until the 1980s, pregnancy in women with diabetic nephropathy was discouraged, and therapeutic abortion was recommended because of the poor fetal outcome.[484] During the last decade, more than 100 pregnancies in IDDM patients with nephropathy have been reported.[485-489] Both the impact of pregnancy on nephropathy and the outcome of gestation appear more encouraging.

The increase in creatinine clearance, which takes place in normal gestation, occurs during the first trimester in only about 56% of pregnant women with diabetic nephropathy.[486,487] In proteinuric patients with initial creatinine clearances ≥50 mL/min, elevated blood pressure of ≥140/90 mm Hg is present in approximately one-third during the first trimester, affecting just over one-half at the end of pregnancy. In women with more reduced renal function, these proportions increase to ~80%.

Pre-eclampsia is reported to occur in 26% of all pregnancies in diabetic women with nephropathy. Its diagnosis is dependent upon the detection of an acute rise in blood pressure, serum creatinine, and proteinuria. Other signs of deranged hepatic and central nervous system function and thrombocytopenia with elevated levels of fibrin-split products may co-exist. Changes in serum uric acid levels have been found to be of no pathognomonic significance in the context of diabetic nephropathy.[485]

A common finding in pregnancy in diabetic nephropathy is an increase in proteinuria, sometimes of massive proportions. Among patients with a creatinine clearance rate >50 mL/min, 16% in the first trimester and 71% in the third trimester excrete >3 g of protein per 24 hours. Pooled data suggest that ~50% of patients develop proteinuria in which the 24-hour excretion is >5 g and that 17% excrete >10 g.[485-489]

Anemia was found to relate significantly to the decreased renal function, and hematocrit values of ≤28%

and/or hemoglobin levels of ≤10 g/dL were seen in 42%.[485,489]

The natural history of nephropathy does not appear to be adversely affected by pregnancy. Following delivery, a marked reduction in proteinuria is common, and in 67% of the 27 patients in whom it was measured within 1 year of delivery, it had returned to or was below preconception values. The rate of decline of creatinine clearance was calculated in 23 patients who were followed up for 6 to 35 months after delivery and was found to be 0.85 mL/min per month.[485] A reduction in renal function after pregnancy was more likely in patients with more severe proteinuria or hypertension during the first trimester. Overall, the impact of pregnancy on the kidney seemed not to be different from that observed for other renal diseases.[490,491]

Fetal survival in a pooled series of five studies was 91.3%.[485–489] The unacceptably high rates of spontaneous abortions and of congenital malformations seen in women with diabetic nephropathy before the 1980s[484,492] have been considerably reduced to ~9.5%. There is ample evidence that normalization of HbA_{1C} prior to conception reduces the frequency of malformations in offspring of women with diabetes in general,[493–495] and the same may apply to women with diabetic nephropathy.[486,496,497] Increases in blood pressure, fetal distress, and premature labor are responsible for a high rate (~55%) of preterm deliveries, a rate similar to that reported for women with nondiabetic renal disease and depressed renal function.[491]

Pregnancy in a woman with diabetic nephropathy should be considered and planned carefully. Its outcome depends to a great extent on the joint efforts of the patient and a team of experts in a specialized center. The ultimate decision should be based on the long-term prognosis for the patient with diabetic nephropathy and the increased risk to the fetus.

Urinary Tract Infections

Urinary tract infections have been considered to be more frequent in patients with diabetes, probably as a result of reports of renal histologic evidence of interstitial inflammation and scarring in 10 to 40% of patients with diabetes.[27,159,396,430,498,499] These histologic aspects could arise from other conditions, such as ischemia, reflux nephropathy, or renal papillary necrosis, and are difficult to distinguish from those of "chronic pyelonephritis."[146,155,396]

Indeed, several surveys have failed to show an increased incidence of urinary infection in patients with diabetes over that in control populations.[500–502] However, some workers have reported that the incidence of bacteriuria in women with diabetes is approximately double that in nondiabetic controls.[502–504] Diabetic nephropathy seems to be associated with an increased frequency of infection only in pregnant diabetic patients.[506,507] A high proportion of urinary tract infections are asymptomatic, and their pathogenic role is not clear. However, in patients with diabetic nephropathy, even asymptomatic infection may be associated with worsening renal function, and every effort should be directed towards its eradication.

Urinary tract infections, when involving the upper urinary tract, can lead to severe complications in the patient with diabetes. Perinephric abscesses, which can be bilateral,[508] are more frequent in patients with diabetes and may have an insidious onset followed by persistent fever and rigors. Urine cultures are frequently negative, and sometimes a tender flank mass can be felt.[509] Computed tomographic (CT) examination may establish the diagnosis.[510] Prolonged antibiotic therapy usually is necessary.

Infections of the kidney with anaerobic gas-forming organisms are distinctly more common in patients with diabetes and have recently been reviewed by Evanoff et al.[511] More than 90% of cases of emphysematous pyelonephritis occur in patients with diabetes. This condition of parenchymal infection is more frequent in women, and in the majority of cases is due to *Escherichia coli*, but *Candida* spp. and *Cryptococcus neoformans* have also been reported. Fever, abdominal pain, nausea, and vomiting in an ill-appearing patient are common presenting features. Elevated white blood cell count and creatinine level and grossly elevated blood glucose level are common, and frank pyuria usually is present. The infection is bilateral in ~10% of cases. Plain abdominal radiographic examination, an intravenous pyelogram, or ultrasound scanning are diagnostic in ~85% of cases, showing gas bubbles extending along the renal pyramids and collecting under the perirenal fascia or, after its rupture, extending into the adjoining retroperitoneal space. A CT scan will be needed in the remaining cases and will define more precisely the location of the gas. Emphysematous pyelonephritis has a guarded prognosis. Medical treatment alone results in a mortality of ~60% when gas is confined to the kidney and in a mortality of over 80% when gas has extended to the perirenal spaces. Nephrectomy can be a life-saving procedure and should not be delayed, but the mortality rate is still ~20%.

Emphysematous pyelitis refers to the presence of gas within the collecting system only, and 50% of cases occur in diabetic patients, particularly women. Its clinical presentation is similar to that of emphysematous pyelonephritis, although renal failure may be absent and glucose control may remain adequate. Radiographic examination by plain film, intravenous pyelogram, or ultrasound shows gas outlining the pelvicaliceal system and sometimes the ureters. Obstruction and dilatation are not uncommon associated features, needing urgent correction. Medical supportive treatment and antibiotic therapy are usually effective, although the overall mortality rate is still ~20%.

Nephropathy Induced by Radiologic Contrast Agents

Diabetic patients with nephropathy are at higher risk of acute exacerbation of their renal function (defined as a ≥1.0 mg/dL [88 μmol/L] rise in serum creatinine) after the administration of both ionic and non-ionic radiographic contrast media. The incidence has in the past been reported to be as high as 76% after intravenous pyelography[512] and 23% after cardiac angiography[513] in patients with prestudy serum creatinine levels of ≥2.0 mg/dL (176 mmol/L). The risk does not seem to be dose dependent, as high-dose pyelography is not associated with more cases of acute renal failure. Patients with IDDM appear more at risk than patients with NIDDM. In more recent studies the reported risk is substantially lower and is proportional to existing renal function at the time of the contrast radiologic investigation.[514,515] In diabetic patients with normal renal function, the risk is minimal.[516] It has been suggested that adequate hydration both before and after contrast radiography[517] and the use of furosemide[518] and mannitol[519] may substantially reduce the incidence of nephropathy induced by contrast agents.

The use of contrast radiography in diabetic patients with renal impairment should therefore be limited whenever possible. For instance intravenous pyelography has almost been superseded by renal tract ultrasonography and isotope imaging. Doppler ultrasound scanning is a useful alternative to angiography in the preliminary investigation of peripheral artery disease. Concomitant use of nephrotoxic agents such as nonsteroidal anti-inflammatory preparations and aminoglycosides should be avoided.

END-STAGE RENAL FAILURE

Recent developments in the treatment of diabetic patients with nephropathy have been successful in delaying the onset of end-stage renal failure (ESRF), but so far no intervention has proved effective in arresting the progression of renal disease. If premature death, mostly from cardiovascular causes, does not occur, then ESRF affects almost all diabetic patients with nephropathy.

The derivation of the number of diabetic patients who develop ESRF is usually based on statistics on all patients entering renal replacement therapy (RRT) programs. These figures may, however, be misleading, as the acceptance of patients with diabetes into RRT programs varies greatly among countries, depending on local practices and resources. In Europe in 1989, the number of patients with diabetes in ESRF who were receiving RRT was calculated to be 18,930.[520] Among the European countries, the Federal Republic of Germany had the highest rate of acceptance for diabetic patients, approaching 22% of the total number of patients receiving RRT. In the United Kingdom, diabetic patients represent approximately 11% of all patients receiving RRT.[521] A survey of six representative health regions in the United Kingdom in 1985 showed that every year approximately 600 patients with diabetes develop ESRF, defined as a serum creatinine level of >500 μmol/L and/or a serum urea level of >25 mmol/L.[6] Among these patients, 78% were considered by their physicians to be suitable for RRT. A review of these patients 2 years later revealed, however, that only 66% of the diabetic patients with ESRF in 1985 had been accepted into a RRT program.[46] One-third of patients died without treatment, renal failure being the cause of death in 50% of the cases. Age was an important

selection criterion for RRT and the mode of treatment. Two-thirds of patients considered unsuitable for RRT were older patients with NIDDM. Blindness alone was not a contraindication to RRT. These figures from the United Kingdom support the view that, at least in some countries, the number of patients receiving RRT does not accurately reflect the number of individuals who develop ESRF and that a number of patients may be excluded from treatment. The proportion of diabetic patients accepted for RRT has increased steadily in the last 15 years. In 1976, only 3% of all patients receiving RRT had diabetes, as compared with 10% in 1985. At the end of 1989, according to the EDTA registry, 7.2% of all patients receiving RRT and 13.7% of all patients commencing treatment had diabetes.[521]

The situation is very different in the United States, where about one-third of all patients receiving RRT have diabetes.[522] In 1982 diabetes mellitus was the second commonest cause of ESRF, and by 1988 it became the commonest cause, accounting for nearly 45 new patients per million population each year. This high percentage is due in part to the large number of patients with Type II diabetes and to the excess incidence of ESRF among the African-American and native American population. Medicare provides payment for services to over 90% of patients with ESRF, and the cost of caring for diabetic patients with ESRF was calculated to be of the order of US $2 billion in 1989.[522] The overall ratio of the number of patients with IDDM vs. the number with NIDDM receiving RRT varies among countries. In 1989 in Finland, 26% of all patients receiving RRT were insulin-dependent as compared with only 3% who did not receive insulin. In the United Kingdom, the corresponding figures were 9% and 4%.[520] In the United States, a survey of all patients (blacks and whites) who developed ESRF from 1974 through 1983 revealed that patients with IDDM were 11.6 times more likely to progress to renal failure than were patients with NIDDM.[34] However, because of the predominance of patients with NIDDM and the high incidence of primary hypertension and diabetic nephropathy among the African-Americans and native Americans, the number of patients with NIDDM with ESRF is approaching that of patients with IDDM with ESRF.

In Europe in 1989, the age group with the most patients receiving RRT was 35 to 44 years for patients with IDDM and 55 to 64 years for patients with NIDDM.[520]

The predominant mode of RRT for diabetic patients of all age groups in both Europe and the United States is hemodialysis, followed by peritoneal dialysis and renal transplantation. For patients in the age group between 35 and 44 years, similar numbers of patients are treated with hemodialysis and transplantation.[521] In the United Kingdom continuous ambulatory peritoneal dialysis (CAPD) is, by far, the commonest form of RRT for all patients with diabetes. Of all the diabetic patients with ESRF who were identified in a survey in the United Kingdom in 1985 and who subsequently received RRT, 95% were treated with dialysis, of whom 60% started with CAPD.[46]

Survival of Patients Receiving Renal Replacement Therapy

A patient with diabetes reaching ESRF usually has developed multiple complications. Severe complications are present in 50% of the patients, with blindness affecting 34% and a previous myocardial infarction present in 17%[46] (Table 40–7). This multisystem pathology is likely to account for the high mortality rate in this group of patients during treatment for renal failure. In Europe overall mortality has been reported to be five- to tenfold higher in diabetic patients than in nondiabetic patients with ESRF. In the age group 35 to 44 years old, the EDTA registry recorded 3-year survival rates of 44% in men and of 66% in women among patients with diabetes as compared with rates of 75% and 87% for patients with nondiabetic renal failure. For patients between 65 and 74 years old, the 5-year survival rate is still better among those with nondiabetic renal failure: 37% vs. 22% in men and 70% vs. 50% in women with and without diabetes, respectively.[521] In the United States, similar findings have been reported, with diabetic patients showing substantially higher mortality due to cardiovascular disease and infection than nondiabetic patients with ESRF. In addition, patients with diabetes have a higher rate of withdrawal from RRT.[522] In the United Kingdom, between 1981 and 1985 the relative risk of age-specific death rate from myocardial infarction among all diabetic patients during the first year of RRT was 89-fold higher than that of the general population.[521] For the age group 35 to 44 years old, this risk soared to a staggering 320-fold. The risk for nondiabetic patients in the same age group was approximately 10 times lower. The differences between diabetic and nondiabetic patients diminished with age, but even by age 66 to 75 years diabetic patients were still three times more likely to die of myocardial infarction than were nondiabetic patients. Survival depends partly on the type of RRT employed (see below), but there is little doubt that the presence of vascular disease before the initiation of RRT is one of the strongest predictors of cardiovascular events during treatment. It is therefore essential for diabetic patients with ESRF to begin RRT in the best possible general medical conditions to achieve long-term survival.

Preparation for Renal Replacement Therapy

Cardiovascular Disease

In 1985 approximately 17% of diabetic patients with ESRF in the United Kingdom had suffered at least one myocardial infarction before entering RRT.[6] In the United States, since 1980 the commonest cause of death in diabetic patients who have undergone renal transplantation has been cardiovascular disease, which accounts for 41% of the deaths of these patients. The high proportion of deaths due to cardiovascular disease is due in part to the longer survival of these patients and the sharp decrease in the early deaths from infection.[522] In one study of 101 patients with IDDM who underwent renal transplantation in the United States between 1980 and 1986, a death rate of 30% was reported over a mean follow-up period of 4 years; 57% of these deaths were from cardiovascular causes.[523] Of the patients who died, 40% had clinical manifestation of vascular diseases before transplantation and 78% suffered new events after transplantation. Only 34% of patients were free of vascular disease both before and after transplantation. Because of this high mortality and morbidity due to cardiovascular disease among diabetic patients receiving RRT, it is important to investigate the extent of vascular damage present before RRT even though the patient may be asymptomatic. Silent myocardial ischemia and infarction may occur more commonly in diabetic patients as a result of autonomic neuropathy.[524]

A resting electrocardiogram does not sufficiently predict coronary heart disease, and an exercise electrocardiogram is often impractical in diabetic patients with peripheral vascular disease and severe neuropathy. Impairment of left ventricular function and left ventricular hypertrophy are well diagnosed by echocardiography. Cardiac radionuclide imaging using thallium 201 is useful as a relatively noninvasive technique for detecting myocardial ischemia that apears as area(s) of hypoperfusion. Some authorities recommend coronary angiography before the commencement of RRT in all patients who have clinical manifestation of ischemic heart disease. Correction of coronary artery disease by balloon angioplasty or coronary vessel bypass surgery, together with effective treatment of hypertension and heart failure before the initiation of RRT, in theory should improve patient survival. However, this remains to be proven by long-term intervention studies.

Visual Loss

Visual loss is the commonest associated complication in diabetic patients with ESRF and was found to affect 35% of patients in a survey in 1985 in the United Kingdom.[46] The introduction of laser photocoagulation in the early 1970s has at least halved the risk of severe visual loss from both proliferative retinopathy and maculopathy.[525] It has also virtually abolished the increased

Table 40–7. Type and Frequency of Complications in Patients with Insulin-Treated and Non-Insulin-Treated Diabetes with Renal Failure

	No. With Complication/Total (%)	
Complications	Insulin-Treated	Non-Insulin-Treated
Disabling stroke	2/112 (1.8)	6/62 (9.7)
Leg amputation	8/113 (7.1)	3/62 (4.8)
Myocardial infarct	19/111 (17.1)	11/62 (17.7)
Severe bilateral vision loss	41/111 (36.9)	19/63 (30.2)

Table is reproduced with permission from reference 6 (Joint Working Party on Diabetic Renal Failure. Renal failure in diabetics in the UK: deficient provision of care in 1985. Diabetic Med 1988;5:77–84; copyright © John Wiley & Sons).

risk of vitreous hemorrhage in patients receiving heparin during hemodialysis. Severe bilateral visual loss, although not a contraindication to RRT, renders the patient more dependent and also limits, although does not exclude, CAPD as one of the choices of RRT.[526] It is therefore recommended that diabetic patients with significant renal impairment and retinopathy be seen regularly in an ophthalmology clinic and that photocoagulation treatment be applied in a timely manner.

Peripheral Vascular Disease

In the United Kingdom about 7% of diabetic patients who started RRT had at least one limb amputation.[6] The risk of limb amputation does not diminish after initiation of RRT[523] as the result of a combination of continuous deterioration of both peripheral neuropathy and peripheral vascular disease. All patients with diminished pedal pulses should have their peripheral vasculature investigated prior to commencing RRT. Doppler ultrasonography of the lower limbs is a useful first-line investigation. If discrete areas of obstruction to blood flow are demonstrated (as opposed to diffuse narrowing affecting the entire arterial tree), angiography is carried out to detail the extent and sites of stenoses in preparation for surgical correction. This avoids unnecessary use of contrast studies, with the added risk of acute renal failure. The importance of foot care and cessation of smoking in patients with peripheral vascular disease cannot be too heavily emphasized.

Insulin Requirement and Use of Oral Hypoglycemic Agents

The insulin requirement tends to fall with the advancement of renal failure as a result of a reduction in insulin metabolism by the kidneys. This reduction may be particularly marked in patients who are anorexic and cachectic from chronic uremia. However, this reduced insulin requirement is partly offset by the peripheral insulin resistance associated with uremia.[527,528] The change in insulin requirement therefore affects each individual differently. The risk of hypoglycemia is increased with long-acting insulin, which should be avoided in patients with ESRF. The use of renally metabolized sulfonylureas, particularly long-acting preparations such as chlorpropamide and glibenclamide, is contraindicated for the same reason. Biguanides should not be used because of the increased danger of lactic acidosis.

The use of measurements of glycosylated hemoglobin to monitor glycemic control may lead to an overestimation of the prevailing glycemia when column chromatography methods are used.[529] This problem is due to the presence of carbamylated hemoglobin, which forms as a result of a condensation of urea-derived cyanate to the N-terminal amino group of hemoglobin. The carbamylated hemoglobin has a chromatographic motility similar to that of glycosylated hemoglobin. A calometric method that is not subjected to artefacts from carbamylation should be employed in this case for the estimation of true levels of glycosylated hemoglobin. Measurement of fruc-

tosamine may be an alternative, but for this assay the plasma protein concentrations must be within the normal range.

Lipid Disturbances

An array of lipid disturbances accompanies ESRF in patients with diabetes and continues during RRT. These disturbances are characterized by raised levels of total cholesterol, LDL cholesterol, total triglycerides, VLDL triglycerides, and apoliproproteins B and Lp(a) and reduced levels of HDL_2 cholesterol.[271,273,274] This constellation of lipid disturbances represents a significant risk factor for atherosclerotic lesions and is most likely to contribute to the increased frequency of cardiovascular complications in this group of patients. Some authors have suggested that renal failure itself may be aggravated by dyslipidemia.[388] Until recently, vigorous treatment of hyperlipidemia in patients with ESRF was often been hampered by the lack of safe and effective drugs. Diet alone is often insufficient, and in the past the potential benefit provided by the use of compounds such as fibric acid and ion-exchange resins had to be balanced against the risk of adverse effects such as myopathy and gastrointestinal disturbances. The introduction of inhibitors of 3-hydroxy-3-methylglutaryl coenzyme A (HMG CoA) reductase may prove to be a safer alternative and at the same time an effective agent for treatment of dyslipidemia in ESRF. Pharmacologic treatment of hyperlipidemia in rats with chronic renal failure has resulted in amelioration of glomerular injury in the animals.[275] Preliminary results showing correction of atherogenic lipid profile in patients with nephrotic syndrome are encouraging,[530] but long-term trials are needed to establish whether these biochemical changes are translated into clinical benefits.

Choice of Renal Replacement Therapy

Hemodialysis

Hemodialysis is the commonest form of RRT in most of the European countries and accounted for 59% of all forms of RRT in the United States in 1989.[522] Recent statistics from the EDTA registry indicate that in Europe in 1988 the 3-year survival rate among patients receiving hemodialysis was 50% and 20% for those diabetic patients starting treatment before and after the age of 50 years, respectively.[520] Mortality appears to be higher in northern than in southern Europe in patients older than 50 years receiving hemodialysis. This disparity is explained in part by the higher incidence of coronary heart disease and by selective removal of fitter patients who are more likely to receive renal transplantation in northern Europe. In one center in the United States, the 4-year survival rate among diabetic patients starting dialysis after 1976 was reported to be 43%, compared with a 75% survival rate for nondiabetic patients of comparable age.[531] Severe dialysis-related problems are more prominent in diabetic patients. Vascular access is a particular difficult problem, and early creation of fistulae is recommended to allow time for the fistulae to mature. Diabetic patients tend to be more fluid overloaded, which in combination with impaired left ventricular function and autonomic neuropathy renders them less able to tolerate the rapid volume fluxes that occur during dialysis. Furthermore, since the blood pressure of diabetic patients with ESRF is exquisitely volume-dependent, interdialysis hypertension and intradialysis hypotension can be a problem. Nowadays, a combination of gentle dialysis followed by ultrafiltration for fluid control often is employed. The use of bicarbonate dialysis in Europe continues to increase rapidly—from 35% in 1988 to 39% in 1989.[520]

Finally, aluminum bone disease is more prevalent among diabetic patients receiving hemodialysis. It is believed that this increased prevalence is due to a reduced rate of bone turn-over in patients with diabetes, a situation that makes them more prone to accumulation of aluminum.[532]

Peritoneal Dialysis

The number of patients treated with peritoneal dialysis represents 15% of total number of patients receiving RRT in Europe[520] and 17% of those in the United States.[522] In United Kingdom CAPD is the first choice of RRT for both diabetic and nondiabetic patients with ESRF. Sixty percent of all diabetic patients who commenced a program of RRT dialysis in 1985 were treated with CAPD.[45] In Europe between 1982 and 1988, the 5-year survival rate among patients receiving CAPD was 80% for those who started dialysis before the age of 50 years and 38% for those who started after 50 years.[533] Lower mortality in diabetic patients receiving CAPD than in those receiving hemodialysis has been reported in Australia and New Zealand.[561] CAPD avoids rapid fluid shifts and intradialysis hypotension, thus making it particularly suitable for diabetic patients. One group of workers reported that two-thirds of the patients no longer required antihypertensive therapy 3 years after commencement of CAPD.[533] Patients also are more hospital-independent, less anemic, and subject to less stringent dietary protein and potassium restriction. There is no evidence to suggest that the rate of peritonitis among patients receiving CAPD is higher among patients with diabetes than among those without diabetes. The use of intraperitoneal insulin by direct injection into the dialysis tubing or the dialysis bags for control of diabetes is a more controversial practice. Some authorities argue against this practice because of the additional risk of infection. Others, however, encourage it because of the improved glycemic control obtained. If insulin is used in conjunction with CAPD, it should be remembered that the insulin requirement is likely to increase three- to fourfold because of the glucose in the dialysate, dilution in the peritoneal cavity, and adhesion of insulin to plastic ware.

Renal Transplantation

Renal transplantation is no doubt the treatment of choice for ESRF, especially for young diabetic patients. However, survival rates for patients receiving different modes of RRT are not strictly comparable because patients selected for transplantation are on the whole younger and in better general health than patients who receive other forms of RRT. In the United Kingdom in 1989, diabetic patients represented 6% of the patients who received renal transplants.[521] Both patient and graft survival have improved over the past years for both liver and cadaveric kidney transplantation. In Europe, 3-year patient and cadaveric graft survival for patients in the 15- to 44-year old group rose from 88% and 55% in 1982 to 95% and 72% in 1988, respectively. In general, 3-year graft survival is 10% greater for living-donor grafts than for cadaveric grafts.[520] Specialized centers in the United States have reported 90% and 40% survival rates at 3 and 10 years, respectively, among diabetic patients, a figure comparable to that for nondiabetic patients.[535] In the United Kingdom, the 3-year survival rate in diabetic patients of similar age were found to be much lower, at 53% in 1985.[536] Bentley et al., in 1986,[537] found that 60% of deaths within the first year of transplantation were caused by infection whereas after 3 years 60% were due to cardiovascular disease. Another, more recent, study in the United States reported a 4-year survival rate of 70% for patients with IDDM, with 57% of deaths caused by cardiovascular disease.[523] In 41% of cases clinical manifestations of macrovascular disease were present before transplantation, and 78% suffered new events after transplantation. Only 34% of diabetic patients who received transplants were free of large-vessel disease both before and after renal transplantation over an average follow-up period of 4 years. Among the different manifestations of macrovascular disease, only peripheral arteriopathy was found to be more frequent after transplantation, and one-fifth of the patients required limb amputation. Pretransplantation coronary and cerebral vascular disease have been shown to predispose to post-transplantation clinical events.[523]

The improved graft survival for cadaveric kidney transplants in the last few years is most likely due to a combination of factors. Improvement in surgical technique has no doubt had an effect on graft survival in both living and cadaveric kidney transplantation. The practice of multiple blood transfusions from multiple donors has also been claimed by some authors to have contributed to the improved survival figures.[538] The introduction of cyclosporine has permitted the dose of steroid used for maintenance immunosuppressant therapy to be dramatically reduced and has certainly contributed to improved cadaveric graft survival. In countries such as France and the United Kingdom, in 1988 only 63% and 71% respective diabetic patients with a functioning renal allograft were taking steroids, compared with 98% and 100% in Spain and Sweden.[520] Unfortunately, cyclosporine is nephrotoxic,[539] and careful titration of drug doses with regular monitoring of drug level and renal function is required.

After successful renal transplantation, the insulin requirement virtually returns to the levels before ESRF, and in theory a patient with NIDDM could return to treatment with oral hypoglycemic agents. In practice, however, this latter event rarely occurs, as strict metabolic control is more difficult to achieve with oral medication alone when the patient is receiving steroid therapy.

Combined Renal and Pancreatic Transplantation

A selected number of centers around the world are now reporting the first series of combined kidney and pancreas transplantation. In Europe a review of all combined transplantation carried out in 1986 revealed a 1-year patient survival of 89% in recipients of the combination graft compared with 90% in recipients of an isolated kidney transplant. Kidney survival was 78% at 1 year for recipients of combined grafts vs. 76% for patients with an isolated kidney transplant.[540] In Minneapolis, Minnesota, 2-year patient, kidney, and pancreas survival rates recently were reported as 89%, 77%, and 65% respectively, compared with a 92% patient survival rate and an 83% kidney graft survival rate in patients who had received a renal transplant alone. Long-term patient survival, however, depends on the extent of coronary atherosclerosis, which is little influenced by the function of the pancreatic graft. Normalization of blood glucose levels appears to have a beneficial effect on peripheral neuropathic symptoms but not on autonomic neuropathy.[541,542] Evidence that successful pancreatic transplantation retards progression of retinopathy is lacking,[543] but the recurrence of diabetic kidney disease in the transplanted kidney appears to be retarded.[292,544] It has recently been suggested that pancreatic transplantation in patients with IDDM who have proteinuria and mildly reduced glomerular function may stabilize renal function.[545] There is little doubt that successful pancreatic transplantation does greatly improve the quality of life of the patient, who no longer needs to administer daily insulin injections. The discussion of the advantages and disadvantages of pancreatic transplantation is beyond the scope of this review and should at present still be considered an experimental procedure. Uncorrected coronary artery disease represents a major exclusion criterion.

REFERENCES

1. Cotunnius D. De ischiade nervosa commentarius. Naples: Simonios, 1764.
2. Rollo J. In: Cases of the diabetes mellitus. 2nd ed. London: Dilly, 1798.
3. Bright R. Cases and observations illustrative of renal disease accompanied with the secretion of albuminous urine. Guy's Hosp Rep 1836;10:338–400.
4. Rayer P. In: Tindall and Cox, eds. Traite des maladies du rein. Vol 2. Paris: Baillière, 1840.
5. Kimmelstiel P, Wilson C. Intercapillary lesions in glomeruli of kidney. Am J Pathol 1936;12:83–97.
6. Joint Working Party on Diabetic Renal Failure. Renal failure in diabetics in the UK: deficient provision of care in 1985. Diabetic Med 1988;5:79–84.
7. Eggers PW. Effect of transplantation on the Medicare end-stage renal disease program. N Engl J Med 1988;318:223–9.
8. Andersen AR, Christiansen JS, Andersen JK, et al. Diabetic nephropathy in Type 1 insulin-dependent diabetes: an epidemiological study. Diabetologia 1983;25:496–501.
9. Krolewski AS, Warram JH, Christlieb AR, et al. The changing natural history of nephropathy in Type 1 diabetes. Am J Med 1985;78:785–94.
10. Kofoed-Enevoldsen A, Borch-Johnsen K, Kreiner S, et al. Declining incidence of persistent proteinuria in Type 1 insulin-dependent diabetic patients in Denmark. Diabetes 1987;36:205–9.
11. Borch-Johnsen K, Andersen PK, Deckert T. The effect of proteinuria on relative mortality in Type 1 insulin-dependent diabetes mellitus. Diabetologia 1985; 28:590–6.
12. Cameron JS. The natural history of glomerulonephritis. In: Kincaid-Smith P, d'Apice AJ, Atkins RC, eds. Progress in glomerulonephritis. New York: Wiley Medical Publications, 1979:1–25.
13. Finn R, Harmer D. Etiological implications of sex ratio in glomerulonephritis. Lancet 1979;2:1194.
14. Pasternack A, Kasanen A, Sourander L, Kaarsalo E. Prevalence and incidence of moderate and severe clinical renal failure in South Western Finland. Acta Med Scand 1985;218:173–80.
15. Danielsen R, Helgason T, Jonasson F. Prognostic factors and retinopathy in Type 1 diabetics in Iceland. Acta Med Scand 1983;213:323–36.
16. Klein R, Klein BEK, Moss SE, et al. The Wisconsin epidemiology study of diabetic retinopathy: proteinuria and retinopathy in a population of diabetic persons diagnosed prior to 30 years of age. In: Friedman EA, L'Esperance FA, eds. Diabetic renal-retinal syndrome. Vol 3. New York: Grune and Stratton, 1986:245–64.
17. Williamson JR, Rowold E, Chang K, et al. Sex steroid dependency of diabetes-induced changes in polyol metabolism, vascular permeability and collagen cross-linking. Diabetes 1986;35:20–27.
18. Kostraba JN, Dorman JS, Orchard TJ, et al. Contribution of diabetes duration before puberty to development of microvascular complications in IDDM subjects. Diabetes Care 1989;12:686–93.
19. Derby L, Laffel LBM, Krolewski AS. Risk of diabetic nephropathy declines with age in Type 1 insulin-dependent diabetes. Diabetologia 1988;31:485A.
20. Deckert T, Poulsen JE, Larsen M. Prognosis of diabetics with diabetes onset before the age of thirty one. Diabetologia 1978;14:363–70.
21. Borch-Johnsen K, Kreiner S. Proteinuria: value as predictor of cardiovascular mortality in insulin-dependent diabetes. BMJ 1987;294:1651–4.
22. Jensen T, Borch-Johnsen K, Kofoed-Enevoldsen A, Deckert T. Coronary heart disease in young Type 1 insulin-dependent diabetic patients with and without diabetic nephropathy: incidence and risk factors. Diabetologia 1987;30:144–8.
23. Krolewski AS, Kosinski EJ, Warram JH, et al. Magnitude and determinants of coronary artery disease in juvenile-onset, insulin-dependent diabetes mellitus. Am J Cardiol 1987;59:750–5.
24. Parving H-H, Hommel E. Prognosis in diabetic nephropathy. BMJ 1989;29:230–3.
25. Mathiesen ER, Borch-Johnsen K, Jensen DV, Deckert T. Increased survival in patients with diabetic nephropathy. Diabetologia 1989;32:884–6.
26. Knowles HC Jr. Long-term juvenile diabetes treated with unmeasured diet. Trans Assoc Am Physicians 1971;84:95–101.
27. Fabre J, Balant LP, Dayer PG, et al. The kidney in maturity onset diabetes mellitus: a clinical study of 510 patients. Kidney Int 1982;21:730–8.
28. Klein R, Klein BEK, Moss S, DeMets DL. Proteinuria in diabetes. Arch Intern Med 1988;148:181–6.

29. Parving H-H, Gall M-A, Skøtt P, et al. Prevalence and causes of albuminuria in non-insulin-dependent diabetic NIDDM patients. Kidney Int 1990;37:243.

30. WHO (World Health Organization Multinational) Study of Vascular Disease in Diabetes. Prevalence of small vessel and large vessel disease in diabetic patients from 14 centres. Diabetologia 1985;28;615–40.

31. Rate RG, Knowler WC, Morse HG, et al. Diabetes mellitus in Hopi and Navajo Indians. Diabetes 1983;32:894–9.

32. Nelson RG, Kunzelman CL, Pettitt DJ, et al. Albuminuria in Type 2 non-insulin-dependent diabetes mellitus and impaired glucose tolerance in Pima Indians. Diabetologia 1989;32:870–6.

33. Haffner SM, Mitchell BD, Pugh JA, et al. Proteinuria in Mexican Americans and non-Hispanic whites with NIDDM. Diabetes Care 1989;12:530–6.

34. Cowie CC, Port FK, Wolfe RA, et al. Disparities in incidence of end-stage renal disease according to race and type of diabetes. N Engl J Med 1989;321:1074–9.

35. Collins VR, Dowse GK, Finch CF, et al. Prevalence and risk factors for micro- and macroalbuminuria in diabetic subjects and entire population of Nauru. Diabetes 1989;38:602–10.

36. Samanta A, Burden AC, Feehally J, Walls J. Diabetic renal disease: differences between Asian and white patients. BMJ 1986;293:366–7.

37. Allawi J, Rao PV, Gilbert R, et al. Microalbuminuria in non-insulin-dependent diabetes: its prevalence in Indian compared with Europid patients. BMJ 1988;296:462–4.

38. Ballard DJ, Humphrey LL, Melton LJ III, et al. Epidemiology of persistent proteinuria in Type II diabetes mellitus. Population-based study in Rochester, Minnesota. Diabetes 1988;37:405–12.

39. Hasslacher C, Ritz E, Tschøpe W, et al. Hypertension in diabetes mellitus. Kidney Int 1988;34(Suppl 25):S133–7.

40. Hasslacher C, Ritz E, Wahl P, Michael C. Similar risks of nephropathy in patients with Type 1 or Type 2 diabetes mellitus. Nephrol Dial Transplant 1989;4:859–63.

41. Sasaki A, Horiuchi N, Hasegawa K, Uehara M. Risk factors related to the development of persistent albuminuria among diabetic patients observed in a long-term follow-up. J of the Jpn Diabetes Soc 1986;29:1017–23.

42. Kunzelman CL, Knowler WC, Pettitt DJ, Bennett PH. Incidence of proteinuria in Type 2 diabetes mellitus in the Pima Indians. Kidney Int 1989;35:681–7.

43. Knowler WC, Bennett PH, Nelson RG. Prediabetic blood pressure predicts albuminuria after development of NIDDM. Diabetes,1988;37(Suppl 1):120A.

44. Pettitt DJ, Saad MF, Bennett PM, et al. Familial predisposition to renal disease in two generations of Pima Indians with Type 2 non-insulin dependent diabetes mellitus. Diabetologia 1990;33:438–43.

45. Humphrey LL, Ballard DJ, Frohnest PP, et al. Chronic renal failure in non-insulin-dependent diabetes mellitus. Ann Intern Med 1989;111:788–96.

46. Joint Working Party on Diabetic Renal Failure. Treatment and mortality of diabetic renal failure patients identified in the 1985 UK survey. BMJ 1989;299:1135–6.

47. Grenfell A, Bewick M, Parsons V, et al. Non-insulin-dependent diabetes and renal replacement therapy. Diabetic Med 1988;5:172–6.

48. Schmitz A, Vaeth M. Microalbuminuria: a major risk factor in non-insulin dependent diabetes. A 10 year follow-up study of 503 patients. Diabetic Med 1988;5:126–34.

49. Morrish NJ, Stevens LK, Head J, et al. A prospective study of mortality among middle-aged diabetic patients (the London cohort of the WHO Multinational Study of Vascular Disease in Diabetics). II. Associated risk factors. Diabetologia 1990;33:542–8.

50. Jarrett RJ, Viberti GC, Argyropoulos A, et al. Microalbuminuria predicts mortality in non-insulin-dependent diabetes. Diabetic Med 1984;1:17–9.

51. Mogensen CE. Microalbuminuria predicts clinical proteinuria and early mortality in maturity onset diabetes. N Engl J Med 1984;310:356–60.

52. Nelson RG, Newman JM, Knowler WC, et al. Incidence of end-stage renal disease in Type 2 non-insulin-dependent diabetes mellitus in Pima Indians. Diabetologia 1988;31:730–6.

53. Pugh JA, Stern MP, Haffner SM, et al. Excess incidence of treatment of end-stage renal disease in Mexican Americans. Am J Epidemiol 1988;127:135–44.

54. Rostand SG, Kirk KA, Rutsky EA, et al. Racial differences in the incidence of treatment for end-stage renal disease. N Engl J Med 1982;306:1276–9.

55. Abdullah MS. Diabetic nephropathy in Kenya. East Afr Med J 1978;55:513–8.

56. Adetuyibi A. Diabetes in the Nigerian African. 1. Review of long-term complications. Trop Geogr Med 1976;28:155–9.

57. Nelson RG, Pettitt DJ, Carraher JM, et al. Effect of proteinuria on mortality in NIDDM. Diabetes 1988;37:1499–504.

58. Cambier P. Application de la théorie de Rehberg à l'étude clinique des affections rénales et du diabète. Ann Med 1934;35:273–99.

59. Fiaschi E, Grassi B, Andres G. La funzione renale nel diabete mellito. Rassegna Fisiopatologica, Clinica e Terapeutica 1952;4:373–410.

60. Stalder G, Schmid R. Severe functional disorders of glomerular capillaries and renal haemodynamics in treated diabetes mellitus during childhood. Ann Paediatr 1959;193:129–38.

61. Ditzel J, Schwartz M. Abnormal glomerular filtration in short-term insulin-treated diabetic subjects. Diabetes 1967;16:264–7.

62. Mogensen CE. Glomerular filtration rate and renal plasma flow in short-term and long-term juvenile diabetes mellitus. Scand J Clin Lab Invest 1971;28:91–100.

63. Schmitz A, Christensen T, Jensen FT. Glomerular filtration rate and kidney volume in normo-albuminuric non-insulin-dependent diabetics: lack of glomerular hyperfiltration and renal hypertrophy in uncomplicated NIDDM. Scand J Clin Lab Invest 1989;49:103–8.

64. Palmisano JJ, Lebowitz HE. Renal function in black Americans with Type 2 diabetes. J Diabetic Complications 1989;3:40–4.

65. Vora J, Thomas DM, Dean J, et al. Renal function and albumin excretion rate in 62 newly presenting non-insulin dependent diabetics NIDDM. Kidney Int 1990;37:245.

66. Loon N, Nelson R, Myers BD. Glomerular barrier abnormality in new onset NIDDM in Pima Indians. Kidney Int 1990;37:513.

67. Wiseman MJ, Viberti GC, Keen H. Threshold effect of plasma glucose in the glomerular hyperfiltration in diabetes. Nephron 1984;48:257–60.

68. Christiansen JS, Gammelgaard J, Tronier B, et al. Kidney function and size in diabetics before and during initial insulin treatment. Kidney Int 1982;21:683–8.

69. Wiseman MJ, Saunders AJ, Keen H, Viberti GC. Effect of blood glucose on increased glomerular filtration rate and

kidney size in insulin-dependent diabetes. N Engl J Med 1985;312:617−21.

70. Schmitz A, Hansen HH, Christensen T. Kidney function in newly diagnosed Type 2 non-insulin-dependent diabetic patients, before and during treatment. Diabetologia 1989;32:434−9.

71. Mogensen CE. Kidney function and glomerular permeability to macromolecules in early juvenile diabetes. Scand J Clin Lab Invest 1971;28:79−90.

72. Christiansen JS, Gammelgaard J, Frandsen M, Parving H-H. Increased kidney size, glomerular filtration rate and renal plasma flow in short-term insulin-dependent diabetics. Diabetologia 1981;20:451−6.

73. Ditzel J, Junker K. Abnormal glomerular filtration rate, renal plasma flow, and renal protein excretion in recent and short-term diabetics. BMJ 1972;2:13−9.

74. Christiansen JS. On the pathogenesis of the increased glomerular filtration rate in short-term insulin-dependent diabetics [Dissertation]. Copenhagen: Laegeforeningens Forlsag, 1984.

75. Mogensen CE, Andersen MJF. Increased kidney size and glomerular filtration rate in early juvenile diabetes. Diabetes 1973;22:706−12.

76. Puig JG, Anton FM, Grande E, et al. Relation of kidney size to kidney function in early insulin-dependent diabetes. Diabetologia 1981;21:363−7.

77. Wiseman M, Viberti GC. Kidney size and GFR in Type 1 insulin-dependent diabetes mellitus revisited. Diabetologia 1983;25:530.

78. Dumler F, Kumar V, Romanski NM, et al. Renal involvement in Type 2 diabetes mellitus: a clinicopathologic study of the Henry Ford Hospital experience. Henry Ford Hosp Med J 1987;35:221−5.

79. Mogensen CE, Andersen MJF. Increased kidney size and glomerular filtration rate in untreated juvenile diabetics: normalization by insulin treatment. Diabetologia 1975; 11:221−4.

80. Feldt-Rasmussen B, Hegedus L, Mathiesen ER, Deckert T. Kidney volume in Type 1 insulin-dependent diabetic patients with normal or increased urinary albumin excretion. Effect of long-term improved metabolic control. Scand J Clin Lab Invest 1991;51:31−6.

81. Christensen CK, Christiansen JS, Christensen T, et al. The effect of six months continuous subcutaneous insulin infusion on kidney function and size in insulin-dependent diabetics. Diabetic Med 1986;3:29−32.

82. Rasch R. Prevention of diabetic glomerulopathy in streptozotocin diabetic rats by insulin treatment. Kidney size and glomerular volume. Diabetologia 1979; 16:125−8.

83. Seyer-Hansen K. Renal hypertrophy in streptozotocin-diabetic rats. Clin Sci Molec Med 1976;51:551−5.

84. Kahn CB, Paman PG, Zic Z. Kidney size in diabetes mellitus. Diabetes 1974;23:788−92.

85. Ellis EN, Steffes MW, Gøetz FC, et al. Relationship of renal size to nephropathy in Type 1 insulin-dependent diabetes. Diabetologia 1985;28:12−5.

86. Kleinman KS, Fine LG. Prognostic implications of renal hypertrophy in diabetes mellitus. Diabetes Metab Rev 1988;4:179−89.

87. Segel MC, Lecky JW, Slasky BS. Diabetes mellitus: the predominant cause of bilateral renal enlargement. Radiology 1984;153:341−2.

88. Mogensen CE, Christensen CK. Predicting diabetic nephropathy in insulin-dependent diabetic patients. N Engl J Med 1984;311: 89−93.

89. Mogensen CE. Early glomerular hyperfiltration in insulin-dependent diabetics and late nephropathy. Scand J Clin Lab Invest 1986;46:201−6.

90. Lervang H-H, Jensen S, Brøchner-Mortensen J, Ditzel J. Early glomerular hyperfiltration and the development of late nephropathy in Type 1 insulin-dependent diabetes mellitus. Diabetologia 1988;31:723−9.

91. Jones SL, Wiseman MJ, Viberti GC. Glomerular hyperfiltration as a risk factor for diabetic nephropathy: five year report of a prospective study. Diabetologia 1991; 34:59−60.

92. Keen H, Chlouverakis C, Fuller JH, Jarrett RJ. The concomitants of raised blood sugar: studies in newly detected hyperglycaemics. II. Urinary albumin excretion, blood pressure and their relation to blood sugar levels. Guy's Hosp Rep 1969;118:247−52.

93. Mogensen CE. Urinary albumin excretion in early and long term juvenile diabetes. Scand J Clin Lab Invest 1971; 28:183−93.

94. Parving H-H, Noer I, Deckert T, et al. 1976. The effect of metabolic regulation on microvascular permeability to small and large molecules in short-term juvenile diabetics. Diabetologia, 12, 161−6.

95. Mogensen CE. Renal function changes in diabetes. Diabetes 1976;25:872−6.

96. Viberti GC, Mackintosh D, Bilous RW, et al. Proteinuria in diabetes mellitus: role of spontaneous and experimental variation of glycaemia. Kidney Int 1982;21:714−20.

97. Mogensen CE, Chachati A, Christensen CK, et al. Microbalbuminurea: an early marker of renal involvement in diabetes. Uremia Invest 1986;9:85−95.

98. Feldt-Rasmussen B, Mathiesen ER. Variability of urinary albumin excretion in incipient diabetic nephropathy. Diabetic Nephropathy 1984;3:101−3.

99. Mathiesen ER, Øxenboll B, Johansen K, et al. Incipient nephropathy in Type 1 insulin-dependent diabetes. Diabetologia 1984;26:406−10.

100. Rowe DJF, Bagga H, Betts PB. Normal variation in the rate of albumin excretion and albumin to creatinine ratios in overnight and daytime urine collections in non-diabetic children. BMJ 1985;291:693−4.

101. Cohen DL, Close CF, Viberti GC. The variability of overnight urinary albumin excretion in insulin-dependent diabetic and normal subjects. Diabetic Med 1987;4:437−40.

102. Chachati A, von Frenckell R, Foidart-Willems J, et al. Variability of albumin excretion in insulin-dependent diabetics. Diabetic Med 1987;4:441−5.

103. Mathiesen ER, Saurbrey N, Hommel E, Parving H-H. Prevalence of microalbuminuria in children with Type 1 insulin-dependent diabetes mellitus. Diabetologia 1986; 29:640−3.

104. Microalbuminuria Collaborative Study Group, U.K. Microalbuminuria in Type 1 (insulin-dependent) diabetic patients: prevalence and clinical characteristics. Diabetes Care (in press).

105. Gardete LM, Silva-Graça, Boavida JM, et al. Microalbuminuria—an early marker of developing microangiopathy. Diabetologia 1987;29:539A.

106. Gatling W, Knight C, Mullee MA, Hill RD. Microalbuminuria in diabetes: a population study of the prevalence and an assessment of three screening tests. Diabetic Med 1988;5:343−7.

107. Parving H-H, Hommel E, Mathiesen E, et al. Prevalence of microalbuminuria, arterial hypertension, retinopathy and neuropathy in patients with insulin-dependent diabetes. BMJ 1988;296:156−60.

108. Marshall SM, Alberti KGMM. Comparison of the preva-

lence and associated features of abnormal albumin excretion in insulin-dependent and non-insulin-dependent diabetes. Q J Med 1989;70:61–71.

109. Mogensen CE, Christensen CK, Vittinghus E. The stages in diabetic renal disease with emphasis on the stage of incipient diabetic nephropathy. Diabetes 1983;32(Suppl 2):64–78.

110. Viberti GC, Pickup JC, Jarrett RJ, Keen H. Effect of control of blood glucose on urinary excretion of albumin and beta-2 microglobulin in insulin-dependent diabetes. N Engl J Med 1979;300:638–41.

111. Mogensen CE, Vittinghus E. Urinary albumin excretion during exercise in juvenile diabetes: a provocation test for early abnormalities. Scand J Clin Lab Invest 1975;35:295–300.

112. Viberti GC, Jarrett RJ, McCartney M, Keen H. Increased glomerular permeability to albumin induced by exercise in diabetic subjects. Diabetologia 1978;14:293–300.

113. Koivisto VA, Huttunen NP, Vierikko P. Continuous subcutaneous insulin infusion corrects exercised-induced albuminuria in juvenile diabetes. BMJ 1981;282:778–9.

114. Viberti GC, Pickup JC, Bilous RW, et al. Correction of exercise-induced microalbuminuria in insulin-dependent diabetics after 3 weeks of subcutaneous insulin infusion. Diabetes 1981;30:818–23.

115. Vittinghus E, Mogensen CE. Graded exercise and protein excretion in diabetic man and the effect of insulin treatment. Kidney Int 1982;21:725–9.

116. Damsgaard EM, Mogensen CE. Microalbuminuria in elderly hyperglycaemic patients and controls. Diabetic Med 1986;3:430–5.

117. Allawi J, Jarrett RJ. Microalbuminuria and cardiovascular risk factors in Type 2 diabetes mellitus. Diabetic Med 1990;7:115–8.

118. Viberti GC, Hill RD, Jarrett RJ, et al. Microalbuminuria as a predictor of clinical nephropathy in insulin-dependent diabetes mellitus. Lancet 1982;1:1430–2.

119. Parving H-H, Øxenboll B, Svendsen PA, et al. Early detection of patients at risk of developing diabetic nephropathy. A longitudinal study of urinary albumin excretion. Acta Endocrinol (Copenh) 1982;100:550–5.

120. Jerums J, Cooper ME, Seeman E, et al. Spectrum of proteinuria in Type 1 and Type 2 diabetes. Diabetes Care 1987;10:419–27.

121. Chavers BM, Bilous RW, Ellis EN, et al. Glomerular lesions and urinary albumin excretion in Type 1 diabetes without overt proteinuria. N Engl J Med 1989;320:966–70.

122. Mattock M, Morrish N, Viberti GC, et al. Microalbuminuria as a predictor of mortality in NIDDM: a prospective study. Diabetes 1992 (in press).

123. Yudkin JS, Forrest RD, Jackson CA. Microalbuminuria as a predictor of vascular disease in non-diabetic subjects. Lancet 1988;2:530–3.

124. Ireland JT, Viberti GC, Watkins PJ. The kidney and renal tract. In: Keen H, Jarrett J, eds. Complications of diabetes. 2nd ed. London: Edward Arnold, 1982:137–78.

125. Bending JJ, Viberti GC, Watkins PJ, Keen H. Intermittent clinical proteinuria and renal function in diabetes: evolution and the effect of glycaemic control. BMJ 1986;292:83–6.

126. Mogensen CE. Progression of nephropathy in long-term diabetics with proteinuria and effect of initial antihypertensive treatment. Scand J Clin Lab Invest 1976;36:383–8.

127. Jones RH, Hayakawa H, Mackay JD, et al. Progression of diabetic nephropathy. Lancet 1979;1:1105–6.

128. Parving H-H, Smidt UM, Friisberg B, et al. A prospective study of glomerular filtration rate and arterial blood pressure in insulin-dependent diabetics with diabetic nephropathy. Diabetologia 1981;20:457–61.

129. Viberti GC, Bilous RW, Mackintosh D, Keen H. Monitoring glomerular function in diabetic nephropathy. Am J Med 1983;74: 256–64.

130. Feldt-Rasmussen B, Mathiesen ER, Deckert T. Effect of two years of strict metabolic control on progression of incipient nephropathy in insulin-dependent diabetes. Lancet 1986;2:1300–4.

131. Viberti GC, Bilous RW, Mackintosh D, et al. Long term correction of hyperglycaemia and progression of renal failure in insulin-dependent diabetes. BMJ 1983;286:598–602.

132. Hasslacher C, Stech W, Wahl P, Ritz E. Blood pressure and metabolic control as risk factors for nephropathy in Type 1 insulin-dependent diabetes. Diabetologia 1985;28:6–11.

133. Nyberg G, Blohne G, Norden G. Impact of metabolic control in progression of diabetic nephropathy. Diabetologia 1987;30:82–6.

134. Viberti GC, Keen H, Dodds R, Bending JJ. Metabolic control and progression of diabetic nephropathy. Diabetologia 1987;30:481–2.

135. Laffel LMB, Krolewski AS, Rand LI, et al. The impact of blood pressure on renal function in insulin-dependent diabetes. Kidney Int 1987;31:207.

136. Walser M, Drew HH, LaFrance ND. Creatinine measurements often yield false estimates of progression in chronic renal failure. Kidney Int 1988;34:412–8.

137. Shemesh O, Golbetz H, Kriss JP, Myers BD. Limitations of creatinine as a filtration marker in glomerulopathic patients. Kidney Int 1985;28:830–8.

138. Walker JD, Bending JJ, Dodds RA, et al. Restriction of dietary protein and progression of renal failure in diabetic nephropathy. Lancet 1989;2:1411–5.

139. Zeller KR, Whittaker E, Sullivan L, et al. Effect of restricting dietary protein on the progression of renal failure in patients with insulin-dependent diabetes mellitus. N Engl J Med 1991;324:78–84.

140. Wiseman MJ, Viberti GC, Mackintosh D, et al. Glycaemia, arterial pressure and micro-albuminuria in Type 1 insulin-dependent diabetes mellitus. Diabetologia 1984;26:401–5.

141. Jensen T, Borch-Johnsen K, Deckert T. Changes in blood pressure and renal function in patients with Type 1 insulin-dependent diabetes mellitus prior to clinical diabetic nephropathy. Diabetes Res 1987;4:159–62.

142. Keen H, Track NS, Sowry GSC. Arterial pressure in clinically apparent diabetics. Diabete Metab 1975;1:159–78.

143. Drury PL. Diabetes and arterial hypertension. Diabetologia 1983;24:1–9.

144. Borch-Johnsen K, Nissen RN, Nerup J. Blood pressure after 40 years of diabetes. Diabetic Nephropathy 1985;4:11–2.

145. Watkins PJ, Blainey JD, Brewer DB, et al. The natural history of diabetic renal disease. A follow-up study of a series of renal biopsies. Q J Med (New Series) 1972;41:437–56.

146. Thomsen AC. The kidney in diabetes mellitus [Dissertation]. Munksgaard, Copenhagen, 1965.

147. Malins J. Clinical diabetes mellitus. London: Eyre & Spottiswoode, 1968:.170.

148. Deckert T, Poulsen JE. Prognosis for juvenile diabetics with late diabetic manifestations. Acta Med Scand 1968;183:351–6.

149. Bilous RW, Viberti GC, Christiansen JS, et al. Dissociation of diabetic complications in insulin-dependent diabetes: a clinical report. Diabetic Nephropathy 1985;4:73–6.

150. Root HF, Mirsky S, Ditzel J. Proliferative retinopathy in diabetes mellitus; review of eight hundred forty seven cases. JAMA 1959;169:903–9.

151. Feldman JN, Hirsch SR, Beyer MB, et al. Prevalence of diabetic nephropathy at time of treatment for diabetic retinopathy. In: Friedman EA, L'Esperance FA, eds. Diabetic renal-retinal syndrome. Vol 2. New York, Grune and Stratton, 1982:9–20.

152. Krolewski AS, Warram JH, Rand LI, Kahn CR. Epidemiologic approach to the etiology of Type 1 diabetes mellitus and its complications. N Engl J Med 1987;317:1390–8.

153. West KM, Erdreich LJ, Stober JA. A detailed study of risk factors for retinopathy and nephropathy in diabetes. Diabetes 1988;29:501–8.

154. Hommel E, Carstensen H, Skøtt P, et al. Prevalence and causes of microscopic haematuria in Type 1 insulin-dependent diabetic patients with persistent proteinuria. Diabetologia 1987;30:627–30.

155. Taft JL, Billson VR, Nankervis A, et al. A clinical-histological study of individuals with diabetes mellitus and proteinuria. Diabetic Med 1990;7:215–21.

156. Hatch FE Jr, Parrish AE. Apparent remission of a severe diabetic on developing the Kimmelstiel-Wilson syndrome. Ann Intern Med 1961;54:544–9.

157. Rifkin H, Parker JG, Polin EB, et al. Diabetic glomerulosclerosis. Medicine 1948;27:429–57.

158. Bell ET. Renal vascular disease in diabetes mellitus. Diabetes 1953;2:376–89.

159. Gellman DD, Pirani CL, Soothill JF, et al. Diabetic nephropathy: a clinical and pathologic study based on renal biopsies. Medicine (Baltimore) 1959;38:321–67.

160. Axelrod L. Response of congestive heart failure to correction of hyperglycaemia in the presence of diabetic nephropathy. N Engl J Med 1975;293:1243–5.

161. DeFronzo RA. Hyperkalaemia and hyporeninaemic hypoaldosteronism. Kidney Int 1980;17:118–34.

162. Campbell IW, Heading C, Tothill P, et al. Gastric emptying in diabetic autonomic neuropathy. Gut 1977;18:462–7.

163. Watkins PJ. Facial sweating after food: a new sign of autonomic diabetic neuropathy. BMJ 1973;1:583–7.

164. White P, Graham CA. The child with diabetes. In: Marble A, White P, Bradley RF, Krall LP, eds. Joslin's diabetes mellitus. 11th ed. Philadelphia: Lea & Febiger, 1971:539–60.

165. Hostetter TH, Troy JC, Brenner BM. Glomerular haemodynamics in experimental diabetes mellitus. Kidney Int 1981;19:410–5.

166. Zatz R, Meyer TW, Rennke HG, Brenner BM. Predominance of haemodynamic rather than metabolic factors in the pathogenesis of diabetic glomerulopathy. Proc Natl Acad Sci USA 1985;82:5963–7.

167. Jensen PK, Christiansen JS, Steven K, Parving H-H. Renal function in streptozocin-diabetic rats. Diabetologia 1981;21:409–14.

168. Michels LD, Davidman M, Keane WF. Determinants of glomerular filtration and plasma flow in experimental diabetic rats. J Lab Clin Med 1981;98:869–85.

169. O'Donnell MP, Kasiske BL, Daniels FX, Keane WF. Effects of nephron loss on glomerular haemodynamics and morphology in diabetic rats. Diabetes 1986;35:1011–5.

170. Wiseman MJ, Mangili R, Alberetto M, et al. Glomerular response mechanisms to glycaemic changes in insulin-dependent diabetics. Kidney Int 1987;31:1012–8.

171. Kroustrup JP, Gundersen HJG, Østerby R. Glomerular size and structure in diabetes mellitus. III. Early enlargement of the capillary surface. Diabetologia 1977;13:207–10.

172. Gøtzsche O, Gundersen HJG, Østerby R. Irreversibility of glomerular basement membrane accumulation despite reversibility of renal hypertrophy with islet transplantation in early experimental diabetes. Diabetes 1981;30:481–5.

173. Hirose K, Tsuchida H, Østerby R, Gundersen HJG. A strong correlation between glomerular filtration rate and filtration surface area in diabetic kidney hyperfunction. Lab Invest 1980;43:434–7.

174. Parving H-H, Rutili F, Granath K, et al. Effect of metabolic regulation on renal leakiness to dextran molecules in short-term insulin-dependent diabetics. Diabetologia 1979;17:157–60.

175. Ballerman BJ, Skorecki KL, Brenner BM. Reduced glomerular angiotensin II receptor density in early untreated diabetes mellitus in the rat. Am J Physiol 1984;247:F110–6.

176. Viberti GC, Wiseman MJ. The kidney in diabetes: significance of the early abnormalities. Clin Endocrinol Metab 1986;15:753–82.

177. Christiansen JS, Frandsen M, Parving H-H. Effect of intravenous glucose infusion on renal function in normal man and in insulin-dependent diabetics. Diabetologia 1981;21:368–73.

178. Mogensen CE. Maximum tubular reabsorption capacity for glucose and renal haemodynamics during rapid hypertonic glucose infusion in normal and diabetic subjects. Scand J Clin Lab Invest 1971;28:101–9.

179. Fox M, Thier S, Rosenberg L, Segal S. Impaired renal tubular function induced by sugar infusion in man. J Clin Endocrinol Metabol 1964;24:1318–27.

180. Brøchner-Mortensen J. The glomerular filtration rate during moderate hyperglycaemia in normal man. Acta Med Scand 1973;194:10–7.

181. Atherton A, Hill DW, Keen H, et al. The effect of acute hyperglycaemia on the retinal circulation of the normal cat. Diabetologia 1980;18:233–7.

182. Blantz RC, Peterson OW, Gushwa L, Tucker BJ. Effect of modest hyperglycaemia on tubuloglomerular feedback activity. Kidney Int 1982;22(Suppl 12):S206–12.

183. Leyssac PP. The renin angiotensin system and kidney function. A review of contributions to a new theory. Acta Physiol Scand 1976;442(Suppl):1–52.

184. Trevisan R, Nosadini R, Fioretto P, et al. Ketone bodies increase glomerular filtration rate in normal man and in patients with Type 1 diabetes mellitus. Diabetologia 1987;30:214–21.

185. Mogensen CE, Christensen NJ, Gundersen HGJ. The acute effect of insulin on renal haemodynamics and protein excretion in diabetics. Diabetologia 1978;15:153–7.

186. Christiansen JS, Frandsen M, Parving H-H. The effect of intravenous insulin infusion on kidney function in insulin-dependent diabetes mellitus. Diabetologia 1981;20:199–204.

187. DeFronzo RA, Cooke CR, Andres R, et al. The effect of insulin on renal handling of sodium, potassium, calcium and phosphate in man. J Clin Invest 1975;55:845–55.

188. Skøtt P, Hother-Nielsen O, Bruun NE, et al. Effects of insulin on kidney function and sodium excretion in healthy subjects. Diabetologia 1989;32:694–9.

189. Parving H-H, Noer I, Mogensen CE, Svendsen PA. Kidney function in normal man during short-term growth-

hormone infusion. Acta Endocrinologica 1978; 89:796–800.

190. Corvilain J, Abramow M. Some effects of human growth hormone on renal haemodynamics and on tubular phosphate transport in man. J Clin Invest 1962; 41:1230–5.

191. Christiansen JS, Gammelgaard J, Ørskov H, et al. Kidney function and size in normal subjects before and during growth hormone administration for one week. Eur J Clin Invest 1981;11:487–90.

192. Christiansen JS, Gammelgaard J, Frandsen M, et al. Kidney function and size in Type 1 insulin-dependent diabetic patients before and during growth hormone administration for one week. Diabetologia 1982;22:333–7.

193. Lundbaek K, Christensen NJ, Jensen VA, et al. Diabetes, diabetic angiopathy, and growth hormone. Lancet 1970;2:131–3.

194. Wiseman MJ, Redmond S House F, et al. The glomerular hyperfiltration of diabetics is not associated with elevated levels of glucagon and growth hormone. Diabetologia 1985;28:718–21.

195. Parving H-H, Noer I, Kehlet H, et al. The effect of short-term glucagon infusion on kidney function in normal man. Diabetologia 1977;13:323–5.

196. Parving H-H, Christiansen JS, Noer I, et al. The effect of glucagon infusion on kidney function in short-term Type 1 insulin-dependent juvenile diabetics. Diabetologia 1980; 19:350–4.

197. Ueda J, Nakanishi H, Miyazaki M, Abe Y. Effects of glucagon on the renal haemodynamics of dogs. Eur J Pharmacol 1977;41:209–12.

198. Uranga J, Frenzalida R, Rapoport AL, Del Castillo E. Effect of glucagon and glomerulopressin on the renal function of the dog. Horm Metab Res 1979;11:275–9.

199. Fioretto P, Trevisan R, Valerio, et al. Impaired renal response to a meat meal in insulin-dependent diabetes: role of glucagon and prostaglandins. Am J Physiol 1990;258:F675–83.

200. Viberti GC, Benigni A, Bognetti E, et al. Glomerular hyperfiltration and urinary prostaglandins in Type 1 diabetes mellitus. Diabetic Med 1989;6:219–23.

201. Esmatjes E, Fernandez MR, Halperin I, et al. Renal hemodynamic abnormalities in patients with short-term insulin-dependent diabetes mellitus: role of renal prostaglandins. J Clin Endocrinol Metabol 1985;60:1231–6.

202. Kasiske BL, O'Donnell MP, Keane WF. Glucose induced increases in renal haemodynamic function. Possible modulation by renal prostaglandins. Diabetes 1985;34:360–4.

203. Jensen PK, Steven K, Blæhr H, et al. Effects of indomethacin on glomerular haemodynamics in experimental diabetes. Kidney Int 1986;29:490–5.

204. Schambelan M, Blake S, Sraer J, et al. Increased prostaglandin production by glomeruli isolated from rats with streptozotocin-induced diabetes mellitus. J Clin Invest 1985;75:404–12.

205. Moel DI, Safirstein RL, McEvoy RC, Hsueh W. Effect of aspirin on experimental diabetic nephropathy. J Lab Clin Med 1987;110:300–7.

206. Christiansen JS, Feldt-Rasmussen B, Parving H-H. Short-term inhibition of prostaglandin synthesis has no effect on the elevated glomerular filtration rate of early insulin-dependent diabetes. Diabetic Med 1985;2:17–20.

207. Hommel E, Mathiesen E, Arnold-Larssen S, et al. Effect of indomethacin on kidney function in Type 1 insulin-dependent diabetic patients with diabetic nephropathy. Diabetologia 1987;30:78–81.

208. Del Castillo E, Fuenzalida R, Uranga J. Increased glomerular filtration rate and glomerulopressin activity in diabetic dogs. Horm Metab Res 1977;9:46–53.

209. Ortola FV, Ballerman BJ, Anderson S, et al. Elevated plasma atrial natriuretic peptide levels in diabetic rats. Potential mediators of hyperfiltration. J Clin Invest 1987;80:670–4.

210. Rave K, Heinemann L, Sawicki P, et al. Increased concentration of atrial natriuretic peptide in Type 1 insulin-dependent diabetic patients with glomerular hyperfiltration. Diabetologia 1987;30:573A.

211. Sawiki PT, Heineman L, Rave K, et al. Atrial natriuretic factor in various stages of diabetic nephropathy. J Diabetic Complications 1988;2:207–9.

212. Solerte SB, Fioravanti M, Spriano P, et al. Plasma atrial natriuretic peptide, renal haemodynamics and microalbuminuria in short-term Type 1 insulin-dependent diabetic patients with hyperfiltration. Diabetologia 1987;30:584A.

213. Jones SL, Perico N, Benigni A, et al. Glomerular filtration rate, extracellular fluid volume and atrial natriuretic factor in insulin-dependent diabetics. Kidney Int 1988;33:268.

214. Hommel E, Mathiesen ER, Giese J, et al. On the pathogenesis of arterial pressure elevation early in the course of diabetic nephropathy. Scand J Clin Lab Invest 1989; 49:537–44.

215. Brøchner-Mortensen J, Ditzel J. Glomerular filtration rate and extracellular fluid volume in insulin-dependent patients with diabetes mellitus. Kidney Int 1982;21:696–8.

216. Feldt-Rasmussen B, Mathiesen ER, Deckert T, et al. Central role for sodium in the pathogenesis of blood pressure changes independent of angiotensin, aldosterone and catecolamines in Type 1 insulin-dependent diabetes mellitus. Diabetologia 1987;30:610–7.

217. Cortes P, Dumler F, Goldman J, Levin NW. Relationship between renal function and metabolic alterations in early streptozotocin-induced diabetes in rats. Diabetes 1987;36:80–7.

218. Seyer-Hansen K, Hansen J, Gundersen HJG. Renal hypertrophy in experimental diabetes. A morphometric study. Diabetologia 1988;18:501–5.

219. Østerby R, Gundersen HJG. Fast accumulation of basement membrane material and the rate of morphological changes in acute experimental diabetic glomerular hypertrophy. Diabetologia 1980;18:493–500.

220. Rasch R. Tubular lesions in streptozotocin-diabetic rats. Diabetologia 1984;27:32–7.

221. Seyer-Hansen K. Renal hypertrophy in experimental diabetes mellitus. Kidney Int 1983;23:643–6.

222. Peterson PA, Evrin PE, Berggård I. Differentiation of glomerular, tubular, and normal proteinuria: determinations of urinary excretion of β_2-microglobulin, albumin, and total protein. J Clin Invest 1969;48:1189–98.

223. Wibell L. Studies of β_2-microglobulin in human serum, urine and amniotic fluid [Dissertation]. Abstracts of Uppsala Dissertations from the Faculty of Medicine, 1974:183.

224. Pappenheimer JR, Renkin EM, Barrero LM. Filtration diffusion and molecular sieving through peripheral capillary membranes. A contribution to the pore theory of capillary permeability. Am J Physiol 1951;167:13–46.

225. Brenner BM, Hostetter TH, Humes HD. Molecular basis of proteinuria of glomerular origin. N Engl J Med 1978; 298:826–33.

226. Venkatachalam MA, Rennke HG. The structural and molecular basis of glomerular filtration. Circ Res 1978; 43:337–47.

227. Deen WM, Satvat B. Determinants of glomerular filtration of proteins. Am J Physiol 1981;241:F162–70.

228. Myers BD, Winetz JA, Chui F, Michaels AS. Mechanisms of proteinuria in diabetic nephropathy: a study of glomerular barrier function. Kidney Int 1982;21:633−41.

229. Viberti GC, Mackintosh D, Keen H. Determinants of the penetration of proteins through the glomerular barrier in insulin-dependent diabetes mellitus. Diabetes 1983; 32(Suppl 2):92−5.

230. Viberti GC, Keen H. The patterns of proteinuria in diabetes mellitus. Relevance to pathogenesis and prevention of diabetic nephropathy. Diabetes 1984; 33:686−92.

231. Westberg NG, Michael AF. Human glomerular basement membrane: chemical composition in diabetes mellitus. Acta Med Scand 1973;194:39−47.

232. Winetz JA, Golbetz HV, Spencer RJ, et al. Glomerular function in advanced human diabetic nephropathy. Kidney Int 1982;21:750−6.

233. Parthasarathy N, Spiro RG. Effect of diabetes on the glycosaminoglycan component of the human glomerular basement membrane. Diabetes 1982;31:738−41.

234. Schober E, Pollack A, Coradello H, Lubec G. Glycosylation of glomerular basement membrane in Type 1 insulin-dependent diabetic children. Diabetologia 1982; 23:485−7.

235. Hostetter TH, Rennke HG, Brenner BM. The case for intrarenal hypertension in the initiation and progression of diabetic and other glomerulopathies. Am J Med 1982;72:375−80.

236. Kanwar YS, Rosenzweig LJ, Linker A, Jakubowski ML. Decreased de novo synthesis of glomerular proteoglycans in diabetes: biochemical and autoradiographic evidence. Proc Natl Acad Sci USA 1983;80:2272−5.

237. Brenner BM. Nephron adaptation to renal injury or ablation. Am J Physiol 1985;249:F234−7.

238. Nakamura Y, Myers BD. Charge selectivity of proteinuria in diabetic glomerulopathy. Diabetes 1988;37:1202−11.

239. Deckert T, Feldt-Rasmussen B, Djurup R, Deckert M. Glomerular size and charge selectivity in insulin-dependent diabetes mellitus. Kidney Int 1988;33:100−6.

240. Bertolatus JA, Abuyousef M, Hunsicker LG. Glomerular sieving of high molecular weight proteins in proteinuric rats. Kidney Int 1987;31:1257−66.

241. Melvin T, Kim Y, Michael AF. Selective binding of IgG$_4$ and other negatively charged plasma proteins in normal and diabetic human kidney. Am J Pathol 1984;115:443−6.

242. Guthrow CE, Morris MA, Day JF, et al. Enhanced nonenzymatic glycosylation of human serum albumin in diabetes mellitus. Proc Natl Acad Sci USA 1979;76:4258−61.

243. Cohen MP, Urdanivia E, Surma M, Ciborowski C.. Nonenzymatic glycosylation of basement membranes in in vitro studies. Diabetes 1981;30:367−71.

244. Williams SK, Devenny JJ, Bitensky MW. Micropinocytic ingestion of glycosylated albumin by isolated microvessels: possible role in pathogenesis of diabetic microangiopathy. Proc Natl Acad Sci USA 1981; 78:2393−7.

245. Ghiggeri GM, Candiano G, Delfino G, Queirolo C. Electrical charge of serum and urinary albumin in normal and diabetic humans. Kidney Int 1985;28:168−177.

246. Williams SK, Siegel RK. Preferential transport of nonenzymatically glycosylated ferritin across the kidney glomerulus. Kidney Int 1985;28:146−52.

247. Shaklai N, Garlick RL, Bunn HF. Nonenzymatic glycosylation of human serum albumin alters its conformation and function. J Biol Chem 1984;259:3812−7.

248. Pillay VKG, Gandhi VC, Sharma BK, et al. Effect of hydration and frusemide given intravenously on proteinuria. Arch Intern Med 1972;130:90−2.

249. Jarrett RJ, Verma NP, Keen H. Urinary albumin excretion in normal and diabetic subjects. Clin Chim Acta 1976;71:55−9.

250. First MR, Patel VB, Pesce RJ, et al. Albumin excretion by the kidney. The effect of osmotic diuresis. Nephron 1978;20:171−5.

251. Hegedüs L, Christensen NJ, Mogensen CE, Gundersen HJG. Oral glucose increases urinary albumin excretion in normal subjects but not in insulin-dependent diabetics. Scand J Clin Lab Invest 1980;40:479−82.

252. Viberti GC, Mogensen CE, Keen H, et al. Urinary excretion of albumin in normal man: the effect of water loading. Scand J Clin Lab Invest 1982;42:147−51.

253. Viberti GC, Strakosch CR, Keen H, et al. The influence of glucose-induced hyperinsulinaemia on renal glomerular function and circulating catecholamines in normal man. Diabetologia 1981;21:436−9.

254. Viberti GC, Haycock GB, Pickup JC, et al. Early functional and morphologic vascular renal consequences of the diabetic state. Diabetologia 1980;18:173−5.

255. Kokko JP. Proximal tubule potential difference. Dependence on glucose, HCO$_3$, and amino-acids. J Clin Invest 1973;52:1362−7.

256. Ditzel J, Brøchner-Mortensen J, Kawahara R. Dysfunction of tubular phosphate reabsorption related to glomerular filtration and blood glucose control in diabetic children. Diabetologia 1982;23:406−10.

257. Watanabe Y, Nunoi K, Maki Y, et al. Contribution of glycaemic control to the levels of N-acetyl-β-D-glucosaminidase and serum NAG in Type 1 insulin-dependent diabetes mellitus without proteinuria. Clin Nephrol 1987;28:227−31.

258. Gibb DM, Tomlinson PA, Dalton NR, et al. Renal tubular proteinuria and microalbuminuria in diabetic patients. Arch Dis Child 1989;64:129−34.

259. Ditzel J, Brøchner-Mortensen J. Tubular reabsorption rates as related to glomerular filtration in diabetic children. Diabetes 1983;32(Suppl 2):28−33.

260. Mauer SM, Steffes MW, Ellis EN, et al. Structural-functional relationships in diabetic nephropathy. J Clin Invest 1984;74:1143−55.

261. Tomlanovich S, Deen WM, Jones HW, et al. Functional nature of glomerular injury in progressive diabetic glomerulopathy. Diabetes 1987;36:556−65.

262. Pinto JR, Bending JJ, Dodds R, et al. Effect of low protein diet on the renal response to meat ingestion in diabetic nephropathy. Eur J Clin Invest 1991;21:175−83.

263. Remuzzi A, Viberti GC, Ruggenenti P, et al. Glomerular response to hyperglycaemia in human diabetic nephropathy. Am J Physiol 1990;259:F545−52.

264. De Cosmo S, Ruggenenti P, Walker JD, et al. Mechanisms of glucose induced glomerular haemodynamic changes in diabetic nephropathy. Diabetologia 1989;32:480A.

265. Kefalides NA. Biochemical properties of human glomerular basement membrane in normal and diabetic kidneys. J Clin Invest 1974;53:403−7.

266. Wahl P, Deppermann D, Hasslacher C. Biochemistry of glomerular basement membrane of the normal and diabetic human. Kidney Int 1982;21:744−9.

267. Rohrbach DH, Wagner CW, Star VL, et al. Reduced synthesis of basement membrane heparan sulfate proteoglycan in streptozotocin-induced diabetic mice. J Biol Chem 1983;258:11676−7.

268. Cohen MP, Surma ML. Effect of diabetes on in vivo metabolism of ^{35}S-labeled glomerular basement membrane. Diabetes 1984;33:8–12.

269. Wu V-Y, Wilson B, Cohen MP. Disturbances in glomerular basement membrane glycosaminoglycans in experimental diabetes. Diabetes 1987;36:679–83.

270. Shimomura H, Spiro RG. Studies on the macromolecular components of human glomerular basement membrane and alterations in diabetes: decreased levels of heparan sulfate proteoglycan and laminin. Diabetes 1987; 36:374–81.

271. Vannini P, Ciavarella A, Flammini M, et al. Lipid abnormalities in insulin-dependent diabetic patients with albuminuria. Diabetes Care 1984;7:151–4.

272. Winocour PH, Durrington PN, Ishola M, et al. Influence of proteinuria on vascular disease, blood pressure, and lipoproteins in insulin dependent diabetes mellitus. BMJ 1987;294:1648–51.

273. Jensen T, Stender S, Deckert T. Abnormalities in plasma concentrations of lipoproteins and fibrinogen in type 1 insulin-dependent diabetic patients with increased albumin excretion. Diabetologia 1988;31:142–5.

274. Winocour PH, Bhatnagar D, Ishola M, et al. Lipoprotein (a) and microvascular disease in Type I (insulin-dependent) diabetes. Diabetic Med 1991;8:922–7.

275. Kasiske BL, O'Donnell MP, Cleary MP, Keane WF. Treatment of hyperlipidaemia reduces glomerular injury in obese Zucker rats. Kidney Int 1988;33:667–72.

276. Jones SL, Close CE, Mattock MB, et al. Plasma lipid and coagulation factor concentrations in insulin dependent diabetics with microalbuminuria. BMJ 1988; 29:487–90.

277. Dullaart RPF, Dikkeschei LD, Doorenbos HH. Alterations in serum lipids and apolipoproteins in male Type 1 insulin-dependent diabetic patients with microalbuminuria. Diabetologia 1989;32:685–9.

278. Mattock MB, Keen H, Viberti GC, et al. Coronary heart disease and urinary albumin excretion rate in Type 2 non-insulin-dependent diabetic patients. Diabetologia 1988;31:82–7.

279. Siperstein MD, Unger RH, Madison LL. Studies of muscle capillary basement membranes in normal subjects, diabetic, and pre-diabetic patients. J Clin Invest 1968;47:1973–99.

280. Williamson JR, Kilo C. Current status of capillary basement-membrane disease in diabetes mellitus. Diabetes 1977;26:65–73.

281. Steffes MW, Sutherland DER, Gøetz FC, et al. Studies of kidney and muscle biopsy specimens from identical twins discordant for Type 1 diabetes mellitus. N Engl J Med 1985;312:1282–7.

282. Becker D, Miller M. Presence of diabetic glomerulosclerosis in patients with haemochromatosis. N Engl J Med 1960;263:367–73.

283. Ireland JT, Patnaik BK, Duncan LJP. Glomerular ultrastructure in secondary diabetics and normal subjects. Diabetes 1967;16:628–35.

284. Brown DM, Andres GA, Hostetter TH, et al. Proceedings of a task force on animals appropriate for studying diabetes mellitus and its complications. Kidney complications. Diabetes 1982;31(Suppl 1):71–81.

285. Lee CS, Mauer SM, Brown DM, et al. Renal transplantation in diabetes mellitus in the rat. J Exp Med 1974;139:793–800.

286. Mauer SM, Steffes MW, Sutherland DER, et al. Studies of the rate of regression of the glomerular lesions in diabetic rats treated with pancreatic islet transplantation. Diabetes 1975;24:280–5.

287. Steffes MW, Brown DM, Basgen JM, et al. Amelioration of mesangial volume and surface alterations following islet transplantation in diabetic rats. Diabetes 1980;29:509–15.

288. Rasch R. Prevention of diabetic glomerulopathy in streptozotocin diabetic rats by insulin treatment. The mesangial regions. Diabetologia 1979;17:243–8.

289. Rasch R. Prevention of diabetic glomerulopathy in streptozotocin diabetic rats. Albumin excretion. Diabetologia 1980;8:413–6.

290. O'Donnell MP, Kasiske BL, Keane WF. Glomerular haemodynamics and structural alterations in experimental diabetes mellitus. FASEB J 1988;2:2339–47.

291. Mauer SM, Steffes MW, Connet J, et al. The development of lesions in the glomerular basement membrane and mesangium after transplantation of normal kidneys into diabetic patients. Diabetes 1983;32:948–52.

292. Mauer SM, Goetz FC, McHugh LE. Long-term study of normal kidneys transplanted into patients with Type 1 diabetes. Diabetes 1989;38:516–23.

293. Brownlee M, Vlassara H, Cerami A. Non-enzymatic glycosylation and the pathogenesis of diabetic complications. Ann Intern Med 1984;101:527–37.

294. Brownlee M, Cerami A, Vlassara H. Advanced glycosylation end-products in tissue and the biochemical basis of diabetic complications. N Engl J Med 1988; 318:1315–21.

295. Stevens VJ, Rouzer CA, Monnier VM, Cerami A. Diabetic cataract formation: potential role of glycosylation of lens crystallins. Proc Natl Acad Sci USA 1978;75:2918–22.

296. Brownlee M, Pongor S, Cerami A. Covalent attachment of soluble proteins by nonenzymatically glycosylated collagen: role in the in situ formation of immune complexes. J Exp Med 1983;158:1739–44.

297. Brownlee M, Vlassara H, Cerami A. Nonenzymatic glycosylation reduces the susceptibility of fibrin to degradation by plasmin. Diabete 1983;32:680–4.

298. Cohen MP, Ku L. Inhibition of fibronectin binding to matrix components by non-enzymatic glycosylation. Diabetes 1984;33:970–4.

299. Cohen MP, Saini R, Klepser H, Vasanthi LG.. Fibronectin binding to glomerular basement membrane is altered in diabetes. Diabetes 1987;36:758–63.

300. Vlassara H, Brownlee M, Cerami A. Novel macrophage receptor for glucose-modified proteins is distinct from previously described scavenger receptors. J Exp Med 1986;164:1301–9.

301. Ludvigson MA, Sorenson RL. Immunohistochemical localization of aldose reductase. II. Rat eye and kidney. Diabetes 1980;29:450–9.

302. Kikkawa R, Umemura K, Haneda M, et al. Evidence for existence of polyol pathway in cultured rat mesangial cells. Diabetes 1987;36:240–3.

303. Burg MB. Role of aldose reductase and sorbitol in maintaining the medullary intracellular milieu. Kidney Int 1988;33:635–41.

304. Cogan DG. Aldose reductase and complications of diabetes. Ann Intern Med 1984;101:82–91.

305. Kador PF, Robinson WG Jr, Kinoshita JH. The pharmacology of aldose reductase inhibitors. Annu Rev Pharmacol Toxicol 1985;25:691–714.

306. Pugliese G, Tilton RG, Speedy A, et al. Modulation of hemodynamics and vascular filtration changes in diabetic rats by dietary myo-inositol. Diabetes 1990;39:312–22.

307. Beyer-Mears A, Ku L, Cohen MP. Glomerular polyol accumulation in diabetes and its prevention by oral sorbinil. Diabetes 33:604–7.

308. Goldfarb S, Simmons DA, Kern EFO. Amelioration of glomerular hyperfiltration in acute experimental diabetes mellitus by dietary myo-inositol supplementation and aldose reductase inhibition. Trans Assoc Am Physicians 1986;99:67–72.

309. Beyer-Mears A Cruz E, Edelist T, Varagianuis E. Diminished proteinuria in diabetes mellitus by sorbinil, an aldose reductase inhibitor. Pharmacology 1986;32:52–60.

310. Daniels BS, Hostetter TH. Aldose reductase inhibition and glomerular abnormalities in diabetic rats. Diabetes 1989;38:981–6.

311. Coco M, Aynedjian HS, Bank N. Effect of galactose and aldose reductase inhibition on renal haemodynamics. Clin Res 1988;36:626A.

312. Mower P, Aynedjian H, Silverman S, et al. Sorbinil prevents glomerular hyperperfusion in diabetic rats. Kidney Int 1989;35:433.

313. Frey J, Zager P, Jackson J, et al. Aldose reductase activity mediates renal prostaglandin production in streptozotocin diabetic rats. Kidney Int 1989;35:292.

314. Jacobson M, Sharma YR, Cotlier E, Hollander JD. Diabetic complications in lens and nerve and their prevention by sulindac or sorbinil: two novel aldose reductase inhibitors. Invest Ophthalmol Vis Sci 1983;24:1426–9.

315. Beyer-Mears A, Cruz E, Dillon P, et al. Diabetic renal hypertrophy diminished by aldose reductase inhibition [Abstract]. Fed Proc 1983;42:505.

316. Rasch R, Østerby R. Lack of influence of aldose reductase inhibitor treatment for 6 months on the glycogen nephrosis in streptozotocin diabetic rats. Diabetologia 1990;32:532A.

317. Tilton RG, Chang K, Pugliese G, et al. Prevention of hemodynamic and vascular albumin filtration changes in diabetic rats by aldose reductase inhibitors. Diabetes 1989;38:1258–70.

318. Pedersen MM, Christiansen JS, Mogensen CE. Reduction of glomerular hyperfiltration in normoalbuminuric IDDM patients by 6 mo of aldose reductase inhibition. Diabetes 1991;40:527–31.

319. Blohmé G, Smith U. Aldose reductase inhibition reduces urinary albumin excretion rate in incipient diabetic nephropathy. Diabetologia 1989;32:467A.

320. Cohen DL, Allawi J, Brophy K, et al. Tolerance, safety and effects of Statil, an aldose reductase inhibitor in Type 2 non-insulin-dependent diabetic patients with microalbuminuria. Diabetologia 1989;32:477A.

321. Brownlee M, Spiro MG. Glomerular basement membrane metabolism in the diabetic rat. In vivo studies. Diabetes 1979;28:121–5.

322. Khalifa A, Cohen MP. Glomerular protocollagen lysil hydroxylase activity in streptozotocin diabetes. Biochim Biophys Acta 1975;386:332–9.

323. Farquhar MG. The glomerular basement membrane: a selective macromolecular filter. In: Hay ED, ed. Cell biology of extracellular matrix. New York: Plenum, 1981:335–78.

324. Spiro RG, Spiro MJ. Effect of diabetes on the biosynthesis of the renal glomerular basement membrane: studies on the glucosyltransferase. Diabetes 1971;20:641–8.

325. Beisswenger PJ, Spiro RG. Studies on the human glomerular basement membrane: composition, nature of the carbohydrate units and chemical changes in diabetes mellitus. Diabetes 1972;22:180–93.

326. Beisswenger PJ. Glomerular basement membrane. Biosynthesis and chemical composition in the streptozotocin diabetic rat. J Clin Invest 1976;58:844–52.

327. Lorenzi M, Cagliero E, Toledo S. Glucose toxicity for human endothelial cells in culture: delayed replication, disturbed cell cycle, and accelerated death. Diabetes 1985;34:621–7.

328. Lorenzi M, Nordberg J, Toledo S. High glucose prolongs cell-cycle traversal of cultured human endothelial cells. Diabetes 1987;36:1261–7.

329. Lorenzi M, Toledo S, Boss GR, et al. The polyol pathway and glucose-6-phosphate in human endothelial cells cultured in high glucose concentrations. Diabetologia 1987;30:222–7.

330. Lorenzi M, Montisano D, Toledo S, et al. High glucose induces DNA damage in cultured human endothelial cells. J Clin Invest 1986;77:322–5.

331. Lorenzi M, Montisano DF, Toledo S, Wong H-CH. Increased single strand breaks in DNA of lymphocytes from diabetic subjects. J Clin Invest 1987;79:653–6.

332. Cagliero E, Maiello M, Boeri D, et al. Increased expression of basement membrane components in human endothelial cells cultured in high glucose. J Clin Invest 1988;82:735–8.

333. Boeri D, Almus FE, Maiello M, et al. Modification of tissue-factor mRNA and protein response to thrombin and interleukin 1 by high glucose in cultured human endothelial cells. Diabetes 1989;38:312–8.

334. Jensen T. Increased plasma level of von Willebrand factor in Type 1 insulin-dependent diabetic patients with incipient nephropathy. BMJ 1989;298:27–8.

335. Jensen T, Feldt-Rasmussen B, Bjerre-Knudsen J, Deckert T. 1989. Features of endothelial dysfunction in early diabetic nephropathy. Lancet 1989;1:461–3.

336. Steffes MW, Brown DM, Mauer SM. Diabetic glomerulopathy following unilateral nephrectomy in the rat. Diabetes 1978;27:35–41.

337. Mauer SM, Steffes MW, Azar S, et al. The effects of Goldblatt hypertension on development of the glomerular lesions of diabetes mellitus in the rat. Diabetes 1978;27:738–44.

338. Berkman J, Rifkin H. Unilateral nodular diabetic glomerulosclerosis Kimmelstiel-Wilson. Report of a case. Metabolism 1973;22:715–22.

339. Béroniade VC, Lefèbvre R, Falardeau P. Unilateral diabetic glomerulosclerosis: recurrence of an experiment of nature. Am J Nephrol 1987;7:55–9.

340. Zatz R, Dunn BR, Meyer TW, et al. Prevention of diabetic glomerulopathy by pharmacologic amelioration of glomerular capillary hypertension. J Clin Invest 1986;77:1925–30.

341. Anderson S, Rennke HG, Brenner BM. Therapeutic advantages of converting-enzyme inhibitors in arresting progressive renal disease associated with systemic hypertension in the rat. J Clin Invest 1986;77:1925–30.

342. Ausiello DA, Kreisberg JI, Roy C, Karnovsky MJ. Contraction of cultured rat glomerular cells of apparent mesangial origin after stimulation with angiotensin II and arginine vasopressin. J Clin Invest 1980;65:754–60.

343. Webb RC, Bohr DF. Recent advances in the pathogenesis of hypertension: consideration of structural, functional, and metabolic vascular abnormalities resulting in elevated arterial resistance. Am Heart J 1981;102:251–64.

344. Leung DYM, Glagov S, Mathews MB. Cyclic stretching stimulates synthesis of matrix components by arte-

rial smooth muscle cells in vitro. Science 1976; 191:475–7.

345. Ross R, Glomset JA. The pathogenesis of atherosclerosis. N Engl J Med 1976;295:369–77.

346. Olson JL, Hostetter TH, Rennke HG, et al. Altered glomerular permselectivity and progressive sclerosis following extreme ablation of renal mass. Kidney Int 1982;22:112–26.

347. Mauer SM, Steffes MW, Chern M, Brown DM. Mesangial uptake and processing of macromolecules in rats with diabetes mellitus. Lab Invest 1979;41:401–6.

348. Velosa JA, Glasser RJ, Nevins TE, Michael AF. Experimental model of focal sclerosis. II. Correlations with immunopathologic changes, macromolecular kinetics, and polyanion loss. Lab Invest 1977;36:527–34.

349. Mauer SM, Steffes MW, Brown DM. The kidney in diabetes. Am J Med 1981;70:603–12.

350. Grond J, Schilthuis MS, Koudstaal J, Elema J. Mesangial function and glomerular sclerosis in rats after unilateral nephrectomy. Kidney Int 1982;22:338–43.

351. Fogo A, Ichikawa I. Evidence for the central role of glomerular growth promoters in the development of sclerosis. Semin Nephrol 1989;9:329–42.

352. Hirose K, Østerby R, Nozawa M, Gunderson HJG. Development of glomerular lesions in experimental long-term diabetes in the rat. Kidney Int 1982;21:689–95.

353. Bank N, Klose R, Aynedjian HS, et al. Evidence against increased glomerular pressure initiating diabetic nephropathy. Kidney Int 1987;31:898–905.

354. Yoshida Y, Fogo A, Shiraga H, et al. Serial micropuncture analysis of single nephron function in subtotal renal ablation. Kidney Int 1988;33851–5.

355. Neugarten J, Feiner HD, Schacht RG, et al. Aggravation of experimental glomerulonephritis by superimposed clip hypertension. Kidney Int 1987;22:257–63.

356. Fogo A, Ichikawa I. Evidence for a central role of glomerular growth promoters in the development of sclerosis. Semin Nephrol 1989;9:392–42.

357. Purkerson ML, Hoffsten PE, Klahr S. Pathogenesis of the glomerulopathy associated with renal infarction in rats. Kidney Int 1976;9:407–17.

358. Purkerson ML, Joist JH, Greenberg JM, et al. Inhibition by anticoagulant drugs of the progressive hypertension and uraemia associated with renal infarction in rats. Thromb Res 1982;26:227–40.

359. Purkerson ML, Joist JH, Yates J, et al. Inhibition of thromboxane synthesis ameliorates the progressive kidney disease of rats with subtotal renal ablation. Proc Natl Acad Sci USA 1985;82:193–7.

360. Purkerson ML, Tollefsen DM, Klahr S. N-desulfated/acetylated heparin ameliorates the progression of renal disease in rats with subtotal renal ablation. J Clin Invest 1988;81:69–74.

361. Olson JL. Role of heparin as a protective agent following reduction of renal mass. Kidney Int 1984;25:376–82.

362. Castellot JJ, Hoover RL, Harper PA, Karnovsky MJ. Heparin and glomerular epithelial cell-secreted heparin-like species inhibit mesangial cell proliferation. Am J Pathol 1985;120:427–35.

363. Fogo A, Yoshida Y, Yared A, Ichikawa I. Importance of angiogenic angiotensin II in the glomerular growth of maturing kidneys. Kidney Int 1990;38:1068–74.

364. Ichikawa I, Yoshida Y, Fogo A, et al. Effect of heparin on the glomerular structure and function of remnant nephrons. Kidney Int 1988;34:638–44.

365. Doi T, Striker LJ, Quaife C, et al. Progressive glomerulo-sclerosis develops in transgenic mice chronically expressing growth hormone and growth hormone releasing factor but not in those expressing insulin-like growth factor-1. Am J Pathol 1988;131:398–403.

366. Seaquist ER, Gøetz FC, Rich S, Barbosa J. Familial clustering of diabetic kidney disease. Evidence for genetic susceptibility to diabetic nephropathy. N Engl J Med 1989;320:1161–5.

367. Viberti GC, Keen H, Wiseman MJ. Raised arterial pressure in parents of proteinuric insulin-dependent diabetics. BMJ 1987;295:515–7.

368. Krolewski AS, Canessa M, Warram JH, et al. Predisposition to hypertension and susceptibility to renal disease in insulin-dependent diabetes mellitus. N Engl J Med 1988;318:140–5.

369. Jensen JS, Mathiesen ER, Norgaard K, et al. Increased blood pressure and erythrocyte sodium-lithium countertransport activity are not inherited in diabetic nephropathy. Diabetologia 1990;33:619–25.

370. Earle K, Walker J, Hill C, et al. Familial clustering of cardiovascular disease in patients with insulin-dependent diabetes and nephropathy. N Engl J Med 1992;326:673–7.

371. Dadone MM, Hasstedt SJ, Hunt SC, et al. Genetic analysis of sodium-lithium countertransport in ten hypertension-prone kindreds. Am J Med 1984;17:565–77.

372. Boerwinkle E, Turner ST, Weinshilboum R, et al. Analysis of the distribution of sodium lithium countertransport in a sample representative of the general population. Genet Epidemiol 1986;3:365–78.

373. Mangili R, Bending JJ, Scott G, et al. Increased sodium-lithium countertransport activity in red cells of patients with insulin-dependent diabetes and nephropathy. N Engl J Med 1988;318:146–50.

374. Walker JD, Bending JJ, Dodds RA, Mattock MB, et al. Restriction of dietary protein and progression of renal failure in diabetic nephropathy. Lancet 1989;2:1411–4.

375. Jones SL, Trevisan R, Tariq T, et al. Sodium-lithium countertransport in microalbuminuric insulin-dependent diabetic patients. Hypertension 1990;15:570–5.

376. Lopes de Faria JB, Jones SL MacDonald F, et al. Sodium lithium countertransport activity and insulin resistance in normotensive IDDM patients. Diabetes 1992;41:610–5.

377. Trevisan R, Nosadini R, Firoetti P, et al. Clustering of risk factors in hypertensive insulin-dependent diabetics with high sodium-lithium countertransport. Kidney Int 1992;41:85–61.

378. Foster DW. Insulin resistance: a secret killer? N Engl J Med 1989;320:733–4.

379. Silberberg JS, Barre PE, Prichard SS, Sniderman AD. Impact of left ventricular hypertrophy on survival in end-stage renal disease. Kidney Int 1989;36:286–90.

380. Sampson MJ, Chambers J, Sprigings D, Drury PL. Intraventricular septal hypertrophy in Type 1 diabetic patients with microalbuminuria or early proteinuria. Diabetic Med 1990;7:126–31.

381. Reaven GM, Hoffman BP. A role for insulin in the aetiology and course of hypertension? Lancet 1987;2:435–7.

382. Mahnensmith RL, Aronson PS. The plasma membrane sodium-hydrogen exchanger and its role in physiological and pathological processes. Circ Res 1985;56:773–88.

383. Trevisan R, Li LK Messant JJ, et al. Na$^+$/H$^+$ antiport activity and cell growth in cultured skin fibrobasts of insulin-dependent diabetic patients with nephropathy. Diabetologia 1990;33:371–7.

384. Ng LL, Simmonds D, Frigh V, et al. Leucocyte Na/H

antiport activity in Type I (insulin-dependent) diabetic patients with nephropathy. Diabetologia 1990; 33:371–7.

385. Amiel SA, Sherwin RS, Simonson DC, et al. Impaired insulin action in puberty. A contributing factor to poor glycaemic control in adolescents with diabetes. N Engl J Med 1986;315:215–9.

386. Parving H-H, Viberti GC, Keen H, et al. Haemodynamic factors in the genesis of diabetic microangiopathy. Metabolism 1983;32:943–9.

387. Feldt-Rasmussen B. Increased transcapillary escape rate of albumin in Type 1 (insulin-dependent) diabetic patients with microalbuminuria. Diabetologia 1986;29:282–6.

388. Moorhead JF, Chan MK, El-Nahas M, Varghese Z. Lipid nephrotoxicity in chronic progressive glomerular and tubulo-interstitial disease. Lancet 1982;2:1309–11.

389. Zavaroni I, Bonori E, Pagliara M, et al. Risk factors for coronary artery disease in healthy persons with hyperinsulinemia and normal glucose tolerance. N Engl J Med 1989;320:702–6.

390. Fahr T. Über Glomerulosklerose. Virchows Arch Pathol Anat Physiol Klin Med 1942;309:16–33.

391. Spühler O, Zollinger HU. Direfe diabetische Glomerulosklerose. Dtsch Arch Klin Med 1943;190:321–79.

392. Kamenetzky SA, Bennet P, Dippe SE, et al. A clinical and histologic study of diabetic nephropathy in the Pima Indians. Diabetes 1974;23:61–8.

393. Tchobroutsky G. Prevention and treatment of diabetic nephropathy. In: Hamburger J, Crosnier J-P, Maxwell MH, eds. Advances in nephrology. Vol 9. Chicago: Year Book Medical Publishers, 1979:63–86.

394. Saito Y, Kida H, Takeda S-I, et al. Mesangiolysis in diabetic glomeruli; its role in the formation of nodular lesions. Kidney Int 1988;34:389–96.

395. Bloodworth JMB. A re-evaluation of diabetic glomerulosclerosis 50 years after the discovery of insulin. Hum Pathol 1978;9:439–53.

396. Heptinstall RH. Diabetes mellitus and gout. In: Heptinstall RH, ed. Pathology of the kidney. 3rd ed. Boston: Little, Brown and Company, 1983:1397–453.

397. Østerby R, Gundersen HJG. Glomerular size and structure in diabetes mellitus. I. Early abnormalities. Diabetologia 1975;11:225–9.

398. Gundersen HJG, Østerby R. Glomerular size and structure in diabetes mellitus. II. Late abnormalities. Diabetologia 1977;13:43–8.

399. Østerby R, Gundersen HJG, Nyberg G, Aurell M. Advanced diabetic glomerulopathy. Quantitative structural characterization of nonoccluded glomeruli. Diabetes 1987; 36:612–9.

400. Schmitz A, Gundersen HJG, Østerby R. Glomerular morphology by light microscopy in non-insulin-dependent diabetes mellitus: lack of glomerular hypertrophy. Diabetes 1988;37:38–43.

401. Mauer SM, Barbosa J, Vernier RL, et al. Development of diabetic vascular lesions in normal kidneys transplanted into patients with diabetes mellitus. N Engl J Med 1976;295:916–20.

402. Rasch R, Holck P. Ultrastructure of the macula densa in streptozotocin diabetic rats. Lab Invest 1988;59:666–72.

403. Westberg NG, Michael AF. Immunohistopathology of diabetic glomerulsclerosis. Diabetes 1972;21:163–74.

404. Miller K, Michael AF. Immunopathology of renal extracellular membranes in diabetes mellitus. Specificity of tubular basement membrane immunofluorescence. Diabetes 1976;25:701–8.

405. Falk RJ, Scheinman JI, Mauer SM, Michael AF. Poly-

406. Glick AD, Jacobson HR, Haralson MA. Evidence for type I collagen synthesis in diabetic glomerulosclerosis. Kidney Int 1990;37:507.

407. Ikeda K, Kida H, Oshima A. Participation of type VI collagen fibres in formation of diabetic nodular lesions. Kidney Int 1990;37:252.

408. Mohan PS, Carter WG, Spiro RG. Occurrence of type VI collagen in extracellular matrix of renal glomeruli and its increase in diabetes. Diabetes 1990;39:31–7.

409. Scheinman JI, Fish AJ, Michael AF. The immunohistopathology of glomerular antigens. The glomerular basement membrane, collagen, and actomyosin antigens in normal and diseased kidneys. J Clin Invest 1974;54:1144–54.

410. Farquhar A, MacDonald MK, Ireland JT. The role of fibrin deposition in diabetic glomerulosclerosis: a light, electron and immunofluorescence microscopy study. J Clin Pathol 1972;25:657–67.

411. Østerby-Hansen R. A quantitative estimate of the peripheral glomerular basement membrane in recent juvenile diabetes. Diabetologia 1965;1:97–100.

412. Østerby R. Early phases in the development of diabetic glomerulopathy. A quantitative electron microscopy study. Acta Med Scand Suppl 1975;574:1–82.

413. Kimmelstiel P, Osawa G, Beres J. Glomerular basement membrane in diabetics. Am J Pathol 1966;45:21–31.

414. Østerby R, Gundersen HJG, Hørlyck A, et al. Diabetic glomerulopathy. Structural characteristics of the early and advanced stages. Diabetes 1983;32(Suppl 2):79–82.

415. Ireland JT, Patnaik BK, Duncan LJP. Effect of pituitary ablation on the renal arteriolar and glomerular lesions in diabetes. Diabetes 1967;16:636–42.

416. Ellis EN, Steffes MW, Chavers B, et al. Observations of glomerular epithelial cell structure in patients with Type 1 diabetes mellitus. Kidney Int 1987;32:736–41.

417. Cohen AH, Mampaso F, Zamboni L Glomerular polocyte degeneration in human renal disease. Lab Invest 1977; 37:30–4.

418. Ireland JT. Diagnostic criteria in the assessment of glomerular capillary basement membrane lesions in newly diagnosed juvenile diabetics. Adv Metab Dis 1970;1:273.

419. Østerby R. A quantitative electron microscopic study of mesangial regions in glomeruli from patients with short-term juvenile diabetes mellitus. Lab Invest 1973; 29:99–110.

420. Kimmelstiel P, Kim OJ, Beres J. Studies on renal biopsies specimens with the aid of the electron microscope. I. Glomeruli in diabetes. Am J Pathol 1962;38:270–7.

421. Dachs S, Churg J, Mautner W, Grishman E. Diabetic nephropathy. Am J Pathol 1964;44:155–68.

422. Østerby R, Parving HH, Hommel E, et al. Glomerular structure and function in diabetic nephropathy. Early to advanced stages. Diabetes 1990;39:1057–63.

423. Ellis EN, Steffes MW, Gøetz FC, et al. Glomerular filtration surface in Type 1 diabetes mellitus. Kidney Int 1986; 29:889–94.

424. Østerby R, Parving H-H, Nyberg, et al. A strong correlation between glomerular filtration rate and filtration surface in diabetic nephropathy. Diabetologia 1988;31:265–70.

425. Thomsen OF, Andersen AR, Christiansen JS, Deckert T. Renal changes in long-term Type 1 insulin-dependent diabetic patients with and without clinical nephropathy; a light microscopic, morphometric study of autopsy material. Diabetologia 1984;26:361–5.

426. Steffes MW, Østerby R, Chavers B, Mauer SM. Mesangial expansion as a central mechanism for loss of kidney function in diabetic patients. Diabetes 1989; 38:1077–81.

427. Inomata S, Nakamoto Y, Inoue M, et al. Relationship between urinary albumin excretion and renal histology in non-insulin-dependent diabetes mellitus: with reference to the clinical significance of microalbuminuria. J Diabetic Complications 1989;3:178–88.

428. Kincaid-Smith P, Whitworth JA. Haematuria and diabetic nephropathy. In: Mogensen CE, ed. The kidney and hypertension in diabetes mellitus. Boston: Martinus Nijhoff, 1988;81–89.

429. Amoah E, Glickman JL, Malchoff CD, et al. Clinical identification of non-diabetic renal disease in diabetic patients with Type 1 and Type 2 disease presenting with renal dysfunction. Am J Nephrol 1988;8:204–11.

430. Kasinath BS, Musais SK, Spargo BH, Katz AI. Non-diabetic renal disease in patients with diabetes mellitus. Am J Med 1983;75:613–7.

431. Silva FG, Pace EH, Burns DK, Krous H. The spectrum of diabetic nephropathy and membranous glomerulopathy: report of two cases and review of the literature. Diabetic Nephropathy 1983;2:28–32.

432. Chihara J, Takebayashi S, Taguchi T, et al. Glomerulonephritis in diabetic patients and its effect on prognosis. Nephron 1986;43:45–9.

433. Bertani T, Olesnicky L, Abu-Regiaba S, et al. Concomitant presence of three different glomerular diseases in the same patient. Nephron 1983;34:260–6.

434. Rao KV, Crosson JT. Idiopathic membranous glomerulonephritis in diabetic patients. Report of three cases and review of the literature. Arch Intern Med 1980; 140:624–7.

435. Kobayashi K, Harada A, Onoyama K, et al. Idiopathic membranous glomerulonephritis associated with diabetes mellitus. Nephron 1981;28:163–8.

436. Okuda S, Oh Y, Onoyama K, et al. Autologous immune-complex nephritis in streptozotocin-induced diabetic rats. Nephron 1984;37:166–73.

437. Jarrett RJ, Keen H, Chakrabarthi R. Diabetes, hyperglycaemia, and arterial disease. In: Keen H, Jarrett, eds. Complications of diabetes. 2nd ed. London: Edward Arnold, 1982:179–204.

438. Parving H-H, Andersen AR, Smidt UM, et al. Effect of antihypertensive treatment on kidney function in diabetic nephropathy. BMJ 1987;294:1443–7.

439. Melbourne Diabetic Nephropathy Study Group. Comparisons between perindopril and nifedipine in hypertensive and normotensive diabetic patients in microalbuminuria. BMJ 1986;302:210–6.

440. Taguma Y, Kitamoto Y, Futaki G, et al. Effect of captopril on heavy proteinuria in azotemic diabetics. N Engl J Med 1985;313:1617–20.

441. Bjørck S, Nyberg G, Mulec H, et al. Beneficial effects of angiotensin converting enzyme inhibition on renal function in patients with diabetic nephropathy. BMJ 1986; 293:471–4.

442. Hommel E, Parving H-H, Mathiesen E, et al. Effect of captopril on kidney function in insulin-dependent diabetic patients with nephropathy. BMJ 1986;293:467–70.

443. Parving H-H, Hommel E, Smidt UM. Protection of kidney function and decrease in albuminuria by captopril in insulin-dependent diabetics with nephropathy. BMJ 1988;297:1086–91.

444. Pinto JR, Walker JD, Turner CD, et al. Renal response to lowering of arterial pressure by angiotensin converting enzyme inhibitor or diuretic therapy in insulin-dependent diabetic patients with nephropathy. Kidney Int 1990; 37:516.

445. Morelli E, Loon N, Meyer T, et al. Effects of converting-enzyme inhibition on barrier function in diabetic glomerulopathy. Diabetes 1990;39:76–82.

446. Ruggenitti P, Viberti GG, Battaglia C. Low-dose enalapril and glomerular selective function in insulin-dependent diabetics. Kidney Int 1990;37:A519

447. Marre M, Chatellier G, Leblanc H, et al. Prevention of diabetic nephropathy with enalapril in normotensive diabetics with microalbuminuria. BMJ 1988; 297:1092–5.

448. Pedersen MM, Schmitz A, Pedersen EB, et al. Acute and long-term renal effects of angiotensin converting-enzyme inhibition in normotensive, normoalbuminuric insulin-dependent diabetic patients. Diabetic Med 1988;5:562–9.

449. Parving H-H, Hommel E, Nielson MD, Giese J. Effect of captopril on blood pressure and kidney function in normotensive insulin-dependent diabetics with nephropathy. BMJ 1985;299:533–6.

450. Bergstrom J. Discovery and rediscovery of low-protein diet. Clin Nephrol 1984;21:29–35.

451. Attman PO, Bucht H, Larsson O, Uddebom G. Protein reduced diet in diabetic renal failure. Clin Nephrol 1983;19:217–20.

452. Barsotti G, Morelli E, Giannoni A, et al. Restricted phosphorus and nitrogen intake to slow the progression of chronic renal failure: a controlled trial. Kidney Int 1983;24(Suppl 16):S278–84.

453. Evanoff GV, Thompson CS, Brown J, et al. The effect of dietary protein restriction on the progression of diabetic nephropathy. A 12-month follow-up. Arch Intern Med 1987;147:492–5.

454. Bending JJ, Dodds RA, Keen H, Viberti GC. Renal response to restricted protein intake in diabetic nephropathy. Diabetes 1988;37:1641–6.

455. Rosenberg ME, Swanson JE, Thomas BL, Hostetter TH. Glomerular and hormonal responses to dietary protein intake in human renal disease. Am J Physiol 1987; 253:F1083–90.

456. Cohen DL, Close CF, Viberti GC. The variability of overnight urinary albumin excretion in insulin-dependent diabetic and normal subjects. Diabetic Med 1987;4:437–40.

457. Wiseman MJ, Bognetti E, Dodds R, et al. Changes in renal function in response to protein restricted diet in Type 1 insulin-dependent diabetic patients. Diabetologia 1987; 30:154–9.

458. Kontessis PS, Jones SJ, Dodds R. Renal, metabolic and hormonal responses to ingestion of animal and vegetable proteins. Kidney Int 1990;38:136–44.

459. Bending JJ, Viberti GC, Bilous RW, Keen H. Eight-month correction of hyperglycaemia in IDDM is associated with a significant and sustained reduction of urinary albumin excretion rates in patients with microalbuminuria. Diabetes 1984;34(Suppl 3):69–73.

460. Kroc Collaborative Study Group. Blood glucose control and the evolution of diabetic retinopathy and albuminuria. A preliminary multicentre trial. N Engl J Med 1984; 311:365–72.

461. Dahl-Jørgensen K, Hanssen KF, Kierulf P, et al. Reduction of urinary albumin excretion after 4 years of continuous subcutaneous insulin infusion in insulin-dependent diabetes mellitus. The Oslo study. Acta Endocrocrinol (Copenh) 1988;117:19–25.

462. Vasquez B, Flock EV, Savage PJ, et al. Sustained reduction

of proteinuria in Type 2 non-insulin-dependent diabetes following diet-induced reduction of hyperglycaemia. Diabetologia 1984;26:127−33.

463. Warram J, Derby L, Laffel L, Krolewski AS. Role of mean arterial pressure in the development of persistent proteinuria. Kidney Int 1990;37:404.

464. Tuttle K, Bruton JL, Perusek MC, et al. Effect of strict glycaemic control on renal hemodynamic response to amino acids and renal enlargement in insulin-dependent diabetes mellitus. N Engl J Med 1991; 324:1626−32.

465. Donadio JV, Ilstrup DM, Holley KE, Romero JC. Platelet-inhibitor treatment of diabetic nephropathy: a 10-year prospective study. Mayo Clin Proc 1988;63:3−15.

466. Mujais SK. Renal papillary necrosis in diabetes mellitus. Semin Nephrol 1984;4:40−7.

467. Mandel EE. Renal medullary necrosis. Am J Med 1952;13:322−7.

468. Lauler DP, Schreiner GE, David A. Renal medullary necrosis. Am J Med 1960;29:132−56.

469. Eknoyan G, Quinibi WY, Grissom RT, et al. Renal papillary necrosis: an update. Medicine 1981;61:55−73.

470. Groop L, Laasonen L, Edgren J. Renal papillary necrosis in patients with IDDM. Diabetes Care 1989;12:198−202.

471. Rundles RW. Diabetic neuropathy: general review with report of 125 cases. Medicine 1945;24:111−60.

472. Martin MM. Diabetic neuropathy. A clinical study of 125 cases. Brain 1953;76:594−624.

473. Frimodt-Möller C. Diabetic cystopathy. I. A clinical study of the frequency of bladder dysfunction in diabetes. Danish Med Bull 1976;23:267−78.

474. Mahony DJ, Laferte RO, Blais DJ. Integral storage and voiding reflexes. Neurophysiologic concept of continence and micturition. Urology 1977;9:95−106.

475. deGroat WC, Booth AM. Physiology of the urinary bladder and urethra. Ann Intern Med 1980;92:32−15.

476. Ellenberg M. Diabetic neurogenic vesical dysfunction. Arch Intern Med 1966;117, 348−54.

477. Kahan M, Goldberg PD, Mandell EE. Neurogenic vesical dysfunction and diabetes mellitus. N Y State J Med 1970;2:2448−2455.

478. Giberd FB. The neurogenic bladder. Clin Obstet Gynecol 1981;8:149−60.

479. Rubinow DR, Nelson JC. Tricyclic exacerbation of undiagnosed diabetic uropathy. J Clin Psychiatry 1982; 943:210−2.

480. Ewing DJ, Clark F. Autonomic neuropathy: its diagnosis and prognosis. Clin Endocrinol Metab 1986;15:855−88.

481. Bradley WE. Diagnosis of urinary bladder dysfunction in diabetes mellitus. Ann Intern Med 1980;92:323−6.

482. Frimodt-Møller C, Mortensen S. Treatment of diabetic cystopathy. Ann Intern Med 1980;92:327−8.

483. Ellenberg M. Development of urinary bladder dysfunction in diabetes mellitus. Ann Intern Med 1980;92:321−3.

484. Pedersen J. The pregnant diabetic and her newborn. 2nd ed. Copenhagen: Munksgaard, 1977.

485. Kitzmiller JL, Brown ER, Phillippe M, et al. Diabetic nephropathy and perinatal outcome. Am J Obstet Gynecol 1981;141:741−51.

486. Jovanovic R, Jovanovic L. Obstetric management when normoglycaemia is maintained in diabetic pregnant women with vascular compromise. Am J Obstet Gynecol 1984;149:617−23.

487. Dicker D, Feldberg D, Peleg D, et al. Pregnancy complicated by diabetic nephropathy. J Perinat Med 1986; 14:299−307.

488. Grenfell A, Brudenell JM, Doddridge MC, Watkins PJ. Pregnancy in diabetic woman who have proteinuria. Q J Med 1986;59:379−86.

489. Reece EA, Coustan DR, Hayslett JP, et al. Diabetic nephropathy: pregnancy performance and fetomaternal outcome. Am J Obstet Gynecol 1988;159:56−66.

490. Katz AI, Davison JM, Hayslett JP, et al. Pregnancy in women with kidney disease. Kidney Int 1980;18:192−206.

491. Hou SH, Grossman SD, Madias NE. Pregnancy in women with renal disease and moderate renal insufficiency. Am J Med 1985;78:185−94.

492. Hare JW, White P. Pregnancy in diabetes complicated by vascular disease. Diabetes 1977;26:953−5.

493. Fuhrmann K, Reiher H, Semmler K, et al. Prevention of congenital malformations in infants of insulin-dependent diabetic mothers. Diabetes Care 1983;6:219−23.

494. Buschard K, Hougaard P, Mølsted-Pedersen L, Kühl C. Type 1 insulin-dependent diabetes mellitus diagnosed during pregnancy: a clinical and prognostic study. Diabetologia 1990;33:31−5.

495. Hanson U, Persson B, Thunell S. Relationship between haemoglobin A_{1C} in early Type 1 insulin-dependent diabetic pregnancy and the occurrence of spontaneous abortion and fetal malformation in Sweden. Diabetologia 1990;33:100−4.

496. Peterson CM, Jovanovic L. Natural history of the diabetic renal-retinal syndrome during pregnancy. In: Friedman EA, L'Esperance FA, eds. Diabetic renal-retinal syndrome. Vol 3. New York: Grune and Stratton, 1986:471−80.

497. Miodovnik M, Mimouni F, St. John Dignan P, et al. Major malformations in infants of IDDM women: vasculopathy and early first-trimester poor glycemic control. Diabetes Care 1988;11:713−8.

498. Young KR, Clancy CF. Symposium on diabetes and obesity. Urinary tract infections complicating diabetes mellitus. Med Clin North Am 1955;59:1665−70.

499. Ditscherlein G. Renal histopathology in hypertensive diabetic patients. Hypertension 1985;7(Suppl 2):29−32.

500. Huvos A, Rocha H. Frequency of bacteriuria in patients with diabetes mellitus. A controlled study. N Engl J Med 1959;261:1213−6.

501. O'Sullivan DJ, Fitzgerald MG, Meynell MJ, Malins JM. Urinary tract infection. A comparative study in the diabetic and general populations. BMJ 1961;1:786−8.

502. Vejlsgaard R. Studies on urinary infections in diabetics. I. Bacteriuria in patients with diabetes mellitus and in control subjects. Acta Med Scand 1966; 179:173−82.

503. Pometta D, Rees SB, Younger D, Kass EH. Asymptomatic bacteriuria in diabetes mellitus. N Engl J Med 1967;276:1118−21.

504. Vejlsgaard R. Studies on urinary infections in diabetics. III. Significant bacteriuria in pregnant diabetics and in matched controls. Acta Med Scand 1973;193:337−41.

505. Forland M, Thomas V, Shelokov A. Urinary tract infections in patients with diabetes mellitus. JAMA 1977; 238:1924−6.

506. Vejlsgaard R. Studies on urinary infections in diabetics. II. Significant bacteriuria in relation to long-term diabetic manifestations. Acta Med Scand 1966;179:183−8.

507. Vejlsgaard R. Studies on urinary infections in diabetics. IV. Significant bacteriuria in pregnancy in relation to age of onset, duration of diabetes, angiopathy and urologic symptoms. Acta Med Scand 1973;193:343−46.

508. Bevan JS, Griffiths GJ, Williams JD, Gibby OM. Bilateral

renal cortical abscesses in a young woman with Type 1 diabetes. Diabetic Med 1989;6:454–7.

509. Thorley JD, Jones SR, Sanford JP. Perinephric abscess. Medicine 1974;53:441–51.

510. Bova JG, Potter JL, Arevalos E, et al. Renal and perirenal infection: the role of computerized tomography. J Urol 1985;133:539–43.

511. Evanoff GV, Thompson CS, Foley R, Weinman EJ. Spectrum of gas within the kidney. Emphysematous pyelonephritis and emphysematous pyelitis. Am J Med 1985;83:149–54.

512. Harkonen S, Kjellstrand CM. Exacerbation of diabetic renal failure following intravenous pyelography. Am J Med 1977;63:939–46.

513. Taliercio CP, Vlietstra RE, Fisher LD, Burnett JC. Risks for renal dysfunction with cardiac angiography. Ann Intern Med 1986;104:501–4.

514. Pafrey PS, Griffiths SM, Barrett BJ, et al. Contrast material-induced renal failure in patients with diabetes mellitus, renal insufficiency, or both: a prospective controlled study. N Engl J Med 1989;320:143–9.

515. Schwab SJ, Hlatkly MA, Piepper KS, et al. Contrast nephrotoxicity: a randomised control trial of a nonionic and ionic radiographic contrast agent. N Engl J Med 1989;320:149–53.

516. Bresiz M, Epstein FH. A closer look at radiocontrast-induced nephropathy. N Engl J Med 1989;320:179–81.

517. Eisenberg R, Bank W, Hedgecock M. Renal failure after major angiography. Am J Med 1980;68:43–6.

518. Heyman S, Brezis M, Greenfield, Rosen S. Protective role of frusemide and saline in radiocontrast-induced acute renal failure. Clin Res 1988;36:520A.

519. Porush JS, Chou SY, Auto HR, et al. Infusion intravenous pyelography and renal failure: effects of hypertonic mannitol and furosemide in patients with chronic renal insufficiency. In: Eliahou HE, ed. Acute renal failure. London: John Libbey, 1982:161–7.

520. EDTA Registry. Combined report on regular dialysis and transplantation in Europe, XX, 1989. Nephrol Dial Transplant 1991;6(Suppl 1):5–35.

521. Geerlings W, Tufveson G, Brunner FD, et al. Combined report on regular dialysis and transplantation in Europe, XXI, 1990. Nephrol Dial Transplant 1991;6(Suppl 4):5–29.

522. USRDS Annual Data Report. Vol 16. Am J Kidney Dis 1990;6(Suppl 2):Dec 1990.

523. Lemmers MJ, Barry JM. Major role for arterial disease in morbidity and mortality after kidney transplantation in diabetic recipients. Diabetes Care 1991;14:295–301.

524. Bennett WM, Kloster F, Rosch J, et al. Natural history of asymptomatic coronary arteriographic lesions in diabetic patients with end-stage renal disease. Am J Med 1978;65:779–84.

525. Diabetic Retinopathy Research Group. Photocoagulation treatment of proliferative retinopathy: clinical application of Diabetic Retinopathy Study (DRS) findings. DRS report no. 8. Ophthalmology (Rochester) 1981;88:7.

526. Flynn CT. Diabetic control by CAPD. In: Friedman EA, L'Esperance FA, eds. Diabetic renal-retinal syndrome. New York: Grune and Stratton, 1980:435–8.

527. Westervelt FB, Schreiner GE. The carbohydrate intolerance of uraemic patients. Ann Intern Med 1962;57:266–76.

528. DeFronzo RA, Alvestrand A, Smith D, et al. Insulin resistance in uraemia. J Clin Invest 1981;67:563–8.

529. Fluckiger R, Harmon W, Meier W, et al. Hemoglobin carbamylation in uremia. N Engl J Med 1981;304:823–7.

530. Rabelink AJ, Hene RJ, Erkelens DW, et al. Lipoprotein profile in hyperlipidaemia in nephrotic syndrome. Lancet 1988;2:1335–8.

531. Matson M, Kjellstrand CM. Long-term follow-up of 369 diabetic patients undergoing dialysis. Arch Intern Med 1988;48:600–4.

532. Andres DL, Kopp JB, Maloney NA, et al. Early deposition of aluminium in diabetic patients on hemodialysis. N Engl J Med 1987;316:292–6.

533. Rottembourg, J, El Shahat Y, Agrafiotis A, et al. Continuous peritoneal dialysis in insulin-dependent diabetic patients: a 40 month experience. Kidney Int 1983;23:40–45.

534. Disney, A.P.S. 1989. Twelth report of the Australian and New Zealand combined Dialysis and Transplantation Registry. Woodville, South Australia: Queen Elizabeth Hospital, 1989.

535. Najarian JS, Kaufman DB, Fryd DS, et al. Long-term survival following kidney transplantation in 100 Type 1 diabetic patients. Transplantation 1989;47:106–13.

536. Cameron JS. Treatment of end stage renal failure due to diabetes in the United Kingdom. J Diabetic Complications (in press).

537. Bentley FR, Sutherland DER, Mauer SM. et al. The status of diabetic renal allograft recipients who survive for ten or more years after renal transplantation. Transplant Proc 1986;17:1573–6.

538. Sutherland DER, Morrow CE, Fryd DS, et al. Improved patient and primary renal allograft survival in uraemic diabetic patients. Transplantation 1982;34:319.

539. Myers BD, Sibley R, Newton L, et al. The long-term course of cyclosporine-associated chronic nephropathy. Kidney Int 1988;33:590–600.

540. Tufveson G, Brynger H, Dimeny E, Renal transplantation in diabetic patients with and without simultaneous pancreatic transplantation. 1986: Date from the EDTA Registry. Nephrol Dial Transplant 1991;6:1–4.

541. Solders G, Wilzeck H, Gunnarsson R, et al. Effects of combined pancreatic and renal transplantation on diabetic neuropathy: a 2 year follow-up study. Lancet 1987;2:1232–5.

542. Kennedy WR, Navarro X, Goetz FC, et al. Effects of pancreas transplantation on diabetic neuropathy. N Engl J Med 1990;322:1031–7.

543. Ramsay RC, Goetz FC, Sutherland DER, et al. Progression of diabetic retinopathy after pancreas transplantation for insulin-dependent diabetes mellitus. N Engl J Med 1990;318:208–14.

544. Bilous RW, Mauer SM, Sutherlane DER, et al. The effects of pancreas transplantation on the glomerular structure of renal allografts in patients with insulin-dependent diabetes. N J Med 1989;32:80–5.

545. Sutherland DER. Who should get a pancreas transplant? Diabetes Care 1980;11:681–5.

Chapter 41

DIABETIC KETOACIDOSIS AND THE HYPERGLYCEMIC, HYPEROSMOLAR NONKETOTIC STATE

ABBAS E. KITABCHI

JOSEPH N. FISHER

MARY BETH MURPHY

MARK J. RUMBAK

In the previous edition of this text, the title of the chapter on this subject was "Coma in Diabetes."[1] The authors discussed both diabetic ketoacidosis and hyperglycemic, hyperosmolar nonketotic comas. However, in general no more than 20% of patients in diabetic ketoacidosis and a somewhat higher percentage of patients in the hyperosmolar nonketotic state present in a comatose condition. In addition, patients presenting with severe hypoglycemia are in a comatose state. Therefore, we have chosen the terminology that most correctly identifies these two hyperglycemic conditions, namely *diabetic ketoacidosis* (DKA) and the *hyperglycemic, hyperosmolar nonketotic state* (HHNS) and will describe each condition under a separate heading with the following subheadings: Definition; Historical Background, Incidence, and Mortality Rate; Precipitating Factors; Etiology and Pathogenesis; and Diagnosis.

Since modes of treatment for DKA and HHNS are similar, we will describe the treatment for both under a single heading. We have incorporated two additional conditions with acidosis in our chapter: alcoholic ketoacidosis and lactic acidosis.

DIABETIC KETOACIDOSIS (DKA)

Definition

One of greatest pitfalls encountered in reporting on the incidence, epidemiology, and mortality rate for DKA has been the lack of a uniformly accepted definition for this condition. The syndrome consists of the triad of hyperglycemia, ketosis, and acidemia,[2] each of which may independently be associated with other clinical conditions (Fig. 41−1). The consensus among most workers in this field is that an arterial pH of less than 7.3, a bicarbonate value of less than 15 meq/L, and a blood glucose level of greater than 250 mg/dL with a moderate degree of ketonemia and ketonuria (as determined by the nitroprusside method) are necessary for the diagnosis. It is important to note that although the majority of patients with DKA present with a blood glucose level higher than 250 to 300 mg/dL some patients arrive at the emergency room having already received insulin and/or a reduction in food intake, both of which can contribute to reduced plasma glucose concentrations, while the remaining parameters still show a moderate degree of metabolic decompensation. Alterations in blood glucose values may also be due to variations in hydration or to reduction in the concentration of counterregulatory hormones such as glucagon and catecholamines, particularly in patients with diabetes of long duration. Therefore, the level of blood glucose should not be a primary factor in determining the severity of DKA.

Historical Background, Incidence, and Mortality Rate

In 1886 Dreschfeld described two types of fatal diabetic complications with coma.[3] One was associated with a fruity odor on the patient's breath and urine, severe dyspnea, and the presence of a strong reducing agent in the urine. This clinical entity is now known as diabetic ketoacidosis (DKA). A second, less common, syndrome, with an insidious onset of symptoms ending in coma, was seen in the older diabetic patient. This condition is now recognized as hyperosmolar, hyperglycemic nonketotic syndrome (HHNS). These syndromes have since been the subject of many reviews.[4−12]

Good studies on the epidemiology of DKA are sparse. In a carefully defined, well-demarcated population, Faich et al. reported an incidence of DKA of 1.6% in Rhode Island, with patients with newly diagnosed diabetes accounting for 20% of those studied.[13] The annual rate of DKA was 14 per 100,000 of total population or 46 per 10,000 patients with diabetes. From data collected by the National Diabetes Data Group, the incidence of DKA appears to be between 3 and 8 episodes per 100 diabetic patients at the onset of diabetes.[7] Murphy et al.[14] recently reported that 5.4% of all emergency room admissions involving diabetic patients were for DKA. Similar studies in New Zealand suggested that 8% of all hospital admissions of diabetic patients were due to DKA.[15] Neither of these latter two studies clearly defined DKA. Because of a lack of recent data on these parameters, we decided to evaluate both the incidence of hospital admissions of patients with diabetes and the percentage of patients admitted with a diagnosis of DKA or HHNS to the Regional Medical Center of Memphis, a county-supported teaching hospital of the University of Tennessee, Memphis. During the period from January 1981 to June 1989, a total of 172,796 patients were admitted to the hospital, for an average annual admission rate of 20,329. The detailed data for DKA and HHNS are presented in Table 41−1. It is interesting to note that 1.1% of all admissions were for the primary diagnosis of diabetes and that 3.9% of other admissions carried the secondary diagnosis of diabetes. Thus, 5% of the total of

OTHER HYPERGLYCEMIC STATES
- Diabetes Mellitus
- Non-Ketotic Hyperosmolar Coma
- Impaired Glucose Tolerance
- Stress Hyperglycemia

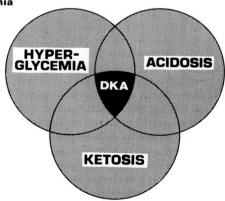

OTHER METABOLIC ACIDOTIC STATES
- Lactic Acidosis
- Hyperchloremic Acidosis
- Salicylism
- Uremic Acidosis
- Drug-Induced Acidosis

OTHER KETOTIC STATES
- Ketotic Hypoglycemia
- Alcoholic Ketosis

Fig. 41−1. Symptom complex in diabetic ketoacidosis (DKA) associated with hyperglycemia, metabolic acidosis, and ketotic states. Reprinted with permission from reference 2 (Kitabchi AE. Metabolic effects in neuropeptides. In: Givens JR, ed. Hormone-secreting pituitary tumors. Chicago: Year Book Medical Publishers, 1982:45−62).

Table 41–1. Data on Inpatient Admissions for Diabetes Mellitus (DM), Diabetic Ketoacidosis (DKA), and Hyperglycemic, Hyperosmolar Nonketotic State (HHNS), with Mortality Rates, at the Regional Medical Center, Memphis, from January 1981 through June 1989.

	No. (%)	Mortality Rate (%)
DIABETES		
Total admissions	172,796	
Average admissions/yr	20,329	
Admissions: primary diagnosis DM	1,908	
Average no. of admissions/yr	225	
% of admissions with primary diagnosis DM	(1.1)	
Admissions: secondary diagnosis DM	6,808	
Average admissions/yr	801	
% admissions with secondary diagnosis DM	(3.9)	
DKA*		
Admissions: primary diagnosis DKA	547	
Average admissions/yr	64	2.7
% of all admissions	(0.3)	
% of all admissions with primary diagnosis DM	(28.7)	
Admissions: secondary diagnosis DKA	118	
Average admissions/yr	14	9.3
% of all admissions	(0.07)	
% of all admissions with primary diagnosis DM	(6.2)	
HHNS†		
Admissions: primary diagnosis HHNS	83	
Average admissions/yr	10	34.9
% of all admissions	(0.05)	
% of all admissions with primary diagnosis DM	(4.4)	
Admissions: secondary diagnosis HHNS	30	
Average admissions/yr	3.5	33.0
% of all admissions	(0.02)	
% of all admissions with primary diagnosis DM	(1.06)	

Data are from A. E. Kitabchi, M. B. Murphy, S. McConnell, and D. Andrews (unpublished).

*Criteria for diagnosis of DKA were a blood glucose level >250 mg/dL, a blood bicarbonate level <15 meq/L, and a pH <7.3 with no ketonemia or ketonuria of moderate degree as determined by the nitroprusside method.

†Criteria for the diagnosis of HHNS were a calculated serum osmolality >330 mOsm/kg, pH >7.3, and bicarbonate >20 meq/L with no ketonemia or ketonuria as determined by the nitroprusside method.

admissions to the hospital were diabetes-related. DKA (primary diagnosis) accounted for 28.7%, with 6.2% having a secondary diagnosis of DKA, for a total of 34.9% of all primary diabetic admissions.

With the advent of continuous subcutaneous insulin infusion devices (CSII) in the early 1970s, the incidence of DKA appeared to increase in both the United States and Great Britain.[8] However, a reduction of the frequency of DKA was noted after both education of the patient and correction of mechanical problems.[16,17] Nevertheless, in a randomized study, the incidence of DKA in a group using the insulin pump was greater than that in a control group using multiple insulin injections.[18]

Prior to the discovery of insulin by Banting and Best in 1922, the mortality rate associated with episodes of DKA was almost 100%.[5] By 1932 the mortality rate among 1007 patients with DKA reported by Bertram from a review of 25 different authors was down to 29%.[19] Further reductions of mortality to 15% in 1955[20] and to 5% in 1960[21] were reported. This decline was thought to reflect the introduction of antibiotic therapy in the mid-1940s, as well as other improvements in patient care. As early as 1951 Harwood reported only one death among 67 patients treated for DKA and credited his success to prompt therapy, continuous observation, subspecialty consultation, and appropriate use of insulin and fluid.[22] However, in the mid-1960s the average mortality rate among patients with DKA remained around 9%, as reflected by the report of Beigelman, who reviewed the outcome of 482 episodes of DKA at a University of California-Los Angeles county hospital between 1965 and 1968.[23] Recent reports of National Institutes of Health (NIH) data analysis suggest that between 1969 and 1973 the mortality rate for DKA in patients with diabetes was 10%.[7] As can be seen from Table 41–1, the mortality rate associated with DKA during the last 8 years at the Regional Medical Center in Memphis was 2.7% for those patients with a primary diagnosis of DKA. This rate has remained remarkably constant from year to year for the last 8 years. It is of interest that during this period both the criteria for diagnosis and the method of therapy for DKA have remained the same. Some factors that explain the decrease in the mortality rate among these patients is the immediate attention given to the patient in the emergency room by the triage nurse and the prompt admission of patients with DKA to the intensive care unit (ICU).

Precipitating Factors

The major precipitating factors for DKA are infection, intercurrent illness, and omission or inadequate insulin therapy (for a review, see Marshall and Alberti[8]). In addition, psychological causes and noncompliance are important contributing factors, particularly in repeated cases of DKA in adolescents.[24–26] A recent factor currently contributing to an increase in the incidence of DKA is the use of CSII devices.[27] CSII does not provide an intermediate or long-acting insulin depot, so plasma insulin levels quickly dissipate if delivery is interrupted. Furthermore, these patients have low levels of circulating insulin with no provision for automatic delivery of large doses of insulin during unexpected stress or infection. Therefore, they are vulnerable to the development of DKA during periods of intercurrent illness and stress of which they may not be aware, such as silent myocardial infarction. An example of such an event was reported for a patient with long-standing diabetes who was receiving CSII, who during hospitalization experienced multiple episodes of atypical myocardial ischemia (as confirmed by measurements of cardiac enzymes and electrocardiography) and developed DKA despite having received CSII.[28] The precipitating factors in this patient therefore consisted of the stress of myocardial ischemia, which led to elevation in levels of counterregulatory hormones, coupled with the relatively low levels of circulating insulin (typically present in patients receiving insulin by CSII). Another factor possibly contributing to repeated episodes of DKA is the presence of large amounts of insulin antibodies, which may decrease the efficacy of intermediate-acting insulin. Treatment of one such patient with two or three daily doses of regular pork insulin prevented further episodes of DKA.[29]

Evaluation of precipitating factors in 202 cases of DKA at the Clinical Research Center (CRC), University of Tennessee, between 1974 and 1985 are summarized in Table 41–2. Infection contributed the greatest percentage of cases (38%), followed by omission of or inadequate insulin (28%). Infection also was reported as the most frequent precipitating cause by Hockaday and Alberti, who noted its occurrence in 56% of their patients.[35] Approximately one-fourth of those admitted for DKA had previously undiagnosed diabetes. Of this group of patients with newly diagnosed diabetes who presented with DKA, analysis revealed that 20 were 16 to 39 years old and 25 were 40 to 73 years old, suggesting that patients in the older group, who might otherwise have been classified as having non-insulin-dependent diabetes mellitus (NIDDM), may present with acute metabolic decompensation of DKA.

Pathogenesis

Etiology

Three major factors contribute to the pathophysiology of DKA: insulin deficiency; increased levels of counterregulatory hormones; and dehydration. Proponents for the role of each factor have marshalled certain evidence from the literature and developed hypotheses for the

Table 41–2. Precipitating Factors for Diabetic Ketoacidosis (DKA) in 202 Patients Admitted to the University of Tennessee–Memphis, Clinical Research Center: 1974–1985.

Precipitating Factor	No. of Patients (%)
Infection	76 (38)
Omission of or inadequate insulin	56 (28)
Unknown	4 (2)
Newly diagnosed diabetes mellitus*	45 (22)
Other†	21 (10)
Total	202 (100)

Data are from Kitabchi et al.[30] Kitabchi et al. (unpublished), Sacks et al.,[31] Fisher et al,[32,33] and Morris et al.[34]

*No other discernable cause of DKA was determined. Of the newly diagnosed patients, 20 were 16 to 39 years old and 25 were 40 to 73 years old.

†Other causes incuded dietary noncompliance (7), alcohol abuse (5), pulmonary embolism (3), emotional stress (2), pancreatitis (2), gastrointestinal obstruction (1), pleural effusion (1), surgery for undescended testicle (1), gunshot wound/60% pancreatectomy (1), lupus treated with steroids (1), acute asthma attack (1), intravenous dextrose in oral surgery (1).

pathogenesis, but until recently the paucity of data has made the development of a strong case for each hypothesis weak.

Insulin Deficiency. The hypothesis that insulin deficiency plays an important role in the pathogenesis of DKA has been difficult to clarify, since the measurement of immunoreactive insulin (IRI) in plasma may not adequately portray insulin secretion. Furthermore, some of the earlier studies demonstrating pancreatic secretory capacity in DKA have included some patients with Type I diabetes during the "honeymoon" period following recovery from DKA.[36,37] Most studies have reported low to normal basal insulin levels in patients with DKA who had received insulin previously.[30,38] Baseline (fasting) IRI levels usually range between 5 to 15 μU/mL in nondiabetic subjects whose fasting blood glucose levels range between 70 and 115 mg/dL. Once such individuals are challenged with a glucose-containing meal, however, their postprandial IRI increases five- to sevenfold (to approximately 100 μU/mL). In patients with previously undiagnosed diabetes presenting with DKA, however, despite having blood glucose levels 300 mg/dL or higher, insulin levels are seldom above 15 μU/mL. Thus, insulin levels are very low and ineffective despite hyperglycemia. However, since IRI is not a measure of the actual state of insulin secretion, a better method of determining the capacity for insulin secretion is necessary. Such studies became available with the advent of the C-peptide assay.

C-peptide is a 31-peptide component of proinsulin that is cleaved during the process of insulin biosynthesis and secreted in equimolar amounts with insulin.[39] In a study by Chupin et al.,[40] baseline and stimulated C-peptide values for 22 patients with DKA were compared with those for 12 patients with HHNS (Table 41–3). This study clearly showed that although levels of insulin were low in both situations, tolbutamide-stimulated C-peptide values of patients with HHNS increased from baseline values of 1.14 to 1.75 nM and those of patients with DKA only increased from 0.21 to 0.25 nM, the latter being an insignificant rise. Thus, there was a clear divergence between IRI and C-peptide in the two groups. We also studied baseline and hourly levels of C-peptide in 37 consecutive cases of patients with DKA who were admitted to the CRC from 1984 to 1985.[41] These studies revealed that on admission the average C-peptide value was 0.1 ± 0.05 nM and the average glucose level was 520 ± 30 mg/dL. At recovery the C-peptide level remained below 0.05 nM. It is interesting that only 4 of 37 patients had C-peptide levels greater than 0.2 nM, a finding suggesting that on admission the majority of these patients were insulinopenic with no significant pancreatic reserve either before or after recovery from DKA.

Increased Counterregulatory Hormones. It is well known that during severe DKA the levels of counterregulatory hormones such as glucagon,[30,42] catecholamines,[43] cortisol,[30,44] and growth hormone[45,46] are increased and tend to return toward normal at recovery (Kitabchi et al., unpublished data).[47] This combined increase in levels of counterregulatory hormones may have an additive effect on glucose production and negative nitrogen balance in nondiabetic obese sub-

Table 41–3. Biochemical Data on Admission in Patients with Diabetes Admitted for Hyperglycemic, Hyperosmolar Nonketotic State (HHNS) or Diabetic Ketoacidosis (DKA).

	Mean ± SEM	
Value	HHNS (n = 12)	DKA (n = 22)
Glucose (mM)	51.6 ± 4.6	34.2 ± 2.0
Na⁺ (mM)	149.0 ± 3.2	134.4 ± 1.0
K⁺ (mM)	3.9 ± 0.2	4.5 ± 0.13
BUN (mM)	23.4 ± 3.8	11.7 ± 1.0
Creatinine (μM)	123.9 ± 6.6	97.3 ± 3.7
pH	7.33 ± 0.03	7.12 ± 0.04
Bicarbonate (mM)	18.0 ± 1.1	9.4 ± 1.4
Lactate (mM)	3.9 ± 0.4	2.4 ± 0.2
3-β-hydroxybutyrate (mM)	1.0 ± 0.2	9.10 ± 0.85
Osmolality*	380.0 ± 5.7	323.3 ± 2.5
IRI (nM)	0.08 ± 0.01	0.07 ± 0.01
C-peptide (nM)	1.14 ± 0.10	0.21 ± 0.03
FFA (nM)	1.5 ± 0.19	1.6 ± 0.16
Glucagon (ng/mL)	1.9 ± 0.2	6.1 ± 1.2
Cortisol (ng/mL)	570.0 ± 49	500.0 ± 61
IRI (nM)†	0.27 ± 0.05	0.09 ± 0.01
C-peptide (nM)†	1.75 ± 0.23	0.25 ± 0.05

Data are from Chupin et al.[40] IRI = immunoreactive insulin.
*According to the formula: 2(Na + K) + urea + glucose (mM).
†Values following intravenous administration of tolbutamide.

jects.[48] In addition, since infection is the most common precipitating event in DKA, other factors may play a role. Schade and Eaton studied the effects of an injected pyrogen on levels of counterregulatory hormones in diabetic subjects and found that levels of these hormones and ketone bodies were increased despite simultaneous insulin infusion.[49] On the other hand, Gerich et al.[50] showed that in insulin-dependent patients, infusion of counterregulatory hormones such as glucagon and growth hormone failed to bring about an elevation of levels of free fatty acids, ketone bodies, and glycerol in the presence of insulin. However, withdrawal of insulin during infusion of glucagon and growth hormone in combination with somatostatin promptly raised the level of these metabolites.[50] One factor that may contribute to a failure of elevation in levels of counterregulatory hormones may be the inability of certain patients with insulin-dependent diabetes mellitus (IDDM) of long duration to respond to stress by increasing levels of counterregulatory hormones. Studies by Bolli et al.[51] indicate that 30 to 40% of patients with IDDM of greater than 15 years' duration may have impaired glucagon and catecholamine responses to stress. When counterregulatory hormone levels are low, the severity of ketoacidosis may be decreased.[52,53] It has therefore been suggested that although insulin deficiency is a crucial etiologic factor in the genesis of DKA, the severity of DKA may depend in part on the presence of "stress" hormones.[4]

In order to investigate the role of insulin and counterregulatory hormones in DKA, Matteri et al.[54] took hourly measurements of metabolites, free insulin, glucose, and counterregulatory hormones in five patients with IDDM during withdrawal of the CSII (experimental period) and compared these values during a control period when the patients received insulin. During both periods, patients were ambulatory and ate regular meals beginning with breakfast. When patients became uncomfortable or had blood glucose values greater than 500 mg/dL, they received an infusion of 200 mL of normal saline and their insulin pump was restarted. This study differs from other insulin-withdrawal protocols in that the patients continued to receive meals. Therefore, a moderate degree of hyperglycemia (400 to 500 mg/dL) was evident by hour 5 or 6 after withdrawal, when the levels of free insulin had become undetectable. This hyperglycemia also was accompanied by an increase in levels of glucagon, norepinephrine, free fatty acids, and ketone bodies; no change in cortisol, growth hormone, or epinephrine levels; and a 50% drop in free insulin levels in 2 hours. This suggests that mild DKA can occur as a result of hypoinsulinemia in the absence of a significant elevation of counterregulatory hormone levels. The importance of increased levels of some counterregulatory hormones in the development of DKA is apparent, however, in patients who develop DKA while receiving CSII during a stressful event. Such events may be seen in patients with IDDM who develop myocardial ischemia, intercurrent illness, or severe infection with concomitant elevation of counterregulatory hormones leading to increased free fatty acid and ketone body production, hyperglycemia, and ultimately ketoacidosis. Therefore, although elevations in counterregulatory hormone levels are not essential to the development of mild ketoacidosis, they can exaggerate the state of acute metabolic decompensation.[55]

Dehydration. Dehydration is inevitably found in severe DKA and results from the osmotic diuresis of hyperglycemia, often being further complicated by fluid deprivation caused by gastrointestinal disturbances. The fluid deficit may be as great as 7 L in severe DKA. As early as 1960, Cohen et al. showed that adequate hydration is an important aspect of DKA therapy and that it can reduce the mortality rate dramatically.[21] Hydration has been shown to reduce hyperglycemia without altering acid-base balance,[29,31,56–58] since most of the glucose is disposed of in the urine.[57,58] Hydration also may improve ketoacidosis secondary to dilution of counterregulatory hormones.[47]

In summary, three factors—insulin deficiency, elevated levels of counterregulatory hormones, and dehydration—are important contributing factors in the development of DKA. Each can contribute to different degrees of decompensation of the metabolic state, depending on the individual patient. The most severe cases of DKA are the result of a combination of prolonged deprivation of insulin, elevation of counterregulatory hormone levels, and severe fluid deprivation.

Alteration of Intermediary Metabolism in DKA

Glucose Metabolism. Glucose ingestion, glycogenolysis, and gluconeogenesis provide three sources of glucose in the blood, whereas oxidation, lipogenesis, and glycogen synthesis provide a means of dissipating this

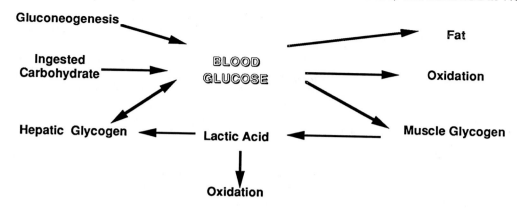

Fig. 41—2. Sources and fate of glucose. Reprinted with permission from reference 2 (Kitabchi AE, Fisher JN. Diabetes mellitus. In: Glew RH, Peters SP, eds. Clinical studies in medical biochemistry. New York: Oxford University Press, 198:102—17).

substrate (Fig. 41—2). Blood glucose levels are maintained within a very narrow range in normal individuals in a fed state, with particularly important control being exerted by insulin and glucagon (Fig. 41—3, left). In the fed state, insulin is the major anabolic hormone responsible for the conversion of substrates into energy stores through its effects on insulin-sensitive tissues. Insulin assimilates amino acids into protein throughout the body in liver and muscle, fatty acids into triglycerides in adipose tissue and liver, and glucose into glycogen in muscle and liver. DKA, on the other hand, is a catabolic state (Fig. 41—3, right) in which the major counterregu-

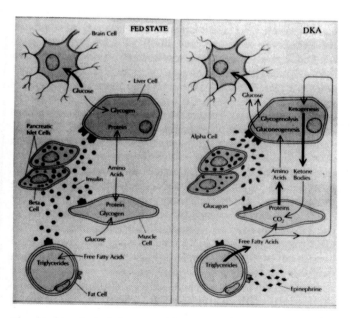

Fig. 41—3. Left: Substrate utilization in the fed state showing the role of insulin in the promotion of fuel storage. Right: Metabolic alterations in diabetic ketoacidosis (DKA). Insulin deficiency and elevation of counterregulatory hormones activate ketogenic, gluconeogenic, glycogenolytic, and lipolytic pathways. Reprinted with permission from reference 166 (Kitabchi AE, Rumbak MJ. The management of diabetic emergencies. Hosp Pract 1989;224:229(6):129—33. Illustration by Ilil Arbel).

latory hormones (glucagon, catecholamines, cortisol, and possibly growth hormone), combined with various degrees of insulin deficiency, lead to an increase in gluconeogenesis (glucose production from noncarbohydrate precursors) and glycogenolysis.

Ketone Body Metabolism. Insulin, the most potent antilipolytic hormone in humans, is effectively reduced during DKA in combination with a relative or absolute elevation in the levels of catabolic hormones such as catecholamines, glucagon, and cortisol. These events favor lipolysis with increased production of free fatty acids, leading to β oxidation by the liver and increased ketogenesis. Glucagon has a multifactorial effect on the promotion of ketogenesis. Glucagon lowers the hepatic level of malonyl coenzyme A (CoA) by blocking the conversion of pyruvate to acetyl CoA through inhibition of acetyl CoA carboxylase,[60] the first rate-limiting enzyme in de novo fatty acid synthesis and production of malonyl CoA. Malonyl CoA usually inhibits carnitine palmitoyltransferase (CPTI), the rate-limiting enzyme for transesterification of fatty acyl CoA to fatty acyl carnitine, allowing further metabolism of fatty acid by β oxidation to ketone bodies in the mitochondria. Although it has been stated that reduction of malonyl CoA prevents the inhibition of CPTI and accelerates the production of β-hydroxybutyric acid and acetoacetic acid, a second mechanism was recently proposed. The K_i of malonyl CoA for CPTI is increased in diabetes, leading to a decrease in the efficacy of inhibition of CPTI activity.[61] Glucagon also stimulates the hepatic level of carnitine by an unknown mechanism; this, together with an increase in CPTI and fatty acyl CoA leads to increased ketogenesis (for review, see McGarry[62]). In addition to the above mechanism, both cyclic adenosine monophosphate (cAMP) and glucagon in the presence of insulin deficiency exert a direct positive effect on ketogenesis that is independent of an increased substrate supply from adipose tissue (i.e., free fatty acids).[63] Beside the ketogenesis in the liver, about 10 to 20% may occur in the kidney. Not only is production of ketone bodies increased in DKA, there is evidence that clearance of ketones is decreased. This decrease may be due to a decreased insulin level, an increased glucocorticoid level, and decreased ketone body utilization by peripheral tissues.

Although some studies suggest both increased ketogenesis and decreased clearance of ketone bodies in DKA,[64–66] at least one study using radioactive tracers indicated that clearance is normal in DKA.[67] Acetone production is also variable in DKA[68] and may contribute up to 50% of the acetoacetate produced.

Generally, the level of β-hydroxybutyric acid is about three times higher than that of acetoacetic acid. β-Hydroxybutyric acid does not react with nitroprusside, whereas acetoacetic acid reacts avidly. Acetone also reacts with nitroprusside but to a much lesser degree. However, acetone does not have acidic properties, and because of its volatility, its level in the blood may vary according to the rate of respiration. Acetone also may serve as a gluconeogenic substrate in starvation and DKA.[69] With improvement in DKA during therapy, conversion of β-hydroxybutyric acid to acetoacetic acid increases because of a higher oxidation state. Figure 41–4 demonstrates the response of these two types of ketone bodies in the serum to insulin therapy in 37 cases of DKA during 12 hours of follow-up. During recovery, the molar ratio of acetoacetic acid to β-hydroxybutyric acid gradually increases. Thus, although both β-hydroxybutyrate and acetoacetate decline during therapy, the relative levels of acetoacetate increases. As expected, therefore, the nitroprusside reactions of urine and blood continue to remain at a plateau despite an improvement in metabolic state (Fig. 41–4, right panels).

Protein and Amino Acid Metabolism. Negative nitrogen balance is another hallmark of DKA, an effect known since the pioneering work of Atchley et al.,[70] Butler et al.,[71] and Nabarro et al.,[72] who found that insulin withdrawal resulted in the loss of 9 to 12 g of nitrogen per day followed by slow recovery during therapy. In addition, levels of gluconeogenic amino acids (glutamine, alanine, threonine, serine, glutamate, glycine) decrease

whereas levels of ketogenic amino acids (leucine, isoleucine, valine) increase during DKA.[73,74] Both an increase in proteolysis and a decrease in protein synthesis have been suggested as reasons for these changes, but the detailed mechanism in humans has not been fully delineated. In experimental animal studies, acidosis appears to increase glucocorticoid production, which leads both to decreased protein synthesis and to increased nonlysosomal proteolysis.[75] It is thus possible that in severe DKA, during which both glucagon and cortisol levels are elevated, synergistic effects of these two hormones enhance amino acidemia and sustain a negative nitrogen balance. In addition, under the influence of glucagon, alanine—the major gluconeogenic amino acid—is converted to glucose in the liver. Therefore, the plasma level of alanine is reduced in DKA as a result of increased gluconeogenesis.[76]

Lipid Metabolism. It has been known for many years that hypertriglyceridemia is frequently found in patients with severe, uncontrolled diabetes (for a review, see Foster and McGarry[6]). Increased levels of chylomicrons and very-low-density lipoproteins (VLDL), demonstrated as lipemia retinalis, may be observed in severe DKA in the presence of increased lipolysis. Thus, in DKA there is the apparent dichotomy of increased lipolysis and hypertriglyceridemia, but the level of serum cholesterol is relatively normal. The increased level of triglycerides is the result of an increase in the secretion of VLDL secreted by the liver in insulin deficiency, coupled with an increase in the level of free fatty acids, which leads to further synthesis of triglycerides. This increase in triglyceride levels occurs despite the fact that VLDL production, relative to the level of free fatty acids, is decreased in patients with DKA as compared with that in nondiabetic subjects; however, an abundance of free fatty acids in DKA ultimately leads to overproduction of VLDL by the liver. Additional mechanisms responsible for hypertriglyceridemia in DKA may be decreased clearance of VLDL.[77]

With regard to lipoproteins in DKA, it is known that levels of intermediate-density lipoprotein (IDL), high-density lipoprotein (HDL), and low-density lipoprotein (LDL) cholesterol are initially low in DKA. However, the level of HDL cholesterol rises with insulin therapy, whereas levels of IDL and LDL cholesterol do not. The mechanisms are not well understood.

Weidman et al.[78] undertook a careful investigation of the plasma lipoprotein profiles in 14 patients in severe DKA and studied the early effect of physiologic doses of insulin on their lipid profiles. Of interest was the finding that during therapy most patients with hypertriglyceridemia responded within 24 hours with reductions in their triglyceride levels through reductions in chylomicron and VLDL levels. Of importance was the finding that treatment of DKA with physiologic doses of insulin significantly reduced the level of apoprotein A_I, as well as the ratio of apoprotein A_I to HDL cholesterol. This suggests that insulin may decrease the secretion of apoprotein A_I into the plasma or increase its catabolism. These studies have been subsequently confirmed by other groups.[79]

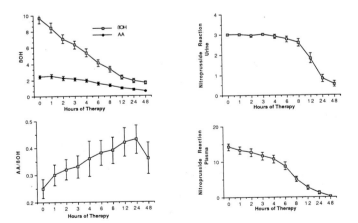

Fig. 41–4. Comparative data in 37 patients with diabetic ketoacidosis with regard to plasma acetoacetic acid (AA) and β-hydroxybutyric acid (βOH) (top left); ratio of AA to βOH (bottom left); and ketone bodies (nitroprusside reaction) in the urine (top right) and plasma (bottom right) before and during low-dose intravenous infusion of insulin for 48 hours (Kitabchi et al., unpublished data).

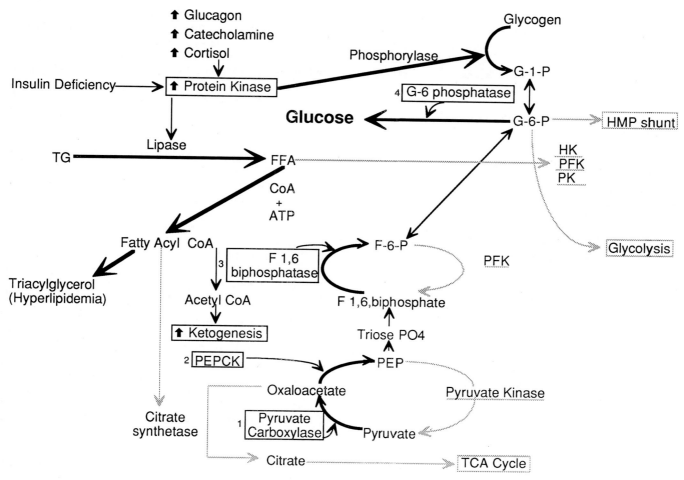

Fig. 41–5. Proposed biochemical changes that occur during diabetic ketoacidosis. These alterations lead to increased gluconeogenesis and lipolysis and decreased glycolysis. ATP = adenosine triphosphate. CoA = coenzyme A; FFA = free fatty acids; F-6-P = fructose-6-phosphate; G-(X)-P = glucose-(X)-phosphate; HK = hexokinase; HMP = hexose monophosphate; PC = pyruvate carboxylase; PFK = phosphofructokinase; PEP = phosphoenolpyruvate; PEPCK = PEP carboxykinase; PK = pyruvate kinase; TCA = tricarboxylic acid; TG = triglycerides. Note: Lipolysis occurs mainly in adipose tissue. Other events occur primarily in the liver (except some gluconeogenesis in the kidney).

Alteration of Biochemical Pathways. Figure 41–5 details the biochemical alterations in DKA. As stated earlier, DKA is a catabolic state characterized by a net reduction of insulin action and an elevation in the concentrations of glucagon, catecholamines, and cortisol, changes leading to an increase in the cAMP-dependent protein kinase activity, which, through a cascade phenomenon, modifies metabolic pathways in three major insulin-sensitive tissues—muscle, fat, and liver—as follows. Increased lipolytic activity in adipose tissue leads to increased production of free fatty acids. As stated earlier, both increased substrate (free fatty acids) and increased levels of glucagon and cAMP, coupled with insulin deficiency, directly lead to increased ketogenesis, independent of the malonyl CoA mechanism. On the other hand, accelerated conversion of fatty acyl CoA to triacylglycerol, as well as decreased clearance of VLDL and chylomicrons, results in hypertriglyceridemia.[80] Increased free fatty acid levels may also directly reduce

glycolysis in the liver by decreasing the rate-limiting enzymes of glycolysis: hexokinase, phosphofructokinase, and pyruvate kinase. The high level of glucagon/insulin also may, through the activity of cAMP-dependent protein kinase, decrease the hepatic level of fructose-1,6-biphosphate. On the other hand, increased gluconeogenesis in DKA is achieved through activation of a series of rate-limiting enzymes—fructose-1,6-bisphosphatase, phosphoenolypyruvate carboxykinase (PEPCK), glucose-6-phosphatase, and pyruvate carboxylase—in the liver. PEPCK is particularly modulated by the inhibitory effects of insulin. In addition, glucagon—through cAMP production, the stimulation of cAMP-dependent protein kinase, and activation of phosphorylase—enhances glycogenolysis in the liver and the breakdown of glycogen to glucose-1-phosphate. Glucagon also enhances conversion of glucose-6-phosphate to glucose by activation of glucose-6-phosphatase in the liver (for review, see Schade et al.[4]). This also reduces the flow of glucose-6-phosphate through the hexose monophosphate shunt. Thus, both glycogenolysis and gluconeogenesis are increased in uncontrolled diabetes and account for a major portion of the hyperglycemia in DKA (Fig. 41–5). Furthermore, insulin deficiency in DKA results not only in increased hepatic output but in decreased uptake of glucose by insulin-sensitive tissues (muscle, fat, and liver), leading to further progression of hyperglycemia. These events are reversed with the institution of insulin therapy.[58]

Renal Function and Acid-Base Balance

DKA is characterized by increased renal excretion of glucose, ketone bodies, and nitrogenous compounds. There is also a nonspecific defect in tubular luminal uptake of low-molecular-weight proteins in DKA that is reversible within 10 to 15 days following metabolic recovery.[81] Studies of Owen and co-workers[82] suggest that a decrease in the plasma glucose concentration during hydration is caused primarily by renal glucose excretion and that the absence of maximal renal tubular reabsorption for both acetoacetate and β-hydroxybutyrate serves to explain the large urinary loss of sodium and potassium during DKA.

The classical investigations of Atchley et al.[70] and Butler et al.[71] provide detailed studies of electrolyte balance in DKA. The usual loss of water in DKA is approximately 5 to 8 L, with an average sodium and potassium loss of about 400 to 700 meq[70] and 250 to 700 meq,[83] respectively. These losses represent a loss of water in excess of sodium, and therefore the fluid lost in DKA more closely resembles hypotonic saline solution than isotonic solution.[5] The increase in plasma anion gap is due to the accumulation of ketone ions as a result of titration of protons from ketoacids by bicarbonate. However, this anion gap may not be correlated with serum bicarbonate.[84] The normal anion gap (Na − Cl + HCO_3) is between 8 and 16 meq/L. In DKA this gap is usually increased because of the presence of ketoacids as unmeasured anions. Thus, in DKA, acidosis ranges from anion gap acidosis to pure hyperchloremic metabolic acidosis (HCMA).[84]

On the basis of prospective and retrospective studies in 196 patients with DKA, Adrogué et al.[84] found no relationship between the initial total level of serum carbon dioxide and the anion gap. The degree of acidosis was independent of renal dysfunction and the severity of metabolic acidosis. However, the initial renal function appeared to be responsible for the variable retention of plasma ketones, i.e., the more severe the dehydration on admission, the greater the ketone retention with less prominent HCMA. They interpreted the results as indicating that recovery from acidosis was slower in those patients admitted with HCMA. However, in those patients who developed HCMA 4 to 8 hours after the initiation of DKA therapy, the retention of chloride was in excess of the retention of sodium and of the excretion of ketones by the kidneys.

Kitabchi et al.[41] investigated the incidence of HCMA in 37 patients with DKA who were treated with three different physiologic doses of insulin (0.07 U/kg of regular insulin by intravenous bolus followed by 0.07 U/kg per hour by continuous infusion; 0.07 U/kg per hour by continuous infusion without a bolus dose; and 0.14 U/kg by continuous infusion without a bolus dose). Twenty-seven percent developed HCMA. Among those patients receiving a bolus injection of insulin (who had a higher initial circulating level of free insulin than patients in the other two groups), only one developed HCMA, whereas in the two groups, a total of nine patients developed HCMA. No significant difference was noted in admission laboratory data; recovery times; or amount of intravenous fluid, sodium, or chloride administered. However, the higher blood urea nitrogen (BUN) values and lower blood pressure in the patients who did not develop HCMA suggests greater dehydration. The contributing factor in the development of HCMA may be a higher intravascular fluid volume and lower initial insulin level during initital therapy.[41]

Pathophysiologic Basis of Clinical Presentation

The effective reduction of insulin, the major anabolic and antilipolytic hormone, along with variably increased levels of counterregulatory hormones such as catecholamines, glucagon, and cortisol, brings about the metabolic derangements in DKA (Fig. 41–6), in which the catabolic state predominates over the anabolic state. Lack of insulin promotes lipolytic activity and inhibits utilization of substrates by insulin-sensitive tissues (i.e., conversion of glucose to glycogen, of amino acids to protein, and of free

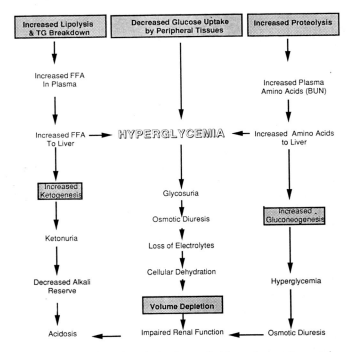

Fig. 41–6. Altered carbohydrate, lipid, and protein metabolism in diabetic ketoacidosis and resultant water and electrolyte imbalances, impaired renal function, and acidosis resulting from insulin deficiency and increase in counterregulatory hormones. TG = triglycerides; FFA = free fatty acids; and BUN = blood urea nitrogen. Adapted from Kitabchi and Murphy.[9]

fatty acids to triglyceride). In the presence of a higher glucagon/insulin ratio and catecholamine levels, the reverse of the anabolic state prevails[85]:

1) Catecholamines stimulate phosphorylase, which catalyzes the conversion of glycogen to glucose-6-phosphate by glyconeogenesis. Glucose-6-phosphate is converted to glucose by glucose-6-phosphatase in the liver.

2) Catecholamines stimulate glycogenolysis in muscle, leading to the liberation of lactate rather than glucose since muscle lacks the enzyme glucose-6-phosphatase.

3) Catecholamines accelerate triglyceride breakdown to glycerol and free fatty acid in adipocytes. Glycerol provides the carbon skeleton for gluconeogenesis. Free fatty acids proceed through fatty acid oxidation and ketogenesis as previously described. Free fatty acids also stimulate hyperglycemia through the gluconeogenic pathway (Fig. 41–5).

It is of note that in addition to providing substrate for ketogenesis in the liver through the action of glucagon and an increased glucagon/insulin ratio, increased levels of free fatty acids provide another source of triglyceride-rich VLDL. Increased ketogenesis and decreased clearance of ketone bodies leads to ketonemia, which, when it surpasses the renal threshold, leads to ketonuria. The two major ketone bodies, β-hydroxybutyric acid and acetoacetic acid, are strong acids that are neutralized to β-hydroxybutyrate and acetoacetate, respectively, before excretion in the urine. This neutralization occurs at the expense of the bicarbonate reserve. This decrease in the bicarbonate reserve leads to manifestations of acidosis, as well as to further losses of sodium in the urine.

In the presence of acidosis, increased glucagon, and increased cortisol and in the absence of adequate insulin, proteolysis is increased and protein synthesis is decreased. Such events transiently increase levels of both ketogenic and gluconeogenic amino acids. The former are utilized in the liver for ketogenesis and the latter for gluconeogenesis in the liver or kidney under the influence of an increased glucagon/insulin ratio. The net result is increased hepatic production of glucose. Further hyperglycemia in DKA is brought about by decreased uptake of glucose in insulin-sensitive tissues, primarily in response to insulin deficiency but also because of the inhibitory effect of catecholamines and free fatty acids on glucose utilization by peripheral tissues. Significant hyperglycemia above the renal threshold results in glycosuria and osmotic diuresis, with a loss of large amounts of fluid and electrolytes. Loss of fluid leads to polydipsia and polyuria. The increase in urinary loss of glucose leads to a loss of calories and ultimately to polyphagia. Thus, the catabolic state in DKA results in increased proteolysis, lipolysis, ketogenesis, gluconeogenesis, and glycogenolysis, changes that lead to acidosis, hyperglycemia, ketosis, severe dehydration, and transient impairment in renal function (Fig. 41–6). These can be promptly reversed with appropriate hydration and physiologic doses of insulin, provided that therapy is initiated early enough.

Diagnosis

The importance of obtaining a history rapidly but thoroughly and performing a rapid physical cannot be overemphasized. However, of 123 patients with DKA presenting to a major medical center, 19.9% were comatose, 13.8% were stuporous, 39.8% were drowsy, and only 41.5% were fully conscious.[30–32] Therefore, if the patient is unable to communicate, a history should be obtained from friends or relatives to assist in the prompt delivery of treatment and identification of the underlying cause.

The classical clinical picture includes a history of polyuria, polydipsia, weight loss, vomiting, abdominal discomfort, Kussmaul respirations, dehydration with loss of skin turgor, soft eyeballs, weakness, acetone odor on the breath, signs of vascular shock, and finally coma. Although the most common precipitating event is infection, many patients are normothermic or hypothermic. The physical examination supports but does not always validate the diagnosis of DKA, because classical symptoms are not always present. For example, many patients do not exhibit Kussmaul respirations even when the pH is less than 7.1, and the presence of acetone on the breath is difficult to assess objectively. In addition, the qualitative analysis of ketones in the urine and blood by the nitroprusside reaction only determines the amount of acetoacetate and, to a lesser extent, the amount of acetone. However, in DKA, β-hydroxybutyrate may be the predominant ketone body. Therefore, the level of ketosis may be underestimated. Coma may or may not be present and has been shown to correlate with serum osmolality. In comatose and stuporous patients, the serum osmolality is generally greater than 330 mOsm/kg of water, whereas in alert patients it is seldom so high[31–33] (Fig. 41–7). Abdominal pain may be the result of DKA rather than an indication of appendicitis or peritoneal inflammation from some other cause. Finally, pneumonia may not be apparent on initial chest films because of dehydration but may become visible following hydration.

As noted at the beginning of this chapter, the syndrome of DKA consists of the triad of hyperglycemia, ketosis, and acidemia, all three of which must be present for diagnosis (Fig. 41–1). The diagnosis of DKA, however, can be confounded by many variables, making it difficult to obtain a clear picture of the acid-base status of the patient. In general, a working diagnosis of DKA can be made if the plasma glucose is greater than 250 mg/dL, serum bicarbonate is less than 15 meq/L, pH is lower than 7.30, and ketonemia (nitroprusside method) is present at a dilution of 1:2. Adrogué et al.[84] reported that 46% of patients admitted for DKA had a predominant anion-gap acidosis, 43% had mixed anion-gap acidosis and HCMA, and 11% had a predominant HCMA. Furthermore, a tendency toward metabolic alkalosis may occur in DKA secondary to nausea and vomiting and the use of diuretics. Respiratory alkalosis, as well as respiratory

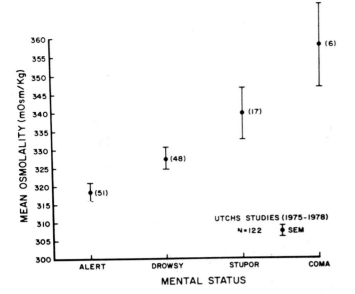

Fig. 41–7. Calculated serum osmolality in 122 ketoacidotic patients, with relation to mental status, at the time of admission. UTCHS = University of Tennessee Center for the Health Sciences. Data are from Kitabchi et al.,[30] Sacks et al.,[31] and Fisher et al.[32] Reprinted with permission from reference 29 (Kitabchi AE, Fisher JN. Insulin therapy of diabetic ketoacidosis; physiologic versus pharmacologic doses of insulin and their routes of administration. In: Brownlee M, ed. Handbook of diabetes mellitus. Vol 5. New York: Garland Press, 1981:95–149).

compensation for acidosis, may coexist with DKA, secondary to fever and infection. Blood glucose values may be lower than 300 mg/dL in a patient with DKA; therefore, strict adherence to this parameter in the differential diagnosis may result in misdiagnosis and undertreatment. Fifteen percent of patients will present with a blood glucose level lower than 300 mg/dL, especially in cases of alcohol use, which inhibits gluconeogenesis, and in pregnancy, in which the fetus is able to use glucose independent of insulin action.[86]

Fluid and electrolyte deficits per kilogram of body weight in DKA typically include 100 mL of water, 7 to 10 meq of sodium, 3 to 5 meq of potassium, 5 to 7 meq of chloride, 1 mmol of phosphorus, and 0.5 to 0.8 meq of magnesium. Serum sodium values vary, depending on the duration of symptoms, and may be factitiously low secondary to hyperglycemia and hyperlipidemia. Hyperglycemia leads to volume changes in the extracellular compartment, which causes underestimation in the laboratory assessment of sodium values. This underestimation is corrected by adding 1.6 meq to the reported sodium value for every 100 mg of glucose over 100 mg.[87] Severe hyperlipidemia leads to falsely low serum sodium values because the assay is volume dependent. Therefore, the elevated levels of lipid displace plasma water and result in incorrect calculation of sodium values.[88]

Initial serum potassium levels vary depending on how long the patient has had symptoms before seeking

assistance. Shifts in the intracellular compartment result in reported deficits of as much as 700 meq. Leukocyte counts may be elevated to 25,000/mm^3 because of stress, but markedly elevated levels should alert the clinician to an underlying infection. Amylase levels are elevated in 66% of patients in DKA because of assay interference by ketoacids and secretion of amylase from nonpancreatic sources such as the parotid gland.[89] However, an abdominal emergency can be the precipitating cause of DKA. Therefore, abdominal complaints should be closely followed and evaluated by additional laboratory tests and early surgical consultation when abdominal complaints or signs persist. In addition, the serum creatinine level is falsely elevated as a result of assay interference by ketoacids. Liver function test values are elevated in as many as one-third of the patients because of liver enlargement and interference by hyperlipidemia in liver enzyme assays.[88] Last, pseudonormoglycemia may be seen with hypertriglyceridemia in DKA.[90]

Physical examination plays a pivotal role in determining the precipitating factor and assists in ruling out other causes of coma. Other metabolic causes of acidosis and coma include lactic acidosis; alcoholic ketosis; intoxication with salicylates, methanol, or ethylene glycol; rhabdomyolysis; hypoglycemia; and HHNS. Table 41–4 provides guides to the differential diagnosis of these clinical conditions.

HYPERGLYCEMIC, HYPEROSMOLAR NONKETOTIC STATE (HHNS)

Definition

The hyperglycemic, hyperosmolar nonketotic state (HHNS) was first described by Sament and Schwartz in 1957[92] and has been the topic of many reviews.[1,2,4,7,87–99] HHNS is defined by extreme hyperglycemia, increased serum osmolarity (calculated as follows: 2(Na)(meq/L) + glucose (mg/dL)/18 + BUN (mg/dL)/2.8, with normal values being 290 ± 5 mOsm/kg water), and severe dehydration without significant ketosis or acidosis. In general, serum is negative for ketones at 1:2 dilution by the nitroprusside method, serum bicarbonate concentration is greater than 20 meq/L, and the arterial pH is greater than 7.3. Hyperglycemia is usually more severe than in DKA, and therefore an arbitrary blood glucose value of greater than 600 mg/dL has been used as one of the diagnostic criteria. There is generally a greater incidence of depressed sensorium in HHNS than in DKA. The occurrence of HHNS is more frequent in the elderly and in patients with newly diagnosed diabetes and often has an insidious onset. HHNS and DKA may represent opposite ends of a spectrum of hyperglycemia with or without acidosis.[9] However, mild mixed ketotic hyperosmolar conditions also may exist.[87]

Incidence and Mortality Rate

Good epidemiologic studies on the incidence of HHNS are sparse. Recent data from Fishbein collected from 1979 to 1981 by an NIH data group[7] suggest an incidence

Table 41–4. Laboratory Evaluation of Metabolic Causes of Acidosis and Coma

	pH	Plasma Glucose	Glycosuria	Total Plasma Ketones*	Anion Gap	Osmolality	Uric Acid	Miscellaneous
Starvation or high fat intake	Normal	Normal	—	Slight ↑	Slight ↑	Normal	Mild ↑ (starvation)	...
DKA	↓↓	↑↑	++	↑↑	↑↑	Normal	Normal	...
Lactic acidosis	↓↓	Normal	—	Normal	↑↑	Normal	Normal	Serum lactate >7 mM
Uremic acidosis	Mild ↓	Normal	—	Normal	Slight ↑	↑ or normal	Normal or ↑	BUN >200 mg/dL
Alcohol ketosis (starvation)	↓ ↑	Normal or ↓	—	Slight to moderate ↑	↑	Normal	↑	...
Salicylate intoxication	↓ ↑†	Normal or ↓	—	Normal	↑	Normal	Normal	Serum salicylate +
Methanol or ethylene glycol intoxication	↓	Normal	—‡	Normal	↑	↑↑	Normal	Serum levels +
Hyperosmolar coma	Normal	↑↑ >500 mg/dL	++	Normal or slight ↑	Normal	↑↑ >330 mOsm/kg	Normal	...
Hypoglycemic coma	Normal	↓↓ <30 mg/dL	—	Normal	Normal	Normal	Normal	...
Rhabdomyolysis	Mild ↓ may be ↓↓	Normal	—	Normal	↑↑	Normal or slight ↑	↑	Myoglobulinurea Hemoglobinuria

Data are from Morris and Kitabchi.[91] DKA = diabetic ketoacidosis; + = positive; – = negative.
*Acetest and Ketostix measure acetoacetic acid only. Thus, misleading low values may be obtained because the majority of "ketone bodies" are β-hydroxybutyrate.
†Respiratory alkalosis/metabolic acidosis.
‡May get false-positive or false-negative urinary glucose caused by the presence of salicylate or its metabolites.

of 10 cases per 100,000 of the general population (which is about one-sixth that of DKA). The actual rate of hospital admissions due to HHNS is difficult to obtain because of the lack of a universally accepted definition, differences in the type of health-care setting, and other factors. The incidence of HHNS as a primary diagnosis at the Regional Medical Center, Memphis, from 1981 to 1989 was 0.05% of all diabetes-related admissions. There is almost unanimous agreement among reviewers on the subject that the mortality rate is far greater for HHNS, which ranges from 40 to 70%, than for DKA, which ranges from 1 to 10%. At the University of Tennessee, during the same 8.5-year period and determined by using a standard written protocol, the mortality rate for HHNS was 34.9% vs. a rate for DKA of 2.7% (Table 41–1).

Precipitating Factors

The typical patient with HHNS has undiagnosed Type II diabetes, is between 57 and 69 years old, and frequently is a nursing-home resident or someone who has delayed seeking medical treatment.[98] In many instances an acute illness, such as gram-negative pneumonia, uremia, vomiting, or acute viral infection, is the precipitating factor. This is exemplified by the findings of a study comparing the profiles of diabetic patients with HHNS with those of diabetic controls without HHNS, which revealed HHNS patients were more likely to be nursing-home residents (28% vs. 15%), newly diagnosed diabetics (36% vs. 7%), demented patients (18% vs. 8%), and to have experienced an acute infection (39% vs. 19%). Since one-third of these patients had no history of diabetes, delayed recognition of hyperglycemic symptoms may have led to severe dehydration. Table 41–5 contrasts the causes and factors contributing to HHNS and DKA.

Pathogenesis

Although the hallmark of HHNS is dehydration and severe hyperglycemia, the biochemical mechanism underlying the pathogenesis of these two components has not been fully elucidated. In general, three major mechanisms have been proposed to account for the greater dehydration and lack of significant ketogenesis in HHNS compared with that in DKA: 1) higher levels of counterregulatory hormones and free fatty acids in DKA vs. HHNS, 2) relatively higher levels of endogenous insulin reserve in HHNS, i.e., insulin adequate to prevent lipolysis but inadequate to inhibit hepatic glucose production and/or stimulate glucose utilization, and 3) inhibition of lipolysis by the hyperosmolar state, thus decreasing ketogenesis.

As to the proposal that levels of counterregulatory hormones are lower in HHNS, an early study by Gerich et al.[99] suggested that levels of free fatty acid, cortisol, and growth hormone were lower in HHNS than in DKA. However, later studies of Chupin et al.[40] comparing 12 cases of HHNS with 22 cases of DKA (Table 41–3), although confirming the higher level of growth hormone, revealed no significant difference in either free fatty acid or cortisol in the two groups. Other studies[102] suggest a higher level of glucagon in DKA than in HHNS.

In considering the differential level of pancreatic secretion of insulin in HHNS vs. DKA, it is important to point out that the majority of hypotheses regarding pancreatic secretion developed before 1980 were based on measurements made by means of insulin assays that 1) did not use a highly selective monoiodinated label in the immunoassay, 2) could not separate proinsulin from insulin, or 3) used a very complex or controversial measurement of free insulin. However, with the development of a more specific indication of insulin secretion through the C-peptide assay, Chupin et al.[40] were able to clearly show a significant difference between the C-peptide levels in patients with HHNS and those in patients with DKA (Table 41–3). With the same level of free fatty acids and cortisol in DKA and HHNS but higher levels of growth hormone and glucagon in DKA and much less circulating insulin in DKA, it appears that the greater ratio of glucagon/insulin in DKA leads to ketogenesis in DKA or, alternatively, that the high level of insulin/glucagon prevents ketogenesis in HHNS. Free fatty acids do not appear to play the determining role, since Chupin et al. found that the levels were the same in DKA and HHNS. It is well known that the half-maximal concentration of insulin for antilipolysis is much less than that for glucose utilization by peripheral tissues both in experimental animal tissues[103] and in humans.[104,105]

The role of the hyperosmolar state in inhibition of lipolysis has been shown by studies of adipocytes of experimental animals.[106] These findings may not be applicable to humans, in whom there are comparable concentrations of free fatty acids in DKA and HHNS, suggesting a similar rate of lipolysis in the two states (Table 41–3). On the other hand decreased glucose utilization in severe hyperglycemic states has been demonstrated in humans.[107]

The vicious cycle generated by HHNS is most commonly initiated in mentally compromised older patients who are unable to recognize thirst or the need for food or fluid and who have a background of mild NIDDM. Often they may have consumed solutions with a high sugar

Table 41–5. Precipitating Factors for Development of Diabetic Ketoacidosis (DKA) and Hyperglycemic, Hyperosmolar Nonketotic State (HHNS)

Precipitating Factor	% of Admissions DKA*	HHNS†
Infection	35	60
Pneumonia	18	35
Septicemia	9	5
Urosepsis	5	5
Abscess	3	10
Gastroenteritis	. . .	5
New-onset diabetes	30	33
Discontinued insulin	20	. . .
Unknown/miscellaneous	15	7

*Data are from Slovis et al.[100]
†Data are from Peden et al.,[101] who also determined that 42% of patients with failure of continuous subcutaneous insulin pump therapy presented with DKA.

content that exaggerated the hyperglycemic state. Hyperglycemia is augmented by accelerated hepatic glucose production, often above 1 kg/day. The glomerular filtration rate may be decreased with increasing age in this group, particularly with dehydration. Increased gluconeogenesis adds to the hyperglycemia that causes polyuria and results in a decreased intravascular space, leading to tachycardia and hypotension. Added to the loss of glucose in the urine are the large losses of electrolytes during the episode, i.e., sodium (7 mg/kg), chloride (5 meq/kg), potassium (10 meq/kg), phosphorus (70 to 140 mmol), calcium (50 to 100 meq), and magnesium (50 to 100 meq).

It is clear from the classical studies of Arief and Carroll,[108] which have since been confirmed,[29,109] that the level of coma is proportional to the level of osmolarity (Fig. 41–7). Furthermore, when a comparison was made of comatose and non-comatose patients with DKA,[110] the comatose patients were found to be older and to have greater hyperglycemia, greater dehydration (higher BUN and lower blood pressure), and higher serum osmolarity. There were no significant differences between the groups with regard to pH, ketone bodies, or serum cortisol, or glucagon (Table 41–6).

Diagnosis

HHNS is diagnosed by finding the following biochemical profile: 1) plasma glucose concentration greater than 600 mg/dL; 2) serum osmolality greater than 330 mOsm/kg; 3) absence or minimal level of serum ketones; 4) arterial pH greater than 7.3; 5) serum bicarbonate greater than 20 meq/L; 6) moderate to severe mental obtundation; and 7) negative or small amounts of urinary ketones.

The clinical presentation of HHNS is similar to that of DKA but reveals a more volume-contracted state without severe acidosis and ketosis. Typically, these are elderly patients with undiagnosed Type II diabetes with debilitating illnesses who have had a protracted history of diabetes out of control, which may have been present for as long as several weeks. Patients with HHNS, in contrast to those with DKA, have a mean rectal temperature on admission of 99.8° F,[95] and higher rectal temperatures correlate with a poorer prognosis in this group of patients. Often patients are comatose or present with neurologic abnormalities such as grand mal or focal seizures, aphasia, homonymous hemianopia, as well as other clinical manifestations suggesting a cerebrovascular accident. These often resolve with treatment.[111,112]

The laboratory profile on admission, from a series of 135 patients with HHNS reported by Wachtel et al.[98] and 130 patients reported by Matz et al.,[95] demonstrated the following mean values: sodium, 143 meq/L; potassium, 5.0 meq/L; HCO_3, 21.6 meq/L; plasma glucose, 998 mg/dL; calculated serum osmolarity, 363 mOsm/L; BUN, 65.8 mg/dL; anion gap, 23.4 meq/L; and creatinine, 2.9 mg/dL. Varying levels of HCO_3 and pH values can be seen in patients with HHNS secondary to inadequate tissue perfusion and resultant lactic acidosis. All laboratory parameters that are subject to change from volume

contraction are affected, such as the leukocyte count, hematocrit, and BUN. Last, hyperlipidemia can occur secondary to the uncontrolled diabetic state.

DKA and HHNS represent points along a spectrum of emergencies caused by poorly controlled diabetes with or without acidosis. Therefore, mixed acid-base patterns occur with various levels of hyperglycemia. The clinician should be aware of the diagnostic criteria and the vagaries of the clinical presentation so as to ensure proper treatment, follow-up, and detection of complications.

TREATMENT

Insulin

> The disease is chronic in its character, and is slowly engendered, though the patient does not survive long when it is completely established, for the marasmus produced is rapid, and death speedy. Life too is odious and painful, the thirst is ungovernable, and the copious potations are more than equaled by the profuse urinary discharge; for more urine flows away, and it is impossible to put any restraint to the patient's drinking or making water. For if he stop for a very brief period, and leave off drinking, the mouth becomes parched, the body dry; the bowels seem on fire, he is wretched and uneasy, and soon dies, tormented with burning thirst.[113]

This poignant description of the patient dying of diabetes by Aretaeus of Cappadocia in the second century remained the norm for almost two millennia until the discovery of insulin. At the beginning of the twentieth century, acidosis accounted for more than 60% of deaths in diabetic patients. This figure was lowered to 41.5% with treatment by undernutrition in the Allen era between 1914 and 1922. With insulin therapy, the figure decreased to 14.5% from 1922 to 1929 and to 4.9% from 1930 to 1936.[114] Not only did the discovery of insulin decrease the incidence of DKA, it provided a rational therapy for the condition should it occur. In the early days of insulin treatment of DKA, small insulin doses were used, undoubtedly more because of the scarcity of the substance than of an appreciation of its physiologic properties. In 1923, Foster treated 15 patients in diabetic coma. Some given as little as 10 units every 2 hours were noted to recover, and the maximal dose given during the first 12 hours was 180 units.[115] The use of relatively small amounts of insulin to treat DKA persisted at some centers,[115–117] but in many, if not most, centers the accepted dogma was that very large doses were necessary to overcome "insulin resistance." This belief stemmed from the earlier reports of Root in 1945[118] and Black and Malins in 1949[119] ascribing a lower mortality among patients who received high-dose insulin for DKA. Unfortunately, their studies were retrospective and failed to take into account many variables in addition to insulin dose. Smith and Martin in 1954[120] and Shaw et al. in 1962[121] performed careful prospective randomized investigations that demonstrated no advantage of high doses compared with moderate doses of insulin in the treatment of DKA (for a review, see Kitabchi and

Table 41–6. Admission Clinical and Biochemical Profile and Response to Therapy Among Comatose and Noncomatose Patients Randomized to Receive High-Dose or Low-Dose Insulin Therapy for Diabetic Ketoacidosis

Parameter, Insulin Dose	Mean ± SEM		P* (Coma vs. No Coma)
	Noncomatose	Comatose	
ADMISSION DATA			
Age (yr)			
Low	34.8 ± 3.5	53.4 ± 8.5	<.02
High	37.2 ± 4.4	46.6 ± 5.1	
Blood pressure (supine) (mm Hg)			
Low			
Systolic	128 ± 5	115 ± 15	
Diastolic	78 ± 3	70 ± 5	<.02 systolic
High			<.02 diastolic
Systolic	138 ± 7	111 ± 7	
Diastolic	81 ± 3	68 ± 5	
Glucose (mg/dL)			
Low	575 ± 36	985 ± 230	<.01
High	559 ± 49	981 ± 121	
HCO$_3$(meq/L)			
Low	8.1 ± 0.5	6.2 ± 0.97	<.02
High	9.1 ± 0.95	6.2 ± 0.84	
pH			
Low	7.14 ± 0.02	7.09 ± 0.05	NS
High	7.16 ± 0.03	7.12 ± 0.03	
BUN(mg/dL)			
Low	29 ± 2	57 ± 10	<.01
High	19 ± 2	52 ± 10	
Osmolality (mOsm/kg; estimated)			
Low	316 ± 4	345 ± 17	<.01
High	310 ± 4	346 ± 14	
Cortisol (μg/dL)			
Low	76 ± 8	81 ± 5	NS
High	64 ± 10	89 ± 11	
Glucagon (pg/mL)			
Low	551 ± 105	749 ± 165	NS
High	381 ± 71	456 ± 80	
Ketones (mM)			
Low	14.6 ± 0.81	13.2 ± 1.1	NS
High	12.8 ± 0.7	15.3 ± 1.8	
RESPONSE TO THERAPY			
(hr to reach indicated value)			
Glucose ≤250 mg/mL			
Low	5.2 ± 0.6	9.5 ± 2.5	<.05
High	4.1 ± 0.9	6.9 ± 1.7	NS
HCO$_3$ ≥15 meg/L			
Low	11.1 ± 1.4	11.2 ± 2.7	NS
High	10.1 ± 2.0	14.6 ± 2.7	NS
pH ≥7.3			
Low	7.8 ± 1.0	10.3 ± 2.4	NS
High	5.4 ± 1.0	9.8 ± 3.2	NS
Mentally alert			
Low	NA	7.0 ± 4.0	NA
High	NA	8.5 ± 4.5	NA

Data are from Morris and Kitabchi.[110] NS = not significant; NA = data not available.

*Coma is defined as responsiveness to deep pain stimuli only. Stupor is defined as responsiveness to light pain and/or incoherent response to verbal stimuli (included in noncomatose group).

†For all comparisons between low-dose and high-dose insulin groups, the differences are not significant. All listed comparisons are between noncomatose and comatose patients.

Fisher[29]), but most authorities continued to advocate the use of very high doses of insulin for DKA therapy through the late 1970s.[122,123]

The rediscovery of and recommendation by Sönksen and colleagues in 1972[124] that low-dose intravenous insulin be used in treating DKA was quickly followed by the publication of many studies that championed low-dose therapy.[125–133] Alberti et al., in 1973, described the successful treatment of 14 patients in DKA with only 5 to 10 units of insulin per hour administered intramuscularly following an initial dose of 16 ± 2 units.[125] In the same year, Genuth reported on a low-dose intravenous protocol,[126] with others[127,128] following suit in 1974. Soler and co-workers compared the efficacy of low-dose intramuscular and intravenous insulin in 18 patients with DKA with the efficacy of an intravenous bolus of 100 units of insulin every 2 to 3 hours in a retrospective group of 25 patients.[129] As pointed out by Alberti, however, these studies suffered from a lack of randomization, a deficiency resulting in comparisons that were not necessarily valid.[130] A prospective randomized study in 1976[30] helped settle this issue.

In this study, 48 patients in moderate to severe DKA were randomly assigned to receive either conventional therapy with high-dose insulin administered subcutaneously and intravenously or low-dose insulin therapy administered intramuscularly. The time required for the plasma glucose level to reach 250 mg/dL or lower was not significantly different in the high- and low-dose groups despite the use of insulin doses of 263 ± 45 units and 46 ± 5 units, respectively (Fig. 41–8). Other biochemical and clinical end points in the two sets of patients were comparable except for the development of hypoglycemia in 25% of patients in the high-dose group and the absence of hypoglycemia in the low-dose group. Furthermore, hypokalemia (potassium, <3.4 meq/L) was observed during treatment in seven of the patients in the high-dose group, but only in one patient in the low-dose group. The authors concluded that low-dose intramuscular insulin is as effective as high-dose insulin as therapy for DKA, without the risk of hypoglycemia and with a decreased incidence of hypokalemia. A number of investigations published subsequently were both prospective and randomized and involved both adults[131,132] and children.[133,134] The results of these studies are summarized in Tables 41–7 and 41–8.

One of the questions raised by these early studies was the optimal route of insulin therapy. Fisher et al.,[32] using a low-dose protocol, prospectively studied 45 patients in DKA, randomly assigning them to receive low-dose insulin therapy intravenously, subcutaneously, or intramuscularly, all other treatment being identical. Times for recovery from DKA (glucose ≤250 mg/dL, bicarbonate

≥15 meq/L, pH ≥7.3) were identical in the three groups. It was noted, however, that during the first 2 hours of therapy the group receiving intravenous therapy showed a more rapid decrease in the levels of plasma glucose (P ≤.01) and ketone bodies (P ≤.05). In fact the groups receiving insulin subcutaneously or intramuscularly actually had an additional rise in quantitative measures of ketone bodies during the first 2 hours of therapy (Fig. 41–9).[32] Fifteen of the 45 patients had never taken insulin previously; thus, it was possible to determine their levels of immunoreactive insulin during therapy. As seen in Fig. 41–10, despite their receiving identical loading doses of insulin—0.33 U/kg body weight followed by 7 U/hour—the group receiving intravenous therapy immediately achieved pharmacologic levels of plasma insulin. Subsequently, the plasma concentration of insulin in the group receiving insulin intravenously leveled out at approximately 100 μU/mL. Thus, an intravenous loading dose of insulin is desirable regardless of the route of subsequent administration. Another observation in that study was that 30 to 40% of the patients in the groups receiving intramuscular and subcutaneous therapy required a second or sometimes a third loading dose to decrease the plasma glucose level by 10% from the baseline value, whereas, 90% of the group receiving intravenous doses had at least a 10% decline in plasma glucose level during the first hour of therapy. A follow-up study by Sacks et al.[31] demonstrated that a priming dose given half intravenously and half intramuscularly was as effective as one given entirely intravenously in lowering the level of ketone bodies within the first hour and that the addition of albumin to the infusate, a routine procedure in previous studies to prevent insulin absorption to tubing and containers, was not necessary.

Fluid and Electrolytes

Patients in DKA are invariably dehydrated—often severely so—and restoration of fluid and electrolyte deficits is of the first priority. As noted by Atchley and colleagues[70] in their classic experiments in the 1930s and confirmed by Martin et al.[83] a generation later, most patients will have normal, or even elevated, plasma concentrations of potassium, magnesium, and phosphorus (and of sodium as well, if the dilutional effect of hyperglycemia is taken into account) at the time of presentation. These initial determinations are misleading, however, since body stores of these elements are almost always depleted.

Potassium deficit is the most serious of the electrolyte disturbances and is usually about 3 to 5 meq/kg body weight, although in some instances a deficit of as much as 10 meq/kg has been noted.[135] Despite having normal or high potassium levels initially, two-thirds of the patients will be hypokalemic by the 12th hour of therapy if replacement potassium is not provided.[83] It is important to make certain that urine output is adequate and that the serum potassium level is not elevated before potassium therapy is initiated. Major alterations of potassium flux across cell membranes may alter electrical activity and can lead to respiratory arrest or fatal cardiac

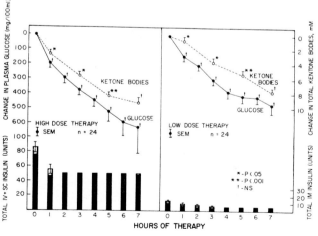

Fig. 41–8. Efficacy of low-dose vs. conventional therapy with insulin for diabetic ketoacidosis. Reprinted with permission from reference 30 (Kitabchi AE, Ayyagari V, Guerra SMO, Medical House Staff. The efficacy of low-dose versus conventional therapy of insulin for treatment of diabetic ketoacidosis. Ann Intern Med 1976; 84:633–8).

Table 41-7. Comparative Studies on the Efficacy of Low-Dose vs. High-Dose Insulin for the Treatment of Diabetic Ketoacidosis in Adults

	Alberti et al.[46,130]		Soler et al.[129]			Kitabchi et al.[30]		Heber et al.[131]		Piters et al.[132]		
	Low IM*†	High†	Low IM	Low IV Infusion	High IV and SC*†	Low IM† Intermittent	High SC and IV† Intermittent	Low IV Infusion	High IV and SC†	Very Low IV Infusion	Low IV Infusion	High IV Bolus
No. of patients	14	37	18	18	25	24	24	10	7	7	9	10
Mean age (yr)	47.5	48.2	44	40	40	38.7	40.3	27	40	‡	‡	‡
Initial insulin dose (U)	14	77	20	0	100	14	87	6	50–300	0	0	50
Subsequent insulin dose (U/time)	5/hr	Variable	10/hr	8/hr	100/2–3	5/hr	15–50/hr	6/hr	50–300/2 hr	2/hr	10/hr	50/2 hr
Serum insulin (μg/mL) Initial	7.1	6.6	...	...	...	23.8	21.2	12.0	...	9	9	9
Highest	93	540	...	...	...	89.3	5448	132	...	25	136	66
Plasma glucose Initial (mg/dL)	637	661	700	680	650	723	697	574	712	671	635	754
Fall (mg/dLh)	76	81	50	73	70	71	99	115	114	46	73	78
Blood pH	7.22	7.09	...	...	...	7.13	7.15	7.14	7.09	7.19	7.14	7.14
Serum HCO$_3$ (meq/L)	10.2	...	<10	<10	<10	7.7	8.1	9	9	7.4	6.2	5.8
Blood ketones (mM)	12.1	10.0	...	...	...	14.3	13.7	...	...	16.4	16.5	18.5
Time (hr) for glucose to reach 250–300 mg/dL	6.5	6.3	9.0	5.9	5.7	6.7	4.5	3.1	3.9	7.0	4.3	3.4
Time (hr) for HCO$_3$ to reach 15–20 meq/L	...	...	12.8	13.6	10.7	11.1	11.6	...	...	>12	8.3	8.9
% Hypoglycemia	0	...	11	...	...	0	25	...	...	...	...	...
% Hypokalemia	...	...	...	...	...	5	29	...	...	...	...	...
% Died	7	5	0	0	0	0	0	0	0	...	...	...

*By intermittent injection.
†High-dose studies retrospectively compared with low-dose studies.
‡Average age of all patients in study was 37 ± 3 years.

Table 41–8. Comparative Studies on Low-Dose vs. High-Dose Insulin Therapy for the Treatment of Diabetic Ketoacidosis (DKA) in Children

| | Edwards et al.[133] | | Burghen et al.[134] | |
	Low IV	High SC	Low IV	High IV
No. of patients	10	10	16	16
Mean age (yr)	. . . (1.8–16)*	. . . (1.8–16)*	12.6 (6.2–15.8)*	13.6 (8.8–15.1)*
Initial insulin dose (U/kg)	None	1.5 (1.0–2.2)*	None	None
Subsequent insulin dose (U/kg/time)	0.1	1.4–1.2	0.1	1
Highest plasma insulin (μg/mL)	50–200	50–300	19–24	. . .
Initial plasma glucose (mg/dL)	533	484	. . .	. . .
Initial blood pH	. . .	. . .	. . .	. . .
Initial serum HCO$_3$ (meq/L)	5.7	4.5	4	3.7
Initial blood β-hydroxybutyrate (mM)	7.2	6.2	7.5	8.5
Fall in glucose (mg/dL·hr)	31†	22†	54	102
Time (hr) for glucose to reach 250–300 mg/dL	. . .	. . .	5.4	3.4
Time (hr) for HCO$_3$ to reach 15–20 meq/L	9.6	9.8	11.7	9.6
No. with hypoglycemia (<100 mg/dL)	1/10	1/10	2/16	12/16
No. with hypokalemia (<3.4 meq/dL)	0	4/10	3/16	10/16
Criteria for admission		DKA	Plasma glucose >300 mg/dL; arterial blood pH <7.30; HCO$_3$ <15 meq/L; serum acetone positive at 1:2 dilution	

*Range.
†In this study, glucose was infused while patients were in hyperglycemic state.
‡And/or patient's serum and urine were clear of acetone.

arrhythmias; therefore, careful monitoring is essential. A rare patient will present with hypokalemia, with the implication of severe depletion in total body potassium and an even more urgent need for potassium replenishment.[136] The causes of the often rapid fall in potassium during therapy are complex, reflecting not only a direct action of insulin on cellular potassium uptake but also alterations in systemic pH (which may be enhanced by bicarbonate therapy), enhancement in renal potassium excretion, and a reduction in the serum glucose concentration and hyperosmolality.[10] The serum potassium should be monitored every 2 hours, or hourly if it falls below 3.0 meq/hour. Serial electrocardiograms may be helpful in providing an early warning of hypokalemia. Generally, potassium replenishment at a rate of 20 to 40 meq/hour is appropriate. Since potassium losses will continue for several hours because of osmotic diuresis, most patients will still have a total body potassium deficit at the completion of therapy for DKA and may require oral potassium supplementation for several days.

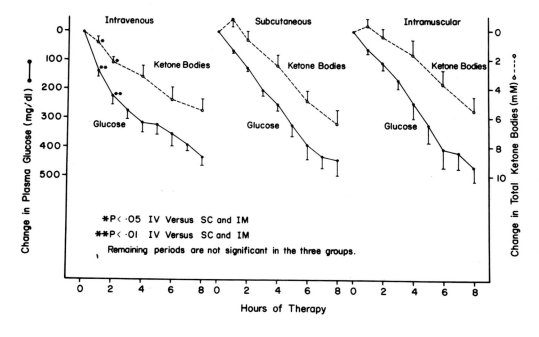

Fig. 41–9. Comparison of the effects of low-dose intravenous, subcutaneous, and intramuscular insulin regimens on changes in plasma glucose and total ketone bodies in patients with diabetic ketoacidosis (15 in each group). Reprinted with permission from reference 32 (Fisher JN, Shahshahani MN, Kitabchi AE. Diabetic ketoacidosis: low-dose insulin therapy by various routes. N Engl J Med 1977;297:238–41).

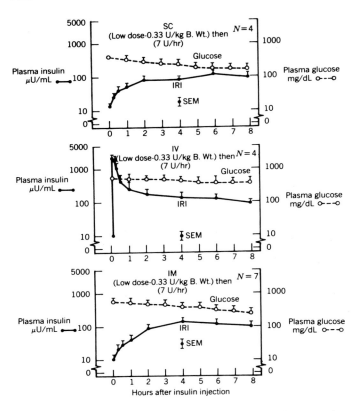

Fig. 41–10. Comparison of the effect of low-dose insulin regimen (7 U/hr) administered by subcutaneous, intravenous, and intramuscular injections on plasma levels of immunoreactive insulin and glucose levels in three groups of patients with diabetic ketoacidosis not previously treated with insulin. Reprinted with permission from John Wiley & Sons, Ltd. from reference 12 (Kitabchi AE. Low-dose insulin therapy in diabetic ketoacidosis; fact or fiction? Diabetes Metab Rev 1989;5:337–63).

Phosphate

More than 50 years ago Guest and Rapoport reported on the occurrence of hypophosphatemia and the depletion of diphosphoglycerate (2,3-DPG) during therapy for DKA.[137] Since that time many treatment regimens have included phosphate therapy.[71,138–140] In the 1960s, Benesch and Benesch[141] and Chanutin and Curnish[142] independently reported studies on the modulation of hemoglobin oxygen affinity by 2,3-DPG. When 2,3-DPG is depleted in erythrocytes, the oxyhemoglobin dissociation curve is shifted to the left, an effect counterbalanced by acidosis. Theoretically, tissue hypoxia may occur following recovery from ketoacidosis as the curve shifts back to the left in response to hypophosphatemia and delayed restoration of 2,3-DPG. In an uncontrolled study in the 1940s, Franks and co-workers administered buffered sodium phosphate to patients in severe DKA and reported a number of improvements, including a more rapid clearing of the mental state and a statistically significant decrease in the mortality rate.[138] More recently, Ditzel[140] described the restoration of 2,3-DPG by

phosphate therapy in DKA and alleged that the striking improvement in the mental status of two patients was due to such treatment. However, neither older uncontrolled[22,83] or more recent randomized studies[33,143] have demonstrated any clear benefit of phosphate therapy. Wilson and co-workers provided either a single dose of 15 mmol of sodium phosphate at 3 hours or doses of 15 mmol of phosphate at 2, 6, and 10 hours or no phosphate replacement in a randomized study of patients in DKA. None of the patients in any of the groups became clinically hypophosphatemic, and the groups showed no differences in rates of clinical or biochemical recovery. Magnesium levels remained stable. but serum calcium levels declined in all three groups.[143]

In a prospective randomized study, we compared the effect of potassium phosphate (8.5 mmol/hour or approximately 6 g of phosphate/24 hours) with no phosphate in 30 patients with DKA, 15 in each group. Although the experimental group had a higher level of 2,3-DPG than did the control group by 48 hours, neither this difference nor the difference in po$_2$50 (partial pressure of O_2 at which 50% of hemoglobin saturated) was significant. The experimental group, however, did exhibit a significantly lower level of plasma ionized calcium at 24 hours.[39] On the basis of these observations, it appears that routine use of phosphate salts in the treatment of DKA is unnecessary. It seems reasonable to make exceptions, however, for patients who are hypoxic for any reason, e.g., anemia, chronic pulmonary disease, or congestive heart failure, in which situation, hypophosphatemia, and low erythrocyte 2,3-DPG might cause them to be further compromised.[144]

Bicarbonate

Bicarbonate therapy in DKA has remained controversial, but most modern investigators recommend against its routine use.[34,145–148] In a scholarly review of the subject analyzing the risks and benefits of bicarbonate therapy, Matz[145] concluded that perhaps the only clear indication for use of bicarbonate in DKA is life-threatening hyperkalemia. As noted, however, most patients with DKA already have a total body deficit of potassium even though the initial serum potassium concentration may be high. The administration of bicarbonate will accelerate the decline in serum potassium level, sometimes with disastrous consequences.[145] In a retrospective analysis of 95 episodes of severe DKA, Lever and Jaspan detected no differences in biochemical or clinical end points between 73 episodes of DKA treated with sodium bicarbonate and 22 episodes not treated with sodium bicarbonate.[146] Hale et al., using a randomized protocol, gave a standard dose of bicarbonate (150 meq) regardless of initial pH. Although they found a faster rise in arterial pH in the treatment group at 120 minutes, the overall responses of patients who did and did not receive bicarbonate treatment were similar.[147] Morris et al., in a prospective randomized study, administered bicarbonate to 10 patients and withheld it from 11 with similar degrees of DKA (pH 6.9 to 7.14). No significant difference was observed between the treatment and the control groups with regard to changes in glucose, ketone bodies, bicarbonate, or blood pH (Fig. 41–11). In some patients cerebrospinal fluid was measured initially and at two other time points (6 to 8 and 12 to 24 hours). A comparison of initial plasma and cerebrospinal fluid values is seen in Table 41–9. It was of note that initial pH and bicarbonate levels were significantly higher in cerebrospinal fluid. Regression analysis of the levels of glucose, bicarbonate, pH, lactate, and ketones showed no significant differences in the slopes of these variables between the two groups.[34]

Table 41–10[33,34] summarizes the results of two prospective randomized studies from the University of Tennessee Clinical Research Center, one on the effect of phosphate therapy and the other on that of bicarbonate in DKA. It is of interest that the time to reach predetermined pH and bicarbonate values was longer in the bicarbonate studies than in the phosphate studies. This is due primarily to the recruitment in the bicarbonate studies of patients who were more acidotic, with pH values ranging from 6.9 to 7.1, whereas the phosphate protocol included any patient with DKA whose pH value was below 7.3.

COMPLICATIONS OF THERAPY

Cerebral Edema

The occurrence of cerebral edema during DKA, while rare, is an event to be feared as it is usually fatal or associated with serious neurologic sequelae.[10] It is most often seen in children and adolescents (in one survey of 69 cases, all but 3 patients were younger than 20 years, with 33% younger than 5 years), with one-half or more being patients presenting with previously undiagnosed diabetes.[149] The etiology of the condition remains spec-

ulative despite its having been observed repeatedly since Dillon et al.[150] called attention to it in 1936. The rarity of the condition has prevented any attempt at a prospective, randomized protocol of study of the many proposed causes in human subjects. The suggested causes have included the too-rapid administration of fluid and correction of osmotic imbalance between the brain and its extracellular fluid,[151] excessive use of bicarbonate,[152] development of hyponatremia,[153] or allowing the blood glucose level to fall rapidly below 200 mg/dL.[154] Retrospective analysis has failed to incriminate any of these putative causes.[149] In studies of healthy anesthetized dogs, Clements et al. observed cerebral edema when induction of hyperglycemia was followed by rehydration with isotonic saline.[155] Although this phenomenon was initially ascribed to glucose and sorbitol accumulation, it has since been demonstrated that polyols can account for only a portion of the osmotic gradient. These "idiogenic osmoles" remain a mystery.[111] Recently, Van Der Meulen et al. proposed the hypothesis that cerebral edema in DKA resulted from the activation of the Na^+/H^+ exchanger,[156] whereby osmotic swelling of brain cells occurred as a result of the accumulation of Na^+ and the anions of weak organic acids. No experimental proof of this theory has yet been published.

Brain edema without overt clinical signs during DKA appears to be a common phenomena. Increased cerebrospinal fluid pressure during treatment of DKA was noted more than 20 years ago,[157] and Fein et al., using serial echoencephalograms, demonstrated a significant decrease in lateral ventricle width in 9 of 11 patients during DKA therapy.[158] Krane et al. studied six children ages 11 to 14 years by obtaining a cranial computed tomographic (CT) scan toward the end of recovery from DKA (blood glucose <250 mg/dL or pH >7.3) and again several days later just before the patient's discharge from the hospital.

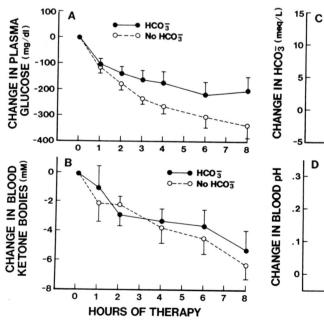

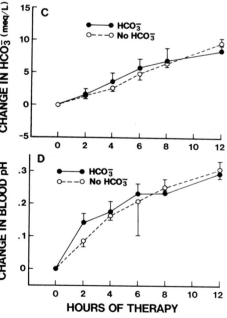

Fig. 41–11. Changes in blood chemistry values during treatment with (*n* = 10) or without (*n* = 11) bicarbonate of patients for diabetic ketoacidosis. No significant difference between the treatment and control groups was seen for any variable measured (to convert concentration of glucose from mg/dL divide by 18). Reprinted with permission from reference 34 (Morris LR, Murphy MB, Kitabchi AE. Bicarbonate therapy in severe diabetic ketoacidosis. Ann Intern Med 1986;105:836–40).

Table 41–9. Comparison of Initial Plasma and Cerebrospinal Fluid Values for Patients with Diabetic Ketoacidosis

Parameters Measured	No. of Patients	Plasma	CSF	P Value
Glucose (mg/dL)	14	5.3 ± 42	368 ± 27	<.001
HCO₃ (meq/L)	12	3.7 ± 0.6	7.7 ± 0.55	<.001
pH	11	7.01 ± 0.03	7.26 ± 0.02	<.001
Total ketones (mM)	11	10.9 ± 1.2	7.6 ± 0.66	<.05
Osmolality (mOsm/kg)	12	324 ± 7.7	320 ± 9.8	NS

Data are from Morris et al.[34]

The earlier scans showed narrowing of the ventricular system of the brain, which in each case was thought to be due to asymptomatic brain swelling.[159] In a subsequent provocative study, Hoffman et al. performed three cranial CT scans on each of nine children in DKA—on admission prior to treatment, 6 to 8 hours after initiation of treatment, and 7 days later.[160] Their finding, in contrast to that of Fein et al., was a reduction in the size of the lateral and third ventricles in the pretreatment, as well as in the 6- to 8-hour scans, in comparison to the 7-day scans. Hoffman et al. concluded that cerebral swelling is usually present in DKA before treatment is begun.

Therapy for cerebral edema remains empiric.[149,161] Rosenbloom pointed out that in approximately one-half of the reported cases "there was a premonitory period when development of cerebral edema could be suspected on the basis of severe headache, incontinence, dramatic change in arousal or behavior, pupillary changes, blood pressure changes, seizures, bradycardia, or disturbed temperature regulation."[149]

When neurologic changes make cerebral edema a strong suspect, immediate treatment with mannitol, 1 to 2 g/kg body weight, is recommended. Intubation with hyperventilation to reduce intracranial pressure is also advised for the comatose patient.

Hyperchloremic Acidosis

It is common for patients recovering from DKA to develop a non-anion-gap hyperchloremic metabolic acidosis.[84,162] Several reasons have been postulated for this phenomenon: 1) ketonuria results in the loss of much of the ketones that would have been used as substrate for bicarbonate regeneration, and this is further accentuated by the enhancement of ketonuria by vigorous fluid therapy; 2) the amount of bicarbonate in the proximal tubule is limited, resulting in greater chloride reabsorption; 3) not only is plasma bicarbonate reduced but so is total buffering capacity in other body compartments. Speculation that hyperchloremic acidosis results from hyporeninemic hypoaldosteronism in diabetic subjects was not substantiated in a small series of patients with DKA.[162] It is important to distinguish this cause of persistently low serum bicarbonate levels in the course of DKA therapy from incompletely treated ketoacidosis since the latter calls for continued vigorous insulin administration. When the plasma glucose has been controlled, the pH is 7.30 or higher, and the patient is clinically recovered, oral intake can be resumed and the rate of insulin administration reduced. It may take several days for the hyperchloremic metabolic acidosis to resolve as bicarbonate production and acid secretion are readjusted by the kidneys.

Other Complications

Pulmonary edema, not associated with left ventricular failure, has been reported on rare occasions in DKA.[163–165] Adult respiratory distress syndrome in this setting may occur in the young, as in the 23-year-old woman who experienced two such episodes reported by Brun-Buisson et al.[165] Hyperventilation, acidosis, and vigorous fluid therapy may contribute to the condition, but only the unusual patient is predisposed, perhaps because of diabetic pulmonary vascular microangiopathy with alteration in alveolocapillary permeability.

Table 41–10. Response to Therapy with Phosphate or Bicarbonate in Diabetic Ketoacidosis

Response to Therapy	Phosphate Treatment			Bicarbonate Treatment		
	No	Yes	P	No	Yes	P
Time (hr) to recovery (mean ± SEM)						
Glucose ≤250 (mg/dL)	3.6 ± 0.8	5.4 ± 1.4	NS	4.2 ± 1.0	4.9 ± 1.3	NS
HCO₃ ≥15 meq/L	10.5 ± 0.8	12.7 ± 1.8	NS	21.0 ± 4.0	21.0 ± 4.3	NS
pH ≥7.3	11.3 ± 1.4	8.3 ± 1.2	NS	15.6 ± 2.5	13.1 ± 2.5	NS
Rate of decline						
Glucose (mg/dL·hr)	93.4	90.8	NS			
Ketone bodies (mM/hr)	0.64	0.8	NS			

Data are from Fisher et al.[33] and Morris et al.[34]

Aspiration of gastric contents resulting in pneumonia or in respiratory or cardiac arrest is an avoidable complication. All patients who are obtunded or have gastric distention should have a nasogastric tube in place attached to suction. Hypokalemia, which may contribute to gastric atony, is also avoidable with careful monitoring and early potassium replenishment. Late hypoglycemia often occurred in the era of high-dose insulin but is seen less frequently now that more-physiologic doses of insulin are prescribed for DKA.

RECOMMENDATIONS FOR TREATMENT OF DKA AND HHNS

The therapeutic recommendations for DKA and HHNS that we have proposed previously[59,166] are summarized in Figures 41–12, 41–13, and 41–14. In both condi-

tions, a rapid but careful history and physical examination is essential, with particular attention to 1) patency of the airway, 2) mental status, 3) cardiovascular and renal status, 4) source of infection, and 5) state of hydration. The initial biochemical evaluation in the emergency room should include assessment of urinary ketones and glucose, blood glucose, and plasma acetone (qualitative utilizing test strips) and immediate measurement of plasma glucose, serum electrolytes, BUN, amylase, complete blood count, urinalysis, and arterial blood gases and pH. If indicated, a chest film, electrocardiogram, and appropriate cultures should be obtained. In both conditions, severe dehydration is the rule. Hydration with up to 1 L of normal saline over the first hour during the wait for laboratory results is almost always appropriate, with subsequent fluid therapy depending on the state of hydration. When the blood glucose level reaches 200 to

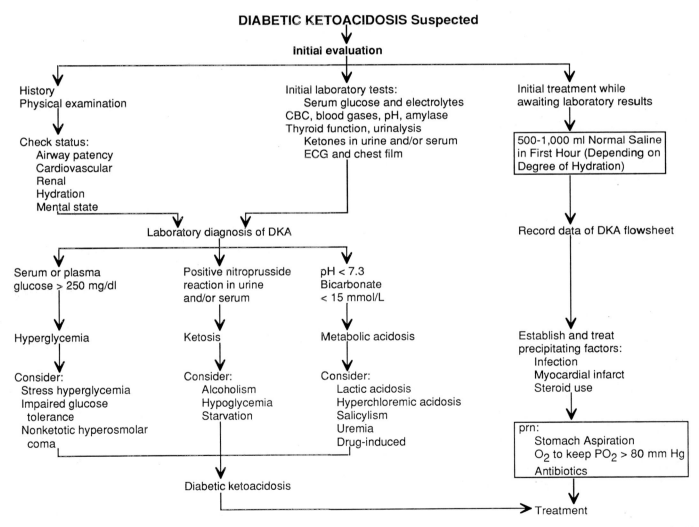

Fig. 41–12. Flow diagram depicting the work-up of a patient with suspected diabetic ketoacidosis (DKA). CBC = complete blood count; ECG = electrocardiogram. Reprinted with permission from reference 59 (Kitabchi AE, Rumbak MJ. Diabetic ketoacidosis: diagnosis; diabetic ketoacidosis: treatment; hyperglycemic hyperosmolar nonketotic coma; and maintenance treatment after hyperglycemic crisis. In: Callahan C, Barton W, Schumaker HM. Decision making in emergency medicine. Philadelphia. BC Decker, 1990:178–85).

THE DEFINITIVE TREATMENT OF DIABETIC KETOACIDOSIS (DKA)

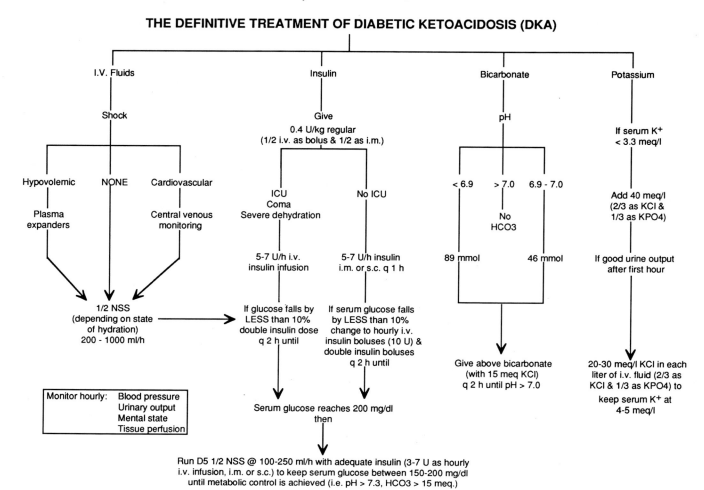

Fig. 41–13. Flow chart depicting the definitive treatment of diabetic ketoacidosis. NSS = normal saline solution; ICU = intensive care unit; D5 = 5% dextrose. Figure is modified from Kitabchi et al.[59]

250 mg/dl the hydrating fluid is changed to 5% dextrose with ½ normal saline solution.

Once the diagnosis of DKA has been confirmed, a loading dose of regular insulin of 0.3 to 0.4 U/kg body weight (half administered intravenously, half intramuscularly) is given. If the patient is in an intensive care unit (ICU), 5 to 7 units of insulin is administered per hour as a continuous insulin infusion until the plasma glucose level reaches 200 mg/dL. If the patient is not in an ICU, it may be more prudent to give subcutaneous or intramuscular insulin since there is a greater chance that therapy will be interrupted or not given on a timely basis, and such administration will at least provide some residual insulin. If the plasma glucose level does not decrease by at least 10% from the initial value, the loading dose is repeated hourly until it does so. As noted already, bicarbonate therapy is probably of no benefit and theoretically may be harmful if given to excess. Thus, we would give no bicarbonate if the pH is greater than 7.0 but would provide small amounts if less than 7.0 to bring the pH up to that level.

Administration of potassium should be begun as soon as the patient's potassium level is less than 5.5 meq/L and urinary output is adequate. If the initial serum potassium value is less than 3.3 meq/L, indicating severe potassium deficiency, 40 meq/L should be added to the hydrating fluid. Thereafter, 20 to 30 meq/L of intravenous fluid is generally sufficient, although many patients will require oral potassium supplementation for several days after treatment for DKA. Initially, the serum potassium should be checked every 2 hours and when the levels have stabilized, every 6 hours. Although, phosphate therapy appears to be of no benefit in hastening recovery from DKA, the use of potassium phosphate salts in a mixture with potassium chloride will decrease the chloride load and thus the tendency to perpetuate acidosis by hyperchloremia.

Dehydration in HHNS is usually more pronounced than in DKA, and it is recommended that fluid replacement approximating 12% of total body weight be provided during the first 12 to 24 hours. Generally, patients with HHNS are more sensitive than those with DKA, and

THE DIAGNOSIS AND TREATMENT OF HYPERGLYCEMIC HYPEROSMOLAR NONKETOTIC STATE (HHNS)

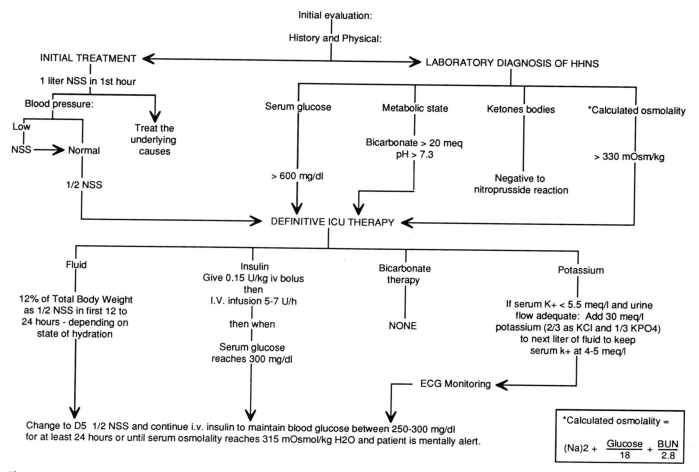

Fig. 41–14. Diagnosis and treatment of hyperglycemic, hyperosmolar nonketotic state (HHNS). ICU = intensive care unit; ECG = electrocardiogram; NSS = normal saline solution; D5 = 5% dextrose; BUN = blood urea nitrogen.

hydration alone will often result in a considerable decline in plasma glucose level. A gradual reduction in hyperglycemia and osmolality should be the goal of therapy. We recommend initiation of a glucose infusion in HHNS when blood glucose reaches 300 mg/dL during therapy, as compared with 200 mg/dL in DKA.

In all patients, other ancillary measures need to be kept in mind, e.g., aspiration of the stomach and continuous nasogastric suction, as well as catheterization of the urinary bladder to continuous closed drainage in unconscious patients; oxygen therapy for a po_2 less than 80 mm Hg; use of a plasma expander for treatment of consistent hypotension; and antibiotic therapy as needed. A flow sheet (Fig. 41–15) is essential to organize and keep a record of therapy. Furthermore, because HHNS carries a poorer prognosis than DKA, we recommend that these patients, as well as obtunded patients, be admitted to an ICU. One should continue to search for precipitating factors such as infection and silent myocardial infarction. The key to successful therapy is the constant monitoring of the patient's condition by knowledgeable and con-

cerned physicians and nurses. Last, once the patient has reached a therapeutic end point, it is important that appropriate orders be written when he or she is transferred out of the ICU to prevent recurrence of hyperglycemia. Suggested maintenance treatment is provided in Fig. 41–16.

ALCOHOLIC KETOACIDOSIS

Clinical Findings

Patients with alcoholic ketoacidosis (AKA) are usually chronic alcohol abusers or binge drinkers. At presentation, they have a history of 2 to 3 days of diminished oral intake because of abdominal pain, nausea, and vomiting. On examination, dry mucous membranes, tachycardia, and postural hypotension reflect dehydration.[167] Presenting symptoms are initially attributed to gastritis, pancreatitis, or hepatitis. The patients are prone to the development of aspiration pneumonia, bacterial infections, subdural and subarachnoid hemorrhages, and rhabdomy-

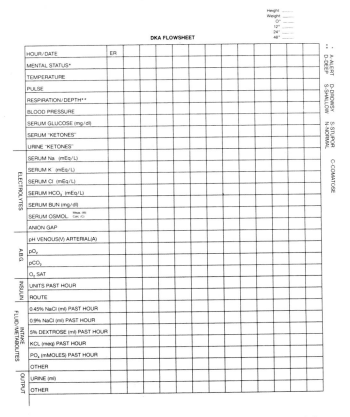

Fig. 41–15. Flow sheet to document serial changes in laboratory/clinical values and supplementary measures during recovery from diabetic ketoacidosis (DKA). Reprinted with permission from reference 9 (Kitabchi AE, Murphy MB. Diabetic ketoacidosis and hyperosmolar hyperglycemic nonketotic coma. Med Clin North Am 1988;72:1545–63).

olysis. Alcohol withdrawal syndrome also may develop.[167,168] Alcohol is not usually detected in the blood at the time of diagnosis because severe abdominal pain, nausea, and vomiting have prevented its ingestion by the patient.[168] The diagnosis is made with a high index of suspicion.

Pathophysiology

The metabolism of ethyl alcohol changes the redox state in the liver, inhibiting gluconeogenesis. The following changes in glycogen metabolism occur. Ethyl alcohol is metabolized to acetaldehyde and then to acetate. As this occurs, oxidized nicotinamide adenine dinucleotide (NAD^+) is reduced to NADH. Reoxidation of NADH to NAD^+ is the result of the conversion of pyruvate to lactate and of oxaloacetate to malate.[169] Pyruvate and oxaloacetate are substrates for gluconeogenesis, and low levels, which occur in AKA, result in decreased gluconeogenesis.[167–169] The entry of acetyl CoA into the Krebs cycle is slowed because of the low level of oxaloacetic acid. Acetyl CoA carboxylase activity is also reduced. The resulting low level of malonyl CoA permits transport of free fatty acids into the mitochondria. Volume depletion and concurrent illnesses all increase levels of the coun-

terregulatory hormones. The high levels of catecholamines decrease insulin secretion. This, together with the increase in transport of fatty acids into the mitochondria, sets the stage for increased ketogenesis. Therefore, acetyl CoA is shunted into the ketogenic pathway, resulting in the production of acetone, acetoacetate, and β-hydroxybutyric acid. Usually acetate, the end product of alcohol metabolism, inhibits this pathway.[170] Therefore, AKA usually occurs with cessation of alcohol intake. Acetoacetic acid produces a persistent toxic effect on the mitochondria, preventing regeneration of NAD^+ from NADH and thereby initiating a vicious cycle.[169,171]

Laboratory Findings

Blood levels of magnesium, potassium, and phosphate are low in AKA because of poor intake and excess losses.[172] Hypocalcemia, when present, may be due to low levels of parathyroid hormone, because the level of magnesium, which is necessary for the release and action or parathyroid hormone, is low. The glucose level is usually low to normal.[173] If, in fact, the glucose level is above 300 mg/dL, the proper diagnosis should be DKA.[170] Lactic acid levels are increased in AKA because of the altered redox state in the liver. Occasionally, if the patient is able to continue to abuse alcohol, the lactic acid level will be greater than the ketone level.[170,172] Even so, if a high serum level of lactate acid is found, concurrent serious illness must be ruled out.[170] Both lactic acid and ketoacids contribute to the increased anion gap. Vomiting and hypokalemia may predispose to an underlying alkalosis, masking the concomitant acidosis. Therefore, pH levels may be low, normal, or high. Because of the altered redox state, the acetoacetic acid is metabolized to

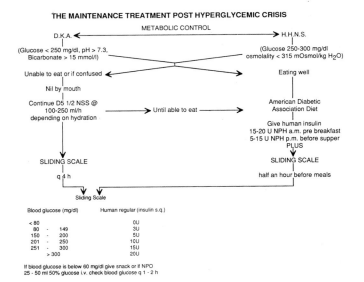

Fig. 41–16. Flow sheet depicting maintenance treatment following hyperglycemic crisis. DKA = diabetic ketoacidosis; HHNS = hyperosmolar hyperglycemic nonketotic state; NSS = normal saline solution; D5 = 5% dextrose. Modified from Kitabchi and Rumbak.[59]

β-hydroxybutyric acid and the nitroprusside reaction (which does not measure this ketone body) may be either low or negative, leading to a false impression. During treatment of this condition, the nitroprusside reaction may become strongly positive as the β-hydroxybutyric acid is metabolized to acetoacetic acid.[172] Table 41–4 outlines the laboratory findings in different acidotic states and coma.

Treatment

Patients with AKA are usually dehydrated. Fluid replacement is necessary to correct the dehydration. The associated electrolyte deficit, except that of phosphate, must be replaced. Phosphate needs to be replaced only if the deficit is significant (<1 mg/dL).[171,173] Glucose is given at a rate of 7 g/hour, which stimulates secretion of endogenous insulin and thus promotes the proper utilization of the glucose and metabolism of the ketone bodies, as well as inhibiting ketogenesis. The serum glucose level may rise above 300 mg/dL following the glucose infusion. Low-dose insulin is then infused, as with DKA.[171,173] The AKA usually responds within 6 to 18 hours. If it does not respond in this time, another cause for the illness should be sought. In a series of 24 patients, the only deaths that occurred were from gastroesophageal hemorrhage and pulmonary edema. Serious underlying illnesses were looked for and aggressively treated.[173]

LACTIC ACIDOSIS

Metabolic acidosis can be divided into a normal or increased anion gap (AG) acidosis. The AG is defined as the difference between the serum concentration of sodium minus that of chloride and bicarbonate: $AG = Na - (Cl + HCO_3)$, with normal values being 8 to 16 mM. Lactic acidosis is a common cause of a high anion-gap acidosis and can itself be divided into two groups.[174] The first, hyperlactemia, is characterized by a persistent elevation in the serum lactate level without a corresponding decrease in the arterial pH. This unbalance is due to a greater production than consumption of lactic acid and is not of much clinical importance. If the tricarboxylic acid (TCA) cycle is functioning, the H^+ produced with lactic acid is quickly metabolized and an elevated lactic acid level can occur without an acidosis.[175] The second type is characterized by a persistently elevated level of lactic acid with an accompanying low arterial pH. This type of lactic acidosis is commonly classified according to whether clinical evidence of tissue hypoxia and diminished perfusion does (type A) or does not (type B) exist (Table 41–11).[174]

Diagnosis

A working criteria for the diagnosis of lactic acidosis is a blood level of lactate of 7 mM or greater with an arterial pH lower than 7.35.[176] There is a gray area between 2 to 6 mM. In patients with an underlying metabolic alkalosis, lactic acidosis may be masked by a pH in the normal range. In addition, a normal pH and anion gap may be found in patients with lactic acidosis who have low serum

Table 41–11. Classification of Lactic Acidosis

Type A: Evidence of clinical tissue hypoperfusion
  1. Anemia
  2. Hemorrhage
  3. Congestive heart failure
  4. Grand mal seizures
  5. Carbon monoxide poisoning
  6. Pheochromocytoma
Type B: No evidence of clinical tissue hypoperfusion
Type B_1: Associated with underlying disease
  1. Diabetes mellitus
  2. Liver disease
  3. Malignancy
  4. Sepsis
  5. Pheochromocytoma
  6. Thiamine deficiency
  7. Uremia
Type B_2: Associated with drugs, toxins, and metabolites
  1. Alcohols (methyl, ethyl, and propyl)
  2. Biguanides
  3. Cyanide
  4. Isoniazid
  5. Salicylate
  6. Acetaminophen
Type B_3: Associated with hereditary disease
  Type 1 glycogen storage disease
Type B_4: Miscellaneous
  Hypoglycemia

albumin levels or high serum globulin levels. Under these conditions, more negative anions are lost than cations. Similarly, a preceding metabolic alkalosis may mask lactic acidosis. Patients with low glycogen stores cannot generate lactic acid and therefore cannot develop lactic acidosis.[174] Table 41–4 helps differentiate lactic acidosis from other significant causes of a metabolic acidosis.

Lactic Acid Metabolism

Under normal resting conditions the heart, brain, skeletal muscle, red blood cells, and skin have the highest rate of glycolysis and produce most of the body's lactic acid.[174] The end product of glycolysis is pyruvic acid. Transamination of alanine also results in the formation of pyruvic acid.[174,177] During anaerobic conditions, lactate is produced from pyruvic acid under the control of the enzyme lactate dehydrogenase: lactate + NAD + H^+ ⇌ pyruvate + NADH. The normal ratio of lactate to pyruvate is 10:1. Significant lactic acidosis can occur only if there is a high rate of glycolysis, a decrease in the extraction of lactic acid (abnormal TCA cycle), or both.[178] Under normal resting aerobic conditions, the liver is able to metabolize up to 15 to 20 mM of lactic acid, keeping the serum levels at less than 1 mM.[179] During exercise lactic acid may increase sixtyfold because of its production by skeletal muscle.[179]

Lactic acid is transported to either the muscle (the lactate shuttle)[177] or to the liver and the kidney (the Cori cycle)[180] to be metabolized via the TCA cycle to carbon dioxide and water. The enzymes pyruvate carboxylase and phosphoenolpyruvate carboxykinase are found exclusively in the liver and the kidney. These enzymes catalyze the conversion of lactic acid to glucose (gluconeogenesis). The liver metabolizes almost two-thirds of the lactate, and the kidney metabolizes one-third.[174]

Factors influencing formation of lactic acid are the concentration of pyruvate, the ratio of NADH/NAD$^+$, and the intracellular pH (pH$_i$).[178] For example, as the liver pH$_i$ falls, so does its ability to remove lactate from the serum.[181] When the pH$_i$ falls below 7.0, the liver becomes a net producer of lactate. A decreased pH$_i$ is also associated with a significantly decreased utilization of lactate in the liver parenchyma.[182] In the myocardium, intracellular acidosis has a strong negative inotropic effect, but for lactic acidosis itself to be negatively inotropic, it must be associated with hypercapnea and hypoxia.[178]

Extracellular pH also may exert a feedback control over net lactic acid metabolism.[183] A mild respiratory or metabolic acidosis virtually abolishes lactic acid accumulation, even when the pH drops by as little as 0.03.[183] In humans, plasma lactic acid levels are transiently and reversibly increased during alkalemia (bicarbonate administration) and decreased during acidemia.[183] Therefore, a lowering of plasma pH is an attempt to protect the organism by impeding lactic acid formation.[183] Under conditions of exercise to the point of exhaustion, the serum pH, by the feedback mechanism, is able to modify net lactic acid production.[183] The effect of pH on lactic acid utilization is not as clear.[183]

Type A Lactic Acidosis

Type A acidosis is by far the more common form of lactic acidosis. For this type to occur, the heart must be unable to deliver an adequate amount of oxygen to the tissues.[182] During hypoxia, a number of adaptive mechanisms occur. When the arterial po$_2$ reaches 40 to 65 mm Hg, oxygen delivery is reduced by 20 to 30% and the major adaption is at the tissue extraction level. The oxygen extraction reserve (OER) is the ability to extract enough oxygen for tissue demands during an insufficiency of oxygen delivery.[178] In this situation, because of the local acidosis and the shape of the hemoglobin-oxygen dissociation curve, an adequate amount of oxygen is given off to the tissues—the so-called shift.[178] Under aerobic conditions, the body as a whole has an OER 300% of oxygen extraction during resting conditions. Because the heart has a much higher resting oxygen requirement per gram of tissue than the body as a whole, the resting oxygen extraction is greater than the OER. The heart muscle, therefore, can only extract 50% of the resting oxygen requirement and the coronary oxygen reserve is easily depleted.[178]

As the arterial po$_2$ drops below 40 mm Hg, circulatory adaptations increasing oxygen delivery must occur if the supply of oxygen to the myocardium is to be adequate.[184] First, the hypoxia acts directly on the local vessels of the brain and the heart, causing a vasodilatory effect.[185] Second, the sympathetic nervous system is stimulated, resulting in increased serum catecholamine levels.[186] This increases the stroke volume and cardiac output and redistributes the blood flow to maintain the cerebral and coronary circulation. These adaptations increase delivery of oxygen to the tissues of the vital organs. In general, these changes are efficient enough to compensate for an arterial po$_2$ as low as 25 to 30 mm Hg, and even at this level, the total body oxygen consumption does not change.[187]

When the arterial blood becomes even more hypoxic, the vasoconstriction increases the systemic vascular resistance and the myocardial oxygen demand. The OER of the myocardium is depleted, and depression of the myocardium occurs.[178] In addition, during sepsis a myocardial depressive factor[188] further depresses the cardiac output. Both of these factors inhibit the cardiac response to stress, decreasing the body's ability to deliver enough oxygen to the tissues and resulting in additional lactic acidosis, resulting in a continuation of the cycle. Significant left ventricular dysfunction follows, with the development of pulmonary edema, which further compromises the pulmonary oxygen exchange.[178]

With the shunt of blood toward the heart and brain and the subsequent low oxygen delivery to the other tissues, the production of lactic acid increases—primarily in the skeletal muscles and the intestinal mucosa.[187] When oxygen delivery to the liver (and, to a lesser extent, to the kidneys) is not adequate, the resultant ischemia and hypoxia cause a drop in the pH$_i$ and these organs become net producers of lactic acid.[187]

Type B Lactic Acidosis

Type B lactic acidosis occurs in the absence of any obvious evidence of tissue hypoperfusion. This type has been subdivided into four categories: type B$_1$, which occurs in association with an underlying disease, e.g., diabetes mellitus, liver disease, malignancy, sepsis, pheochromatosis, and thiamine deficiency; type B$_2$, which is due to certain drugs or toxins, e.g., biguanides, the alcohols, salicylates, acetaminophen, epinephrine, cyanide, nitroprusside, isoniazid, and propylene glycol; type B$_3$, which occurs as a result of genetic deficiencies affecting key enzymes; and type B$_4$, which is the miscellaneous category, e.g., hypoglycemia.

Examples of Types of Lactic Acidosis in Different Disease States

Diabetes Mellitus. The incidence of any type of lactic acidosis in persons with DKA is less than 10%[188] and it is usually due to tissue hypoxia because of sepsis, congestive heart failure, or dehydration.[188] Persons with diabetes have many risk factors for type A lactic acidosis, as they have a high incidence of both macro- and microvascular disease, low levels of 2,3-diphosphoglycerate, and an increased blood viscosity.[179] Type B lactic acidosis is usually cited as a major cause of lactic acidosis in diabetic patients,[188] but since the discontinuation of biguanides in the United States, the incidence of type B lactic acidosis has been rare indeed, even in patients with DKA.[189] Theoretically, diabetic individuals may be predisposed to type B lactic acidosis, as insulin deficiency is associated with low levels of muscle pyruvate dehydrogenase (PDH), which may disinhibit alanine production and thus permit formation of lactate.[174] Diabetic patients may also be predisposed to overproduction of lactic acid during exercise.[174,189] In diabetic rats, lactate oxidation is significantly reduced, and in normal rabbits infusion of ketoacid and bicarbonate produces lactic acidosis.[174,190] In spite of the theoretical reasons for this occurrence, the clinical incidence of lactic acidosis is low.[190] Therefore, if lactic acidosis is found in diabetic patients, it should be investigated and treated as type A lactic acidosis until it has been proven otherwise.

Liver Disease. Lactic acidosis in chronic liver disease is usually the result of increased lactic acid production due to sepsis, hypoperfusion, seizures, alkalosis, or ethanol ingestion.[174] In the majority of cases of severe acute liver failure, patients will present with type B lactic acidosis, caused in part by porto-systemic shunting.[174] However, whenever hyperlactemia is accompanied by a metabolic acidosis, tissue underperfusion must be suspected.

Malignancy. Type A lactic acidosis is the most common cause of lactic acidosis of malignancy and is due to an overproduction of lactic acid from ischemia in the neoplastic bed.[191] Type B lactic acidosis is thought to be due to a "factor" produced by the tumor that inhibits phosphate dehydrogenase and increases lactate production.[174] Precipitation of lactic acidosis may occur iatrogenically as a result of glucose administration or hyperalimentation.[174] When bicarbonate is administed as therapy, it overwhelms lactic acid utilization because it induces alkalemia.[174,191] The lactic acidosis of malignancy is the only lactic acidosis in which lactic acid is spilled into the urine with bicarbonate, with the development of a hyperchloremic acidosis in addition to the high anion gap acidosis of lactic acid.[174]

Sepsis. Sepsis has been noted to cause lactic acidosis in the absence of tissue hypoperfusion. Sepsis or endotoxicosis may depress oxidative metabolism in response to a cytotoxic effect caused by an inhibition of the H^+ mitochondrial-cytoplasmic shuttle. This increases the $NADH/NAD^+$ ratio, impairing ATP formation and favoring the development of lactic acidosis.[174] During multi-organ failure syndrome, lactic acidosis may be a consequence of ATP requirements not being met by glycolysis rather than of oxidative phosphorylation.[192] However, type A lactic acidosis is also common in sepsis, as described above. The lactic acidosis of sepsis is therefore both type A and B.

Biguanide Toxicity. The incidence of type B lactic acidosis is low with the biguanides (10 times lower with metformin than with phenformin). Usually lactic acidosis occurs when the drug is given to a patient with concomitant hepatic, renal, or cardiac dysfunction or associated drug ingestion.[174] Sixty-six percent of patients with phenformin toxicity present in frank shock (type A lactic acidosis),[174,178] and those with an admission systolic blood pressure of less than 100 mm Hg rarely recover.[178] Type B lactic acidosis of biguanide toxicity is thought to be due to the inhibition of mitochondrial metabolism.[174,178]

Treatment of Lactic Acidosis

The treatment of lactic acidosis has always focused on the correction of the arterial pH.[193] It has been said that the lactic acidosis per se is responsible for the reduced cardiac output, decreased response to catecholamines, abnormal hepatic metabolism, and increased arrhythmias, the factors that could account for the poor survival rate.[193] However, other factors may be responsible, including primarily the underlying disease, organ failure, or epinephrine administration.[194] Contrary to previous beliefs, lactic acid infusion increases the cardiac output by 20 to 30% and decreases the systemic vascular resistance.[178] The doctrine that if acidosis is bad, bicarbonate must be good is not valid, since bicarbonate therapy has not reduced the mortality rate due to lactic acidosis over the last 30 years.[195]

The arguments against the use of bicarbonate are as follows. Pulmonary edema, hypertonicity, and rebound alkalosis occur directly with the administration of bicarbonate, as does hypocalcemia and a shift of the hemoglobin-oxygen dissociation curve.[195] In low flow states such as shock, the arterial pH does not reflect the mixed venous pco_2 or the pH and may fall if hyperventilation is part of the resuscitation.[196] The carbon dioxide that is produced when bicarbonate is given is readily diffusable into the cells, thus depressing the pH_i, following which the molar equivalent of H^+ diffuses into the cell to sustain this low pH_i. During full cardiopulmonary resuscitation, the pH_i can reach 6.1 and the intracellular carbon dioxide pressure rises to 300 mm Hg.[196]

Direct administration of bicarbonate into the atria or intracoronary vessels results in significant, although transient, myocardial depression.[196] Fourteen critically ill patients with significant lactic acidosis and a mean arterial pH of 7.22 were studied in the only double-blind, prospective, controlled trial of bicarbonate administration.[197] Bicarbonate administration markedly increased the arterial pH initially but produced no hemodynamic advantage over that attained with an equal salt load in the control group. There was also no documented increased sensitivity to catecholamines as determined by cardiac output responses in the bicarbonate group vs. the control group. The bicarbonate decreased the amount of ionized calcium and induced an arterial hypercapnea.

Alternate buffers such as Carbicarb (a mixture of equimolar amounts of sodium bicarbonate and sodium carbonate) have been used because they generate 30% less carbon dioxide than does bicarbonate. However, trials of these compounds in the treatment of lactic acidosis in humans are still lacking. Tromethamine (THAM) is no longer considered better than bicarbonate. Dichloroacetate decreases lactic acid production by increasing the activity of phosphate dehydrogenase-limiting lactic acid production. Dichloroacetate has not been shown to prolong survival in lactic acidosis—probably because it does not improve the tissue hypoxia.

Even dialysis does not improve survival or hemodynamics because it does not treat the underlying cause.[195]

The modern aim of treatment of lactic acidosis is directed more toward the underlying disease. Replacement of thiamine and magnesium and other vitamins are indicated when they are deficient. During florid septic shock, increasing oxygen delivery without increasing metabolism is the goal. Maintenance of cardiac output is, therefore, of paramount importance.

REFERENCES

1. Vignati L, Asmal AC, Black WL, et al. Coma in diabetes. In: Marble A, Krall LP, Bradley RF, et al. Joslin's diabetes mellitus. 12th ed. Philadelphia, Lea & Febiger, 1985:526–52.
2. Kitabchi AE, Fisher JN. Diabetes mellitus. In: Glew RH, Peters SP, eds. clinical studies in medical biochemistry. New York: Oxford University Press, 1987:102–17.
3. Dreschfeld J. The Bradshawe lecture on diabetic coma. BMJ 1886;2:358–63.
4. Schade DS, Eaton RP, Alberti KGGM, Johnston DG. Diabetic coma: ketoacidotic and hyperosmolar. 1st ed. Albuquerque: University of New Mexico Press, 1981.
5. Keller U. Diabetic ketoacidosis: current views on pathogenesis and treatment. Diabetologia 1986;29:71–7.
6. Foster DW, McGarry JD. The metabolic derangements and treatment of diabetic ketoacidosis. N Engl J Med 1983;309:159–69.
7. Fishbein HA. Diabetic ketoacidosis, hyperosmolar nonketotic coma, lactic acidosis and hypoglycemia. In: Harris MI, Hamman RF, eds. Diabetes in America (National Diabetes Group). Diabetes data compiled 1984. Washington, DC: US Department of Health and Human Services, 1985:1–22.
8. Marshall SM, Alberti KGGM. Diabetic ketoacidosis. Diabetes Ann 1987;3:498–526.
9. Kitabchi AE, Murphy MB. Diabetic ketoacidosis and hyperosmolar hyperglycemic nonketotic coma. Med Clin North Am 1988;72:1545–63.
10. Kreisberg RA. Diabetic ketoacidosis. In: Rifkin H, Porte D, eds. Diabetes mellitus: theory and practice. 4th ed. Amsterdam: Elsevier, 1990:591–603.
11. Halperin ML, Goldstein MB, Bear RA, Josse RG. Diabetic comas. In: Arieff AI, DeFronzo RA, eds. Fluid, electrolyte, and acid-base disorders. Vol 2. New York: Churchill-Livingstone, 1985:933–67.
12. Kitabchi AE. Low-dose insulin therapy in diabetic ketoacidosis: fact or fiction? Diabetes Metab Rev 1989;5:337–63.
13. Faich GA, Fishbein HA, Ellis SE. The epidemiology of diabetic acidosis: a population-based study. Am J Epidemiol 1983;117:551.
14. Murphy C, Faulkenberry EH, Rumpel JD. The use of a county hospital emergency room by diabetic patients. Diabetes Care 1985;8:48.
15. Scott RS, Brown IJ, Clifford P. Use of health services by diabetic persons. II. Hospital admissions. Diabetes Care 1985;8:43–7.
16. Kitabchi AE, Fisher JN, Burghen GA, et al. Evaluation of a portable insulin infusion pump for outpatient management of brittle diabetes. Diabetes Care 1979;2:421–4.
17. Mecklenburg RS, Guinn TS, Sannar CA, Blumenstein BA. Malfunction of continuous subcutaneous insulin infusion systems: a one-year prospective study of 127 patients. Diabetes Care 1986;9:351–5.
18. Davies AG, Price DA, Houlton CA, et al. Continuous subcutaneous insulin infusion in diabetes mellitus: a year's prospective trial. Arch Dis Child 1984;59:1027–33.
19. Bertram F. Pathogenese und Prognose des Coma Diabeticum. Ergeb Inn Med Kinderheilkd 1932;43:258–365.
20. Skillman TG, Wilson R, Knowles HC Jr. Mortality of patients with diabetic acidosis in a large city hospital. Diabetes 1956;7:109–13.
21. Cohen AS, Vance VK, Runyan JW Jr, Hurwitz D. Diabetic acidosis: an evaluation of the cause, course and therapy of 73 cases. Ann Intern Med 1960;52:55–86.
22. Harwood R. Diabetic acidosis: results of treatment in 67 consecutive cases. N Engl J Med 1951;245:1–9.
23. Beigelman PM. Severe diabetic ketoacidosis (diabetic "coma"): 482 episodes in 257 patients' experiences of three years. Diabetes 1971;20:490–500.
24. Orr DP, Golden MP, Myers G, Marrero DG. Characteristics of adolescents with poorly controlled diabetes referred to a tertiary care center. Diabetes Care 1983;6:170–5.
25. White K, Kolman ML, Wexler P, et al. Unstable diabetes and unstable families: a psychosocial evaluation of diabetic children with recurrent ketoacidosis. Pediatrics 1984;73:749–55.
26. Flexner CW, Weiner JP, Saudek CD, Dans PE. Repeated hospitalization for diabetic ketoacidosis: the game of 'sartoris'. Am J Med 1984;76:691–5.
27. Kitabchi AE, Fisher JN, Matteri R, Murphy MB. The use of continuous insulin delivery systems in the treatment of diabetes mellitus. Adv Intern Med 1983;28:449–90.
28. Kitabchi AE, Fisher JN, Burghen GA, et al. Problems associated with continuous subcutaneous insulin infusion. Horm Metab Res Suppl 1982;12:271–6.
29. Kitabchi AE, Fisher JN. Insulin therapy of diabetic ketoacidosis: physiologic versus pharmacologic doses of insulin and their routes of administration. In: Brownlee M, ed. Handbook of diabetes mellitus. Vol 5. New York, Garland Press, 1981:95–149.
30. Kitabchi AE, Ayyagari V, Guerra SMO, Medical House Staff. The efficacy of low dose versus conventional therapy of insulin for treatment of diabetic ketoacidosis. Ann Intern Med 1976;84:633–8.
31. Sacks HS, Shahshahani M, Kitabchi AE, et al. Similar responsiveness of diabetic ketoacidosis to low-dose insulin by intramuscular injection and albumin-free infusion. Ann Intern Med 1979;90:36–42.
32. Fisher JN, Shahshahani MN, Kitabchi AE. Diabetic ketoacidosis: low-dose insulin therapy by various routes. N Engl J Med 1977;297:238–47.
33. Fisher JN, Kitabchi AE. A randomized study of phosphate therapy in the treatment of diabetic ketoacidosis. J Clin Endocrinol Metab 1983;57:177–80.
34. Morris LR, Murphy MB, Kitabchi AE. Bicarbonate therapy in severe diabetic ketoacidosis. Ann Intern Med 1986;105:836–40.
35. Hockaday TDR, Alberti KGMM. Diabetic coma. Br J Hosp Med 1972;7:183–98.
36. Genuth SM. Clinical remission in diabetes mellitus: studies of insulin secretion. Diabetes 1970;19:116–21.
37. Block MB, Mako ME, Steiner DF, Rubenstein AH. Diabetic ketoacidosis: evidence for C-peptide and proinsulin secretion following recovery. J Clin Endocrinol Metab 1972;35:402–6.
38. Kipnis DM. Insulin secretion in diabetes mellitus. Ann Intern Med 1968;69:891–901.
39. Kitabchi AE, Duckworth WC, Stentz FB. Insulin synthesis, proinsulin and C-peptides. In: Rifkin H, Porte D, eds. Diabetes mellitus: theory and practice. 4th ed. Amsterdam: Elsevier, 1990.

40. Chupin M, Charbonnel B, Chupin F. C-peptide blood levels in keto-acidosis and in hyperosmolar non-ketotic diabetic coma. Acta Diabet Lat 1981;18:123–8.

41. Kitabchi AE, Murphy MB, Matteri R, Spencer J. Contributing factors in the development of hyperchloremic metabolic acidosis during the treatment of diabetic ketoacidosis [Abstract no. 167]. Diabetes 1991;40(Suppl 1):42A.

42. Müller WA, Faloona GR, Unger RH. Hyperglucagonemia in diabetic ketoacidosis: its prevalence and significance. Am J Med 1973;54:52–7.

43. Christensen NJ. Plasma norepinephrine and epinephrine in untreated diabetics during fasting and after insulin administration. Diabetes 1974;23:1–8.

44. Jahnke K, Buro F. Das Coma diabeticum. Verh Dtsch Ges Inn Med 1970;76:359–70.

45. Unger R. High growth hormone levels in diabetic ketoacidosis: a possible cause of insulin resistance. JAMA 1965;191:945–7.

46. Alberti KGM, Hockaday TD. Diabetic coma: serum growth hormone before and during treatment. Diabetologia 1973;9:13–9.

47. Waldhäusl W, Kleinberger G, Korn A, et al. Severe hyperglycemia: effects of rehydration on endocrine derangements and blood glucose concentration. Diabetes 1979;8:577–84.

48. Gelfand RA, Matthews DE, Bier DM, Sherwin RS. Role of counterregulatory hormones in the catabolic responses to stress. J Clin Invest 1984;74:2238–48.

49. Schade DS, Eaton RP. The temporal relationship between endogenously secreted stress hormone and metabolic decompensation in diabetic man. J Clin Endocrinol Metab 1980;50:131–6.

50. Gerich JE, Lorenzi M, Bier DM, et al. Effects of physiologic levels of glucagon and growth hormone on human carbohydrate and lipid metabolism: studies involving administration of exogenous hormone during suppression of endogenous hormone secretion with somatostatin. J Clin Invest 1976;57:875–84.

51. Bolli G, De Feo P, Compagnucci P, et al. Abnormal glucose counterregulation in insulin-dependent diabetes mellitus: interaction of antiinsulin antibodies and impaired glucagon and epinephrine secretion. Diabetes 1983;32:134–41.

52. Barnes AJ, Bloom SR, Alberti GMM, et al. Ketoacidosis in pancreatectomized man. N Engl J Med 1977;296:1250–3.

53. Barnes AJ, Kohner EM, Bloom SR, et al. Importance of pituitary hormones in the aetiology of diabetic ketoacidosis. Lancet 1978;1:1171–4.

54. Matteri R, Murphy MB, Kitabchi AE. Metabolic dysfunction during pump withdrawal in brittle diabetics [Abstract no. 269]. Diabetes 1982;31(Suppl 2):68A.

55. Schade DS, Eaton RP. The controversy concerning counterregulatory hormone secretion: a hypothesis for the prevention of diabetic ketoacidosis? Diabetes 1977;26:596–601.

56. Page MM, Alberti KGMM, Greenwood R, et al. Treatment of diabetic coma with continuous low-dose infusion of insulin. BMJ 1974;2:687–90.

57. Clements RS Jr, Vourganti B. Fatal diabetic ketoacidosis: major causes and approaches to their prevention. Diabetes Care 1978;1:314–25.

58. Luzi L, Barrett EJ, Groop LC, et al. Metabolic effects of low-dose insulin therapy on glucose metabolism in diabetic ketoacidosis. Diabetes 1988;37:1470–7.

59. Kitabchi AE, Rumbak MJ. Diabetic ketoacidosis: diagnosis; diabetic ketoacidosis: treatment; hyperglycemic hyperosmolar nonketotic coma; and maintenance treatment after

hyperglycemic crisis. In: Callahan ML, Barton CW, Schumaker HM, eds. Decision making in emergency medicine. Philadelphia: BC Decker, 1990:178–85.

60. Cook GA, King MT, Veech RL. Ketogenesis and malonyl coenzyme A content of isolated rat hepatocytes J Biol Chem 1978;253:2529–31.

61. Cook GA, Gamble MS. Regulation of carnitine palmitoyltransferase by insulin results in decreased activity and decreased apparent K_i values for malonyl-CoA. J Biol Chem 1987;262:2050–5.

62. McGarry JD. Lilly lecture 1978: new perspectives in the regulation of ketogenesis. Diabetes 1979;28:517–23.

63. Heimberg M, Weinstein I, Kohout M. The effects of glucagon dibutyryl cyclic adenosine 3′,5′-monophosphate, and concentration of free fatty acid on hepatic lipid metabolism. J Biol Chem 1969;244:5131–9.

64. Ruderman NB, Goodman MN. Inhibition of muscle acetoacetate utilization during diabetic ketoacidosis. Am J Physiol 1974;226:136–43.

65. Miles JM, Rizza RA, Haymond MW, Gerich JE. Effects of acute insulin deficiency on glucose and ketone body turnover in man: evidence for the primacy of overproduction of glucose and ketone bodies in the genesis of diabetic ketoacidosis. Diabetes 1980;29:926–30.

66. Féry F, Balasse EO. Ketone body production and disposal in diabetic ketosis: a comparison with fasting ketosis. Diabetes 1985;34:326–32.

67. Nosadini R, Avogaro A, Trevisan R, et al. Acetoacetate and 3-hydroxybutyrate kinetics in obese and insulin-dependent diabetic humans. Am J Physiol 1985;248:R611–20.

68. Owen OE, Trapp VE, Skutches CL, et al. Acetone metabolism during diabetic ketoacidosis. Diabetes 1982;31:242–8.

69. Reichard GA Jr, Skutches CL, Hoeldtke RD, Owen OE. Acetone metabolism in humans during diabetic ketoacidosis. Diabetes 1986;35:668–74.

70. Atchley DW, Loeb RE, Richards DW Jr, et al. A detailed study of electrolyte balances following the withdrawal and reestablishment of insulin therapy. J Clin Invest 1933;12:297–326.

71. Butler AM, Talbot NB, Burnett CH, et al. Metabolic studies in diabetic coma. Trans Assoc Am Physicians 1947;60:102–9.

72. Nabarro JDN, Spencer AG, Stowers JM. Metabolic studies in severe diabetic ketosis. Q J Med 1952;21:225–48.

73. Felig P, Marliss E, Ohman JL, Cahill GF Jr. Plasma amino acid levels in diabetic ketoacidosis. Diabetes 1970;19:727–9.

74. Blackshear PJ, Alberti KGMM. Sequential amino acid measurements during experimental diabetic ketoacidosis. Am J Physiol 1975;228:205–11.

75. May RC, Kelly RA, Mitch WE. Metabolic acidosis stimulates protein degradation in rat muscle by a glucocorticoid-dependent mechanism. J Clin Invest 1986;77:614–21.

76. Genuth SM, Castro J. Effect of oral alanine on blood beta-hydroxybutyrate and plasma glucose, insulin, free fatty acids, and growth hormone in normal and diabetic subjects. Metabolism 1974;23:375–86.

77. Woodside WF, Heimberg M. The metabolism of oleic acid by the perfused rat liver in experimental diabetes induced by anti-insulin serum. Metabolism 1978;27:1763–77.

78. Weidman SW, Ragland JB, Fisher JN, et al. Effects of insulin on plasma lipoproteins in diabetic ketoacidosis: evidence for a change in high density lipoprotein composition during treatment. J Lipid Res 1985;23:171–82.

79. Joven J, Rubiés-Prat J, De La Figuera M, et al. High density lipoprotein changes during treatment of diabetic ketoacidosis. Diabete Metab 1985;11:102–5.

80. Weinstein I, Patel TB, Heimberg M. Secretion of triglyceride and ketogenesis by livers from spontaneous diabetic BB Wistar rats. Biochem Biophys Res Commun 1991;176:1157–62.

81. Sacks H, Rabkin R, Kitabchi AE. Reversible hyperinsulinuria in diabetic ketoacidosis in man. Am J Physiol 1981;241:E396–405.

82. Owen OE, Licht JH, Sapir DG. Renal function and effects of partial rehydration during diabetic ketoacidosis. Diabetes 1981;30:510–8.

83. Martin HE, Smith K, Wilson ML. The fluid and electrolyte therapy of severe diabetic acidosis and ketosis: a study of twenty-nine episodes (twenty-six patients). Am J Med 1958;24:376–89.

84. Adrogué HJ, Wilson H, Boyd AE, et al. Plasma acid-base patterns in diabetic ketoacidosis. N Engl J Med 1982;307:1603–10.

85. Bessman SP, Renner VJ. Biphasic hormonal nature of stress. In: Crowley RA, Trump BF, eds. Pathophysiology of shock, anoxia, and ischemia. Baltimore: Williams and Wilkins, 1982:60–5.

86. Narins RG, Jones ER, Stom MC, et al. Diagnostic strategies in disorders of fluid, electrolyte and acid-base homeostasis. Am J Med 1982;72:496–520.

87. Katz MA. Hyperglycemia-induced hyponatremia-calculation of expected serum sodium depression. N Engl J Med 1973;289:843–44.

88. Young DS, Thomas DW, Friedman RB, Pestaner LC. Effects of drugs on clinical laboratory tests. Clin Chem 1972;18:1041–2.

89. Vinicor F, Lehrner LM, Karn RC, Merritt AD. Hyperamylasemia in diabetic ketoacidosis: sources and significance. Ann Intern Med 1979;91:200–4.

90. Rumbak MJ, Hughes TA, Kitabchi AE. Pseudonormoglycemia in diabetic ketoacidosis in a patient with hypertriglyceridemia. Am J Emerg Med 1991;9:61–3.

91. Morris LE, Kitabchi AE. Coma in the diabetic. In: Schnatz JD, ed. Diabetes mellitus: problems in management. Menlo Park, CA: Addison-Wesley Publishing,1982:234–51.

92. Sament S, Schwartz MB. Severe diabetic stupor without ketosis. S Afr Med J 1957;31:893–4.

93. Arieff AI, Carroll HJ. Nonketotic hyperosmolar coma with hyperglycemia: clinical features, pathophysiology, renal function, acid-base balance, plasma-cerebrospinal fluid equilibria and the effects of therapy in 37 cases. Medicine (Baltimore) 1972;51:73–94.

94. Marshall SM, Alberti KGMM. Hyperosmolar nonketotic diabetic coma. Diabetes Ann 1988;4:235–47.

95. Matz R. Hyperosmolar nonacidotic diabetes (HNAD). In: Rifkin H, Porte D, eds. Diabetes mellitus: theory and practice. 4th ed. Amsterdam: Elsevier, 1990:604–16.

96. Carroll P, Matz R. Uncontrolled diabetes mellitus in adults: experience in treating diabetic ketoacidosis and hyperosmolar nonketotic coma with low-dose insulin and a uniform treatment regimen. Diabetes Care 1983;6:579–85.

97. Halperin ML, Marsden PA, Singer GG, West ML. Can marked hyperglycemia occur without ketosis? Clin Invest Med 1985;8:253–6.

98. Wachtel TJ, Silliman RA, Lamberton P. Predisposing factors for the diabetic hyperosmolar state. Arch Intern Med 1987;147:499–501.

99. Gerich JE, Martin MM, Recant LL. Clinical and metabolic characteristics of hyperosmolar nonketotic coma. Diabetes 1971;20:228–38.

100. Slovis CM, Mark VG, Slovis RJ, Bain RP. Diabetic ketoacidosis and infection: leukocyte count and differential as early predictors of infection. Am J Emerg Med 1987;5:1–5.

101. Peden NR, Braaten JT, McKenry JB. Diabetic ketoacidosis during long-term treatment with continuous subcutaneous insulin infusions. Diabetes Care 1984;7:1–5.

102. Lindsey CA, Faloona GR, Unger RH. Plasma glucagon in nonketotic hyperosmolar coma. JAMA 1974;229:1771–3.

103. Yu SS, Kitabchi AE. Biological activity of proinsulin and related polypeptides in the fat tissue. J Biol Chem 1973;248:3753–61.

104. Schade DS, Eaton RP. Dose response to insulin in man: differential effects on glucose and ketone body regulation. J Clin Endocrinol Metab 1977;44:1038–53.

105. Nurjhan N, Campbell PJ, Kennedy FP, et al. Insulin dose-response characteristics for suppression of glycerol release and conversion of glucose in humans. Diabetes 1986;35:1326–31.

106. Turpin BP, Duckworth WC, Solomon SS. Simulated hyperglycemic hyperosmolar syndrome: impaired insulin and epinephrine effects upon lipolysis in the isolated rat fat cell. J Clin Invest 1979;63:403–9.

107. Bratusch-Marrain PR, DeFronzo RA. Impairment of insulin-mediated glucose metabolism by hyperosmolality in man. Diabetes 1983;32:1028–34.

108. Arieff AI, Carroll HM. Cerebral edema and depression of sensorium in nonketotic hyperosmolar coma. Diabetes 1974;23:525–31.

109. Fulop M, Rosenblatt A, Kreitzer SM, Gerstenhabner B. Hyperosmolar nature of diabetic coma. Diabetes 1975;24:594–9.

110. Morris LR, Kitabchi AE. Efficacy of low-dose insulin therapy for severely obtunded patients in diabetic ketoacidosis. Diabetes Care 1980;3:53–6.

111. Guisado R, Arieff AI. Neurologic manifestations of diabetic comas: correlation with biochemical alterations in the brain. Metabolism 1975;24:665–79.

112. Maccario M. Neurological dysfunction associated with nonketotic hyperglycemia. Arch Neurol 1968;19:525–34.

113. Turnebum A. Of the causes and signs of acute and chronic disease, 1554. Reynolds TF, translator. London: William Pickering, 1837.

114. Root Howard F. Diabetic acidosis and coma. In: Joslin EP, Root HF, White P, Marble A, eds. The treatment of diabetes mellitus. 10th ed. Philadelphia, Lea & Febiger, 1959.

115. Foster NB. The treatment of diabetic coma with insulin. Am J Med Sci 1923;166:699–709.

116. Katsch G. Insulin be Handlung des diabetischen Koma. Dtsch Gesundheitwes 1946;1:651–5.

117. Menzel R, Zander E, Jutzi E. Treatment of diabetic coma with low-dose injections of insulin. Endokrinologie 1976;67:230–9.

118. Root HF. The use of insulin and the abuse of glucose in the treatment of diabetic coma. JAMA 1975;127:557–64.

119. Black AB, Malins JM. Diabetic ketosis: a comparison of results of orthodox and intensive methods of treatment based on 170 consecutive cases. Lancet 1949;1:56–9.

120. Smith K, Martin HE. Response of diabetic coma to various insulin dosages. Diabetes 1954;3:287–95.

121. Shaw CE Jr, Hurwitz GE, Schmukler M, et al. A clinical and laboratory study of insulin dosage in diabetic acidosis: comparison with small and large doses. Diabetes 1962;11:23–30.

122. Steinke J, Soeldner JS. Diabetes mellitus. In: Thorn GW, Adams RD, Braunwald E, et al, eds. Harrison's principles of internal medicine. Vol 1. 8th ed. New York: McGraw-Hill, New York, 1977:563–83.

123. Larner J, Haynes RC Jr. Insulin and oral hypoglycemic drugs: glucagon. In: Goodman LS, Gilman A, eds. The pharmacological basis of therapeutics. 5th ed. New York: Macmillan Publishing, 1975:1507–33.

124. Sönksen PH, Srivastava MC, Tompkins CV, Nabarro JDN. Growth-hormone and cortisol responses to insulin infusion in patients with diabetes mellitus. Lancet 1972; 2:155–60.

125. Alberti KGMM, Hockaday TDR, Turner RC. Small doses of intramuscular insulin in the treatment of diabetic "coma". Lancet 1973;5:515–22.

126. Genuth SM. Constant intravenous insulin infusion in diabetic ketoacidosis. JAMA 1973;223:1348–51.

127. Kidson W, Casey J, Kraegen E, Lazarus L. Treatment of severe diabetes mellitus by insulin infusion. BMJ 1974;2:691–4.

128. Semple PF, White C, Manderson WG. Continuous intravenous infusion of small doses of insulin in treatment of diabetic ketoacidosis. BMJ 1974;2:694–8.

129. Soler NG, Wright AD, FitzGerald MG, Malins JM. Comparative study of different insulin regimens in management of diabetic ketoacidosis. Lancet 1975;2:1221–4.

130. Alberti KGMM. Comparison of different insulin regimens in diabetic ketoacidosis [Letter]. Lancet 1976;1:83.

131. Heber D, Molitch ME, Sperling MA. Low-dose continuous insulin therapy for diabetic ketoacidosis: prospective comparison with "conventional" insulin therapy. Arch Intern Med 1977;137:1377–80.

132. Piters KM, Kumar D Pei E, Bessman AN. Comparison of continuous and intermittent intravenous insulin therapies for diabetic ketoacidosis. Diabetologia 1977; 13:317–21.

133. Edwards GA, Kohaut EC, Wehring B, Hill LL. Effectiveness of low-dose continuous intravenous insulin infusion in diabetic ketoacidosis: a prospective comparative study. J Pediatr 1977;91:701–5.

134. Burghen GA, Etteldorf JN, Fisher JN, Kitabchi AE. Comparison of high-dose and low-dose insulin by continuous intravenous infusion in the treatment of diabetic ketoacidosis in children. Diabetes Care 1980;3:15–20.

135. Beigelman PM. Potassium in severe diabetic ketoacidosis [Editorial]. Am J Med 1973;54:419–20.

136. Abramson E, Arky R. Diabetic acidosis with initial hypokalemia; therapeutic implications. JAMA 1966;196;401–3.

137. Guest GM, Rapoport S. Role of acid-soluble phosphorus compounds in red blood cells in experimental rickets, renal insufficiency, pyloric obstruction, gastroenteritis, ammonium chloride acidosis and diabetic acidosis. Am J Dis Child 1939;58:1072–89.

138. Franks M, Berris RF, Kaplan NO, Myers GB. Metabolic studies in diabetic acidosis. II. The effect of the administration of sodium phosphate. Arch Intern Med 1948;81:42–55.

139. Nabarro JDN, Spencer AG, Stowers JM. Treatment of diabetic ketosis. Lancet 1952;1:983–9.

140. Ditzel J. Effect of plasma inorganic phosphate on tissue oxygenation during recovery from diabetic ketoacidosis. Adv Exp Med Biol 1973;37A:163–72.

141. Benesch R, Benesch RE. The effect of organic phosphates from the human erythrocyte on the allosteric properties of hemoglobin. Biochem Biophys Res Comm 1967; 26:162–7.

142. Chanutin A, Curnish RR. Effect of organic and inorganic phosphates on the oxygen equilibrium of human erythrocytes. Arch Biochem Biophys 1967;121:96–102.

143. Wilson HK, Keuer SP, Lea AS, et al. Phosphate therapy in diabetic ketoacidosis. Arch Intern Med 1982;142:517–20.

144. Kreisberg RA. Phosphorus deficiency and hypophosphatemia. Hosp Pract 1977;12(3):121–8.

145. Matz R. Diabetic acidosis: rationale for not using bicarbonate. NY State J Med 1976;76:1299–303.

146. Lever E, Jaspan JB. Sodium bicarbonate therapy in severe diabetic ketoacidosis. Am J Med 1983;75:263–8.

147. Hale PJ, Crase J, Nattrass M. Metabolic effects of bicarbonate in the treatment of diabetic ketoacidosis. BMJ 1984;289:1035–8.

148. Barnes HV, Cohen RD, Kitabchi AE, Murphy MB. When is bicarbonate appropriate in treating metabolic acidosis including diabetic ketoacidosis? In: Gitnick G, Barnes HV, Duffy TP, et al., eds. Debates in medicine. Chicago: Yearbook Medical Publishers, 1990.

149. Rosenbloom AL. Intracerebral crises during treatment of diabetic ketoacidosis. Diabetes Care 1990;13:22–33.

150. Dillon ES, Riggs HE, Dyer WW. Cerebral lesions in uncomplicated fatal diabetic acidosis. Am J Med Sci 1936;192:360–5.

151. Duck SC, Wyatt DT. Factors associated with brain herniation in the treatment of diabetic ketoacidosis. J Pediatr 1988;113:10–4.

152. Ohman JL Jr, Marliss EB, Aoki TT, et al. The cerebrospinal fluid in diabetic ketoacidosis. N Engl J Med 1971; 284:283–90.

153. Duck SC, Weldon VV, Pagliara AS, Haymond MW. Cerebral edema complicating therapy for diabetic ketoacidosis. Diabetes 1976;25:111–5.

154. Felts PW. Diabetic ketoacidosis. In: Sussman KE, Metz RJS, eds. Diabetes mellitus. 4th ed. New York: American Diabetes Association, 1975:1611–9.

155. Clements RS Jr, Prockop LD, Winegrad AI. Acute cerebral oedema during treatment of hyperglycaemia: an experimental model. Lancet 1968;2:384–6.

156. Van Der Meulen JA, Klip A, Grinstein S. Possible mechanism for cerebral oedema in diabetic ketoacidosis. Lancet 1987;2:306–8.

157. Clements RS Jr, Blumenthal SA, Morrison AD, Winegrad AI. Increased cerebrospinal-fluid pressure during treatment of diabetic ketosis. Lancet 1971;2:657–61.

158. Fein IA, Rackow EC, Sprung CL, Grodman R. Relation of colloid osmotic pressure to arterial hypoxemia and cerebral edema during crystalloid volume loading of patients with diabetic ketoacidosis. Ann Intern Med 1982; 96:570–5.

159. Krane EJ, Rockoff MA, Wallman JK, Wolfsdorf JI. Subclinical brain swelling in children during treatment of diabetic ketoacidosis. N Engl J Med 1985;312:1147–51.

160. Hoffman WH, Steinhart CM, Gammal TE, et al. Cranial CT in children and adolescents with diabetic ketoacidosis. AJNR 1988;9:733–9.

161. Ellis EN. Concepts of fluid therapy in diabetic ketoacidosis and hyperosmolar hyperglycemic nonketotic coma. Pediatr Clin North Am 1990;37:313–21.

162. Wall BM, Jones GV, Kaminska E,.et al. Causes of hyperchloremic acidosis during treatment of diabetic ketoacidosis [Abstract]. Clin Res 1990;38:960A.

163. Powner D, Snyder JV, Grenvik A. Altered pulmonary capillary permeability complicating recovery from diabetic ketoacidosis. Chest 1975;68:253–6.

164. Sprung CL, Rackow EC, Fein IA. Pulmonary edema: a

complication of diabetic ketoacidosis. Chest 1980; 77:687–8.

165. Brun-Buisson CJL, Bonnet F, Bergeret S, et al. Recurrent high-permeability pulmonary edema associated with diabetic ketoacidosis. Crit Care Med 1985;13:55–6.

166. Kitabchi AE, Rumbak MJ. The management of diabetic emergencies. Hosp Pract 1989;24(6):129–33.

167. Fulop M, Ben-Ezra J, Bock J. Alcoholic ketosis. Alcoholism 1986;10:610–5.

168. Halperin ML, Hammeke M, Josse RG, Jungas RL. Metabolic acidosis in the alcoholic: a pathophysiologic approach. Metabolism 1983;32:308–15.

169. Krebs HT. The effects of ethanol on the metabolic activities of the liver. Adv Enzyme Regul 1968;6:467–80.

170. Lefèvre A, Adler H, Lieber S. Effect of ethanol on ketone metabolism. J Clin Invest 1970;49:1775–82.

171. Silverberg JD, Kreisberg RA. Hyperglycemic disorders. Probl Crit Care 1990;4:355–8.

172. Kreisberg RA. Acid-base and electrolyte disturbances in the alcoholic. Probl Crit Care 1987;1:66–72.

173. Miller PD, Heinig RE, Waterhouse C. Treatment of alcoholic acidosis: the role of dextrose and phosphorus. Arch Intern Med 1978;138:67–72.

174. Mizock BA. Lactic acidosis. Dis Mon 1989;35:233–300.

175. Krebs HA, Woods HF, Alberti KGMM. Hyperlactataemia and lactic acidosis. Essays Med Biochem 1975;1:81–103.

176. Cohen RD, Woods HF. Clinical and biochemical aspects of lactic acidosis. Oxford: Blackwell Scientific Publications, 1976.

177. Brooks GA. Lactic production under fully aerobic conditions: the lactate shuttle during rest and exercise. Fed Proc 1986;29:45.

178. Arieff AI. Pathogenesis of lactic acidosis. Diabetes Metab Rev 1989;5:637–49.

179. Kreisberg RA. Lactate homeostasis and lactic acidosis. Ann Intern Med 1980;92:227–37.

180. Madias NE. Lactic acidosis. Kidney Int 1986;29:752–74.

181. Lloyd MH, Iles RA, Simpson BR, et al. The effect of simulated metabolic acidosis on the intracellular pH and lactate metabolism in the isolated perfused rat liver. Clin Sci Molec Med 1973;45:543–9.

182. Cohen RD, Woods HF. Lactic acidosis revisited. Diabetes 1983;32:181–91.

183. Hood VL, Tannen RL. pH control of lactic acid and keto acid production: a mechanism of acid-base regulation. Miner Electrolyte Metab 1983;9:317–25.

184. Baim DS, Rothman MT, Harrison DC. Simultaneous measurement of coronary venous blood flow and oxygen saturation during transient alterations in myocardial oxygen supply and demand. Am J Cardiol 1982; 49:743–52.

185. Daugherty RM Jr, Scott JB, Dabney JM, Haddy FJ. Local effects of O_2 and CO_2 on limb, renal, and coronary vascular resistances. Am J Physiol 1967;213:1102–10.

186. Heistad DD, Abboud FM. Cirulatory adjustments to hypoxia. Circulation 1980;61:463–70.

187. Arieff AI, Graf H. Pathophysiology of type A hypoxic lactic acidosis in dogs. Am J Physiol 1987;253:E271–6.

188. Kreisberg RA. Pathogenesis and management of lactic acidosis. Annu Rev Med 1984;35:181–93.

189. Fulop M, Hoberman HD, Rascoff JH, et al. Lactic acidosis in diabetic patients. Arch Intern Med 1976;136:987–90.

190. Kreisberg RA. Lactic acidosis: an update. J Intensive Care 1987;2:76–8.

191. Kopec IC, Groeger JS. Life-threatening fluid and electrolyte abnormalities associated with cancer. Crit Care Clin 1988;4:81–105.

192. Stoner HB. Metabolism after trauma and in sepsis. Circ Shock 1986;19:75–87.

193. Narins RG, Cohen JJ. Bicarbonate therapy for organic acidosis: the case for its continued use. Ann Intern Med 1987;106:615–8.

194. Oliva PB. Lactic acidosis. Am J Med 1970;48:209–25.

195. Cooper DJ, Worthley LIG. Buffer therapy for patients who have lactic acidosis. Intensive Crit Care Dig 1990;9:30–4.

196. Rumbak MJ. Lactic acidosis [Letter]. Ann Intern Med 1990;113:254–5.

197. Cooper DJ, Walley KR, Wiggs BR, Russell JA. Bicarbonate does not improve hemodynamics in critically ill patients who have lactic acidosis: a prospective controlled clinical study. Ann Intern Med 1990;112:492–8.

Chapter 42

OCULAR COMPLICATIONS OF DIABETES MELLITUS

LLOYD M. AIELLO

JERRY D. CAVALLERANO

Ocular complications in diabetes are frequent, distressing and destined to become one of the challenging problems of the future.

These prophetic words of Dr. Howard Root opened the chapter on ocular complications in the 1935 edition of Joslin's *The Treatment of Diabetes Mellitus.*[1] Indeed, as insulin increased the life span of persons with diabetes, diabetic retinopathy became a major cause of severe visual loss in the United States and in other industrialized countries of Europe and the Americas. By the 1960s, diabetic retinopathy was recognized as the leading cause of new, severe visual loss in the United States among persons 21 to 74 years old. Diabetic retinopathy is still neither preventable nor curable.

Dedicated efforts by researchers and patients, however, have established treatment and surgical modalities that

can reduce the 5-year risk of severe visual loss (visual acuity less than 5/200) from proliferative diabetic retinopathy (PDR) to less than 5% and the 5-year risk of moderate visual loss (vision reduced to 20/200) from diabetic macular edema to 12% or less.

Ongoing research efforts now hold out the promise that soon diabetic retinopathy might be curable or preventable and that research on diabetic macular edema and proliferative retinopathy will be conducted by the study of medical history books. Presently, however, clinical goals must concentrate on identifying eyes at risk of visual loss and ensuring that appropriate and timely laser surgery is offered to reduce the risk.

SIGNIFICANCE OF APPROACHING/REACHING HIGH-RISK PROLIFERATIVE DIABETIC RETINOPATHY AND CLINICALLY SIGNIFICANT MACULAR EDEMA

In 1967, the first evidence of the effectiveness of scatter (panretinal) laser photocoagulation surgery in the treatment of diabetic retinopathy was promulgated in the ophthalmologic and medical communities.[2] Since these promising beginnings, dramatic strides have been made in controlling diabetic retinopathy and macular edema

---

The reports of the Early Treatment Diabetic Retinopathy Study,[17–29] which form the basis of the discussion of diabetic retinopathy, are widely quoted and paraphrased and set the standards of care for patients with diabetic retinopathy. Frequently used terms and abbreviations are given in Table 42–1. Portions of this chapter appear in *Principles and Practices of Ophthalmology: The Harvard System.* Philadelphia: WB Saunders (in press) and the *Journal of the American Optometric Association* 1990;61:533–43 (used with permission).

Table 42–1. Abbreviations of Commonly Used Terms

CSME	Clinically significant macular edema
DRS	Diabetic Retinopathy Study
DRVS	Diabetic Retinopathy Vitrectomy Study
ETDRS	Early Treatment Diabetic Retinopathy Study
FPD	Fibrous proliferations on or within 1 DD of disc margin
FPE	Fibrous proliferations elsewhere—not FPD
H/Ma	Hemorrhages and/or microaneurysms
HE	Hard exudates
IRMA	Intraretinal microvascular abnormalities
MVL	Moderate visual loss: a doubling of the visual angle (e.g., 20/40 to 20/80 at two consecutive, completed 4-month follow-up visits)
NPDR	Nonproliferative diabetic retinopathy
NVD	Neovascularization of the disc: new vessels on or within 1 disc diameter of disc margin
NVE	Neovascularization elsewhere: new vessels elsewhere in the retina outside of disc and 1 disc diameter from disc margin
PDR	Proliferative diabetic retinopathy
SE	Soft exudates (cotton-wool spots)
SVL	Severe visual loss: visual acuity equal to or less than 5/200 at two consecutive, completed 4-month follow-up visits
VB	Venous beading

through the effective use of scatter (panretinal) laser and other surgical techniques. The value of these techniques has received strong support from the findings of three major, nationwide randomized and controlled clinical trials: the Diabetic Retinopathy Study (DRS),[3-16] the Early Treatment Diabetic Retinopathy Study (ET-DRS),[17-29] and the Diabetic Retinopathy Vitrectomy Study (DRVS).[30-34] Scientists can now offer the hope that, by the year 2000, proper diagnosis and treatment will virtually eliminate the 5-year risk of severe visual loss from PDR for the 7 million Americans who have diagnosed diabetes mellitus.

Nevertheless, diabetic retinopathy remains a leading cause of blindness in the United States for persons between the ages of 20 and 74 years. This blindness usually results from nonresolving vitreous hemorrhage, traction retinal detachment, or diabetic macular edema. However, the 5-year risk of severe visual loss can be reduced to less than 5% if a person with diabetic retinopathy approaching or just reaching high-risk proliferative retinopathy, as defined below, undergoes scatter (panretinal) laser photocoagulation surgery. Furthermore, people with clinically significant diabetic macular edema (CSME) can have the risk of moderate visual loss reduced by 50% or more, to approximately 12% or less, if they have appropriate focal laser surgery. Since diabetic retinopathy is often asymptomatic in its most treatable stages, early detection of diabetic retinopathy through regularly scheduled ocular examination becomes critical.

This chapter will review prognostic implications of the lesions of diabetic retinopathy and the risks of progression of retinopathy, placing particular emphasis on identifying patients at risk of visual loss and in need of laser surgery. The laser treatment techniques are described in only general terms in this chapter but are carefully detailed in ETDRS reports 3 and 4.[19,20] Nonret-

inal ocular complications of diabetes mellitus and alterations in visual function also are discussed.

EPIDEMIOLOGY OF DIABETIC RETINOPATHY

An estimated 14 million Americans have diabetes mellitus, but only one-half of these cases have been diagnosed.[35,36] Among the population with diabetes, 10 to 15% have insulin-dependent diabetes mellitus (IDDM or Type I), which is usually diagnosed before the age of 40 years. The majority of diabetic patients, however, have non-insulin-dependent diabetes mellitus (NIDDM or Type II), which is usually diagnosed after the age of 40 years. These patients may or may not be treated with insulin. While those with Type I diabetes experience a high incidence of severe ocular complications and are more likely to develop significant ocular problems during their lifetimes, those with Type II diabetes account for the majority of clinical cases of diabetic eye disease because of their larger overall number.

Diabetic retinopathy is a highly specific vascular complication of both Type I and Type II diabetes, and the duration of diabetes is a significant risk factor for the development of retinopathy. After 20 years of diabetes, nearly all patients with IDDM and more than 60% with NIDDM have some degree of retinopathy. Laser surgery and other surgical modalities help minimize the risk of moderate and severe visual loss from diabetes mellitus and, in some cases, restore useful vision for those who have suffered visual loss. These surgical modalities, particularly laser treatments, are most effective if initiated when a person approaches or just reaches high-risk PDR or before a person has lost visual acuity from diabetic macular edema.[25]

The 5-year risk of severe visual loss from high-risk proliferative diabetic neuropathy may be as high as 60%, and the risk of moderate visual loss from CSME may be as high as 25 to 30%. Since proliferative retinopathy and macular edema may cause no ocular or visual symptoms when the retinal lesions are most amenable to treatment, the goal is to identify eyes at risk of visual loss and ensure that patients are referred for laser surgery at the most appropriate time. Even minor errors in diagnosis of the level of retinopathy can result in a significant increase in a person's risk of visual loss.

Furthermore, collateral health and medical problems present a significant risk for the development and progression of diabetic retinopathy (Table 42–2). These factors include pregnancy,[37-39] chronic hyperglycemia,[40-43] hypertension,[44] renal disease,[42] and hyperlipidemia.[45,46] Patients with these conditions require careful medical evaluation and follow-up for the progression of diabetic retinopathy.

CLINICAL TRIALS OF DIABETIC RETINOPATHY: SCIENTIFIC BASIS FOR MANAGEMENT

The results of three nationwide randomized clinical trials have determined in large part the strategies for appropriate clinical management of patients with diabetic retinopathy.

Table 42–2. Medical Problems Presenting Significant Risk for Development of Diabetic Retinopathy or Affecting Its Course

Condition	Comment
RISK INDICATORS OF DIABETIC NEUROPATHY	
1. Joint contractures	1. Association of retinopathy and contractures has been established. Eye examination is indicated. Care of joint contractures is important.
2. Neuropathy	2. Peripheral neuropathy may result in difficulty in handling contact lenses. Neuropathy in lower extremities may alter mobility; therefore, restoration and maintenance of as much vision as possible is important.
CONDITIONS THAT MAY AFFECT COURSE OF DIABETIC NEPHROPATHY	
1. Hypertension	1. Appropriate medical treatment is indicated for prevention of cardiovascular disease, stroke, and death. Hypertension itself may result in hypertensive retinopathy superimposed on diabetic retinopathy.
2. Elevated lipids	2. Appropriate management to normalize lipids is important. Proper diet and drug treatment may result in less retinal vessel leakage and hard exudate.
3. Proteinuria; elevated creatinine	3. Aggressive management of renal disease is indicated to avoid renal retinopathy, which may increase risk of progression of diabetic retinopathy and of neovascular glaucoma.
4. Cardiovascular disease	4. Increased risk of peripheral vascular disease, particularly coronary vascular disease, is often associated with an increase in the attenuation and arteriosclerotic closure of the arterial system of the retina. A decreased risk of hemorrhage into the vitreous may result, but there also may be a decrease in retinal function with associated decrease in vision. Aggressive management of cardiovascular risk factors theoretically could relieve some of the ischemic process in the retina.
5. Clinical trials	5. There are no clinical trials that have shown specifically that control of systemic conditions that may affect the eyes (i.e., 1–4 above) prevents the progression of diabetic retinopathy. However, clinical experience suggests that appropriate treatment of these problems is beneficial.

Diabetic Retinopathy Study

The DRS (Table 42–3) conclusively demonstrated that scatter (panretinal) photocoagulation significantly reduces the risk of severe visual loss from PDR, particularly when high-risk PDR is present.

Early Treatment Diabetic Retinopathy Study

The ETDRS provided valuable information concerning the timing of scatter (panretinal) laser surgery for advancing diabetic retinopathy and conclusively demonstrated that focal photocoagulation for CSME reduces the risk of moderate visual loss by 50% or more (Table 42–4). Furthermore, the ETDRS demonstrated that both early scatter (panretinal) laser surgery (before high-risk PDR) and deferral of treatment "until and as soon as high-risk PDR developed are effective in reducing the risk of severe visual loss." Scatter laser surgery, therefore,

Table 42–3. Diabetic Retinopathy Study (DRS)

Major Eligibility Criteria
1. Visual acuity ≥20/100 in each eye.
2. PDR in at least one eye or severe NPDR in both eyes.
3. Both eyes suitable for photocoagulation.
Major Design Features
1. One eye of each patient assigned randomly to photocoagulation (scatter [panretinal], local [direct confluent treatment of surface new vessels], and focal [for macular edema] as appropriate); other eye assigned to follow-up without photocoagulation
2. The eye assigned to treatment then randomly assigned to argon laser or xenon arc
Major Conclusions
1. Photocoagulation reduced risk of SVL by ≥50% (SVL = visual acuity <5/200 at two consecutively completed 4-month follow-up visits)
2. Modest risks of decrease in visual acuity (usually only one line) and constriction of visual field (risks greater with xenon than argon)
3. Treatment benefit outweighs risks for eyes with high-risk PDR (50% 5-year rate of SVL in such eyes without treatment reduced to 20% by treatment)

Table was prepared by Matthew D. Davis, M.D., and the ETDRS Research Group for the Diabetes 200 Program of the American Academy of Ophthalmology. For abbreviations, see Table 42–1.

Table 42–4. Early Treatment Diabetic Retinopathy Study (ETDRS)

Major Eligibility Criteria
1. Visual acuity ≥20/40 (≤20/400 if reduction caused by macular edema)
2. Mild NPDR to non-high-risk PDR, with or without macular edema
3. Both eyes suitable for photocoagulation
Major Design Features
1. One eye of each patient assigned randomly to early photocoagulation and the other to deferral (careful follow-up and photocoagulation if high-risk PDR develops)
2. Patients assigned randomly to aspirin or placebo
Major Conclusions
1. Focal photocoagulation (direct laser for focal leaks and grid laser for diffuse leaks) reduced risk of MVL (doubling of the visual angle) by ≥50% and increased the chance of a small improvement in visual acuity
2. Both early scatter with or without focal photocoagulation and deferral followed by low rates of severe visual loss (5-year rates in deferral subgroups 2–10%; in early photocoagulation groups, 2–6%)
3. Focal photocoagulation should be considered for eyes with CSME
4. Scatter photocoagulation not indicated for mild to moderate NPDR but should be considered as retinopathy approaches high-risk PDR and usually should not be delayed when this high-risk stage is present

Table was prepared by Matthew D. Davis, M.D., and the ETDRS Research Group for the Diabetes 200 Program of the American Academy of Ophthalmology. For abbreviations, see Table 42–1.

should be considered as an eye approaches the high-risk stage and "usually should not be delayed if the eye has reached the high-risk proliferative stage."[25]

Diabetic Retinopathy Vitrectomy Study

The DRVS provided guidelines to most opportune time for vitrectomy surgery for patients with Type I and Type II diabetes who suffered from vitreous hemorrhage[30,31,34] or from severe PDR in eyes with useful vision (Table 42–5).[32,33] Early vitrectomy for eyes with recent severe vitreous hemorrhage and a visual acuity of less than 5/200 was beneficial, especially for patients with Type I diabetes. Furthermore, the chance of achieving visual acuity 10/20 or better was increased by early vitrectomy in eyes with severe proliferating neovascular retinopathy, again especially for patients with Type I diabetes.

DIAGNOSIS, CLASSIFICATION AND MANAGEMENT OF DIABETIC RETINOPATHY

Retinal Lesions

The processes by which diabetes mellitus results in retinopathy and maculopathy are not fully understood. It is apparent in studies with laboratory animals, however, that insulin deficiency itself, even in animals not genetically diabetic, is sufficient to cause diabetic retinopathy.[47] The elevated blood glucose level is accompanied by and

Table 42–5. Diabetic Retinopathy Vitrectomy Study (DRVS)

RECENT SEVERE VITREOUS HEMORRHAGE (GROUP H)
Major Eligibility Criteria
1. Visual acuity ≥5/200
2. Vitreous hemorrhage consistent with visual acuity, duration 1–6 months
3. Macula attached by ultrasound
Major Design Features
1. In most patients, only one eye eligible
2. Eligible eye(s) assigned randomly to early vitrectomy or conventional management (vitrectomy if center of macula detaches or if vitreous hemorrhage persists for 1 year; photocoagulation as needed and as possible)
Major Conclusions
1. Chance of recovery of visual acuity ≥10/20 increased by early vitrectomy, at least in patients with Type I diabetes, who were younger and had more severe PDR (in most severe PDR group, ≥10/20 at 4 years in 50% of early vitrectomy group vs. 12% in conventional management group)
VERY SEVERE PDR WITH USEFUL VISION (GROUP NR)
Major Eligibility Criteria
1. Visual acuity ≥10/200
2. Center of macula attached
3. Extensive, active, neovascular or fibrovascular proliferations
Major Design Features
1. Same as Group H (except conventional management included vitrectomy after a 6-month waiting period in eyes that developed severe vitreous hemorrhage)
Major Conclusions
1. Chance of visual acuity ≥10/20 increased by early vitrectomy, at least for eyes with very severe new vessels

Table was prepared by Matthew D. Davis, M.D., and the ETDRS Research Group for the Diabetes 200 Program of the American Academy of Ophthalmology. For abbreviations, see Table 42–1.

Table 42–6. Proliferative Diabetic Nephropathy at 1-Year Visit, by Severity of Individual Lesion

Lesion	Grade	PDR in 1 Year
H/Ma	Present in 2–5 fields	9%
	Very severe	57%
IRMA	None	9%
	Moderate in 2–5 fields	57%
VB	Absent	15%
	Present in 2–5 fields	59%

Data are from the ETDRS.[28] See Table 42–1 for abbreviations.

probably causes structural, physiologic, and hormonal changes that affect the retinal capillaries, causing the capillaries to become functionally less competent.[48–50]

Six basic pathophysiologic processes are recognized in the development of diabetic retinopathy: 1) loss of pericyte function of retinal capillaries; 2) outpouching of capillary walls to form microaneurysms; 3) closure of retinal capillaries and arterioles; 4) breakdown of the blood/retinal barrier with increased vascular permeability of retinal capillaries; 5) proliferation of new vessels and fibrous tissue; 6) contraction of vitreous and fibrous proliferation with subsequent vitreous hemorrhage and retinal detachment due to traction.

These pathophysiologic processes result in the various lesions of diabetic retinopathy. Loss of function of intramural pericytes of retinal capillaries, either preceding or secondary to the development of nonperfusion of retinal capillaries, results in weakness of the capillary wall.[15,19,20] These changes, resulting in microaneurysm formation, are the earliest signs of diabetic retinopathy.

Various individual retinal lesions identify the risk of progression of retinopathy and visual loss (Table 42–6). The early clinical signs of diabetic retinopathy are microaneurysms, which are saccular outpouchings of retinal capillaries (Fig. 42–1). Ruptured microaneu-

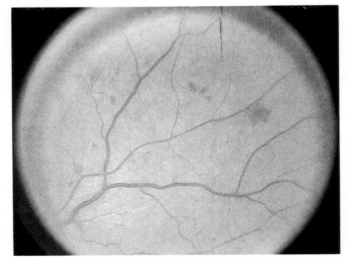

Fig. 42–1. Standard photograph 2A of the modified Airlee House classification of diabetic retinopathy demonstrating a moderate degree of hemorrhage and/or microaneurysms.

rysms, leaking capillaries, and intraretinal microvascular abnormalities result in intraretinal hemorrhages. The clinical appearance of these hemorrhages reflects the retinal architecture of the retinal level where the hemorrhage occurs. Hemorrhages in the nerve-fiber layer assume a more flame-shaped appearance, coinciding with the structure of the nerve-fiber layer that runs parallel to the retinal surface. Hemorrhages deeper in the retina, where the arrangement of cells is more or less perpendicular to the surface of the retina, assume a pinpoint or dot shape and are more characteristic of diabetic retinopathy.

Intraretinal Microvascular Abnormalities

Intraretinal microvascular abnormalities (IRMA) (Fig. 42–2) represent either new vessel growth within the retina or, more likely, pre-existing vessels with endothelial cell proliferation that become "shunts" through areas of nonperfusion. IRMA may be seen adjacent to cotton-wool spots. Multiple IRMA mark a severe stage of nonproliferative retinopathy, and frank neovascularization is likely to appear on the surface of the retina or optic disc within a short time.

Venous Caliber Abnormalities

Venous caliber abnormalities (Fig. 42–3) are indicators of severe retinal hypoxia. These abnormalities can be venous dilation, venous beading, or loop formation. There are large areas of nonperfusion adjacent to the veins. Treatment with scatter (panretinal) photocoagulation may cause these abnormal veins to become less dilated and more regular.

Proliferative Retinopathy

Proliferative retinopathy (Fig. 42–4) is marked by proliferating endothelial cell tubules. The rate of growth

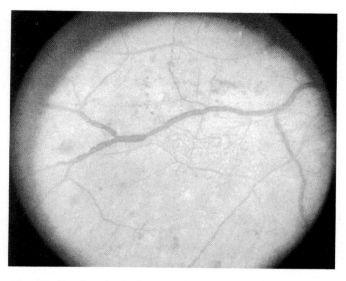

Fig. 42–3. Standard photograph 6B of the modified Airlee House classification of diabetic retinopathy demonstrating venous beading.

of these new vessels is variable. These vessels grow either at or near the optic disc (neovascularization of the disc [NVD]) or elsewhere in the retina (neovascularization elsewhere [NVE]). Translucent fibrous tissue often appears adjacent to the new vessels. This fibroglial tissue appears opaque and becomes adherent to the adjacent vitreous.

Patients with high-risk PDR require immediate scatter laser photocoagulation. High-risk PDR is characterized by any one or more of the following lesions: 1) NVD approximately one-fourth to one-third the disc area or more in size (i.e., greater than or equal to NVD in standard photo 10A; Fig. 42–4). (In 1968 the Airlee

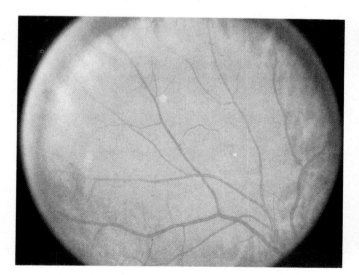

Fig. 42–2. Standard photograph 8A of the modified Airlee House classification of diabetic retinopathy demonstrating intraretinal microvascular abnormalities.

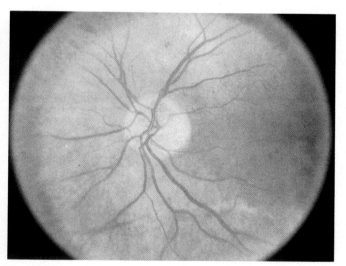

Fig. 42–4. Standard photograph 10A of the modified Airlee House classification of diabetic retinopathy demonstrating neovascularization of the optic disc covering approximately one-fourth to one-third of the disc area.

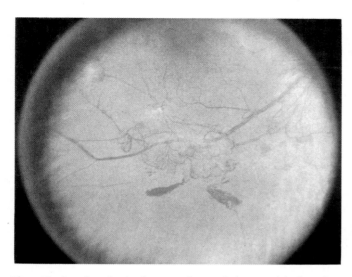

Fig. 42–5. Standard photograph 7 of the modified Airlee House classification of diabetic retinopathy demonstrating neovascularization elsewhere in the retina greater than one-half disc area with fresh hemorrhage present.

House Symposium of Diabetic Retinopathy designated specific "standard photographs" to document levels and severity of diabetic retinopathy; these photographic standards were subsequently modified by the DRS and ETDRS research groups.[9]); 2) NVD less than one-fourth the disc area in size if fresh vitreous or preretinal hemorrhage is present; 3) NVE greater than or equal to one-half the disc area in size if fresh vitreous or preretinal hemorrhage is present (Fig. 42–5).

Attention therefore must be paid to the presence or absence of new vessels, the location of new vessels, the severity of new vessels, and the presence or absence of preretinal or vitreous hemorrhages.[5]

Levels of Diabetic Retinopathy

It is crucial to consider scatter (panretinal) laser surgery as retinopathy approaches or reaches the high-risk stage of PDR. An eye is considered to be approaching the high-risk stage when there are retinal signs of severe or very severe nonproliferative proliferative diabetic retinopathy (NPDR), with or without early PDR (see below), or new vessels not quite fulfilling the definition of high-risk PDR (see below) associated with any level of NPDR. The baseline level of retinopathy indicates the risk of progression from the NPDR stage to early PDR and to high-risk PDR (Tables 42–6, 42–7, and 42–8).[28]

Nonproliferative Diabetic Retinopathy

Diabetic retinopathy is broadly classified as nonproliferative diabetic retinopathy (NPDR) and proliferative diabetic retinopathy (PDR). Diabetic macular edema can occur with either NPDR or PDR and is discussed separately. Accurate diagnosis of a patient's "diabetic retinopathy level" is critical since the risk of progression to PDR and high-risk PDR varies depending on specific NPDR level (Table 42–8, Fig. 42–6).

Mild NPDR is marked by at least one retinal microaneurysm, but hemorrhages and microaneurysms are less than those in the ETDRS standard photograph 2A in all four retinal quadrants (Fig. 42–1 and Table 42–7). No other retinal lesion or abnormality associated with diabetes is present. Those with mild NPDR have a 5% risk of progression to PDR within 1 year and a 15% risk of progression to high-risk PDR within 5 years (Table 42–8).

Moderate NPDR (Table 42–7) is characterized by hemorrhages and/or microaneurysms (H/Ma) greater than those pictured in the ETDRS standard photograph 2A in at least one field but less than four retinal quadrants, with or without venous beading and IRMA to a mild degree. The risk of progression to PDR within 1 year is 12 to 27%, and the risk of progression to high-risk PDR within 5 years is 33% (Table 42–8).

Patients with mild or moderate NPDR generally are not candidates for scatter (panretinal) laser surgery and can be followed safely at 6- to 12-month intervals as determined by the examiner. The presence of macular edema, even with mild or moderate degrees of NPDR, requires follow-up in a shorter period, and if CSME is present, focal laser treatment is advisable (Table 42–8). Coincident

Table 42–7. Levels of Retinopathy

NONPROLIFERATIVE DIABETIC RETINOPATHY
A. Mild NPDR
   At least one microaneurysm
   Definition not met for B, C, D, E, or F (see below)
B. Moderate NPDR
   H/Ma greater than standard photograph 2A (Fig. 42–1) or
   SE, VB, and IRMA definitely present
   Definition not met for C, D, E, or F (see below)
C. Severe NPDR
   H/Ma greater than standard photograph 2A (Fig. 42–1) in all 4 quadrants or
   VB in 2 or more quadrants (Fig. 42–3) or
   IRMA greater than standard photograph 8A (Fig. 42–2) in at least 1 quadrant
D. Very-severe NPDR
   Any two or more of C above
   Definition not met for E or F
   PROLIFERATIVE DIABETIC RETINOPATHY (PDR)
   Composition of PDR (at least one of the following)
   1. NVD or NVE
   2. Preretinal or vitreous hemorrhage
   3. Fibrous tissue proliferation
E. Early PDR
   New vessels
   Definition not met for F
F. High-risk PDR
   1. NVD ≥1/3–1/4 disc area (Fig. 42–4) or
   2. NVD and vitreous or preretinal hemorrhage or
   3. NVE ≥1/2 disc area and preretinal or vitreous hemorrhage (Fig. 42–5)
   CLINICALLY SIGNIFICANT DIABETIC MACULAR EDEMA
   1. Thickening of the retina located ≤500 μm from the center of the macula or
   2. HE with thickening of the adjacent retina located ≤500 μm from the center of the macula or
   3. A zone of retinal thickening, 1 disc area or larger in size located ≤1 disc diameter from the center of the macula

Definitions are from ETDRS.[26,28] See Table 42–1 for abbreviations.

Table 42–8. General Management Recommendations

LEVEL OF RETINOPATHY	NATURAL COURSE		EVALUATION		TREATMENT STRATEGIES		
	Rate of Progression to		Color Fundus Photo	FA	PRP	Focal	F/U (mo)
	PDR 1 Yr	HRC 5 Yr					
1. Mild NPDR	5%	15%					
No macular edema			No	No	No	No	12
Macular edema*			Yes	Occ	No	No	4–6
CSME			Yes	Yes	No	Yes	2–4
2. Moderate NPDR	12–27%	33%					
No macular edema			Yes	No	No	No	6–8
Macular edema*			Yes	Occ	No	No	4–6
CSME			Yes	Yes	No	Yes	2–4
3. Severe NPDR	52%	60%					
No macular edema			Yes	No	Rarely	No	3–4
Macular edema*			Yes	Occ	OccAF	Occ	2–3
CSME			Yes	Yes	OccAF	Yes	2–3
4. Very severe NPDR	75%	75%					
No macular edema			Yes	No	Occ	No	2–3
Macular edema*			Yes	Occ	OccAF	Occ	2–3
CSME			Yes	Yes	OccAF	Yes	2–3
5. Non-high-risk PDR		75%					
No macular edema			Yes	No	Occ	No	2–3
Macular edema*			Yes	Occ	OccAF	Occ	2–3
CSME			Yes	Yes	OccAF	Yes	2–3
6. High-risk PDR							
No macular edema			Yes	No	Yes	No	2–3
Macular edema*			Yes	Yes	Yes	Usually	1–2
CSME			Yes	Yes	Yes	Yes	1–2

HRC = high-risk characteristics; FA = fluorescein angiogram; PRP = scatter (panretinal) photocoagulation; F/U = follow-up; Occ = occasionally; OccAF = occasionally after focal. For all other abbreviations, see Table 42–1.
*Not CSME.

medical problems or pregnancy will influence the period of re-evaluation.

Severe NPDR, based on the severity of H/Ma, IRMA, and venous beading, is characterized by any one of the

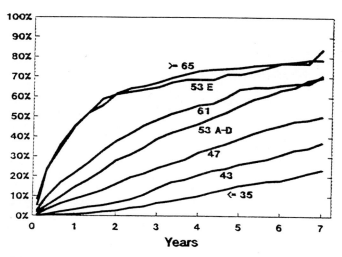

Fig. 42–6. Life-table cumulative event rates of high-risk proliferative retinopathy by level of retinopathy severity at baseline in eyes assigned to deferral of photocoagulation in the ETDRS: level ≥35, mild NPDR; level 43, moderate NPDR; level 47, moderate to severe NPDR; level 53 A–D, severe NPDR; level 53 E, very severe NPDR; level 61, early PDR; level 65, PDR less than high-risk PDR.[27] See table 42–1 for abbreviations.

following lesions (Table 42–7): 1) H/Ma greater than in standard photo 2A (Fig. 42–1) in four quadrants or 2) venous beading (Fig. 42–3) in two or more quadrants or 3) IRMA greater than standard photo 8A (Fig. 42–2) in at least one quadrant.

Eyes with severe NPDR have a 52% risk of developing PDR within 1 year and a 60% risk of developing high-risk PDR within 5 years. These patients require follow-up evaluation in 2 to 4 months. Treatment of CSME is strongly indicated because of the risk of the development of PDR and high-risk PDR; some eyes with macular edema, even if it is not clinically significant, may require focal treatment in preparation for impending scatter (panretinal) laser surgery, which may also be indicated, as determined by the clinical judgment of the retinal specialist (Table 42–8).

Eyes with very severe NPDR (Table 42–7) have two or more lesions of severe NPDR but no frank neovascularization and a 75% risk of developing PDR within 1 year. Patients with very severe NPDR may be candidates for scatter (panretinal) laser surgery, and macular edema, if present, may require treatment. Very close follow-up evaluation at 2- to 3-month intervals is important (Table 42–8).

Early Proliferative Diabetic Retinopathy

Diabetic retinopathy marked by new vessel growth on the optic disc (NVD) or elsewhere (NVE) on the retina or by fibrous-tissue proliferation is designated PDR. Early PDR does not meet the definition of high-risk PDR (Table

42−7). Eyes with early PDR (less than high risk) have a 75% risk of developing high-risk PDR within a 5-year period. These eyes may require scatter (panretinal) laser surgery; and macular edema, even if not clinically significant, may benefit from focal treatment before scatter is initiated (Table 42−8).

In patients with early PDR (less than high-risk PDR), early scatter (panretinal) laser surgery should be considered if any of the associated findings are present: 1) any new vessels accompanied by severe or very severe NPDR; 2) elevated new vessels 3) or NVD.

In the presence of macular edema, patients with severe NPDR or worse should be considered for focal treatment of macular edema whether or not the macular edema is clinically significant, in preparation for the impending future need of scatter laser photocoagulation (Table 42−8).

Role of Clinical Fluorescein Angiography in Management of Diabetic Retinopathy

Fluorescein angiography of the macula in the presence of CSME is fundamental for the detection of treatable lesions as described below. However, its use for identifying lesions such as NVE or feeder vessels on NVD is not necessary since scatter (panretinal) laser surgery is the method of choice for the treatment of diabetic retinopathy as it approaches or reaches the high-risk stage.

Angiographic risk factors for progression of NPDR to PDR have been identified.[27,29] Analysis of data for the untreated (deferred) eyes in the ETDRS indicates that the following lesions are independently related to outcome: 1) fluorescein leakage, 2) capillary loss on fluorescein angiography, 3) capillary dilatation on fluorescein angiography; and 4) the following color fundus photographic risk factors: IRMA; venous beading; and H/Ma. Hard and soft exudates have an inverse relationship to progression.

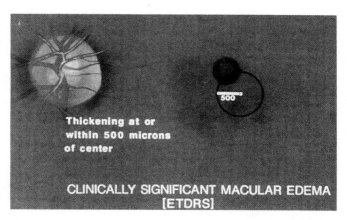

Fig. 42−7. Schematic showing clinically significant macular edema with thickening of the macular <500 μm from the center of the macula (schematic courtesy Robert Murphy, M.D.)

It is widely accepted that capillary loss as documented on fluorescein angiography is a risk factor for progression of NPDR to PDR.[27,29,48−50] However, capillary dilatation on fluorescein angiography, fluorescein leakage, capillary loss on fluorescein angiography, and the ETDRS color fundus photographic retinopathy are all closely correlated. Although the fluorescein angiography abnormalities provide additional prognostic information, the color fundus photographic grading of retinopathy levels of both eyes gives the same prognostic results.[28,29] Therefore, the increase in power to predict progression from NPDR to PDR by fluorescein angiography is "not of significant clinical importance to warrant routine fluorescein angiography."[29]

Periodic follow-up retinal examinations, however, are necessary. The appropriate interval can be determined by skillful grading of seven standard-field stereo color fundus

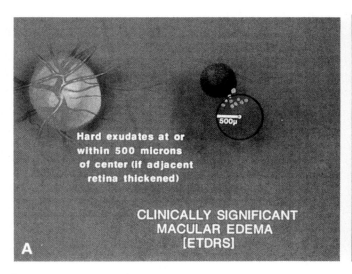

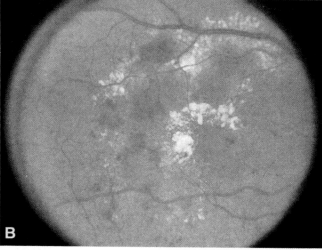

Fig. 42−8. A: Schematic showing clinically significant macular edema (CSME) with hard exudates at or within 500 μm from the center of the macula, with thickening of the retina adjacent to the exudates (schematic courtesy Robert Murphy, M.D.). B: Clinical appearance of hard exudates <500 μm from the center of the macula. There is thickening of the adjacent retina, not appreciated without stereoscopic observation.

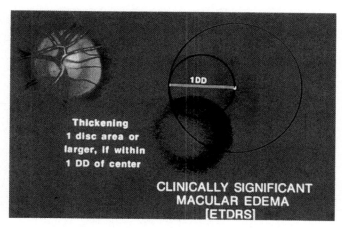

Fig. 42–9. Schematic showing area of thickening one disc area in size, part of which is within one disc diameter of the center of the macula (schematic courtesy Robert Murphy, M.D.).

photographs and/or of retinal examination by an ophthalmologist experienced in the management of diabetic eye disease. Since the level of diabetic retinopathy derived from color fundus photography is predictive enough to establish frequency of follow-up, since fluorescein angiography classification cannot "identify all cases destined to progress," and since initiation of scatter (panretinal) laser photocoagulation should be considered as diabetic retinopathy approaches (before or just as it reaches) the high-risk stage, "periodic follow-up of all patients with diabetic retinopathy continues to be of fundamental clinical importance."[29] Table 42–8 summarizes the appropriate use of fundus photography and fluorescein angiography in monitoring and treating diabetic retinopathy and macular edema.

Diabetic Macular Edema

Diabetic macular disease may be present at any level of retinopathy (Table 42–8) and alters the structure of the macula, significantly affecting its function, in any of the following ways: 1) macular edema, that is, a collection of intraretinal fluid in the macula with or without lipid exudates and with or without cystoid changes; 2) nonperfusion of parafoveal capillaries with or without intraretinal fluid; 3) traction in the macula by fibrous tissue proliferation causing dragging of the retinal tissue, surface wrinkling, or detachment of the macula; 4) intraretinal or preretinal hemorrhage in the macula; 5) lamellar or full-thickness retinal hole formation; 6) combination of the above.

Clinically, macular edema is retinal thickening within 2 disc diameters of the center of the macula (not fluorescein leakage without thickening). Retinal thickening or hard exudates with adjacent retinal thickening that threaten or involve the center of the macula are considered to be clinically significant. CSME as defined by the ETDRS includes any one of the following lesions (Table 42–7); 1) retinal thickening at or within 500 μm from the center of the macula (Fig. 42–7); 2) hard exudates at or within 500 μm from the center of the macula, if there is thickening of the adjacent retina (Fig. 42–8); or 3) an area or areas of retinal thickening at least one disc area in size, at least part of which is within 1 disc diameter of the center of the macula (Fig. 42–9).

In managing CSME, there are particular retinal lesions identified on fluoroscein angiography that are amenable to treatment. These "treatable lesions" associated with macular edema include 1) focal leaks more than 500 μm from the center of the macula thought to be causing retinal thickening and/or hard exudates (Fig. 42–10); 2) focal leaks 300 to 500 μm from the center of the macula thought to be causing retinal thickening and/or hard

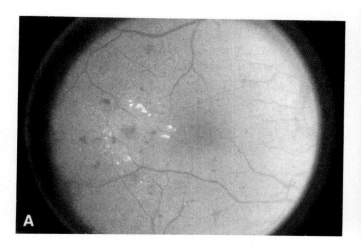

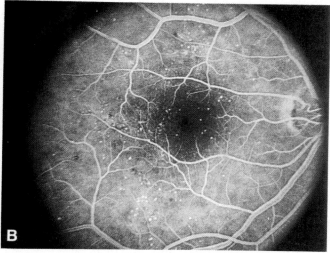

Fig. 42–10. A: Clinical picture showing macular edema >500 μm from the center of the macula (edema not appreciated without stereoscopic evaluation). B: Fluorescein angiogram showing focal leaks from microaneurysms >500 μm from the center of the macula.

exudates, if the treating ophthalmologist does not believe that treatment is likely to destroy the remaining
perifoveal capillary network (Fig. 42–11); and visual
acuity is 20/40 or worse; 3) areas of diffuse leakage (Fig.
42–12) from extensive numbers of microaneurysms or
from many IRMAs; or 4) avascular zones, other than the
normal foveal avascular zone, not previously treated (Fig.
42–12B).

Focal laser surgery for CSME consists of "direct" laser
treatment, "grid" laser treatment, or "combination" focal
laser and grid laser treatment. These treatment methods
are described in detail elsewhere.[18,20] Table 42–8 summarizes the management recommendations for CSME at
the various retinopathy levels.

LASER PHOTOCOAGULATION

Timing of Photocoagulation

The 3-year risk of moderate visual loss from macular
edema in the ETDRS without focal laser treatment was
30%. Focal laser surgery for CSME reduced this risk to
15%,[17] a reduction in risk of approximately 50%. Focal
treatment also increased the chance of improvement in
visual acuity of one line or more. On the other hand,
scatter (panretinal) laser surgery was not effective in
managing diabetic macular edema and in some cases may
have had a deleterious effect on the progression of
macular edema.

Eyes with CSME and retinopathy approaching high-risk
PDR are best treated first with focal photocoagulation for
the macular edema 6 to 8 weeks before initiating scatter
(panretinal) laser surgery. Eyes with mild or moderate
NPDR and CSME respond best to prompt focal photocoagulation, with scatter treatment delayed unless very
severe NPDR or high-risk PDR occurs. Delaying scatter
photocoagulation while focal treatment is being completed is unlikely to increase the risk of severe visual loss,
provided the retinopathy is not progressing rapidly and
careful follow-up can be maintained. Delaying scatter
photocoagulation while focal treatment is completed in
eyes with high-risk PDR usually is not advisable.

Focal treatment was not attended by adverse effects on
central visual field or color vision in comparison with
eyes assigned to deferral of focal treatment in the
ETDRS.[18] Any harmful effects of early photocoagulation
reflected by constriction of the peripheral visual fields
seem to be due mostly to scatter photocoagulation.
Because the principal benefit of treatment is the prevention of a further decrease in visual acuity, focal laser
surgery should be considered in all eyes with CSME,
especially if the center of the macula is threatened or
involved, even if visual acuity is normal.

The DRS demonstrated in 1976 that scatter (panretinal) photocoagulation was effective in reducing the risk
of severe visual loss from high-risk PDR. One question of
concern for the ETDRS was whether earlier scatter
photocoagulation, before the development of high-risk
PDR, justified the side effects and risks of laser surgery
(Table 42–9), since the DRS did not provide a clear

choice between prompt treatment or deferral of treatment unless there was progression to high-risk PDR.

In the ETDRS, early treatment, compared with "deferral" of photocoagulation until the development of high-
risk PDR,[22] was associated with a small reduction in the
incidence of severe visual loss, but 5-year rates of severe
visual loss were low for both the early treatment group
and the group assigned to "deferral" of treatment (2.6%
and 3.7%, respectively). Provided that careful follow-up
can be maintained, scatter laser surgery is not recommended for eyes with mild or moderate NPDR.[25] When
retinopathy is more severe (i.e., severe or very severe
NPDR and early PDR), scatter photocoagulation should
be "considered and usually should not be delayed if the
eye has reached the high-risk proliferative stage."[25]

As retinopathy approaches the high-risk stage (very
severe NPDR or early PDR), the benefits and risks of early
photocoagulation may be roughly balanced; the benefit of
a reduction of the risk of severe visual loss from early
photocoagulation may be more important in an eye that
has almost a 50% risk of reaching high-risk stage within 1
year. Initiating scatter photocoagulation early in at least
one eye seems particularly appropriate when both of a
patient's eyes are approaching the high-risk stage, because optimal timing of photocoagulation may be difficult
if both eyes need photocoagulation simultaneously. Also,
prompt scatter photocoagulation should be considered
for eyes with neovascularization in the anterior chamber
angle, whether or not high-risk PDR is present.[25]

Treatment Program

The treatment program (Table 42–8) for diabetic
retinopathy consists of 1) initial scatter laser photocoagulation surgery as the diabetic retinopathy approaches or
reaches the high-risk stage, 2) careful follow-up at
4-month intervals following the treatment, 3) re-treat-
ment of persistent or recurrent treatable lesions, 4) focal
laser photocoagulation treatment for macular edema
prior to scatter (panretinal) photocoagulation to reduce
the risk of progression of macular edema secondary to
scatter photocoagulation (see above).

As high-risk PDR is reached, the major threat for SVL is
traction retinal detachment; a lesser threat is the vitreous
hemorrhage. The primary goal of the scatter laser surgery
is the prevention of traction retinal detachment, particularly involving the macula.

Various strategies are involved in follow-up treatment.
The ocular lesions to be considered for follow-up
photocoagulation include new flat neovascularization or
elevated neovascularization; new, persistent, or recurrent
CSME; and, rarely, feeder vessels to NVD. The treatment
methods include additional scatter laser treatment, local
laser to NVE, focal laser for CSME, pars plana vitrectomy
for recurrent hemorrhages with fibrovascular proliferation causing traction, or perhaps merely continued
observation. Further scatter treatment may be placed
between previously placed laser scars as long as these
scars do not become confluent and the extent of the
scatter treatment is not such as to totally destroy retinal
function.

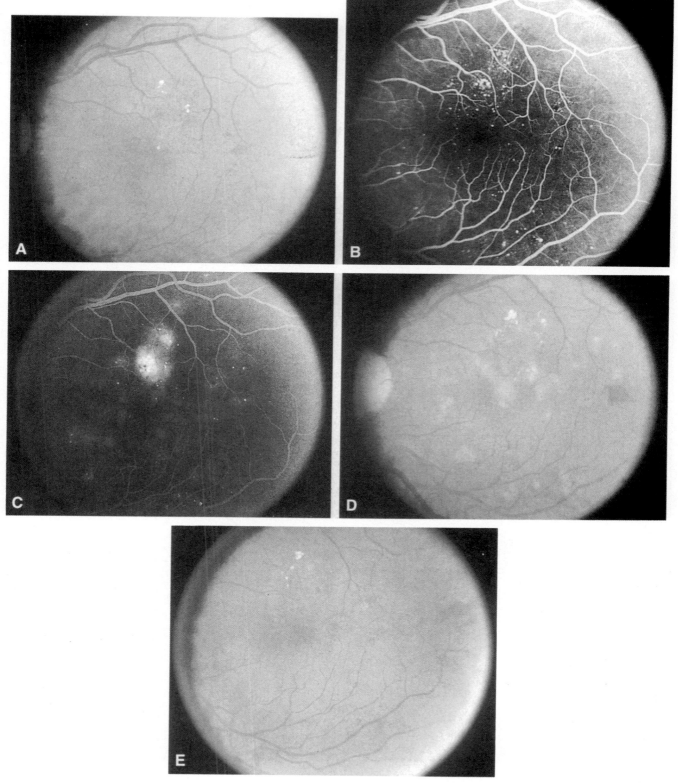

Fig. 42–11.　A: There is a small area of retinal thickening just above the center of the macula (poorly appreciated without stereopsis), detectable monocularly because of blurring of the choroidal pattern. Several microaneurysms are visible within the thickened area. There is a little hard exudate around the edges of the edematous patch, some of which extends almost to the center of the macula. Thickening extends to within 500 μm of the center of the macula (clinically significant macular edema). Visual acuity was 20/15. B: In the 17- to 18-second phase of the fluorescein angiogram, microaneurysms and slightly dilated capillaries are visible in the area of thickening. C: The 7-minute phase of the angiogram shows leakage into the retina from the two groups of microaneurysms noted in B. D: Treatment has been applied to most of the microaneurysms. E: Four months later the appearance of the retina is satisfactory, with flattening of the center of the macula and disappearance of the thickening noted before the treatment. Visual acuity remains at 20/15.

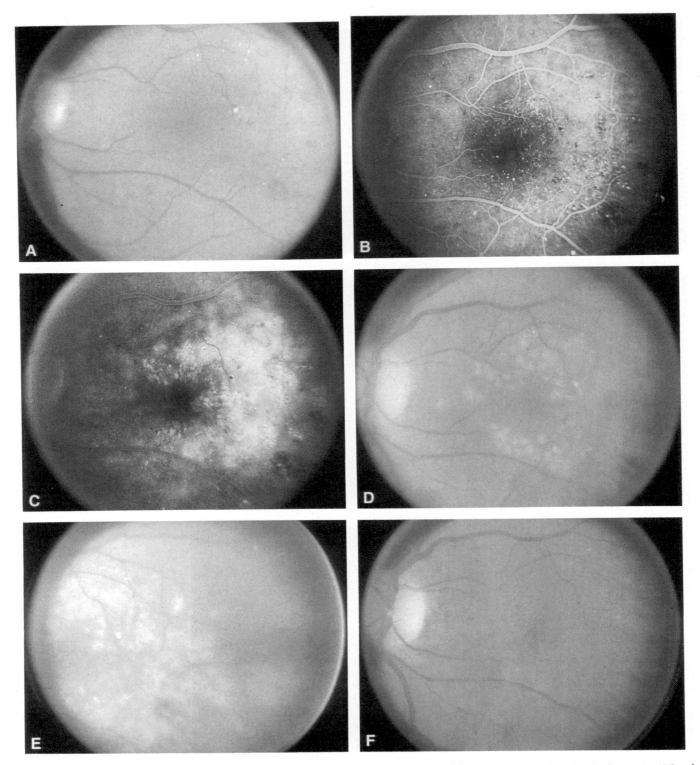

Fig. 42–12. A: Clinical picture showing retinal thickening temporal to the center of the macula extending just to the center. Visual acuity is 20/40. B: Early phase of the angiogram shows capillary loss adjacent to the foveal avascular zone, capillary dilation, and scattered microaneurysms. C: The 7-minute phase of the angiogram shows extensive small cystoid spaces temporal to the center of the macula and above and below it. The center appears uninvolved. D: The microaneurysms have been treated focally and, in addition, laser burns have been applied in a grid pattern in the areas of diffuse leakage. E: The temporal extent of the grid laser treatment. F: Four months later hemorrhages and hard exudates have decreased and the retinal thickening can no longer be detected. Visual acuity was 20/25. G: The 7-minute phase of the angiogram showing disappearance of most of the cystoid space visible in C.

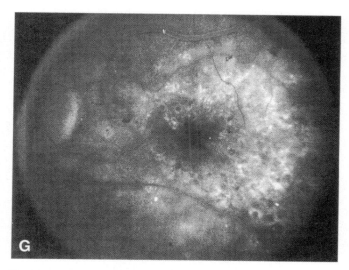

Fig. 42–12. Continued

While laser surgery often is considered painless, in younger patients some pain may be associated with the treatment. There also may be some discomfort or pain in all patients when the peripheral retina is treated. Complications and side effects of laser photocoagulation are summarized in Table 42–9.

In summary, scatter treatment significantly reduces the risk of severe visual loss from PDR. Both early scatter treatment prior to development of high-risk PDR and deferral of treatment until the development of high-risk PDR reduce the risk of severe visual loss. The rates of

Table 42–9. Complications and Side Effects of Scatter (Panretinal) Laser Photocoagulation

1. Field constriction and night blindness
   Depends upon extent of scatter
2. Foveal burn
   Landmarks may be difficult to identify
3. Macular edema
   About 10% risk of mild visual loss
4. Foveal traction
   Occurs with remission
   Occurs with burns applied over blood
5. Serous and/or choroidal detachment
   Acute angle-closure glaucoma possible
6. Anterior segment
   Posterior synechiae
   Cornea and lens burns
   Internal ophthalmoplegia
   Uncommon with multiple sessions, light to moderately intense burns, and use of laser instead of xenon
7. Pain
   Younger diabetic patients: more painful
   Peripheral retina: more painful
   Reassurance
   Retrobulbar anesthesia rarely needed
8. Retrobulbar hemorrhage due to retrobulbar anesthesia injection
   Laser surgery can continue
   More frequent without sedation
   Watch central retinal artery
9. Loss of follow-up
   Importance of patient/doctor relationship

severe visual loss are low for each group. Consequently, it is recommended that scatter laser treatment not be used for mild to moderate NPDR. For severe NPDR and early PDR, scatter treatment is appropriate when close follow-up is unlikely or the disease process is progressing rapidly.

NONRETINAL OCULAR COMPLICATIONS

Clinical Significance

The potentially devastating effects of diabetes on the retina and the attendant threat of visual loss are generally well recognized. All structures of the eye, however, are susceptible to the deleterious effects of diabetes (Table 42–10). Some of these effects are of little consequence and go unnoticed by both the patient and the doctor. Other effects, while not sight-threatening, result in uncomfortable vision or other symptoms interfering with normal visual function. Still other effects, while perhaps most prevalent with diabetes, must be fully evaluated to rule out potentially life-threatening underlying causes other than diabetes.

Complications

Mononeuropathies

Mononeuropathies of the third, fourth, or sixth cranial nerves occasionally arise in association with diabetes.[51] These nerve palsies are usually of serious concern to the patient and present a significant diagnostic challenge, since misdiagnosis may result in a life-threatening lesion remaining untreated. On the other hand, a full neurologic evaluation, including computed tomography, magnetic resonance imaging, and other tests, may prove unwarranted and unnecessary. In one review of cranial nerve palsies treated in a diabetic patient population in 1967, 42% of mononeuropathies were not diabetic in origin.[52] This finding underscores the danger of routinely attributing mononeuropathies, even in a diabetic person, to the diabetic condition itself without carefully ruling out other potential causes. The percentage of all extraocular muscle palsies attributable to diabetes mellitus is estimated at 4.5 to 6%.[53–55]

Histopathologic studies of diabetic third-nerve palsies suggest that they are secondary to ischemic infarction of the nutrient vessels to the oculomotor nerve within the cavernous sinus or subarachnoid space.[56–57] By extension, vascular infarct with resulting ischemia to any of the cranial nerves serving the extraocular muscles is generally accepted as the cause of diabetes-related cranial nerve palsies.

The trochlear or fourth cranial nerve is the least likely to be affected by diabetes[51,53,54] (Table 42–11). Palsies of the oculomotor or third cranial nerve are more frequent and are usually accompanied by a ptosis of the affected eye, which may block or mask a horizontal and vertical diplopia. The ptosis itself, however, is usually sufficient to cause a person to seek medical evaluation. Characteristically, the affected eye has an exotropic and hypotropic posture (down and out). Pain may be associ-

Table 42–10. Nonretinal Complications of Diabetes Mellitus

Structure	Complication	Management
Extraocular muscles	Mononeuropathy	1. Examination to rule out other causes 2. Consultation with internist or diabetologist 3. Neurologic referral 4. Patient education 5. Follow-up 6 weeks or as indicated
Cornea	Decreased sensitivity Recurrent erosion Abrasion Ulceration	1. Artificial tears 2. Patient education 3. Careful contact lens-patient selection
Iris	Rubeosis iridis Neovascular glaucoma	1. Referral for possible panretinal photocoagulation 2. Management of glaucoma
Lens	Diabetic cataract Premature cataract Refractive fluctuations	1. Optimal refractive correction 2. Surgical referral 3. Control of blood glucose level

ated with the onset of the palsy, which is usually acute.[52,58–61] The pupil is usually unaffected or spared in diabetic third-nerve palsy, although there may be pupillary involvement in up to 20% of diabetes-induced third-nerve palsies.[62,63] Pupil involvement suggests pressure on the nerve by a mass lesion or aneurysm and is sufficient reason to arrange immediate consultation for neurologic evaluation. In one series, 19.2% of all oculomotor nerve palsies were associated with diabetes.[64]

Paralysis of the abducens or sixth cranial nerve occurs at least as often as third-nerve palsy in diabetes.[51,53,54] Patients with sixth-nerve palsies usually complain of horizontal diplopia, sometimes only on extreme lateral gaze to the side of the affected eye. The affected eye is esotropic and usually cannot be moved past the midline. The sixth cranial nerve has a lengthy path, and there are myriad causes of abducens nerve insult, many of which are life-threatening.

Mononeuropathies also may be the initial presenting sign of new-onset diabetes. Diabetes should therefore be considered in the differential diagnosis of any mononeu-

ropathy affecting the extraocular muscles, even in patients who do not claim a history of diabetes. Diabetes-induced third-, fourth-, and sixth-nerve palsies are usually self-limited and should begin to clear spontaneously in 2 to 6 months, although more or less time may be needed and the palsies may recur.

Treatment involves patching one eye to eliminate diplopia, if symptoms warrant, and a mild analgesic if needed. In monocular patients, or in patients with poor vision in one eye, the maintenance of vision, especially when ptosis obstructs the visual axis of the better seeing eye, may present a challenge. Taping of the lid or the use of a ptosis crutch may be required, although the problem of corneal drying is significant.

Periorbital and Orbital Structures

Waite and Beetham reported a slightly higher frequency of xanthelasma in their diabetic patients than in their nondiabetic patients.[51] The xanthelasma are usually of no clinical significance. A far more serious complication is orbital infection, usually at the apex of the orbit, with fungi of the order Mucorales (see Chapter 47). Although rare, mucormycosis (also called phycomycosis) is a fungal infection that develops in the adjacent periorbital sinuses in predisposed persons.[65,66] Schwartz and co-workers found that 80% of their patients with the disorder had diabetes; most had diabetic ketoacidosis.[66] The condition is frequently fatal, and prompt diagnosis is crucial. The patient typically has internal and external ophthalmoplegia, as well as decreased vision, proptosis, and ptosis. Treatment of the diabetic condition and aggressive treatment of the infectious organism with amphotericin B may result in recovery, although the survival rate still remains at only 57%.[67,68]

Conjunctiva and Lacrimal System

Changes in the microcirculation of the bulbar conjunctiva of diabetic persons have been identified. In one series, microaneurysms of the bulbar conjunctiva were observed before cataract surgery in 63.6% of 22 eyes of diabetic patients.[69] Histologically, these conjunctival microaneurysms show a thickened basement membrane,

Table 42–11. Diabetic Nerve Palsies

Cranial Nerve	Symptoms and Signs
III (oculomotor)	1. Complete or partial ptosis 2. Horizontal and vertical diplopia 3. Affected eye "down and out" 4. Possible supraorbital pain 5. Pupillary sparing (80% of cases) 6. Decreased sursumduction and adduction
IV (trochlear)	1. Vertical diplopia with associated esotropia 2. Vertical deviation increases in downward gaze or when head is tilted to side of affected muscle 3. Vertical deviation decreases with abduction of the affected eye 4. Esotropia increases with downward gaze
VI (abducens)	1. Lateral or horizontal diplopia 2. Esotropia of the affected eye 3. Decreased abduction 4. Possible head turn in the direction of the affected eye

proliferation of endothelium, and lamellated hyaline deposits similar to the retinal microaneurysms in diabetic retinopathy.[70] Diurnal variations in the dilation of conjunctival veins have also been noted.[71] Insulin use itself appears to affect the composition of tears, sometimes resulting in a decrease in their lysozyme content.[72]

Conjunctivitis and other disorders of the conjunctiva and lacrimal system need to be treated aggressively. Mild infections or marginal dry-eye syndromes potentially can cause serious ocular injuries, particularly in the presence of neuropathies or compromised corneal integrity.

Cornea

The cornea of the diabetic person is often more susceptible to injury and slower to heal after injury than is the cornea of a nondiabetic person. A potential threat to corneal integrity is the measured reduction of corneal sensitivity in the diabetic individual.[73] Measured corneal sensitivity was significantly lower in poorly controlled diabetic dogs than in nondiabetic dogs and diabetic dogs with good blood glucose control.[74] The decrease in corneal sensitivity was also more marked with increased duration of diabetes in the dogs with poorly controlled diabetes.

The reduction of corneal sensitivity results in elevated tactile corneal thresholds.[75] This reduction usually affects both eyes symmetrically and is the result of diffuse polyneuropathy of the trigeminal nerve and its branches. Other studies have suggested that panretinal photocoagulation can reduce corneal sensitivity caused by inadvertent thermal injury to the sensory nerves to the cornea between the choroid and the sclera.[76] The reduction of corneal sensitivity may predispose a person to the development of neurotrophic corneal ulcerations.[77] Furthermore, there is mounting evidence supporting the clinical impression that once corneal abrasions develop the cornea in the diabetic patient is slower to heal than the cornea in the nondiabetic patient. The corneal tissue most likely responsible for this delayed wound healing is the basement membrane of the epithelium.[78-80]

Waite and Beetham found disorders in the deeper layers of the cornea as well,[51] and subsequent research has verified the presence of these wrinkles in Descemet's membrane layer in diabetic persons.[81,82] Subsequent studies demonstrated increased corneal thickness in diabetic individuals compared with that in nondiabetic control individuals,[83,84] changes representing minimal corneal swelling, possibly as the result of increased corneal hydration.

Potential corneal complications affect contact-lens wear for diabetic patients. The diabetic person may be a poor candidate for contact lenses, since discomfort from a poorly fitting or damaged lens may be absent because of a reduction in corneal sensitivity. Corneal abrasions or minor erosions that may be detected in an otherwise healthy cornea may develop into significant ulcerations. Long-term (2-week) extended-wear contact lenses should be used with extreme caution and careful monitoring and reserved only for patients with optimal conditions and specific needs, such as aphakia. All diabetic contact-lens users need to be properly educated to be aware of potential problems, early signs of lens rejection and infection, or corneal abrasion. The risk of corneal abrasion and the delay of corneal wound healing apparent in diabetic persons because of irregularities in the corneal basement epithelium dictate careful and selective contact-lens wear, although diabetes itself is not a contraindication for the use of rigid or soft contact lenses. Many of the programmed-replacement or flexible-wear lenses provide adequate safeguards for successful adaptation to contact-lens wear.

The tendency for corneal abrasion may necessitate the use of artificial tears, particularly in dry environments. Patients with diabetes should be alerted to the potential side effects of contact lenses, and follow-up evaluations need to be frequent and thorough. The necessity of wearing safety glasses and goggles for appropriate work and sport environments should be emphasized. For ocular examination and treatment, care must be exercised to avoid corneal insult when treating or examining the retina with a corneal contact fundus lens, particularly if the patient has had a corneal abrasion in the past.

Iris

Diabetic complications affecting the iris have been well documented and the subject of much study. Glycogen deposits in the pigment epithelial cells of the iris can cause thickening of ocular tissue and depigmentation of the epithelial layer of the iris.[51] Similar glycogen deposition occurs in the retina, optic nerve, epithelium of the lens capsule, and the ciliary body.[51,85,86] The most serious diabetic complication affecting the iris is rubeosis iridis, a growth of new blood vessels on the iris (Fig. 42–13). Usually these vessels are first observed at the pupillary border and may resemble grape clusters in appearance. If rubeosis progresses, a fine network of vessels may grow over the iris tissue and into the filtration angle of the eye. Fibrous tissue accompanying the new vessels may contract and pull the underlying pigmented layer of the iris forward through the pupillary opening, resulting in ectropion uveae. Fibrovascular growth in the filtration angle may result in peripheral anterior synechiae. Closure of the angle by the fibrovascular network results in neovascular glaucoma, although intraocular pressure may be elevated prior to angle involvement because of protein and cellular leakage from the proliferating vessels.[87,88] This glaucoma is difficult to manage and requires aggressive treatment.

Usually rubeosis iridis is first seen around the pupillary margin, although the vessels can grow initially in or near the filtration angle. Evaluation with a slit-lamp biomicroscope is necessary to observe and evaluate these vessels. The development of neovascular glaucoma in one eye is strongly correlated with the development of the same condition in the patient's other eye.

Diabetes is the second leading cause of neovascular glaucoma, accounting for 32.2% of cases, as opposed to 36.1% of cases resulting from retinal venous obstructive disease.[89] This neovascularization of the anterior segment occurs in 4 to 7% of diabetic eyes and may be

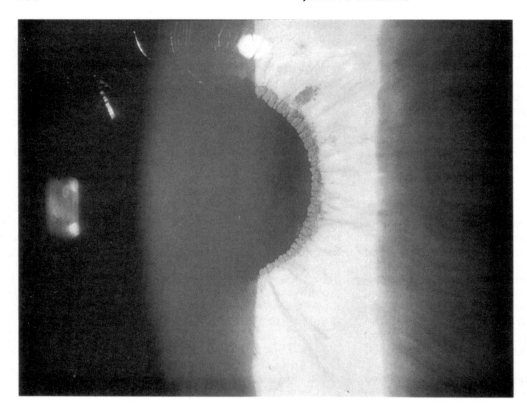

Fig. 42–13. Rubeosis iridis around the pupillary margin.

present in up to 40 to 60% of eyes with proliferative retinopathy.[90–92]

Treatment for rubeosis iridis and neovascular glaucoma includes scatter (panretinal) laser photocoagulation; goniophotocoagulation with a green or yellow laser; topical antiglaucoma medications; systemic antiglaucoma medications; antiglaucomatous filtration surgery, including Molteno valve implants; or a combination of the above therapies.[2,93–97]

Glaucoma

Open-angle glaucoma is 1.4 times more common in the diabetic population than in the nondiabetic population.[98–101] The prevalence of glaucoma increases with age and duration of diabetes, but medical therapy for open-angle glaucoma is generally effective. Choice of treatment of open-angle glaucoma in diabetic individuals must be influenced by the patient's general medical condition. Caution must be exercised with the use of topical β-adrenergic blockers in masking hypoglycemic symptoms or affecting concurrent cardiovascular disease. Acetozolamide or other carbonic anhydrase inhibitors may be used if needed, but since these medications can cause a metabolic acidosis, electrolyte monitoring should be done more frequently. The presence of renal disease may influence how these and other pressure-lowering drugs may be used, and close cooperation with the internist is important.

Argon laser trabeculoplasty may normalize intraocular pressures in some if medical therapy proves ineffective.

Narrow-angle glaucoma or acute angle-closure glaucoma is comparatively rare. Narrow-angle glaucoma does not seem to be more common in persons with diabetes than in the general population, but investigations suggest the shallower the anterior chamber of the patient's eye, the more likely the patient is to respond abnormally to an oral glucose tolerance test.[102] The postulated mechanism for this association is autonomic dysfunction within the anterior segment of the eye resulting in a hypersensitivity to both sympathetic and parasympathetic autonomic mediators, with the iris-lens diaphragm moving forward and closing the angle.

In acute angle-closure glaucoma, the outflow angle in the anterior chamber of the eye formed by the iris plane and the posterior corneal surface becomes closed, blocking outflow to the outflow channels of the trabecula meshwork. The result is a dramatic and rapid rise in intraocular pressure, with ocular pain, decreased vision, colored halos around lights, and frequently nausea and vomiting. Angle-closure glaucoma should be considered as part of the differential diagnosis for a diabetic patient presenting with nausea and vomiting.

Angle-closure glaucoma is considered a medical emergency. Treatment consists of attempts to break the angle closure medically with miotic drops and to lower the pressure with either systemic or topical medications. A peripheral iridectomy or laser iridotomy can restore the normal aqueous outflow in the eye if the angle closure is broken. Since pupil dilation can trigger an angle-closure attack, care needs to be exercised before dilation of any pupil.

Lens

Diabetic effects on the crystalline lens can result in transitory refractive changes and cataracts.

Refractive Changes. Refractive changes related to fluctuation of blood glucose levels are readily acknowledged by all clinicians, and diabetes has also been found to affect accommodation ability.

Blood Glucose Levels. The mechanism of such refractive changes due to fluctuations in blood glucose levels is only poorly understood. Myopic shifts with elevations of blood glucose levels or as an initial symptom or sign of undiagnosed diabetes are common in the phakic eye.[51] These myopic shifts can be of several diopters or more and are the result of osmotic swelling of the crystalline lens.

Sudden refractive shifts are frequently the presenting symptom for a person with new diabetes. Patients who were able to see clearly at a distance either with or without their glasses may complain that their distance vision is now blurry. On the other hand, those who required reading glasses or who were experiencing difficulty with close work may now find they can read more easily without their glasses, misinterpreting the change as "an improvement" in their eyes. Patients with uncontrolled or poorly controlled blood glucose levels should be encouraged to postpone the purchase of eyeglasses until their blood glucose levels have stabilized. This stabilization may take 4 to 6 weeks to occur, although the effects of a rise in blood glucose level on refractive state are generally recognized as being more sudden. Any coexisting physical condition that impacts on blood glucose level, such as infection or stress, is reason not to prescribe glasses, especially if a person recognizes recent or sudden fluctuations in vision.

The proposed cause of such refractive shifts in phakic eyes invariably involves fluid absorption by the crystalline lens. The galacticol and sorbitol pathways have been implicated, and rat models have shown that osmotic changes caused by the accumulation of galacticol in the lenses of rats fed with galactose leads to lens swelling and premature cataract development.[2,93–97,103–110] The sorbitol pathway, however, is most likely beneficial in protecting the lens against glucose-generated osmotic changes.[108]

Accommodation. While discussions of refractive changes associated with diabetes most frequently are directed to myopic shifts related to elevated blood glucose levels, there is evidence that diabetes alters accommodative ability. Waite and Beetham demonstrated transitory paresis of accommodation in 21% of the diabetic patients in their study.[51] This paresis was most predominant in the 20- to 50-year-old group and resolved with improvement of the diabetic condition. Transient accommodative paralysis accompanied with hyperopia may be associated with either a rise or fall in blood glucose levels, most frequently after insulin treatment has been started, and may be present even in young individuals.[111]

Reduced accommodative ability, as well as diminished pupillary response, has been demonstrated following panretinal argon laser photocoagulation.[111] It is postulated that this internal ophthalmoplegia following panretinal laser photocoagulation is the result of direct injury to the parasympathetic motor fibers to the ciliary body and the iris. These fibers enter the globe at the posterior pole and course forward between the sclera and the choroid. As the fibers course forward, the choroid becomes thinner, providing less protection against the heat generated in the retinal pigment epithelium from the laser surgery. Unlike the paresis of accommodation associated with uncontrolled diabetes, the internal ophthalmoplegia associated with scatter (panretinal) photocoagulation surgery is generally irreversible, since the laser burns cause permanent damage to the underlying parasympathetic nerve fibers.

Diabetic persons frequently demonstrate presbyopia at an earlier age than nondiabetic persons, and the loss of accommodative ability frequently progresses more rapidly for diabetic persons. Consequently, it is not uncommon for myopic contact-lens wearers, who need to accommodate more through contact lenses than through spectacle lenses, or hyperopic individuals to demonstrate difficulty in reading or in close tasks. Identifying these problems may be difficult because of refractive changes secondary to fluctuating blood glucose levels. These changes in accommodation are irreversible with age.

Cataracts. Cataracts occur earlier in life and progress more rapidly in the presence of diabetes.[112–114] Cataracts are 1.6 times more common in people with diabetes than in those without diabetes.[108,109] This increased risk of cataract development for the diabetic person occurs both in persons with earlier-onset diabetes and those with later-onset diabetes. Many factors affect cataract development, including duration of diabetes and retinopathy status in the patient with earlier-onset diabetes, as well as the use of diuretics and the level of glycosylated hemoglobin.[109] In patients with later-onset diabetes, age of the patient, as well as severity of retinopathy, use of diuretics, lower intraocular pressure, smoking, and lower diastolic blood pressure, may be risk factors. Fortunately, cataract extraction with and without lens implantation is 90 to 95% successful in restoring useful vision, but the surgery is not without potential complications unique to diabetes, such as delayed wound healing, acceleration of diabetic retinopathy, iris or retinal neovascularization, and macular edema. Cataracts obscuring retinal examination may need to be surgically removed to permit retinal examination and, in some cases, appropriate laser photocoagulation surgery.

Reversible lenticular opacities related to diabetes mellitus have also been reported.[115–122] These reversible cataracts can occur in different layers of the lens and are most frequently related to poor metabolic control of diabetes. The so-called true diabetic cataracts are usually bilateral and are characterized by dense bands of white, subcapsular spots that are snow-flake in appearance, or fine, needle-shaped opacities[123,124] (Fig. 42–14). Since these diabetic cataracts are related to prolonged periods of severe hyperglycemia and untreated diabetes mellitus, they are rarely seen in the United States and other industrialized countries.

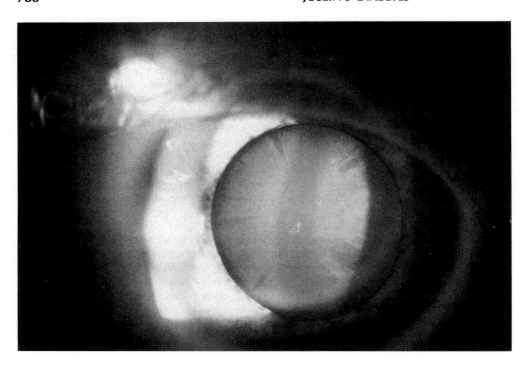

Fig. 42–14. Diabetic cataract in a 16-year-old girl.

Management of diabetic cataract involves the same treatment strategies as those for age-related cataracts. For visual impairment not requiring surgery, optimal refraction is mandatory. Glare-control lenses and the use of sunglasses may relieve cataract-induced visual symptoms. Surgically, intraocular lens implants provide the most natural postsurgical refractive correction, depending on retinopathy status.[125]

Vitreous

Problems with the vitreous in the diabetic patient are intimately related to retinal disease.[126–133] PDR is associated with an increased incidence of posterior vitreous detachment, although frequently a partial vitreous detachment rather than a total posterior vitreous detachment is present.[126] Partial vitreous detachment may result in vitreous hemorrhage, an increase in retinal neovascularization, and tractional retinal detachment.[134]

Optic Disc

Although the optic disc is usually discussed only in relation to proliferative diabetic retinopathy and neovascularization at the disc, it can be affected in a variety of other ways by diabetes.

Optic disc edema unrelated to anterior ischemic optic neuropathy or other neurologic disorders can occur with diabetes mellitus.[135,136] The condition seems to be related to a vasculopathy of the most superficial layer of capillaries of the optic disc[137] and is more common in younger patients with Type I diabetes. Although transient optic disc edema usually leaves little or no lasting effect on visual acuity or visual fields, especially in younger patients, some residual disc pallor

may follow resolution of the disc edema. One or both eyes may be affected.

Diabetic papillopathy must be distinguished from other causes of disc swelling, such as true papilledema from increased intracranial pressure; other pseudopapilledema, such as optic nerve head drusen; toxic optic neuropathies; neoplasm of the optic nerve; and hypertension.[138,139]

Optic disc pallor can occur following spontaneous remission of proliferative retinopathy or remission following scatter (panretinal) laser photocoagulation. This disc pallor does not result in a change of the cup/disc ratio. Since diabetes poses an increased risk for the development of open-angle glaucoma and anterior ischemic optic neuropathy, the disc pallor following remission of retinopathy or panretinal photocoagulation must be considered when evaluating the optic-nerve head for open-angle glaucoma or low-tension glaucoma.[139]

FUTURE HORIZONS

Present strategies for dealing with diabetic retinopathy address retinopathy that is already established. The Diabetes Control and Complications Trial (DCCT), a nationwide clinical trial testing very tight control of blood glucose levels vs. standard control of blood glucose levels, is investigating the effect of tight control on the development of retinopathy itself. The DCCT determined that very tight control of blood glucose levels reduces the risks of renal and retinal complications of diabetes. The results of the DCCT firmly establish the benefit of very tight control for patients with IDDM.

Another multicentered clinical trial, the Sorbinil Retinopathy Trial (Table 42–12), tested whether a daily dose of sorbinil, an aldose reductase inhibitor (ARI),

Table 42–12. Sorbinil Retinopathy Study (SRT)

SRT Evaluating
  Effect on onset and progression of diabetic retinopathy
  Effect on neuropathy and nephropathy
  Safety and tolerance of sorbinil
SRT Design Features
  Type I diabetic subjects for 1–15 years
  Randomized sorbinil/placebo treatment
  Follow-up for 3 years
  Dose 250 mg daily
SRT Results (250 mg)
  No effect on onset of diabetic retinopathy
  No effect on progression of diabetic retinopathy
  Hypersensitivity in 7%
  Slightly lower microaneurysm count
  No effect on blood pressure or glycosylated hemoglobin
Limitations of SRT
  Diabetic retinopathy not early enough
  Duration of SRT too short
  Dosage (250 mg) too low
  Unknown effect on retina
  Pharmacokinetics still unclear

reduces the complications of diabetic retinopathy. Over a 3-year period the drug had no clinically important effect on the course of diabetic retinopathy in adults with IDDM of moderate duration.[140] The group taking sorbinil, however, did show a slightly lower number of microaneurysms. Forthcoming reports will address the effect of sorbinil on diabetic neuropathy and diabetic nephropathy.

There were complications of the use of the drug in the study population. Nearly 7% of the initial 202 participants had adverse reactions, including toxic epidermal necrolysis, erythema multiforme, and Stevens-Johnson syndrome. It is unlikely that sorbinil will be used prophylactically because of the hypersensitivity reactions and similarities in outcome for the sorbinil-treated and control groups. Other ARIs, notably tolrestat, which has a chemical structure different from that of sorbinil, are presently under investigation in the United States and Canada. Discouraging results of the Sorbinil Retinopathy Trial suggest that further research on the pharmokinetics and side effects of ARIs is necessary before further human clinical trials are undertaken.

Other research is addressing mechanisms contributing to altered retinal blood flow and retinal vascular complications in diabetes.[141,142] Various metabolic and hormonal factors are suspected in the initiation and progression of retinal vascular abnormalities. Retinal blood flow is decreased in diabetic patients with less than 5 years of diabetes. Furthermore, a direct relationship between decreased retinal blood flow and the activation of protein kinase C in the rat model has been shown. Identifying the biochemical alterations associated with hyperglycemia and functional changes in retinal circulation may provide approaches to the prevention or amelioration of the course of diabetic retinopathy.

Ongoing investigations are addressing the modulation of retinal blood flow by vasoactive agents such as angiotensin II, histamine, and oxygen. Inhibition of these processes with insulin therapy or islet-cell transplants may normalize retinal blood flow in diabetes. The prevalence of the presence of antipericyte antibodies, a reflection of pericyte degeneration, may be related to early development of diabetic retinopathy.

GUIDELINES

Until modalities are in place to prevent or cure diabetic retinopathy and other complications, the emphasis must be placed on identification, careful follow-up, and timely laser photocoagulation for patients with diabetic retinopathy and diabetic eye disease. Proper care will result in reduction of personal suffering for those involved, as well as in a substantial cost savings for the involved individuals and their families and the country as a whole.[143–145] Therefore, strict guidelines have been established for the ocular care of people with diabetes (Tables 42–8 and 42–13).

All diabetic patients should be informed of the possibility of developing retinopathy with or without symptoms and the associated threat of visual loss. The natural course and treatment of diabetic retinopathy should be discussed, and the importance of routine examination should be stressed. Patients should be informed of the possible relationship between level of control of diabetes and the subsequent development of ocular and other medical complications as the rationale for their partnership with the health-care team. Patients should be informed that diabetic nephropathy, as manifest by proteinuria, requires aggressive early treatment with proper diet and blood pressure control, especially with ACE inhibitors, to avoid superimposed renal retinopathy (and the possible associated risk of neovascular glaucoma). The association of joint contractures, hypertension, cardiovascular disease, elevated lipid levels, and neuropathy with onset and progression of diabetic retinopathy should be discussed.

Diabetic women contemplating pregnancy should have a complete eye examination before they conceive. Pregnant women with diabetes should have their eyes examined early in each trimester of their pregnancy or more frequently, as indicated by level of retinopathy, and 3 to 6 months after delivery. Since pregnancy may exacerbate existing retinopathy and be associated with

Table 42–13. Eye Examination Schedule

Type of Diabetes	Recommendation Time for First Examination	Routine Minimal Follow-Up
Type I (IDDM)	5 years after onset or during puberty	Yearly
Type II (NIDDM)	At time of diagnosis	Yearly
During pregnancy	Prior to pregnancy for counseling	
	Early in first trimester	
	Each trimester or more frequently as indicated	
	3–6 months post partum	

*Abnormal findings will dictate more frequent follow-up examinations (see Table 42–8).

hypertension, careful medical and ocular observation is crucial during pregnancy. In women with proliferative retinopathy, cesarean delivery may be preferable to vaginal delivery to reduce the risk of vitreous hemorrhage. Close communication among the various members of the health-care team is essential.

Patients with diabetic retinopathy, even in its mildest form, must be informed of the availability and benefits of early and timely laser photocoagulation therapy in reducing the risk of visual loss. The management program outlined in Table 42–8 is fundamental. Furthermore, patients with visual impairment of any degree, legal blindness, or total blindness should be informed of the availability of visual, vocational, and psychosocial rehabilitation programs.

CONCLUSIONS

In its earliest stages, diabetic retinopathy usually causes no symptoms. Visual acuity may be excellent at the time of diagnosis, and a patient may deny the presence of retinopathy. It is crucial at this stage for a patient's physician to initiate a careful program of education and medical and ocular follow-up.

If retinal disease progresses, visual acuity may be compromised by macular edema or episodes of vitreous hemorrhage. Difficulties in the work or home environment may result. Although denial may continue, anger may ensue. Fear of blindness and other complications of diabetes, including death, also may develop. If visual acuity drops to 20/200 or worse, a patient may remain in a state of uncertainty until his or her retinopathy is in quiescence secondary to laser treatment, vitreoretinal surgery, or the natural history of the disease process. Anger and fear continue. Once the retinopathy is in remission and vision is stable, a patient is in a position to accept his or her situation and to make the appropriate psychological and social adjustments. At this time, visual and vocational rehabilitation may be successful.

Communication among all members of a patient's health-care team is of paramount importance in dealing with the physical and psychological stresses of visual loss from diabetes. Faced with their inability to prevent or cure diabetic retinopathy, the main concern of doctors must be the early detection of diabetic retinopathy. Patient access, careful follow-up, and timely laser photocoagulation are fundamental to the successful elimination of blindness in people with diabetes mellitus.

REFERENCES

1. Joslin EP. The treatment of diabetes mellitus. 5th ed. Philadelphia: Lea & Febiger, 1935:411.
2. Aiello LM, Beetham WP, Balodimos MC, et al. Ruby laser photocoagulation in treatment of diabetic proliferating retinopathy: preliminary report. In: Goldberg MF, Fine SL, eds. Symposium on the treatment of diabetic retinopathy. US Public Health Service. Publication no. 1890. Washington, DC: US Government Printing Office, 1969:437–63.
3. The Diabetic Retinopathy Study Research Group. Preliminary report on effects of photocoagulation therapy. Am J Ophthalmol 1976;81:383–96.
4. The Diabetic Retinopathy Study Research Group. Photocoagulation treatment of proliferative diabetic retinopathy: the second report of Diabetic Retinopathy Study findings. Ophthalmology 1978;85:82–106.
5. The Diabetic Retinopathy Study Research Group. Four risk factors for severe visual loss in diabetic retinopathy: the third report from the Diabetic Retinopathy Study. Arch Ophthalmol 1979;97:654–5.
6. The Diabetic Retinopathy Study Research Group. Photocoagulation treatment of proliferative diabetic retinopathy: a short report of long range results. Diabetic Retinopathy Study (DRS) report number 4. Amsterdam: Excerpta Medica, 1980.
7. Diabetic Retinopathy Study Research Group. Photocoagulation treatment of proliferative diabetic retinopathy: relationship of adverse treatment effects to retinopathy severity. Diabetic Retinopathy Study report number 5. Dev Ophthalmol 1981;2:248–61.
8. Diabetic Retinopathy Study Report Research Group. Report 6. Design, methods, and baseline results. Invest Ophthalmol Vis Sci 1981;21:149–209.
9. Diabetic Retinopathy Study Research Group. Report 7. A modification of the Airlie House classification of diabetic retinopathy. Invest Ophthalmol Vis Sci 1981;21:210–26.
10. The Diabetic Retinopathy Study Research Group. Photocoagulation treatment of proliferative diabetic retinopathy: clinical application of Diabetic Retinopathy Study (DRS) findings, DRS report number 8. Ophthalmology 1981;88:583–600.
11. Diabetic Retinopathy Study Research Group. Report 9. Assessing possible late treatment effects in stopping clinical trials early: a case study by F Ederer, MJ Podgor. Controlled Clin Trials 1984;5:373–81.
12. Rand LI, Prud'homme GJ, Ederer F, Canner PL, Diabetic Retinopathy Research Group. Factors influencing the development of visual loss in advanced diabetic retinopathy: Diabetic Retinopathy Study report no. 10. Invest Ophthalmol Vis Sci 1985;26:983–91.
13. Kaufman SC, Ferris FL III, Swartz M, Diabetic Retinopathy Study Research Group. Intraocular pressure following panretinal photocoagulation for diabetic retinopathy: Diabetic Retinopathy report no. 11. Arch Ophthalmol 1987;105:807–9.
14. Ferris FL III, Podgor MJ, Davis MD, the Diabetic Retinopathy Study Research Group. Macular edema in diabetic retinopathy study patients: Diabetic Retinopathy Study report number 12. Ophthalmology 1987;94:754–60.
15. Kaufman SC, Ferris FL III, et al, the DRS Research Group. Factors associated with visual outcome after photocoagulation for diabetic retinopathy: Diabetic Retinopathy Study report #13. Invest Ophthalmol Vis Sci 1989;30:23–8.
16. The Diabetic Retinopathy Study Research Group. Indications for photocoagulation treatment of diabetic retinopathy: Diabetic Retinopathy Study report no. 14. Int Ophthalmol Clin 1987;27:239–53.
17. Early Treatment Diabetic Retinopathy Study Research Group. Photocoagulation for diabetic macular edema; Early Treatment Diabetic Retinopathy Study report number 1. Arch Ophthalmol 1985;103:1796–806.
18. Early Treatment Diabetic Retinopathy Study Research Group. Treatment techniques and clinical guidelines for photocoagulation of diabetic macular edema: Early Treatment Diabetic Retinopathy Study report number 2. Ophthalmology 1987;94:761–74.
19. The Early Treatment Diabetic Retinopathy Study Research Group. Techniques for scatter and local photocoagulation treatment of diabetic retinopathy: Early Treatment Dia-

betic Retinopathy Study report no. 3. Int Ophthalmol Clin 1987;27:254–64.

20. The Early Treatment Diabetic Retinopathy Study Research Group. Photocoagulation for diabetic macular edema: Early Treatment Diabetic Retinopathy Study report no. 4. Int Ophthalmol Clin 1987;27:265–72.

21. The Early Treatment Diabetic Retinopathy Study Research Group. Case reports to accompany Early Treatment Diabetic Retinopathy Study reports 3 and 4. Int Ophthalmol Clin 1987;27:273–333.

22. Kinyoun J, Barton F, Fisher M, et al, the ETDRS Research Group. Detection of diabetic macular edema: ophthalmoscopy versus photography—Early Treatment Diabetic Retinopathy Study report number 5. Ophthalmology 1989;96: 746–51.

23. Early Treatment Diabetic Retinopathy Study Research Group. Early Treatment Diabetic Retinopathy Study design and baseline patient characteristics: ETDRS report number 7. Ophthalmology 1991;98(5)(Suppl):741–56.

24. Early Treatment Diabetic Retinopathy Study Research Group. Effects of aspirin treatment on diabetic retinopathy: ETDRS report number 8. Ophthalmology 1991; 98(5)(Suppl):757–65.

25. Early Treatment Diabetic Retinopathy Study Research Group. Early photocoagulation for diabetic retinopathy: ETDRS report number 9. Ophthalmology 1991;98(5) (Suppl):766–85.

26. Early Treatment Diabetic Retinopathy Study Research Group. Grading diabetic retinopathy from stereoscopic color fundus photographs—an extension of the modified Airlie House classification: ETDRS report number 10. Ophthalmology 1991;98(5)(Suppl):786–806.

27. Early Treatment Diabetic Retinopathy Study Research Group. Classification of diabetic retinopathy from fluorescein angiograms: ETDRS report number 11. Ophthalmology 1991;98(5)(Suppl):807–22.

28. Early Treatment Diabetic Retinopathy Study Research Group. Fundus photographic risk factors for progression of diabetic retinopathy: ETDRS report number 12. Ophthalmology 1991;98(5)(Suppl):823–33.

29. Early Treatment Diabetic Retinopathy Study Research Groups. Fluorescein angiographic risk factors for progression of diabetic retinopathy: ETDRS report number 13. Ophthalmology 1991;98(5)(Suppl):834–40.

30. The DRVS Research Group. Two-year course of visual acuity in severe proliferative diabetic retinopathy with conventional management: Diabetic Retinopathy Vitrectomy Study (DRVS) report #1. Ophthalmology 1985;92: 492–502.

31. The Diabetic Retinopathy Vitrectomy Study Research Group. Early vitrectomy for severe vitreous hemorrhage in diabetic retinopathy: two-year results of a randomized trial: Diabetic Retinopathy Vitrectomy Study report 2. Arch Ophthalmol 1985;103:1644–52.

32. The Diabetic Retinopathy Vitrectomy Study Research Group. Early vitrectomy for severe proliferative diabetic retinopathy in eyes with useful vision: results of a randomized trial—Diabetic Retinopathy Vitrectomy Study report 3. Ophthalmology 1988;95:1307–20.

33. The Diabetic Retinopathy Vitrectomy Study Research Group. Early vitrectomy for severe proliferative diabetic retinopathy in eyes with useful vision: clinical application of results of a randomized trial—Diabetic Retinopathy Vitrectomy Study report 4. Ophthalmology 1988;95: 1321–34.

34. The Diabetic Retinopathy Vitrectomy Study Research Group. Early vitrectomy for severe vitreous hemorrhage

in diabetic retinopathy. Four-year results of a randomized trial: Diabetic Retinopathy Study report 5. Arch Ophthalmol 1990;108:958–64.

35. Klein R, Klein BEK, Moss SE, et al. The Wisconsin Epidemiologic Study of Diabetic Retinopathy. II. Prevalence and risk of diabetic retinopathy when age at diagnosis is less than 30 years. Arch Ophthalmol 1984; 102:520–6.

36. Klein R, Klein BEK, Moss SE, et al. The Wisconsin Epidemiologic Study of Diabetic Retinopathy. III. Prevalence and risk of diabetic retinopathy when age at diagnosis is 30 or more years. Arch Ophthalmol 1984; 102:527–32.

37. Moloney JBM, Drury MI. The effect of pregnancy on the natural course of diabetic retinopathy. Am J Ophthalmol 1982;93:745–56.

38. Serup L. Influence of pregnancy on diabetic retinopathy. Acta Endocrinol Suppl 1986;277:122–4.

39. Phelps RL, Sakol P, Metzger BE, et al. Changes in diabetic retinopathy during pregnancy: correlations with regulation of hyperglycemia. Arch Ophthalmol 1986;104: 1806–10.

40. The Kroc Collaborative Study Group. Blood glucose control and the evolution of diabetic retinopathy and albuminuria; a preliminary multicenter trial. N Engl J Med 1984;311:365–72.

41. Grunwald JE, Riva CE, Martin DB, et al. Effect of an insulin-induced decrease in blood glucose on the human diabetic retinal circulation. Ophthalmology 1987;94: 1614–20.

42. Chase HP, Jackson WE, Hoops SL, et al. Glucose control in the renal and retinal complications of insulin-dependent diabetes. JAMA 1989;261:1155–60.

43. Brinchmann-Hansen O, Dahl-Jørgensen K, Hanssen KF, et al, Oslo Study Group. Effects of intensified insulin treatment on various lesions of diabetic retinopathy. Am J Ophthalmol 1985;100:644–53.

44. Krolewski AS, Canessa M, Warram JH, et al. Predisposition to hypertension and susceptibility to renal disease in insulin-dependent diabetes mellitus. N Engl J Med 1988: 318;140–5.

45. Stern MP, Patterson JK, Haffner SM, et al. Lack of awareness and treatment of hyperlipidemia in Type II diabetes in a community survey. JAMA 1989:262:360–4.

46. Chantry KH, Klein ML, Chew EY, Ferris III FL, Early Treatment Diabetic Retinopathy Study Research Group. Association of serum lipids and retinal hard exudates in patients enrolled in the Early Treatment Diabetic Retinopathy Study [Abstract]. Invest Ophthalmol Vis Sci 1989; 30(3)(Suppl):434.

47. Engerman RL, Kern TS. Is diabetic retinopathy preventable? Int Ophthalmol Clin 1987;27:225–9.

48. Bresnick GH. Background diabetic retinopathy. In: Ryan SJ, ed. Retina. Vol 2. Medical retina. St Louis: CV Mosby, 1989;327–66.

49. Shimizu K, Kobayashi Y, Muraoka K. Midperipheral fundus involvement in diabetic retinopathy. Ophthalmology 1981;88:601–12.

50. Niki T, Muraoka K, Shimizu K. Distribution of capillary nonperfusion in early-stage diabetic retinopathy. Ophthalmology 1984;91:1431–9.

51. Waite JH, Beetham WP. The visual mechanism in diabetes mellitus: a comparative study of 2002 diabetics and 457 non-diabetics for control. N Engl J Med 1935; 212:367–79, 429–43.

52. Zorrilla E, Kozak GP. Ophthalmoplegia in diabetes mellitus. Ann Intern Med 1967;67:968–76.

53. Rucker CW. Paralysis of the third, fourth, and sixth cranial nerves. Am J Ophthalmol 1958;46:787–94.

54. Rush JA, Younge BR. Paralysis of cranial nerves III, IV, and VI: cause and prognosis in 1,000 cases. Arch Ophthalmol 1981;99:76–9.

55. Rucker CW. The causes of paralysis of the third, fourth, and sixth cranial nerves. Am J Ophthalmol 1966; 61:1293–8.

56. Asbury AK, Aldredge H, Hershberg R, Fisher CM. Oculomotor palsy in diabetes mellitus: a clinico-pathological study. Brain 1970;93:555–66.

57. Weber RB, Daroff RB, Mackey EA. Pathology of oculomotor nerve palsy in diabetics. Neurology 1970;20:835–8.

58. Jackson WPU. Ocular nerve palsy with severe headache in diabetics. BMJ 1955;:408–9.

59. Waind APB. Ocular nerve palsy associated with severe headache. BMJ 1956;1:901–2.

60. Lincoff HA, Cogan DG. Unilateral headache and oculomotor paralysis not caused by aneurysm. Arch Ophthalmol 1957;57:181–9.

61. King FP. Paralyses of the extraocular muscles in diabetes. Arch Intern Med 1959;104:318–22.

62. Goldstein JE, Cogan DG. Diabetic ophthalmoplegia with special reference to the pupil. Arch Ophthalmol 1960; 64:592–600.

63. Eareckson VO, Miller JM. Third-nerve palsy with sparing of pupil in diabetes mellitus: a subsequent identical lesion of the opposite eye. Arch Ophthalmol 1952;47:607–10.

64. Green WR, Hackett ER, Schlezinger NS. Neuro-ophthalmologic evaluation of oculomotor nerve paralysis. Arch Ophthalmol 1964;72:154–67.

65. Baum JL. Rhino-orbital mucormycosis: occurring in an otherwise apparently healthy individual. Am J Ophthalmol 1967;63:335–9.

66. Schwartz JN, Donnelly EH, Klintworth GK. Ocular and orbital phycomycosis. Surv Ophthalmol 1977;22:3–28.

67. Blitzer A, Lawson W, Meyers BR, Biller HF. Patient survival factors in paranasal sinus mucormycosis. Laryngoscope 1980;90:635–48.

68. Fleckner RA, Goldstein JH. Mucormycosis. Br J Ophthalmol 1969;53:542–58.

69. Funahashi T, Fink AI. The pathology of the bulbar conjunctiva in diabetes mellitus. I. Microaneurysms. Am J Ophthalmol 1963;55:504–11.

70. Henkind P. The eye in diabetes mellitus: signs, symptoms, and their pathogenesis. In: Mausolf FA, ed. The eye and systemic disease. 2nd ed. St Louis: CV Mosby, 1980: 187–203.

71. Ditzel J, Beaven DW, Renold AE. Early vascular changes in diabetes mellitus. Metabolism 1960;9:400–7.

72. Moses RA, ed. Adler's physiology of the eye: clinical applications. 6th ed. St Louis: CV Mosby, 1975:22.

73. Ishida N, Rao GN, del Cerro M, Aquavella JV. Corneal nerve alterations in diabetes mellitus. Arch Ophthalmol 1984;102:1380–4.

74. MacRae SM, Engerman RL, Hatchell DL, Hyndiuk RA. Corneal sensitivity and control of diabetes. Cornea 1982;1:223–6.

75. Schwartz DE. Corneal sensitivity in diabetics. Arch Ophthalmol 1974;91:174–8.

76. Rogell GD. Corneal hypesthesia and retinopathy in diabetes mellitus. Ophthalmology 1980;87:229–33.

77. Hyndiuk RA, Kazarian EL, Schultz RO, Seideman S. Neurotrophic corneal ulcers in diabetes mellitus. Arch Ophthalmol 1977;95:2193–6.

78. Hatchell DL, Pederson HJ, Faculjak ML. Susceptibility of the corneal epithelial basement membrane to injury in diabetic rabbits. Cornea 1982;1:227–31.

79. Kenyon K, Wafai Z, Michels R, et al. Corneal basement membrane abnormality in diabetes mellitus [Abstract]. Invest Ophthalmol Vis Sci 1978;17(Suppl):245.

80. Khodadoust AA, Silverstein AM, Kenyon KR, Dowling JF. Adhesion of regenerating corneal epithelium: the role of basement membrane. Am J Ophthalmol 1968;65:339–48.

81. Henkind P, Wise GN. Descemet's wrinkles in diabetes. Am J Ophthalmol 1961;52:371–4.

82. Pardos GJ, Krachmer JH. Comparison of endothelial cell density in diabetics and a control population. Am J Ophthalmol 1980;90:172–4.

83. Busted N, Olsen T, Schmitz O. Clinical observations on the corneal thickness and the corneal endothelium in diabetes mellitus. Br J Ophthalmol 1981;65:687–90.

84. Olsen T, Busted N. Corneal thickness in eyes with diabetic and nondiabetic neovascularisation. Br J Ophthalmol 1981;65:691–3.

85. Hoffmann M. Concerning diseases of the ocular nerves in diabetes mellitus. Arch Ophthalmol 1914;43:39–49.

86. Yanoff M, Fine BS, Berkow JW. Diabetic lacy vacuolation of iris pigment epithelium: a histopathologic report. Am J Ophthalmol 1970;69:201–10.

87. Gartner S, Henkind P. Neovascularization of the iris (rubeosis iridis). Surv Ophthalmol 1978;22:291–312.

88. Zirm M. Protein glaucoma—overtaxing of flow mechanisms? Preliminary report. Ophthalmologica 1982; 184:155–61.

89. Brown GC, Magargal LE, Schachat A, Shah H. Neovascular glaucoma: etiologic considerations. Ophthalmology 1984; 91:315–20.

90. Pavan PR, Folk JC. Anterior neovascularization. Int Ophthalmol Clin 1984;24:61–70.

91. Madsen PH. Rubeosis of the iris and haemorrhagic glaucoma in patients with proliferative diabetic retinopathy. Br J Ophthalmol 1971;55:368–71.

92. Ohrt V. The frequency of rubeosis iridis in diabetic patients. Acta Ophthalmol (Copenh) 1971;49:301–7.

93. Krill AE, Archer D, Newell FW. Photocoagulation in complications secondary to branch vein occlusion. Arch Ophthalmol 1971; 85:48–60.

94. Wand M, Dueker DK, Aiello LM, Grant WM. Effects of panretinal photocoagulation on rubeosis iridis, angle neovascularization, and neovascular glaucoma. Am J Ophthalmol 1978;86:332–9.

95. Pavan PR, Folk JC, Weingeist TA, et al. Diabetic rubeosis and panretinal photocoagulation: a prospective, controlled, masked trial using iris fluorescein angiography. Arch Ophthalmol 1983;101:882–4.

96. Simmons RJ, Dueker DK, Kimbrough RL, Aiello LM. Goniophotocoagulation for neovascular glaucoma. Trans Am Acad Ophthalmol Otolaryngol 1977;83:80–9.

97. Aiello LM, Wand M, Liang G. Neovascular glaucoma and vitreous hemorrhage following cataract surgery in patients with diabetes mellitus. Ophthalmol 1983; 90:814–20.

98. Armstrong JR, Daily RK, Dobson HL, Girard LJ. The incidence of glaucoma in diabetes mellitus: a comparison with the incidence of glaucoma in the general population. Am J Ophthalmol 1960;50:55–63.

99. Cristiansson J. Glaucoma simplex in diabetes mellitus. Acta Ophthalmol 1965;43:224–34.

100. Becker B, Bresnick G, Chevrette L, et al. Intraocular pressure and its response to topical corticosteroids in diabetes. Arch Ophthalmol 1966;76:477–83.

101. Klein BEK, Klein R, Moss SE. Intraocular pressure in diabetic persons. Ophthalmology 1984;91:1356–60.

102. Mapstone R, Clark CV. Prevalence of diabetes in glaucoma. BMJ 1985;291:93–5.

103. Gwinup G, Villarreal A. Relationship of serum glucose concentration to changes in refraction. Diabetes 1976; 25:29–31.

104. Kinoshita JH, Merola LO, Satoh K, Dikmak E. Osmotic changes caused by the accumulation of dulcitol in the lenses of rats fed with galactose. Nature 1962; 194:1085–7.

105. Chylack LT Jr, Kinoshita JH. A biochemical evaluation of a cataract induced in a high-glucose medium. Invest Ophthalmol 1969;8:401–12.

106. Kinoshita JH. Mechanisms initiating cataract formation. Invest Ophthalmol Vis Sci 1974;13:713–24.

107. Harding RH, Chylack LT Jr, Tung WH. The sorbitol pathway as a protector of the lens against glucose-generated osmotic stress [Abstract]. Invest Ophthalmol Vis Sci 1981;20(Suppl):34.

108. Bursell S-E, Karalekas DP, Craig MS. The effect of acute changes in blood glucose on lenses in diabetic and non-diabetic subjects using quasi-elastic light scattering spectroscopy. Curr Eye Res 1989;8:821–33.

109. Bursell S-E, Baker RS, Weiss JN, et al. Clinical photon correlation spectroscopy evaluation of human diabetic lenses. Exp Eye Res 1989;49:241–58.

110. Marmor MF. Transient accommodative paralysis and hyperopia in diabetes. Arch Ophthalmol 1973;89:419–21.

111. Rogell GD. Internal ophthalmoplegia after argon laser panretinal photocoagulation. Arch Ophthalmol 1979; 97:904–5.

112. Klein BEK, Klein R, Moss SE. Prevalence of cataracts in a population-based study of persons with diabetes mellitus. Ophthalmology 1985;92:1191–6.

113. Ederer F, Hiller R, Taylor HR. Senile lens changes and diabetes in two population studies. Am J Ophthalmol 1981;91:381–95.

114. Epstein DL. Reversible unilateral lens opacities in a diabetic patient. Arch Ophthalmol 1976;94:461–3.

115. Lawrence RD, Oakley W, Barne IC. Temporary lens changes in diabetic coma and other dehydrations. Lancet 1942;2:63–5.

116. Lawrence RD. Temporary cataracts in diabetes. Br J Ophthalmol 1946;30:78–81.

117. Roberts W. Rapid lens changes in diabetes mellitus. Am J Ophthalmol 1950;33:1283–5.

118. Neuberg HW, Griscom JH, Burns RP. Acute development of diabetic cataracts and their reversal: a case report. Diabetes 1958;7:21–6.

119. Jackson RC. Temporary cataracts in diabetes mellitus. Br J Ophthalmol 1955;39:629–31.

120. Turtz CA, Turtz AI. Reversal of lens changes in early diabetes. Am J Ophthalmol 1958;46:219–20.

121. Brown CA, Burman D. Transient cataracts in a diabetic child with hyperosmolar coma. Br J Ophthalmol 1973; 57:429–33.

122. O'Brien CS, Molsberry JM, Allen JH. Diabetic cataract: incidence and morphology in 126 young diabetic patients. JAMA 1934;103:892–7.

123. Rosen E. Diabetic needles. Br J Ophthalmol 1945; 29:645–53.

124. Straatsma BR, Pettit TH, Wheeler N, Miyamasu W. Diabetes mellitus and intraocular lens implantation. Ophthalmology 1983;90:336–43.

125. Jalkh A, Takahashi M, Topilow HW, et al. Prognostic value of vitreous findings in diabetic retinopathy. Arch Ophthalmol 1982;100:432–4.

126. Tagawa H, McMeel JW, Furukawa H, et al. Role of the vitreous in diabetic retinopathy. I. Vitreous changes in diabetic retinopathy and in physiologic aging. Ophthalmology 1986;93:596–601.

127. Tagawa H, McMeel JW, Trempe CL. Role of the vitreous in diabetic retinopathy. II. Active and inactive vitreous changes. Ophthalmology 1986;93:1188–92.

128. Nasrallah FP, Jalkh AE, van Coppenolle FV, et al. The role of the vitreous in diabetic macular edema. Ophthalmology 1988;95:1335–9.

129. Smith JL. Asteroid hyalitis: incidence of diabetes mellitus and hypercholesteremia. JAMA 1958;168:891–3.

130. Bard LA. Asteroid hyalitis: relationship to diabetes and hypercholesterolemia. Am J Ophthalmol 1964; 58:239–42.

131. Smith JL. Asteroid hyalitis and diabetes mellitus. Trans Am Acad Ophthalmol Otolaryngol 1965;69:269–78.

132. Luxenberg M, Sime D. Relationship of asteroid hyalosis to diabetes mellitus and plasma lipid levels. Am J Ophthalmol 1969;67:406–13.

133. Davis MD. Vitreous contraction in proliferative diabetic retinopathy. Arch Ophthalmol 1965;74:741–51.

134. Tolentino FI, Lee P-F, Schepens CL. Biomicroscopic study of vitreous cavity in diabetic retinopathy. Arch Ophthalmol 1966;75:238–46.

135. Lubow M, Makley TA Jr. Pseudopapilledema of juvenile diabetes mellitus. Arch Ophthalmol 1971;85:417–22.

136. Pavan PR, Aiello LM, Wafai MZ, et al. Optic disc edema in juvenile-onset diabetes. Arch Ophthalmol 1980; 98:2193–5.

137. Appen RE, Chandra SR, Klein R, Myers FL. Diabetic papillopathy. Am J Ophthalmol 1980;90:203–9.

138. Barr CC, Glaser JS, Blankenship G. Acute disc swelling in juvenile diabetes: clinical profile and natural history of 12 cases. Arch Ophthalmol 1980;98:2185–92.

139. Johns KJ, Leonard-Marti T, Feman SS. The effect of panretinal photocoagulation on optic nerve cupping. Ophthalmology 1989;96:211–6.

140. Sorbinil Retinopathy Trial Research Group. A randomized trial of sorbinil, an aldose reductase inhibitor in diabetic retinopathy. Arch Ophthalmol 1990;108:1234–44.

141. de la Rubia Sanchez G, Oliver-Pozo J, Shiba T, King GL. Modulation of endothelin-1 (ET-1) receptor on retinal pericytes by elevated glucose levels [Abstract no. 3110]. Invest Ophthalmol Vis Sci 1991;32(4)9 (Suppl):1302.

142. Shiba T, Bursell S-E, Clermont A, et al. Protein kinase C (PKC) activation is a causal factor for the alteration of retinal blood flow in diabetes of short duration [Abstract no. 582]. Invest Ophthalmol Vis Sci 1991;32(4):75.

143. Javitt JC, Aiello LP, Bassi LJ, et al. Detecting and treating retinopathy in patients with Type I diabetes mellitus: savings associated with improved implementation of current guidelines. Ophthalmology 1991;98:1565–74.

144. Awh CC, Cupples HP, Javitt JC. Improved detection and referral of patients with diabetic retinopathy by primary care physicians: effectiveness of education. Arch Intern Med 1991;151:1405–8.

145. Huse DM, Oster G, Killen AR, et al. The economic costs of non-insulin-dependent diabetes mellitus. JAMA 1989; 262:2708–13.

Chapter 43

THE NERVOUS SYSTEM AND DIABETES

DANIEL TARSY
ROY FREEMAN

Disorders of the nervous system associated with diabetes have long been recognized. Rollo[1] is credited with having recorded this association in 1798, and until the middle of the nineteenth century, diabetes itself was attributed to a primary disorder of the central nervous system. It was Marchal de Calvi[2] in 1864 who first suggested that diabetes might be the cause rather than the effect of neuropathy. Most neurologic complications associated with diabetes involve the peripheral nervous system, and it is these that will be emphasized in this chapter. The diabetic neuropathies include several distinctive clinical syndromes with differing clinical manifestations, anatomic distributions, clinical course, and possibly underlying pathophysiology.[3] Pavy's[4] description in 1885 of neuropathic symptoms is noteworthy for its completeness:

> The usual account given by these patients of their condition is that they cannot feel properly in their legs, that their feet are numb, that their legs seem too heavy—as one patient expressed it, 'as if he had 20 pound weights on his legs, and a feeling as if his boots were a good deal too large for his feet'. Darting or 'lightning' pains are often complained of. Or there may be hyperesthesia, so that a mere pinching up of the skin gives rise to great pain; or, it might be, the patient is unable to bear the contact of the seam of a dress against the skin on account of the suffering it causes.

The authors acknowledge Dr. Simeon Locke's contribution to this chapter in previous editions of the textbook.

> Not infrequently there is deep-seated pain, located, as the patient describes it, in the marrow of the bones, which are tender on being grasped; and I have noticed that these pains are generally worse at night. With this there is the usual loss or impairment of the patellar tendon reflex.

CLASSIFICATION

Because of incomplete information concerning the etiology and pathophysiology of the diabetic peripheral neuropathies, current classifications are based primarily on clinical manifestations.[5] Many patients do not manifest a single type of diabetic neuropathy but rather a mixture of neuropathic features often dominated by one or another subtype. Historical classifications begin with Leyden[6] who described hyperesthetic, paralytic, and ataxic forms of neuropathy. Jordan,[7] on the basis of observations of patients treated at the Joslin Clinic, recognized three types of neuropathy: 1) a "hyperglycemic" type dominated by sensory symptoms, without neurologic signs, that usually was reversed by treatment of diabetes; 2) a chronic "circulatory-degenerative" type with advanced sensory, motor, and reflex abnormalities associated with arterial insufficiency of the legs; and 3) a "neuritic" type characterized by more acute neuropathic symptoms and signs. In a similar classification Treusch[8] described 1) diabetes with pain in which control of diabetes improved symptoms, 2) ischemic neuropathy, 3) diabetic polyneuritis, and 4) visceral neuritis. Goodman et al.[9] listed 1) functional neuropathy with uncontrolled diabetes without neurologic deficit, 2) organic neuropathy with neurologic signs, and 3) post-treatment neuropathy. These classifications all suffer the disadvantage of mixing clinical and uncertain pathophysiologic criteria. Locke[10] proposed a simpler anatomic classification system in which lesions of nerve roots produce *radiculopathy,* lesions of mixed nerves produce *neuropathy,* lesions of multiple individual nerves produce *mononeuropathy multiplex,* and involvement of the distal portion of multiple nerves produces *polyneuropathy.* More recent classifications continue to emphasize topographic body distribution[11-13] and are summarized by Dyck's classification[5] into 1) symmetric distal polyneuropathy with sensory, autonomic, and motor involvement; 2) symmetric proximal neuropathy; 3) asymmetrical focal neuropathy including cranial, truncal, limb plexus, multifocal entrapment, and ischemic neuropathies; and 4) asymmetric neuropathy combined with symmetric distal polyneuropathy. Perhaps the simplest and most useful current classification divides the diabetic neuropathies into symmetrical polyneuropathies (sensory, motor, and autonomic) and focal neuropathies (mononeuropathy, mononeuropathy multiplex, plexopathy, radiculopathy, and cranial neuropathy).[3]

Diabetic Polyneuropathy

Predominantly sensory or sensorimotor distal polyneuropathy is the most common of the diabetic neuropathies. Estimated prevalence among patients with diabetes varies widely—from 10 to 100%[3,14]—mainly because of differences in definition, patient selection, diagnostic criteria, and sensitivity of methods of detection.[13,14] Prevalence is typically low if ascertainment is based on subjective symptoms and physical findings and high if based on quantitative sensory testing[15] or electrophysiologic measurements.[14] The best available data are from Pirart,[16] who, in a large cohort of patients, found clinical evidence of neuropathy in 8% of patients at the time of diagnosis, which increased to 50% after 25 years of follow-up. Palumbo et al.[17] followed 995 patients with adult-onset diabetes for up to 20 years and found an accumulated incidence rate of polyneuropathy of 4% at 5 years and 15% at 20 years.

Sensory symptoms and signs are commonly associated with mild distal weakness and features of autonomic neuropathy. Numbness and paresthesia begin in the toes and gradually ascend to involve the feet and lower legs. Sensory deficit usually occurs symmetrically in the distal territory of overlapping nerves, but not infrequently asymmetric patterns of sensory loss in root or nerve distribution are found in the extremities. Because distal portions of longer nerves are affected first, the feet and lower legs are involved before the hands, producing the typical "stocking and glove" pattern of sensory deficit. Impaired touch and two-point discrimination in the fingertips may interfere with the reading of braille.[18] In more severe cases distal portions of thoracic intercostal nerves are affected, producing an asymptomatic midline sensory loss in a teardrop distribution over the anterior thorax and abdomen.[19] This differs from focal thoracic

truncal radiculopathy[20-22] in being a painless, bilateral, and persistent form of neuropathy.

In most patients symptoms of polyneuropathy are mild and consist of numbness or paresthesia of the toes and feet often described as like "walking on pebbles or having cotton bunched up under the toes." In more severe cases, symptoms include superficial burning paresthesia and deep, aching pains that are typically more severe at night, dysesthesia (contact-induced paresthesia) of the skin to touch, and paroxysmal jabbing pains. It has been suggested that polyneuropathy occurs in predominantly small- or large-fiber forms.[13] Although this distinction is rarely absolute, small-fiber neuropathy is characterized clinically by pain, a pseudosyringomyelic dissociated pattern of pain and temperature deficit with preserved vibration and position sense, preserved tendon reflexes and strength, painless foot ulcers and neuropathic joint degeneration, and autonomic neuropathy. Sensory and motor nerve conduction velocities are only mildly slow, since routine measurements are dependent on conduction in the surviving large myelinated nerve fibers. In one study, sural nerve biopsy of two patients with clinical small-fiber neuropathy showed changes confined to unmyelinated and small myelinated fibers.[23] Another pathologic study[24] of sural nerve biopsy specimens in five patients with clinical evidence of small-fiber polyneuropathy revealed severe loss of unmyelinated and small myelinated axons, which appeared to occur earlier than in larger myelinated fibers. However, Dyck et al.[25] failed to find a discrete separation between patients with small- or large-fiber neuropathies but instead found a continuum of small- to large-fiber involvement in which polar cases represented extremes of a normal distribution.

Although selective large-fiber neuropathy might be expected to cause muscle weakness, painless loss of vibration and position sense, and impaired tendon reflexes, pathologic[24,26] and quantitative sensory studies[15] have not demonstrated pure loss of large fibers in diabetic peripheral neuropathy.[5] However, patients with disproportionate large-fiber involvement may manifest muscle weakness, atrophy of the intrinsic foot muscles, and weakness of the extensors and flexors of the toes and ankles with foot drop. When these deficits are combined with proprioceptive deficit in the toes and feet, a "pseudotabetic" gait ataxia may result. Neuropathy of this severity often coexists with diabetic retinopathy and nephropathy. Marked distal muscle weakness with sparing of sensation does occasionally occur but often is due to mononeuropathy multiplex involving the peroneal or ulnar nerves. Pure motor polyneuropathy with few or no sensory symptoms or signs is rarely due to diabetes and should trigger a search for alternative causes of muscle weakness such as motor neuron disease, primary muscle disease, spinal cord disease, or other potentially treatable causes of peripheral neuropathy.

Once established, sensory and sensorimotor distal neuropathy is a permanent condition; although the course of painful manifestations is highly variable, it may last for months to years and may be exacerbated by intercurrent illness, infection, and depression. In one report, 36 patients with pain for at least 12 months showed no significant change in symptoms over a mean follow-up period 4.7 years.[27] Acute painful neuropathy[28] is a variant of sensory polyneuropathy in which severe burning pain of the extremities is combined with deep aching pain in proximal muscles, jabs of pain radiating from the feet to the legs, and striking hypersensitivity or allodynia of the extremities and trunk to touch, clothing, or bedsheets often likened to sunburn. Objective sensory deficit is surprisingly mild in comparison with the painful paresthesia and dysesthesia. Depression, anorexia, and weight loss are often so prominent that the term "diabetic neuropathic cachexia" was coined by Ellenberg.[29] This syndrome often correlates poorly with severity of diabetes or presence of other diabetic microangiopathic complications. Prognosis is generally good, with gradual recovery over a period of months.

"Hyperglycemic" neuropathy refers to widespread paresthesias of the extremities and trunk that occasionally occur in patients with newly diagnosed diabetes and that rapidly improve with control of hyperglycemia. Similar symptoms sometimes appear following recovery from ketoacidosis.[30] The unique reversibility of this form of neuropathy and the diffuse rather than distal distribution of paresthesia suggest a pathophysiologic basis different from that for later-appearing diabetic sensory neuropathy. Sensory neuropathy sometimes appears for the first time coincident with treatment with insulin or oral hypoglycemic agents[31,32] and has been referred to as treatment-induced neuropathy. Although the cause is unknown, it has been suggested that improved glycemic control may initiate regenerating axonal sprouts, which generate ectopic nerve impulses.[30] There is usually gradual improvement as treatment continues and glycemic control is maintained.

Foot ulceration and neuropathic arthropathy are two of the more dreaded neurologic complications of diabetic neuropathy and are discussed in greater detail elsewhere in this volume (Chapters 50 and 53). Foot ulcers usually occur in patients with either small- or large-fiber neuropathy. Painless ulcers in weight-bearing areas occur on a background of insensitivity to pain, impaired proprioception, atrophy of intrinsic foot muscles, disturbed sweating, impaired capillary blood flow caused by autonomic neuropathy, and noninflammatory edema.[33] Neuropathic arthropathy (Charcot joints) is a rarer complication. This occurs primarily in the metatarsophalangeal and metatarsal-tarsal joints and is believed to be due to a combination of impaired deep pain, proprioceptive sensibility, and autonomic neuropathy. In addition, recurrent trauma may cause pathologic fractures of the metatarsal bones with progressive external rotation and eversion deformities of the foot.

Proximal Motor Neuropathy

Diabetic amyotrophy was originally described by Bruns[34] in 1890 and again by Garland and Taverner[35] in 1953 as *diabetic myelopathy*. Because clinical and pathologic evidence for spinal cord involvement was not forthcoming, this syndrome was subsequently designated *diabetic amyotrophy*,[36] a deliberately noncommittal term with regard to localization of the disease process. An array of terms have subsequently been used for this syndrome, including *femoral neuropathy*,[37] *asymmetric motor neuropathy*,[38] *subacute proximal diabetic neuropathy*,[39] *proximal mononeuropathy multiplex*,[40] and *diabetic polyradiculopathy*.[41] Asbury[42] has recommended that the term *diabetic amyotrophy* be dropped because of its ambiguity and that the term *proximal motor neuropathy* be used instead. This neuropathy typically occurs with a peak incidence in the sixth decade in patients with adult-onset, Type II, diabetes. Although many patients are only mildly diabetic at the time of diagnosis, a number of authors have emphasized an association with poor glycemic control.[36,43,44] The clinical picture is one of acute or subacute pain, weakness, and atrophy of the pelvic girdle and thigh musculature. The iliopsoas and quadriceps are always involved, producing weakness of hip flexion and knee stabilization within several weeks of onset of pain. As a result, buckling of the knee and difficulty climbing stairs are typical symptoms. In some cases coexistent weakness of the glutei, hamstrings, thigh adductors, and—less commonly—the peroneal and tibial muscles is present, indicative of the more widespread distribution of the disorder.[44-46] Despite its designation as a motor neuropathy, sensory symptoms and signs are commonly present in the form of paresthesia and sensory findings of the anterior thigh and anteromedial aspect of the lower leg in anterior femoral cutaneous and saphenous nerve distribution. Deep, aching pain is prominent and is localized to the hip, buttock, and anterior thigh. Pain is unrelieved by rest, is typically worse at night than during the day, and is not increased with straight leg raising or other mechanical maneuvers. The process is typically unilateral in onset, but subsequent involvement of the opposite leg occasionally occurs within several months. The knee jerk is nearly always reduced or absent on the affected side, whereas ankle jerks may be preserved unless compromised by coexistent distal polyneuropathy. Despite early reports to the contrary,[35,36] signs of myelopathy are absent and plantar responses are usually flexor. Pain, sensory abnormalities, and weakness in thoracic root distribution occasionally occur concomitantly,[22,41] but isolated shoulder girdle involvement is distinctly uncommon[41] and, when present, usually occurs in patients with marked leg weakness.[36,39,43,45,47] Weight loss is nearly always present and may be compounded by anorexia caused by reactive depression or the use of narcotic analgesics. Differentiation from compressive lumbar nerve root disease and neoplastic infiltration of lumbosacral plexus may be difficult, and laminectomies and laparotomies have occasionally been carried out in such patients in search of a structural cause. As originally pointed out by Root and Rogers[48] and more recently discussed by Hirsh,[49] the absence of mechanical signs and symptoms, lack of back pain, prominent nocturnal pain with failure to respond to bed rest, and muscular atrophy and weakness involving more than one lumbar root usually distinguishes proximal motor neuropathy from nerve root compression. Prognosis is usually good, with most patients showing resolution of pain followed later by gradual return of strength over a period of 6 to 18 months.[41,43,44] Patients with unilateral and relatively focal pain and weakness seem to improve more rapidly and completely than patients with more widespread involvement. Because of the severe pain and disability associated with this syndrome, the ability to reassure affected patients of a favorable prognosis provides them great psychological relief.

There has been considerable debate concerning the etiology and proper classification of proximal motor neuropathy.[42] Subramony and Wilbourn[50] have emphasized the heterogeneity of the syndrome in that some patients with proximal motor neuropathy have clinical and electromyographic evidence of distal polyneuropathy while others appear to have a more localized process. The finding of slow nerve-conduction velocities in femoral and distal nerves[50–54] and of features of demyelination in nerve biopsy specimens in these patients indicates that "diabetic amyotrophy" is a form of diabetic neuropathy with a predilection for proximal nerves rather than a primary disorder of anterior horn cells or muscle. On the basis of extensive clinical and electrophysiologic experience, Bastron and Thomas[41] at the Mayo Clinic concluded that the disorder is a polyradiculopathy that has considerable overlap with the thoracic root syndromes associated with diabetes. Pathologic studies in patients with severe neuropathy of the lower extremities but not necessarily root syndromes also have shown axonal and demyelinative lesions in nerve roots, particularly of the lumbar region.[55,56] A vascular etiology has been proposed for the more acute cases.[40,42] In one study[40] numerous small-vessel infarcts were described in the lumbosacral plexus and proximal nerve trunks of a patient who exhibited the rapid appearance of painful proximal, asymmetric leg weakness. Although acute cases of unilateral or asymmetric proximal neuropathy may be explained on this basis,[57] the broad spectrum of clinical presentations, including a subacute or chronic course, prominent weight loss, and the remarkable sparing of distal muscles, has in the past suggested a "metabolic" rather than a vascular basis[39,42,46,58] for at least some forms of proximal motor neuropathy. It has been suggested, for example, that the major abnormality in diabetic amyotrophy may lie in the intramuscular motor terminals of proximal nerves.[45,46] Muscle biopsy has shown a pattern of single-fiber atrophy with a distribution that does not conform to a pattern of motor-unit atrophy or ischemic change.[39,43,45,46] Motor point biopsies of motor endplate from proximal muscles have shown ballooned subneural elements, beaded and thickened terminal axons, and spherical axonal swelling suggesting primary involvement of intramuscular branches of proximal nerves or their terminal portions.[46] However, grouped fiber atrophy suggesting a more proximal neuropathic process has also been demonstrated,[39,46] and the specificity of these motor endplate ultrastructural abnormalities for proximal motor neuropathy as distinct from other forms of diabetic peripheral neuropathy has not been demonstrated.

Thoracic Radiculopathy

This entity, also known as thoracoabdominal neuropathy, did not gain attention in the English-language literature until the late 1970s.[20,21] Similar to painful proximal motor neuropathies of the legs, this disorder usually occurs in middle-aged patients and often in those who have relatively mild diabetes. In many cases patients with this syndrome have had previous or concomitant painful lumbar root syndromes in the lower extremities. Onset of pain is usually acute, and the pain may be located in the back, chest, or abdomen in either a root, posterior ramus, or intercostal nerve distribution.[59] The character of the pain resembles that of herpes zoster and is usually deep and aching with some elements of superficial sharp or burning pain. Changes in pain with alterations of position or physical activity are variable. Paresthesia and cutaneous hypersensitivity are usually present but may be mild or absent, sometimes causing failure to recognize the neuropathic basis for the pain. The pain is usually unilateral but is sometimes bilateral, may be distributed over more than one dermatomal segment, and often does not have a classic girdling radicular distribution. Impaired light touch and hypersensitivity to pin stimulation may be present in the area of pain but are often absent. In severe cases, weakness and laxity of segmental paraspinal and abdominal muscles are present and abdominal hernia may even occur.[60,61] Electromyography of paraspinal, intercostal, and abdominal muscles is diagnostically helpful and usually shows changes of acute denervation.[21,62,63] As with proximal lower extremity motor neuropathy, weight loss may be prominent, and because of the frequent absence of definite neuropathic symptoms and signs, exhaustive unfruitful searches for an intrathoracic or intraabdominal neoplasm often are undertaken. The finding of electromyographic abnormalities usually leads to the correct diagnosis. Cases in which the distribution of symptoms and signs conforms to a single thoracic root should be evaluated with x-ray and magnetic resonance imaging (MRI) studies of the thoracic spine to exclude a compressive radiculopathy. The prognosis is usually better than for the lower extremity radiculopathies, with gradual recovery within a matter of months to a year.[20]

Similar to other diabetic mononeuropathies and radiculopathies, the etiology of thoracic radiculopathy is obscure, although the acute onset and spontaneous recovery suggest a focal ischemic process. The observation that thoracic radiculopathy, proximal asymmetric motor neuropathy, and cranial mononeuropathy occur among middle-aged patients with Type II diabetes, often appear in the same patient, improve spontaneously, and have a tendency to recur suggests a common pathophysiologic mechanism. Although no pathologic studies of patients with thoracic radiculopathy have been published, postmortem studies of patients with diabetic polyneuropathy do show axonal and demyelinative lesions of nerve roots.[54,55]

Diabetic Mononeuropathy

Mononeuropathy is particularly common in persons with diabetes and may occur on the basis of focal ischemia, entrapment, or trauma to superficially placed nerves.[64] Any of the major peripheral nerves may be affected. When several nerves are involved simultaneously, the disorder is referred to as *mononeuropathy multiplex.* Many patients with diabetic polyneuropathy have electrophysiologic or clinical evidence of superimposed focal mononeuropathy at various common sites of entrapment or nerve injury such as the median nerve at the wrist, ulnar nerve at the elbow, peroneal nerve at the fibular head, radial nerve above the elbow, and lateral cutaneous nerve of the thigh.[3] This may be because nerves affected by segmental demyelination are known to be particularly sensitive to the effects of compression and anoxia. Differential diagnosis of mononeuropathy or mononeuropathy multiplex includes vasculitis, paraproteinemic neuropathy, amyloidosis, acromegaly, hypothyroidism, sarcoidosis, Lyme disease, and bleeding into peripheral nerves caused by coagulation defects.

Carpal tunnel syndrome caused by median-nerve entrapment in the wrist is particularly common among persons with diabetes and produces symptoms and signs similar to those in persons without diabetes. Occasionally, however, distal median-nerve mononeuropathy may occur in the absence of the usual pain and sensory symptoms of carpal tunnel syndrome. Although entrapment is still possible in such cases, coexistent distal ulnar neuropathy[65] and bilateral involvement should suggest distal polyneuropathy rather than nerve entrapment. Nerve-conduction studies showing prolonged distal latencies in multiple nerves rather than limited to the median nerve will serve to distinguish distal polyneuropathy from entrapment. Peroneal mononeuropathy typically produces sudden painless foot drop and, in addition to vascular factors, may be due to trauma because of the superficial location of the nerve at the fibular head. Ulnar mononeuropathy is probably also related to the vulnerable position of the nerve at the elbow. In this case, symptoms usually appear insidiously and may be due to chronic trauma rather than to acute injury or entrapment.

Cranial Neuropathy

Cranial neuropathies also belong to the category of mononeuropathies. The majority of cranial neuropathies affect the third and sixth cranial nerves,[66,67] while the fourth cranial nerve is rarely affected alone.[67] Onset of diplopia is followed by complete ophthalmoplegia within several days. In cases of third nerve involvement, there may be complete ptosis but the pupil is typically spared. Ocular pain accompanies ophthalmoplegia in about 50% of cases. Unlike painful ophthalmoplegia associated with temporal arteritis,[68] eye muscle weakness occurs in a specific nerve distribution rather than from ischemic muscle involvement. The suggestion that pain may be due to involvement of the first and second divisions of the trigeminal nerve in the cavernous sinus is supported by the occasional presence of sensory impairment in this distribution.[67] However, a more likely explanation is that pain originates from ischemia of pain-sensitive terminals in the sheath of the third nerve.[69] Differentiation from a neoplastic or vascular lesion in the orbital fissure, cavernous sinus, infarction at the base of the brain, or focal midbrain infarction[70] should be made with brain-imaging studies such as MRI. A vascular cause of diabetic ophthalmoplegia is strongly supported by three postmortem studies[71-73] in which focal swelling together with axonal and demyelinative lesions were identified in the precavernous or cavernous sinus portions of the third nerve. Extensive hyaline thickening of nutrient vessels of the third nerve without vascular occlusion was found in all three cases. Sparing of the pupil may be a consequence of the relatively intact peripherally located pupillomotor fibers supplied by cavernous sinus blood and spared by the centrally placed nerve lesion. However, compressive lesions of the third nerve within the cavernous sinus also frequently spare the pupil[74] and should be excluded by brain-imaging studies. Recovery without residual weakness always occurs and is usually complete within 3 months, supporting the notion that focal demyelination without axonal destruction is the responsible lesion.[72]

Convincing evidence that other cranial nerve palsies occur with increased frequency in diabetes is lacking. In one uncontrolled study, impaired olfaction was reported in 35 of 58 diabetic patients who gave no evidence of abnormalities of the nasal mucosa.[75] Optic disc edema indistinguishable in appearance from papilledema with associated hemorrhages of the nerve fiber layer and cotton-wool spots has been described in juvenile-onset diabetes.[76,77] This usually is associated with only mild impairment in visual acuity and a favorable prognosis. This condition is of obscure etiology but is believed to be due to a vasculopathy of the most superficial capillary layer of the disc and adjacent retina.[76,77] Anterior ischemic optic neuropathy may occur in diabetes but is more closely associated with hypertension. This is an ischemic infarction of the anterior optic nerve that produces acute edema of the optic disc, profound visual loss, and subsequent development of optic atrophy. Optic atrophy and nerve deafness are associated with diabetes in Wolfram's syndrome and will be discussed below. Facial paralysis due to seventh nerve palsy may occur with increased frequency in patients with diabetes,[78] and the prognosis for recovery may be worse than in patients without diabetes.[79] In view of the high frequency of this neuropathy in the general population, its designation as a diabetic mononeuropathy remains uncertain.

ELECTRODIAGNOSIS

The electrodiagnostic examination provides objective information about the physiologic state of the nerve, nerve root, neuromuscular junction, and muscle. Electrodiagnostic techniques can localize the neuropathologic processes associated with diabetes as focal or multiple mononeuropathies, plexopathies, polyradiculopathies, or polyneuropathies. The electrodiagnostic examination can be used to confirm a clinical diagnosis, quantify the pathophysiologic process, and provide a measure of disease progression or response to therapeutic intervention.[80,81]

The amplitude of the evoked sensory and motor action potential of the standard nerve-conduction study provides an index of the number of functioning axons in the large myelinated nerves and the number of muscle fibers innervated. The area and configuration of the action potential may be a superior measure of axon function, particularly if there is temporal dispersion caused by a pathologic process that produces asynchronous conduction velocities. These parameters correlate well with clinical deficits. The distal latency and conduction velocity depend on fiber size, myelination, and internodal length. They do not correlate well with symptoms or neurologic deficits. Needle electromyography (EMG) assesses electrical activity generated by muscle fibers at rest and with activity. Early EMG abnormalities seen with axonal neuropathic processes include the appearance of fibrillations and positive sharp-waves, followed by abnormalities of the motor-unit potential such as prolonged duration, polyphasia, and increased amplitude.

The standard protocol for the evaluation of a diabetic polyneuropathy should include unilateral evaluation of at least one motor and one sensory nerve from both an upper and a lower extremity, with measurements of the amplitudes of the evoked muscle or sensory action potential, the distal latency, and segmental conduction velocities. The presence of focal or asymmetric deficits and suspected nerve entrapments requires the testing of additional nerves. The EMG examination permits the localization of processes to the nerve roots and plexuses.[82]

Reduction in the amplitude of the sensory nerve action potential is the earliest abnormality in diabetic polyneuropathy and may be present before there are demonstrable abnormalities in the clinical examination.[15,51,53] This is most likely a reflection of loss of distal myelinated nerve fibers.[83,84] The abnormalities are maximal in the lower extremities and can be demonstrated initially in the sural, superficial, peroneal, or plantar nerves. With disease progression the upper extremities become affected and the sensory action potentials may become unrecordable in the lower extremities unless special techniques such as near-nerve needle recordings are used.

The nerve conduction velocity may be decreased slightly at time of diagnosis and usually declines progressively with increased disease duration. Nerve conduction velocity may show a slight improvement with the institution of therapy and declines with the withdrawal of therapy,[85,86] suggesting a reversible metabolic component. Involvement of the proximal segment of nerves, which occurs with disease progression, has been demonstrated with the use of F-wave ratios (a ratio of proximal to distal motor latencies)[87] and somatosensory evoked potentials.[88] Findings of denervation on electromyography, particularly in the intrinsic foot muscles, are an early sign of axonal injury and can precede abnormalities in nerve conduction velocity.[53] Electromyographic signs of

reinnervation, such as prolonged, high-amplitude, polyphasic motor units, occur with further progression of the disease.

Entrapment neuropathies and traumatic focal neuropathies are a frequent complication of diabetes and are diagnosed by demonstrating a focal slowing of nerve conduction known as conduction block. Common sites of compression or chronic injury include the median nerve in the carpal tunnel, the ulnar nerve at the elbow, and the peroneal nerve at the knee. Since these nerve entrapments and chronic injuries usually are superimposed on a diabetic polyneuropathy, their assessment requires side-to-side comparisons and comparisons between conduction velocities in different nerves in the same limb. The presence of bilateral mononeuropathy in the same nerve often complicates diagnosis.

The electrodiagnosis of diabetic proximal motor neuropathy rests on needle electromyography more than on nerve conduction studies. The electromyogram usually reveals fibrillation potentials in proximal lower extremity muscles, particularly the quadriceps, iliopsoas, adductor, and gracilis muscles. There are usually fibrillation potentials in paraspinal muscles extending through multiple spinal levels. Abnormalities of motor unit potentials are typically mild.

Electrodiagnostic examination is of particular help in separating pain caused by thoracic, abdominal, or pelvic disease from pain caused by diabetic truncal neuropathies or radiculopathies, in which sensory findings on the trunk may be subtle or absent. Patients with diabetic thoracoabdominal neuropathies or radiculopathies will demonstrate fibrillations at multiple segmental levels in paraspinal muscles, rectus abdominus, and the external oblique muscles.[21,63]

When the electrodiagnostic evaluation is used to chart disease progression or to monitor the response of therapeutic interventions, it becomes particularly important that techniques be standardized. This includes careful attention to sites of stimulating and recording electrodes, methods of measuring amplitude latency and conduction velocity, and techniques of controlling or correcting for limb temperature. Since multiple measures are made over time, it is important to introduce the appropriate statistical corrections when analyzing results so as to avoid drawing spurious conclusions. Furthermore, even if statistically significant changes in nerve conduction occur, these changes may not necessarily be clinically significant.[81]

PATHOLOGY OF PERIPHERAL NEUROPATHY

The pathophysiologic basis of diabetic distal polyneuropathy remains uncertain and will be reviewed in detail by Simmons elsewhere in this volume (Chapter 39). Two major prevailing theories relate the metabolic effects of chronic hyperglycemia and the effect of ischemia on peripheral nerves. The metabolic hypothesis suggests that hyperglycemia produces several effects, including increased tissue levels of sorbitol and fructose, decreased concentrations of nerve myoinositol, decreased Na^+/K^+ adenosine triphosphatase (ATPase) activity, nonenzymatic glucosylation of proteins, and abnormalities of axonal flow, some or all of which may be responsible for pathologic changes in nerve fibers.[3,89] Alternatively, the vascular hypothesis proposes that hyperglycemia-related metabolic alterations produce an interposed change in tissues and the microvasculature that are then responsible for ischemic pathologic changes in nerve fibers.[25]

Early investigators[90] emphasized macrovascular findings in peripheral nerves and, on the basis of studies of limbs amputated for arteriosclerotic gangrene, attributed the neuropathic changes to arteriosclerotic occlusive disease of the vasa nervorum. Lundbaeck[91] suggested a specific diabetic vascular disease different from arteriosclerosis, while Fagerberg[92] described the presence of material positive for periodic acid-Schiff staining, stenosis, and hyalinization of intraneural vessels. Other authors have suggested the possible role of microvascular changes in capillary endothelial basement membranes, with thickening of the perivascular space, which is known to be more frequent in diabetic neuropathy than other acquired neuropathies.[83,93,94] Whether such changes are etiologically important for diabetic neuropathy is uncertain. It has been suggested that defective blood supply of peripheral nerve occurs in diabetic neuropathy that produces alterations in the nerve microenvironment such as endoneurial hypoxia that are responsible for progressive nerve injury.[95]

Investigators[55,56,93,96] less impressed with the severity of vasa nervorum involvement have argued against a correlation between vascular lesions and severity of neuropathy and favor a metabolic basis for damage to myelin and axons of peripheral nerves and nerve roots. At one time considerable debate existed concerning whether segmental demyelination or axonal degeneration is the primary abnormality in diabetic neuropathy. Some investigators[56,97] suggested a primary degeneration of motor and sensory nerve cell bodies with secondary degeneration of peripheral nerves and nerve root axons and centripetal degeneration of the posterior columns in spinal cord. According to this scheme, dysfunction of the nerve cell body causes the initial manifestations to appear at the periphery because of a "dying back" process that begins distally and spreads proximally.[24,98] Chopra and colleagues[93,99] held that segmental demyelination, presumably the result of a metabolic disturbance of Schwann cell function, was the primary abnormality. Thomas and Lascelles,[96] in studies of teased-fiber preparations, emphasized segmental demyelination and remyelination as the main pathologic change but also identified axonal degeneration in severe cases. Said et al.[24] found evidence of both primary and secondary demyelination, while Behse et al.,[83] finding loss of large and small myelinated fibers and unmyelinated fibers, concluded that axonal degeneration and Schwann-cell damage proceed independently of each other. More recently, Dyck and colleagues[25,100] confirmed that a reduction in the number of myelinated fibers is the characteristic finding in the diabetic peripheral nerve but is a secondary response to axonal degeneration rather than part of a primary process of demyelination and remyelination.

In recent years the pendulum has swung back, and there has been increasing pathologic evidence that microvascular abnormalities may underlie diabetic neuropathy. Dyck has pointed out that previous conclusions concerning primary metabolic neuronal abnormalities reflect studies compromised by severe limitations in tissue sampling.[100] He has remedied this with a more systematic study of the spatial distribution of pathologic abnormalities along the length of peripheral nerve in a population of diabetic patients and nondiabetic controls.[25,100] In postmortem studies, nerve tissue was obtained from the fifth lumbar roots, segmental nerves in lumbar and sacral plexus, and proximal and distal portions of sciatic, tibial, peroneal, and sural nerves of patients with diabetic neuropathy and control subjects to determine the proximal-to-distal pattern of nerve-fiber damage. The number of myelinated fibers was counted in each level of nerve. In patients with diabetic neuropathy, a pattern of multifocal nerve-fiber loss was found to begin in proximal segmental nerves and to become worse distally. Dorsal roots were more affected than ventral roots. Even mildly affected nerves were associated with proximal fiber loss. The early proximal involvement and multifocal pattern of nerve-fiber loss that was observed was felt to be incompatible with both a dying-back neuropathy and a primary metabolic disorder of Schwann cells.[101] Instead, these findings were felt to correlate best with a multifocal pathologic process of nerve beginning proximally and affecting multiple levels of nerve.[101] Distal worsening of nerve-fiber degeneration was attributed to the cumulative effect of multiple random lesions along the course of the nerve.[19,101] The strong similarity of this pattern of nerve-fiber loss to previously described patterns in necrotizing vasculitis[102] and experimental studies of microsphere embolization[100] suggested that ischemia is responsible for diabetic neuropathy. Thickening of capillary walls and occlusive disease of small arteries and arterioles that supply peripheral nerve are more pronounced in patients with diabetic neuropathy than in age-matched controls,[25,103] and a correlation between microvascular disease in peripheral nerve and severity of diabetic neuropathy has recently been established.[104] In another postmortem study of proximal, intermediate, and distal portions of peripheral nerve in diabetes, Johnson et al.[105] found focal, fascicular nerve lesions characterized by reduced density of myelinated axons that occasionally had a wedge-shaped, superficial location within the nerve. More-common lesions were multifocal areas of reduced density of myelinated nerve fibers similar to the lesions described by Dyck et al.[101] Most were located in proximal portions of lumbosacral plexus and posterior tibial nerve. As in the experience of Dyck et al.,[102] both types of lesions were similar to those described by Johnson and Beggs in patients with vasculitis.[106] Frequent vascular abnormalities such as thick-walled endoneurial and epineural vessels also were noted, but no intravascular thrombi were identified that could be correlated with particular focal nerve lesions. Timperley et al.[107] also described endothelial cell hyperplasia in endoneurial blood vessels of the sural nerve with plugging of the vascular lumen by necrotic cellular material in patients with severe diabetic neuropathy.

On the basis of the careful study of a very small number of cases, the pathologic basis of diabetic mononeuropathy and mononeuropathy multiplex is presumed to be ischemic infarction of nerve. Raff and Asbury[40] described a patient with an acute and rapidly progressive asymmetric neuropathy who was found to have numerous microinfarcts in the proximal portions of the obturator, femoral, sciatic, and tibial nerves. The occurrence of infarcts in bridging interfascicular bundles was similar to the distribution of microinfarcts in other ischemic mononeuropathies.[94] Although fibrosis and hyalinization of small arterioles and capillaries were prominent, most infarcts did not relate to identifiable vascular occlusions, and some question has been raised as to whether the identified nerve lesions were infarcts or normal structures known as Raynaud's corpuscles.[100,101] Pathologic studies of three cases of diabetic oculomotor nerve palsy have also been carried out.[71-73] All three demonstrated a localized zone of central fascicular nerve injury associated with hyaline thickening of vessels but an absence of an identifiable vascular occlusion.

The pathologic basis of diabetic autonomic neuropathy is incompletely understood. A number of investigators have identified abnormalities in paravertebral sympathetic ganglia, including neurons distended by lipid-rich material,[108-110] vacuolar degeneration of neurons produced by dilatation of endoplasmic reticulum,[110] and mononuclear-cell infiltration of autonomic nerve bundles and ganglia.[110] Loss of myelinated nerve fibers has been described in sympathetic communicating rami,[111,112] vagus nerve,[111,113] postganglionic sympathetic nerves,[114] splanchnic nerves,[112] and nerves to the bladder wall.[115]

MECHANISM OF PAINFUL DIABETIC NEUROPATHY

Pain is one of the more distressing and difficult to manage symptoms of diabetic neuropathy and occurs in both focal neuropathy and symmetric polyneuropathy. In polyneuropathy the incidence, severity, and duration of pain are quite variable, whereas in focal mononeuropathy and radiculopathy, pain is usually more severe but temporary. A pathophysiologic basis for the pain of diabetic neuropathy has not been established. Brown et al.[23] described axonal degeneration predominantly involving small myelinated and unmyelinated fibers in sural nerve biopsies of two patients with painful distal diabetic neuropathy. Since small myelinated and unmyelinated fibers mediate pain sensation, it was proposed that pain results from increased ectopic activity in the regenerating small-fiber nerve sprouts. However, the fact that pain is not prominent in other predominantly small-fiber peripheral neuropathies has cast doubt on this hypothesis. Said et al.,[24] for example, found similar small-fiber abnormalities with axonal sprouting in five patients with clinical features of small-fiber diabetic neuropathy, but only two of these patients had painful manifestations. Dyck et al.[116] found that painful diabetic neuropathy was correlated with acute breakdown of myelinated nerve fibers but not

with differential involvement of small and large nerve fibers. Archer et al.[28] found acute degeneration with regeneration in nerve fibers of all diameters in patients with acute and severe painful polyneuropathy. In a population of patients with more chronic polyneuropathy, some of whom had pain, Behse et al.[83] found loss of both small and large fibers. Britland et al.[117] found uniform degeneration and regeneration in large and small myelinated fibers and in small unmyelinated fibers in patients with either acute or chronic painful neuropathy as well as in patients with painless neuropathy and neurotrophic foot ulcers. There were no differences in the extent of unmyelinated fiber pathology or acute axonal degeneration in patients with and without pain, but fibers with disproportionately large Schwann cells relative to axon diameter occurred exclusively in patients with painful neuropathy, raising the possibility that axonal atrophy may play a role in pain production.[118]

The gate-control theory of pain[119] suggested that loss of inhibition mediated by large fibers may increase transmission of nociceptive pain information in small fibers. However, the fact that the ratio of intact large to small fibers is not consistently altered in diabetic neuropathy[116] and that peripheral neuropathies characterized by predominantly large-fiber involvement are not uniformly associated with pain fails to support a gate mechanism in painful diabetic neuropathy. Asbury and Fields[69] have proposed that pain in diabetic neuropathy may be due to regenerative sprouting of small unmyelinated and myelinated axons. The concept that dysesthetic pain is due to volleys of impulses originating from damaged and regenerating afferent fibers is derived from studies of experimental traumatic neuromas. Transection injury of peripheral nerve in rodents[120] causes sprouting of small primary afferents into the neuroma, which show increased spontaneous activity, increased sensitivity to mechanical stimulation, and increased sensitivity to topical epinephrine and sympathetic efferent activity.[121-123] Whether regenerating axonal sprouts in diabetic neuropathy show similar characteristics is unknown, but Britland et al.[117] found similar sprouting of myelinated and unmyelinated axons in patients with diabetic neuropathy both with and without painful manifestations.

Pain in focal mononeuropathies or radiculopathies may be similar to the dysesthetic pain of distal polyneuropathy but usually includes a more deep-seated dull, aching pain, which Asbury and Fields[69] have suggested is due to activation of pain receptors of nervi nervorum in the sheath of swollen or chemically irritated nerve trunks. This may also be the basis of the ocular pain that occurs in 50% of patients with diabetic oculomotor palsies and the deeply localized thigh, hip, and trunk pain of diabetic radiculopathies.

MANAGEMENT OF DIABETIC NEUROPATHY

Treatment of Hyperglycemia

Management of diabetic neuropathy, whether painful or painless, begins with treatment of hyperglycemia.

Although the precise relationship between poor diabetic control and peripheral neuropathy is uncertain, clinical consensus favors maintenance of strict control of blood glucose levels in patients with or without diabetic neuropathy.[12,124] In experimental models of diabetes produced by streptozocin or alloxan,[125] reductions in nerve conduction velocity occur acutely and can, at least in early stages, be restored by treatment with insulin.[126]

There is also evidence that high blood glucose levels may alter pain threshold. Morley et al.[127] found that glucose infusions in normal subjects lower the pain threshold and tolerance levels and that persons with diabetes have lower pain thresholds and tolerance levels than do persons without diabetes. In experimental animals hyperglycemia reduces the analgesic effect of morphine, suggesting a possible effect of glucose on opiate receptors.[128,129] The acute painful paresthesias that sometimes accompany hyperglycemia in early untreated diabetes and subside with glucose control and the painful paresthesias that occasionally occur immediately following treatment of hyperglycemia may relate to an effect of glucose level and glucose flux on nociceptive receptors.[130]

The American Neurological Association[124] has reviewed the available evidence that the development and severity of neuropathy is related to glycemic control. First, uncontrolled retrospective studies have shown that patients with poor diabetic control develop all diabetic complications, including neuropathy, earlier and more severely than do patients with better control.[16,131,132] Second, severity of hyperglycemia measured by fasting glucose and glycosylated hemoglobin levels in patients with newly diagnosed diabetes was inversely correlated with motor but not sensory conduction velocity.[133] Third, in patients with newly diagnosed diabetes, improvement in blood glucose and glycosylated hemoglobin levels after treatment with oral hypoglycemic agents[134] or insulin[86,132,135] was associated with improvement in motor but not sensory nerve conduction velocities. Newer methods of providing continuous insulin by subcutaneous infusion[136–138] and pancreatic transplantation[139] in patients with well-established diabetes have also demonstrated improvement in at least some measures of peripheral nerve function and in pain scores, although improvement has been relatively mild and, in the case of pancreatic transplantation, not always demonstrable.[140] Finally, comparisons of conventional treatment with strict control of blood glucose levels accomplished by multiple insulin injections, home blood glucose monitoring, and frequent adjustments in insulin dosage have been carried out. Service et al.[141] treated 33 patients with either "rigorous" or "conventional" treatment. After 3 years, no significant difference in glucose control or severity of peripheral nerve function was found, possibly because 13 of 33 patients failed to meet criteria for either rigorous or conventional control by the conclusion of the study. Holman et al.[142] randomized 74 insulin-dependent diabetic patients to continuance of their usual care of diabetes or to treatment with a more-intensive program of insulin and blood glucose

monitoring. After 2 years, sensory nerve function, as measured by vibration threshold, was significantly better preserved in the strictly controlled group than in the conventionally treated group. Here too, some crossover occurred between groups over the course of the trial. In an uncontrolled study, Reeves et al.[143] studied 10 patients with relatively mild peripheral neuropathy who were intensively treated over a period of 6 months and found a progressive improvement in motor and sensory conduction velocities, with some results coming into the normal range. The Diabetes Control and Complications Trial (DCCT),[144,145] which is currently still in progress, has randomized 1441 patients to receive either intensive or standard therapy. Feasibility of adherence to the study protocol and prescribed regimens has been established,[144] and the study will terminate in 1993, by which time the range of follow-up will be 5 to 10 years.

Treatment of Metabolic Abnormalities

Specific treatment with aldose reductase inhibitors, which is directed at the presumed pathophysiologic basis of diabetic neuropathy, has been under investigation for a number of years. In animal models persistent hyperglycemia causes increased conversion of glucose to sorbitol by aldose reductase.[146] Accumulation of sorbitol, depletion of myoinositol, and reduced Na^+/K^+-ATPase activity in peripheral nerve have been proposed as causes of diabetic peripheral neuropathy. Electrophysiologic, morphologic, and biochemical studies of the effect of aldose reductase inhibitors in streptozocin-diabetic rats have shown prevention and reversal of peripheral neuropathy.[147] Alrestatin was the first aldose reductase inhibitor to be used in humans, but it produced equivocal results and a high incidence of adverse reactions.[148,149] Tolrestat was developed to replace alrestatin[150] and in 8-week and 1-year double-blind, placebo-controlled studies was associated with improvement in neuropathic symptoms and nerve conduction velocities.[151,152]

Sorbinil is a longer-acting aldose reductase inhibitor that has undergone more thorough clinical investigation. Judzewitsch et al.[153] found a small but statistically significant improvement in motor and sensory nerve conduction velocity in a group of 39 asymptomatic patients with abnormal nerve-conduction velocities in a crossover trial comparing 9 weeks of sorbinil treatment with 9 weeks of placebo. In a similar crossover study of 15 patients, Young et al.,[154] found improvement in pain, tendon reflexes, and amplitude of sural nerve action potentials but worsening in sensory impairment and no change in vibration perception, motor nerve conduction velocity, and tests of autonomic function. In another crossover study, Lewin et al.[155] found no improvement in electrophysiologic or clinical measures of peripheral neuropathy in 12 patients treated with sorbinil for 4 weeks. Jaspan et al.[156] reported beneficial effects of sorbinil in a single-blind, uncontrolled, and poorly standardized study in which eight of 11 patients were relieved of pain while smaller numbers of patients showed improved strength, sensation, nerve conduction velocity, and autonomic function. In longer studies, Fagius et al.[157] randomized 27 patients to receive sorbinil and 28 patients to receive placebo for 6 months and found no major clinical improvement and only minor short-term improvement in similar electrophysiologic and clinical measures of peripheral and autonomic nerve function, whereas Martyn et al.[158] found no improvement in clinical or electrophysiologic measures of peripheral and autonomic function in 22 patients with asymptomatic diabetic polyneuropathy treated with sorbinil and placebo for 6 months each. Preliminary reports of more recent multicenter trials[159,160] have indicated more favorable results. In a multicenter, placebo-controlled, double-blind trial of 202 patients with painful diabetic neuropathy, a significant difference in clinical measures of neuropathy in favor of sorbinil over placebo was found.[159] A 12-month placebo-controlled, double-blind trial in 217 patients with diabetic neuropathy also showed that sorbinil-treated patients more frequently exhibited clinically significant improvement in quantitative neurologic tests and in scored neurologic signs than patients treated with placebo.[160] Results of a multicenter study of sorbinil vs. placebo over a period of 2 to 3 years in the prevention of diabetic complications, including peripheral neuropathy, are currently pending.

If aldose reductase inhibitors are effective in the treatment of diabetic neuropathy, what is their mechanism of action? Endoneurial edema caused by the increased osmotic gradient resulting from increased nerve sorbitol levels has been proposed as a possible contributing factor. Recent neuropathologic and neurochemical studies have shown that patients with diabetic neuropathy have higher than normal amounts of glucose, fructose, and sorbitol and normal amounts of myoinositol in peripheral nerve[161] and that levels of sorbitol are inversely related to the density of myelinated nerve fibers.[162] In two studies involving a total of 22 patients, treatment with sorbinil for 1 year was associated with a significant reduction in nerve sorbitol concentration[161,162] and increased regeneration of myelinated nerve fibers[162] in biopsied sural nerve before and after treatment. MRI spectroscopy of peripheral nerve has shown increased water content in the sciatic nerve of galactose-fed rats with endoneurial edema that can be prevented by feeding of sorbinil.[163] Use of MRI spectroscopy in diabetic patients with symptomatic neuropathy has shown an increased water content in the sural nerve of seven of 11 patients as compared with normal nerve hydration in two of 11 diabetic patients with asymptomatic neuropathy.[164] Diabetic patients with symptomatic neuropathy treated with sorbinil or tolrestat for more than 2 years showed reduction in neuropathic symptoms and had normal nerve hydration.[164]

Unfortunately, sorbinil has been associated with a relatively high frequency of hypersensitivity reactions, with rash, fever, lymphadenopathy, and abnormal liver chemistries occurring in approximately 10% of patients.[165] In view of the intriguing pathologic and spectroscopic findings discussed above, as well as the more recent encouraging clinical studies with sorbinil,

further evaluation of newer aldose reductase inhibitors with fewer adverse effects is anticipated.

Improved function in experimental and human diabetic nerves following treatment with aldose reductase inhibitors has also been attributed to increased myoinositol concentrations. Myoinositol is an important constituent of the phospholipids that make up cell membranes and other cellular structures. Myoinositol concentration is reduced in peripheral nerves of diabetic animals and is normalized by aldose reductase inhibitors and myoinositol supplementation.[166] However, despite an earlier report of reduced nerve myoinositol levels in diabetic neuropathy,[167] more recent biochemical and pathologic studies have indicated that the nerve myoinositol concentration is not reduced in diabetic patients with or without neuropathy.[161,168] Moreover, human treatment studies with myoinositol have given either negative or barely significant results.[166]

Gangliosides are complex glycolipids that are essential components of neuronal cell membranes and have been shown to enhance nerve-fiber regeneration and sprouting in tissue culture preparations.[169] Several double-blind controlled studies lasting between 6 weeks and 6 months have shown slight but inconsistent improvement in neuropathic symptoms and nerve conduction velocities,[170-172] and further studies of long-term treatment are needed. There is no evidence that treatment with vitamins is of any value in diabetic neuropathy.[150]

Treatment of Painful Neuropathy

Pain control is often the major management problem in patients with either focal neuropathy or polyneuropathy. As discussed above, several types of pain and discomfort may occur. Patients with distal sensory polyneuropathy usually describe tingling or burning paresthesia of the feet, lower legs, and hands often associated with dysesthesia manifest by hypersensitivity to touch, clothing, or bedsheets. Patients with proximal motor neuropathy usually describe deep, aching pain in the thigh, hip, or lower trunk, sometimes associated with superficial paresthesia and dysesthesia of the anterolateral thighs. Brief, lancinating pains of the extremities or trunk occasionally occur, which, by analogy with tabes dorsalis or Fabry's disease, are likely due to disturbances in dorsal root ganglia or dorsal roots. Pain is typically more severe in the evening and at night, either because of reduced environmental stimulation or because of other, unidentified, diurnal variations. Bed cradles and support stockings worn at night are sometimes of value in alleviating symptoms.

Treatment of pain requires attempts at strict control of blood glucose levels, use of analgesics, and treatment of associated reactive or underlying depression. In mild to moderate painful neuropathy, regular use of simple analgesics such as acetaminophen or ibuprofen may suffice. Since painful diabetic neuropathy may persist for months and occasionally years, continued use of narcotics should be avoided except as a last resort. When non-narcotic analgesics are effective, they should be taken on a carefully timed, regular basis throughout the day, as in the management of cancer pain, not after pain has been allowed to build in repeated crescendo fashion. We have often found analgesics such as propoxyphene with acetaminophen, for example, to be helpful when given according to a regular dosing schedule. Since the pain of diabetic neuropathy is characteristically worse at night, regular dosing of an analgesic in the early evening and again before sleep may reduce analgesic requirements at night and improve sleep.

Anticonvulsants such as phenytoin, carbamazepine, and benzodiazepines have all been used to treat painful diabetic neuropathy. Despite initial reports of efficacy,[173] phenytoin has usually been ineffective in controlled studies[174] and general clinical experience. Carbamazepine was effective in one controlled study[175] but is usually no more effective than phenytoin.[12] Benzodiazepines such as diazepam and clonazepam are also ineffective.[176,177] Despite negative results in treatment of chronic neuropathic pain, anticonvulsants are worthwhile in patients with lancinating and paroxysmal pain, being effective for such pain in an estimated 50% of patients.[13]

Depression, anxiety, and insomnia are common accompaniments of chronic painful neuropathy.[29,177] These may occur as a direct result of the pain or may exist as predisposing factors that enhance the pain. In severe forms of diabetic neuropathy with anorexia and weight loss, pain usually precedes the appearance of depression.[29] Similar to other painful neuropathies, such as postherpetic neuralgia or tic douloureux, in painful diabetic neuropathy disappearance of pain usually is followed by resolution of depressive symptoms. In one study of painful diabetic neuropathy, a high incidence of psychologic and somatic symptoms of depression were identified.[177] Treatment with amitriptyline or imipramine, 100 mg daily, produced remission of pain with concomitant relief of depression over a mean period of 10 weeks, a time course compatible with the antidepressant effect of these drugs. In more recent double-blind crossover studies, both amitriptyline,[178] at doses of up to 150 mg daily, and imipramine,[179,180] at doses of up to 100 mg daily, have been found to be superior to placebo. It is important to note that this effect was not necessarily associated with a concomitant improvement in mood. Efficacy of tricyclic antidepressants for pain may relate to potentiation of endogenous serotonin-mediated analgesic systems of the central nervous system.[181] With both amitriptyline and imipramine, patients receiving higher doses or achieving higher blood levels of tricyclic metabolites have shown the greatest improvement.[178,179,182] Care should be taken to avoid anticholinergic side effects such as urinary retention and impotence, especially in patients with autonomic neuropathy.

The combination of a potent phenothiazine such as fluphenazine given together with an antidepressant for management of painful diabetic neuropathy has also been recommended, but this recommendation has been based on relatively few studies that have either been uncontrolled[183] or shown only partial reduction in pain.[184] In one double-blind, placebo-controlled study, the combination of amitriptyline and fluphenazine was no more effective than placebo.[185] On the other hand, the use of a low dose of a sedative phenothiazine such as promazine or thorazine at night together with analgesic medication may be helpful. In resistant cases the addition of a more potent phenothiazine to treatment with a tricyclic antidepressant may be indicated but should not exceed 3 months' duration because of the risk of tardive dyskinesia.[186]

In recent preliminary studies, intravenous lidocaine[187] and its structural analogue oral mexilitene[188] were more effective than placebo in double-blind, crossover trials in patients with painful diabetic neuropathy. Topical capsaicin, a substance P antagonist, has been used with some success in the management of postherpetic neuralgia.[189] However, in preliminary reports, topical capsaicin has had only mildly beneficial effects compared with placebo in alleviating the pain of diabetic neuropathy.[190,191] Pentoxifylline, a drug that increases red blood cell flexibility and improves microvascular blood flow, appeared to be effective against painful diabetic neuropathy in one open study[192] but ineffective in a follow-up brief randomized double-blind study.[193]

DIABETIC AUTONOMIC NEUROPATHY

Diabetes is the commonest cause of autonomic peripheral neuropathy and is responsible for a significant proportion of the mortality and morbidity associated with that disease. With the possible exception of pain, the autonomic manifestations of diabetes are responsible for the most troublesome and disabling features of diabetic peripheral neuropathy. A broad spectrum of symptoms occurs, affecting cardiovascular, gastrointestinal, urogenital, thermoregulatory, sudomotor, and pupillomotor function. The recent availability of sensitive, specific, and reproducible noninvasive tests of autonomic function has enhanced our understanding of the prevalence, pathophysiology, and clinical manifestations of this disorder.[194]

Cardiovascular System

An increased resting heart rate has frequently been observed in diabetic patients.[195,196] With the progression of disease, some patients display a fixed heart rate that, like the rate of the transplanted heart, responds only minimally to physiologic stimuli. The initial tachycardia is due to a vagal cardiac neuropathy that may be followed by a decrease in heart rate and ultimately a fixed heart rate resulting from the progression of dysfunction of the cardiac sympathetic nervous system.[197–199]

Orthostatic hypotension, defined as a fall in systolic blood pressure of 20 to 30 mm Hg or diastolic blood pressure of 10 to 15 mm Hg, occurs in diabetes as a consequence of efferent sympathetic vasomotor denervation, causing reduced vasoconstriction of the splanchnic and other peripheral vascular beds. Diminished cardiac acceleration and cardiac output (particularly in association with exercise) may play a lesser role in the development of this disorder.[200,201] Patients typically present with lightheadedness and presyncopal symptoms.

Complaints less easily recognized as hypotensive in origin, such as weakness, fatigue, visual blurring, and neck pain, may also be present. Many patients, however, remain asymptomatic despite significant falls in blood pressure. Fluctuations in the amount of orthostatic hypotension are frequently observed and may reflect postprandial blood pooling, the hypotensive role of insulin, and changing patterns of fluid retention caused by renal failure and congestive heart failure.[202] The rise in plasma norepinephrine levels is typically less than expected relative to the fall in blood pressure. Less frequently an increase in norepinephrine is observed that may reflect low blood volume or decreased red blood cell mass.[203,204]

Endeavors at treatment include nonpharmacologic approaches such as the patient's eating a high-sodium diet, raising the head of the bed during sleep, and wearing supportive hose. These measures usually help only the mildly afflicted. Pharmacologic treatments include the use of mineralocorticoid fludrocortisone, direct and indirect sympathomimetic agents, β-blockers with or without intrinsic sympathomimetic activity, pressor agents, prostaglandin synthesis inhibitors, antihistamines, and antiserotonergic agents.[205-207] Therapy should be initiated with fludrocortisone (0.1 to 0.5 mg). A pressor, sympathomimetic agent, or prostaglandin synthetase inhibitor can be added to the drug regimen of those patients who remain symptomatic. Most diabetic patients with orthostatic hypertension will respond to these interventions. Refractory patients may require a combination of several of these agents or even the addition of further agents (see Table 43–1). These medications may be used singly or in combination, although the orthostatic hypotension that is associated with diabetes only rarely demands such extensive therapy.

Other cardiovascular abnormalities have included a cardiomyopathy in patients without ischemic heart disease manifesting as impaired myocardial contractility and decreased left ventricular diastolic filling observed by radionuclear ventriculography.[208] This may be a consequence of autonomic neuropathy, intrinsic myocardial disease, or decreased cardiac catecholamine responsivity. Silent cardiac ischemia[209,210] and prolongation of the Q-T interval have also been observed.[211,212]

Several authors have drawn attention to the increased frequency of sudden death in patients with autonomic neuropathy. Proposed etiologies have included cardiorespiratory arrest caused by cardiac arrhythmias, silent cardiac ischemia, sleep apnea, and an abnormal response to hypoxia, particularly in association with pulmonary infection, surgery, and anesthesia.[213,214]

The laboratory evaluation of cardiovascular autonomic neuropathy includes measures of heart-rate variation at rest and in response to deep respiration, the Valsalva maneuver, and postural change. These tests primarily provide an index of vagal cardiac function. The blood pressure response to postural change (active standing or passive tilting), immersion in cold water, mental stress tests, and isometric exercise also is determined. These tests assess predominantly sympathetic function. Combinations of such tests provide a sensitive measure of autonomic function and have been used by many investigators for evaluating patients with autonomic failure.[215-217] Other, more specialized, techniques have been reported and include spectral analysis of the heart rate,[218] measures of baroreceptor function,[219] long-term cardiac monitoring,[220,221] and measures of cardiovascular responses to pharmacologic agents.[217]

Clinical studies using these noninvasive measures of cardiovascular function have demonstrated a strong correlation with symptoms.[222,223] Abnormal measures of cardiovascular autonomic function also have correlated with abnormal autonomic function in other organ systems, including abnormal pupillomotor function,[224,225] gastrointestinal function,[226] and norepinephrine production.[227] Although these cardiovascular tests are sensitive, abnormalities in sudomotor function of the lower extremities and impotence may precede any detectible cardiovascular autonomic neuropathy.[222,228]

Among unselected diabetic patients, 20 to 40% display abnormalities in cardiovascular autonomic function.[229,230] Abnormalities have been found in teenagers and patients tested shortly after diagnosis.[135,231,232] A pattern of initial parasympathetic cardiac dysfunction followed by sympathetic dysfunction has been observed. This may be a consequence of the nerve-length dependence of a neuropathic process or a reflection of the sensitivity of the tests of cardiac autonomic function. Low et al.[228] addressed the latter possibility in a study comparing distal sweating with heart-rate variation in patients with diabetic neuropathy. He demonstrated that distal abnormalities in sweating, a function mediated by the sympathetic nervous system, occurred with a fre-

Table 43–1. Pharmacologic Agents for Treatment of Orthostatic Hypotension

Mineralocorticoids
  Fludrocortisone
Sympathomimetic agents
  Ephedrine
  Phenylephrine
  Methylphenidate
  Phenylpropanolamine
  Tyramine (with monoamine oxidase inhibition)
  Midodrine
  Clonidine
  Yohimbine
  DL-dihydrophenylserine (DL-DOPS)
Nonspecific pressor agents
  Dihydroergotamine
  Caffeine
  Somatostatin analogues
Dopamine blocking agents
  Metoclopramide
β-Adrenergic blocking agents
  Propranolol
  Pindolol
  Xamoterol
Prostaglandin synthetase inhibitors
  Indomethacin
  Ibuprofen
  Naproxen
Other agents
  Desmopressin acetate (DDAVP)

quency equal to that of heart-rate variation test abnormalities.

Several important pitfalls are associated with the use of cardiovascular tests of autonomic function. Many measures of autonomic function decline with age, and age-based norms should be used. A combination of tests is recommended to avoid reliance on a single measure of autonomic function. The use of such a battery will improve diagnostic discrimination by assessing different afferent and efferent autonomic pathways. Performance of several tests also minimizes the likelihood of misdiagnosis caused by the limitations in reproducibility inherent to all tests. Variation in clinical methodologies, such as whether a test is done when the patient is lying or sitting or whether an absolute difference or a ratio is measured, in addition to the age dependence of many tests of autonomic function, emphasizes the need for laboratory-based normal values.

Urogenital System

Bladder symptoms associated with autonomic neuropathy include hesitancy, poor stream, increase in interval between micturition, and a sense of inadequate bladder emptying. These symptoms may be followed by urinary retention and overflow incontinence.[233,234] Sensory abnormality of the detrusor muscle is the earliest bladder autonomic abnormality to occur, producing impaired bladder sensation and an increase in the threshold for initiation of the micturition reflex. A decrease in detrusor activity (detrusor areflexia) follows, which leads to incomplete bladder emptying, increased postmicturition residual volume, decreased peak urinary flow rate, and ultimately to urinary retention.[233,235] These changes predispose to the development of urinary tract infections, including pyelonephritis, which may accelerate or exacerbate renal failure.

Evaluation of diabetic cystopathy includes the measurement of postmicturition urinary residual volume, intravenous pyelography and urography with measurement of the urinary flow rate, cystometry, and urethral sphincter electromyography.[233,235] The goal of treatment is the improvement of bladder emptying and includes the institution of regular voiding patterns, intermittent catheterization, the use of cholinergic agonists such as carbachol and bethanechol, and, under very rare circumstances, bladder-neck surgery.[234]

Impotence is a frequent and disturbing symptom in male diabetic patients and can have an autonomic, sensory, vascular, or psychogenic etiology (see Chapter 46). The reported incidence has ranged from 30 to 75%.[236-238] Impotence may be the earliest symptom of diabetic autonomic neuropathy.[239] A significant proportion of diabetic patients, presenting with impotence alone, will develop other autonomic symptoms and abnormalities on autonomic testing when studied prospectively.[223]

Erectile function is mediated predominantly by the parasympathetic nervous system. Impotence caused by autonomic neuropathy progresses gradually but is usually permanent 2 years after onset. Sympathetically mediated ejaculatory failure may precede the appearance of impotence, although impotence can occur with a retained ability to ejaculate and experience orgasm. Retrograde ejaculation will occur if bladder-neck closure fails, a function also controlled by the sympathetic nervous system.[240,241]

Clinical and laboratory testing includes the evaluation of nocturnal penile tumescence and rigidity,[242] circumferential measures of penile expansion,[243,244] penile blood pressure measures,[245] penile vascular ultrasonography,[246] nerve conduction studies of the dorsal nerve of the penis,[247] and measurement of the latency of the bulbocavernosus reflex.[248] Therapy for this problem entails the use of mechanical devices,[249] penile prosthetic implants,[250] or the autoinjection of papaverine[251] and other vasoactive substances into the corpus cavernosum.[252-254]

Gastrointestinal Tract

Gastrointestinal autonomic neuropathy results in disordered gastrointestinal motility, secretion, and absorption (see Chapter 51). In one study, up to 76% of unselected diabetic subjects acknowledged gastrointestinal symptoms.[255] Autonomic dysfunction occurs throughout the gastrointestinal tract, producing several specific clinical syndromes.

Diabetic gastroparesis may manifest as nausea, postprandial vomiting, bloating, belching, loss of appetite, and early satiety. Food residue is retained in the stomach because of an absence of or decrease in gastric peristalsis compounded by lower intestinal dysmotility. A gastric splash may be elicited on clinical examination. Gastroparesis may impair the establishment of adequate glycemic control.[256,257] Investigations include upper gastrointestinal x-ray examination, gastroscopy, studies of gastric motility, and scintigraphic studies of gastric emptying. A difference between the rates of emptying of liquids and solids is commonly observed.[226,258] Frequent small meals and pharmacotherapy with dopamine antagonists such as metoclopromide[259] and domperidone[260] or cisapride[261] are standard approaches to the treatment of this disorder. A recent study has proposed the use of erythromycin, which may act as an agonist upon motilin receptors, as a gastrokinetic agent.[262]

Diarrhea and other lower gastrointestinal tract symptoms also may occur. Diabetic diarrhea manifests as a profuse, watery, typically nocturnal diarrhea, which can last for hours or days and frequently alternates with constipation. Abdominal discomfort is commonly associated. Fecal incontinence, caused by anal sphincter incompetence or reduced rectal sensation, is another manifestation of diabetic autonomic neuropathy.[263,264]

The pathogenesis of diabetic diarrhea includes abnormalities in gastrointestinal motility,[265] decreased gut transit time,[266] reduced (α_2-adrenergic receptor-mediated) fluid absorption,[267] bacterial overgrowth,[268] pancreatic insufficiency, coexistent celiac disease,[269] and abnormalities in bile salt metabolism.[270] The pathophysiology of diabetic constipation is poorly understood but may reflect loss of the postprandial gastrocolic reflex.[255]

The treatment of diabetic diarrhea entails symptomatic treatment with loperamide, diphenoxylate, or codeine phosphate, antibiotic treatment (tetracycline) for bacterial overgrowth,[271] clonidine treatment for reduced α_2-adrenergic receptor-mediated intestinal absorption.[267]

Abnormalities in esophageal motility have also been demonstrated. Although usually asymptomatic, this may result in symptoms such as heartburn, dysphagia, and an increased predisposition to esophageal ulceration. These symptoms may be relieved by domperidone.[272]

Sweating Abnormalities

Abnormalities of sweating initially appear in a stocking distribution. These abnormalities are correlated and associated with other deficits of autonomic function, including orthostatic hypotension, cardiac vagal abnormalities, and absence of sympathetic activation on microneurographic studies.[273–275] A decrease in pain perception frequently accompanies loss of distal sweating.[276]

Unusual patterns of sweating abnormalities include the focal loss of sweating associated with diabetic truncal neuropathy and gustatory sweating, an abnormal production of sweating after eating, particularly spicy food, which may manifest over the face, head, neck, shoulders, and chest.[277] Therapy with anticholinergic agents may be successful, although high doses that produce side effects are frequently required.

Testing of the eccrine sweat glands has provided a useful means of assessing and localizing sympathetic nervous system function in patients with autonomic disorders. Thermoregulatory sweating can be tested by raising the body temperature with an external heating source. The sweat response is assessed by measuring the color change of an indicator such as iodine with starch, quinizarin, or alizarin red.[278,279] Skin bioelectric recordings measuring skin conductance, skin resistance, or the sympathetic skin potential provide alternate measures of sudomotor function.[280,281] These tests measure both central and peripheral aspects of the afferent sympathetic nervous system. Postganglionic sudomotor function can be determined by measuring sweat output after iontophoresis or intradermal injection of cholinergic agonists such as pilocarpine, nicotine, or acetylcholine. These agents either stimulate sweat glands directly[282] or affect a neighboring population of sweat glands via an axonal reflex.[274]

Neuroglycopenia and Hypoglycemic Unawareness

Hypoglycemia is the commonest complication of the treatment of diabetes and limits attempts to attain a euglycemic state. The incidence of significant hypoglycemic events is increased two to three times in patients receiving intensive insulin therapy.[144] Because the brain is unable to synthesize glucose and has limited ability to store glucose, hypoglycemia produces an array of neurologic symptoms. Typical symptoms include those attributable to neuroglycopenia, such as cognitive dysfunction, encephalopathy, seizures, hemiplegia, and coma,[283] and those due to systemic epinephrine release, such as anxiety, hunger, restlessness, diaphoresis, and tachycar-

dia.[284] Microneurographic studies have demonstrated an increase in sympathetic nervous system outflow accompanying hypoglycemia.[285] The physiologic response to hypoglycemia involves the dissipation of insulin and the activation of glucose counterregulatory systems, which include the release of glucagon, epinephrine, growth hormone, and cortisol.[286,287] A selective defect in glucagon secretion in response to hypoglycemia develops after several years in all persons with diabetes. Many diabetic individuals also develop a deficient epinephrine response in association with loss of hypoglycemic warning symptoms.[286,287] Absent hypoglycemic warning symptoms were previously attributed to an autonomic neuropathy.[288,289] Recent studies, however, have associated a reduced hypoglycemic threshold for activation of the counterregulatory system and the awareness of hypoglycemia with strict glycemic control.[290,291] By contrast, the hypoglycemic threshold for neuroglycopenic symptoms such as seizures and cognitive dysfunction may not be altered by prior treatment.[292]

CENTRAL NERVOUS SYSTEM

Cerebrovascular Disease

Central nervous system neurons are not directly affected in diabetes mellitus. Their involvement reflects associated disease of the large and small arteries of the brain or results from the metabolic derangements caused by prolonged hypoglycemia, anoxia, or ketoacidosis. Cerebral infarction has been claimed to occur one and a half to two times more frequently in persons with diabetes than in persons without diabetes.[17,293,294] Whether diabetes is uniquely responsible for an increased risk of cerebrovascular disease distinct from the risk produced by frequently associated hypertension and hyperlipidemia is uncertain. Prospective data from the Framingham Study indicate an increased risk of cerebral infarction in individuals with an even slight intolerance to glucose intolerance.[295] In a community-based study in Rochester, Minnesota,[17] the observed frequency of transient ischemic attack was three times greater than expected and the frequency of stroke was 1.7 times greater than expected. The coexistence of hypertension further increased the frequency of transient ischemic attack or stroke in the diabetic population. Obesity, clinical coronary heart disease, and an abnormal electrocardiogram were not associated with a significantly increased frequency of transient ischemic attack or stroke. In the Honolulu Heart Program, the relative risk of thromboembolic stroke for patients with diabetes was twofold higher than the rate for those without diabetes,[294] an effect independent of risk factors associated with hypertension and coronary artery disease.

It has been suggested that in brain infarction elevated blood glucose concentration at the time of stroke may be harmful to the ischemic brain. In laboratory models of stroke, glucose given prior to the creation of ischemia was followed by more severe brain injury and cerebral edema than that in animals given saline injection prior to brain ischemia.[296] It has been proposed that excessive accumulation of lactic acid in the ischemic brain may be the pathophysiologic basis for this phenomenon.[296] In one study[297] diabetic patients were found to have a higher early mortality rate than nondiabetic patients after stroke. In more recent studies, a more indirect association between hyperglycemia and stroke morbidity and mortality was suggested whereby glucose concentration was an epiphenomenon reflecting stroke severity rather than exerting a direct harmful effect on damaged brain neurons.[298]

Ketoacidosis

The clinical manifestations of ketoacidotic coma are no different from those of coma from any cause and may simulate an acute neurosurgical emergency.[299] Cerebral edema with intracranial hypertension is a well-known complication of diabetic ketoacidosis.[300] However, the pathophysiologic basis of cerebral edema in diabetic ketoacidosis is poorly understood. Cerebral edema, especially in the pediatric population, often appears in delayed fashion after improvement in hyperglycemia and ketoacidosis have already taken place.[301] In spite of laboratory improvement, progression to coma followed by acute respiratory arrest may occur. In other patients the neurologic condition often deteriorates following temporary improvement in level of consciousness.[302] It is known that subclinical cerebral edema occurs in many conscious adults treated for ketoacidosis. Elevated cerebrospinal fluid (CSF) pressure appears after improvement in hyperglycemia and may persist for several hours, as determined by serial measurements of CSF pressure.[303]

Posner and colleagues[304] found that mental confusion and coma occur when the pH of CSF falls below 7.15. Not only is the pH of CSF more important than the blood pH in the genesis of diabetic coma but improvement in the CSF pH lags behind that of the blood pH during treatment.[305] Posner et al. suggested that rapid and excessive administration of sodium bicarbonate may be responsible for the cerebral edema that is sometimes seen in patients treated for diabetic ketoacidosis. Presumably the use of alkali, especially by rapid direct intravenous injection, slows down the increase of CSF pH or, paradoxically, causes the CSF pH to fall further. However, in more recent clinical studies, use of bicarbonate, rate of hydration, tonicity of intravenous fluids, and the rate of correction of hyperglycemia could not be implicated in the pathogenesis of cerebral edema.[306]

Nonketotic Hyperglycemia

The syndrome of nonketotic hyperglycemic coma usually occurs in elderly patients with non-insulin-dependent diabetes. In addition to stupor, lethargy, coma, and generalized seizures, a number of focal neurologic manifestations have been described. Most notable of these are continuous focal epileptic seizures lasting several hours to several days and often associated with transient postictal focal neurologic deficits lasting for 5 to 10 days.[307,308] Occasionally, focal neurologic deficits such as hemiparesis may occur that last for several days and are unassociated with focal seizures.[307,308] More recently, other focal seizure manifestations, including epilepsia partialis continua,[309] movement-induced focal seizures,[310] and tonic postures of one arm with head rotation and speech arrest[311] occurring in alert patients have been described. Seizures occurring with nonketotic hyperglycemia are typically poorly responsive to anticonvulsant medications and eventually will respond only to correction of the hyperosmolar state. It has been suggested that an underlying cerebral cortical ischemic infarction predisposes to focal neurologic manifestations of an abnormal osmotic state,[308] and in several cases, computed tomographic scan and postmortem evidence for focal cerebral infarction in appropriate brain locations has been identified.[309]

Spinal Syndromes

Although diabetic amyotrophy initially was referred to incorrectly as diabetic myelopathy,[35] spinal cord disease as a direct result of diabetes is uncommon, despite early reports to the contrary.[312] Apparent clinical signs of spinal cord disease, as well as pathologic evidence of spinal degeneration, particularly in the posterior columns,[312] result from retrograde centripetal changes secondary to peripheral neuropathy and pathologic changes in dorsal root ganglia. Diabetic patients with peripheral neuropathy do, in fact, display slowing of conduction velocities in the dorsal columns of the spinal cord, as measured by somatosensory evoked potential techniques.[313,314] Pathologic examination of the spinal cord generally fails to reveal unequivocal change.[315,316] As in other patients with arteriosclerosis, anterior spinal artery thrombosis may occur in patients with diabetes. Infarction of the anterior two-thirds of the spinal cord may evolve subacutely or acutely and be associated with weakness and impairment of pain and temperature sensitivity below the level of the lesion, with relative preservation of vibration and position sense. Usually the level of involvement is related to one of the major radicular arteries that supply the spinal cord. When cervical spondylosis occurs in persons with diabetes, it may be particularly disabling because of associated vascular involvement, which produces increased susceptibility to compression-induced ischemia.

Wolfram Syndrome

Wolfram syndrome, also known as DIDMOAD syndrome,[317] refers to a disorder defined by the presence of diabetes mellitus (DM) and bilateral optic atrophy (OA) associated with various combinations of diabetes insipidus (DI), deafness (D), dilation of the genitourinary tract, hypogonadism, and a variety of neurologic abnormalities, including ataxia, insomnia, and psychiatric disturbances. Family studies have indicated autosomal recessive inheritance,[318] and sporadic cases are not uncommon.[319] Insulin-dependent diabetes mellitus usually appears in early childhood, whereas optic atrophy, diabetes insipidus, deafness, and neurologic manifestations of the syndrome follow later in childhood or early adulthood.

Optic atrophy appears in the first or second decade and may be associated with partial loss of vision, blindness, impaired color vision, pupillary abnormalities, and defects in peripheral or central visual fields.[318,319] Pathologic studies have demonstrated several abnormalities in the visual system, including atrophy of the lateral geniculate nucleus of the thalamus,[320,321] atrophy of the optic nerves and optic tracts,[318,320,321] and degeneration of the retinal ganglion cell layer. Sensorineural deafness or abnormal audiograms are present in at least 39% of patients.[318] Diabetes insipidus occurs in at least one-third of patients, with a median age at onset of 12 years, and may be responsive to vasopressin or chlorpropamide.[318] Neuronal loss in the paraventricular and supraoptic nuclei of the hypothalamus and atrophy of the posterior pituitary have been described.[322,323] Ataxia may occur later in life, producing gait disturbance with relative sparing of limb coordination. Vertical nystagmus, likely the result of central vestibulocerebellar abnormalities, and vertical, rotatory, and horizontal nystagmus, possibly related to peripheral vestibular dysfunction, have also been described.[318,319,321] Pathologic changes in the cerebellar system have been described, including olivopontocerebellar atrophy[321-324] and degeneration of Purkinje cells.[320] Other, less common, neurologic abnormalities include insomnia,[318,319] abnormalities of temperature regulation,[325] seizures,[318] dysphagia,[321] and respiratory failure caused by dysfunction of the pontomedullary brainstem. A higher-than-expected incidence of depression and psychotic behavioral disturbances was recently described, and these disturbances are believed to have an organic neurologic basis.[326] Differential diagnosis is limited and includes Refsum's syndrome, which produces diabetes mellitus, deafness, retinitis pigmentosa, ataxia, nystagmus, peripheral neuropathy, and ichthyosis; Laurence-Moon-Beidl syndrome, which produces retinitis pigmentosa, deafness, obesity, hypogonadism, and impaired intelligence; Friedreich's ataxia, which may be associated with diabetes mellitus and optic atrophy; and Leber's optic atrophy.

REFERENCES

1. Rollo, sited by Marton MM. Diabetic neuropathy: a clinical study of 150 cases. Brain 1953;76:594–624.
2. Marchal de Calvi CJ. Recherches sur les accidents diabétiques. Paris: P. Asselin, 1864.
3. Greene DA, Sima AAF, Albers JW, et al. Diabetic neuropathy. In: Rifkin H, Porte D Jr, eds. Ellenberg and Rifkin's diabetes mellitus: theory and practice. 4th ed. New York: Elsevier, 1989.
4. Pavy FW. Introductory address to the discussion on the clinical aspect of glycosuria. Lancet 1885;2:1033–35.
5. Dyck PJ, Karnes J, O'Brien PC. Diagnosis, staging, and classification of diabetic neuropathy and association with other complications. In: Dyck PJ, Thomas PK, Asbury AK, et al, eds. Diabetic neuropathy. Philadelphia: WB Saunders, 1987:36–44.
6. Leyden E. Beiträge zur Klinik des Diabetes Mellitus. Wein Med Wochenschr 1893;43:926.
7. Jordan WR. Neuritic manifestations in diabetes mellitus. Arch Intern Med 1936;57:307–66.
8. Treusch JV. Diabetic neuritis: a tentative working classification. Proc Mayo Clin 1945;20:393–402.
9. Goodman JI, Barmoel S, Frankel L, et al. The diabetic neuropathies. Springfield: Charles C Thomas, 1953.
10. Locke S. The peripheral nervous system in diabetes mellitus. Diabetes 1964;13:307–11.
11. Bruyn GW, Garland H. Neuropathies of endocrine origin. In: Vinken PJ, Bruyn GW, eds. Handbook of clinical neurology. Vol 8. Diseases of nerves. Part II. Amsterdam: North-Holland Publishing Co, 1970:29–71.
12. Thomas PK, Eliasson SJ. Diabetic neuropathy. In: Dyck PJ, Thomas PK, Lambert EH, Bunge R, eds. Peripheral neuropathy. Vol 2. 2nd ed. Philadelphia: WB Saunders, 1984:1773–810.
13. Brown MJ, Asbury AK. Diabetic neuropathy. Ann Neurol 1984;15:2–12.
14. Melton IJ, Dyck PJ. Clinical features of the diabetic neuropathies: epidemiology. In: Dyck PJ, Thomas PK, Asbury AK, et al, eds. Diabetic neuropathy. Philadelphia: WB Saunders, 1987:27–35.
15. Dyck PJ. Detection, characterization, and staging of polyneuropathy: assessed in diabetics. Muscle Nerve 1988;11:21–32.
16. Pirart J. Diabetes mellitus and its degenerative complications: a prospective study of 4,400 patients observed between 1947 and 1973. Diabetes Care 1978;1:168.
17. Palumbo PJ, Elveback LR, Whisnant JP. Neurologic complications of diabetes mellitus: transient ischemic attack, stroke and peripheral neuropathy. Adv Neurol 1978;19:593–601.
18. Heinrichs RW, Moorhouse JA. Touch-perception thresholds in blind diabetic subjects in relation to the reading of braille type. N Engl J Med 1969;280:72–5.
19. Waxman SG, Sabin TD. Diabetic truncal polyneuropathy. Arch Neurol 1981;38:46–7.
20. Ellenberg M. Diabetic truncal mononeuropathy—a new clinical syndrome. Diabetes Care 1978;1:10–3.
21. Longstreth GF, Newcomer AD. Abdominal pain caused by diabetic radiculopathy. Ann Intern Med 1977;86:166–8.
22. Sun SF, Streib EW. Diabetic thoracoabdominal neuropathy: clinical and electrodiagnostic features. Ann Neurol 1981;9:75–9.
23. Brown MJ, Martin JR, Asbury AK. Painful diabetic neuropathy. A morphometric study. Arch Neurol 1976;33:164–71.
24. Said G, Slama G, Selva J. Progressive centripetal degeneration of axons in small fibre diabetic polyneuropathy: a clinical and pathological study. Brain 1983;106:791–807.
25. Dyck PJ, Lais A, Karnes JL, et al. Fiber loss is primary and multifocal in sural nerves in diabetic polyneuropathy. Ann Neurol 1986;19:425–9.
26. Young RJ, Zhou YQ, Rodriguez E, et al. Variable relationship between peripheral somatic and autonomic neuropathy in patients with different syndromes of diabetic polyneuropathy. Diabetes 1986;35:192–7.
27. Boulton AJM, Armstrong WD, Scarpello JHB, Ward JD. The natural history of painful diabetic neuropathy—a 4-year study. Postgrad Med J 1983;59:556–9.
28. Archer AG, Watkins PJ, Thomas PK, et al. The natural history of acute painful neuropathy in diabetes mellitus. J Neurol Neurosurg Psychiatry 1983;46:491–9.
29. Ellenberg, M. Diabetic neuropathic cachexia. Diabetes 1974;23:418–23.
30. Thomas PK, Brown MJ. Diabetic polyneuropathy. In: Dyck PJ, Thomas PK, Asbury AK, et al, eds. Diabetic neuropathy. Philadelphia: WB Saunders, 1987:56–65.

31. Caravati CM. Insulin neuritis: a case report. Va Med Monthly 1933;59:745–6.

32. Ellenberg M. Diabetic neuropathy precipitating after institution of diabetic control. Am J Med Sci 1958; 236:466–71.

33. Edmunds ME, Watkins PJ. Management of the diabetic foot. In: Dyck PJ, Thomas PK, Asbury AK, et al, eds. Diabetic neuropathy. Philadelphia: WB Saunders, 1987:208–15.

34. Bruns L. Ueber neuritische Lähmungen beim Diabetes Mellitus. Berl Klin Wochenschr 1890;27:509–15.

35. Garland H, Taverner D. Diabetic myelopathy. BMJ 1953; 1:1405–13.

36. Garland JT. Diabetic amyotrophy. BMJ 1955;2:1287–90.

37. Calverley JR, Mulder DW. Femoral neuropathy. Neurology 1960;10:963–7.

38. Sullivan JF. The neuropathies of diabetes. Neurology 1958; 8:243–9.

39. Williams IR, Mayer RF. Subacute proximal diabetic neuropathy. Neurology 1976;26:108–16.

40. Raff MC, Asbury AK. Ischemic mononeuropathy and mononeuropathy multiplex in diabetes mellitus. N Engl J Med 1968;279:17–22.

41. Bastron JA, Thomas JE. Diabetic polyradiculopathy: clinical and electromyographic findings in 105 patients. Mayo Clin Proc 1981;56:725–32.

42. Asbury AK. Proximal diabetic neuropathy [Editorial]. Ann Neurol 1977;2:179–80.

43. Hamilton CR Jr, Dobson HL, Marshall J. Diabetic amyotrophy: clinical and electronmicroscopic studies in six patients. Am J Med Sci 1968;256:81–90.

44. Casey EB, Harrison MJG. Diabetic amyotrophy: a follow-up study. BMJ 1972;1:656–9.

45. Locke S, Lawrence DG, Legg MA. Diabetic amyotrophy. Am J Med 1963;34:775–85.

46. Chokroverty S, Reyes MG, Rubino FA, Tonaki H. The syndrome of diabetic amyotrophy. Ann Neurol 1977; 2:181–94.

47. Riley DE, Shields RW Jr. Diabetic amyotrophy with upper extremity involvement [Abstract no. PP230]. Neurology 1984;34(Suppl 1):216.

48. Root HF, Rogers MH. Diabetic neuritis with paralysis. N Engl J Med 1930;202:1049–53.

49. Hirsh LF. Diabetic polyradiculopathy simulating lumbar disc disease: report of four cases. J Neurosurg 1984; 60:183–304.

50. Subramony SH, Wilbourn AJ. Diabetic proximal neuropathy. Clinical and electromyographic studies. J Neurol Sci 1982;53:293–304.

51. Gilliatt RW, Willison RG. Peripheral nerve conduction in diabetic neuropathy. J Neurol Neurosurg Psychiatry 1962; 25:11–8.

52. Chopra JS, Hurwitz LJ. Femoral nerve conduction in diabetes and occlusive vascular disease. J Neurol Neurosurg Psychiatry 1968;31:28–33.

53. Lamontagne A, Buchthal F. Electrophysiological studies in diabetic neuropathy. J Neurol Neurosurg Psychiatry 1970; 33:442–52.

54. Chokroverty S. Proximal nerve dysfunction in diabetic proximal amyotrophy: electrophysiology and electron microscopy. Arch Neurol 1982;39:403–7.

55. Dolman CL. The morbid anatomy of diabetic neuropathy. Neurology 1963;13:135–42.

56. Greenbaum D, Richardson PC, Salmon MV, Urich H. Pathological observations on six cases of diabetic neuropathy. Brain 1964;87:201–14.

57. Asbury AK. Focal and multifocal neuropathies of diabetes. In: Dyck PJ, Thomas PK, Asbury AK, et al, eds. Diabetic neuropathy. Philadelphia: WB Saunders, 1987:45–55.

58. Locke S, Tarsy D. The nervous system and diabetes. In: Marble A, Krall LP, Bradley RF, et al, eds. Joslin's diabetes mellitus. 12th ed. Philadelphia: Lea & Febiger, 1985: 665–85.

59. Stewart JD. Diabetic truncal neuropathy: topography of the sensory deficit. Ann Neurol 1989;25:233–8.

60. Boulton AJM, Angus E, Ayyar DR, et al. Diabetic thoracic polyradiculopathy presenting as abdominal swelling. BMJ 1984;289:798–99.

61. Parry GJ, Floberg J. Diabetic truncal neuropathy presenting as abdominal hernia. Neurology 1989;39:1488–90.

62. Kikta DG, Breuer AC, Wilbourn AJ. Thoracic root pain in diabetes: the spectrum of clinical and electromyographic findings. Ann Neurol 1982;11:80–5.

63. Streib EW, Sun SF, Paustian FF, et al. Diabetic thoracic radiculopathy: electrodiagnostic study. Muscle Nerve 1986;9:548–53.

64. Fraser DM, Campbell IW, Ewing DJ, Clarke BF. Mononeuropathy in diabetes mellitus. Diabetes 1979;28:96–101.

65. Jung Y, Hohmann TC, Gerneth JA, et al. Diabetic hand syndrome. Metabolism 1971;20:1008–15.

66. Ross AT. Recurrent cranial nerve palsies in diabetes mellitus. Neurology 1962;12:180–5.

67. Zorrilla E, Kozak GP. Ophthalmoplegia in diabetes mellitus. Ann Intern Med 1967;67:968–76.

68. Barricks ME, Traviesa DB, Glaser JS, Levy IS. Ophthalmoplegia in cranial arteritis. Brain 1977;100:209–21.

69. Asbury AK, Fields HL. Pain due to peripheral nerve damage: an hypothesis. Neurology 1984;34:1587–90.

70. Breen LA, Hopf HC, Farris BK, Guttmann L. Pupil-sparing oculomotor nerve palsy due to midbrain infarction. Arch Neurol 1991;48:105–6.

71. Dreyfus PM, Hakim S, Adams RD. Diabetic ophthalmoplegia. Report of case, with postmortem study and comments on vascular supply of human oculomotor nerve. Arch Neurol Psychiatry 1957;77:337–49.

72. Asbury AK, Aldredge H, Hershberg R, Fisher CM. Oculomotor palsy in diabetes mellitus: a clinicopathological study. Brain 1970;93:555–66.

73. Weber RB, Daroff RB, Mackey EA. Pathology of oculomotor nerve palsy in diabetics. Neurology 1970;20:835–8.

74. Nadeau SE, Trobe JD. Pupil sparing in oculomotor palsy: a brief review. Ann Neurol 1983;13:143–8.

75. Jørgensen MB, Buch NH. Studies on the sense of smell and taste in diabetics. Acta Otolaryngol 1961;53:539–45.

76. Pavan PR, Aiello LM, Wafai MZ, et al. Optic disc edema in juvenile-onset diabetes. Arch Ophthalmol 1980;98: 2193–5.

77. Lubow M, Makley TA Jr. Pseudopapilledema of juvenile diabetes mellitus. Arch Ophthalmol 1971;85:417–22.

78. Korczyn AD. Bell's palsy and diabetes mellitus. Lancet 1971;1:108–10.

79. Adour KK, Wingerd J. Idiopathic facial paralysis (Bell's palsy): factors affecting severity and outcome in 446 patients. Neurology 1974;24:1112–6.

80. Daube JR. Electrophysiologic testing in diabetic neuropathy. In: Dyck PJ, Thomas PK, Asbury AK, et al, eds. Diabetic neuropathy. Philadelphia: WB Saunders, 1987:162–76.

81. Dyck PJ, O'Brien PC. Meaningful degrees of prevention or improvement of nerve conduction in controlled clinical trials of diabetic neuropathy. Diabetes Care 1989;12: 649–52.

82. American Diabetes Association., American Academy of

Neurology. Consensus statement: report and recommendations of the San-Antonio conference on diabetic neuropathy. Diabetes Care 1988;11:592–7.

83. Behse F, Buchthal F, Carlsen F. Nerve biopsy and conduction studies in diabetic neuropathy. J Neurol Neurosurg Psychiatry 1977;40:1072–82.

84. Dorfman LJ, Cummins KL, Reaven GM, et al. Studies of diabetic polyneuropathy using conduction velocity distribution (DCV) analysis. Neurology 1983;33:773–9.

85. Gregersen G. Diabetic neuropathy: influence of age, sex, metabolic control and duration of diabetes on motor conduction velocity. Neurology 1967;17:972–80.

86. Ward JD, Barnes CG, Fisher DJ, Jessop JD. Improvement in nerve conduction following treatment in newly diagnosed diabetics. Lancet 1971;1:428–31.

87. Kimura J, Yamada T, Stevland NP. Distal slowing of motor nerve conduction velocity in diabetic polyneuropathy. J Neurol Sci 1979;42:291–302.

88. Noël P. Sensory nerve conduction in the upper limbs at various stages of diabetic neuropathy. J Neurol Neurosurg Psychiatry 1973;36:786–96.

89. Gabbay KH. The sorbitol pathway and the complications of diabetes. N Engl J Med 1973;288:831–6.

90. Woltman HW, Wilder RM. Diabetes mellitus: pathologic changes in the spinal cord and peripheral nerves. Arch Intern Med 1929;44:576–603.

91. Lundbaeck K. Diabetic angiopathy: a specific vascular disease. Lancet 1954;1:377–9.

92. Fagerberg S-E. Neuropathie diabétique. World Neurol 1961;2:509–19.

93. Chopra JS, Hurwitz LJ, Montgomery DAD. The pathogenesis of sural nerve changes in diabetes mellitus. Brain 1969;92:391–418.

94. Asbury AK, Johnson PC. Pathology of peripheral nerve. Major problems in pathology. Vol 9. Philadelphia: WB Saunders, 1978.

95. Low PA, Tuck RR, Takeuchi M. Nerve microenvironment in diabetic neuropathy. In: Dyck PJ, Thomas PK, Asbury AK, et al, eds. Diabetic neuropathy. Philadelphia: WB Saunders, 1987:266–78.

96. Thomas PK, Lascelles RG. The pathology of diabetic neuropathy. Q J Med (New Series) 1966;35:489–509.

97. Olsson Y, Säve-Söderbergh J, Sourander P, et al. A patho-anatomical study of the central and peripheral nervous system in diabetes of early onset and long duration. Pathol Europ 1968;3:62–79.

98. Coërs C, Hildebrand J. Latent neuropathy in diabetes and alcoholism. Electromyographic and histological study. Neurology 1965;15:19–38.

99. Chopra JS, Sawhney BB, Chakravorty RN. Pathology and time relationship of peripheral nerve changes in experimental diabetes. J Neurol Sci 1977;32:53–67.

100. Dyck PJ. Pathology. In: Dyck PJ, Thomas PK, Asbury AK, et al, eds. Diabetic neuropathy. Philadelphia: WB Saunders, 1987:223–36.

101. Dyck PJ, Karnes JL, O'Brien P, et al. The spatial distribution of fiber loss in diabetic polyneuropathy suggests ischemia. Ann Neurol 1986;19:440–9.

102. Dyck PJ, Conn DL, Okazaki H. Necrotizing angiopathic neuropathy: three-dimensional morphology of fiber degeneration related to sites of occluded vessels. Mayo Clin Proc 1972;47:461–75.

103. Dyck PJ, Hansen S, Karnes J, et al. Capillary number and percentage closed in human diabetic sural nerve. Proc Natl Acad Sci USA 1985;82:2513–7.

104. Yasuda H, Dyck PJ. Abnormalities of endoneurial mi-

crovessels and sural nerve pathology in diabetic neuropathy. Neurology 1987;37:20–8.

105. Johnson PC, Doll SC, Cromey DW. Pathogenesis of diabetic neuropathy. Ann Neurol 1986;19:450–7.

106. Johnson PC, Beggs JL. Vasculitic neuropathy [Abstract no. 115]. J Neuropathol Exp Neurol 1985;44:345.

107. Timperley WR, Boulton AJM, Davies-Jones GAB, et al. Small vessel disease in progressive diabetic neuropathy associated with good metabolic control. J Clin Pathol 1985;38:1030–8.

108. Appenzeller O, Richardson EP Jr. The sympathetic chain in patients with diabetic and alcoholic polyneuropathy. Neurology 1966;16:1205–9.

109. Hensley GT, Soergel KH. Neuropathologic findings in diabetic diarrhea. Arch Pathol 1968;85:587–97.

110. Duchen LW, Anjorin A, Watkins PJ, MacKay JD. Pathology of autonomic neuropathy in diabetes mellitus. Ann Intern Med 1980;92:301–3.

111. Olsson Y, Sourander P. Changes in the sympathetic nervous system in diabetes mellitus. A preliminary report. J Neurovisc Relat 1968;31:86–95.

112. Low PA, Walsh JC, Huang CY, McLeod JG. The sympathetic nervous system in diabetic neuropathy, a clinical and pathological study. Brain 1975;98:341–56.

113. Kristensson K, Nordborg C, Olsson Y, Sourander P. Changes in the vagus nerve in diabetes mellitus. Acta Pathol Microbiol Scand [A] 1971;79:684–5.

114. Martin MM. Involvement of autonomic nerve fibres in diabetic neuropathy. Lancet 1953;1:560–5.

115. Faerman I, Glocer L, Celener D, et al. Autonomic nervous system and diabetes: histological and histochemical study of the autonomic nerve fibers of the urinary bladder in diabetic patients. Diabetes 1973;22:225–37.

116. Dyck PJ, Lambert EH, O'Brien PC. Pain in peripheral neuropathy related to rate and kind of fiber degeneration. Neurology 1976;26:466–71.

117. Britland ST, Young RJ, Sharma AK, Clarke BF. Association of painful and painless diabetic polyneuropathy with different patterns of nerve fiber degeneration and regeneration. Diabetes 1990;39:898–908.

118. Thomas PK, Scadding JW. Treatment of pain in diabetic neuropathy. In: Dyck PJ, Thomas PK, Asbury AK, et al, eds. Diabetic neuropathy. Philadelphia: WB Saunders, 1987:216–22.

119. Melzack R, Wall PD. Pain mechanisms: a new theory. Science 1965;150:971–9.

120. Devor M, Wall PD. Type of sensory nerve fibre sprouting to form a neuroma. Nature 1976;262:705–8.

121. Wall PD, Gutnick M. Ongoing activity in peripheral nerves: the physiology and pharmacology of impulses originating from a neuroma. Exp Neurol 1974; 43:580–93.

122. Scadding JW. Development of ongoing activity, mechanosensitivity, and adrenaline sensitivity in severed peripheral nerve axons. Exp Neurol 1981;73:345–64.

123. Devor M, Jänig W. Activation of myelinated afferents ending in neuroma by stimulation of the sympathetic supply in the rat. Neurosci Lett 1981 24:43–7.

124. Committee on Health Care Issues, American Neurological Association. Does improved control of glycemia prevent or ameliorate diabetic polyneuropathy? Ann Neurol 1986;19:288–90.

125. Eliasson SG. Properties of isolated nerve fibres from alloxanized rats. J Neurol Neurosurg Psychiatry 1969;32:525–9.

126. Jakobsen J. Early and preventable changes of peripheral

nerve structure and function in insulin-deficient diabetic rats. J Neurol Neurosurg Psychiatry 1979;42:509–18.

127. Morley GK, Mooradian AD, Levine AS, Morley JE. Mechanisms of pain in diabetic peripheral neuropathy: effect of glucose on pain perception in humans. Am J Med 1984;77:79–82.

128. Simon GS, Dewey WL. Narcotics and diabetes. I. The effects of streptozotocin-induced diabetes on the antinociceptive potency of morphine. J Pharmacol Exp Ther 1981;218:318–23.

129. Raz I, Hasdai D, Seltzer Z, Melmed RN. Effect of hyperglycemia on pain perception and on efficacy of morphine analgesia in rats. Diabetes 1988;37:1253–9.

130. Anonymous. Pain perception in diabetic neuropathy [Editorial]. Lancet 1985;1:83–4.

131. Fagerberg S-E. Diabetic neuropathy. Acta Med Scand 1959;164(Suppl 345):1–81.

132. Gregersen G. Variations in motor conduction velocity produced by acute changes of the metabolic state in diabetic patients. Diabetologia 1968;4:273–7.

133. Graf RJ, Halter JB, Halar E, et al. Nerve conduction abnormalities in untreated maturity-onset diabetes: relation to levels of fasting plasma glucose and glycosylated hemoglobin. Ann Intern Med 1979;90:298–303.

134. Porte D Jr, Graf RJ, Halter JB, et al. Diabetic neuropathy and plasma glucose control. Am J Med 1981;70:195–200.

135. Fraser DM, Campbell IW, Ewing DJ, et al. Peripheral and autonomic nerve function in newly diagnosed diabetes mellitus. Diabetes 1977;26:546–50.

136. Boulton AJ, Drury J, Clarke B, Ward JD. Continuous subcutaneous insulin infusion in the management of painful diabetic neuropathy. Diabetes Care 1982;5:386–90.

137. Troni W, Carta Q, Cantello R, et al. Peripheral nerve function and metabolic control in diabetes mellitus. Ann Neurol 1984;16:178–83.

138. Bertelsmann FW, Heimans JJ, Van Rooy JCG, et al. Peripheral nerve function in patients with painful diabetic neuropathy treated with continuous subcutaneous insulin infusion. J Neurol Neurosurg Psychiatry 1987;50:1337–41.

139. Kennedy WR, Navarro X, Goetz FC, et al. Effects of pancreatic transplantation on diabetic neuropathy. N Engl J Med 1990;322:1031–7.

140. Solders G, Wilczek H, Gunnarsson R, et al. Effects of combined pancreatic and renal transplantation on diabetic neuropathy: a two-year follow-up study. Lancet 1987;2:1232–5.

141. Service FJ, Daube JR, O'Brien PC, et al. Effect of blood glucose control on peripheral nerve function in diabetic patients. Mayo Clin Proc 1983; 58:283–9.

142. Holman RR, Dornan TL, Mayon-White V, et al. Prevention of deterioration of renal and sensory-nerve function by more intensive management of insulin-dependent diabetic patients. A two-year randomized prospective study. Lancet 1983;1:204–8.

143. Reeves ML, Seigler DE, Ayyar DR, Skyler JS. Medial plantar sensory response. Sensitive indicator of peripheral nerve dysfunction in patients with diabetes mellitus. Am J Med 1984;76:842–6.

144. The DCCT Research Group. Factors in the development of diabetic neuropathy: baseline analysis of neuropathy in the feasibility phase of Diabetes Control and Complications Trial (DCCT). Diabetes 1988;37:476.

145. The DCCT Research Group. Diabetes Control and Complications Trial (DCCT): update. Diabetes Care 1990;13:427–33.

146. Greene DA, Chakrabarti S, Lattimer SA, Sima AAF. Role of sorbitol accumulation and myo-inositol depletion in paranodal swelling of large myelinated nerve fibers in the insulin-deficient spontaneously diabetic Bio-Breeding rat: reversal by insulin replacement, an aldose reductase inhibitor and myo-inositol. J Clin Invest 79:1479, 1987.

147. Tomlinson DR, Moriarty RJ, Mayer JH. Prevention and reversal of defective axonal transport and motor nerve conduction velocity in rats with experimental diabetes by treatment with the aldose reductase inhibitor sorbinil. Diabetes 1984;33:470–6.

148. Fagius J, Jameson S. Effects of aldose reductase inhibitor treatment in diabetic polyneuropathy: a clinical and neurophysiological study. J Neurol Neurosurg Psychiatry 1981;44:991–1001.

149. Handelsman DJ, Turtle JR. Clinical trial of an aldose reductase inhibitor in diabetic neuropathy. Diabetes 1981;30:459–64.

150. Harati Y. Diabetic peripheral neuropathies. Ann Intern Med 1987;107:546–59.

151. Boulton AJM, the Tolrestat in Neuropathy Study Group. Effects of tolrestat, a new aldose reductase inhibitor, on nerve conduction and paraesthetic symptoms in diabetic neuropathy [Abstract no. 61]. Diabetologia 1986;29:521A.

152. The Tolrestat in Painful Neuropathy Study Group. Objective (nerve conduction) and subjective (painful symptom) improvement in diabetic neuropathy following administration of tolrestat, a new aldose reductase inhibitor [Abstract no. 436]. Diabetologia 1986;29:588A.

153. Judzewitsch RG, Jaspan JB, Polonsky KS, et al. Aldose reductase inhibition improves nerve conduction velocity in diabetic patients. N Engl J Med 1983;308:119–25.

154. Young RJ, Ewing DJ, Clarke BF. A controlled trial of sorbinil, an aldose reductase inhibitor, in chronic painful diabetic neuropathy. Diabetes 1983;32:938–42.

155. Lewin IG, O'Brien IAD, Morgan MH, Corrall RJM. Clinical and neurophysiological studies with the aldose reductase inhibitor, sorbinil, in symptomatic diabetic neuropathy. Diabetologia 1984;26:445–8.

156. Jaspan J, Maselli R, Herold K, Bartkus C. Treatment of severely painful diabetic neuropathy with an aldose reductase inhibitor: relief of pain and improved somatic and autonomic nerve function. Lancet 1983;2:758–62.

157. Fagius J, Brattberg A, Jameson S, Berne C. Limited benefit of treatment of diabetic polyneuropathy with an aldose reductase inhibitor: a 24-week controlled trial. Diabetologia 1985;28:323–9.

158. Martyn CN, Reid W, Young RJ, et al. Six-month treatment with sorbinil in asymptomatic diabetic neuropathy: failure to improve abnormal nerve function. Diabetes 1987;36:987–90.

159. Jaspan J, Malone J, Nikolai T, et al. Clinical response to sorbinil in painful diabetic neuropathy [Abstract no. 56]. Diabetes 1989;38(Suppl 2):14A.

160. The Sorbinil Neuropathy Study Group. Clinical response to Sorbinil treatment in diabetic neuropathy [Abstract no. 55]. Diabetes 1989;38(Suppl 2):14A.

161. Dyck PJ, Zimmerman BR, Vilen TH, et al. Nerve glucose, fructose, sorbitol, myo-inositol, and fiber degeneration and regeneration in diabetic neuropathy. N Engl J Med 1988;319:542–8.

162. Sima AAF, Bril V, Nathaniel V, et al. Regeneration and repair of myelinated fibers in sural-nerve biopsy specimens from patients with diabetic neuropathy treated with sorbinil. N Engl J Med 1988;319:548–55.

163. Griffey RH, Eaton RP, Gasparovic C, Sibbitt W. Galactose

neuropathy: structural changes evaluated by nuclear magnetic resonance spectroscopy. Diabetes 1987;36: 776–8.

164. Griffey RH, Eaton RP, Sibbitt RR, et al. Diabetic neuropathy: structural analysis of nerve hydration by magnetic resonance spectroscopy. JAMA 1988;260:2872–8.

165. Zimmerman BR. Aldose reductase inhibitors. In: Dyck PJ, Thomas PK, Asbury AK, et al, eds. Diabetic neuropathy. Philadelphia: WB Saunders, 1987:190–3.

166. Gregersen G. Myoinositol supplementation. In: Dyck PJ, Thomas PK, Asbury AK, et al, eds. Diabetic neuropathy. Philadelphia: WB Saunders, 1987:188–9.

167. Mayhew JA, Gillon KRW, Hawthorne JN. Free and lipid inositol, sorbitol and sugars in sciatic nerve obtained post-mortem from diabetic patients and control subjects. Diabetologia 1983;24:135.

168. Hale PJ, Nattrass M, Silverman SH, et al. Peripheral nerve concentrations of glucose, fructose, sorbitol, and myo-inositol in diabetic and non-diabetic patients. Diabetologia 1987;30:464–7.

169. Gorio A, Carmignoto G, Facci L, Finesso M. Motor nerve sprouting induced by ganglioside treatment: possible implications for gangliosides on neuronal growth. Brain Res 1980;197:236–41.

170. Abraham RR, Abraham RM, Wynn V. A double-blind placebo-controlled trial of mixed gangliosides in diabetic peripheral and autonomic neuropathy. Adv Exp Med Biol 1984;174:607–24.

171. Hallett M, Harrington H, Tyler HR, et al. Trials of ganglioside therapy for amyotrophic lateral sclerosis and diabetic neuropathy. Adv Exp Med Biol 1984;174:575–9.

172. Horowitz SH. Ganglioside therapy in diabetic neuropathy. Muscle Nerve 1986;9:531–6.

173. Ellenberg M. Treatment of diabetic neuropathy with diphenylhydantoin. NY State J Med 1968;68:2653–5.

174. Saudek CD, Werns S, Reidenberg MM. Phenytoin in the treatment of diabetic symmetrical polyneuropathy. Clin Pharmacol Ther 1977;22:196–9.

175. Rull JA, Quibrera R, Gonzalez-Millán H, Lozano-Castañeda O. Symptomatic treatment of peripheral diabetic neuropathy with carbamazepine (Tegretol): double-blind cross-over study. Diabetologia 1969;5:215–8.

176. Gade GN, Hofeldt FD, Treece GL. Diabetic neuropathic cachexia: beneficial response to combination therapy with amitriptyline and fluphenazine. JAMA 1980;243:1160–1.

177. Turkington RW. Depression masquerading as diabetic neuropathy. JAMA 1980;243:1147–50.

178. Max MB, Culnane M, Schafer SC, et al. Amitriptyline relieves diabetic neuropathy pain in patients with normal or depressed mood. Neurology 1987;37:589–96.

179. Kvinesdal B, Molin J, Frøland A, Gram LF. Imipramine treatment of painful diabetic neuropathy. JAMA 1984; 251:1727–30.

180. Young RJ, Clarke BF. Pain relief in diabetic neuropathy: the effectiveness of imipramine and related drugs. Diabetic Med 1985;2:363–6.

181. Basbaum AI, Fields HL. Endogenous pain control mechanisms: review and hypothesis. Ann Neurol 1978;4: 451–62.

182. Sindrup SH, Gram LF, Skjold T, et al. Concentration-response relationship in imipramine treatment of diabetic neuropathy symptoms. Clin Pharmacol Ther 1990;47: 509–15.

183. Davis JL, Lewis SB, Gerich JE, et al. Peripheral diabetic neuropathy treated with amitriptyline and fluphenazine. JAMA 1977;238:2291–2.

184. Gomez-Perez FJ, Rull JA, Dies H, et al. Nortriptyline and fluphenazine in the symptomatic treatment of diabetic neuropathy: a double-blind cross-over study. Pain 1985; 23:395–400.

185. Mendel CM, Klein RF, Chappell DA, et al. A trial of amitriptyline and fluphenazine in the treatment of painful diabetic neuropathy. JAMA 1986;255:637–9.

186. Tarsy D, Baldessarini RJ. Tardive dyskinesia. Annu Rev Med 1984;35:605–23.

187. Kastrup J, Petersen P, Dejgård A, et al. Intravenous lidocaine infusion—a new treatment of chronic painful diabetic neuropathy? Pain 1987;28:69–75.

188. Dejgård A, Petersen P, Kastrup J. Mexiletine for treatment of chronic painful diabetic neuropathy. Lancet 1988; 1:9–11.

189. Watson CPN, Evans RJ, Watt VR. Post-herpetic neuralgia and topical capsaicin. Pain 1988;33:333–40.

190. Chad DA, Aronin N, Lundstrom R, et al. Does capsaicin relieve the pain of diabetic neuropathy? Pain 1990; 42:387–8.

191. Tandon R, Aronin N, Chad D, et al. Topical capsaicin in painful diabetic neuropathy. Neurology 1990;40(Suppl 1):380.

192. Cohen KL, Harris S. Pentoxifylline and diabetic neuropathy [Letter]. Ann Intern Med 1987;107:600.

193. Cohen KL, Lucibello FE, Chomiak M. Lack of effect of clonidine and pentoxifylline in short-term therapy of diabetic peripheral neuropathy. Diabetes Care 1990; 13:1074–7.

194. Ewing DJ, Clarke BF. Diabetic autonomic neuropathy: present insights and future prospects. Diabetes Care 1986;9:648–65.

195. Wheeler T, Watkins PJ. Cardiac denervation in diabetes. BMJ 1973;4:584–6.

196. Sundkvist G, Almér L-O, Lilja B. Respiratory influence on heart rate in diabetes mellitus. BMJ 1979;1:924–5.

197. Lloyd-Mostyn RH, Watkins PJ. Defective innervation of heart in diabetic autonomic neuropathy. BMJ 1975; 3:15–7.

198. Bennett T, Hosking DJ, Hampton JR. Cardiovascular control in diabetes mellitus. BMJ 1975;2:585–7.

199. Ewing DJ, Campbell IW, Clarke BF. Heart rate changes in diabetes mellitus. Lancet 1981;1:183–6.

200. Hilsted J, Galbo H, Christensen NJ. Impaired cardiovascular responses to graded exercise in diabetic autonomic neuropathy. Diabetes 1979;28:313–9.

201. Hilsted J, Parving H-H, Christensen NJ, et al. Hemodynamics in diabetic orthostatic hypotension. J Clin Invest 1981;68:1427–34.

202. Page MM, Watkins PJ. Provocation of postural hypotension by insulin in diabetic autonomic neuropathy. Diabetes 1976;25:90–5.

203. Cryer PE, Silverberg AB, Santiago JV, Shah SD. Plasma catecholamines in diabetes: the syndromes of hypoadrenergic and hyperadrenergic postural hypotension. Am J Med 1978;64:407–16.

204. Tohmeh JF, Shah SD, Cryer PE. The pathogenesis of hyperadrenergic postural hypotension in diabetic patients. Am J Med 1979;67:772–8.

205. Thomas JE, Schirger A, Fealey RD, Sheps SG. Orthostatic hypotension. Mayo Clin Proc 1981;56:117–25.

206. Onrot J, Goldberg MR, Hollister AS, et al. Management of chronic orthostatic hypotension. Am J Med 1986;80:454–64.

207. Anonymous. Management of orthostatic hypotension [Editorial]. Lancet 1987;1:197–8.

208. Zola B, Kahn JK, Juni JE, Vinik AI. Abnormal cardiac function in diabetic patients with autonomic neuropathy in the absence of ischemic heart disease. J Clin Endocrinol Metab 1986;63:208–14.

209. Faerman I, Faccio E, Milei J, et al. Autonomic neuropathy and painless myocardial infarction in diabetic patients: histologic evidence of their relationship. Diabetes 1977; 26:1147–58.

210. Nesto RW, Phillips RT. Asymptomatic myocardial ischemia in diabetic patients. Am J Med 1986;80(Suppl 4C):40–7.

211. Kahn JK, Sisson JC, Vinik AI. QT interval prolongation and sudden cardiac death in diabetic autonomic neuropathy. J Clin Endocrinol Metab 1987;64:751–4.

212. Bellavere F, Ferri M, Guarini L, et al. Prolonged QT period in diabetic autonomic neuropathy: a possible role in sudden cardiac death? Br Heart J 1988;59:379–83.

213. Ewing DJ, Campbell IW, Clarke BF. Mortality in diabetic autonomic neuropathy. Lancet 1976;1:601–3.

214. Page M, Watkins PJ. Cardiorespiratory arrest and diabetic autonomic neuropathy. Lancet 1978;1:14–6.

215. Bennett T, Farquhar IK, Hosking DJ, Hampton JR. Assessment of methods for estimating autonomic nervous control of the heart in patients with diabetes mellitus. Diabetes 1978;27:1167–74.

216. Ewing DJ, Borsey DQ, Bellavere F, Clarke BF. Cardiac autonomic neuropathy in diabetes: comparison of measures of R-R interval variation. Diabetologia 1981;21: 18–24.

217. McLeod JG, Tuck RR. Disorders of the autonomic nervous; system. Part 2. Investigation and treatment. Ann Neurol 1987;21:519–29.

218. Freeman R, Saul JP, Roberts MS, et al. Spectral analysis of heart rate in diabetic autonomic neuropathy: a comparison with standard tests of autonomic function. Arch Neurol 1991;48:185–90.

219. Eckberg DL, Harkins SW, Fritsch JM, et al. Baroreflex control of plasma norepinephrine and heart period in healthy subjects and diabetic patients. J Clin Invest 1986;78:366–74.

220. Ewing DJ, Borsey DQ, Travis P, et al. Abnormalities of ambulatory 24-hour heart rate in diabetes mellitus. Diabetes 1983;32:101–5.

221. Ewing DJ, Neilson JMM, Travis P. New method for assessing cardiac parasympathetic activity using 24 hour electrocardiograms. Br Heart J 1984;52:396–402.

222. Ewing DJ, Campbell IW, Clarke BF. The natural history of diabetic autonomic neuropathy. Q J Med (New Series) 1980;49:95108.

223. Mackay JD, Page MM, Cambridge J, Watkins PJ. Diabetic autonomic neuropathy: the diagnostic value of heart rate monitoring. Diabetologia 1980;18:471–8.

224. Pfeifer MA, Cook D, Brodsky J, et al. Quantitative evaluation of cardiac parasympathetic activity in normal and diabetic man. Diabetes 1982;31:339–45.

225. Smith SA, Smith SE. Reduced pupillary light reflexes in diabetic autonomic neuropathy. Diabetologia 1983;24: 330–2.

226. Campbell IW, Heading RC, Tothill P, et al. Gastric emptying in diabetic autonomic neuropathy. Gut 1977; 18:462–7.

227. Ewing DJ, Bellavere F, Espi F, et al. Correlation of cardiovascular and neuroendocrine tests of autonomic function in diabetes. Metabolism 1986;35:349–52.

228. Low PA, Zimmerman BR, Dyck PJ. Comparison of distal sympathetic with vagal function in diabetic neuropathy. Muscle Nerve 1986;9:592–6.

229. Sundkvist G. Autonomic nervous function in asymptomatic diabetic patients with signs of peripheral neuropathy. Diabetes Care 1981;4:529–34.

230. Niakan E, Harati Y, Comstock JP. Diabetic autonomic neuropathy. Metabolism 1986;35:224–34.

231. Young RJ, Ewing DJ, Clarke BF. Nerve function and metabolic control in teenage diabetics. Diabetes 1983; 32:142–7.

232. Pfeifer MA, Weinberg CR, Cook DL, et al. Autonomic neural dysfunction in recently diagnosed diabetic subjects. Diabetes Care 1984;7:447–53.

233. Bradley WE. Diagnosis of urinary bladder dysfunction in diabetes mellitus. Ann Intern Med 1980;92:323–6.

234. Frimodt-Møller C, Mortensen S. Treatment of diabetic cystopathy. Ann Intern Med 1980;92:327–8.

235. Ellenberg M. Development of urinary bladder dysfunction in diabetes mellitus. Ann Intern Med 1980;92:321–3.

236. McCulloch DK, Campbell IW, Wu FC, et al. The prevalence of diabetic impotence. Diabetologia 1980; 18:279–83.

237. Ellenberg M. Impotence in diabetes: the neurologic factors. Ann Intern Med 1971;75:213–9.

238. Kaiser FE, Korenman SG. Impotence in diabetic men. Am J Med 1988;85(Suppl 5A):147–52.

239. Kolodny RC, Kahn CB, Goldstein HH, Barnett DM. Sexual dysfunction in diabetic men. Diabetes 1974;23:306–9.

240. DeGroat WC, Booth AM. Physiology of male sexual function. Ann Intern Med 1980;92:329–31.

241. Krane RJ, Siroky MB. Neurophysiology of erection. Urol Clin North Am 1981;8:91–101.

242. Karacan I. Diagnosis of erectile impotence in diabetes mellitus: an objective and specific method. Ann Intern Med 1980;92:334–7.

243. Anders EK, Bradley WE, Krane RJ. Nocturnal penile rigidity measured by the snap-gauge band. J Urol 1983; 129:964–6.

244. Barry JM, Blank B, Boileau M. Nocturnal penile tumescence monitoring with stamps. Urology 1980;15:171–2.

245. Abelson D. Diagnostic value of the penile pulse and blood pressure: a Doppler study of impotence in diabetics. J Urol 1975;113:636–9.

246. Lue TF, Hricak H, Marich KW, Tanagho EA. Vasculogenic impotence evaluated by high-resolution ultrasonography and pulsed Doppler spectrum analysis. Radiology 1985; 155:777–81.

247. Bradley WE, Lin JTY, Johnson B. Measurement of the conduction velocity of the dorsal nerve of the penis. J Urol 1984;131:1127–9.

248. Ertekin C, Akyürekli O, Gürses AN, et al. The value of somatosensory-evoked potentials and bulbocavernosus reflex in patients with impotence. Acta Neurol Scand 1985; 71:48–53.

249. Witherington R. Vacuum constriction device for management of erectile impotence. J Urol 1989; 141:320–2.

250. Beaser RS, Van der Hoek C, Jacobson AM, et al. Experience with penile prostheses in the treatment of impotence in diabetic men. JAMA 1982;248:943–8.

251. Virag R. Intracavernous injection of papaverine for erectile failure [Letter]. Lancet 1982;2:938.

252. Zorgniotti AW, Lefleur RS. Auto-injection of the corpus cavernosum with a vasoactive drug combination for vasculogenic impotence. J Urol 1985;133:39–41.

253. Stackl W, Hasun R, Marberger M. Intracavernous injection of prostaglandin E1 in impotent men. J Urol 1988; 140:66–8.

254. Zentgraf M, Baccouche M, Jünemann KP. Diagnosis and

therapy of erectile dysfunction using papaverine and phentolamine. Urol Int 1988;43:65–75.

255. Feldman M, Corbett DB, Ramsey EJ, et al. Abnormal gastric function in longstanding insulin-dependent diabetic patients. Gastroenterology 1979;77:12–7.

256. Loo FD, Palmer DW, Soergel KH, et al. Gastric emptying in patients with diabetes mellitus. Gastroenterology 1984; 86:485–94.

257. Kassander P. Asymptomatic gastric retention in diabetics (gastroparesis diabeticorum). Ann Intern Med 1958;48: 797–812.

258. DePonti F, Fealey RD, Malagelada JR. Gastrointestinal syndromes due to diabetes mellitus. In: Dyck PJ, Thomas PK, Asbury AI, et al, eds. Diabetic neuropathy. Philadelphia: WB Saunders, 1987:155–61.

259. Brownlee M, Kroopf SS. Metoclopramide for gastroparesis diabeticorum [Letter]. N Engl J Med 1974;291:1257–8.

260. Watts GF, Armitage M, Sinclair J, Hill RD. Treatment of diabetic gastroparesis with oral domperidone. Diabetic Med 1985;2:491–2.

261. Feldman M, Smith HJ. Effect of cisapride on gastric emptying of indigestible solids in patients with gastroparesis diabeticorum: a comparison with metoclopramide and placebo. Gastroenterology 1987;92:171–4.

262. Janssens J, Peeters TL, Vantrappen G, et al. Improvement of gastric emptying in diabetic gastroparesis by erythromycin: preliminary studies. N Engl J Med 1990; 322:1028–31.

263. Read NW, Harford WV, Schmulen AC, et al. A clinical study of patients with fecal incontinence and diarrhea. Gastroenterology 1979;76:747–56.

264. Schiller LR, Santa Ana CA, Schmulen AC, et al. Pathogenesis of fecal incontinence in diabetes mellitus: evidence for internal anal sphincter dysfunction. N Engl J Med 1982;307:1666–71.

265. Whalen GE, Soergel KH, Geenen JE. Diabetic diarrhea. A clinical and pathophysiological study. Gastroenterology 1969;56:1021–32.

266. Scarpello JHB, Greaves M, Sladen GE. Small intestinal transit in diabetics. BMJ 1976;2:1225–6.

267. Fedorak RN, Field M, Chang EB. Treatment of diabetic diarrhea with clonidine. Ann Intern Med 1985;102: 197–9.

268. Scarpello JHB, Hague RV, Cullen DR, Sladen GE. The ^{14}C-glycocholate test in diabetic diarrhoea. BMJ 1976; 2:673–5.

269. Walsh CH, Cooper BT, Wright AD, et al. Diabetes mellitus and coeliac disease: a clinical study. Q J Med (New Series) 1978;47:89–100.

270. Molloy AM, Tomkin GH. Altered bile in diabetic diarrhoea. BMJ 1978;2:1462–3.

271. Green PA, Berge KG, Sprague RG. Control of diabetic diarrhea with antibiotic therapy. Diabetes 1968;17: 385–7.

272. Maddern GJ, Horowitz M, Jamieson GG. The effect of domperidone on oesophageal emptying in diabetic autonomic neuropathy. Br J Clin Pharmacol 1985;19:441–4.

273. Goodman JI. Diabetic anhidrosis. Am J Med 1966;41: 831–5.

274. Low PA, Caskey PE, Tuck RR, et al. Quantitative sudomotor axon reflex test in normal and neuropathic subjects. Ann Neurol 1983;14:573–80.

275. Fagius J. Microneurographic findings in diabetic polyneuropathy with special reference to sympathetic nerve activity. Diabetologia 1982;23:415–20.

276. Kennedy WR, Sakuta M, Sutherland D, Goetz FC. The sweating deficiency in diabetes mellitus: methods of quantitation and clinical correlation. Neurology 1984;34: 758–63.

277. Watkins PJ. Facial sweating after food: a new sign of diabetic autonomic neuropathy. BMJ 1973;1:583–7.

278. List CF, Peet MM. Sweat secretion in man. 1. Sweating responses in normal persons. Arch Neurol Psychiatry 1938;39:1228–37.

279. Guttman L. The management of the quinizarin sweat test (Q.S.T.), Postgrad Med J 1947;23:353–66.

280. Low PA. Quantitation of autonomic responses. In: Dyck PJ, Thomas PK, Lambert EH, Bunge R, eds. Peripheral neuropathy. Vol 1. 2nd ed. Philadelphia: WB Saunders, 1984: 1139–65.

281. Shahani BT, Halperin JJ, Boulu P, Cohen J. Sympathetic skin response: a method of assessing unmyelinated axon dysfunction in peripheral neuropathies. J Neurol Neurosurg Psychiatry 1984;47:536–42.

282. Kennedy WR, Sakuta M, Sutherland D, Goetz FC. Quantitation of the sweating deficiency in diabetes mellitus. Ann Neurol 1984;15:482–8.

283. Malouf R, Brust JCM. Hypoglycemia: causes, neurological manifestations and outcome. Ann Neurol 1985;17: 421–30.

284. Maddock RK, Krall LP. Insulin reactions: manifestations and need for a recognition of long-acting insulin reactions. Arch Intern Med 1953;91:695–703.

285. Fagius J, Niklasson F, Berne C. Sympathetic outflow in human muscle nerves increases during hypoglycemia. Diabetes 1986;35:1124–9.

286. Cryer PE. Glucose counterregulation in man. Diabetes 1981;30:261–4.

287. Cryer PE, Gerich JE. Glucose counterregulation, hypoglycemia and intensive insulin therapy in diabetes mellitus. N Engl J Med 1985;313:232–41.

288. Hilsted J, Madsbad S, Krarup T, et al. Hormonal, metabolic, and cardiovascular responses to hypoglycemia in diabetic autonomic neuropathy. Diabetes 1981;30:626–33.

289. Hoeldtke RD, Boden G, Shuman CR, Owen OE. Reduced epinephrine secretion in hypoglycemia unawareness in diabetic autonomic neuropathy. Ann Intern Med 1982;96: 459–62.

290. Simonson DC, Tamborlane WV, DeFronzo RA, Sherwin RS. Intensive insulin therapy reduces counterregulatory hormone responses to hypoglycemia in patients with Type I diabetes. Ann Intern Med 1985;103:184–90.

291. Amiel SA, Tamborlane WV, Simonson DC, Sherwin RS. Defective glucose counterregulation after strict glycemic control of insulin dependent diabetes mellitus. N Engl J Med 1987;316:1376–83.

292. Widom B, Simonson DC. Glycemic control and neuropsychologic function during hypoglycemia in patients with insulin-dependent diabetes mellitus. Ann Intern Med 1990;112:904–12.

293. Alex M, Baron EK, Goldenberg S, et al. An autopsy study of cerebrovascular accident in diabetes mellitus. Circulation 1962;25:663–73.

294. Abbott RD, Donahue RP, MacMahon SW, et al. Diabetes and the risk of stroke: the Honolulu Heart Program. JAMA 1987;257:949–52.

295. Kannel WB. Current status of the epidemiology of brain infarction associated with occlusive arterial disease. Stroke 1971;2:295–318.

296. Pulsinelli WA, Waldman S, Rawlinson D, Plum F. Moderate hyperglycemia augments ischemic brain damage: a neuropathologic study in the rat. Neurology 1982; 32:1239–46.

297. Oppenheimer SM, Hoffbrand BI, Oswald GA, Yudkin JS.

Diabetes mellitus and early mortality from stroke. BMJ 1985;291:1014–5.

298. Woo J, Lam CWK, Kay R, et al. The influence of hyperglycemia and diabetes mellitus on immediate and 3-month morbidity and mortality after acute stroke. Arch Neurol 1990;47:1174–7.

299. Anderson JM. Diabetic ketoacidosis presenting as neurosurgical emergencies. BMJ 1974;3:22–3.

300. Young E, Bradley RF. Cerebral edema with irreversible coma in severe diabetic ketoacidosis. N Engl J Med 1967;276:665–9.

301. Krane EJ, Rockoff MA, Wallman JK, et al. Subclinical brain swelling in children during treatment of diabetic ketoacidosis. N Engl J Med 1985;312:1147–51.

302. Winegrad AI, Kern EFO, Simmons DA. Cerebral edema in diabetic ketoacidosis. N Engl J Med 1985;312:1184–5.

303. Clements RS Jr, Blumenthal SA, Morrison AD, Winegrad AI. Increased cerebrospinal-fluid pressure during treatment of diabetic ketosis. Lancet 1971;2:671–5.

304. Posner JB, Swanson AG, Plum F. Acid-based balance in cerebrospinal fluid. Arch Neurol 1965;12:479–96.

305. Posner JB, Plum F. Protection of CSF pH and of brain function during severe metabolic acidosis. Trans Am Neurol Assoc 1966;91:38–43.

306. Rosenbloom AL. Intracerebral crises during treatment of diabetic ketoacidosis. Diabetes Care 1990;13:22–33.

307. Maccario M. Neurological dysfunction associated with nonketotic hyperglycemia. Arch Neurol 1968;19:525–34.

308. Daniels JC, Chokroverty S, Barron KD. Anacidotic hyperglycemia and focal seizures. Arch Intern Med 1969;124:701–6.

309. Singh BM, Strobos RJ. Epilepsia partialis continua associated with nonketotic hyperglycemia: clinical and biochemical profile of 21 patients. Ann Neurol 1980;8:155–60.

310. Aquino A, Gabor AJ. Movement-induced seizures and nonketotic hyperglycemia. Neurology 1980;30:600–4.

311. Venna N, Sabin TD. Tonic focal seizures in nonketotic hyperglycemia of diabetes mellitus. Arch Neurol 1981;38:512–4.

312. Williamson RT. Changes in the posterior columns of the spinal cord in diabetes mellitus. BMJ 1894;1:398–400.

313. Cracco J, Castells S, Mark E. Conduction velocity in peripheral nerve and spinal afferent pathways in juvenile diabetics [Abstract]. Neurology 1980;30:370–1.

314. Gupta PR, Dorfman LJ. Spinal somatosensory conduction in diabetes [Abstract]. Neurology 1980;30:414–5.

315. Skanse B, Gydell K. A rare type of femoral-sciatic neuropathy in diabetes mellitus. Acta Med Scand 1959;155:463–8.

316. Matthews WB. Discussion on some clinical, genetic and biochemical aspects of metabolic disorders of the nervous system. Proc R Soc Med 1958;51:859–63.

317. Anonymous. Didmoad (Wolfram) syndrome [Editorial]. Lancet 1986;1:1075–6.

318. Cremers CWRJ, Wijdeveld PGAB, Pinckers AJLG. Juvenile diabetes mellitus, optic atrophy, hearing loss, diabetes insipidus, atonia of the urinary tract and bladder, and other abnormalities (Wolfram syndrome). Acta Paediatr Scand 1977;264(Suppl 264):3–16.

319. Lessell S, Rosman NP. Juvenile diabetes mellitus and optic atrophy. Arch Neurol 1977;34:759–65.

320. Barron KD, Shuman S, Dentinger MP. Necrobiosis of neurons of lateral geniculate body in Wolfram's syndrome [Abstract]. Neurology 1983;33(Suppl 2):119.

321. Khardori R, Stephens JW, Page OC, Dow RS. Diabetes mellitus and optic atrophy in two siblings: a report on a new association and a review of the literature. Diabetes Care 1983;6:67–70.

322. Carson MJ, Slager UT, Steinberg RM. Simultaneous occurrence of diabetes mellitus, diabetes insipidus, and optic atrophy in a brother and a sister. Am J Dis Child 1977;131:1382–5.

323. Karp M, Laron Z, Sandbank U. Wolfram syndrome [Letter]. Am J Dis Child 1978;132:818–9.

324. Samanta A, Burden AC, Hearnshaw JR, et al. Didmoad syndrome in a brother and sister [Abstract no. 438]. Diabetologia 1986;29:588A.

325. Marquardt JL, Loriaux L. Diabetes mellitus and optic atrophy: with associated findings of diabetes insipidus and neurosensory hearing loss in two siblings. Arch Intern Med 1974;134:32–7.

326. Swift RG, Sadler DB, Swift M. Psychiatric findings in Wolfram syndrome hemozygotes. Lancet 1990;336:667–9.

Chapter 44

HYPERTENSION

A. RICHARD CHRISTLIEB
ANDRZEJ S. KROLEWSKI
JAMES H. WARRAM

Since the last edition of this text, the specialty of hypertension associated with diabetes mellitus has become recognized. The first International Symposium on High Blood Pressure Associated with Diabetes Mellitus was held in Bern in 1984, the second in Paris in 1988, and the third in Boston in 1991. A great deal of new data have accumulated as a result of the efforts of numerous investigators now interested in this specialty. For example, the data are sufficient to provide a foundation for understanding the pathophysiology of both the hypertension associated with diabetic nephropathy and the hypertension without accompanying nephropathy. Our knowledge regarding the relationship between hypertension in the person with diabetes and subsequent cardiovascular complications has been enhanced. With the advent of new antihypertensive drugs and the achievement of a better understanding of the complications of older antihypertensive drugs, treatment can be recommended on a more rational basis. In this chapter we will review the current status of hypertension associated with diabetes mellitus.

PREVALENCE OF HYPERTENSION IN PATIENTS WITH DIABETES MELLITUS

Hypertension is frequently associated with diabetes mellitus. The prevalence of hypertension in the diabetic population appears to be twice that in the nondiabetic population and would be higher were it not for attrition caused by early mortality.[1,2] It is estimated that 2.5 to 3 million Americans have both diabetes mellitus and hypertension.[3] However, the prevalence of hypertension in persons with insulin-dependent diabetes mellitus (IDDM) differs from that in persons with non-insulin-dependent diabetes mellitus (NIDDM).

Two studies assessing the natural history of diabetes mellitus in patients with IDDM with the onset of diabetes during youth have demonstrated that hypertension in these patients generally parallels the occurrence of renal disease, which is at present approximately 30%.[4,5] Considering that at most only 10% of the diabetic population has IDDM, this translates to fewer than 100,000 patients. Therefore, most hypertension associated with diabetes mellitus occurs in patients with NIDDM. Further, the prevalence increases with increasing age.

NIDDM in the United States is more common in the black population than in the white population. It is therefore interesting that the prevalence of hypertension in these two populations is about equal—70% among blacks with NIDDM and 63% among whites with NIDDM as compared with a prevalence of 41% and 32% in nondiabetic blacks and whites, respectively.[6] Although the prevalence of high blood pressure in blacks and whites increases with age in the general population throughout the whole age range, among those with diabetes the increase occurs only until the age of 54 years. After this, the prevalence of high blood pressure in whites remains steady and in blacks declines. Excessive mortality in the diabetic population presumably accounts for these changes in rates.

PATHOGENESIS AND PATHOPHYSIOLOGY OF HYPERTENSION

Surgically curable forms of hypertension must be considered in any hypertensive patient, including the hypertensive patient with diabetes. Among hypertensive patients, the frequencies of occurrence of these forms of hypertension, even that due to renal arterial stenosis,[7] are similar in the diabetic and nondiabetic populations. Recommendations regarding the evaluation and treatment for surgically curable hypertension have recently been outlined.[8] In the evaluation of patients with diabetes, once it has been deemed that none of these surgically curable forms of hypertension is present, the hypertension can be classified into four types: 1) renal hypertension associated with the diabetic renal disease; 2) essential hypertension that occurs in patients without nephropathy; 3) isolated systolic hypertension; and 4) supine hypertension with orthostatic hypotension. For each of these forms of hypertension, the pathogenesis and treatment differ. Therefore, they will be reviewed independently.

Hypertension Associated with Renal Disease

Retrospective studies of inception cohorts of young patients with IDDM have revealed that only approximately 30% ever will develop nephropathy.[4,5,9] All of these patients with IDDM who develop nephropathy develop hypertension. The prevalence of nephropathy in patients with NIDDM 20 years after diagnosis is 20 to 40%, and this nephropathy often is accompanied by hypertension.[10] Because the renal disease and hypertension are so intimately related, they will be discussed together.

The earliest clinical manifestation of nephropathy is so-called microalbuminuria, which can be defined as the presence of small but elevated concentrations of albumin in the urine.[11,12] During the period of microalbuminuria, i.e., before the presence of gross albuminuria, there is a modest increase in the blood pressure that does not reach hypertensive levels.[11] This period of microalbuminuria can be considered a transitional stage toward the development of hypertension since most patients with IDDM and many with NIDDM are hypertensive when gross albuminuria does appear. As renal disease progresses, virtually all patients with IDDM become hypertensive. It is interesting that the incidence of diabetic nephropathy in patients with IDDM appears to be decreasing over time,[4,5,13] and the incidence of hypertension is decreasing in a parallel fashion.

Such observations suggest an etiologic relationship between the nephropathy and the hypertension. Whether hypertension initiates early nephropathy or vice versa has been the subject of debate for some time and has been discussed in recent reviews.[12,14,15] Several lines of evidence suggest that hypertension is the initiating event for nephropathy. First, the blood pressure in patients with IDDM surviving for 40 years or more without nephropathy is lower than that in the general population,[16] suggesting that low blood pressure is protective against nephropathy. Second, a parental history of hypertension is four times more frequent in patients with nephropathy than in those without nephropathy,[17–19] suggesting a possible genetic predisposition to hypertension. Third, an increase in sodium/lithium countertransport by the red blood cell has been reported in patients with nephropathy.[17,20] Such an increase is considered a marker for essential hypertension.

Other evidence, however, is compatible with a primary function of the renal disease and renal mechanisms for the development of hypertension. First, although mild increases in blood pressure are observed with high levels of microalbuminuria, the blood pressure remains unchanged with low levels of microalbuminuria, a finding that suggests the renal disease precedes the elevations in blood pressure.[21] Similarly, in a prospective study of 200 patients, an increase in microalbuminuria was noted before any increase in blood pressure occurred.[22] Second, long-term essential hypertension in patients with IDDM usually does not lead to nephropathy.[15]

In view of these contradictory data, the question regarding the etiologic primacy of hypertension or nephropathy remains to be answered. However, the bulk of the evidence favors the pathogenicity of a genetic predisposition to hypertension in the development of nephropathy, as suggested previously.[17]

In patients with NIDDM, hypertension frequently is present at the time of diagnosis of diabetes. However, the presence of hypertension at diagnosis does not predict the development of nephropathy.[23] Further, in patients with NIDDM, microalbuminuria itself does not necessarily predict nephropathy. In this older age group, many other forms of renal disease may be present.

Regardless of whether or not hypertension is involved in the pathogenesis of nephropathy, it is clear that nephropathy accelerates the hypertension and that hypertension accelerates the nephropathy.

Hypertension without Renal Disease

The pathogenesis of the hypertension that accompanies diabetes in patients without renal disease has features similar to that in nondiabetic patients with essential hypertension. However, hypertension is observed with twice the frequency in this diabetic population. The excess of hypertension can be explained if one assumes that mechanisms responsible for increasing blood pressure occur more frequently in the diabetic population than in the nondiabetic population.

Hypertensive patients in the general population have an increased chance of being glucose intolerant and of developing NIDDM as compared with the normotensive population.[24] It is not surprising then that an excess of hypertension is present in individuals with newly diagnosed NIDDM.[25] Blood pressure continues to increase progressively with longer duration of diabetes mellitus and is independent of obesity, treatment modality, and postprandial glucose levels. From these observations, it appears that the excess of hypertension in patients with

NIDDM may be the result of factors preceding clinical manifestations of the disease as well as those operating in the presence of diabetes.

It is now recognized that hypertension, diabetes mellitus, and obesity bear a relationship characterized by resistance to insulin-stimulated glucose uptake, glucose intolerance, and hyperinsulinemia.[26,27]

NIDDM is closely related to insulin resistance, a condition influenced by both age and obesity. Before the clinical onset of NIDDM, most patients compensate for insulin resistance by increasing the secretion of endogenous insulin. Three reports in the mid-1980s suggested an association between the level of insulin and blood pressure in patients with NIDDM.[28-30] Many reports have confirmed this observation and in addition have demonstrated that insulin resistance may be a primary defect in both diabetic and nondiabetic subjects with hypertension.[31]

In one important study, obese normotensive patients had normal glucose tolerance whereas obese hypertensive patients had glucose intolerance.[32] It is interesting that the plasma insulin responses of the hypertensive subjects were threefold higher than those of the normotensive subjects. In addition, in the hypertensive patients, the insulin response correlated highly with blood pressure. More recently, insulin resistance with hyperinsulinemia in nonobese, nondiabetic patients with essential hypertension was reported.[33] Again, the degree of insulin resistance was related to blood pressure. These findings have been confirmed in a large patient population.[34]

That hyperinsulinemia is probably a connecting link between insulin resistance and hypertension was best demonstrated in a study of purportedly normal individuals.[35] Subjects were grouped into those with normal insulin levels and those with elevated insulin levels. Those with hyperinsulinemia not only had higher glucose levels after an oral glucose challenge but also had higher systolic and diastolic blood pressures. Similar data were reported for a large population of both black and white young adults.[36] Racial differences do exist, however, in that no relationship between insulin and hypertension was observed in Pima Indians.[37]

Evidence that an elevation in blood pressure per se is not a cause of the insulin-resistant state has been conveyed by studies comparing normal subjects, patients with essential hypertension, and patients with renal vascular hypertension.[38] Whereas patients with essential hypertension had elevated insulin levels, patients with renovascular hypertension had levels similar to those of the controls.

It appears, therefore, that the evidence is sufficient to implicate insulin resistance and hyperinsulinemia in the pathogenesis of both hypertension associated with NIDDM and essential hypertension. Although this cannot explain the pathogenesis of hypertension in all hypertensive individuals, it may explain much of the excess hypertension found in the population with NIDDM.

The regulation of blood pressure is multifactorial. Further, the association of insulin resistance with NIDDM and obesity is not universal.[39] Several pieces of evidence suggest that the defect causing insulin resistance may be genetically determined.[27,39] For example, hyperinsulinemia and NIDDM are more prevalent in Mexican-Americans than in the rest of the population. Nondiabetic members of families with NIDDM are more often hyperinsulinemic than those of families with no history of NIDDM.[40] Nondiabetic offspring of parents with NIDDM have systolic and diastolic blood pressures higher than those of nondiabetic offspring without parental diabetes.[41] In view of these observations, it was proposed that insulin resistance itself is under genetic control but that the insulin resistance can lead to NIDDM and/or hypertension only in the presence of other specific genes. By this theory, the Pima Indians would lack the "hypertensive gene."[37]

Systolic Hypertension

Isolated systolic hypertension may be defined as a systolic blood pressure of 160 mm Hg or greater with normal or low diastolic blood pressures. Elevated systolic pressure can be present in several conditions, such as anemia, hyperthyroidism, and Paget's disease, in which arteriovenous shunting occurs.

When these conditions are not present, isolated systolic hypertension results from a loss of major arterial elasticity associated with the atherosclerotic process. It is this elastic property of major vessels (compliance) that allows for the occurrence of sudden changes in volume during the phases of the cardiac cycle. The large arteries normally will expand during systole in order to accept the abrupt increase in intra-arterial volume resulting from cardiac systole. This expansion limits the degree to which systolic pressure will be elevated. The vessels then contract as blood passes through the arteriolar system, thus maintaining intra-arterial volume and pressure. With the progression of atherosclerosis in the patient with diabetes, the large arteries lose their elasticity and gradually become rigid. Any given volume of blood ejected from the left ventricle will enter an arterial system that, to a greater or lesser degree, is incapable of expansion. The systolic pressure will thus be increased.

The diastolic pressure is determined by the degree of resistance in the arteriolar system. Vasoconstriction of resistance vessels will increase, and vasodilatation will decrease the diastolic pressure. The mean blood pressure is determined by both the systolic and the diastolic pressure. Therefore, for the mean blood pressure to remain normal in the presence of an elevated systolic pressure, peripheral vascular resistance must decrease, thus lowering the diastolic pressure. In isolated systolic hypertension, this condition prevails.

Orthostatic Hypotension

Orthostatic hypotension is common in patients with diabetes mellitus—both those with and those without supine elevations in the blood pressure. Sometimes it is observed in patients with diabetic nephropathy, especially in its early stages, at which time autonomic neuropathy frequently is present.

Maintenance of the erect blood pressure involves the integrity of multiple blood pressure homeostatic mechanisms. Among these are the baroceptor reflexes, various vasoactive hormones, cardiac output, and blood volume. Because these mechanisms compensate for one another, it is unlikely that a compromise in the function of any one will result in orthostatic hypotension. However, should several of the mechanisms be compromised simultaneously, as may occur in the diabetic population, an inability to maintain the erect posture will ensue. Baroceptor reflexes are frequently blunted in patients with neuropathy. Circulating catecholamine levels generally are low. However, some diabetic patients with orthostatic hypotension may have normal or elevated levels of circulating catecholamines, but vascular resistance limits their effectiveness. The RAA system is difficult to stimulate. In patients with nephropathy, hypoalbuminemia secondary to urinary protein losses may occur prior to any clinically significant compromise in renal function. Contraction of the plasma volume ensues. Severe coronary heart disease or diabetic cardiomyopathy may result in decreased myocardial contractility and a decrease in cardiac output. Therefore, in the diabetic population, any of these mechanisms responsible for the maintenance of upright blood pressure may be compromised. The combined deficiency of some of these mechanisms in any given individual may then result in orthostatic hypotension.

MECHANISMS OF BLOOD PRESSURE REGULATION

Blood pressure regulation is directly related to changes in cardiac output and peripheral vascular resistance (PVR). Cardiac output is influenced by a host of factors, including blood volume, which in turn is influenced by sodium; and PVR is influenced by arteriolar luminal diameter, which in turn is under the control of many hormonal influences, including relative activities of vasopressor and vasodepressor hormones.

Sodium retention is characteristic of both IDDM and NIDDM. Insulin levels are elevated in each type of diabetes—in IDDM by the supraphysiologic doses of exogenous insulin necessary to treat most patients and in NIDDM by the high endogenous levels secreted to overcome the insulin resistance. Even mild elevations in insulin levels[42] can increase proximal and distal renal tubular sodium reabsorption and result in the high total-body levels of exchangeable sodium observed in diabetes.[43,44]

Several mechanisms can account for the sodium retention in diabetes. Of major importance is the proximal tubular glucose-sodium cotransporter.[45,46] This cotransporter system is not dependent on insulin and becomes operative in the presence of hyperglycemia of sufficient magnitude to cause glomerular hyperfiltration of glucose.

Insulin receptors are present throughout the nephron, being most numerous in the proximal tubule.[47] In addition, the kidney does not share the insulin resistance of other body tissues.[48] Therefore, insulin can stimulate renal tubular Na^+/K^+-ATPase[49] and also the Na^+/H^+ antiporter system,[50] resulting in renal sodium retention.

In patients with renal disease, exchangeable sodium is increased even before the stage of microalbuminuria, and in subjects with overt nephropathy, mean blood pressure and exchangeable sodium are positively correlated.[51] Elevations in the systemic pressure could represent one mechanism of enhancement of renal perfusion and thereby could increase sodium excretion.

The level of exchangeable sodium also is increased in patients with NIDDM.[52] Although not studied in NIDDM, in obese patients without diabetes, weight loss is associated with an improvement in insulin sensitivity, a decrease in plasma insulin levels, natriuresis, and a decrease in blood pressure that correlates with a decrease in insulin levels.[53] These observations suggest a prominent role for insulin in sodium homeostasis and, secondarily, in blood pressure regulation.

One would expect that the sodium excess would distribute in the body so as to increase extracellular fluid (ECF) volume and plasma volume and that the increased plasma volume would increase cardiac output and, secondarily, the blood pressure. ECF volume tends to be increased.[44,51] However, plasma volume may be either normal or even decreased in patients with NIDDM and patients with progressing renal disease.[43,44,51,54,55] The latter is consistent with the increased vascular permeability and hypoalbuminuria in established renal disease. Only in late-stage renal disease, when free-water clearance is compromised, would one expect volume expansion. Therefore, there is no evidence that sodium retention is involved in the genesis of hypertension in diabetes through an expansion in plasma volume and an increase in cardiac output.

Other pathogenetic mechanisms must be implicated in the hypertension. At the cellular level, including that of vascular smooth muscle cells, insulin can alter transmembranous electrolyte exchange systems and thus change the intracellular electrolyte composition. Na^+/K^+-ATPase is stimulated by insulin, with the usual result being an extrusion of sodium from the cell.[27,44,56] In the presence of insulin resistance, the Na^+/K^+-ATPase may not function normally, a situation resulting in an excess of intracellular sodium, which could lead to vasoconstriction.

Another cellular system, the Na^+/H^+ antiporter system, is stimulated by insulin and can thereby augment intracellular accumulation of sodium in the presence of insulin resistance with hyperinsulinemia. It was previously mentioned that red blood cell sodium-lithium countertransport activity is increased in patients with nephropathy.[17,20] This countertransport system is purported to be one mode of operation of the Na^+/H^+ antiporter system, and the elevated activity provides indirect evidence that intracellular sodium may be increased even in IDDM. Indeed, increased leukocyte Na^+/H^+ antiport activity has been reported in patients with IDDM with nephropathy.[57] Further, increased activity of the Na^+/H^+ antiporter system is associated with increased activity of the calcium exchange system, a process that results in an elevation in level of intracellular calcium.[58,59]

These elevated levels of intracellular sodium and calcium render resistance vessels more responsive to endogenous vasopressors, thus resulting in augmented

PVR and an increase in the blood pressure. Enhanced vascular responsiveness to exogenous vasopressors has been demonstrated in diabetic patients.[52,60-62] Further, increased responsiveness to angiotensin II (A-II) has been reported in hypertensive patients with NIDDM both when they are on a high-sodium diet and when they are on a low-sodium diet, a finding consistent with their sodium retention.[62]

Other mechanisms leading to increased vascular tone have recently been reviewed.[57] The intracellular alkalinization associated with Na^+/H^+ antiporter activity could enhance vascular contractility directly by increasing calcium/calmodulin interaction. An elevated intracellular pH also could stimulate a response to growth factors, leading to cell proliferation, vascular medial thickening, and narrowing of the arteriole lumen, changes increasing vascular resistance and sustaining the hypertension. Stimulation of the sympathetic nervous system by insulin provides another mechanism through which insulin may induce hypertension. Even physiologic increases in plasma insulin levels can markedly increase activity of the sympathetic nervous system.[63-65] Further, there is a correlation between plasma insulin concentrations and incremental increases in plasma norepinephrine levels.[63] Although these observations are from short-term studies, circumstantial evidence suggesting a long-term effect derives from studies showing that with weight reduction a decrease in norepinephrine level goes along with decreases in plasma insulin levels and blood pressure.[66] Mechanisms to explain the elevation in blood pressure with increased sympathetic activity include arteriolar vasoconstriction, elevations in cardiac output, and renal sodium retention.

Not only can insulin stimulate overactivity of the sympathoadrenal system, overactivity of the sympathoadrenal system can cause alterations in glucose metabolism. Catecholamine-induced hyperglycemia results from glycogenolysis and gluconeogenesis. Further, inhibition of glucose uptake occurs with infusions of epinephrine at levels comparable to those observed in association with stress.[67] Therefore, excessive catecholamine levels can cause insulin resistance and hyperinsulinemia and conceivably could be an initiating event in the pathogenesis of hypertension in NIDDM. Further studies are needed to assess the effect of physiologic levels of epinephrine over time.

Results of several studies have shown that insulin modulates blood flow to skeletal muscle.[68] It is of interest that studies of both obese nondiabetic patients and obese patients with NIDDM have revealed a blunted ability to increase blood flow in response to hyperglycemia in association with hyperinsulinemia.[69,70] The resultant decrease in blood flow can be attributed to decreased peripheral vascular perfusion and would contribute to lower rates of glucose uptake, i.e., manifesting as insulin resistance. This resistance to the vasodilatory affect of insulin might also be the mechanism involved in increasing the blood pressure.

While there is much evidence to suggest that hyperinsulinemia is the common pathway linking insulin resistance in hypertension, some data inconsistent with this view have been reviewed.[71] Catecholamine activity does not increase in patients with autonomic neuropathy, in whom insulin can block calcium currents and even induce hypertension. Prolonged insulin infusions in dogs are accompanied by renal sodium retention, but the blood pressure remains unchanged. Renal sodium retention may be explained by hyperglycemia via activation of the proximal tubular glucose-sodium cotransporter and may not be insulin related, at least in patients with glucosuria. In view of these potential inconsistencies, Resnick and colleagues have suggested that hypertension and insulin resistance may be different clinical manifestations of a common underlying cellular defect by which the level of cytosolic free calcium is increased and the level of intracellular free magnesium is decreased.[71-73] Hypertension or diabetes mellitus may predominate depending on differences in genetic and/or environmental influences.

Should hyperinsulinemia be the major pathogenetic defect in initiating the hypertensive process in patients with NIDDM, it is unlikely that it sustains the hypertension indefinitely. With increasing insulin resistance, the pancreas must secrete higher levels of insulin. Eventually, its reserve capacity is exhausted and plasma insulin levels fall. Other mechanisms must then sustain the hypertension. Hypertrophy of arteriolar smooth muscle established by factors associated with the hyperinsulinemia, as discussed previously, would increase PVR and sustain the hypertension.

No discussion of mechanisms for the hypertension would be complete without a review of the role of vasoactive hormones. Excesses of vasopressor hormones or deficiencies of vasodepressor hormones could be implicated in initiating and/or sustaining the hypertension. Of the vasopressor and vasodepressor hormonal systems, the renin-angiotensin-aldosterone (RAA) system has been investigated most extensively. This system is intimately involved in salt and volume regulation and also in governing vascular tone and can be influenced by insulin.[74] The function of this system in patients with diabetes has recently been reviewed.[75] An understanding of this system is important not only because of its role in the pathogenesis of nephropathy and hypertension but also because of the potential role of the RAA system in other complications and the implications for the treatment of hypertension.

It may be helpful to review briefly the physiology of the RAA system. The enzyme renin is cleaved from prorenin in the juxtaglomerular cells of the renal afferent arterioles and also in other body tissues, including the vascular system. These juxtaglomerular cells act as baroreceptors, such that a decrease in pressure or a decrease in volume will stimulate renin release. The concentration of sodium in the renal tubule at the level of the macula densa, sympathetic nervous system activity of the kidney, and prostaglandins can also affect renin release. Renin then acts on its substrate, angiotensinogen, to cleave a decapeptide known as angiotensin I (A-I). A-I is in turn converted to an octapeptide, angiotensin II (A-II), by angiotensin-converting enzyme (ACE), with most of the systemic conversion occurring in the lung. A-II is a potent vasoconstrictor and is also a major stimulus for aldosterone release. Aldosterone in turn acts in the renal distal tubule to retain sodium and excrete potassium.

Prorenin has no known effects on the vascular system. Recently, elevated levels of prorenin were found to be present in patients with IDDM who later developed microangiopathy.[76,77] The significance of this association is unknown, and, indeed, elevated prorenin levels may merely be a marker for microvascular disease. However, in that levels of glycosylated hemoglobin were higher in the patients with microangiopathy, abnormal glycosylation of intracellular prorenin may prevent the formation of renin. An impairment of renin formation is present in many diabetic patients with nephropathy and neuropathy. Glycosylated prorenin therefore could be a precipitating factor for hyporeninemic hypoaldosteronism.[77]

Renin activity is most often normal in diabetic patients without nephropathy but may be decreased in diabetic patients with hypertension and no nephropathy just as it is in nondiabetic patients with essential hypertension.[55,78] Normal or decreased levels of both renin and aldosterone have been reported in patients with diabetic nephropathy.[51,78–79] Several mechanisms decreasing renin release in these patients include deficient conversion of prorenin to renin as discussed above, destruction of the juxtaglomerular cells by hyalinization,[82] decreased sympathetic stimulation of renin release as a result of associated neuropathy,[83,84] and volume expansion secondary to inappropriately low sodium and water excretion as nephropathy advances or possibly to the increased osmolality of plasma that may occur with hyperglycemia.[54] The latter may be involved in the acceleration of the systemic hypertension in advanced nephropathy. Renin itself has no specific function other than to cleave A-I. However, inhibitors of renin eventually may prove beneficial therapeutically.[85,86]

A-II appears to be involved in the pathogenesis of both the hypertension and the nephropathy of diabetes. Conversion of A-I to A-II can be prevented with inhibitors of ACE. These drugs have been observed to lower systemic blood pressure, although not consistently, in both patients with and those without nephropathy.[87–89] In that levels of renin and A-II are often low in patients with nephropathy[51,78] ineffectiveness of ACE inhibitors might be expected. However, since vascular reactivity to A-II is increased in some patients with diabetes,[52,60–62] an elevated systemic blood pressure may be maintained with less than normal levels of this hormone, especially in the presence of sodium excess, which generally enhances vascular reactivity.

Increased intraglomerular pressure appears to be involved in the pathogenesis and progression of nephropathy[90,91] and therefore of the hypertension. Factors increasing this pressure include elevated systemic pressures and A-II-mediated constriction of the efferent arterioles. ACE inhibitors induce relaxation of the efferent arterioles and thus reduce intraglomerular pressure and hyperfiltration. Microalbuminuria, progression of the renal disease, and incidence of hypertension are thereby decreased.[92–94]

A-II is a major stimulus for aldosterone secretion. Hyporeninemic hypoaldosteronism in diabetic patients with nephropathy is a clinically important complication related to the RAA system.[79,95,96] Perhaps the hypoaldosteronism serves as a compensatory mechanism to counteract enhanced sodium reabsorption in individuals predisposed to hypertension, thus minimizing increases in blood pressure.[97] Clinically, the hypoaldosteronism can lead to life-threatening hyperkalemia. The primary controlling mechanisms for potassium homeostasis include mineralocorticoid activity and the effect of insulin on driving glucose and potassium into cells. Hyperkalemia can appear in patients without renal disease if aldosterone is deficient. In the presence of renal disease, hyperkalemia can be exaggerated. Diabetes further complicates this situation. Acute infusions of glucose will result in hyperkalemia when levels of both aldosterone and insulin are deficient.[98] Similarly, patients with hypoaldosteronism can develop severe hyperkalemia in the absence of adequate insulin, such as that occurring in hyperosmolar nonketotic states. These observations emphasize both the independent and the combined effects of insulin and aldosterone in regulating serum potassium levels and emphasize the necessity for good glycemic control in patients with nephropathy and hypoaldosteronism.

Other vasopressor and vasodepressor peptides are involved in the pathophysiology of the hypertension associated with diabetes mellitus. The data regarding these hormones are limited. Prostaglandins are involved in stimulating renin release,[99] but their role in the pathogenesis of the hypertension remains unknown. However, nonsteroidal anti-inflammatory drugs that inhibit prostaglandin synthesis decrease renin levels and thereby can aggravate hyperkalemia that is caused by hyporeninemic hypoaldosteronism.[100–102]

Atrial natriuretic peptide (ANP) interacts with various other hormones in controlling salt and water balance and therefore is involved primarily in the regulation of extracellular fluid and also in blood pressure homeostasis. In patients with IDDM, with their increased level of exchangeable total body sodium, infusions of ANP have an augmented natriuretic effect associated with increased renal plasma flow and glomerular filtration rate.[103] These observations suggest that the renal vasculature is more sensitive to ANP in patients with IDDM. In another study, however, patients with IDDM without nephropathy were challenged with a saline infusion. In the control subjects the levels of endogenous ANP increased in association with natriuresis, whereas in the diabetic subjects levels of ANP did not change.[104] The enhanced response to ANP infusions may therefore be secondary to elevations in ANP receptor populations because of low levels of endogenous ANP. Such defective mechanisms in ANP dynamics may accentuate sodium retention.

Endothelin has a potent vasoconstrictor effect on the microcirculation, acting on both efferent and afferent renal arterioles.[105] In addition, it modulates other endocrine systems, including catecholamines, aldosterone, and ANP, and can inhibit renin release. Circulating levels of endothelin are increased in patients with essential hypertension, suggesting a role in the hypertensive process. Studies are needed to assess the role of endothelin in the renal disease and hypertension associated with diabetes mellitus.

COMPLICATIONS OF HYPERTENSION IN PATIENTS WITH DIABETES MELLITUS

Hypertension is one of the primary risk factors for cardiovascular diseases, including coronary artery disease (CAD), stroke, heart failure, and renal disease. The effect of hypertension on vascular complications in patients with diabetes mellitus must be considered in conjunction with other major risk factors including the diabetes itself,[106] which accelerates the progression of macrovascular and microvascular disease and is often associated with early mortality. Adverse cardiovascular effects also are associated with the renal disease and hyperinsulinemia that frequently accompany diabetes. The latter has recently been reviewed.[107,108] The adverse consequences of the diabetes are illustrated by a sample of patients from the Joslin Clinic who were 40 to 54 years of age at the time of diagnosis of diabetes mellitus. Only 35% of men and 45% of women survived to age 70 years, whereas in a similar population of nondiabetics in the Framingham Study, 68% of men and 82% of women survived to that age.[109] CAD accounted for most of these deaths among diabetics, and the contribution of hypertension to CAD was significant. In another group of patients from the Joslin Clinic who were followed for 12 years after the diagnosis of diabetes, mortality due to CAD increased with increasing systolic and diastolic blood pressures.

These findings from the Joslin Clinic population have been confirmed with data from other populations. Over a 10-year period of follow-up of a large population of patients with NIDDM in Warsaw, Poland, 702 deaths occurred, although only 395 were expected on the basis of mortality rates for the general population in that area.[110] Heart disease, including CAD, and stroke were responsible for 80% of the excess deaths. In addition, the risk of death caused by disease of the major blood vessels was strongly related to the blood pressure. Mortality rates were twice as high among patients whose systolic pressure was between 160 and 200 mm Hg or diastolic pressure was between 95 and 115 mm Hg than among normotensive diabetics, after adjustments were made for other possible risk factors. In diabetic patients with even higher pressures, the relative risk for cardiovascular death, as compared with rates in normotensive diabetics, increased to 2.5 for men and 5.0 for women.

The presence of subclinical albuminuria (microalbuminuria) in IDDM precedes overt renal disease and also appears to be a marker for CAD. Thirty percent of patients with IDDM will develop nephropathy, and all of these patients become hypertensive. Further, all of these hypertensive patients will progress to end-stage renal failure; 50% will die of the renal failure, and the remainder will die of CAD in the presence of renal failure.[4] An additional 20% of patients with IDDM die of

CAD between the ages of 30 and 55 years without evidence of renal disease.[111] Only rarely is hypertension observed in long-term survivors without nephropathy or coronary heart disease.

Patients with NIDDM, because they generally are older than those with IDDM, are exposed to renal disease of various etiologies. Therefore, in patients with NIDDM, the presence of microalbuminuria or even overt proteinuria does not necessarily implicate diabetes in the renal disease. Regardless of the etiology, only approximately 8% of these patients ever advance to end-stage renal disease.[112] This small percentage may be accounted for in large part by those who die early as a result of cardiac or other macrovascular events.

An association between hypertension and diabetic retinopathy has been proposed.[113,114] However, this association may well be spurious and the result of the frequent occurrence of eye lesions in patients with diabetic nephropathy. When the blood pressure of patients with proliferative retinopathy who have no nephropathy is compared with that of patients with no retinopathy, no difference is observed.[25] Therefore, one can conclude that factors associated with nephropathy accelerate retinopathy. Any possible role of blood pressure in this process remains to be determined.

BENEFITS OF ANTIHYPERTENSIVE THERAPY

When one considers the major adverse effect of hypertension in accelerating the macrovascular and renal complications of diabetes, antihypertensive therapy should not only be effective in lowering the blood pressure but also not adversely affect diabetic control, other risk factors, or preexisting diabetic complications. No reliable data are available for assessment of the effect of antihypertensive therapy on the progression of macrovascular disease in patients with diabetes. However, such studies in the general population have demonstrated beneficial effects. Vascular complications of hypertension in diabetic patients are similar to those in nondiabetic patients except for the accelerated rate of their development in the diabetic patient. In view of the similarities of these complications, the results of antihypertensive therapy in the general hypertensive population may be applicable to the diabetic hypertensive population.

The benefit of antihypertensive therapy in reducing the rate of stroke, heart failure, progression of renal disease, hypertensive retinopathy, and rupture from dissecting aortic aneurysms is unquestioned.[115–118] However, none of the studies of antihypertensive therapy for mild hypertension have demonstrated an unequivocal reduction in the morbidity or mortality of CAD. Some explanations for these results include the small sample size in the trials, the short duration of the trials, the possibility that adverse metabolic effects of antihypertensive drugs offset the benefits of the reduction in blood pressure, and the use of antihypertensive therapy in the control populations. The small sample size found in individual trials was obviated by analyzing the combined results of 11 such trials.[117] No significant reduction in CAD events was apparent. In a subsequent analysis of 14 trials involving 37,000 individuals with a mean duration of therapy of 5 years and a mean lowering of the diastolic pressure of 5 to 6 mm Hg, CAD events were reduced by 14%.[118] However, as pointed out by Kaplan,[119] the three trials added to the original analysis included patients with moderate to severe hypertension. Therefore, the question regarding the benefit of antihypertensive therapy in preventing CAD in patients with mild hypertension remains.

β-Adrenergic blocking drugs were prescribed as part of the antihypertensive program in many of these trials. Despite the lack of a beneficial effect in reducing CAD events in hypertensive patients, these agents have a demonstrated beneficial short-term and long-term benefit when administered without regard to blood pressure status following a myocardial infarction.[120] In addition, the use of β-blockers obviates the circadian variation in myocardial infarction,[121] and their use prior to a myocardial infarction improves long-term survival.[122] It is probable that similar effects will be observed in patients with diabetes.

Antihypertensive therapy is beneficial for patients with diabetic nephropathy, delaying the onset of end-stage renal disease. Circumstantial evidence in support of such renal protection derives from studies involving Goldblatt hypertension in the diabetic rat model.[123] Kidneys with stenosis of one renal artery have decreased pressure beyond the stenosis. Histologic examination of these "protected kidneys" showed minimal diabetic changes as compared with those in unprotected kidneys.

Mogensen was the first to show clearly that antihypertensive therapy can delay the rate of the deterioration of the glomerular filtration rate in humans.[124] Other investigators have confirmed these observations and have also demonstrated that albuminuria can be decreased with antihypertensive therapy consisting of the administration of a diuretic, hydralazine, and a β-adrenergic blocker.[125,126]

Trials of ACE inhibitors in diabetic patients with severe proteinuria and various degrees of renal failure have shown that these agents also significantly decrease the degree of proteinuria and the rate of decline of the glomerular filtration rate.[87] However, the degree of reduction in the blood pressure was variable. More recent studies have focused on the role of ACE inhibitors in decreasing both blood pressure and microalbuminuria at this very early stage of renal disease.[127–130] Originally it was thought that this renal effect may be specific for the ACE inhibitors that decrease glomerular efferent arteriolar tone and thus decrease intraglomerular pressure. Indeed, when the calcium channel blocker nifedipine was compared with captopril, both effectively decreased blood pressure. However, microalbuminuria decreased with captopril but increased with nifedipine.[129] In a subsequent report, however, both nifedipine and perindopril decreased microalbuminuria.[131] Recent reports suggest that both diltiazem and nicardipine improve renal function and also can reduce urinary albumin excretion even at the stage of microalbuminuria.[132–134]

The data concerning the use of ACE inhibitors in diabetic patients with microalbuminuria or overt nephropathy support an intrarenal role for locally produced A-II. Further, the variability of blood pressure reduction with ACE inhibition in these patients supports the observation that systemic plasma renin activity and A-II are usually not increased and may not be involved in the etiology of their hypertension. The early results with ACE inhibitors are encouraging. Several trials are currently in progress to confirm possible specific effects of therapy with ACE inhibitors on amelioration of glomerular injury.

MEDICATIONS FOR HYPERTENSION

Some of the newer medications for hypertension may have potential benefits, as compared with the benefits of older drugs, in the treatment of the hypertensive diabetic patient. Diuretics and β-adrenergic blocking drugs have been first-line therapy for years. They were used in most of the clinical trials discussed above in which lowering the blood pressure had no beneficial effect on CAD. Such drugs have many deleterious effects, including adverse influences on glucose and lipid metabolism, that could in part account for these negative results. Further, they might accelerate the vascular disease of diabetes. ACE inhibitors, calcium channel blockers, and α-adrenergic inhibitors do not adversely effect lipid or glucose metabolism in humans.[135–139] Indeed, ACE inhibitors may improve glucose metabolism through increasing insulin sensitivity[135] and/or via increasing blood flow to skeletal muscle.[136] Further, when ACE inhibitors are used in conjunction with diuretics, the adverse metabolic effects of the diuretics are minimized.[140,141] In addition, other cardiovascular risk factors are not adversely affected by ACE inhibitors. For example, these agents have been shown to cause regression of left ventricular hypertrophy[142] and also may decrease cellular growth and proliferation of smooth muscle cells.[143] One further benefit of ACE inhibitors is a reported improvement in the patient's feeling of well-being.[144,144a,145]

Impotence in association with the use of ACE inhibitors, calcium blockers, and α-adrenergic inhibitors is rare. An additional purported benefit of calcium channel blockers is the prevention of atherosclerosis through retardation of plaque formation.[146] Recent studies with doxazosin showed reductions in total cholesterol and triglyceride levels.[137,139] In addition, doxazosin reduced the left ventricular mass index over a 12-week period.[147] With any of the antihypertensive medications, side effects can occur regardless of whether diabetes is present. Many adverse effects, however, are peculiar to the patient with diabetes.[148] Frequently encountered adverse effects of the various classes of antihypertensive agents are reviewed in Table 44–1 and described briefly below.

Diuretics

Diuretics have been shown to adversely effect the cardiovascular risk factors of hypercholesterolemia and glucose intolerance. Elevations in cholesterol levels persist as long as diuretic therapy continues.[149] The

Table 44–1. Possible Adverse and Beneficial Effects of Antihypertensive Drugs Used in Patients with Diabetes Mellitus

Drug Class*	Possible Adverse Effects and Precautions†	Possible Benefits
Adrenergic antagonists		
Cardioselective β-blockers	Obscure hypoglycemic symptoms; impotence, hypertriglyceridemia, ↓ HDL cholesterol, heart failure, renal excretion (except metoprolol), same as noncardioselective in high doses	Effective in coronary heart disease
Noncardioselective β-blockers	Same as cardioselective, plus delayed recovery from hypoglycemia, deterioration of glucose control (NIDDM), hyperosmolar coma, hypertension if hyperglycemic, aggravated peripheral vascular disease, ↑ potassium (hyperaldonsteronism)	Effective in coronary heart disease
Combined α- and β-blockers	Same as noncardioselective blockers	. . .
Peripheral adrenergic inhibitors	Orthostatic hypotension, impotence, sodium retention	. . .
Central adrenergic inhibitors	Same as peripheral inhibitors	. . .
α₁-Adrenergic inhibitors	Orthostatic hypotension, sodium retention	Rarely cause impotence, no adverse effects on glucose or lipids
ACE inhibitors	Severe hyperkalemia (hypoaldonsteronism); further compromise of renal function in renal failure	Rarely cause impotence, no effect on glucose or lipids, minimize adverse metabolic effects of diuretics, rarely cause orthostatic hypotension, ↓ albuminuria, may ↓ rate of renal deterioration
Calcium channel blockers	Orthostatic hypotension (occasionally), glucose intolerance (?)	Rarely cause impotence, no adverse effects on lipids
Direct vasodilators	Aggravate of coronary disease, sodium retention	Rarely cause orthostatic hypertension, rarely cause impotence, no effect on glucose or lipids
Diuretics		
Thiazide	↑ glucose (NIDDM), impotence, hypotension, hypercholesterolemia, ineffective in renal failure, may accelerate renal failure	Minimize sodium retention when used with sodium-retaining drugs
Loop	Same as thiazides (except regarding renal failure)	Effective in renal failure, impotence unusual
Potassium-sparing	Severe hyperkalemia (renal failure and hypoaldosteronism), impotence	. . .

Reprinted with permission from reference 148 (Christlieb AR. Treatment selection considerations for the hypertensive diabetic patient. Arch Intern Med 1990;150:1167–74; copyright 1990, American Medical Association).
*ACE = angiotensin-converting enzyme.
† High-density lipoprotein; NIDDM = non-insulin-dependent diabetes mellitus.

results of the Lipid Research Clinics Coronary Primary Prevention Trial[150] demonstrated that for every 1% reduction in serum cholesterol level, mortality decreased 2%. Although no verifying studies are available, it can be anticipated that even small elevations in serum cholesterol are of potential clinical importance.

Both thiazide and loop diuretics produce modest elevations in the fasting glucose levels.[151] It appears that both peripheral insulin resistance and diuretic-induced hypokalemia that suppresses insulin secretion are involved.[135,151,152] Restoration of normokalemia with potassium replacement or the use of potassium-sparing diuretics generally can return insulin secretion and glucose levels to baseline values. This complication is observed primarily in patients with NIDDM who do not rely on exogenous insulin.

Diuretic-induced abnormalities in electrolytes may increase the risk of sudden death in patients with underlying cardiac disease. No reduction in cardiac-related mortality with antihypertensive treatment was observed in the Multiple Risk Factor Intervention Trial.[153] In fact, an excessive mortality was observed in hypertensive patients with abnormal electrocardiograms at baseline. The hypokalemia and hypomagnesemia that developed in these participants may have increased the risk for ventricular arrhythmias and sudden death.

Diuretics, when used alone, have been reported to accelerate the progression of renal disease and to increase cardiovascular-related mortality.[154–156] One explanation for this observation might be that diuretic-induced stimulation of the renin-angiotensin system, producing elevated levels of renin and A-II, has adverse effects on the cardiovascular system.[157] However, early studies that used diuretics in conjunction with other antihypertensive agents did offer protection against the progression of renal disease.[11,126] Therefore, one must question whether diuretics should be used as the only antihypertensive drug in such patients. It may be that these agents are beneficial when used in conjunction with other agents or that other agents offset their detrimental effects.

β-Adrenergic Blocking Agents

β-Adrenergic blockers have the potential for causing several adverse effects in the patient with diabetes. Cardioselective β-blockers administered in small doses may have fewer adverse effects than noncardioselective β-blockers (Table 44–1). However, as doses of the cardioselective β-blockers increase, they produce many of the side effects of noncardioselective β-blockers.

The adverse effect of β-adrenergic blockade on glucose metabolism is mediated in part through a reduction in the effects of catecholamines. Stimulation of pancreatic β-adrenergic receptors by catecholamines enhances insulin release. Hyperglycemia can result when β-adrenergic blockade inhibits this insulin release. Usually this response is of little clinical significance. However, hyperosmolar nonketotic coma has occurred with propranolol therapy.[158] When β-blockers are used in conjunction with diuretics, the adverse effect on glucose is enhanced.[159]

During hypoglycemia, catecholamine stimulation of β_2 receptors may contribute to the increased release of glucagon. When these receptors are inhibited, glycogenolysis and gluconeogenesis are impaired, and the result is a delay in the recovery from hypoglycemia. This delay can be of clinical significance, especially in patients receiving intensive insulin therapy. Finally, catecholamine-induced symptoms of hypoglycemia can be blunted or even abolished with β-adrenergic blockade. These symptoms include anxiety, palpitations, and tremors.

β-Adrenergic blockers tend to increase the level of triglyceride and decrease that of high-density lipoprotein. This adverse effect is minimal for β-adrenergic blockers that have intrinsic sympathomimetic activity or α-adrenergic blocking activity. The cardioprotective effect of β-adrenergic blockers in patients with coronary heart disease has already been mentioned. However, because of the ability of drugs to precipitate heart failure, they must be used with caution in patients with borderline cardiac compensation.

Although β-adrenergic blockers are used as antihypertensive agents, under certain conditions they can elevate the blood pressure. The vasoconstrictor α-adrenergic receptors are unopposed during β-adrenergic blockade. Thus, catecholamines released during hypoglycemia can produce elevations in the blood pressure.[160] Hypertensive crises have been reported in association with both propranolol and metoprolol under these conditions.[161,162] Peripheral vascular disease may also be aggravated through the same mechanism.

Central Adrenergic Inhibitors

The central adrenergic inhibitors are associated with a greater decrease in the standing blood pressure than in the supine blood pressure. Therefore, orthostatic hypotension frequently occurs, especially in patients with diabetes with autonomic neuropathy. Impotence and fluid retention are quite common. The latter can be controlled with diuretics, but therapy with the combination of a central adrenergic inhibitor and a diuretic may be accompanied by greater degrees of orthostatic hypotension.

α-Adrenergic Blocking Agents

Orthostatic hypotension following the first dose of an α-adrenergic blocking agent has been well described. However, in patients with diabetes mellitus, the orthostatic hypotension may be persistent. It is advisable to start with small doses, with frequent monitoring of the blood pressure in both the supine and upright positions. A long-acting α-adrenergic blocker, doxazosin, was recently released. Because of the attributes of this group of drugs, including the absence of adverse metabolic effects, rare impotence, unaltered cardiac output, and a beneficial effect on peripheral blood flow, this newer drug deserves adequate trials in patients with diabetes. The accompanying fluid retention can be controlled with concomitant use of diuretics.

Angiotensin-Converting Enzyme Inhibitors

ACE inhibitors can precipitate hyperkalemia and also further compromise renal function both in patients with and those without hyporeninemic hypoaldosteronism. Although hypoaldosteronism is most frequently encountered in patients with nephropathy, it does occur in patients with neuropathy.[79] Replacement of mineralocorticoids with fludrocortisone acetate therapy can normalize the potassium levels. Many patients, however, require doses of mineralocorticoids that promote sodium retention and exacerbate the hypervolemia associated with nephropathy.

In patients receiving mineralocorticoid replacement therapy, ACE inhibitors may be considered for antihypertensive treatment but the risk of hyperkalemia is not completely abolished.

Calcium Channel Blockers

Because calcium plays an important regulatory role in the release of insulin and glucagon, calcium channel blockers might be expected to decrease glucose tolerance by impairing insulin secretion. However, data in support of such an effect are not conclusive. In both nondiabetic subjects and in patients with impaired glucose tolerance, nifedipine caused small but significant increases in plasma glucose concentrations.[163–165] No effects on glucose or insulin concentrations were observed with felodipine,[166] and improved glucose was observed in some patients treated with verapamil.[167] It appears that the different calcium channel blockers may vary in their effects.

Vasodilators

Vasodilators act by decreasing peripheral vascular resistance directly. They do not dilate the venous side of the circulation and therefore do not decrease venous return to the heart. Therefore, cardiac output is often elevated. The resultant increase in cardiac effort could precipitate angina pectoris or aggravate preexisting angina. The use of these drugs in patients with active coronary disease must be weighed against the beneficial effect of lowering the blood pressure. When a β-adrenergic blocker is used in conjunction with a vasodilator, the increase in cardiac work will be minimized. This adverse effect of vasodilators does not apply to patients with significant autonomic neuropathy, who are unable to increase cardiac work significantly. Fluid retention is almost universal with vasodilator drugs, an effect necessitating the concomitant use of a diuretic.

SPECIAL CONSIDERATIONS IN TREATMENT

Many patients with diabetes mellitus have autonomic neuropathy with accompanying orthostatic hypotension. Therefore, the importance of determining the blood pressure both supine and upright (immediately upright and after 1 to 2 minutes upright) must be stressed. The goal of antihypertensive treatment should be that of reaching the desired blood pressure level when the patient is in the upright position.

It remains unknown to what degree the blood pressure should be decreased in hypertensive patients in either the general or diabetic population. Insurance statistics for the general population have shown a direct correlation between level of blood pressure and mortality. More recently, it was concluded from a combined analysis of nine major prospective observational studies with 420,000 individuals that "for the large majority of individuals, whether conventionally hypertensive or normotensive, a lower blood pressure should eventually confer a lower risk of vascular disease."[168]

Much attention has been paid to the "J-curve phenomenon" i.e., a point beyond which therapeutic reduction of the blood pressure in hypertensive patients is no longer beneficial and may even be deleterious. In a review of existing studies, no consistent J-shaped relationship was found between treatment of hypertension and stroke.[169] However, there was a consistent J-shaped relationship for cardiac events in relation to diastolic blood pressure levels that appeared to be more marked in patients with preexisting cardiac disease. Quite consistently, the J appeared below a diastolic blood pressure of 85 mm Hg. Therefore, it may be prudent to consider lowering the diastolic pressure only to 85 mm Hg in patients with heart disease. This observation presents somewhat of a dilemma in that treatment of the stroke-prone patient with coronary artery disease could be compromised by not decreasing the blood pressure below 85 mm Hg. Further, in patients with isolated systolic hypertension, the diastolic blood pressure often is below this level before treatment is initiated.

Several possible mechanisms have been invoked to explain this J-curve phenomenon,[169] including increased oxygen demands accompanying left ventricular hypertrophy that cannot be met with lower blood pressures because of near-capacity oxygen extraction, loss of autoregulation in coronary arteries, increased blood viscosity as a result of low flow, and ischemia-producing ventricular dysrhythmias.

In consideration of the accelerated rate of progression of vascular disease associated with hypertension in patients with diabetes, and until data are available that establish the optimal degree of reduction in blood pressure, one should follow the recommendations of the Working Group on Hypertension in Diabetes.[170] These guidelines propose that patients with a blood pressure of 140/90 mm Hg or greater require antihypertensive treatment and, further, that the blood pressure should be reduced to below 140/90 mm Hg if such treatment is tolerated.

Regarding the treatment of isolated systolic hypertension, the results of the Systolic Hypertension in the Elderly Program (SHEP) have recently been published.[171] In this study 4736 subjects aged 60 years and older were randomized to received stepped-care treatment with chlorthalidone and atenolol or a placebo. The average systolic blood pressure over 5 years was 143 mm Hg in the treatment group vs. 155 mm Hg in the placebo group. The incidence of stroke was reduced by 36% and that of total coronary heart disease events by 25%.

In view of these results, it appears that aggressive antihypertensive therapy is indicated in this group of patients to decrease the systolic blood pressure to 140 to 160 mm Hg, as tolerated by the patient.

APPROACH TO TREATMENT OF HYPERTENSION

It is important for the physician who takes care of the hypertensive patient with diabetes to be knowledgeable not only about therapy for hypertension but also about therapy for diabetes. Diet, maintenance of ideal body weight, exercise when indicated, and either oral glucose-lowering agents or insulin should be used together to achieve the best possible control of the blood glucose level. Control should be monitored not only by blood glucose determinations but also by measurement of glycosylated hemoglobin. Before antihypertensive therapy with drugs is initiated, the same nonpharmacologic approaches mentioned above for diabetes should be prescribed. In addition, restriction of alcohol intake to 1 ounce daily, mild-to-moderate sodium restriction, and discontinuation of tobacco use are essential.[148,170] Should nonpharmacologic therapy alone fail to maintain the blood pressure at the desired level, such therapy should be continued with the addition of antihypertensive drugs to the regimen.

Hypertension with Diabetic Complications

It is clear that decreasing the blood pressure with antihypertensive medications has beneficial effects on the complications of hypertension and diabetes. However, recent data suggest that certain drugs may negate these benefits and that others may accelerate the progression of certain complications such as diabetic nephropathy. Therefore, it is important to assess whether diabetic complications are present before initiating hypertensive therapy. In Table 44–2, guidelines for individualization of therapy are presented together with information on the drugs that should be avoided in the treatment of patients with various diabetic complications. Those agents that have no inherent adverse metabolic effects should be considered as first-line therapy. If a drug reduces the blood pressure but not to the desired level, the dosage of that drug can be increased or a second drug can be added. If the first drug selected is not effective, another can be tried.

Hypertension with Nephropathy

Earlier in this chapter, the potential specific effects of ACE inhibitors in the preservation of renal function in patients with nephropathy were discussed. Long-term data either confirming or refuting the early clinical data should be forthcoming. However, the current data, excepting patients with hypoaldosteronism, are sufficiently convincing to warrant a recommendation for ACE inhibitors as initial therapy for hypertension in diabetic patients with nephropathy (Fig. 44–1). Because certain calcium channel blockers appear to have similar beneficial characteristics, these can be used as alternative first-line therapy. In patients with hypoaldosteronism, ACE inhibitors may aggravate hyperkalemia severely; thus, a calcium channel blocker would be preferred. If Step 1 therapy does not produce a sufficient decrease in blood pressure, a diuretic should be added as Step 2 therapy. Step 3 agents can be added as necessary. Because of the negative inotropic activity of calcium channel blockers, appropriate caution is advised when they are used (particularly verapamil) with β-adrenergic blockers.

Consistent with the course of the nephrotic syndrome, edema will eventually be evident. Should edema be present when the diagnosis of hypertension is made, a diuretic should be included in Step 1 therapy. If edema occurs later, a diuretic should be added. Thiazide diuretics are ineffective when serum creatinine levels are above 2.5 to 3 mg/100 dL. At that point, a loop diuretic, used either alone or in combination with metolazone, can be prescribed. Volume depletion with worsening of renal failure can occur with excessive diuresis. Therefore, it should be emphasized that the maintenance of a trace of edema is advisable to avoid volume depletion. Electrolytes and renal function should be monitored at appropriate intervals.

Hypertension without Nephropathy or Other Complications

In 1988, the Working Group on Hypertension and Diabetes[170] recommended a stepped-care approach to therapy, with the use of diuretics, β-adrenergic blockers, ACE inhibitors, calcium channel blockers, and α_1-adrenergic blockers as Step 1 drugs. Since that time, knowledge of the potential adverse as well as the beneficial effects of antihypertensive drugs in patients with diabetes has expanded. With this increase in knowledge, revision of the Working Group's recommendations seems appropriate. Such a revision was first proposed by Kaplan and associates,[172] adopted by the American Diabetes Association,[173] and later outlined more specifically.[148] This approach, which is presented in Figure 44–2, is applicable to diabetic patients with either essential hypertension or isolated systolic hypertension without complications. (For the treatment of patients with complications, refer to Table 44–2.)

Table 44–2. Concurrent Medical Conditions in Diabetic Patients That May Influence Choice of Hypertensive Drug

Condition	Drugs of Choice*	Drugs to Avoid
Cardiac		
Coronary heart disease	ACE inhibitor, calcium channel blocker, cardioselective β-blocker, diuretic	None
Heart failure	ACE inhibitor, diuretic, vasodilator	β-Blocker, calcium channel blocker
Left ventricular hypertrophy	ACE inhibitor, α-blocker, cardioselective β-blocker	Hydralazine
Metabolic		
Frequent hypoglycemia	ACE inhibitor, calcium channel blocker	β-Blocker
Hyperlipidemia	ACE inhibitor, α-blocker, calcium channel blocker	β-Blocker, diuretic
Hypoaldosteronism	Calcium channel blocker, α-blocker	ACE inhibitor, β-blocker, potassium-sparing diuretic
Neuropathic		
Impotence	ACE inhibitor, α-blocker, calcium channel blocker, vasodilator	β-Blocker, central or peripheral adrenergic inhibitor, diuretic
Orthostatic hypotension	ACE inhibitor, calcium channel blocker, vasodilator	α-Blocker, central or peripheral adrenergic inhibitor
Renal		
Nephropathy	ACE inhibitor, calcium channel blocker	None
Vascular		
Peripheral vascular disease	ACE inhibitor, α-blocker, calcium channel blocker	β-Blocker

Reprinted with permission from reference 148 (Christlieb AR. Treatment considerations for the hypertensive diabetic patient. Arch Intern Med 1990;150:1167–74; copyright 1990, American Medical Association).
*ACE = angiotensin-converting enzyme.

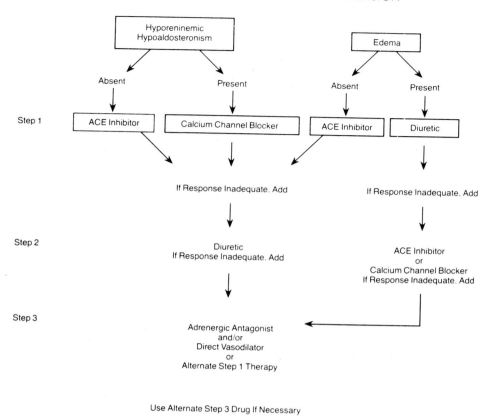

Fig. 44—1. Proposed treatment approach for hypertensive diabetic patients with nephropathy. ACE = angiotensin-converting enzyme. Reprinted with permission from reference 148 (Christlieb AR. Treatment selection considerations for the hypertensive diabetic patient. Arch Intern Med 1990;150: 1167—74; copyright 1990, American Medical Association).

An ACE inhibitor or a calcium channel blocker can be used as initial Step 1 therapy. Unless there are specific indications for the use of diuretics and β-blockers (Table 44—2), these agents are removed from the Step 1 therapy proposed by the Working Group on Hypertension in Diabetes[170] because of their adverse metabolic and/or electrolyte effects. α-Adrenergic inhibitors might be considered good choices for Step 1 therapy in view of the paucity of side effects. However, because of their propensity for producing or aggravating orthostatic hypotension and for promoting sodium retention, they have been moved to Step 3.

When choosing an ACE inhibitor or a calcium channel blocker, one should consider features that may influence patient adherence to the therapeutic program. For example, ACE inhibitors and calcium channel blockers with either a short or a long half-life are available. Drugs with a rapid onset and short duration of action such as captopril can be advantageous because the blood pressure response can be assessed while the patient is in the physician's office. This is helpful in the treatment of patients who are already receiving other antihypertensive medications, especially diuretics. Further, short-acting drugs are often best for patients with supine hypertension and orthostatic hypotension when given once daily prior to bedtime. For most patients, the longer-acting preparations will promote better patient compliance.

Once therapy is initiated, gradual increases in dosage should be made until the desired reduction in blood pressure is achieved. If there is no response, the alternate Step 1 drug can be substituted. If the response is partial, the alternate Step 1 drug can be added or small doses of a diuretic can be added as Step 2. These combinations will control the hypertension sufficiently in most patients. As discussed previously, the adverse metabolic effects of diuretics are minimized when they are used in conjunction with ACE inhibitors.[140,141] Further, the stimulation of A-II production produced by treatment with a diuretic will be blocked by the ACE inhibitor.

Any Step 3 drug can be either added or substituted. Again, caution is advised if a β-adrenergic blocker is used concomitantly with a calcium channel blocker. In severe refractory hypertension, a vasodilator can be added as Step 4. However, because volume retention and increased cardiac work are frequently associated with the use of vasodilators, they should be used in conjunction a diuretic and a β-adrenergic blocker.

Orthostatic Hypotension

Supine hypertension with orthostatic hypotension is probably the most difficult blood pressure abnormality to treat in the patient with diabetes. Occasionally, the orthostatic hypotension can be of sufficient severity to prevent the patient from maintaining an upright position. In patients with less difficulty remaining upright, antihypertensive medications to control the supine blood pressure may result in exacerbation of the orthostatic hypotension. If orthostatic hypotension is associated with hypoaldosteronism, renal sodium wasting may occur and

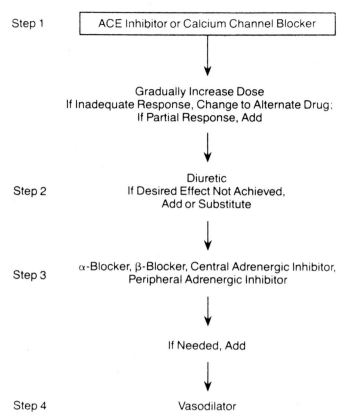

Step 1 | ACE Inhibitor or Calcium Channel Blocker |

Gradually Increase Dose
If Inadequate Response, Change to Alternate Drug:
If Partial Response, Add

Step 2   Diuretic
If Desired Effect Not Achieved,
Add or Substitute

Step 3   α-Blocker, β-Blocker, Central Adrenergic Inhibitor,
Peripheral Adrenergic Inhibitor

If Needed, Add

Step 4   Vasodilator

Fig. 44–2. Proposed treatment approach for diabetic patients with essential or isolated systolic hypertension. ACE = angiotensin-converting enzyme. Reprinted with permission from reference 148 (Christlieb AR. Treatment selection considerations for the hypertensive diabetic patient. Arch Intern Med 1990;150:1167–74; copyright 1990, American Medical Association).

result in sodium depletion. Blunted vascular responsiveness to endogenous vasopressor hormones and some degree of volume depletion will ensue. To treat the hypoaldosteronism, mineralocorticoid replacement with fludrocortisone acetate may be necessary. Although initially it may appear paradoxical to add a mineralocorticoid to the therapeutic program for a patient with any form of hypertension, it must be remembered that this is replacement therapy for a hormone deficiency in such patients. Restoration of normal mineralocorticoid activity will increase vascular reactivity and plasma volume and, in some patients, will decrease the degree of orthostatic hypotension. The use of elastic support stockings during the day and the placement of 8- to 10-inch blocks under the head of the bed at night may minimize the morning orthostatic drop in blood pressure and lower the nocturnal supine hypertension. To decrease the blood pressure further during the night, the patient may take a short-acting ACE inhibitor such as captopril, a short-acting calcium channel blocker such as nifedipine, or the vasodilator hydralazine in a single-dose shortly before retiring. Ephedrine is beneficial in some patients as a

means of increasing the orthostatic blood pressure during the day.

It must be recognized that despite these maneuvers and pharmacologic manipulations, supine hypertension with orthostatic hypotension may be alleviated only minimally. As with many of the other neuropathic problems in the diabetic patient, orthostatic hypotension generally improves with time. Frequently this occurs with the onset or progression of diabetic nephropathy.

Hypertensive Emergencies

Hypertensive emergences are life-threatening disorders characterized by rapid elevations in the blood pressure, arteriolar spasm, necrotizing arteriolitis, and end-organ damage. Urgencies and emergencies such as malignant hypertension, hypertensive encephalopathy, rapidly progressive renal failure, and left ventricular failure may occur during the natural history of hypertension in the patient with diabetes. Classical malignant hypertension, however, is distinctly rare in the hypertensive diabetic patient with nephropathy probably because the RAA system is frequently suppressed. For most emergencies immediate hospitalization and treatment are necessary. Diagnostic evaluation for surgically curable forms of hypertension should be delayed until the blood pressure is adequately controlled.

Principles of treatment of hypertensive emergencies in the diabetic patient are similar to those in the nondiabetic patient. Treatment with parenterally administered antihypertensive drugs should be started as soon as possible, with oral antihypertensive drugs instituted when permitted by the patient's condition. A comprehensive review of hypertensive emergencies together with up-to-date treatment recommendations has recently been published.[174] The reader is referred to this review for the particulars of diagnosis and treatment of patients with hypertensive emergencies.

CONCLUSIONS

Hypertension in the patient with diabetes is of several types, with different mechanisms responsible for the elevation in arterial pressure. Understanding these mechanisms and the mode of action of the various antihypertensive drugs will provide the physician with the necessary knowledge to approach antihypertensive therapy rationally. Adverse effects of these drugs that are peculiar to the patient with diabetes necessitate special precautions in their use.

REFERENCES

1. Christlieb AR. Diabetes and hypertensive vascular disease: mechanisms and treatment. Am J Cardiol 1973; 32:592–606.
2. Christlieb AR, Warram JH, Krolewsky AS, et al. Hypertension: the major risk factor in juvenile-onset insulin-dependent diabetics. Diabetes 1981;30(Suppl 2):90–6.
3. Consensus statement. Am J Kidney Dis 1989;13:2–6.
4. Krolewski AS, Warram JH, Christlieb AR, et al. The

changing natural history of nephropathy in Type I diabetes. Am J Med 1985;78:785–94.

5. Andersen AR, Christiansen JS, Andersen JK, et al. Diabetic nephropathy in Type I (insulin-dependent) diabetes: an epidemiological study. Diabetologia 1983;25:496–501.

6. Harris MI. Noninsulin-dependent diabetes mellitus in black and white Americans. Diabetes Metab Rev 1990; 6:71–90.

7. Munichoodappa C, D'Elia JA, Libertino JA, et al. Renal artery stenosis in hypertensive diabetics. J Urol 1979; 121:555–8.

8. Gifford RW Jr, Kirdendall W, O'Connor DT, Weidman W. Office evaluation of hypertension: a statement for health professionals by a writing group of the Council for High Blood Pressure Research, American Heart Association. Hypertension 1989;13:283–93.

9. Noth RH. Diabetic nephropathy: hemodynamic basis and implications for disease management. Ann Intern Med 1989;110:795–813.

10. Krolewski AS, Warram JH, Christlieb AR. Onset, course, complications, and prognosis of diabetes mellitus. In: Marble A, Krall LP, Bradley RF, et al, eds. Joslin's diabetes mellitus. 12th ed. Philadelphia: Lea & Febiger, 1985:251–77.

11. Mogensen CE. Microalbuminuria as a predictor of clinical diabetic nephropathy. Kidney Int 1987;31:673–89.

12. Mogensen CE. Prevention and treatment of renal disease in insulin-dependent diabetes mellitus. Sem Nephrol 1990;10:260–73.

13. Kofoed-Enevoldsen A, Borch-Johnsen K, Kreiner S, et al. Declining incidence of persistent proteinuria in Type I (insulin-dependent) diabetic patients in Denmark. Diabetes 1987;36:205–9.

14. Selby JV, FitzSimmons SC, Newman JM, et al. The natural history and epidemiology of diabetic nephropathy: implications for prevention and control. JAMA 1990; 263:1954–60.

15. Feldt-Rasmussen B, Nørgaard K, Jensen T, et al. The role of hypertension in the development of nephropathy in Type I (insulin-dependent) diabetes mellitus. Acta Diabetol Lat 1990;27:173–9.

16. Borch-Johnsen K, Nissen H, Henriksen E, et al. The natural history of insulin dependent diabetes mellitus in Denmark. I. Long-term survival with and without late diabetic complications. Diabetic Med 1987;4:201–10.

17. Krolewski AS, Canessa M, Warram JH, et al. Predisposition to hypertension and susceptibility to renal disease in insulin-dependent diabetes mellitus. N Engl J Med 1988; 318:140–5.

18. Viberti GC, Keen H, Wiseman MJ. Raised arterial pressure in parents of proteinuric insulin-dependent diabetics. BMJ 1987;295:515–7.

19. Barzilay J, Warram JH, Bak M, et al. Predisposition to hypertension: risk factor for nephropathy and hypertension in IDDM. Kidney Int 1992;41:723–30.

20. Mangili R, Bending JJ, Scott G, et al. Increased sodium-lithium countertransport activity in red cells of patients with insulin-dependent diabetes and nephropathy. N Engl J Med 1988;18:146–50.

21. Deckert T, Feldt-Rasmussen B, Borch-Johnsen K, et al. Albuminuria reflects widespread vascular damage: the Steno hypothesis. Diabetologia 1989;32:219–26.

22. Mathiesen ER, Rønn B, Jensen T, et al. Relationship between blood pressure and urinary albumin excretion in development of microalbuminuria. Diabetes 1990; 39:245–9.

23. Ballard DJ, Humphrey LL, Melton LJ III, et al. Epidemiology of persistent proteinuria in Type II diabetes mellitus: population-based study in Rochester, Minnesota. Diabetes 1988;37:405–12.

24. Medalie JH, Papier CM, Goldbourt U, Herman JB. Major factors in the development of diabetes mellitus in 10,000 men. Arch Intern Med 1975;135:811–17.

25. Krolewski AS, Warram JH, Cupples A, et al. Hypertension, orthostatic hypotension and the microvascular complications of diabetes. J Chronic Dis 1985;38:319–26.

26. Reaven GM. Banting Lecture 1988. Role of insulin resistance in human disease. Diabetes 1988;37:1595–607.

27. DeFronzo RA, Ferrannini E. Insulin resistance: a multifaceted syndrome responsible for NIDDM, obesity, hypertension, dyslipidemia, and atherosclerotic cardiovascular disease. Diabetes Care 1991;14:173–94.

28. Christlieb AR, Krolewsky AS, Warram JH, Soeldner JS. Is insulin the link between hypertension and obesity? Hypertension 1985;7(Suppl II):54–7.

29. Lucas CP, Estigarribia JA, Darga LL, Reaven, G. Insulin and blood pressure in obesity. Hypertension 1985;7:702–6.

30. Modan M, Halkin H, Almog S, et al. Hyperinsulinemia: a link between hypertension, obesity, and glucose intolerance. J Clin Invest 1985;75:809–17.

31. Reaven GM. Insulin resistance, hyperinsulinemia, hypertriglyceridemia, and hypertension: parallels between human disease and rodent models. Diabetes Care 1991; 14:195–202.

32. Manicardi V, Camellini L, Bellodi G, et al. Evidence for an association of high blood pressure and hyperinsulinemia in obese man. J Clin Endocrinol Metab 1986;62:1302–4.

33. Ferrannini E, Buzzigoli G, Bonadonna R, et al. Insulin resistance in essential hypertension. N Engl J Med 1987; 317:350–7.

34. Pollare T, Lithell H, Berne C. Insulin resistance is a characteristic feature of primary hypertension independent of obesity. Metabolism 1990;39:167–74.

35. Zavaroni I, Bonora E, Pagliara M, et al. Risk factors for coronary artery disease in healthy persons with hyperinsulinemia and normal glucose tolerance. N Engl J Med 1989;320:703–6.

36. Manolio TA, Savage PJ, Burke GL, et al. Association of fasting insulin with blood pressure and lipids in young adults: the Cardia study. Arteriosclerosis 1990;10:430–6.

37. Saad MF, Knowler WC, Pettitt DJ, et al. Insulin and hypertension: relationship to obesity and glucose tolerance in Pima Indians. Diabetes 1990;39:1430–5.

38. Marigliano A, Tedde R, Sechi LA, et al. Insulinemia and blood pressure: relationships in patients with primary and secondary hypertension, and with or without glucose metabolism impairment. Am J Hypertens 1990;3:521–6.

39. Ferrannini E, Haffner SM, Stern MP. Essential hypertension: an insulin-resistant state. J Cardiovasc Pharmacol 1990; 15(Suppl 5):S18–25.

40. Haffner SM, Stern MP, Hazuda HP, et al. Increased insulin concentrations in nondiabetic offspring of diabetic parents. N Engl J Med 1988;319:1297–301.

41. Haffner SM, Stern MP, Hazud HP, et al. Parental history of diabetes is associated with increased cardiovascular risk factors. Arteriosclerosis 1989;9:929–33.

42. DeFronzo RA, Cooke CR, Andres R, et al. The effect of insulin on renal handling of sodium, potassium, calcium, and phosphate in man. J Clin Invest 1975;55:845–55.

43. Weidmann P, Beretta-Piccoli C, Keusch G, et al. Sodium-volume factor, cardiovascular reactivity and hypotensive mechanism of diuretic therapy in mild hypertension

associated with diabetes mellitus. Am J Med 1979;67: 779–84.

44. Weidmann P, Ferrari P. Central role of sodium in hypertension in diabetic subjects. Diabetes Care 1991;14:220–32.

45. Ullrich KJ. Renal tubular mechanisms of organic solute transport. Kidney Int 1976;9:134–48.

46. Crane RK. The gradient hypothesis and other models of carrier-mediated active transport. Rev Physiol Biochem Pharmacol 1977;78:99–159.

47. Butlen D, Vadrot S, Roseau S, Morel F. Insulin receptors along the rat nephron [^{125}I] insulin binding in microdissected glomeruli and tubules. Pflugers Arch 1988; 412:604–12.

48. Rocchini AP, Katch V, Kveselis D, et al. Insulin and renal sodium retention in obese adolescents. Hypertension 1989;14:367–74.

49. Jørgensen PL. Sodium and potassium ion pump in the kidney tubules. Physiol Rev 1990;60:864–917.

50. Goldstein DA, Massry SG. Diabetic nephropathy: clinical course and effect of hemodialysis. Nephron 1978; 20:286–96.

51. Feldt-Rasmussen B, Mathiesen ER, Deckert T, et al. Central role for sodium in the pathogenesis of blood pressure changes independent of angiotensin, aldosterone and catecholamines in Type I (insulin-dependent) diabetes mellitus. Diabetologia 1987;30:610–7.

52. Weidmann P, Beretta-Piccoli C, Trost BN. Pressor factors and responsiveness in hypertension accompanying diabetes mellitus. Hypertension 1985;7(Suppl II):33–42.

53. Sowers JR, Nyby M, Stern N, et al. Blood pressure and hormone changes associated with weight reduction in the obese. Hypertension 1992;4:686–91.

54. De Chatel R, Weidmann P, Flammer J, et al. Sodium, renin, aldosterone, catecholamines and blood pressure in diabetes mellitus. Kidney Int 1977;12:412–21.

55. Christlieb AR, Assal J-P, Katsilambros N, et al. Plasma renin activity and blood volume in uncontrolled diabetes: ketoacidosis, a state of secondary aldosteronism. Diabetes 1975;24:190–3.

56. Hilton PJ. Na$^+$ transport in hypertension. Diabetes Care 1991;14:233–9.

57. Ng LL, Simmons D, Frighi V, et al. Leucocyte Na$^+$/H$^+$ antiport activity in Type 1 (insulin-dependent) diabetic patients with nephropathy. Diabetologia 1990;33:371–7.

58. Dominiczak AF, Bohr D.F. Vascular smooth muscle in hypertension. J Hypertens 1989;7(3)(Suppl):S107–16.

59. Erne P, Hermsmeyer K. Intracellular vascular muscle Ca^{2+} modulation in genetic hypertension. Hypertension 1989; 14:145–51.

60. Christlieb AR, Janka H-U, Kraus B, et al. Vascular reactivity to angiotensin II and to norepinephrine in diabetic subjects. Diabetes 1976;25:268–74.

61. Drury PL, Smith GM, Ferriss JB. Increased vasopressor responsiveness to angiotensin II in Type I (insulin-dependent) diabetic patients without complications. Diabetologia 1984;27:174–9.

62. Tuck M, Corry D, Trujillo A. Salt-sensitive blood pressure and exaggerated vascular reactivity in the hypertension of diabetes mellitus. Am J Med 1990;88:210–6.

63. Rowe JW, Young JB, Minaker KL, et al. Effect of insulin and glucose infusions on sympathetic nervous system activity in normal man. Diabetes 1981;30:219–25.

64. Landsberg L, Kreiger DR. Obesity, metabolism, and the sympathetic nervous system. Am J Hypertens 1989;2 (Suppl):125S-32S.

65. Daly PA, Landsberg L. Hypertension in obesity and NIDDM: role of insulin and sympathetic nervous system. Diabetes Care 1991;14:240–8.

66. Tuck ML. Role of salt in the control of blood pressure in obesity and diabetes mellitus. Hypertension 1991:17 (Suppl I):135–42.

67. Deibert DC, DeFronzo RA. Epinephrine-induced insulin resistance in man. J Clin Invest 1980;65:717–21.

68. Laakso M, Edelman SV, Brechtel G, Baron AD. Decreased effect of insulin to stimulate skeletal muscle blood flow in obese man: a novel mechanism for insulin resistance. J Clin Invest 1990;85:1844–52.

69. Laakso M, Edelman SV, Olefsky JM, et al. Kinetics of in vivo muscle insulin-mediated glucose uptake in human obesity. Diabetes 1990;39:965–74.

70. Baron AD, Laakso M, Brechtel G, Edelman SV. Reduced capacity and affinity of skeletal muscle for insulin-mediated glucose uptake in noninsulin-dependent diabetic subjects: effects of insulin therapy. J Clin Invest 1991; 87:1186.

71. Resnick LM. Hypertension and abnormal glucose homeostasis: possible role of divalent ion metabolism. Am J Med 1989;87(Suppl 6A):17S–22S.

72. Resnick LM, Gupta RK, Gruenspan H, et al. Hypertension and peripheral insulin resistance: possible mediating role of intracellular free magnesium. Am J Hypertens 1990; 3:373–9.

73. Resnick LM, Gupta RK, Bhargava KK, et al. Cellular ions in hypertension, diabetes, and obesity: a nuclear magnetic resonance spectroscopic study. Hypertension 1991; 17:951–7.

74. Trovati M, Massucco P, Anfossi G, et al. Insulin influences the renin-angiotensin-aldosterone system in humans Metabolism 1989;38:501–3.

75. Bjørck S, Aurell M. Diabetes mellitus, the renin-angiotensin system, and angiotensin-converting enzyme inhibition. Nephron 1990;55(Suppl 1):10–20.

76. Luetscher JA, Kraemer FB, Wilson DM. Prorenin and vascular complications of diabetes. Am J Hypertens 1989; 2:382–6.

77. Wilson DM, Luetscher JA. Plasma prorenin activity and complications in children with insulin-dependent diabetes mellitus. N Engl J Med 1990;323:1101–6.

78. Christlieb AR, Kaldany A, D'Elia JA. Plasma renin activity and hypertension in diabetes mellitus. Diabetes 1976; 25:969–74.

79. Christlieb AR, Kaldany A, D'Elia JA, Williams GH. Aldosterone responsiveness in patients with diabetes mellitus. Diabetes 1978;27:732–7.

80. O'Hare JA, Ferriss JB, Brady D, et al. Exchangeable sodium and renin in hypertensive diabetic patients with and without nephropathy. Hypertension 1985;7(Suppl II):43–8.

81. Tomita K, Matsuda O, Ideura T, et al. Renin-angiotensin-aldosterone system in mild diabetic nephropathy. Nephron 1982;31:361–7.

82. Schindler AM, Sommers SC. Diabetic sclerosis of the renal juxtaglomerular apparatus. Lab Invest 1966;15:877–84.

83. Christlieb AR, Munichoodappa C, Braaten JT. Decreased response to plasma renin activity to orthostasis in diabetic patients with orthostatic hypotension. Diabetes 1974;23:835–40.

84. Fernandez-Cruz A, Noth RH, Lassman, et al. Low plasma renin activity in normotensive patients with diabetes mellitus: relationship to neuropathy. Hypertension 1981;3:87–92.

85. Kleinert HD. Renin inhibitors: discovery and development—an overview and perspective. Am J Hypertens 1989;2:800–8.

86. Van den Meiracker AH, Admiraal PJJ, Man in't Veld AJ, et al. Prolonged blood pressure reduction by orally active renin inhibitor RO 42–5892 in essential hypertension. BMJ 1990;301:205–10.

87. Taguma Y, Kitamoto Y, Futaki G, et al. Effect of captopril on heavy proteinuria in azotemic diabetics. N Engl J Med 1985;313:1617–20.

88. Bjørck S, Nyberg G, Mulec H, et al. Beneficial effects of angiotensin converting enzyme inhibition on renal function in patients with diabetic nephropathy. BMJ 1986; 293:471–4.

89. Hommel E, Parving H-H, Mathiesen E, et al. Effect of captopril on kidney function in insulin-dependent diabetic patients with nephropathy. BMJ 1986;293:467–70.

90. Hostetter TH, Troy JL, Brenner BM. Glomerular hemodynamics in experimental diabetes mellitus. Kidney Int 1981;19:410–5.

91. Hostetter TH, Rennke HG, Brenner BM. The case of intrarenal hypertension in the initiation and progression of diabetic and other glomerulopathies [Editorial]. Am J Med 1982;72:375–80.

92. Scherstén B. Effects of antihypertensive therapy on kidney function in diabetic patients. Drugs 1988;35(Suppl 5):59–61.

93. Williams GH. Converting-enzyme inhibitors in the treatment of hypertension. N Engl J Med 1988;319:1517–25.

94. Tuck M. Management of hypertension in the patient with diabetes mellitus: focus on the use of angiotensin converting enzyme inhibitors. Am J Hypertens 1988;1 (Suppl):384S–8S.

95. DeLeiva A, Christlieb AR, Melby JC, et al. Big renin and biosynthetic defect of aldosterone in diabetes mellitus. N Engl J Med 1976;295:639–43.

96. Tuck ML, Sambhi MP, Levin L. Hyporeninemic hypoaldosteronism in diabetes mellitus: studies of the autonomic nervous system's control of renin release. Diabetes 1979;28:237–41.

97. Christlieb AR. Renin-angiotensin-aldosterone system in diabetes mellitus. Diabetes 1976;25:820–5.

98. Goldfarb S, Cox M, Singer I, Goldberg M. Acute hyperkalemia induced by hyperglycemia: hormonal mechanisms. Ann Intern Med 1976;84:426–32.

99. Oates JA, FitzGerald GA, Branch RA, et al. Clinical implications of prostaglandin and thromboxane A2 formation. N Engl Med 1988;319:761–7.

100. Tan SY, Shapiro R, Franco R, et al. Indomethacin induced prostaglandin inhibition of hyperkalemia. Am Intern Med 1979;90:783–5.

101. Kaufman JS, Peck M, Hamburger RJ, Flamenbaum W. Isolated hypoaldosteronism and abnormalities in renin, kallikrein, and prostaglandin. Nephron 1986;43:203–10.

102. Rimmer JM, Horn JF, Gennari J. Hyperkalemia as a complication of drug therapy. Arch Intern Med 1987; 147:867–9.

103. Predel H-G, Schulte-Vels O, Sorger M, et al. Atrial natriuretic peptide in patients with diabetes mellitus Type I: effects on systemic and renal hemodynamics and renal excretory function. Am J Hypertens 1990; 3:674–81.

104. Trevisan R, Fioretto P, Semplicini A, et al. Role of insulin and atrial natriuretic peptide in sodium retention in insulin-treated IDDM patients during isotonic volume expansion. Diabetes 1990;39:289–98.

105. Lerman A, et al. Endothelin: a new cardiovascular regulatory peptide. Mayo Clin Proc 1990;65:1441.

106. Kannel WB, McGee DL. Diabetes and cardiovascular disease: the Framingham Study. JAMA 1979;241:2035–8.

107. Black HR. The coronary artery disease paradox: the role of hyperinsulinemia and insulin resistance and implications for therapy. J Cardiovasc Pharmacol 1990;15(Suppl 5): S26–38.

108. Krolewski AS, Warram JH, Valsania P, et al. Evolving natural history of coronary artery disease in diabetes mellitus. Am J Med 1991;90(Suppl 2A):56S–61S.

109. Lerner DJ, Kannel WB. Patterns of coronary heart disease morbidity and mortality in the sexes: a 26-year follow-up of the Framingham population. Am Heart J 1986; 111:383–90.

110. Janeczko D, Czyzyk A, Kopczynski J, Krzyzanowski M. Risk differentials of 10-year cardiovascular mortality among Type I (insulin-dependent) and Type II (non-insulin-dependent) diabetic patients [Abstract no. 233]. Diabetologia 1987;29:552A.

111. Krolewski AS, Kosinski EJ, Warram JH, et al. Magnitude and determinants of coronary artery disease in juvenile-onset, insulin-dependent diabetes mellitus. Am J Cardiol 1987;59:750–5.

112. Tung P, Levin SR. Nephropathy in non-insulin-dependent diabetes mellitus. Am J Med 1988;85(Suppl 5A):131–6.

113. Constable IJ, Knuiman MW, Welborn TA, et al. Assessing the risk of diabetic retinopathy. Am J Ophthalmol 1984; 97:53–61.

114. Klein R, Klein BEK, Moss SE, et al. The Wisconsin epidemiologic study of diabetic retinopathy. II. Prevalence and risk of diabetic retinopathy when age at diagnosis is less than 30 years. Arch Ophthalmol 1984; 102:520–6.

115. Veterans Administration Cooperative Study Group on Antihypertensive Agents. Effects of treatment on morbidity in hypertension: results in patients with diastolic blood pressures averaging 115 through 129 mm Hg. JAMA 1967; 202:1028–34.

116. Weinberger MH. Cardiovascular risk factors and antihypertensive therapy. Am J Med 1988;84(Suppl 4A):24–9.

117. MacMahon SW, Cutler JA, Furberg CD, Payne GH. The effects of drug treatment for hypertension on morbidity and mortality from cardiovascular disease: a review of randomized controlled trials. Progr Cardiovasc Dis 1986; 29(Suppl 1):99–118.

118. Collins R, Peto R, MacMahon S, et al. Blood pressure, stroke, and coronary heart disease: Part 2, short-term reductions in blood pressure: overview of randomised drug trials in their epidemiological context. Lancet 1990;335:827–38.

119. Kaplan NM. Dredging the data on antihypertensive therapy. Am J Hypertens 1991;4:19–7.

120. Yusuf S, Wittes J, Friedman L. Overview of results of randomized clinical trials in heart disease. 1. Treatment following myocardial infarction. JAMA 1988;260: 2088–93.

121. Willich SN, Linderer T, Wegscheider K, et al. Increased morning incidence of myocardial infarction in the ISAM Study: absence with prior β-adrenergic blockage. Circulation 1989;80:853–8.

122. Nidorf SM, Parsons RW, Thompson PL, et al. Reduced risk of death at 28 days in patients taking a β blocker before admission to hospital with myocardial infarction. BMJ 1990;300:71–44.

123. Mauer SM, Steffes MW, Azar S, et al. The effects of

Goldblatt hypertension on development of the glomerular lesions of diabetes mellitus in the rat. Diabetes 1978; 27:738–44.

124. Mogensen CE. Antihypertensive treatment of inhibiting the progression of diabetic nephropathy. In: Ditzel J, ed. Diabetes and diabetes treatment. Proceedings of the Third Nordic Symposium on Diabetes. Denmark: Nordisk Insulin Laboratories, 1979.

125. Hasslacher CH, Stech W, Wahl P, Ritz E. Blood pressure and metabolic control as risk factors for nephropathy in Type I (insulin-dependent) diabetes. Diabetologia 1985; 28:6–11.

126. Parving H-H, Andersen AR, Smidt UM, et al. Effect of antihypertensive treatment on kidney function in diabetic nephropathy. BMJ 1987;294:1443–7.

127. Marre M, Chatellier G, Leblanc H, et al. Prevention of diabetic nephropathy with enalapril in normotensive diabetics with microalbuminuria. BMJ 1988;297:1092–5.

128. Marre M, Leblanc H, Suarez L, et al. Converting enzyme inhibition and kidney function in normotensive diabetic patients with persistent microalbuminuria. BMJ 1987; 294:1448–52.

129. Mimran A, Insua A, Ribstein J, et al. Comparative effect of captopril and nifedipine in normotensive patients with incipient diabetic nephropathy. Diabetes Care 1988; 11:850–3.

130. Brichard SM, Santoni JP, Thomas JR, et al. Long term reduction of microalbuminuria after 1 year of angiotensin converting enzyme inhibition by perindropil in hypertensive insulin-treated diabetic patients. Diabete Metab 1990; 16:30–6.

131. Melbourne Diabetic Nephropathy Study Group. Comparison between perindopril and nifedipine in hypertensive and normotensive diabetic patients with microalbuminuria. BMJ 1981;302:210–6.

132. Baba T, Murabayashi S, Takebe K. Comparison of the renal effects of angiotensin converting enzyme inhibitor and calcium antagonist in hypertensive Type 2 (non-insulin-dependent) diabetic patients with microalbuminuria: a randomized controlled trial. Diabetologia 1989;32:40–4.

133. Stornello M, Valvo EV, Scapellato L. Hemodynamic, renal, and humoral effects of the calcium entry blocker nicardipine and converting enzyme inhibitor captopril in hypertensive Type II diabetic patients with nephropathy. J Cardiovasc Pharmacol 1989;14:851–5.

134. Bakris GL. Effects of diltiazem or lisinopril on massive proteinuria associated with diabetes mellitus. Ann Intern Med 1990;112:707–8.

135. Pollare T, Lithell H, Berne C. A comparison of the effects of hydrochlorothiazide and captopril on glucose and lipid metabolism in patients with hypertension. N Engl J Med 1989;321:868–73.

136. Kodama J, Katayama S, Tanaka K, et al. Effect of captopril on glucose concentration: possible role of augmented postprandial forearm blood flow. Diabetes Care 1990; 13:1109–11.

137. Wessels F. Double-blind comparison of doxazosin and enalapril in patients with mild or moderate essential hypertension. Am Heart J 1991;121:299–303.

138. Klauser R, Prager R, Gaube S, et al. Metabolic effects of isradipine versus hydrochlorothiazide in diabetes mellitus. Hypertension 1991;17:15–21.

139. Talseth T, Westlie L, Daae L. Doxazosin and atenolol as monotherapy in mild and moderate hypertension: a randomized, parallel study with a three-year follow-up. Am Heart J 1991;121:280–5.

140. Prince MJ, Stuart CA, Padia M, et al. Metabolic effects of hydrochlorothiazide and enalapril during treatment of the hypertensive diabetic patient: enalapril for hypertensive diabetics. Arch Intern Med 1988;148:2363–8.

141. Weinberger MH. Influence of an angiotensin-converting enzyme inhibitor on diuretic-induced metabolic effects in hypertension. Hypertension 5(Suppl 3):132–8.

142. Lombardo M, Zaini G, Pastori F, et al. Left ventricular mass and function before and after antihypertensive treatment. J Hypertens 1983;1:215–9.

143. Keane WF, Shapiro BE. Renal protective effects of angiotensin-converting enzyme inhibition. Am J Cardiol 1990; 65:491–53I.

144. Schoenberger JA, Testa M, Ross AD, et al. Efficacy, safety, and quality-of-life assessment of captopril antihypertensive therapy in clinical practice. Arch Intern Med 1990; 150:301–6.

144a. Breckenridge A. Angiotensin converting enzyme inhibitors and quality of life. Am J Hypertens 1991;4 (Suppl):79S–82S.

146. Gotto AM Jr. Calcium channel blockers and the prevention of atherosclerosis. Am J Hypertens 1990;3 (Suppl):342S–6.

147. Monsalve P, Vera O, Acuña FP, et al. Echocardiographic assessment of doxazosin on left ventricular mass in patients with essential hypertension. Am Heart J 1991; 121:356–61.

148. Christlieb AR. Treatment selection considerations for the hypertensive diabetic patient. Arch Intern Med 1990; 150:1167–74.

149. Weidmann P, Gerber A, Mordasini R. Effects of antihypertensive therapy on serum lipoproteins. Hypertension 5(Suppl 3):120–31.

150. Lipid Research Clinics Program. The Lipid Research Clinics Coronary Primary Prevention Trial results. II. The relationship of reduction in incidence of coronary heart disease to cholesterol lowering. JAMA 1984;251:365–74.

151. Amery A, Birkenhäger W, Brixko P, et al. Glucose intolerance during diuretic therapy in elderly hypertensive patients: a second report from the European Working Party on High Blood Pressure in the Elderly (EWPHE). Postgrad Med J 1986;62:919–24.

152. Rowe JW, Tobin JD, Rosa RM, Andres R. Effect of experimental potassium deficiency on glucose and insulin metabolism. Metabolism 1980;29:498–502.

153. Multiple Risk Factor Intervention Trial Research Group. Baseline rest electrocardiographic abnormalities, antihypertensive treatment, and mortality in the Multiple Risk Factor Intervention Trial. Am J Cardiol 1985;55:1–15.

154. Walker WG, Hermann J, Yin D, et al. Diuretics accelerate diabetic nephropathy in hypertensive insulin-dependent and noninsulin dependent subjects. Trans Assoc Am Physicians 1987;C305–15.

155. Klein R, Moss SE, Klein BEK, DeMets D.L. Relation of ocular and systemic factors to survival in diabetes. Arch Intern Med 1989;149:266–72.

156. Warram JH, Laffel LMB, Valsenia P, et al. Excess mortality associated with diuretic therapy. Arch Intern Med 1991;151:1350–6.

157. Alderman MH, Madhavan S, Ooi WL, et al. Association of the renin-sodium profile with the risk of myocardial infarction in patients with hypertension. N Engl J Med 1991;324:1098–104.

158. Podolsky S, Pattavina, C.G. Hyperosmolar nonketotic diabetic coma: a complication of propranolol therapy. Metabolism 1973;22:685–93.

159. Fuh MMT, Sheu WH, Shen DC, et al. Metabolic effects of diuretic and beta-blocker treatment of hypertension in patients with non-insulin-dependent diabetes mellitus. Am J Hypertens 1990;3:387–90.

160. Ryan JR, LaCorte W, Jain A, McMahon FG. Hypertension in hypoglycemic diabetics treated with β-adrenergic antagonists. Hypertension 1985;7:443–6.

161. McMurtry RJ. Propranolol, hypoglycemia, and hypertensive crisis [Letter]. Ann Intern Med 1974;80:669–70.

162. Shepherd AMM, Lin MS, Keeton TK. Hypoglycemia-induced hypertension in a diabetic patient on metoprolol. Ann Intern Med 1981;94:357–8.

163. Charles S, Ketelslegers JM, Buysschaert M, Lambert AE. Hyperglycaemic effect of nifedipine. BMJ 1981;283:19–20.

164. Palumbo G, Barantini E, Pozzi F, et al. Long-term nifedipine treatment and glucose homeostasis in hypertensive patients. Curr Ther Res 1988;43:171–9.

165. Guigliano D, Torella R, Cacciapuoti F, et al. Impairment of insulin secretion in man by nifedipine. Eur J Clin Pharmacol 1980;18:395–8.

166. Hedner T, Elmfeldt D, Von Schenck H, et al. Glucose tolerance in hypertensive patients during treatment with the calcium antagonist, felodipine. Br J Clin Pharmacol 1987;24:145–9.

167. Kendall MJ, Horton RC, Chellingsworth MC. Calcium antagonists and glycaemic control. J Clin Hosp Pharm 1986;11:175–80.

168. MacMahon S, Peto R, Cutler J, et al. Blood pressure, stroke, and coronary heart disease. Part 1, prolonged differences in blood pressure:prospective observational studies corrected for the regression dilution bias. Lancet 1990;335:765–74.

169. Farnett L, Mulrow CD, Linn WD, et al. The J-curve phenomenon and the treatment of hypertension: is there a point beyond which pressure reduction is dangerous? JAMA 1991;265:489–95.

170. Working Group on Hypertension in Diabetes. Statement on hypertension in diabetes mellitus: final report. Arch Intern Med 1987;147:830–42.

171. SHEP Cooperative Research Group. Prevention of stroke by antihypertensive drug treatment in older persons with isolated systolic hypertension: final results of the systolic hypertension in the elderly program (SHEP). JAMA 1991;265:3255–64.

172. Kaplan NM, Rosenstock J, Raskin P. A differing view of treatment of hypertension in patients with diabetes mellitus. Arch Intern Med 1987;147:1160–2.

173. American Diabetes Asociation. Consensus statement: role of cardiovascular risk factors in prevention and treatment of macrovascular disease in diabetes. Diabetes Care 1989;12:573–9.

174. Calhoun DA, Oparil S. Treatment of hypertensive crisis. N Engl J Med 1990;323:1177–83.

Chapter 45

HEART DISEASE IN DIABETES

RICHARD W. NESTO
STUART W. ZARICH
RICHARD M. JACOBY
MASOOR KAMALESH

Heart disease was thought to be associated with diabetes as early as 1883, when Vergely recommended testing the urine of patients with angina for glucose.[1] Over the years, the survival rate among patients with diabetes has increased substantially, largely in response to 1) the discovery of insulin, which reduced the mortality related to ketoacidosis; 2) the development of antibiotics for effective treatment of infections; and 3) the availability of various methods of managing renal failure. These developments have resulted in a relative increase in morbidity and mortality from cardiovascular disease, as indicated by the Joslin Clinic[2] and Framingham studies.[3,4] The mortality due to diabetes decreased from the late 1960s through the 1970s, when it reached a plateau, although age-adjusted death rates for persons with diabetes increased by 3% between 1987 and 1988. As of 1988, however, diabetes ranked as the seventh leading cause of death in the United States. Since these statistics are based on underlying cause of death, they underestimate the overall impact of diabetes on mortality.[5]

This chapter reviews the major areas of cardiovascular involvement in diabetes. The principal clinical expressions of diabetes-related cardiac disease are 1) atherosclerotic coronary artery disease; 2) cardiomyopathy, including preclinical systolic and diastolic left ventricular dysfunction; and 3) autonomic nervous system dysfunction.

CORONARY ARTERY DISEASE

Asymptomatic Hyperglycemia

Although relatively uncommon in comparison to other major cardiovascular risk factors, diabetes has a tremendous impact on mortality due to coronary artery disease. For a prevalence of diabetes of only 2.8%, the nonadditive population-attributable risk (i.e., percentage of mortality attributable to diabetes) is 5.1% as compared with hypertension, for which the overall prevalence is 29.7% and the population-attributable risk is 32.9%.[6] In other words, mortality due to coronary artery disease in diabetes is expressly linked to the prevalence of diabetes in the population, whereas hypertension, although more prevalent in the general population, has less of an impact on mortality due to coronary artery disease. Thus, any small change in the prevalence of diabetes will have a profound effect on mortality from coronary artery disease.

The relation of asymptomatic hyperglycemia to cardiovascular risk has been addressed by the Paris Prospective Study,[7] the Tecumseh Study,[8] and the Chicago Heart Association Detection Project.[9] These studies strongly suggest that asymptomatic hyperglycemia is an independent risk factor for coronary artery disease. In the Tecumseh Study, 921 men and 937 women aged 40 years and older who were without coronary artery disease at entry were followed for a minimum of 12 years. Although diabetes was a statistically significant independent risk factor for mortality due to coronary artery disease for both sexes (17.8 deaths per 1000 persons with diabetes as opposed to 5.9 per 1000 persons without diabetes), an elevated blood glucose (1 hour after a 100-g oral glucose challenge) in those individuals without a diagnosis of diabetes also was associated with excess mortality due to coronary artery disease. It is of interest that this study showed no excess mortality in women over that in men. It was concluded that hyperglycemia following glucose challenge may identify individuals who have other cardiac risk factors, such as obesity, high blood pressure, hyperlipidemia, and hyperinsulinemia. Similar findings were noted in the Chicago Heart Association Detection Project, which compiled 9-year follow-up data for 11,230 white men and 8030 white women aged 35 through 64 years at entry.[9] Both diabetes and asymptomatic hyperglycemia were associated with increased mortality from coronary artery disease. The extent of association was greater in women than in men with regard to relative risk, while absolute excess risk for both diabetes and asymptomatic hyperglycemia was greater for men. More recently, Wilson et al. reported on the relation of nonfasting blood glucose levels to the incidence of coronary artery disease in the Framingham Heart Study.[10] Age-adjusted incidence of coronary artery disease was associated with blood glucose levels in nondiabetic women who did not develop diabetes during follow-up. No such association was seen in men. Multivariate analysis confirmed the independent association of blood glucose levels with subsequent coronary artery disease in nondiabetic women. This study suggests that hyperglycemia in the original Framingham cohort is an independent risk factor for coronary artery disease in women but not in men.

Glycemic Control

Whether or not treatment for hyperglycemia affects cardiovascular morbidity and mortality has been a subject of debate. The Framingham Study[11] has shown that a reduction in risk of coronary artery disease in the patient with diabetes depends more on the control of obesity, correction of hypertension, cessation of cigarette smoking, and improvement in the ratio between low-density lipopolysaccharide (LDL) and high-density lipopolysaccharide (HDL) than on the control of hyperglycemia. Waller et al. studied the extent of atherosclerosis in the coronary arteries of 229 patients with diabetes and found that the type of treatment received by patients (diet, insulin, or oral agents) or their adherence to the therapeutic regimen did not correlate with number of severe narrowings of the coronary arteries.[12] The results of three prospective studies[7-9] suggest a nonlinear relationship between atherosclerosis with a threshold phenomenon (relationship between coronary atherosclerosis and response to oral glucose load is not linear) in the upper range of the distribution of blood glucose values after an oral glucose load. Multivariate analysis showed that the association of blood glucose levels to cardiovascular disease was not independent of the other major risk variables. Hence, it is not clear whether stringent control of blood glucose levels directly reduces the risk of the development of cardiac disease in persons with diabetes.

Lipid and Lipoprotein Abnormalities

Lipid abnormalities represent an important cardiovascular risk factor.[11] A recent review examined this subject as it relates to diabetes.[13] In Type II diabetes, increased levels of very-low-density lipopolysaccharide (VLDL) and decreased levels of LDL are typical (see Chapter 38). Obesity, which is frequent in persons with Type II diabetes, contributes to these lipoprotein abnormalities. Obesity is less frequent in persons with diabetes, whose lipoprotein metabolism is influenced by their insulin deficiency. In these patients, elevations in VLDL levels correlate well with the degree of diabetic control, and extreme elevations in VLDL levels sometimes are seen in diabetic ketoacidosis.

The Framingham Study highlights the profound effects lipoprotein abnormalities have on the incidence of coronary artery disease[11] in diabetic as compared with nondiabetic subjects. Female but not male diabetic subjects had higher serum cholesterol levels than nondiabetic subjects. Even among men who developed atherosclerotic cardiovascular disease, the total cholesterol levels were lower than those in nondiabetic men. Levels of HDL were consistently lower in diabetic patients of either sex than in subjects without diabetes. In the general population, and presumably also in the diabetic population, the risk of coronary artery disease at any total serum cholesterol level is greatly influenced by the ratio of LDL- to HDL-cholesterol. Thus, for any LDL value, risk is inversely related to the amount of HDL-cholesterol. Multivariate analysis suggests that the protective influence of HDL is twice that of the atherogenic influence of LDL-cholesterol in the general population.

Hyperinsulinemia

Hyperinsulinemia, which is particularly common in patients with non-insulin-dependent diabetes mellitus (NIDDM) with insulin resistance, appears to be a risk factor for atherogenesis. Hyperinsulinemia, even in the presence of normal glucose tolerance, is associated with other risk factors for coronary artery disease, including low HDL levels and hypertension.[14,15] Hyperinsulinemia also may play a role in promoting atherosclerosis by causing proliferation of smooth muscle cells and synthesis of cholesterol, as well as by increasing levels of growth hormone.[16] Hyperglycemia alone has been suggested as a risk factor for atherosclerosis but has not been proven to be an independent risk factor for the development of coronary artery disease.

Data from the Framingham Heart Study demonstrate the increased incidence and poor prognosis of cardiac disease in diabetes. Mortality related to cardiovascular disease is more than doubled in diabetic men and more than quadrupled in diabetic women over that in their nondiabetic counterparts.[17] The incidence of angina relative to that in men and women without diabetes is 60% higher in diabetic men and 90% higher in diabetic women. The relative risk of myocardial infarction is 50% higher in men with diabetes and 150% higher in women with diabetes than in their nondiabetic counterparts. Similarly, sudden death is 50% more frequent in diabetic men and 300% more frequent in diabetic women than in age-matched nondiabetic controls.[18] The Joslin Study demonstrated that the cumulative mortality due to coronary artery disease for persons with insulin-dependent diabetes (IDDM) is 35% by age 55 years, far higher than the corresponding rate (4 to 8%) for persons without diabetes.[19]

Diabetes is an independent risk factor for the development of coronary artery disease.[20] Various diagnostic methods indicate that the overall prevalence of coronary artery disease is as high as 55% for adults with diabetes, as compared with a prevalence of 2 to 4% for the general population. Not only is coronary atherosclerosis more prevalent in diabetic than nondiabetic persons, it is clearly more extensive.[21] Coronary angiography or autopsy reveals a higher incidence of double- and triple-vessel disease and a relatively lower incidence of single-vessel disease in diabetic than in nondiabetic patients.[20,22] The incidence of severe disease of the left main coronary artery is also significantly higher in diabetic than nondiabetic patients (13% vs. 6%).[12] In one large autopsy study, 91% of persons with adult-onset diabetes without clinical evidence of coronary artery disease had severe narrowing of at least one major coronary artery and 83% had severe involvement of two or three vessels.[12] Whether coronary atherosclerosis is actually more "diffuse" or is merely expressed as a greater number of discrete stenoses has been the subject of some debate.[23] In the above-mentioned autopsy study, among persons who died of coronary artery disease, those with diabetes had more numerous stenoses than did those without diabetes, but the appearance of other arterial segments was similar in the two groups. Another autopsy study, however, found that persons with juvenile-onset diabetes may have a more "diffuse" form of coronary artery disease, with at least one-half of the overall length of their epicardial coronary arteries narrowed by at least 50%, as compared with nondiabetics, in whom less than 1% of the length was similarly involved.[24]

Diabetic patients with symptomatic peripheral vascular disease are likely to harbor significant coronary artery disease that may not be clinically apparent. One study, using dipyridamole thallium scanning, demonstrated a 47% incidence of asymptomatic myocardial ischemia and a 37% incidence of prior "silent" infarction in a group of diabetic patients with symptomatic peripheral vascular disease but without clinical evidence of coronary artery disease.[25] The Framingham Study also showed a significant relation between cardiovascular events and intermittent claudication in persons with diabetes. Both the risk of congestive heart failure and that of coronary artery disease were significantly increased when both intermittent claudication and diabetes were present over the risk with either alone.[11]

Clinical Presentation

As a result of a blunted appreciation for pain among diabetics, myocardial ischemia or infarction may be associated with only mild symptoms and go unrecognized or may be entirely asymptomatic and thus truly silent. Although 25% of the myocardial infarctions in the Framingham Study were "silent," symptoms referable to the unrecognized infarction could be elicited in nearly one-half of these cases.[26] The remaining infarctions (or approximately 12% of the total) were considered truly asymptomatic. Unrecognized infarction tends to be more common in persons with diabetes[27] and accounts for 39% of their infarctions as compared with 22% of those in persons without diabetes.[28] While there has generally been a trend toward a higher prevalence of silent infarction in persons with diabetes, the limited statistical power of most studies has hindered efforts to prove this conclusively. These data parallel the observation that the presence of a myocardial scar in the absence of an antemortem history of infarction is found at autopsy three times more frequently in persons with diabetes than in those without diabetes.[29]

As might be inferred from the above, persons with diabetes may also lack angina during ischemia. The incidence of painless ST depression during exercise tolerance tests in nondiabetic patients is more than double that seen in nondiabetic patients (75% vs. 35%).[30] Nesto et al. demonstrated that angina is less common in diabetic than nondiabetic patients during ischemia assessed by exercise thallium scintigraphy.[31] Patients with diabetes who do experience angina become aware of their symptoms later in the course of ischemia than do patients without diabetes.[32] The delay in time from the onset of ST depression to angina may be twice as long in patients with diabetes than in patients without diabetes and correlates with the extent of autonomic nervous dysfunction. Neuropathy of efferent autonomic pathways also may indicate damage to afferent autonomic fibers responsible for the transmission of sensory impulses relating to perception of myocardial ischemia. Both the presence of histologic damage to cardiac afferent nerve fibers in persons with diabetes[33] and physiologic evidence of damage to afferent and efferent nerves[34-36] suggest that neuropathy involving these fibers exists and may play a role in blunting ischemic pain.

When persons with diabetes seek medical attention because of acute myocardial infarction, they frequently do so because of atypical symptoms. Accurate diagnosis of infarction based on historical grounds may therefore be difficult. Atypical symptoms such as confusion, dyspnea, fatigue, or nausea and vomiting may be the presenting complaint in 32 to 42% of diabetic patients with myocardial infarction, as compared with 6 to 15% of nondiabetic patients.[37] In some cases such symptoms may mimic those associated with either hypo- or hyperglycemia and result in a delay in triage for the patient.[38]

The atypical presenting symptoms seen in the diabetic patient may lower the clinician's suspicion of infarction, leading to less than optimal care. Soler et al. found that 35% of diabetic patients with acute myocardial infarction were admitted initially to the general wards rather than to the coronary care unit.[39] More than 75% of those diabetic patients assigned to ward care lacked typical chest pain, whereas nearly all of those admitted to the coronary care unit exhibited severe chest pain.[39] A comparison of the electrocardiogram at presentation with a tracing done previously may be extremely helpful in establishing a diagnosis when suspicion of acute infarction exists in the absence of typical symptoms.

Atypical symptoms may alter the patient's perception of the nature of his or her illness and interfere with the decision to seek medical care. Uretsky et al. examined a group of patients, both with and without diabetes, in whom acute myocardial infarction was associated with atypical symptoms.[40] These patients were older than patients with more classical symptoms and generally lacked a previous history of angina. They did not seek medical care until a mean of 12 hours following the onset of symptoms, and at least one-third waited more than 24 hours. Thirty-five percent of patients with atypical presenting symptoms showed cardiogenic shock, and 50% died in the hospital. It seems plausible that a delay in receiving appropriate care could contribute to the observed increase in morbidity and mortality in diabetic patients with myocardial infarction.

Autonomic Neuropathy

The development of symptomatic autonomic neuropathy in patients with diabetes is an ominous sign, with mortality over 50% 3 years after its onset.[41] Sudden death, presumably cardiac-related, is responsible for up to one-third of these deaths. Generally, parasympathetic nerve fibers are affected first, leading to a relative increase in sympathetic tone that results in resting tachycardia and attenuation of the expected increase in heart rate and blood pressure with exercise.[42,43] An absence of parasympathetic tone may also be responsible for exaggerated or inappropriate coronary vasoconstriction, which may produce or worsen ischemia.[44] Sympathetic nervous system dysfunction is usually evident within 5 years of the diagnosis of parasympathetic dysfunction. Postural hypotension is the principal clinical manifestation of sympathetic dysfunction. Thus, autonomic neuropathy may lead to ischemia or infarction by several routes: by increasing myocardial demand for oxygen by increasing resting heart rate; by reducing myocardial blood flow by increasing coronary vascular tone at the site of a coronary stenosis; and by reducing coronary perfusion pressure during orthostatic hypotension.[45]

The importance of intact autonomic function during cardiovascular stress (as during a myocardial infarction) is exemplified in diabetic patients undergoing general anesthesia. The increased morbidity seen in diabetic patients during general anesthesia may be due to an inability to counteract the hemodynamic effects of the induction of anesthesia because of impaired cardiovascular reflexes. Burgos et al.[46] has shown that 35% of diabetic patients required vasopressors intraoperatively compared with only 5% of nondiabetic patients ($P < .05$). Furthermore, the diabetic patients who required vasopressor support had significantly greater autonomic impairment than did those who did not require it.

Autonomic neuropathy may be responsible for sudden death in persons with diabetes.[35,47] Although some of these deaths may be due to arrhythmia secondary to a silent myocardial infarction, autopsy studies have demonstrated a surprising absence of significant coronary artery disease in some diabetic patients who died unexpectedly.[47,48] A relation exists between diabetic cardiac autonomic neuropathy and a prolonged QT interval on the electrocardiogram,[48-51] which may predispose to life-threatening ventricular arrhythmia. It has been proposed that the combination of relatively heightened sympathetic tone and the prolongation of QT interval might increase the likelihood of arrhythmias leading to sudden death.[52,53] Although a search for other causes of prolongation of QT interval in these patients is not well documented, it is quite possible that other factors such as acute ischemia, electrolyte disturbances (hypokalemia), metabolic abnormalities (hypomagnesemia, hypocalcemia, hypophosphatemia), and drug toxicity (digoxin) could have contributed to the sudden death in these patients by altering the threshold for life-threatening arrhythmia.

Course of Acute Infarction

Overall in-hospital mortality for diabetic patients is much higher than for nondiabetic patients experiencing myocardial infarction and may be as high as 28%.[54] Mortality is 18% with a first infarction but increases substantially to 41% in those patients with prior infarction. Approximately 5% of patients presenting with acute myocardial infarction have previously undiagnosed diabetes mellitus. These patients have the same poor prognosis as the previously diagnosed diabetic patient with acute infarction.[55]

Diabetic women have a particularly poor prognosis, with an overall in-hospital mortality of 37% as compared with 19% for diabetic men.[54] In one study, the increased mortality in women was thought to be attributable to their high incidence of severe congestive heart failure and cardiogenic shock.[56] Why this particular patient group experiences an increased frequency of congestive heart failure and shock is not known. In this regard, obese diabetic women may be at particular risk, with an in-hospital mortality of 43% in one study.[57]

In contrast to younger persons without diabetes, who generally seem to tolerate infarction better than do the elderly, younger persons with diabetes constitute a particularly high-risk group. Czyzk et al. found that diabetic patients between the ages of 45 and 64 years experience 3.2 times the mortality of nondiabetic patients of similar age with acute myocardial infarction,[58] and Singer et al. found that, overall, younger diabetic patients experience a poorer outcome than do their nondiabetic counterparts.[59]

Diabetic patients who sustain a myocardial infarction are more likely than nondiabetic patients to encounter complications. Recurrent infarction, cardiogenic shock, atrioventricular and intraventricular conduction abnormalities, chronic congestive heart failure, and myocardial rupture are all more common in the diabetic patient.[60-63] In addition, some studies have found anterior infarction to be more common,[60,62,64,65] and this may offer a partial explanation for the generally poorer prognosis.

Clinically significant (class III or IV) congestive heart failure develops in 44% of diabetic women and in 25% of diabetic men with acute myocardial infarction and is thought to be the cause of death in 22% of diabetic women and 6% of diabetic men.[54] The increased incidence of congestive heart failure in diabetic patients, and in diabetic women in particular, is seen despite the similar magnitude of the infarcts in diabetic and nondiabetic patients.[56] This increase in congestive heart failure occurs despite the similarity of left ventricular ejection fractions in diabetic and nondiabetic patients.[61] Several factors may be responsible for these observations. Diabetic patients are likely to have antecedent hypertension, which may impair systolic and/or diastolic function. In addition, congestive heart failure out of proportion to the size of a myocardial infarction could be the result of subclinical diabetic cardiomyopathy.[66] Reflex adaptation to hemodynamic stress secondary to infarction may be impaired by autonomic effector dysfunction. The greater extent of coronary artery disease in the diabetic patient might also limit the availability of collateral blood flow to the infarct zone. Finally, metabolic responses to ischemia particular to the diabetic could affect contractile performance.

Under conditions of myocardial ischemia, glycemic control becomes particularly important. During ischemia, the heart shifts from aerobic metabolism, with fatty acids as the primary fuel source, to anaerobic metabolism, which depends on glucose. Glucose transport into cells is therefore crucial. Insulin favors glucose uptake, whereas ketones and high levels of free fatty acids, found during insulinopenia, inhibit its transport. An excess of catecholamines, often present with infarction, may further worsen myocardial metabolism in the diabetic patient by decreasing the insulin secretory reserve and favoring lipolysis and myocardial uptake of free fatty acids. Moreover, there is some evidence that free fatty acids may be toxic to myocardial cells.[66] Several studies have shown that elevated levels of plasma glucose during myocardial infarction may be associated with a poor outcome.[39,60,61] These data must be interpreted with caution since hyperglycemia or diabetic ketoacidosis may be the result of increased sympathetic tone caused by more extensive infarction. Diabetic ketoacidosis occurs in approximately 4% of diabetic patients with infarcts[54] and may be the presenting symptom. When diabetic ketoacidosis complicates infarction, mortality is higher and may approach 85%.[62]

The increased in-hospital mortality in the diabetic patient with infarction tends to occur during days 2 through 7 of hospitalization. During this period the mortality is more than three times that for the nondiabetic patient and most prominent in patients with IDDM.[58] Much of the excess mortality during this interval is due to congestive heart failure, although arrhythmias and conduction abnormalities are significant contributors as well. Some, but not all, studies[67] have documented an increase in atrioventricular[61] and intraventricular[62] conduction abnormalities in diabetic patients. In one study, diabetic patients with second- and third-degree atrioventricular block and left bundle branch block experienced a 47% in-hospital mortality—three times that experienced by nondiabetic patients with similar blocks.[58] Four prognostic variables in the immediate period following acute myocardial infarction in diabetic patients were found to be independent predictors of poor prognosis. In order of descending importance they were 1) Q-wave acute myocardial infarction; 2) prior acute myocardial infarction; 3) female gender; and 4) insulin treatment prior to hospitalization.[54]

Course following Nonfatal Myocardial Infarction

Mortality within 6 months after discharge from the hospital following nonfatal myocardial infarction in diabetic patients is especially high, approximating 60% among those with a previous myocardial infarction. Mortality at 5 years following the first myocardial infarction reaches 79%.[61,68,69] While early postinfarction mortality usually is due to congestive heart failure, cardiogenic shock, or conduction disturbances, late mortality tends to be due to recurrent myocardial infarction. One explanation for the enhanced morbidity and mortality may be persistent ischemia or ongoing myocardial damage following myocardial infarction. Technetium pyrophosphate scintigraphy has been performed in diabetic and nondiabetic patients in the acute phase of myocardial infarction and then 3 month later.[70] Sixty-two percent of diabetic patients were found to have persistently positive technetium pyrophosphate scans at 3 months as compared with 12% of nondiabetic patients. Complications following hospital discharge were more frequent in both diabetic and nondiabetic patients with chronic abnormalities in technetium pyrophosphate uptake and included congestive heart failure and recurrent myocardial infarction. Diabetic patients with persistently abnormal technetium scintigrams exhibited marked myocardial myocytolysis at autopsy, signifying ongoing myocardial necrosis.[70]

In patients with diabetes, as in those without diabetes, certain characteristics identify patients at high risk for future cardiac events. Prognostic indicators associated with a poor outcome following hospital discharge in patients who survive the phase of hospitalization in the coronary care unit include 1) the presence of cardiac symptoms at least 1 month preceding the infarction, 2) pulmonary rales during the initial phase of hospitalization, 3) greater than 10 ventricular premature beats per hour before hospital discharge, and 4) at least a moderately reduced left ventricular ejection fraction (<40%) by radionuclide ventriculography.[68]

Special Management Considerations

Thrombolysis Therapy

Thrombolytic therapy for myocardial infarction has been shown to reduce infarct size and improve survival in patients presenting soon after the onset of Q-wave infarction. Atypical symptoms commonly associated with myocardial ischemia or infarction in patients with diabetes not only may cause a delay in their seeking medical care but may make it difficult to determine the time of onset of infarction. These factors peculiar to the diabetic patient may interfere with the decision to initiate thrombolytic therapy. Denying treatment with a thrombolytic agent on this basis is unfortunate, as the decrease in mortality associated with thrombolytic therapy in these patients is similar to that seen in nondiabetic patients.[71] Since a high incidence of hemorrhagic complications associated with increased mortality in elderly diabetic patients has been reported, in this group thrombolytic therapy should probably be limited to patients with life-threatening myocardial infarction.[72] One might presume that the presence of proliferative retinopathy would represent a relative contraindication to the use of thrombolytic agents in many diabetic patients. However, no retinal hemorrhages were seen in the 121 diabetic patients treated with thrombolytic agents in the TAMI (thrombolysis in acute myocardial infarction) trial.[71]

Invasive Management

Myocardial revascularization should be strongly considered for diabetic patients with acute myocardial infarction who manifest signs of ongoing ischemia despite medical therapy. Coronary-artery bypass is as effective in relieving anginal symptoms in diabetic patients as in nondiabetic patients, although the long-term survival rate following bypass remains consistently lower in diabetic than nondiabetic patients.[73,74] Even though diabetic patients may need a larger number of bypass grafts because of their more extensive atherosclerosis, their late graft patency is similar to that for nondiabetic patients.[74] Perioperative mortality appears to be higher in the diabetic patient than in the nondiabetic patient (7.1% vs. 4.5%), and morbidity due to poor sternotomy healing and renal failure, resulting in prolonged hospitalization, is more common in diabetic patients.[74]

Percutaneous transluminal coronary angioplasty is an effective tool for relieving ischemic symptoms in diabetic patients whose coronary anatomy is suitable, although the most important independent predictor of restenosis following angioplasty is diabetes.[75] Diabetes is also an independent variable predicting restenosis after a second coronary angioplasty at a given site.[76] Despite its possible shortcomings, coronary artery angioplasty is an attractive treatment option because of its low associated morbidity and brief convalescence period and the avoidance of the potential problems associated with bypass surgery. Unfortunately, no prospective controlled trials comparing coronary angioplasty with coronary artery bypass surgery in diabetic patients have been performed.

Secondary Prevention

β-Adrenergic Blockade

β-Adrenergic blockers have been shown to reduce mortality following myocardial infarction. In the Timolol in Myocardial Infarction Study, administration of timolol (a cardioselective β-adrenergic blocker) was associated with a substantial reduction in overall mortality, including total cardiac-related death, sudden death, and nonfatal reinfarction.[77] In the placebo group in this study, the mortality rate in the diabetic patients was twice that in the nondiabetic patients. In the treatment group, the mortality rates in the diabetic and nondiabetic patients were similar, suggesting that timolol was at least as effective at reducing mortality following infarction in diabetic patients as in nondiabetic patients. With the use of timolol, cardiac-related death was reduced by 67% in diabetic patients and by 40% in nondiabetic patients and nonfatal reinfarction was reduced by 83% in diabetic patients vs. 34% in nondiabetic patients. Of importance, timolol was tolerated equally well by the two patient groups. Another study, which examined the use of β-adrenergic blockers in 281 diabetic patients following acute myocardial infarction, found a decrease in 1-year mortality from 17% to 10% following hospital discharge.[78] The use of a β-adrenergic blocker was found to be an independent predictor of 1-year survival after a coronary event in diabetic patients whether or not pulmonary congestion was present on a chest roentgenogram.

The potential benefits of β-adrenergic blockers are counterbalanced by adverse effects particular to the diabetic patient. These agents may attenuate reflex tachycardia, mask "warning" symptoms of hypoglycemia, and potentiate insulin-induced hypoglycemia by inhibiting glycogenolysis. For these reasons, many clinicians have been reluctant to use β-adrenergic blockers in patients with diabetes. On the contrary, β-adrenergic blockers are usually well tolerated and may be of particular benefit. Many of the above-mentioned complications seen with the use of β-adrenergic blockers are encountered with doses higher than those that provide secondary protection against cardiac-related death.

Aspirin

Aspirin has a significant, proven value in reducing short-term mortality following myocardial infarction by 23% and in reducing reinfarction by about 50%.[79] Overall, aspirin has been shown to reduce cardiovascular mortality by 13% and nonfatal reinfarction by about 30%.[79] Diabetic patients have heightened platelet reactivity,[80–83] which may play a role not only in the acceleration of progression of atherosclerosis but also in the development of an occlusive thrombus at the site of coronary plaque rupture. Theoretically, aspirin should be particularly beneficial in diabetic patients because of this increased platelet reactivity.

There has been some concern, however, that aspirin may potentiate the development of retinal hemorrhage in diabetic patients (see Chapter 42). The safety of long-term aspirin use in diabetic patients with early retinopathy was demonstrated in the DAMAD study, in which 267 diabetic patients with early retinopathy received aspirin (325 mg tid) and none experienced a worsening of retinal hemorrhage.[84] These data may not be applicable to diabetic patients with more severe retinopathy, for whom the safety of aspirin has not been determined.

Risk-Factor Modification

Attention must also be focused on the modification of risk factors to reduce progressive atherosclerosis and the risk of reinfarction. Hypertension should be controlled, preferably with agents tailored to improve any systolic or diastolic left ventricular dysfunction. Hyperlipidemia and obesity should be managed aggressively. These efforts may be most justified in diabetic women, who experience a particularly high late cardiac-related mortality after surviving myocardial infarction.[57,62]

Cigarette smoking is an important factor promoting coronary atherosclerosis. Despite their increased risk of coronary artery disease, diabetic patients are as likely as the general public to be smokers.[85] Cigarette smoking is an independent predictor of mortality in patients with IDDM and is particularly dangerous in women with IDDM, more than doubling their risk of cardiac-related mortality.[85]

Factors Favoring Myocardial Infarction in Patients with Diabetes

Acute infarction most often involves interruption of myocardial blood flow because of an underlying atherosclerotic plaque with further luminal compromise by thrombus.[86] Progression of atherosclerosis may occur via repeated plaque rupture and thrombosis in a repetitive cycle of injury and healing that results in luminal narrowing.[87] Diabetes is associated with an increased propensity for both atherosclerotic plaque formation and intraluminal thrombosis, developments leading to an increased likelihood of infarction.

Accelerated Atherosclerosis and Plaque Rupture

Several factors may relate to atherosclerosis development and favor plaque rupture leading to infarction. These may include dyslipidemias, hypertension, hyperinsulinemia, and abnormal blood viscosity. Elevated serum lipid levels induce vascular damage and promote atherosclerosis. Pathologic studies of coronary vessels of patients after infarction indicate that lipid-rich plaques may be more likely than fibrous plaques to rupture.[87] Diabetic and hypertensive patients appear to have a greater number of such fissured plaques than do nondiabetic patients.[88] Despite a preponderance of lipid abnormalities in diabetic patients, the independent contribution of total cholesterol to coronary artery disease is approximately the same in diabetic and nondiabetic patients.[89] The average total cholesterol level in the Framingham Study was 245 mg/dL and was similar in diabetic and nondiabetic subjects.[11] Persons with diabetes have higher levels of VLDL and triglycerides and lower levels of HDL than persons without diabetes, whereas levels of total and LDL-cholesterol are not substantially different in the two groups.[90] The significance of the altered lipid profile in persons with diabetes as it relates to risk of coronary artery disease has not yet been defined.

Hypertension has been associated with an increased tendency toward plaque fissuring, a major precursor to myocardial infarction,[88] and hypertension is more common in persons with diabetes,[11] being found in over 50% of diabetic persons over 45 years old.[89] The prevalence of hypertension is especially high in diabetic women and is a frequent accompaniment to diabetic nephropathy. Cardiovascular mortality in diabetic nephropathy is up to 37 times that in the general population; this increase probably is due, at least in part, to the associated hypertension.[91-93]

Hyperinsulinemia, particularly common in patients with NIDDM with insulin resistance, appears to be a risk factor for atherogenesis. Hyperinsulinemia even in the presence of normal glucose tolerance is associated with an increase in risk factors for coronary artery disease, including low HDL levels and hypertension.[94] Hyperinsulinemia also may play a role in promoting atherosclerosis by causing the proliferation of smooth muscle cells and synthesis of cholesterol as well as by increasing levels of growth factors.[95] Hyperglycemia alone has been suggested as a risk factor for atherosclerosis, although the level of hyperglycemia itself has not been shown to be an independent risk factor for the development of coronary artery disease.

Persons with diabetes are known to exhibit elevated viscosity of plasma and whole blood because of the high levels of plasma proteins, increased red cell aggregation, and decreased red cell deformability.[96,97] These effects are particularly evident during periods of metabolic derangement such as diabetic ketoacidosis and appear to improve with better glycemic control. It seems likely that increased shear forces caused by high viscosity could accentuate the tendency toward plaque rupture. In addition, these rheologic effects could contribute to infarct extension by impeding coronary blood flow, particularly in areas where blood flow is low.

Hematologic Abnormalities

Occlusive thrombus formation is likely a dynamic process that depends on a balance between those factors that favor clotting and those that oppose it. In diabetes, abnormalities relating to platelet function, coagulation, fibrinolysis, and endothelial function favor intraluminal thrombosis.

Platelet aggregation is an essential step in occlusive thrombus formation. Spontaneous platelet aggregation has recently been shown to predict recurrent infarction following myocardial infarction.[98] Spontaneous and induced platelet aggregation have been shown to be higher in persons with diabetes[80-83] than in those without diabetes and correlates with an increase in cardiovascular events.[80] Platelets in diabetic patients synthesize thromboxane A$_2$ in abnormally high amounts,[99-102] a behavior favoring platelet aggregation and vascular spasm. Elevated thromboxane levels are most often found in diabetic patients with poor glycemic control or with vascular complications.[82] Platelet consumption is higher in diabetic than nondiabetic subjects,[82] and two platelet-specific proteins, β-thromboglobulin and platelet factor 4, which are thought to reflect platelet activation in vivo, may be elevated in persons with diabetes.[82,97] Levels of plasma fibrinogen are known to be elevated in persons with diabetes[82,103] and have been shown to correlate with myocardial infarction and sudden death in diabetic men.[80] Levels of factor VIII and factor VIII ristocetin cofactor antigen are elevated in diabetic patients as well.[97] Fibrinopeptide A reflects thrombin activity in vivo, and levels may also be elevated in persons with diabetes.[97,104] Endothelial dysfunction or damage in persons with diabetes results in deficient production of prostacyclin[105,106] and elevated levels of the procoagulant von Willebrand factor.[97] Endogenous fibrinolysis has also been found to be deficient in diabetic patients.[103,104]

Circadian Differences

In the population at large, there is a significant morning peak in time of onset of Q-wave infarction[107] that parallels the circadian variation of platelet aggregability. In the diabetic patient, however, this morning increase is somewhat blunted and Q-wave infarction occurs more evenly throughout the day.[108] It is intriguing to speculate that the absence of a prominent morning increase in infarction may be explained by the consistently heightened platelet reactivity seen in diabetic patients throughout the day.[109] Non-transmural infarcts in diabetic patients exhibits two relative peaks, the first occurring from noon to 6 p.m. and the second, from 8 p.m. to midnight.[110] The reason for this distribution remains unclear. Similarly, silent ischemia in diabetic patients shows a morning increase that persists throughout waking hours and parallels the circadian variation in heart rate.[110]

Diabetic patients with autonomic neuropathy have been found to have a relative decrease in vagal tone (thus a relative increase in sympathetic tone) at the same time during the day that the frequency of sudden death has been reported to be particularly high.[53] It has been suggested that this relative increase in sympathetic tone may be responsible, at least in part, for sudden death in persons with diabetes.

DIABETIC CARDIOMYOPATHY

Clinical, epidemiologic, and pathologic data support the presence of a specific cardiomyopathy related to diabetes mellitus.[111,112] Despite the use of the term "diabetic" cardiomyopathy, considerable debate exists about the exact nature and cause of cardiac dysfunction attributable to diabetes mellitus. Diabetes mellitus is commonly associated with conditions such as coronary atherosclerosis and hypertension, which may impair myocardial performance.[3] Separating these potential causes from those directly related to the metabolic derangements of diabetes is difficult and is responsible for the confusion and skepticism regarding the existence of a true diabetic cardiomyopathy.

Clinical and Epidemiologic Studies

The existence of a diabetic cardiomyopathy was first suggested by Rubler et al.[113] in 1972 on the basis of postmortem findings in four diabetic adults who had congestive heart failure in the absence of atherosclerotic, valvular, congenital, hypertensive, or alcoholic heart disease. All patients demonstrated electrocardiographic evidence of left ventricular hypertrophy, and at autopsy Kimmelstiel-Wilson disease was found in association with myocardial enlargement, hypertrophy, and fibrosis. The causal role of diabetes mellitus in the development of congestive heart failure was delineated more conclusively in the Framingham Heart Study.[4] In this prospective study of 5000 individuals over an 18-year follow-up period, the frequency of congestive heart failure was more than twice as high in diabetic men than in the nondiabetic cohort, while it was increased fivefold in diabetic women. This excessive risk persisted after accounting for age, hypertension, obesity, hypercholesterolemia, and coronary artery disease, factors that commonly coexist with long-standing diabetes. Diabetic women were especially vulnerable, having congestive heart failure at twice the frequency experienced by men irrespective of coronary artery disease status. This excessive risk of heart failure was confined to those with hyperglycemia severe enough to warrant insulin therapy, whereas patients treated with diet or oral hypoglycemic agents had no increased risk of congestive failure. The role of severity or duration of diabetes in the development of congestive heart failure was not addressed in this study.

Further support for the existence of a diabetic cardiomyopathy was provided by Hamby et al.,[114] who noted an increased incidence of diabetes in patients with idiopathic cardiomyopathy. Sixteen (22%) of 73 patients with idiopathic cardiomyopathy were diabetic, compared with only 11% in an age- and sex-matched cohort without cardiomyopathy. The duration of diabetes in affected subjects was quite variable, ranging from less than 1 year to 11 years. In contrast to the Framingham Study, in this study one of 16 diabetic patients with cardiomyopathy was insulin-dependent. Autopsy findings of four diabetic subjects revealed patent epicardial coronary arteries, but pathologic changes compatible with diabetic vasculopathy were noted in the smaller intramyocardial vessels.

Regan et al.[115] described the angiographic and hemodynamic findings in patients with adult-onset diabetes without hypertensive or valvular disease. Four of 17 patients experienced episodes of congestive heart failure despite the absence of coronary artery disease on angiography. Lactate production by the coronary sinus did not occur with atrial pacing, suggesting that coronary flow reserve was not diminished. Since no myocardial ischemia could be demonstrated, abnormalities of the small arteries or capillaries were thought to be responsible for a restriction in myocardial perfusion. Hemodynamic findings included a modest elevation of left ventricular end-diastolic pressure and a reduction of both stroke volume and ejection fraction. Ventricular compliance also was found to be significantly diminished. Of interest, a similar impairment of left ventricular compliance was discovered in eight diabetic subjects without evidence of congestive failure, D'Elia et al.[116] found similar evidence for diastolic or systolic dysfunction in 59% of a diabetic cohort with renal failure in the absence of significant coronary artery disease.

Preclinical Cardiomyopathy

Preclinical cardiac abnormalities have been recognized in diabetic patients with the use of a variety of techniques. In 1966, Karlefors[117] noted that asymptomatic diabetic men had a lower cardiac output during supine exercise than did nondiabetic controls. These findings appeared to be independent of the duration of diabetes. In a subsequent study,[118] Carleström and Karlefors noted that patients with newly diagnosed juvenile-onset diabetes had lower stroke volumes during exercise. Cardiac output, however, was maintained as a result of higher heart rates. Of interest is the reversal of these hemodynamic derangements after insulin therapy.

Noninvasive evaluation of cardiac performance through the measurement of systolic time intervals and the use of phonocardiography, M-mode and two-dimensional echocardiography, and Doppler echocardiography also has documented subclinical left ventricular dysfunction in diabetic individuals. Systolic time intervals have long been used in assessing left ventricular performance. A prolonged pre-ejection period (PEP) and a shortened left ventricular ejection time (LVET) were noted in four studies in both patients with Type I and Type II diabetes without evidence of clinical heart disease.[119-122] Low-dose ethanol provoked similar abnormalities in young asymptomatic diabetic subjects but not in a control cohort.[123] These findings were associated with the presence of microvascular disease in one study[122] but were not related to duration of disease or treatment in several other studies.[119,121]

Echocardiography and phonocardiography also were employed in the aforementioned studies, with diminished fractional shortening and ejection fractions reported in 6 (15%) of 40 diabetic patients and prolonged isovolumic relaxation in diabetic individuals compared with that in controls. Sanderson et al.,[124] using digitized M-mode echocardiography, similarly evaluated the diastolic function in young asymptomatic diabetic individuals, most of whom had retinopathy. Only 25% of diabetic subjects had normal timing and patterns of mitral valve opening in relationship to changes in the dimensions of the left ventricular wall. There is extensive evidence from a series of investigations for increased PEP/LVET ratios, impaired isovolumic relaxation, and other diastolic and systolic left ventricular abnormalities in a large number of

diabetic patients.[125-128] In studies using digitized M-mode echocardiography, asymptomatic diabetic subjects were consistently found to have impaired left ventricular relaxation. These abnormalities correlated to a large degree with the duration of diabetes and the extent of microvascular complications. Left ventricular dysfunction occurred in both subjects with IDDM and those with NIDDM, but were more frequent in the former. Of interest is the finding that left ventricular hypertrophy was seen only in diabetic subjects with concomitant hypertension. Hypertensive diabetic patients had a greater incidence of clinical congestive failure (28% vs. 3% in normotensive diabetic patients), abnormal PEP/LVET ratios, and diminished fractional shortening. Patients with markedly elevated PEP/LVET ratios showed no improvement in systolic performance after 4 months of treatment for hyperglycemia. However, treatment of diabetes resulted in a fall in the PEP/LVET ratio in a group of 54 patients whose PEP/LVET ratios were only modestly increased prior to treatment.

In many of these earlier reports, however, left ventricular dysfunction may not have been due solely to diabetes mellitus. Left ventricular diastolic function can be affected by age, ischemia, hypertension, and by a variety of other factors.[129,130] In several of these earlier reports, many of these asymptomatic diabetic patients were older or may have had coexistent illnesses known to affect ventricular function. Subsequent studies have focused on younger patients and have excluded subjects at risk for cardiac dysfunction independent of that presented by diabetes mellitus.

Airaksinen et al.[131] used digitized M-mode echocardiography to study 36 young (mean age, 25 years) women with IDDM who were free of clinical cardiac disease or hypertension. Abnormal diastolic function identified by a prolongation of early diastolic rapid filling was noted in 19 of these women (53%). An interesting relationship was found between the duration of early filling and serum triglyceride concentration. Diabetic subjects with severe microvascular complications had thicker left ventricular walls and smaller end-diastolic diameters and stroke volumes than did healthy control subjects.

Significant abnormalities of systolic function were detected in a series of echocardiographic studies of 25 diabetic children and adolescents.[132,133] Ejection fraction and percent fractional shortening were diminished, while end-systolic volumes and dimensions were elevated. Lababidi and Goldstein[134] studied a larger group of 107 young asymptomatic patients with IDDM and found increased left ventricular systolic and diastolic dimensions and decreased interventricular septal excursion compared with these values in control subjects. These abnormalities were not related to the duration of diabetes or to glucose control as assessed by levels of hemoglobin A_{1C}.

The response of the left ventricle to exercise provides a means of detecting latent cardiac dysfunction, and this test has been used extensively in diabetic patients. Diminished stroke volume with exercise in diabetic individuals was first documented via invasive monitoring and indicator-dye dilution techniques[117,118] as previously mentioned. More recent studies[135-138] have used gated radionuclide ventriculography to assess left ventricular function at rest and with exercise. Nuclear studies are considered a more direct and reliable way to assess ejection fraction than is the measurement of systolic time intervals (especially as elevated PEP/LVET ratios also may reflect changes in loading conditions) and require fewer geometric assumptions than does echocardiography and also are well suited for serial studies.

Thirty young diabetic men (aged 21 to 35 years) without evidence of coronary artery disease or hypertension were studied by Vered et al.[135] with exercise radionuclide ventriculography. Ejection fraction was normal at rest in all subjects but either failed to increase appropriately or actually decreased with exercise in 43% of the diabetic subjects. Inducible ischemia was not responsible for this impaired contractile response, as no patient developed angina, electrocardiographic signs of ischemia, or regional abnormalities in wall motion. In four patients with abnormal ejection-fraction responses to exercise, thallium studies indicated normal myocardial perfusion.

In a similar study by Mildenberger et al.,[136] 35% of 20 young asymptomatic diabetic subjects, as compared with only 1 of 18 controls, had an abnormal ejection fraction response during exercise radionuclide ventriculography despite a normal ejection fraction at rest. In both of the aforementioned studies, the exercise ejection fraction response did not correlate with duration of diabetes or microvascular complications.

Diabetic patients with autonomic neuropathy form a subgroup at particular high risk for death, with many sudden deaths (presumably due to cardiovascular events).[41] Hilsted et al.[139] documented impaired stroke volumes during exercise in a select group of diabetic patients with autonomic neuropathy. In a recent study[137] of 30 patients with long-standing diabetes mellitus who were free of clinical, electrocardiographic, or thallium scan evidence of ischemic heart disease, 11 (37%) of 30 patients had abnormal left ventricular performance as assessed by resting and exercise radionuclide ventriculography, and the majority had autonomic dysfunction. The presence of systolic dysfunction did not correlate with the duration of diabetes or microvascular complications.

Abnormalities of left ventricular diastolic function have also been detected by radionuclide ventriculography in a similar group of young asymptomatic diabetic subjects free of clinical heart disease.[140] Twenty-one percent of 28 diabetic subjects had abnormal diastolic filling, as judged by abnormally low peak filling rates or prolonged time to peak filling, compared with healthy controls. Left ventricular diastolic filling was impaired in those individuals with autonomic neuropathy as compared with that in diabetic individuals free of autonomic neuropathy. The severity of the autonomic neuropathy (reflected by lower scores in tests of autonomic functioning and levels of plasma norepinephrine) was related to the degree of diastolic dysfunction. The presence of orthostatic hypotension had the strongest association with diastolic filling abnormalities.

A recent study[138] using exercise radionuclide ejection fraction response clearly confirms the above finding. In a group of 20 young diabetic subjects, 35% had an abnormal response to exercise as compared with only 1 of 20 control individuals. There were no ischemic changes on electrocardiographic monitoring, and the double product (product of blood pressure and heart rate) did not differ between the groups. No correlation was found between the exercise ejection fraction response and fasting blood sugar level, hemoglobin A_{1C} value, incidence of microvascular changes, duration of diabetes, or insulin usage.

Doppler echocardiography has been used with increasing frequency to assess left ventricular diastolic function.[141-143] Evaluation of early and late components of transmitral flow velocities has been shown to be a reliable means of identifying abnormalities in diastolic filling. We recently used Doppler-derived mitral inflow patterns to compare diastolic function in a group of 21 young asymptomatic subjects with Type I diabetes and 21 age-matched control subjects.[144] No patient in either group had clinical, electrocardiographic, or echocardiographic evidence of ischemic, valvular, or hypertensive heart disease. Nearly 30% of diabetic subjects had at least two Doppler-derived parameters of left ventricular filling that were abnormal compared with those in controls. As in many other studies, diastolic abnormalities did not correlate with the duration of diabetes or with microvascular complications. Mitral inflow velocities have also been assessed by Doppler echocardiography in 60 patients with adult-onset diabetes.[145] Patients with known hypertension or positive exercise electrocardiography were excluded from analysis. Diabetic individuals with retinopathy had a significantly higher late-to-early diastolic peak mitral flow velocity than either diabetic patients without retinopathy or control subjects.

In summary, noninvasive evaluation of cardiac function in diabetic individuals supports the existence of a diabetic cardiomyopathy. Abnormalities of both systolic and diastolic left ventricular function can be demonstrated by virtually all techniques employed. Many carefully designed studies have excluded other predisposing factors that may alter cardiac function. However, the data at hand do not clearly relate the type, duration, and severity of diabetes or the presence of microvascular disease to the time of onset or the degree of ventricular dysfunction. The role of coexistent conditions such as hypertension in the potentiation of diabetes-induced myocardial disease also awaits elucidation, and the effect of metabolic control on myocardial abnormalities needs clarification.

Pathologic Studies

Numerous histopathologic studies in humans have explored the association of diabetes with a myopathic state. Early postmortem studies in diabetic subjects without overt congestive heart failure documented a higher incidence of intramural periodic acid-Schiff (PAS)-positive material and hyaline thickening with and without endothelial cell proliferation in both the intramural and extramural portions of coronary arteries.[146,147] No correlation was found between the presence of PAS-positive lesions and antemortem blood pressure. Zoneraich et al.[148] also found evidence of intramural involvement, with significant proliferative changes and wall thickening, in young persons with juvenile diabetes. In the latter study, small-vessel disease was evident in 72% of normotensive diabetic patients but in only 12% of nondiabetic subjects.

Similar pathologic features have been found in diabetic subjects with congestive heart failure without significant coronary atherosclerosis. Rubler et al.[113] noted substantial myocardial hypertrophy and fibrosis in their original series of four patients with diabetic cardiomyopathy. Endothelial and subendothelial proliferation were also prominent, suggesting that small-vessel disease may be involved in the pathogenesis of myocardial dysfunction. Zoneraich[149] recently reviewed an extensive body of literature concerning the role of small-vessel disease in diabetic cardiomyopathy. Of interest is the possible role of small-vessel disease in diabetic patients with angina pectoris and normal coronary angiograms; two such patients have recently been found to have identical small-vessel changes by right ventricular endomyocardial biopsy.[150]

Many alterations in myocardial small vessels are qualitatively similar to those seen in other organs of diabetic patients. Such alterations include increased thickening of the capillary basement membranes of the myocardium and microaneurysms in autopsy specimens as well as in tissue analyzed at the time of coronary artery bypass surgery.[151,152] Basement-membrane thickening was more severe in those with overt diabetes than in those with simple glucose intolerance. Such microvascular damage within the myocardium may represent part of the spectrum of vasculopathy typically found in diabetic patients, as microaneurysms are not typically encountered in individuals with cardiomyopathy nor are they associated with other specific myocardial lesions.[152]

Interstitial infiltration with PAS-positive material and fibrosis, however, may be associated with systolic and diastolic abnormalities. In this context, Regan et al.[115] noted minimal changes in intramural locations of the coronary arteries in nine diabetic subjects without coronary atherosclerosis. Similar findings were noted in diabetic patients with and without overt congestive heart failure. No patient had significant coronary artery disease. Perivascular and interstitial fibrosis and accumulation of PAS-positive material were observed along with degeneration and fragmentation of myocytes. Diminished left ventricular compliance (elevated end-diastolic pressure at reduced diastolic volume) was noted in all patients and was felt to be associated with interstitial changes and not with small-vessel disease. Patients with congestive heart failure had similar, though more extensive, findings.

Factor et al.[153] have emphasized that the combination of diabetes and hypertension may lead to more severe interstitial fibrosis and myocellular damage than that seen with diabetes or hypertension alone. In nine hypertensive diabetic patients with severe congestive heart failure and minimal obstructive coronary artery disease, dense interstitial connective tissue was seen throughout the myocardium. Myocytolysis and scarring were more prominent than in patients with isolated diabetes or hypertension. Of interest was the similar extent of small-vessel changes in the three groups despite significant differences in interstitial scarring, suggesting that interstitial disease is responsible for the mechanical dysfunction and not "small-vessel disease," which may be an incidental finding.

Pathogenesis

There is conflicting evidence regarding the relative importance of small-vessel disease, interstitial fibrosis, microvascular changes, and metabolic derangements in the pathogenesis of diabetic cardiomyopathy. The relationship of type, duration, and severity of diabetes to myocardial abnormalities remains somewhat nebulous as well. Also, myocardial disease may or may not be related to the degree and extent of other microvascular complications. However, several attractive hypotheses exist regarding the pathogenesis of diabetic cardiomyopathy.

As mentioned, diabetic autonomic neuropathy has been associated with an extremely high mortality rate, with many of the deaths being sudden and unexpected.[41] Simple testing of cardiovascular reflexes is a good guide to prognosis in diabetic autonomic neuropathy. Recently, plasma catecholamine levels were found to be significantly reduced in diabetic subjects with cardiac autonomic neuropathy and the reduced levels noted to be correlated with abnormalities of diastolic function.[140] Histologic evidence of diabetic cardiac autonomic neuropathy has been noted in diabetic individuals with painless infarction.[33] Sympathetic stimulation not only improves left ventricular contractility but increases left ventricular relaxation rates and results in an earlier onset of ventricular relaxation, perhaps by facilitating calcium uptake by the sarcoplasmic reticulum. Thus, left ventricular systolic and diastolic dysfunction could be related to diminished sympathetic stimulation in many diabetic subjects.

Previous studies have documented the association of sympathetic nervous system dysfunction with congestive heart failure. Myocardial catecholamine depletion frequently occurs in patients with heart failure,[154] and postmortem studies in diabetic subjects have revealed reduced cardiac concentrations of norepinephrine.[155] Altered norepinephrine turnover and metabolism have also been noted in rats with streptozotocin-induced diabetes and found to be reversible by insulin therapy.[156] Once autonomic dysfunction is clearly detected in diabetic patients, 5-year survival is only 44% as compared with 85% in age- and sex-matched control individuals with diabetes.[41] Although the relationship of autonomic nervous system dysfunction to enhanced mortality is established, the cause-and-effect nature of the relationship is not completely clear (especially with regard to cardiac risk). Similarly, a relationship between cardiac microvascular alterations and growth hormone has recently been suggested. Experimentally, growth hormone enhances production of procollagen in arterial myomedial cell cultures[157] and increases glomerular capillary membrane thickness in streptozotocin-diabetic rats.[158]

Growth hormone—deficient diabetic dwarfs have been noted to lack the microvascular changes associated with diabetes despite their having metabolic changes similar to those in patients with diabetes.[159] Growth hormone would thus appear to be involved in the pathogenesis of angiopathy in the diabetic patients. In a canine alloxan model of mild diabetes,[160] however, no association was seen between an elevation in levels of collagen in the left ventricular free wall and elevated levels of growth hormone. Perhaps enhanced responsiveness of collagen to growth hormone account for some of the interstitial changes seen in diabetes.

Finally, the correlation between the extensive myocardial alterations in a diabetic-hypertensive rat model[161] and clinical and pathologic findings in a comparable human population[153] needs to be explored. The authors of the aforementioned studies suggested that diabetes might somehow sensitize the myocardium to subsequent hypertension. Hypertension is more common in diabetic subjects, perhaps in relation to widespread arteriolar hyalinization.[162] Hypertension has also been correlated with other microvascular complications (nephropathy and retinopathy),[163,164] and its treatment may retard progression of renal disease and retinal complications.

Superimposed hypertension therefore may interact with the ensuing diabetic myocardial and vascular alterations to result in progressive myocyte damage. Factor and Sonnenblick[165] recently presented experimental evidence for microvascular hyperreactivity (spasm) in a hypertensive-diabetic rat model. Transient spasm of the myocardial microcirculation therefore may lead to focal myocellular necrosis and scarring. Verapamil therapy in the Syrian hamster model of hereditary cardiomyopathy prevents such microvascular spasm and subsequent myocellular necrosis. These observations provide hope that in the future similar preventive therapy could be applied to patients with diabetic cardiomyopathy.

The diagnosis of a diabetic cardiomyopathy can be entertained only after the exclusion of coronary artery disease and other conditions such as hypertension, valvular disease, and alcohol abuse, known to cause myocardial dysfunction. In this regard, hemochromatosis also needs to be considered in diabetic patients with heart disease. Similarly, uremia itself may lead to systolic dysfunction[166] and should be considered in a diabetic patient with advanced nephropathy.

Treatment

Treatment of congestive heart failure in the diabetic patient should follow the same guidelines as in nondiabetic patients, with a few notable exceptions. Treatment of hypertension and hypercholesterolemia, along with avoidance of excessive alcohol intake and cessation of smoking, are advised for all patients. Patients with NIDDM requiring thiazide diuretics or β-adrenergic-blocking agents may run the risk of impaired insulin secretion, resulting in worsening of hyperglycemia. Conversely, in patients requiring insulin, the use of β-adren-

ergic blockers can cause more severe episodes of hypoglycemia. The former problem may be improved by the use of cardioselective β-adrenergic blockers.

Similarly, arterial reflexes may be impaired in diabetic persons with autonomic dysfunction. Thus preload- and afterload-reducing agents (veno-dilators and arterial dilators, respectively) should be used cautiously in diabetic patients. Although altered myocardial sensitivity to cardiac glycosides has not been established clinically, isolated muscle from diabetic rats has shown a greater tendency to contracture when exposed to ouabain.[167]

Finally, the role of intensive treatment of hyperglycemia in the primary prevention or reversal of myocardial dysfunction remains to be elucidated. The results of clinical and experimental studies are equivocal, although encouraging results of metabolic control in improving myocardial function have been presented. These studies suffer from inadequacy of sample size, variation in patient populations, and variation in duration of treatment. An editorial on microvascular complications and diabetes reviews these problems thoroughly.[168] Maintenance of metabolic control in diabetic patients is crucial, but we cannot support intensive insulin treatment with its attendant increased risk of hypoglycemia in patients with myocardial dysfunction until the benefit-to-risk ratio for such treatment is better known.

REFERENCES

1. Vergely P. De l'angine de poitrine dans ses rapports avec le diabète. Gaz Hebd Med Chir (Paris) (Series 2) 1883; 20:364–8.
2. Kessler II. Mortality experience of diabetic patients: a twenty-six year follow-up study. Am J Med 1971;51: 715–24.
3. Garcia MJ, McNamara PM, Gordon T, Kannell WB. Morbidity and mortality in diabetics in the Framingham population: sixteen year follow-up study. Diabetes 1974; 23:105–11.
4. Kannel WB, Hjortland M, Castelli WP. Role of diabetes in congestive heart failure: the Framingham study. Am J Cardiol 1974;34:29–34.
5. Centers for Disease Control. Trends in diabetes mellitus mortality. MMWR 1988;37:769–73.
6. Centers for Disease Control Chronic disease reports: coronary heart disease mortality—United States, 1986. MMWR 1989;38:285–8.
7. Eschwege E, Richard JL, Thibult N, et al. Coronary heart disease mortality in relation with diabetes, blood glucose and plasma insulin levels. The Paris Prospective Study, ten years later. Horm Metab Res Suppl 1985;15:41–6.
8. Butler WJ, Ostrander LD Jr, Carman WJ, Lamphiear DE. Mortality from coronary heart disease in the Tecumseh study. Long-term effect of diabetes mellitus, glucose tolerance and other risk factors. Am J Epidemiol 1985: 121:541–7.
9. Pan W-H, Cedres LB, Liu K, et al. Relationship of clinical diabetes and asymptomatic hyperglycemia to risk of coronary heart disease mortality in men and women. Am J Epidemiol 1986;123:504–16.
10. Wilson PWF, Cupples LA, Kannel WB. Is hyperglycemia associated with cardiovascular disease? The Framingham Study. Am Heart J 1991;121:586–90.

11. Kannel WB. Lipids, diabetes and coronary artery disease: insights from the Framingham Study. Am Heart J 1985; 110:1100–17.

12. Waller BF, Palumbo PJ, Lie JT, Roberts WC. Status of the coronary arteries at necropsy in diabetes mellitus with onset after age 30 years: analysis of 229 diabetic patients with and without clinical evidence of coronary heart disease and comparison to 183 control subjects. Am J Med 1980;69:498–506.

13. Howard BV. Lipoprotein metabolism in diabetes mellitus. J Lipid Res 1987:28;613–28.

14. Modan M, Halkin H, Almog S, et al. Hyperinsulinemia: a link between hypertension, obesity and glucose intolerance. J Clin Invest 1985;75:809–18.

15. Orchard TJ, Becker DJ, Bates M, et al. Plasma insulin and lipoprotein concentration—an atherogenic association. Am J Epidemiol 1983;118:326–47.

16. Stout RW. Insulin and atheroma: an update. Lancet 1987; 1:1077–9.

17. Kannel WB, McGee DL. Diabetes and cardiovascular disease: the Framingham Study. JAMA 1979;241:2035–8.

18. Fein FS. Heart disease in diabetes. Cardiovasc Rev Rep 1982;3:877–93.

19. Krowlewski AS, Kosinski EJ, Warram JH, et al. Magnitude and determinants of coronary artery disease in juvenile-onset, insulin-dependent diabetes mellitus. Am J Cardiol 1987;59:750–5.

20. Fein F, Scheuer J. Heart disease. In: Rifkin H, Porte D Jr. Diabetes mellitus: theory and practice. New York: Elsevier, 1990:812–23.

21. Robertson WB, Strong JB. Atherosclerosis in persons with hypertension and diabetes mellitus. Lab Invest 1968; 5:538–51.

22. Hamby RI, Sherman L, Mehta J, Aintablian A. Reappraisal of the role of the diabetic state in coronary artery disease. Chest 1976;2:251–7.

23. Dortimer AC, Shenoy PN, Shiroff RA, et al. Diffuse coronary artery disease in diabetic patients: fact or fiction? Circulation 1978;57:133–6.

24. Crall FV Jr, Roberts WC. The extramural and intramural coronary arteries in juvenile diabetes mellitus: analysis of nine necropsy patients aged 19 to 38 years with onset of diabetes before age 15 years. Am J Med 1978;64:221–30.

25. Nesto RW, Watson FS, Kowalchuk GJ, et al. Silent myocardial ischemia and infarction in diabetics with peripheral vascular disease; assessment by dipyridamole thallium-201 scintigraphy. Am Heart J 1990;120:1073–7.

26. Kannel WB, Abott RD. Incidence and prognosis of unrecognized myocardial infarction. N Engl J Med 1984; 311:1144–7.

27. Niakan E, Harati Y, Rolak LA, et al. Silent myocardial infarction and diabetic cardiovascular autonomic neuropathy. Arch Intern Med 1986;146:2229–30.

28. Margolis JR, Kannel WB, Feinleib M, et al. Clinical features of unrecognized myocardial infarction—silent and symptomatic: eighteen year follow-up: the Framingham Study. Am J Cardiol 1973;32:1–7.

29. Cabin HS, Roberts WC. Quantitative comparison of extent of coronary narrowing and size of healed myocardial infarct in 33 necropsy patients with clinically recognized and in 28 with clinically unrecognized ("silent") previous acute myocardial infarction. Am J Cardiol 1982; 50:677–81.

30. Murray DP, O'Brien T, Mulrooney R, O'Sullivan DJ. Autonomic dysfunction and silent myocardial ischaemia on exercise testing in diabetes mellitus. Diabetic Med 1990;7:580–4.

31. Nesto RW, Phillips RT, Kett KG, et al. Angina and exertional myocardial ischemia in diabetic and nondiabetic patients: assessment by exercise thallium scintigraphy. Ann Intern Med 1988;108:170–5.

32. Ambepityia G, Kopelman PG, Ingram BD, et al. Exertional myocardial ischemia in diabetes: a quantitative analysis of anginal perceptual threshold and the influence of autonomic function. J Am Coll Cardiol 1990;15:72–7.

33. Faerman I, Faccio E, Milei J, et al. Autonomic neuropathy and painless myocardial infarction in diabetic patients: histologic evidence of their relationship. Diabetes 1977; 6:1147–58.

34. Watkins PJ, Mackay JD. Cardiac denervation in diabetic neuropathy. Ann Intern Med 1980;2:304–7.

35. Lloyd-Mostyn RH, Watkins PJ. Defective innervation of heart in diabetic autonomic neuropathy. BMJ 1975; 3:15–7.

36. Langer A, Freeman MR, Josse RG, et al. Silent ischemia in asymptomatic diabetic patients and its association with autonomic dysfunction and pain threshold [Abstract]. J Am Coll Cardiol 1990;15(Suppl A):119A.

37. Nesto RW, Phillips RT. Asymptomatic myocardial ischemia in diabetic patients. Am J Med 1986;80(Suppl 4C):40–7.

38. Pladziewicz DS, Nesto RW. Hypoglycemia-induced silent myocardial ischemia. Am J Cardiol 1989:63;1531–2.

39. Soler NG, Bennett M, Pentecost BL, et al. Myocardial infarction in diabetics. Q J Med 1975;173:125–32.

40. Uretsky BF, Farquhar DS, Berezin AF, Hood WB Jr. Symptomatic myocardial infarction without chest pain: prevalence and clinical course. Am J Cardiol 1977; 40:498–503.

41. Ewing DJ, Campbell IW, Clarke BF. The natural history of diabetic autonomic neuropathy. Q J Med 1980; 49:95–108.

42. Kahn JK, Zola B, Juni JE, Vinik AI. Decreased exercise heart rate and blood pressure response in diabetic subjects with cardiac autonomic neuropathy. Diabetes Care 1986;9:4:389–94.

43. Hilsted J, Galbo H, Christensen N. Impaired cardiovascular responses to graded exercise in diabetic autonomic neuropathy. Diabetes 1979;28:313–9.

44. Kosinski EJ, Krolewski AS, Adams KG, et al. Effect of diabetic autonomic neuropathy on coronary blood flow regulation [Abstract no. 89]. Circulation 1984:70(Suppl): II–23.

45. Almog C, Pik A. Acute myocardial infarction as a complication of diabetic neuropathy. JAMA 1978;239:2782.

46. Burgos LG, Ebert TJ, Assiddao C, et al. Increased intraoperative cardiovascular morbidity in diabetics with autonomic neuropathy. Anesthesiology 1989;70:591–7.

47. Ewing DJ, Campbell IW, Clarke BF, Mortality in diabetic autonomic neuropathy. Lancet 1976;1:601–3.

48. Ewing DJ, Campbell IW, Clarke BF. Assessment of cardiovascular effects in diabetic autonomic neuropathy and prognostic implications. Ann Intern Med 1980; 92:308–11.

49. Ewing DJ, Boland O, Neilson JM, et al. Autonomic neuropathy, QT interval lengthening and unexpected deaths in male diabetic patients. Diabetologia 1991; 34:182–5.

50. Bellavere F, Ferri M, Guarini L, et al. Prolonged QT period in diabetic autonomic neuropathy: a possible role in sudden cardiac death? Br Heart J 1988;59:379–83.

51. Jermendy G, Tóth L, Vörös P, et al. Cardiac autonomic neuropathy and QT interval length. A follow-up study in diabetic patients. Acta Cardiol 1991;46:189–200.

52. Kahn JK, Sisson JC, Vinik AI. QT interval prolongation and sudden cardiac death in diabetic autonomic neuropathy. J Clin Endocrinol Metab 1987;64:751–4.

53. Bernardi L, Ricordi L, Rossi M, et al. Impairment of modulation of sympathovagal activity in diabetes: an explanation for sudden death? [Abstract] Circulation 1989;80(Suppl 2):1564.

54. Savage MP, Krolewski AS, Kenien GG, et al. Acute myocardial infarction in diabetes mellitus and significance of congestive heart failure as a prognostic factor. Am J Cardiol 1988;62:665–9.

55. Oswald GA, Corcoran S, Yudkin JS. Prevalence and risks of hyperglycaemia and undiagnosed diabetes in patients with acute myocardial infarction. Lancet 1984;1:1264–7.

56. Jaffe AS, Spadaro JJ, Schechtman K, et al. Increased congestive heart failure after myocardial infarction of modest extent in patients with diabetes mellitus. Am Heart J 1984;108:31–7.

57. Tansey MJB, Opie LH, Kennelly BM. High mortality in obese women diabetics with acute myocardial infarction. BMJ 1977;1:1624–6.

58. Czyzk A, Krolewski AS, Szablowska S, et al. Clinical course of myocardial infarction among diabetic patients. Diabetes Care 1980;3:526–9.

59. Singer DE, Moulton AW, Nathan DM. Diabetic myocardial infarction: interaction of diabetes with other preinfarction risk factors. Diabetes 1989;38:350–7.

60. Rytter L, Troelsen S, Beck-Nielsen H. Prevalence and mortality of acute myocardial infarction in patients with diabetes. Diabetes Care 1985;8:230–4.

61. Stone PH, Muller JE, Hartwell T, et al. The effect of diabetes mellitus on prognosis and serial left ventricular function after acute myocardial infarction: contribution of both coronary disease and diastolic left ventricular dysfunction to the adverse prognosis. J Am Coll Cardiol 1989;14:49–57.

62. Partamian JO, Bradley RF. Acute myocardial infarction in 258 cases of diabetes: immediate mortality and five-year survival. N Engl J Med 1965;273:455–61.

63. Hands ME, Rutherford JD, Muller JE, et al, The MILIS Study Group. The in-hospital development of cardiogenic shock after myocardial infarction: incidence, predictors of occurrence, outcome and prognostic factors. J Am Coll Cardiol 1989;14:40–6.

64. Dash H, Johnson RA, Dinsmore RE, et al. Cardiomyopathic syndrome due to coronary artery disease. II. Increased prevalence in patients with diabetes mellitus: a matched pair analysis. Br Heart J 1977;39:740–7.

65. Zarich SW, Nesto RW. Diabetic cardiomyopathy. Am Heart J 1989;118:1000–12.

66. Leland OS, Maki PC. Heart disease and diabetes mellitus. In: Marble A, Krall LP, Bradley R, et al, eds. Joslin's diabetes mellitus. 12th ed. Philadelphia: Lea & Febiger, 1985:553–82.

67. Kereiakes DJ. Myocardial infarction in the diabetic patient. Clin Cardiol 1985;8:446–50.

68. Smith JW, Marcus FI, Serokman R, Multicenter Postinfarction Research Group. Prognosis of patients with diabetes mellitus after acute myocardial infarction. Am J Cardiol 1984;54:718–21.

69. Schechtman K, Capone RJ, Kleiger RE, et al. Differential risk patterns associated with 3 month as compared with 3 to 12 month mortality and reinfarction after non-Q wave myocardial infarction. J Am Coll Cardiol 1990;15:940–7.

70. Nicod P, Lewis SE, Corbett JC, et al. Increased incidence and clinical correlation of persistently abnormal technetium pyrophosphate myocardial scintigrams following acute myocardial infarction in patients with diabetes mellitus. Am Heart J 1982;103:822–9.

71. Granger CB, Aronson L, Wall TC. The impact of diabetes on survival in acute myocardial infarction: the TAMI experience [Abstract]. J Am Coll Cardiol 1990;15(Suppl A):198A.

72. Lew AS, Hod H, Cercek B, et al. Mortality and morbidity rates of patients older and younger than 75 years with acute myocardial infarction treated with intravenous streptokinase. Am J Cardiol 1987;59:1–5.

73. Salomon NW, Page US, Okies JE, et al. Diabetes mellitus and coronary artery bypass: short-term risk and long-term prognosis. J Thorac Cardiovasc Surg 1983;85:264–71.

74. Lawrie GM, Morris GC Jr, Glaeser DH. Influence of diabetes mellitus on the results of coronary bypass surgery: follow-up of 212 diabetic patients ten to 15 years after surgery. JAMA 1986;256:2967–21.

75. Benchimol D, Benchimol H, Bonnet J, et al. Risk factors for progression of atherosclerosis six months after balloon angioplasty of coronary stenosis. Am J Cardiol 1990;65:980–5.

76. Deligonul U, Vandormael M, Kern M, Galan K. Repeat coronary angioplasty for restenosis: results and predictors of follow-up clinical events. Am Heart J 1989;117:997–1002.

77. Gundersen T, Kjekshus J. Timolol treatment after myocardial infarction in diabetic patients. Diabetes Care 1983;6:285–90.

78. Kjekshus J, Gilpin E, Cali G, et al. Diabetic patients and beta-blockers after acute myocardial infarction. Eur Heart J 1990;11:43–50.

79. Fuster V, Cohen M, Halperin J. Aspirin in the prevention of coronary disease [Editorial]. N Engl J Med 1989;321:183–5.

80. Breddin HK, Krzywanek HJ, Althoff P, et al. PARD: platelet aggregation as a risk factor in diabetics: results of a prospective study. Horm Metab Res Suppl 1985;15:63–8.

81. Sagel J, Colwell JS, Crook L, Laimins M. Increased platelet aggregation in early diabetes mellitus. Ann Intern Med 1975;82:733–8.

82. Ostermann H, van de Loo J. Factors of the hemostatic system in diabetic patients: a survey of controlled studies. Haemostasis 1986;16:386–416.

83. Colwell JA, Lopes-Virella MF. A review of the development of large-vessel disease in diabetes mellitus. Am J Med 1988;85(Suppl 5A):113–9.

84. DAMAD Study Group. Effect of aspirin alone and aspirin plus dipyridamole in early diabetic retinopathy: a multicenter randomized controlled clinical trial. Diabetes 1989;38:491–8.

85. Moy CS, LaPorte RE, Dorman JS, et al. Insulin dependent diabetes mellitus mortality: the risk of cigarette smoking. Circulation 1990;82:37–43.

86. Muller JE, Tofler GH, Stone PH. Circadian variation and triggers of onset of acute cardiovascular disease. Circulation 1989;79:733–43.

87. Davies MJ, Thomas AC. Plaque fissuring—the cause of acute myocardial infarction, sudden ischaemic death and crescendo angina. Br Heart J 1985;53:363–73.

88. Davies MJ, Bland JM, Hangartner JRW, et al. Factors influencing the presence or absence of acute coronary artery thrombi in sudden ischaemic death. Eur Heart J 1989;10:203–8.

89. Assmann G, Schulte H. The Prospective Cardiovascular Münster (PROCAM) Study: prevalence of hyperlipidemia in persons with hypertension and/or diabetes mellitus and

the relationship to coronary heart disease. Am Heart J 1988;116:1713–24.

90. Brand FN. Abbott RD, Kannel WD. Diabetes, intermittent claudication and risk of cardiovascular events: the Framingham Study. Diabetes 1989;38:504–9.

91. Jensen T, Borch-Johnsen K, Kofoed-Enevoldsen A, Deckert T. Coronary heart disease in young Type 1 insulin-dependent diabetic patients with and without diabetic nephropathy: incidence and risk factors. Diabetologia 1987;30:144–8.

92. Borch-Johnsen K, Kreiner S. Proteinuria: value as a predictor of cardiovascular mortality in insulin dependent diabetes mellitus. BMJ 1987;294:1651–4.

93. Nelson RG, Pettitt DJ, Carraher MJ, et al. Effect of proteinuria on mortality in NIDDM. Diabetes 1988; 37:1499–504.

94. Zavaroni I, Bonora E, Pagliara M, et al. Risk factors for coronary artery disease in healthy persons with hyperinsulinemia and normal glucose tolerance. N Engl J Med 1989;320:702–6.

95. Serrano-Rios M, Perez A. Saban-Ruiz J. Cardiac complications in diabetes. World book of diabetes in practice. Vol 2. New York: Elsevier Science Publishers, 1986:169–78.

96. MacRury SM, Lowe GD. Blood rheology in diabetes mellitus. Diabetic Med 1990;7:285–91.

97. Rosove MH, Frank HJL, Harwig SSL. Plasma β-thromboglobulin, platelet factor 4, fibrinopeptide A, and other hemostatic functions during improved, short-term glycemic control in diabetes mellitus. Diabetes Care 1984; 7:174–9.

98. Trip MD, Cats VM, Van Capelle FJL, Vreeken J. Platelet hyperreactivity and prognosis in survivors of myocardial infarction. N Engl J Med 1990;322:1549–54.

99. Ziboh VA, Maruta H, Lord J, et al. Increased biosynthesis of thromboxane A_2 by diabetic platelets. Eur J Clin Invest 1979;9:223–8.

100. Butkus A, Skrinska VA, Schumacker OP. Thomboxane production and platelet aggregation in diabetic subjects with clinical complications. Thromb Res 1980; 19:211–23.

101. Lagarde M, Burtin M, Berciaud P, et al. Increase of platelet thromboxane A_2 formation and of its plasmatic half-life in diabetes mellitus. Thromb Res 1980;19:823–30.

102. Davì G, Catalano I, Averna M, et al. Thromboxane biosynthesis and platelet function in Type II diabetes mellitus. N Engl J Med 1990;322:1769–74.

103. Badawi H, El-Sawy M, Mikhail M, et al. Platelets, coagulation and fibrinolysis in diabetic and non-diabetic patients with quiescent coronary heart disease. Angiology 1970;21:511–9.

104. Small M, Lowe GDO, MacCuish A, Forbes C. Thrombin and plasmin activity in diabetes mellitus and their association with glycaemic control. Q J Med 1987;65:1025–31.

105. Dembińska-Kieć A, Kostka-Trabka E, Grodzińska L, et al. Prostacyclin and blood glucose levels in humans and rabbits. Prostaglandins 1981;21:113–21.

106. Johnson M, Harrison HE, Raftery AT, Elder JB. Vascular prostacyclin may be reduced in diabetes in man [Letter]. Lancet 1979;1:325–6.

107. Hjalmarson A, Gilpin EA, Nicod P, et al. Differing circadian patterns of symptom onset in subgroups of patients with acute myocardial infarction. Circulation 1989;80:267–75.

108. ISIS-2 (Second International Study of Infarct Survival) Collaborative Group. Morning peak in the incidence of myocardial infarction: experience in the ISIS-2 trial. Eur Heart J 1992;13:594–8.

109. Stubbs ME, Jimenez AH, Yamane M, et al. Platelet hyper-reactivity in diabetics: relation to time of onset of acute myocardial infarction [Abstract]. J Am Coll Cardiol 1990;15(Suppl A):2:119A.

110. Nesto RW, Zarich SW, Freeman R, et al. Ambulant ischemia in diabetics with coronary artery disease: does autonomic nervous system dysfunction affect time of onset of ischemia? Circulation 1991;84(Suppl II):II–727.

111. Fein FS, Sonnenblick EH. Diabetic cardiomyopathy. Prog Cardiovasc Dis 1985;27:255–70.

112. Regan TJ. Congestive heart failure in the diabetic. Annu Rev Med 1983;34:161–8.

113. Rubler S, Dlugash J, Yuceoglu YZ, et al. New type of cardiomyopathy associated with diabetic glomerulosclerosis. Am J Cardiol 1972;30:595–602.

114. Hamby RI, Zoneraich S, Sherman L. Diabetic cardiomyopathy. JAMA 1974;229:1749–54.

115. Regan TJ, Lyons MM, Ahmed SS, et al. Evidence for cardiomyopathy in familial diabetes mellitus. J Clin Invest 1977;60:885–99.

116. D'Elia JA, Weinrauch LA, Healy RW, et al. Myocardial dysfunction without coronary artery disease in diabetic renal failure. Am J Cardiol 1979;43:193–9.

117. Karlefors T. Haemodynamic studies in male diabetics. Acta Med Scand Suppl 1966;449:45–73.

118. Carlström S, Karlefors T. Haemodynamic studies on newly diagnosed diabetics before and after adequate insulin treatment. Br Heart J 1970;32:355–8.

119. Ahmed SS, Jaferi GA, Narang RM, Regan TJ. Preclinical abnormality of left ventricular function in diabetes mellitus. Am Heart J 1975;89:153–8.

120. Zoneraich S, Zoneraich O, Rhee JJ. Left ventricular performance in diabetic patients without clinical heart disease: evaluation by systolic time intervals and echocardiography. Chest 1977;72:748–51.

121. Rynkiewicz A, Semetkowska-Jurkiewicz E, Wyrzykowski B. Systolic and diastolic time intervals in young diabetics. Br Heart J 1980;44:280–3.

122. Seneviratne BIB. Diabetic cardiomyopathy: the preclinical phase. BMJ 1977;1:1444–6.

123. Rubler S, Sajadi MRM, Araoye MA, Holford FD. Noninvasive estimation of myocardial performance in patients with diabetes: effect of alcohol administration. Diabetes 1978;27:127–34.

124. Sanderson JE, Brown DJ, Rivellese A, Kohner E. Diabetic cardiomyopathy? An echocardiographic study of young diabetics. BMJ 1978;1:404–7.

125. Shapiro LM, Leatherdale BA, Coyne ME, et al. Prospective study of heart disease in untreated maturity onset diabetics. Br Heart J 1980;44:342–8.

126. Shapiro LM, Howat AP, Calter MM. Left ventricular function in diabetes mellitus. I. Methodology and prevalence and spectrum of abnormalities. Br Heart J 1981; 45:122–8.

127. Shapiro LM, Leatherdale BA, MacKinnon J, Fletcher RF. Left ventricular function in diabetes mellitus. II. Relation between clinical features and left ventricular function. Br Heart J 1981;45:129–32.

128. Shapiro LM. Echocardiographic features of impaired ventricular function in diabetes mellitus. Br Heart J 1982; 47:439–44.

129. Kitabatake A, Inoue M, Asao M, et al. Transmitral blood flow reflecting diastolic behavior of the left ventricle in health and disease: a study by pulsed Doppler technique. Jpn Circ J 1982;46:92–102.

130. Harizi RC, Bianco JA, Alpert JS. Diastolic function of the heart in clinical cardiology. Arch Intern Med 1988; 148:99–109.

131. Airaksinen J, Ikäheimo M, Kaila J, et al. Impaired left ventricular filling in young female diabetics: an echocardiographic study. Acta Med Scand 1984;216:509–16.

132. Friedman NE, Levitsky LL, Edidin DV, et al. Impaired myocardial performance in children with Type I (insulindependent) diabetes mellitus [Abstract no. 88]. Diabetes 1980;29(Suppl 2):22A.

133. Friedman NE, Levitsky LL, Edidin DV, et al. Echocardiographic evidence for impaired myocardial performance in children with Type I diabetes mellitus. Am J Med 1982; 73:846–50.

134. Lababidi ZA, Goldstein DE. High prevalence of echocardiographic abnormalities in diabetic youths. Diabetes Care 1983;6:18–22.

135. Vered Z, Battler A, Segal P, et al. Exercise-induced left ventricular dysfunction in young men with asymptomatic diabetes mellitus (diabetic cardiomyopathy). Am J Cardiol 1984;54:633–7.

136. Mildenberger RR, Bar-Shlomo B, Druck MN, et al. Clinically unrecognized ventricular dysfunction in young diabetic patients. J Am Coll Cardiol 1984;4:234–8.

137. Zola B, Kahn JK, Juni JE, Vinik AI. Abnormal cardiac function in diabetic patients with autonomic neuropathy in the absence of ischemic heart disease. J Clin Endocrinol Metab 1986;63:208–14.

138. Arvan S, Singal K. Knapp R, Vagnucci A. Subclinical left ventricular abnormalities in young diabetics. Chest 1988; 93:1031–4.

139. Hilsted J, Galbo H, Christensen NJ, et al. Haemodynamic changes during graded exercise in patients with diabetic autonomic neuropathy. Diabetologia 1982;22:318–23.

140. Kahn JK, Zola B, Juni JE, Vinik AI. Radionuclide assessment of left ventricular diastolic filling in diabetes mellitus with and without cardiac autonomic neuropathy. J Am Coll Cardiol 1986;7:1303–9.

141. Rokey R, Kuo LC, Zoghbi WA, et al. Determination of parameters of left ventricular diastolic filling with pulsed Doppler echocardiography: comparison with cineangiography. Circulation 1985;71:543–50.

142. Spirito P, Maron BJ, Bonow RO. Noninvasive assessment of left ventricular diastolic function: comparative analysis of Doppler echocardiographic and radionuclide angiographic techniques. J Am Coll Cardiol 1986;7:518–26.

143. Friedman BJ, Drinkovic N, Miles H, et al. Assessment of left ventricular diastolic function: comparison of Doppler echocardiography and gated blood pool scintigraphy. J Am Coll Cardiol 1986;8:1348–54.

144. Zarich SW, Arbuckle BE, Cohen LR, et al. Diastolic abnormalities in young asymptomatic diabetic patients assessed by pulsed Doppler echocardiography. J Am Coll Cardiol 1988;12:114–20.

145. Takenaka K, Sakamoto T, Amano K, et al. Left ventricular filling determined by Doppler echocardiography in diabetes mellitus. Am J Cardiol 1988;61:1140–3.

146. Blumenthal HT, Alex M, Goldenberg S. A study of lesions of the intramural coronary artery branches in diabetes mellitus. Arch Pathol 1960;70:13–28.

147. Ledet T. Histological and histochemical changes in the coronary arteries of old diabetic patients. Diabetologia 1968;4:268–72.

148. Zoneraich S, Silverman G, Zoneraich O. Primary myocardial disease, diabetes mellitus and small vessel disease. Am Heart J 1980;10:754–5.

149. Zoneraich S. Small-vessel disease, coronary artery vasodilator reserve and diabetic cardiomyopathy [Editorial]. Chest 1988;94:5–7.

150. Mosseri M, Yarom R, Gotsman MS, Hasin Y. Histologic evidence for small-vessel coronary artery disease in patients with angina pectoris and patent large coronary arteries. Circulation 1986;74:964–72.

151. Fischer VW, Barner HB, Leskiw ML. Capillary basal laminar thickness in diabetic human myocardium. Diabetes 1979;28:713–9.

152. Factor SM, Okun EM, Minase T. Capillary microaneurysms in the human diabetic heart. N Engl J Med 1980; 302:384–8.

153. Factor SM, Minase T, Sonnenblick EH. Clinical and morphological features of human hypertensive-diabetic cardiomyopathy. Am Heart J 1980;99:446–58.

154. Chidsey CA, Braunwald E, Morrow AG. Catecholamine excretion and cardiac stores of norepinephrine in congestive heart failure. Am J Med 1965;39:442–51.

155. Neubauer B, Christensen NJ. Norepinephrine, epinephrine, and dopamine content of the cardiovascular system in long-term diabetics. Diabetes 1976;25:6–10.

156. Ganguly PK, Dhalla KS, Innes IR, et al. Altered norepinephrine turnover and metabolism in diabetic cardiomyopathy. Circ Res 1986;59:684–93.

157. Ledet T, Vuust J. Arterial procollagen type I, type III, and fibrinectin: effects of diabetic serum glucose, insulin, ketone and growth hormone studied in rabbit aortic myomedial cell cultures. Diabetes 1980;29:964–70.

158. Østerby R, Seyer-Hansen K, Gundersen H, Lundbaek K. Growth hormone enhances basement membrane thickening in experimental diabetes: a preliminary report. Diabetologia 1978;15:487–9.

159. Merimee TJ. A follow-up study of vascular disease in growth-hormone-deficient dwarfs with diabetes. N Engl J Med 1978;298:1217–22.

160. Regan TJ, Altszuler N, Eaddy C, Bakth S. Relation of growth hormone and myocardial collagen accumulation in experimental diabetes. J Lab Clin Med 1987;110:274–8.

161. Factor SM, Bhan R, Minase T, et al. Hypertensive-diabetic cardiomyopathy in the rat: an experimental model of human disease. Am J Pathol 1981;102:219–28.

162. Christlieb AR. Diabetes and hypertensive vascular disease: mechanisms and treatment. Am J Cardiol 1973; 32:592–606.

163. Knowler WC, Bennett PH, Ballintine EJ. Increased incidence of retinopathy in diabetes with elevated blood pressure: a six-year follow-up study in Pima Indians. N Engl J Med 1980;302:645–50.

164. Mogensen CE. Progression of nephropathy in long-term diabetics with proteinuria and effect of initial antihypertensive treatment. Scand J Clin Lab Invest 1976; 36:383–8.

165. Factor SM, Sonnenblick EH. Hypothesis: is congestive cardiomyopathy caused by a hyperreactive myocardial microcirculation (microvascular spasm)? Am J Cardiol 1982;50:1149–52.

166. Hung J, Harris PJ, Uren RJ, et al. Uremic cardiomyopathy-effect of hemodialysis on left ventricular function in end-stage renal failure. N Engl J Med 1980;302:547–51.

167. Fein FS, Aronson RS, Nordin C, et al. Altered myocardial response to ouabain in diabetic rats: mechanics and electrophysiology. J Mol Cell Cardiol 1983;15:769–84.

168. The DCCT Research Group. Are continuing studies of metabolic control and microvascular complications in insulin-dependent diabetes mellitus justified? The Diabetes Control and Complications Trial. N Engl J Med 1988; 318:246–50.

Chapter 46

ERECTILE DYSFUNCTION AND DIABETES

IRWIN GOLDSTEIN
IÑIGO SAENZ DE TEJADA

Male sexual dysfunctions are classified into dysfunctions of libido, problems with emission/ejaculation/orgasm, impotence, and priapism. Erectile dysfunction or impotence is the most common of the various sexual dysfunctions, and since multiple advances have been realized in the physiologic and biochemical mechanisms involving penile erection and in clinical techniques of improving erectile dysfunction, this chapter will be devoted primarily to the sexual dysfunction of impotence.

Erectile dysfunction or impotence is the consistent inability to achieve or sustain an erection of sufficient rigidity to permit satisfactory sexual intercourse.[1] It has been estimated from data collected in 1948 that 10 million American males, or approximately 1 in 10 men, have impotence.[1,2] New epidemiologic research in a random, community-based population of aging men suggests that the prevalence of impotence among men 39 to 70 years old is greater than 50%.[3] Contemporary studies indicate, therefore, that impotence afflicts over 30 million American men.

The prevalence of impotence is particularly high in certain groups of patients. In the above study,[3] aging, treated hypertension, treated heart disease, and treated diabetes were among several physiologic variables found to strongly predict impotence. The prevalence of self-assessed complete impotence was more than three times higher among men with diabetes than among men without diabetes. Other studies have demonstrated this higher prevalence of impotence among men with diabetes than in the general male population. Depending on the investigators and the study population, the reported prevalence of impotence in diabetic men has ranged from 35 to 75%.[4-10] Impotence is an age-dependent disorder[2,11,12] that affects the diabetic male an average of 10 to 15 years earlier than his nondiabetic counterpart.

Impotence in men with diabetes develops insidiously over a period of months or years.[7] Patients frequently describe diminished penile rigidity and reduced ability to sustain an erection. Impotence, however, is not always a late progressive complication of the disease but can occur early in its natural history. Libido may persist despite poor erectile performance.[6,7]

ANATOMY OF THE PENIS

The penis has two paired corpora cavernosa and a corpus spongiosum, which surrounds the urethra and distally forms the glans penis. Each corpus cavernosum is surrounded by a thick fibrous sheath, the tunica albuginea, which encases the sponge-like cavernosal tissue. The erectile tissue consists of multiple, interconnected lacunae lined by vascular endothelium. The walls of the lacunae, the trabeculae, are composed of thick bundles of smooth muscle and a fibroelastic frame.[13]

Blood reaches the corpora cavernosa through the cavernosal arteries, which are terminal branches of the hypogastric arteries. Multiple muscular helicine arteries branch off each cavernosal artery and open directly into the lacunar spaces. Blood is drained from the corporal bodies through subtunical venules located between the periphery of the erectile tissue and the tunica albuginea. Subtunical venules coalesce to form larger emissary veins that pierce the tunica albuginea.[14,15]

The peripheral innervation of the penis consists of sympathetic nerves arising from the 11th thoracic to the 2nd lumbar spinal cord segments and from parasympathetic and somatic nerves arising from the 2nd, 3rd, and

4th sacral spinal cord segments. Somatic innervation is via the pudendal nerve, which is composed of efferent fibers innervating the striated musculature of the perineum and of afferent fibers from the penile and perineal skin.[16]

PHYSIOLOGY OF ERECTION

Mechanism of Erection

Penile erections are elicited by local sensory stimulation of the genital organs (reflexogenic erections) and by central psychogenic stimuli received by or generated within the brain (psychogenic erections).[16,17] A variety of stimuli processed in several regions of the brain—including the thalamic nuclei, the rhinencephalon, and the limbic structures—can elicit supraspinal erectile responses. The medial preoptic-anterior hypothalamic area appears to integrate input from these diverse regions and to send projections to the thoracolumbar sympathetic and sacral parasympathetic centers of the spinal cord. The pudendal nerve, which is the afferent limb for reflexogenic erections, collects somatic sensation from the genital skin. The autonomic nerve fibers that arise from the sacral parasympathetic center (S_2-S_4) make up the efferent limb for this reflex, innervating the penile smooth muscle. Reflexogenic and psychogenic erectile mechanisms probably act synergistically in the control of penile erection.[16-23]

Erection follows relaxation of arterial and trabecular smooth muscle.[24] Dilation of the cavernosal and helicine arteries increases blood flow into the lacunar spaces. Relaxation of the trabecular smooth muscle dilates the lacunar spaces, accommodating a larger volume of blood and thus engorging the penis. The expansion of the relaxed trabecular walls against the tunica albuginea compresses the plexus of subtunical venules.[14,24,25] This results in increased resistance to the outflow of blood with increased lacunar space pressure, making the penis rigid. The reduction of venous outflow by the mechanical compression of subtunical venules is known as the corporal veno-occlusive mechanism (Fig. 46–1).

Detumescence results following contraction of penile smooth muscle. Activation of sympathetic constrictor nerves causes an increase in the tone of the smooth muscle of the helicine arteries and the trabeculae, resulting in a reduction of arterial inflow, a collapse of the lacunar spaces with decompression of subtunical venules,[14,24,25] an increase in venous outflow from the lacunar space, and a return of the penis to the flaccid state.

Neurogenic and Endothelium-Mediated Control of Penile Smooth Muscle

Little information is available concerning the neurogenic and endothelial control of the tone of penile blood vessels. Histochemical studies of the cavernosal and helicine arteries have demonstrated the presence of adrenergic nerves and acetylcholinesterase-containing (probably cholinergic) nerves, as well as nerves immunoreactive to vasoactive intestinal polypeptide (VIP) and neuropeptide Y.[26-30] Contraction of the cavernosal

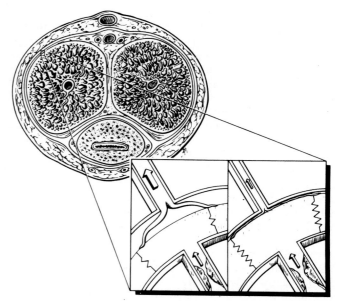

Fig. 46–1. Schematic cross-section of the penis including two corporal bodies and a corpus spongiosum. The left and right inserts depict enlargements of the subtunical space between the trabeculae and the tunica albuginea. Erection tissue drainage passes via subtunical venules into emissary veins that drain through the tunica. When the penis is in the flaccid state (left insert), the contracted corporal smooth muscle allows blood to drain from the erectile tissue to the subtunical venules under conditions of low outflow resistance. When the penis is in the erect state (right insert), following activation of efferent autonomic nerves, the elevated pressure in the lacunar space expands the trabecular structures against the tunica albuginea. The expanded volume of the corporal tissue both mechanically compresses and physically stretches the subtunical venules, greatly increasing the resistance to flow through these venous channels. The resultant restriction of venous outflow through the subtunical venules is called the corporal veno-occlusive mechanism.

artery in humans is controlled by adrenergic nerves via α-adrenoreceptors,[31] while the neurogenic dilator response is attributed to a nonadrenergic, noncholinergic neurotransmitter (NANC).[32]

Several investigators have proposed VIP as the nonadrenergic noncholinergic neurotransmitter in penile smooth muscle, a suggestion supported by the observation that VIP-immunoreactive fibers densely innervate the trabecular smooth muscle and that VIP elicits relaxation of the trabecular smooth muscle.[28,30] Cholinergic nerves appear to modulate the other two neuroeffector systems and not to affect the trabecular smooth muscle directly.[33,34]

Recent studies have shown that NANC-mediated relaxation in the corpus cavernosum is associated with release of nitric oxide and accumulation of cyclic guanosine monophosphate (cGMP).[35] Nitric oxide may act as a neurotransmitter in the peripheral nervous system in various organs, accounting for NANC neurogenic inhibitory responses.[36,37] Nitric oxide synthase has been localized in the peripheral autonomic nerves of several organs containing smooth muscle.[38] In preparations of human corpus cavernosum in which the endothelium has been removed, the NANC-mediated neurogenic relaxation is inhibited by substances that interfere with the synthesis or the effects of nitric oxide. Such evidence strongly supports the possibility that a nitric oxide-like substance mediates NANC-mediated relaxation in trabecular smooth muscle.[39]

The relaxation induced by various vasodilators (i.e., acetylcholine, bradykinin) and physical stimuli (i.e., shear stress) requires the presence of functional endothelium.[32,33] This phenomenon, first described in the rabbit aorta by Furchgott and Zawadzki,[40] has also been demonstrated in the corpus cavernosum vascular bed.[32,38] In human corpus cavernosum the endothelium-derived relaxing factor (EDRF) released by acetylcholine has the chemical properties of nitric oxide,[39] which is proposed to be the EDRF in various vascular beds.[41]

Nitric oxide stimulates guanylate cyclase, with accumulation of cGMP and a resultant relaxation in smooth muscle.[35,42] This pathway appears to be of key importance for relaxation of trabecular smooth muscle (Fig. 46–2).

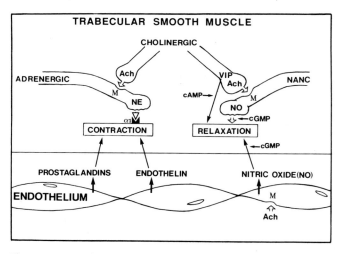

Fig. 46–2. Schematic diagram of the neurogenic and endothelium-derived mechanisms that exert local control of corporal smooth muscle tone. Neurogenic mechanisms involve three neuroeffector systems: adrenergic (constrictor) using norepinephrine (NE) as a neurotransmitter; cholinergic (dilator) using acetylcholine (Ach) and/or vasoactive intestinal polypeptide (VIP) as a neurotransmitter; and nonadrenergic, noncholinergic (NANC) (dilator) using nitric oxide (NO) as a neurotransmitter. Endothelium-derived vasoactive substances such as nitric oxide (dilator), prostaglandins (both constrictor and dilator), and endothelin (constrictor) also may contribute to the control of trabecular smooth muscle tone; cGMP = cyclic guanosine monophosphate.

PATHOPHYSIOLOGY OF DIABETES-RELATED IMPOTENCE

While impotence in diabetic men can be primarily psychogenic, several reports have documented that a primarily organic origin is more common.[6,7] In diabetic patients the erectile disorder is rarely reversible, lending support to an organic cause.[9,43] Organic impotence can be differentiated from psychogenic impotence by monitoring nocturnal erections associated with rapid eye movement (REM), and diabetic men have been found to have a decrease in such REM-associated erections,[44] again supporting an organic basis to their impotence.

Vasculopathy and neuropathy are common complications associated with the natural history of diabetes mellitus. It is hypothesized that cavernosal artery insufficiency, corporal veno-occlusive dysfunction, and/or autonomic neuropathy are the major organic pathophysiologic mechanisms leading to persistent erectile impairment in diabetes mellitus.[46] The role of hormonal abnormalities in the pathophysiology of organic-based impotence is controversial.

Neurogenic Impotence

Penile autonomic neuropathy has a major role in the pathophysiology of erectile dysfunction in patients with diabetes. The incidence of peripheral and autonomic neuropathy is significantly higher in impotent than in potent diabetic men.[6,47] Erectile failure is a common feature of diabetic autonomic neuropathy[48] and may precede the appearance of neuropathy.[49]

Until recently, clinical tests of the integrity of the autonomic nerves to the corpora have been performed exclusively by indirect testing, such as tests of nocturnal penile tumescence. Since diabetic patients commonly have associated hemodynamic abnormalities, indirect testing is not reliable as a technique for accurately documenting cavernosal nerve integrity.[50]

The presence of bladder areflexia and bladder or bowel dysfunction provides indirect support for the impairment of the motor efferent autonomic cavernosal nerves since the bladder and penis receive autonomic innervation from a common origin.[6,51] Ellenberg[6] found that 82% of impotent patients with diabetes had evidence of neuropathic bladder by cystometric diagnosis, while only 10% of age-matched potent patients with diabetes had bladder involvement. Vascular reflexes such as beat-to-beat variation in heart rate provide another indirect measurement of autonomic parasympathetic neuropathy (see Chapter 39). Several studies have also documented abnormal vascular reflexes in the diabetic patient with impotence.[52]

The possibility of direct testing of the autonomic innervation of the corpora is now being investigated by recording the electrical activity of the corporal smooth muscle by the use of intracavernosal electromyographic needles or surface electrodes on the penile shaft.[53] With use of single-potential analysis, waveforms of a defined duration, amplitude, and polyphasity can be recorded in normal subjects.[54] In patients with peripheral neuropathy secondary to diabetes, the single-potential analysis of cavernous electrical activity may reveal potentials that are of abnormal duration and amplitude.[54,55] Since this technique is at the initial development phase and is available in only a few centers, further investigations will be needed for its validation as a test of the autonomic nervous system.

Several tests are used in the evaluation of the presence of neuropathy in the sensory afferent nerves from the penile skin and the motor efferent nerves to the perineal skeletal musculature. These tests include perineal electromyography, sacral latency testing, evaluation of dorsal nerve somatosensory-evoked potential, and testing of vibration-perception sensitivity.[56-59] An abnormal result in somatic testing may suggest but does not prove the co-existence of autonomic neuropathy in the corpora cavernosa. Faerman et al.[60] reported morphologic alterations in the unmyelinated nerves in the corpus cavernosum of the impotent men with diabetes. Ultrastructural studies of penile nerves in rats with long-term streptozotocin-induced diabetes reveal axonal degeneration with loss of axonal filaments, tubules, and mitochondria.[61] The most prominent finding we observed in the penile nerves of impotent patients with diabetes was a thickening of the Schwann and perineurial cell basement membranes.[62]

The nerves in diabetic patients can exhibit biochemical abnormalities, which are subject to some degree of improvement with strict glycemic control.[63] Excessive nonenzymatic glycosylation of myelin proteins and polyol pathway activity, as well as abnormal metabolism of myoinositol and its phospholipid derivatives, have been proposed as possible biochemical mechanisms in the pathogenesis of diabetic neuropathy.[64]

Melman et al. were the first to report diminished levels of norepinephrine in the tissues of patients with diabetes.[65] Norepinephrine depletion was most severe in insulin-dependent patients. These results were corroborated by Lincoln et al., who also found diminished levels of norepinephrine and a marked reduction in acetylcholinesterase-positive fibers in corpus cavernosum tissue of patients with diabetes.[66] These findings suggest the possibility of a depletion in the number of cholinergic nerves in corpus cavernosum of patients with diabetes. Diabetic impotent men have a functional impairment of the neurogenic dilator mechanism of penile smooth muscle[67] (Fig. 46–3). Corporal tissue from impotent men with diabetes accumulates and releases less acetylcholine than corporal tissue from impotent men without diabetes.[68] Since penile smooth muscle relaxation is necessary for erection and the cholinergic neuroeffector system facilitates this smooth muscle relaxation, the dysfunction of penile cholinergic nerves may be contributory to the development of impotence in diabetic men. The duration of diabetes is negatively correlated to the ability of the cholinergic nerves to synthesize acetylcholine.[68] Therefore, patients with long-standing diabetes were more likely to present with penile autonomic neuropathy.

Several studies have reported a decrease in the tissue levels of VIP and the number of VIP-like immunoreactive

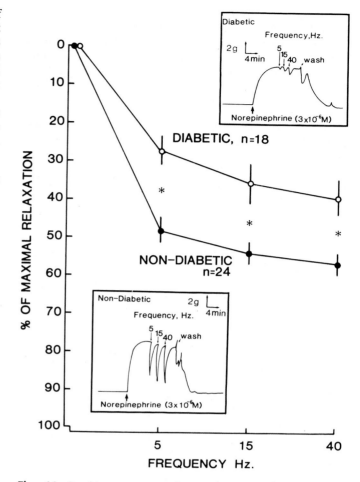

Fig. 46–3. Human corporal erectile tissue from diabetic impotent patients reveals electrical field stimulation relaxation responses to 5, 15, and 40 Hz that average 28 to 35% of maximal relaxation, responses that are significantly diminished in comparison to those in nondiabetic tissues. This finding suggests a functional impairment of the neurogenic dilator mechanism of penile smooth muscle in diabetic impotent men.

fibers in human corpus cavernosum from patients with diabetes.[66,69] Similar findings have been in rats with streptozotocin-induced diabetes.[70]

Vasculogenic Impotence

Vascular disease, of either large or small vessels, has long been recognized as a major contributor to the morbidity and mortality of diabetes.[71,72] Diabetic microangiopathy produces alterations and decompensation of local microvascular blood flow.[73] There is progressive venule dilation, periodic arteriolar vasoconstriction, and sclerosis of the walls of the arterioles, capillaries, and venules.[74] Endothelial cell metabolism and function, thickened basement membrane of the vessel wall, oxygen transport, blood-flow properties, and hemostasis also are altered in diabetic microangiopathy.[75] Similarly, large-vessel disease is strongly associated with diabetes. Intimal, medial, and luminal changes observed in obliterative atherosclerosis have been well documented.[76]

Atherosclerotic vascular disease and erectile dysfunction are strongly related. Arteriosclerosis is the most common organic disorder leading to impotence.[77] Forty to fifty percent of men with clinically significant peripheral arterial disease complain of impotence, and in 80% of these cases, the primary cause of the impotence is organic.[78] Erectile dysfunction develops when more than 50% of the major arterial supply to the penis is involved in atherosclerotic occlusive disease.[79] Atherosclerosis has also been observed to have an adverse effect on the ultrastructure of corpus cavernosum in 40 to 45% of men with diabetic impotence, with the percentage of altered cells increasing with increasing severity of symptoms and clinical findings.[80-83]

Postmortem examination of impotent diabetic men has revealed numerous penile arterial vascular abnormalities, including fibrous proliferation of the intima, medial fibrosis, calcification, and narrowing and obliteration of the lumen. Such vascular alterations in the penile arteries impede blood flow to the cavernous bodies at the time of erection and are thus in part responsible for the erectile dysfunction.[84]

Impotent diabetic men may also have associated vascular risk factors, such as cigarette smoking, hypertension, and hyperlipidemia.[1] Cigarette smoking is a statistically significant independent risk factor in the development of angiographically confirmed atherosclerotic arterial occlusive disease to the hypogastric-cavernous arterial bed. Five, ten, and twenty pack-year (1 pack, or 20 cigarettes, per day for 1 year) histories of exposure to cigarette smoking are associated with 15%, 30% and 70% incidence, respectively, of arterial occlusive disease within the common penile artery.[84] Hypertension also was noted in 45% of impotent men, while hyperlipidemia or other disturbances of lipid metabolism were found in 40 to 50% of impotent men.[78]

Diabetes-associated vascular disease affects the physiology of erection by many routes—at the level of large inflow vessels, the penile microvasculature, the lacunar space endothelium, and the penile fibroelastic frame. One mechanism of diabetes-induced, atherosclerosis-associated erectile dysfunction is the lowering of arterial perfusion pressure and arterial inflow to the lacunar spaces of the corpora cavernosa.[86-88] The clinical consequences of these hemodynamic changes are a diminished rigidity of the erect penis and a prolongation of the time to maximal erection. Another mechanism is interference with corporal veno-occlusion. In all organically impotent men, the incidence of corporal veno-occlusive dysfunction may be as high as 86%.[89]

Corporal veno-occlusive dysfunction associated with diabetes can be due to a structural alteration in the fibroelastic components of the trabeculae.[1] Loss of compliance of the fibroelastic frame of the penis may be the result of altered synthesis of collagen, elastin, or tissue cellularity[90-92] or alterations in the reactivity of the smooth muscle of the corpus cavernosum and the endothelial cells of the lacunar space.[93] Functional studies in isolated human corporal tissue have demonstrated decreased endothelium-dependent relaxation of the penile smooth muscle and loss of compliance of the penile fibroelastic frame. These may result in an inability of the trabeculae to expand against the tunica albuginea and compress the subtunical venules. The clinical consequences of such hemodynamic alterations is excessive outflow of lacunar blood, which prevents the attainment of adequate penile rigidity and duration of erection.

Vascular Testing in Diabetes-Related Impotence

Noninvasive and invasive vascular testing of impotent diabetic patients has been performed in numerous series.[94,95] These include studies of the penile brachial index, penile plethysmography, cavernosal artery systolic occlusion pressure in the erect state, recordings of the change in the diameter of the cavernosal artery in the flaccid and erect state, and selective internal pudendal arteriography in the erect state. The incidence of suspected vascular pathology by such vascular testing has ranged from 33 to 87%.[11]

Pharmacocavernosography of the erect penis in impotent men with diabetes typically shows a diffuse abnormality of draining veins in a diffuse pattern,[50,96,97] including the dorsal, cavernosal and crural veins, corpus spongiosum, and glans penis. It has been inferred from the diffuse pattern of abnormal vein visualization seen in patients with diabetes that the primary basis of the pathology is a pan-cavernosal pathology such as poor compliance or abnormal smooth muscle function (Fig. 46–4). The diffuse diabetic pattern is different from the pharmacocavernosographic pattern of abnormal visualization of veins in impotent patients with Peyronie's disease,[97] following trauma,[50] or as a consequence of a penile fracture.[98] The focal cavernosal pathology of these latter disorders is reflected by the focal site-specific abnormalities seen on pharmacocavernosography.

Endocrinologic Impotence

Studies in the 1940s through the 1960s demonstrated abnormal endocrinologic factors, primarily hypogonadotropic hypogonadism, in association with diabetic impotence. These conclusions were based on the presence of both pituitary gonadotropin and 17-ketosteroids in the urine and on the documentation of infiltration of testicular interstitial matrix with collagen-like material and abnormalities in the seminiferous tubules in testicular biopsy material.[5]

Endocrine studies of diabetic men done since the advent of radioimmunoassay analyses have had variable results.[6,7,51,99,100] Total serum testosterone values are not consistently altered in impotent men with diabetes. In some series, values have been normal or low or the magnitude of the increase following stimulation with human chorionic gonadotropin was attenuated in diabetic men. In one series, a deficit of gonadal function was inferred from high urinary excretion of luteinizing hormone and low serum-free testosterone levels. In another study,[101] a decrease in concentration of luteinizing hormone followed a lowering of the blood sugar level in impotent diabetic men but not in potent controls,

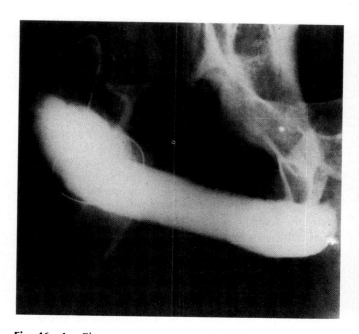 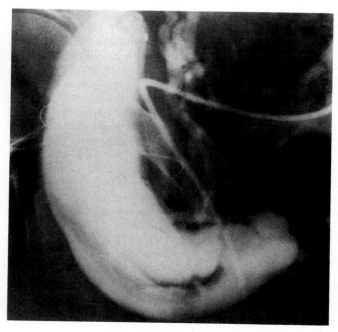

Fig. 46—4. Pharmacocavernosography following administration of intracavernosal vasoactive agents in an impotent nondiabetic patient with normal corporal veno-occlusion (left) and in an impotent diabetic patient with abnormal "diffuse" corporal veno-occlusion (right). In the nondiabetic patient, no veins draining the corporal body are visualized. In the diabetic patient, numerous veins draining the corporal body are visualized, including the dorsal vein (downward arrow) and corpus spongiosum (curved arrow).

suggesting that hyperglycemia may be responsible for these endocrine abnormalities.

The etiologic significance of the hypothalamic-pituitary-testicular axis in erectile dysfunction is unclear. Androgens influence the growth and development of the male reproductive tract and secondary sexual characteristics.[102] Their effect on libido and sexual behavior is well established,[103] but the effect of androgens on normal erectile physiology is poorly understood. Androgen receptor sites have been demonstrated in the sacral parasympathetic nucleus and on neurons on the hypothalamus and limbic system, suggesting possible hormonal regulation of these centers involved in erection. In animals castration has also been found to reduce the size of some motor neurons, dendritic length, the number of chemical synapses onto the somatic and dendritic membranes, and the gap junctions between motor neurons in the spinal nuclei.[104–106]

Patients with castration levels of testosterone can achieve erections comparable in quality to those achieved by men with normal levels of testosterone in response to visual sexual stimulation.[107] This observation suggests that the neurovascular mechanisms that control erection are functional in the presence of low levels of androgens. On the other hand, it has been shown that hypogonadal men have decreased nocturnal penile erectile activity and show improved activity when they receive androgen replacement.[103]

Thyroid disease, pituitary disorders, adrenal disease, and hyperprolactinemia, in addition to hypogonadism, may all be associated with erectile dysfunction in men

with diabetes. One study found serum prolactin to be similar in normal and diabetic patients, while another study reported an above-average incidence of hyperprolactinemia in diabetic patients.[99,108] In patients with hyperprolactinemia, declining libido and impotence can be early symptoms. Hyperprolactinemia is associated with low circulating levels of testosterone, which appear to be secondary to the inhibition by elevated prolactin levels of normal pulsation of gonadotropin-releasing hormone. In approximately one-half of impotent patients with hyperprolactinemia and low testosterone levels, potency is not restored by normalization of serum testosterone levels, implying that prolactin may have an antagonistic effect on the peripheral action of testosterone.[1] Hyperthyroid states are commonly associated with diminished libido and, less frequently, with impotence. Impotence in hypothyroid states has been reported and may be secondary to associated low levels of testosterone secretion and elevated levels of prolactin.[108] Although endocrine-related impotence does not play a major role in the overall pathogenesis of diabetic impotence, a recognized hormonal abnormality may be amenable to medical treatment; thus, endocrine screening is recommended for impotent diabetic patients.

EVALUATION OF THE IMPOTENT DIABETIC PATIENT

The initial evaluation for impotence begins with a sexual, psychosocial, and medical history; a physical examination; and routine laboratory tests. The impressions discovered on the initial evaluation may subsequently be corroborated by a series of diagnostic examinations, such as neurologic, psychologic, hormonal, and vascular testing. There are many noninvasive and invasive tests of erectile function: e.g., nocturnal penile tumescence testing, penile Doppler ultrasonography, and penile biothesiometry. Additional diagnostic evaluations, such as response to visual sexual stimulation, cavernosal electrical activity, gravity cavernosometry, determination of corporal blood po$_2$, and cavernosal tissue biopsy have only recently been introduced. Most tests of erectile function are evolving, and their standardization and reliability have not been fully determined.[1]

After the initial evaluation of impotence, additional testing should be tailored to the individual patient. In general, there is no universally agreed upon diagnostic algorithm for the evaluation of all impotent patients. As a general rule, for the impotent patient with diabetes, sophisticated invasive testing should be considered only under unusual conditions.

As the organic diagnostic evaluation has become more intricate and sophisticated, primary organic factors influencing erectile performance in patients with diabetes are being found with increasing frequency. It should be stressed that the secondary psychologic reaction to these organic factors must not be ignored. Successful management of the impotent diabetic patient who has primary organic and secondary psychologic impotence demands attention to both dysfunctions.

TREATMENT OF DIABETES-RELATED IMPOTENCE

The options available for the treatment of diabetic erectile dysfunction will be discussed in the order of their invasiveness and will include nonhormonal and hormonal oral agents, vacuum erection devices, intracavernosal injections of vasoactive agents, implantation of penile prostheses, and surgical procedures directed toward the amelioration of arterial insufficiency and corporal veno-occlusive dysfunction.

Nonhormonal Therapy

The most widely used oral nonhormonal medication for the treatment of impotence has been yohimbine hydrochloride, an α_2-adrenergic blocking agent. Yohimbine has long been considered an aphrodisiac, and a report of its effect on erectile dysfunction was first published 25 years ago.[110] In a prospective double-blind placebo-controlled study in patients with predominantly organic disease, including patients with diabetes-related impotence, the rate of response to yohimbine was not statistically increased over that to placebo. However, 21% of the patients who received yohimbine achieved a complete response.[111,112]

Hormonal Therapy

Men with diabetic impotence who have hypogonadotropic or hypergonadotropic hypogonadism or hyperprolactinemia should receive hormonal therapy. Indiscriminate use of testosterone in impotent diabetic men should be avoided. Diabetic patients should be considered for testosterone replacement therapy only if the diagnosis of hypogonadism is based on several repeat determinations of low serum testosterone levels in early-morning specimens. In these cases, testosterone replacement is used to maintain normal serum levels of testosterone and restore potency and libido. Because of the relatively unpredictable serum levels obtained following oral administration of testosterone, testosterone enanthate should be administered intramuscularly in doses of 200 to 300 mg every 2 to 3 weeks. The amount and frequency of administration will vary with the individual and can be titrated.[113]

Testosterone may induce a marked increase in libido without exerting a positive effect on erectile capabilities in diabetic patients who do not have hypogonadal disorders. Oral preparations also may have hepatotoxic effects and produce abnormalities in serum lipid levels.[114] Lastly, many older impotent diabetic men may have adenocarcinoma of the prostate, and testosterone may increase the rate of growth of the adenocarcinoma.[115] Before testosterone replacement therapy is initiated in diabetic men older than 50, it would seem prudent to determine levels of prostate-specific antigen in serum and perhaps to perform transrectal ultrasound studies.

The treatment of hyperprolactinemia in patients with diabetes is 1) the cessation of medication causing hyperprolactinemia (e.g., estrogens, α-methyldopa), 2) the administration of bromocryptine, or 3) the surgical ablation or extirpation of a pituitary prolactin-secreting tumor. Treatment with exogenous testosterone to supplement the diminished levels of serum testosterone usually seen with this disorder does not appear to reverse the erectile dysfunction.[116,117]

Vacuum Constrictor Devices

Vacuum constrictive devices are a new and viable therapeutic option for diabetic patients with erectile dysfunction because of the absence of significant complications associated with the use of these devices and their high degree of acceptance among patients who elect to use them.[118-120] As a general rule, this treatment option should be offered to most patients with diabetic impotence. A variety of external penile appliances are now available for the management of diabetic impotence. The majority have three common components: a vacuum chamber, a vacuum pump that creates negative pressure within the chamber, and a constrictor or tension band that is applied to the base of the penis after erection is achieved. While standing, the patient places his penis in the chamber, which is attached to a pump mechanism that can produce a negative pressure within the chamber, thereby drawing blood into the penis to produce an erection-like state. When adequate tumescence and rigidity have been achieved, the patient transfers a constrictor band at the base of the chamber to the base of the penis, thereby "trapping" blood within the penis (Fig. 46–5).

Vacuum-induced erection is significantly different from a physiologically induced erection. The latter type is achieved by the initial relaxation of the corporal smooth

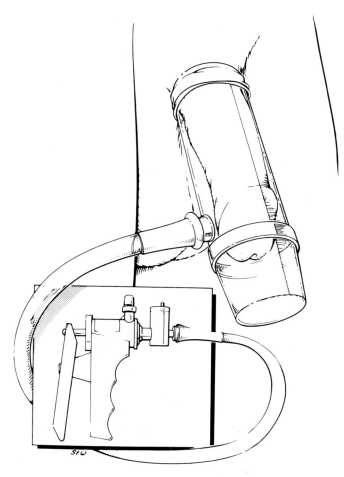

Fig. 46–5. Although many different devices are manufactured, the majority have three components in common: a vacuum chamber, a vacuum pump that creates negative pressure within the chamber, and a constrictor or tension band that is applied to the base of the penis after erection is achieved.

of the corpora.[122] In humans, vacuum constrictive devices may induce an expansion of penile diameter equal to or greater than that attained during a physiologically induced erection, presumably secondary to the entrapment of blood in extracorporeal tissues. Venous drainage from the corpora proximal to the constrictor device is not altered.[123]

Theoretically, in almost all impotent men so treated, the vacuum constrictor devices should create penile rigidity sufficient for vaginal penetration. Men with diabetic impotence who have had a penile prosthesis explanted may also be treated successfully with a vacuum constrictor device.[124] However, patients with significant intracorporeal scarring, such as those with severe Peyronie's disease, postpriapism, or previously infected penile implants, may not be able to develop adequate rigidity. Patients who do not obtain sufficient penile rigidity from intracavernosal pharmacotherapy alone could be candidates for a vacuum constrictor device used in conjunction with self-injection therapy.

To date the complications from the use of these devices have been minor and self-limited.[118–121] They have included difficulty with ejaculation, penile pain, ecchymoses, hematomas, and petechiae. Patients taking aspirin or warfarin are more likely to develop vascular complications. Many of the devices manufactured have a valve that limits the vacuum pressure (less than 250 mm Hg), a feature that might decrease the complication rate. Patient acceptance and satisfaction with vacuum constrictive devices in all types of impotence, including diabetic impotence, has been reported to be 68% to 83%. The reasons for discontinuation of this treatment have included premature loss of penile tumescence and rigidity, penile pain, pain during ejaculation, and inconvenience.[125]

Intracavernosal Injection of Vasoactive Agents

One of the most important advances in the treatment of impotence over the past decade has been self-administration by intracavernosal injection of vasoactive agents that either relax the corporal smooth musculature directly or block adrenergic tone of the corporal smooth muscle.[126] The pioneering work in this area involved the use of papaverine hydrochloride,[127] a direct smooth-muscle relaxant; or phenoxybenzamine[128] or phentolamine mesylate,[129] both α-adrenergic blocking agents. As the use of these agents became more clinically widespread, several issues became apparent. Intracavernosal injection of phentolamine alone was not as effective as papaverine in producing an erection. In addition, injection of papaverine alone was not as effective as injection of papaverine and phentolamine together. More recently, the synthetic prostanoid prostaglandin El, a direct smooth-muscle relaxant, has been successful when injected intracavernosally.[130] A variety of solutions containing the above agents are presently being used in clinical practice.[131]

The mechanism of action of papaverine hydrochloride and prostaglandin El is direct relaxation of smooth muscle. Therefore, injected intracavernosally they will maximize arterial inflow as well as corporal veno-

musculature, thus allowing for engorgement of blood into the lacunar spaces. With vacuum-induced erection, corporal smooth muscle relaxation does not occur initially and blood is simply trapped in both the intra- and extracorporeal compartments of the penis. Venous stasis and decreased arterial inflow are observed from the constricting band at the base of the penis to the glans penis distally. This may result in penile distension, edema, and cyanosis if the device is used for too long. In most cases, manufacturers recommend that the vacuum-induced erection be maintained for less than 30 minutes. Second, a physiologically induced erection will cause rigidity along the entire length of the corpora, whereas a vacuum-induced erection causes rigidity only distal to the constricting band, permitting the penis to pivot at its base.

In monkeys, increases in cross-sectional corporal area secondary to vacuum-induced erections were found to be only 50% of those induced by intracavernosal papaverine (see below). This limited corporal expansion may be secondary to the continued smooth muscle contraction occlusion by relaxing the arterial and trabecular smooth musculature, respectively. Phentolamine, on the other hand, blocks adrenergically induced muscle tone and therefore does not, by itself, initiate erections but does prolong the erectile response.[132]

Intracavernosal injections will work best in patients with diabetic impotence whose arterial inflow and corporal veno-occlusion mechanism are normal. These would include diabetic patients with purely neurogenic impotence or those with psychogenic impotence. Patients with diabetic impotence caused by arterial insufficiency also may respond by virtue of the long-acting and maximal dilator effects provided by this therapy. Diabetic patients whose impotence is caused by significant corporal veno-occlusive dysfunction, however, would be those least likely to respond to such therapy.[133]

In general, intracavernosal pharmacotherapy, like vacuum constrictor therapy, can be offered to most patients with organic diabetic impotence. Those diabetic patients with poor manual dexterity, poor visual acuity, or morbid obesity or those in whom a transient hypotensive episode may have deleterious consequences (e.g., patients with unstable cardiovascular disease and transient ischemic attacks) should be offered this option only after careful consideration. Diabetic patients taking aspirin or warfarin have been treated successfully with intracavernosal injections. Patients with significant psychiatric disease or who might misuse or abuse this therapy should be excluded from treatment. Once patients are offered intracavernosal pharmacotherapy, they should be informed of the risks and complications of this form of therapy and that it will not affect orgasm or ejaculation and is used solely for restoration of erectile capabilities. The usual therapeutic goal is the achievement of an erection rigid lasting 30 minutes to 1 hour that is rigid enough for satisfactory vaginal penetration.[133]

Diabetic patients who enter a program for pharmacologic treatment of inadequate erectile response should first be asked to read and sign a detailed informed consent form that states the known complications of this treatment and discusses the possibility of long-term side effects. A dosage-determination phase defines the lowest dose required for the achievement of an appropriate erectile response. Diabetic patients with purely neurogenic impotence would first be given an extremely low dose since they are the patients most likely to respond. Patients with vascular disease will usually first be given a higher dose, which is subsequently increased by increments. To minimize pain and bleeding, an insulin syringe with a 27- to 30-gauge needle usually is used. Patients also are taught to compress the site of injection for 3 minutes following injection. After an appropriate dose has been determined, the patient is instructed in proper injection techniques. When patients are in the more sexually stimulating home environment, it is very common for them to decrease the dose from that determined in the office. The patient also is instructed in sterile technique. Patients are told not to administer an injection more frequently than once a day.

Approximately 4000 impotent patients throughout the world, including many with diabetic impotence, who

have been treated with papaverine alone or in combination with phentolamine have been followed up.[134] Reported side effects have included hematomas, burning pain after injection, urethral damage, cavernositis or local infections, fibrotic changes of the corpora cavernosa, curvature, and prolonged erections or priapism. Cavernositis or infection has been extremely rare. Burning pain at the time of injection has been most common with prostaglandin El and appears to be less of a problem when prostaglandin El is mixed with other agents. Hematomas were noted in a small percentage of patients undergoing autoinjection therapy; these usually resolve within a few days without any permanent sequelae.

The two most important complications are prolonged erections and localized fibrotic changes of the corpora cavernosum. Prolonged erections usually occur during the dosage-determination phase and have been reported in 2.3 to 15% of all patients treated. Patients must be cautioned to call their physician if an erection persists for 4 hours or longer. In the majority of patients, these prolonged erections will detumesce on their own; however, some patients will require an intracavernosal injection of an α-adrenergic agonist such as epinephrine, phenylephrine, or metaraminol. An initial intracavernosal injection of 200 μg of phenylephrine has been successful and may be repeated as necessary until detumescence.[135] Following the dosage-determination phase, the complication of prolonged erection is quite rare (less than 1% of injections) and, if treated according to the protocol described above, should not produce any permanent sequelae.

The most frequent side effect (reported in 1.5 to 60% of patients treated for 1 year) of intracavernosal pharmacologic therapy is the formation of painless fibrotic nodules within the corpora cavernosa, which sometimes leads to penile curvature. In one series, the development of fibrotic nodules was related to the frequency of injection and the duration of treatment.[136] The complications of corporal fibrosis and prolonged erections have been seen less frequently in men treated with prostaglandin El alone. We feel that the formation of cavernosal fibrotic nodules is to some extent secondary to trauma and bleeding within the corpus and for this reason stress the importance of application of compression over the injection site for 3 minutes.

In addition, attempts to decrease the amount of fluid injected are encouraged. The goal of therapy is the injection of less than 0.5 mL of drug mixture intracavernosally. Diabetic patients injecting 1 mL or more of the papaverine and phentolamine mixture can reduce this volume by adding prostaglandin El—thus the use of a three-drug mixture.

There have been several cases of diffuse fibrosis of the corpora following intracavernosal injections. These have almost invariably been associated with markedly prolonged erections. A patient with diffuse fibrosis following the administration of a test dose of intracavernosal papaverine that led to a prolonged erection lasting more than 36 hours was treated successfully with intracavernosal injection of a combination of papaverine and phentolamine.[137] Therefore, the degree of corporal scarring and fibrosis required to obviate the positive results of intracavernosal pharmacotherapy has not been determined.

Systemic side effects of this treatment have included vasovagal episodes and syncope, which are probably related to hypotension. These side effects are infrequent and usually occur during the dosage-determination phase. It would be expected that diabetic patients with significant corporal veno-occlusive dysfunction will exhibit an increase in systemic distribution of intracavernosal agents and therefore be more susceptible to this side effect. As mentioned above, diabetic patients for whom transient hypotensive episodes may have significant deleterious effects should be carefully evaluated before receiving this therapy. Intracavernosal pharmacotherapy with papaverine has been associated with hepatotoxicity. In the first 201 patients we treated, only three cases (1.5%) of abnormal liver function tests were reported during a mean follow-up period of 26 months.[135] Others have seen essentially no changes in liver function during this therapy, while one series reported at least one chemical abnormality of liver function in 40% of patients.

Penile Prostheses

The urologic subspecialty of erectile dysfunction developed in the early 1970s, following the development of an intracorporeal penile prosthesis by Small and Carrion[138] and Scott et al.[139] Through the 1970s and early 1980s, the development of penile prostheses proceeded along two distinct lines: the malleable or rigid prosthesis and the multicomponent inflatable prosthesis. Self-contained inflatable devices were introduced more recently. Last, modifications of the three-piece inflatable device subsequently led to the introduction of a two-piece inflatable device.

Initially, the postoperative complication rate following placement of malleable devices was relatively low and implantation was relatively simple. Therefore, the rates of component failure and reoperation were kept to a minimum. With these devices, the length and girth of the penis do not change in the "tumescent" and "detumescent" phases, which at times results in an aesthetically less desirable "detumescent" phase. The inflatable devices, unlike the malleable devices, are based on hydraulic principles, thus allowing the patient to inflate and deflate the device to simulate tumescent and nontumescent phases. This provided an improved aesthetic result, especially in the "detumescent" phase, but initially was coupled with a relative increase in component failure and reoperation. Activation of the multicomponent inflatable device allows for an increase in penile girth during the "tumescent" phase.[50]

Subsequent improvements of inflatable devices have markedly reduced the likelihood of reoperation and component failure (Fig. 46–6). Self-contained inflatable devices have been designed to preserve the aesthetic qualities of an inflatable device and combine them with ease of surgical implantation and a potential decrease in component failure. Further ease of implantation of an inflatable device was attained with the introduction of

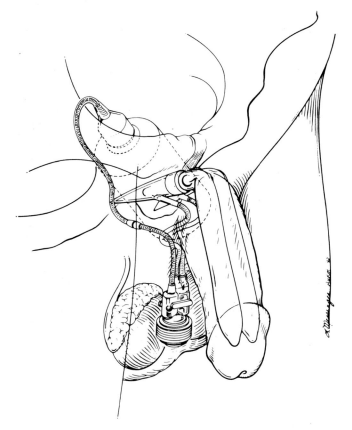

Fig. 46–6. Inflatable devices are based on hydraulic principles, thus allowing the patient to inflate and deflate the device to simulate tumescent and nontumescent phases. The multicomponent device depicted, a Mentor Alpha-1, allows for an increase in penile girth during the simulated tumescent phase. The three components consist of a reservoir placed in the retropubic space, two penile cylinders placed in the corpora cavernosa, and a pump apparatus with inflate and deflate mechanisms placed in the scrotum. The advantage of this device is its lack of connectors or connector components between the pump and the cylinders, the known high-pressure portion of a hydraulic device.

two-piece inflatable devices. The second- and third-generation prostheses have been designed to increase aesthetic results, increase penile girth at times, decrease the likelihood for component failure, and, when possible, facilitate implantation.

With the advent of newer treatments such as intracavernosal pharmacotherapy and vacuum erection devices, many physicians now consider the implantation of a penile prosthesis the last treatment option for impotence. Thus, penile implantation is offered to diabetic patients with organic impotence after other, nonsurgical, forms of therapy, such as vacuum constrictive devices or intracavernosal pharmacotherapy, have been attempted and failed. Patients whose impotence is thought to be psychogenic and who have not responded to appropriate psychological or behavioral sex therapy and have no psychological contraindications for therapy may be treated in the same manner.

Certainly, appropriate counseling of diabetic patients before implantation of a prosthesis is essential to the success of this surgery. The purpose of the prosthesis is to simulate an erection by providing penile rigidity sufficient for intercourse. The ability of the patient to ejaculate and have an orgasm is not altered by the implantation of a prosthesis but in some cases may be restored. In addition, diabetic patients undergoing the surgery should be informed of the potential complications of prosthetic surgery, as well as of their frequencies and sequelae. The postoperative complications of penile implant surgery usually are relegated to those of component failure, postoperative infection, or device erosion. Probably the most significant complication of prosthetic surgery is infection. The best defense against infection is prophylaxis. We request that patients scrub their genitalia and perineum for 10 minutes each day for 7 days with chlorhexidine digluconate soap (e.g., Hibiclens) before surgery.[50] Patients also are given intravenous perioperative antibiotics, and surgical technique must be meticulous. The incidence of infections following penile prosthetic surgery ranges between 1 and 9%.[140]

Following implantation, the time frame for the presentation of infection will vary depending on the organism involved. Infections with more virulent and aggressive bacteria will usually present within the first few postoperative days, with the patient presenting with fever, pain, and swelling overlying the prosthesis accompanied by purulent wound drainage. However, a group of patients will complain of prolonged pain overlying the device but will have not obvious purulent drainage from the wound. Prolonged pain, fixation of the pump or tubing to the overlying scrotal skin, and elevated white blood cell count and sedimentation rate may all be helpful in diagnosing a possible infection by less virulent organisms.

The reoperative rate for penile prosthetic surgery has been reported to be between 3 and 44%, with newer series showing a markedly lower rate.[141] Penile prostheses have been accepted by patients and physicians worldwide, with over 80% of patients reporting satisfaction after prosthetic surgery.[50]

Vascular Surgery

Arterial Procedures

The aim of arterial reconstructive surgery for impotence is to increase blood flow to the penis by bypassing arterial obstruction. Microvascular bypass procedures were introduced for the treatment of erectile dysfunction in the early 1970s.[151] These procedures showed that bringing a new source of blood to the corporal tissue could restore potency, albeit for a short time.

Contemporary procedures of penile microvascular arterial bypass involve anastomosis of either the inferior epigastric artery or a dorsal artery to an isolated deep dorsal penile vein segment, the proximal dorsal penile artery, or some combination of the above.[143] It appears that patient selection for these procedures is most critical and strongly influences the results of this surgery. The best candidates appear to be younger men with discrete lesions in the pudendal artery, the common penile artery, or both as a result of pelvic or perineal trauma, rather than older men with more generalized arteriosclerotic occlusive disease involving the hypogastric system.[143,144] Surgical technique and adherence to principles of vascular and microvascular surgery, especially those that result in preservation of endothelium, are also essential for anastomotic patency.

Diabetic patients are thus only rarely considered good candidates for the procedure. Those who are considered should have undergone some form of sophisticated arterial examination as well as pharmacocavernosometry, pharmacocavernosography, and pudendal arteriography.

Venous Procedures

At present, most diabetic patients who show evidence of corporal veno-occlusive dysfunction by pharmacocavernosometry and cavernosography should not be considered for surgical and/or radiologic options to increase venous outflow resistance.[144,152] In diabetic patients, the dysfunction may be related to a pancavernosal alteration in corporal tissue compliance. In such patients, cavernosography may reveal a more generalized corporal veno-occlusive dysfunction with visualization of the glans, corpus spongiosum, dorsal vein, and cavernosal vein. The available procedures—crural plication, ligation, or excision of the deep dorsal vein of the penis; ligation of cavernosal veins; spongiolysis; or a combination of the above, including the radiologic administration of coils or sclerosing agents—have not demonstrated long-term success in impotent diabetic patients.[146,147] Complications reported from the various procedures, especially those involving proximal penile dissection, include diminished penile sensation and shortened penile length.

REFERENCES

1. Krane RJ, Goldstein I, Saenz de Tejada I. Impotence. N Engl J Med 1989;321:1648–59.
2. Kinsey AC, Pomeroy W, Martin C. Age and sexual outlet. In: Kinsey AC, Pomeroy W, Martin, C, eds. Sexual behavior in the human male. Philadelphia: WB Saunders, 1948:218.
3. Goldstein I. The effect of AIDS-related diseases on the development of impotence [Abstract]. In: National Institutes of Health Consensus Development Conference on Impotence, Bethesda, MD, December 7–9, 1992.
4. Rubin A, Babbott D. Impotence and diabetes mellitus. JAMA 1958;168:498–500.
5. Schöffling K, Federlin K, Ditschuneit H, et al. Disorders of sexual function in male diabetics. Diabetes 1963; 12:519–27.
6. Ellenberg M. Impotence in diabetes: the neurologic factor. Ann Intern Med 1971;75:213–9.
7. Kolodny RC, Kahn CB, Goldstein HH, Barnett DM. Sexual dysfunction in diabetic men. Diabetes 1974;23:306–9.
8. Renshaw DC. Impotence in diabetics. Dis Nerv Syst 1975; 36:369–71.
9. McCulloch DK, Campbell IW, Wu FC, et al. The prevalence of diabetic impotence. Diabetologia 1980; 18:279–83.

10. Lester E, Grant AJ, Woodroffe FJ. Impotence in diabetic and non-diabetic hospital outpatients. BMJ 1980;281: 354–5.

11. Goldstein I, Siroky MB, Krane RJ. Impotence in diabetes mellitus. In: Krane RJ, Siroky MB, Goldstein I, eds. Male sexual dysfunction. Boston: Little, Brown and Co, 1983: 77–86.

12. Masters WH, Johnson VE. Human sexual inadequacy. Boston: Little, Brown and Co, l970.

13. Goldstein AMB, Meehan JP, Zakhary R, et al. New observations on microarchitecture of corpora cavernosa in man and possible relationship to mechanism of erection. Urology 1982;20:259–66.

14. Lue TF, Tanagho EA. Functional anatomy and mechanism of penile erection. In: Tanagho EA, Lue TF, McClue RD, eds. Contemporary management of impotence and infertility. Baltimore: Williams & Wilkins, 1988:39–50.

15. Puech-Leão P, Reis JMSM, Glina S, Reichelt AC. Leakage through the crural edge of corpus cavernosum: diagnosis and treatment. Eur Urol 1987;13:163–5.

16. de Groat WC, Steers WD. Neuroanatomy and neurophysiology of penile erection. In: Tanagho EA, Lue TF, McClue RD, eds. Contemporary management of impotence and infertility. Baltimore: Williams & Wilkins, 1988:3–27.

17. Weiss HD. The physiology of human penile erection. Ann Intern Med 1972;76:793–9.

18. Hart BL, Leedy MG. Neurological bases of male sexual behavior: a comparative analysis. In: Adler N, Pfaff D, Goy RW, eds. Handbook of behavioral neurobiology. Vol 7. Reproduction. New York: Plenum, 1985:373–422.

19. MacLean PD, Ploog DW. Cerebral representation of penile erection. J Neurophysiol 1962;25:29–55.

20. MacLean PD, Denniston RH, Dua S. Further studies on cerebral representation of penile erection: caudal thalamus, midbrain, and pons. J Neurophysiol 1963; 26:274–93.

21. Dua S, MacLean PD. Localization for penile erection in medial frontal lobe. Am J Physiol 1964;207:1425–34.

22. Saper CB, Loewy AD, Swanson LW, Cowan WM. Direct hypothalamo-autonomic connections. Brain Res 1976; 117:305–12.

23. Swanson LW, Sawchenko PE. Hypothalamic integration: organization of the paraventricular and supraoptic nuclei. Annu Rev Neurosci 1983;6:269–324.

24. Saenz de Tejada I, Goldstein I, Blanco R, et al. Smooth muscle of the corpora cavernosae: role in penile erection. Surg Forum 1985;36:623–4.

25. Lue TF, Tanagho EA. Physiology of erection and pharmacological management of impotence. J Urol 1987; 137:829–36.

26. McConnell J, Benson GS. Innervation of human penile blood vessels. Neurourol Urodynam 1982;1:199–210.

27. Benson GS, McConnell J, Lipshultz LI. Neuromorphology and neuropharmacology of the human penis: an in vitro study. J Clin Invest 1980;65:506–13.

28. Benson GS. Penile erection: in search of a neurotransmitter. World J Urol 1983;1:209–12.

29. Adrian TE, Gu J, Allen JM, et al. Neuropeptide Y in the human male genital tract. Life Sci 1984;35:2643–8.

30. Polak JM, Gu J, Mina S, Bloom SR. Vipergic nerves in the penis. Lancet 1981;2:217–9.

31. Hedlund H, Andersson K-E. Comparison of the responses to drugs acting on adrenoreceptors and muscarinic receptors in human isolated corpus cavernosum and cavernous artery. J Auton Pharmacol 1985;5:81–8.

32. Kimoto Y, Ito Y. Autonomic innervation of the canine penile artery and vein in relation to neural mechanisms involved in erection. Br J Urol 1987;59:463–72.

33. Saenz de Tejada I, Blanco R, Goldstein I, et al. Cholinergic neurotransmission in human corpus cavernosum. I. Responses of isolated tissue. Am J Physiol 1988; 254:H459–67.

34. Blanco R, Saenz de Tejada I, Goldstein I, et al. Cholinergic neurotransmission in human corpus cavernosum. II. Acetylcholine synthesis. Am J Physiol 1988;254:H468–72.

35. Ignarro LJ, Bush PA, Buga GM, et al. Nitric oxide and cyclic GMP formation upon electrical field stimulation cause relaxation of corpus cavernosum smooth muscle. Biochem Biophys Res Comm 1990;170:843–50.

36. Gillespie JS, Liu X, Martin W. The effects of L-arginine and N⁶-monomethyl L-arginine on the response of the rat anococcygeus muscle to NANC nerve stimulation. Br J Pharmacol 1989;98:1080–2.

37. Bult H, Boeckxstaens GE, Pelckmans PA, et al. Nitric oxide as an inhibitory non-adrenergic non-cholinergic neurotransmitter. Nature 1990;345:346–7.

38. Bredt DS, Hwang PM, Snyder SH. Localization of nitric oxide synthase indicating a neural role for nitric oxide. Nature 1990;347:768–70.

39. Kim N, Azadzoi KM, Goldstein I, Saenz de Tejada I. A nitric oxide-like factor mediates nonadrenergic-noncholinergic neurogenic relaxation of penile corpus cavernosum smooth muscle. J Clin Invest 1991;88:112–8.

40. Furchgott RF, Zawadzki JV. The obligatory role of endothelial cells in the relaxation of arterial smooth muscle by acetylcholine. Nature 1980;288:373–6.

41. Palmer RMJ, Ferrige AG, Moncada S. Nitric oxide release accounts for the biological activity of endothelium-derived relaxing factor. Nature 1987;327:524–6.

42. Vane JR, Änggärd EE, Botting RM. Regulatory functions of the vascular endothelium. N Engl J Med 1990;323:27–36.

43. Jensen SB. Sexual dysfunction in insulin-treated diabetics: a six-year follow-up study of 101 patients. Arch Sex Behav 1986;15:271–83.

44. Karacan I, Salis PJ, Catesby J, et al. Nocturnal penile tumescence and diagnosis in diabetic impotence. Am J Psychiatry 1978;135:191–7.

45. Deutsch S, Sherman L. Previously unrecognized diabetes mellitus in sexually impotent men. JAMA 1980; 244:2430–2.

46. Saenz de Tejada I, Goldstein I. Diabetic penile neuropathy. Urol Clin North Am 1988;15:17–22.

47. Campbell IW. Diabetic autonomic neuropathy. Br J Clin Pract 1976;30:153.

48. Fairburn CG, McCulloch DK, Wu FC. The effects of diabetes on male sexual function. Clin Endocrinol Metab 1982;11:749–67.

49. McCullock DK, Young RJ, Prescott RS. The natural history of impotence in diabetic men. Diabetologia 1980;18:279.

50. Goldstein I, Krane RJ. Diagnosis and therapy of erectile dysfunction. In: Walsh PC, Retik AB, Stamey TA, Vaughan ED Jr, eds. Campbell's urology. 6th ed. Philadelphia: WB Saunders 1992:3033–72.

51. Faerman I, Vilar O, Rivarola MA, et al. Impotence and diabetes: studies of androgenic function in diabetic impotent males. Diabetes 1972;21:23–30.

52. Nisen HO, Alfthan OS, Lindstrom BL, et al. Single breath beat-to-beat variation testing in the diagnosis of autonomic neuropathy in impotence. Int J Impotence Res 1990;2(Suppl 2):136.

53. Wagner G, Gerstenberg T, Levin RJ. Electrical activity of corpus cavernosum during flaccidity and erection of the

human penis: a new diagnostic method. J Urol 1989; 142:723–5.

54. Stief CG, Djamilian M, Schaebsdau F, et al. Single potential analysis of cavernous electric activity—a possible diagnosis of autonomic impotence? World J Urol 1990;8:75.

55. Buvat J, Quittelier E, Lemaire A, et al. Electromyography of the human penis, including single potential analysis during flaccidity and erection induced by vasoactive agents. Int J Impotence Res 1990;2(Suppl 2):85.

56. Ertekin C, Akjürekli Ö, Gürses AN, Turgut H. The value of somatosensory-evoked potentials and bulbocavernosus reflex in patients with impotence. Acta Neurol Scand 1985;71:48–53.

57. Newman HF. Vibratory sensitivity of the penis. Fertil Steril 1970;21:791–3.

58. Goldstein I. Electromyography: evoked-response evaluations. In: Barrett DM, Wein AJ, eds. Controversies in neuro-urology, New York: Churchill Livingstone, 1984; 3D:117–29.

59. Padma-Nathan H, Goldstein I. Neurologic assessment of the impotent male. In: Montague DK, ed. Disorders of male sexual functions. Chicago: Year Book Medical Publications, 1987:86–94.

60. Faerman I, Glocer L, Fox D, et al. Impotence and diabetes: histological studies of the autonomic nervous fibers of the corpora cavernosa in impotent diabetic males. Diabetes 1974;23:971–6.

61. Fani K, Lundin AP, Beyer MM, et al. Pathology of the penis in long-term diabetic rats. Diabetologia 1983;25:424–8.

62. Saenz de Tejada I, Andry C, Blanco R, et al. Ultrastructural studies of autonomic nerves within the corpus cavernosum of impotent diabetic patients. In: Virag H, Virag R, eds. Proceedings of the First World Meeting on Impotence. Paris: Les Editions du Ceri, 1986:210–4.

63. Porte D Jr, Graf RJ, Halter JB, et al. Diabetic neuropathy and plasma glucose control. Am J Med 1981;70:195–200.

64. Clements RS Jr. Peripheral nerve biochemistry in diabetes. Clin Physiol 1985;5(Suppl 5):19–22.

65. Melman A, Henry DP, Felten DL, O'Connor B. Effect of diabetes upon penile sympathetic nerves in impotent patients. South Med J 1980;73:307–9.

66. Lincoln J, Crowe R, Blacklay PF, et al. Changes in the vipergic, cholinergic and adrenergic innervation of human penile tissue in diabetic and non-diabetic impotent males. J Urol 1987;137:1053–9.

67. Saenz de Tejada I, Goldstein I, Azadzoi K, et al. Impaired neurogenic and endothelium-mediated relaxation of penile smooth muscle from diabetic men with impotence. N Engl J Med 1989;320:1025–30.

68. Blanco R, Saenz de Tejada I, Goldstein I, et al. Dysfunctional penile cholinergic nerves in diabetic impotent men. J Urol 1990:144:278–80.

69. Gu J, Polak JM, Lazarides M, et al. Decrease of vasoactive intestinal polypeptide (VIP) in the penises from impotent men. Lancet 1984;2:315–8.

70. Crowe R, Lincoln J, Blacklay PF, et al. Vasoactive intestinal polypeptide-like immunoreactive nerves in diabetic penis: a comparison between streptozotocin-treated rats and man. Diabetes 1983;32:1075–7.

71. Ruzbarsky V, Michal V. Morphologic changes in the arterial bed of the penis with aging: relationship to the pathogenesis of impotence. Invest Urol 1977;15:194–9.

72. Herman A, Adar R, Rubinstein Z. Vascular lesions associated with impotence in diabetic and nondiabetic arterial occlusive disease. Diabetes 1978;27:975–81.

73. Jager E. Beitrage zur Pathologie des Auges. Vienna 1855.

74. Ashton N. Vascular changes in diabetes with particular reference to the retinal vessels: preliminary report. Br J Ophthalmol 1949:33:407–20.

75. McMillan DE. Deterioration of the microcirculation in diabetes. Diabetes 1975;24:944–57.

76. Colwell JA, Halushka PV, Sarji KE, et al. Vascular disease in diabetes: pathophysiological mechanisms and therapy. Arch Intern Med 1979;139:225–30.

77. Jünemann K-P, Persson-Jünemann C, Alken P. Pathophysiology of erectile dysfunction. Semin Urol 1990;8:80–93.

78. Virag R, Bouilly P, Frydman D. Is impotence an arterial disorder? A study of arterial risk factors in 440 impotent men. Lancet 1985;1:181–4.

79. Rosen MP, Greenfield AJ, Walker TG, et al. Arteriogenic impotence: findings in 195 impotent men examined with selective internal pudendal angiography. Radiology 1990; 174:1043–8.

80. Wetterauer U, Stief CG, Kulvelis F, et al. Ultrastructural changes of the cavernous tissue in erectile dysfunction. Proceedings of the Sixth Biennial International Symposium on Corpus Cavernosum Revascularization and Third Biennial World Meeting on Impotence. Boston, October 1988:11.

81. Persson C, Diederichs W, Lue TF, et al. Correlation of altered penile ultrastructure with clinical arterial evaluation. J Urol 1989;142:1462–8.

82. Jevtich MJ, Khawand NY, Vidic B. Clinical significance of ultrastructural findings in the corpora cavernosa of normal and impotent men. J Urol 1990;143:289–93.

83. Mersdorf A, Goldsmith PC, Diederichs W, et al. Ultrastructural changes in impotent penile tissue: a comparison of 65 patients. J Urol 1991;145:749–58.

84. Michal V, Pospíchal J. Phalloarteriography in the diagnosis of erectile impotence. World J Surg 1978;2:239–48.

85. Rosen MP, Greenfield AJ, Walker TG, et al. Cigarette smoking: an independent risk factor for atherosclerosis in the hypogastric-cavernous arterial bed of men with arteriogenic impotence. J Urol 1991;145:759–63.

86. Mottonen M, Nieminen K. Relation of atherosclerotic obstruction of the arterial supply of corpus cavernosum to erectile dysfunction. Proceedings of the Sixth Biennial International Symposium on Corpus Cavernosum Revascularization and Third Biennial World Meeting on Impotence. Boston, October 1988:12.

87. Aboseif SR, Breza J, Orvis BR, et al. Erectile response to acute and chronic occlusion of the internal pudendal and penile arteries. J Urol 1989;141:398–402.

88. Takagane H, Matsuzaka J, Aoki H, et al. Hemodynamic studies of penile erection in dogs: blood flow changes in the corpus cavernosum caused by arterial ligation. Proceedings of the Sixth Biennial International Symposium on Corpus Cavernosum Revascularization and Third Biennial World Meeting on Impotence. Boston, October 1988:13.

89. Rajfer J, Rosciszewski A, Mehringer M. Prevalence of corporeal venous leakage in impotent men. J Urol 1988; 140:69–71.

90. Fischer GM, Swain ML, Cherian K. Increased vascular collagen and elastin synthesis in experimental atherosclerosis in the rabbit: variation in synthesis among major vessels. Atherosclerosis 1980;35:11–20.

91. Pietilä K, Nikkari T. Enhanced synthesis of collagen and total protein by smooth muscle cells from atherosclerotic rabbit aortas in culture. Atherosclerosis 1980;37:11–9.

92. Ehrhart LA, Holderbaum D. Aortic collagen, elastin and non-fibrous protein synthesis in rabbits fed cholesterol and peanut oil. Atherosclerosis 1980;37:423–32.

93. Azadzoi KM, Saenz de Tejada I. Hypercholesterolemia impairs endothelium-dependent relaxation of rabbit corpus cavernosum smooth muscle. J Urol 1991; 146:238–40.

94. Abelson D, Diagnostic value of the penile pulse and blood pressure: a Doppler study of impotence in diabetics. J Urol 1975;113:636–9.

95. Karacan I. Diagnosis of erectile impotence in diabetes mellitus: an objective and specific method. Ann Intern Med 1980;92:334–7.

96. Goldstein I, Krane RJ, Greenfield AJ, Padma-Nathan H. Vascular diseases of the penis: impotence and priapism. In: Pollack HM, ed. Clinical urography. Vol 3. Philadelphia: WB Saunders, 1990:2231–52.

97. Gasior BL, Levine FJ, Howannesian A, et al. Plaque-associated corporal veno-occlusive dysfunction in idiopathic Peyronie's disease: a pharmacocavernosometric and pharmacocavernosographic study. World J Urol 1990; 8:90–6.

98. Penson DF, Seftel AD, Krane RJ, et al. The hemodynamic pathophysiology of impotence following blunt trauma to the erect penis. J Urol (in press).

99. Jensen SB, Hagen C, Frøland A, Pedersen PB. Sexual function and pituitary axis in insulin treated diabetic men. Acta Med Scand Suppl 1979;624:65–8.

100. Murray FT, Wyss HU, Thomas RG, et al. Gonadal dysfunction in diabetic men with organic impotence. J Clin Endocrinol Metab 1987;65:127–35.

101. Ziedler A, Gelfand R, Tamagna E, et al. Pituitary gonadal function in diabetic male patients with and without impotence. Andrologia 1982;14:62–8.

102. Wilson JD, George FW, Griffin JE. The hormonal control of sexual development. Science 1981;211:1278–84.

103. Kwan M, Greenleaf WJ, Mann J, et al. The nature of androgen action on male sexuality: a combined laboratory-self-report study on hypogonadal men. J Clin Endocrinol Metab 1983;57:557–62.

104. Sar M, Stumpf WE. Androgen concentration in motor neurons of cranial nerves and spinal cord. Science 1977;197:77–9.

105. Sar M, Stumpf WE. Distribution of androgen target cells in rat forebrain and pituitary after [$_3$H]-dihydrotestosterone administration. J Steroid Biochem 1977;8:1131–5.

106. Murray FT, Klimberg IW. Organic impotence. In: Bardin CW, ed. Current therapy in endocrinology and metabolism. Vol 3. Philadelphia: BC Decker, 1988:252–62.

107. Bancroft J, Wu FCW. Changes in erectile responsiveness during androgen replacement therapy. Arch Sex Behav 1983;12:59–66.

108. Mooradian AD, Morley JE, Billington CJ, et al. Hyperprolactinaemia in male diabetics. Postgrad Med J 1985; 61:11–4.

109. Pogach LM, Vaitukaitis JL. Endocrine disorders associated with erectile dysfunction. In: Krane RJ, Siroky MB, Goldstein I, eds. Male sexual dysfunction. Boston: Little, Brown and Co, 1983:63–76.

110. Margolis R, Prieto P, Stein L, Chinn S. Statistical summary of 10,000 male cases using Afrodex in treatment of impotence. Curr Ther Res 1971;13:616–22.

111. Morales A, Condra M, Owen JA, et al. Is yohimbine effective in the treatment of organic impotence? Results of a controlled trial. J Urol 1987;137:1168–72.

112. Morales A, Condra MS, Owen JE, et al. Oral and transcutaneous pharmacologic agents in the treatment of impotence. Urol Clin North Am 1988;15:87–93.

113. Snyder PJ, Lawrence DA. Treatment of male hypogonadism with testosterone enanthate. J Clin Endocrinol Metab 1980;51:1335–9.

114. Wilson JD, Griffin JE. The use and misuse of androgens. Metabolism 1980;29:1278–95.

115. Jackson JA, Waxman J, Spiekerman AM. Prostatic complications of testosterone replacement therapy. Arch Intern Med 1989;149:2365–6.

116. Carter JN, Tyson JE, Tolis G, et al. Prolactin-secreting tumors and hypogonadism in 22 men. N Engl J Med 1978; 299:847–52.

117. Franks S, Jacobs HS, Martin N, Nabarro JDN. Hyperprolactinaemia and impotence. Clin Endocrinol 1978; 8:277–87.

118. Nadig PW, Ware JC, Blumoff R. Noninvasive device to produce and maintain an erection-like state. Urology 1986;27:126–31.

119. Nadig PW. Vacuum erection devices. A review. World J Urol 1990;8:114–7.

120. Witherington R. Vacuum constriction device for management of erectile impotence. J Urol 1989;141:320–2.

121. Witherington R. External penile appliances for management of impotence. Semin Urol 1990;8:124–8.

122. Diederichs W, Kaula NF, Lue TF, Tanagho EA. The effect of subatmospheric pressure on the simian penis. J Urol 1989;142:1087–9.

123. Wespes E, Schulman CC. Hemodynamic study of the effect of vacuum device on human erection. Int J Impotence Res 1990;2(Suppl 2):337.

124. Moul JW, McLeod DG. Negative pressure devices in the explanted penile prosthesis population. J Urol 1989; 142:729–31.

125. Sidi AA, Becher EF, Zhang G, Lewis JH. Patient acceptance of and satisfaction with an external negative pressure device for impotence. J Urol 1990;144:1154–6.

126. Juenemann K-P, Lue TF, Fournier GR Jr, Tanagho EA. Hemodynamics of papaverine- and phentolamine-induced penile erection. J Urol 1986;136:158–61.

127. Virag R. Intracavernous injection of papaverine for erectile failure [Letter]. Lancet 1982;2:938.

128. Brindley GS. Pilot experiments on the actions of drugs injected into the human corpus cavernosum penis. Br J Pharmacol 1986;87:495–500.

129. Zorgniotti AW, Lefleur RS. Auto-injection of the corpus cavernosum with a vasoactive drug combination for vasculogenic impotence. J Urol 1985;133:39–41.

130. Stackl W, Hasun R, Marberger M. Intracavernous injection of prostaglandin E1 in impotent men. J Urol 1988; 140:66–8.

131. Lee LM, Stevenson RWD, Szasz G. Prostaglandin E1 versus phentolamine/papaverine for the treatment of erectile impotence: a double-blind comparison. J Urol 1989; 141:549–50.

132. Azadzoi KM, Payton T, Krane RJ, Goldstein I. Effects of intracavernosal trazodone hydrochloride: animal and human studies. J Urol 1990;144:1277–82.

133. Padma-Nathan H, Goldstein I, Payton T, Krane RJ. Intracavernosal pharmacotherapy: the pharmacologic erection program. World J Urol 1987;5:160–5.

134. Zentgraf M, Baccouche M, Jünemann KP. Diagnosis and therapy of erectile dysfunction using papaverine and phentolamine. Urol Int 1988;43:65–75.

135. Padma-Nathan H, Goldstein I, Krane RJ. Treatment of prolonged or priapistic erections following intracavernosal papaverine therapy. Semin Urol 1986;4:236–8.

136. Levine SB, Althof SE, Turner LA, et al. Side effects of self-administration of intracavernous papaverine and

phentolamine for the treatment of impotence. J Urol 1989; 141:54–7.

137. Lakin MM, Montague DK. Intracavernous injection therapy in post-priapism cavernosal fibrosis. J Urol 1988; 140:828–9.

138. Small MP, Carrion HM. A new penile prosthesis for treating impotence. Contemp Surg 1975;7(2):29–33.

139. Scott FB, Bradley WE, Timm GW. Management of erectile impotence: use of implantable inflatable prosthesis. Urology 1973;2:80–2.

140. Carson CC. Infections in genitourinary prostheses. Urol Clin North Am 1989;16:139–47.

141. Kessler R. Surgical experience with the inflatable penile prosthesis. J Urol 1980;124:611–2.

142. Michal V, Kramář R, Pospíchal J, Hejhal L. Direct arterial anastomosis on corporal cavernosa penis in therapy of erectile impotence. Rozhl Chir 1973;52:587–90.

143. Levine FJ, Goldstein I. Vascular reconstructive surgery in the management of erectile dysfunction. Int J Impotence Res 1990;2:59–78.

144. Levine FJ, Greenfield AJ, Goldstein I. Arteriographically determined occlusive disease within the hypogastric cavernous bed in impotent patients following blunt perineal and pelvic trauma. J Urol 1990;144:1147–53.

145. Sharlip ID. The role of vascular surgery in arteriogenic and combined arteriogenic and venogenic impotence. Semin Urol 1990;8:129–37.

146. Bar-Moshé O, Vandendris M. Treatment of impotence due to perineal venous leakage by ligation of crura penis. J Urol 1988;139:1217–9.

147. Lewis RW. Venous surgery for impotence. Urol Clin North Am 1988;15;115–21.

Chapter 47

INFECTION AND DIABETES

DEBORAH E. SENTOCHNIK
GEORGE M. ELIOPOULOS

It is commonly believed that the incidence of infection is higher in persons with diabetes mellitus and that such infections in the diabetic person result in complications and death more frequently than would be anticipated in otherwise healthy individuals.[1,2] Older studies, upon which much of this information is based, focus particularly on infections of the urinary tract, respiratory tree, and the extremities and derive their data from autopsy cases. However, in these studies the degree to which infection at these sites actually contributed to the cause of death is frequently not clear, and control groups are typically lacking. More recent studies, while documenting excess mortality among patients with diabetes, have ascribed this largely to cardiovascular disease rather than to uncontrolled infection.[3,4] For example, pneumonia did not cause an increase in the mortality rate over that in age- and sex-matched controls, and infections of the urinary tract and extremities were not further categorized.[3,4]

In diabetes mellitus, a number of factors greatly complicate efforts to assess risk of infection and resulting complications. The most basic is the problem of determining an appropriate estimate of the population at risk,

which may be difficult to obtain for diabetes and is rarely if ever presented. Furthermore, in diabetes, as with other chronic diseases in which the natural history may span decades in any individual, historical controls are of limited utility, given the expected improvements in the general health of a population, the development of more effective diagnostic techniques, earlier medical intervention, and the availability of expanded therapeutic options, including the availability of more active and better tolerated antimicrobial agents. A number of variables, including duration of illness, severity of noninfectious complications, concurrent illnesses, level of glucose control, and even degree of medical supervision, result in a very heterogeneous group of individuals at risk even within a more narrowly defined time frame. Finally, some infections that may be particular to diabetics, such as emphysematous cholecystitis, are so uncommon that information regarding risk factors and management options is limited.

Despite these limitations, much is known both about those uncommon infections that occur predominantly in patients with diabetes mellitus and about the more common infections that, while not restricted to those with diabetes, will often complicate the general management of this group of patients. To acknowledge such limitations in advance is to underscore the need for careful individualization in the approach to diagnosis and therapy for any diabetic patient with suspected or proven infection.

DIABETES AND THE IMMUNE SYSTEM

Defining altered host responses in diabetes has long been hampered both by the complexity of the systems in question and by the as yet rather elementary approaches available for evaluating these responses. In vivo the various arms of the immune system are highly dynamic and interdependent. It is thus simplistic to study any single component of it "in vacuo." Historically, however, methodologic constraints did in fact limit such studies to individual aspects of host defenses, such as leukocyte adherence or phagocytosis, exclusive of other components of the system. Even more recent has been an increase in the appreciation of complex interactions not only among the various cellular elements of the immune system itself but also among the elements of the immune system and other body components such as the vascular endothelium. As the approaches to the investigation of these issues evolve, it becomes increasingly more difficult to compare studies. It is for these reasons that, even after decades of investigation, questions about whether diabetes itself results in specific immunologic defects and how such defects might predispose to infection are still actively debated.[5]

Function of Polymorphonuclear Leukocytes

Mobilization and Chemotaxis

Using the Rebuck skin window technique, which was to remain the standard for many years, Perillie et al.[6] studied polymorphonuclear leukocyte (PMN) chemotaxis in 10 patients with well-controlled diabetes, 6 patients with diabetic ketoacidosis, 4 patients with nondiabetic uremic acidosis, and 10 healthy controls. An abrasion was created on the volar forearm, and sterile cover slips were serially applied over the next several hours. Mobilization of PMNs to the area of inflammation was graded by microscopic examination of the cover slip after staining. There was a diminished early (24-hour) response by the PMNs of all acidotic patients. This response time became normal in the 4 diabetic patients whose acidosis was corrected. In an ambitious analysis of leukocyte function, Brayton et al.[7] examined chemotaxis with use of a modified Rebuck technique in 18 patients with fairly well controlled diabetes, 5 of whom were acidotic at the time of study. At 2 and 4 hours, mobilization of the PMNs of all diabetic subjects was diminished. However, at later time points, no differences were seen between the mobilization responses of the PMNs of diabetic subjects and those of healthy controls. The PMNs of acidotic uremic patients had a chemotactic response similar to that of controls at all time points.

Mowat and Baum[8] studied chemotaxis of PMNs from 31 diabetic patients with various degrees of glycemic control in vitro with use of a modified tissue culture chamber. A chemotactic index (CI) was derived by comparing the original number of PMNs with the number that had completely crossed a filter barrier in response to chemoattractants. A lower CI (i.e., diminished response) was found in the PMNs of all patient with diabetes, without any correlation being seen between CI and type of therapy or fasting blood glucose levels. Incubation of the PMNs from 11 controls with glucose at concentrations of 100 to 900 mg/dL did not change the CI of the PMNs. Incubation of the PMNs of diabetic patients with insulin at concentrations of 10 to 100 μU/mL improved the CI of PMNs of the diabetic patients if glucose was also present. Molenaar et al.[9] employed a bacterial factor from Escherichia coli as a chemoattractant and found a lower CI for the PMNs of 52 first-degree relatives of 15 patients with diabetes as compared with the CI of controls. Not all the diabetic subjects had PMNs with a depressed CI, but the average CI was lower than that for the PMNs of their relatives. A later study,[10] in which a similar technique was used (Boyden's modified chamber) but the cells also were washed free of plasma, found no difference in the CI of the PMNs of control subjects and those of patients with insulin-dependent diabetes (IDDM) with various degrees of glucose control or duration of disease.

Shortly after the above studies were conducted, there was a shift to the sub-agarose technique for assaying chemotaxis. This technique yields more reproducible results and corrects for chemokinetic movement. Measurements are made of the migration from a center well in an agarose plate toward a chemoattractant (zymogen-activated plasma) and of random migration toward a control well. With this technique, the average CI of the PMNs of 58 diabetic patients was found to be depressed.[11] Chemically defined chemotactic activity of PMNs under agarose was investigated by Naghibi et al.[12] for 26 patients receiving oral hyperglycemic agents, daily insulin injections, or continuous insulin infusion before an intensive control regimen and in 11 of these patients after institution of the intensive regimen. Chemotaxis of the PMNs of all groups was comparable to that of control PMNs.

Phagocytosis

Bybee and Rogers[13] studied leukocyte phagocytosis in 31 patients with well-controlled diabetes, 7 patients with diabetic acidosis, and a control group. Washed PMNs and an equal number of Staphylococcus aureus or Staphylococcus epidermidis were incubated together for 60 minutes in 10% human serum. Phagocytosis was considered to be present if at least one bacterium was ingested. There was no quantitation of the number of organisms engulfed per cell. Only the PMNs of ketotic diabetic patients were found to exhibit diminished phagocytosis. This defect was corrected if acidosis was reversed but not if the cells were incubated with normal serum. Control PMNs functioned normally if they were incubated with serum from acidotic diabetic patients. However, serum factors may have been diluted out, given that a 10% concentration of serum was employed.

Bagdade et al.[14] used a similar system, but with 90% serum, to examine phagocytosis of *Streptococcus pneumoniae* type 25 by leukocytes from eight patients who were not acidotic but had poorly controlled diabetes. Decreased phagocytosis was especially notable when fasting blood glucose levels were greater than 250 mg/dL. After glucose was controlled, phagocytic activity improved but did not attain control values. In contrast to the findings of Bybee and Rogers,[13] the activity of control PMNs was diminished when the cells were incubated with serum from diabetic patients, whereas the activity of PMNs from diabetic patients was increased when they were incubated with normal serum. The work of Rayfield et al.[15] supports the possibility of an opsonization defect in the PMNs of individuals with diabetes. Normal PMNs had decreased uptake of radiolabeled *Escherichia coli* or *Staphylococcus aureus* in the presence of serum from diabetic patients.

Using the lysostaphin assay technique, which allows one to differentiate between phagocytosis and intracellular killing, Tan et al.[16] demonstrated a defect in phagocytosis of *Staphylococcus aureus by* the PMNs of 31 patients with adult-onset diabetes. The presence of the defect showed no correlation with level of glycemic control or history of recurrent infections. The addition of normal serum had no effect. Using shorter observation periods, Nolan et al.[17] found that PMNs from 17 patients with poorly controlled diabetes ingested a smaller proportion of an inoculum of 10^6 *S. aureus* after 20 minutes (the interval during which the majority of engulfment takes place under normal physiologic conditions) than did control PMNs. This difference vanished at 60 minutes. Davidson et al.[18] measured engulfment of *Candida guilliermondii* over a 45-minute period by PMNs from 11 patients with moderately well controlled diabetes. The ratio of white cells to organisms was such that 90% of the control cells would have ingested at least one yeast cell in 30 minutes. Phagocytosis was diminished in the PMNs of the diabetic patients, regardless of levels of glycosylated hemoglobin 1C (HbA_{1C}). The diminished uptake appeared consistent throughout the population of cells from any individual. A defect in opsonization was suggested, since experiments in which the PMNs from diabetic subjects were mixed with normal plasma and vice versa demonstrated a defect in both the PMNs and plasma of these patients. In addition, when pre-opsonized yeast particles were added to serum from diabetic patients that contained PMNs from control subjects, engulfment was at normal levels.

Adherence

Comparatively few papers have specifically addressed the question of adherence in the leukocytes of patients with diabetes. Peterson et al.[19] found that the PMNs of six of seven patients with poorly controlled diabetes exhibited impaired adherence to a glass-wool column.[20] Adherence improved 1 to 2 months later when glycemic control had improved. However, no control patients were examined. Bagdade et al.[21] showed an enhancement of adherence of PMNs to a nylon-fiber column following an improvement in the control of blood glucose levels. Adherence increased from 53% to 74% of control values. In another study, Bagdade and Walters[22] demonstrated a direct relationship between degree of control and PMN adherence.

Andersen et al.[23] pointed the study of adhesion in a dramatic new direction by devising a more physiologic system. Noting that vascular endothelium is not a passive participant in the inflammation cascade, they examined the ability of PMNs from 26 patients with diabetes and from age-matched controls to bind to bovine aortic endothelium. The PMNs of 60% of the diabetic patients had severely depressed function that did not correlate with HbA_{1C} levels. PMN-PMN aggregation was not defective. No quantitative defect in fibronectin was seen, but a qualitative defect could not be excluded.

Bactericidal Activity

Early studies, such as that of Dziatkowiak et al.,[24] compared the number of live *Staphylococcus aureus* in a granulocyte with the total number of bacteria engulfed to calculate the proportion of organisms killed. Several studies[16] demonstrated diminished killing by the PMNs of diabetic patients while others did not. Repine et al.,[25] took a more quantitative and functional approach. Instead of using a single low ratio of bacteria to PMNs, they used five different ratios (1:1 to 100:1). Study patients included infected and noninfected individuals with and without diabetes. Cells were incubated with *Staphylococcus aureus* for 1 hour, after which colonies were counted. The rates of intracellular killing of bacteria by PMNs from uninfected controls and by PMNs of persons with well-controlled diabetes were comparable. PMNs from uninfected patients with poorly controlled diabetes functioned less well, especially when the higher ratios of bacteria to white cells were used. Although the functioning of PMNs from infected patients with well-controlled diabetes was on a par with the functioning of those from uninfected controls, the PMNs from the infected diabetic patients did not display the increase in killing activity seen in the PMNs of infected patients without diabetes. The bactericidal function of PMNs from infected patients with poorly controlled diabetes was the lowest of all the groups. Naghibi et al.,[12] using a single low ratio of bacteria to PMNs, found depressed bactericidal function of the PMNs of patients against *Pseudomonas aeruginosa*, but they did not study any infected patients. Serum from diabetic patients had an inhibitory effect on PMNs from both normal controls and diabetic subjects before and after intensive glucose management. Bactericidal activity of PMNs from the diabetic patients remained depressed even after intensive management.

In recent years, the significance of products of oxidative metabolism in cell killing has been appreciated. Stimulated PMNs have a burst of oxidative metabolism that produces superoxide anions and other oxygen-derived species that are operative in bacterial killing. These reactions produce chemiluminescence, a sensitive indicator of oxidative metabolism that correlates with antimicrobial activity. Shah et al.[26] looked at the superoxide anion production and chemiluminescence of PMNs from diabetic patients, examining the cells in both the resting state and in response to soluble and particulate stimuli. In resting PMNs from diabetic patients, chemiluminescence of cells placed in serum from diabetic patients was comparable to that of cells placed in control serum. Superoxide production was higher in autologous diabetic than in normal serum. The significance of these findings taken together is unclear. When stimulated, the PMNs from diabetic patients showed a blunted response with regard to both superoxide production and chemiluminescence. Cross-incubation serum studies effected no change, suggesting that an intracellular defect rather than an inhibitory serum factor is present. Winocour et al.[27] found no difference between the chemiluminescence response to zymosan stimulation of the PMNs of elderly control subjects and that of diabetic patients receiving oral hypoglycemic agents. They did not test the PMNs of younger patients.

Oberg et al.[28] took biochemical evaluation even further by measuring bactericidal proteins within the PMNs of 55 patients with IDDM. The only abnormality found was a markedly increased level of elastase, suggesting that any deficit in killing was not the result of an insufficiency in the granular content of the cells. No functional assays were undertaken. Collier et al.[29] have suggested that elastase may promote an interaction between endothelial cells and PMNs.

The PMNs of diabetic patients have shown a decreased prostaglandin E and thromboxane B2 response to stimulation by zymosan or killed *Staphylococcus aureus.*[30] The synthesis and release of leukotriene B4 by these cells were also diminished compared with that of the PMNs of sex- and age-matched controls.[31] The significance of these findings is not known.

Monocyte Function in Diabetes

Geisler et al.[32] found a decrease in the total number of circulating monocytes in 14 diabetic patients. These cells displayed diminished phagocytosis of *Candida albicans* but not of latex particles or sheep red blood cells. Glass et al.[33] proposed that monocytes from diabetic patients have a diminished activity of "lectin-like" receptors necessary for the recognition of cell-wall components of microorganisms. Attachment of *Staphylococcus epidermidis* to these monocytes was impaired, but that of coated sheep red blood cells, which are recognized by the Fc receptor, was normal. It could not be assessed whether the proportion of monocytes with the "lectin-like" receptors was reduced, each receptor had a lower affinity, or each monocyte had fewer receptors. Katz et al.[34] described subpopulations of monocytes with a reduced ability to phagocytose *Listeria monocytogenes.* Impaired monocyte chemotaxis has also been reported.[35] Monocytes from diabetic patients have been found to exhibit increased adhesion to fibronectin. While this property may play a role in the genesis of atherosclerosis,[36] its relationship to antimicrobial function is not known. The metabolic activity in response to ingestion of zymosan particles of the monocytes from diabetic patients is increased, as reflected by higher levels of chemiluminescence, superoxide production, and hexose monophosphate shunt activity than the levels in control monocytes.[37] The consequences of this increased activity have not been evaluated.

Cell-Mediated Immunity

A recent study of cell-mediated immunity in 99 patients with well-controlled diabetes in which multiple intradermal skin test antigens were used was unable to demonstrate any defect in responses as compared with those of controls.[38] However, reports of defects of cell-mediated immunity in vitro abound. Unfortunately, results are piecemeal both because of the complex interrelationships involved in the cell-mediated immune system and because of the evolution of study techniques over time.

MacCuish et al.[39] found that lymphocyte transformation in response to the mitogen phytohemagglutinin (PHA) was diminished in patients with poorly controlled diabetes. Meanwhile, Casey et al.[40,41] determined that the transformation of lymphocytes of diabetic patients in response to PHA was normal regardless of the patient's glycemic control but that the response to a staphylococcal antigen was decreased. These authors did not mention any ketotic patients. In a study by Speert and Silva,[42] the lymphocytes of children with diabetic ketoacidosis had a decreased mitogenic response that reverted to normal when metabolic derangements were corrected. There may be a diminished release of migration-inhibition factor by T lymphocytes from diabetic patients.[43,44] T-lymphocyte subsets have been studied with regard to the possibility of an autoimmune basis of diabetes mellitus. While alterations of the ratio of CD4 to CD8 lymphocyte ratio during the evolution and progression of diabetes have been noted,[45–47] no relationship of these changes to infection has been detected. No agreement has been reached as to whether the number and function of T and B cells in diabetic patients is increased, decreased, or normal as compared with the those in controls.[10]

Interleukin-2 is a polypeptide hormone produced by T cells that governs their clonal expansion and reactivity. An acquired defect in the production of interleukin-2 has been demonstrated in patients with IDDM,[48] as have increased levels of receptors for this cytokine.[49] Decreased responsiveness of natural killer cells from patients with IDDM to interferon has been observed.[50] The implications of these abnormalities with regard to defense against infection remain speculative at the present time.

Miscellaneous Factors

Abnormalities in the microvascular circulation of individuals with diabetes may result in decreased tissue perfusion.[51] While it is intuitively clear how such abnormalities might facilitate the acquisition of infection and impair response to therapy, it is unclear what role microvascular defects actually play in the pathogenesis of infections relatively specific for diabetic patients, such as mucormycosis, malignant external otitis, or emphysematous cholecystitis. Reviews of these topics often mention the arteriolar narrowing seen on pathologic examination, but comparisons with control specimens have not been reported. It appears that the white blood cells of diabetic patients may play a role in producing damage to the capillary and venular endothelium.[52,53]

INFECTIONS STRONGLY ASSOCIATED WITH DIABETES

Mucormycosis

The Organism and Host Response

The term *mucormycosis* connotes a variety of infections caused by fungi belonging to the order Mucorales, members of the class Zygomycetes.[54,55] *Zygomycosis* and *phycomycosis* are synonyms that have been rendered obsolete by ongoing reclassification. *Rhizopus* spp. (especially *Rhizopus oryzae* and *Rhizopus arrhizus*) are the most commonly isolated pathogens, followed by *Mucor* spp. *Cunninghamella*[56] and other species have also been found to cause disease. These molds produce large, thick-walled, non-septate hyphae that branch at more or less right angles. Ubiquitous in the environment, these organisms are most often found in decaying matter. Humans commonly inhale the spores, which have a low virulence potential. The ability of the spores to germinate successfully is dependent on specific host factors. Most information regarding pathogenesis comes from studies in rabbit and mouse models. After inhalation of spores, normal animals do not become ill, whereas diabetic animals develop a rapidly progressive pulmonary disease.[57] Alveolar macrophages from normal mice, but not those from diabetic mice, will ingest the spores and inhibit their germination into the invasive hyphal forms. Experimentally, neither hyperglycemia nor metabolic acidosis alone is sufficient to permit infection,[58] despite the propensity for the development of certain mucormycosis syndromes among acidotic diabetic patients. In contrast to normal human serum, the serum of diabetic patients with ketoacidosis does not inhibit the growth of *Rhizopus oryzae*.[59] It has been proposed that acidosis disrupts the ability of transferrin to bind iron, a deficiency that results in the release of free iron into the serum and perhaps an interference in the host defenses against *Rhizopus*,[60] an iron-requiring organism.[61] Credence has been lent to the proposed role of iron regulation in host defense by the increasing recognition of the occurrence of deferoxamine-associated mucormycosis in patients undergoing dialysis. In this situation, it appears that *Rhizopus* may be able to utilize the iron mobilized by the chelating agent, a capability that has been demonstrated in other organisms.[61]

Clinical Syndromes

Mucormycosis may present as a rhinocerebral, pulmonary, cutaneous, gastrointestinal, or disseminated form of the disease. Rhinocerebral mucormycosis was first recognized about 50 years ago.[62] It occurs almost exclusively in persons with diabetes and is one of the most fulminant forms of fungal disease affecting that population. The typical patient presents with ketoacidosis. Fungal elements gain entry through the nasopharynx, where tissue invasion may result in nasal discharge that may be blood-tinged. Close inspection of the infected region may reveal necrotic areas with black eschar involving the nasal mucosa or hard palate. The patient is likely to have fever and to remain lethargic even after metabolic derangements are corrected. Commonly, by the time the diagnosis is suspected, headache and/or facial pain already reflect extension of the process into the paranasal sinuses and possibly into the orbit of the eye. Occasional patients present with a dramatic, rapid onset of ocular proptosis and vision loss caused by invasion of the orbit. Rapid progression of clinical findings is the result of invasion of blood vessels, with vascular occlusion and subsequent necrosis of tissues dependent on the affected vessels. Progression of thrombosis can include the cavernous sinus[63] and the internal carotid artery.[64] Invasion of the brain results in meningoencephalitis and/or abscess formation with deterioration of neurologic function.

Progression usually occurs over a matter of hours to days and is invariably fatal if not treated early. Diagnosis must be established by demonstration of characteristic invasion of tissues by hyphal elements in biopsy specimens. A careful search for evidence of vascular invasion must be conducted. Culture results will often be negative. Spinal fluid findings are nonspecific.[65] Sinus films may show mucosal thickening and clouding with some spotty destruction of the orbit.[66] Computed tomographic (CT) scans, with special orbital views, can help define the extent of involvement, although the extent estimated by this method may underestimate the actual extent of involvement determined at surgery.[67] Angiography has been used to define the degree of large vessel involvement. The role of magnetic resonance imaging (MRI) has not yet been defined, but this technique may prove a useful adjunct in assessment of tissue or large vessel involvement. Extension beyond the orbit carries a very poor prognosis.

Aggressive surgical management is mandatory in all situations; radical debridement sometimes necessitates orbital exenteration. Repeated debridement may be necessary. Concomitantly, underlying metabolic disorders must be addressed. Amphotericin B remains the standard antifungal therapy and must be used in conjunction with surgery.[54,68,69] Aggressive antifungal therapy should be used, and while the exact duration of treatment and the total dose administered are not well defined, it is reasonable to aim for a total dose of at least 2 g. The new azoles have no defined role in therapy.[70] CT scans may be useful for following the response to treatment, and repeat biopsy may be necessary.[71] With optimal therapy, mortality remains at 50%, despite some reports of more encouraging results.[72] The nature of the almost universal neurologic residua depends on what anatomic structures have been compromised by the time the infection is brought under control.

The remaining forms of mucormycosis do not have a predilection for a specific host, although the pulmonary disease may have a distinctive presentation in diabetic patients. In contrast to the fatal pneumonia and extensive thrombosis that is typical in immunocompromised patients, diabetic patients have been noted to develop endobronchial and large-airway lesions that may follow a less fulminant course. The main complication of pulmonary mucormycosis is massive hemoptysis. Lesions may respond to aggressive local resection in combination with intravenous therapy with amphotericin B.[73-76]

Malignant External Otitis

In 1968, Chandler described a series of patients with a disorder termed *malignant external otitis* (MEO).[77] Occasionally referred to as *progressive, invasive,* or *necrotizing external otitis,* these names attest to the destructive nature of the process. These terms connote a slowly progressive cellulitis that begins in the soft tissues of the external auditory canal. As it penetrates more deeply into the subcutaneous tissue, this process may spread via the fissures of Santorini (clefts in the cartilaginous floor of the external canal) into the mastoid air cells. Access to the temporal bone (osteomyelitis) occurs through the cartilaginous/osseous junction in the outer ear canal.[78] Almost all cases are due to *Pseudomonas aeruginosa* even though this is not a normal colonizer of the ear in any patient group.[79] The vast majority of patients are elderly, and 75 to 90% have diabetes. There does not appear to be a distinct relationship between MEO and ketoacidosis or magnitude of hyperglycemia.[80]

Typically, patients will present with a two- to several-week history of external otitis unresponsive to local therapy. The evolution into MEO, with localized invasion of soft tissue and osseous structures, is heralded by unrelenting, severe otalgia often accompanied by purulent discharge.[81] It is unusual for patients to appear systemically ill or to have a fever and an elevated white blood cell count. One of the hallmarks of MEO that distinguishes it from simple external otitis is the finding of granulation tissue, usually at the junction of the cartilaginous and osseous portion of the canal, in more than 90% of cases. A swollen, reddened, moist-appearing canal is usual. The tympanic membrane is normal in the rare cases in which it can be visualized. The extent to which the process has progressed toward the base of the skull is reflected clinically by progressive involvement of cranial nerves. The facial nerve is impaired at presentation in up to 50% of cases,[78,82] the result of swelling of the soft tissue surrounding the styloid foramen where the nerve exits the skull or of direct invasion of the bone at the foramen itself. The function of cranial nerves IX, X, XI can be affected next as the jugular foramen becomes involved.[82,83] Finally, the hypoglossal canal can be destroyed. In the most extreme cases, contralateral cranial nerves are compromised as the destructive process erodes the base of the skull. Meningitis may result by extension into the subarachnoid space.

The relative value of several radiologic imaging procedures in delineating the extent of destruction has recently been reviewed.[82] Plain films of the ear canal are of limited sensitivity and specificity and are useful primarily to confirm a suspicion of advanced disease with skeletal destruction. While technetium scanning is highly sensitive, it is of low specificity, as is gallium scanning. CT scanning, with special views, is currently the imaging modality of choice,[84] although tumors cannot be reliably distinguished from MEO. MRI may prove to be of higher sensitivity and specificity, but comparative studies do not yet exist.[84]

In Chandler's original series,[77] the mortality rate from MEO was 50%. A more recent review of this entity cited a current mortality rate of 20%.[80] Cure rates since 1985 may have reached 90%.[85] The improvement in survival may be attributable in part to the development of more effective antipseudomonal antibiotics. As important, however, is the likelihood that increased awareness by physicians of this entity has, over time, led to earlier recognition of affected patients and thus to the possible control of infection with antibiotic therapy and local debridement and to a diminished need for the more radical surgical procedures necessitated by more advanced disease.

Standard antibiotic regimens for treatment of MEO have included the administration of an antipseudomonal penicillin plus an aminoglycoside for a prolonged period[82,86] (4 to 6 weeks or more). With the advent of newer, potentially less toxic antipseudomonal agents, new regimens are evolving. Monotherapy with the third-generation cephalosporin ceftazidime for 4 to 6 weeks, much of it as home therapy, realized a rate of favorable response of 92% in a series of 20 patients, 30% of whom presented with ipsilateral facial palsy.[87] Follow-up was 1 year with no recurrences. While the results are encouraging, it is of note that two of the patients in this series did not even need debridement, indicating that some presented with the extreme of mild disease. In another study, 21 of 23 patients with MEO were successfully treated with 6 weeks of oral therapy with ciprofloxacin.[88] However, only 65% of the patients in this study had diabetes. As the authors themselves pointed out, one must use extreme caution in extrapolating these results to clinical practice, as this approach makes the treatment of a serious infection dependent on patient compliance and employs the oral route, with the attendant concerns about adequacy of drug absorption in some patients. In addition, even when the patient is at home, close medical supervision is still necessary, as repeated debridement may be required.[89] While emergence of resistance has not been an obvious problem in studies employing monotherapy, the issue should be addressed with regard to patients for whom therapy fails.

Emphysematous Pyelonephritis

Severe bacterial urinary tract infection in the diabetic patient may result in emphysematous pyelonephritis. The precise definition of this rare entity varies among authors. The most rigorous definition includes a requirement for the presence of gas within the renal parenchyma, which may enter the perinephric space by extension. Gas can occur in the calices, collecting system, or bladder, but if it is limited to these sites, these entities are distinct from true emphysematous pyelonephritis and carry different prognoses. The differential diagnosis includes iatrogenic manipulation with introduction of air and fistula formation arising from the digestive system. The first reference to emphysematous pyelonephritis is usually cited in 1898,[90] although in retrospect, it appears that this patient probably had gas only in the collecting system. Only about 65 cases have been reported.[91–95] Between 85% and 100% of patients have had diabetes mellitus, although diabetic ketoacidosis has been uncommon. Up to 40% of patients may have had concomitant obstruction, which is present in almost all nondiabetic patients with emphysematous pyelonephritis. At presentation, it is not possible clinically to distinguish emphysematous from uncomplicated acute pyelonephritis unless gas has spread beyond the bounds of perirenal tissues to cause subcutaneous crepitation. Pneumaturia is distinctly unusual.

Plain radiographs,[96] ultrasound, or abdominal CT scans[97] will reveal gas within the renal parenchyma. A plain x-ray film may show a mottled renal parenchyma with gas bubbles, often in a radial distribution. As the infection advances, gas may be seen outside the renal cortex either outlining the kidney or forming thin crescents, although this classic finding is unusual. Abdominal CT scanning is especially useful for documenting the spread of gas beyond Gerota's fascia.[92,97] About 10% of patients have bilateral involvement.[93] Radiologic evaluation should be undertaken if a suspected case of acute pyelonephritis does not respond to adequate antibiotic therapy within a few days. CT scans may also uncover previously unsuspected abscesses.

The usual causative organisms are typical urinary pathogens, including *Escherichia coli*, *Klebsiella pneumoniae*, *Proteus mirabilis*, and *Enterobacter aerogenes*. There are case reports implicating other organisms; anaerobes are typically not found. It is not clear why the microbes involved produce gas in a specific clinical situation. The presence of glycosuria, while providing a substrate for production of gas by fermentation, is clearly not the sole factor, given the rarity of emphysematous pyelonephritis and the frequency of glycosuria.

While it is clear that therapy with antibiotics directed at the offending organisms and management of underlying diabetes are imperative, the role of surgical intervention is much less well defined. The lack of prospective, controlled studies is understandable given the rarity of the syndrome. Obstruction should always be sought and relieved as necessary. Some authors suggest following the resolution of gas radiographically and proceeding with nephrectomy only if the patient fails to respond to appropriate antibiotics.[93] Others have recommended total nephrectomy as soon as the diagnosis is made, citing the possibility of rapid clinical deterioration in some patients.[92] A reasonable approach might be to try medical management with local drainage if obstruction is documented but to consider nephrectomy if clinical improvement does not occur. This may be especially appropriate if the affected kidney is shown to be nonfunctioning, as is the case in about half the patients.[94]

The duration of antibiotic therapy is not addressed in various reviews, but a several-week course would appear prudent. Reported mortality rates range from 10 to 40%.[92,93,98] At autopsy, 50% of 42 patients had severe acute and chronic necrotizing pyelonephritis with multiple cortical abscesses; 20% had papillary necrosis, and 20% had intrarenal vascular thrombi.[95] In one fourth of the cases, the kidney could not even be identified. Currently, this rare entity may carry a better prognosis if a high index of clinical suspicion is maintained and leads to early imaging studies.

Emphysematous Cholecystitis

Emphysematous cholecystitis is a rare complication of acute cholecystitis in which air is found in the lumen and wall of the gallbladder, with possible extension to the pericholecystic space. It was first diagnosed at surgery in 1908, with the first preoperative diagnosis made by abdominal roentgenography in 1931.[99] In 1975, Mentzner et al.[100] published their comprehensive study, which encompassed the 161 cases reported to date in the literature and three cases of their own. More than one-third of the patients in this series had diabetes. In contrast to acute cholecystitis, for which almost three-fourths of the patients are female, males account for three-fourths of the cases of emphysematous cholecystitis. Perforation and gangrene of the gallbladder are 30 times and 3 times more common, respectively, and mortality is 10 times higher in patients younger than 60 years old but only two times higher for those older than 60 than in patients with acute cholecystitis. Diabetes does not appear to be an independent factor relative to a worse prognosis. Cholelithiasis is present about half of the time.

Patients present with pain in the right upper quadrant, nausea and vomiting, and fever. During the next 48 hours, gas develops within the gallbladder lumen and wall, with progression into the surrounding tissues in the next 48 hours.[101] Even during this time, one cannot reliably distinguish acute uncomplicated cholecystitis from emphysematous cholecystitis at the bedside. Diagnosis is established by roentgenographic documentation of gas in the aforementioned areas. On plain films, one may initially see a globular shadow representing the air-filled gallbladder. Soon afterwards, intramural—usually submucosal—air may be visualized.[99] Air may sometimes be seen only in the biliary radicles.[102] Air under the diaphragm suggests perforation and is a poor prognostic sign.[99] Differential diagnosis of these radiographic findings includes the presence of enterovesicular fistula. Ultrasonography has proven a useful tool, although plain films must still be obtained to rule out a porcelain gallbladder or a heavily calcified stone as the source of high-density echoes.[103,104] It is likely that CT and MRI could be useful, but no data yet exist.

Given the high complication rate of emphysematous cholecystitis, it is important to consider this diagnosis during the first few days of observation of a patient with acute cholecystitis. It has been recommended that cholecystectomy be performed as soon as the diagnosis is established.[101] Typically, a crepitant gangrenous gallbladder is found at surgery. Cultures are positive 50 to 90% of the time, a frequency much higher than that for simple acute cholecystitis. *Clostridium perfringens* is isolated from 25 to 50% of positive cultures, along with more typical enteric organisms such as *Escherichia coli*. Antibiotic coverage should include anaerobes as well as both gram-positive and gram-negative facultative organisms.

The issue of elective cholecystectomy in diabetic patients remains controversial. Because of the perceived increased risk of mortality among diabetic patients with acute disease, for many years it was recommended that those with cholelithiasis undergo prophylactic cholecystectomy.[105,106] However, a recent retrospective controlled study suggests diabetes mellitus alone is not correlated with a higher mortality rate during an episode of acute cholecystitis.[106] In a decision-analysis model, it was found—under a broad range of assumptions—that, when managed expectantly (i.e, observed without surgery), diabetic patients with asymptomatic gallstones did no worse than nondiabetic patients.[107] Other work suggests a higher rate of infectious complications following cholecystectomy for acute cholecystitis among diabetic than nondiabetic patients.[108] In treatment of acute cholecystitis, the trend has been toward expeditious (within 24 hours) surgery.[101,109] The outcome of this approach, in contrast to that of surgery following a "cooling-off" period, has not been rigorously examined in relation to patients with diabetes.

INFECTIONS CAUSED BY THERAPEUTIC INTERVENTIONS

Insulin Therapy

Standard self-administered insulin injections result in abscesses remarkably rarely. Preservatives added to insulin have antibacterial activity. Before the 1970s, glass syringes stored in methylated industrial spirit were used. The inadvertent substitution of surgical spirit, which contains a larger number of additives, has more often, although still rarely, been associated with abscess formation.[110,111] In many parts of the world, disposable syringes have largely replaced glass syringes. Manufacturers and many medical practitioners recommend discarding plastic syringes after a single use. However, repeated use of syringes for a month or more has not been reported to result in an increased rate of infection if the syringe is refrigerated between uses, if the needle is wiped with alcohol, or if the syringe-needle unit is soaked in alcohol between uses.[112]

In an investigation of the actual insulin injection practices of a group of diabetic patients, no injection-site infections or significant bacterial contamination of equipment was found. This was despite a lack of "traditional practices" such as wiping the vial and skin or even washing the hands before injection.[112,113] One-half the patients re-used their syringes many times. In a preliminary study of jet insulin injectors, for which cleaning every 2 weeks is recommended, no significant growth was seen in cultures of any of the injectors from 19 patients.[114] On the other hand, continuous subcutaneous insulin infusion (CSI) is commonly associated with infectious complications, typically in the form of abscesses at the needle site.[115,116] This is among the most common reasons cited by patients for discontinuing this form of therapy.[117] No association between the staphylococcal carrier state and infection at the injection site has been shown.[118]

Penile Implants

Men with diabetes make up one-fourth to one-third of the approximately 17,000 patients each year who undergo penile implant procedures for impotence. The implant apparatuses available range from rigid rods placed in the paired corpora cavernosa to the new, more commonly used, inflatable devices.[119,120] Included among the inflatable implants are those with multiple components placed in the scrotum, abdominal wall, and corpora cavernosa that have been available since 1973 and several similar types of succeeding units. The most recent kinds of implants are contained entirely in the corpora cavernosa. All types are inserted with a single incision. There is no correlation between type of prosthesis or incision with infection rate.[119,120] The infection rate ranges from 0.8 to 8%, with most series having an average of 2 to 3%. This is an improvement from the 15% rate seen before antibiotic prophylaxis was routine. In several recent series, no increased incidence of infection in diabetic patients was noted.[121,122] *Staphylococcus epidermidis* is the infecting organism in 40 to 80% of the infections, with coliforms being isolated in most of the others. Infection is thought to originate at the time of surgery primarily as a result of contamination with microorganisms of the skin or colorectal area. Rarely, late infection caused by hematogenous seeding has been reported.[122]

Evidence of infection is seen 2 weeks to 2 years after implantation, with the gram-negative organisms tending to present in the earlier part of the range. Systemic signs and symptoms are usually absent. The degree of local findings can be subtle, such as tenderness with manipulation, mechanical malfunction, mild hyperemia or erosion over the mechanism, or formation of periprosthetic adhesive tissue. More dramatic evidence of infection, such as pain, swelling, induration, fistula formation, or extrusion of the device, tends to occur with infections with gram-negative organisms, although not exclusively. Findings at surgical exploration can range from minor adhesions to gross purulence. Immediate therapy consists of removal of the prosthesis, therapy with broad-spectrum intravenous antibiotics, and postoperative drainage. Although what constitutes optimal ensuing therapy is controversial, most authors suggest a waiting period of 3 to 6 months before reimplantation is attempted.[119] The rate of infection is increased for implants after the first procedure.

Prevention of infection of penile prostheses focuses on the time of surgery. As with all procedures incorporating prosthetic material, concurrent infection, particularly of the urinary tract, is a contraindication to surgery. Antibiotic prophylaxis, an appropriately clean operating room environment, extensive skin preparation, and copious intraoperative irrigation have all been recommended as means of decreasing the chance of infection.[120]

Organ Transplantation

Renal transplantation is an option for a number of diabetic patients with end-stage renal disease. For a general population of individuals undergoing renal transplantation, 1-year patient survival is greater than 95%, and 1-year graft survival is greater than 85%.[123] Although methods of immunosuppression have improved greatly over the years, permitting the use of lower doses of immunosuppressive drugs, infection is still a significant problem in this population. The sources of infection can be the endogenous flora, reactivated latent infection, infection with opportunistic pathogens, or primary transmission from the donor allograft.[124,125] Rubin et al. proposed a now classic timetable for infections occurring in renal transplant recipients.[126] In the first month following transplantation, these patients present with the same kinds of infectious complications seen in any postoperative patient: i.e., wound, urinary tract, pulmonary, and intravenous catheter bacterial infections. Opportunistic infections are unlikely during the early part of this period. Cumulative immunosuppression is at its height 1 to 6 months after transplantation, and it is during this period that the patient is at greatest risk of opportunistic infections, such as those due to cytomegalovirus, *Pneumocystis carinii,* and *Aspergillus,* among others. After these first 6 months, the recipient is susceptible to chronic forms of viral disease contracted earlier in his course, some opportunistic infections, and diseases found in the community. For further information, the reader is directed to in-depth reviews of the large body of data on this topic.[123,126,127]

To date, little has been written concerning infectious complications of pancreatic transplantation with or without concomitant renal transplantation.[128,129] Since the course of immunosuppression follows essentially the same pattern as that for renal transplantation, it would be expected that the time frame for infectious complications of the two would be similar. Different immediate postoperative complications might be expected, given that anastomotic sites frequently involve bowel.[128] It is likely that these postoperative complications will become less frequent as more technical skill is acquired, as has occurred with renal transplantation.[123] A study of heart transplantation in carefully selected diabetic patients revealed no increased risk of infection.[129]

Infections Associated with Dialysis

Continuous Ambulatory Peritoneal Dialysis

Continuous ambulatory peritoneal dialysis (CAPD) is an increasingly common modality of therapy for end-stage renal disease in patients with diabetes. Like any indwelling foreign body, the silastic catheters inserted into the peritoneum carry a risk of infection. On the average, one to two episodes of catheter-related peritonitis per patient per year can be anticipated, although it appears that some patients suffer multiple episodes while others have fewer than the expected number.[131–133] The rate of CAPD-related infection does not appear to be greater in diabetic than in nondiabetic patients.[134,135]

This is also true for patients receiving chronic intermittent peritoneal dialysis,[136] for which the overall risk of infection is lower than that for CAPD.

The source of infection[132] can be intraluminal, from touch contamination of the apparatus at insertion, a break in the tubing or attachment site that permits ingress of bacteria, or contamination at bag changes caused by poor technique. Contamination of dialysate is another potential route of entry of microorganisms. Infection also can occur by the periluminal route, for the skin never makes a complete seal with the catheter at the exit site. Both these routes can result in infection with organisms of the endogenous skin flora. Coagulase-negative staphylococci account for 40% of the cases of peritonitis in patients undergoing CAPD.[137] Other gram-positive organisms, such as *Staphylococcus aureus* and streptococci, are responsible for another 30%. Gram-negative organisms are seen in almost 30% of cases, often reflecting a third route of infection, i.e., that of contamination of the peritoneum and then the catheter from an intestinal source. Such contamination can occur without an overt disruption in the bowel mucosa. A bowel source is suggested by findings of multiple organisms or anaerobes in the dialysate. It is very rare for blood cultures to be positive as the result of CAPD peritonitis. Positive blood cultures should prompt a search for a source that has led to hematogenous seeding. Fungi, especially *Candida* spp., account for almost 5% of cases of CAPD-associated peritonitis, with the rate no higher in patients with diabetes.[138] *Mycobacterium tuberculosis* is seen in fewer than 3% of cases. A number of unusual causes of CAPD peritonitis have been seen.[139]

Patients with exit-site infections may be unaware of any problems until an examiner notes erythema at the site. Serous or purulent discharge may be present. Infections in the subcutaneous tunnel can be very difficult to diagnose, especially when no concurrent exit-site infection is present, as signs may be absent early in the course of infection. Ultrasound imaging may be helpful in finding a localized collection around the tunnel, but one may not be present. Either an exit-site or tunnel infection may exist without causing peritonitis, but each increases the risk of peritoneal infection. Patients with peritonitis may have very mild symptoms of abdominal discomfort with or without a low-grade fever, but almost all will note a cloudy dialysate. Some individuals may present with acute illness and appear septic, particularly if they have *Staphylococcus aureus* infection. Regardless of patient presentation, CAPD peritonitis is documented by noting more than 100 cells/mm^3 (mostly PMNs) in the dialysate, which normally contains 50 to 100 cells/mm^3 with a predominance of macrophages. For infection to be documented definitively, an organism must be demonstrated in the dialysate, either by gram staining or culture.[133] Culture of large volumes of dialysate (50 to 100 mL) can greatly improve yield. The gram stain is positive in fewer than 50% of cases, even when concentrated dialysis fluid is examined. Noninfectious causes of cloudy dialysate should not result in increased cell counts. With treatment, patients should improve clinically, culture results become negative, and cell counts fall dramatically in 4 to 5 days. It should be kept in mind that cell counts can vary with the time that dialysate is permitted to dwell within the peritoneum. Sequential sampling for evaluation of cellular response should be performed at comparable time points of the dialysis cycle. If resolution of infection is delayed, a tunnel infection or other complicating factor should be ruled out. If cultures remain negative and the patient is not improving, the possibility of tuberculosis should be considered.

The route of delivery, type of antibiotic, and duration of therapy have not been studied in a prospective, controlled manner, and conventional regimens can vary by institution. Empiric initial coverage should include both gram-positive and gram-negative organisms. At some centers, the majority of patients are treated as outpatients.[133] A number of antibiotics can be mixed into each dialysis bag.[140] Oral or intravenous therapy is sometimes used. The duration of therapy is typically 10 days for gram-positive infections and 14 days for gram-negative infections. For recurrences of infection that occur within 2 weeks, 2 to 4 weeks of therapy is used. Catheter removal is generally included in the treatment for fungal and mycobacterial peritonitis.[131] The traditional approach of removal of the catheter for patients with pseudomonal infection has not been re-evaluated since the advent of more effective and less toxic antipseudomonal agents. Catheter removal may be needed in other cases of infection that are refractory to treatment with appropriate antibiotics alone.

Hemodialysis

Many diabetic patients with end-stage renal disease undergo hemodialysis, which may be carried out with "temporary" access through a subclavian or femoral catheter that is either in place for days to months or by means of new access with each dialysis procedure. The attendant risks and the principles of management of infections of these lines are the same as those for any deep intravascular access lines.

Permanent access for hemodialysis can be attained with an arteriovenous shunt—an external connection between the radial artery and cephalic vein. More common now, however, is the use of an arteriovenous fistula, which can be accomplished in several ways. If vessels are of sufficient caliber and patency, an autologous graft can be surgically created between the radial artery and the cephalic vein. A bovine heterograft can be placed between the vessels, or prosthetic material—either polytetrafluoroethylene (PTFE) or Dacron—can be used as a graft. The native arteriovenous fistula carries the lowest rate of infection (2 to 13%).[132,141,142] Infectious complications occur most frequently with the bovine heterografts (1 to 20%). The rate of infections for prosthetic grafts falls somewhere between the rates for native and bovine grafts.[132,141,143]

Standard vascular surgery prophylaxis is used for placement of fistulas. The expected 1% of fistulas that become infected perioperatively typically suffer only a delay in maturation. The true incidence of late infections[141,143] is difficult to determine because many series focus on hospitalized patients, whereas many of these infections are successfully treated on an outpatient basis. Localized graft infections typically manifest as tenderness, warmth, and erythema over the graft—perhaps with exudate. Findings may, however, be much more subtle, consisting of hemorrhage or mechanical malfunction caused by infection-related destruction of the anastomotic site. As many as one-third of patients who present with bacteremia caused by access-site infection have an unremarkable fistula on examination. Blood cultures (not obtained through the access site) and cultures of any pus are the keys to bacteriologic diagnosis. Grafts can also be infected by hematogenous spread of microorganisms from a distant site of infection.

Staphylococcus aureus is estimated to cause up to 80% of graft infections,[143] with gram-negative organisms and coagulase-negative staphylococci being responsible for much of the remainder. When bacteremia is associated with graft-site infection, *S. aureus* is implicated 40 to 70% of the time.[141,145] Endocarditis, osteomyelitis, or septic pulmonary emboli caused by distant seeding increase mortality and the rate of primary treatment failure.[145,146] Mortality rates among patients with grafts is also higher if the identifiable focus for the bacteremia is other than the graft.[144] It is generally agreed that patients with *S. aureus* bacteremia related to graft infection should receive a prolonged course of antibiotic therapy, e.g., 6 weeks.[132,144] How to manage the graft itself, particularly if it is prosthetic, is controversial. While excision of the graft is the approach most likely to prove curative, the desire to preserve the graft is often paramount. There have been attempts at partial removal and patch repair of the graft,[147,148] but there are no prospective studies of various surgical approaches.

INFECTIONS POSSIBLY RELATED TO DIABETES

Urinary Tract Disease

Bacteriuria

An association between urinary tract infection and diabetes mellitus was noted in autopsy series in the 1940s.[149] Since then, numerous studies have been published regarding the prevalence of bacteriuria in persons with diabetes. The number of studies documenting an increased prevalence and the number that have not are approximately equal. Those studies that did demonstrate an increase did so almost exclusively in adult women. Reports have varied regarding presence and/or type of controls, clinical setting, definition of diabetes, and definition of infection, making it difficult to compare studies. Three recent papers examining the prevalence of asymptomatic bacteriuria in diabetic outpatients found a prevalence of approximately 9% in women, i.e., two- to fourfold higher than that in controls.[149–151] It is of note that these investigations can only remark on *prevalence*, as subjects were tested at one point in time. Therefore, it cannot be determined whether diabetic women are more prone to episodes of bacteriuria or if they simply experience the same frequency of bacteriuria as nondiabetic women but that episodes persist for more prolonged periods.

Lower urinary tract disease in diabetic patients is of concern because of the perception that these patients have more-complicated infections of the upper urinary tract. The incidence of bacteremia due to the Enterobacteriaceae also is increased in diabetic patients, presumably because of the increased incidence of urinary tract infections.[152] Information relating disease in the urinary tract specifically to asymptomatic or symptomatic bacteriuria is lacking. It is also not known how often asymptomatic bacteriuria progresses to symptomatic bacteriuria. Thus, the benefit, if any, of treating asymptomatic episodes in this population is not clear. Some of the presumed predisposing factors that have been examined include age, neurogenic bladder, duration of diabetes, and degree of glycemic control. Results do not all agree, and since several of the conditions may be closely interrelated, it is often not possible to demonstrate definitively any independent associations. Although it might appear intuitive that the presence of a large post-voiding residual volume of urine would predispose an individual to bacteriuria, there is no consistent evidence of such a causal relationship.[152] Although diabetic women have been documented to have an increased frequency of anatomic abnormalities, as detected by intravenous pyelography,[153] comparative studies are lacking, and frequently it is difficult to know whether an abnormality is the result of previous infections. A neurogenic bladder can predispose to infection because of the high likelihood of use of instrumentation for diagnosis and/or therapy in these patients. It is not known whether the risk of infection posed by instrumentation is higher than usual in diabetic patients. The distribution of organisms found in the urine of diabetic patients is similar to that in other populations.

Pyelonephritis and Renal Papillary Necrosis

While the precise incidence of pyelonephritis in diabetic individuals as compared with that in persons who are not diabetic is not well documented, diabetic patients have been shown to be at increased risk for renal papillary necrosis, which is often, although not always, a result of pyelonephritis. One study has shown that diabetic patients with proteinuria are more apt to develop infections with P-fimbriated strains of *Escherichia coli*, which are more likely than nonfimbriated strains to cause ascending infection.[154] There is a suggestion from work done in a diabetic rat model that polyuria facilitates the ascent of bacteria from the bladder by creating vesicoureteral reflux.[154]

Infection may be both a cause and an effect of renal papillary necrosis. The majority of patients who are symptomatic for this entity have concomitant pyelonephritis.[156] In addition to the colicky flank pain that is possible from the passing of a papillary fragment, there may be fever, chills, flank tenderness, and pyuria. Renal papillary necrosis should be suspected in diabetic patients with frequently relapsing or difficult-to-eradicate pyelonephritis as well as in those who have a particularly fulminant presentation of pyelonephritis accompanied by hematuria. Diabetes is estimated to be present in 30 to 50% of patients with renal papillary necrosis. Of note is evidence for other risk factors, such as analgesic use, in these patients.[157,158] Autopsy series of persons with diabetes have noted renal papillary necrosis in about 5%.[156] A recent study of diabetic outpatients with and without asymptomatic bacteriuria found mild or moderate papillary necrosis by intravenous pyelography in 18 of 76 patients but in none of 34 nondiabetic control subjects.[156] The percentage of patients who had experienced more than three urinary tract infections was higher in those with papillary necrosis. Women account for 80% of patients with papillary necrosis among both diabetic and nondiabetic patients.

Eradication of infection is a requirement for effective treatment. Catheter drainage or percutaneous nephrostomy is preferred over initial nephrectomy for obstruction and pyelonephrosis. Debris may be dislodged with irrigation or direct urologic manipulations.[157] The appropriate duration of antibiotic therapy, which should be directed at usual urinary pathogens, has not been clearly established.

Renal Abscesses

It has been stated that renal abscesses occur with twice the frequency in diabetic as in nondiabetic persons.[159,160] However, controls have often been compiled retrospectively or merely extrapolated from diagnoses at discharge. Renal parenchymal abscesses can be divided into renal carbuncles (cortical abscesses) and corticomedullary abscesses. Carbuncles are formed from multiple interconnecting cortical microabscesses. More than 90% of them are due to *Staphylococcus aureus*, and almost all result from hematogenous seeding of the kidney from a distant focus. Only rarely are they due to ascending urinary tract infection.[162] Corticomedullary abscesses are typically associated with some underlying abnormality of the urinary tract such as reflux or obstruction, often in association with instrumentation.[159] Bacteriologic studies usually reveal the involvement of gram-negative enteric organisms that commonly cause urinary tract infections, such as *Escherichia coli*, *Klebsiella* spp., and *Proteus* spp. Patients with parenchymal abscesses can present with flank pain, fever, chills, or abdominal pain. Nausea and vomiting are common. Dysuria may be absent, and urinalysis may reveal no abnormalities. A flank mass can be palpated about half the time. Blood cultures may be positive. CT is currently the most accurate way of diagnosing and following parenchymal abscesses.[162] Ultrasound can also be helpful. There is a chance that these abscesses will resolve with antibiotic therapy alone, but if no clinical improvement is seen within a few days, if a collection is large, or if obstructive uropathy is present, prompt drainage is required.[161] Drainage may initially be attempted with a percutaneous catheter. A prolonged course of antibiotic therapy is generally required. Open incision and drainage may be needed for those who do not respond to closed drainage.

Perinephric Abscess

Diabetes is routinely mentioned as a major contributing factor in perinephric abscess. Various series report that 14 to 75% of patients with perinephric abscess also have diabetes mellitus.[161] Frequently, however, many patients in these series have also had previous urinary tract infection, undergone urologic surgery, or had other risk factors, and it cannot be determined which of these individuals have had concomitant diabetes.

A perinephric abscess consists of purulent material between Gerota's fascia and the capsule of the kidney and most often results from rupture of a renal parenchymal abscess. Rarely, it may be the result of contiguous extension of a local process such as osteomyelitis or intra-abdominal infection. The bacteria isolated from the abscess thus reflect the source of the infection. *Staphylococcus aureus* (usually from a renal carbuncle) and gram-negative enteric organisms (as from rupture of a corticomedullary abscess) are the most common. As with any abscess, presentation may be fulminant or the course may be indolent and the presentation delayed.[163,164] Fever and flank tenderness are the most common signs. Urinalysis can reveal abnormalities if ascending urinary tract infection is the underlying cause. A high clinical suspicion is usually needed to make the diagnosis. Often a patient with undiagnosed perinephric abscess will be treated for pyelonephritis without the symptoms resolving within 4 to 5 days. This delay in response should prompt radiologic evaluation, preferably with an abdominal CT scan, which can reveal suggestive or even characteristic findings. Perinephric abscesses can track along any of several fascial planes, leading to peritoneal, retroperitoneal, or pleural space collections. The utility of CT scanning in the diagnosis of perinephric abscesses may be responsible for a recent decrease in the mortality rate from 50% to one of 0 to 5%.[163] In contrast to parenchymal abscesses, perinephric abscesses mandate drainage in combination with a prolonged course of antibiotics. Placement of a catheter for closed drainage, often under CT guidance, may suffice, but open drainage may be needed for collections that resolve slowly or are multiloculated. Surgery is also indicated if a patient is failing to improve with closed drainage of the abscess.

Fungal Infections

Oral Candidiasis

Although persons with diabetes are often said to experience an increased incidence of oral candidiasis,[165] most papers address the issue of colonization only. Hill et al.,[166] using the direct swab technique, found that a level of HbA_{1c} of 12% or greater correlated with yeast colonization. Analyzing a much larger group of patients (412), Fisher et al.[167] found no correlation between level of glycemic control and yeast colonization as determined by the oral rinse technique. Both these studies and others

have documented an increased rate of candidal carriage as well as an overall increase in colony counts in diabetic patients who wear dentures as compared with those who do not. A study of the incidence of overt denture stomatitis[168] failed to show any difference between the incidence in diabetic and nondiabetic persons with dentures. Bartholomew et al.[165] examined cytologically the oral mucosa of a group of 60 diabetic inpatients and 57 age- and sex-matched controls, none of whom had clinically apparent oral candidiasis. Almost 75% of the diabetic patients, vs. 35% of controls, were colonized. Although no difference was found between the incidence of antibiotic usage in diabetic patients who were colonized and those who were not, there were no control patients receiving antibiotics.

Treatment of clinically overt oral candidiasis in patients with diabetes is the same as that for nondiabetic patients. Clotrimazole troches offer an alternative to nystatin solutions. For refractory cases, systemic therapy with ketoconazole or fluconazole is an option. Fluconazole has proven useful in therapy for the entity of chronic mucocutaneous candidiasis, which in rare cases is associated with diabetes mellitus and which typically affects the mouth, nails, skin, and vagina.[169]

Vulvovaginal Candidiasis

While there is an often-repeated anecdotal association between diabetes and vulvovaginal candidiasis, no prospective controlled trials have addressed the issue and the confounding effect of concomitant antibiotic use has not been factored out in most studies. A study of the vaginal microbial flora of diabetic and nondiabetic women showed no difference in the isolation of *Candida albicans*.[170] Most experts agree with the statement of Sobel[171] that vulvovaginal candidiasis is "unlikely to be the only manifestation of occult diabetes"; none of 85 women with recurrent vaginal candidiasis who were referred to that author for evaluation of diabetes mellitus had an abnormal 2-hour glucose tolerance test.[171] The incidence of candidal vulvovaginitis increases during pregnancy, a change that may be due to an estrogenic effect that results in an increase in vaginal glycogen stores. This change in ambient glycogen levels has also been postulated to occur in persons with diabetes.[172] Therapy with intravaginally administered miconazole results in a 90% cure rate after 1 week. Oral ketoconazole or fluconazole therapy may be useful in refractory cases.

Fungal Urinary Tract Infection

Candida albicans and, less commonly, *Candida* (formerly *Torulopsis*) *glabrata* are found in the urine of a small percentage of healthy women.[173] Use of antibiotics or an indwelling urinary catheter are frequent predisposing conditions to increased colonization with these fungi. Although there is debate concerning how many colonies are indicative of urinary tract infection, 10^5 colonies/mL of urine is generally considered significant, although true infection can occur with even lower colony counts. Lower urinary tract infection is typically antecedent to ascending infection. Most patients have the previously mentioned risk factors and/or an abnormal urinary tract. It is not clear precisely what role diabetes itself plays. A review of *Candida glabrata* infections noted that three of nine patients with "significant urinary tract infections" had undergone urologic surgery and, oftentimes, had been treated with antibiotics.[174] Discontinuation of antibiotics or removal of an indwelling catheter may be sufficient to clear candidal organisms from the urine. More often, however, since many of these patients have residual urinary tract abnormalities that may hinder clearance, local instillation of amphotericin B, either intermittently or with constant irrigation, has been necessary. Of the oral antifungal agents available, fluconazole, is the most promising since it is excreted primarily in the urine.

Pyelonephritis due to candidal organisms is often a result of hematogenous spread in systemic candidiasis,[175] for which diabetes is not a risk factor. Manifestations of upper urinary tract disease related to initial cystitis can manifest as fungus balls,[176] which are aggregates of pseudohyphae that can be found in the renal pelvis or ureters and appear as irregular, radiolucent filling defects.[177] Fungus balls may be found more frequently in diabetic patients. Removal of the obstructing mass, either by closed methods such as with a basket or by an open surgical procedure, is required. The antifungal therapy in this situation is not well worked out. Whereas bladder irrigation may suffice for patients with fungus balls confined to the bladder, systemic therapy is required in most other situations. A long course of amphotericin B, with or without flucytosine, has been a standard approach. The difficulties in utilizing such regimens are obvious. The role of newer agents has not been thoroughly investigated, although the newer azoles appear promising.

A form of fungal ball that is particularly unusual and difficult to deal with is the renal aspergilloma.[178] Eleven cases have been reported in the literature; six of the affected patients had diabetes, although only three patients had diabetes without any complicating factors such as immunosuppression. Patients typically give no evidence of disseminated aspergillosis and present with symptoms suggestive of renal colic associated with kidney stones or sloughed renal papillae. Retrograde pyelography is the most informative radiologic test. The recovery of aspergillus from fungal urine cultures is higher than the recovery when routine (bacterial) culture techniques are used. The cornerstone of therapy is the removal of the obstructing mass. The means by which the fungal ball is removed can range from spontaneous evacuation by the patient to multiple open procedures, and possibly even nephrectomy, when the mass is not expelled or otherwise removed. Amphotericin B has been used in this setting, but the precise role of amphotericin therapy and the optimal regimens for its use are still unclear.

Staphylococcus aureus Infections

It has generally been maintained that the frequency of carriage of *S. aureus* by persons with diabetes, particularly those who use daily insulin injections, is higher than that in diabetic subjects using oral hypoglycemic agents and in nondiabetic subjects. However, studies addressing this issue are often difficult to evaluate and even more difficult to compare because of the lack of consistent control groups and stratification of patients. Smith et al.[179] found a 75% rate of nasal carriage in diabetic children as compared with a 44% rate in hospitalized nondiabetic children. Healthy adults and diabetic patients receiving oral hypoglycemic agents had a 35% carriage rate, while diabetic patients using insulin had a 53% carriage rate. The idea that the use of needles could be an important factor was examined by Tuazon et al.,[180] who found a 35% rate of carriage of *S. aureus* in both intravenous drug abusers and insulin-using diabetic patients but an 11% rate in diabetic patients receiving only oral hypoglycemic therapy and in nondiabetic subjects who did not receive injections. Chandler and Chandler[181] reported a higher rate of carriage of *S. aureus* in diabetic patients than in nondiabetic subjects, but statistical analysis was minimal, all diabetics being considered as one entity regardless of therapy, which ranged from dietary therapy alone to daily insulin injections. A population-based study by Boyko et al. did not demonstrate an increased prevalence of *S. aureus* carriage among patients with non-insulin-dependent diabetes, regardless of the form of therapy they were receiving.[181] Lipsky et al.[183] considered a number of factors, including recent hospitalizations, level of glycemic control, type of therapy, age, and recent antibiotic use, in a group of diabetic outpatients. Of the 44 controls, 11% had nasal colonization with *S. aureus*, whereas 30.5% of the 59 diabetic patients were colonized. The rate of colonization was no different for those who injected insulin and those who did not. However, the level of glycemic control was inversely related to *S. aureus* colonization, i.e., the higher the glucose levels, the higher the rate of colonization. This factor has typically not been looked at as a distinct variable in earlier studies. Overall, one of the few definitive statements that can be made regarding this issue is that certain groups of diabetic persons may have an increased rate of staphylococcal carriage and that this increase may be related to the level of glycemic control or to injection therapy. Suspicion regarding a role for the latter is based on evidence for higher carriage rates among intravenous drug abusers and patients receiving hemodialysis. It may well be, however, that use of injections is simply a confounding factor when studying the diabetic population.

What are the consequences of an increased rate of carriage of *S. aureus*? In all populations, the rate of postoperative wound infection may be higher among carriers.[184] While diabetics are often categorized as being at high risk for staphylococcal infection in general, investigations of this issue are not abundant. For many years, the "definitive" work was that of Greenwood,[185] who in 1927 found a 2.4% rate of erysipelas, furuncles, and carbuncles in a diabetic population. His study included neither cultures nor controls. A paper published in 1942 documented no increased rate of infection.[186] Although extensive reviews of staphylococcal infections may include a number of diabetic patients,[187] the insufficiency of the data presented makes it impossible to derive a denominator for the number of diabetic patients at risk. A recently published study of the rate of *S. aureus* carriage in a population of patients receiving CAPD noted a 77% carriage rate among those with diabetes as compared with a 36% rate among those without diabetes.[188] All carriers had a higher rate of exit-site infections, but only diabetics had a higher rate of tunnel infections.

While many series have examined the incidence and outcome of staphylococcal bacteremia,[189] it is again impossible to draw conclusions about the proportional risk in the diabetic population. Studies are often retrospective and without controls.[190] For the same reason, it is difficult to determine the role of diabetes as a risk factor for the development of endocarditis in the setting of staphylococcal bacteremia. Diabetes is often found as a comorbid condition in those who appear more likely to have a poor outcome with endocarditis.[191] Cooper and Platt[192] did not find an increased mortality among diabetic patients with *S. aureus* endocarditis as compared with nondiabetics with *S. aureus* endocarditis or with diabetic patients with *S. aureus* bacteremia without endocarditis. Of note is that all cases of endocarditis due to a primary focus of infection occurred in the diabetic group. Five of six of the diabetic patients with endocarditis had chronic infection with *S. aureus* in an extremity—in distinction to the situation in which the primary focus is an intravenous catheter, which is usually quickly identified as the source and removed and for which a short course (2 to 3 weeks) of intravenous therapy is often adequate. The risk for diabetic patients with bacteremia related to a promptly removed focus is not known, and a conservative course of therapy (4 to 6 weeks) is reasonable.

Soft Tissue Infections

Consideration of soft tissue infections is complicated by confusing nomenclature and a lack of uniform terminology.[193,194] One approach has been to use definitions based on the anatomic structures (tissues and tissue planes) involved, but this cannot always be ascertained reliably unless surgical exploration is undertaken. In addition, because of the close relationship of various tissues and potential spaces of the soft tissues, various designations often reflect progressive stages of a single infection. Classification by causative organisms has also been used, but any organism may cause a variety of clinical syndromes, depending on what other microbes are present and what level of tissue is infected. Progress in culture techniques has revealed that polymicrobial infection with a broader spectrum of organisms than has previously been appreciated often is present. To further confound the issue, eponyms frequently are used. In recent years there has been debate about the utility of any of the present designations. Obviously, the point of classification should be to organize in a rational fashion the features of an illness so as to permit accurate communication and judgments about progression, prognosis, and intervention. An attempt has been made here to use the most common terms found in the literature. The reader is referred to any standard surgery or infectious disease text for additional information on this extensive topic.

Necrotizing Fasciitis

In recent series,[195–198] 20 to 80% of patients with necrotizing fasciitis had diabetes. In the most general terms, necrotizing fasciitis is any necrotizing soft tissue infection that spreads along fascial planes, either with or without overlying cellulitis. It is sometimes categorized bacteriologically as type 1 or type 2, with type 1 referring to an infection involving at least one anaerobe and one or more facultative anaerobes such as streptococci or Enterobacteriaceae (basically, organisms of the intestinal flora) and type 2 referring specifically to an infection with group A streptococci alone or in combination with *Staphylococcus aureus.* Persons with diabetes are prone to type 1 infection. It is most common on the extremities, especially the legs, but can also affect the perineum, abdominal wall, and perianal region. It can also occur almost anywhere as a postoperative wound infection. At presentation, patients are almost universally febrile with systemic signs of moderate to severe toxicity. Initially, examination of the involved site may reveal only edema, warmth, and tenderness. However, as the infection progresses, causing necrosis of the subcutaneous tissues, the vessels supplying the overlying skin become thrombosed, resulting in overlying bullae, gangrene, ulcerations, or discoloration accompanied by anesthesia. Sometimes a small area of overt skin injury belies a large area of underlying fascial necrosis. Underlying musculature becomes involved less frequently (myonecrosis) because of its richer blood supply. Crepitation is reported in about 50% of patients. In one study, plain films were done for all patients with a diagnosis of necrotizing fasciitis. Gas was found in 19 of 26 patients, only 5 of whom had physical signs of gas when examined. Gas was visualized in 17 of the 21 diabetic patients in the study.[199] It is unclear what impact this had on management.

The cornerstone of management of necrotizing fasciitis is a high index of clinical suspicion and prompt surgical exploration, with debridement of all the tissues found to be involved. Repeated explorations and ensuing debridement are usually necessary.[194–196,199] Grafting may ultimately be necessary. Antibiotic coverage should be aimed at enteric gram-negative organisms, anaerobes, and streptococci. The diagnosis carries a high mortality rate that worsens with delay in surgical intervention and when underlying disease is present. In the most thorough recent report on this subject, there was a 75% overall mortality rate but an 85% rate among those with diabetes. Other reports agree with this general trend. A delay of more than 12 hours from the time of presentation to surgical intervention or localization of the process in the groin and perianal region increases the mortality rate. Since there are no controlled studies, it is difficult to surmise from the literature what specific clinical findings correlate well with an operative diagnosis of necrotizing fasciitis.

Fournier's Gangrene

Fournier's gangrene,[200-202] first described in 1883, is a rare, anatomically based subclassification of necrotizing fasciitis that occurs around the male genitalia. It is generally associated with some form of perirectal or urologic disease, often in combination with diabetes. Infection in the periurethral area can spread through the vascular corpus spongiosum to penetrate the tunica albugenea, thus spreading to involve Buck's fascia of the penis. It can then progress along dartos fascia of the scrotum and penis, a direct extension of Colles scrotal fascia, which in turn is an extension of Scarpa's fascia of the anterior abdominal wall. Perirectal infections can have their entry point at Colles fascia and then follow the same tract. Penetration of Colles fascia can result in spread to the buttocks and thigh.[201] The typical bacteriologic finding is a mixture of gram-negative bacteria, anaerobes, and possibly streptococci, again reflecting intestinal organisms. Cellulitis is evident relatively early because of the lack of subcutaneous tissue in the penis and scrotum. There is much pain, with swelling, erythema, crepitation, and possible breakdown of the skin with overlying bullae, along with signs of systemic toxicity. Progression is rapid, particularly if the abdominal fascial planes become involved. The testicles are spared because they have a blood supply separate from the fascial and cutaneous circulation of the scrotum. Wide surgical debridement of devitalized tissue is necessary, whereas orchiectomy is not.[201,202] Fortunately, the scrotal skin has excellent regenerative properties, and skin grafting may not be necessary. The mortality rate is high, remaining in the 40 to 50% range even with aggressive management. Incidence of diabetes mellitus in series (there are only about 400 cases in the literature) ranges from 0 to 40%. Whether diabetes increases the risk of death from this syndrome is unknown.

The counterpart of Fournier's gangrene in the female carries no eponym and is less well described, but it involves the vulva and perineum.[203] Predisposing factors may include diabetes and pelvic surgical procedures, including episiotomy and pudendal block. Early recognition and surgical debridement are again paramount.

Synergistic Necrotizing Cellulitis

Some sources consider synergistic necrotizing cellulitis as a distinct category of necrotizing soft tissue infection cellulitis that preferentially affects diabetic patients.[204] Several authors suggest it may be the severe end of the spectrum of type 1 necrotizing fasciitis that occurs in those with underlying illnesses. The flora is generally made up of one or more species of gram-negative aerobic (or facultative) bacteria and an obligate or facultative anaerobe. A "synergistic" relationship between the infecting organisms has been postulated, given the occurrence of two organisms with differing oxygen requirements. However, the flora may simply reflect the source of the cellulitis, such as the bowel. The role of anaerobes in typical necrotizing fasciitis has come to be appreciated more in the last 10 years. Swartz[205] considers synergistic necrotizing cellulitis to be a variant of necrotizing fasciitis

with prominent involvement of skin and muscle as well as of the subcutaneous tissues and fascia. There is classically thin, brown, and malodorous "dishwater pus" seen coming from small ulcers in the skin with surrounding blue-gray gangrene. Normal-appearing skin between the ulcers belies extensive necrosis of underlying muscles and intervening tissue. Early recognition and therapy with broad-spectrum antibiotics combined with wide surgical debridement, including debridement of necrotic muscle, are imperative.[204,205] As might be surmised from the aggressive nature of this infection, mortality rates are higher than those for a typical necrotizing fasciitis.

Nonclostridial Anaerobic Cellulitis

Although clostridial infection of soft tissue does not occur with increased frequency in the diabetic population, nonclostridial cellulitis,[206] which can present in a similar fashion, does. Many non-spore-forming anaerobes have been found mixed with facultative bacteria such as streptococci, enteric gram-negative organisms, or staphylococci. While the bacteriologic composition of the infection is comparable to that of synergistic necrotizing cellulitis, nonclostridial anaerobic cellulitis sharply contrasts with this entity in its lack of muscle involvement. The cellulitis typically occurs around a lower-extremity wound. Extensive gas is found on radiologic examination, and crepitation is typically palpable. Other skin findings are minimal. There is moderate systemic toxicity. Antibiotic therapy is aimed at a mixed anaerobic and aerobic infection. Surgical debridement of necrotic tissue with exploration to exclude involvement of deeper tissues is undertaken as necessary.

Tuberculosis

The purported relationship between diabetes and tuberculosis dates back to Roman times. Autopsies in the eighteenth and nineteenth centuries were supportive of this association as well, although the tubercle bacillus was not discovered until 1882.[207] However, as in so many conditions frequently thought to be associated with diabetes, the actual increased risk is difficult to assess because of the lack of controlled prospective studies. In addition, studies have tended to draw from populations that may, for other reasons, have a higher incidence of tuberculosis. Such groups at increased risk might include clinic populations and hospitalized patients. In an extensive recent review of the epidemiology of tuberculosis, Rieder et al.[208] have drawn on three large surveys from the 1950s that included some form of control group and/or information on the population. The combined data suggest a relative risk of tuberculosis in individuals with diabetes that is 2.0 to 3.6 times that in those without diabetes. No studies have been published on this topic since the 1960s in either the United States or England. The relative infrequency of tuberculosis presently seen in many clinical settings in the United States makes it difficult to assess whether an association presently exists between tuberculosis and diabetes. In a recent study from Papua New Guinea, the frequency of occurrence of tuberculosis in diabetic patients was found to be 11 times the expected rate in the general population.[209] Diabetes does not alter the basic guidelines for prophylaxis and treatment of tuberculosis,[210] but it is still listed as an indication for tuberculosis testing.[211]

GENERAL CARE OF THE DIABETIC PATIENT WITH REGARD TO INFECTION AND IMMUNIZATION

Generally speaking, the selection of antibiotics for the treatment of infections in diabetic patients is influenced by the same factors that affect the choice of drugs for any other individual. An extra measure of caution should be applied when considering potentially nephrotoxic drugs. Because many diabetic patients have or are at risk for diabetic nephropathy, it would be especially desirable to prevent the added insult of toxic injury. When such drugs must be employed, careful attention should be directed to measures of renal function, drug dosing, and measurement of serum levels of drug if applicable. By the same token, consideration should be given to possible difficulties in the use of potentially ototoxic (auditory and/or vestibular components) antibiotics in patients with visual loss due to diabetic retinopathy. In this group, difficulties with hearing or balance may have greater significance than in the general population. When orally administered antibiotics are used in patients with diabetic complications, the possible effects of gastroenteropathy on the reliability of drug absorption should be kept in mind.

Hyperbaric oxygen therapy has been used for some of the severe diabetic infections, particularly mucormycosis and necrotizing fasciitis. Studies have not been controlled, and numbers have been small. A recent review on hyperbaric oxygen therapy notes that while necrotizing fasciitis is an "accepted indication," for such therapy, what benefit it provides, if any, is poorly understood.[212]

Prevention of infection by general hygienic measures is as important in diabetic patients as in anyone else, if not more so. This is especially true concerning care of the feet, an area that merits special attention in relation to persons with diabetes (Chapter 53).

Immunizations

Diabetic patients should receive immunizations according to the guidelines set forth by the Centers for Disease Control (CDC).[213] None of the available toxoids or vaccines are contraindicated solely on the basis of diabetes.[213] There are two vaccines for which diabetics should be given special consideration, the influenza vaccine and the pneumococcal vaccine.[214] The influenza vaccine, a combination of inactivated viral strains that is modified annually,[215] is 70 to 90% effective if the circulating virus is homologous to the vaccine strains. Immunization with influenza vaccine is particularly important for the elderly, who suffer excess morbidity and mortality from the complications of influenza.[216] In one study, when patients with diabetes who had influenza were stratified by age into those older and those younger than 45 years, those older than 45 years had excess morbidity and mortality if they also had cardiovascular disease.[217] Not enough data were presented to ascertain

the extent of increased risk, if any, that occurs on the basis of diabetes alone. At present, several high-priority groups are targeted for influenza vaccination. The most recent CDC guidelines specifically include persons with diabetes.[215] Good antibody responses have been documented in individuals with well-controlled diabetes[218] receiving either insulin or oral therapy.[219,220] However, it has been suggested that a defect in glycosylation of IgG noted in vitro may result in a decreased response to influenza vaccine.[221] Efficacy of the vaccine in the diabetic population per se has not been rigorously analyzed.

The pneumococcal vaccine available since 1984 is a 23-valent vaccine containing capsular polysaccharide antigens of at least 85 to 90% of those strains responsible for invasive disease.[222] This formulation has replaced an earlier 14-valent vaccine. The vaccine appears to be effective in individuals with diabetes.[223] While the techniques of measuring antibody responses to pneumococcal vaccine are often controversial,[224] it appears that people with diabetes do have an adequate antibody response.[225] It is not clear whether diabetes alone increases the risk of pneumococcal disease or its complications. Diabetes has often been present in patients with serious pneumococcal infection but usually as a comorbid condition.[225] Diabetic patients with cardiac disease may be at some increased risk for serious pneumococcal infection, and pneumococcal vaccination is suggested in these cases as for cardiopulmonary disease in general.[213–215,226]

The hepatitis B vaccine is worth noting in connection with diabetes in that some question exists about whether adequate antibody levels are achieved after the usual dosing schedule of 0, 1, and 6 months.[227–229] Studies are under way to determine the populations, if any, that would benefit from booster doses.

REFERENCES

1. Robbins SL, Tucker AW Jr. The cause of death in diabetes: a report of 307 autopsied cases. N Engl J Med 1944; 231:865–8.
2. Seymour A, Phear D. The causes of death in diabetes mellitus. A study of diabetic mortality in the Royal Adelaide Hospital from 1956 to 1960. Med J Aust 1963; 1:890–4.
3. Sasaki A, Horiuchi N, Hasegawa K, Uehara M. Mortality and causes of death in Type 2 diabetic patients: a long-term follow-up study in Osaka District, Japan. Diabetes Res Clin Prac 1989;7:33–40.
4. Kessler II. Mortality experience of diabetic patients: a twenty-six year follow-up study. Am J Med 1971; 51:715–24.
5. Rubin RH. Defects in host defense mechanisms. In: Rubin RR, Young LS eds. Clinical approach to infection in the compromised host. 2nd ed. New York: Plenum Medical Book Company, 1988.
6. Perillie PE, Nolan JP, Finch SC. Studies of the resistance to infection in diabetes mellitus: local exudative cellular response. J Lab Clin Med 1962;59:1008–15.
7. Brayton RG, Stokes PE, Schwartz MS, Louria DB. Effect of alcohol and various diseases on leukocyte mobilization

phagocytosis and intracellular bacterial killing. N Engl J Med 1970;282:123–8.

8. Mowat AG, Baum J. Chemotaxis of polymorphonuclear leukocytes from patients with diabetes mellitus. N Engl J Med 1971;284:621–7.

9. Molenaar DM, Palumbo PJ, Wilson WR, Ritts RE Jr. Leukocyte chemotaxis in diabetic patients and their nondiabetic first-degree relatives. Diabetes 1976; 25:880–3.

10. Valerius NH, Eff C, Hansen NE, et al. Neutrophil and lymphocyte function in patients with diabetes mellitus. Acta Med Scand 1982;211:463–7.

11. Tater D, Tepaut B, Bercovici JP, Youinou P. Polymorphonuclear cell derangements in Type I diabetes. Horm Metab Res 1987;19:642–7.

12. Naghibi M, Smith RP, Baltch AL, et al. The effect of diabetes mellitus on chemotactic and bactericidal activity of human polymorphonuclear leukocytes. Diabetes Res Clin Pract 1987;4:27–35.

13. Bybee JD, Rogers DE. The phagocytic activity of polymorphonuclear leukocytes obtained from patients with diabetes mellitus. J Lab Clin Med 1964;64:1–13.

14. Bagdade JD, Root RK, Bulger RJ. Impaired leukocyte function in patients with poorly controlled diabetes. Diabetes 1974;23:9–15.

15. Rayfield EJ, Ault MJ, Keusch GT, et al. Infection and diabetes: the case for glucose control. Am J Med 1982; 72:439–50.

16. Tan JS, Anderson JL, Watanakunakorn C, Phair JP. Neutrophil dysfunction in diabetes mellitus. J Clin Lab Med 1975;85:26–33.

17. Nolan CM, Beaty HN, Bagdade JD. Further characterization of the impaired bactericidal function of granulocytes in patients with poorly controlled diabetes. Diabetes 1978;27:889–94.

18. Davidson J, Sowden JM, Fletcher J. Defective phagocytosis in insulin controlled diabetics: evidence for a reaction between glucose and opsonizing proteins. J Clin Pathol 1984;37:783.

19. Peterson CM, Jones RL, Koenig RJ, et al. Reversible hematologic sequelae of diabetes mellitus. Ann Intern Med 1977;86:425–9.

20. Sohnle PG. Neutrophil adherence in diabetes mellitus [Editorial]. J Lab Clin Med 1988;111:263–4.

21. Bagdade JD, Stewart M, Walters E. Impaired granulocyte adherence: a reversible defect in host defense in patients with poorly controlled diabetes. Diabetes 1978; 27:677–81.

22. Bagdade JD, Walters E. Impaired granulocyte adherence in mildly diabetic patients: effects of tolazamide treatment. Diabetes 1980;29:309–11.

23. Andersen B, Goldsmith GH, Spagnuolo PJ. Neutrophil adhesive dysfunction in diabetes mellitus: the role of cellular plasma factors. J Lab Clin Med 1980; 111:275–85.

24. Dziatkowiak H, Kowalska M, Denys A. Phagocytic and bactericidal activity of granulocytes in diabetic children. Diabetes 1982;31:1041–3.

25. Repine JE, Clawson CC, Goetz FC. Bactericidal function of neutrophils from patients with acute bacterial infections and from diabetics. J Infect Dis 1980;142:869–75.

26. Shah SV, Wallin JD, Eilen SD. Chemiluminescence and superoxide anion production by leukocytes from diabetic patients. J Clin Endocrinol Metab 1983;57:402–9.

27. Winocour PH, Lenton J, Puxty JA, Anderson DC. Leukocyte microbicidal activity assessed by chemiluminescence in elderly non-insulin dependent diabetes mellitus. Diabetes Res 1988;9:73–5.

28. Öberg G, Hällgren R, Moberg L, Venge P. Bactericidal proteins and neutral proteases in diabetes neutrophils. Diabetalogica 1986;29:426–9.

29. Collier A, Jackson M, Bell D, et al. Neutrophil activation detected by increased neutrophil elastase activity in Type I (insulin-dependent) diabetes mellitus. Diabetes Res 1989;10:135–8.

30. Qvist R, Larkins RG. Diminished production of thromboxane B_2 and prostaglandin E by stimulated polymorphonuclear leukocytes from insulin treated diabetic subjects. Diabetes 1983;32:622–6.

31. Jubiz W, Draper RE, Gale J, Nolan G. Decreased leukotriene B_4 synthesis by polymorphonuclear leukocytes from male patients with diabetes mellitus. Prostaglandins Leukotrienes Med 1984;14:305–11.

32. Geisler G, Almdal T, Bennedsen J, et al. Monocyte functions in diabetes mellitus. Acta Pathol Microbiol Immunol Scand 1982;90C:33–7.

33. Glass EJ, Stewart J, Matthews DM, et al. Impairment of monocyte "lectin-like" receptor activity in Type I (insulin-dependent) diabetic patients. Diabetologia 1987; 30:228–31.

34. Katz S, Klein B, Elian I, et al. Phagocytic activity of monocytes from diabetic patients. Diabetes Care 1983; 6:479–82.

35. Hill HR, Augustine NH, Rallison ML, Santos JI. Defective monocyte chemotactic response in diabetes mellitus. Clin Immunol 1983;3:70–7.

36. Setiadi H, Wautier J-L, Courilon-Mallet A, et al. Increased adhesion to fibronectin and MO-I expression by diabetic monocytes. J Immunol 1987;138:3230–4.

37. Kitahara M, Eyre HJ, Lynch RE, et al. Metabolic activity of diabetic monocytes. Diabetes 1980;29:251–6.

38. Pozzilli P, Pagani S, Arduini P, et al. In vivo determination of cell mediated immune response in diabetic patients using a multiple intradermal antigen dispenser. Diabetes Res 1987;6:5–8.

39. MacCuish AC, Urbaniak SJ, Campbell CJ, et al. Phytohemagglutinin transformation and circulating lymphocyte subpopulations in insulin-dependent diabetic patients. Diabetes 1974;25:908–12.

40. Casey JI, Heeter BJ, Klyshevich KA. Impaired response of lymphocytes of diabetic subjects to antigen of Staphylococcus aureus. J Infect Dis 1987;136:495–501.

41. Casey J, Sturm C Jr. Impaired response of lymphocytes from non-insulin-dependent diabetics to staphage lysate and tetanus antigen. J Clin Microbiol 1982; 15:109–14.

42. Speert DP, Silva J Jr. Abnormalities of in vitro lymphocyte response to mitogens in diabetic children during acute ketoacidosis. Am J Dis Child 1978;132:1014–7.

43. Kolterman OG, Olefsky JM, Kurahara C, Taylor K. A defect in cell-mediated immune function in insulin-resistant diabetic and obese subjects. J Lab Clin Med 1980; 96:535–43.

44. Topliss D, How J, Lewis M, et al. Evidence for cell-mediated immunity and specific suppressor T-lymphocyte dysfunction in Graves' disease and diabetes mellitus. J Clin Endocrinol Metab 1983;57:700–5.

45. Pozzilli P, Visalli N, Cavallo MG, et al. Normalization of the CD4/CD8 lymphocyte ratio and increased B lymphocytes in long standing diabetic patients following therapy with thymopentin. Diabetes Res 1987;6:51–6.

46. Faustman D, Eisenbarth G, Daley J, Beitmeyer J. Abnormal

T-lymphocyte subsets in Type I diabetes. Diabetes 1989; 38:1462–8.

47. Fisher BM, Smith JG, McCruden DC, Frier BM. Responses of peripheral blood cells and lymphocyte subpopulations to insulin-induced hypoglycaemia in human insulin-dependent (Type I) diabetes. Eur J Clin Invest 1987; 17:208–13.

48. Kaye WA, Adri MN, Soelder JS, et al. Acquired defect in interleukin-2 production in patients with Type I diabetes mellitus. N Engl J Med 1986;315:920–4.

49. Giordano C, Galluzzo A, Marco A, et al. Increased soluble interleukin-2 receptor levels in the sera of Type I diabetic patients. Diabetes Res 1988;8:135–8.

50. Negishi K, Gupta S, Chandy KG, et al. Interferon responsiveness of natural killer cells in Type I human diabetes. Diabetes Res 1988;7:49–52.

51. McMillan DE. The microcirculation: changes in diabetes mellitus. Mayo Clin Proc 1988;63:517–20.

52. Vermes I, Steinmetz ET, Zeyen LJJM, van der Veen EA. Rheological properties of white blood cells are changed in diabetic patients with microvascular complications. Diabetologia 1987;30:434–6.

53. Williamson JR, Tilton RG, Chang K, Kilo C. Basement membrane abnormalities in diabetes mellitus: relationship to clinical microangiopathy. Diabetes Metab Rev 1988; 4:339–70.

54. Lehrer RI (moderator-UCLA conference). Mucormycosis. Ann Intern Med 1980;93:93–108.

55. Rippon JW. Zygomycosis. In: Medical mycology: the pathogenic fungi and the pathogenic Actinomycetes. Philadelphia: WB Saunders, 1988:681–713.

56. Brennan RO, Crain BJ, Proctor AM, Durack DT. *Cunninghamella*: a newly recognized cause of rhinocerebral mucormycosis. Am J Clin Pathol 1983;80:98–102.

57. Waldorf AR, Ruderman N, Diamond RD. Specific susceptibility to mucormycosis in murine diabetes and bronchoalveolar macrophage defense against *Rhizopus*. J Clin Invest 1984;74:150–60.

58. Waldorf AR. Host-parasite relationship in opportunistic mycoses. Crit Rev Microbiol 1986;13:133–72.

59. Gale GR, Welch AM. Studies of opportunistic fungi: inhibition of *Rhizopus oryzae* by human serum. Am J Med Sci 1961;241:604–12.

60. Artis WM, Fountain JA, Delcher HK, Jones HE. A mechanism of susceptibility to mucormycosis in diabetic ketoacidosis: transferrin and iron availability. Diabetes 1982; 31:1109–14.

61. Daly AL, Velazquez LA, Bradley SF, Kauffman CA. Mucormycosis: association with deferoxamine therapy. Am J Med 1989;87:468–71.

62. Gregory JE, Golden A, Haymaker W. Mucormycosis of the central nervous system: a report of three cases. Bull Johns Hopkins Hosp 1943;73:405–19.

63. Marr TJ, Traisman HS, Davis T, Kernahan D. Rhinocerebral mucormycosis and juvenile diabetes mellitus: report of a case with recovery. Diabetes Care 1978;1:250.

64. Lowe JT Jr, Hudson WR. Rhinocerebral phycomycosis and carotid internal artery thrombosis. Arch Otolaryngol 1975;101:100–3.

65. Rubin RH. Fungal infection in the compromised host. In: Rubin RH, Young LS, eds. Clinical approach to infection in the compromised host. New York: Plenum Medical Book Co, 1988.

66. Oakley LA, Fisher JF, Dennison JH. Bread mold infection in diabetes: the life-threatening condition of rhinocerebral zygomycosis. Postgrad Med 1986;80(2):93–96.

67. Greenberg MR, Lippman SM, Grinnell VS, et al. Computed tomographic findings in orbital mucor. West J Med 1985;143:102–3.

68. Abramson E, Wilson D, Arky RA. Rhinocerebral phycomycosis, in association with diabetic ketoacidosis: report of two cases and a review of clinical and experimental experience with amphotericin B therapy. Ann Intern Med 1967;66:735–42.

69. Gallis HA, Drew RH, Pickard WW. Amphotericin B: 30 years of clinical experience. Rev Infect Dis 1990; 12:308–29.

70. Saag MS, Dismukes WE. Azole antifungal agents: emphasis on new triazoles. Antimicrob Agents Chemother 1988; 32:1–8.

71. Hamill R, Oney LA, Crane LR. Successful therapy for rhinocerebral mucormycosis with associated bilateral brain abscesses. Arch Intern Med 1983;143:581–3.

72. Parfrey NA. Improved diagnosis and prognosis of mucormycosis: a clinicopathologic study of 33 cases. Medicine (Baltimore) 1986;65:113–23.

73. Hansen LA, Prakash UBS, Colby TV. Pulmonary complications in diabetes mellitus. Mayo Clin Proc 1989; 64:791–9.

74. Bigby TD, Serota ML, Tierney LM Jr, Matthay MA. Clinical spectrum of pulmonary mucormycosis. Chest 1986; 89:435–9.

75. Johnson GM, Baldwin JJ. Pulmonary mucormycosis and juvenile diabetes [Letter]. Am J Dis Child 1981; 135:567–8.

76. Donohue JF. Endobronchial mucormycosis [Letter]. Chest 1983;83:585.

77. Chandler JR. Malignant external otitis. Laryngoscope 1968;78:1257–94.

78. Zaky DA, Bentley DW, Lowy K, et al. Malignant external otitis: a severe form of otitis in diabetic patients. Am J Med 1976;61:298–302.

79. Salitt IE, Miller B, Wigmore M, Smith JA. Bacterial flora of the external canal in diabetics and non-diabetics. Laryngoscope 1982;92:672–3.

80. Doroghazi RM, Nadol JP Jr, Hyslop NE Jr, et al. Invasive external otitis: report of 21 cases and review of the literature. Am J Med 1981;71:603–13.

81. Petton SI, Klein JO. The draining ear. Infect Dis Clin North Am 1988;2:117.

82. Rubin J, Yu VL. Malignant external otitis: insights into pathogenesis clinical manifestations diagnosis and therapy. Am J Med 1988;85:391–8.

83. Corey JP, Levandowski RA, Panwalker AP. Prognostic implications of therapy for necrotizing external otitis. Am J Otol 1985;6:353–8.

84. Gherini SG, Brackmann DE, Bradley WG. Magnetic resonance imaging and computerized tomography in malignant external otitis. Laryngoscope 1986;96:542–8.

85. Babiatzki A, Sandé J. Malignant external otitis. J Laryngol Otol 1987;101:205–10.

86. Kraus DH, Rehm SJ, Kinney SE. The evolving treatment of necrotizing external otitis. Laryngoscope 1988;98:934–9.

87. Johnson MP, Ramphal R. Malignant external otitis: report on therapy with ceftazidime and review of therapy and prognosis. Rev Infect Dis 1990;12:173–80.

88. Lang R, Goshen S, Kitzes-Cohen R, Sadé J. Successful treatment of malignant external otitis with oral ciprofloxacin: report of experience with 23 patients. J Infect Dis 1990;161:537–40.

89. Leggett JM, Prendergast K. Malignant external otitis: the use of oral ciprofloxacin. J Laryngol Otol 1988;102:53–4.

90. Kelly HA, MacCallum WG. Pneumaturia. JAMA 1898; 31:375.

91. Freiha FS, Messing EM, Gross DM. Emphysematous pyelonephritis. JCE Urol 1979;18:9.

92. Ahlering TE, Boyd SD, Hamilton CL, et al. Emphysematous pyelonephritis: a 5-year experience with 13 patients. J Urol 1985;134:1086–8.

93. Zabbo A, Montie JE, Popowniak KL, Weinstein AJ. Bilateral emphysematous pyelonephritis. Urology 1985; 25:293–6.

94. Michaeli J, Mogle P, Perlberg S, et al. Emphysematous pyelonephritis. J Urol 1984;131:203–8.

95. Cook DJ, Achong MR, Dobranowski J. Emphysematous pyelonephritis: complicated urinary tract infection in diabetes. Diabetes Care 1982;12:229–32.

96. Ouellet LM, Brook MP. Emphysematous pyelonephritis: an emergency indication for the plain abdominal radiograph. Ann Emerg Med 1988;17:722–4.

97. Vas W, Carlin B, Salimi Z, et al. CT diagnosis of emphysematous pyelonephritis. Comput Radiol 1985;9:37–9.

98. Lowe FC, Walther JM. Case profile: emphysematous pyelonephritis. Urology 1986;28:532–3.

99. Sarmiento RV. Emphysematous cholecystitis: report of four cases and review of the literature. Arch Surg 1966;93:1009–14.

100. Mentzer RM Jr, Golden GT, Chandler JG, Horsley JH III. A comparative appraisal of emphysematous cholecystitis. Am J Surg 1975;129:10–5.

101. Schwartz SI. Gallbladder and extrahepatic biliary system. In: Schwartz SI, Shires GT, Spencer FC, Husser WC, eds. Principles of surgery. 5th ed. New York: McGraw Hill, 1989:1381–412.

102. Ruby ST, Gladstone A, Treat M, Weber CJ. Emphysematous cholecystitis: a case report. JAMA 1983;249:248–9.

103. Nemcek AA Jr, Gore RM, Vogelzang RL, Grant J. The effervescent gallbladder: a sonographic sign of emphysematous cholecystitis. AJR Am J Roentgenol 1980; 150:575–93.

104. Hunter ND, Macintosh PK. Acute emphysematous cholecystitis: An ultrasonic diagnosis. AJR Am J Roentgenol 1980;134:592–3.

105. Walsh DB, Eckhauser FE, Ramsburgh SR, Burney RB. Risk associated with diabetes mellitus in patients undergoing gallbladder surgery. Surgery 1982;91:254–7.

106. Ransohoff DF, Miller GL, Forsythe SB, Hermann RE. Outcome of acute cholecystitis in patients with diabetes mellitus. Ann Intern Med 1987;106:829–32.

107. Friedman LS, Roberts MS, Brett AS, Marton KI. Management of asymptomatic gallstones in the diabetic patient: a decision analysis. Ann Intern Med 1988;109:913–9.

108. Hickman MS, Schwesinger WH, Page CP. Acute cholecystitis in the diabetic: a case-control study of outcome. Arch Surg 1988;123:409–11.

109. Sharp KW. Acute cholecystitis. Surg Clin North Am 1988;68:269–79.

110. Insulin injections and infections [Editorial]. BMJ 1981; 282:340.

111. Swift PGF, Hearnshaw JR. Insulin injections and infections [Letter]. BMJ 1981;282:1323.

112. Borders LM, Bingham PR, Riddle MC. Traditional insulin-use practices and the incidence of bacterial contamination and infection. Diabetes Care 1984;7:121–7.

113. Poteet GW, Reinert B, Ptak HE. Outcome of multiple usage of disposable syringes in the insulin-requiring diabetic. Nurs Res 1987;36(6):350–2.

114. Price JP, Kruger DF, Saravolatz LD, Whitehouse FW. Evaluation of the insulin jet injector as a potential source of infection. Am J Infect Control 1989;17:258–63.

115. Brink SJ, Stewart C. Insulin pump treatment in insulin-dependent diabetes mellitus: children, adolescents, and young adults. JAMA 1986;255:617–21.

116. Chantelau E, Lange G, Sonnenberg GE, Berger M. Acute cutaneous complications and catheter needle colonization during insulin-pump treatment. Diabetes Care 1987; 10:478–82.

117. Bell DS, Ackerson C, Cutter G, Clements RS Jr. Factors associated with discontinuation of continuous subcutaneous insulin infusion. Am J Med Sci 1988;295:23–8.

118. van Faassen I, Razenberg PPA, Simoons-Smit AM, van der Veen EA. Carriage of Staphylococcus aureus and inflamed infusion sites with insulin pump therapy. Diabetes Care 1989;12:153–5.

119. Carson CC. Infections in genitourinary prostheses. Urol Clin North Am 1989;16:139–47.

120. Blum MD. Infections of genitourinary prostheses. Infect Dis Clin North Am 1989;3:259–74.

121. Montague DK. Periprosthetic infections. J Urol 1987; 138:68–9.

122. Carson CC, Robertson CN. Late hematogenous infection of penile prostheses. J Urol 1988;139:50–2.

123. Rubin RH. Infection in the renal and liver transplant patient. In: Rubin RH, Young LS, eds. Clinical approach to infection in the compromised host. 2nd ed. New York: Plenum Press, 1988:577.

124. Gottesdiener KM. Transplanted infections: donor-to-host transmission with the allograft. Ann Intern Med 1989; 110:1001–16.

125. Bowen PH II, Lobel SA, Caruana RJ, et al. Transmission of human immunodeficiency virus (HIV) by transplantation: clinical aspects and time course analysis of viral antigenemia and antibody production. Ann Intern Med 1988; 108:46–8.

126. Rubin RH, Wolfson JS, Cosimi AB, Tolkoff-Rubin NE. Infection in the renal transplant recipient. Am J Med 1981;70:405–11.

127. Peterson PK, Andersen RC. Infection in renal transplant recipients: current approaches to diagnosis, therapy, and prevention. Am J Med 1986;81(Suppl 1A):2–10.

128. Perkins JD, Fromme GA, Narr BJ, et al. Pancreas transplantation at Mayo. II. Operative and perioperative management. Mayo Clin Proc 1990;65:483–95.

129. Perkins JD, Frohnert PP, Service FJ, et al. Pancreas transplantation at Mayo. III. Multidisciplinary management. Mayo Clin Proc 1990;65:496–508.

130. Rheuman MJ, Rheuman B, Icenogle T, et al. Diabetes and heart transplantation. J Heart Transplant 1988;7:356–8.

131. Peterson PK, Keane WF. Infections in chronic peritoneal dialysis patients. Curr Clin Topics Infect Dis 1985;6:239.

132. Steigbigel RT, Cross AS. Infections associated with hemodialysis and chronic peritoneal dialysis. Curr Clin Topics Infect Dis 1984;5:124–45.

133. Vas SI. Infections of continuous ambulatory peritoneal dialysis catheters. Infect Dis Clin North Am 1989; 3:301–28.

134. Amair P, Khanna R, Leibel B, et al. Continuous ambulatory peritoneal dialysis in diabetics with end-stage renal disease. N Engl J Med 1982;306:625–30.

135. Madden MA, Zimmerman SW, Simpson DP. Continuous ambulatory peritoneal dialysis in diabetes mellitus: the risks and benefits of intraperitoneal insulin. Am J Nephrol 1982;2:133–9.

136. Kraus ES, Spector DA. Characteristics and sequelae of

peritonitis in diabetics and nondiabetics receiving chronic intermittent peritoneal dialysis. Medicine (Baltimore) 1983;62:52–7.

137. Vas SI, Law L. Microbiological diagnosis of peritonitis in patients on continuous ambulatory peritoneal dialysis. J Clin Microbiol 1985;21:522–3.

138. Kerr CM, Perfect JR, Craven PC, et al. Fungal peritonitis in patients on continuous ambulatory peritoneal dialysis. Ann Intern Med 1983;99:334–7.

139. Arfania D, Everett D, Nolph K, Rubin J. Uncommon causes of peritonitis in patients undergoing peritoneal dialysis. Arch Intern Med 1981;141:61–4.

140. Bunke CM, Aronoff GR, Luft FC. Pharmacokinetics of common antibiotics used in continuous ambulatory peritoneal dialysis. Am J Kidney Dis 1983;3:114–7.

141. Kherlakian GM, Roedersheimer LR, Arbaugh JJ, et al. Comparison of autogenous fistula versus expanded polytetrafluoroethylene graft fistula for angioaccess in hemodialysis. Am J Surg 1986;152:238–43.

142. Vas SI. Infections associated with peritoneal and hemodialysis. In: Bisno AL, Waldvogel FA, eds. Infections associated with indwelling medical devices. Washington DC: American Society for Microbiology, 1989;215–48.

143. Winsett OE, Wolma FJ. Complications of vascular access for hemodialysis. South Med J 1985;78:513–7.

144. Quarles LD, Rutsky EA, Rostand SG. *Staphylococcus aureus* bacteremia in patients on chronic hemodialysis. Am J Kidney Dis 1985;6:412–9.

145. Cross AS, Steigbigel RT. Infective endocarditis and access site infections in patients on hemodialysis. Medicine (Baltimore) 1976;55:453–66.

146. Francioli P, Masur H. Complications of *Staphylococcus aureus* bacteremia: occurrence in patients undergoing long-term hemodialysis. Arch Intern Med 1982;142:1655–8.

147. Munda R, First MR, Alexander JW, et al. Polytetrafluoroethylene graft survival in hemodialysis. JAMA 1983;249:219–22.

148. Tanchajja S, Mohaideen AH, Avram MM, Eisenberg MM. Management of infection associated with prosthetic graft exposure in angioaccess. Vasc Surg 1985;19:117–21.

149. Bryan CS, Reynolds KL, Metzger WT. Bacteremia in diabetic patients: comparison of incidence and mortality with nondiabetic patients. Diabetes Care 1985;8:244–9.

150. Keane EM, Boyko EJ, Reller LB, Hamman RF. Prevalence of asymptomatic bacteriuria in subjects with NIDDM in San Luis Valley of Colorado. Diabetes Care 1988;11:708–12.

151. Schmitt JK, Fawcett CJ, Gullickson G. Asymptomatic bacteriuria and hemoglobin A$_1$. Diabetes Care 1986;9:518–20.

152. Sawers JS, Todd WA, Kellett HA, et al. Bacteriuria and autonomic nerve function in diabetic women. Diabetes Care 1986;9:460–4.

153. Forland M, Thomas VL. The treatment of urinary tract infections in women with diabetes mellitus. Diabetes Care 1985;8:499–506.

154. Brauner A, Östenson CG. Bacteremia with P-fimbriated *Escherichia coli* in diabetic patients: correlation between proteinuria and non-p-fimbriated strains. Diabetes Res 1987;6:61–5.

155. Levison ME, Pitsakis PG. Effect of insulin treatment on the susceptibility of the diabetic rat to *Escherichia coli*-induced pyelonephritis. J Infect Dis 1984;150:554–60.

156. Groop L, Laasonen L, Edgren J. Renal papillary necrosis in patients with IDDM. Diabetes Care 1989;12:198–202.

157. Eknoyan G, Qunibi WY, Grissom RT, et al. Renal papillary necrosis: an update. Medicine (Baltimore) 1982; 61:55–73.

158. Mujais SK. Renal papillary necrosis in diabetes mellitus. Semin Nephrol 1984;4:40–7.

159. Saiki J, Vaziri ND, Barton C. Perinephric and intranephric abscesses: a review of the literature. West J Med 1982; 136:95–102.

160. Plevin SN, Balodimos MC, Bradley RF. Perinephric abscess in diabetic patients. J Urol 1979;103:539–43.

161. Patterson JE, Andriole VT. Renal and perirenal abscesses. Infect Dis Clin North Am 1987;1:907.

162. Bova JG, Potter JL, Arevalos E, et al. Renal and perirenal infection: the role of computerized tomography. J Urol 1985;133:375–8.

163. Hutchison FN, Kaysen GA. Perinephric abscess: the missed diagnosis. Med Clin North Am 1988;72:993–1014.

164. Edelstein H, McCabe RE. Perinephric abscess: modern diagnosis and treatment in 47 cases. Medicine (Baltimore) 1988;67:118–31.

165. Bartholomew GA, Rodu B, Bell DS. Oral candidiasis in patients with diabetes mellitus: a thorough analysis. Diabetes Care 1987;10:607–12.

166. Hill LVH, Tan MH, Pereira LH, Embil JA. Association of oral candidiasis with diabetic control. J Clin Pathol 1989; 42:502–5.

167. Fisher BM, Lamey P-J, Samaranayake LP, et al. Carriage of Candida species in the oral cavity in diabetic patients: relationship to glycaemic control. J Oral Pathol 1987; 16:282–4.

168. Phelan JA, Levin SM. A prevalence study of denture stomatitis in subjects with diabetes mellitus or elevated plasma glucose levels. Oral Surg Oral Med Oral Pathol 1986;62:303–5.

169. Jorizzo JL. Chronic mucocutaneous candidosis: an update. Arch Dermatol 1982;118:963–5.

170. Williams DN, Knight AH, King H, Harris DM. The microbial flora of the vagina and its relationship to bacteriuria in diabetic and non-diabetic women. Br J Urol 1975; 47:453–7.

171. Sobel JD. Vulvovaginal candidiasis—What we do and do not know [Editorial]. Ann Intern Med 1984;101:390–2.

172. Rein MF, Holmes KK. Nonspecific vaginitis vulvovaginal candidiasis and trichomaniasis. Curr Clin Topics Infect Dis 1983;4:281.

173. Roy JB, Geyer JR, Mohr JA. Urinary tract candidiasis: an update. Urology 1984;23:533–7.

174. Frye KR, Donovan JM, Drach GW. Torulopsis glabrata urinary infections: a review. J Urol 1988;139:1245–9.

175. Frangos DN, Nyberg LM Jr. Genitourinary fungal infections. South Med J 1986;79:455–9.

176. Fisher J, Mayhall G, Duma R, et al. Fungus balls of the urinary tract. South Med J 1979;72:1281–4.

177. Urinary tract candidosis. Lancet 1988;2:1000–2.

178. Bibler MR, Gianis JT. Acute ureteral colic from an obstructing renal aspergilloma. Rev Infect Dis 1987; 9:790–4.

179. Smith JA, O'Connor JJ. Nasal carriage of Staphylococcus aureus in diabetes mellitus. Lancet 1966;2:776–7.

180. Tuazon CU, Perez A, Kishaba T, Sheagren JN. *Staphylococcus aureus* among insulin-injecting diabetic patients: an increased carrier rate. JAMA 1975;231:1272.

181. Chandler PT, Chandler SD. Pathogenic carrier rate in diabetes mellitus. Am J Med Sci 1977;273:259–63.

182. Boyko EJ, Lipsky BA, Sandoval R, et al. NIDDM and prevalence of nasal *Staphylococcus aureus* colonization:

San Luis Valley diabetes study. Diabetes Care 1989; 12:189–92.

183. Lipsky BA, Pecoraro RE, Chen MS, Koepsell TD. Factors affecting staphylococcal colonization among NIDDM outpatients. Diabetes Care 1987;10:483–6.

184. Tuazon CU. Skin and skin structure infections in the patient at risk: carrier state of *Staphylococcus aureus.* Am J Med 1984;76(Suppl 5A):166–71.

185. Greenwood AM. A study of the skin in five hundred cases of diabetes. JAMA 1927;89:774–9.

186. Williams JR. Does diabetes mellitus predispose the patient to the pyogenic skin infections? A study of the etiologic relationship of furunculosis and carbuncle. JAMA 1942; 118:1357.

187. Musher DM, McKenzie SO. Infections due to *Staphylococcus aureus.* Medicine (Baltimore) 1977;56:383–409.

188. Luzar MA, Coles GA, Faller, et al. *Staphylococcus aureus* nasal carriage and infection in patients on continuous ambulatory peritoneal dialysis. N Engl J Med 1990; 322:505–9.

189. Mylotte JM, McDermott C, Spooner JA. Prospective study of 114 consecutive episodes of *Staphylococcus aureus* bacteremia. Rev Infect Dis 1987;9:891–907.

190. Cluff LE, Reynolds RC, Page DL, Breckenridge JL. Staphylococcal bacteremia and altered host resistance. Ann Intern Med 1968;69:859–73.

191. Watanakunakorn C, Baird IM. Prognostic factors in Staphylococcus aureus endocarditis and results of therapy with a penicillin and gentamicin. Am J Med Sci 1977; 273:133–9.

192. Cooper G, Platt R. *Staphylococcus aureus* bacteremia in diabetic patients: endocarditis and mortality. Am J Med 1982;73:658–62.

193. Freischlag JA, Ajalat G, Busuttil RW. Treatment of necrotizing soft tissue infections: a need for a new approach. Am J Surg 1985;149:751–5.

194. Dellinger EP. Severe necrotizing soft-tissue infections: multiple disease entities requiring a common approach. JAMA 1981;246:1717–21.

195. Rouse TM, Malangoni MA, Schulte WJ. Necrotizing fasciitis: a preventable disaster. Surgery 1982;92:765–70.

196. Ahrenholz DH. Necrotizing soft-tissue infections. Surg Clin North Am 1968;68:199–214.

197. Gozal D, Ziser A, Shupak A, et al. Necrotizing fasciitis. Arch Surg 1986;121:233–5.

198. Freeman HP, Oluwole SF, Ganepola GAP, Dy E. Necrotizing fasciitis. Am J Surg 1981;142:377–83.

199. Fisher JR, Conway MJ, Takeshita RT, Sandoval MR. Necrotizing fasciitis: importance of roentgenographic studies for soft-tissue gas. JAMA 1979;241:803–6.

200. O'Dell K, Shipp J. Fournier's syndrome in a ketoacidotic diabetic patient after intrascrotal insulin injections because of impotence. Diabetes Care 1983;6:601–3.

201. Spirnak JP, Resnick MI, Hampel N, Persky L. Fournier's gangrene: report of 20 patients. J Urol 1984; 131:289–91.

202. Lamb RC, Juler GL. Fournier's gangrene of the scrotum: a poorly defined syndrome or a misnomer? Arch Surg 1983;118:38–40.

203. Addison WA, Livengood CH III, Hill GB, et al. Necrotizing fasciitis of vulvar origin in diabetic patients. Obstet Gynecol 1984;63:473–9.

204. Stone HH, Martin JD Jr. Synergistic necrotizing cellulitis. Ann Surg 1972;175:702–11.

205. Swartz MN. Subcutaneous tissue infections and abscesses. In: Mandell GL, Douglas RG Jr, Bennett JE, eds. Principles and practice of infectious disease. 3rd ed. New York: Churchill Livingstone, 1990:808–18.

206. Bessman AN, Wagner W. Nonclostridial gas gangrene: report of 48 cases and review of the literature. JAMA 1975;233:958–63.

207. Oscarsson PN, Silwer H. Incidence of pulmonary tuberculosis among diabetics: search among diabetics in the county of Kristianstad. Acta Med Scand Suppl 1958; 335:23–48.

208. Rieder HL, Cauthen GM, Comstock GW, Snider DE Jr. Epidemiology of tuberculosis in the United States. Epidemiol Rev 1989;11:79–98.

209. Patel MS. Bacterial infections among patients with diabetes in Papua New Guinea. Med J Aust 1989;150:25–8.

210. American Thoracic Society/Centers for Disease Control. Treatment of tuberculosis and tuberculosis infection in adults and children. Am Rev Respir Dis 1986;134:355–63.

211. Centers for Disease Control. Screening for tuberculosis and tuberculosis infection in high-risk populations, and the use of preventive therapy for tuberculous infection in the United States: recommendations of the Advisory Committee for Elimination of Tuberculosis. MMWR 1990; 39:1–12.

212. Grim PS, Gottlieb LJ, Boddie A, Batson E. Hyberbaric oxygen therapy. JAMA 1990;263:2216–20.

213. Recommendations of the Immunization Practices Advisory Committee (ACIP). General recommendations on immunization 1989. MMWR 1989;38:205–27.

214. ACP Task Force on Adult Immunization. Guide for adult immunization. 2nd ed. Philadelphia: American College of Physicians, 1990.

215. Centers for Disease Control. Prevention and control of influenza. Recommendations of the Immunization Practices Advisory Committee (ACIP). MMWR 1990;39:1–15.

216. Barker WH, Mullooly JP. Pneumonia and influenza deaths during epidemics: implications for prevention. Arch Intern Med 1982;142:85–9.

217. Diepersloot RJA, Bouter KP, Beyer WEP, et al. Humoral immune response and delayed type hypersensitivity to influenza vaccine in patients with diabetes mellitus. Diabetologica 1987;30:397–401.

218. Lederman MM, Rodman HM, Schacter BZ, et al. Antibody response to pneumococcal polysaccharides in insulin-dependent diabetes mellitus. Diabetes Care 1982;5:3–96.

219. Pozzilli P, Gale EAM, Visalli N, et al. The immune response to influenza vaccination in diabetic patients. Diabetologica 1986;29:850–84.

220. Feery BJ, Hartman LJ, Hampson AW, Proietto J. Influenza immunization in adults with diabetes mellitus. Diabetes Care 1983;6:475–8.

221. Kaneshige H. Nonenzymatic glycosylation of serum IgG and its effect on antibody activity in patients with diabetes mellitus. Diabetes 1987;36:822–38.

222. Fedson DS. Pneumococcal vaccine. In: Plotkin SA, Mortimer EA Jr, eds. Vaccines. Philadelphia: WB Saunders, 1988:271–99.

223. Bolan G, Broome CV, Facklam RR, et al. Pneumococcal vaccine efficacy in selected populations in the United States. Ann Intern Med 1986;104:1–6.

224. Spika JS, Fedson DS, Facklam RR. Pneumococcal vaccination: controversies and opportunities. Infect Dis Clin North Am 1990;4:11–27.

225. Beam TR Jr, Crigler ED, Goldman JK, Schiffman G. Antibody response to polyvalent pneumococcal polysaccharide vaccine in diabetics. JAMA 1980;244:2621–4.

226. Centers for Disease Control. Pneumococcal polysaccha-

ride vaccine. Recommendations of the Immunization Practices Advisory Committee (ACIP). MMWR 1989; 38:64.

227. Centers for Disease Control. Protection against viral hepatitis. Recommendations of the Immunization Practices Advisory Committee (ACIP). MMWR 1990;39:1—26.

228. Pozzilli P, Arduini P, Visalli N. Reduced protection against hepatitis B virus following vaccination in patients with Type I (insulin-dependent) diabetes. Diabetologica 1987; 30:817—9.

229. Hadler SC. Vaccines to prevent hepatitis B and hepatitis A virus infections. Infect Dis Clin North Am 1990;4:29—46.

Chapter 48

DIABETES AND PREGNANCY

JOHN W. HARE

Diabetes is a chronic disease whose phenotype ordinarily affects only the proband. A special situation occurs when the proband is gravid, for the fetus is an obligate parasite of the mother and necessarily engulfed by the maternal metabolic milieu.

It is important to note that the overwhelmingly important clinical issue is the fuel mixture available to the fetus. The mixture is dependent not only on the mother's intermediary metabolism but also on her circulatory state and its effect on the uterine-placental delivery of oxygen to the fetus.

Diabetes may develop in the mother before or during pregnancy. If it antedates pregnancy (pregestational), the embryo is subjected to metabolic insult from the moment of conception. Thus, its entire intrauterine life, from organ anlage and growth to lean and fat tissue distribution, as well as the fetal insulin secretion, is adversely influenced by the mother's diabetes. If diabetes develops during pregnancy (gestational), the period of adverse influence is truncated. Gestational diabetes typically occurs in the latter half of pregnancy and has no effect on embryonic growth and thus is not a cause of congenital defects. Both categories of maternal diabetes affect fetal growth and development in mid- to late pregnancy. They may cause macrosomia and contribute to fuel-mediated teratogenesis resulting in developmental defects with lifelong consequences, including obesity and impaired intellect.[1]

The following section discusses the classification of diabetes in pregnancy from the broad prospective of gestational and pregestational diabetes. These two categories are subdivided according to the etiology of gestational diabetes and the pathophysiology of pregestational diabetes.

CLASSIFICATION

Gestational Diabetes

Gestational diabetes is defined as diabetes that is discovered during pregnancy. This does not necessarily mean that diabetes developed during pregnancy but it usually does. Several possibilities are listed in Table 48–1. By far the most common possibility is the unmasking of incipient Type II diabetes by the metabolic demands of the pregnancy—which outstrip the pregnant woman's β-cell secretory reserve. An ever-increasing secretion of insulin is needed to conduct the maternal metabolic symphony. This need is driven by placental secretion of peptide and ring-structured hormones. Women who are unable to meet this demand develop mild diabetes, typically during the latter half of pregnancy.[2] Once the woman delivers, her hormone levels rapidly revert to normal and diabetes disappears. Because of an inherent β-cell defect, these women are likely to develop Type II diabetes one or two decades later. If men were to become pregnant, they would experience a similar syndrome. Women with incipient Type II diabetes that appears as gestational diabetes have about a

Table 48–1. Classification of Gestational Diabetes

Incipient Type II
Preexisting Type II
Incipient Type I
Newly overt Type I

Gestational diabetes is defined as diabetes discovered during pregnancy.

889

50% chance of developing Type II diabetes during middle age.[3]

Some women have undiagnosed Type II diabetes before pregnancy. Their pregnancy brings them to the attention of a physician, who then discovers their diabetes, often in the first trimester. Because the diabetes is discovered during pregnancy, these women are considered to have gestational diabetes, but their diabetes will persist post partum. In fact, the failure of gestational diabetes to disappear during the puerperium suggests that it was present before pregnancy.

Before Type I diabetes becomes clinically overt, there is a period of active autoimmunity and, in the late stages, very subtle defects in β-cell secretion. The defects may not be identified except by intravenous glucose tolerance testing.[4] However, if pregnancy is superimposed at this point, mild diabetes may develop. In some sense, this is not different clinically from incipient Type II diabetes but has a different etiology. The diabetes also may disappear after delivery but is likely to reappear in months or years rather than decades because of the shorter natural history of the development of Type I diabetes. Many of these women are not obese and may be younger than women with the more common incipient Type II diabetes.

Finally, both Type I diabetes and pregnancy occur in young women. Clearly, the onset of Type I diabetes during pregnancy may be coincidental. A Danish Study[5] showed that the incidence of Type I diabetes was tripled in the third trimester, suggesting that pregnancy may hasten the onset of Type I diabetes, probably through alterations in the immune system. Because the incidence of Type I diabetes is low, even the tripling of its incidence during pregnancy does not make it a common event.

Gestational diabetes is typically asymptomatic, and the diagnosis must be sought actively. The American Diabetes Association suggests that all women be screened between gestational weeks 24 and 28.[6] This screening is accomplished by giving 50 g of glucose orally at any time of day. Fasting is not necessary. One hour later, the plasma glucose level should not exceed 140 mg/dL. If it is higher, a 3-hour glucose tolerance test must be performed to confirm the presence or absence of gestational diabetes. Pregnant women are challenged with 100-g of glucose for this test. The diagnosis is established if any two values during the glucose tolerance test exceed the upper limit of normal (Table 48–2). Once the diagnosis is made, the initial treatment is dietary, with insulin therapy added if dietary measures fail to normalize the glucose levels. The aim of therapy is to prevent the complications of gestational diabetes. The most devastating of these is stillbirth, and the most common is macrosomia. It has recently been recognized that macrosomia may predispose infants to childhood obesity and probably to adult obesity.[7]

Pregestational Diabetes

Women whose diabetes antedates childbearing almost invariably have Type I diabetes. They may have Type II diabetes, particularly if they are obese, have short-term diabetes, or are pregnant relatively late in life. However,

Table 48–2. Glucose Tolerance Tests during Pregnancy

Time	Upper Limits of Normal for Plasma Glucose Levels (mg/dL)†
Fasting	105
After glucose challenge*	
1 hr	190
2 hr	165
3 hr	145

*Oral glucose load of 100 g.
†Diagnosis of gestational diabetes is made if any two values exceed these levels.

the typical onset of Type II diabetes after age 40 makes it a far less common variety of pregestational diabetes.

In recent years, the perinatal survival rates of offspring of women with Type I diabetes have approached but not equaled those of offspring of their nondiabetic peers. Improved techniques of fetal surveillance and assessment of fetal pulmonary maturity have greatly reduced, if not practically eliminated, respiratory distress as a cause of neonatal death. There has always been a small but significant death rate due to congenital anomalies, but in the past this was overshadowed by the severalfold higher death rate caused by respiratory distress. With the near elimination over the last 10 to 15 years of respiratory distress as a cause of neonatal mortality, congenital anomalies have emerged as the leading cause. The rate of congenital anomalies in the offspring of nondiabetic women is about 2%. The rate in infants of diabetic women is about 10%; a third to half of their infants die. The defects are related to disordered maternal metabolism during the first trimester. This has been shown clinically most easily by the relationship of glycohemoglobin levels to the rate of anomalies. There is additional evidence that the circulating products of intermediary metabolism, and perhaps hypoglycemia, may be teratogenic.[8–10] Determining a glycohemoglobin level is a particularly good practical way of assessing risk for the development of an anomaly. The levels of glycohemoglobin also are related to the rate of spontaneous abortion.[9,11]

Leslie et al.[12] suggested in an aside in a paper in 1978 that high glycohemoglobin levels during the first trimester were associated with congenital anomalies in three patients, although they did not state the levels in their patients. The following year Mills et al.[13] reviewed the anomalies most commonly associated with maternal diabetes: neural tube, renal, and cardiac. They noted that differentiation of the anlage of these organs occurs very early in gestation and that damage is likely done between weeks 3 and 6 after conception. In 1981, a paper from the Joslin Clinic[8] related the first-trimester glycohemoglobin levels to the rate of congenital anomalies. In that study, 116 patients were grouped into two equal groups: those with the better diabetes control those with the worse control. The offspring of the group with the better control had a malformation rate of only 3.4%, and the offspring of the group with the worse control had a rate of 22.4%. Other papers have buttressed the thesis that progressively higher levels of glycohemoglobin are associated with progressively higher rates of malformation as well as of spontaneous abortion.[9,14] A major disclaimer to this view was published in 1987, when Mills et al. published the results of a multicenter study, stating in the title of that paper that they found a lack of a relationship between glycohemoglobin levels and malformation rates.[15] The malformation rate among the offspring of the women in their study group, who had prospectively entered the study before conception or very soon thereafter, was 4.9%. Although the authors were unable to correlate glycohemoglobin levels within this group with the presence or absence of anomalies, the entire group was by and large in good control. Another group of diabetic women entered their study later and had ordinary clinical care. Their levels of glycohemoglobin were unknown. The anomaly rate among their offspring was 9%, which is what one might expect in an unselected diabetic population. These results can be interpreted to mean that good treatment during the early stages of diabetic pregnancy reduces the rate of anomalies but does not eliminate the excess above the nondiabetic rate.

Two papers have shown that early institution of good control is beneficial. One by Führmann[16] demonstrated that with vigorous intervention and therapy early in pregnancy the malformation rate could be reduced to that of the population at large. Unfortunately, no glycohemoglobin determinations were done. Kitzmiller et al.[17] also showed that early education and intensive management could reduce the malformation rate to values in the offspring of nondiabetic women. In his study, the malformation rate among the offspring of the late-entry diabetic group was 10.9%—again, what one would expect in an unselected population of diabetic mothers. His early-entry population had a rate of only 1.2%. which is equal to that of nondiabetic women.

Rates of spontaneous abortion for women with diabetes are similar to those for nondiabetic women but rise when the first-trimester glycohemoglobin is high.[9,11]

The most important message of the past decade for both patient and practitioner is that poor control of diabetes very early in pregnancy has deleterious consequences and that women who may become pregnant should be assiduous about the management of their diabetes prior to conception so as to deter the occurrence of preventible abortions and malformations.

Clinical Classification

Almost 50 years ago Priscilla White drew upon her two-decade experience in treating pregnant women with diabetes at the Joslin Clinic to formulate the world's most widely used system of classification for the mother's clinical condition,[18] assigning each category a letter.[18] An updated version of the White classification is shown in Table 48–3. Class A, her original first category, identified women whose diabetes, whether gestational or pregestational, is treated with diet alone. The later separate categorization of gestational and pregestational diabetes in 1980 diminished the utility of class A.[19] Furthermore,

Table 48–3. White Classification of Diabetes during Pregnancy (Revised)

Gestational diabetes	Abnormal glucose tolerance test but euglycemia maintained by diet alone or diet alone insufficient, insulin required
Class A	Diet alone sufficient, any duration or age at onset
Class B	Age at onset ≥20 yr and duration <10 yr
Class C	Age at onset 10–19 yr or duration 10–19 yr
Class D	Age at onset <10 yr or duration ≥20 yr or background retinopathy or hypertension (not preeclampsia)
Class R	Proliferative retinopathy or vitreous hemorrhage
Class F	Nephropathy with proteinuria >500 mg/day
Class RF	Criteria for both classes R and F coexist
Class H	Arteriosclerotic heart disease clinically evident
Class T	Prior renal transplantation

Table is from Hare and White.[19]
Women in classes below A require insulin therapy. Women in classes R, F, RF, H, and T have no criteria for age at diabetes onset or duration of diabetes but usually have long-term diabetes. The development of a complication moves the patient to the next class.

during the 1980s the lowering of the acceptable glycemic levels for diet-treated pregnant women to normality, and, if this was not achieved, the requisite institution of insulin therapy essentially eliminated the use of this category. Since 1980 we have had no patients in class A at the Joslin Clinic because women with pregestational diabetes invariably need insulin during pregnancy.

All women in the class B category and below are treated with insulin. A patient who starts with dietary management but then receives insulin changes classes. Although women with gestational diabetes may undergo this therapeutic progression, they are no longer placed in the class A or class B category but rather are called gestationally diabetic and further identified as treated with diet or with diet and insulin.

The underlying presumption for all subsequent classes was that vascular disease adversely affected maternal or fetal outcome; moreover, the vascular disease did not need to be clinically overt. Since the development of vascular disease may be related to age of onset and duration of diabetes, these factors determine classes B, C, and D. Class B includes women who have had diabetes for less than 10 years and were 20 years or older at its onset. Women with pregestational Type II diabetes, as well as those with short-term Type I diabetes, fall into this category. All subsequent classes include only women with Type I diabetes. Class C comprises both women with 10 to 20 years of uncomplicated diabetes and those with onset of diabetes before age 20, however short the duration of their diabetes. Class D is a transitional class that includes not only women with diabetes of more than 20 years' duration or diabetes onset before age 10 but also those with background retinopathy or hypertension (without renal disease). Class E was once used for women with pelvic vascular calcification, which was often discovered at the time of x-ray pelvimetry. Since x-ray examination of pregnant women is now avoided, pelvimetry is no longer done and the class E designation is no longer used. Class G, that of adverse obstetrical history unrelated to vascular disease, is also no longer used. Class F indicates nephropathy defined as proteinuria of more than 500 mg/day and has serious prognostic import for both mother and fetus. These women often have hypertension. Their proteinuria is often sufficiently heavy to cause the nephrotic syndrome with edema. Thus, the diagnosis of preeclampsia must be entertained (see below). Prematurity and low birth weight were common in infants of women in Class F.

Class T, which includes women with prior renal transplantation, is really a variant of class F. Class R, which identifies women with proliferative retinopathy, includes those with neovascularization with or without vitreous hemorrhage. The modern use of laser photocoagulation for preproliferative changes has tended to make proper categorization of women with retinopathy difficult. When laser therapy was used only for proliferative retinopathy, a history of its use indicated that the woman was in class R. Now, prior laser therapy may mean only that the woman has had preproliferative changes, but we have tended to include these women in class R. Since many women with nephropathy also have proliferative retinopathy, a combined FR category is commonly used.

Class H includes women with coronary artery disease. Its early description was of women with a myocardial infarction, but it is now appropriate to include women who have only angina or myocardial dysfunction (congestive heart failure) even if no infarction has occurred. Further discussion of maternal, retinal, renal, and cardiac disease is included in the section on complications.

From the above discussion, one can see how the classification has evolved, with the addition of new classes (H and T) and the elimination of others (A, E, and G). As a happy consequence of improved prenatal, perinatal, and neonatal care over the past two decades, distinctions between the White classes have been blurred. Uncomplicated maternal diabetes has subsumed classes B and C, and the rates of maternal and neonatal success for some women in class D are so high that no distinction can be made between classes B, C, and D. Once vascular disease develops in the mother, outcomes

are adversely affected and differences between classes can be discerned.

We have collected data for pregnancies in insulin-treated women (essentially all with Type I diabetes) for over 7 years from 1983 to 1989.[20] The women were followed at the Joslin Clinic and delivered at the Brigham and Women's Hospital, with the data collected including glycohemoglobin levels, gestational age at delivery, incidence of prematurity, birth weight and birth-weight ratios (observed birth weight divided by the median birth weight for that gestational week), Apgar scores (Table 48–4), and in some cases the incidence of respiratory disease in the newborn. In a subset of these women, the relationship between maternal hypertension and prematurity was highlighted.[21] Prematurity often was related to preeclampsia, which in turn was related to maternal hypertension and/or microvascular disease.

Glycohemoglobin levels, which correlate so strongly with rates of abortion and malformation, were virtually the same in all classes but class B, for which the levels were lower than those in classes D and F. The intuitive explanation for this finding is that patients with shorter-term diabetes tend to be in better control because they are more likely to have residual β-cell function.

When all the women in this same series whose infants were malformed were compared with those women whose infants were not malformed, the duration of diabetes tended to be longer and the glycohemoglobin levels tended to be lower in the women with nonmalformed infants.[9] This finding presumably reflects maternal experience and awareness of the importance of good early control in preventing malformations.

Gestational age at delivery was only partially related to White class. Prematurity was also more common in women with renal disease, especially those in class FR (Table 48–4). Hypertension is more frequent in this group than in classes B, C, and D. Over one-half of the women in class FR delivered prematurely. In fact, one-sixth to one-fourth of all women in the other classes delivered prematurely. In other words, premature delivery is common in women with diabetes but is especially so when the mother's diabetes is complicated by nephropathy. Prematurity (less than 37 weeks) was strongly correlated (in a subset of these women) with hyperten-

Table 48–4. Outcome of 559 Insulin-Treated Pregnancies

White Class (n)	First Trimester HbA₁ (%)	Gestational Age at Delivery (wks)	Birth Weight (g)	Birth-Weight Ratio	5-Min Apgar
B (138)	9.9 ± 0.4*	37.6 ± 0.4	3730 ± 150	1.27 ± 0.04	8.7 ± 0.2
C (169)	10.1 ± 0.4	37.6 ± 0.4	3620 ± 140	1.23 ± 0.04	8.5 ± 0.2
D (128)	10.8 ± 0.4	37.4 ± 0.4	3640 ± 160	1.25 ± 0.05	8.5 ± 0.2
R (51)	10.2 ± 0.6	37.0 ± 1.1	3520 ± 250	1.23 ± 0.07	8.6 ± 0.3
F (22)	11.6 ± 1.0	37.0 ± 0.7	2960 ± 370‡	1.04 ± 0.10	8.6 ± 0.6
FR (51)	10.8 ± 0.6	34.8 ± 0.7†	2440 ± 250§	0.99 ± 0.07‖	7.8 ± 0.4¶

*Lower than D, F; P < .05.
†Lower than all others; P < .01.
‡Lower than all but R; P < .01.
§Lower than all others; P < .01.
‖Lower than all others; P < .01.
¶Lower than B, C; P < .01.

sive disorders of pregnancy as well as with long-term (over 20 years) diabetes.[21]

Birth weight either in absolute terms or corrected for gestational age and expressed as a birth-weight ratio is clearly related to maternal nephropathy, with these values being lower in both classes F and FR. Absolute birth weights in class FR were lower than those in other classes, and those in class F were lower than those in classes B, C, and D. The effect of maternal renal disease is even more evident when a correction is made for gestational age and the data are expressed as a birth-weight ratio, with the birth-weight ratios being lower in classes F and FR than in all other classes.

Macrosomia, defined as an absolute birth weight greater than 4 kg, was very common in our population despite the virtual absence of deliveries at or beyond 40 weeks of gestation. Roughly one-third of infants born of mothers without renal disease weighed over 4 kg (Table 48–5). Fewer than 4% infants of mothers in classes F and FR weighed over 4 kg.

If macrosomia is defined as a birth weight that is large for gestational age (above the 90th percentile for that gestational week), well over 50% of all infants, save those born to mothers with renal disease, were overlarge. Moreover, the percentage of infants who were small for gestational age (below the 10th percentile for that gestational week) was equal to or less than 2% in classes B, C, D, and R and was less than 5% in class F. Only in class FR did the complication of one condition (diabetes) by another (nephropathy) exert a counterbalance and bring the extremes (large for gestational age vs. small for gestational age) near the expected 10% incidence: 15.7% vs. 11.8%, respectively. We have preliminary data indicating that birth weight is reduced even when microalbuminuria is present.[22] After delivery, the infants of class FR mothers tended to have Apgar scores at 5 minutes that were significantly lower than those of infants of mothers in classes B and C. Respiratory distress and transient tachypnea of the neonate was higher in a subset of these patients.[23]

Perinatal mortality is fortunately so uncommon that no one class was found to have more deaths than any other.

In this 7-year series, one woman died during pregnancy. Her death occurred during the first trimester after two episodes of pulmonary edema. She was classed as FR and had a competent porcine prosthetic aortic valve that had been placed after an episode of endocarditis some years before. She died suddenly and at autopsy was found to have a high-grade occlusion of her left anterior descending coronary artery. Thus, she should have been placed in class H.

Maternal retinopathy is believed to be aggravated by pregnancy (see below). Thus, in terms of maternal outcome, class R status is important.

In summary, White classes A, E, and G are no longer used at the Joslin Clinic and gestational diabetes is now a separate classification. Classes F and FR have significant deleterious effects on fetal outcome, and classes R and H are important with regard to the mother's health. Classes B and C cannot be distinguished from one another. For that matter it is unlikely that any modest effect of class D (e.g., premature delivery) would be seen in mothers free of any evidence of microvascular disease such as microalbuminuria.

The type of diabetes (I or II) makes no difference with regard to outcome. The degree of control does but is unrelated to class designation. The late Jørgen Pedersen's special note about noncompliance worsening the neonatal prognosis is worthwhile but not related to vascular disease.[24] Pedersen also recognized the deleterious effect of pyelonephritis, an observation which is no doubt valid, but this complication has been rare in our patient population, as has ketoacidosis. Thus, although we acknowledge Pedersen's concern, neither condition has been included in our classification.

Thus, the White classification, after nearly half a century of useful application, appears to be in need of significant revision. Because of improvements in care, uncomplicated diabetes does not need to be further subdivided. White's original premise that the presence of maternal vascular disease is relevant to outcome is confirmed by our recent data. Congenital malformation, the most significant cause of neonatal mortality, is related to maternal metabolism but not to White class. The same is true for any late consequences of fuel-mediated teratogenesis (such as obesity in childhood).

A new classification of maternal diabetes that embraces and emphasizes Dr. White's perceptive analysis of her patients' disease is proposed in Table 48–6. In this new scheme, vascular disease includes hypertension as well as microvascular disease (retinopathy and nephropathy) and macrovascular disease (coronary artery disease). Autonomic neuropathy is identified as a significant complication. Gestational diabetes remains a separate category. In its simplest form the classification of pregestational diabetes should recognize the presence or absence of maternal vascular disease. If vascular disease is present, further subdivision according to the nature of the complication in order. Hypertension may occur alone or predate pregnancy or be induced by pregnancy. It also may also appear as a comorbid factor with nephropathy.

TREATMENT

Diet

All cases of diabetes during pregnancy are treated with diet. No oral agents are used during pregnancy. Therefore, a woman with Type II diabetes treated with an oral agent prior to pregnancy must discontinue taking this

Table 48–5. Percentage of Infants of Mothers in White Classes Weighing >4 kg at Birth: 1983–1989

Class (n)	Percentage >4 kg
B (138)	35
C (169)	30
D (128)	32
R (51)	29
F (22)	0
FR (51)	4

Table 48–6. Classification of Diabetes Mellitus and Pregnancy

Category	Abbreviation
Uncomplicated	DM
Complicated	DM+
Microvascular disease	
Retinopathy	
Background	BDR
Proliferative	PDR
Nephropathy	
Overt, macroalbuminuria	K-W
Microalbuminuria	MA
Hypertension	
Preexisting	HTN
Pregnancy-induced	PIH
Preeclampsia/toxemia	PET
Macrovascular disease	
Coronary artery disease	CAD
Autonomic neuropathy	AN
Discovered during gestation*	GDM

*See Table 48–1 for types of GDM.

drug. It is nearly certain that insulin therapy will be necessary. Initially, gestational diabetes is treated with diet, but insulin therapy may become necessary. If diet does not result in normalization of glucose levels, with fasting plasma glucose values of less than 105 mg/dL and 2-hour postprandial values of less than 120 mg/dL, insulin therapy is used.

The basis for a caloric prescription during pregnancy is not as clearcut as once thought. An assessment of fetal nutritional demands and a calculation of caloric need suggest that the mother must ingest about 300 or 400 additional calories. Some physicians prefer to alter the dietary prescription each trimester, using a formula of 30 kcal/kg of body weight. Others prefer to prescribe 35 to 38 kcal/kg of maternal (including the conceptus) body weight early in pregnancy and to alter the prescription only if the mother and nutritionist agree that more or less caloric intake is necessary.[25] If the woman is obese, the prescriptions are based on desired body weight—not on observed weight. Recent reexamination of the question has suggested that pregnant woman may require less than 300 or 400 additional calories per day.[26] This is particularly true if the woman is obese. Moreover, the amount of weight that should be gained has not been clarified. Normal weight gains vary substantially during pregnancy, ranging from as little as 5 or 10 kg to as much as 25 or 30 kg. Women who eat several balanced meals a day probably do not require vitamin supplements, although they are prescribed routinely. Supplemental iron and calcium are probably beneficial.

Although the total daily caloric needs may be the subject of some disagreement, there is a consensus that the normal distribution of food intake for pregnant women with diabetes should be continued, i.e., three meals and snacks as appropriate for her insulin program. Consistent with prescriptions for nutrition in diabetes in recent years, diets during pregnancy, as well as during the nonpregnant state, tend to include a substantial amount of carbohydrates, particularly those foods high in fiber, and minimal amount of fat.

All pregnant women should be seen by a nutritionist who can obtain a diet history and provide an appropriate meal plan. This history should take into account relevant social and ethnic factors.

Insulin Programs

In general, insulin treatment of the diabetic pregnant woman is no different from the vigorous management of diabetes with insulin in the nonpregnant woman. The only real difference is the necessity to respond to the changing insulin requirements during the pregnancy. Some women have more insulin reactions during the first trimester and may require less insulin. Placental growth and attendant secretion of peptide and steroid hormones proceeds during the second and third trimester. The insulin requirement commonly increases, and women who have had a relatively simple insulin program may require a more complex one.[27]

Self-monitoring of blood glucose is essential because of the need for close management of diabetes during pregnancy. Glucose levels may be measured pre- or postprandially or even at both times. It is our routine practice to have the woman take a glucose measurement before breakfast and 2 hours after breakfast, lunch, and supper. The last measurement often is close to her bedtime. Women who use multiple doses of regular insulin with each meal must take measurements before all of these meals.

The insulin program should be designed to achieve excellent control, with a monthly glycohemoglobin value in or near the normal range. Although we have no objection to relatively simple insulin prescriptions, we often find that a more complicated or intensive regimen is required. Many of our patients use multiple-dose insulin regimens with regular insulin before each meal and intermediate-acting insulin at bedtime. Some use programs with ultralente insulin given twice daily in conjunction with premeal regular insulin, and others use intermediate-acting insulin given once or twice daily in conjunction with premeal regular insulin. A small minority of our patients use insulin pumps to provide continuous subcutaneous infusion.

Glycemic Standards

The ideal goal of treatment during pregnancy is the achievement of normal blood glucose and glycohemoglobin levels. Attainment of this goal is hindered by the occurrence of maternal hypoglycemia. It is virtually impossible for patients with Type I diabetes to obtain euglycemia without paying a significant price in terms of the occurrence of hypoglycemia. It may be possible to achieve a normal glycohemoglobin level, but only by balancing hyperglycemic episodes with hypoglycemic ones, in addition to the times the patient has values in the normal range. Although it makes intuitive sense that control resulting in normal glycohemoglobin levels is best for the fetus, published data do not show any further benefit once the glycohemoglobin levels are within 1 or

2% of the normal range—which is not to say that outcomes are normalized. In fact, diabetic women, even those with good to excellent control, continue to experience rates of perinatal morbidity, mortality, and malformations greater than those for the nondiabetic population. However, as a practical point, the best outcomes in diabetic pregnancies are achieved when glycohemoglobin levels approach or reach normal values. The attainment of normal glycohemoglobin levels may not demonstrably improve matters, presumably because, as stated above, this is not synonymous with euglycemia. As a general rule, our glycemic goals have both upper and lower limits for glucose levels (Table 48–7). The glycohemoglobin level should be no more than 1 to 2% above normal values.

Late in the third trimester, the insulin dose may diminish, particularly the pre-supper or bedtime dose, because fetal siphonage of maternal glucose and amino acids continues around the clock. This phenomenon is operative throughout pregnancy but is more noticeable during the last weeks of pregnancy when the conceptus is bigger and the nocturnal drain of maternal metabolites is quantitatively larger. Doses of insulin taken during the day and before meals are typically not affected.

During labor a substantial amount of glucose is consumed by the contracting uterus and perhaps by skeletal muscle as well. Even in women with clearcut Type I diabetes, the requirement for insulin may disappear.[28] It is possible that additional hormonal effects occur during labor, but this is speculative.[29] At any rate, the insulin dose given on the day of labor should be sharply reduced if administered subcutaneously or intravenously. If the intravenous route is chosen, insulin should be infused at a rate of 0 to 2 units/hour in combination with 5% dextrose at a rate of 100 to 150 mL/hour. Hourly monitoring of blood glucose is necessary. If spontaneous labor ensues after the usual dose of subcutaneous insulin has been given, glucose levels must also be measured hourly and the physician should be alert to the need for an increased infusion of glucose if hypoglycemia occurs.

After delivery, the woman's insulin requirement is markedly diminished, coincident with a marked increase in insulin sensitivity.[30] This alteration in dosage requirements persists for as briefly as a day or two or for as long as a week or two. The postpartum insulin requirement is usually a fraction of the prepregnancy requirement. This point needs emphasis because the insulin requirement during pregnancy is typically increased substantially and may well be double that before pregnancy. If the postpartum insulin dose is less than one-half the prepregnancy dose, it will be less than one-fourth the late-pregnancy dose. If the delivery has been vaginal and the mother begins eating right away, the insulin requirement tends to return to prepregnancy levels in only a few days. If the delivery has been by cesarean section and full nutritional replenishment is delayed, the insulin requirement tends to return to prepregnancy levels 5 to 7 days after delivery and occasionally even later.

The mother should also be told that pregnancy increases not only her insulin requirement but also the stability of her diabetes,[31] the reason such good control is achievable in the latter half of pregnancy. Once she has delivered and her insulin requirement has returned to prepregnancy levels, any inherent instability her diabetes had previously will reassert itself. It will be almost impossible for her to achieve the same degree of even control she had during late pregnancy. She should be urged to recall what her diabetes was like 9 months before and not to become discouraged if she is unable to achieve the control that she had in the last weeks of pregnancy.

COMPLICATIONS

Complications of diabetes are related to the duration of the disease and are believed to be related to the degree of control. Because of the relationship of complications to duration of diabetes, many young women with diabetes are free of complications during pregnancy. However, microvascular and macrovascular complications may be present and may affect maternal and fetal outcome. Many patients with diabetes live in fear of the development of complications and, knowing that they are at risk because of their diabetes, wonder when misfortune will strike. Dr. Donald Barnett at the Joslin Clinic has termed this "the Hiroshima syndrome," making the analogy between the situation among Japanese exposed to radiation from the atom bomb who wonder when or if they will develop late effects of exposure and patients with diabetes exposed to a noxious metabolic stimulus who wonder when or if they will develop complications.

Hypoglycemia and Ketoacidosis

The most common complication of diabetes is hypoglycemia. As discussed earlier, it may be a particular problem during pregnancy because of the tight control sought. If hypoglycemia is frequent and incapacitating, the management program must be relaxed a bit.

Fortunately, ketoacidosis is rare in our patient population. If it occurs during midpregnancy, it is frequently lethal to the fetus. The rarity of ketoacidosis during pregnancy is no doubt due to the improved degree of control permitted by self-monitoring of blood glucose and frequent doses of insulin. We ask our patients to monitor a morning urine sample for ketones on a daily basis. Because this detects starvation ketosis, it is a way of ensuring the adequacy of nutritional intake, but it also allows the patient to quickly detect developing ketoacidosis.

Table 48–7. Glycemic Goals during Pregnancy

Time	Glucose (mg/dL)*
Fasting	60–100
1-hr postprandial	100–140
2-hr postprandial	80–120
Nocturnal	80–100
During labor	60–100
Glycohemoglobin	Normal (<1–2% above) or nearly so

*Capillary blood or venous plasma.

Neuropathy

Neuropathy, a common complication of diabetes, can occur in the pregnant patient, but little has specifically been written about this problem during pregnancy.[32] Peripheral neuropathy is the most common type of diabetic neuropathy. Usually it is predominantly sensory and is typically symmetrical, affecting mainly the lower limbs. It may occasionally affect the intercostal nerves and be unilateral, with pain in the lower thoracic or upper abdominal region. During pregnancy it may need to be differentiated from a surgical or obstetrical complication. Peripheral neuropathy may also occur in the upper extremities, and carpal tunnel syndrome may complicate diabetes. Carpal tunnel syndrome may also be related specifically to pregnancy; thus, if it develops during pregnancy, treatment should be conservative because it may disappear after delivery.

Visceral neuropathy, which is autonomic, may affect the stomach, bowel, or bladder. If it affects the stomach during pregnancy, causing gastroparesis, the consequences can range from being uncomfortable and disconcerting to devastating. We have occasionally had patients who became malnourished because of their inability to eat as a result of constant nausea and vomiting.[32] Nausea and vomiting are common in early pregnancy and may persist throughout pregnancy as hyperemesis gravidarum. Gastropathy during pregnancy may mimic hyperemesis gravidarum, with the two conditions at times being difficult to distinguish. Gastropathy is most commonly diagnosed by upper gastrointestinal x-ray examination or by a gastric emptying study, both of which should be avoided during pregnancy because of the risk of radiation exposure to the fetus.

If a woman has gastropathy before pregnancy, it will probably worsen, permitting the physician to anticipate her difficulty with eating during pregnancy. If gastropathy is not known to exist before pregnancy and protracted nausea and vomiting persist during pregnancy, the distinction between gastropathy and hyperemesis gravidarum will be a clinical one. In either situation, it may be difficult to maintain adequate maternal nutrition. The most severe cases require parenteral nutrition.

Retinopathy

Pregnancy probably aggravates retinopathy. However, although the effect of pregnancy on retinopathy has been debated for many years, the considerable body of literature on the question has not fully resolved the issue. No one center has extensive experience because of the relative infrequency of proliferative retinopathy during pregnancy. Moreover, the effect of pregnancy on proliferative retinopathy has been harder to discern because of the trend towards earlier treatment of preproliferative changes. The weight of opinion is that pregnancy accelerates the progression of retinopathy and may cause the initiation of retinopathy if it was not present before pregnancy. It may be worth noting that the debate centers around whether retinopathy is worsened by pregnancy or whether progression during pregnancy represents the natural history of the disease that would

have occurred without pregnancy. No one has suggested that pregnancy improves retinopathy.

Intensive insulin therapy, with dramatic improvement in control, has been purported to worsen retinopathy. This situation occurs even in anticipation of pregnancy when women who have not had particularly good control are enrolled in antenatal clinics, with sudden emphasis placed on their diabetes control. Phelps et al. suggested that any worsening of retinopathy during pregnancy is a consequence of the sudden improvement in metabolic control.[33] Their paper examined 38 pregnancies in 35 women. As is commonly the case, the study sample was small. Moreover, neither consistent results of self-monitoring of blood glucose or glycohemoglobin values were available, so the best available measurement was the decrement in fasting plasma glucose level from the time of enrollment in the study to delivery. A larger study by Klein et al. prospectively examined 171 pregnant diabetic women and 298 nonpregnant women for progression of retinopathy.[34] They concluded that pregnancy more than doubled the risk for progression of retinopathy. Although glycosylated hemoglobin levels were measured in this study, the prepregnancy levels were not known. Thus, it was impossible to know the decrement during pregnancy. These authors did note that women with higher levels of glycosylated hemoglobin during pregnancy were more likely to show progression than were women with lower levels.

Some older series are of interest. Jervell et al. followed 274 pregnancies in the 1970s.[35] One-fourth of these women were noted to have progression of their retinopathy. Moloney and Drury found that their patients had worsening of both background and proliferative retinopathy during pregnancy and improvement post partum.[36] Both studies were done before the advent of self-monitoring of blood glucose and the clinical capability of achieving really strict control. Although in these studies, control may have improved during pregnancy, it was surely not to the degree achieved in today's patients, suggesting that pregnancy per se was operative in the worsening retinopathy.

It is the clinical opinion of physicians and ophthalmologists at the Joslin Clinic that retinopathy of all types tends to progress during pregnancy and to revert post partum to the level noted before pregnancy. A corollary to this theory is that the long-term prognosis for retinopathy is unaffected by pregnancy except in the circumstance of vitreous hemorrhage, with subsequent scarring and irretrievable visual loss.

At the Joslin Clinic, we ask that all pregnant women be examined each trimester in our ophthalmology unit. We are less insistent if little or no retinopathy is present in women who are known to have short-term diabetes: women with gestational diabetes, if it is clear their diabetes developed during pregnancy, or women with Type I diabetes of less than 5 years' duration. Women with little or no retinopathy in the second trimester are not likely to develop any significant change in the third trimester.

Before becoming pregnant, many women who have been treated with laser photocoagulation for proliferative or preproliferative retinopathy seek the advice of a physician as to the wisdom and safety of having a child. There is not much firm evidence available on which to base advice. We generally feel that if the woman has had quiescent retinopathy for 6 to 12 months, it is probably safe for her to become pregnant and that retinopathy will not reactivate. Women who have active retinopathy are advised to first receive treatment and wait until retinopathy becomes quiescent for the prescribed 6 to 12 months. Some women who are nearing the end of their reproductive years and whose vision is not particularly threatened by actively progressing retinopathy may elect not to wait.

Occasionally, florid retinopathy arises in early pregnancy. The decision arises as to whether termination of the pregnancy is advisable. We believe that once florid changes develop, no good is done by terminating the pregnancy (L. M. Aiello, personal communication).

Nephropathy

Nephropathy, typically accompanied by hypertension, is the complication of diabetes that has the greatest effect on the outcome of pregnancy. It may be present before or develop during pregnancy and is associated with low birth weight and prematurity. The rate of perinatal mortality is greatest for women with nephropathy than for women in any other of the White classes and has been so for many years. A review of 50 years of experience at the Joslin Clinic, from 1924 to 1974,[37] indicated that the perinatal survival rate among offspring of women in White classes F and FR was always lower than that for other patients in our population. During this 50-year period, nephropathy in the women studied was defined by the presence of overt proteinuria. At various times proteinuria has been defined as the daily excretion of 300, 400, or 500 mg of protein in the urine. Women who do not have overt proteinuria in early pregnancy but develop it later in pregnancy probably have preeclampsia. Women who have modest proteinuria with diabetic nephropathy in early pregnancy commonly will have more severe proteinuria—often in the nephrotic range—as pregnancy progresses.[38] Because these women will also have edema and hypertension, it will be difficult to distinguish them from patients with preeclampsia or pregnancy-induced hypertension. Perinatologists at the Brigham and Women's Hospital tend to consider all these patients to have a pregnancy-associated hypertensive disorder and do not try to make a clinical distinction.

When nephropathy is present in nonpregnant diabetic patients, treatment with a low-protein diet and antihypertensive agents (angiotensin-converting enzyme [ACE] inhibitors in particular) is prescribed. Women who are pregnant may not be best served by a low-protein diet, and there is evidence that ACE inhibitors are teratogenic. Therefore, during pregnancy dietary protein is not restricted and antihypertensive agents other than ACE inhibitors (but not diuretics) are used.

There have been several small reviews of diabetes in pregnancy complicated by nephropathy. Kitzmiller et al.

from the Joslin Clinic[38] reviewed 26 pregnancies and noted a perinatal mortality of over 10%, which was more than double the rate in non-nephropathic pregnancies. They noted a dramatic increase in proteinuria in the third trimester. Many women excreted 5 to 10 g of protein per day in the third trimester. One woman went from excreting 2 g of protein daily during the first trimester to excreting 20 g during the third trimester.

A common question has been whether or not pregnancy actually worsens the course of renal disease and hastens renal failure. In this series, 13 women had mild azotemia; six of them had either a spontaneous or therapeutic abortion, and seven delivered. These two small groups were compared. Two of the six who aborted progressed to complete renal failure within 2 years, as did three of the seven who delivered. These numbers are too small to permit any real conclusion to be drawn but do suggest that the renal disease progressed to complete renal failure independent of completion of a pregnancy.

A serum creatinine concentration of 3 mg/dL is incompatible with fetal life.[39] Women who begin pregnancy with a creatinine level of 2 mg/dL or higher are likely to have considerable difficulty completing the pregnancy successfully. Renal function may or may not deteriorate during pregnancy, as evidenced by the serum creatinine value. However, the typical rise in glomerular filtration rate tends not to occur in diabetic pregnancies complicated by renal disease.

A series by Hayslet and Reece examined 31 pregnancies in which renal disease was present.[40] Nearly two-thirds of these women did not have overt proteinuria prior to pregnancy. All 31 women had retinopathy, and two-thirds had proliferative changes. Nearly one-half of the women had a decline in renal function during pregnancy, but in all of these women, function returned to first-trimester levels after delivery, again suggesting that pregnancy does not ultimately influence renal function. These authors also noted that almost 75% of the women excreted less than 3 g of protein per day during the first trimester but that almost 75% excreted more than 3 g per day during the third trimester. After delivery, proteinuria—like creatinine clearance—returned to the first-trimester levels.

When patients with renal disease develop a nephrotic syndrome associated with edema and hypertension (which is difficult to distinguish from preeclampsia), the first treatment we prescribe is 2 hours of bed rest at home twice a day in the morning and afternoon. Antihypertensive agents normally used in pregnancy may be prescribed, and diuretics are avoided. It is often the case that a woman finds it difficult to rest at home for the prescribed periods and requires hospitalization. This is particularly true of women who have small children at home. Women who have jobs outside the home often must cease working.

Despite the relatively high success rates of pregnancies in women with renal disease, the high risks to their fetuses cannot be overemphasized. The presence of even microgram quantities of albumin in the urine may be associated with low birth weights, as is the case for the presence of overt proteinuria.[22]

Finally, there have been a few case reports of pregnancies in women who have undergone renal transplantation. One small series of nine patients included two women from the Joslin Clinic.[41] Eight of the ten fetuses survived (one twin gestation) as did eight of nine mothers. The woman who died did so suddenly during the 21st gestational week. The cause of death was not identifiable either clinically or at autopsy. It should be emphasized that of the nine women, six had preeclampsia and seven of nine fetuses developed fetal distress. None of the nine women went beyond gestational week 36. Prematurity and hypertension have also been noted in individual case reports. Thus, women with prior renal transplantation are likely to complete a pregnancy successfully, but the clinical picture is much like that for women with overt renal disease, even if the transplanted kidney is functioning normally.

Heart Disease

Fortunately, coronary artery disease during pregnancy is rare. Of course, it may occur in relatively young adults with Type I diabetes, but its development typically requires a diabetes duration of many years. Most women have completed childbearing by the time they are at risk. Unfortunately, this is not always the case. Occasionally, angina, myocardial infarction, or congestive heart failure are seen in pregnant diabetic women. Earlier series have particularly grim conclusions about outcome, suggesting that as many as three-fourths of these women die.[42] One of the difficulties with other case reports is that some deaths occurred post partum. Thus, some women were retrospectively considered to be in White class H. Some women may have only angina during pregnancy and may not be at such high risk. There are also a few case reports of women who have successfully completed pregnancy after coronary artery bypass.[43,44] Because the number of women with coronary artery disease is so small, it is difficult to collect any sizeable series. Moreover, cases have been collected over years during which therapeutic modalities have improved. For example, most of the cases of pregnancies in diabetic women with coronary artery disease were described before balloon angioplasty became available and many were reported before coronary artery bypass surgery became routine. Most reported cases preceded the use of newer medical therapies such as calcium channel or selective β-adrenergic blockers.

Women with coronary artery disease and good myocardial function probably can complete a successful pregnancy more easily than has previously been believed. It remains impossible to give reliable advice because the experience upon which to base a prediction is so inadequate. However, the presence of coronary artery disease must be taken seriously.

REFERENCES

1. Freinkel N. Of pregnancy and progeny. Diabetes 1980;29: 1023–35.
2. Buchanan TA. Glucose metabolism during pregnancy: normal physiology and implications for diabetes mellitus. Isr J Med Sci 1991;27:432–41.
3. O'Sullivan JB, Mahan CM. Criteria for the oral glucose tolerance test in pregnancy. Diabetes 1964;13:278–85.
4. Eisenbarth GS. Type I diabetes mellitus: a chronic autoimmune disease. N Engl J Med 1986;314:1360–8.
5. Buschard K, Buch I, Mølsted-Pedersen L, et al. Increased incidence of true Type I diabetes acquired during pregnancy. BMJ 1987;294:275–9.
6. Freinkel N. Summary and recommendations of the Second International Workshop. Conference on gestational diabetes mellitus. Diabetes 1985;34(Suppl 2):123–6.
7. Metzger BE, Silverman BL, Freinkel N, et al. Amniotic fluid insulin concentration as a predictor of obesity. Arch Dis Child 1990;65:1050–2.
8. Miller E, Hare JW, Cloherty JP, et al. Elevated maternal hemoglobin A_{1c} in early pregnancy and major congenital anomalies in infants of diabetic mothers. N Engl J Med 1981;304:1331–4.
9. Greene MF, Hare JW, Cloherty JP, et al. First-trimester hemoglobin A_1 and risk for major malformation and spontaneous abortion in diabetic pregnancy. Teratology 1989;39:225–31.
10. Buchanan TA, Schemmer JK, Freinkel N. Embryotoxic effects of brief maternal insulin-hypoglycemia during organogenesis in the rat. J Clin Invest 1986;78:643–79.
11. Mills JL, Simpson JL, Driscoll SG, et al. Incidence of spontaneous abortion among normal women and insulin-dependent diabetic women whose pregnancies were identified within 21 days of conception. N Engl J Med 1988;319:1617–23.
12. Leslie RDG, Pyke DA, John PN, White JM. Haemoglobin A_1 in diabetic pregnancy. Lancet 1978;2:958–9.
13. Mills JL, Baker L, Goldman AS. Malformations in infants of diabetic mothers occur before the seventh gestational week: implications for treatment. Diabetes 1979;28: 292–3.
14. Ylinen K, Aula P, Stenman U-H, et al. Risk of minor and major fetal malformations in diabetics with high haemoglobin A_{1c} levels in early pregnancy. BMJ 1984;289: 345–6.
15. Mills JL, Knopp RH, Simpson JL, et al. Lack of relation of increased malformation rates in infants of diabetic mothers to glycemic control during organogenesis. N Engl J Med 1988;318:671–6.
16. Führmann K, Reiher H, Semmler K, et al. Prevention of congenital malformations in infants of insulin-dependent diabetic mothers. Diabetes Care 1983;6:219–23.
17. Kitzmiller JL, Gavin LA, Gin GD, et al. Preconception care of diabetes: glycemic control prevents congenital anomalies. JAMA 1991;265:731–6.
18. White P. Pregnancy complicating diabetes. Am J Med 1949;7:609–16.
19. Hare JW, White P. Gestational diabetes and the White classification. Diabetes Care 1980;3:394.
20. Hare JW, Greene MF. Classification of diabetes in pregnancy. In: Shafrir E, Hod M, eds. Diabetes and pregnancy: presentations, discussions and conclusions. London, Smith-Gordon, 1993 (in press).
21. Greene MF, Hare JW, Krache M, et al. Prematurity among insulin-requiring diabetic gravid women. Am J Obstet Gynecol 1989;161:106–11.
22. Laffel LMB, Greene MF, Wilkins-Haug L. First trimester urinary albumin excretion predicts birth weight in diabetic pregnancies [Abstract no. 474]. Diabetes 1992;41(Suppl 1): 133A.
23. Hare JW, Greene MF. Perinatal outcome by White class: 1983–1987 [Abstract no 954]. Diabetes 1988;37(Suppl 1): 250A.

24. Pedersen J. Foetal mortality. In: The pregnant diabetic and her newborn. Baltimore: Williams & Wilkins, 1967: 108–27.

25. Holman SR. Nutritional management. In: Hare JW, ed. Diabetes complicating pregnancy: the Joslin Clinic method. New York: Alan R. Liss, 1989:69–80.

26. Bertorelli AM. Calorie requirements in gestational diabetes: a review. Diabetes Care Educ 1992;13:7–9.

27. Hare JW. Medical management. In: Hare JW, ed. Diabetes complicating pregnancy: the Joslin Clinic method. New York: Alan R Liss, 1989:33–51.

28. Jovanovic L, Peterson CM. Insulin and glucose requirements during the first stage of labor in insulin-dependent diabetic women. Am J Med 1983;75:607–12.

29. Hanif K, Goren HJ, Hollenberg MD, Lederis K. Oxytocin action: mechanisms for insulin-like activity in isolated rat adipocytes. Mol Pharmacol 1982;22:381–8.

30. Tulchinsky D. The postpartum period. In: Tulchinsky D, Ryan KJ, eds. Maternal-fetal endocrinology. Philadelphia: WB Saunders, 1980:144–66.

31. Lev-Ran A, Goldman JA. Brittle diabetes in pregnancy. Diabetes 1977;26:926–30.

32. Hare JW. Diabetic neuropathy and coronary heart disease. In: Reece EA, Coustan DR, eds. Diabetes mellitus in pregnancy: principles and practice. New York: Churchill Livingstone, 1989:515–22.

33. Phelps RL, Sakol P, Metzger BE, et al. Changes in diabetic retinopathy during pregnancy: correlations with regulation of hyperglycemia. Arch Ophthalmol 1986;104:1806–10.

34. Klein BEK, Moss SE, Klein R. Effect of pregnancy on progression of diabetic retinopathy. Diabetes Care 1990; 13:34–40.

35. Jervell J, Moe N, Skjaeraasen J, et al. Diabetes mellitus and pregnancy: management and results at Rikshospitalet, Oslo, 1970–1977. Diabetologia 1979;16:151–5.

36. Moloney JBM, Drury MI. The effect of pregnancy on the natural course of diabetic retinopathy. Am J Ophthalmol 1982;93:745–56.

37. Hare JW, White P. Pregnancy in diabetes complicated by vascular disease. Diabetes 1977;26:953–5.

38. Kitzmiller JL, Brown ER, Phillippe M, et al. Diabetic nephropathy and perinatal outcome. Am J Obstet Gynecol 1981;141:741–51.

39. Katz AI, Davison JM, Hayslett JP, et al. Pregnancy in women with kidney disease. Kidney Int 1980;18:192–206.

40. Hayslett JP, Reece EA. Effect of diabetic nephropathy on pregnancy. Am J Kidney Dis 1987;9:344–9.

41. Ogburn PL Jr, Kitzmiller JL, Hare JW, et al. Pregnancy following renal transplantation in class T diabetes mellitus. JAMA 1986;255:911–5.

42. Silfen SL, Wapner RJ, Gabbe SG. Maternal outcome in class H diabetes mellitus. Obstet Gynecol 1980;55:749–51.

43. Hare JW. Complicated diabetes complicating pregnancy. Baillieres Clin Obstet Gynaecol 1991;5:349–67.

44. Reece EA, Egan JFX, Coustan DR, et al. Coronary artery disease in diabetic pregnancies. Am J Obstet Gynecol 1986;154:150–1.

Chapter 49

SKIN MANIFESTATIONS OF DIABETES MELLITUS

BONNIE T. MACKOOL
MARK H. LOWITT
JEFFREY S. DOVER

An estimated 30% of patients with diabetes develop a skin manifestation of their disease.[1] Several skin conditions are specific to diabetes, but most of them also occur in the nondiabetic population. The clinical manifestations and complications of skin disease are frequently more severe in the setting of diabetes. The literature abounds with studies that attempt to identify and understand the pathophysiology of cutaneous disorders in the diabetic patient, but many remain poorly understood. In this chapter, we identify and describe the characteristic skin conditions associated with diabetes, incorporating discussions of clinical presentation, pathology, pathogenesis, and treatment (Table 49–1).

CUTANEOUS INFECTIONS IN DIABETES

Candidiasis

Candidal infections of mucosal membranes, genitalia, and nail folds are generally accepted to be more prevalent in patients with poorly controlled diabetes than in the nondiabetic population,[2–5] although data from controlled studies in support of this contention are lacking. Women are more prone than men to these infections.[3]

Although yeast infections may be the initial presentation of diabetes, they generally occur in patients already known to be diabetic.[4] In individuals with diabetes, the ratio of epidermal glucose to blood glucose is higher than in persons without diabetes,[6] a condition that may result in an environment more favorable to the growth of yeast and fungi.[7]

Oral Mucosal Candidiasis

Distinctive forms of oral mucosal candidiasis include thrush (curd-like white colonies) over intra-oral surfaces; atrophic candidiasis, which manifests as bright red atrophy of the hard palate or tongue, sore mouth, and angular cheilitis (perleche), which presents as superficial or deep erosions along the labial commissures. Antifungal creams or troches usually are required to eradicate infection.

Candidal Paronychia

The frequency of candidal paronychia, the inflammation surrounding the nail that is caused by a candidal infection, is increased in persons with diabetes. In one study of 250 women with diabetes, 9.6% had clinical evidence of candidal paronychia as compared with 3.4% of 500 nondiabetic controls.[8] Typical candidal paro-

Table 49–1.   Skin Manifestations of Diabetes

Cutaneous infections	**Skin conditions with strong but**
Candidiasis	**unexplained association with**
Dermatophytosis	**diabetes**
Phycomycosis	Diabetic dermopathy
Erythrasma	Diabetic bullae
Malignant external otitis	Rubeosis
Neurologic lesions	Vitiligo
Charcot joint	Acanthosis nigricans
Compensatory hyperhidrosis	Perforating disorders
Neuropathic ulcer	Generalized pruritus
Disorders of collagen	**Cutaneous reactions to diabetic**
Necrobiosis lipoidica	**treatment**
Granuloma annulare	Insulin-induced disorders
Scleredema diabeticorum	Insulin allergy
Waxy skin	Insulin lipodystrophy
Metabolic diseases	Insulin-induced
Porphyria cutanea tarda	lipohypertrophy
Yellow skin	Hypoglycemic agents
Xanthomatosis	Hypersensitivity reactions
Hemochromatosis	Disulfiram reactions
Lipodystrophy	
Glucagonoma syndrome	

Table is adapted from Fine and Moschella.[80]

nychia begins with erythema, swelling, and pain at the lateral nail fold, leading to its separation from the nail margin. The posterior nail fold then becomes involved, and the cuticle may separate from the nail plate.[9] Purulent drainage may be mistaken for bacterial infection. Candidal paronychia is characterized by intermittent exacerbations with episodic indolent periods, a course that may result in a rippled appearance of the nail plate. Patients with occupations in which their hands are frequently immersed in water are more prone to this condition.[10] Practical treatment includes keeping the hands as dry as possible. The wearing of cotton gloves under rubber or vinyl gloves can protect hands during dishwashing. Topical antifungal solutions are usually adequate for treatment; however, patients with refractory cases may require oral imidazole therapy.

Candidal Vulvitis

Candidal vulvovaginitis is characterized by pruritus, vulvar erythema, and occasionally fissuring and pustules.[9] Glycosuria may promote growth of *Candida albicans.* Certain case studies have shown that the severity of pruritus is proportional to the degree of glycosuria.[11] Broad-spectrum antibiotics, birth-control pills, and topical corticosteroids are also common causes of candidal vulvovaginitis. Antifungal vaginal suppositories or creams are necessary to eradicate infection.

Monilial Balanitis

Men with monilial balanitis present with diffuse or focal erythema of the glans penis, often in association with pain or pruritus. White discharge in association with erosions or pustules is commonly seen, particularly under the foreskin of uncircumcised patients. Men with balanitis and phimosis, especially if middle-aged or elderly, should be evaluated for diabetes. In one retrospective study,

among 100 men who required circumcision for phimosis, 35% were diabetic. For most of these patients, diabetes had not been diagnosed previously.[5] Administration of topical imidazoles is the treatment of choice. If phimosis is present, a cotton-tipped applicator may be used to gently introduce the anticandidal preparation underneath the foreskin.[9]

Dermatophyte Infections

Tinea pedis (athlete's foot) is more prevalent in persons with diabetes than in the general population.[2] Although innocuous in most people, tinea can create fissures and portals of entry that may lead to severe bacterial infections in those with diabetes. Web spaces are pruritic, scaly, erythematous, and macerated. Vesicles and pustules may also be present. A "moccasin" distribution of scaling extending from the soles onto the lateral part of the feet is another variant of tinea pedis. Longstanding tinea pedis may involve the nails, which develop a thick, yellowish-brown, roughened nail plate and subungual debris. KOH scraping identifies branching, septate hyphae.[10] Patients with tinea involving hands or fingernails may inoculate other body sites as well.

Topical treatment with antifungal drugs is difficult because penetration of these agents is relatively poor. For severe fungal infections of skin, hair, or nails, administration of an oral antifungal agent is the treatment of choice. A minimum of 6 months of treatment for fingernail infections and of up to 18 months for toenail infections is generally required. Blood counts and liver function must be monitored during treatment. Preventive foot care, including careful drying, wearing cotton socks, and wearing sandals in public shower facilities may help prevent infection.

Phycomycetes Infections

The phycomycetes are a group of fungi found on decaying vegetation and foods that have a high sugar content. Although rarely pathogenic, the genera most commonly involved in human infection include *Rhizopus, Mucor,* and *Absidia.*[12] In the clinical setting, any disease caused by these organisms is referred to as *mucormycosis.*

Several major clinical syndromes, involving the rhinocerebral, thoracic, gastrointestinal, and cutaneous systems, are described.[13] Rhinocerebral disease is that most closely associated with diabetes. The fungal organism colonizes the nasal turbinates and sinuses but can invade the orbit and brain, particularly in the setting of diabetic ketoacidosis. Characteristically black crusty or purulent material is present on the turbinates, septae, or palate, and mucormycosis may initially be mistaken for bacterial sinusitis. Cutaneous mucormycosis occurs when the organisms colonize burned or skin-grafted tissues or nonhealing leg ulcers in patients with diabetes.[14]

The diagnosis can be confirmed by skin biopsy or potassium iodide tissue preparation of sputum or skin, which may demonstrate the large, broad, nonseptate hyphae characteristic of phycomycetes.[12] Debridement of necrotic tissue, intravenous administration of amphotericin B, correction of acid-base imbalance, and control of hyperglycemia are the necessary components of treatment.[15] The more invasive forms of disease are frequently fatal.

Bacterial Infections

Although patients with well-controlled diabetes do not have increased susceptibility to most bacterial infections, evidence suggests that patients with poorly controlled diabetes may have more frequent or more severe bacterial infections than experienced by the rest of the population.[16] Several authors have described abnormalities in leukocyte function associated with diabetes, including diminished chemotaxis,[17] depressed phagocytosis,[18,19] and decreased bactericidal activity,[20-22] decreased leukocyte migration,[23] and an altered early granulocyte phase of the local cellular inflammatory response.[24]

Bacterial infections of the lower extremities are a particular risk for patients with diabetes who have vascular disease or neuropathy.[16] Careful foot care and early treatment of dermatophytosis is essential in minimizing potential bacterial portals of entry.

Malignant External Otitis

Malignant external otitis is a severe necrotizing bacterial infection that occurs almost exclusively in patients with diabetes.[25] Beginning in the external auditory canal, the infection invades local soft tissues and ultimately leads to osteomyelitis of the temporal bone, occasionally progressing to fatal meningitis. *Pseudomonas aeruginosa* is the causative agent in virtually all cases. Symptoms can include unremitting ear pain, purulent otic discharge, and cranial nerve palsies. A tender ear and mastoid area with granulation tissue or polyps in the external auditory canal are typical physical findings. More than 20% of patients have bilateral disease.[26] Extended therapy with antipseudomonal agents is necessary, and surgical debridement may also be required.

Erythrasma

Erythrasma is a superficial infection usually affecting intertriginous areas of the skin that is caused by *Corynebacterium minutissimum*. Carriage of fluorescent diphtheroids on clinically normal skin is more common in patients with poorly controlled diabetes than in persons without diabetes. Obesity may be an additional contributing factor, especially in those with adult-onset diabetes.[27]

Reddish-brown, slightly scaly patches typically occur in intertriginous areas such as the axillae, groin, and web spaces and can be pruritic or asymptomatic. Erythrasma is commonly limited to the toe webs, manifesting with white discoloration and maceration. Frequently the diagnosis is missed, and not infrequently toe web involvement is misdiagnosed as tinea pedis. The characteristic coral red fluorescence under Wood's light is diagnostic. The red glow seen is from a porphyrin-like substance produced by the bacteria.[28] Gram stain or culture of affected skin scrapings shows gram-positive rods and thread-like filaments traversing the stratum corneum.[29] Topical imidazole antifungal agents, topical antibiotics, or systemic erythromycin or tetracycline each provide effective treatment for the disorder.

NEUROPATHIC AND ISCHEMIC DIABETIC SKIN DISEASE

Diabetic Polyneuropathy

Diabetic neuropathy is usually bilateral and more severe in the lower extremities than the upper extremities.[30] Dry shiny skin and ulceration on pressure points, particularly on structurally deformed feet, is common. Skin hypoesthesia is one of the most important signs of polyneuritis.[30] Lack of thermal sensitivity may lead to burns, callouses, and subsequent ulceration.[31] Abnormalities of motor function are much less obvious than sensory defects. Paralysis of the intrinsic muscles of the feet, the most common motor alteration, results in atrophy of the interosseus muscles, which is demonstrated by the "fan sign"—the inability to separate the toes. Such alteration in motor function causes the foot to adopt unusual position resulting in claw toe or hammer toe deformities or to the Charcot joint. In the latter, the tarsal and metatarsal bones are gradually destroyed and joint spaces are obliterated.[30,32] As autonomic neuropathy progresses, sweat glands become inactivated. Patients with diabetes may exhibit a compensatory hyperhidrosis of the trunk or face in response to anhidrosis of the lower body.[33] Dry and thickened skin of the anhidrotic diabetic foot is prone to the development of fissures, which may serve as portals of entry for bacteria and fungi. Unperceived chronic pressure to the toenails results in thickening, abnormal curvature, and hypertrophy of the nail plate. Ingrown toenails may lead to infection.[10]

Peripheral Vascular Disease

Peripheral vascular disease (PVD) in diabetic patients can be diffuse and early in onset. The predilection for atherosclerosis and microangiopathy plays a role in the vessel occlusion that occurs in diabetes.[34] Some authors consider microangiopathy to play a part in diabetic vascular disease, while others disagree.[34,35] The skin of the lower extremities in diabetic patients with PVD is thin, smooth, cold, and often mottled in the dependent position.[36] Hair is either sparse or absent. Other signs of PVD include pallor or cyanosis with elevation, dependent rubor, and delayed capillary refill.

Diabetic Ulcers

Neuropathic ulcers develop most frequently in areas of high pressure and repeated trauma, such as the toes, heels, and metatarsal heads[31] (Plate II, A). The patient may present with pain, paresthesia, or anesthesia of the legs and feet. Only occasionally is the ulcer completely asymptomatic in presentation.[32]

Venous ulcers tend to occur on the medial malleoli in association with superficial varicosities and yellow-brown skin discoloration and are seldom painful. Rest and leg elevation ease venous ulcers by controlling edema and reducing venous hypertension.

Arterial ulcers are typically painful (except when accompanied by neuropathy) and occur more distally, on the tips of the toes and on the heel.[37] Ulcers of arterial origin may respond to the control of hypertension and diabetes as well as to increased exercise, which promotes collateral circulation. Cessation of smoking can be critical. Aggressive treatment of infection, administration of antiplatelet agents or anticoagulants, and surgical revascularization are important treatment modalities in severe cases.

DISORDERS OF COLLAGEN

Necrobiosis Lipoidica

Necrobiosis lipoidica is an unusual skin disorder that is strongly associated with diabetes mellitus. The entity was first described in 1929[38] and was named *necrobiosis lipoidica diabeticorum* (NLD) in 1932.[39] Because of the significant minority of cases of NLD in patients without diabetes, most investigators now choose to call this condition simply *necrobiosis lipoidica* (NL).

Typical lesions of NL occur on the pretibial skin as irregular ovoid plaques with a violaceous indurated periphery and a yellow central atrophic area (Plate II, B, C). Overlying superficial telangiectasia and scattered hyperkeratotic plugs often are noted.[40] The lesions can start as small firm reddish-brown papules, which slowly enlarge. They are usually multiple and bilateral, with ulceration seen in approximately 35%. Ulcers are often secondary to minor trauma or are iatrogenically induced by intralesional injection of corticosteroids. It is curious that the ulcers only rarely lead to infection. Patients may complain of pruritus, dysesthesia, or pain at the site of lesions. More frequently, however, the lesions of NL are asymptomatic, and it is the cosmetic disability that is of greatest concern to the patient. Although most commonly found on the lower legs (85% of cases involve only the legs), other locations include the hands, fingers, forearms, face, and scalp.[41] Lesions in these locations are often annular, erythematous, or brown and can coalesce to form larger serpiginous plaques, which demonstrate little or no atrophy.

Muller and Winkelmann's classic papers in 1966 demonstrate the close association between NL and diabetes.[41,42] Sixty-five percent of their 171 patients with NL had diabetes. Of the remainder available for study, 42% (8/19) demonstrated abnormal glucose tolerance, with abnormal oral glucose tolerance tests or cortisone glucose tolerance tests. Among those with normal glucose tolerance, 55% had family histories positive for glucose intolerance. Despite the high prevalence of diabetes in patients with NL, it is relatively uncommon in diabetes, the reported prevalence being 3 per 1000 diabetic patients. The female-to-male ratio is 3:1, with an average age of onset of 30 years in diabetic patients. Fifty percent of patients with NL demonstrate other diabetes-related end-organ damage.[41]

Two major histologic patterns of NL have been described. The "necrobiotic" pattern reveals large areas of necrobiotic collagen within the dermis, with irregularly shaped, often anuclear, collagen fibers. A characteristic cellular infiltrate consisting of histiocytes, fibroblasts, and lymphoid cells surrounds the necrobiotic areas. Giant cells often are present, and blood vessels show endothelial proliferation and infiltration with a periodic acid-Schiff (PAS)-positive material. In the second type of NL, or the "granulomatous" pattern, the lesions contain little or no necrobiotic material. The epithelioid and giant cells assume a more typically granulomatous configuration, and vascular changes are rare.[40]

Despite extensive investigation, the etiology of NL remains largely unknown. Evidence suggests that NL and glycemic control are not related[43] and that genetic factors do not play a large role.[44] Vascular etiologies for NL have been entertained; however, vascular changes are absent in one-third of biopsy samples. A link with diabetic microangiopathy has been suggested, yet the caliber of the affected vessels in NL is usually larger than that of vessels affected in diabetes. The abnormal collagen found in NL has invited speculation on a direct etiologic relationship of NL to the collagen itself, as a result of accelerated aging of collagen in diabetes,[45] abnormal collagen cross-linking, or overhydrated collagen produced in response to osmotic effects generated by the end-products of the aldose reductase (polyol) pathway.[46] Abnormal leukocyte mobility has been implicated as well.[47] Immune complex disease has been considered as a cause of NL. Ullman and Dahl reported deposition of C3, fibrinogen, and immunoglobulins around dermal blood vessels in 9 of 12 patients with NL,[48] but subsequent reports only partially confirm these results.[49] A recent review of NL addresses these theories in greater detail.[49]

Clinically, early NL can be difficult to distinguish from granuloma annulare. As the lesions enlarge, however, NL becomes more distinct, with the epidermal change, atrophy, and yellow color seen developing. Included in the differential diagnosis for NL are diabetic dermopathy, sarcoidosis, rheumatoid nodules, morphea, stasis dermatitis, and erythema nodosum.

A consistently effective treatment for NL has yet to be found. Potent topical corticosteroids applied to the inflammatory rim of lesions are thought to help control disease progression, although no controlled studies have been published. Other agents employed, with variable results, include fibrinolytic agents such as stanozolol and pentoxifylline; and aspirin, dipyridamole, ticlopidine, nicotinamide, and clofazimine, but none have ever been demonstrated to be effective in blinded studies. Ulcerative NL usually responds to routine ulcer treatment, but surgical intervention occasionally becomes necessary.

Granuloma Annulare

Granuloma annulare (GA) is characterized by an annular configuration of flesh-colored or pale red papules and plaques that occur in a localized or generalized (disseminated) pattern (Plate II, D). Most studies find no association between diabetes and localized GA,[50–52] but a link between disseminated GA and diabetes has repeatedly been demonstrated.[53,54] In one recent study, 21% of 100 patients with generalized GA were found to be diabetic.[55]

The lesions of GA may vary in size from a few millimeters to 5 centimeters.[56] Localized GA is most characteristically located on the dorsa of the hands and feet. A single lesion is present in half of the patients with GA.[57] The papules develop and enlarge slowly in a centrifugal fashion over a period of months to years. Only 15% of patients develop more than 10 lesions. Generalized GA is characterized by a symmetrical eruption of hundreds of tiny papules, which can occur all over the body surface. Localized GA eventually undergoes spontaneous resolution—usually within 2 years. Lesions often recur at the same site, however. Resolution in patients with generalized GA is less likely.[57] Ulceration and scar formation are rare.[56]

Localized GA appears most commonly in children and young adults, affecting twice as many females as males. Generalized GA is, however, more likely to occur in older women.[56] GA can have a histologic appearance similar to that of NL, with granulomatous foci of degenerated collagen in the upper dermis and palisading histiocytes. Unlike NL lesions, however, GA lesions generally contain abundant mucin, fewer giant cells, and less extensive collagen degeneration.[40] The etiology of GA is unknown. IgG and C3 have been found in blood vessels of involved skin, suggesting an immunologic role. The differential diagnosis includes tinea corporis, sarcoidosis, NL, secondary or tertiary syphilis, annular lichen planus, and insect bites.

Treatment of GA is often unsatisfactory, but fortunately the disease is usually asymptomatic and self-limited. Topical or intralesional corticosteroids are sometimes of benefit in the treatment of localized disease. Treatment of disseminated GA is also difficult. Therapy can include the use of systemic corticosteroids, potassium iodide, antimalarial agents, nicotinic acid, and dapsone, although controversy exists as to their efficacy.[57] One recent study reported complete clearance of disease in all five patients treated with oral psoralen plus ultraviolet A (PUVA) irradiation.[58]

Scleredema Diabeticorum

Scleredema diabeticorum is a diffuse, nonpitting induration of skin characteristically occurring on the upper back, neck, and shoulders. In one study of 484 patients with diabetes, 2.5% were affected.[59] Erythema and induration typically begin on the posterior and lateral neck and may extend to the upper back and extremities, including the hands, resulting in extreme limitation of movement. The indurated areas are typically erythematous and finely papular. Patients may perceive decreased light touch and pain in the involved areas. In one report, eight of 13 patients with scleredema diabeticorum had persistent disease lasting up to 20 years.[60]

In contrast, another form of scleredema occurs in younger, nondiabetic patients after streptococcal infection. This subset of scleredema tends to resolve spontaneously within a period of months in 85% of patients.[29]

Male diabetics are more often affected than female diabetics (ratio 4:1).[61] Most patients are middle-aged. Both patients with insulin-dependent (IDDM) and non-insulin-dependent diabetes (NIDDM) are affected, but in most instances, diabetes is longstanding. Patients are generally obese, exhibiting a high frequency of diabetic retinopathy, neuropathy, hypertension, and ischemic heart disease. The etiology of scleredema diabeticorum is unknown.[62]

Histologic examination reveals a dermis that is approximately three times thicker than normal.[34] Thickened collagen bundles with deposition of hyaluronic acid are present in the dermis, and much of the underlying subcutaneous fat appears to be replaced by thickened collagen as well. The differential diagnosis includes scleroderma, eosinophilic fasciitis, the eosinophilia myalgia syndrome, and lymphedema. No specific treatment exists.[63] Scleredema does not respond to increased glycemic control.[61]

Waxy Skin

Persons with juvenile-onset IDDM can develop waxy, tight skin, also known as diabetic thick skin, in association with limited joint mobility.[64,65] Rosenbloom et al. studied more than 300 patients with IDDM and found 30% to have elements of this syndrome. Biopsy specimens of wrist skin reveal a markedly thickened dermis, with sparse glands and hair follicles. Increased collagen cross-linking, perhaps related to elevated nonenzymatic glycosylation, has been offered as an explanation.[66,67] One group of authors observed some resolution of these changes in association with improved glycemic control.[68]

METABOLIC DISEASES

Porphyria Cutanea Tarda

Porphyria cutanea tarda (PCT) is a disorder of heme synthesis characterized by a sporadic cutaneous eruption and uroporphyrinuria. It is estimated that 25% of men between the ages of 45 and 75 years who have PCT have diabetes.[69] Men are more frequently affected than women. The classic clinical picture includes vesicles, bullae, and erosions over the dorsal hands and arms and other sun-exposed areas. The primary lesions heal slowly, leaving scarring and milia (tiny epidermal inclusion cysts). Patients also are noted to exhibit skin fragility and hypertrichosis. The enzymatic defect, a deficiency of uroporphyrinogen decarboxylase, leads to excessive serum concentrations of uroporphyrins, which accumulate in tissues. These compounds are excreted in the urine, which fluoresces pink under a Wood's light. The iron concentration in serum is frequently increased. Uroporphyrinogen decarboxylase deficiency occurs in both a familial (autosomal dominant) form and a sporadic/induced form, which is triggered by alcohol, estrogens, or any of several hepatotoxic aromatic hydrocarbons. Treatments of choice include avoidance of alcohol, serial phlebotomy, and administration of antimalarial agents.[70]

Yellow Skin

As many as 10% of patients with diabetes may have yellow discoloration of the skin. The yellow color may be caused by the concentration of carotene in areas of prominent sebaceous activity (face, forehead, and axilla) and areas of thick stratum corneum (palms, soles, and bony prominences). These patients, unlike those with jaundice of hyperbilirubinemia, do not exhibit scleral icterus.[71]

Early reports linked hypercarotenemia with diabetes, citing elevated levels of carotene in more than 50% of patients with diabetes.[72] These studies may have been conducted when the recommended diet for patients with diabetes included large amounts of foods with a high carotene content. More recently, Hoerer et al. used spectrophotometry to compare the skin color and levels of serum carotene in diabetic and nondiabetic individuals.[73] They found the group with diabetes had yellower skin than the group without diabetes but found no correlation between skin color and carotene level. The explanation for the higher incidence of yellow skin among patients with diabetes is unclear and remains controversial.

Xanthomatosis

Eruptive Xanthoma

Eruptive xanthomas occur in 1 per 1000 patients with diabetes.[72] Lesions are small, firm, nontender, pinkish-yellow papules with erythematous areolas, most commonly occurring in crops on the knees, elbows, back, buttocks, and trunk (Plate II, E). Persistent papules may coalesce to form larger plaques.

In IDDM, decreased lipoprotein lipase activity results in elevated serum triglyceride levels. Cutaneous eruptive xanthomas form when the serum triglyceride level rises above 1000 mg/dL.[72] Lipids accumulated in the serum may be deposited extracellularly in the form of cholesterol or triglycerides in the dermis or subcutaneous tissue. This deposition creates a cutaneous xanthoma.

The histologic appearance of cutaneous xanthomas is characterized by the presence of macrophages containing lipid particles (foam cells). Foam cells are mixed with inflammatory cells in the superficial dermis. Fully developed eruptive xanthomas contain more triglycerides and free fatty acids than cholesterol. As xanthomas resolve, this ratio reverses.[74,75]

Lesions are indistinguishable from those in other conditions that produce hypertriglyceridemia. Chronic biliary cirrhosis, nephrotic syndrome, chronic pancreatitis, and myxedema may cause secondary eruptive xanthomas. Xanthomas and diabetes also are associated with hemochromatosis and total lipodystrophy. Prompt control of hyperlipidemia can result in disappearance of the papules. Weight reduction, carbohydrate restriction, and treatment with clofibrate may be necessary.[76]

Xanthelasma

Xanthelasma is a distinctive type of xanthoma that occurs on the eyelids. Lesions begin as small yellow-orange macules, which thicken to form oval foamy plaques. Xanthelasma is most common in middle-aged women and is particularly associated with hyperlipoproteinemia, hepatobiliary disorders, and diabetes. Although 50% or more of patients may be normolipemic, it is considered appropriate to obtain serum lipid profiles in these patients. Surgical removal is frequently successful, although recurrences are common. Xanthelasma does not usually regress when diabetes is controlled.[16]

Hemochromatosis

Hemochromatosis is a disorder of iron storage in which increased gastrointestinal absorption of iron leads to deposition of excessive iron in tissues. The most significant complications result from deposition in the liver, heart, joints, pancreas, and skin. Diabetes is found in 65% of patients, particularly those with family histories of diabetes. In 90% of patients, skin involvement is manifested by diffuse bronzed hyperpigmentation, which is due to cutaneous deposition of melanin and hemosiderin. Therapy includes phlebotomy and use of iron-chelating agents.[77]

Lipodystrophy

Progressive lipodystrophy, a rare disorder characterized by complete absence of subcutaneous fat, is associated with diabetes.[78] Most cases involve the face, back, upper trunk, and upper extremities. Onset is insidious, and discomfort is absent. In the most common partial type, the cheeks are hollowed with prominent malar eminences. Muscles and veins are prominent in affected areas.[78] Approximately 20% of these patients develop diabetes.[79] Generalized lipodystrophy is an autosomal recessive disorder with onset at puberty and results in an acromegalic appearance.[80] Decreased binding of insulin to its receptor has been shown,[81] but the complete molecular basis for the insulin resistance is unknown. Diabetic patients with progressive lipodystrophy are frequently insulin-resistant or require high doses of insulin. Diabetic control does not improve or alter lipodystrophy. Autologous fat transplantation has been reported to be successful in some cases.

Glucagonoma Syndrome

In 1942, Becker et al. first described the characteristic eruption of glucagonoma in a patient with an islet-cell type of pancreatic carcinoma.[82] Their report represents the classic clinical presentation of the syndrome, with its symmetric confluent areas of macular, erythematous, and vesicular eruptions with exfoliation and superficial necrosis. It was not until 1966 that McGavran et al. documented the hyperglucagonemia resulting from a functioning islet-cell tumor.[83] Wilkinson later called the characteristic skin changes of this glucagon-secreting A α-cell carcinoma "necrolytic migratory erythema."[84] The eruption occurs most severely in intertriginous and periorificial areas. Individual lesions last from 7 to 14 days, heal centrally, and are found in various stages of development. Other associated cutaneous findings include glossitis, conjunctivitis, periorbital crusting, ridging and thickening of nails, and paronychia.[85]

Approximately two-thirds of patients with glucagonoma have cutaneous abnormalities, and approximately 67% have fasting hyperglycemia. Neither the presence or the severity of hyperglycemia appears to be related to the degree of skin manifestations. Anemia and weight loss frequently occur.[86]

The eruption may precede by years all other symptoms of pancreatic carcinoma.[87] Removal of the carcinoma prior to metastasis results in complete cure and clearing of cutaneous symptoms.[88,89] Unfortunately, most glucagonomas have already metastasized at the time of clinical diagnosis. The cutaneous eruption, which may wax and wane spontaneously, is typically misdiagnosed and resembles many dermatoses, including pemphigus foliaceus, bullous pemphigoid, vasculitis, and psoriasis.[86]

Histopathologically, upper layers of the epidermis show abrupt necrolysis, with subsequent cleft or vesicle formation. Pale and eosinophilic keratinocytes with pyknotic nuclei are present. Neutrophils later invade the necrotic portion, with subsequent crust formation.[40]

Extreme fasting hyperglucagonemia (>500 pg/mL) is present in most cases. Hypoaminoacidemia occurs, in part secondary to the consumption of large quantities of amino acids by enhanced gluconeogenesis. Initial work-up includes a determination of fasting plasma glucagon concentration by radioimmunoassay followed by an abdominal computed tomographic scan. Celiac and hepatic arteriography may also be required.[86]

Hyperglucagonemia or the presumed secondary hypoaminoacidemia may be responsible for the skin changes, a possibility suggested by the improvement of cutaneous lesions following systemic administration of amino acids.[86,90] Various chemotherapeutic agents have been employed when surgery has failed or was not an option; the agents have included streptozotocin, phenoxybenzamine, and diaminotriazenocinidazole carbaramide.

OTHER SKIN CONDITIONS STRONGLY ASSOCIATED WITH DIABETES

Diabetic Dermopathy

The lesions of diabetic dermopathy (DD), also known as pigmented pretibial patches or shin spots, are by some reports the most common cutaneous finding in diabetes.[91] Early lesions are small, flat-topped, dull, red papules that are typically painless. Over several weeks, the lesions progress to atrophic hyperpigmented irregular patches approximately 5 to 12 mm in diameter. Lesions can be linear, grouped, or individual and frequently appear in crops. Individual lesions resolve over 1 to 2 years, but the emergence of new lesions makes the course appear stationary.[16] The lesions are most commonly located on the anterior shins, as well as on the forearms, anterior thighs, and feet, with a propensity to appear over bony prominences.[8]

The histologic appearance of the early lesions includes epidermal and papillary dermal edema with extravasated erythrocytes and a mild lymphohistiocytic infiltrate. Older, more atrophic lesions show capillary basement membrane thickening, with deposition of PAS-positive material in the intima of dermal arterioles. Scattered hemosiderin deposits are reported. There is no edema or necrobiosis.

Melin found DD in 50% of male patients and in 29% of females with diabetes who were older than 50 years of age.[92] There is controversy as to whether DD is more common with increasing duration and severity of diabetes. Association of DD with diabetic retinopathy, neuropathy, and nephropathy has been noted. The lesions are not specific to diabetes, however. Similar lesions have been noted in 1.5% of medical students and in 30% of randomly selected endocrinology patients.[93] The etiology is unknown. Because of the appearance of DD over bony prominences, trauma is thought to play a role. In a study of 19 patients with preexisting DD treated with local heat or cold, 16 developed new lesions.[94] Melin could not, however, reproduce the disease with repetitive blows from a rubber mallet. Generally no treatment other than the protection of susceptible areas from repetitive trauma is indicated.

Diabetic Bullae

Spontaneous bullous formation is a rare but distinct cutaneous sign of diabetes. Known as diabetic bullae, bullous diabeticorum, or idiopathic bullae of diabetes, it is a diagnosis made by exclusion. Kramer, in 1930, described asymptomatic blisters on the extremities of diabetic patients.[95] Diabetic bullae generally are found bilaterally on the hands, feet, and distal extremities of diabetic patients, particularly those with neuropathy and/or retinopathy.[96] The lesions are typically asymptomatic and nonhemorrhagic, ranging in size from small vesicles to bullae 3 to 5 cm in diameter. Notably, there is no surrounding erythema.

The etiology of diabetic bullae is unclear. Proposed causes include mechanical trauma, exposure to ultraviolet light, immune-mediated vasculitis,[29] and altered calcium and magnesium levels related to renal failure, changes leading to facilitated epidermal and dermal separation with trauma. The histology of this disorder is not well defined, as both epidermal and subepidermal blistering have been reported. Diabetic bullae may represent more than one entity, a diversity that may explain different histologic presentations.

The differential diagnosis includes localized bullous pemphigoid, porphyria cutanea tarda, drug-induced blistering, and blisters of renal failure. Direct immunofluorescence of perilesional skin is normal in diabetic bullae, distinguishing it from bullous pemphigoid. It is essential to make this distinction to avoid the unnecessary use of glucocorticoids in diabetic patients.[97] Treatment is symptomatic, with compresses or incision and drainage if necessary. Lesions generally resolve spontaneously within several weeks.

Rubeosis

Rubeosis is a descriptive term for the rosy facial coloration found in many patients with diabetes. This appearance tends to be more pronounced in lighter-skinned individuals. The cause remains unknown, but erythema may result from the decreased ability of the thickened dermal vessels to vasoconstrict.[98] Some authors believe that improved diabetic control may lessen the erythema. Protection from the sun and avoidance of topical irritants, dietary vasodilators such as alcohol, or substances that cause facial flushing by their increased temperature, such as coffee or tea, may be helpful.

Vitiligo

Vitiligo is an acquired condition of skin characterized by symmetrical circumscribed macular depigmentation in a localized or generalized pattern. Lesions occur typically around the nostrils, mouth, genitals, and the extensor surface of the hands. Other frequent locations include axillae, nipples, shins, and elbows. Dermatomal patterns occur rarely. Overlying hair can be white or normally pigmented. The amelanotic macules progressively enlarge, and skin depigmentation can be almost complete. In 50% of cases, onset is before the age of 20 years.

Vitiligo is associated with diabetes mellitus. Dawber found vitiligo present in 4.8% of patients with adult-onset diabetes, as compared with 0.7 to 1% of the general population.[99] An increased frequency in patients with IDDM has been reported as well. Of 2000 patients with vitiligo, however, 3.1% had diabetes.

The pathogenesis of vitiligo is unclear, but there is substantial evidence implicating an autoimmune process. Vitiligo can occur in association with states of polyglandular hypofunction, including Addison's disease, Hashimoto's thyroiditis, hypoparathyroidism, gonadal failure, diabetes mellitus, pernicious anemia, celiac sprue, and myasthenia gravis. Elevated titers of anti-thyroid, anti-adrenal, and anti-gastric antibody activity have been found in children with diabetes and vitiligo.[100] It is therefore surprising that the prevalence would be increased in adult-onset diabetes (NIDDM), which is not thought to be an autoimmune disease.

The condition is asymptomatic but can be difficult for the patient emotionally. Management includes the use of cosmetics to cover depigmented areas and avoidance of sun, although minimal spontaneous repigmentation in sun-exposed areas has been reported. PUVA therapy has been used successfully for repigmentation, although over 200 courses of treatment may be needed for an improvement rate of 50 to 70%.[101] In exceptional cases, and only with diffuse involvement, bleaching agents may be applied to surrounding skin. This treatment is irreversible, prolonged, and requires thorough evaluation of potential psychosocial ramifications for the patient. The course of vitiligo associated with diabetes is not affected by glycemic control.

Acanthosis Nigricans

Acanthosis nigricans is a cutaneous condition characterized by the presence of confluent areas of mid- to dark brown epidermal thickening with a characteristic "velvety" texture. The lesions appear most commonly in the axillae, neck, groin, and intertriginous areas. Histologically, the lesions are notable for marked hyperkeratosis and papillomatosis, with mild acanthosis and hyperpigmentation.

A childhood form of the condition, which often occurs during adolescence, is usually benign. In adulthood the condition can be associated with obesity, endocrinopathies, insulin resistance, and malignancy. Acanthosis nigricans associated with obesity is usually benign. The lesions may reverse with weight loss. Familial acanthosis nigricans with autosomal dominant inheritance has been reported as well.[102] Several endocrine disorders, including Addison's disease, polycystic ovarian disease, Cushing disease, acromegaly, and diabetes mellitus, are associated with benign acanthosis nigricans. Kahn et al. described two syndromes linking diabetes mellitus, glucose intolerance, and insulin resistance to acanthosis nigricans.[103] In patients with "type A" insulin resistance, the resistance is due to a reduction in the number of cellular insulin receptors, whereas in patients with "type B" insulin resistance, the basis of the resistance is thought to be the presence of antibodies to the receptor.[103] Acanthosis nigricans also occurs in association with the use of certain drugs, including diethylstilbestrol, nicotinic acid, and corticosteroids. When acanthosis nigricans occurs out of the setting of any of the previous conditions, underlying malignancy must be suspected.[104] The most commonly associated tumors are adenocarcinoma, particularly of gastric origin. Squamous cell carcinoma, undifferentiated carcinoma, and lymphoma have also been associated with acanthosis nigricans. In two-thirds of cases, the lesions of acanthosis nigricans parallel the course of the malignancy.

Treatment of acanthosis nigricans is directed primarily at identification and treatment of the underlying condition, if known. Locally, the lesions can be peeled with 5 to 10% salicylic acid in petrolatum.

Perforating Disorders

The perforating disorders are a group of diseases in which dermal material perforates through the epidermis out to the surface of the skin. The four classic members of this group are reactive perforating collagenosis, Kyrle's disease, perforating folliculitis, and elastosis perforans serpiginosa. All but the last appear to be associated with diabetes, occurring most commonly in patients with coexisting nephropathy. These diseases are occasionally seen in patients with renal disease without diabetes and are rarely noted in healthy individuals.

Reactive perforating collagenosis is characterized by follicular plugs over the extremities, particularly the knees and elbows.[105] Kyrle's disease affects a similar subpopulation of older patients with severe diabetes and renal disease. Keratin plugs are surrounded by erythema and are found in various stages of development (Plate II, F, G). Lesions occur preferentially on the extremities, buttocks, and sacral region.[106] Perforating folliculitis produces similar, but slightly smaller and more numerous, lesions that are most often on the extremities. Pruritus, the most common complaint, can be extremely resistant to treatment.

Generalized Pruritus

The frequency of generalized pruritus in diabetes is unknown; however, many believe that it is increased in the diabetic population. Pruritus without primary lesions in a diabetic patient requires a thorough work-up to rule out known causes of pruritus. Patients with systemic disease (renal disease, liver disease, hypo- or hyperthyroidism, iron-deficiency anemia) or lymphoreticular malignancies (Hodgkin's disease) may present initially with pruritus. Each of these, as well as a primary dermatologic cause of itching, should first be ruled out before the pruritus is attributed to diabetes.

CUTANEOUS REACTIONS TO THERAPY FOR DIABETES

Insulin-Induced Disorders

Insulin allergy may be secondary to exposure to the insulin molecule or to additives or protein contaminants in the commercial preparation.[107,108] Local reactions to insulin include erythema, pruritus, and induration at the injection site; edema; subcutaneous nodules; or urticaria.[109] Serious immediate generalized reactions such as angioedema, bronchial constriction, dyspnea, cardiovascular collapse, and anaphylaxis have occurred, but are rare, and necessitate discontinuation of insulin therapy.[107,110] Delayed reactions, which are usually local at the site of injection, occur approximately 2 weeks after initiation of treatment. Injections that are too superficial may cause cutaneous reactions. These allergic reactions are much less common now that more highly purified insulins are used. When reactions occur in patients using bovine and/or porcine insulin, the first approach is to switch to human insulin. However, occasional cases of insulin allergy have occurred even in association with human insulin.[107]

Atrophy of subcutaneous fat (insulin lipodystrophy) may occur, resulting in atrophic areas at insulin injection sites 6 to 24 months after initiation of therapy. Women are more prone than men to this reaction. Improvement has been achieved by injection of purified insulin into atrophic areas.[111] In some reported cases, lipodystrophy disappeared in patients treated with human insulin for whom lipoatrophy had not been improved by administration of purified porcine insulin.[112] Insulin-induced lipohypertrophy is more common in males than in females and is caused by repetitive injections into the same site, a presumed local anabolic effect of insulin. The condition clears spontaneously with rotation of the insulin site.[110]

Hypoglycemic Agents

The most common adverse effects of hypoglycemic drugs, which are sulfur-based compounds, are gastrointestinal and dermatologic.[113] Cutaneous hypersensitivity reactions are similar for the various oral hypoglycemic drugs. Serious cutaneous reactions include a diffuse exfoliative dermatitis, generalized erythema multiforme, which may progress to Stevens-Johnson syndrome and toxic epidermal necrolysis.[114] Cross-reactivity with other sulfonylurea agents may occur, as well as with other sulfur-based drugs such as thiazides, furosemide, and sulfa antibiotics. Thus, when substitution is necessary, it must be done cautiously.

Topically applied preparations may sensitize a person to sulfanilamides. Fisher reported two cases of a widespread contact dermatitis in patients receiving oral hypoglycemic agents who had previously been sensitized with topical agents containing the *para*-amino group.[115]

A disulfiram-like reaction may follow the ingestion of alcohol in patients receiving sulfonylurea agents,[113] and as many as 10 to 30% of patients taking oral sulfonylurea agents experience such a reaction.[116] Chlorpropamide is the most common offending agent.[117] Patients should be warned about this potential side effect, and symptoms to be aware of include flushing, diaphoresis, mild headache, nausea, vomiting, and tachycardia. Symptoms usually occur 15 minutes after ingestion and subside within an hour.

REFERENCES

1. Halprin KM, Ohkawara A, Adachi K. Glucose entry into the human epidermis. I. The concentration of glucose in the human epidermis. J Invest Dermatol 1967;49:559–60.
2. Alteras I, Saryt E. Prevalence of pathogenic fungi in the toe-webs and toe-nails of diabetic patients. Mycopathologia 1979;67:157–9.
3. Sonck CE, Somersalo O. The yeast flora of the anogenital region in diabetic girls. Arch Dermatol 1963; 88:846–52.
4. Muller SA. Dermatologic disorders associated with diabetes mellitus. Mayo Clin Proc 1966;41:689–703.
5. Cates JL, Finestone A, Bogash M. Phimosis and diabetes mellitus. J Urol 1973;110:406–407.
6. Peterka ES, Fusaro RM. Cutaneous carbohydrate studies. III. Comparison of the fasting glucose content of the skin of the back, arm, abdomen and thigh. J Invest Dermatol 1966;47:410–1.
7. Knight L, Fletcher J. Growth of *Candida albicans* in saliva: stimulation by glucose associated with antibiotics, corticosteroids, and diabetes mellitus. J Infect Dis 1971;123: 371–7.
8. Stone OJ, Mullins JF. Incidence of chronic paronychia. JAMA 1963;186:71–3.
9. Huntley AC. The cutaneous manifestations of diabetes mellitus. J Am Acad Dermatol 1982;7:427–55.
10. Greene RA, Scher RK. Nail changes associated with diabetes mellitus. J Am Acad Dermatol 1987;16:1015–21.
11. Vallance-Owen J. Diabetes mellitus. Br J Dermatol 1969; 81(Suppl 2):9–13.
12. Utz JP, Shadomy HJ. Deep fungal infections. In: Fitzpatrick TB, Eisen AZ, Wolff K, et al, eds. Dermatology in general medicine. Vol 2. 3rd ed. New York: McGraw-Hill, 1987: 2248–75.

13. Rippon JW. Systemic mycoses. In: Rose NR, Barron AL, Crane LR, Menna JH, eds. Microbiology: basic principles and clinical application. New York: MacMillan, 1983:299–310.

14. Tomford JW, Whittlesey D, Ellner JJ, Tomashefski JF Jr. Invasive primary cutaneous phycomycosis in diabetic leg ulcers. Arch Surg 1980;115:770–1.

15. Bennett JE. Fungal infections. In: Wilson JD, Braunwald E, Isselbacher KJ, et al, eds. Harrison's principles of internal medicine. Vol 1. 12th ed. New York: McGraw-Hill, 1991: 743–51.

16. Freinkel RK, Freinkel N. Cutaneous manifestations of endocrine disorders. In: Fitzpatrick TB, Eisen AZ, Wolff K, et al, eds. Dermatology in general medicine. Vol 2. 3rd ed. New York: McGraw-Hill, 1987:2063–81.

17. Mowat AG, Baum J. Chemotaxis of polymorphonuclear leukocytes from patients with diabetes mellitus. N Engl J Med 1971;284:621–7.

18. Davidson NJ, Swoden JM, Fletcher J. Defective phagocytosis in insulin controlled diabetics: evidence for a reaction between glucose and opsonising proteins. J Clin Pathol 1984;37:783–6.

19. Rayfield EJ, Ault MJ, Keusch GT, et al. Infection and diabetes: the case for glucose control. Am J Med 1982;72: 439–50.

20. Repine JE, Clawson CC, Goetz FC. Bactericidal function of neutrophils from patients with acute bacterial infections and from diabetics. J Infect Dis 1980;142:869–75.

21. Bagdade JD, Root RK, Bulger RJ. Impaired leukocyte function in patients with poorly controlled diabetes. Diabetes 1974;23:9–15.

22. Nolan CM, Beaty HN, Bagdade JD. Further characterization of the impaired bactericidal function of granulocytes in patients with poorly controlled diabetes. Diabetes 1978;27:889–94.

23. Kontras SB, Bodenbender JG. Studies of the inflammatory cycle in juvenile diabetes. Am J Dis Child 1968;116: 130–4.

24. Perillie PE, Nolan JP, Finch SC. Studies of the resistance to infection in diabetes mellitus: local exudative cellular response. J Lab Clin Med 1962;59:1008–15.

25. Harter DH, Petersdorf RG. Bacterial meningitis and brain abscess. In: Wilson JD, Braunwald E, Isselbacher KJ, et al, eds. Harrison's principles of internal medicine. Vol 2. 12th ed. New York: McGraw-Hill, 1991:2023–31.

26. Zaky DA, Bentley DW, Lowy K, et al. Malignant external otitis: a severe form of otitis in diabetic patients. Am J Med 1976;61:298–302.

27. Somerville DA, Lancaster-Smith M. The aerobic cutaneous microflora of diabetic subjects. Br J Dermatol 1973; 89:395–400.

28. Gilgor RS. Cutaneous infections in diabetes mellitus. In: Jelinek JE, ed. The skin in diabetes. Philadelphia: Lea & Febiger, 1986.

29. Sibbald RG, Schachter RK. The skin and diabetes mellitus. Int Dermatol 1984;23:567–84.

30. Faerman I, Jadzinsky M, Podolsky S. Diabetic neuropathy and sexual dysfunction. In: Podolsky S, ed. Clinical diabetes: modern management. New York: Appleton-Century-Crafts, 1980.

31. Phillips TJ, Dover JS. Leg ulcers. J Am Acad Dermatol 1991;25:965–87.

32. Levin M, O'Neal ME. The diabetic foot. St Louis: Mosby, 1987.

33. Hurley HJ. The eccrine sweat glands. In: Moschella SL, Hurley HJ, eds. Dermatology. Vol 2. 2nd ed. Philadelphia. WB Saunders, 1985.

34. Danowski TS, Bahl VK, Fisher ER. Macrovascular and microvascular disease and their prevention. In: Podolsky S, ed. Clinical diabetes and modern management. New York: Appleton-Century-Crafts, 1980.

35. LoGerfo FW, Coffman JD. Vascular and microvascular disease of the foot in diabetes: implications for foot care. N Engl J Med 1984;311:25: 1615–9.

36. Haroon TS. Diabetes and skin: a review. Scott Med J 1974;19:257–67.

37. Edwards EA, Coffman JD. Cutaneous changes in peripheral vascular disease. In: Fitzpatrick TB, Eisen AZ, Wolff K, et al, eds. Dermatology in general medicine. Vol 2. 3rd ed. New York: McGraw-Hill, 1987:1997–2022.

38. Oppenheim M. Eigentumlich disseminierte Degeneration des Bindegewebes der Haut bie einem Diabetiker. Zentralbl Haut Geschlechtskr 1929–1930;32:179.

39. Urbach E. Beitrage zu einer physiologischen und pathologischen Chemie der Haut. X. Mitteilung. Eine neue diabetische Stoffwechseldermatose: Nekrobiosis Lipoidica Diabeticorum. Arch Dermatol Syph 1932;166:273–85.

40. Lever WF, Shaumburg-Lever G. Histopathology of the skin. 7th ed. Philadelphia: JB Lippincott, 1990.

41. Muller SA, Winkelmann RK. Necrobiosis lipoidica diabeticorum: a clinical and pathological investigation of 171 cases. Arch Dermatol 1966;93:272–81.

42. Muller SA, Winkelmann RK. Necrobiosis lipoidica diabeticorum: results of glucose-tolerance tests in nondiabetic patients. JAMA 1966;195:433–6.

43. Dandona P, Freedman D, Barter S, et al. Glycosylated haemoglobin in patients with necrobiosis lipoidica and granuloma annulare. Clin Exp Dermatol 1981;6:299–302.

44. Soler NG, McConnachie PR. HLA antigens and necrobiosis lipoidica diabeticorum—a comparison between insulin-dependent diabetics with and without necrobiosis. Postgrad Med J 1983;59:759–62.

45. Hamlin CR, Kohn RR, Luschin JH. Apparent accelerated aging of human collagen in diabetes mellitus. Diabetes 1975;24:902–4.

46. Eaton RP. The collagen hydration hypothesis: a new paradigm for the secondary complications of diabetes mellitus [Editorial]. J Chronic Dis 1986;39:763–6.

47. Gange RW, Black MM, Carrington P. Defective neutrophil migration in granuloma annulare, necrobiosis lipoidica, and sarcoidosis. Arch Dermatol 1979;115:32–5.

48. Ullman S, Dahl MV. Necrobiosis lipoidica: an immunofluorescence study. Arch Dermatol 1977;113:1671–3.

49. Lowitt MH, Dover JS. Necrobiosis lipoidica. J Am Acad Dermatol 1991;25:735–48.

50. Mobacken H, Gisslen H, Johannisson G. Granuloma annulare: cortisone-glucose tolerance test in a non-diabetic group. Acta Derm Venereol 1970;50:440–4.

51. Meier-Ewert H, Allenby CF. Granuloma annulare and diabetes mellitus. Arch Dermatol Forsch 1971;241: 194–8.

52. Williamson DM, Dykes JRW. Carbohydrate metabolism in granuloma annulare. J Invest Dermatol 1972;58:400–4.

53. Haim S, Friedman-Birnbaum R, Haim N, et al. Carbohydrate tolerance in patients with granuloma annulare: study of fifty-two cases. Br J Dermatol 1973;88:447–51.

54. Eng AM. Erythematous generalized granuloma annulare. Arch Dermatol 1979;115:1210–1.

55. Dabski K, Winkelmann RK. Generalized granuloma annulare: histopathology and immunopathology. Systematic review of 100 cases and comparison with localized granuloma annulare. J Am Acad Dermatol 1989;20:28–39.

56. Wells RS, Smith MA. The natural history of granuloma annulare. Br J Dermatol 1963;75:199–205.

57. Dahl MV, Goltz RW. Granuloma annulare. In: Fitzpatrick TB, Eisen AZ, Wolff K, et al, eds. Dermatology in general medicine. Vol 2. 3rd ed. New York: McGraw-Hill, 1987: 1018–22.

58. Kerker BJ, Huang CP, Morison WL. Photochemotherapy of generalized granuloma annulare. Arch Dermatol 1990; 126:359–61.

59. Cole GW, Headley J, Skowsky R. Sclerederma diabeticorum: a common and distinct cutaneous manifestation of diabetes mellitus. Diabetes Care 1983;6:189–92.

60. Cohn BA, Wheeler CE Jr, Briggaman RA. Scleredema adultorum of Buschke and diabetes mellitus. Arch Dermatol 1970;101:27–35.

61. Fleischmajer R, Faludi G, Krol S. Scleredema and diabetes mellitus. Arch Dermatol 1970;101:21–6.

62. Jelinek JE. Collagen disorders in which diabetes and cutaneous features coexist. In: Jelinek JE, ed. The skin in diabetes. Philadelphia: Lea & Febiger, 1988.

63. Parker SC, Fenton DA, Black MM. Scleredema. Clin Exp Dermatol 1989;14:385–6.

64. Rosenbloom AL, Silverstein JH, Kubilis PS, Riley WJ. Limited joint mobility (L.J.M.) in insulin-dependent diabetes indicates high risk for microvasculopathy (MVP) [Abstract no. 925]. Pediatr Res 1980;14:580.

65. Barta L. Flexion contractures in a diabetic child (Rosenbloom syndrome). Eur J Pediatr 1980;135:101–2.

66. Chang KF, Uitto J, Rowold EA, et al. Increased collagen cross-linkages in experimental diabetes. Diabetes 1980; 29:778–81.

67. Schnider SL, Kohn RR. Effects of age and diabetes mellitus on the solubility and nonenzymatic glucosylation of human skin collagen. J Clin Invest 1981;67:1630–5.

68. Lieberman LS, Rosenbloom AL, Riley WJ, Silverstein JH. Reduced skin thickness with pump administration of insulin [Letter]. N Engl J Med 1980;303:940–1.

69. Grossman ME, Poh-Fitzpatrick MB. Porphyria cutanea tarda: diagnosis and management. Med Clin North Am 1980;64(5):807–27.

70. Poh-Fitzpatrick MB. Porphyrin-sensitized cutaneous photosensitivity: pathogenesis and treatment. Clin Dermatol 1985;3:41–82.

71. Leung AKC. Carotenemia. Adv Pediatr 1987;34:223–48.

72. Huntley AC. Diabetes mellitus and miscellaneous metabolic conditions affecting the skin. In: Jelinek JE, ed. The skin in diabetes. Philadelphia: Lea & Febiger, 1986.

73. Hoerer E, Dreyfuss F, Herzberg M. Carotenemia, skin colour and diabetes mellitus. Acta Diabetol Lat 1975;12: 202–7.

74. Baes H, Van Gent CM, Pries C. Lipid composition of various types of xanthoma. J Invest Dermatol 1968; 51:286–93.

75. Parker F, Bagdade JD, Odland GF, Bierman EL. Evidence for the chylomicron origin of lipids accumulating in diabetic eruptive xanthomas: a corrective lipid biochemical, histochemical, and electron microscopic study. J Clin Invest 1970;49:2172–87.

76. Brewer HB Jr, Fredrickson DS. Dyslipoproteinemias and xanthomatoses. In: Fitzpatrick TB, Eisen AZ, Wolff K, et al, eds. Dermatology in general medicine. Vol 2. 3rd ed. New York: McGraw-Hill, 1987:1722–38.

77. Powell LW, Isselbacher KJ. Hemochromatosis. In: Wilson JD, Braunwald E, Isselbacher KJ, et al, eds. Harrison's principles of internal medicine. Vol 2. 12th ed. New York: McGraw-Hill, 1991:1835–34.

78. Taylor WB, Honeycutt WM. Progressive lipodystrophy and lipoatrophic diabetes: review of the literature and case reports. Arch Dermatol 1961;84:31–6.

79. Murray I. Lipodystrophy. BMJ 1952;2:1236–9.

80. Fine J, Moschella SL. Diseases of nutrition and metabolism. In: Moschella SL, Hurley HJ, eds. Dermatology. Vol 2. 2nd ed. Philadelphia: WB Saunders, 1985.

81. Oseid S, Beck-Nielsen H, Pedersen O, et al. Decreased binding of insulin to its receptor in patients with congenital generalized lipodystrophy. N Engl J Med 1977;296: 245–8.

82. Becker SW, Kahn D, Rothman S. Cutaneous manifestations of internal malignant tumors. Arch Dermatol Syph 1942; 45:1069–80.

83. McGavran MH, Unger RH, Recant L, et al. A glucagon-secreting alpha-cell carcinoma of the pancreas. N Engl J Med 1966;274:1408–13.

84. Wilkinson DS. Necrolytic migratory erythema with carcinoma of the pancreas. Trans St. John's Hosp Dermatol Soc 1973;59:244–50.

85. Leichter SB. Clinical and metabolic aspects of glucagonoma. Medicine (Baltimore) 1980;59:100–13.

86. Stacpoole PW. The glucagonoma syndrome: clinical features, diagnosis and treatment. Endocr Rev 1984;2: 347–61.

87. Domen RE, Shaffer MB Jr, Finke J, et al. The glucagonoma syndrome: report of a case. Arch Intern Med 1980;140: 262–3.

88. Kahan RS, Perez-Figaredo RA, Neimanis A. Necrolytic migratory erythema: distinctive dermatosis of the glucagonoma syndrome. Arch Dermatol 1977;113: 792–7.

89. Sweet RD. A dermatosis specifically associated with a tumour of pancreatic alpha cells. Br J Dermatol 1974;90: 301–8.

90. Norton JA, Kahn CR, Schiebinger R, et al. Amino acid deficiency and the skin rash associated with glucagonoma. Ann Intern Med 1979;91:213–5.

91. Bernstein JE, Medenica M, Soltani K, Griem SF. Bullous eruption of diabetes mellitus. Arch Dermatol 1979;115: 324–5.

92. Melin H. An atrophic circumscribed skin lesion in the lower extremities of diabetics. Acta Med Scand 1964; 176(Suppl 423):1–75.

93. Danowski TS, Sabeh G, Sarver ME, et al. Shin spots and diabetes mellitus. Am J Med Sci 1966;251:570–5.

94. Lithner F. Cutaneous reactions of the extremities of diabetics to local thermal trauma. Acta Med Scand 1975; 198:319–25.

95. Kramer DW. Early or warning signs of impending gangrene in diabetes. Med J Rec 1930;132:338–42.

96. Kurwa A, Roberts P, Whitehead R. Concurrence of bullous and atrophic skin lesions in diabetes mellitus. Arch Dermatol 1971;103:670–5.

97. Jelinek JE. Cutaneous markers of diabetes mellitus and the role of microangiopathy. In: Jelinek JE, ed. The skin in diabetes. Philadelphia: Lea & Febiger, 1986.

98. Ditzel J. Functional microangiopathy in diabetes mellitus. Diabetes 1968;17:388–9.

99. Dawber RPR, Bleehen SS, Vallance-Owen J. Vitiligo and diabetes mellitus [Letter]. Br J Dermatol 1971;84:600.

100. Macaron C, Winter RJ, Traisman HS, et al. Vitiligo and juvenile diabetes mellitus. Arch Dermatol 1977;113: 1515–7.

101. Parrish JA, Fitzpatrick TB, Shea C, et al. Photochemotherapy of vitiligo: use of orally administered psoralens and a high-intensity long-wave ultraviolet system. Arch Dermatol 1976;112:1531–4.

102. Tasjian D, Jarratt M. Familial acanthosis nigricans. Arch Dermatol 1984;120:1351–4.

103. Kahn CR, Flier JS, Bar RS, et al. The syndromes of insulin resistance and acanthosis nigricans: insulin-receptor disorders in man. N Engl J Med 1976;294:739–45.

104. Haynes HA. Cutaneous manifestations of internal malignancy. In: Braunwald E, Isselbacher KJ, Petersdorf RG, et al, eds. Harrison's principles of internal medicine. Vol 2. 11th ed. New York: McGraw-Hill, 1987:1588–93.

105. Poliak SC, Lebwohl MG, Parris A, et al. Reactive perforating collagenosis associated with diabetes mellitus. N Engl J Med 1982;306:81–4.

106. Wolff-Schreiner EC. Kyrle's disease. In: Fitzpatrick TB, Eisen AZ, Wolff K, et al, eds. Dermatology in general medicine. Vol 1. 3rd ed. New York: McGraw-Hill, 1987:541–5.

107. Shore RN, Shelley WB, Kyle GC. Chronic urticaria from isophane insulin therapy: sensitivity associated with non-insulin components in commercial preparations. Arch Dermatol 1975;111:947.

108. Grammer LC, Chen PY, Patterson R. Evaluation and management of insulin allergy. J Allergy Clin Immunol 1983;71:2:250–4.

109. Lieberman P, Patterson R, Metz R, Lucena G, et al. Allergic reactions to insulin. JAMA 1971;215:1106–12.

110. Gilgor RS, Lazarus GS. Skin manifestations of diabetes mellitus. In: Ellenberg M, Rifkin H, eds. Diabetes mellitus theory and practice. 3rd ed. New Hyde Park, NY: Medical Examination Publishing, 1983:879–93.

111. Ferland L, Ehrlich RM. Single-peak insulin in the treatment of insulin-induced fat atrophy. J Pediatr 1975;86:741–3.

112. Valenta LJ, Elias AN. Insulin-induced lipodystrophy in diabetic patients resolved by treatment with human insulin. Ann Intern Med 1985;102:6:790–1.

113. Peters AL, Davidson MB. Use of sulfonyluric agents in older diabetic patients. Clin Geriatr Med 1990;6:903–21.

114. Bruinsma W. A guide to drug reaction. Amsterdam: Excerpta Medica, 1973:99.

115. Fisher AA. Systemic contact dermatitis from Orinase and Diabinase in diabetics with para-amino hypersensitivity. Cutis 1982;29:551–65.

116. Fitzgerald MG, Gaddie R, Malins JM, et al. Alcohol sensitivity in diabetics receiving chlorpropamide. Diabetes 1962;11:40–3.

117. Groop L, Eriksson CJP, Huupponen R, et al. Roles of chlorpropamide, alcohol and acetaldehyde in determining the chlorpropamide-alcohol flush. Diabetologia 1984;26:34–8.

Chapter 50

JOINT AND BONE MANIFESTATIONS OF DIABETES MELLITUS

SUSAN F. KROOP
LEE S. SIMON

Although the other complications of diabetes mellitus are better recognized as causes of morbidity and mortality, the musculoskeletal syndromes associated with diabetes mellitus may be very debilitating. Overall, changes in the connective tissue of patients with diabetes are probably due to disturbances in the structural macromolecules of the extracellular matrix. Many of these rheumatologic manifestations of diabetes mellitus have been reviewed in the last several years.[1-3] A wide range of musculoskeletal syndromes have been described in association with diabetes (Table 50–1). In general, these are syndromes commonly or uniquely associated with diabetes mellitus. There are also common rheumatic diseases with an increased incidence in the diabetic population.

RHEUMATIC SYNDROMES UNIQUELY OR COMMONLY ASSOCIATED WITH DIABETES MELLITUS

Adhesive Capsulitis of the Shoulder

Adhesive capsulitis of the shoulder is a common problem manifested by diffuse shoulder pain associated with a loss of motion in all directions and little or no evidence of intra-articular disease.[4] The joint capsule is thickened and adherent to the humeral head. Arthroscopy reveals marked reduction in the volume of the glenohumeral joint. Increased uptake of ^{99m}Tc-methylene diphosphonate by the periarticular tissue has been demonstrated, suggesting the presence of inflammation.[5] Bone demineralization follows. Although patients may recover spontaneously within 3 years, the syndrome may recur, and some patients with severe disease may become disabled.[3]

The association of adhesive capsulitis and diabetes mellitus has been well documented. Bridgman identified adhesive capsulitis in 11% of 800 diabetic patients compared with an incidence of 2.5% in 600 control patients. Alternatively, abnormal glucose tolerance tests were seen in 28% of patients with adhesive capsulitis compared with 12% of age- and sex-matched controls attending a rheumatology clinic.[6]

The treatment of patients is directed toward increasing the range of motion of the tightened joint. Early physical therapy, including exercises, heat, and ultrasound, may be helpful. Splinting may lead to further restriction of motion. Treatment of pain during physical therapy is important. Treatment includes the use of nonsteroid anti-inflammatory drugs (NSAIDs) as both anti-inflammatory agents and analgesics. Although there are no long-term studies concerning the use of local glucocorticoid injections in this setting, intra-articular injections may occasionally be useful in decreasing pain and increasing motion. Rarely, patients may require manipulation of the

Table 50–1. Musculoskeletal Syndromes Associated with Diabetes Mellitus

Rheumatic syndromes uniquely or commonly associated with diabetes
  mellitus
    Adhesive capsulitis
    Shoulder-hand syndrome
    Diabetic hand syndrome
    Dupuytren's disease
    Neuroarthropathy
    Hyperostosis
Common rheumatic diseases associated with diabetes mellitus
    Osteoarthritis
    Gout and hyperuricemia
    Calcium pyrophosphate deposition arthropathy
Osteopenia
Osteolysis of forefoot
Migratory osteolysis of hip and knee

shoulder while they are under general anesthesia to increase the range of motion. In severe cases of adhesive capsulitis, the patient may not recover full motion and may become disabled.

Shoulder-Hand Syndrome

Shoulder-hand syndrome (SHS) is characterized by adhesive capsulitis of the shoulder associated with pain, swelling, tenderness, dystrophic skin, and vasomotor instability in the hand. It is one of a family of disorders that includes reflex sympathetic dystrophy syndrome, major and minor causalgia, Sudeck's atrophy, and algodystrophy. Doury et al. described these syndromes as consisting of severe pain disproportionate to the findings of the physical examination in association with articular or periarticular swelling.[7] Steinbrocker and Argyros described three stages of this syndrome. During the first stage, which lasts 3 to 6 months, there is pain, tenderness, swelling, and vasomotor changes, including temperature and color changes. The second stage, which also may last 3 to 6 months, is characterized by trophic skin changes characterized by shiny skin with loss of normal wrinkling. The final stage is characterized by atrophy of skin and subcutaneous tissue, tendon contractures, and progressive osteopenia. Spontaneous improvement may occur, although permanent loss of function of the affected limb may occur as well.[8,9]

Trauma is the most common condition predisposing to SHS, but diabetes; cerebrovascular disease; myocardial infarction; post-thoracotomy state; hyperthyroidism; hyperlipidemia; electrocution; medications, including barbiturates, isoniazid, ethionamide, and cycloserine; and previous exposure to radioiodine have all been associated with the onset of this syndrome.[3] In one study of 108 patients with SHS or related conditions, 7.4% had diabetes mellitus.[7] The prevalence of diabetes mellitus actually may be greater in patients with this syndrome, since glucose tolerance tests were not performed in all cases.

Radiologic findings in SHS typically include a diffuse, patchy osteopenia. Measurements of bone mineral density demonstrate loss of up to one-third of the bone mass. Three-phase bone scintigraphy reveals asymmetric uptake and increased blood flow and, in most cases, pooling in phases 1 and 2. The phase 3 images are characterized by increased uptake in the periarticular tissues. A small percentage of patients may show decreased uptake on bone scintigraphs.

Treatment of patients with SHS is most effective when begun early in the development of the syndrome. Analgesic medication and range-of-motion exercises should be prescribed. If these are ineffective, systemic glucocorticoid therapy or sympathetic blockade should be considered. In patients with diabetes, regional sympathetic ganglion block with a long-acting anesthetic agent, performed by an anesthesiologist, is the preferred treatment method since the use of systemic glucocorticoids may cause difficulties in the maintenance of glucose control. Steinbrocker and Argyros reviewed 146 patients with SHS and found some improvement in up to 80%

treated with glucocorticoids or regional sympathetic blockade.[9] Intra-articular steroids may also be used, but no controlled trials exist and experience with this technique is limited. Patients are candidates for surgical sympathectomy if the above approaches provide only temporary relief of symptoms. Recently, interest has increased in the use of α-adrenergic blockade and other vasoactive drugs in the treatment of SHS.

Diabetic Hand Syndrome

Diabetic hand syndrome (DHS), also termed cheiropathy, stiff hand syndrome, diabetic stiff hand, diabetic contractures, or syndrome of limited joint mobility, was first described by Jung et al.[10] in adults with diabetes and by Grgic et al.[11] in a pediatric population with diabetes and short stature. A comprehensive review of this syndrome was recently published.[12] The syndrome has since been described in juveniles with Type I diabetes and normal stature and in adults with Type I or Type II diabetes.[13-17] The reported prevalence of DHS in diabetes varies from 8 to 53%.[18-25] Most studies suggest a prevalence of about 35% in patients with diabetes.[26-29] It is more common in patients with Type I diabetes and may be associated with duration of disease. The onset of DHS may not be related to the patient's sex, insulin dosage, or quality of the metabolic control.

Clinically, patients complain of stiffness, loss of dexterity, and weakness of their hands. The skin on the hands is thick, tight, and waxy. There is evidence of recurrent tenosynovitis and decreased range of motion of the small joints of the hands. The patient may exhibit the prayer sign, i.e., when asked to hold the palms of the hands together, the patient is unable to bring both the fingers and palms together because of flexor tendon contractures. Limitation of flexion and extension occurs predominantly in the proximal interphalangeal and metacarpophalangeal joints. Decreased grip strength results. Sclerodactyly and thick skin may be present. Raynaud's phenomenon, digital ulcers, or other systemic manifestations of scleroderma or other autoimmune diseases are not present. Laboratory evaluation is unrevealing, and radiographs of the hands may be normal or show diffuse osteopenia.

Pathologically, a biopsy of the thickened skin reveals dermal fibrosis with increased collagen deposition in the dermis and loss of sebaceous glands and other secondary skin appendages.[27,28]

Much has been reported about the relationship of DHS with the age of the patient, the duration of diabetes, and the presence of diabetic retinopathy.[10,27,30] In general, DHS is more common in patients with long-standing diabetes and microvascular disease. The presence of DHS may indicate that the patient is at high risk for microvascular disease. In patients with diabetes for 16 years, the prevalence of observed microvascular lesions was three- to fourfold higher in those with hand contractures than in those without contractures.[27,30-33] In addition, a form of restrictive lung disease has been described in patients with DHS in which total and vital lung capacity is decreased.[18,22-24] These patients are usually asymptomatic but may experience dyspnea secondary to hypoxemia. It is likely that in some instances similar abnormalities in connective tissue occur in the hand and the lung.

The limitation of joint movement probably results from dermal and subcutaneous sclerosis.[28,34,35] In addition, the fibrous thickening of the flexor tendon sheaths contributes to the loss of mobility. The pathogenesis of these altered connective tissues remains obscure. Some investigators have documented increased cross-linking of collagen, which leads to increased resistance to collagenase and the resultant decrease in turnover.[36-38] Increased nonenzymatic glycosylation of collagen, which might increase intermolecular cross-linking, has been demonstrated as well.[39-45] Other possible factors include increased hydration of collagen, swelling of the connective tissue through the aldose reductase pathway, and microangiopathy leading to increased collagen synthesis.

Therapy for the diabetic hand syndrome should include dynamic splinting and an attempt to increase range of motion through exercise. It is unclear without prospective studies whether an increase in exercise will prevent the onset of limited joint mobility or will restore joint mobility that has been lost. Aspirin or NSAIDs may be helpful in controlling pain and stiffness. There are case reports in the literature suggesting that better glycemic control may lead to a decrease in skin thickness.[46] Finally, aldose reductase inhibitors are being used on an experimental basis, and one report of three patients demonstrated a reversal of hand symptoms in patients with contractures.[47]

Dupuytren's Disease

Dupuytren's disease is common in the general population and increases in incidence as the population ages.[3,48] It causes a focal flexion contracture with a thickened band of palmar fascia. Flexion deformities along with tethering of the skin are noted. Knuckle pads (Garrod's pads), as well as heel-pad nodules, may be noted.[3] Pain and loss of motion result. Dupuytren's contracture, in which a low-grade inflammatory reaction producing nodularity may occur, often is associated with diabetes. Contractures may involve the third, fourth, or fifth flexor tendons. It has been suggested that 25% of patients with Dupuytren's contractures have diabetes.[2,49] In addition, studies have shown that from 21 to 63% of patients with diabetes have the contractures, in contrast to 5 to 22% of the normal population.[2] Noble et al. reported the development of this complication in more than 50% of patients with diabetes and an increase in incidence with duration of diabetes and also demonstrated that a high proportion—as high as 16% of adults with diabetes—have Dupuytren's contracture at the time of diagnosis of diabetes.[50]

The pathogenesis of Dupuytren's disease remains unknown. Occasionally, a history of occupational or other trauma may precede its onset. Investigators have described the occurrence of modified fibroblasts (myofibroblasts), which resemble smooth muscle cells and are contractile within tendon nodules.[51,52] Proliferation of these cells with subsequent contraction might subject neighboring fascial structures to intermittent tension, resulting in hypertrophy. These same cells have also been reported in the nodules of patients with Ledderhose's disease and may be present in the abnormal tissues of patients with Peyronie's disease.[53,54] In addition, studies have documented the deposition of increased amounts of type III collagen in the palmar aponeurosis and in diseased fascia. It appears that as more type III collagen is deposited the disease becomes more severe. The greatest proportion of the type III collagen is found in the nodules. It is unknown whether onset is linked to impaired glucose tolerance[55-57] or whether good glucose control in the diabetic patient will limit onset of this problem.[58-61]

Treatment includes aggressive physical therapy, including dynamic splinting and exercises. NSAIDs may be helpful in decreasing pain. Intralesional glucocorticoid injections may provide relief of pain as well as increased range of motion. Occasionally, surgical release of the contracture is necessary.

NEUROARTHROPATHY

Diabetes mellitus is one of the major causes of Charcot joints. The usual presentation is that of a patient with long-standing diabetes, often complicated by hypertension, proteinuria, and retinopathy, who develops joint swelling or deformity after the age of 50. The foot is most commonly involved, followed in frequency by the ankle and knee. Rarely, upper extremity joints are involved. Unilateral painless foot swelling is the most common presentation. Warmth and erythema may be present. When they are present, the differential diagnosis includes gout, pseudogout, osteomyelitis, or septic arthritis. Typically, there are few systemic symptoms and no documented fever and leukocytosis. Radiographically, there are destructive changes of the tarsometatarsal and metatarsophalangeal joints. Involvement of the tarsal and proximal metatarsal bones may occur and lead to osteoporosis, osteolysis, and bone fragmentation.

Patients with diabetic peripheral sensory neuropathy have a loss of pain and proprioceptive sensations distally. This loss of the normal afferent signals reduces the protection of the joint from microtrauma, which may result in progressive joint destruction.[2,3] In addition, ischemia secondary to both large and small vessel disease may play an etiologic role. Whitehouse and Wechstein[62] have suggested that this osteopathy represents a healing phase of local osteomyelitis.

Management of diabetic neuroarthropathy is difficult. Lumbar sympathectomy, arthrodesis, immobilization, and special footwear have been of little value. Minimizing trauma, maintenance of good muscle strength, use of appropriate shoes, and regular inspection of the skin and nails to avoid secondary infection may be helpful. Splinting may exacerbate the problem and may lead to skin ulceration, perforation, and secondary osteomyelitis.

Spinal neuroarthropathy characterized by usually symmetric extensive new bone formation (hyperostosis) also occurs. The vertebral changes include sclerosis and altered bony trabeculae. These changes result in an inability of the vertebrae to withstand normal stresses, with resultant collapse. Typically, local pain and tenderness may occur in association with irritation of the nerve root.

Although not a true neuroarthropathy, the carpal tunnel syndrome (CTS) is a frequent cause of hand pain in diabetic patients. Entrapment of the median nerve within the carpal tunnel results in hand pain and numbness in the second to fourth fingers, particularly at night. Diabetes mellitus is one of the systemic diseases most frequently associated with CTS. In one study, diabetes was present in 16.6% of patients with CTS.[3] Other sensory peripheral neuropathies, such as ulnar neuropathy, may coexist with CTS and may be associated with the diabetic hand syndrome discussed above. Therapy for CTS includes the use of NSAIDs and splinting. If these are ineffective, local glucocorticoid injection or surgical release of the retinaculum may be indicated.

HYPEROSTOSIS

Although patients with Type I diabetes have a tendency to develop osteopenia[63] (see below), patients with Type II diabetes seem to make more bone or to develop hyperostosis. In one study of 428 diabetic patients, 25% had hyperostosis of different areas, including spine involvement, hyperostosis frontalis interna, calcification of the pelvic ligaments, and osteitis condensans ilii.[3] New bone formation has also been noted around the hips, knees, and wrists.[2,3,64] In Morgagni syndrome, hyperostosis frontalis interna is accompanied by Type II diabetes.[3]

The most common form of new bone formation in diabetes is disseminated idiopathic skeletal hyperostosis (DISH) or ankylosing hyperostosis of the spine. This syndrome occurs in 2 to 4% of the normal population over the age of 40; in contrast, the prevalence is 13% in patients with diabetes.[65,66] In patients with diabetes between the ages of 60 and 69, the prevalence increases to more than 20%.[66] The presence of DISH is also associated with obesity, independent of diabetes. No correlation has been found between the degree of diabetic control and the extent of the hyperostosis.

Typically, a patient with DISH may complain of some mild back pain and stiffness, but range of motion is preserved. Occasionally, the abnormality may be an incidental radiographic finding. Sparing of the posterior spinal joints probably accounts for the preservation of good back motion.[67] The syndrome is characterized by asymmetric osteophytes or bony outgrowths that extend vertically along the anterolateral surface of the vertebral bodies, particularly on the right. Anterior bridges between vertebrae and sclerosis of the underlying bony cortex are seen. Unlike patients with ankylosing spondylitis, these patients rarely complain of early morning stiffness and loss of back motion. In addition, the sacroiliac joints are spared. Radiographically, the vertebral body osteoporosis seen in ankylosing spondylitis is absent. Although early reports suggested an association between DISH and the histocompatibility antigen HLA-B27, this has not been confirmed.[2,68,69] The thoracic spine is most commonly involved in DISH, followed by the cervical spine and the lumbar spine. If extensive involvement of the anterior cervical spine occurs, it may result in dysphagia and disturbance of esophageal function.

In addition to the spinal involvement of DISH, widespread osseous changes may be detected elsewhere. These changes are most common around the acetabulum, where formation of fluffy new bone occurs, but similar changes around the knees and wrists have been documented. In addition, some of the changes in the spine can be internal within the canal as well as external. Changes have been noted around the apophyseal joints; these changes may impinge on emerging nerve roots, while the intervertebral discs may be relatively normal. Thus, there may be symptoms of radicular irritation as well as mild localized pain. Degenerative arthritis of the hips has frequently been noted. However, this is a common occurrence in this particular age group with or without DISH. It is unclear whether a progressive degenerative disease of the hip is a unique phenomenon in this syndrome or is just an associated clinical event.

The explanation for the association of diabetes and new bone formation is unclear. Levels of growth hormone are normal in these patients. An abnormal or exaggerated serum insulin response to glucose challenge has been documented in some patients with ankylosing hyperostosis without diabetes.[70,71] It is probable that insulin and/or insulin-like growth factors may be important in promoting new bone formation in patients with adult-onset diabetes, obesity, or both of these disorders.

COMMON RHEUMATIC DISEASES ASSOCIATED WITH DIABETES MELLITUS

Osteoarthritis

Osteoarthritis, or degenerative joint disease, is the most common rheumatic disease in the general population. It may be asymptomatic or mild, but severe involvement leading to pain, stiffness, and limitation of motion in the hips, knees, spine, and, less commonly, other joints may be a source of major disability and morbidity. It is difficult to establish a relationship between common diseases such as osteoarthritis and diabetes, but several studies have documented a positive correlation.[3] Several investigators have suggested that the prevalence of osteoarthritis is higher in young and middle-aged diabetic patients and that joint damage starts at an earlier age and is much more severe in diabetic than in control patients.[3]

Insulin has been demonstrated to stimulate cartilage growth and proteoglycan biosynthesis. These effects are likely mediated through somatomedin (insulin-like growth factor 1).[72-79] Although insulin may alter the extracellular matrix present in bone and cartilage, the significance of such changes, particularly as a cause of osteoarthritis, has not been determined. Treatment of osteoarthritis is directed toward the control of pain with acetaminophen or NSAIDs as well as physical therapy-guided exercise programs for the strengthening of muscles and tendons.

Gout and Hyperuricemia

Gout is a heterogeneous disorder characterized by hyperuricemia and arthritis induced by the accumulation of urate crystals. Acute gouty arthritis is characterized by severe joint pain, redness, warmth, and tenderness usually affecting a lower-extremity joint. Gout is a recognized but relatively uncommon complication of diabetic ketoacidosis.[3] Diabetic patients who have uncontrolled glucose metabolism associated with ketoacidosis will develop hyperuricemia as a result of competitive inhibition of tubular excretion of urate in the kidney by organic acids. Dehydration and increased protein catabolism also play a role.

There is also a possible correlation between chronically stable diabetes and onset of gout symptoms.[80,81] Previous studies have demonstrated an increased incidence of hyperuricemia in individuals with stable diabetes and of hyperglycemia in patients with gout. It is likely that a significant proportion of this latter group are patients with gout who are obese with relative states of insulin resistance leading to abnormal glucose tolerance. In addition, many of these studies did not make age-correlations. It is now known that glucose tolerance decreases with age. Thus, age may be a link between gout and diabetes. Unfortunately, no prospective studies with age-, sex-, and weight-matched controls have been performed, but it appears that the risk of gout in non-obese diabetic patients is no greater than that in the normal population.[3] Paradoxically, the new onset of frank diabetes has been accompanied by a decrease in serum urate levels and a reduction in the frequency and severity of attacks in patients with preexisting gout.[3,82] In general, obesity may be the most important factor linking hyperglycemia with hyperuricemia, as obesity is known to precipitate hyperglycemia, hyperuricemia, and hyperlipidemia.[83,84]

Acute gouty attacks may be treated with indomethacin, other NSAIDs, or colchicine. Long-term prophylaxis with allopurinol or a uricosuric agent may be necessary in some clinical settings.

Calcium Pyrophosphate Deposition Disease

Pseudogout is an inflammatory arthritis caused by the deposition of calcium pyrophosphate dihydrate crystals in synovial structures. It may present as an acute monoarticular arthritis, a chronic polyarticular inflammatory arthritis, or as asymptomatic chondrocalcinosis, defined as linear deposition of calcium pyrophosphate crystals in cartilage, which appear calcified on plain radiographs. Calcium pyrophosphate deposition disease (CPDD) arthropathy is suggested by the radiologic finding of chondrocalcinosis in a patient with acute or chronic inflammatory arthritis and the identification by polarizing light microscopy of weakly positive birefringent rhomboid-shaped crystals in synovial fluid. Acute inflammatory arthritis secondary to CPDD, or pseudogout, without radiographic evidence of chondrocalcinosis has been reported, particularly in the small joints.[2]

In 1962 McCarty et al. demonstrated the apparent clinical association of CPDD arthropathy with diabetes. However, this observation has not been confirmed.[86] Alexander et al. were unable to document the association in 105 consecutive patients with CPDD arthropathy.[86] The incidence of CPDD arthropathy in diabetic patients has been reported to range between 8 and 73%,[3] compared with an incidence of 0.2% in the normal population.[87] This discrepancy must be attributable to variations in the diagnostic criteria used in the studies as well as to intervening variables such as age and osteoarthritis.

It is possible that the simultaneous occurrence of CPDD arthropathy and diabetes may represent no more than the chance association of two relatively common abnormalities in elderly patients. Alternatively, it is also possible that diabetic patients with chondrocalcinosis may be more susceptible than diabetic patients to symptomatic articular disease such as pseudogout. Certainly, an elderly patient presenting with CPDD arthropathy should be tested for subclinical diabetes. The corollary is true as well; pseudogout should be considered in each diabetic patient who presents with articular symptoms.

Symptomatic CPDD arthropathy may be managed with systemic anti-inflammatory drugs such as NSAIDs, colchicine, or prednisone. Aspiration of the affected joints alone and/or the intra-articular injection of glucocorticoids may also be effective. McCarty et al. suggested that control of hyperglycemia in diabetic patients did not appear to influence the frequency or severity of recurrent attacks of CPDD arthropathy.[85,87]

OSTEOPENIA

There is controversy about the incidence of osteopenia and osteoporosis in patients with diabetes. Several studies support the relationship between insulin-dependent diabetes (IDDM) and reduced bone mass.[88–93] In children, objective measurements of forearm bone mineral density reveal an 8% reduction in cortical bone density and a 14% reduction in trabecular bone density in patients with diabetes compared with these values in age- and sex-matched controls.[89] A similar reduction in bone mass occurs in adults.[91] The decrease in bone density is detectable early in the disease.[89] In adults, the rate of bone loss is maximal at or soon after diagnosis of diabetes and is correlated with the serum level of endogenous insulin.[94] As insulin levels fall, the incidence of osteopenia increases. However, the relationship between the degree of metabolic control in patients with IDDM and the degree of osteopenia has not been well documented. In patients with non-insulin-dependent diabetes (NIDDM), results of forearm bone density studies are conflicting.[88,95–97] As discussed previously, hyperostosis, not osteopenia, may occur in this patient population.

Although patients with diabetes may have osteopenia, the evidence regarding the consequences of this osteopenia is confusing. The incidence of diabetes among patients with femoral neck fractures appears to be greater than expected by chance, the relative risk values reported being 1.16 to 3.4.[98-102] However, there is no good evidence about the incidence of vertebral compression fractures in patients with diabetes.[103]

The role of insulin in normal bone turnover remains a puzzle. Insulin is an anabolic hormone, and the effects of insulin and insulin-like growth factors have been well documented.[104-111] Insulin stimulates nucleotide synthesis by osteoblasts *in vitro*, promotes the intracellular accumulation of amino acids in membranous bone, and can restore levels of circulating somatomedin in experimental diabetes.[107-109] Insulin-like growth factors have also been shown to promote synthesis of bone collagen[104,105,108,110] and to increase the deposition of calcium in the skeleton.[106,111] These findings suggest that when circulating insulin levels are decreased, the synthesis of a good bone matrix will be inadequate and the bone will not calcify. It is possible that in NIDDM, with its insulin resistance, hyperinsulinemia will stimulate bony overgrowth. This suggestion is supported by recent data demonstrating that bone mineral density is increased, not decreased, in patients with NIDDM who have increased levels of endogenous insulin but decreased sensitivity to insulin.[112]

OSTEOLYSIS OF FOREFOOT

A distinct clinical syndrome has been described in patients with diabetes that is characterized by patchy or generalized osteoporosis of the distal metatarsal and proximal phalanges in association with variable amounts of pain and erythema.[3,113-115] Because of the appearance of the forefoot, both cellulitis and osteomyelitis need to be considered in the differential diagnosis and excluded by laboratory, radiographic, and microbiologic data. Diabetic patients with this syndrome do not necessarily have small-vessel vascular disease or neuropathy. Osteopenia may be accompanied by juxta-articular erosions mimicking rheumatoid arthritis or gout.[113,114] Articular surfaces are initially spared, but progressive osteolysis may cause disappearance of adjacent bone. At any stage during this process, the syndrome may resolve spontaneously and normal bony architecture may be partially or completely restored. The cause of this condition is unknown. Severe disease with osteoporosis and subsequent fracture or fragmentation of the bone may be confused with neuropathic joint disease. Because the syndrome resolves spontaneously, no specific treatment is recommended.

MIGRATORY OSTEOLYSIS OF HIP AND KNEE

The syndrome of migratory osteolysis of the hip and knee is characterized by local areas of decreased bone density or osteopenia associated with significant local pain. The pain may last for up to 1 year and usually resolves without sequelae. Typically, the patient is a woman over 50 years of age who presents with severe pain involving initially one joint in the lower extremity. The painful joint is usually a large weight-bearing joint, but any joint can be affected. The pain is out of proportion to the physical findings. There are few signs of inflammation, although an effusion may be present. However, the joint fluid is usually not inflammatory when aspirated. There may be a recent history of pain similar in type that may have affected a different joint in the lower extremity and resolved spontaneously.

Blood tests are usually not helpful. Radiographs of the joint may reveal a small localized area of osteopenia, but the bone scan will show significantly increased uptake over the affected area.

The etiology of this syndrome remains obscure. In a study of 34 patients with involvement of the hip, five were diabetic and all had an exaggerated serum triglyceride response following alcohol ingestion.[3] Doury et al.[7] made an association between diabetes and migratory osteolysis of the knee; however, both of these syndromes are typically seen in patients older than 50 years, the age at which the incidence of Type II diabetes increases. Patients are typically remarkably sensitive to low-dose glucocorticoid treatment, which may exacerbate the insulin resistance and thus worsen the diabetes. In Europe the use of calcitonin has gained popularity. However, because calcitonin induces a decrease in the output of endogenous insulin in vitro, this therapy should be used with caution.[3]

REFERENCES

1. Gray RG, Gottlieb NL. Rheumatic disorders associated with diabetes mellitus: literature review. Sem Arthritis Rheum 1976;6:19–34.
2. Holt PJL. Rheumatological manifestations of diabetes mellitus. Clin Rheum Dis 1981;7:723–46.
3. Crisp AJ, Heathcoate JG. Connective tissue abnormalities in diabetes mellitus. J R Coll Physicians 1984;18:132–41.
4. Bruckner FE. Frozen shoulder (adhesive capsulitis) [Editorial]. J R Soc Med 1982;75:688–9.
5. Stodell MA, Nicholson R, Scott J, Sturrock RD. Radioisotope scanning in the painful shoulder. Rheumatol Rehabil 1980;19:163–6.
6. Bridgman JF. Periarthritis of the shoulder and diabetes mellitus. Ann Rheum Dis 1972;31:69–71.
7. Doury P, Dirheimer Y, Pattin S. Algodystrophy: diagnosis and therapy of a frequent disease of the locomotor apparatus. Berlin: Springer-Verlag, 1981.
8. Steinbrocker O. The shoulder-hand syndrome: associated painful homolateral disability of the shoulder and hand with swelling and atrophy of the hand. Am J Med 1947;3:402–7.
9. Steinbrocker O, Argyros TG. The shoulder-hand syndrome: present status as a diagnostic and therapeutic entity. Med Clin North Am 1958;42:1533–53.
10. Jung Y, Hohmann TC, Gerneth JA, et al. Diabetic hand syndrome. Metabolism 1971;20:1008–15.
11. Grgic A, Rosenbloom AL, Weber FT, et al. Joint contractures—common manifestation of childhood diabetes mellitus. J Pediatr 1976;88:584–88.
12. Kapoor A, Sibbitt WL Jr. Contractures in diabetes mellitus: the syndrome of limited joint mobility. Sem Arthritis Rheum 1989;18:168–80.
13. Lundbaek K. Stiff hands in long-term diabetes. Acta Med Scand 1957;158:447–51.

14. Pastan RS, Cohen AS. The rheumatologic manifestation of diabetes mellitus. Med Clin North Am 1978;62:829–39.

15. Campbell RR, Hawkins SJ, Maddison PJ, Reckless JPD. Limited joint mobility in diabetes mellitus. Ann Rheum Dis 1985;44:93–7.

16. Slama G, Letanoux M, Thibult N, et al. Quantification of early subclinical limited joint mobility in diabetes mellitus. Diabetes Care 1985;8:329–32.

17. Eaton RP. The collagen hydration hypothesis: a new paradigm for the secondary complications of diabetes mellitus. J Chronic Dis 1986;39:763–6.

18. Schuyler MR, Niewoehner DE, Inkley SP, Kohn R. Abnormal lung elasticity in juvenile diabetes. Am Rev Respir Dis 1976;113:37–41.

19. Eversmeyer WH. Digital sclerosis in adult insulin-dependent diabetes [Letter]. Arthritis Rheum 1983;26:932.

20. Rosenbloom AL, Silverstein JH, Riley WJ, Maclaren NK. Limited joint mobility in childhood diabetes: family studies. Diabetes Care 1983;6:370–3.

21. Rosenbloom AL. Skeletal and joint manifestations of childhood diabetes. Pediatr Clin North Am 1984;31:569–86.

22. Buckingham BA, Uitto J, Sandborg C, et al. Scleroderma-like changes in insulin-dependent diabetes mellitus: clinical and biochemical studies. Diabetes Care 1984;7:163–9.

23. Buckingham B, Perejda AJ, Sandborg C, et al. Skin, joint and pulmonary changes in Type I diabetes mellitus. Am J Dis Child 1986;140:420–3.

24. Schnapf BM, Banks RA, Silverstein JH, et al. Pulmonary function in insulin-dependent diabetes mellitus with limited joint mobility. Am Rev Respir Dis 1984;130:930–2.

25. Larkin JG, Frier BM. Limited joint mobility and Dupuytren's contracture in diabetic, hypertensive, and normal populations. BMJ 1986;292:1494.

26. Traisman HS, Traisman ES, Marr TJ, Wise J. Joint contractures in patients with juvenile diabetes and their siblings. Diabetes Care 1978;1:360–1.

27. Rosenbloom AL, Silverstein JH, Lezotte DC, et al. Limited joint mobility in childhood diabetes mellitus indicates increased risk for microvascular disease. N Engl J Med 1981;305:191–4.

28. Seibold JP. Digital sclerosis in children with insulin dependent diabetes mellitus. Arthritis Rheum 1982;25:1357–61.

29. Starkman H, Brink S. Limited joint mobility of the hand in Type I diabetes mellitus. Diabetes Care 1982;5:534–6.

30. Lawson PM, Maneschi F, Kohner EM. The relationship of hand abnormalities to diabetes and diabetic retinopathy. Diabetes Care 1983;6:140–3.

31. Rosenbloom AL, Silverstein JH, Lezotte DC, et al. Limited joint mobility in diabetes mellitus of childhood: natural history and relationship to growth impairment. J Pediatr 1982;101:874–8.

32. Fitzcharles MA, Duby S, Waddell RW, et al. Limitation of joint mobility (cheiroarthropathy) in adult noninsulin-dependent diabetic patients. Ann Rheum Dis 1984;43:251–7.

33. Starkman HS, Gleason RE, Rand LI, et al. Limited joint mobility (LJM) of the hand in patients with diabetes mellitus: relation to chronic complications. Ann Rheum Dis 1986;45:130–5.

34. Robertson JR, Earnshaw PM, Campbell IW. Tenolysis in juvenile diabetic cheiroarthropathy. BMJ 1979;2:971–2.

35. Sherry DD, Rothstein RRL, Petty RE. Joint contractures preceding insulin-dependent diabetes mellitus. Arthritis Rheum 1982;11:1362–4.

36. Harris ED Jr, Farrell ME. Resistance to collagenase: a characteristic of collagen fibrils cross-linked by formaldehyde. Biochim Biophys Acta 1972;278:133–41.

37. Vater CA, Harris ED Jr, Siegel RC. Native cross-links in collagen fibrils induce resistance to human synovial collagenase. Biochem J 1979;181:639–45.

38. Chang K, Uitto J, Rowold EA, et al. Increased collagen cross-linkages in experimental diabetes: reversal by β-aminopropionitrile and D-penicillamine. Diabetes 1980;29:778–81.

39. Berenson GS, Radhakrishnamurthy B, Dalferes ER Jr, et al. Connective tissue macromolecular changes in rats with experimentally induced diabetes and hyperinsulinism. Diabetes 1972;21:733–43.

40. Sharma C, Dalferes ER Jr, Radhakrishnamurthy B, et al. Glycoprotein biosynthesis during inflammation in normal and streptozotocin-induced diabetic rats. Inflammation 1985;9:273–83.

41. Tenni R, Tavella D, Donnelly P, et al. Cultured fibroblasts of juvenile diabetics have excessively soluble pericellular collagen. Biochem Biophys Res Comm 1980;92:1071–5.

42. Rosenberg H, Modrak JB, Hassing JM, et al. Glycosylated collagen. Biochem Biophys Res Comm 1979;91:498–501.

43. Schnider SL, Kohn RR. Glucosylation of human collagen in aging and diabetes mellitus. J Clin Invest 1980;66:1179–81.

44. Schnider SL, Kohn RR. Effects of age and diabetes mellitus on the solubility and nonenzymatic glycosylation of human skin collagen. J Clin Invest 1981;67:1630–5.

45. Perejda AJ, Uitto J. Nonenzymatic glycosylation of collagen and other proteins: relationship to development of diabetic complications. Coll Relat Res 1982;2:81–8.

46. Lieberman LS, Rosenbloom AL, Riley WJ, Silverstein JH. Reduced skin thickness with pump administration of insulin [Letter]. N Engl J Med 1980;303:940–1.

47. Eaton RP, Sibbitt WL Jr, Harsh A. The effect of an aldose reductase inhibiting agent on limited joint mobility in diabetic patients. JAMA 1985;253:1437–40.

48. Mikkelsen OA. The prevalence of Dupuytren's disease in Norway: a study in a representative population sample of the municipality of Haugesund. Acta Chir Scand 1972;138:695–700.

49. Davies JS, Finesilver EM. Dupuytren's contracture—with a note on the incidence of the contracture in diabetes. Arthritis Surg 1932;24:933–89.

50. Noble J, Heathcote JG, Cohen H. Diabetes mellitus in the aetiology of Dupuytren's disease. J Bone Joint Surg [Br] 1984;66B:322–5.

51. Gabbiani G, Majno G. Dupuytren's contracture: fibroblast contraction? An ultrastructural study. Am J Pathol 1972;66:131–46.

52. Gabbiani G, Majno G, Ryan GB. The fibroblast as a contractile cell: the myo-fibroblast. In: Kulonen E, Pik-karainen J, eds. Biology of fibroblast. New York: Academic Press, 1973:139–54.

53. Luck JV. Dupuytren's contracture: a new concept of the pathogenesis correlated with surgical management. J Bone Joint Surg 1959;41A:635–64.

54. Somers KD, Dawson DM, Wright GL Jr, et al. Cell culture of Peyronie's disease plaque and normal penile tissue. J Urol 1982;127:585–8.

55. Revach M, Cabilli C. Dupuytren's contracture and diabetes mellitus. Isr J Med Sci 1972;8:774–5.

56. Spring M, Fleck H, Cohen BD. Dupuytren's contracture: warning of diabetes? N Y State J Med 1970;70:1037–41.

57. Ravid M, Dinai Y, Sohar E. Dupuytren's disease in diabetes mellitus. Acta Diabetol Lat 1977;14:170–4.

58. Bazin S, Le-Lous M, Duance VC, et al. Biochemistry and histology of the connective tissue of Dupuytren's disease lesions. Eur J Clin Invest 1980;10:9–16.

59. Brickley-Parsons D, Glimcher MJ, Smith RJ, et al. Biochemical changes in the collagen of the palmar fascia in patients with Dupuytren's disease. J Bone Joint Surg [Am] 1981; 63A:787–97.

60. Ehrlich HP, Brown H, White BS. Evidence for type V and I trimer collagens in Dupuytren's contracture palmar fascia. Biochem Med 1982;28:273–84.

61. Aumailley M, Krieg T, Razaka G, et al. Influence of cell density on collagen biosynthesis in fibroblast cultures. Biochem J 1982;206:505–10.

62. Whitehouse FW, Wechstein M. On diabetic osteopathy: a radiographic study of 21 patients. Diabetes Care 1978;1: 303–4.

63. Forgács S, Rosinger A, Vertes L. Diabetes mellitus and osteoporosis. Endokrinologie 1976;67:343–50.

64. Teotia SPS, Teotia M, Singh RK, Teotia NP. Hyperostosis and diabetes mellitus. J Indian Med Assoc 1978;71:117–8.

65. Julkunen H, Heinonen OP, Knekt P, Maatela J. The epidemiology of hyperostosis of the spine together with its symptoms and related mortality in a general population. J Scand Rheumatol 1975;4:23–7.

66. Julkunen H, Kärävä R, Viljanen V. Hyperostosis of the spine in diabetes mellitus and acromegaly. Diabetologia 1966;2: 123–6.

67. Vernon-Roberts B, Pirie CJ, Trenwith V. Pathology of the dorsal spine in ankylosing hyperostosis. Ann Rheum Dis 1974;33:281–8.

68. Forgács S, Halmos T, Salamon F. Bone changes in diabetes mellitus. Isr J Med Sci 1972;8:782–3.

69. Resnick D, Shapiro RF, Wiesner KE, et al. Diffuse idiopathic skeletal hyperostosis (DISH). Semin Arthritis Rheum 1978;7:153–87.

70. Julkunen H, Heinonen OP, Pyörälä K. Hyperostosis of the spine in an adult population: its relation to hyperglycaemia and obesity. Ann Rheum Dis 1971;30:605–12.

71. Littlejohn GO, Smythe HA. Marked hyperinsulinemia after glucose challenge in patients with diffuse idiopathic skeletal hyperostosis. J Rheumatol 1981;8:965–8.

72. Phillips LS, Young HS. Nutrition and somatomedin. II. Serum somatomedin activity and cartilage growth activity in streptozotocin-diabetic rats. Diabetes 1976;25: 516–27.

73. Weiss RE, Reddi AH. Influence of experimental diabetes and insulin on matrix-induced cartilage and bone differentiation. Am J Physiol 1980;238:E200–7.

74. Weiss RE, Gorn AH, Nimni ME. Abnormalities in the biosynthesis of cartilage and bone proteoglycans in experimental diabetes. Diabetes 1981;30:670–7.

75. Axelsson I, Lorentzon R, Pita JC. Biosynthesis of rat growth plate proteoglycans in diabetes and malnutrition. Calcif Tissue Int 1983;35:237–42.

76. Caterson B, Baker JR, Christner JE, et al. Diabetes and osteoarthritis. Ala J Med Sci 1980;17:292–9.

77. Stuart CA, Furlanetto RW, Lebovitz HE. The insulin receptor of embryonic chicken cartilage. Endocrinology 1979;105:1293–302.

78. Foley TP Jr, Nissley SP, Stevens RL, et al. Demonstration of receptors for insulin and insulin-like growth factors on swarm rat chondrosarcoma chondrocytes: evidence that insulin stimulates proteoglycan synthesis through the insulin receptor; J Biol Chem 1982;257:633–9.

79. Axelsson I, Pita JC, Howell DS, et al. Kinetics of proteoglycans and cells in growth plate of normal, diabetic, and malnourished rats. Pediatr Res 1990;27:41–4.

80. Whitehouse FW, Cleary WJ Jr. Diabetes mellitus in patients with gout. JAMA 1966;197:73–6.

81. Boyle JA, McKiddie M, Buchanan KD, et al. Diabetes mellitus and gout: blood sugar and plasma insulin responses to oral glucose in normal weight, overweight, and gouty patients. Ann Rheum Dis 1969;28:374–8.

82. Herman JB, Goldbourt U. Uric acid and diabetes: observations in a population study. Lancet 1982;2:240–5.

83. Yano K, Rhoads GG, Kagan A. Epidemiology of serum uric acid among 8000 Japanese-American men in Hawaii. J Chronic Dis 1977;30:171–84.

84. Berkowitz D. Gout, hyperlipidemia, and diabetes interrelationships. JAMA;1966:197:77–80.

85. McCarty DJ, Silcox DC, Coe F, et al. Diseases associated with calcium pyrophosphate dihydrate crystal deposition: a controlled study. Am J Med 1974;56:704–14.

86. Alexander GM, Dieppe PA, Doherty M, Scott DG. Pyrophosphate arthropathy: a study of metabolic associations and laboratory data. Ann Rheum Dis 1982;41:377–81.

87. McCarty DJ, Silcox DC. Gout and pseudogout. Geriatrics 1973;28(June):110–20.

88. Levin ME, Boisseau VC, Avioli LV. Effects of diabetes mellitus on bone mass in juvenile and adult onset diabetes. N Engl J Med 1976;294:241–5.

89. Shore RM, Chesney RW, Mazess RB, et al. Osteopenia in juvenile diabetes. Calcif Tissue Int 1981;33:455–7.

90. Rosenbloom AL, Lezotte DC, Weber FT, et al. Diminution of bone mass in childhood diabetes. Diabetes 1977;26: 1052–5.

91. McNair P, Madsbad S, Christiansen C, et al. Osteopenia in insulin treated diabetes mellitus: its relation to age at onset, sex, and duration of disease. Diabetologia 1978; 15:87–9.

92. Wiske PS, Wentworth SM, Norton JA Jr, et al. Evaluation of bone mass and growth in young diabetics. Metabolism 1982;31:848–54.

93. Selby PL. Osteopenia and diabetes. Diabetic Med 1988; 5:423–8.

94. McNair P, Christiansen C, Christensen MS, et al. Development of bone mineral loss in insulin-treated diabetes: a 1½ years follow-up study in sixty patients. Eur J Clin Invest 1981;11:55–9.

95. Meema HE, Meema S. The relationship of diabetes mellitus and body weight to osteoporosis in elderly females. Can Med Assoc J 1967;96:132–9.

96. DeLeeuw I, Abs R. Bone mass and bone density in maturity-type diabetics measured by the ^{125}I photon-absorption technique. Diabetes 1977;26:1130–5.

97. Ishida H, Seino Y, Matsukura Y, et al. Diabetic osteopenia and circulating levels of vitamin D metabolites in Type 2 (noninsulin-dependent) diabetes. Metabolism 1985;34: 797–801.

98. Paganini-Hill A, Ross RK, Gerkins VR, et al. Menopausal estrogen therapy and hip fractures. Ann Intern Med 1981; 95:28–31.

99. Gallagher JC, Melton LJ, Riggs BL. Examination of prevalence rates of possible risk factors in a population with a fracture of the proximal femur. Clin Orthop 1980;153: 158–65.

100. Hutchinson TA, Polansky SM, Feinstein AR. Post-menopausal oestrogens protect against fractures of hip and distal radius: a case-control study. Lancet 1979;2: 705–9.

101. Menczel J, Makin M, Robin G, et al. Prevalence of diabetes mellitus in Jerusalem: its association with presenile osteoporosis. Isr J Med Sci 1972;8:918–9.

102. Alffram P-A. An epidemiologic study of cervical and

trochanteric fractures of the femur in an urban population. Acta Orthop Scand Suppl 1964;65:9–109.

103. Nabarro JDN. Compression fractures of the dorsal spine in hypoglycaemic fits in diabetes. BMJ 1985;291:1320.

104. Canalis E. The hormonal and local regulation of bone formation. Endocrinol Rev 1983;4:62–77.

105. Raisz LG, Kream BE. Regulation of bone formation. N Engl J Med 1983;309:29–35,83–9.

106. Locatto ME, Fernández MC, Abranzón H, et al. Calcium metabolism of rats with varying degrees of insulinopenia. Bone Miner 1990;8:119–30.

107. Puche RC, Romano MC, Locatto ME, Ferretti JL. The effect of insulin on bone resorption. Calcif Tissue Res 1973; 12:8–15.

108. Hahn TJ, Downing SJ, Phang JM. Insulin effects on amino acid transport in bone: dependence on protein synthesis and Na$^+$. Am J Physiol 1971;220:1717–23.

109. Phillips LS, Orawski AT. Nutrition and somatomedin. III. Diabetic control, somatomedin, and growth in rats. Diabetes 1977;26:864–9.

110. Canalis E. Effect of hormones and growth factors on alkaline phosphatase activity and collagen synthesis in cultured rat calvariae. Metabolism 1983;32:14–20.

111. Dixit PK, Stern AMK. Effect of insulin on the incorporation of citrate and calcium into the bones of alloxan-diabetic rats. Calcif Tissue Int 1979;27:227–32.

112. Weinstock RS, Goland RS, Shane E, et al. Bone mineral density in women with Type II diabetes mellitus. J Bone Miner Res 1989;4:97–101.

113. Schwarz GS, Berenyi MR, Siegel MW. Atrophic arthropathy and diabetic neuritis. Am J Roentgenol 1969;106:523–9.

114. Clouse ME, Gramm HF, Legg M, Flood T. Diabetic osteoarthropathy: clinical and roentgenographic observations in 90 cases. J Am Roentgenol 1974;121:22–34.

115. Lithner F, Hietala S-O, Steen L. Skeletal lesions and arterial calcifications of the feet in diabetics. Acta Med Scand Suppl 1984;687:47–54.

Chapter 51

EFFECTS OF DIABETES MELLITUS ON THE DIGESTIVE SYSTEM

ROGER J. MAY

RAJ K. GOYAL

All parts of the digestive system are affected by diabetic mellitus, and digestive system dysfunctions are important contributors to the morbidity of this disease.[1-5] Symptoms related to diabetic involvement of the gut are common but frequently are not severe. Feldman and Schiller questioned 136 unselected patients at a hospital diabetes clinic about the presence of gastrointestinal symptoms. Three-fourths of all patients had digestive symptoms.[3] Frequent gastrointestinal symptoms were constipation (60%), abdominal pain (34%), nausea and vomiting (29%), diarrhea (22%), and fecal incontinence (20%). The true prevalence of diabetic involvement of the gut is probably even greater since asymptomatic abnormalities of gut function frequently occur in these patients.

PATHOGENESIS OF DIGESTIVE SYSTEM DYSFUNCTION

The digestive system dysfunction in diabetes may result from diabetes per se or, more often, from complications associated with diabetes mellitus. Diabetic neuropathy plays an important role in motor and secretory abnormalities in the gastrointestinal tract, in nausea and vomiting, and in the syndrome of abdominal pain. Diabetic angiopathy and vascular complications are important in the pathogenesis of intestinal ischemia as well as in the severity and outcome of cholecystitis and biliary tract surgery. Defects in immune mechanisms in diabetes are related to an increased incidence of esophageal candidiasis, and decreased resistance to infection accounts for the many pyogenic complications in the digestive tracts of these patients. Hormonal abnormalities play important roles in pathogenesis of exocrine pancreatic insufficiency in diabetes. Moreover, some of the digestive system abnormalities in diabetes may not be causally related to diabetes but may reflect a common association of diabetes with these abnormalities; the increased incidence of gallstones and fatty liver are due to associated obesity and hyperlipidemia in patients with Type II diabetes, and the incidence of celiac disease is increased in diabetes because of a common gene that predisposes to both the conditions.

ENTERIC NEUROPATHY IN DIABETES

The gastrointestinal tract is richly innervated by nerves, which can be divided into intrinsic and extrinsic nerves.[6,7] The intrinsic nerves constitute the enteric nerve system (ENS). The extrinsic nerves contain sensory (afferent) and motor (efferent) fibers and are carried along sympathetic, parasympathetic, and somatic pathways to the central nervous system (CNS) (Fig. 51–1). In diabetes mellitus, any one or several of the various components of the nerve elements that control the gut function may be involved. Diabetic enteric neuropathy is responsible for many of the gastrointestinal abnormalities in these patients. The wide spectrum of possible enteric neuropathies may explain the wide range of gastrointestinal dysfunction in the diabetic patient.

Parasympathetic Innervation

The vagal efferents provide parasympathetic innervation to the entire gut down to the right half of the transverse colon. The left half of the colon and the rectum are innervated by sacral parasympathetic efferents. Parasympathetic efferents are thinly myelinated or unmyelinated fine axons. They are preganglion cholinergic fibers that terminate on enteric neurons. The parasympathetic influence on the gut includes precise and localized motor and secretory control activity. Separate parasympathetic fibers may control inhibitory and excitory neurons in the enteric plexus. Parasympathetic influence is most dominant in the most proximal regions of the gut (esophagus and stomach) and in the most distal regions (distal colon, rectum, and anal canal), providing these regions with prominent dual control by the CNS as well as the ENS. In the middle regions of the gut (small bowel), control by the ENS dominates, with extrinsic parasympathetic efferents playing a minor role. The parasympathetic afferents mediate a large variety of reflex activity, including nausea, vomiting, and satiety. They do not seem to be

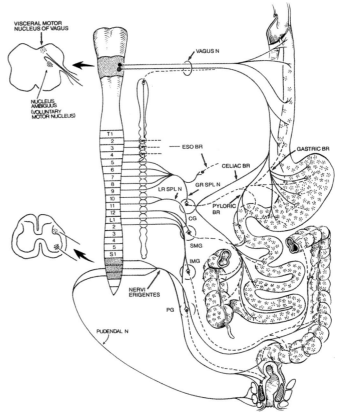

Fig. 51–1. Efferent innervation of the gastrointestinal tract. The α motor neurons are shown in black. They innervate skeletal muscle at either end of the gut. The α motor neurons to the pharynx and upper esophagus are present in the nucleus ambiguous, and their axons are carried in the vagus nerve. The α motor neurons to the external anal sphincter are present in Onuf's nucleus, and their axons are carried in the pudendal nerve. The sympathetic pathway, shown in blue, consists of cell bodies of preganglionic neurons located in spinal-cord segments T2 through L2. The preganglionic fibers, shown in solid blue lines, are carried in the greater splanchnic nerve (GR SPL N), lesser splanchnic nerve (LR SPL N), and smallest splanchnic nerve (not labeled) to terminate in the celiac ganglion (CG), superior mesenteric ganglion (SMG), inferior mesenteric ganglion (IMG), and pelvic ganglion (PG). The postganglionic sympathetic neurons, shown in broken blue lines, are distributed in a segmental fashion to the gastrointestinal tract. The parasympathetic pathway, shown in green, consists of vagal and sacral outflows. The vagal pathway, shown in solid green lines, consists of preganglionic parasympathetic axons whose cell bodies are present in the dorsal motor nucleus of vagus. The vagal parasympathetic fibers supply the gastrointestinal tract up to the right half of the colon. Sacral preganglionic parasympathetic fibers arising from neurons in spinal cord segments S2 to S4 (nervi erigentes) supply the left half of the colon, including the rectum and the internal anal sphincter. The postganglionic parasympathetic nerves and fibers, shown in green broken lines, are present intramurally in the gut wall. The enteric nervous system is shown in red. Sympathetic and parasympathetic nerves make extensive contacts with neurons in the enteric nervous system. In diabetes mellitus one or more components of efferent or afferent innervation (not shown) may be involved (see text). Reprinted with permission from reference 7 (Goyal RK, Crist J. Neurology of the gut. In: Sleisenger MH, Fordtran JS, eds. Gastrointestinal disease: pathophysiology, diagnosis, management. Philadelphia: WB Saunders, 1989:21–52).

involved with painful sensations from the gut. These fibers are also thinly myelinated or nonmyelinated fine fibers.

Morphologic studies of vagal abnormalities in diabetes have had variable results. In experimental animal studies, Diani et al. reported marked abnormalities in the vagus nerve in nonketonuric and ketonuric diabetic Chinese hamsters.[8] This analysis of axons from the ventral division of the vagus nerve demonstrated that in the diabetic animals the diameter of the nonmyelinated axons was reduced and the numerical and volume density of myelinated fibers was also markedly decreased. In an autopsy study of diabetic patients, Smith demonstrated sparse changes in the vagus nerve.[9] In sections obtained at both the cervical and diaphragmatic levels of the vagus, she observed that a small number of fibers had undergone segmental demyelination. A larger number of fibers showed Wallerian changes of degeneration. More severe pathologic changes of the vagus nerve were described by Duchen et al. in an autopsy study of four patients with prolonged diabetes.[10] Sections taken from the cervical vagus demonstrated severe loss of myelinated axons with an associated excess of collagen. Guy et al. described severe pathologic changes in a segment of the abdominal vagus removed during gastric surgery from a patient with severe gastroparesis.[11] These changes included a severe reduction in unmyelinated axons; the remaining axons were characterized by a small diameter with an associated increase in surrounding collagen. In contrast to the findings of the above studies, Yoshida et al. found no abnormalities by morphologic analysis of sections of the abdominal vagus nerve in five diabetic patients, two of whom had symptomatic gastroparesis.[12]

Functional studies provide evidence of parasympathetic efferent denervation of the gut in diabetes. Patients with long-standing diabetes have been found to have an impairment of the cephalic phase of gastric acid secretion.[13,14] In such patients, sham feeding or insulin-induced hypoglycemia is associated with a diminished secretory response, a finding indicative of decreased vagal influence on the stomach. Moreover, the rise in serum levels of pancreatic polypeptide with sham feeding is also impaired in patients with advanced diabetes, indicating deficient parasympathetic innervation of the pancreas.[14]

Sympathetic Innervation

The preganglionic neurons of sympathetic efferents are located in the spinal cord (T5 to L3), and the corresponding postganglionic neurons are located in the various sympathetic ganglia. The sympathetic efferent fibers entering the gut are postganglion adrenergic fibers, and they exert most of their actions indirectly via the enteric neurons. The sympathetic efferents exert inhibitory effects on the gut except in the sphincters, which are contracted by the sympathetic nerves.

In a pathologic study of autopsy findings in diabetic patients, Duchen et al. found several abnormalities in the pattern of sympathetic innervation.[10] In the intermediolateral columns of the spinal cord, where the sympathetic neurons arise, cell numbers appeared reduced at several thoracic levels. In addition, in the cervical and celiac sympathetic ganglia, neurons were observed to be distended or vacuolated with enlarged club-shaped neural processes. Chang et al. demonstrated that rats with experimentally induced diabetes have a deficiency in adrenergic-mediated absorption of fluid and electrolyte in the ileum and colon, presumably secondary to deficient sympathetic innervation.[15,16]

Sympathetic afferents are involved in many sympathetic reflexes, in nausea and vomiting, and in gastrointestinal pain. Specific information on sympathetic afferent dysfunction in the gut of diabetics is lacking. However, it is possible that sensory neuropathy may be involved in the syndrome of abdominal pain, nausea and vomiting, and impaired perception of rectal distension.

Enteric Nervous System

The enteric plexus, which consists of the myenteric and submucous plexuses, forms the enteric nervous system (ENS), which is the "local brain" of the gut (Fig. 51–2).[16] The ENS resembles the CNS in that it contains sensory, motor, and integrating-command interneurons and program generators. Moreover, ENS neurons, like CNS neurons, employ a large variety of neurotransmitters, including acetylcholine, neuropeptides such as cholecystokinin (CCK), galanin, calcitonin gene-related peptide (CGRP), gastrin-releasing peptide (GRP), enkephalins, somatostatin, substance P, vasoactive intestinal polypeptide (VIP), purines such as adenosine triphosphate (ATP) and adenosine, and possibly amino acids such as γ-aminobutyric acid (GABA); there are no intrinsic adrenergic neurons in the gut.

Previous pathologic studies of diabetic patients in which conventional sections were used found the morphology of the myenteric plexus to be normal. More recent pathologic studies that used tangential sections demonstrated mild abnormalities in these patients. Smith described the myenteric plexus of the esophagus as being mostly normal, with only a small number of neurons with swollen irregular processes.[9] She also described the lymphocytic infiltration of a large number of nonneuronal cells in the plexus. Duchen et al. confirmed this finding in sections from a wider distribution of the gut.[10] He also described infiltration of the ganglia with inflammatory cells, especially around unmyelinated axons. In contrast, Yoshida et al., who prepared extensive sections from the stomachs of diabetic patients, described the myenteric plexus as being completely normal with no evidence of morphologic change or inflammatory infiltrate.[12]

Rats with streptozotocin-induced diabetes show distinctive and contrasting changes in the nerves in the ileum and proximal colon.[17,18] In the ileum, immunohistochemical studies showed degeneration of adrenergic and serotonin-containing nerves, apparently intact cholinergic nerves, decreased stores of CGRP, an apparent increase in VIP, and apparently unchanged stores of substance P. In contrast, in the proximal colon the local stores of all these neurotransmitters appeared to be within normal limits or increased. It is noteworthy that the diabetic rats had diarrhea.[18] The diminished adrener-

A

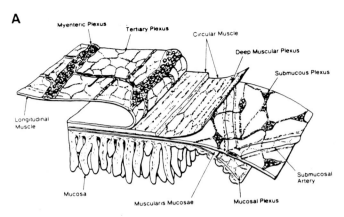

B

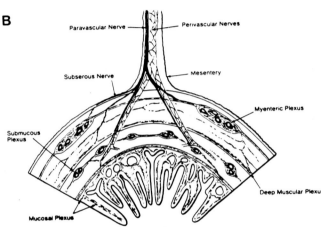

Fig. 51—2. Diagrammatic representation of the enteric plexuses as they are seen in whole mounts of intestine (A) and in transverse section (B). The diagrams show the general arrangement in the small intestine of all mammals. Neuropathy of the enteric plexuses may be involved in some gastrointestinal disorders associated with diabetes (see text). Reprinted with permission from reference 6 (Furness JB, Costa M. The enteric nervous system. London: Churchill Livingstone, 1987).

gic innervation of the ileum might well have contributed to the diarrhea by impairing fluid and electrolyte absorption in this segment.

Functional studies have suggested defects in cholinergic innervation in diabetic rats. Nowalk et al. measured the contraction of longitudinal and circular strips of intestine in response to electrical-field stimulation in rats with streptozotocin-induced diabetes.[19] Only in strips of longitudinal muscle from the ileum were significant differences seen among the three groups of rats. The amplitude of contraction was highest in control rats, lowest in diabetic rats, and intermediate in insulin-treated diabetic rats. These changes were seen in the atropine-sensitive contractions, suggesting impaired cholinergic neuromuscular transmission in the distal small bowel in diabetic rats.

Somatic Innervation

Each end of the gastrointestinal tube (pharynx, upper esophagus, and external anal sphincter) is composed of striated muscle fibers that are innervated by somatic nerves. Moreover, the parietal peritoneum and abdominal wall receive somatic sensory innervation. Both sensory and motor neuropathy are well-known complications of diabetes. They may cause, on one hand, abnormalities in pharyngeal swallowing and, on the other, external anal sphincter dysfunction during defecation. Sensory neuropathy and radiculopathy may be responsible for unexplained abdominal pain in diabetics.

ABDOMINAL PAIN IN DIABETES

Both acute and chronic abdominal pain can present in a rather unique fashion in patients with diabetes mellitus. Syndromes of acute and chronic abdominal pain can masquerade as disorders of intra-abdominal or pelvic pathology and must be recognized to permit the institution of appropriate therapy.

Acute Abdominal Pain

It has long been recognized that abdominal pain, tenderness, and vomiting are frequently present in patients presenting with diabetic ketoacidosis.[20,21] Unexplained abdominal pain in the setting of diabetic metabolic decompensation tends to be generalized or epigastric in location. The mechanism of acute abdominal pain is not clear. Hyperamylasemia can occur but is not correlated with the presence of pancreatitis. It has been suggested that abdominal pain and vomiting might be due to the gastric dilatation and intestinal ileus that can occur secondary to the metabolic acidosis. Theoretically, the pain could be due to stretching of the hepatic capsule in response to hepatic steatosis; abrupt hepatic distention, however, is unlikely to be due to steatosis. Finally, acute pain may simply be due to activation of nociceptors in response to metabolic derangements.

Campbell et al. reviewed the clinical findings and outcome in 211 episodes of metabolic decompensation in 140 diabetic patients over an 8-year period.[20] Severe abdominal pain and tenderness that necessitated diagnostic evaluation occurred in 46 patients. In 17 patients, the abdominal pain could be attributed to an underlying disorder (e.g., pyelonephritis, appendicitis) considered to have precipitated the metabolic decompensation. In the other 29 patients, the abdominal pain remained unexplained and was attributed to the ongoing ketoacidosis. Patients with unexplained abdominal pain were less than 40 years of age and, with only three exceptions, had a plasma bicarbonate level less than 10 mEq/L. The authors suggested that acute abdominal pain in diabetic patients older than 40 years of age or with plasma bicarbonate levels greater than 10 mEq/L should not be attributed to the metabolic decompensation and that a search should be undertaken for an underlying abdominal or pelvic disorder. In all patients, gastrointestinal, renal, or pelvic diseases should be excluded, especially in those with fever, localized abdominal pain or tenderness, or abnormal laboratory findings. The acute abdominal pain associated with diabetic ketoacidosis resolves with correction of the metabolic abnormalities. It is important to recognize this entity so as to avoid unnecessary and harmful exploration laparotomy in these patients.

Chronic Abdominal Pain

Chronic abdominal pain can occur as a result of diabetic sensory neuropathy and can masquerade as serious intra-abdominal pathology, especially when it is associated with weight loss. Thoracic radiculopathy is an important cause of chronic pain in diabetic patients. Longstreth and Newcomer described the syndrome of chronic abdominal pain and weight loss caused by thoracic radiculopathy in four middle-aged or elderly patients with adult-onset diabetes mellitus.[21] These patients initially underwent investigations focused on possible malignancy. Some had even undergone laparotomy in a search for possible carcinoma of the pancreas. In the affected patients, the pain tended to be asymmetric rather than bilateral and most often affected the left upper abdomen and often radiated into or from the lower thoracic spine. At times both the upper abdomen and lower chest were involved in the pattern of symptoms. The pain was described as a pressure discomfort or sharp pain and at times had neuropathic qualities such as "burning" or "stabbing." Two of the patients had associated paresthesias over the abdominal wall. The onset of the pain was gradual, being at first intermittent, later more frequent, and finally constant. It is especially noteworthy that the pain was not brought on or affected by either eating or defecation, a possible clue that the pain did not originate from the gastrointestinal tract. Marked weight loss—up to 19 kg—occurred in three of the patients and presumably was caused by pain-induced anorexia. Two patients had evidence of either recent or ongoing femoral neuropathy with symptoms of pain in one or both thighs. The diagnosis of thoracic radiculopathy secondary to diabetes was confirmed by electromyographic demonstration of either unilateral or bilateral denervation of the paraspinal muscles in the middle thoracic to upper lumbar region. In these patients, the pain gradually resolved, and both appetite and weight increased after intervals of 6 to 20 months. A combination of nonsteroidal anti-inflammatory drugs and tricyclic antidepressants has been used in other syndromes of radiculopathy and/or peripheral neuropathy and is worth a trial in this syndrome.

GUT SMOOTH MUSCLE IN DIABETES

In general, the intestinal smooth muscle in diabetes is normal and functionally intact.[22] Although the primary disorder of gut motility appears to be one of hypomotility or even atony, experimental observations strongly argue that these changes are the result of deficient innervation. When cholinergic agonists are administered, contractions are of normal amplitude.[23,24] Yoshida et al. confirmed the morphologic health of gastric smooth muscle in their study.[12] Their extensive review of many sections obtained from all parts of the stomach demonstrated normal smooth muscle without evidence of degeneration or vacuolization. In contrast, Duchen et al.[10] and Guy et al.,[11] in a small number of patients, described a distinctive

morphologic abnormality of intestinal smooth muscle. Both investigators observed eosinophilic or hyaline-like bodies (rounded or club-shaped) lying in or replacing smooth muscle cells. The extensive autopsy studies of Duchen et al. described the presence of these smooth muscle bodies throughout the gastrointestinal tract and, in addition, in the smooth muscle of the bladder.[10] The significance of these hyaline bodies is unclear, but the preponderance of clinical data indicate that the intestinal smooth muscle is functionally healthy.

PHARYNX AND ESOPHAGUS IN DIABETES

Pharyngeal and esophageal motor abnormalities are frequently found in persons with diabetes. However, these motor abnormalities rarely produce significant symptoms. The incidence of reflux esophagitis and candida esophagitis may be increased in diabetic patients.

Pharyngeal Motility

Borgström et al., in barium studies, evaluated "swallowing complaints" in 18 diabetic patients, 16 of whom had evidence of autonomic neuropathy.[25] Videofluoroscopy of the pharynx demonstrated motor abnormalities in 14 patients. These included defective epiglottic mobility, defective closure of the laryngeal vestibule, and weakness of the pharyngeal musculature. When symptoms of pharyngeal dysphagia are present, swallowing therapy may be helpful in the management of these patients.

Esophageal Motility

Several prospective studies have demonstrated that abnormalities of esophageal motility and transit are quite common among diabetic patients with neuropathy but are usually asymptomatic.[25–35] Maddern et al.[32] and Horowitz et al.[36,37] performed scintigraphic studies of esophageal emptying of a solid bolus and found delayed emptying in 42% of patients with insulin-dependent diabetes (IDDM) and in 30% of patients with Type II diabetes (non-insulin-dependent; NIDDM) who were receiving oral hypoglycemic agents.

Manometric studies of esophageal motility are an even more sensitive measure of esophageal motor dysfunction. Hollis et al. studied esophageal motility in patients with diabetes and found that 56% had abnormal esophageal motility.[34] Abnormalities were more common in patients with diabetic neuropathy. Among those with evidence of peripheral sensory neuropathy but not of autonomic neuropathy, 80% had abnormalities in esophageal motility. All four patients in this study who had evidence of autonomic neuropathy showed abnormalities of esophageal motility. In patients with peripheral neuropathy alone, esophageal motility showed 1) contractions of low or normal amplitude, 2) some slowing of conduction velocity of peristaltic contractions, 3) an increased frequency of dropped swallows, and 4) a mild delay of transit. Nevertheless, in patients with peripheral neuropathy alone, the majority of swallows are associated with normal peristalsis. In diabetic patients with autonomic neuropathy, there is an increased frequency of multipeaked and simultaneous contractions. A similar finding was observed by Loo et al.[33] In a study of 14 patients with IDDM who had both peripheral and autonomic neuropathy, all showed evidence of abnormal esophageal motility (Fig. 51–3). In 12 patients, all swallows were associated with multipeaked peristaltic waves of normal duration and amplitude. In the other two patients, the majority of swallows were associated with these waves. All patients were asymptomatic. In scintigraphic studies of esophageal transit, multipeaked contractions usually are associated with normal esophageal transit, but simultaneous contractions are associated with delayed transit.[28]

The overwhelming majority of patients in manometric and scintigraphic studies are free of esophageal symptoms. Even patients with motility patterns compatible with diffuse esophageal spasm were often asymptomatic.[34] Among patients who did complain of dysphagia, the symptom was mild and often correlated with prolonged esophageal transit associated with simultaneous contractions.[28] Chest pain was a rare symptom.

The mechanism of the esophageal motor abnormalities in diabetes remains unclear. Loo et al. reported that the administration of atropine inhibited the development of the second esophageal peak.[33] It has been suggested that the presumed loss of vagal innervation of the esophagus is the mechanism of abnormal peristalsis, although the experimental demonstration of this theory has not been documented. In contrast, Clouse et al. suggested that the

esophageal motor abnormalities observed in diabetic patients were due to coincident psychiatric disease (depression and anxiety disorders) rather than to neuropathy.[30] Psychiatric illness, as defined by testing, was present in 87% of those diabetic patients with motor abnormalities but in only 21% of those with normal motility. According to the investigators, log-linear analysis suggested that the association was independent of neuropathy. In this study the vast majority of patients were without esophageal symptoms.

Reflux Esophagitis

In diabetic patients the lower esophageal sphincter generally demonstrates normal pressures and relaxation.[34] Although these studies do describe some patients with symptoms of gastroesophageal reflux, it is not clear if incidence of reflux in diabetic patients is increased over the incidence in a matched control population.[38] In patients with symptomatic diabetic gastroparesis, the combination of gastric distention and increased gastric residual volume may make gastroesophageal reflux a more common occurrence.[39] Treatment of reflux esophagitis in patients with diabetes is no different from that in patients without diabetes.[39]

Candida Esophagitis

One important esophageal complication of diabetes is candida esophagitis.[40] Presumably, the impaired immunity associated with diabetes causes these patients to be more susceptible to this disorder. In addition, the stasis of esophageal contents associated with abnormal motor function could contribute to the susceptibility to this infection. Extensive esophageal candidiasis may be asymptomatic or may be associated with symptoms of odynophagia (pain on swallowing) or dysphagia. The presence or absence of oral candidiasis has no reliable predictive value for the presence of candida esophagitis. The technique of barium swallow is a relatively insensitive means of detecting this disorder; with advanced esophageal candidiasis, a single- or double-contrast barium swallow may demonstrate extensive mucosal abnormalities indicative of esophagitis. Fiberoptic esophagoscopy is much more sensitive and often demonstrates innumerable scattered white plaques over variable lengths of the esophagus. Esophageal brushings obtained through the endoscope can confirm the diagnosis.

Therapy includes the consumption of oral nystatin solution as a swish and swallow (1 to 3 million units every 6 hours) or clotrimazole troches (10 mg allowed to dissolve in the mouth) five times a day. A more reliable therapy is ketoconazole at a dosage of 200 mg once a day. Because this drug requires the presence of gastric acid for its dissolution and absorption, it should not be administered with antacids or other agents that inhibit gastric acid secretion. Indeed, if a patient with esophageal candidiasis fails to respond to a standard dose of ketoconazole, achlorhydria should be suspected and additional measures are called for, such as increasing the dose or dissolving the medication in a small volume of 0.1 N HCl

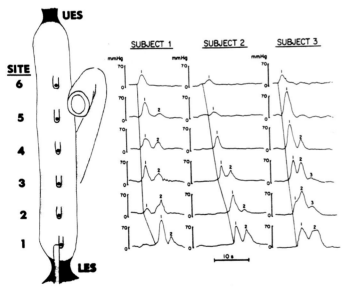

Fig. 51–3. Examples from esophageal manometric recordings in three diabetic patients with neuropathy. The numbers identify each discrete contraction wave at a given site. The dashed line demonstrates the peristaltic progression of the lead pressure wave. LES = lower esophageal sphincter; UES = upper esophageal sphincter. Reprinted with permission from reference 33 (Loo FD, Dodds WJ, Soergel KH, et al. Multipeaked esophageal peristaltic pressure waves in patients with diabetic neuropathy. Gastroenterology 1985:88;485–91).

and having the patient sip the solution through a straw to avoid injury to the teeth. Most recently, fluconazole was shown to be more effective than ketoconazole.[41] Fluconazole is administered at a dose of 200 mg on the first day and 100 mg once daily thereafter.

Dysphagia in Diabetes

Although minor pharyngeal esophageal motor abnormalities are quite common in diabetes, they are usually asymptomatic.[25] Because this is a disorder associated with few, if any, symptoms, a specific therapy is generally not needed. In general, prokinetic agents (metoclopramide or domperidone), which have been shown to enhance esophageal contractions, have not been shown to improve esophageal transit in patients with delayed transit, as demonstrated by scintigraphic techniques.[32] Only in one study was the acute administration of oral cisapride found to improve esophageal transit in patients with baseline slowing of transit.[37] It is not known if the relative lack of esophageal symptoms in diabetic patients is due to changes in sensory threshold caused by associated sensory neuropathy involving the esophagus. Feldman and Schiller reported that 27% of the unselected diabetic patients complained of some dysphagia.[3] In general, significant dysphagia in a diabetic patient should not be explained by the diabetic pharyngeal or esophageal motility abnormalities, and a search for another associated cause of dysphagia should be made.

STOMACH IN DIABETES

Gastric Motor Activity

The normal motor activity of the stomach has at least four functions. First, the stomach acts as a reservoir to accommodate the large volume of solid and liquid contained in a meal. Second, the stomach acts to pulverize solids and mix them with gastric acid such that they are reduced to a particle size compatible with optimal digestion. Third, the stomach empties only liquids and pulverized solids into the duodenum during the postprandial digestive period. Fourth, the stomach empties all the food residues, including indigestible material, during the interdigestive period. The stomach achieves these ends through three distinctly different regions of motor activity, i.e., the proximal stomach, the distal stomach, and the pyloric sphincter, and by coordinating its contractions with those of the duodenum (Fig. 51–4). In diabetes all of these functions may be impaired (Table 51–1).

Proximal Stomach

The proximal stomach consists of the fundus and the orad third of the gastric body. The proximal stomach exhibits tonic contractions, producing prolonged pressure elevations lasting 1 to 6 minutes.[42] These contractions press gastric contents aborally toward the distal stomach and the duodenum and play an important role in gastric emptying. They are stimulated by excitatory fibers in the vagus and by hormones such as motilin.

Normally, the proximal stomach relaxes with each swallow ("receptive relaxation") and also as the volume of swallowed food builds up ("accommodation").[43,44] With receptive relaxation and accommodation, the stomach can accommodate increasing volumes without increasing gastric pressure, an ability that enhances its function as a reservoir. Receptive relaxation is mediated by inhibitory fibers in the vagus nerve, while accommodation is due to inhibitory neurohormonal influences. The resting tone of the fundus in diabetic patients is comparable to that in normal subjects, but fundic contractions, as measured by a motility index, are reduced in diabetic patients.[45] The status of the receptive relaxation or accommodation in diabetic patients is not known.

Distal Stomach

Normally, during the digestive period, contraction waves arise in the pacemaker region (in the greater curvature region of the stomach) and sweep distally to the gastroduodenal junction, carrying part of the gastric contents ahead of the wave[46] (Fig. 51–4). Most motility studies in patients with diabetic gastroparesis show decreased numbers as well as reduced amplitude of contractions.[23,24,45] Some patients have only reduced amplitude of contraction but normal high frequency,[24] whereas others have both reduced amplitude and frequency,[23] resulting in a marked reduction of motility index. The motility index is the product of amplitude of

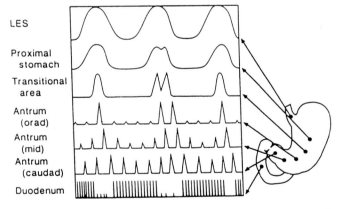

Fig. 51–4. Phasic pressure patterns in proximal stomach, distal stomach, and proximal duodenum during a period of motor activity. Note broad-base fundic pressure waves that propagate into distal stomach and gradually transform themselves into peaked antral waves. Antral waves that are coordinated with fundic waves are of higher amplitude than those interposed. Antral waves coordinated with fundic waves are also associated with quiescence in duodenum (noticeable during periods of duodenal regular motor activity). Diabetic gastroparesis is associated with abnormalities of one or more of these activities (see text). LES = lower esophageal sphincter. Reprinted with permission from reference 42 (Malagelada J-R, Aspiroz F. Determinants of gastric emptying and transit in the small intestine. In: Handbook of physiology. The gastrointestinal system. Vol 1. Motility and circulation. Bethesda: American Physiological Society, 1989:909–37).

Table 51—1.   Gastric Motor Abnormalities in Diabetes Mellitus

Gastric contractions
  1. Reduced amplitude of fundic contractions
  2. Reduced amplitude of antral contractions
  3. Reduced frequency of antral contractions
  4. Absence of IMMCs*
  5. Periods of sustained high-frequency, nonpropagated contractions
  6. Pylorospasm
Electrogastrographic findings
  1. Tachygastria
  2. Bradygastria
  3. Flat pattern
  4. Absence of postprandial increase in the strength of slow waves
Delay in gastric emptying
  1. Liquids: variable
  2. Digestible solids: frequent
  3. Undigestible solids: very frequent

*IMMC = antral interdigestive migrating motor complex.

contraction and number of contractions over a certain time period.

In the indigestive period, four phases of variable motor activity occur in a cyclic fashion.[46] During phase I, few if any contractions occur in the stomach. During phase II, intermittent random contractions are propagated distally over short distances. This is followed by phase III, which is a brief complex of rhythmic (3 cycles/minute), strong propulsive contractions. Phase III originates in the proximal stomach and migrates through the distal stomach. This succession of cycles has been termed the interdigestive migrating motor complex (IMMC), and the period of an entire cycle is approximately 100 minutes.

Vagal innervation of the stomach is essential for the interdigestive cyclic motor activity. With vagotomy, fasting motor activity in the stomach is abolished and the IMMC originates in the duodenum distal to the stomach.[46] The cyclical release of motilin from endocrine cells in the duodenum and jejunum plays an important role in initiating IMMCs in the stomach.[47] This cyclical motilin release is mediated by vagal cholinergic influences in the dog, but perhaps not in humans.[48] Malagelada et al. demonstrated that diabetic patients with symptomatic gastroparesis had no antral IMMCs but had normal IMMCs in the duodenum. In diabetic patients without symptoms of gastroparesis, IMMC activity was present in both the antrum and the duodenum.[45] Achem-Karam et al. confirmed that IMMC activity was absent in the antrum of symptomatic patients with diabetic gastroparesis and that, in some of these patients, activity was also absent in the duodenum.[49]

The decreased motor activity in the distal stomach in diabetic patients may be due to both autonomic neuropathy and diabetic hyperglycemia. Fox and Behar suggested that this decreased activity is due to decreased cholinergic transmission; when such patients were treated with parenteral bethanechol, the amplitude and frequency of contractions increased to normal levels.[23] In studies in normal subjects, Barnett and Owyang demonstrated that experimentally induced hyperglycemia re-

duced antral motor activity and even abolished the gastric component of the IMMC.[50] They also observed that with increasing hyperglycemia, levels of serum motilin fell. Since motilin is postulated to be a physiologic regulator of gastric IMMC activity, the authors suggested that the hyperglycemic reduction in motor activity might in part be due to a hyperglycemic reduction in levels of serum motilin.. The investigators observed, however, that gastric IMMC activity was reduced at levels of blood glucose that had no effect on the serum motilin level. Hence they suggested that hyperglycemia per se might also decrease antral motor activity independent of changes in serum motilin levels. These authors also observed that the serum motilin levels were elevated in diabetic patients, arguing therefore that the absence of gastric IMMC activity in these patients was not due to a deficiency of circulating serum motilin.[50]

In contrast to the general pattern of decreased gastric motor activity, occasional diabetic patients demonstrate fasting patterns of ectopic and aberrant antral motility. In some patients episodes of sustained high-frequency activity (3 cycles/minute) that is neither propagated nor associated with IMMC activity have been observed in the antrum.[24] These motor abnormalities also cause gastric stasis. It has been suggested that this phenomenon is related to intestinal motor aberrations created by sympathetic denervation.

Pylorus

The gastric pylorus is a thick-walled, narrow channel that can actively change its opening size under the influence of excitatory and inhibitory nerves. The pylorus is not a usual sphincter, since under basal conditions its resting pressure is not elevated.[46] The opening size of the pylorus determines not only the rate of gastric emptying but also the size of the food particles that are permitted to leave the stomach. Soon after a meal, as the peristaltic waves in the stomach and antrum carry pieces of food toward it, the pylorus opens partially so that only liquids or small particles pass through, and solid chunks of food are trapped in the antrum to be ground by powerful antral contractions. If the pylorus does not open or relax, gastric emptying of liquids as well as of ground and unground solids is inhibited and gastric stasis occurs. It has been reported that luminal contents in the small bowel may inhibit gastric emptying by enhancing pyloric closure via neurohormonal reflexes.[46] Wider opening of pylorus is also essential for movement of large pieces of food during the IMMC.

Careful manometric studies have shown that diabetic patients have increased fasting and postprandial pyloric motor activity.[51] In addition, these patients demonstrate episodes of "pylorospasm" characterized by prolonged periods of increased tonic and phasic motor activity in this region.[51] It has been suggested that pyloric motor activity and pylorospasm could act as a "brake" on gastric emptying and hence could contribute to the morbidity and disability of gastroparesis. The increased pyloric motor activity might be due to an increase in cholinergic or noncholinergic excitatory nerve activity or to a decrease in adrenergic or nonadrenergic activity with resultant decreased pyloric inhibition.

Duodenum

Normally, duodenal activity is coordinated with antral and pyloric activity.[46] During the period of enhanced gastric emptying, the duodenal and pyloric activities are inhibited with each antral peristalsis. The inhibition is followed by contractions that form a peristaltic sequence with antral contractions. Such a duodenal inhibition can be called receptive relaxation of the duodenum and is due to inhibitory neural influences. Impairment of this duodenal relaxation results in antroduodenal incoordination, and this acts to inhibit gastric emptying. However, the importance, if any, of antroduodenal incoordination in diabetic gastroparesis is not known.

Duodenal mucosal afferents also play an important role in reflex modulation of gastric emptying of liquids based on the composition of liquid meal emptied from the stomach.[46] Thus, liquid meals of high caloric densities, high fat content, high osmolality, and acid pH stimulate duodenal receptors to inhibit gastric emptying. No information is available on duodenogastric reflexes in diabetic gastroparesis.

Electrogastrography

The electrical activity in different parts of the stomach is quite different and is related to the different patterns of mechanical activity in these regions. The electrical activity of the distal part of the stomach is prominent and can be recorded clinically with the use of cutaneous electrodes. This procedure of recording of gastric electrical activity is called electrogastrography (Fig. 51–5).[52] The electrical activity of the distal stomach is characterized by cyclical depolarizations (slow wave) that occur at a rate of about 3 cycles/minute. These cycles originate in a region of the greater curvature of the gastric body (gastric pacemaker) and move distally toward the pylorus at an accelerating rate of 0.5 to 4 cm/second. When the depolarizations become larger under the influence of neurotransmitters or hormones, action potentials cause gastric contractions (Fig. 51–6). When the amplitude of slow wave depolarizations decreases, no action potentials are produced by the normal exposure to excitatory neurotransmitters or hormones and no associated contractions occur.[46] The decreased amplitude of depolarization may be associated with abnormal rhythms (dysrhythmia) of gastric slow waves such as tachygastria (increased slow-wave frequency), bradygastria (decreased slow-wave frequency), or gastric arrhythmia (irregular slow-wave frequencies) (Fig. 51–7).[52] Gastric slow-wave frequencies and amplitude of depolarizations (also described as power of the slow waves) can be monitored with cutaneous electrogastrograms.

Some patients with diabetic gastroparesis have gastric dysrhythmia. In one study, 9 of 10 patients with diabetic gastroparesis had runs of tachygastria as compared with only one subject from a comparable control group.[52] Similarly, in another study of six patients with diabetic gastroparesis, one had tachygastria, two had bradygastria, and the remaining three had flat-line patterns on cutaneous gastrograms.[53] Normally, after a meal the amplitude of depolarizations of the slow wave increases and more slow waves are associated with contractions. In one study, patients with diabetic gastroparesis had normal

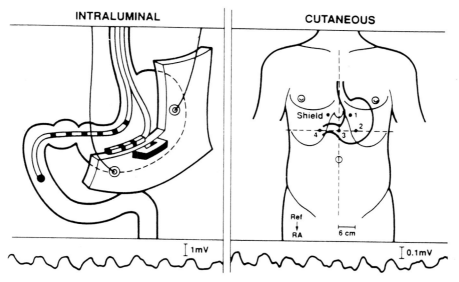

Fig. 51–5. Recording of gastric electrical activity by electrographic techniques. Intraluminal electrogastrographic techniques use an internal electrode system that is apposed to the stomach wall by an external magnet placed on the abdominal wall. Cutaneous techniques involve placement of skin electrodes over the region of the stomach. Each technique records a sinusoidal waveform, but the intraluminal signal is 10 times stronger than the cutaneous signal. Reprinted with permission from reference 52 (Hasler W, Owyang C. Peptide-induced gastric arrhythmias: a new cause of gastroparesis. Regul Pept Lett 1990:2:6–12).

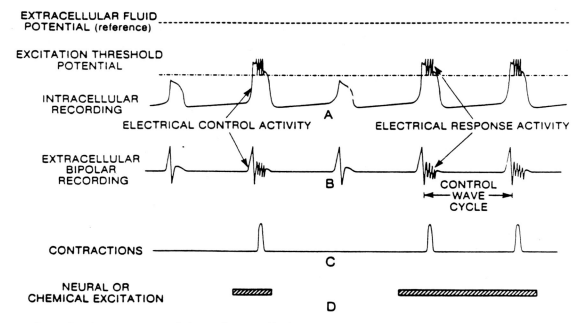

EXTRACELLULAR FLUID
POTENTIAL (reference)

EXCITATION THRESHOLD
POTENTIAL

INTRACELLULAR
RECORDING

ELECTRICAL CONTROL ACTIVITY   ELECTRICAL RESPONSE ACTIVITY

A

EXTRACELLULAR
BIPOLAR
RECORDING

B   CONTROL
←WAVE→
CYCLE

CONTRACTIONS

C

NEURAL OR
CHEMICAL EXCITATION

D

Fig. 51–6. Relationship between intracellular and extracellular electrical activities and contractile activity. Resting membrane potential in intracellular recordings is negative with respect to extracellular fluid potential (reference). Intracellularly recorded monophasic depolarizations are recorded as biphasic or triphasic depolarizations by extracellular bipolar electrodes. In intracellular recordings, bursts of electrical response activity appear during depolarized phase of control potential, but in extracellular recordings they appear after initial large depolarization of control potential. However, their temporal relationship to contractile activity is the same in both types of recordings. Membrane potential depolarizations that do not exceed the excitation threshold level are not superimposed with a bout of electrical response activity and are not accompanied by a contraction. Neurochemical stimulation (rectangles) increases the amplitude of electrical control activity oscillation and results in a burst of electrical response activity and a contraction during depolarization. An understanding of the electromechanical relationships of the gastrointestinal smooth muscle is necessary for evaluation of the importance of abnormalities in electromyographic studies of the gastrointestinal tract in diabetes mellitus. Reprinted with permission from reference 46 (Sarna SK. In vivo myoelectric activity: methods, analysis and interpretation. In: Handbook of physiology. The gastrointestinal system. Vol 1. Motility and circulation. Bethesda: American Physiological Society, 1989:817–63).

slow-wave cycles but lacked the normal postprandial increase in strength of the slow waves.[52]

Gastric Emptying

Diabetic gastroparesis is associated with delayed gastric emptying of all constituents of food, i.e., liquids,[54–56] digestible solids,[37,53,57–59] and indigestible solids.[60] Moreover, the delay is not the same for all of these constituents. Simultaneous investigations of gastric emptying of liquids and digestible solids have been carried out with the use of dual markers: a ^{99}Tc-labeled solid phase and ^{111}In-labeled liquid phase.[61] Gastric emptying of indigestible solids has been determined by studying the emptying of radiopaque markers from the stomach with serial abdominal x-ray studies.[62] Figure 51–8 shows patterns of gastric emptying of liquids and solids in one patient with diabetic gastroparesis and in a normal control.

Emptying of Liquids

Gastric emptying of liquids is normally influenced by the composition of the liquid meal, whose characteristics, e.g., acidity, caloric and nutritional content, and osmolal-

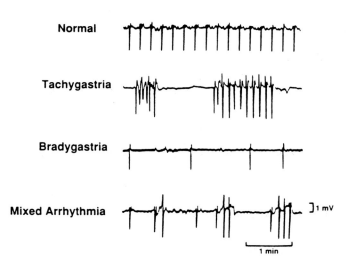

Normal

Tachygastria

Bradygastria

Mixed Arrhythmia   ] 1 mV

1 min

Fig. 51–7. Examples of normal and dysrhythmic slow wave recordings using serosally placed electrodes on canine stomach. Similar patterns of dysrhythmic slow waves are observed on external electrogastrographs in diabetic patients (see text). Reprinted with permission from reference 52 (Hasler W, Owyang C. Peptide-induced gastric arrhythmias: a new cause of gastroparesis. Regul Pept Lett 1990:2;6–12).

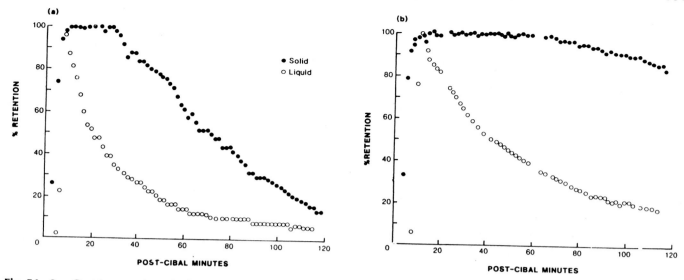

Fig. 51–8. Gastric emptying of solids and liquids in one control subject (a) and a diabetic patient with autonomic neuropathy (b). Note that emptying of solids is slower than that of liquids and both solid and liquid emptying are slower in the diabetic patient. Reprinted with permission from reference 63 (Horowitz M, Harding PE, Chatterton BE, et al. Acute and chronic effects of domperidone on gastric emptying in diabetic autonomic neuropathy. Dig Dis Sci 1985:30;1–9).

ity, elicit different responses from duodenal receptors and, in turn, from reflexes responsible for emptying.[46] Hence, the liquid emptying varies in different studies because of their use of meals ranging from simple solutions (water, 10% dextrose, and orange juice) to complex nutritional solutions that truly justify the term "liquid meal."[47] Moreover, even with a standardized meal, gastric emptying of liquids in diabetic patients is variable. Keshavarzian et al. demonstrated rapid emptying of liquids in diabetic patients and suggested that it was due to diminished receptive relaxation in the diabetic stomach.[56] In contrast, Loo et al.[57] and Wright et al.[59] demonstrated normal emptying of liquids in diabetic patients. Finally, Horowitz et al.[37,63] and Snape et al.[54] demonstrated delayed emptying of liquids in diabetic patients. The delayed gastric emptying of liquids may be due to reduced fundic motor activity and antral motility. Another factor that could affect gastric emptying is hyperglycemia. MacGregor et al. demonstrated that in normal subjects experimentally induced hyperglycemia is associated with a slowing of the gastric emptying of liquid meals containing fat and protein; hyperglycemia may cause a reflex decrease in vagal excitatory tone of the stomach with a resulting delay in gastric emptying.[64] However, there was no correlation between the degree of delay of emptying of liquids and the delay in emptying of solids.[37]

Emptying of Digestible Solids

Normally, in the postprandial period, digestible solids are emptied more slowly than liquids because the emptying of solids depends on their being pulverized to a size sufficient (<2 mm) to pass through the sieve created by the contracted pyloric sphincter.[46] In diabetic patients, the gastric emptying of solids is frequently

delayed. Horowitz et al. studied gastric emptying among unselected diabetic patients. Delayed emptying of solids was present among 58% of patients with Type I diabetes[37] and among 30% of those with Type II diabetes.[36] Clinically, a variety of different meals are used for measurement of gastric emptying of solids. Because both the physical state of the labeled meal and its nutritional composition determine the rate of emptying in control subjects, the degree of sensitivity of different test meals in detecting abnormalities in diabetes varies.

The most sensitive technique for the measurement of gastric emptying involves the use of chicken liver labeled with ^{99}Tc-sulfur colloid by either in vivo or in vitro methods.[37,47,57] The labeled liver is then cooked and incorporated into a complex meal. This technique appears to yield the most stable bonding of the radionuclide to solids. In normal subjects, the labeled meal is emptied in two phases, a lag phase, which appears to correlate with antral grinding of the meal, and a post-lag phase of emptying, which represents the passage of the dispersed chyme from the stomach. A less-sensitive technique binds the ^{99}Tc-sulfur colloid with cooked eggs, either scrambled or in an egg salad sandwich.[58,61] This test meal usually empties in a single linear phase since the binding of label to solid is not as stable, and some of the label begins emptying early with the liquid phase.

Emptying of Indigestible Solids

Indigestible solids, such as dietary fiber, normally do not empty during the postprandial period of motor activity because of the functional sieving produced by the pyloric sphincter.[46] Such ingredients of food are emptied during the interdigestive period by phase III activity of the IMMC. Since gastric IMMC activity is impaired and often absent in symptomatic diabetic patients, the emp-

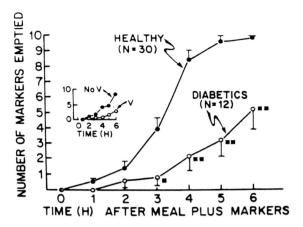

Fig. 51–9. Emptying of solid radiopaque markers in 30 healthy subjects and 12 diabetic patients. Emptying of solid radiopaque markers was significantly delayed in diabetics (P < .01 vs. controls at 3 hours; P < .001 at 4, 5, and 6 hours). The insert shows that emptying of solid markers was slower in seven diabetic patients with vomiting (V) than in five diabetic patients with no vomiting (no V) (P < .05 at 6 hours). Reprinted with permission from reference 62 (Feldman M, Smith HJ, Simon TR. Gastric emptying of solid radiopaque markers: studies in healthy subjects and diabetic patients. Gastroenterology 1984:87;895–902).

tying of indigestible solids from the stomach is delayed in these patients.[47,65]

Feldman et al. studied the emptying of indigestible solids in normal and diabetic subjects[62] using a combination of a high-carbohydrate test meal and indigestible solids fashioned from a radiopaque nasogastric tube. Patients consumed the test meal and the radiopaque markers (1.0 cm length) at the outset of the study, and the emptying of markers from the stomach was assessed with plain abdominal films. Normal subjects emptied all of the markers within 6 hours, a rate faster than that of the diabetic patients (Fig. 51–9). The gastric emptying study using the radiopaque marker identified diabetic patients

with symptoms of gastroparesis more accurately than did a scintigraphic technique using a meal of ^{99}Tc-labeled scrambled eggs. It is important to realize that scintigraphic and radiopaque-marker gastric emptying studies are measuring two different gastric emptying phenomena.[47] The scintigraphic-meal study assesses the competence of the postprandial motor pattern in dispersing and emptying a meal. The radiopaque-marker study measures both the lag time at which the interdigestive motor pattern reappears after a meal and the efficiency with which phase III motor activity empties the markers. Patients who lack IMMC activity in the stomach and demonstrate delayed gastric emptying of radiopaque markers are more likely to have abnormal gastric emptying of dietary fiber and would be susceptible to the formation of gastric bezoars.[66] If the pyloric sphincter fails to open widely because of either a motility abnormality[51] or partial mechanical stenosis, gastric stasis of indigestible food also would occur.

Nausea and Vomiting in Diabetes

Nausea and vomiting are common complaints in diabetic patients, occurring in almost one-third.[45] Nausea and vomiting are common symptoms during acute ketoacidosis, and in most patients they subside with treatment of the acute metabolic abnormality. Sometimes they occur in a chronic pattern of daily symptoms that wax and wane in severity. In a minority of symptomatic diabetic patients, the pattern is paroxysmal; such patients may have varying periods with minimal or no symptoms, only to be unexpectedly disabled by the sudden onset of severe nausea and vomiting necessitating hospitalization for dehydration and ketoacidosis.

The symptoms of nausea and vomiting are frequently the manifestations of delayed gastric emptying in diabetic patients. However, it is important to appreciate that the cause-and-effect relationship between gastric stasis and motor abnormalities and nausea and vomiting is quite complex and is not the same in all diabetic patients (Fig. 51–10). This is exemplified by a poor correlation

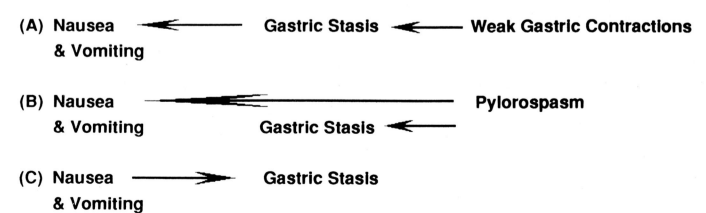

Fig. 51–10. Relationship between nausea and vomiting and gastric stasis in diabetic patients. The cause-and-effect relationship between nausea and vomiting and gastric stasis in diabetic patients is quite complex. On one hand, gastric motor abnormalities in diabetic patients with or without gastric stasis can lead to nausea and vomiting; on the other hand, nausea and vomiting per se can cause gastric stasis.

between the symptoms of nausea and vomiting and delayed gastric emptying in patients with diabetes.[47]

In some diabetic patients, delayed gastric emptying with gastric stasis is the primary problem and could lead to nausea and vomiting by stimulating gastric afferents carried via vagal and sympathetic nerves to the vomiting center in the brainstem. In nondiabetic patients, nausea and vomiting are common when gastric distention is associated with obstruction and vigorous gastric contractions. In some patients, atonic dilation of stomach, even when massive, may not be associated with nausea and vomiting. If gastric stasis and distention are primary causes of nausea and vomiting in diabetic gastroparesis, these symptoms should respond to gastric decompression brought about either by vomiting or by insertion of a nasogastric tube.

In other diabetic patients, nausea and vomiting are associated with episodes of pyloric spasm or intense disorganized antral contractions.[51] These abnormalities may cause both gastric stasis and the symptoms of nausea and vomiting. Pylorospasm and antral motor disorders respond to treatments that inhibit abnormal contractions rather than to the use of prokinetic agents.

In still other diabetic patients, nausea and vomiting may be due to an unknown cause unrelated to gastroparesis, and nausea and vomiting may cause rather than result from delayed gastric emptying. The vomiting reflex, regardless of activation by central or peripheral mechanisms, produces dysrhythmia of gastric slow waves and inhibition of antral contractions and characteristic retropropulsive motor activities in the small bowel. It is well known that stimulation of vestibular system by circular vection involving rotation of a drum with alternating dark and light vertical stripes around a subject placed inside the drum leads to development of symptoms of motor sickness. Such a stimulation also causes tachygastria.[67] Tachygastria is associated with weakened contractions and delayed gastric emptying.[47] If delayed gastric emptying represents gastrointestinal motor response to nausea and vomiting, treatment should be directed toward searching and treating for the underlying cause of nausea and vomiting and primary use of antiemetics.

Diabetic Gastroparesis

Many patients with abnormal gastric emptying have no specific symptoms and may be found to have a gastric bezoar or a largely dilated stomach with retained contents. Frequently, however, these patients have symptoms of anorexia, early satiety, and postprandial abdominal fullness and discomfort. In some patients these symptoms can limit oral nutrition and be a contributor to morbidity. Obviously, gastroparesis contributes to poor diabetic control both because of unpredictable oral intake and because of poor absorption of nutrients as a result of delayed gastric emptying. Usually, the most disturbing symptoms are those of nausea and vomiting. When nausea and vomiting are prominent symptoms, some determination should be made as to whether or not gastroparesis is the primary cause of these symptoms. However, such a

determination is not usually easy to make. In general, abdominal pain is not a common feature of diabetic gastroparesis. Although some patients may develop vague upper abdominal discomfort from excessive gastric dilation, when patients complain of marked upper or mid-abdominal pain, a search should be made for other gastrointestinal and abdominal diseases.

Simple studies such as a plain abdominal film and an upper gastrointestinal series will help identify patients with gastric bezoar and major problems of gastric stasis. Barium studies and esophagogastroduodenoscopy will help exclude mechanical causes of gastric outlet obstruction. Medications such as antidepressants with anticholinergic properties are a potential cause of gastric stasis and should be excluded as a possible cause by a careful history.

Treatment of Diabetic Gastroparesis

The main principles of treatment of diabetic gastroparesis are 1) correction of underlying pathophysiology when possible and avoidance of drugs that impair gastric emptying; 2) dietary adjustments; 3) use of gastric prokinetic agents, which enhance gastric emptying; 4) treatment of associated conditions; 5) feeding jejunostomy; and 6) surgery.

Correction of Underlying Pathogenesis

In situations in which severe episodes of protracted vomiting are associated with dehydration and diabetic ketoacidosis, hospitalization is mandatory. In such cases it is essential that the patient be fasted, and the passage of nasogastric tube may also be necessary. Intravenous fluid should be administered, and insulin should be given as indicated by the serum levels of glucose and ketones.

Dietary Adjustments

In all patients with symptomatic gastroparesis, dietary adjustments should be undertaken. The recommended diet should be low in fiber and fat and administered in frequent small feedings. It may be necessary to obtain caloric counts to quantitate the adequacy of nutritional intake. If caloric intake is inadequate, it can be supplemented with high-calorie liquid supplements. Since liquids are emptied more easily from the gastroparetic stomach, these will be better tolerated. Some patients may even find it more practical to ingest the majority of their nutrition as liquid supplements.

Gastric Prokinetic Agents

Gastric prokinetic agents are a group of drugs characterized by their ability to enhance gastric emptying and reduce gastric stasis.[47] The pharmacology of these drugs, including the mechanisms of receptor interaction and prokinetic action, is not yet fully defined. A wide variety of pharmacologic agents may have gastric prokinetic effects.

Metoclopramide. Metoclopramide is lipid-soluble and readily crosses the blood-brain barrier.[68] The only gastric prokinetic agent available for clinical use in the

United States, it has powerful central antiemetic and peripheral gastric prokinetic actions.

Pharmacology. Metoclopramide is a dopamine D_2 receptor antagonist, a $5HT_3$ receptor antagonist, an acetylcholine releaser, and a cholinesterase inhibitor. It also has some local anesthetic and antiarrhythmic properties and has direct stimulating action on smooth muscle. Its prokinetic activities in the gut are thought to reflect a combination of an antagonism of the inhibitory effects of dopamine on gastric motility and an enhancement of cholinergic activity in the gastroduodenum, which can be blocked by anticholinergic agents.[69] When administered parenterally or orally, metoclopramide can increase the amplitude and frequency of fundic[45] and antral contractions[45,58] and induce associated pyloric and duodenal coordination. This drug may not initiate gastric IMMC activity. Achem-Karam et al. observed that parenteral administration of metoclopramide initiated gastric IMMC activity in diabetic patients if it was given more than 30 minutes after the previous cycle of IMMC activity.[49] Malagelada et al. could not induce such activity with this drug in diabetic patients.[45] Chaussade et al. also failed to initiate such activity with metoclopramide, although it was their practice to administer metoclopramide less than 30 minutes after the previous cycle of IMMC activity.[70] The IMMC-like activity produced by metoclopramide does not show the full distal migration characteristic of the normal IMMC.

In clinical studies, metoclopramide enhances the rate of gastric emptying of both solids[57,58] and liquids (Fig. 51–11).[54,55] and reduces symptoms in diabetic patients. However, there is no correlation between the degree of reduction of symptoms and the magnitude of enhancement of gastric emptying.[54,55,58] Even some patients with complete relief of nausea and vomiting may not demonstrate normalization or even improvement in gastric emptying. For example, Snape et al. reported that with metoclopramide the rate of liquid emptying at 60 minutes in diabetic patients increased from 32.8% to 56.8%; control subjects emptied 79.4% of the meal in

this period.[54] Seventy percent of the patients were symptomatically improved with metoclopramide treatment, and 50% experienced complete relief of symptoms with only minimal changes in the rate of emptying. A similar observation was made by Ricci et al., who observed that metoclopramide therapy was successful in reducing clinical symptoms but that it failed to improve gastric emptying in one-half of the patients.[58] This phenomenon may reflect the beneficial antiemetic effects of this drug independent of its prokinetic activity.

Even when metoclopramide therapy is effective in reducing symptoms and in promoting gastric emptying, these effects may be short-lived. Schade et al. studied the effects of acute and chronic therapy with metoclopramide on gastric emptying in diabetic patients (Fig. 51–11).[55] After receiving metoclopramide intravenously, 10 diabetic subjects with evidence of delayed emptying of liquids demonstrated an enhanced rate of emptying to a level comparable to that of normal subjects. The patients responded similarly to an oral dose of metoclopramide. When gastric emptying was reassessed in eight patients after 1 month of therapy with metoclopramide, in six patients the rate of gastric emptying had returned to the delayed pretreatment level. Nevertheless, all eight patients continued to experience symptomatic improvement. Other patients may initially improve with metoclopramide therapy but then experience a return of their symptoms after 1 or 2 months of treatment.

Metoclopramide is an effective antiemetic agent independent of its gastric prokinetic effects and is able to produce a striking reduction in the incidence of nausea and vomiting from other causes, including chemotherapy. Hence, in some studies of the effects of metoclopramide on the symptoms of diabetic gastroparesis, it is unclear whether its beneficial effects are due to its prokinetic activity or to its antiemetic activity.

Pharmacokinetics. The onset of action of metoclopramide is 1 to 30 minutes after intravenous injection, 10 to 15 minutes after intramuscular injection, and 30 to 60

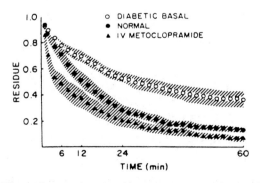
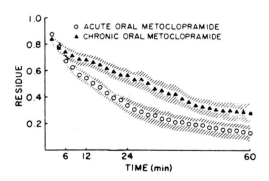

Fig. 51–11. Effect of metoclopramide on gastric emptying of liquids. Left: Residue curves for gastric liquid emptying in normal control subjects, diabetic subjects without metoclopramide treatment, and in diabetic subjects after intravenous administration of 10 mg of metoclopramide. Note that metoclopramide enhanced the rate of emptying and reduced gastric residue. Right: shows residue curve following a single 10-mg oral dose of metoclopramide and the response to the same dose after 1 month of chronic administration. Note that the beneficial effect of acute metoclopramide administration is lost with chronic therapy. Reprinted with permission from reference 55 (Schade RR, Dugas MC, Lhotsky DM, et al. Effect of metoclopramide on gastric liquid emptying in patients with diabetic gastroparesis. Dig Dis Sci 1985;30;10–5).

minutes after oral intake. The duration of action is 1 to 2 hours.[71,72]

Dosage and Administration. Metoclopramide is available as 5- and 10-mg tablets and as an injectable solution containing 5 mg/mL. It also is available as rectal suppositories.[73] The usual dose is 10 mg orally 15 to 30 minutes before meals and at bedtime. It is also available as a syrup for use in children. Oral therapy may not be effective in acute stages of the disease. In such circumstances it can be administered by slow intravenous injection, intramuscularly, or subcutaneously. Higher doses may be used if tolerated. In patients with renal failure, downward adjustment of the dose is necessary.

Side Effects and Drug Interactions.[68,69] As a dopamine antagonist that is capable of crossing into the CNS, metoclopramide is associated with many CNS adverse effects, which are seen in up to 20% of subjects. These include drowsiness, restlessness, anxiety, and depression. Dystonic symptoms, including tardive dyskinesia, oculogyric crises, opisthotonos, trismus, and torticollis, may occur. Parkinson-like symptoms, including tremor, rigidity, and akinesia, may be produced. Metoclopramide therapy may increase the risk of seizures in patients with underlying seizure disorders. In addition, its antidopaminergic activity enhances the release of prolactin and, in female patients, can lead to breast enlargement, nipple tenderness, galactorrhea, and amenorrhea. It also raises levels of aldosterone and thyrotropin and reduces levels of luteinizing hormone, follicle-stimulating hormone, and growth hormone. This drug should not be used in patients with pheochromocytoma, Parkinsonism, or seizure disorder. It should be used with care and in smaller doses in infants, children, and the elderly because of the greater incidence of side effects in these patients. Metoclopramide enhances the side effects of other D_2 receptor antagonists, such as the phenothiazines, and its prokinetic effects are annulled by the concomitant use of drugs with antimuscarinic properties. It enhances the effects of monoamine oxidase inhibitors.

Domperidone.[74] Domperidone is a benzimidazole derivative. Its use remains investigational in the United States, but it is available for clinical practice in both Canada and Europe.

Pharmacology. Domperidone is a D_2 receptor antagonist, but unlike metoclopramide it may not release acetylcholine from cholinergic nerves. However, it is a cholinesterase inhibitor. It does not cross as readily as metoclopramide into the CNS and hence is associated with a lower incidence of neurologic side effects. Domperidone enhances the frequency and amplitude of antral and duodenal contractions, enhances antroduodenal coordination, and enhances the rate of gastric emptying of both solids and liquids. In clinical studies in diabetic patients with gastroparesis, treatment with domperidone is associated with an improvement in both the rate of gastric emptying and the severity of clinical symptoms. However, as with metoclopramide, there is no correlation between the degree of improvement in symptoms and the magnitude of enhancement of gastric emptying.[53,63,71] Koch et al. studied the effect of domperidone treatment on symptoms of gastroparesis, the rate of

gastric emptying of a radionuclide-labeled solid meal, and gastric electrical activity as assessed by electrogastrography (EGG).[53] The six subjects studied had moderate to severe symptoms, delayed gastric emptying of solids, and abnormal EGG results. After 6 months of treatment with domperidone, all six patients reported improvement in their symptoms. However, the mean rate of gastric emptying was not significantly improved, and two patients showed no change or even a decrease in the rate. It is interesting that all six patients demonstrated a normalization of the gastric electrical activity on EGG. The observed discordance between the improvement in clinical symptoms and the lack of improvement in the rate of gastric emptying is analogous to that seen with metoclopramide. Horowitz et al. studied the acute and chronic effects of domperidone therapy on gastric emptying in diabetic patients.[63] With acute administration, domperidone did enhance the rate of emptying of both solids and liquids in these patients. After 4 weeks of treatment, however, oral therapy with domperidone enhanced the rate of emptying of liquids but not that of solids. As in other studies, clinical symptoms improved acutely and remain improved with chronic therapy.[75]

Pharmacokinetics. Peak plasma concentrations of domperidone are reached within 10 to 30 minutes after oral or intramuscular administration and from 1 to 3 hours after insertion of a rectal suppository. The bioavailability of intramuscularly administered domperidone is 90% in contrast to 15% for the orally administered drug.[70]

Dosage and Administration. The recommended dose of domperidone is 20 to 40 mg orally 60 minutes before meals and at bedtime. The usual total dose is 40 to 120 mg/day. It is also available as suppositories.[70] However, its intravenous use is not recommended in view of reports of associated cardiac arrhythmias.

Side Effects. Because domperidone does not cross the blood-brain barrier and enter into the CNS as readily as metoclopramide, the incidence of neurologic side effects is much lower with domperidone than with metoclopramide.[70] However, since both the chemoreceptor trigger zone and the site of prolactin release are located outside the blood-brain barrier, it acts as an antiemetic and causes hyperprolactinemia. In 10 to 15% of female patients, it causes breast enlargement, nipple tenderness, galactorrhea, and amenorrhea. The high incidence of these side effects is related to the higher doses of domperidone used. Other side effects include dry mouth, skin rash, itching, headache, diarrhea, and nervousness. Cardiac arrhythmias have been reported with intravenous administration. Domperidone is useful for the treatment of gastroparesis in patients with coincident Parkinson's disease, as it does not exacerbate the extrapyramidal symptoms of Parkinson's disease.

Cisapride.[76] Cisapride is a benzamide derivative that is chemically distinct from domperidone and metoclopramide.[71,76] The drug remains under investigation in the United States but is available for clinical therapy in both Canada and Europe.

Pharmacology. Cisapride has no antidopaminergic properties but enhances the release of acetylcholine in the intestinal myenteric plexus. It also has $5HT_3$-receptor antagonistic and $5HT_4$-agonistic properties. It enhances the amplitude of contractions throughout the gut, including the stomach and small and large bowels, and therefore its prokinetic effect extends through the entire gut. The increased gastroduodenal activity is associated with enhanced gastroduodenal coordination.[77] In therapeutic doses it has no effect on gastric acid secretion. In diabetic patients, it improves the rate of gastric emptying of both digestible and indigestible solids and liquids.[37,60,62,78,79] There is no correlation between the degree of cisapride-mediated improvement in clinical symptoms and the magnitude of enhancement of gastric emptying.[79,80] In contrast to the time-dependent deterioration of the beneficial effect of metoclopramide and domperidone, chronic therapy with cisapride is associated with continued enhancement of gastric emptying (Fig. 51–12). Horowitz et al. studied the effects of acute and chronic treatment with cisapride on the rates of gastric emptying of both solids and liquids in diabetic patients.[37] With acute therapy, cisapride not only reduced clinical symptoms but improved the rate of emptying of both solids and liquids. With chronic therapy with cisapride over 4 weeks, the pattern of symptomatic improvement continued; moreover, the enhanced rate of gastric emptying persisted. Of interest is the inverse relationship of the magnitude of improvement of gastric emptying to the rate of emptying with placebo; i.e., the patients who showed the greatest degree of improvement with cisapride were those with the slowest rate of emptying at baseline. Recently, Horowitz and Roberts reported that in one diabetic patient treated with cisapride for 14 months the rate of gastric emptying not only was still improved but was enhanced somewhat over earlier rates during treatment.[81]

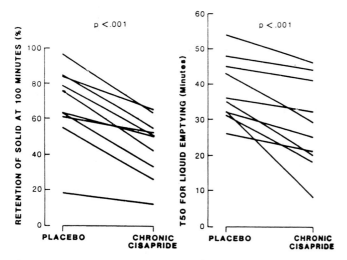

Fig. 51–12. Effect of administration of cisapride (10 mg qid) for 4 weeks on solid (percentage retention at 100 minutes) and liquid (50% emptying time, T50) gastric emptying. Reprinted with permission from reference 37 (Horowitz M, Maddox A, Harding PE, et al. Effect of cisapride on gastric and esophageal emptying in insulin-dependent diabetes mellitus. Gastroenterology 1987:92;1899–907).

Side Effects and Drug Interactions. Cisapride is associated with a low incidence of side effects. Since this drug lacks antidopaminergic properties, it does not have neurologic side effects. Infrequently reported side effects include headache, abdominal cramps, and diarrhea, reflecting the effect of this drug on the distal bowel.[71] Its prokinetic effect on the gut is blocked by agents with antimuscarinic properties.

Pharmacokinetics. The half-life of cisapride after intravenous administration is 19.4 hours. Bioavailability after oral administration is 35 to 40%. Plasma levels after ingestion of a 10-mg tablet peak at 1.5 to 2.0 hours.[71]

Dosage and Administration. Cisapride is available in Europe and Canada as 10-mg tablets for oral use. It is not available as suppositories or for parenteral use. The recommended dosage is 10 to 20 mg three times a day taken 30 to 60 minutes before meals.[71,79]

Motilin Agonists and Erythromycin (Motilides).
Erythromycin is a macrolide antibiotic.

Pharmacology. Erythromycin is known to have many gastrointestinal side effects. Itoh observed that, in the dog stomach, erythromycin in doses 2000 times smaller than the usual antibacterial doses induced typical phase II and phase III contractions that migrated to the duodenum and upper jejunum.[82] The contractile pattern induced by erythromycin was similar to a spontaneous or motilin-induced migrating motor-activity front. Erythromycin also caused endogenous release of motilin in the dog; therefore, the authors suggested that the action of erythromycin in inducing IMMCs is mediated indirectly by release of motilin.[82] Subsequent studies of isolated rabbit duodenum showed that erythromycin is a motilin agonist, interacting directly with motilin receptors.[83] Omura et al. have identified erythromycin derivatives, EM523 and EM536, that have no antibiotic activity but are up to 3000 times more potent than erythromycin in inducing IMMCs in the dog.[83]

Otterson and Sarna[84] studied in detail the motor effects of erythromycin on gastrointestinal motility. They found that erythromycin initiated IMMCs only when administered in very small doses (1 mg/kg intravenously) and not with larger doses. Larger doses (up to 25 mg/kg intravenously) initiated retrograde giant contractions and "vomiting complexes," periods of generalized inhibition of all activity, and giant peristaltic contractions. These higher doses also produced increased coordinated antroduodenal activity. Tomomasa et al. showed that erythromycin also induced migrating motor complexes in humans.[85] Moreover, Doty et al. observed that when control subjects were treated with intravenous erythromycin, 63.2% of the particles recovered from the duodenum were larger than 0.5 mm compared with only 7.7% of the particles of that size obtained from untreated control subjects.[86] Whether this abnormality in gastric emptying affects digestion and absorption remains unknown. In a recent study, the erythromycin derivative EM523 also was found to induce migrating motor complexes in a human volunteer, a finding suggesting that erythromycin derivatives may find an important place in the therapy for gastroparesis.[87]

In clinical studies, erythromycin enhanced gastric emptying of both liquids and solids in normal subjects as well as in diabetic subjects.[88,89] Janssens et al. reported that gastric emptying of liquid and solid meals in diabetic patients was shortened after intravenous administration of erythromycin (200 mg).[88] Two hours after a solid meal, the mean retention in the stomach was 63 ± 9% with a placebo and 4 ± 1% with erythromycin. This compares with 9 ± 3% retention in controls (Fig. 51–13). When this drug was administered orally over a period of 4 weeks, however, the effects on the rate of emptying of solids and liquids were significant but not of the magnitude observed with acute intravenous administration. To date, there are no controlled studies documenting a beneficial effect of intravenous or oral erythromycin therapy on symptoms of gastroparesis. Only a few anecdotal reports attest to the possible beneficial activity. It is not clear if the lack of lack of efficacy of oral therapy is related to the failure of absorption of erythromycin because of gastroparesis or to the occurrence of tachyphylaxis with chronic therapy.

Pharmacokinetics. After intravenous administration of erythromycin lactobionate, peak serum levels are reached 15 to 30 minutes after initiation of the infusion. The peak action following intravenous administration lasts for about 1 hour. Oral erythromycin succinate does not achieve as high a serum level as erythromycin stearate.

Dosage and Administration. Erythromycin is available for oral use as erythromycin stearate and erythromycin ethylsuccinate and for intravenous use as erythromycin lactobionate. The lactobionate is administered as an infusion over a 30-minute period at a dose of 200 mg diluted in normal saline. Lower doses (60 to 100 mg) may be effective. For oral use erythromycin stearate is used at doses of 250 mg administered three times a day 30 to 60 minutes before each meal.

Side Effects. Erythromycin administration has long been known to cause nausea, vomiting, and abdominal cramping in 80 to 95% of healthy subjects. These side effects of erythromycin in humans appear to be variants of those reported in dogs.

Treatment of Associated Conditions

If gastric bezoar is present, it can be disrupted with a water prick during endoscopy.[90] Alternatively, the patient is instructed to consume 1 to 2 L of clear liquids or a cellulase solution (0.5 g/dL of water) over a 24-hour period for 2 days or is administered an infusion of metoclopramide, 40 mg, over a 24-hour period for 3 days.[91,92] Some patients with diabetic gastroparesis have associated depression. These patients need sympathetic support, psychotherapy, and, if appropriate, antidepressant therapy. Because of the negative effects of drugs with anticholinergic properties on both gastroparesis and the action of prokinetic agents, antidepressive agents should be carefully selected and should include agents with minimal anticholinergic properties, such as desipramine (Norpramin), trazodone (Desyrel), and fluoxetine (Prozac). Some patients may also benefit from behavioral therapy.

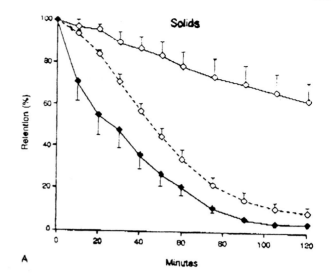

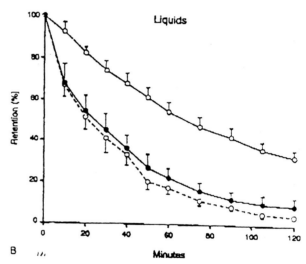

Fig. 51–13. Effect of erythromycin on gastric emptying of solids and liquids in diabetic gastroparesis. Top: Rate of emptying of the solid part of the test meal, expressed as the mean (±SE) percentage of isotope remaining in the stomach at various times after the ingestion of the meal, in 10 patients with diabetes after intravenous administration of placebo or 200 mg of erythromycin and in 10 healthy subjects. Bottom: Rate of emptying of the liquid part of the test meal, expressed as the percentage of isotope remaining in 10 patients with diabetes after the administration of placebo or erythromycin and in 10 healthy subjects. Diabetic subjects: placebo, open diamonds and open circles linked by solid lines; erythromycin, solid diamonds and solid circles linked by solid lines. Healthy controls: open diamonds and open circles linked by broken lines. Reprinted with permission from reference 88 (Janssens J, Peeters TL, Vantrappen G, et al. Improvement of gastric emptying in diabetic gastroparesis by erythromycin: preliminary studies. N Engl J Med 1990:322;1028–31).

Feeding Jejunostomy

The endoscopic placement of both percutaneous gastrostomies and jejunostomies may be useful in some diabetic patients with gastroparesis and malnutrition.[93,94] These procedures are successful if the tubes are carefully placed and maintained. It should be recognized that feeding jejunostomies, whether surgically or endoscopically placed, are useful palliative measures that can greatly improve hydration and nutrition. These devices relieve the patient of the need to eat and drink and thereby reduce the clinical symptoms of gastroparesis.

Surgery

In general, surgery is of no proven benefit in diabetic gastroparesis. The reported conservative gastric operations, such as loop gastroenterostomy and vagotomy and pyloroplasty, have been unsuccessful. Guy et al., who reported on two patients with gastroparesis, stressed that these patients were the only diabetic patients to have undergone elective surgery for gastroparesis in a 10-year period at their institution.[11] In these two patients, clinical improvement, but not complete relief of symptoms, was observed only after extensive operations resulting in subtotal gastrectomy, truncal vagotomy, and Roux en Y gastrojejunostomy. Reardon et al. reported their experience with surgery in a single patient.[95] Their patient failed to respond to a pyloroplasty but did seem to benefit from the placement of both a surgical gastrostomy, which aided in decompressing the stomach, and a jejunostomy, which was successfully employed for enteral feedings. They suggested that symptomatic and nutritional benefit in these patients resulted from the placement of a feeding jejunostomy. These experiences coincide with the observations of Karlstrom and Kelly, who suggested that the surgical management of states of gastric retention (postsurgical, idiopathic, and diabetic) will likely require a subtotal or near total gastrectomy with Roux en Y gastrojejunostomy.[96] In general, such surgery for diabetic gastroparesis should not be undertaken lightly.

SMALL BOWEL IN DIABETES

Motor and Electrical Activity

Normally, the fasting pattern of small-bowel motility is characterized by the presence of the cyclic interdigestive migrating motor complex (IMMC).[97] In the small bowel, as in the stomach, the IMMC is characterized by periods of motor silence (phase I), random motor activity (phase II), and intense motor activity (phase III). In the small bowel, phase III activity consists of high frequency (10 to 12 contractions/minute) complexes that are propagated distally through the entire small intestine. The highest frequency of contractions is determined by the rate of slow waves (pace-setter potential) in the small bowel. In normal subjects approximately 80% of phase III activity originates in the stomach, whereas 10 to 20% of such activity originates in the duodenum. In each case the initiated complex then travels distally. After a meal, small-bowel motility consists of randomly occurring nonpropulsive or segmental contractions.[97] Interspersed among the segmental contractions are some peristaltic contractions that propagate aborally for distances of several centimeters and cause periodic slow shifts of intestinal contents distally. Another type of small-bowel contraction is called a "giant contraction," as it is 1.5 to 2 times the amplitude and 4 to 6 times the duration of a normal contraction of the small bowel.[97] The giant contractions occur without regard to the intestinal slow waves. Normally, these giant contractions are present only in the distal small bowel. Abnormally, retrogradely propagated giant contractions occur during nausea and vomiting, and antegradely propagated giant contractions occur with a variety of pharmacologic manipulations that cause diarrhea.

Camilleri and Malagelada analyzed gastrointestinal motility by manometric studies in 14 diabetic patients with gastroparesis but no diarrhea. All of the patients had long histories of IDDM.[24] Striking abnormalities of both fasting and fed motor activity in the small bowel were observed: 1) Migrating motor complexes were noted in the small bowel in most of the patients, although 60% of the observed phase III complexes did not have an antral component; among the control subjects, only 8% of phase III complexes failed to originate in the antrum. 2) In 28% of the patients, the amplitude and frequency of duodenal and jejunal contractions was decreased. 3) In addition, in 64% of the patients, there were striking periods of marked phasic pressure activity that were not propagated; these complexes consisted of both short bursts and long periods of high frequency (10 to 12 contractions/minute) activity that were often isolated and not propagated distally as is characteristic of phase III activity. 4) After the test meal, 50% of the patients failed to develop the typical fed motor pattern; instead, these patients had a persistence of the long and short bursts of high frequency activity. The appearance of abnormal complexes was thought to be due to sympathetic denervation that might result in the loss of an inhibitory "brake," thus allowing the appearance of ectopic and uncoordinated high-frequency motor activity. The small-bowel motor patterns observed in the diabetic patients were similar to those observed in dogs following experimental ganglionectomy of the celiac and superior mesenteric plexuses.[98]

Dooley et al. studied fasting gastrointestinal motility in 12 diabetic patients with unexplained diarrhea and evidence of autonomic neuropathy.[99] In 16% of the patients, phase III activity was completely absent at all levels of the antrum, duodenum, and jejunum. In 81% of the patients, phase III activity had no antral component, whereas in 62.5% the proximal duodenum was not involved by the complex. In 12.5% of the patients, the observed phase III activity originated in the jejunum without antral or duodenal components. Furthermore, in three patients, phase III activity was abnormally propagated; in one of these patients, phase III activity appeared simultaneously in the small-bowel leads, and in the other two patients, the complex was conducted at an excessively rapid rate.

Small-Bowel Transit and Bacterial Overgrowth

Dooley et al., using the lactulose-hydrogen breath test, studied oral-cecal transit times.[99] Transit was prolonged in the diabetic patients (173 ± 20 minutes) compared with the time in control subjects (93 ± 10 minutes), but it is unclear to what extent the prolonged transit reflected delayed gastric emptying as opposed to delayed small-bowel transit. In those diabetic patients with delayed transit, there was no correlation between abnormal motility and individual transit times. It was of interest that 25% of the diabetic patients with diarrhea had evidence of bacterial overgrowth of the small bowel and improved clinically with antibiotic therapy. Two of the three patients in this study who had bacterial overgrowth did have phase III activity. However, the conduction of the complexes through the entire jejunum and ileum was not studied.

Wegener et al. incorporated lactulose into a radionuclide-labeled meal so that gastric emptying and small-bowel transit could be assessed simultaneously.[100] These authors studied 43 patients with IDDM who had been hospitalized for various diabetic complications; 60% had clinical evidence of autonomic neuropathy, 30% had vomiting, and 14% complained of diarrhea. The oral-cecal transit times of the diabetic patients were not significantly different from those of a large number of control subjects. However, more diabetic patients had delayed small-bowel transit (23%) compared with control subjects (3.6%), and even when patients with delayed gastric emptying were excluded, this trend among diabetic patients persisted. Although all six patients with diarrhea had delayed gastric emptying and evidence of autonomic neuropathy, there was no consistent pattern of rapid or delayed transit in these patients. Keshavarzian and Iber examined oral-cecal transit by the hydrogen breath-test technique in diabetic patients with and without peripheral neuropathy and autonomic neuropathy. Of the 25 patients studied, 12% had diarrhea and 16% had nausea without vomiting.[101] In both the diabetic and control subjects, the transit of a liquid meal to the cecum was more rapid than that of a solid meal. There was no significant difference between the transit times for either meal in control and diabetic patients. No significant differences in transit times were seen between diabetic patients with and without autonomic neuropathy and peripheral neuropathy. Sixteen percent of patients demonstrated rapid transit and 16% demonstrated slow transit, and there was no striking correlation between the clinical complaint of diarrhea and abnormal transit.

Gluten-Sensitive Enteropathy

Diabetes mellitus per se has no demonstrable effect on mucosal morphology or absorption in the small bowel. However, gluten-sensitive enteropathy (GSE) can coexist with diabetes and may be a cause of or contributor to diarrhea in such patients. Shanahan et al. undertook HLA subtyping in patients with diabetes mellitus, GSE, and both disorders.[102] HLA haplotypes B8 and DR3 were more prevalent in patients with GSE alone and patients with both diabetes and GSE. Therefore, some patients are at increased risk for developing both IDDM and GSE as a result of autoimmune features associated with their HLA status. In this study of 24 patients with both disorders, the diagnosis of GSE was made after the onset of clinical diabetes in more than one-half of the patients. Therefore,

when patients with diabetes and diarrhea show evidence of malabsorption and poor diabetic control, one should consider the possible coexistence of GSE and perform a small-bowel biopsy.

Intestinal Fluid Secretion

In streptozotocin-treated diabetic rats, net secretion of fluid and electrolytes by the intestine is increased. This increase is thought to be due to sympathetic denervation.[15] Sympathetic nerves release norepinephrine, which acts on α_2-adrenergic receptors present on the enterocytes.[103] The villous enterocyte responds to stimulation of the α_2-adrenergic receptor by stimulating intracellular Ca^{++}-mediated electroneutral NaCl absorption, and the crypt enterocyte responds to stimulation of the α_2-adrenergic receptor by stimulating intracellular Ca^{++}-mediated Cl^- secretion.[103] However, the adrenergic influences cause net fluid absorption. In the absence of adrenergic influence, a net secretion of fluid and electrolytes occurs in the small bowel, particularly in the postprandial state. In some patients with diabetic diarrhea, this secretory defect may be corrected by an agonist of α_2-adrenergic reception such as clonidine.[104]

COLON IN DIABETES

Colonic Motility

The normal colonic motor activity consists of short-duration contractions (<10 seconds), long-duration contractions (>1 minute), and peristaltic contractions (which are >1 minute in duration and two to three times larger in amplitude than other colonic contractions).[105] The short-duration contractions occur as a result of spikes associated with colonic slow waves.[105] They occur irregularly at a frequency of 3 to 12/minute, corresponding with the frequency of colonic slow waves. Long-duration contractions and giant contractions occur without regard to slow waves or spikes. The short- and the long-duration contractions occur singly or in trains and may be propagated or nonpropagated (segmental). The propagated wave may be propagated antegrade (peristaltic) or retrograde (retroperistaltic).[104] Segmental and retropulsive contractions form the main activity of the right colon. An increase in segmental contractions in the left side of the colon is associated with constipation, and a decrease is associated with diarrhea. Peristaltic short- and long-duration contractions are responsible for slow caudal shifts of colonic contents. The giant peristaltic contractions propagate at velocities of 2 to 3 cm/second and are responsible for rapid shifts of large volumes of colonic contents.[105] These movements are called "mass movements." Giant peristaltic contractions occur that sweep over the entire colon during defecation, but they also occur without associated defecation when they travel over a small segment of the colon. Mass movements are induced in the left side of the colon as a reflex response to stimulation such as eating (gastrocolonic reflex). These reflexes, mediated by neurohormonal influences and parasympathetic nerves, play an important role in giant peristaltic contractions and associated mass movements.

Information available on colonic electrical activity and motility in diabetics is limited. Battle et al. studied colonic myoelectric and motor activity in the sigmoid colon in 12 patients with IDDM; although 11 of the patients had clinical evidence of autonomic neuropathy, six had no or mild constipation and six patients had severe constipation as defined by a stool frequency of two or fewer stools per week.[106] After subjects consumed a 1000-calorie meal, both the myoelectric spike activity and the motor response were greater in the control than in the diabetic subjects (Fig. 51–14). Those patients with severe constipation had no postprandial response at all, whereas the six patients with mild constipation had a distinct but reduced postprandial response. In these latter diabetic patients, the myoelectric response was delayed until 60 to 90 minutes after the meal, in contrast to the physiologic response, which occurred during the first 30 minutes after the meal.

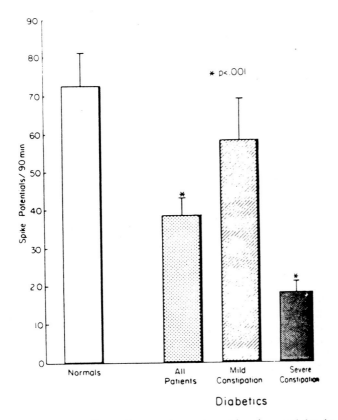

Fig. 51–14. Effect of a meal on sigmoid colon activity in diabetic patients. Note that the cumulative spike potential response after ingestion of a 1000-calorie meal is decreased in patients with diabetes mellitus. This decrease is most marked in patients who have severe constipation. Asterisk indicates significant ($P < .001$) decrease in response in various patient groups as compared with normal controls. Reprinted with permission from reference 106 (Battle WM, Snape WJ Jr, Alavi A, et al. Colonic dysfunction in diabetes mellitus. Gastroenterology 1980:79;1217–21).

Constipation and Colonic Dilation

There are no studies of comprehensive motor activity of the entire colon in diabetes. The constipation in diabetes is considered to be a complication of autonomic dysfunction of the gut, although no correlation was noted between the rate of gastric emptying of a liquid meal and the postprandial colonic spike activity.[106] Despite the decreased colonic motility, intramuscular administration of the cholinesterase inhibitor neostigmine stimulated colonic myoelectric activity to a normal level. Whereas the administration of neostigmine and metoclopramide are associated with increased colonic motor activity, neither agent has been shown to consistently improve the clinical pattern of constipation, probably because they increase the frequency of segmental contractions but do not promote overall colonic transit. Some diabetic patients with both gastroparesis and constipation may experience an improvement in their constipation during treatment with metoclopramide. Whether this beneficial effect reflects a direct action of metoclopramide on the colon or an indirect effect by increasing oral intake and promoting colonic bulk remains unclear. In clinical practice, constipation in a diabetic patient is treated conservatively with the usual methods using bulk agents (such as psyllium) and stool softeners. If these agents fail, laxatives used prudently can be quite helpful. Recently, cisapride was shown to have prokinetic properties in some but not all patients with idiopathic or diabetic constipation.[107] The eventual long-term role of cisapride, if any, in the management of diabetic constipation remains to be defined.

Infrequently, colonic dysfunction in diabetic patients may lead to more severe colonic disorders. Berenyi and Schwarz described 13 patients with autonomic dysfunction and marked sigmoid dilation.[108] Surprisingly, the majority of these patients experienced diarrhea. Diabetes was present in 9 of the 13 patients and was thought to be the underlying cause of the observed autonomic dysfunction.

DIABETIC DIARRHEA

Clinical Features

Diabetic diarrhea is a clinical syndrome of unexplained diarrhea in patients with IDDM.[109] By definition, "diabetic diarrhea" occurs in diabetic patients without an identifiable underlying gastrointestinal disorder and is therefore a diagnosis of exclusion. The clinical characteristics are quite variable, and presumably the underlying pathogenetic mechanisms are numerous and heterogeneous. Therefore, the pathophysiologic basis of so-called diabetic diarrhea is not the same in different patients, and hence they do not all respond to a common treatment. The vast majority of patients with this disorder have long-standing diabetes mellitus with its associated complications.[109] Almost all have evidence of both peripheral and autonomic neuropathy, and, indeed, autonomic neuropathy is thought to be an underlying mechanism. In the majority of affected patients, the pattern of diarrhea is intermittent, lasting weeks to months, with intervening periods of either normal stool frequency or constipation. Although original reports emphasized a predominantly nocturnal pattern of diarrhea, more recent series have described a variable pattern, with the majority of patients experiencing a persistent or predominantly daytime pattern.[109] Fecal incontinence is quite common. In diabetic diarrhea, stool weight can vary from 200 to 1600 g/day. Coincident steatorrhea can occur in 40 to 50% of patients,[109–111] is usually mild, and generally is not a cause of progressive weight loss. In a diabetic patient, the documentation of steatorrhea does not exclude the diagnosis of diabetic diarrhea but should prompt a careful exclusion of underlying jejunal and pancreatic disease.

Pathogenesis

Suggested mechanisms of diabetic diarrhea have included pancreatic exocrine insufficiency, altered intestinal motility, bacterial overgrowth, altered composition of the bile-salt pool and bile-salt excretion, and increased intestinal secretion as a result of autonomic neuropathy.[109]

Role of Exocrine Pancreatic Insufficiency

Given the high incidence of impaired pancreatic exocrine function in IDDM, exocrine insufficiency in steatorrhea would seem to be a possible mechanism of diabetic diarrhea. Because of the high capacity for enzyme secretion of the exocrine pancreas, however, the observed 50 to 60% reduction in bicarbonate and enzyme secretion does not impair luminal digestion and hence does not result in steatorrhea.[112,113] In patients with diabetic diarrhea, duodenal intubation studies have demonstrated either modest or no reduction in exocrine function.[109] Furthermore, empiric trials of pancreatic enzyme supplements have routinely been ineffective in reducing the volume of diarrhea in these patients.

Role of Abnormal Small-Bowel Motility and Bacterial Overgrowth

Abnormal small-bowel motility in diabetes may be associated with bowel stasis and bacterial overgrowth.[114] Clearance of luminal bacteria by normal small-bowel motility is sufficient to prevent the development of pathologic concentrations of bacteria. Normally, bacteria are present in the proximal small bowel in very low concentrations, and the concentration increases only with the stasis caused by obstruction or motility disorders. The interdigestive migrating motor complex (IMMC) has been found to be absent in intestine in some patients with diabetic diarrhea. Vantrappen et al. suggested that the absence of the IMMC correlated with the presence of bacterial overgrowth.[115]

In clinical studies, the prevalence of bacterial overgrowth in diabetic patients with diarrhea has ranged from 20 to 43%.[99,116] In one study, however, none of 11 patients had clinically significant bacterial overgrowth.[104] In patients with bacterial overgrowth, steatorrhea often is present as a result of impaired micelle formation caused by bacterial deconjugation and hydroxylation of bile salts.[104] The presence of bacterial overgrowth can be documented by 1) culture of jejunal contents,[116] 2) [14C]glycocholate[117] or [14C]xylose breath tests,[114] or 3) the glucose- or lactulose-hydrogen breath tests.[114] In clinical practice, one may alternatively observe the effect of an empiric trial of antibiotics (tetracycline or metronidazole) on the pattern of diarrhea and clinical symptoms. In patients with more complex forms of bacterial overgrowth that prove resistant to empiric antibiotic therapy, jejunal intubation studies should be performed so that accurate antibiotic sensitivity determinations can be done.

Autonomic neuropathy, by causing alterations in small-bowel motility, might result in rapid intestinal transit, which in turn may lead to diarrhea in affected diabetic patients. In contrast, however, careful studies suggest that transit through the small intestine in patients with diabetic diarrhea is delayed—not accelerated.[99,101] This slowing of transit has been documented both by breath tests[99,101] and by luminal sampling via multilumen tubes.[111] Although small-bowel motility is abnormal in diabetic patients with diarrhea, no specific pattern of abnormal motility was found to correlate with rapid or delayed transit.[99] It seems unlikely, therefore, that diabetic diarrhea is due to rapid intestinal transit. Rather, the demonstration of slow intestinal transit in this population is presumably the basis for the increased incidence of bacterial overgrowth.

Bile-Salt Malabsorption

Altered bile-salt circulation and kinetics through the gut have been suggested as possible causes of or contributors to diabetic diarrhea.[118] Bile salts usually are absorbed efficiently in the terminal ileum, and the passage of increased amounts of bile salts into the colon results in increased colonic secretion of fluid and electrolytes.[119] Observations in diabetic subjects suggest that increased amounts of bile salts escape ileal absorption and pass into the colon. Studies of kinetics and turnover of the bile-salt pool in diabetic patients with diarrhea indicate that metabolism of endogenous bile salts by intestinal bacteria is increased.[118] Although these results could be caused by abnormal contact between the bile salts and bacteria in the small bowel as a result of overgrowth, they more likely reflect the action of colonic bacteria on bile salts. In addition, the size of the bile-salt pool has been described as reduced and the fraction of the bile-salt pool that is excreted has been found to be increased.[118] Although bile-salt malabsorption does occur in diabetic patients with diarrhea, this phenomenon does not appear to be the mechanism of the diarrhea. For example, Schiller et al. found that increased fecal excretion of bile salts is a nonspecific finding in several forms of both clinical and experimental diarrhea and does not prove a pathogenetic basis of the bile-salt excretion in the diarrhea.[120] Indeed, there are no clinical data attesting to the efficacy of agents that bind bile salts (e.g., cholestyramine) in halting diabetic diarrhea.

Impaired Intestinal Fluid Absorption

Diarrhea in diabetic patients might also result from impaired intestinal absorption of fluid and electrolytes secondary to autonomic neuropathy. In experimental studies, Chang and Field demonstrated that a component of fluid and electrolyte absorption in the ileum and colon is mediated by α_2-adrenergic receptors.[103,104] Adrenergic-mediated fluid and electrolyte transport does not play a physiologic role in jejunal absorption. Studying the pathogenesis of diarrhea in rats with streptozotocin-induced chronic diabetes, Chang et al. demonstrated a decrease in sympathetic tone in the ileal and colonic mucosa that was presumably secondary to sympathetic denervation caused by autonomic neuropathy. The resulting reduction in absorption of fluid and electrolytes in these segments of the intestine produced clinical diarrhea.[15] In vitro studies also demonstrated that the impaired sympathetic tone in the ileum and colon was accompanied by adrenergic-denervation hypersensitivity, presumably as a result of an increase in the number of α_2-adrenergic receptors.[16] In the diabetic rat, administration of clonidine, an α_2-adrenergic agonist, can correct this defect in ileal and colonic absorption.[16]

Few clinical studies have directly examined intestinal fluid and electrolyte absorption in diabetic patients. Whalen et al. studied fluid and electrolyte absorption in the jejunum and ileum of 13 diabetic patients with unexplained diarrhea.[111] Under fasting conditions, the absorption of fluid and electrolytes in the jejunum and ileum of these patients was comparable to that of controls. Following the administration of a test meal, however, the volume of the test meal in the ileum was greater in diabetic than control subjects, suggesting that the ileal absorption of the fluid from the test meal was impaired. Indirect evidence of impaired sympathetic innervation of the gut in diabetic subjects with diarrhea also comes from the study of Fedorak et al.[110] In three patients with diabetic diarrhea, therapy with clonidine strikingly reduced the volume of diarrhea, presumably by stimulating intestinal adrenergic receptors. The prevalence of these different pathogenetic disorders (including impaired absorption) in a population of diabetic patients with diarrhea is not known. However, at least some fraction of diabetic patients appear to experience diarrhea related to the impaired fluid and electrolyte absorption in the ileum and colon caused by sympathetic denervation.

Diagnostic Studies

Diabetic patients with chronic intermittent or persistent diarrhea should undergo a careful evaluation.[109] A 72-hour stool collection should be made to assess the volume of stool as well as the magnitude of fecal excretion of fat. Evidence of bacterial overgrowth should be sought. In patients with steatorrhea, disorders of jejunal malabsorption, and pancreatic insufficiency should be carefully excluded. If the outlined evaluation fails to identify a definite source of diarrhea, it is likely that increased fecal-fluid excretion is due to impaired intestinal absorption of fluid and electrolytes.

Therapy

If the outlined evaluation identifies a specific cause of the diarrhea, specific therapy should be undertaken. If diagnostic studies for the presence of bacterial overgrowth are not available, it is reasonable to undertake an empiric trial of antibiotics. In patients for whom diagnostic studies are unrevealing and antibiotic therapy is unhelpful, trials of symptomatic therapy with diphenoxylate/atropine or loperamide are reasonable. Since diarrhea in these patients is episodic, symptomatic therapy can be used during periods of symptoms and later discontinued. In patients for whom symptomatic therapy is unsuccessful, a trial of clonidine is reasonable.[110,121-123] Regrettably, few data are available to guide the clinician in the dosage and schedule of clonidine. Furthermore, no data exist on the rate of success of clonidine therapy in diabetic patients with unexplained diarrhea. Fedorak et al. reported beneficial results with high doses of clonidine (0.5 to 0.6 mg) administered every 12 hours, but these were associated with side effects of excessive sedation. Since experimental studies suggest that a state of adrenergic hypersensitivity may exist, it is hoped that lower doses will be effective and better tolerated.[16] In diabetic patients with coincident diarrhea, autonomic neuropathy, and orthostatic hypotension, clonidine therapy does not appear to exacerbate the orthostatic hypotension, presumably because of the underlying neuropathy. At least one observer recommended topical administration of clonidine with a transdermal preparation.[123]

When diarrhea is severe and unresponsive to clonidine therapy, one should consider therapy with the somatostatin analogue octreotide.[124,125] Although the specific mechanism of somatostatin action in diabetic diarrhea is unknown, this drug has been demonstrated to both reduce intestinal mucosal secretion and enhance mucosal absorption under physiologic conditions[126,127] and in several intestinal disorders.[128,129] Octreotide must be administered parenterally, either subcutaneously in divided doses or intravenously through a constant-infusion pump. When administered in this fashion, octreotide has been demonstrated to produce striking reductions in the volume of diabetic diarrhea in a small number of patients.[124,125] Of interest, in this setting octreotide was also helpful in the management of refractory orthostatic hypotension.[125]

ANORECTAL FUNCTION IN DIABETES

Fecal Incontinence

Clinical Features

Fecal incontinence denotes the inability to retain stool and prevent its involuntary passage and can occur with or without the patient's knowledge. Although infrequent patients experience incontinence even with solid stool, the majority of affected individuals suffer this problem with liquid stool. The prevalence of fecal incontinence among diabetic patients is approximately 20%.[3] This figure, however, is likely an underestimate, since many embarrassed patients complain of diarrhea rather than incontinence. Diabetic patients frequently have both diarrhea and fecal incontinence. Almost one-third of affected patients have mild steatorrhea, which does not correlate with the volume of the diarrhea. Among diabetic patients, the frequency of incontinence varies from several episodes daily to a few episodes yearly and worsens during periods of diarrhea. On physical examination both continent and incontinent diabetic patients appear to have reduced resting and squeeze pressures in the anal canal. One should remember, however, that the subjective assessment of sphincter function on rectal examination correlates poorly with actual manometric measurements of sphincter pressure.[130]

Quantification

Schiller et al. assessed the anal continence mechanism for liquids and solids in diabetes. The continence mechanism for liquids was assessed by determining the volume of saline infused into the rectum that a person could hold without leaking. Both the intrarectal saline volume at which the first leak occurred and the total volume retained were much lower in incontinent diabetic patients than in continent diabetic patients or control subjects. Moreover, the volume at first leak showed a better correlation with clinical continence than did the strength of anal sphincter squeeze measured manometrically.[130] The anal continence mechanism for solids was determined by measuring the applied weight required to pull a solid sphere through the contracted sphincter. Diabetic patients with fecal incontinence expelled the spheres at lower applied weights than did the control subjects (Table 51–2).[131]

Pathogenesis

At the junction of the distal rectum and the pelvic floor, the anal canal extends as a slit-like lumen 2.5 to 5.0 cm through the diaphragm of the pelvis musculature.[132] One of the muscles of the diaphragm, the puborectalis, forms a sling of fibers that originates from both sides of the pubis symphysis and passes backwards to the posterior wall of the anorectal junction. This sling of voluntary striated muscle is innervated by branches of the sacral nerve (S3, S4), and its tonic contraction creates a relatively acute angle of 80 to 100 degrees at the anorectal junction (anorectal angle) that is thought to be a major contributor to the continence of solid stool.

The internal anal sphincter consists of a thickening of the rectal circular muscle that extends the length of the anal canal. It is composed of involuntary smooth muscle whose tonic contraction is due to intrinsic myogenic activity and a variety of neurohormonal influences. Sympathetic innervation via the hypogastric nerve (L5) results in contraction of the sphincter. The parasympathetic innervation via the pelvic nerves (S1, S2, S3) exerts both excitatory and inhibiting influences. The excitatory neurons are both cholinergic and noncholinergic. The inhibitory neurons are nonadrenergic, noncholinergic, and possibly involve nitric oxide and vasoactive intestinal peptide as neurotransmitters. It is estimated that the tonic contraction of the internal anal sphincter results in approximately 80% of the resting closure of the anal canal. With rectal distention the sphincter relaxes transiently (anorectal inhibitory reflex). Although the inhibitory reflex could "allow" incontinence of stool, sensation mediated by rectal distention results in both reflex and voluntary contraction of the external anal sphincter, resulting in closure of the anal canal.

The external anal sphincter consists of at least three bundles of striated muscle that surround the anal canal and act as a single unit. It is a voluntary muscle with innervation by the pudendal nerve (S2, S3, S4). Whereas the external sphincter demonstrates some tonic activity at rest (contributing to closure), its voluntary contraction is a major mechanism for continence of stool and flatus. The fibers of the pudendal nerve are cholinergic and exert their effect at the motor end-plate via nicotinic receptors. With rectal distention, the external anal sphincter contracts reflexly to close the anal canal (sphincteric reflex).

Rectal sensation is mediated by afferent pelvic splanchnic fibers passing to the sacral cord (S2, S3) and alerts the

Table 51–2. Effect of Diabetes on Anal-Sphincter Pressure and Anal Continence: Incontinent Diabetic Patients Have Sphincter Hypotension, Decreased Squeeze-Pressure Increment, and Marked Incontinence of Liquids

	Nondiabetic Controls (n = 35)	Incontinent Diabetics (n = 16)	Continent Diabetics (n = 14)
Basal pressure (mm Hg)	63 ± 4	37 ± 4	54 ± 5
Squeeze increment (mm Hg)	111 ± 13	75 ± 10	99 ± 18
Continence of solid sphere			
Weight held with sphincter relaxed (g)	685 ± 32	532 ± 52	624 ± 48
Weight held with sphincter contracted (g)	1065 ± 37	799 ± 64	951 ± 55
Continence of infused saline			
Saline infused before first leak (mL)	1253 ± 71	410 ± 107	1222 ± 424
Total saline held (mL)	1423 ± 39	715 ± 115	1328 ± 86

Table is reprinted with permission from reference 131 (Schiller LR, Santa Ana CA, Schmulen AC, et al. Pathogenesis of fecal incontinence in diabetes mellitus: evidence for internal-anal-sphincter dysfunction. N Engl J Med 1982;307:1666–71).

subject to rectal distention produced by stool or flatus. The stimulus of rectal distention causes one consciously or reflexly to contract the external anal sphincter and puborectalis.

Under physiologic conditions, the internal anal sphincter provides resting closure of the anal canal and some protection against rectal leakage and fecal stress incontinence. As stool passes into the rectum, distention of the rectum alerts one to contract both the external anal sphincter, which tightens the closure of the anal canal and the puborectalis, which further closes the anorectal angle. Contractions of the external anal sphincter and puborectalis nullify the relaxation of the internal sphincter associated with rectal distention. These mechanisms maintain continence until defecation is appropriate.

In diabetic patients with fecal incontinence, anorectal testing has demonstrated 1) decreased basal anal pressure,[131] 2) decreased rectal sensation,[133] and 3) an elevated threshold for the external anal sphincteric reflex[133] with a normal internal anal sphincter inhibitory reflex (Fig. 51–15).

The observed basal hypotonia of the anal canal is presumably caused by dysfunction of the internal anal sphincter secondary to diabetic autonomic neuropathy. Diabetic patients with fecal incontinence not only show evidence of autonomic neuropathy but also suffer from diarrhea, suggesting a distinctive pattern of sympathetic denervation of the gut that results in both impaired fluid absorption and dysfunction of the internal sphincter.[131]

Altered rectal sensation in diabetic patients is presumably a manifestation of sensory neuropathy and is not observed in patients with fecal incontinence related to other disorders. Since rectal sensation mediates the afferent limb of the sphincteric reflex, it is not surprising that the threshold for reflex contraction of the external

anal sphincter is also elevated. In diabetic patients, however, the threshold for anorectal inhibitory reflex is comparable to that for control subjects.[133] In this setting, fecal incontinence can occur since an amount of rectal distention that will induce relaxation of the internal sphincter may fail either to initiate reflex contraction of the external sphincter or to alert the subject to contract the sphincter voluntarily.

The voluntary squeeze pressures of the anal canal are also reduced in diabetic patients with fecal incontinence.[131] In these patients, squeeze pressures are lower than those of both continent diabetic patients and control subjects, but statistically significant differences exist only in comparisons between the incontinent patients and control subjects. This decrease in anal squeeze pressure is presumably the cause of the impaired rectal continence of infused saline and solid spheres in incontinent patients. The pathogenesis of this impairment in diabetic patients is unclear since anal squeeze pressures are mediated directly by the striated muscle of the external sphincter and indirectly by the somatic fibers of the pudendal nerve. Clarification of this question will require electromyographic studies of the external anal sphincter and the puborectalis as well as terminal motor latency studies of the pudendal nerve in diabetic patients.

Treatment

In diabetic patients, fecal incontinence usually occurs in relation to liquid stool. Since the success of attempts to develop continence is much greater if the patient has solid stools, every effort should be made to identify and treat the underlying cause of diarrhea. In some patients, trials of clonidine can be undertaken to control so-called diabetic diarrhea. In patients with functional diarrhea, the

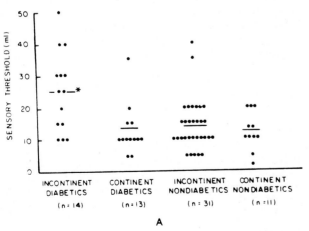

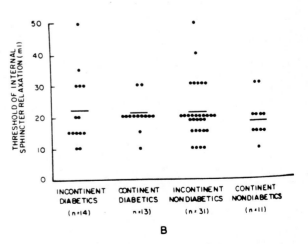

A   B

Fig. 51–15. Anorectal sensory thresholds and thresholds of internal anal sphincter relaxation in four groups of subjects. The mean threshold of rectal sensation (A) was significantly higher in the incontinent diabetic patients than in the other three groups of patients (P < .02), as indicated by the asterisk. There were no significant differences in thresholds of internal-sphincter relaxation (B). Note that in all groups except the incontinent diabetic patients the sensory threshold was lower than the threshold for internal anal sphincter relaxation. These observations suggest that fecal incontinence in diabetic patients may be due to an increase in the sensory threshold above the threshold for internal anal sphincter relaxation. (Reprinted with permission from reference 133 (Wald A, Tunuguntla AK. Anorectal sensorimotor dysfunction in fecal incontinence and diabetes mellitus: modification with biofeedback therapy. N Engl J Med 1984:310;1282–7).

use of antidiarrheal agents, such as loperamide and diphenoxylate/atropine, is helpful. If these measures are unsuccessful in achieving fecal continence, the performance of anorectal manometry is recommended. Basal anal-canal pressure, sensory threshold pressure for rectal distention, and internal anal-sphincter relaxation and external anal-sphincter contraction responses to rectal distention should be studied. If manometric studies demonstrate an elevated sensory threshold for rectal distention, biofeedback training can be helpful in obtaining symptomatic relief.

Biofeedback training in incontinent diabetic patients employs a balloon catheter to achieve both rectal sensory and external sphincter conditioning (Fig. 51–16). Using this technique, Wald and Tunuguntla reported improvement in 73% of diabetic patients, who achieved a reduction in fecal soiling without any striking change in stool frequency.[133] Improvement in fecal control correlated with the ability to improve both the sensory threshold and the threshold for phasic external-sphincter contraction. Most important, the manometric improvements did result in clinically meaningful improvements in lifestyle, as patients experienced a greater freedom of activity once the risk and frequency of rectal incontinence was reduced. Long-term testing demonstrated that the improvements in sensory and sphincter thresholds was sustained during periods of follow-up exceeding 1 year. Presumably, enhancement of sensory perception results from recruitment of adjacent neurons that mediate rectal sensation. By relearning the appropriate physi-

ologic response to rectal distention, patients thereby regain improved control over rectal function.

BILIARY SYSTEM IN DIABETES

Diabetic patients have physiologic reasons for being at increased risk for the formation of cholesterol gallstones.[134] First, in these patients, total body cholesterol synthesis is increased independent of obesity. Second, some diabetic patients do have diminished gallbladder motility, which could result in enhanced formation of cholesterol crystals.[135] Although older epidemiologic studies suggested an increased risk of gallstones in diabetic patients, these studies failed to differentiate the effects of obesity and hypertriglyceridemia from those of diabetes per se. Recent careful studies have suggested that diabetes per se does not predispose to secretion of abnormal bile.[135]

Lithogenic Bile

Under physiologic conditions, the liver secretes bile that is unsaturated with respect to cholesterol, and the relative amounts of bile salts and lecithin in the bile are capable of maintaining cholesterol in a stable solution.[136] Pathologic disorders that result in either a decrease in bile-salt secretion or an increase of cholesterol secretion will result in the formation of bile that is supersaturated with respect to cholesterol. Cholesterol crystals and eventually gallstones can develop from such lithogenic bile. Risk factors leading to the

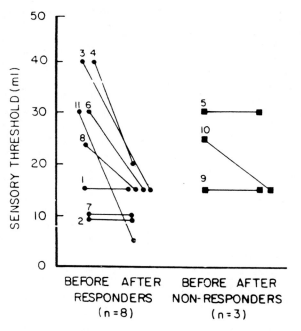

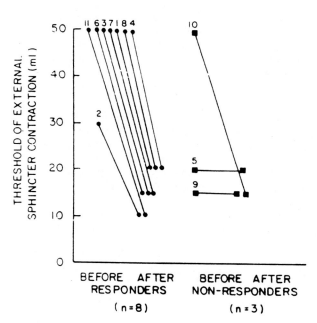

Fig. 51–16. Effect of biofeedback conditioning of rectal sensation on anorectal sensory threshold and threshold of external anal sphincter contraction in eight responders (decreased frequency of fecal incontinence) and three nonresponder diabetic patients. Left: Normalization of rectal sensory thresholds to less than 20 mL occurred in all but one patient with thresholds above 20 mL. No improvement in the sensory threshold was noted in patient 5. Right: Thresholds of external sphincter contraction showing strong association between improvement of the external sphincter response and reestablishment of bowel control. Reprinted with permission from reference 133 (Wald A, Tunuguntla AK. Anorectal sensorimotor dysfunction in fecal incontinence and diabetes mellitus: modification with biofeedback therapy. N Engl J Med 1984:310;1282–7).

secretion of lithogenic bile include 1) increasing age, 2) obesity, 3) hypertriglyceridemia, and 4) decreased size of the bile-salt pool.[135]

Haber et al. examined the lipid composition of bile in diabetic patients and in controls matched for obesity.[137] Patients with Type I and Type II diabetes were matched to nondiabetic control subjects by age, gender, and obesity index. The analyses demonstrated no significant difference between the cholesterol saturation of bile in diabetic patients and that of appropriately matched control subjects. The bile of patients with Type I diabetes was unsaturated with respect to cholesterol. Patients with Type II diabetes had a higher body-mass index and more-saturated bile than did patients with Type I diabetes. Thus, the risk of lithogenic bile is greater in patients with Type II diabetes than in those with Type I diabetes and is related to concurrent obesity rather than to diabetes itself.

Gallbladder Emptying

Earlier studies, using radiographic cholecystography, suggested that emptying of the gallbladder was delayed or impaired in diabetic patients.[138,139] More recent studies, however, using ultrasonography and scintigraphy, yielded contradictory results. Stone et al. used radionuclide cholescintigraphy to analyze gallbladder emptying in response to intravenous cholecystokinin octapeptide (CCK-OP). Stimulated gallbladder emptying was lower in diabetic patients than in controls (55% vs. 74%).[140] Furthermore, the most severe impairment of gallbladder emptying occurred in diabetic patients with associated autonomic neuropathy. Keshavarzian et al. found contrasting results in an examination of fasting gallbladder volume and postprandial emptying using ultrasonography.[141] Among the diabetic patients, both fasting and postprandial gallbladder volumes were comparable to the respective values in controls. No effect of autonomic neuropathy on gallbladder emptying could be demonstrated.

It is difficult to reconcile the differences in gallbladder motor function reported in these two studies. Obvious methodologic differences between ultrasonography and cholescintigraphy exist, but no data identifying which technique is a better measure physiologically are available. Similarly, the two studies used different methods for inducing gallbladder emptying—maximally effective doses of CCK-OP vs. a test meal. It appears, therefore, that no consistent pattern of gallbladder motor dysfunction exists in diabetic patients.

Gallstones

Prevalence

In keeping with these contrasting observations about gallbladder function among diabetic patients, recent studies have also yielded contradictory results concerning the prevalence of gallstones in this population. The results of both autopsy studies[142,143] and epidemiologic studies[144,145] have conflicted. For example, a large case-control study from Canada failed to find any association between cholesterol cholelithiasis and clinical diabetes.[146] Hence, if diabetes does affect the prevalence of gallstones, the effect is small.

Treatment

The surgical approach to the management of asymptomatic gallstones has been changing greatly. As pointed out by Pellagrini, several observations have discouraged the routine use of surgery in nondiabetic patients with asymptomatic gallstones.[147] Among such patients, relatively few develop symptoms during periods of follow-up as long as 20 years. In addition, life-threatening complications of gallstone disease are rarely the first manifestation. Milder symptoms of biliary colic usually arise first and prompt a timely surgical referral before the appearance of acute cholecystitis and cholangitis. Furthermore, long-term follow-up of many patients with mild symptoms indicates that the majority remain free of serious complications. Finally, autopsy studies indicate that more than 90% of patients with gallstone disease die of unrelated cause.

The role of surgery in diabetic patients with asymptomatic gallstones has been controversial. In the past, it was believed that diabetic patients with cholelithiasis should undergo surgery, even if asymptomatic, to avoid the increased morbidity and mortality presumed to occur in diabetic patients. This aggressive perspective originated with Rabinowitch in 1932, who suggested that patients with diabetes and cholecystitis fared worse than patients without diabetes.[148] A subsequent study by Eisele in 1943 supported this observation.[149] In 1961, Turrill et al. reported that the mortality rate after surgery for gallstones was fivefold higher in diabetic patients.[150] Deaths in that series occurred primarily in diabetic patients undergoing emergency surgery. When the analysis was limited to patients in the fifth and sixth decades of life who underwent emergency cholecystectomy, the mortality among diabetic patients was reported to be twentyfold higher than that among nondiabetic patients. In a contemporary study, Mundth also reported increased morbidity and mortality associated with emergency surgery for gallstones among diabetic patients and recommended elective surgery for gallstones when possible, since the mortality among diabetic patients with elective surgery was comparable to that of among nondiabetic patients.[151] Both Turrill and Mundth even recommended that all diabetic patients undergo screening with oral cholecystography and that all patients with gallstones undergo elective surgery.[150,151]

More recent analyses of the morbidity and mortality of gallstone surgery among diabetic patients criticized the conclusions of these earlier studies with respect to several issues: first, modern morbidity and mortality rates are much lower as a result of the use of antibiotics and improvements in medical and surgical care; second, earlier studies failed to report the prevalence of concurrent medical disorders among the diabetic patients (e.g., atherosclerosis) that might affect the rate of postoperative complications independent of diabetes; and finally, studies such as that of Mundth failed to include a contemporary control group that was analyzed over a comparable period.

Within the last 10 years, four retrospective studies examined the morbidity and mortality among diabetic patients with surgical gallstone disease more critically.[152–155] Diabetic patients undergoing surgery tended to be older than nondiabetic patients and have more concurrent medical disorders, especially cardiovascular disease. There was a trend towards increased surgical mortality among the diabetic patients, but this difference was statistically significant in only one study. It is interesting that in a review of a 21-year period at one institution, the case-fatality rate among diabetic patients with surgical gallstone disease decreased over the course of the study, presumably as a result of improvements in medical and surgical care.[152]

In both diabetic and nondiabetic patients, morbidity and mortality were increased in the setting of emergency surgery and with preoperative evidence of cardiovascular and renal disease. In none of the studies was diabetes per se a risk factor for increased operative mortality. Analyses indicated that the presence of preoperative concurrent medical disorders predicted postoperative morbidity and mortality more accurately than did the presence of diabetes. In reviewing earlier surgical studies, Walsh et al. suggested that 50 to 80% of the diabetic patients in those studies showed evidence of occlusive vascular disease, which might have accounted for the observed increase in morbidity and mortality independent of diabetes.[155]

There was a trend towards increased postoperative complications among diabetic patients, but it is unclear whether this risk is related to diabetes or to concurrent medical disorder. Hickman et al. observed that with emergency cholecystectomy the incidence of postoperative infectious complications was higher in diabetic patients, an increase that could not be explained by any pattern of concurrent medical disorders.[153] In contrast, Sandler et al., applying regression analysis, demonstrated that the twofold higher rate of postoperative complications in diabetic patients was related to coincident medical problems rather than to diabetes per se. Furthermore, the increased incidence of postoperative complications among diabetic patients occurred with both emergency and elective cholecystectomy.[154]

In summary, the current data do not support elective cholecystectomy in diabetic patients with asymptomatic gallstones. Nevertheless, since emergency cholecystectomy for acute cholecystitis is associated with increased morbidity and possibly increased mortality, one should consider elective surgery in those diabetic patients with concurrent biliary symptoms, especially if serious medical disorders do not coexist. Laparoscopic cholecystectomy may provide a safer and preferable alternative to abdominal cholecystectomy.[156]

EXOCRINE PANCREAS AND DIABETES

Diabetes in Pancreatic Disease

It is well known that primary disorders of the exocrine pancreas can affect islet cell function and result in states of glucose intolerance or in distinct diabetes mellitus. For example, with acute pancreatitis of any etiology, hyperglycemia can result and is recognized as a prognostic sign of severity of pancreatitis.[157] In this setting, hyperglycemia is thought to be secondary to increased circulating levels of glucagon and epinephrine rather than to islet destruction with actual insulin deficiency.[158] Indeed, individuals who are not diabetic before an episode of acute pancreatitis will again achieve normal glucose control after resolution of the episode. In contrast, both diabetes and glucose intolerance are recognized complications of advanced chronic pancreatitis. The advanced stages of pancreatic injury and fibrosis result in damage to the islets, with resulting insulin deficiency and chronic diabetes.[159]

Exocrine Pancreas in Diabetes

Well-recognized changes in pancreatic exocrine morphology and function have been identified in idiopathic diabetes mellitus. In Type I diabetes, there is widespread islet atrophy and fibrosis with associated atrophy and fibrosis in the surrounding exocrine tissue.[160] Careful studies of pancreatic histology in patients who died shortly after initial presentation of Type I diabetes are of interest.[161] In these patients, the effects of Type I diabetes on the endocrine and exocrine pancreas are halted at a relatively early stage. In parts of the diabetic pancreas where the islets remain intact and concentrations of insulin in β-cells determined immunohistochemically are normal, the surrounding exocrine tissue appears normal. In contrast, in those areas where the islets have atrophied, the surrounding acinar tissue also is atrophied. These observations support the hypothesis that insulin and other islet-cell peptides have trophic effects on the surrounding acinar cells and are consistent with a microcirculatory architecture of the pancreas.[162] Blood traveling through islet capillaries supplies surrounding exocrine tissue and exposes the acinar cells to high concentrations of islet-cell peptides. Both insulin and pancreatic polypeptide appear to have trophic effects on acinar glands, whereas glucagon and somatostatin may have inhibitory effects.[163] By this theory, islet dysfunction resulting in either decreased levels of trophic hormones or increased levels of inhibitory peptides could result in exocrine dysfunction.[161,163]

In Type II diabetes, the changes in the islets are less extensive, with variable reduction of the β-cells; there is hyalinosis of the islets of varying extent and severity. The associated changes in the surrounding exocrine tissue are less extensive than those seen in Type I diabetes but are easily demonstrated nevertheless. As indicated by ultrasound examination, the overall size of the pancreas is smaller than in control subjects.[164] On histologic study, the reduction in gland size correlates with atrophy and fibrosis of exocrine tissue.

Careful studies of pancreatic exocrine function in diabetes have demonstrated a surprisingly high prevalence of dysfunction.[111,165] Exocrine function has traditionally been measured by duodenal intubation and collection of pancreatic secretions following stimulation of the gland with both cholecystokinin and secretin. More recently, exocrine function was measured indirectly by assessing serum levels of immunoreactive trypsin, which were shown to correspond with exocrine secretions into the duodenal lumen.[166] Both direct[111,165] and indirect measures[166] of exocrine function identify moderate degrees of exocrine deficiency in 65 to 80% of patients with Type I diabetes. With direct studies, both amylase and bicarbonate secretion were found to be reduced 55 to 65%.[111,165] Despite the marked reduction in exocrine function in a large fraction of the diabetic population, steatorrhea caused by exocrine insufficiency is quite rare owing to the large secretory capacity of the exocrine pancreas.[167] Both direct and indirect studies of exocrine function found a significant correlation between the declining endogenous insulin secretion, as measured by C-peptide concentration, and amylase and bicarbonate output.[165,166] In some studies the reduction in exocrine function worsened with time and corresponded to the progressive decline in concentrations of C-peptide.[165] This correlation is thought to represent the causal effect of insulin deficiency on exocrine function and would support the hypothesis of the trophic effects of insulin on exocrine function. Hence, with a decline in the release of endogenous insulin in Type I diabetes, the surrounding acinar cells atrophy, with resulting exocrine dysfunction. In Type II diabetes for which insulin therapy is not required, there is also a demonstrable decrease in exocrine secretion but of a magnitude smaller than that observed in Type I diabetes and insulin-dependent Type II diabetes.[165]

Although the presence of autonomic neuropathy could reduce pancreatic exocrine secretion as a result of reduced secretomotor action, careful secretory studies have suggested that this is not the case.[111] In patients with IDDM, the decreased exocrine secretion cannot be corrected with supramaximal concentrations of cholecystokinin and secretin. In addition, when bethanechol was administered simultaneously with cholecystokinin and secretin, the additional cholinergic stimulation also failed to correct the decrease in exocrine secretion. These data are seen to indicate a reduction in or atrophy of the acinar cell mass rather than an alteration in the secretomotor activity of the nerves or hormones on the pancreas.

Hyperamylasemia and Pancreatitis

Hyperamylasemia has been reported in 46 to 79% of patients with diabetic ketoacidosis.[168] Abdominal pain and tenderness occur in up to 45%, and a history of vomiting exists in up to 73%.[168] In the past, this constellation of symptoms and findings was attributed to acute pancreatitis. However, more recent careful analyses have indicated that acute pancreatitis is rarely present in diabetic ketoacidosis and hence is not a common cause of the abdominal symptoms and hyperamylasemia. Hyperamylasemia is often not present at the initial presentation with ketoacidosis but can develop later during hospitalization.[168] The magnitude of serum amylase elevation is variable, but the level reaches up to six times higher than

normal, which is an elevation often considered specific for acute pancreatitis.[169] However, there is no correlation between hyperamylasemia and the abdominal symptoms, and hyperamylasemia occurs with equal frequency in patients with and without these symptoms. In the vast majority of patients with ketoacidosis and hyperamylasemia, isoamylase testing has demonstrated that the major contributor to the elevation is a salivary-type, rather than a pancreatic, isoamylase. Simultaneous lipase levels are usually normal. The source of the salivary-type isoamylase is unclear, since all forms of isoamylase other than pancreatic isoamylase are assayed as the salivary-type isoenzyme. Hyperamylasemia may be a consequence of acidemia per se rather than a specific consequence of diabetic acidosis. Eckfeldt et al. collected serum from 33 patients with metabolic or respiratory acidosis in the absence of diabetic acidosis or renal failure.[170] The total serum amylase level was elevated in 36% of these patients, and five patients had marked elevations in a range usually considered diagnostic of acute pancreatitis. There was a trend toward a greater prevalence of hyperamylasemia with worsening acidosis, but the difference was not statistically significant. As in other studies of hyperamylasemia, the majority of patients had a salivary-type isoamylase of unknown origin and almost all affected patients had normal lipase levels.

The cause of the abdominal symptoms in diabetic ketoacidosis remains uncertain but is likely not related to pancreatitis. Alternate explanations for the pain have included intestinal ileus or gastric dilatation caused by the underlying acidosis. In patients presenting with diabetic ketoacidosis and hyperamylasemia, for whom a reasonable question exists regarding the presence of pancreatitis, examination of the lipase level and studies of pancreatic morphology by abdominal imaging should be helpful.

Although there is no known association between diabetes mellitus and pancreatitis, two important associations should be recognized. First, the incidence of gallstones may be increased in Type II diabetes mellitus because of coincident obesity.[137] In this setting acute pancreatitis secondary to the passage of gallstones can occur.[171] Second, Type IV hyperlipoproteinemia occurs more frequently in Type II diabetes. In susceptible patients high dietary fat intake might turn Type IV hyperlipoproteinemia into Type V hyperlipoproteinemia, which is associated with an increased risk of acute pancreatitis.[171]

LIVER IN DIABETES MELLITUS

Increased Hepatic Glycogen

It is surprising that hepatic glycogen is increased in some diabetic patients, since adequate serum levels of insulin are necessary to stimulate glycogen synthesis. Nevertheless, in some patients with Type I diabetes, increased hepatic glycogen does occur and results in or contributes to clinical hepatomegaly.[172] Among these patients, the disorder is observed with increased frequency in patients with "brittle" diabetes who are prone to hypoglycemia. In these patients, intermittent excesses in insulin therapy appear to achieve the serum levels necessary to stimulate glycogen synthesis in the liver. Although increased hepatic glycogen can cause hepatomegaly, it does not produce clinical liver dysfunction as typified by abnormal laboratory testing or clinical symptoms.[173]

Diabetic Fatty Liver

Hepatic steatosis is defined as the accumulation of lipid by the liver, usually in the form of triglyceride, such that the weight of lipid exceeds 5% of the total weight of the liver.[172,174] Histologic studies indicate that diabetic hepatic steatosis can produce either microvesicular or macrovesicular deposition of fat. In general, with marked fatty infiltration, there is macrovesicular fatty deposition with some hepatocellular destruction.[175] Hepatocyte necrosis is usually mild and is not associated with an inflammatory infiltrate.

It is difficult to estimate accurately the incidence of this lesion in diabetes since a percutaneous liver biopsy is necessary for proper identification. The medical literature reports a wide range in incidence, differences that are probably due to the large variation in body weight of patients as well as to the effect of the type of diabetes on this disorder. In Type I diabetes the incidence of hepatic steatosis is low (4 to 17%).[172,176] In these patients, hepatic steatosis is related to inadequate serum levels of insulin and hence to poor diabetic control. Increased mobilization of fatty acids from peripheral adipose tissue results in an increased hepatic concentration of fatty acids and enhanced hepatic synthesis of triglyceride and very-low-density lipoprotein (VLDL).[172] Both hyperlipidemia and hepatic steatosis are readily reversible with appropriate insulin therapy. Because of this reversibility, the incidence of hepatic steatosis in Type I diabetes remains relatively low.

In Type II diabetes, the incidence of hepatic steatosis is high (21 to 78%) and is related primarily to concurrent obesity rather than to the duration of the diabetes or the adequacy of control.[172,177] It is difficult to differentiate the effect of diabetes from that of obesity in the pathogenesis of fatty liver in this setting. In patients with morbid obesity, without coincident diabetes, the incidence of fatty liver can be as high as 94%.[175,178]

In Type II diabetes, the pathogenesis of hepatic steatosis is multifactorial.[172,175] Increased serum and hepatic fatty acids found in these patients result in an increased rate of hepatic triglyceride synthesis that exceeds a relatively normal rate of hepatic secretion of VLDL. In Type II diabetes, hepatic steatosis is less readily reversible and is managed more effectively by the introduction of a low-calorie, low-carbohydrate diet with achievement of weight loss.

In general, the hepatic steatosis of diabetes produces asymptomatic hepatomegaly and few if any clinical symptoms. The results of laboratory studies of hepatic function and injury tend to be normal. Mild elevation of these test values have been documented in up to 18% of unselected patients with either Type I or Type II diabetes. Laboratory abnormalities are more likely with the measurement of the alkaline phosphatase and γ-glutamyltranspeptidase.[174,179] Diagnostic imaging studies can document the presence of hepatic steatosis; an abdominal computed tomographic (CT) scan can show decreased hepatic density caused by fatty infiltration, and abdominal ultrasonography demonstrated a reflective or "bright" pattern in 23% of unselected patients in one series.[174,180]

The natural history of hepatic steatosis of diabetes is controversial. In general this lesion is benign and not prone to progression to a more severe hepatic injury. Indeed, it is rare to document actual cirrhosis as a consequence of hepatic steatosis.[171]

Diabetic Steatonecrosis

A more severe histologic lesion has been described in some patients with diabetic fatty liver. Steatonecrosis ("nonalcoholic steatohepatitis" or "fatty liver hepatitis") produces changes similar to those seen in alcoholic hepatitis or following ileojejunal bypass in obese patients.[172,177,181] The histologic findings are of moderate steatosis with macrovesicular fatty change. There are findings of both periportal and pericentral fibrosis. Hepatocellular degeneration and necrosis can occur, with intracellular hyalin bodies identical to Mallory bodies. Although chronic inflammatory cells may infiltrate the portal areas, there is no infiltration by polymorphonuclear cells, a finding that may distinguish this lesion from that of alcoholic hepatitis. In the latter lesion, infiltration by polymorphonuclear cells is common and almost pathognomonic in the setting of the other histologic findings. In some patients with diabetic steatonecrosis, bridging fibrosis between portal tracts and central veins may exist.

As might be expected, steatonecrosis is more common in patients with Type II diabetes, particularly in middle-aged, obese women.[177] Although it usually presents as asymptomatic hepatomegaly with abnormal values in liver function tests, in rare cases the patient presents with complaints of fatigue and with ascites. Laboratory studies can demonstrate marked elevations of the sedimentation rate as well as mild to moderate elevations in alkaline phosphatase and γ-glutamyltranspeptidase levels; elevations of transaminases tend to be mild. In general, the levels of bilirubin, albumin, and globulin are normal.

In initial reports, the finding of pericentral fibrosis raised concerns regarding the progression of this lesion to more severe liver disease. In other disorders, sclerosis of the terminal hepatic venules represents an index of progressive liver injury that may signal the eventual development of cirrhosis.[182] In steatonecrosis, however, progression to more severe liver disease seems quite uncommon. In one study, bridging fibrosis was found in those patients with diabetes of longer duration.[177] Actual cirrhosis proved to be quite rare. In a study that provided long-term follow-up of 35 patients with nonalcoholic steatohepatitis, the hepatic histology in 91% of the patients remained stable or changed only slowly.[183] Only 9% of the patients demonstrated deterioration of the histologic lesion, and cirrhosis was found in only two patients.

Steatonecrosis in a patient with Type I diabetes mellitus has been reported.[181] Although this patient presented with mild jaundice and hepatosplenomegaly, liver biopsy did not demonstrate cirrhosis. With improved diabetic control, the liver function test became normal, hepatosplenomegaly resolved, and serial imaging studies by abdominal CT scan demonstrated a return of hepatic density to near normal values.

REFERENCES

1. Yang R, Arem R, Chan L. Gastrointestinal tract complications of diabetes mellitus: pathophysiology and management. Arch Intern Med 1984;44:1251–6.
2. O'Reilly D, Long RG Diabetes and the gastro-intestinal tract. Dig Dis 1987;5:57–64.
3. Feldman M, Schiller LR. Disorders of gastrointestinal motility associated with diabetes mellitus. Ann Intern Med 1983;98:378–84.
4. Rothstein RD. Gastrointestinal motility disorders in diabetes mellitus. Am J Gastroenterol 1990;5:782–5.
5. Keshavarzian A, Iber FL. Gastrointestinal involvement in insulin-requiring diabetes mellitus. J Clin Gastroenterol 1987;9:685–92.
6. Furness JB, Costa M. The enteric nervous system. London: Churchill Livingstone, 1987.
7. Goyal RK, Crist JR. Neurology of the gut: pathophysiology, diagnosis, management. In: Sleisenger MH, Fordtran JS, eds. Gastrointestinal disease. 4th ed. Vol 1. Philadelphia: WB Saunders, 1989:21–52.
8. Diani A, West C, Vidmar T, et al. Morphometric analysis of the vagus nerve in non-diabetic and ketonuric diabetic Chinese hamsters. J Comp Pathol 1984;94:495–504.
9. Smith B. Neuropathology of the oesophagus in diabetes mellitus. J Neurol Neurosurg Psychiatry 1974;37:1151–4.
10. Duchen LW, Anjorin A, Watkins PJ, Mackay JD. Pathology of autonomic neuropathy in diabetes mellitus. Ann Intern Med 1980;92:301–3.
11. Guy RJC, Dawson JL, Garrett JR, et al. Diabetic gastroparesis from autonomic neuropathy: surgical considerations and changes in cagus nerve morphology. J Neurol Neurosurg Psychiatry 1984;47:686–91.
12. Yoshida MM, Schuffler MD, Sumi SM There are no morphologic abnormalities of the gastric wall or abdominal vagus in patients with diabetic gastroparesis. Gastroenterology 1988;94:907–14.
13. Feldman M, Corbett DB, Ramsey EJ, et al. Abnormal gastric function in longstanding insulin-dependent patients. Gastroenterology 1979;77:12–7.
14. Buysschaert M, Donckier J, Dive A, et al. Gastric acid and pancreatic polypeptide responses to sham feeding are impaired in diabetic subjects with autonomic neuropathy. Diabetes 1985;34:1181–5.
15. Chang EB, Bergenstal RM, Field M. Diarrhea in streptozocin-treated rats: loss of adrenergic regulation of intestinal fluid and electrolyte transport. J Clin Invest 1985;75:1666–70.
16. Chang EG, Fedorak RN, Field M. Experimental diabetic diarrhea in rats: intestinal mucosal denervation hypersensitivity and treatment with clonidine. Gastroenterology 1986;91:564–9.
17. Belai A, Burnstock G. Selective damage of intrinsic calcitonin gene-related peptide-like immunoreactive enteric nerve fibers in streptozotocin-induced diabetic rats. Gastroenterology 1987;92:730–4.
18. Lincoln J, Bokor JT, Crowe R, et al. Myenteric plexus in streptozotocin-treated rats: neurochemical and histochemical evidence for diabetic neuropathy in the gut. Gastroenterology 1984;86:654–61.
19. Nowak JTV, Harrington B, Kalbfleisch JH, Amatruda JM. Evidence for abnormal cholinergic neuromuscular transmission in diabetic rat small intestine. Gastroenterology 1986;91:124–32.
20. Campbell IW, Duncan LJP, Innes JA, et al. Abdominal pain in diabetic metabolic decompensation: clinical significance. JAMA 1985;233:166–8.
21. Longstreth GF, Newcomer AF. Abdominal pain caused by diabetic radiculopathy. Ann Intern Med 1977;86:166–8.
22. Conklin J, Goyal RK. Gastrointestinal smooth muscle. In: Sleisenger MH, Fordtran JS, eds. Gastrointestinal disease. 4th ed. Vol 1. Philadelphia: WB Saunders, 1989:53–78.
23. Fox S, Behar J. Pathogenesis of diabetic gastroparesis: a pharmacologic study. Gastroenterology 1980;78:757–63.
24. Camilleri M, Malagelada J. Abnormal intestinal motility in diabetics with the gastroparesis syndrome. Eur J Clin Invest 1984;14:420–7.
25. Borgström PS, Olsson R, Sundkvist G, Ekberg O. Pharyngeal and oesophageal function in patients with diabetes mellitus and swallowing complaints. Br J Radiol 1988;61:817–21.
26. Sundkvist G, Hillarp B, Lilja B, Edberg O. Esophageal motor function evaluated by scintigraphy, video-radiography and manometry in diabetic patients. Acta Radiol 1989;30:17–9.
27. Westin L, Lilja B, Sundkvist G. Oesophagus scintigraphy in patients with diabetes mellitus. Scand J Gastroenterol 1986;21:1200–4.
28. Keshavarzian A, Iber FL, Nasrallah S. Radionuclide esophageal emptying and manometric studies in diabetes mellitus. Am J Gastroenterol 1987;82:625–31.
29. Steffey DL, Wahl RL, Shapiro B. Diabetic oesophagoparesis: assessment by solid phase radionuclide scintigraphy. Nucl Med Commun 1986;7:165–71.
30. Clouse RE, Lustman PJ, Reidel WL. Correlation of esophageal motility abnormalities with neuropsychiatric status in diabetics. Gastroenterology 1986;90:1146–54.
31. Channer KS, Jackson PC, O'Brien I, et al. Oesophageal function in diabetes mellitus and its association with autonomic neuropathy. Diabetic Med 1985;2:378–82.
32. Maddern GJ, Horowitz M, Jamieson GG. The effect of domperidone on oesophageal emptying in diabetic autonomic neuropathy. Br J Clin Pharmacol 1985;19:441–4.
33. Loo FD, Dodds WJ, Soergel KH, et al. Multipeaked esophageal peristaltic pressure waves in patients with diabetic neuropathy. Gastroenterology 1985;88:485–91.
34. Hollis JB, Castell DO, Braddom RL. Esophageal function in diabetes mellitus and its relation to peripheral neuropathy. Gastroenterology 1977;73:1098–102.
35. Russell COH, Gannan R, Coatsworth J, et al. Relationship among esophageal dysfunction, diabetic gastroenteropathy and peripheral neuropathy. Dig Dis Sci 1983;28:289–93.
36. Horowitz M, Harding PE, Maddox AE, et al. Gastric and oesophageal emptying in patients with Type 2 diabetes mellitus. Diabetologia 1989;32:151–9.
37. Horowitz M, Maddox A, Harding PE, et al. Effect of cisapride on gastric and esophageal emptying in insulin-dependent diabetes mellitus. Gastroenterology 1987;92:1899–907.
38. Parkman HP, Schwartz SS. Esophagitis and gastroduodenal disorders associated with diabetic gastroparesis. Arch Intern Med 1987;147:1477–80.

39. Holloway RH, Hongo M, Berger K, McCallum RW. Gastric distention: a mechanism for postprandial gastroesophageal reflux. Gastroenterology 1985;89:779–84.

40. McDonald GB. Esophageal diseases caused by infection, systemic illness, and trauma. In: Sleisenger MH, Fordtran JS, eds. Gastrointestinal disease: pathophysiology, diagnosis, management. 4th ed. Vol 1. Philadelphia, WB Saunders, 1989:640–56.

41. Laine L, Conteas C, Debruin M, Multicenter Study Group. A prospective, randomized trial of fluconazole vs. ketoconazole for candida esophagitis [Abstract]. Gastroenterology 1990;98(Suppl):A458.

42. Malagelada J-R, Azpiroz F. Determinants of gastric emptying and transit in the small intestine. In: Handbook of physiology. Section 6. The gastrointestinal system. Vol 1. Part 2. Motility and circulation. Bethesda: American Physiological Society, 1989:817–67.

43. Jansson G. Extrinsic nervous control of gastric motility: an experimental study in the cat. Acta Physiol Scand [Suppl] 1969;326:1–42.

44. Scratcherd T, Grundy D. Nervous afferents from the upper gastrointestinal tract which influence gastrointestinal motility. In: Wienbeck M, ed. Motility of the digestive tract. New York: Raven Press, 1982:7–17.

45. Malagelada J-R, Rees WDW, Mazzotta LJ, et al. Gastric motor abnormalities in diabetic and postvagotomy gastroparesis: effect of metoclopramide and bethanechol. Gastroenterology 1980;78:286–93.

46. Sarna SK. In vivo myoelectric activity: methods, analysis, and interpretation. In: Handbook of Physiology. Section 6. The gastrointestinal system. Vol 1. Part 2. Motility and circulation. Bethesda: American Physiological Society, 1989:817–63.

47. Lin H, Meyer J. Disorders of gastric emptying. In: Yamada T, ed. Textbook of gastroenterology. Vol 1. Philadelphia: Lippincott, 1991:1213–40.

48. Vantrappen G, Janssens J, Peeters TL, et al. Motilin and the interdigestive migrating motor complex in man. Dig Dis Sci 1979;24:497–500.

49. Achem-Karam SR, Funakoshi A, Vinik AI, Owyang C. Plasma motilin concentration and interdigestive migrating motor complex in diabetic gastroparesis: effect of metoclopramide. Gastroenterology 1985;88:492–9.

50. Barnett JL, Owyang C. Serum glucose concentration as a modulator of interdigestive gastric motility. Gastroenterology 1988;94:739–44.

51. Mearin F, Camilleri M, Malagelada J-R. Pyloric dysfunction in diabetics with recurrent nausea and vomiting. Gastroenterology 1986;90:1919–25.

52. Hasler W, Owyang C. Peptide-induced gastric arrythmias: a new cause of gastroparesis. Regul Pept Lett 1990;2:6–12.

53. Koch KL, Stern RM, Stewart WR, Vasey MW. Gastric emptying and gastric myoelectrical activity in patients with diabetic gastroparesis: effect of long-term domperidone treatment. Am J Gastroenterol 1989;84:1069–75.

54. Snape WJ Jr, Battle WM, Schwartz SS, et al. Metoclopramide to treat gastroparesis due to diabetes mellitus: a double-blind controlled trial. Ann Intern Med 1982;96:444–6.

55. Schade RR, Dugas MC, Lhotsky DM, et al. Effect of metoclopramide on gastric liquid emptying in patients with diabetic gastroparesis. Dig Dis Sci 1985;30:10–5.

56. Keshavarzian A, Iber FL, Vaeth J. Gastric emptying in patients with insulin-requiring diabetes mellitus. Am J Gastroenterol 1987;82:29–35.

57. Loo FD, Palmer DW, Soergel KH, et al. Gastric emptying in patients with diabetes mellitus. Gastroenterology 1984;86: 485–94.

58. Ricci DA, Saltzman MB, Meyer C, et al. Effect of metoclopramide in diabetic gastroparesis. J Clin Gastroenterol 1985;7:25–32.

59. Wright RA, Clemente R, Wathen R. Diabetic gastroparesis: an abnormality of gastric emptying of solids. Am J Med Sci 1985;289:240–2.

60. Feldman M, Smith HJ. Effect of cisapride on gastric emptying of indigestible solids in patients with gastroparesis diabeticorum: a comparison with metoclopramide and placebo. Gastroenterology 1987;92:171–4.

61. Ricci DA, McCallum RW. Diagnosis and treatment of delayed gastric emptying. Adv Intern Med 1988;33: 357–84.

62. Feldman M, Smith HJ, Simon TR. Gastric emptying of solid radiopaque markers: studies in healthy subjects and diabetic patients. Gastroenterology 1984;87:895–902.

63. Horowitz M, Harding PE, Chatterton BE, et al. Acute and chronic effects of domperidone on gastric emptying in diabetic autonomic neuropathy. Dig Dis Sci 1985;30:1–9.

64. MacGregor R, Gueller R, Watts HD, Meyer JH. The effect of acute hyperglycemia on gastric emptying in man. Gastroenterology 1976;70:190–6.

65. Isal J-F, Bergman JF, Dahan R, Caulin C. Gastric emptying of solid radiopaque markers in diabetic patients [Letter]. Gastroenterology 1985;88:1094.

66. Brady PG, Richardson R. Gastric bezoar formation secondary to gastroparesis diabeticorum. Arch Intern Med 1977; 137:1729.

67. Thompson DG, Richelson E, Malagelada J-R. Perturbation of gastric emptying and duodenal motility through the central nervous system. Gastroenterology 1982;83; 1200–6.

68. McCallum RW. Metoclopramide: pharmacology and clinical applications. Ann Intern Med 1983;98:86–95.

69. Pinder RM, Brogden RN, Sawyer PR, et al. Metoclopramide: a review of its pharmacological properties and clinical use. Drugs 1976;12:81–131.

70. Chaussade S, Grandjouan S, Couturier D. Motilin and diabetic gastroparesis: effect of MTC [Letter]. Gastroenterology 1986;90:2039–40.

71. Brown CK, Khanderia U. Use of metoclopramide, domperidone, and cisapride in the management of diabetic gastroparesis. Clin Pharm 1990;9:357–65.

72. Trapnell BC, Mavko LE, Birskovich LM, Falko JM. Metoclopramide suppositories in the treatment of diabetic gastroparesis. Arch Intern Med 1986;146:2278–9.

73. O'Connell ME, Awni WM, Goodman M, et al. Bioavailability and disposition of metoclopramide after single- and multiple-dose administration in diabetic patients with gastroparesis. J Clin Pharmacol 1987;27:610–4.

74. Brogden RN, Carmine AA, Heel RC, et al. Domperidone: a review of its pharmacological activity, pharmacokinetics and therapeutic efficacy in the symptomatic treatment of chronic dyspepsia and as an antiemetic. Drugs 1982; 24:364–400.

75. Heer M, Müller-Duysing W, Benes I, et al. Diabetic gastroparesis: treatment with domperidone—a double-blind placebo-controlled trial. Digestion 1983;27:214–7.

76. McCallum RW, Prakash C, Campoli-Richards DM, Goa KL. Cisapride: a preliminary review of its pharmacodynamic and pharmacokinetic properties and therapeutic use as a prokinetic agent in gastrointestinal motility disorders. Drugs 1988;36:652–81.

77. Johnson AG. The effects of cisapride on antroduodenal co-ordination and gastric emptying: a double-blind

controlled trial. Scand J Gastroenterol Suppl 1989;165: 36–43.

78. Havelund T, ster-Jørgensen E, Eshøy O, et al. Effects of cisapride on gastroparesis in patients with insulin-dependent diabetes mellitus. Acta Med Scand 222:339–343, 1987.

79. Champion MC. Management of idiopathic, diabetic and miscellaneous gastroparesis with cisapride. Scand J Gastroenterol Suppl 1989;165:44–53.

80. Brogna A, Ferrara R, Scornavacca G, et al. Cisapride and gastric emptying of a solid meal in dyspeptic diabetics without autonomic neuropathy and in healthy volunteers. Eur J Clin Pharmacol 1989;37:411–3.

81. Horowitz M, Roberts AP. Long-term efficacy of cisapride in diabetic gastroparesis. Am J Med 1990;88:195–6.

82. Itoh Z, Nakaya M, Suzuki T, et al. Erythromycin mimics exogenous motilin in gastrointestinal contractile activity in the dog. Am J Physiol 1984;247:G688–94.

83. Omura S, Tsuzuki K, Sunazuka T, et al. Macrolides with gastrointestinal motor stimulating activity [Letter]. J Med Chem 1987;30:1941–3.

84. Otterson MF, Sarna SK. Gastrointestinal motor effects of erythromycin. Am J Physiol 1990;259:G355–63.

85. Tomomasa T, Kuroume T, Arai H, et al. Erythromycin induces migrating motor complex in human gastrointestinal tract. Dig Dis Sci 1986;31:157–61.

86. Doty Je, Sanders Sl, Gu YG, Lin HC. Erythromycin accelerates gastric emptying of solids at the expense of sieving [Abstract]. Gastroenterology 1990;98(Suppl 5): A345.

87. Itoh Z. Molilide as motillin receptor agonist: a new class of prokinetic agents originated from macrolides. Regul Pept Lett 1990;2:12–5.

88. Janssens J, Peeters Tl, Vantrappen G, et al. Improvement of gastric emptying in diabetic gastroparesis by erythromycin: preliminary studies. N Engl J Med 1990;322: 1028–31.

89. Annese V, Janssens J, Vantrappen G, et al. Erythromycin accelerates gastric emptying by inducing antral contractions and improved antraduodenal coordination. Gastroenterology 1992;102:823–8.

90. Lange V. Gastric phytobezoar: an endoscopic technique for removal. Endoscopy 1986;18:195–8.

91. Smith BH, Mollot M, Berk JE. Use of cellulase for phytobezoar dissolution. Am J Gastroenterol 1980;73: 257–59.

92. Delpre G, Glanz I, Neeman A, et al. New therapeutic approach in postoperative pytobezoars. J Clin Gastroenterol 1984;6:231–7.

93. Ponsky JL, Aszodi A. Percutaneous endoscopic jejunostomy. Am J Gastroenterol 1984;79:113–6.

94. Van Stiegmann G, Liechty RD. Endoscopic jejunal feeding tube through decompressing gastrostomy. Surg Gynecol Obstet 1985;160:173–5.

95. Reardon TM, Schnell GA, Smith OJ, Schubert TT. Surgical therapy of diabetic gastroparesis. J Clin Gastroenterol 1989;11:204–7.

96. Karlstrom L, Kelly KA. Roux-y gastrectomy for chronic gastric atony. Am J Surg 1989;157:44–9.

97. Weisbrodt NW. Motility of the small intestine. In: Johnson LR, ed. Physiology of the gastrointestinal tract. 2nd ed. Vol 1. New York: Raven Press, 1987:631–63.

98. Marlett JA, Code CF. Effects of celiac and superior mesenteric galionectomy on interdigestive myoelectric motor complex in dogs. Am J Physiol 1979;237:E432–6.

99. Dooley CP, El Newihi HM, Zeidler A, Valenzuela JE. Abnormalities of the migrating motor complex in diabet-

ics with autonomic neuropathy and diarrhea. Scand J Gastroenterol 1988;23:217–23.

100. Wegener M, Börsch G, Schaffstein J, et al. Gastrointestinal transit disorders in patients with insulin-treated diabetes mellitus. Dig Dis 1990;8:23–36.

101. Keshavarzian A, Iber FL. Intestinal transit in insulin-requiring diabetics. Am J Gastroenterol 1986;81: 257–60.

102. Shanahan F, McKenna R, McCarthy CF, Drury MI. Coeliac disease and diabetes mellitus: a study of 24 patients with HLA typing. J Q Med 1982;51:329–35.

103. Chang EB, Field M, Miller RJ. α_2-adrenergic receptor regulation of ion transport in rabbit ileum. Am J Physiol 1982;242:G237–42.

104. Chang EB, Field M, Miller RJ. Enterocyte α_2-adrenergic receptors: yohimbine and P-aminoclonidine binding relative to ion transport. Am J Physiol 1983;244:G76–82.

105. Christensen J. Motility of the colon. In: Johnson LR, ed. Physiology of the gastrointestinal tract. Vol 2. 2nd ed. New York: Raven Press, 1987:665–93.

106. Battle WM, Snape WJ Jr, Alavi A, et al. Colonic dysfunction in diabetes mellitus. Gastroenterology 1980;79:1217–21.

107. Reynolds JC. Prokinetic agents: a key in the future of gastroenterology. Gastroenterol Clin N Am 1989;18: 437–57.

108. Berenyi MR, Schwarz GS. Megasigmoid syndrome in diabetes and neurologic disease: review of 13 cases. Am J Gastroenterol 1967;47:311–20.

109. Ogbonnaya KI, Arem R. Diabetic diarrhea. Arch Intern Med 1990;150:262–7.

110. Fedorak RN, Field M, Chang EB. Treatment of diabetic diarrhea with clonidine. Ann Intern Med 1985;102: 197–9.

111. Whalen GE, Soergel KH, Geenen JE, et al. Diabetic diarrhea: a clinical and pathophysiological study. Gastroenterology 1969;56:1021–32.

112. El Newihi H, Dooley CP, Saad C, et al. Impaired exocrine pancreatic function in diabetics with diarrhea and peripheral neuropathy. Dig Dis Sci 1988;33:705–10.

113. Lankisch PG, Creutzfeldt W. Therapy of exocrine and endocrine pancreatic insufficiency. Clin Gastroenterol 1984;13:985–99.

114. Simon GL, Gorbach SL. Intestinal flora and gastrointestinal function. In: Johnson LR, ed. Physiology of the gastrointestinal tract. Vol 1. 2nd ed. New York: Raven Press 1987: 1729–47.

115. Vantrappen G, Janssens J, Hellemans J, Ghoos Y. The interdigestive motor complex of normal subjects and patients with bacterial overgrowth of the small intestine. J Clin Invest 1977;59:1158–66.

116. Goldstein F, Wirts CW, Kowlessar OD. Diabetic diarrhea and steatorrhea: microbiologic and clinical observations. Ann Intern Med 1970;72:215–8.

117. Scarpello JHB, Hague RV, Cullen DR, Sladen GE. The ^{14}C-glycholate and test in diabetic diarrhoea. BMJ 1976; 2:673–5.

118. Molloy AM, Tomkin GJ. Altered bile in diabetic diarrhoea. BMJ 1978;2:1462–3.

119. Mekhjian HS, Phillips SF, Hofmann AF. Colonic secretion of water and electrolytes induced by bile acids: perfusion studies in man. J Clin Invest 1971;50:1569–77.

120. Schiller LR, Bilhartz LE, Santa Ana CA, Fordtran JS. Comparison of endogenous and radiolabeled bile acid excretion in patients with idiopathic chronic diarrhea. Gastroenterology 1990;98:1036–43.

121. Roof LW. Treatment of diabetic diarrhea with clonidine [Letter]. Am J Med 1987;83:603–4.

122. Migliore A, Barone C, Manna R, Greco AV. Diabetic diarrhea and clonidine [Letter]. Ann Intern Med 1988; 109:170–1.

123. Sacerdote A. Topical clonidine for diabetic diarrhea [Letter]. Ann Intern Med 1986;105:139.

124. Tsai S-T, Vinik AI, Brunner JF. Diabetic diarrhea and somatostatin [Letter]. Ann Intern Med 1986;104:894.

125. Dudl RJ, Anderson DS, Forsythe AB, et al. Treatment of diabetic diarrhea and orthostatic hypotension with somatostatin analogue SMS 201–995. Am J Med 1987;83: 584–8.

126. Dharmsathaphorn K, Sherwin RS, Dobbins JW. Somatostatin inhibits fluid secretion in the rat jejunum. Gastroenterology 1980;78:1554–8.

127. Dharmsathaphorn K, Racusen L, Dobbins JW. Effect of somatostatin on ion transport in the rat colon. J Clin Invest 1980;l66:813–20.

128. Maton PN, O'Dorisio TM, Howe BA, et al. Effects of a long-acting somatostatin analogue (SMS 201–995) in a patient with pancreatic cholera. N Engl J Med 1985; 312:17–21.

129. Kvols LK, Moertel CG, O'Connell M, et al. Treatment of the malignant carcinoid syndrome: evaluation of a long-acting somatostatin analogue. N Engl J Med 1986;315: 663–6.

130. Read NW, Harford WV, Schmulen AC, et al. A clinical study of patients with fecal incontinence and diarrhea. Gastroenterology 1979;76:747–56.

131. Schiller LR, Santa Ana CA, Schmulen AC, et al. Pathogenesis of fecal incontinence in diabetes mellitus: evidence for internal-anal-sphincter dysfunction. N Engl J Med 1982; 307:1666–71.

132. Schiller LR. Fecal incontinence. In: Sleisenger MH, Fordtran JS, eds. Gastrointestinal disease: pathophysiology, diagnosis, management. Vol 1. 4th ed. Philadelphia: WB Saunders, 1989:317–31.

133. Wald A, Tunuguntla AK. Anorectal sensorimotor dysfunction in fecal incontinence and diabetes mellitus: modification with biofeedback therapy. N Engl J Med 1984; 310:1282–7.

134. Apstein MD. Pathophysiology of gallstones and other diseases of the biliary tract. In: Chopra S, May RJ, eds. Pathophysiology of gastrointestinal diseases. Boston: Little Brown, 1989:489–528.

135. Diehl AK. Epidemiology and natural history of gallstone disease. Gastroenterol Clin N Am 1991;20:1–19.

136. Erlinger S. Physiology of bile secretion and enterohepatic circulation. In: Johnson LR, ed. Physiology of the gastrointestinal tract. Vol 2. 2nd ed. New York: Raven Press, 1987:1557–80.

137. Haber GB, Heaton KW. Lipid composition of bile in diabetics and obesity-matched controls. Gut 1979;20: 518–22.

138. Gitelson S, Schwartz A, Fraenkel M, et al. Gall-bladder dysfunction in diabetes mellitus: the diabetic neurogenic gall-bladder. Diabetes 1963;12:308–12.

139. Gitelson S, Oppenheim D, Schwartz A. Size of the gallbladder in patients with diabetes mellitus. Diabetes 1969;18:493–8.

140. Stone BG, Gavaler JS, Belle SH, et al. Impairment of gallbladder emptying in diabetes mellitus. Gastroenterology 1988;95:170–6.

141. Keshavarzian A, Dunne M, Iber FL. Gallbladder volume and emptying in insulin-requiring male diabetics. Dig Dis Sci 1987;32:824–8.

142. Newman H, Northup J. The autopsy incidence of gallstones. Int Abstr Surg 1959;109:1–13.

143. Zahor Z, Sternby NH, Kagan A, et al. Frequency of cholelithiasis in Prague and Malmö: an autopsy study. Scand J Gastroenterol 1974;9:3–7.

144. Diehl AK, Elford J. Gallstone disease in diabetics: analysis using multiple-cause mortality tables. Public Health 1981; 95:261–3.

145. Strom BL, Tamragouri RN, Morse ML, et al. Oral contraceptives and other risk factors for gallbladder disease. Clin Pharmacol Ther 1986;39:335–41.

146. Honoré LH. The lack of a positive association between symptomatic cholesterol cholelithiasis and clinical diabetes mellitus: a retrospective study. J Chronic Dis 1980; 33:465–9.

147. Pellegrini CA. Asymptomatic gallstones: does diabetes mellitus make a difference? [Editorial] Gastroenterology 1986;91:245–7.

148. Rabinowitch IM. On the mortality resulting from the surgical treatment of chronic gall-bladder disease in diabetes mellitus. Ann Surg 1932;96:70–4.

149. Eisele HE. Results of gallbladder surgery in diabetes mellitus. Ann Surg 1943;118:107–15.

150. Turrill FL, McCarron MM, Mikkelsen WP. Gallstones and diabetes: an ominous association. Am J Surg 1961;102: 184–90.

151. Mundth ED. Cholecystitis and diabetes mellitus. N Engl J Med 1962;267:642–6.

152. Ransohoff DF, Miller GL, Forsythe SB, Hermann RE. Outcome of acute cholecystitis in patients with diabetes mellitus. Ann Intern Med 1987;106:829–32.

153. Hickman M, Schwesinger WH, Page CP. Acute cholecystitis in the diabetic: a case-control study of outcome. Arch Surg 1988;123:409–11.

154. Sandler RS, Maule WF, Baltus ME. Factors associated with postoperative complications in diabetics after biliary tract surgery. Gastroenterology 1986;91:157–62.

155. Walsh DB, Eckhauser FE, Ramsburgh SR, Burney RB. Risk associated with diabetes mellitus in patients undergoing gallbladder surgery. Surgery 1982;91:254–57.

156. Wetter LA, Way LW. Surgical therapy for gallstone disease. Gastroenterol Clin N Am 1991;20:157–69.

157. Ranson JHC, Rifkind KM, Roses DF, et al. Prognostic signs and the role of operative management in acute pancreatitis. Surg Gynecol Obstet 1974;139:69–81.

158. Drew SI, Joffe B, Vinik A, et al. The first 24 hours of acute pancreatitis: changes in biochemical and endocrine homeostasis in patients with pancreatitis compared with those in control subjects undergoing stress for reasons other than pancreatitis. Am J Med 1978;64: 795–803.

159. Stasiewicz J, Adler M, Delcourt A. Pancreatic and gastrointestinal hormones in chronic pancreatitis. Hepatogastroenterology 1980;27:152–60.

160. Anonymous. Pancreatic abnormalities in type 2 diabetes mellitus [Editorial]. Lancet 1987;2:1497–8.

161. Foulis AK, Frier BM. Pancreatic endocrine-exocrine function in diabetes: an old alliance disturbed. Diabetic Med 1984; 1:263–6.

162. Foulis AK, Stewart JA. The pancreas in recent-onset type I (insulin-dependent) diabetes mellitus: insulin content of islets, insulitis, and associated changes in the exocrine acinar tissue. Diabetologia 1984;26:456–61.

163. Henderson JR, Daniel PM, Fraser PA. The pancreas as a single organ: the influence of the endocrine upon the exocrine part of the gland. Gut 1981;22:158–67.

164. Fonseca V, Berger LA, Beckett AG, Dandona P. Size of the pancreas in diabetes mellitus: a study based on ultrasound. BMJ 1985;291:1240–1.

165. Frier BM, Saunders JHB, Wormsley KG, Bouchier IAD. Exocrine pancreatic function in juvenile-onset diabetes mellitus. Gut 1976;17:685–91.

166. Dandona P, Freedman DB, Foo Y, et al. Exocrine pancreatic function in diabetes mellitus. J Clin Pathol 1984; 37:302–6.

167. Solomon TE. Control of exocrine pancreatic secretion. In: Johnson LR, ed. Physiology of the gastrointestinal tract. Vol 2. 2nd ed. New York: Raven Press, 1987:1173–208.

168. Vinicor F, Lehrner LM, Karn RC, et al. Hyperamylasemia in diabetic ketoacidosis: sources and significance. Ann Intern Med 1979;91:200–4.

169. McMahon M. Diagnostic assessment in acute pancreatitis. In: Glazer G, Ranson J, eds. Acute pancreatitis. London: Bailliere Tindal, 1988:251–74.

170. Eckfeldt J, Leatherman JW, Levitt MD. High prevalence of hyperamylasemia in patients with acidemia. Ann Intern Med 1989;104:362–3.

171. Soergel KH. Acute pancreatitis. In: Sleisenger MH, Fordtran JS, eds. Gastrointestinal disease: pathophysiology, diagnosis, management. Vol 2. 4th ed. Philadelphia: WB Saunders, 1989:1814–41.

172. Stone BG, Van Thiel DH. Diabetes mellitus and the liver. Semin Liver Dis 1985;5:8–28.

173. Manderson WG, Mckiddie MT, Manners DJ, et al. Liver glycogen accumulation in unstable diabetes. Diabetes 1968;17:13–6.

174. Foster KJ, Griffith AH, Dewbury K, et al. Liver disease in patients with diabetes mellitus. Postgrad Med J 1980; 56:767–72.

175. Schaffner F, Thaler H. Nonalcoholic fatty liver disease. Prog Liver Dis 1986;8:283–98.

176. Wasastjerna C, Reissell P, Karjalainen J, Ekelund P. Fatty liver in diabetes: a cytological study. Acta Med Scand 1972;191:225–8.

177. Falchuk KR, Fiske SC, Haggitt RC, et al. Pericentral hepatic fibrosis and intracellular hyalin in diabetes mellitus. Gastroenterology 1980;78:533–41.

178. Marubbio AT Jr, Buchwald H, Schwartz MZ, et al. Hepatic lesions of pericellular fibrosis in morbid obesity and after jejunoileal bypass. Am J Clin Pathol 1976;66:684–91.

179. Silverman JF, Pories WJ, Caro JF. Liver pathology in diabetes mellitus and morbid obesity. Clinical, pathological and biochemical considerations. Pathol Annu 1989; 24(part 1):275–302.

180. Pamilo M, Sotaniemi EA, Suramo I, et al. Evaluation of liver steatotic and fibrous content by computerized tomography and ultrasound. Scand J Gastroenterol 1983;18: 743–7.

181. Lenaerts J, Verresen L, Van Steenbergen W, Fevery J. Fatty liver hepatitis and type 5 hyperlipoproteinemia in juvenile diabetes mellitus: case report and review of the literature. J Clin Gastroenterol 1990;12:93–7.

182. Van Waes L, Lieber CS. Early perivenular sclerosis in alcoholic fatty liver: an index of progressive liver injury. Gastroenterology 1977;73:646–50.

183. Powell EE, Hanson R, Searle J, et al. The natural history of nonalcoholic steatohepatitis (NASH): an analysis of 35 patients followed for up to 20 years [Abstract no. 766]. Hepatology 1988;8:1410.

Chapter 52

SURGERY AND DIABETES

JOANNE J. PALMISANO

HISTORICAL OVERVIEW

An improvement in the mortality rates following surgery among persons with diabetes was noted in the original textbook on the treatment of diabetes mellitus, published in 1916, by Dr. Elliott P. Joslin, who based his observations on 1000 surgical interventions in patients with diabetes.[1] This allowance for exercising less conservatism in selecting patients with diabetes for surgical intervention predates the discovery and widespread use of insulin.

With the recognition that diabetes mellitus involved an impairment in the normal utilization of carbohydrates, it became common practice to "prepare" a person with diabetes for surgery by instituting a sudden and severe restriction of dietary carbohydrate and fat in an effort to suppress glycosuria. Up to 24 hours of fasting, save for liquids in the form of coffee, tea, and water, was included in this dietetic regimen both before and after the operation. Oral intake of a carbohydrate-restricted and fat-free diet following surgery was reinstituted only if the urine was free of glucose and ketones. Not infrequently, large doses of sodium bicarbonate were given postoperatively, causing stomach upset and preventing normalization of oral intake of nourishment. These measures favored the depletion of glycogen stores and subsequent development of ketoacidosis. The common use of chloroform and ether anesthesia further complicated this risk, with their potential to precipitate acid/base disturbances.[2,3]

Given the metabolic consequences of these dietary manipulations, it is unlikely they were the reason for improved surgical outcome. More likely, the wider use of aseptic technique; improved methods of anesthesia, including the more general use of nitrous oxide rather than chloroform or ether; and improvements in general medical care before and after surgery had much to do with the reduction in perioperative mortality among all individuals, persons with diabetes included.

With the discovery of insulin in 1922 and the advent of its wider use in practice after 1923, persons with insulin-dependent diabetes (IDDM) were more likely to survive with the disease for many years. These individuals, previously denied all but the most urgent surgery, were offered almost the same procedures as patients without diabetes.

With the use of insulin, emphasis shifted to the provision of a large amount of carbohydrate throughout the perioperative period. The incidence of acidosis following surgery declined considerably. In their 1928 monograph, *Diabetic Surgery,* Drs. Leland S. McKittrick and Howard F. Root speculated that the improved outcome of surgery in the diabetic patient that followed the discovery of insulin might well have been related to the abandonment of the practice of starvation before surgery.[4] The use of dietary carbohydrate as vegetable broths, gruel, orange juice, and custards, along with the administration of small doses of crystalline insulin before meals three to four times daily during the preoperative period, formed the basis of preparation for surgery. Glucose was monitored four times daily by urine testing and confirmed on occasion with blood glucose analysis. The dosage of crystalline insulin, with its rapid action and short duration (5 to 7 hours), often was based on a "sliding scale" determined by the results of glucose testing of these single urine specimens. Treatment with insulin was more aggressive if the urine was found to contain ketones. Intravenous glucose was used only in cases of gastric surgery in which oral intake was prohibited or of postoperative shock or persistent vomiting.

Hagedorn's discovery that the action of insulin could be extended by combining it with protamine[5] led to the development of protamine zinc insulin (PZI) in 1935, the first long-acting preparation of depot insulin. Most persons with diabetes for whom dietary therapy was inadequate were now free of multiple daily injections of crystalline insulin. One single morning injection of PZI or, later, of neutral protamine Hagedorn (NPH) insulin sufficed to control hyperglycemia and glycosuria. Shortly after 1936, modern practice was established, with the administration of a portion of the usual daily dose of these longer-acting preparations before surgery supplemented with crystalline insulin during the postoperative period.[3]

As was true for the general surgical population, the surgical mortality of persons with diabetes improved considerably after 1923. Improvements in anesthesia, the use of intravenous fluid and transfusion therapy, and the availability of antibiotics all served to better surgical outcome. Surgery for carbuncles and other abscesses declined. One-third to one-half of all previous surgical deaths had followed major amputations and were related to uncontrollable sepsis. Along with advances in antibiotic therapy, the development of the transmetatarsal amputation by McKittrick in 1944 led to a significant reduction in the number of major amputations and to an overall improvement in operative mortality. In this modern era of insulin treatment, diabetic coma following surgery was far less common than it had been in the past. Arteriosclerotic heart disease with congestive failure or myocardial infarction became the primary cause of perioperative mortality, most frequently following surgery for gangrene of the lower extremity.[3] These same cardiovascular complications remain the primary cause of perioperative mortality among patients with diabetes today.

TREATMENT OBJECTIVES

The question of how tightly to control hyperglycemia during the preoperative and postoperative periods is controversial. The goal of tight glycemic control as a means of minimizing the risk of long-term complications of diabetes is immaterial to the discussion of glucose control in the person with diabetes undergoing a major surgical procedure.

The combination of surgical stress and insulin deficiency in the diabetic patient can precipitate ketoacidosis, although this is a rare occurrence. Excessive hyperglycemia does predispose to osmotic diuresis, volume depletion, and electrolyte disturbances. Insulin is a necessary hormone in protein metabolism and, as such, helps limit the catabolic consequences of surgery.

Treatment objectives center on the establishment and maintenance of reasonable glucose control so as to avoid the acute metabolic disturbances of hypoglycemia, severe hyperglycemia, and ketosis, all of which complicate perioperative care. As with the nondiabetic surgical patient, the principles of proper fluid management and electrolyte balance must be applied.

Members of the operative team must understand the management goals in the care of the patient with diabetes and work together to realize these objectives. Diabetes management is best performed by a physician with special expertise in diabetes. Concurrent care by a diabetologist, if available, contributes to quality of care and minimizes possibilities of error.[6]

INFLUENCE OF DIABETES ON OPERATIVE RISK AND WOUND HEALING

The time-worn aphorism that postoperative morbidity is higher in persons with diabetes is not supported by clinical studies. When persons with diabetes who are undergoing major vascular and abdominal procedures are carefully matched with their nondiabetic counterparts for age, sex, weight, type of surgery, and presence of coexisting organic disease, no difference is found in the incidence of postoperative cardiopulmonary, vascular, or infectious-wound complications.[7-10] Further, there is little evidence that maintenance of near-normal blood glucose levels, rather than moderate hyperglycemia, is associated with a superior outcome.

The conventional postulate that optimal perioperative glycemic control enhances the chance of successful wound healing in IDDM is supported only by experimental studies in animal models of diabetes. These studies implicate hyperglycemia and insulin deficiency as factors contributing to impaired deep-wound healing. Deficient formation of granulation tissue and collagen, poor tensile strength of deep surgical wounds, and deficient capillary ingrowth into the wound have been demonstrated.[11-13]

It is inferred that the diabetic patient is more susceptible to infection since hyperglycemia has been shown to contribute to impairment of humoral host defense mechanisms (see Chapter 47). Deficiencies in neutrophil function, including chemotaxis, phagocytosis, and bactericidal activity, and abnormalities in the action of complement have been demonstrated in vitro in studies using neutrophils from diabetic subjects with poor glycemic control.[14-18] Most of these manifestations of neutrophil dysfunction have been related to levels of hyperglycemia in which the blood glucose is >12 mmol/L and are reversible with the establishment of normal or improved glucose control.

Whether these defects actually influence host defense mechanisms is controversial. Not all deficiencies in humoral response have been demonstrated in any one system or, for that matter, in the neutrophils of all diabetic subjects studied. There exists no strong evidence for a clinical correlation of these in vitro defects with an increased frequency of or susceptibility to infection in diabetic subjects. Neuropathy and large-vessel occlusive disease, common complications of long-standing diabetes, inevitably do affect wound healing. Surgical success and adequate healing more likely correlate with the presence or absence of these factors then with any specific level of blood glucose during the postoperative period.

PREOPERATIVE EVALUATION

In planning for surgery, attention should be directed toward ensuring that the general physical condition of the patient is as good as possible. With the changes imposed by shorter hospital stays, the physician has little time for careful study and correction of related medical problems before surgery. The importance of preadmission outpatient assessment cannot be overemphasized, as it allows for identification and treatment of potential complicating conditions, particularly cardiac, pulmonary, renal, and hematologic disease.

Assessment of Cardiac Risk

Cardiovascular disease is the leading cause of mortality in persons with diabetes. Mortality due to cardiovascular disease increases sharply with age and duration of diabetes. Among persons with diabetes, the mortality rate among those aged 75 years or older is 30 to 50 times higher than that among those aged 44 years or younger.[19] Ischemic heart disease constitutes the bulk of cardiovascular complications in this group. Persons with diabetes appear to have shared the decline in overall mortality related to cardiovascular disease seen in the general population of the United States during the past decade. But although mortality due to major cardiovascular events has declined, among persons with diabetes the number of hospitalizations for ischemic heart disease and stroke have increased, exceeding 390,000 in 1987, the last year for which surveillance data are available.

Both persons with IDDM and those with non-insulin-dependent diabetes (NIDDM), especially those with peripheral vascular disease, may have significant coronary atherosclerosis with no symptoms. Claudication may restrict activity to levels insufficient to stress the heart. Silent myocardial ischemia in the person with diabetes may lead to underestimation of the presence of coronary disease and deflect an adequate preoperative assessment of cardiac risk.

Assessment of cardiac risk is a major focus during the preoperative evaluation of the patient with diabetes. Preparation of the patient for major surgery should include a thorough history and physical examination with attention to cardiac risk factors. Obviously, particular attention should be paid to a history of previous cardiac disease and current cardiac symptoms.

Patients with a history of recent myocardial infarction are at the greatest risk of postoperative death due to a cardiovascular event. In patients without a history of previous myocardial infarction, the risk for infarction in the postoperative period is approximately 0.13%. In patients who have experienced an infarction more than 6 months before surgery, the risk of reinfarction after major noncardiac surgery increases to 4 to 6%. If myocardial infarction has occurred in the preceding 3 to 6 months, the rate of reinfarction during the postoperative period increases significantly, with some studies reporting an incidence of up to 38%.[20–22] Only emergency surgery that cannot be postponed should be performed on patients who have had a myocardial infarction 3 to 6 months previously.

If cardiac disease is suggested by history, physical examination, or electrocardiography, tests to detect the presence of significant ischemic heart disease can be helpful in the preoperative assessment of the patient with diabetes before major elective surgery. If cardiac disease is suspected from auscultation, echocardiography can be used to document the presence of significant aortic or mitral valve disease. Myocardial imaging with thallium 201 of the patient at rest and during exercise has a sensitivity of 80% and a specificity of 90% for detecting the presence of coronary artery disease.[23] The administration of dipyridamole along with thallium 201 may increase diagnostic accuracy.[24,25] The thallium stress test is more efficient than the traditional graded exercise tolerance test in detecting the presence of coronary artery disease and is our choice for the preoperative screening of the patient with diabetes who is at risk for a cardiovascular event.

Multiple gated acquisition (MUGA) scans, also known as gated blood-pool scans, are also useful as predictors of cardiac risk.[26] The MUGA scan has the added advantage of providing an assessment of myocardial-wall kinetics and ventricular ejection fraction. This test has a high sensitivity (89%) and specificity (86%) for detection of transmural myocardial infarction when performed within 2 to 4 days after the onset of chest pain.[27]

In the patient with diabetes and a history of myocardial infarction or unstable angina, the risk of postoperative cardiac complications may be lessened if coronary angiography is performed and, if necessary, coronary artery bypass surgery or angioplasty is performed before other surgery.[28] In the vast majority of situations, however, it is reasonable and safe to proceed with surgery after suitable preparation, including the administration or adjustment of appropriate cardiac medication (see Chapter 45).

Assessment of Renal Disease

Renal disease is common in patients with long-standing diabetes. Parameters of renal function, including serum creatinine, blood urea nitrogen, and urinalysis, should be measured. A 24-hour urine collection for estimation of creatinine clearance and quantitation of protein may be indicated as well. Caution should be exercised in the use of iodine-containing angiographic fluids and contrast agents as these are well-recognized nephrotoxins in the patient with significant renal insufficiency. Recent data by Parfrey et al.[29] indicate that diabetic patients with normal renal function are at no increased risk for acute renal failure when such studies are performed. Both diabetic and nondiabetic patients with significant renal insufficiency (serum creatinine level ≥1.7 mg/dL) were shown to be at increased risk for renal failure induced by contrast material. All patients undergoing such studies, even those whose renal-function parameters are normal, should be kept well hydrated. Monitoring of electrolytes and serum creatinine before and after the procedure is essential. The additional use of furosemide and mannitol is recommended to help prevent acute renal damage when such studies must be performed in the patient with significant renal insufficiency.

Treatment of Hypertension

Hypertension is a common accompaniment of diabetes. All reasonable efforts should be made to bring the blood pressure into control before surgery. As a general rule, antihypertensive medications are given on schedule on the day of surgery. Patients undergoing outpatient day surgery should be instructed to take their usual antihypertensive medications the night before and the morning of surgery.

DIABETES TREATMENT DURING AND AFTER SURGERY

Perioperative glycemic goals are arbitrary, and there is no consensus on the ideal protocol for the management of hyperglycemia in the patient with diabetes undergoing major surgery. Management is considered satisfactory when the blood glucose levels in the perioperative period range between 8 and 13 mmol/L, but levels as high as 15 mmol/L have not been shown to increase postoperative risk. When perioperative glucose values are less than 8 mmol/L, careful vigilance is necessary to avoid hypoglycemia.

For elective procedures, we believe it is worthwhile to obtain good glucose control before surgery. For some patients, this may call for the institution of insulin therapy, and for others, for a change in their usual insulin regimen. In the outpatient setting, it takes weeks or months to adjust insulin to effectively lower the glycohemoglobin level in a poorly controlled patient. It is therefore no surprise that the establishment of good glycemic control can hardly be addressed in the day or two before surgery. Persons with diabetes are commonly admitted to the hospital on the day of surgery for elective minor procedures. Hospital admission may occur at most one to two days before planned major surgery. For this reason, outpatient preoperative assessment, including an attempt to maximize glucose control, is desirable despite its difficulties.

The widespread availability of capillary blood glucose monitoring has greatly enhanced our ability to control the patient's blood glucose level during the perioperative period. The almost instantaneous knowledge of the blood glucose level from bedside monitoring makes planning insulin therapy much simpler. Urine glucose levels are unreliable indicators and should be abandoned as a monitoring technique in hospitals. The frequency of monitoring is a decision to be made on an individual basis. Patients who are metabolically unstable will need to be monitored more closely than patients whose glucose levels are in reasonable control.

Patients with diabetes are a heterogenous group who require individualization of their treatment plans. Knowledge of a patient's previous glycemic control, best determined by the glycohemoglobin or fructosamine test, can be of help in determining preoperative insulin requirements. Alterations in nutrition, variable glucose infusion rates, surgical stress, and postoperative pain and immobility are factors that influence postoperative insulin requirements. For these reasons insulin often is required during the perioperative period by the patient with poorly controlled NIDDM who is receiving oral agents for diabetes management.

What follows are some basic guidelines for a simple but comprehensive approach to perioperative management of the patient with diabetes undergoing surgery.

Conventional Use of Subcutaneous Insulin

The perioperative management of the majority of insulin-requiring patients can be accomplished without the use of an insulin infusion. If the procedure can be done in the early morning and the patient can eat immediately afterward, one-half to two-thirds of the usual morning dose of insulin should be given as intermediate-acting (NPH or lente) insulin before surgery. The balance of the patient's usual morning dose of insulin, including short-acting (regular) insulin if necessary, can then be administered after the procedure, just before the first meal. This approach is particularly useful for outpatient surgery performed early in the day. If the patient normally receives insulin at night, the dose must be decreased if the second half of the morning insulin dose was given late in the day. On the day of surgery, intravenous infusion of glucose should be started early, before the patient is sent to the operating room.

For patients whose surgery is scheduled later in the day or for whom the time of the next meal is uncertain, some modifications may be needed. Again, a portion of the usual morning dose of intermediate-acting insulin should be given and intravenous infusion of glucose equivalent to 5 g/hour should be started simultaneously. Intraoperative insulin is rarely necessary. During the postoperative period, a smaller portion of the balance of the morning dose of intermediate-acting insulin is administered. This is supplemented with the administration of small doses of regular insulin every 3 to 4 hours, with the amount based on an immediate blood glucose reading (bedside capillary blood glucose monitoring is ideally suited for this). This method allows for reasonable control of glucose with the avoidance of hypoglycemia. The glucose infusion is discontinued when the patient can take food or fluids by mouth and resumes taking intermediate-acting insulin.

For patients taking long-acting insulin (ultralente) in a schedule with regular insulin before meals, a switch from long-acting insulin to intermediate-acting insulin a day or two before planned surgery is recommended. The use of sliding scales for determining the dose of subcutaneous insulin creates enormous problems, particularly when the dose is based on a blood glucose value that is several hours old because of delays in the reporting of results from the laboratory. The 2- to 3-hour "time-to-peak" of subcutaneously administered regular insulin results in an additional delay, destabilizing the feedback loop. The result is the introduction of major fluctuations in blood glucose levels. Although this approach relies on guesswork and is generally unsuccessful, it has been vertically transmitted through generations of house staff and has become entrenched as a treatment practice.

There is no place for the use of intravenous insulin injections since intravenously administered insulin has a very short half-life (<15 minutes) and serves no valuable role in the maintenance of postoperative glucose control.

There are some legitimate uses of the sliding scale for subcutaneous insulin injections. For example, one technique used to initiate insulin therapy in a patient not previously receiving insulin is to begin with an arbitrary dose of 12 to 16 units of intermediate-acting insulin and to use a sliding scale for the dosage of regular insulin (1 unit for every 2.2 mmol/L increment the glucose level is above the baseline value of 9 mmol/L) as determined by bedside glucose monitoring before meals. This retrospective method could be used on a short-term basis with the incorporation of the previous days "catch-up" insulin dose into the basic daily dose. Attention must be paid to the kinetics of the various insulins, which are confounded by erratic absorption of insulin in response to fluid shifts during the postoperative period. Thus, if a 3-unit "catch-up" dose is required at the evening meal, the dose of intermediate-acting insulin is raised by 3 units the following morning. With close attention paid to this process, it is possible to discontinue the sliding scale in a few days in most patients with diabetes, it having served its purpose in helping the physician estimate insulin requirements. Exceptions will include patients with significant insulin resistance, for whom the sliding-scale approach may not provide for an increase in the dose of insulin that is adequate to effectively lower the blood glucose level to the desired range.

Intravenous Infusion of Low-Dose Insulin

Some authors advocate constant intravenous infusion of low-dose regular insulin during the perioperative period rather than conventional subcutaneous administration of a portion of the usual dose of intermediate-acting insulin before surgery.[30-32] Only a few prospective randomized studies in a small number of patients have compared these two methods, but it appears from the available studies that, for most surgical procedures, similar glucose control can be attained with the two approaches.[33-35] Glucose levels can always be well controlled with continuous intravenous infusion of low-dose insulin. This approach requires close attention by the physician and other health personnel as well as use of an additional vascular access. To permit appropriate adjustment of insulin and glucose infusion rates, it is necessary to monitor blood glucose levels rapidly and frequently. Bedside capillary glucose monitoring gives instant results and is recommended for this purpose.

Although some authors suggest an insulin infusion for all surgical patients, the actual use of this practice is limited. Intravenous insulin infusion was used in only 5% of cases in a teaching hospital survey.[36] We restrict its use to special situations. In cases of peripheral vascular constriction (hypotension, shock), this technique assures insulin delivery. This method is strongly recommended for the patient who requires emergency surgery during ketoacidosis. It may be appropriate for the brittle diabetic, the pregnant patient with IDDM, the patient requiring stress doses of corticosteroid, the patient with sepsis, and the patient undergoing transplantation surgery or cardiopulmonary bypass. Although used only in specific situations, it is reassuring to know that when achievement of glycemic control through the conventional approach is difficult, it can be achieved smoothly and rapidly with this method.

Various protocols for intravenous insulin infusion have been published.[30,37-39] In general, rates of insulin infusion are 0.5 to 5.0 U/hour. It is important that insulin and glucose infusions be correlated; current recommendations call for the infusion of 0.25 to 0.35 U of insulin per gram of glucose, with individual adjustments made for the level of insulin resistance. Caution must be exercised in the intravenous infusion of insulin, as unrecognized hypoglycemia is a potentially serious related complication, especially in patients under the influence of anesthetic agents who cannot inform caregivers of symptoms. The reader is referred to the excellent review by Alberti and Marshall[39] for a more detailed discussion of the published algorithms for the adjustments of insulin infusion rates.

Patients with NIDDM Receiving Oral Hypoglycemic Agents

Surgical patients receiving oral hypoglycemic agents fall into three categories: 1) those with good glycemic control; 2) those with poor glycemic control that will improve when infection clears or steroid therapy is discontinued; and 3) those who actually require insulin, therapy with oral agents having failed to control hyperglycemia.

For patients in the first group, it is usually sufficient to administer the oral agent with a small amount of water on the morning of surgery. In patients with a history of tight control and a borderline fasting blood glucose level, the oral agent can be withheld and then resumed when they begin eating again. Long-acting oral agents like chlorpropamide should be stopped 24 hours before surgery. Alternatively, chlorpropamide can be discontinued several days before surgery is planned in favor of a shorter-acting sulfonylurea.

The second group of patients need insulin therapy temporarily during the perioperative period. There need be no hesitancy in shifting such patients from oral compounds to insulin. If oral intake will not be restricted, placing the patient on a sliding scale of regular insulin in addition to the oral agent is a reasonable approach. It minimizes the disruption to the patient's program and usually provides more reasonable glycemic control than that achieved by discontinuing the oral agents entirely.

Patients in the second group whose oral intake will be restricted for a prolonged period must be started on insulin. A reasonable approach is the administration of intermediate-acting insulin once or twice daily in small doses, supplementing it with a sliding scale of regular insulin based on glucose monitoring every 6 hours. Achievement of blood glucose levels in the range of 8 mmol/L to 13 mmol/L is a satisfactory goal for this approach. Human insulin is the preferred product for this temporary use of insulin, as it will allow future reintroduction of insulin without concern about antibody interference.

Patients in the third group have an absolute need for insulin therapy, having failed to respond to adequate doses of oral hypoglycemic agents. If glycemic control is poor (glucose >17 mmol/L), the use of an intravenous low-dose insulin infusion can provide control until after surgery. However, it is possible to proceed with surgery even with the glucose in this range by administering intermediate-acting and regular insulin preoperatively and following the outlined approach for obtaining good glucose control with insulin following surgery.

Dietary Management

Nutritional support is important in assuring proper wound healing, and adequate intake of calories, protein, vitamins, and minerals must be assured. All too often, the patient with diabetes is assigned a standard 1800-calorie diabetic diet without attention being paid to estimated caloric need, usual caloric intake, body weight, or activity requirement. Individualized dietary prescriptions are recommended for the hospitalized adult patient with diabetes. A dietary prescription calling for a significantly reduced caloric intake is usually inappropriate in the perioperative period, even for the obese patient. Hospitalization is an ideal opportunity to obtain a nutritional assessment and to assist the patient in developing an appropriate dietary plan.

In the event that the diabetic patient requires parenteral nutrition because of increased protein loss caused by severe complications or of an inability to tolerate sufficient oral intake, standard protocols of oral or intravenous hyperalimentation can be used. Diabetes is controlled with the administration of small amounts of intermediate-acting insulin given daily or every 12 hours supplemented by regular insulin included in the solution given intravenously. The use of intermediate-acting insulin in this fashion provides an important platform upon which regular insulin is superimposed and frequently eliminates the need for additional sliding-scale coverage with regular insulin.

SUMMARY AND CONCLUSIONS

Persons with diabetes should be at no greater risk than their nondiabetic counterparts for poor surgical outcomes. Coexisting complications such as neuropathy and large-vessel occlusive disease will have an impact on rates of wound healing, but no studies in humans support the long-held belief that the level of the blood glucose in the perioperative period directly affects surgical success.

Cardiovascular disease is the leading cause of mortality among persons with diabetes. Assessment of cardiac risk, including appropriate testing to uncover significant coronary artery disease, is essential in the preoperative evaluation of the patient with diabetes who is to undergo a major surgical procedure.

Perioperative glycemic goals are carefully planned to avoid osmotic diuresis, ketosis, and electrolyte disturbances. Care must be exercised to avoid hypoglycemia.

Several options are available for the administration of insulin in preparation for surgery. Good glycemic control is attainable with either conventional subcutaneous insulin therapy or a low-dose infusion of regular insulin. Patients with NIDDM receiving oral agents often require supplemental insulin in the perioperative period. There need be no hesitancy in shifting such patients from oral agents to insulin if necessary.

Dietary management should be based on a sound nutritional assessment of the patient's caloric needs. Diet prescriptions, therefore need to be individualized.

Most important, members of the operative team need to understand the management goals for the patient with diabetes and cooperate to achieve these objectives. Concurrent care by the diabetologist enhances quality of care and minimizes possibilities of error.

REFERENCES

1. Joslin EP. The treatment of diabetes mellitus. Philadelphia: Lea & Febiger, 1916.
2. Joslin EP. The treatment of diabetes mellitus. 2nd ed. Philadelphia: Lea & Febiger, 1917:438–48.
3. Wheelock FC Jr, Root HF. Surgery and diabetes. In: Joslin EP, Root HF, White P, Marble, A, eds. The treatment of diabetes mellitus. 10th ed. Philadelphia: Lea & Febiger, 1959.
4. McKittrick LS, Root HF. Diabetic surgery. Philadelphia: Lea & Febiger, 1928:66.
5. Hagedorn HC, Jensen BN, Krarup NB, Wodstrup I. Protamine insulinate. JAMA 1936;106:177–80.
6. American Diabetes Association. Position statement: concurrent care. Diabetes Care 1989;12:504.
7. Hjortrup A, Sørensen C, Dyremose E, et al. Influence of diabetes mellitus on operative risk. Br J Surg 1985; 72:783–5.
8. Walsh DB, Eckhauser FE, Ramsburgh SR, Burney RB. Risk associated with diabetes mellitus in patients undergoing gallbladder surgery. Surgery 1982;91:254–7.
9. Lawrie GM, Morris GC Jr, Glaeser DH. Influence of diabetes mellitus on the results of coronary bypass surgery: follow-up of 212 patients ten to 15 years after surgery. JAMA 1986;256:2967–71.
10. Clement R, Rousou JA, Engelman RM, Breyer RH. Perioperative morbidity in diabetics requiring coronary artery bypass surgery. Ann Thorac Surg 1988;46:321–3.
11. Yue DK, McLennan S, Marsh M, et al. Effects of experimental diabetes, uremia, and malnutrition on wound healing. Diabetes 1987;36:295–9.
12. Yue DK, Swanson B, McLennan S, et al. Abnormalities of granulation tissue and collagen formation in experimental diabetes, uraemia and malnutrition. Diabetic Med 1986; 3:221–5.
13. Gottrup F, Andreassen TT. Healing of incisional wounds in stomach and duodenum: the influence of experimental diabetes. J Surg Res 1981;31:61–81.
14. Robertson HD, Polk HC Jr. The mechanism of infection in patients with diabetes mellitus: a review of leukocyte malfunction. Surgery 1974;75:123–8.
15. Bagdade JD, Stewart M, Walters E. Impaired granulocyte adherence: a reversible defect in host defense in patients with poorly controlled diabetes. Diabetes 1978; 27:677–81.
16. Molenaar DM, Palumbo PJ, Wilson WR, Ritts RE Jr. Leukocyte chemotaxis in diabetic patients and their non-

diabetic first-degree relatives. Diabetes 1976;25(Suppl 2):880–3.

17. Mowat AG, Baum J. Chemotaxis of polymorphonulear leukocytes from patients with diabetes mellitus. N Engl J Med 1971;284:621–7.

18. Hostetter MK. Handicaps to host defense: effects of hyperglycemia on C3 and *Candida albicans.* Diabetes 1990; 39:271–5.

19. Division of Diabetes Translation. Diabetes surveillance, 1980–1987. Atlanta, GA: Centers for Disease Control, US Department of Health and Human Services, April 1990.

20. Tarhan S, Moffitt EA, Taylor WF, Giuliani ER. Myocardial infarction after general anesthesia. JAMA 1972; 220:1451–4.

21. Goldman L, Caldera DL, Southwick FS, et al. Cardiac risk factors and complications in non-cardiac surgery. Medicine (Baltimore) 1978;57:357–70.

22. Rose SD, Corman LC, Mason DT. Cardiac risk factors in patients undergoing noncardiac surgery. Med Clin North Am 1979;63:1271–88.

23. Ritchie JL, Trobaugh GB, Hamilton GW, et al. Myocardial imaging with thallium-201 at rest and during exercise: comparison with coronary arteriography and resting and stress electrocardiography. Circulation 1977;56:66–71.

24. Okada RD, Dai Y, Boucher CA, Pohost GM. Serial thallium-201 imaging after dipyridamole for coronary disease detection: quantitative analysis using myocardial clearance. Am Heart J 1984;107:475–81.

25. Cutler BS, Leppo JA. Dipyridamole thallium 201 scintigraphy to detect coronary artery disease before abdominal aortic surgery. J Vasc Surg 1987;5:91–100.

26. Borer JS, Kent KM, Bacharach SL, et al. Sensitivity, specificity and predictive accuracy of radionuclide cineangiography during exercise in patients with coronary artery disease: comparison with exercise electrocardiography. Circulation 1979;60:572–80.

27. Sanford CF, Corbett J, Nicod P, et al. Value of radionuclide ventriculography in the immediate characterization of patients with acute myocardial infarction. Am J Cardiol 1982;49:637–44.

28. Scher KS, Tice DA. Operative risk in patients with previous coronary artery bypass. Arch Surg 1976;111:807–9.

29. Parfrey PS, Griffiths SM, Barrett BJ, et al. Contrast material-induced renal failure in patients with diabetes mellitus, renal insufficiency or both: a prospective controlled study. N Engl J Med 1989;320:143–9.

30. Alberti KGMM, Gill GV, Elliot MJ. Insulin delivery during surgery in the diabetic patient. Diabetes Care 1982; 5(Suppl1):65–77.

31. Hirsch IB, McGill JB. Role of insulin in management of surgical patients with diabetes mellitus. Diabetes Care 1990;13:980–91.

32. Watts NB, Bebhart SSP, Clark RV, Phillips LS. Postoperative management of diabetes mellitus: steady-state glucose control with bedside algorithm for insulin adjustment. Diabetes Care 1987;10:722–8.

33. Goldberg NJ, Wingert TD, Levin SR, et al. Insulin therapy in the diabetic surgical patient: metabolic and hormone response to low dose insulin infusion. Diabetes Care 1981;4:279–84.

34. Pezzarossa A, Taddei F, Cimicchi MC, et al. Perioperative management of diabetic subjects: subcutaneous versus intravenous insulin administration during glucose-potassium infusion. Diabetes 1988;11:52–8.

35. Taitelman U, Reece EA, Bessman AN. Insulin in the management of the diabetic surgical patient: continuous intravenous infusion vs subcutaneous administration. JAMA 1977;237:658–60.

36. Farkas-Hirsch R, Boyle PJ, Hirsch I: Glycemic control in the surgical patient with IDDM [Abstract]. Diabetes 1989; 38(Suppl 2):39A.

37. Schade DS. Surgery and diabetes. Med Clin North Am 1988;72:1531–43.

38. Sperling MA, ed. Physician's guide to insulin-dependent (type I) diabetes: diagnosis and treatment. Alexandria, VA: American Diabetes Association, 1988.

39. Alberti KGMM, Marshall SM. Diabetes and surgery. In: Alberti KGMM, Krall LP, eds. The diabetes annual/4. New York: Elsevier, 1988.

Chapter 53

FOOT LESIONS IN PATIENTS WITH DIABETES: CAUSE, PREVENTION, AND TREATMENT

GEOFFREY HABERSHAW

The greatest fears of the diabetic patient are loss of eyesight and amputation. In the United States, 50,000 major nontraumatic amputations (above-knee and below-knee) are performed each year, 30,000 of them involving patients with diabetes. The circumstances have never been better for the preservation of the diabetic lower extremity. The greater attention given to the life-styles of the diabetic patient, including the maintenance of tight blood glucose control, diet, weight control, and exercise, better prepares the person with diabetes to delay and/or prevent complications. Never before have so many effective drugs been available to help eradicate the severe infections of the lower extremities of the diabetic patient. Distal arterial bypass surgery has advanced at a startling rate over the past decade. The use of computerized digital subtraction angiography, the valvulotome, and the angioscope are just a few of the major advances that have made it possible to routinely bypass below the level of the trifurcation in the proximal calf. These procedures have given the patient the opportunity to leave the hospital with both limbs intact and with another chance. Many of these feet have been violated initially by infection and ischemia; incision and drainage; bypass surgery; and, finally, partial foot amputation or surgical reconstruction. The challenge is to get these patients back on their feet. It is an equal challenge to keep these patients out of the hospital to begin with.

OUTPATIENT MANAGEMENT

Two major factors contribute to the problems encountered by the person with diabetes: peripheral polyneuropathy and macrovascular disease.[1] It is no longer acceptable to blame diabetic foot problems on microangiopathy. Infection in the presence of polyneuropathy and/or ischemia does all of the damage. The importance of good routine foot care cannot be overemphasized. The responsibility of identifying foot problems lies with the primary-care physician, who should check the feet of each diabetic patient at each visit. Treatment may then be initiated for any identified problem. Following patients in the hospital setting allows for a readily available team approach, using the services of an internist, surgeon, and podiatrist. The physiotherapist, nutritionist, and other specialists are called on as indicated. The main function of the team is to protect the high-risk foot. Inpatient management of any of the complications of the diabetic patient provides an excellent opportunity for continuing the education of the patient and his or her family about diabetes.

Patients with diabetes who do not have signs and symptoms of peripheral neuropathy or occlusive arterial disease should be able to care for their own feet. Regular visits for foot care become necessary when these complications begin to manifest. Other conditions that preclude self-care of the feet are impairment of vision, severe arthritis, inability to reach the feet, toenails that are too difficult to cut, for example. The podiatrist must be consulted when self-care is no longer feasible.

BREAKS IN THE SKIN

Skin integrity is of utmost importance in the diabetic patient with neuropathy and/or ischemia. Any break in the skin, no matter how small, can permit the introduction of bacteria, which can cause severe infection in a short period. Common sources of breaks in the skin are fissures, blisters, toenails, trauma, and corns and calluses.

Fissures are most commonly caused by dry skin. The most common location is along the edges of the heels, adjacent to the thickened nails, and on the medial plantar edges of the big toe joint. The ability of the skin to hold moisture is hereditarily determined. Those diabetic patients with peripheral neuropathy tend to develop cornified, thickened skin, perhaps as a result of glycosylation of the protein elements of the skin. Ischemia will cause the skin to become thinner and less resilient and cause the skin, in turn, to become dry and prone to cracking. Moisture must be restored to the skin mechanically in the form of the application of dry-skin creams. The vehicles in lotions may have a drying effect and should be avoided. Creams such as Eucerin and Nivea are particularly good. Cream should be applied starting at the heel and progressing toward the toes. Care must be taken not to allow excess cream to accumulate between the toes. This will macerate the skin, which is then at risk of infection. Very difficult dry skin may respond to the use of Bag-Balm, which is available in most pharmacies. Fissures that do not respond to frequent local applications may be treated under occlusion. The desired cream is applied over the fissured area. Clear plastic wrap is placed over the site and is held in place by a carefully applied sock. The patient may then retire to sleep or at least to remain sedentary for a few hours while the occlusive dressing is in place.

Any chronic or acute dermatitis of the skin may permit fissures to develop. The most common of these conditions are fungal infections, which are particularly frequent in diabetic populations. These infections are rarely cured but are easily controlled with locally applied antifungal solutions and creams such as ciclopirox (prescription only), clotrimazole, tolnaftate, haloprogin (prescription only), and undecylinic acid. Even when the fungally induced dermatitis has resolved, it is wise to continue use of the antifungal agent of choice two to three times per week.

Maceration of the skin between the toes because of perspiration or incomplete drying after bathing also can cause fissuring. Careful drying between the toes after bathing is important. Small pledgets of lambswool placed between the toes will keep the interdigital spaces dry. Care should be taken not to cerclage the toes with the wool, so as not to compromise circulation.

Blisters are caused most frequently by friction from shoes, a sudden increase in activity, wrinkles in socks, and foreign bodies in shoes. Heat, intense cold, or chemical irritants may also cause blistering. Small blisters that are not on the weight-bearing surface and do not show surrounding cellulitis or clouding of the fluid may be left alone, but only under the following circumstances: 1) if all friction and pressure is relieved from the site, 2) if a dressing is applied daily with application of an antiseptic, such as ¼-strength povidone-iodine (10% povidine-iodine diluted 3:1 with sterile water), or a topical antibiotic ointment, such as Bacitracin or Neosporin. Changing conditions, or lesions on the bottom of the feet, in weight-bearing areas or covering large areas of the dorsum of the foot should be unroofed and treated as ulcers. Refraining from weight-bearing, administration of broad-spectrum antibiotics, and twice-a-day application

of the mentioned topical agents are then necessary. Patients not able to stay off their feet or those with compromised circulation should be considered for admission to the hospital.

Soaking of the feet by the diabetic patient, especially those with open lesions, is never tolerated. Water macerates the skin and will inhibit the effective growth of granulation tissue. Soaking will also potentially spread existing infection or cause new infection of the open wound. Water that would not harm those with intact sensation and circulation may burn the patient with neuropathy and/or ischemia. For the same reasons, foot fixers, heating pads, electric blankets, and hot-water bottles should never be used. The diabetic patient should avoid all sources of excessive heat or cold. Patients should be advised not to walk barefoot either indoors or outdoors.

Everyone's toenails undergo dystrophic changes with advancing age. Some of the reasons for these changes are hereditary, and others are due to insidious trauma from shoes, acute trauma that injures the nail root, circulatory changes, dry-skin changes, mycotic infections, and psoriasis. The nails are skin appendages and are subject to the same changes as skin. As the nails begin to change shape and thicken, the adjacent skin is at risk of breaking and becoming infected.

When the nails are of normal thickness and shape, they should be cut straight across. Cutting down the side of the nail should be done only if the area is painful or is threatening infection. Self-care should be encouraged until it is not feasible, as previously mentioned. At that time, regular visits (every 6 to 12 weeks) to the podiatrist become necessary. Nails that are thickened because of trauma or fungal infection need to be thinned as much as possible. Left alone a thickened nail will stimulate the development of a blister beneath the nail, which may become infected and lead to abscess and osteomyelitis. A Dremel drill with a side-cutting burr is used to thin the nails. Two circumstances necessitate the surgical removal of part or all of the nail plate and matrix (root): involvement of the nail that causes continual pain not relieved by regular local care and the presence of chronic or chronically recurrent infection despite nonsurgical measures to alleviate infection. Chemical matrixectomy with phenol or sodium hydroxide, for example, may safely be performed in the diabetic patient who has no signs or symptoms of peripheral neuropathy or arterial occlusive disease. If either or both of these are present, a sharp nail procedure, such as Winograd, Frost, or Suppan matrixectomy, must be performed. Prophylactic oral antibiotics should always be used before nail surgery in diabetic patients.

CORNS AND CALLUSES

The development of corns and calluses is a normal response of the skin to friction. They arise in predictable patterns over bony prominences that come in contact with the shoe on the top and bottom of the foot. Under normal circumstances, these lesions become painful as their thickness increases. Keeping the callus or corn thin would then restore comfort. The presence of neuropathy can mask the pain and allow a blister to develop under the lesion. The blister may then break to the outside, become infected, and lead to an ulceration, with potential abscess formation or osteomyelitis.

Calluses and corns require special care. Feet that have arches that are too high (pes cavus) or too low (pes planus) are prone to development or corns and calluses. Hammertoes and metatarsal deformity usually are present. The corns and calluses should never be cut with a sharp instrument except by a podiatrist. Medicated (acidimpregnated) pads should never be used in the diabetic patient. Appropriate shoeing, regular local care, and, if necessary, surgical repair of the deformed, boney structure are the preferred methods of treatment.

SHOEING FOR THE NEUROPATHIC FOOT

All shoes are bad for our feet, but we must wear them because of where we live and what we walk on. As bipeds, the amount of force on each of our feet is twice that of our quadruped ancestors. As members of an industrialized society, we spend most of our time on hard, unforgiving surfaces such as asphalt and cement, making the wearing of shoes necessary. If shoes are inherently bad for everyone, they are worse for the diabetic patient with neuropathy. Shoes that do not fit properly, are excessively worn, or are improperly selected for a given activity are all potential sources of skin breakdown.

When one walks barefoot on a soft surface, two things happen. First, the surface cushions the foot, with this response transferring to the remainder of the musculoskeletal system. Second, the foot sinks into the surface, providing inherent support for the longitudinal and transverse arches of the foot. These two benefits cannot be attained barefoot on cement. Shoes, then, provide a threefold benefit: cushioning, support, and protection of the skin against puncture by foreign bodies.

Considering that shoes are potential sources of skin breakdown for patients with neuropathy, special guidelines about their shoes are necessary. One major rule must be followed by all patients with signs and symptoms of neuropathy—simply, that they change their chosen shoes and socks every 3 to 4 hours during the active part of their day. There are three reasons for this frequent changing: 1) the patient or family members get to inspect the feet several times a day, and the earlier a skin break is found the better; 2) pressure points are changed by changing to a different pair of shoes, even if the shoes are of the same type; 3) all shoes begin to lose cushioning and support after 3 to 4 hours of use, and changing them will lessen the longitudinal and transverse friction and shear against the skin and, it is hoped, prevent blistering, infection, and ulceration. This simple maneuver will significantly reduce the patient's chances of developing neuropathic ulceration. Neuropathic patients should be able to wear the shoes they prefer, provided that they are willing to change them frequently and do not have any deformity that precludes the use of a certain shoe. The modern-day running and walking shoes are excellent for

the support and cushioning they provide but are good for only 3 to 4 hours at a time. If deformities such as bunions and hammertoes are present, extra-depth shoes should be considered (Fig. 53–1). Molded shoes are expensive, clumsy, and are usually not aesthetically pleasing (Fig. 53–2) and are reserved for patients with a deformed foot that will not fit into a shoe with a regular last, for example, patients with post-Charcot foot.

Shoes must be kept in good repair. If the counter of the shoe is allowed to wear over and the sole is worn on one side, the foot will slide in the shoe with each step. Friction increases and the likelihood of skin breakdown is greater. Patients must inspect their shoes for foreign bodies before they put them on. Stones, staples, nails, etc., are potentially harmful items that may be found and should be shaken from shoes before they injure the foot of the neuropathic patient. Shoes do not cause ulcerations of the feet of the neuropathic patient: diabetes, neuropathy, and ischemia do. We and our neuropathic patients must wear shoes. Thus, good habits must be taught and enforced.

ORTHOTIC APPLIANCES FOR THE NEUROPATHIC PATIENT

Orthotic devices for the neuropathic patient have three major functions: to decrease pressure over specific bony prominences; to provide additional cushioning; and to provide additional support. Rigid orthotic aides (made, for example, of Rohadur [an opaque plastic], steel, fiberglass) should be avoided in these patients because of the greater potential for skin irritation. Soft appliances made of materials such as plastazote, PPT (Professional Protective Technology, Langer Laboratories, NY), and Spenco (neoprene rubber; Spenco Industries, Waco, TX) appear to work best. They must be used in shoes roomy enough for both the appliance and the foot. Shoes such as

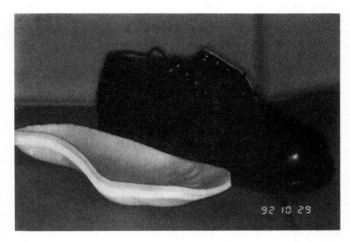

Fig. 53–1. Extra-depth shoes and full-length orthotic appliance. The extra room in this shoe allows for the insertion of an orthotic appliance—in this case a Plastazote orthotic. This combination allows room for the digital deformities that may occur as a result of the neuropathy and cushioning for prominent metatarsal beads.

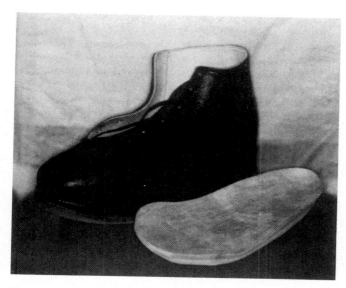

Fig. 53–2. Molded shoe and full-length orthotic appliance. These shoes are used for patients who have a deformed foot, as after Charcot fracture. The soft appliance is usually 0.75 inches thick and is replaced regularly.

running or walking shoes are best. Full-length orthotic appliances may be used in extra-depth or molded shoes. Soft orthotic appliances may need to be repaired or replaced every few months to maintain maximal cushioning and support. Neuropathic patients who will benefit the most from orthotic aides will be those who are threatened with an open lesion on the foot or who have recently had one that has healed. Not all neuropathic patients need orthotic devices.

SOCKS

Cotton and wool continue to be the best materials for socks. Combinations of these with synthetic fibers will prolong the life of socks. Patients with severe sensory neuropathy should be in the habit of changing their socks when they change their shoes during the day. Socks are available that have padded soles for more efficient dissipation of shear forces (some manufacturers are Thorlo and Head). These socks do work but are expensive and take up additional room in the toe box of the shoe. They will work best with walking, running-type, or extra-depth shoes. Patients with a foot deformity, such as post-Charcot joint, are encouraged to wear a thin sock under their regular sock. This provides for an interface of friction between the socks instead of the skin, minimizing the chance of blistering. Colored socks may be worn without fear by the diabetic patient; however, the use of white socks is preferable when there is any interruption of the skin. The cleanliness of a colored sock is always in question. It is also easier to follow the presence of drainage on a white sock.

NEUROPATHIC ULCERATION

Ulcerations may occur in the neuropathic foot for three reasons: 1) active injury—caused by high force, i.e., 700 to 1000 lb/in^2 against the skin, usually caused by a foreign body such as a needle or piece of glass that punctures or cuts the skin; 2) low pressure—characterized by decubitus ulceration 2 to 3 lb/in^2 over a long period, occurring most frequently in the immobilized, bedridden patient but not in the feet of the ambulatory population. 3) repetitive moderate stress—caused by moderate force of 30 to 40 lb/in^2, which is the most common cause of neuropathic ulceration.[2]

Repetitive moderate stress is responsible for the development of calluses and corns. These lesions develop (as mentioned previously) as a result of structural deformity in conjunction with the dynamic factors of pronation (flattening) of the foot and supination (high arch position) of the foot. Excesses in motion of the foot in pronation or supination during the gait cycle can create a shear force against the skin sufficient in itself to allow breakdown. The presence of structural deformity will accelerate the breakdown process and allow for development of neuropathic ulceration. In patients who have peripheral neuropathy, development of an intrinsic muscular atrophy also is common (Fig. 53–3). The intrinsic musculature functions to hold the toes in a straightened position against the powerful motion of the long extensors and flexors. When the intrinsic musculature becomes atrophied in response to the motor component of peripheral neuropathy, the muscles will no longer support the digits. This will result in accelerated hammertoe deformity and prominent metatarsal heads, which will further contribute to the shearing of the skin and increase the likelihood of blistering and ulceration. It is important to identify this foot before it breaks down and to support it appropriately with soft orthotic appli-

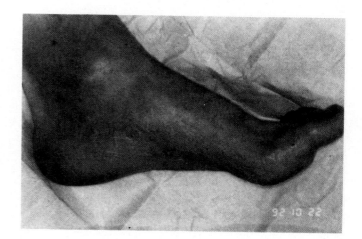

Fig. 53–3. Intrinsic muscular atrophy. Peripheral neuropathy will affect the motor nerves to the intrinsic musculature of the foot and cause them to atrophy. Without functional intrinsic muscles, the toes will curl up and become hammered. The metatarsal beads (ball of the foot) become more prominent and at risk of skin breakdown because of increased pressure.

ances in shoes that will provide for the progressive digital deformities.

EVALUATION OF ULCERATION AND OFFICE MANAGEMENT

The ability to manage a patient with neuropathic ulceration (Fig. 53–4) as an outpatient is dependent on four main factors. First, ulceration on the plantar of the foot must be managed with a regimen of non-weight-bearing. This means the use of crutches or a walker. The use of pads, casts, braces, or other devices is of only secondary benefit. There is some merit to these techniques, and they will be discussed later.

Second, spreading infection must be absent. All open wounds in the skin will harbor bacterial growth and must be considered colonized. There is no evidence that oral antibiotics aid in healing colonized skin. Such colonization, however, must be distinguished from spreading infection, the usual signs of which will be cellulitis, excessive drainage, foul odor, edema, and constitutional signs. For the patient to be safely managed as an outpatient, the ulcer must not undermine, hide abscess, or probe deeply into tendon, capsule, joint spaces, or bone. Bone scans are not necessary to evaluate ulceration, as will be discussed later. The use of a sterile probe is all that is required for effective evaluation of an ulceration in the office. Disposable debridement sets that include scissors, forceps, and a probe are available. The probe is used to determine the severity of ulceration according to depth.

Third, there must be adequate arterial flow to the involved foot. Palpable dorsalis pedis and posterior tibial pulses preclude the necessity for further testing. Absence of palpable pulses necessitates noninvasive arterial stud-

ies. If these show abnormalities, progression to a further vascular work-up is necessary.[3–5]

Fourth, the patient's diabetes must be adequately controlled so that his or her immune system will be able to handle local infection and reparative tissue (i.e., scar, collagen, protein) can be synthesized.

When these factors have been thoroughly considered, the patient may be treated as an outpatient. Being realists, practitioners, treating real patients with painless openings on the bottom of their feet, realize that patients are going to walk despite the practitioner's injunction that patient not bear weight. However, the more convincing the practitioner's presentation, the more likely the patient will remain off his or her feet.

Every time the ulceration hits the ground or floor, the healing process is slowed down or reversed. Some techniques are available for lessening the force on these lesions when they happen to hit the ground. These techniques can lessen the total force on the ulcerated site but cannot eliminate the force. Only non-weight-bearing will accomplish this.

Total-contact casting is one technique that can dampen the force. Plaster applied very close to the skin, covering the entire foot up to below the knee, will dissipate forces up the entire leg when the foot hits the ground and also will control edema. Swelling in the extremity will certainly hinder wound healing and must be controlled. The disadvantages of the total-contact casting technique are that it covers the entire ulceration, inhibiting daily wound inspection and care and presenting the possibility that abrasions caused by the closely applied plaster may go undetected by the neuropathic patient. The technique is also time-consuming and cumbersome and may require additional personnel and supplies. Although this technique is very effective in experienced hands, it is not the choice of the New England Deaconess Hospital and Joslin Diabetes Center unless the felted foam dressing fails.

Felted Foam Dressings

Application of felted foam dressings is simply a method of dispersing friction and shear forces at the ulcerated site using an accommodative pad. Our studies show that between 50 and 70% of the forces are dissipated from the ulcer site with the use of this technique. The advantages are that the felted foam dressing can be applied in less than 5 minutes and requires minimal supplies and no extra personnel. The ulcerated site may be inspected and debrided as many times a day as necessary without disturbing the bandage. It does not help to control edema in the extremity. This disadvantage can easily be overcome by use of elastic (e.g., Ace) bandages applied firmly but not tightly. Supplies include ¼-inch felted foam, rubber cement, scissors, 2-inch latex-impregnated self-adhering gauze (e.g., Fabco), 2 × 2-inch gauze pads, and an antiseptic of choice, such as ¼-strength povidone-iodine.

The foam pad is prepared for application by cutting it to follow the contour of the metatarsal parabola, with an accommodation made for the ulcer (Fig. 53–5). Rubber

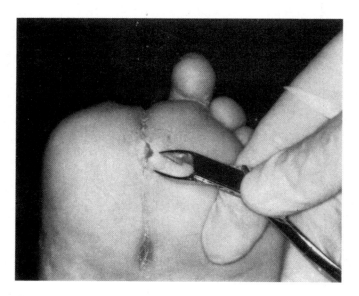

Fig. 53–4. Mild neuropathic ulceration. Patients with ulcerations that do not undermine, have no spreading infection, and are on feet with adequate circulation may be treated as outpatients. Local debridement (shown in photograph) is done on a weekly basis to allow for healing from the inside out.

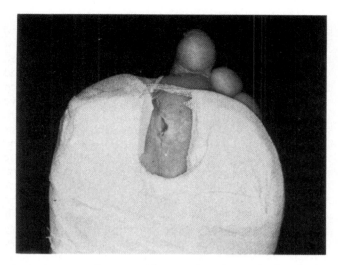

Fig. 53–5. Application of foam pad. Pad is applied to the foot with rubber cement and then wrapped with 2-inch latex-impregnated self-adhering gauze. A window is cut in the gauze, and antiseptic is applied to the ulcerated site. The window is then covered with 2 × 2-inch gauze pad.

cement is then applied to the felted side of the pad onto the foot, plantar and dorsal, but not on the ulcerated site. The Fabco is then wrapped around the foot in a recurrent fashion—not encircling the foot. This will ensure that the circulation will not be interrupted if the foot swells. A small hole is then cut through the Fabco. The antiseptic of choice is then applied with a cotton-tip swab and covered with an all-gauze pad. The patient is then fitted for a postoperative shoe and told to remain at home and not to bear weight on the foot. The pad should be replaced in 7 to 10 days and kept dry. A sock is worn over the pad and removed only when the gauze pad is changed—usually twice a day. This prevents the Fabco from unraveling. If healing of the ulcer continues to progress after 7 to 10 days of use, the pad is reapplied as long as the ulcer is healing. If there is no progress, treatment is changed, which frequently necessitates the patient's hospitalization.

The rubber cement used to hold the pad has certainly not caused any systemic problems. With prolonged use—approximately 6 weeks—an eczema may develop that is caused by the occlusive nature of the cement, not the cement itself. Because of the volatile nature of rubber cement, it should only be used in well-ventilated areas. Felted foam is used because of its resiliency and cushioning effect. It is much softer than 1/4-inch felt, returns to its original shape after weight-bearing, and is less likely to mat and cause further irritation of the skin. This technique is certainly not a panacea, but it has allowed many patients to heal without being hospitalized.

RECONSTRUCTIVE SURGERY FOR THE DIABETIC PATIENT

The use of reconstructive surgery has evolved as a response to help lower the incidence of amputations of the lower extremity in the diabetic patient.[6] Reconstruc-

tive surgery is indicated under four circumstances: 1) the ulceration fails to heal; 2) infection has been adequately drained and treated but the ulcer will not close; 3) arterial flow is adequate initially or has been restored by bypass and the ulcer fails to heal; 4) pressure-relieving techniques are not successful.

Such indications include chronically recurrent ulceration that threatens the foot with more severe infection and ulceration. These operations help preserve tissue that will disperse forces of ambulation and avoid submitting the patient to the psychological impact of amputation.

Procedures other than amputation are always preferred. It is better to perform arthroplasty than toe amputation, metatarsal head resection than ray amputation, or panmetatarsal head resection than transmetatarsal amputation.[6] Acute infection must be adequately drained.[8] Incisions and tissue that is removed to drain infection should, whenever possible, be made with consideration of its affect on the walking foot. For example, debridement of both peroneal tendons on the lateral side of the foot will necessitate eventual release or transfer of the tibialis posterior tendon on the medial side of the foot. If this is not done, the foot will forcibly invert, leading to fracture of the ankle and eventually to loss of the limb. Osteomyelitis may be locally removed and closed primarily or left open partially or totally, depending on the findings at surgery.

CHARCOT JOINT DISEASE

First described in 1868 by French neurologist J. M. Charcot,[9] this bizarre pattern of bone destruction was first noted in patients with tabes dorsalis. No external cause was seen. Of particular note was the absence of pain with such severe destruction.

Charcot joint may develop in persons with any condition that adversely affects the posterior column of the spinal cord, including diabetes mellitus, alcoholism, cerebral palsy, spina bifida, Hansen's disease, hereditary insensitivity to pain, myelodysplasia, poliomyelitis, syringomyelia, and syphilis.[10]

Prevalence

The most comprehensive study to date of Charcot joint disease in patients with diabetes was at the Joslin Diabetes Center in 1970. A survey of 68,000 consecutive diabetic patients found 101 cases of Charcot disease, making the prevalence about 1 in 680.[11] The true prevalence may be higher, since cases may have been overlooked because of the difficulty in recognizing the early stages of the disease before overt destruction is evident.[12,13]

Pathophysiology

Two popular theories had evolved to describe the cause of Charcot disease. The French theory, espoused by Charcot, postulated that a spinal cord lesion occurred that allowed trophic changes in the joints. This theory was based on the observation that changes in the joints were always preceded by sclerotic changes in the spinal cord. The German theory, described by Volkman and Verchow, proposed a theory of microtrauma,[14] i.e., that the cause was repeated unperceived trauma to insensitive joints.

A vascular influence has recently been proposed. Autosympathectomy in neuropathic patients leads to peripheral vasodilation and an increase of arterial-venous shunting. This may lead to abnormal bone sensitivity, with resorption and, thereby, weakening of the bone architecture.

At present, it is appropriate to accept that each of these theories has merit and in combination help explain the pathophysiology of Charcot disease.[15–19]

Diagnosis

Charcot disease usually will present as a unilateral swelling of the foot, which is not necessarily ulcerated or deformed.[20] The swollen foot will be warm on palpation and crepitus may be noted with manipulation of the foot. If the foot is deformed, obvious changes may be seen on routine radiographs. If the foot is not deformed, plain radiographs may be negative. If ulceration is present and radiographic changes are seen, there may be confusion about the presence of osteomyelitis. Absence of exposed bone on investigation with a sterile steel probe and of synovial fluid drainage is usually all that is necessary to disprove a diagnosis of osteomyelitis. Phasic and comparative bone scans are no more effective than this probe technique at ruling out osteomyelitis.[21] Bone biopsy is the most effective way of ruling out osteomyelitis. We do not recommend this technique because of the possibility of introducing infection into a particularly susceptible location. Triphasic bone scanning may be useful if there are no ulcerations and the plain radiograph is negative for fracture. The scan will be markedly positive in the later phases of the scan, indicating ligamentous damage and/or microfracture. This may then serve as a starting point for treatment.

The patient may remember trauma, but more often will not. A recently infected foot of a patient who has resumed weight-bearing is particularly susceptible to the development of Charcot disease. Partial foot amputation or reconstructive foot surgery may precipitate Charcot disease in response to altered foot mechanics.[11] Arterial bypass surgery mobilizes patients who have been unable to stress the extremities because of ischemia. Resumption of activity may allow for joint disruption and make fracture more likely.[19]

Pain can be absent or much less severe than expected for the extent of destructive changes. Deep pressure sensation may be intact, causing patients to describe a dull achiness. Bounding pedal pulses usually are present. Care must be taken to rule out deep venous thrombosis and inflammatory arthritis. Initial presentation is usually unilateral but progresses to bilateral involvement in 20 to 30% of the cases.

Patterns of Destruction

Although there have been other descriptions of destructive patterns, we have chosen to identify Charcot disease in one of three locations: the forefoot, phalanges, and metatarsalphalangeal joints; the midfoot or arch; and the rear foot, ankle, and heel.[22] Forefoot and midfoot fractures heal nicely if they are diagnosed and treated early. As a rule, the closer the fracture is to the heel and ankle, the greater the potential for complications. When the ankle and/or heel bone fracture, the foot may move medially or laterally in relation to the leg. It then becomes difficult to keep weight-bearing and shoe gear from ulcerating the skin. Amputation of the foot may be necessary if the foot becomes flail and the ankle cannot be reconstructed. There are three characteristic observations on plain radiographs. There is initially a *development phase*, with the presence of boney fragmentation and osseous debris adjacent to the involved joints. If ambulation continues, subluxation of the joints may occur in response to continued ligamentous and boney damage. After treatment begins, the *coalescence phase* begins, extending over approximately 3 to 4 months. This phase is characterized by subchondral sclerosis or increased density in areas of previous radiolucency. Osseous debris is resorbed and new bone is laid down on dead trabeculae. The *reconstructive phase* takes place over the next several months. During this time, joint fusion ensues.

Treatment

The mainstay for treatment of Charcot joint disease is that of keeping the patient from bearing weight on the foot. There is no substitute for non-weightbearing. Fracture biology dictates that fractures be as free from motion as possible for maximal efficiency in healing. Treatment time is based on the resolution of clinical and radiographic signs. The minimal treatment time is 8 to 12 weeks, during which a bivalved non-weight-bearing cast is used to keep the foot and ankle stabilized. This type of cast is used because it may be removed several times a day to inspect skin and to permit care of any abrasions that may have developed. The patient is seen regularly to observe for resolution of crepitus, decrease in temperature, and decrease in swelling. The new radiographs are compared with new radiographs each month to watch for coalescence of the fracture sites. When clinical signs improve and stability can be demonstrated, slow resumption of protective weight-bearing with crutches or walker may begin. This protective weight-bearing continues for at least two-thirds of the time the patient was non-weight-bearing. Protection for the contralateral limb is important. Thirty to forty percent of patients may develop Charcot disease on the opposite side. Soft, firm orthotic appliances such as those constructed of Plastazote should be used in an athletic shoe for maximal protection of the contralateral limb.

Surgical fusion of joints should be done only if all other forms of treatment have failed to protect the foot. In that fusion may be successful, it is better to attempt it before progressing to amputation. Boney prominences that may chronically ulcerate the skin may develop either medially or laterally. Exostectomy should be performed in the surgical suite to relieve pressure on the skin when nonsurgical means fail to work. Molded shoes are necessary when the normal shape of the foot has been altered by the fracture. Molded Plastazote insoles should also be used and should be replaced on a regular basis. These patients require close follow-up every 6 to 8 weeks for routine diabetic foot care. They should be instructed to call if any new swelling or break in the skin develops. After patients have had Charcot disease and are walking again, it is advisable that they do not walk for exercise. The mechanics of the foot are so disrupted by this process that skin irritation is likely if the extremity is overused. Rather, the patient should swim or use a stationery bicycle or a rowing machine. Walking should be done for necessary life activities as in work and play.

REFERENCES

1. LoGerfo FW. Vascular disease, matrix abnormalities, and neuropathy: implications for limb salvage in diabetes mellitus. J Vasc Surg 1987;5:793–6.
2. Bauman JH, Brand PW. Plantar pressures and trophic ulceration. J Bone Joint Surg [Br] 1963;45.
3. Gibbons GW, Wheelock FC, Hoar CS, et al. Predicting success of forefoot amputations in diabetics by noninvasive testing. Arch Surg 1979;114:1034–6.
4. LoGerfo, FW, Gibbons GW, Pomposelli FB, et al. Trends in the care of the diabetic foot: expanded role of arterial reconstruction. Arch Surg 1992;127:517–21.
5. Pomposelli FB, Jepsen SJ, Gibbons GW, et al. Efficacy of the dorsal pedis bypass for limb salvage in diabetic patients: short-term observations. J Vasc Surg 1990;11:745–52.
6. Giurini JM, Habershaw GM, Chrzan JS. Panmetatarsal head resection in chronic neuropathic ulceration. J Foot Surg 1987;26:249–52.
7. Wheelock FC Jr. Transmetatarsal amputations and arterial surgery in diabetic patients. N Engl J Med 1961; 264:316–320.
8. Gibbons GW. The diabetic foot: amputations and drainage of infection. J Vasc Surg 1987;5:791–3.
9. Charcot J-M. Sur quelques arthropathies qui paraissent dépendre d'une lésion du cerveau ou de la moelle épinière. Arch Physiol Norm Pathol 1868;1:161–78.
10. Jordan WR. Neuritic manifestations in diabetes mellitus. Arch Intern Med 1936;57:307–66.
11. Sinha S, Munichoodappa CS, Kozak GP. Neuro-arthropathy (Charcot joints) in diabetes mellitus: clinical study of 101 cases. Medicine (Baltimore) 1972;51:191–210.
12. Frykberg RG, Kozak GP. Neuropathic arthropathy in the diabetic foot. Am Fam Physician 1978;17(5):105–13.
13. Bailey CC, Root HP. Neuropathic foot lesions in diabetes mellitus. N Engl J Med 1947;236:397–401.
14. Delano PJ. The pathogenesis of Charcot's joint. Am J Roentgenol 1946;56:189–200.
15. Eloesser L. On the nature of neuropathic affections of the joints. Ann Surg 1917;66:201–7.
16. Edmonds ME, Roberts VC, Watkins PJ. Blood flow in the diabetic neuropathic foot. Diabetologia 1982;22:9–15.
17. Scarpello JHB, Martin TRP, Ward JD. Ultrasound measurements of pulse-wave velocity in the peripheral arteries of diabetic subjects. Clin Sci 1980;58:53–7.
18. Boulton AJ, Scarpello JHB, Ward JD. Venous oxygenation in the diabetic neuropathic foot: evidence of arteriovenous shunting? Diabetologia 1982;22:6–8.
19. Edelman SV, Kosofsky EM, Paul RA Kozak GP. Neuro-osteoarthropathy (Charcot's joints) in diabetes mellitus following revascularization surgery: three case reports and a review of the literature. Arch Intern Med 1987; 147:1504–8.
20. Friedman SA, Rakow RB. Osseous lesions of the foot in diabetic neuropathy. Diabetes 1971;20:302–7.
21. Edmonds ME, Clarke MB, Newton S, et al. Increased uptake of bone radiopharmaceutical in diabetic neuropathy. Q J Med 1985;57:843–55.
22. Harris JR, Brand PW. Patterns of disintegration of the tarsus in the anaesthetic foot. J Bone Joint Surg [Br] 48:4–16.

Chapter 54

VASCULAR DISEASE OF THE LOWER EXTREMITIES IN DIABETES MELLITUS: ETIOLOGY AND MANAGEMENT

FRANK W. LOGERFO

GARY W. GIBBONS

In patients with diabetes mellitus, problems involving the lower extremities are common, affecting one out of four patients. The prospect of possible amputation terrifies patients with diabetes and justifiably so, with two-thirds of all nontraumatic major amputations being performed in this population. Time lost from work, lost wages, and sometimes even dismissal from employment, have important personal and social consequences. Despite improvements in health care, more in-hospital days still are spent treating problems involving the lower extremities than any other complication of diabetes.

Unfortunately, misconceptions persist regarding proper diagnosis and treatment of lower-extremity problems in diabetes, and these misunderstandings may contribute to unnecessary amputation. Education of both patients and health-care providers is essential to optimization of treatment and prognosis. Foremost is the need to realize the three predisposing factors responsible for the development of lower-extremity problems in diabetes: ischemia, peripheral neuropathy, and an altered response to infection.

The most common proximate event initiating the final pathway to ulceration is minor trauma. The foot can survive neuropathy, ischemia, and an altered response to infection quite well with a strict foot-care regimen. Seemingly minor trauma can upset this delicate balance and rapidly lead to severe infection or gangrene. Thus, early recognition and prompt reporting of an injury are essential. To prevent amputation, it is necessary to establish a treatment plan aimed at all three of the primary pathologic situations. Essential to this program is a team approach combining vascular, general and orthopedic surgeons, cardiologists, endocrinologists, podiatrists, infectious disease experts, orthotists, physical therapists, nurses, and social workers.

ISCHEMIA AND VASCULAR DISEASE

Approximately 80 to 90% of foot lesions are accompanied by significant ischemia. One of the most important advances in the management of the diabetic foot in recent years has been in the success of arterial reconstruction to restore normal perfusion. This is fundamental to limb salvage since the well-perfused foot is more resistant to pressure necrosis, neuropathic ulcerations, and infection.

Optimal management of ischemia is dependent on an understanding of the somewhat unique characteristics of occlusive vascular disease as it occurs in association with diabetes mellitus. One harmful misconception is the idea that diabetic patients have a microvascular occlusive disease that impairs perfusion, a concept that arose from an uncontrolled observational study demonstrating the presence of periodic acid-Schiff (PAS)-positive material in small vessels.[1] Subsequent controlled studies failed to demonstrate any small-vessel occlusive disease associated with the diabetic state on the basis of histologic findings,[2] arterial casting,[3] or vascular resistance.[4] The muscle capillaries of patients with diabetes mellitus do have a thickened basement membrane, but the capillaries are not narrowed.[5] The thickening of the basement membrane is associated with albumin leakage[6] but does not impair diffusion of oxygen.[7] Further details of this lesion are discussed elsewhere in this book (Chapter 38). However, the important point to remember is that patients with diabetes mellitus do not have an occlusive lesion in the microcirculation.[1]

The pattern of macrovascular (atherosclerotic) occlusive disease in diabetes is unique. There is a predilection for occurrence of atherosclerosis in the tibial and peroneal arteries. However, this predilection is confined to the segment between the knee and ankle. The foot arteries in patients with diabetes are actually less involved with atherosclerosis than are those of persons without diabetes.[2,3] It is therefore incorrect to use the term "small-vessel disease" to describe any aspect of vascular occlusive disease in diabetic patients. The involvement of the tibial arteries is not a reflection of their small diameter, since the even smaller arteries in the foot are relatively spared. An understanding of this pattern of occlusion is extremely important in clinical management since it is the basis for highly successful arterial reconstruction.[8]

In summary, there are two clinically important characteristics of vascular disease in diabetes mellitus. First, no occlusive lesion is present in the microcirculation that could lead to inadequate perfusion or failure of an arterial graft. Second, the tibial vessel occlusive disease often ends at the ankle, sparing the foot vessels and permitting distal arterial reconstruction.

The clinical presentation of diabetic patients with peripheral vascular disease is somewhat altered by the frequent presence of neuropathy. The details of neuropathy and its role in the development of foot lesions are discussed elsewhere in this book (Chapters 50 and 53). Diabetic patients often present with foot ulcers or small areas of gangrene when relatively mild ischemia is present in combination with neuropathy. When skin necrosis occurs, it should not be ascribed solely to neuropathy until the possibility of coexisting ischemia has been carefully evaluated.

A thorough physical examination of the diabetic patient with lower-extremity complaints is essential. The peripheral pulses at all levels should be palpated. Although patients with diabetes have a propensity for development of atherosclerotic occlusion of the tibial arteries, it is not unusual to encounter atherosclerosis of the aorto-iliac region (evidenced by diminished femoral pulses) or other vessels of the lower extremity. In fact, despite the tibial vessel problem, the most common site of arterial occlusion in the diabetic patient (as in nondiabetic patients) is the superficial femoral artery.[9] Such patients have normal femoral pulses but no popliteal or distal pulses and often, in addition, have occlusion of both the femoral and tibial arteries. Patients who have only tibial vessel disease present with normal femoral and popliteal pulses but with no palpable foot pulses (dorsalis pedis or posterior tibial). More than 80% of patients who present with these physical features have diabetes mellitus.[10] Forty percent of diabetic patients presenting with ulceration or gangrene of the lower extremity have palpable popliteal pulses. Surprisingly, the results of arterial reconstruction in this group are excellent, with long-term salvage of the limb in more than 90%.[11,12]

Examination of the skin, especially careful visualization of all the areas between the toes, is essential in determining whether there is ongoing infection. Evaluation of the tissue around an ulcer, with a search for evidence of edema, capillary refill, pallor, and dependent rubor and the measurement of venous filling time and skin temperature, helps give clues as to the degree of ischemia. Probing the base of an ulceration will give some indication of the involvement of bony structures in the infectious and ischemic process. Plain x-ray films of any lower extremity with an ulcer or with a history of a healed ulcer but continuation of symptoms should be undertaken as part of the initial evaluation. Careful examination of these films for evidence of bony involvement, either fracture (? Charcot foot) or osteomyelitis, or evidence of deep soft-tissue infection with gas is required.

NEURO-OSTEO-ARTHROPATHY

The sensory-motor neuropathy of diabetes may lead to severe osteo-arthropathy (Charcot foot). The joint capsules weaken and the bones fracture or become crushed in weight-bearing areas. An inflammatory response ensues, creating a red, swollen foot that is not painful. This can present a clinical dilemma because the changes may be indistinguishable from those of osteomyelitis on plain films, bone scan, computed tomography, or magnetic resonance imaging.[13] Thus, patients may be treated as if they have extensive osteomyelitis and undergo inappropriate amputation. Alternatively, patients with lesser degrees of osteo-arthropathy may mistakenly be treated with antibiotics. The "successful" outcome may lead to the misguided notion that osteomyelitis can and should be treated with antibiotics without debridement or amputation. This situation can be complicated by the presence of both osteo-arthropathy and osteomyelitis in patients with foot ulcers and severe neuropathy. Clinical examination is more valuable than any diagnostic test. If a probe can be inserted through the ulcer to bone, osteomyelitis may be presumed, and generally the involved segment of bone should be removed. Pressure-point necrosis can be managed by custom foot gear or by joint resection, osteotomy, or ostectomy. In all such cases, coexistent ischemia should be first corrected by arterial reconstruction.

NONINVASIVE VASCULAR TESTING

A number of noninvasive techniques have been developed to measure arterial circulation. Measurement of arterial pressures at different levels of the extremity using a pneumatic cuff and a flow sensor—usually a Doppler ultrasound sensor—is the most commonly used technique. After the cuff has been inflated at the proximal level, it is slowly deflated, and the sensor over the distal vessels identifies the pressure at which flow resumes. This pressure is recorded for several points on the lower extremity, usually the high thigh, low thigh, calf, and ankle.

A common anatomic finding in diabetic patients is the presence of medial calcinosis of peripheral arteries. The artery is less compressible, and the indirect measurement of pressure within the vessel is artificially increased when compression is the basis for measurement. An additional measurement of the toe blood pressure in the diabetic patient has proven valuable, especially for a foot lesion. Toe digital arteries are less likely to be calcified, so that occlusive-pressure measurements more reliably reflect pressure within the digital artery. The measurement of the toe blood pressure in the diabetic patient compared with that in the nondiabetic patient reinforces the tenet that diabetes does not cause "small-vessel disease," since both groups have the same pressures in the small vessels of the foot.[14,15]

When the tibial vessels are noncompressible, other methods may be used to assess perfusing pressure. The most popular of these is pulse volume recording, a form of plethysmography.[16] Plethysmography measures the changes in volume over time. Cuffs are placed at segmental levels on the extremity, and the instrument records changes in the pressure of the cuff; these changes reflect changes in the cuff volume, which in turn reflect momentary changes in limb volume. These changes in limb volume have been correlated with direct measurements of intra-arterial pressure, with good correlation over clinically relevant ranges. The drawback of this technique is the absence of quantitative information in a standardized form.

Examination of the Doppler waveform, specifically its phasic nature, is another test that can provide the experienced examiner with a qualitative view of the degree of stenosis.[17] Semiquantitative information may be obtained by the analysis of the Doppler ultrasound waveform, but the use of these ultrasound-derived analyses has not received wide acceptance. There is a paucity of other truly noninvasive techniques for quantitating flow. Semi-invasive techniques, including radioisotope flow studies, have been used to demonstrate physiologic significance of vascular lesions but have also not achieved widespread acceptance.

Recently, transcutaneous oxygen tension ($tcPo_2$) measurements have been used in both healthy patients and those with occlusive disease as a noninvasive means of determining limb perfusion.[7,18] The $tcPo_2$ measurements of patients with occlusive disease are significantly lower than those of normal subjects. This measurement has been used to determine the possibility of ulcer healing and optimal amputation healing. Surprisingly, diabetic patients with ulcers often have higher $tcPo_2$ levels than do nondiabetic patients with ulceration, and ulcers and amputations of diabetic patients often fail to heal despite $tcPo_2$ levels that would be adequate for healing in a nondiabetic patient.

In summary, the most important steps in evaluating ischemia in the diabetic foot are careful clinical evaluation and examination of pulses. When the pulses are absent, the value or accuracy of noninvasive testing in confirming the diagnosis of ischemia is limited. When a diabetic patient presents with a foot lesion and absent pulses, decisions are based primarily on clinical considerations, and noninvasive testing is only complementary to sound clinical evaluation and judgment. If the ulcer is superficial, a trial of conservative therapy is warranted. However, for enlarging ulcers or deep ulcers involving a bone, joint, or tendon, arteriography is indicated.

ARTERIOGRAPHY

Arteriography is the foundation for successful arterial reconstruction. The above-mentioned pattern of infrageniculate vascular occlusive disease warrants special consideration. If, during an angiogram, the infrageniculate arteries are all noted to be occluded, the angiographer must persist and demonstrate clearly the status of the foot vessels. We have found that digital subtraction arteriography is helpful in this situation, permitting successful visualization of the foot arteries while limiting the volume of contrast agents required.

One of the concerns that arises in patients with diabetes is the possibility of the development of renal failure induced by the contrast agent. Patients with diabetes who have a normal serum creatinine level do not appear to be at an increased risk of contrast agent-induced renal failure. However, diabetic patients with an elevated creatinine level do appear to be at a slightly greater risk as compared with nondiabetic patients with equivalent creatinine levels. This contrast agent-induced renal failure is nearly always reversible and does not necessitate dialysis.[19] The incidence of renal failure can be minimized by hydration prior to angiography.[20,21] The additional use of furosemide and/or mannitol does not appear to offer protection beyond that of simple hydration. Nonionic contrast agents do not offer any clinical advantage over standard contrast agents as far as the incidence of contrast agent-induced renal failure is concerned.[22] Pre-angiographic hydration, the use of selective femoral and/or digital subtraction arteriography, and demonstration of the foot arteries even when the leg arteries are occluded provide the fundamentals for arteriography in patients with diabetes mellitus.

ARTERIAL RECONSTRUCTION

The pattern of vascular disease and the associated problems of neuropathy and infection in diabetes generally require some special attention. When a patient presents with evidence of infection, adequate drainage and antibiotic therapy is a first priority. If arteriography is necessary, it should be performed as soon as infection is under control—usually within 72 hours of admission.

Because of the pattern of atherosclerosis in diabetic patients, it is often necessary to perform arterial reconstruction to the distal tibial, peroneal, or pedal arteries. Surprisingly, the results of vein-bypass grafts to these distal vessels are now as good as or better than bypass grafts to the popliteal artery.[23] The widespread use of in situ vein grafts may in part be responsible for these improved results. Not all agree, and excellent results with reversed vein grafts have been reported as well.[24] There seems to be uniform agreement that prosthetic arterial grafts do not perform well when used for arterial reconstruction to these distal vessels.

We have found vein grafts to the dorsalis pedis artery to be extremely useful in revascularization of the diabetic foot,[25,26] probably because they restore maximal pulsatile flow to the foot circulation. More-proximal grafts such as femoropopliteal or even femorotibial grafts also improve arterial flow to the foot. However, because frequently the distal tibial arteries are occluded, these more-proximal procedures may not connect directly to the foot arteries. The surgeon often is faced with a decision as to whether to bypass to a more proximal artery or to bypass to the dorsalis pedis. In general, the preferred procedure is that which will establish maximal pulsatile flow to the forefoot. As mentioned earlier, because of concomitant neuropathy and infection, it is important to restore optimal perfusion to the foot to achieve and maintain skin integrity. In this regard, there is a difference in the approach to arterial reconstruction in patients with diabetes. In nondiabetics, more-proximal arterial reconstructions to the profunda or popliteal artery may restore perfusion adequate to obtain wound healing. Awareness of this difference, along with an understanding of the management of foot infection, will lead to successful salvage of the diabetic foot.

The rate of limb salvage on a modern vascular surgery service should be no different for diabetic and nondiabetic patients.[23] For the primary physician caring for diabetic patients with ischemic problems of the lower extremities, these guidelines follow from the foregoing information:

1. Ischemia should not be attributed to microvascular occlusive disease, a lesion that does not occur in the extremities of patients with diabetes mellitus.
2. The presence of neuropathy and/or infection should not preclude evaluation and treatment of ischemia.
3. When foot pulses are absent and a foot lesion is present, arteriography should be performed.
4. Arteriography must include the arteries in the foot before arterial reconstruction can be excluded as a possibility.
5. Whenever possible, the surgical procedure should be designed to restore normal arterial pressure to the foot arteries.
6. The results of distal arterial reconstruction in the diabetic patient should be as good as those in the nondiabetic patient.

With the implementation of these guidelines, in recent years we have reduced the amputation rate for all patients (including those with severe infection) admitted to our service for diabetic foot from 40 to 13%.[27] This reduction can be attributed in large part to our success with vein grafts to the dorsalis pedis artery, which now constitute almost 30% of all our bypass procedures in patients with diabetes. Bypass to the pedal arteries has resulted in a rate of limb salvage of 91% and a rate of graft patency of 87% at 3 years.[26] This high success rate has not been adversely affected by the presence of deep infection of the foot.[28] Many factors have contributed to these improved results, including better magnification, lighting, and suture materials. We have found angioscopy to be especially helpful in optimizing preparation of the vein graft and in assessing technical success.[29]

Alternative management of ischemia with the use of hyperbaric oxygen has its advocates.[30] However, the absence of a deficit in $tcPo_2$[7] associated with diabetic foot ulcers as compared with nondiabetic foot ulcers leaves little rationale for this approach. Any marginal benefit must be justified in a controlled prospective trial. Even if such benefits were found, they would be superseded by the established and long-term benefits of modern arterial reconstruction. Drug therapy has focused primarily on pentoxifylline, for which, again, there is little rationale. Without there being a deficit in tissue oxygen delivery or an increase in microcirculatory resistance, there is little reason to impugn stiffness of the red cell membrane as a factor contributing to ischemia. Prospective clinical trials with long-term follow-up are necessary before the use of drug therapy in the management of ischemia is justified.

It must be remembered that ischemia is only one component of the total problem. Incision, drainage, and surgical debridement continue to be misunderstood in regard to patients with diabetes. It is sometimes thought that large incisions in diabetic patients will not heal and thus that incisions and debridements should be made through very small incisions with the use of drains and other means of achieving control of infection, when in fact just the opposite is true. Diabetic patients do not tolerate undrained infection and are a compromised host, especially when very hyperglycemic. Without aggressive insulin therapy, hyperglycemia will continue until all infection is debrided and drained. The incision must be long enough, wide enough, and deep enough to ensure complete drainage of pus or debridement of necrotic tissue.[31] A diabetic patient will heal as well as a nondiabetic patient if the infection is completely resolved and the circulation is adequate. All calluses and crusted areas must be initially debrided and carefully examined for a deeper limb-threatening infection. Again, because of neuropathy the diabetic patient does not demonstrate the usual pain response associated with a deeper infection lying beneath what appears to be a benign callus or crusted area. This is especially true for diabetic patients who have continued to bear weight on the extremity. Because of neuropathy, many of these initial debridements and inspections can be done at bedside, with little or no anesthesia. In general, drains placed through small stab wounds do not adequately drain infection for most diabetic patients.

Local wound care can also present problems. Soaks, heat in any form, or whirlpools have led to complications in our experience and are not recommended. Because of neuropathy they can cause extensive burns. They also can lead to maceration of ischemic tissue and may play a role in the spread of bacteria. We prefer to pack plain gauze dressings moistened with diluted isotonic antiseptic solution into the wound from one to three times per day. This provides mechanical debridement and permits one to inspect the wound constantly to make sure that debridement and drainage are adequate. Full-strength solutions and astringents are to be avoided. The use of growth factors to accelerate healing holds promise for the future,[32] but only in conjunction with arterial reconstruction.

Proper choice of antibiotics is essential in the treatment of limb-threatening foot infections. Polymicrobial infections are the rule.[31] Anaerobes will be present in the mixed infections of one-half to two-thirds of these patients, and the initial use of broad-spectrum intravenous antibiotics is indicated. Changes in antibiotic are made on the basis of the results of antibiotic sensitivity testing and the response of the wound to treatment. We prefer not to use oral antibiotics for serious limb-threatening infections. A course of antibiotics with little or no surgical debridement has generally failed in our experience, and we do not recommended such treatment for routine use.

Once sepsis is controlled, patients with ischemia are evaluated and undergo appropriate arterial reconstruction as described in this chapter. Revisions of previously performed surgical debridements or amputations can then be performed, and once healing is assured, the patient can begin to bear weight. Protective footwear is essential in the progression of weight bearing and for the protection of sensitive high-risk areas.

AMPUTATIONS

In the past, transmetatarsal amputation was the primary approach to the management of deep ulcerations or gangrene of the toes or forefoot.[33] With the improvements in the understanding of vascular disease and in the success of distal bypass, the role of this operation has diminished. Once arterial circulation has been restored, it is possible to perform foot-sparing surgery. For example, when a metatarsal phalangeal joint is infected, it may be possible to simply remove the joint rather than perform a ray or transmetatarsal amputation. Full revascularization of the foot opens up the possibility of many similar minor procedures that preserve as much foot function as possible. In general, revascularization should be carried out before any minor amputations or foot surgery. The greatest assurance of forefoot healing can be obtained by restoring circulation first whenever possible. Thus, the established success of arterial reconstruction has reduced the need for amputations at all levels[27] and has involved techniques for optimal preservation of the foot.

When patients have severe neuropathy and/or infection, amputation may be necessary even in the presence of intact circulation. Transmetatarsal amputation results in minimal interference with ambulation and lifestyle. For more extensive gangrene, transtarsal (Chopart's) or Syme's amputation[34] are useful. Below-knee amputation is necessary in patients who have extensive gangrene or for whom lesser amputations have failed.

When foot pulses are not palpable, the use of noninvasive tests, including tcPo$_2$, may be helpful in predicting amputation level. However, clinical judgment remains very important. If necrosis is progressing, even in the presence of adequate tcPo$_2$, an attempt at transmetatarsal amputation may be ill-advised. On the other hand, if a foot wound has developed healthy-looking granulation tissue, a low tcPo$_2$ would not preclude an attempt at transmetatarsal amputation. Similar arguments apply to other levels of amputation. The combined presence of ischemia, neuropathy, and infection adds complexity to the clinical decision regarding level of amputation. As a practical matter, in this milieu noninvasive tests are useful but not definitive.

REFERENCES

1. Goldenberg S, Alex M, Joshi RA, Blumenthal HT. Nonatheromatous peripheral vascular disease of the lower extremity in diabetes mellitus. Diabetes 1959;8:261–73.
2. Strandness DE, Priest RE Jr, Gibbons GE. Combined clinical and pathologic study of diabetic and nondiabetic peripheral arterial disease. Diabetes 1964;13:366–72.
3. Conrad MC. Large and small artery occlusion in diabetics and nondiabetics with severe vascular disease. Circulation 1967;36:83–91.
4. Barner HB, Kaiser GC, Willman VL. Blood flow in the diabetic leg. Circulation 1971;43:391–4.
5. Siperstein MD, Unger RH, Madison LL. Studies of muscle

6. Parving H-H, Noer I, Deckert T, et al. The effect of metabolic regulation on microvascular permeability to small and large molecules in short-term juvenile diabetics. Diabetologia 1976;12:161–6.
7. Wyss CR, Matsen FA III, Simmons CW, Burgess EM. Transcutaneous oxygen tension measurements on limbs of diabetic and nondiabetic patients with peripheral vascular disease. Surgery 1984;95:339–46.
8. Auer AI, Hurley JJ, Binnington HB, et al. Distal tibial vein grafts for limb salvage. Arch Surg 1983;118:597–602.
9. Gensler SW, Haimovici H, Hoffert P, et al. Study of vascular lesions in diabetic, nondiabetic patients: clinical, arteriographic, and surgical considerations. Arch Surg 1965; 91:617–22.
10. Sidawy AN, Menzoian JO, Cantelmo NL, LoGerfo FW. Effect of inflow and outflow sites on the results of tibioperoneal vein grafts. Am J Surg 1986;152:211–4.
11. Stonebridge PA, Tsoukas AI, Pomposelli FB Jr, et al. Popliteal-to-distal bypass grafts for limb salvage in diabetics. Eur J Vasc Surg 1991;5:265–9.
12. Cantelmo NL, Snow JR, Menzoian JO, LoGerfo FW. Successful vein bypass in patients with an ischemic limb and a palpable popliteal pulse. Arch Surg 1986;121:217–20.
13. Sammarco GJ. Diabetic arthropathy. In: Sammarco GJ, ed. The foot in diabetes. Philadelphia: Lea & Febiger, 1991: 153–79.
14. Ramsey DE, Manke DA, Sumner DS. Toe blood pressure: a valuable adjunct to ankle pressure measurement for assessing peripheral arterial disease. J Cardiovasc Surg 1983; 24:43–8.
15. Bone GE, Pomajzl MJ. Toe blood pressure by photoplethysmography: an index of healing in forefoot amputation. Surgery 1981;89:569–74.
16. Darling RC, Raines JK, Brener BJ, Austen WG. Quantitative segmental pulse volume recorder: a clinical tool. Surgery 1972;72:873–87.
17. Yao JST, Ricco J-B. Arterial survey with Doppler ultrasonography. In: Rutherford RB, ed. Vascular surgery. 2nd ed. Philadelphia: WB Saunders, 1984:81–92.
18. Franzeck UK, Talke P, Bernstein EF, et al. Transcutaneous PO$_2$ measurements in health and peripheral arterial occlusive disease. Surgery 1982;91:156–63.
19. Parfrey PS, Griffiths SM, Barrett BJ, et al. Contrast material-induced renal failure in patients with diabetes mellitus, renal insufficiency or both: a prospective controlled study. N Engl J Med 1989;320:143–9.
20. Eisenberg RL, Bank WO, Hedgock MW. Renal failure after major angiography can be avoided by hydration. AJR Am J Roentgenol 1981;136:859–61.
21. Kerstein MD, Puyau FA. Value of periangiography hydration. Surgery 1984;96:919–22.
22. Stacul F, Carraro M, Magnaldi S, et al. Contrast agent nephrotoxicity: comparison of ionic and nonionic contrast agents. AJR Am J Roentgenol 1987;149:1287–9.
23. Hurley JJ, Auer AI, Hershey FB, et al. Distal arterial reconstruction: patency and limb salvage in diabetics. J Vasc Surg 1987;5:796–802.
24. Taylor LM Jr, Edwards JM, Phinney ES, Porter JM. Reversed vein bypass to infrapopliteal arteries: modern results are superior to or equivalent to in-situ bypass for patency and for vein utilization. Ann Surg 1987;205:90–7.
25. Pomposelli FB Jr, Jepsen SJ, Gibbons GW, et al. Efficacy of the dorsal pedal bypass for limb salvage in diabetic patients: short-term observations. J Vasc Surg 1990;11: 745–52.

capillary basement membranes in normal subjects, diabetic, and prediabetic patients. J Clin Invest 1968;47:1973–99.

26. Pomposelli FB Jr, Jepsen SJ, Gibbons GW, et al. A flexible approach to infrapopliteal vein grafts in patients with diabetes mellitus. Arch Surg 1991;126:724–9.

27. LoGerfo FW, Gibbons GW, Pomposelli FB Jr, et al. Trends in the care of the diabetic foot: expanded role for arterial reconstruction. Arch Surg 1992 (in press).

28. Tannenbaum GA, Pomposelli FB Jr, Marcaccio EJ, et al. Safety of vein bypass grafting to the dorsalis pedis artery in diabetic patients with foot infections. J Vasc Surg 1992 (in press).

29. Miller A, Stonebridge PA, Jepsen SJ, et al. Continued experience with intraoperative angioscopy for monitoring infrainguinal bypass grafting. Surgery 1991;109:286–93.

30. Gorman DF. Oxygen therapy in the diabetic foot. In: Frykberg RG, ed. The high risk foot in diabetes mellitus. New York: Churchill Livingstone, 1991:441–7.

31. Gibbons GW. The diabetic foot: amputations and drainage of infection. J Vasc Surg 1987;5:791–3.

32. Krupski WC, Reilly LM, Perez S, et al. A prospective randomized trial of autologous platelet-derived wound healing factors for treatment of chronic non-healing wounds: a preliminary report. J Vasc Surg 1991;14:526–36.

33. McKittrick LS, McKittrick JB, Risley TS. Transmetatarsal amputation for infection or gangrene in patients with diabetes mellitus. Ann Surg 1949;130:826–42.

34. Wagner WF Jr. A classification and treatment program for diabetic, neuropathic and dysvascular foot problems. In: American Association of Orthopedic Surgery Instructional Course Lectures. Vol 28. AAOS, 1979:143–50.

HYPOGLYCEMIA

LLOYD AXELROD
LYNNE L. LEVITSKY

Hypoglycemia, a low level of glucose in the circulation, is not a disease but a laboratory finding that is often associated with characteristic signs and symptoms. Hypoglycemia occurs in a large number of clinical disorders of diverse cause in which normal homeostatic mechanisms fail to maintain the circulating glucose level within the normal range. These disorders have in common signs and symptoms that reflect inadequate glucose delivery to the brain and compensatory activation of the sympathetic nervous system. The purpose of this chapter is to provide a systematic approach to the diagnosis and management of hypoglycemic disorders in children and adults.

GLUCOSE HOMEOSTASIS

Under normal circumstances, the brain is dependent upon the oxidation of glucose for energy. When the circulating glucose level falls, the brain is unable to function and symptoms of hypoglycemia ensue (see below). The brain also can use ketone bodies (β-hydroxybutyrate and acetoacetate) for energy. In general, the uptake of ketone bodies by the brain is proportional to the arterial concentration of these substances.[1,2] During the fed state, the plasma levels of the ketones are not high enough to provide the energy needs of the brain, so the brain is entirely dependent upon glucose for energy. During a fast, it takes many hours for the circulating ketone levels to increase sufficiently to provide an alternate source of energy to the brain. Thus, except in the fasting state, the brain is totally dependent on glucose for energy. Insulin suppresses ketosis by inhibiting triglyceride lipolysis (thereby reducing circulating levels of free fatty acids) and promoting the utilization of ketones in peripheral tissues such as skeletal muscle. Thus, in insulin-mediated forms of hypoglycemia, insulin not only lowers the circulating glucose level but also decreases the availability of alternate substrates for the brain. Conversely, the availability of ketones explains, at least in part, the observation that normal persons who are fasting or starving tolerate remarkably low levels of circulating glucose (e.g., blood glucose levels of 25 mg/dL (1.39 mM)) without developing symptoms or signs of hypoglycemia.

Because of the dependence of the brain on glucose in most circumstances, it is not surprising that a redundant set of mechanisms has evolved to maintain the level of circulating glucose within normal limits and to prevent hypoglycemia. Glucose homeostasis involves a balance between glucose production and glucose utilization. Hypoglycemia occurs when glucose production is reduced and/or glucose utilization is increased. Both glucose production and glucose utilization require a complex interplay of hormone actions and metabolic processes. Dysfunction of the organs involved in glucose homeostasis and disturbances in the secretion or action of the hormones that regulate these processes can result in hypoglycemia.

Normally, glucose enters the circulation in three ways: it may be ingested as simple or complex carbohydrates; it may be derived from hepatic glycogen by the process of glycogenolysis; or it may be produced in the liver (and in the renal cortex during prolonged fasting) from nonglucose precursors (amino acids, glycerol, and lactate) by the process of gluconeogenesis. The absorption of ingested carbohydrates requires the presence of enzymes that digest complex carbohydrates in the intestinal lumen, the presence of an intact gastrointestinal tract with normally functioning mechanisms for the hydrolysis of oligosaccharides, the active transport of glucose and galactose, and the facilitated diffusion of fructose from the lumen into the small intestinal epithelial cell.

Hepatic glycogenolysis depends upon the availability of stored glycogen. The normal adult liver contains up to 70 g of glycogen after a meal. During a fast the breakdown of hepatic glycogen can provide glucose to the circulation of the adult for about 24 to 48 hours.[3] This process is stimulated by glucagon secreted by the α-cells of the pancreatic islets and by catecholamines (epinephrine and norepinephrine) secreted by the enterochromaffin system.

During the fasting state, hepatic glycogen is gradually depleted over 24 to 48 hours,[3] after which maintenance of the circulating glucose level is completely dependent upon gluconeogenesis. Gluconeogenesis requires the availability of sufficient substrate, an intact liver (and renal cortex) to convert the substrates to glucose, and a hormonal environment that promotes these conversions. Quantitatively, the amino acids are the principal substrates for hepatic gluconeogenesis. Among the amino acids, alanine is by far the most important. During the fasting state, hepatic gluconeogenesis is dependent upon the availability of alanine and other amino acids derived from skeletal muscle. Lactate derived from skeletal muscle and other sources and glycerol derived from triglyceride lipolysis in adipose tissue are additional substrates for hepatic gluconeogenesis. Glutamine is the principal substrate for gluconeogenesis in the renal

cortex. The rate of gluconeogenesis is increased by glucagon and by cortisol. Thus, gluconeogenesis requires the secretion of adrenocorticotropic hormone (ACTH) by the anterior pituitary and cortisol by the adrenal cortex. Cortisol promotes the maintenance of a normal circulating glucose level by multiple mechanisms. It promotes the release of amino acid substrate from skeletal muscle, increases the activity of the rate-limiting enzymes of gluconeogenesis in the liver, increases glucagon secretion, and induces resistance to the action of insulin.[4]

Changes in the rate of glucose utilization may alter the circulating glucose level. Insulin promotes glucose utilization by its actions on skeletal muscle and adipose tissue. Glycogen synthesis in skeletal muscle is the principal pathway of insulin-mediated glucose disposal in normal subjects and patients with non-insulin-dependent diabetes mellitus (NIDDM).[5] Changes in insulin secretion or insulin action at the receptor level or beyond may alter glucose utilization. Glucose utilization increases during exercise, during lactation, and when the availability of fat-derived substrates (free fatty acids and ketones) for peripheral tissues is diminished.

Despite some redundancy of the mechanisms that defend the circulating glucose level and assure glucose availability to the brain, hypoglycemia can occur when a disease process involves virtually any process (nutrient absorption, storage, or release), organ (gastrointestinal tract, skeletal muscle, liver, pituitary, adrenal cortex), or hormone (insulin, glucagon, cortisol, catecholamines, growth hormone, thyroid hormone) involved in this regulatory system. Hypoglycemia also can occur when exogenous substances such as ethanol or certain medications interfere with the normal function of these processes, organs, and hormones. Thus, the redundancy of these defense mechanisms provides the basis for the diversity of the disorders that cause hypoglycemia.

SIGNS AND SYMPTOMS OF HYPOGLYCEMIA

Hypoglycemia induces both adrenergic and neuroglycopenic symptoms. The glycemic threshold for epinephrine release is higher than that for induction of neuroglycopenic symptoms in most studies, but there may be individual variation.[6] This may lead to discrepancies among individuals in their response to hypoglycemia. Symptoms and signs related to epinephrine release include pallor, sweating, tachycardia, widened pulse pressure, nausea, anxiety, and hunger. In adults, sweating is often an especially prominent symptom. Neuroglycopenic symptoms include disturbed mentation, behavioral change, headache, paresthesias, blurred vision, cortical blindness, hemiplegia, aphasia, hypothermia, coma, and seizures. Because the brain oxidizes glucose to meet its energy requirements, it is not surprising that the symptoms of neuroglycopenia and those of hypoxia are virtually indistinguishable. Although it is generally assumed that children tolerate lower levels of blood glucose than do adults, the glycemic threshold for epinephrine release in normal prepubertal children is higher than that in normal adults.[7] Symptoms are less specific in the neonate than in the older child and adult and may include irritability, jitteriness, changes in tone, cyanosis, tachypnea, and lethargy, in addition to frank coma or seizures.

Since the symptoms of hypoglycemia are related to fuel deprivation in the central nervous system, the response to hypoglycemia also depends upon the peripheral availability and transport of alternative fuels for the central nervous system such as ketone bodies and lactate.[8,9] The uptake of ketones and lactate is normally facilitated by the same transport system, which is more active in infants than in adults. The epinephrine response to hypoglycemia is mediated by hypothalamic neurons.[10] However, it is not clear that alternative fuels are available to all areas of the brain.[11] Altered cerebral energy requirements also influence manifestations of hypoglycemia. Chronic hypoglycemia may enhance cerebral glucose extraction.[12,13] Areas of cortical activation take up more glucose than other areas. In animal studies, seizure activity increases glucose requirements because of an increased need for fuel during rapid neuronal firing.[14] On the other hand, cerebral blood flow increases during hypoglycemia in experimental animals, and this may increase cerebral availability of fuel.[15,16] The net effect of increased cerebral glucose extraction and decreased cerebral fuel availability on the manifestations of hypoglycemia may be variable.

DEFINITION OF HYPOGLYCEMIA

Hypoglycemia may be defined by the use of statistical population norms, evidence of physiologic counterregulation, measures of acute neurologic change, or measures of long-term outcome. Long-term outcome depends upon the severity of neuroglycopenia, the duration of the neuroglycopenic episode, and the availability of alternate fuels.

The normal response of the plasma glucose level to fasting is different in adult men and women (Fig. 55–1).[17] In adult men, a normal fasting plasma glucose level is 55 mg/dL (3.1 mM) at 24 hours and 50 mg/dL (2.8 mM) at 48 and 72 hours. In premenopausal women, a normal fasting plasma glucose level is 35 mg/dL (1.9 mM) at 24 hours, but no normal value can be established at 48 or 72 hours because of the wide range of responses.[17]

In the adult, the appearance of neurologic symptoms during a fast is used to indicate that the hypoglycemia has a pathologic basis (e.g., an insulinoma or tumor-induced hypoglycemia) because the availability of alternative fuels such as ketones normally prevents neurologic symptoms during a fast. Because ketosis normally develops during a fast, the absence of ketosis also suggests that hypoglycemia is due to a pathologic condition during a fast.[19] In children, the range of diagnostic possibilities is wider and this rule cannot be followed. Adults and children develop certain counterregulatory responses at different glucose levels. When insulin is used to induce hypoglycemia, epinephrine release is noted at mean plasma glucose levels below 56 mg/dL (3.1 mM) in normal adults and at mean values of 68 mg/dL (3.8 mM) in normal children.[7]

More effort has been devoted to the definition of hypoglycemia in children than in adults. Hypoglycemia in adults is usually accompanied by characteristic symptoms, whereas hypoglycemia in infants and children is often more difficult to recognize and may produce long-term neurologic damage more readily. Statistical norms (values more than two standard deviations below the mean) were initially used to define hypoglycemia in the neonate but offer little assistance in determining whether a blood glucose level is associated with the short- or long-term effects of neuroglycopenia.[20] The classic studies of Cornblath and colleagues suggested that a replicate blood glucose value persistently below 20 mg/dL (1.1 mM) is abnormal in the low-birth-weight infant in the first 24 hours of life and that a value less than 30 mg/dL (1.7 mM) is abnormal in the full-term infant or older low-birth-weight infant.[20] These values are based on studies of infants who were fasted for prolonged periods (24 to 72 hours), a practice that is discordant with the present care of the preterm infant. Further, these studies report glucose levels in whole blood rather than in plasma. More recent examinations of blood glucose values in the neonatal period suggest that the criteria of Cornblath et al. would define 8% of the newborn population as hypoglycemic, while 20% would have blood glucose values below 40 mg/dL (2.2 mM).[21] A review of 36 textbooks of pediatrics showed a wide variation in the definition of hypoglycemia—from blood glucose values of less than 1 mM to values of less than 2.5 mM in both full-term normal weight babies and in low-birth-weight infants.[22] A long-term follow-up study suggested that even moderate hypoglycemia (blood glucose level of less than 2.6 mM) if noted on repeated occasions may be associated with an adverse developmental outcome.[23] However, this study is difficult to analyze because of confounding management variables.

The acute neurologic or physiologic response to hypoglycemia in the neonate might help to define hypoglycemia. Neural dysfunction measured as altered sensory-evoked potentials during spontaneous or fasting hypoglycemia was noted in a small group of infants with blood glucose values ranging from 0.7 to 2.5 mM.[24] Plasma epinephrine levels were increased in over half the preterm neonates with blood glucose values below 45 mg/dL (2.5 mM). Increased cerebral blood flow was associated with these low blood glucose values.[25] This increase could enhance glucose extraction. These studies suggest that a blood glucose value below 45 mg/dL (2.5 mM) may provoke acute adrenergic and neuroglycopenic responses. Larger studies using similar techniques are needed to define this range more precisely.

CLASSIFICATION OF HYPOGLYCEMIC DISORDERS

Many clinical entities cause hypoglycemia. They may be classified in several different ways: as reactive (those in which hypoglycemia occurs in response to a nutrient challenge) or fasting, as insulin-mediated or insulin-independent, and as disorders of decreased glucose production or increased glucose utilization. These classifications are not mutually exclusive and may be used in a

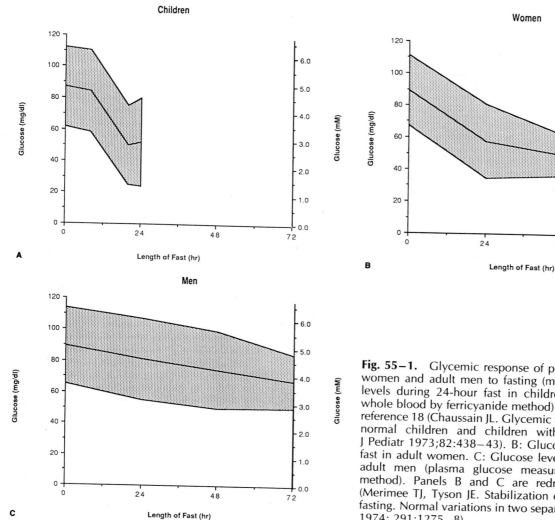

Fig. 55–1. Glycemic response of prepubertal children, adult women and adult men to fasting (mean ±2 SD). A: Glucose levels during 24-hour fast in children (glucose measured in whole blood by ferricyanide method). Panel A is redrawn from reference 18 (Chaussain JL. Glycemic response to 24 hour fast in normal children and children with ketotic hypoglycemia. J Pediatr 1973;82:438–43). B: Glucose levels during 72-hour fast in adult women. C: Glucose levels during 72-hour fast in adult men (plasma glucose measured by glucose oxidase method). Panels B and C are redrawn from reference 17 (Merimee TJ, Tyson JE. Stabilization of plasma glucose during fasting. Normal variations in two separate studies. N Engl J Med 1974; 291:1275–8).

coordinated manner (Figs. 55–2, 55–3, 55–4). From a clinical viewpoint, it is most efficient to classify hypoglycemic disorders as reactive or fasting hypoglycemia. Within the category of fasting hypoglycemia, it is helpful to separate insulin-mediated from insulin-independent entities. It is less helpful to classify the fasting hypoglycemic disorders as conditions due to decreased glucose production or those due to increased glucose utilization because this is often difficult to ascertain clinically and because some entities are due both to decreased production and to increased utilization. Nevertheless, in certain circumstances it quickly becomes evident that the patient requires unusually large quantities of glucose to prevent hypoglycemia [e.g., more than 1.9 to 2.4 mg/(kg · min) in an adult or 12 mg/(kg · min) in an infant]. In these patients, increased glucose utilization is a prominent aspect of the pathogenesis of hypoglycemia. Fasting hypoglycemic disorders due to exogenous substances are important clinically. Hypoglycemia arising as a consequence of the therapeutic use of insulin or oral hypoglycemic agents in diabetic patients, the most common exogenous cause of hypo-

glycemia, is considered elsewhere in this volume (see Chapter 28 on iatrogenic hypoglycemia and Chapter 29 on oral hypoglycemic agents).

APPROACH TO THE ADULT PATIENT WITH HYPOGLYCEMIA

Although the manifestations of hypoglycemia are often characteristic, they are nonspecific. Thus, the physician's first responsibility is to determine whether or not the patient's symptoms are due to hypoglycemia. The diagnosis of hypoglycemia requires the presence of symptoms consistent with hypoglycemia, the finding of a low circulating glucose level at the time of symptoms, and the correction of the patient's symptoms by the administration of food or glucose (Whipple's triad). These criteria must be applied rigorously. When they are not met, the diagnosis of hypoglycemia must be regarded with suspicion. However, on occasion it is not possible to fulfill all of these criteria. For example, it may not be possible to obtain a glucose value during the occurrence of symptoms be-

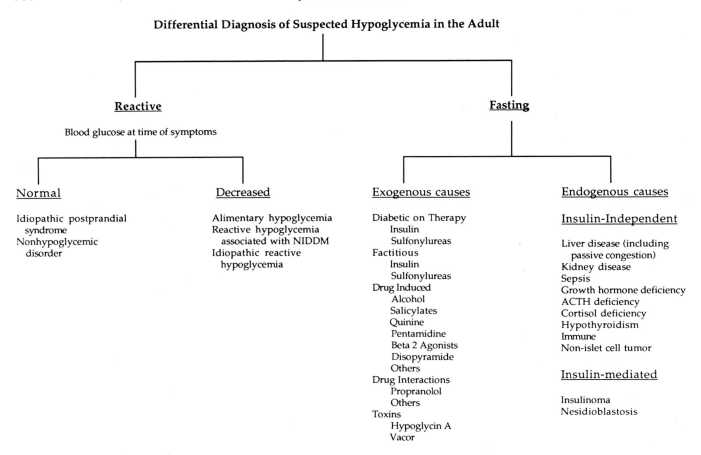

Fig. 55—2. Differential diagnosis of suspected hypoglycemia in the adult.

cause the symptoms occur far from a medical facility. Moreover, a glucose value obtained after cessation of symptoms may not be abnormal as a result of the activation of normal compensatory mechanisms. While the symptoms and signs of hypoglycemia characteristically respond in a rapid and gratifying way to the administration of glucose, this is not invariable. The neurologic manifestations of hypoglycemia may persist for hours or days after correction of hypoglycemia or may be permanent. In these exceptional circumstances the presumptive diagnosis of hypoglycemia may be made by careful consideration of the pertinent findings and exclusion of other possible causes of the patient's symptoms.

The approach to the patient with hypoglycemia depends in large measure upon the history and the physical examination (Fig. 55—2). The use of laboratory tests is governed by the history and the physical findings. During the clinical evaluation, it is essential to determine whether the patient's hypoglycemia is reactive or occurs in the fasting state, keeping in mind that patients with a form of hypoglycemia that typically occurs in the fasting state (an insulinoma, for example) may occasionally have postprandial symptoms. If the history indicates the presence of fasting hypoglycemia, it is essential to address immediately the possibility that the hypoglycemia is due to an exogenous cause, e.g., factitious use of insulin or an oral hypoglycemic agent or use of ethanol or certain

medications. This approach will frequently prevent unnecessary testing and save both time and money. Clinical evaluation may reveal the symptoms and signs of disorders such as congestive heart failure, liver disease, kidney disease, sepsis, pituitary insufficiency, or adrenal insufficiency, thereby focusing and narrowing the diagnostic process.

The differential diagnosis of hypoglycemia varies according to the setting in which it is encountered. In the emergency room of a large municipal hospital serving a socioeconomically deprived urban community, diabetes mellitus, alcoholism, and sepsis, alone or in combination, accounted for 90% of all visits for symptomatic hypoglycemia.[26] In patients hospitalized at a university hospital, treatment of diabetes mellitus was the most common cause of hypoglycemia, followed by renal insufficiency unrelated to diabetes mellitus.[27] The remaining episodes of hypoglycemia were due to liver disease, infections, shock, pregnancy, and neoplasia (usually with liver metastases and malnutrition).[27]

MEASUREMENT OF THE CIRCULATING GLUCOSE LEVEL

To establish or exclude the diagnosis of hypoglycemia, it is necessary to have an accurate measurement of the circulating glucose level. It is important to know whether

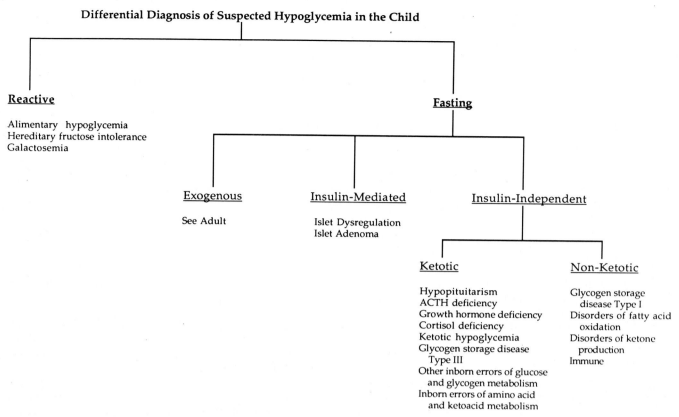

Differential Diagnosis of Suspected Hypoglycemia in the Child

Reactive

Alimentary hypoglycemia
Hereditary fructose intolerance
Galactosemia

Fasting

Exogenous

See Adult

Insulin-Mediated

Islet Dysregulation
Islet Adenoma

Insulin-Independent

Ketotic

Hypopituitarism
ACTH deficiency
Growth hormone deficiency
Cortisol deficiency
Ketotic hypoglycemia
Glycogen storage disease
  Type III
Other inborn errors of glucose
  and glycogen metabolism
Inborn errors of amino acid
  and ketoacid metabolism

Non-Ketotic

Glycogen storage
  disease Type I
Disorders of fatty acid
  oxidation
Disorders of ketone
  production
Immune

Fig. 55–3. Differential diagnosis of suspected hypoglycemia in the child.

the glucose was measured in whole blood or in plasma, and the observed values should be compared with the appropriate standards. Whole blood glucose levels are lower than plasma glucose levels because the concentration of glucose is much lower in erythrocytes than in plasma. Blood glucose measurements may approach plasma glucose values when the patient is severely anemic. In general, glucose levels should not be measured in serum because erythrocytes consume glucose; an artifactually low glucose level can be observed if the sample is stored at room temperature. Blood for the measurement of whole blood or plasma glucose levels is usually collected in a tube containing oxalate and fluoride, an inhibitor of glycolysis, to prevent this artifact of collection and storage. Glucose values are frequently measured with whole blood obtained by a capillary finger stick and applied to a reagent strip by visual inspection or use of a glucose meter. The glucose value in capillary blood is 7 to 8% higher than that in venous blood. Because the glucose level is measured immediately, consumption of glucose by the erythrocytes is not a problem with these methods. Nevertheless, artifactually low glucose levels may result from use of a glucose meter. Application of an insufficient quantity of blood to the reagent strip, failure to clean the window of certain meters, or malfunction of the meter commonly lead to aberrant values. Visual inspection of a reagent strip to which blood has been applied may not be a reliable way to distinguish normal from low glucose values because

the human eye cannot always make such distinctions accurately. Many glucose meters are more reliable in the normal or hyperglycemic range than in the hypoglycemic range. For these reasons, a glucose meter may be used to exclude the presence of hypoglycemia, but low values must be interpreted with caution and confirmed when possible by a glucose determination performed in a chemistry laboratory. In severely hypotensive patients, glucose values obtained by capillary finger stick are frequently lower than venous glucose values.[28] This discrepancy may lead to the erroneous diagnosis of hypoglycemia when blood is obtained by capillary finger stick.

REACTIVE HYPOGLYCEMIA

Reactive hypoglycemia refers to a group of disorders in which hypoglycemia and its manifestations occur after the consumption of food and not during the fasting state (Figs. 55–2 and 55–3).

In the adult patient, the entities included in the category of reactive hypoglycemia are alimentary hypoglycemia, reactive hypoglycemia associated with NIDDM, and idiopathic reactive hypoglycemia. It is essential to distinguish patients with these disorders from patients with postprandial symptoms who do not have reactive hypoglycemia. Such patients are said to have the idiopathic postprandial syndrome. In children the causes of

Differential Diagnosis of Hypoglycemia in the Neonate

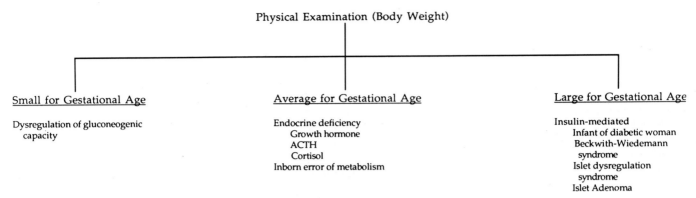

Fig. 55—4. Differential diagnosis of hypoglycemia in the neonate.

reactive hypoglycemia include alimentary hypoglycemia following gastric surgery, hereditary fructose intolerance, and galactosemia. Insulin-mediated hypoglycemia may produce postprandial as well as fasting hypoglycemia.

Alimentary Hypoglycemia

Alimentary hypoglycemia usually occurs in patients who have had gastric surgery. It is typically encountered in patients who have had a total gastrectomy but may also occur after a partial gastrectomy (with or without a gastric emptying procedure). On rare occasions, patients who have had no gastric surgery also develop alimentary hypoglycemia.[29] Alimentary hypoglycemia is the most serious form of reactive hypoglycemia in the adult. In contrast to the other forms of reactive hypoglycemia in the adult, in alimentary hypoglycemia symptoms may include seizures or coma and the disorder may be lethal. Typically, the patient develops adrenergic or neurologic symptoms of hypoglycemia 30 to 60 minutes after eating. Alimentary hypoglycemia appears to reflect loss of the normal gastric reservoir function, rapid absorption of glucose, a normal β-cell response to hyperglycemia, and persistence of the effect of insulin after disposal of the ingested glucose. Under ordinary circumstances, the stomach empties gradually so that the gastric contents are delivered gradually to the small intestine where glucose is absorbed. When the stomach is no longer able to function as a reservoir, the gastric contents are delivered rapidly into the small intestine, increasing the rate of glucose absorption. Consequently, hyperglycemia develops rapidly, often within 30 minutes of the glucose load. This hyperglycemia constitutes an insulinogenic stimulus to the normal β-cells of the pancreas. The effect of the secreted insulin may persist after disposal of the glucose load, with consequent hypoglycemia. Other factors may contribute. It has been suggested that the enteroinsular axis is disturbed as a consequence of gastric surgery and that there is an increase in the secretion of an enteric hormone that stimulates insulin secretion. While it is difficult to exclude this hypothesis, there is no convincing evidence to support it.

The diagnosis of alimentary hypoglycemia should be entertained in any patient with a history of gastric surgery who has symptoms consistent with hypoglycemia, including seizures and coma, approximately 30 minutes to 2 hours after a meal. It is sometimes necessary to distinguish alimentary hypoglycemia from the dumping syndrome, another complication of gastric surgery.

The diagnosis of alimentary hypoglycemia can sometimes be made by measurement of the circulating glucose level when symptoms occur in a patient with an appropriate history. In some instances it may be necessary to perform an oral glucose tolerance test. The characteristic pattern is marked hyperglycemia in the first 30 to 60 minutes after ingestion of glucose followed by hypoglycemia 30 minutes to 2 hours after ingestion. The test must be supervised carefully because of the severity of symptoms that may occur in this setting and the test stopped by administration of intravenous glucose if severe symptoms occur.

The use of multiple small feedings (e.g., a six-meal diet) with no concentrated sweets is usually effective. Compliance may be a problem, especially if the patient does not understand or accept the relationship between the dietary pattern and the occurrence of symptoms.

Reactive Hypoglycemia Associated with Non-Insulin-Dependent Diabetes Mellitus

Rarely, a patient with NIDDM who may otherwise be asymptomatic presents with the symptoms and signs of hypoglycemia 3 to 5 hours after meals.[30] This appears to occur in patients with a relatively mild degree of diabetes, e.g., a fasting circulating glucose level below 250 mg/dL (13.9 mM). The pathophysiology is not well studied. Although the pancreatic β-cells of patients with NIDDM have an impaired ability to respond to a hyperglycemic stimulus,[31,32] the magnitude of the hyperglycemia is apparently sufficient to provoke a delayed increase in insulin secretion. The effect of the secreted insulin may persist after disposal of the ingested glucose, leading to the appearance of hypoglycemia several hours after the glucose load.

Diagnosis may require the performance of an oral glucose tolerance test. The characteristic findings are the presence of hyperglycemia in the first 2 to 3 hours after the ingestion of glucose sufficient to make the diagnosis of diabetes mellitus, followed by the appearance of hypoglycemia and its symptoms and signs 3 to 5 hours after the glucose challenge.

Reactive hypoglycemia in NIDDM is encountered only rarely in clinical practice, and only a few cases have been reported despite the high incidence and prevalence of NIDDM.[30] Possibly, many patients pass through this phase of NIDDM without reporting symptoms. The treatment of this aspect of NIDDM is the treatment of the underlying disease with a diet that includes no concentrated sweets, weight reduction if appropriate, and multiple small feedings.

Idiopathic Reactive Hypoglycemia and the Idiopathic Postprandial Syndrome

In the last two decades, generous attention has been lavished on the possible relationship between a wide range of nonspecific postprandial symptoms and postprandial hypoglycemia in patients with no history of gastric surgery and no evidence of NIDDM. In the past, idiopathic (or functional) reactive hypoglycemia was thought to be characterized by adrenergic and mild neuroglycopenic symptoms several hours after a meal, occurrence of the symptoms at the time of demonstrable hypoglycemia, and relief of symptoms by food or glucose. It is now clear that most patients to whom this label has been attached do not have a disorder of glucose metabolism. Although the diagnosis of idiopathic reactive hypoglycemia has been abused, it is premature to write its obituary.

In many ways, the diagnosis and treatment of idiopathic reactive hypoglycemia in the United States are indicative of a sociologic phenomenon as much as of a medical disorder. An industry based on "hypoglycemia" arose involving physicians, paramedical personnel, elements of the pharmaceutical industry, professional and lay authors, and the media. Its essential premise was that many symptoms commonly encountered in daily life such as fatigue, depression, inability to concentrate, sweating, palpitations, nervousness, and sexual dysfunction are attributable to hypoglycemia. An additional premise was that "the medical establishment" refused to accept this diagnosis for self-serving motives. Frequently (but not always) the diagnosis was made without benefit of a blood glucose determination. Consequently, patients presented to physicians with a diagnosis ("hypoglycemia") rather than a complaint and were distrustful when the diagnosis was questioned. A variety of dietary and pharmacologic approaches were employed. Although this phenomenon has abated in recent years it has not disappeared.

Among responsible professionals the diagnosis of idiopathic reactive hypoglycemia was based on certain plausible but invalid assumptions: that the occurrence of a low blood glucose value after an oral glucose tolerance test is abnormal, that such a value implies the occurrence

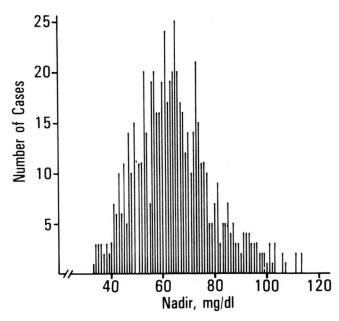

Fig. 55–5. The frequency distribution of nadir plasma glucose values during an oral glucose tolerance test in 650 asymptomatic patients. The median nadir was 64 mg/dL (3.6 mM). Ten percent of the patients had nadir values of ≤47 mg/dL (2.6 mM); 2.5% had values of ≤39 mg/dL (2.2 mM). Reprinted with permission from reference 33 (Lev-Ran A, Anderson RW. The diagnosis of postprandial hypoglycemia. Diabetes 1981;30: 996–9; copyright © of the American Diabetes Association).

of low blood glucose values after a mixed meal, and that these putative low blood glucose values cause symptoms. However, systematic clinical investigation has disproved these assumptions and has provided support for the following generalizations.

1) Normal subjects may have a low circulating glucose level after an oral glucose load; for example, in one study of 650 normal subjects who were free of symptoms before and during a 100-g oral glucose tolerance test, 10% had plasma glucose nadir values of 47 mg/dL (2.6 mM) or below and 2.5% had values of 39 mg/dL (2.2 mM) or less (Fig. 55–5).[33]

2) Those who have low circulating glucose values after an oral glucose tolerance test frequently have normal glucose levels after a mixed meal.

3) Symptoms after an oral glucose load occur without hypoglycemia.

4) Patients who complain of "hypoglycemia" frequently have an emotional basis for their complaints.

In a group of patients undergoing evaluation for reactive hypoglycemia, scores on the Minnesota Multiphasic Personality Inventory were significantly different from those in a matched group of general medical patients. Both men and women had a pattern characteristic of persons who express emotional problems as somatic complaints and are resistant to psychological intervention or interpretation of their symptoms.[34] Nevertheless, some studies have identified patients who appear to have true reactive hypoglycemia. In one study,

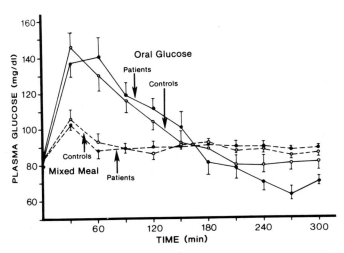

Fig. 55—6. Mean (±SE) plasma glucose values during an oral glucose tolerance test (solid lines) or after a mixed meal (dashed lines) in patients evaluated because of postprandial symptoms (closed circles) and control subjects (open circles). Reprinted with permission from reference 35 (Charles MA, Hofeldt F, Shackelford A, et al. Comparison of oral glucose tolerance tests and mixed meals in patients with apparent idiopathic postabsorptive hypoglycemia: absence of hypoglycemia after meals. Diabetes 1981;30:465—70; copyright © of the American Diabetes Association).

a small fraction of patients (5 of 118) who were evaluated for possible hypoglycemia exhibited hypoglycemia during an oral glucose tolerance test and had symptoms of hypoglycemia after a glucose challenge and after meals.[33] In another study of 18 patients evaluated for hypoglyce-

mia and 16 control subjects, signs and symptoms consistent with hypoglycemia developed after an oral glucose load at comparable rates in the two groups (Fig. 55—6).[35] After mixed meals, hypoglycemia did not occur in either group despite the occurrence of symptoms or signs of hypoglycemia in 14 of 18 patients. Nevertheless, the nadir plasma glucose values during the oral glucose tolerance test were lower in the patients than in the control group (Fig. 55—6). In a recent study, the blood glucose levels were measured in 28 patients while they were experiencing their typical symptoms and in 17 normal subjects (Fig. 55—7).[36] Five patients (18%) had symptoms of hypoglycemia that were associated with blood glucose levels of 2.8 mM (50 mg/dL) or less.[36] Symptoms were more often relieved by food in association with low than with normal blood glucose levels. Thus, it appears that idiopathic reactive hypoglycemia does exist but is an uncommon or rare disorder. The popular attraction of this diagnosis in the United States appears to be waning. If so, the ratio of patients with idiopathic reactive hypoglycemia to patients without this disorder in the population of patients who are evaluated for possible reactive hypoglycemia should increase in the future.

The etiology and pathophysiology of idiopathic reactive hypoglycemia are uncertain. The rate of glucose disposal during a euglycemic hyperinsulinemic glucose clamp study was increased in a study of patients with idiopathic reactive hypoglycemia, suggesting that increased insulin sensitivity is a feature of this disorder.[37] The basis for the increased insulin sensitivity is not known.

Because the finding of a low glucose value after an oral glucose challenge is nonspecific and occurs commonly in normal persons, the performance of an oral glucose

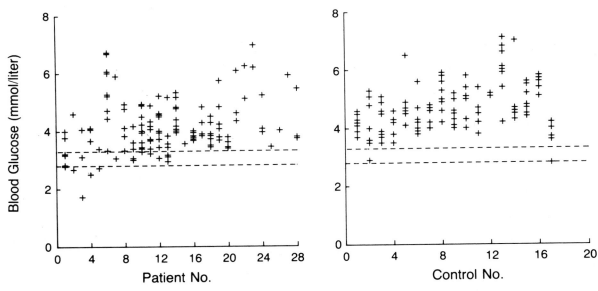

Fig. 55—7. Individual blood glucose values during the occurrence of symptoms in 28 patients with suspected hypoglycemia and 17 normal (control) subjects. The lower dashed line denotes the level 2.8 mM (50 mg/dL) and the upper line, the level 3.3 mM (60 mg/dL). Reprinted with permission from reference 36 (Palardy J, Havrankova J, Lepage R, et al. Blood glucose measurements during symptomatic episodes in patients with suspected postprandial hypoglycemia. N Engl J Med 1989;321:1421—5).

tolerance test is not indicated in the evaluation of the patient who may have idiopathic reactive hypoglycemia. In such a patient, the blood glucose level should be determined during spontaneously occurring symptomatic episodes.[36,38,39] It may be helpful to lend or prescribe a glucose meter to the patient for this purpose, keeping in mind that the accuracy of some glucose meters is decreased in the hypoglycemic range of values.

The evaluation of the patient who is suspected of having idiopathic reactive hypoglycemia presents a diagnostic and therapeutic challenge. In many instances the diagnosis of reactive hypoglycemia will be excluded but important emotional or organic disorders will be found.[33,34] In a minority of patients, idiopathic reactive hypoglycemia will be detected.

The management of idiopathic reactive hypoglycemia involves a diet with no concentrated sweets and sometimes the use of multiple small feedings (six small meals a day). There is no evidence that a high-protein diet is of any value. Such a diet is often high in fat and calories. Consequently, one risks exchanging the control of symptoms for an atherogenic diet and increased body weight. Anticholinergic drugs have been recommended but are generally not needed.

HYPOGLYCEMIA DUE TO EXOGENOUS CAUSES

Diabetic Patients Receiving Insulin or an Oral Hypoglycemic Agent

The most common cause of hypoglycemia in clinical practice is hypoglycemia caused by insulin or an oral hypoglycemic agent in patients with diabetes mellitus. This subject is addressed elsewhere in this volume (see Chapter 28 on iatrogenic hypoglycemia).

Factitious Hypoglycemia

One of the most elusive causes of hypoglycemia is factitious hypoglycemia caused by the surreptitious administration of insulin or an oral hypoglycemic agent.[40] Typically, factitious hypoglycemia occurs in a medical or paramedical worker who understands the ability of the abused medication to induce hypoglycemia and its clinical manifestations and has access to the medication. The patient may go to great lengths to conceal the use of the medication and to conceal the medication itself. Patients who surreptitiously inject insulin may do so in unusual parts of the body such as the axilla, the buccal mucosa, or the areolae of the nipples. The patient usually will deny the use of the abused medication when asked directly about this possibility. Factitious hypoglycemia may also occur in a relative of a diabetic patient treated with insulin or a sulfonylurea or as a result of attempted homicide. Occasionally, factitious hypoglycemia is due to the inadvertent administration of insulin to the wrong patient in a hospital or other institution or to the inadvertent substitution of a sulfonylurea for another medication by a pharmacist, patient, or relative. The patient with factitious hypoglycemia is frequently misdi-

agnosed and treated for an insulinoma because the hypoglycemia is insulin-mediated, in response either to the injection of insulin or to the ingestion of a sulfonylurea, which stimulates insulin secretion. Factitious hypoglycemia must be excluded in any patient thought to have an insulinoma; failure to do so may result in an unnecessary laparotomy.[40]

The diagnosis depends on consideration of this possibility in all patients with insulin-mediated or otherwise unexplained hypoglycemia, especially in those with knowledge of, or access to, a medication that causes hypoglycemia. When factitious hypoglycemia is suspected but denied by the patient, one must seek objective evidence to support or exclude the diagnosis.

The most helpful approach is to determine the circulating levels of glucose, insulin, and C-peptide when symptoms occur. In the patient with factitious hypoglycemia caused by exogenous insulin, the C-peptide level, a measure of endogenous insulin secretion, is low and discordant with the inappropriately elevated insulin level at the time of hypoglycemia. In contrast, in a patient with an insulinoma, the C-peptide and insulin levels are elevated concordantly during an episode of hypoglycemia. When antibodies to insulin are present (see below), the insulin level may be spuriously high (e.g., above 1,000 µU/mL) or spuriously low (e.g., absent), depending upon the method of phase separation used in the insulin radioimmunoassay.[41]

Other laboratory investigations that have been recommended are of limited value. In the past, methods have been developed to identify the species of origin of the circulating insulin at the time of hypoglycemia, an approach known as speciation, based on the idea that exogenous insulin of animal (beef or pork) origin could be distinguished from endogenous human insulin. With the widespread availability of human insulin for the treatment of diabetes, speciation is of little value. While this approach may be helpful in the patient who injects animal insulin surreptitiously, identification of the circulating insulin as human insulin does not exclude the diagnosis of factitious hypoglycemia. Similarly, the identification of antibodies to insulin has been advocated on the theory that nondiabetic patients who have not received insulin should not have antibodies to insulin in the circulation, while patients who administer insulin surreptitiously should have such antibodies. This approach is neither sensitive nor specific. Antibodies to insulin frequently do not develop in patients who inject modern highly purified animal or human insulin preparations. Such antibodies occur spontaneously on rare occasion in patients with autoimmune hypoglycemia (see below). Also, low levels of antibodies to insulin often presage the development of insulin-dependent diabetes mellitus (IDDM).

On rare occasion it may be necessary to search the hospital room of a patient who is thought to have factitious hypoglycemia to find evidence of surreptitious injection of insulin such as vials of insulin or insulin syringes. In general, a room search can only be justified when there is strong clinical suspicion of factitious hypoglycemia supported by objective evidence (e.g., discordant C-peptide and insulin levels during an episode of symptomatic hypoglycemia) and the patient consistently denies the surreptitious use of insulin. The search should be performed when the patient is out of the room (because the room belongs to the hospital, not to the patient) and in the presence of at least one reliable witness (a physician, nurse, or administrator). A room search should be performed only after careful consideration and consultation with the appropriate hospital authorities.

Less commonly, factitious hypoglycemia is due to abuse of a sulfonylurea. When this is suspected it may be helpful to measure the level of one or more sulfonylureas in the circulation, preferably at the time of symptomatic hypoglycemia.

The psychopathology of factitious hypoglycemia is not well understood. On occasion, the patient will admit to a motive of secondary gain. For example, a patient who grew up with a sibling with a chronic illness equated being sick with receiving parental love. Some patients respond to psychotherapy, but in the majority insight is limited. Factitious disease may recur and the patient may later commit suicide.[40] Management involves a firm and supportive confrontation after the diagnosis is established and then psychiatric care.[40]

Hypoglycemia Caused by Drugs and Toxins

Except in the diabetic patient treated with insulin or a sulfonylurea or the patient with alcohol-induced hypoglycemia, drugs are an uncommon cause of hypoglycemia. Important factors predisposing to drug-induced hypoglycemia are age (the very young and the very old), decreased caloric intake (acutely or chronically), and impairment of renal or hepatic function.[42] Approximately 80% of reported patients with drug-induced hypoglycemia had one or more of these risk factors.[42] While many drugs have been reported to cause hypoglycemia, it is not clear that all of the implicated medications do so.[42] The following substances are well-established causes of hypoglycemia.

Alcohol-Induced Hypoglycemia

This characteristically occurs in an alcoholic who has been drinking but not eating for several days.[43] Because the symptoms of alcohol intoxication and the symptoms of hypoglycemia are similar, alcohol-induced hypoglycemia is easily overlooked, with potentially catastrophic consequences. In the absence of food, maintenance of the circulating glucose level depends on glycogenolysis and gluconeogenesis. In the patient who is not eating, hepatic glycogen stores are depleted in 1 to 2 days.[3] Thereafter, maintenance of a normal glucose level depends on gluconeogenesis.[43] Alcohol consumption predictably results in the inhibition of gluconeogenesis. Ethanol is metabolized in the liver by alcohol dehydrogenase to acetaldehyde, which is transformed by acetaldehyde dehydrogenase to acetic acid. Hydrogen ions are liberated at each of these steps, resulting in generation of

reduced nicotinamide adenine dinucleotide (NADH) and an increase in the ratio of NADH to NAD. The increased NADH/NAD ratio inhibits gluconeogenesis at several critical steps, including the conversion of lactate to pyruvate, several steps in the tricarboxylic acid cycle (including the conversion of glutamate to α-ketoglutarate), and the conversion of glycerol to glucose.[43] Inhibition of the generation of pyruvate from lactate and amino acids is probably the most important site of action quantitatively, the administration of pyruvate having been found to overcome the ethanol-induced inhibition of gluconeogenesis in the perfused rat liver.[44] Ethanol is a common cause of hypoglycemia in some emergency rooms[26] but not others,[45] a difference that may reflect the prevalence of alcohol abuse in the community. Nevertheless, it is surprising that alcohol-induced hypoglycemia is not more frequent in view of the predictable effect of ethanol metabolism on gluconeogenesis. While the explanation for this is not clear, it may be that ingestion of alcohol results not only in inhibition of gluconeogenesis but also in decreased glucose disposal.[43]

Salicylates

The ingestion of salicylates can cause hypoglycemia in children and adults. This may occur in response to a large therapeutic dose such as that used to treat rheumatoid arthritis or to an overdose. In the past, salicylates were a leading cause of hypoglycemia in children under 5 years of age, but the incidence of salicylate-induced hypoglycemia in children appears to be declining because of the decreased use of salicylates in children as a result of efforts to prevent Reye's syndrome. The mechanism of salicylate-induced hypoglycemia is unknown.

Quinine

The occurrence of quinine-induced hypoglycemia in patients with malaria has only recently been appreciated.[46] In normal subjects quinine in therapeutic doses stimulates insulin secretion and causes a modest fall in the circulating glucose level that is not sufficient to cause symptoms.[46] In patients who are treated with quinine for falciparum malaria, symptomatic hypoglycemia may occur as a result of quinine-induced insulin secretion and probably also the consumption of glucose by the malarial parasites.[46] Hypoglycemia may easily be overlooked in these patients, in whom neurologic symptoms may be attributed to cerebral malaria. The blood glucose level should be monitored closely, and hypoglycemia should be treated orally or with intravenous glucose, depending on the patient's condition.

Pentamidine

Pentamidine, a biguanide derivative used in the treatment of *Pneumocystis carinii* pneumonia, causes insulin-mediated hypoglycemia because of a toxic effect on the pancreatic β-cells, as a result of which insulin is released into the circulation. Hypoglycemia may be followed by hyperglycemia or permanent diabetes mellitus if the damage is severe. Pentamidine-induced hypoglycemia occurs after systemic use of this agent. The occurrence of hypoglycemia appears to be related to the cumulative dose of this agent.[47] Mild, asymptomatic hypoglycemia may occur after inhalation of pentamidine aerosol at the doses used in some regimens (e.g., every 2 weeks) for prophylaxis of *Pneumocystis carinii* pneumonia in patients infected with human immunodeficiency virus (HIV).[48]

β2-Adrenergic Agonists

Ritodrine and other β2-adrenergic agonists used as tocolytic therapy for spontaneous early labor can cause insulin-mediated hypoglycemia in the neonate and, in rare cases, in the mother.[42] Insulin secretion is stimulated by β-adrenergic agonists in humans. Hypoglycemia occurs during prolonged use of these agents during pregnancy. Hypoglycemia is not known to occur during use of β2-adrenergic agents in other settings, such as reactive airways disease.

Disopyramide

Disopyramide, an antiarrhythmic agent, causes hypoglycemia on rare occasion.[42]

Drug Interactions

A small number of patients have been described in whom hypoglycemia was attributed to the potentiation of the effects of a sulfonylurea agent by a second medication. The mechanism of this interaction is thought to be the prolongation of the hypoglycemic activity of the sulfonylurea by the second agent. It is often difficult to assess the contribution of the various other medications to the hypoglycemia. Furthermore, some of these agents have been reported to cause hypoglycemia only rarely. Thus, the claim that they cause hypoglycemia is open to question.[42] Drugs implicated in this type of interaction include phenylbutazone, sulfa antibiotics, and bishydroxycoumarin (but not warfarin).[42]

β-Adrenergic Antagonists

Propranolol does not cause hypoglycemia in an otherwise healthy person but may do so in patients who are predisposed by virtue of an intercurrent problem such as liver disease, congestive heart failure, and congenital heart disease (so-called tetralogy spells).[42] In fact, propranolol may cause or exacerbate hyperglycemia in a patient with NIDDM because insulin secretion is enhanced by β-adrenergic activity. However, in a patient receiving exogenous insulin (in whom endogenous insulin secretion is presumably diminished or absent), propranolol has different effects. It may block the adrenergic symptoms of hypoglycemia so that the patient loses the early warning provided by these symptoms and develops neuroglycopenic symptoms as the first manifestation of hypoglycemia. In addition, propranolol may retard the return of the plasma glucose level to normal after an insulin reaction because of increased disposal of glucose

peripherally, principally in skeletal muscle. (Catecholamines decrease the peripheral disposal of glucose in this tissue.) Although these effects of propranolol are serious, they are uncommon. Thus, in a patient who takes insulin, the use of propranolol or another β-adrenergic antagonist is relatively but not absolutely contraindicated. If both insulin and a β-adrenergic antagonist are used, tight control of diabetes should be avoided. The use of a relatively selective β1-adrenergic antagonist such as metoprolol may avert or decrease the risk that the recovery from hypoglycemia will be delayed.[42]

Hypoglycemia Due to Toxins

Two known toxins produce potentially lethal forms of hypoglycemia.

Hypoglycin A. Hypoglycemia may occur after the ingestion of the unripe akee fruit. The akee fruit is commonly consumed in Jamaica. When eaten while unripe, it causes Jamaican vomiting sickness. Hours to days after consumption of the unripe fruit, the patient may experience severe weakness, vomiting, seizures, coma, and death. The manifestations are largely attributable to hypoglycemia. An ingredient of the unripe akee fruit, hypoglycin A, decreases gluconeogenesis by inhibiting fatty acid oxidation.

Pyriminil (Vacor). This rat poison is a pancreatic islet β-cell toxin. Like other such toxins (e.g., pentamidine), it may cause hypoglycemia as a result of the unregulated release of insulin from the damaged β-cells, followed by the appearance of hyperglycemia.

ENDOGENOUS CAUSES OF HYPOGLYCEMIA

Liver Disease

Fasting hypoglycemia occurs in patients with extensive destruction of the liver from many different causes.[51] The hypoglycemia may be confused with or may exacerbate hepatic encephalopathy. Hypoglycemia does not occur until more than 80% of the liver mass has been destroyed.[51]

Hypoglycemia may occur in patients with fulminant hepatic failure caused by a variety of infections (hepatitis A, B, and C), drugs, and toxins but occurs only rarely in patients with portal or biliary cirrhosis.[51] Hypoglycemia also occurs in patients with severe congestive heart failure of any cause. The mechanism is not known but possible explanations include a deficiency of substrate for gluconeogenesis because of muscle wasting in patients with cardiac cachexia and alterations in hepatic function caused by impaired hepatocellular function or decreased hepatic blood flow.[51]

Kidney Disease

Hypoglycemia is not uncommon in patients with renal disease. A large percentage of hospitalized patients who develop hypoglycemia have chronic renal failure.[27] The cause of hypoglycemia in patients with renal failure varies considerably from patient to patient.[52] Hypoglycemia may be related to decreased caloric intake (acutely and chronically), to decreased clearance of a sulfonylurea or insulin, and to decreased renal gluconeogenesis. The kidneys are the next major site after the liver for insulin clearance and gluconeogenesis.

Hypoglycemia in patients receiving dialysis is a form of reactive hypoglycemia and is due to the use of a high glucose concentration in the dialysis fluid.[52] This form of hypoglycemia can occur in diabetic and nondiabetic patients and after peritoneal dialysis or hemodialysis.[52] The hypoglycemia may be related to enhanced glucose-induced insulin secretion and to decreased clearance of insulin by the kidneys.[52] Conversely, hypoglycemia may occur because of the omission of glucose from the dialysis fluid.[52]

Sepsis

Sepsis is a frequent cause of hypoglycemia in hospitalized patients. Although the mechanism of hypoglycemia in patients with sepsis is not known, animal studies support the hypothesis that the sepsis is mediated by endotoxin.[53] Interleukin-1 and tumor necrosis factor-α are potential mediators of endotoxin-induced hypoglycemia.

Endocrine Deficiency Disorders

Growth Hormone Deficiency

Growth hormone deficiency may be caused by congenital deficiency of its hypothalamic-releasing factor (growth hormone-releasing hormone), primary deficiency of growth hormone itself, anatomic abnormalities such as space-occupying pituitary or hypothalamic lesions, radiation, or trauma. Individuals who cannot respond to growth hormone (Laron dwarfs) also behave as if growth hormone is deficient.[54] Growth hormone antagonizes insulin action and stimulates lipolysis.[55] Since fasting hypoglycemia in growth hormone-deficient young children is usually seen in patients with decreased body mass for height, deficiencies in energy substrate and gluconeogenic substrate are likely to be contributory factors. Isolated growth-hormone deficiency does not cause hypoglycemia in adults. Growth hormone-deficient children have a decreased fasting rate of glucose production and decreased circulating levels of ketones.[56,57] Nonetheless, hypoglycemic growth hormone-deficient children usually have ketonemia.

Growth hormone is necessary for the counterregulatory response to hypoglycemia. Adults with growth-hormone deficiency induced experimentally by a somatostatin analogue exhibit decreased glucose production and increased glucose utilization in spite of normal counterregulatory responses of other hormones during insulin-induced hypoglycemia over a relatively prolonged period (12 hours).[58] In contrast, growth hormone-deficient children display diminished epinephrine and norepinephrine release when hypoglycemia is induced acutely.[59] Uncommonly, hypoglycemia is associated with every-other-day injections of growth hormone in young children deficient in growth hormone. The explanation is not clear. One hypothesis is that this is a result of

persistent insulin-like effects of insulin-like growth factor-I (IGF-I) generated in response to growth hormone after the insulin-antagonist effects of the growth hormone itself have waned.[60] It is treated by administering growth hormone daily.

Cortisol Deficiency

Cortisol contributes to the maintenance of normal fasting levels of blood glucose by assuring an adequate supply of gluconeogenic precursor, by stimulating key gluconeogenic enzymes and thereby enhancing gluconeogenesis, by stimulating glucagon secretion, and by inducing insulin resistance.[4] Further, cortisol facilitates the glycogenolytic effects of glucagon and epinephrine.[61] It is necessary for glycemic counterregulation after prolonged induction of hypoglycemia (for 12 hours) by exogenous insulin.[62] Although cortisol-deficient adults may become hypoglycemic after fasting, hypoglycemia is more commonly seen after relatively short fasts in cortisol-deficient infants and children because of the inability of young children to maintain fasting euglycemia without adequate gluconeogenesis.

In children, hypoglycemia may be associated with adrenal insufficiency of all etiologies, including primary adrenal insufficiency and congenital adrenal hyperplasia,[63] but is more likely to be seen as an isolated presenting event in individuals with relatively normal mineralocorticoid function. Therefore, ACTH deficiency and the inherited syndrome of ACTH unresponsiveness are particularly likely to be accompanied by fasting hypoglycemia.[64] Hypoglycemia may be a manifestation of withdrawal of glucocorticoid therapy for a nonendocrine condition in children.

Hypopituitarism

Theoretically, the deficiency of multiple pituitary hormones should lead to more severe, more frequent fasting hypoglycemia than should an isolated deficiency of either ACTH or growth hormone alone. In fact, individuals with a deficiency in growth hormone alone and individuals with deficiencies in both growth hormone and ACTH have similarly diminished fasting rates of glucose production and a similar incidence of fasting hypoglycemia. Young, thin individuals are at greatest risk for hypoglycemia, suggesting that the body mass to height ratio and age are the critical variables.[65] Children with multiple pituitary hormone deficiencies (growth hormone, ACTH, thyroid-stimulating hormone, luteinizing hormone, follicle-stimulating hormone) as a result of deficient release of hypothalamic-releasing hormones may present with hypoglycemia in the newborn period. Hypoglycemia may be transient but may recur during stressful periods of decreased intake when the children are slightly older. If neonates are cortisol-deficient, they may have associated hyperbilirubinemia (usually conjugated).[66] If the children are gonadotropin-deficient, boys will have microphallus without hypospadias. Because levels of growth hormone are normally quite high in the neonate and IGF-I levels are very low in the neonate and the small child, interpretation of laboratory data for these children requires the use of age-specific normal values.

Hypothyroidism

Hypothyroidism probably leads to impaired glyco-genolysis, but other aspects of glucose homeostasis in hypothyroidism are not well studied. In adults with severe hypothyroidism, fasting blood glucose levels are lower than those in normal subjects.[67] Although hypoglycemia may be the primary cause of coma in myxedema, this is exceedingly rare.[68,69] Mild hypothyroidism does not lead to hypoglycemia. Severe congenital hypothyroidism would be a remarkable cause of hypoglycemia in the United States in this era of neonatal screening for hypothyroidism. Abnormal thyroid function studies in a hypoglycemic infant or child are more likely to be either a concomitant of associated multiple tropic hormone deficiencies or a manifestation of the sick euthyroid syndrome in a malnourished or otherwise severely ill child.

Immune Hypoglycemia

Hypoglycemia occurs in two distinct antibody-mediated disorders. In one, antibodies are directed at the insulin receptor. In the other, antibodies are directed at insulin itself.

Hypoglycemia from Antibodies to the Insulin Receptor

Patients with hypoglycemia from antibodies to the insulin receptor typically have fasting hypoglycemia, do not have acanthosis nigricans (in contrast to patients with antireceptor antibody-mediated insulin resistance), and may have an associated autoimmune disorder such as systemic lupus erythematosus.[70] Glucocorticoid therapy may correct the hypoglycemia, apparently by inhibiting the hypoglycemic effects of the antibodies to the insulin receptor.[70] Because of the high mortality rate associated with this entity, several approaches have been employed to reduce the antibody titer, including plasmapheresis and immunosuppression with alkylating agents and glucocorticoids. The effectiveness of these treatments has not been evaluated in controlled studies.

Antibodies to the insulin receptor cause insulin resistance in some patients and hypoglycemia in others. The explanation for this difference is not known but may reflect the balance between antibodies with an agonistic effect and those with an antagonistic effect on the insulin receptor and may reflect the titer of antibodies to the insulin receptor.[70] Low antibody titers presumably lead to low levels of receptor occupancy, thereby causing hypoglycemia, while high antibody titers may lead to high levels of occupancy, thereby causing insulin resistance.[70]

Insulin secretion is decreased in this entity, but some patients have inappropriately high levels of circulating insulin because of decreased insulin clearance by receptor-mediated endocytosis, the predominant mechanism of insulin clearance from the circulation.[70]

Hypoglycemia from Antibodies to Insulin

Hypoglycemia may arise from autoantibodies to insulin in patients who have not previously been immunized with exogenous insulin. Typically, the hypoglycemia is reactive, but fasting hypoglycemia also occurs. The majority of patients reported have been Japanese. The diagnosis depends upon the identification of antibodies to insulin in the circulation and is supported by the presence of another autoimmune disease such as Graves' disease, rheumatoid arthritis, or systemic lupus erythematosus.[70] Antibodies to insulin may also be found in patients who surreptitiously inject insulin, in patients with Type I diabetes who have not yet received exogenous insulin, in patients with other autoimmune diseases, in normal subjects following viral infections, and, rarely, in otherwise normal persons.[70] C-peptide levels are not suppressed because insulin is secreted endogenously, in contrast to the occurrence of such suppression in patients who inject insulin surreptitiously.[70] The pathogenesis of hypoglycemia appears to reflect an equilibrium between insulin bound to the antibodies and free insulin.[70] After a meal the level of free insulin rises, some becoming bound to the antibodies. In the postabsorptive state, insulin dissociates from the antibodies, retarding the decrease in the free insulin level and causing hypoglycemia. Hypoglycemia due to antibodies to insulin is usually a self-limited condition.[70]

Hypoglycemia has been described in a patient with multiple myeloma. This hypoglycemia was a response to the production of a monoclonal insulin-binding antibody by clonally proliferated plasma cells.[71] The patient exhibited recurrent postprandial hypoglycemia and spuriously elevated levels of circulating insulin, as in patients with antibodies to insulin. Unlike other patients with antibodies to insulin, in whom antibodies are typically polyclonal, the patient with multiple myeloma produced a monoclonal insulin-binding antibody with a low affinity for insulin and a very high binding capacity.[71]

Non–Islet Cell Tumors

In the syndrome of tumor-induced hypoglycemia, patients with a non-islet cell tumor exhibit the clinical manifestations of hypoglycemia.[72–74] The hypoglycemia may be the presenting manifestation of the tumor or may herald a recurrence. Because the symptoms of neuroglycopenia are more prominent than the symptoms of adrenergic activity, the clinical findings resemble those of an insulinoma. The non-islet cell tumors most commonly associated with hypoglycemia are characteristically large (weighing as much as several kilograms), slow-growing, mesenchymal tumors (such as sarcomas, fibromas, mesotheliomas, or hemangiopericytomas) located in the retroperitoneum or the thorax. Hypoglycemia may also be associated with hepatomas, renal cell carcinomas, adrenocortical carcinomas, or, rarely, a variety of other neoplasms.

While it was known that the hypoglycemia is not insulin-mediated, the pathogenesis of tumor-induced hypoglycemia was a mystery until recently. The evidence suggested the existence of a humoral mediator,

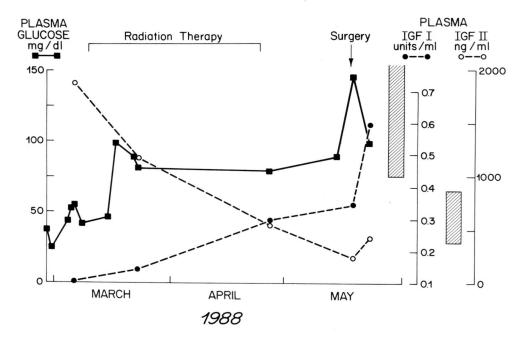

Fig. 55–8. Concentrations of plasma glucose and insulin-like growth factors (IGF) I and II in a patient with hypoglycemia induced by a large retroperitoneal fibrosarcoma. Before treatment, the plasma IGF-II level was elevated and the plasma IGF-I level was decreased. After radiation therapy and surgery the plasma IGF-II and IGF-I levels returned to normal. Reprinted with permission from reference 74 (Ron D, Powers AC, Pandian MR, et al. Increased insulin-like growth factor II production and consequent suppression of growth hormone secretion: a dual mechanism for tumor-induced hypoglycemia. J Clin Endocrinol Metab 1989;68: 701–6; © the Endocrine Society).

one that inhibits hepatic glucose output and increases the peripheral utilization of glucose. Recent studies indicate that the mediator of tumor-induced hypoglycemia at least in mesenchymal tumors is insulin-like growth factor II (IGF-II), a substance that exhibits a high degree of structural homology to proinsulin. The available evidence satisfies many of the criteria for the existence of a hormone-mediated paraneoplastic syndrome, including evidence of increased expression of the gene for the hormone by the tumor, the presence of the hormone in the tumor, and secretion of the hormone by tumor explants in vitro.[73] In some but not all patients, the level of circulating IGF-II is elevated before treatment and returns to normal after treatment of the tumor in association with resolution of the hypoglycemia (Fig. 55–8).[73,74] Secretion of growth hormone is suppressed before treatment and returns to normal afterwards, supporting the theory that the IGF-II secreted by the tumor is biologically active, since IGF-II suppresses secretion of growth hormone in vitro (Fig. 55–9). Even when the level of circulating IGF-II is elevated before treatment, the magnitude of the elevation is modest.

Several explanations have been proposed to explain the absence, or the limited extent, of the elevation in the level of circulating IGF-II in patients in whom other evidence supports a role for IGF-II in the pathogenesis of tumor-induced hypoglycemia. Approximately 75% of the IGF-II in the circulation is present as part of a 150-kd complex that includes a growth hormone-dependent IGF-II-binding protein and an acid-labile complexing component.[75] It is probable that only the free IGF-II and not the complex that it forms exerts the insulin-like activity of the peptide. Consequently, hypoglycemia may occur when the free IGF-II level is elevated even though the level of the carrier complex and of total circulating

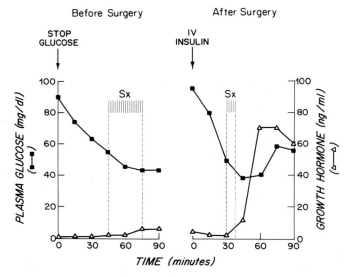

Fig. 55–9. Serum growth hormone responses to hypoglycemia in a patient with a pleural mesothelioma associated with hypoglycemia before and after surgical removal of the tumor. The serum growth hormone response to hypoglycemia induced by temporary interruption of an intravenous glucose infusion was blunted preoperatively, when the plasma level of insulin-like growth factor II (IGF-II) was elevated and the plasma IGF-I level was low. Postoperatively, when the plasma IGF-II and IGF-I levels had returned to normal, hypoglycemia induced during a standard intravenous insulin tolerance test was associated with a normal growth hormone response and spontaneous resolution of the hypoglycemia. Reprinted with permission from reference 74 (Ron D, Powers AC, Pandian MR, et al. Increased insulin-like growth factor II production and consequent suppression of growth hormone secretion: a dual mechanism for tumor-induced hypoglycemia. J Clin Endocrinol Metab 1989; 68:701–6; © the Endocrine Society).

IGF-II remain normal, especially when secretion of growth hormone is depressed.[73] In at least some patients with tumor-induced hypoglycemia, the 150-kd complex is absent and IGF-II circulates as part of several smaller complexes, perhaps because of abnormalities in the secretion of the acid-labile complexing component and because of binding of IGF-II to proteins other than the normal growth hormone-dependent binding proteins.[75] Because the 150-kd complex crosses the capillary poorly and the smaller complexes may enter the interstitial fluid more easily, the fraction of IGF-II reaching its target cells may increase.[75] Also, in some patients, IGF-II circulates in a high-molecular-weight form that may be biologically active but undetectable in some assays.[76] The high-molecular-weight component has a reduced affinity for circulating binding proteins, may circulate as an unbound molecule, and may therefore have increased biologic activity in vivo as compared with lower-molecular-weight forms of IGF-II.[76]

The increased production of IGF-II may cause hypoglycemia by a dual mechanism: 1) increased glucose utilization by the tumor or the host mediated by the insulin-like actions of IGF-II and 2) inhibition of growth hormone secretion, which may account for the decreased hepatic glucose output in this condition (Fig. 55–10).[73,74]

The utility of measuring IGF-II in the circulation in the diagnosis of tumor-induced hypoglycemia is not established. Although an elevated level may be helpful, the value may be normal or only minimally elevated in this condition. Because a low plasma IGF-I value is normally associated with a low plasma IGF-II value, an apparently normal IGF-II value in the presence of a low plasma IGF-I value supports the diagnosis of tumor-induced hypoglycemia in patients with insulin-independent, nonketotic fasting hypoglycemia.[77]

Insulinoma

Insulinomas are discussed elsewhere in the textbook (see Chapter 56).

Nesidioblastosis

Nesidioblastosis describes a diffuse proliferation and budding of pancreatic islet cells from pancreatic ducts. Although it was once thought that this is the pathologic basis for insulin-mediated hypoglycemia in infants, quantitative immunohistochemical studies have demonstrated that these findings occur in normal infants. Therefore, the finding of nesidioblastosis is not sufficient to explain excessive insulin release.[78] Idiopathic hyperinsulinism is now considered to be a syndrome of islet dysregulation (see Hyperinsulinism section in Special Considerations in Infants and Children).

A small number of adult patients have been described in whom insulin-mediated hypoglycemia was associated with the histologic findings of nesidioblastosis.[79] Because nesidioblastosis is not a normal finding in adults, this association may be functionally important. However, the pathophysiologic significance of this observation is unknown.[80] For example, it may reflect a response to an unidentified stimulatory factor, enhanced responsiveness of the endocrine pancreas to normal stimuli,[80] or the absence of a normal inhibitory factor. Nesidioblastosis may occur in factitious hypoglycemia caused by the surreptitious ingestion of a sulfonylurea.

SPECIAL CONSIDERATIONS IN INFANTS AND CHILDREN

Pathophysiology of Hypoglycemia in Children

In childhood, postprandial hypoglycemia may be a result of gastrointestinal surgery and rapid gastric emptying, hereditary fructose intolerance, or galactosemia. Both fasting and postprandial hypoglycemia may accompany organic hyperinsulinism. All other causes of hypoglycemia in children present in the fasting state.

Glucose production and utilization correlate directly with brain mass from infancy to adulthood (Fig. 55–11). Because the ratio of brain mass to body mass is larger in the child than in the adult, the balance between glucose need and glucose production is more precarious in younger persons than in adults. The normal glucose utilization rate is approximately 6 to 8 mg/(kg·min) in the fasting infant, 4 to 6 mg/(kg·min) in the child and 2 mg/(kg·min) in the adult.[81] On the other hand, in the newborn child the average energy needs are 120 to 150 kcal/(kg·24 hr) or 20 to 27 mg/(kg·min) of glucose if all energy needs are supplied by glucose. Thus, hypoglyce-

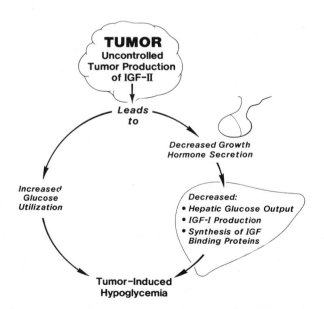

Fig. 55–10. The pathogenesis of tumor-induced hypoglycemia. Increased production of insulin-like growth factor II (IGF-II) by the tumor increases peripheral utilization of glucose and decreases pituitary secretion of growth hormone. The decreased growth hormone secretion results in a reduction of 1) hepatic glucose output, 2) hepatic IGF-I production, and 3) hepatic synthesis of IGF-binding proteins.

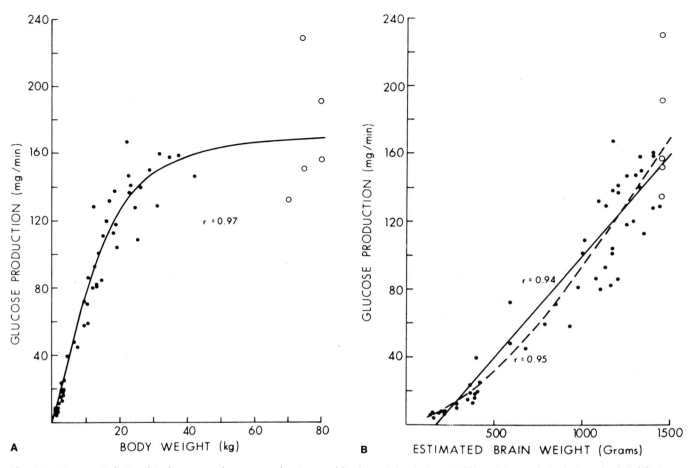

Fig. 55–11. A: Relationship between glucose production and body weight during childhood (closed circles) and adult life (open circles). The solid line depicts the cubic expression $Y = 0.0014X^3 - 0.214X^2 + 10.411X - 9.084$. B: Relationship between glucose production and estimated brain weight during childhood (closed circles) and adult life (open circles). The solid line represents the linear regression $Y = 0.122X - 22.75$, while the dashed line depicts the quadratic function $Y = 0.000041X^2 + 0.05X - 5.64$. Reprinted with permission from reference 81 (Bier DM, Leake RD, Haymond MW, et al. Measurement of "true" glucose production rates in infancy and childhood with 6,6-dideuteroglucose. Diabetes 1977;26:1016–23; copyright © of the American Diabetes Association).

mia may result not only from the inability to generate enough glucose to meet the normal age-appropriate glucose utilization rate but also from the inadequate provision of other energy substrates. Children have decreased fat stores and muscle mass compared with those in adults. Consequently, children may not be able to generate sufficient glucose from glycerol, to produce and recycle gluconeogenic amino acids, or to make available free fatty acids for the energy needs of peripheral tissues. Furthermore, hypoglycemic low-birth-weight infants may be unable to utilize available gluconeogenic substrates and may have lower rates of glucose production than normal infants. Diminished lipid oxidation in the immediate postnatal period has been implicated in this impairment because infusion of medium-chain fatty acids increases the rate of glucose production and restores normoglycemia.[82] The intrahepatic oxidation of fatty acids provides the energy required to sustain gluconeogenesis.

Specific Entities

Hyperinsulinism

In the newborn child, hyperinsulinism may be transient and related to prenatal stimulation of the pancreatic islets, may be a manifestation of chronic islet dysregulation, or may be caused by an anatomic lesion. Although some infants with insulin-mediated hypoglycemia have single or multiple islet cell adenomas, most do not have a specific anatomic abnormality.[80] Hyperinsulinism in utero is associated with increased body weight and an infant who is large for gestational age. The infant of the poorly controlled diabetic woman is chronically exposed to fluctuating and frequently high blood glucose levels, which lead to early and enhanced activation of fetal islet insulin release.[83] In addition, transplacental passage of antibody-bound maternal exogenous insulin may contribute to fetal and early neonatal hyperinsulinism.[84] Persistent hypoglycemia in infants of diabetic women should provoke reevaluation of the diagnosis. Hyperinsulinism and increased insulin content of pancreatic islets may be seen in hypoglycemic infants with severe erythroblastosis fetalis.[85] The mechanism is unclear. Children with the exophthalmos-macroglossia-gigantism (Beckwith-Wiedemann) syndrome often have associated transient hyperinsulinism.[86]

The nomenclature of chronic hyperinsulinism in childhood has undergone revision with the recognition that idiopathic hyperinsulinism in childhood (previously labeled nesidioblastosis) is a syndrome of islet dysregulation. Nesidioblastosis is a term used to describe an anatomic lesion characterized by increased budding of new islets from exocrine pancreatic ducts. Although the insulin-secreting islet mass is increased in proportion to the pancreatic mass in these infants in comparison to adults, the relative islet mass is not always different from that of the normal infant of the same age. The pancreas of the normal newborn infant may consist of as much as 10% islet tissue (Plate III). Insulin secretion is increased in these infants on a functional basis; it is not under appropriate substrate control.[87] It has been suggested that the number of somatostatin-secreting cells in the islets of these children is diminished; however, there is measurable somatostatin release from the cultured islets of patients with this entity.[78,88] Infants with this disorder may respond completely or partially to therapy with diazoxide or a long-acting somatostatin analogue, but they usually require pancreatectomy to prevent recurrent hypoglycemia and severe neurologic impairment.[89,90] Islet dysregulation may be familial and may occur somewhat more frequently in infants of diabetic women.[91,92]

Leucine-sensitive hypoglycemia is not a separate disease entity but is hypoglycemia induced by an amino acid challenge in an individual with organic hyperinsulinism. Insulin-mediated hypoglycemia caused by islet-cell tumors is considered elsewhere in this textbook (see Chapter 56 on islet cell tumors).

Substrate-Limited or Ketotic Hypoglycemia

The most common cause of hypoglycemia in the fasting child is substrate-limited or physiologic-variant fasting hypoglycemia.[93] At the conclusion of a 36-hour fast, the blood glucose values of normal children form a Gaussian distribution. This distribution includes some children who withstand fasting very poorly and become ketotic rapidly as they utilize limited body stores of other energy sources.[18] Children with ketosis and fasting hypoglycemia have in the past been said to have "ketotic hypoglycemia." These children are characteristically 18 months to 2 years old at the time of initial diagnosis. They are more often boys with decreased muscle and body fat mass. Hypoglycemic episodes occur with illness or poor intake and usually occur in the early morning hours. Episodes of spontaneous hypoglycemia cease by midchildhood.[94] Some of these children exhibit a deficient epinephrine response to hypoglycemia. Although it has

been suggested that epinephrine deficiency is etiologic, this is likely to be a secondary phenomenon related to the frequent occurrence of modest hypoglycemia and exhaustion of epinephrine release.[95]

The term "substrate-limited" hypoglycemia has been proposed to explain the inadequate hepatic glucose output. All of these children have low levels of alanine. During hypoglycemic episodes hepatic glycogen stores are depleted but gluconeogenesis from infused precursors is not inhibited. These children become hypoglycemic because of a failure of gluconeogenic reserves to meet cerebral glucose needs.

The same mechanism leads to hypoglycemia in children with diarrhea who do not receive proper caloric supplementation and in children who are fasted for prolonged periods to prepare them for surgical anesthesia.[96,97]

Inborn Errors of Intermediary Metabolism

Inborn errors of intermediary metabolism may lead to hypoglycemia because the specific enzymatic defect directly affects glycogenesis, glycogenolysis, or gluconeogenesis; secondarily affects glycogenolysis or gluconeogenesis; or prevents production or utilization of fat-derived substrates by peripheral tissues, increasing the demand for glucose beyond normal synthetic capacity (Table 55–1).

Table 55–1. Inborn Errors of Metabolism Associated with Hypoglycemia

Primary defects in glycogenesis or glycogenolysis
  Hepatic glycogen synthase deficiency
  Glucose-6-phosphatase deficiency (glycogen storage disease Type Ia)
  Glucose-6-phosphate translocase or pyrophosphate translocase deficiency (glycogen storage disease Type Ib)
  Debrancher enzyme deficiency (amylo-1,6-glucosidase deficiency, glycogen storage disease Type III)
  Brancher enzyme deficiency (amylo-1,4→1,6 transglucosidase deficiency, glycogen storage disease Type IV)
  Phosphorylase deficiency (glycogen storage disease Type VI)
  Phosphorylase b kinase deficiency
Primary defects in gluconeogenesis
  Pyruvate carboxylase deficiency
  Phosphoenolpyruvate carboxykinase deficiency (?)
  Fructose 1,6-diphosphatase deficiency
Secondary defects in glycogenolysis or gluconeogenesis
  Hereditary fructose intolerance (fructose-1-phosphate aldolase deficiency)
  Galactosemia (galactose-1-phosphate uridyl transferase deficiency)
  Defects in glycerol metabolism
  Maple syrup urine disease (defects in branched-chain ketoacid dehydrogenase)
  Methylmalonic aciduria (methylmalonyl CoA isomerase deficiency)
  Phenylketonuria with severe dietary restriction
Disorders of fatty acid utilization and ketogenesis
  Hydroxymethylglutaryl CoA lyase deficiency
  Glutaric aciduria Type II (multiple acyl CoA dehydrogenase deficiency) (also inhibits gluconeogenesis)
  Carnitine palmitoyl transferase deficiency (infantile type), acyl CoA dehydrogenase deficiencies (short, medium, and long chain)
Disorders of ketone utilization
  Acetoacetyl CoA thiolase deficiency

Defects in Glycogenesis or Glycogenolysis. These rare and largely autosomal recessive disorders are produced by enzyme defects in the metabolic pathways of glycogen synthesis or glycogenolysis.

The only defect of glycogen synthesis leading to hypoglycemia that has been delineated is hepatic glycogen synthase deficiency. Although the existence of this defect was initially debated, there are now several carefully investigated cases in which absence of glycogen synthase activity in the liver has been associated with minimal hepatic glycogen stores, hypoglycemia and metabolic acidosis after fasting, and a variable hyperglycemic response to carbohydrate feedings.[98]

In contrast, a wide variety of defects in glycogenolysis cause hypoglycemia. Glucose-6-phosphatase deficiency (Von Gierke's disease or Type Ia glycogen storage disease) is clinically characterized by hypoglycemia after relatively short-term fasting, massive hepatomegaly, a cherubic facies, nephromegaly, severe hyperlipidemia, growth failure, and lactic acidosis. It is the result of absence of glucose-6-phosphatase in liver, kidney, and intestinal mucosa.[99] Individuals with a similar clinical appearance and neutropenia may have normal glucose-6-phosphatase activity when activity is assayed on frozen tissue, but they have a similar functional defect. Some are deficient in a microsomal membrane translocase for glucose-6-phosphate. Others are deficient in a translocase for pyrophosphate.[100] Patients with glucose-6-phosphatase deficiency may maintain normal neurologic function in spite of exceedingly low blood glucose levels. Lactate may serve as an additional central nervous system energy source in these individuals.[9] Debrancher enzyme deficiency (glycogen storage disease Type III, amylo-1,6-glucosidase deficiency) tends to produce milder hypoglycemic symptoms. It is characterized by hepatomegaly and the other symptoms associated with glucose-6-phosphatase deficiency, although it also may affect muscle. Hypoglycemia in these patients tends to improve with age, but they may have more severe hepatotoxic manifestations, including cirrhosis, as they get older. They have ketoacidosis upon fasting, rather than lactic acidosis. This disorder is common in North African populations.[101] Both Types I and III glycogen storage disease are amenable to therapy with frequent or continuous feeding regimens.[102] Glycogen storage disease Type IV (brancher enzyme deficiency, amylo-1,4→1,6 transglucosidase deficiency) leads to the production of an abnormal and toxic glycogen and hepatic cirrhosis. Fasting hypoglycemia may occur since this abnormal glycogen cannot be mobilized to a normal extent. These patients may be treated like patients with Types I and III glycogen storage disease, with limited success.[103] Hepatic phosphorylase deficiency (Type VI glycogen storage disease) and phosphorylase b kinase deficiency (in most cases an X-linked disorder only expressed in males) produce fasting hypoglycemia and variable mild hepatomegaly.[101] Frequent feedings are sometimes required.

Primary Defects in Gluconeogenesis. Three defects in enzymes of gluconeogenesis have been associated with hypoglycemia. Deficiency of pyruvate carboxylase, the first enzymatic step of gluconeogenesis, leads to variable degrees of fasting hypoglycemia, severe lactic acidosis, and elevated levels of other gluconeogenic intermediates (pyruvate, alanine). Children may have progressive psychomotor retardation and seizures.[104] Deficiency of another enzyme involved in a rate-limiting step of gluconeogenesis, hepatic phosphoenolpyruvate carboxykinase, appears to cause severe hypoglycemia in the newborn period. Documentation of this defect is not yet complete, since all studies in the few patients described are not in accord with the presence of this defect.[98] Hepatic fructose 1,6-diphosphatase deficiency leads to failure of hydrolysis of fructose 1,6-diphosphate to fructose-6-phosphate. Children with this disorder develop fasting hypoglycemia and metabolic acidosis. Dietary therapy to inhibit gluconeogenesis by continuous provision of adequate quantities of exogenous glucose appears to be effective.[105]

Secondary Defects in Glycogenolysis and Gluconeogenesis. A number of defects in glycogenolysis or gluconeogenesis secondary to other enzymatic defects have been described. For example, the hypoglycemia following fructose ingestion in hereditary fructose intolerance (fructose-1-phosphate aldolase deficiency) is due not only to fructose-1-phosphate-induced inhibition of hepatic phosphorylase but also to inhibition of fructose-1,6-diphosphatase by this toxic phosphorylated intermediate.[98,105] Galactose ingestion in galactosemia (galactose-1-phosphate uridyl transferase deficiency) occasionally induces hypoglycemia. Galactose-1-phosphate rapidly inhibits phosphoglucomutase, thereby inhibiting glycogenolysis.[106] Hypoglycemia is more common in individuals with previously induced galactosemic liver damage. Rare individuals with poorly described defects in glycerol metabolism may develop hypoglycemia after glycerol ingestion, as will patients with fructose-1,6-diphosphatase deficiency.[107]

Amino Acid and Ketoacid Disorders. Disorders of metabolism of branched-chain amino acids may be associated with fasting hypoglycemia. In maple syrup urine disease (caused by defects in branched-chain ketoacid dehydrogenase), hypoglycemia is ascribed to defective gluconeogenesis from amino acids because of decreased transamination of branched-chain amino acids.[108] Methylmalonic aciduria (methylmalonyl CoA isomerase deficiency) can lead to hypoglycemia because of inhibition of gluconeogenesis at several regulatory steps leading to the production of oxaloacetate.[109]

When low-phenylalanine diets were introduced for the treatment of children with phenylketonuria, the severely restricted nature of the diets led to the occurrence of hypoglycemia in association with severe malnutrition.[110]

Disorders of Fatty Acid and Ketone Utilization and Ketogenesis. Defects in the ability to utilize fatty acids or ketones lead to hypoglycemia because the failure in utilization of nonglucose sources of energy increases the utilization of glucose.

Children who are unable to utilize ketones may present in a manner similar to those with "ketotic" or substrate-limited hypoglycemia. These defects include acetoacetyl CoA thiolase deficiency.[111]

Children with the inability to utilize fatty acids and produce ketones present with hypoketotic, hypoinsulinemic hypoglycemia. Hypoglycemia results from an increased systemic need for glucose in the face of inability to oxidize fatty acids or produce ketones.[112] Hydroxymethylglutaryl CoA lyase deficiency induces a block in the last enzymatic step of leucine catabolism. Patients are severely hypoglycemic because they cannot produce acetoacetate and β-hydroxybutyrate to spare glucose utilization.[113]

Variable defects in gluconeogenesis secondary to increased concentrations of inhibitory metabolites have also been identified. For instance, multiple acyl CoA dehydrogenase deficiency (glutaric aciduria Type II) leads to increased production of glutaryl CoA and ethylmalonic acid, both of which interfere with the malate shuttle. Further, decreased production of acetyl CoA and reducing equivalents interfere with gluconeogenesis by inhibiting pyruvate carboxylase and other steps in the gluconeogenic pathway.[114] Carnitine palmitoyl transferase deficiency of the infantile type and the acyl-CoA dehydrogenase deficiencies (short, medium, and long chain) induce hypoglycemia primarily because of decreased free fatty acid oxidation and ketone body production. Secondary carnitine deficiency may result from these disorders. Primary carnitine deficiency has been postulated to be a cause of hypoketotic hypoglycemia, but the existence of this disorder is still in doubt.[112]

Hepatic Failure and Renal Failure

Hypoglycemia occurs in children with hepatic failure, as it does in adults.[115] Hypoglycemia is clinically significant in children with renal failure only after transplantation.[116] The pathophysiologic considerations and the principles of management in children are similar to those in adults.

Toxins

The spectrum of agents that cause hypoglycemia in children is different from that in adults. This reflects in part differences in exposure to the potential toxins and in part age-related differences in response. Thus, children experience hypoglycemia caused by salicylate toxicity more frequently than do adults when they ingest a salicylate. On the other hand, salicylate-induced hypoglycemia appears to occur less frequently than in the past as a consequence of the reduced use of salicylates in children because of the association of salicylates with Reye's syndrome. Children are more susceptible to the hypoglycemic effects of drugs and toxins than are adults because of their susceptibility to fasting hypoglycemia. Children have developed alcohol-induced hypoglycemia from the use of alcohol rubs to reduce fever and from accidental ingestion of mouthwash.[117,118]

Evaluation of the Child with Hypoglycemia

Reactive hypoglycemia is so uncommon in the child that a history suggestive of hypoglycemia in the postprandial state is best managed by providing parents access to use of a glucose meter to test their child during symptomatic episodes unless there is strong reason to suspect the existence of reactive hypoglycemia, such as previous abdominal surgery[119] or the remarkable signs and symptoms associated with the inborn errors of carbohydrate metabolism that lead to postprandial hypoglycemia. This resolves the diagnostic suspicion in almost every case. This approach is quite similar to that in the adult with comparable postprandial symptoms. Tolerance tests or challenges should be undertaken only after careful deliberation because in some disorders (galactosemia, hereditary fructose intolerance) they may precipitate fulminant symptoms and they are not required for diagnosis.

Fasting hypoglycemia must be investigated vigorously in each child because of the risk of severe neurologic damage from repetitive hypoglycemia in the young child. A blood sample obtained at the time of a spontaneous episode of hypoglycemia may initiate the evaluation. Blood levels of glucose, insulin, growth hormone, cortisol, ketone bodies, and lactate will facilitate establishment of a diagnosis. It is important to recognize that relatively low levels of insulin may be associated with hyperinsulinism in the young child. Therefore, a sensitive assay capable of distinguishing insulin concentrations of 1 μU/mL will aid in diagnosis. Children with the islet dysregulation syndrome may have hyperinsulinism with persistent circulating insulin levels of 4 to 5 μU/mL in the face of blood glucose values below 30 mg/dL (1.7 mM). Plasma and urine samples obtained at this time may be stored frozen for more detailed analysis at a later time. In the infant, physical examination helps determine the course of the investigation. The large infant with frequent, severe episodes of hypoglycemia is most likely to be hyperinsulinemic. Simultaneous measurements of insulin and blood glucose at the time of episodes may easily make the diagnosis. Hepatomegaly and/or metabolic acidosis suggest an inborn error of metabolism. In these children, measurement of blood levels of lactate, pyruvate, amino acids, acetoacetate, and β-hydroxybutyrate and of urinary levels of amino acids and ketoacids is essential. Further diagnostic studies will depend upon the nature of the inborn error suspected. In many cases, peripheral tissues (blood, skin fibroblasts) may be sampled for the enzymatic defect. In others, e.g., those in whom glucose-6-phosphatase deficiency is suspected, a liver biopsy will be necessary. Infants with a history of prolonged jaundice and male infants with microphallus should be investigated carefully for deficiencies of pituitary hormones. When possible, growth-hormone deficiency should be confirmed using one standard provocative test such as levodopa administration, clonidine administration, arginine infusion, or growth-hormone measurement after a diagnostic fast, in addition to measurement of growth hormone during a spontaneous episode of hypoglycemia.[120]

If initial studies do not establish a diagnosis, a diagnostic fast should be conducted. The duration of the fast depends upon the age of the child. After the age of 3 years, a 36-hour fast is reasonable. During the course of the fast and toward the termination of the fasting period, blood and urine should be obtained as described above. A 12-hour urine sample obtained toward the latter part of the fast may be analyzed for organic acids. Blood samples obtained at the beginning and end of the fast may be analyzed for carnitine. Fasting carnitine levels may be in the normal range in fatty acid oxidation disorders and should be repeated in the fed state.[112] The fast should be terminated when the child develops a blood glucose level of 40 mg/dL (30 mg/dL in an infant). The fast must be conducted with care. In rare cases, children with inborn errors of fatty acid oxidation have developed cerebral edema with fasting. At termination, a glucagon tolerance test may be performed to assess the capacity for glycogenolysis if it is deemed likely to provide useful information. Occasionally, a glucagon tolerance test performed in the fed state may provide useful information in a patient with a glycogen storage disease.

Therapy for Hypoglycemia in the Child

Children with hyperinsulinemia may respond to oral diazoxide and/or to cyclic somatostatin.[121,122] Long-acting zinc glucagon has occasionally proved useful in management.[98] Unless diazoxide is immediately and continuously effective, pancreatectomy is the treatment of choice because of the risk of severe neurologic damage.[89] Blood glucose levels must be maintained in the normal or hyperglycemic range with continuous intravenous glucose infusion, glucocorticoids, and the appropriate pharmacologic agents until surgery is successful. Hyperinsulinism secondary to islet dysregulation may recur. Hypoglycemia may not be resolved by 95% pancreatectomy. There are anecdotal reports of regrowth of pancreatic tissue discovered on repeat surgical exploration.

Substrate-limited or physiologic hypoglycemia of childhood may be treated with frequent feedings and attention to the onset of ketosis. Hormonal deficiency disorders are treated with replacement therapy.

The inborn errors of metabolism must be treated with frequent and appropriate feedings, which will bypass or decrease the activity of the gluconeogenic pathway in most cases. The availability of blood glucose monitoring equipment and the ease with which urinary ketones may be monitored have made appropriate parental surveillance easier.

REFERENCES

1. Ruderman NB, Ross PS, Berger M, Goodman MN. Regulation of glucose and ketone-body metabolism in brain of anaesthetized rats. Biochem J 1974;138:1–10.
2. Owen OE, Morgan AP, Kemp HG, et al. Brain metabolism during fasting. J Clin Invest 1967;46:1589–95.
3. Rothman DL, Magnusson I, Katz LD, et al. Quantitation of hepatic glycogenolysis and gluconeogenesis in fasting humans with ^{13}C NMR. Science 1991;254:573–6.
4. Axelrod L. Side effects of glucocorticoid therapy. In: Schleimer RP, Claman HN, Oronsky AL, eds. Anti-inflammatory steroid action: basic and clinical aspects. San Diego: Academic Press, 1989:377–408.
5. Shulman GI, Rothman DL, Jue T, et al. Quantitation of muscle glycogen synthesis in normal subjects and subjects with non-insulin-dependent diabetes by ^{13}C nuclear magnetic resonance spectroscopy. N Engl J Med 1990;322:223–8.
6. Mitrakou A, Ryan C, Veneman T, et al. Hierarchy of glycemic thresholds for counterregulatory hormone secretion, symptoms, and cerebral dysfunction. Am J Physiol 1991;260:E67–74.
7. Jones TW, Boulware SD, Kraemer DT, et al. Independent effects of youth and poor diabetes control on responses to hypoglycemia in children. Diabetes 1991;40:358–63.
8. Kraus H, Schlenker S, Schwedesky D. Developmental changes of cerebral ketone body utilization in human infants. Hoppe-Seyler's Z Physiol Chem 1974;355:164–70.
9. Fernandes J, Berger R, Smit GPA. Lactate as a cerebral metabolic fuel for glucose-6-phosphatase deficient children. Pediatr Res 1984;18:335–9.
10. Field JB. Hypoglycemia: definition, clinical presentations, classification and laboratory tests. Endocrinol Metab Clin North Am 1989;18:27–43.
11. Hawkins RA, Biebuyck JF. Ketone bodies are selectively used by individual brain regions. Science 1979;205:325–27.
12. Pelligrino DA, Segil LJ, Albrecht RF. Brain glucose utilization and transport and cortical function in chronic vs acute hypoglycemia. Am J Physiol 1990;259:E729–35.
13. Shapiro ET, Cooper M, Chen C-T, et al. Change in hexose distribution volume and fractional utilization of [^{18}F]-2-deoxy-2-fluoro-D-glucose in brain during acute hypoglycemia in humans. Diabetes 1990;39:175–80.
14. Young RSK, Cowan BE, Petroff OAC, et al. In vivo ^{31}P and in vitro ^{1}H nuclear magnetic resonance study of hypoglycemia during neonatal seizure. Ann Neurol 1987;22:622–8.
15. Hollinger BR, Bryan RM. β-Receptor-mediated increase in cerebral blood flow during hypoglycemia. Am J Physiol 1987;253:H949–55.
16. Anwar M, Vannucci RC. Autoradiographic determination of regional cerebral blood flow during hypoglycemia in newborn dogs. Pediatr Res 1988;24:41–5.
17. Merimee TJ, Tyson JE. Stabilization of plasma glucose during fasting: normal variations in two separate studies. N Engl J Med 1974;291:1275–8.
18. Chaussain JL. Glycemic response to 24 hour fast in normal children and children with ketotic hypoglycemia. J Pediatr 1973;82:438–43.
19. Teale JD, Marks V. The measurement of insulin, C-peptide and β-hydroxybutyrate in the differential diagnosis of spontaneous hypoglycemia. In: Andreani D, Marks V, Lefebvre PJ, eds. Hypoglycaemia. Serono Symposia. Vol 38. New York: Raven Press, 1987:281–2.
20. Cornblath M, Schwartz R. Disorders of carbohydrate metabolism in infancy. 3rd ed. Boston: Blackwell, 1991.
21. Sexson WR. Incidence of neonatal hypoglycemia: a matter of definition. J Pediatr 1984;105:149–50.
22. Koh THHG, Eyre JA, Aynsley-Green A. Neonatal hypoglycaemia—the controversy regarding definition. Arch Dis Child 1988;63:1386–98.
23. Lucas A, Morley R, Cole TJ. Adverse neurodevelopmental outcome of moderate neonatal hypoglycemia. BMJ 1988;297:1304–8.
24. Koh THHG, Aynsley-Green A, Tarbit M, Eyre JA. Neural dysfunction during hypoglycaemia. Arch Dis Child 1988;63:1353–8.

25. Pryds O, Christensen NJ, Friis-Hansen B. Increased cerebral blood flow and plasma epinephrine in hypoglycemic, preterm neonates. Pediatrics 1990;85:172–6.

26. Malouf R, Brust JCM. Hypoglycemia: causes, neurological manifestations, and outcome. Ann Neurol 1985; 17:421–30.

27. Fischer KF, Lees JA, Newman JH. Hypoglycemia in hospitalized patients. Causes and outcomes. N Engl J Med 1986;315:1245–50.

28. Atkin SH, Dasmahapatra A, Jaker MA, et al. Fingerstick glucose determination in shock. Ann Intern Med 1991; 114:1020–4.

29. Permutt MA, Kelly J, Bernstein R, et al. Alimentary hypoglycemia in the absence of gastrointestinal surgery. N Engl J Med 1973;288:1206–10.

30. Seltzer HS, Fajans SS, Conn JW. Spontaneous hypoglycemia as an early manifestation of diabetes mellitus. Diabetes 1956;5:437–42.

31. Perley MJ, Kipnis DM. Plasma insulin responses to oral and intravenous glucose: studies in normal and diabetic subjects. J Clin Invest 1967;46:1954–62.

32. Porte D Jr. Banting Lecture 1990. β-Cells in type II diabetes mellitus. Diabetes 1991;40:166–80.

33. Lev-Ran A, Anderson RW. The diagnosis of postprandial hypoglycemia. Diabetes 1981;30:996–9.

34. Johnson DD, Dorr KE, Swenson WM, Service FJ. Reactive hypoglycemia. JAMA 1980;243:1151–5.

35. Charles MA, Hofeldt F, Shackelford A, et al. Comparison of oral glucose tolerance tests and mixed meals in patients with apparent idiopathic postabsorptive hypoglycemia: absence of hypoglycemia after meals. Diabetes 1981; 30:465–70.

36. Palardy J, Havrankova J, Lepage R, et al. Blood glucose measurements during symptomatic episodes in patients with suspected postprandial hypoglycemia. N Engl J Med 1989;321:1421–5.

37. Tamburrano G, Leonetti F, Sbraccia P, et al. Increased insulin sensitivity in patients with idiopathic reactive hypoglycemia. J Clin Endocrinol Metab 1989;69: 885–90.

38. Nelson RL. Oral glucose tolerance test: indications and limitations. Mayo Clin Proc 1988;63:263–9.

39. Service FJ. Hypoglycemia and the postprandial syndrome [Editorial]. N Engl J Med 1989;321:1472–4.

40. Grunberger G, Weiner JL, Silverman R, et al. Factitious hypoglycemia due to surreptitious administration of insulin: diagnosis, treatment, and long-term follow-up. Ann Intern Med 1988;108:252–7.

41. Service FJ. Hypoglycemic disorders. Pathogenesis, diagnosis, and treatment. Boston: GK Hall Medical Publishers, 1983.

42. Seltzer HS. Drug-induced hypoglycemia: a review of 1418 cases. Endocrinol Metab Clin North Am 1989;18: 163–83.

43. Madison LL. Ethanol-induced hypoglycemia. Adv Metab Dis 1968;3:85–109.

44. Krebs HA, Freedland RA, Hems R, Stubbs M. Inhibition of hepatic gluconeogenesis by ethanol. Biochem J 1969; 112:117–24.

45. Williams HE. Alcoholic hypoglycemia and ketoacidosis. Med Clin North Am 1984;68:33–8.

46. White NJ, Warrell DA, Chanthavanich P, et al. Severe hypoglycemia and hyperinsulinemia in falciparum malaria. N Engl J Med 1983;309:61–6.

47. Waskin H, Stehr-Green JK, Helmick CG, Sattler FR. Risk factors for hypoglycemia associated with pentamidine therapy for Pneumocystis pneumonia. JAMA 1988; 260:345–7.

48. Murphy RL, Lavelle JP, Allan JD, et al. Aerosol pentamidine prophylaxis following Pneumocystis carinii pneumonia in AIDS patients: results of a blinded dose-comparison study using an ultrasonic nebulizer. Am J Med 1991; 90:418–26.

49. Tanaka K, Kean EA, Johnson B. Jamaican vomiting sickness: biochemical investigation of two cases. N Engl J Med 1976; 295:461–7.

50. Bressler R. The unripe akee-forbidden fruit [Editorial]. N Engl J Med 1976;295:500–1.

51. Arky RA. Hypoglycemia associated with liver disease and ethanol. Endocrinol Metab Clin North Am 1989; 18:75–90.

52. Arem R. Hypoglycemia associated with renal failure. Endocrinol Metab Clin North Am 1989;18:103–21.

53. Naylor JM, Kronfeld DS. In vivo studies of hypoglycemia and lactic acidosis in endotoxic shock. Am J Physiol 1985;248:E309–16.

54. Brook CGD, Hindmarsh PC, Smith PJ, Stanhope R. Clinical features and investigation of growth hormone deficiency. Clin Endocrinol Metab 1986;15:479–93.

55. Davidson MB. Effect of growth hormone on carbohydrate and lipid metabolism. Endocr Rev 1987;8:115–31.

56. Bougnères P-F, Artavia-Loria E, Ferre P, et al. Effects of hypopituitarism and growth hormone replacement therapy on the production and utilization of glucose in childhood. J Clin Endocrinol Metab 1985;61:1152–7.

57. Wolfsdorf JI, Sadeghi-Nejad A, Senior B. Hypoketonemia and age-related fasting hypoglycemia in growth hormone deficiency. Metabolism 1983;32:457–62.

58. DeFeo P, Perriello G, Torlone E, et al. Demonstration of a role for growth hormone in glucose counterregulation. Am J. Physiol 1989;256:E835–43.

59. Voorhess ML, MacGillivray MH. Low plasma norepinephrine responses to acute hypoglycemia in children with isolated growth hormone deficiency. J Clin Endocrinol Metab 1984;59:790–3.

60. Press M, Notarfrancesco A, Genel M. Risk of hypoglycaemia with alternate-day growth hormone injections. Lancet 1987;1:1002–4.

61. Kraus-Friedmann N. Hormonal regulation of hepatic gluconeogenesis. Physiol Rev 1984;64:170–259.

62. DeFeo P, Periello G, Torlone E, et al. Contribution of cortisol to glucose counterregulation in humans. Am J Physiol 1989;257:E35–42.

63. Artavia-Loria E, Chaussain JL, Bougnères PF, Job JC. Frequency of hypoglycemia in children with adrenal insufficiency. Acta Endocrinol 1986;113(Suppl 279):275–8.

64. Moshang T, Rosenfield RL, Bongiovanni AM, et al. Familial glucocorticoid insufficiency. J Pediatr 1973;82:821–6.

65. Hopword NJ, Forsman PJ, Kenny FM, Drash AL. Hypoglycemia in hypopituitary children. Am J Dis Child 1975; 129:918–9.

66. Copeland KC, Franks RC, Ramamurthy R. Neonatal hyperbilirubinemia and hypoglycemia in congenital hypopituitarism. Clin Pediatr 1981;26:523–6.

67. Clausen N, Lins P-E, Adamson U, et al. Counterregulation of insulin-induced hypoglycemia in primary hypothyroidism. Acta Endocrinol 1986;111:516–21.

68. Forester CF. Coma in myxedema. Arch Intern Med 1963;111:734–43.

69. Hermansen K, Johannsen LGK, Rasmussen OB. Hypoglycemic coma in severe primary hypothyroidism. Acta Med Scand 1985;218:345–6.

70. Taylor SI, Barbetti F, Accili D, et al. Syndromes of autoimmunity and hypoglycemia: autoantibodies directed against insulin and its receptor. Endocrinol Metab Clin North Am 1989;18:123−43.

71. Redmon B, Pyzdrowski KL, Elson MK, et al. Hypoglycemia due to a monoclonal insulin-binding antibody in multiple myeloma. N Engl J Med 1992;326:994−8.

72. Daughaday WH, Emanuele MA, Brooks MH, et al. Synthesis and secretion of insulin-like growth factor II by a leiomyosarcoma with associated hypoglycemia. N Engl J Med 1988;319:1434−40.

73. Axelrod L, Ron D. Insulin-like growth factor II and the riddle of tumor-induced hypoglycemia [Editorial]. N Engl J Med 1988;319:1477−9.

74. Ron D, Powers AC, Pandian MR, et al. Increased insulin-like growth factor II production and consequent suppression of growth hormone secretion: a dual mechanism for tumor-induced hypoglycemia. J Clin Endocrinol Metab 1989;68:701−6.

75. Daughaday WH, Kapadia M. Significance of abnormal serum binding of insulin-like growth factor II in the development of hypoglycemia in patients with non-islet-cell tumors. Proc Natl Acad Sci USA 1989;86:6778−82.

76. Shapiro ET, Bell GI, Polonsky KS, et al. Tumor hypoglycemia: relationship to high molecular weight insulin-like growth factor-II. J Clin Invest 1990;85:1672−9.

77. Teale JD, Marks V. Inappropriately elevated plasma insulin-like growth factor II in relation to suppressed insulin-like growth factor I in the diagnosis of non-islet cell tumour hypoglycaemia. Clin Endocrinol (Oxf) 1990;33:87−98.

78. Rahier J, Fält K, Müntefering H, et al. The basic structural lesion of persistent neonatal hypoglycaemia with hyperinsulinism: deficiency of pancreatic D cells or hyperactivity of B cells? Diabetologia 1984;26:282−9.

79. Fong T-L, Warner NE, Kumar D. Pancreatic nesidioblastosis in adults. Diabetes Care 1989;12:108−14.

80. Rahier J. Relevance of endocrine pancreas nesidioblastosis to hyperinsulinemic hypoglycemia [Editorial]. Diabetes Care 1989;12:164−6.

81. Bier DM, Leake RD, Haymond MW, et al. Measurement of "true" glucose production rates in infancy and childhood with 6,6-dideuteroglucose. Diabetes 1977;26:1016−23.

82. Bougneres PF, Castaño L, Rocchiccioli F, et al. Medium chain fatty acids increase glucose production in normal and low birthweight newborns. Am J Physiol 1989;256:E692−7.

83. Schwartz R. Hyperinsulinemia and macrosomia [Editorial]. N Engl J Med 1990;323:340−2.

84. Menon RK, Cohen RM, Sperling MA, et al. Transplacental passage of insulin in pregnant women with insulin-dependent diabetes mellitus: its role in fetal macrosomia. N Engl J Med 1990;323:309−15.

85. Barrett CT, Oliver TK Jr. Hypoglycemia and hyperinsulinism in infants with erythroblastosis fetalis. N Engl J Med 1968;278:1260−3.

86. Jones KL. Smith's recognizable patterns of human malformation. 4th ed. Philadelphia: WB Saunders, 1988:136.

87. Jaffe R, Hashida Y, Yunis EJ. Pancreatic pathology in hyperinsulinemic hypoglycemia of infancy. Lab Invest 1980;42:356−65.

88. Upp JR Jr, Ishizuka J, Lobe TE, et al. Somatostatin secretion in cultured human islet cells from patients with nesidioblastosis: a compensatory mechanism? J Pediatr Surg 1987;22:1185−6.

89. Jacobs DG, Haka-Ikse K, Wesson DE, et al. Growth and development in patients operated on for islet cell dysplasia. J Pediatr Surg 1986;21:1184−9.

90. Schiller M, Krausz M, Meyer S, et al. Neonatal hyperinsulinism-surgical and pathologic considerations. J Pediatr Surg 1980;15:16−20.

91. Schwartz SS, Rich BH, Lucky AW, et al. Familial nesidioblastosis: severe neonatal hypoglycemia in two families. J Pediatr 1979;95:44−53.

92. Gabbay KH. Case records of the Massachusetts General Hospital: case 30−1978. N Engl J Med 1978;299:241−8.

93. Haymond MW, Karl IE, Pagliara AS. Ketotic hypoglycemia: an amino acid substrate limited disorder. J Clin Endocrinol Metab 1974;38:521−30.

94. Colle E, Ulstrom RA. Ketotic hypoglycemia. J Pediatr 1962;64:632−51.

95. Christensen NJ. Hypoadrenalinemia during insulin hypoglycemia in children with ketotic hypoglycemia. J Clin Endocrinol Metab 1974;38:107−12.

96. Bennish ML, Azad AK, Rahman O, Phillips RE. Hypoglycemia during diarrhea in childhood. Prevalence, pathophysiology and outcome. N Engl J Med 1990;322:1357−63.

97. Payne K, Ireland P. Plasma glucose levels in the perioperative period in children. Anesthesia 1989;39:868.

98. Haymond MW. Hypoglycemia in infants and children. Endocrinol Metab Clin North Am 1989;18:211−52.

99. Schwenk WF, Haymond MW. Optimal rate of enteral glucose administration in children with glycogen storage disease type I. N Engl J Med 1988;314:682−5.

100. Burchell A. Molecular pathology of glucose-6-phosphatase. FASEB J 1990;4:2978−88.

101. Hers H-G, Van Hoof F, de Barsy T. Glycogen storage disease. In: Scriver CR, Beaudet AL, Sly WS, Valle D, eds. Metabolic basis of inherited disease. 6th ed. New York: McGraw Hill, 1989:425−52.

102. Wolfsdorf JI, Keller RJ, Landy H, Crigler JF Jr. Glucose therapy for glycogenosis type I in infants: comparison of intermittent uncooked cornstarch and continuous overnight glucose feedings. J Pediatr 1990;117:384−91.

103. Greene HL, Ghishan FK, Brown B, et al. Hypoglycemia in type IV glycogenosis: hepatic improvement in two patients with nutritional management. J Pediatr 1988;112:55−8.

104. Wolf B, Feldman GL. The biotin-dependent carboxylase deficiencies. Am J Hum Genet 1982;34:699−716.

105. Gitzelmann R, Steinmann B, Van Den Berghe G. Disorders of fructose metabolism. In: Scriver CR, Beaudet AL, Sly WS, Valle D, eds. Metabolic basis of inherited disease. 6th ed. New York: McGraw-Hill, 1989:399−424.

106. Segal, S. Disorders of galactose metabolism. In: Scriver CR, Beaudet AL, Sly WS, Valle D, eds. Metabolic basis of inherited disease. 6th ed. New York: McGraw-Hill, 1989:453−80.

107. Fort P, Wapnir RA, DeRosas F, Lifshitz F. Long-term evolution of glycerol intolerance syndrome. J Pediatr 1985;106:453−6.

108. Haymond MW, Karl IE, Feigin RD, et al. Hypoglycemia and maple syrup urine disease: defective glyconeogenesis. Pediatr Res 1973;7:500−8.

109. Halperin ML, Schiller CM, Fritz IB. The inhibition by methylmalonic acid of malate transport by the dicarboxylate carrier in rat liver mitochondria: a possible explanation for hypoglycemia in methylmalonic aciduria. J Clin Invest 1971;50:2276−82.

110. Dodge PR, Mancall EL, Crawford JD, et al. Hypoglycemia complicating treatment of phenylketonuria with a phenyl-

alanine-deficient diet: report of two cases. N Engl J Med 1959;260:1104–11.

111. Leonard JV, Middleton B, Seakins JWT. Acetoacetyl CoA thiolase deficiency presenting as ketotic hypoglycemia. Pediatr Res 1987;21:211–3.

112. Stanley CA. New genetic defects in mitochondrial fatty acid oxidation and carnitine deficiency. Adv Pediatr 1987;34:59–88.

113. Duran M, Schutgens RBH, Ketel A, et al. 3-Hydroxy-3-methylglutaryl coenzyme A lyase deficiency: postnatal management following prenatal diagnosis by analysis of maternal urine. J Pediatr 1979;95:1004–7.

114. Dusheiko G, Kew MC, Joffe BI, et al. Recurrent hypoglycemia associated with glutaric aciduria type II in an adult. N Engl J Med 1979;301:1405–9.

115. Russell GJ, Fitzgerald JF, Clark JH. Fulminant hepatic failure. J Pediatr 1987;111:313–9.

116. Wells TG, Ulstrom RA, Nevins TE. Hypoglycemia in pediatric renal allograft recipients. J Pediatr 1988; 113:1002–7.

117. Moss MH. Alcohol-induced hypoglycemia and coma caused by alcohol sponging. Pediatrics 1970;46:445–7.

118. Leung AKC. Ethyl alcohol ingestion in children: a 15-year review. Clin Pediatr 1986;25:617–9.

119. Rivkees SA, Crawford JD. Hypoglycemia pathogenesis in children with dumping syndrome. Pediatrics 1987; 80:937–42.

120. Kaplan SA. Disorders of the anterior pituitary. In: Kaplan SA, ed. Clinical pediatric endocrinology. Philadelphia: WB Saunders, 1990.

121. Landau H, Perlman M, Meyer S, et al. Persistent neonatal hypoglycemia due to hyperinsulinism: medical aspects. Pediatrics 1982;70:440–6.

122. DeClue TJ, Malone JI, Bercu BB. Linear growth during long-term treatment with somatostatin analog (SMS 201–995) for persistent hyperinsulinemic hypoglycemia of infancy. J Pediatr 1990;116:747–50.

Chapter 56

ENDOCRINE TUMORS OF THE PANCREAS

STEPHEN G. GILBEY
ROBERT C. TURNER
DAVID WYNICK
STEPHEN R. BLOOM

GENERAL PRINCIPLES

Endocrine cells are present throughout the gut and form part of the diffuse neuroendocrine system, formerly known as APUD (amine precursor uptake and decarboxylation). The peptide products of these cells are in many cases also present in the nervous system and have been called brain-gut peptides, although their roles may differ greatly depending on the site of production. Thus, a polypeptide such as somatostatin may act as a neurotransmitter, a modulator of peptide release, or a classical hormone, depending on its site of production.

Peptide Secretion

Pancreatic islet cell tumors may produce entopic peptides that normally are produced by the islet or ectopic peptides that normally are not. Some "function-less" tumors do not secrete peptides or else secrete biologically inactive peptides. Islet cells are versatile: tumors may produce multiple peptide hormones. Metastases from a primary tumor that produces predominantly one peptide hormone may produce another with a completely different clinical syndrome, and in families with multiple endocrine neoplasia type 1 (MEN1), different members of the same family may have tumors that produce different hormones.

The clinical syndromes associated with biologically active peptides may, as in the case of gastrin and vasoactive intestinal polypeptide, have played an important role in establishing the biologic effects of these peptides, thus contributing to their identification and purification. Other products, such as pancreatic polypeptide,[1] have been discovered by chance and do not appear to have significant biologic effects even when produced in large quantities.

Tumor Classification

Histochemical techniques been important in determining the location and function of these cells. Neuroendocrine tumor cells share common features (Fig. 56–1), being round or polygonal cells with clear, finely granulated cytoplasm, a low level of mitotic activity, and characteristic patterns of staining following silver impregnation.

Immunocytochemical techniques involving the use of antibodies to a wide range of neuroendocrine markers and peptide products[2,3] have greatly advanced the ability of histopathologists to both recognize islet cell tumors and characterize them according to their products. Nonspecific markers such as neuron-specific enolase,[4] the chromogranins,[5] and the peptide 7B2[6] can be detected in tissue biopsy specimens with the use of immunohistochemical techniques. In the case of chromogranins[7] or pancreastatin, a peptide derived by proteolytic cleavage of chromogranins,[8,9] tumor production can be detected by measuring circulating concentrations in the plasma. More recently, the availability of hybridization histochemistry and in situ hybridization techniques have allowed detection and quantification of particular gene products within cells. Thus, tumors can be screened for the production and storage of a wide range of peptide products.

Despite the common characteristics of islet cell tumors, their clinical presentation varies considerably. For instance, most insulinomas are small and benign, whereas the majority of other hormone-secreting tumors have metastasized by the time of presentation.[10] Different hormone-producing tumors also show characteristic patterns of localization within the pancreas.[11]

Diagnosis

Islet cell tumors are slow-growing and are compatible with relatively prolonged patient survival. A nonfunctioning islet cell tumor may be an incidental finding during the investigation of a patient with few symptoms and a pancreatic mass, with or without metastases in the liver or elsewhere (Fig. 56–2). Not infrequently in the past, patients were given an erroneous clinical diagnosis of carcinoma of the pancreas, with the diagnosis being reassessed because of their surprisingly long survival. Alternatively, patients may present with a characteristic clinical syndrome of diarrhea, hypoglycemia, or recurrent ulceration.

In patients with nonfunctioning tumors, the diagnosis is made histologically. In patients with suspected hormone syndromes, accurate and reliable measurement of circulating tumor products is an essential preliminary investigation. The clinical significance of raised plasma concentrations of gut peptides will then require confirmation—for instance by demonstrating hyperacidity in association with hypergastrinemia, together with the exclusion of other possible causes of a raised level of circulating peptides (e.g., renal failure).

If biochemical criteria for a hormone-secreting tumor are satisfied, radiologic assessment of tumor site and extent are necessary, primarily to assess the feasibility of surgical cure. Because of the highly vascular nature of these endocrine tumors, highly selective angiography, in combination with ultrasound and computed tomographic (CT) scanning, has proved the most sensitive method of locating tumors. Endoscopic ultrasound may be helpful,[12] while the use of intraoperative ultrasound[13] has made extensive preoperative assessment less essential in the localization of small pancreatic insulinomas. Portal vein

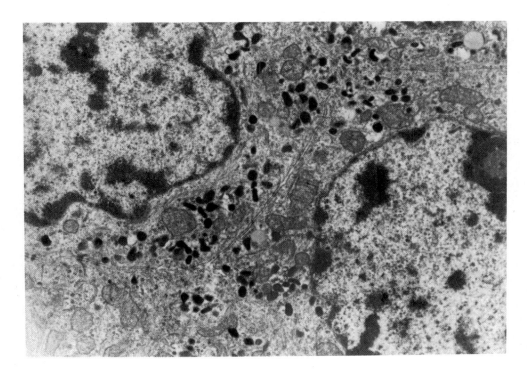

Fig. 56–1. Electron micrograph of a neuroendocrine tumor illustrating numerous electron-dense pleomorphic secretory granules (courtesy of Professor J.M. Polak, Royal Postgraduate Medical School).

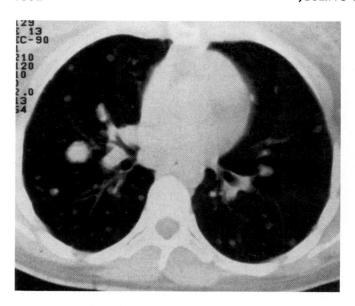

Fig. 56–2. Computed tomographic scan showing lung metastases from a nonfunctioning pancreatic neuroendocrine tumor in a 27-year-old woman. The patient had presented with hepatomegaly and weight loss.

sampling to detect hormone gradients has been used extensively with variable results.

Treatment

The aims of treatment are to effect a curative resection of the tumor if possible or to attenuate the clinical effects of the tumor syndrome either by reducing hormone output or by blocking its effects.

Surgery

The main indication for surgery is removal of the primary tumor with the hope of providing a cure. The availability of effective medical therapy for excess-hormone syndromes, the morbidity and mortality associated with pancreatic surgery, and the recognition that removal of the primary tumor or debulking of metastases may not improve prognosis have all resulted in a more critical appraisal of the indications for surgery in patients with metastatic disease. Major procedures that were once almost routine, such as total gastrectomy in patients with gastrinoma or "blind" subtotal or total pancreatectomy in patients for whom a presumed tumor could not be found at laparotomy, are now performed with decreasing frequency.

Octreotide Therapy

Somatostatin was first discovered in porcine hypothalami in 1973 and was identified as a factor inhibiting the release of growth hormone. Somatostatin is widely distributed in the nervous system and the gut[14] and acts as a peptidergic neurotransmitter within the nervous system, a paracrine modulator within endocrine organs, and an endocrine hormone released into the circulation

in the hypothalamo-pituitary system. A common precursor (pro-SS) is processed into 28- and 14-amino acid somatostatins (SS14 and SS28), which are produced in varying proportions by different tissues.[15] Somatostatin inhibits multiple endocrine functions (Table 56–1), as well as the secretion of gastric acid and enzymes and bicarbonate from the exocrine pancreas.[16]

Native somatostatin has a half-life in the circulation of 2 to 3 minutes, limiting its clinical use. An eight-amino-acid analogue, octreotide (formerly SMS 201-995), has been developed that preserves the four-peptide sequence (Phe-Trp-Lys-Thr) identified as necessary for the biologic activity of somatostatin. Octreotide has, however, a prolonged half-life (90 to 115 minutes intravenously) and can be given subcutaneously.

Octreotide reduces hormone production by islet cell tumors, may also inhibit the peripheral action of circulating peptide products, and has proven to be of immense clinical value in the treatment of some hormone-secreting tumors.[17,18] Gradual loss of the effectiveness of octreotide may occur. The cause of this loss of efficacy is not clear but may be an increase in tumor burden, desensitization (as yet poorly characterized), or a combination of these.[19] In these circumstances the dose of octreotide can be increased from a typical starting dose of 100 μg subcutaneously three times daily to much higher doses, with dosage limited only by inconvenience and cost. A study of 10 patients with pancreatic endocrine tumors treated with octreotide for 13 to 54 months showed, however, that resistance to octreotide treatment eventually culminated in a complete loss of response, which was associated with a very poor survival.[20]

Adverse effects of octreotide treatment are relatively few. Abdominal discomfort may occur following injection, and long-term use may lead to an increased risk of gallstone formation—probably as a consequence of cholestasis.[21] Diarrhea due to pancreatic exocrine insufficiency may occur and will respond to enzyme supplementation. Glucose intolerance is a theoretical concern but is rarely clinically important.

The primary use of octreotide in patients with gut hormone tumors is for the relief of symptoms. There is no convincing evidence that octreotide treatment reduces the size of islet cell tumors or their metastases or prolongs life. However, octreotide treatment may be

Table 56–1. Endocrine Actions of Somatostatin

Organ: Action	Clinical Application
Pituitary	
Inhibition of GH and prolactin secretion	Acromegaly
Nervous system	
Modulation of neurotransmitter effects	?
Pancreas	
Inhibition of insulin and glucagon production	Islet cell tumors
Inhibition of exocrine secretion	Pancreatic fistula
Gastrointestinal tract	
Inhibition of hormone production/actions	Carcinoid syndrome
Decreased splanchnic blood flow	GI hemorrhage
Adrenal gland	
Decreased aldosterone production	?

lifesaving in some circumstances: patients with VIPoma crisis showed a reduction of diarrhea almost to normal in 24 hours and a resolution of electrolyte imbalance within 48 hours.[22] Similarly, octreotide premedication before hepatic embolization can prevent acute crises caused by the massive release of tumor products during this procedure.

Octreotide Imaging

The action of somatostatin is mediated through cell membrane receptors. Distinctive subtypes of somatostatin receptor may have different affinities for the different forms of endogenous somatostatin. In vitro studies of resected tumors and cell lines have shown that pancreatic tumors express somatostatin receptors.[32] Radiolabeling of these receptors in vivo and their imaging by means of scanning techniques have recently been achieved by Lamberts' group in Holland.[24,25] They used an analogue of octreotide in which tyrosine was substituted at the 3 position to allow labeling with iodine 123. Their published work has shown that 1) this method can be used to visualize, with radioisotope scanning, tumors and their metastases that express somatostatin receptors and 2) positive labeling correlates with tumor response to somatostatin. In vitro studies on resected tumors that did not take up the labeled somatostatin showed that, on the whole, these did not express somatostatin receptors.[26] If radioisotopic labeling of somatostatin and the use of this technique can be reproduced by other centers, the potential for its future use is considerable. Diagnosis of small primary tumors may be improved, as may evaluation of the sites and extent of metastases. The uptake of somatostatin may serve as a way of selecting patients likely to respond to octreotide. The method could also be used to direct specific treatment (e.g., ablative doses of radioiodine) at the tumor and metastases.

Hepatic Embolization

Hepatic metastases may be responsible for most of the circulating hormone in patients with islet cell tumors. Hepatic metastases are supplied by the systemic arterial system, while hepatic metabolism can be sustained by the portal circulation (Fig. 56–3). Hence selective hepatic arterial embolization, using a variety of exogenous materials, provides a useful alternative to surgical debulking of hepatic metastases as palliative treatment. Experience suggests that embolization (Fig. 56–4) is preferable to ligation of the hepatic artery, as occlusion of distal, smaller vessels during embolization may delay collateral formation.[27] Morbidity from this procedure exists even when performed by experienced hands, and deaths have occurred. Hazards include infection, inadvertent emboli-

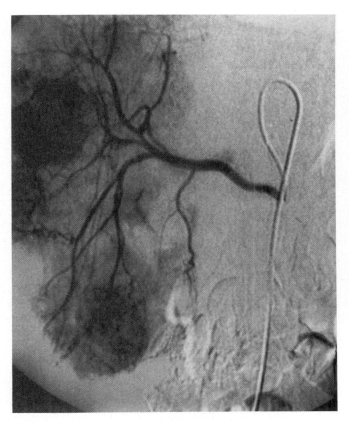
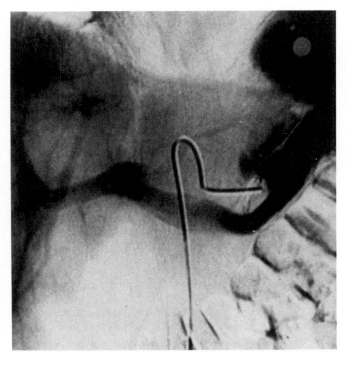

Fig. 56–3. Left: The hepatic arteriogram shows numerous highly vascular metastases in a patient with the carcinoid syndrome. Right: The portal venogram demonstrates the absence of a portal venous supply to the metastases, giving rise to the apparently "empty" areas within the liver (courtesy of Dr. James Jackson, Royal Postgraduate Medical School).

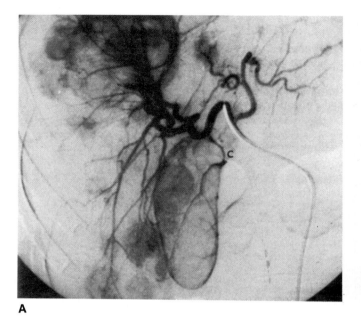

A

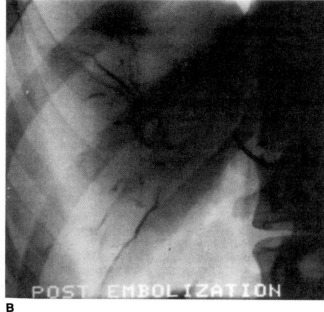

B

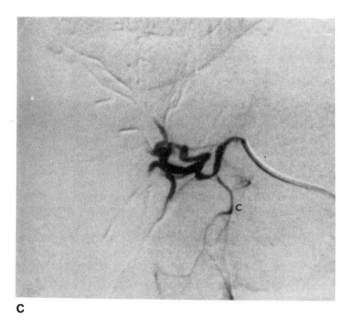

C

Fig. 56–4. A: A hepatic arteriogram demonstrates vascular metastases (c = cystic artery). B: A plain radiograph following hepatic arterial embolization showing radioopaque embolization material within branches of the hepatic artery. C: Hepatic arteriogram immediately following embolization, demonstrating that the hepatic blood supply has been occluded while the cystic artery (c) remains patent (courtesy of Dr. James Jackson, Royal Postgraduate Medical School).

zation of other arteries,[28] morbidity caused by outpouring of vasoactive tumor products during the procedure, postprocedure renal failure due to the required load of contrast dye, and hepatic necrosis when embolization of a very large tumor mass is attempted at one sitting. Careful monitoring of blood pressure and fluid balance is necessary during the procedure, which in the author's unit is covered by octreotide, mainly to prevent abrupt blood pressure changes caused by a massive efflux of peptides during and immediately after the procedure. Prophylaxis with a broad-spectrum antibiotic is advisable. Successful embolization results in pyrexia for up to 10 days following the procedure; hence diagnosis of intercurrent infection can be difficult.

Occlusion of the portal vein with inadequate collateral formation is a contraindication to embolization. Replacement of over 50% of liver by tumor and/or evidence of grossly deranged liver function may make the procedure unacceptably hazardous. Collaterals develop after a variable time interval, and the tumor metastases regrow. Sequential embolization may be undertaken when appropriate. Ajani and colleagues[29] reported the results of embolization in 22 patients with islet cell tumors: 9 with gastrinomas, 2 with glucagonoma, and 11 with "functionless" tumors. The patients had a total of 97 embolizations (range, 1 to 12) at intervals of 1 to 8 months. Twelve of the 20 patients who were evaluated for response showed a partial remission, and 4 showed minor evidence of remission (<50% reduction in measurable tumor). One patient died of hepatic necrosis, and all patients experienced morbidity (nausea, vomiting, abdominal pain, fever), which generally resolved by the 10th day after embolization.

Cytotoxic Treatment

The islet cell toxin streptozotocin, usually in combination with fluorouracil, has been used extensively for islet cell tumors, with claims of up to 50 to 70% response as judged either by hormone secretion in functioning tumors such as gastrinomas or by tumor size in nonfunctioning tumors.[30] Other chemotherapeutic agents have been used with varying results.[31-33] The regimen used at the author's hospital is streptozotocin, 500 mg/m^2, and fluorouracil, 400 mg/m^2, administered together as an intravenous bolus on alternate days over 10 days. Renal, hepatic, and bone marrow function are closely monitored. The course is repeated every 2 to 3 months, and normally three to four courses would be given followed by a 6-month wait to assess reduction in tumor bulk.

Oberg and colleagues[34,35] and others[36] have reported limited success with interferon, with 25% of patients showing a reduction in hormone secretion but less than 10% showing a decrease in tumor bulk. However, interferon has also been associated with many adverse effects, including autoimmune hemolytic anemia, leukopenia with associated influenza-like symptoms, and liver fibrosis.

The indication for palliative treatment is the relief of symptoms when other measures have failed. There is little or no evidence that embolization or chemotherapy improves long-term survival.

INSULINOMAS

The insulinoma syndrome was first described in 1927 in a physician with recurrent hypoglycemia. The syndrome of hypoglycemia with inappropriately elevated plasma concentrations of insulin is now known to be due to insulin-secreting tumors, almost all of which originate in the pancreas. Insulinomas are the most common islet cell tumors. They have a prevalence[37] of approximately one per million, are more common in women, and present most frequently between the ages of 40 and 60 years (younger when in association with MEN1).[38] They may, however, present at any age, although they are very rare in those younger than 5 years old.

Insulinomas are usually very small at the time of presentation (90% are <2 cm in diameter), presumably because small tumors can cause significant hypoglycemia.[39] In one series[40] 80% of tumors were solitary with no evidence of metastases, 11% were multiple, and 6% were malignant; 10% were associated with MEN1, and these were predominantly multiple. These figures emerged from a major tertiary referral center and may present an overestimate of the prevalence of multiple tumors. In this author's experience, multiple tumors constitute 5% or less of all insulinoma. The diagnosis of malignancy is based on the presence of metastases or of local invasion of capsule, blood vessels, or lymph nodes at the time of excision.[41] Metastasis is usually to the liver or local lymph nodes but can occur to a wide variety of organs.

Clinical Features

Recurrent hypoglycemia is the predominant feature of insulinoma and the basis of nearly all its symptomatology. Unlike normal β-cells, insulinoma cells do not switch off insulin production in response to low blood glucose concentrations. Thus, clinical hypoglycemia occurs, particularly following periods without food or after exercise. Classically, patients present with difficulty in waking after an overnight fast, symptoms that are relieved by a warm drink with sugar at breakfast. Very rarely, postprandial hypoglycemia may occur. Insulinomas rarely induce unpredictable hypoglycemia unless blood glucose levels are chronically low. Symptoms may be insidious and present for many years before diagnosis. The most common symptoms are from neuroglycopenia, with diplopia, blurred vision, and weakness, together with confusion or abnormal behavior, episodes of unconsciousness, and, rarely, grand mal seizures.[40] Adrenergic symptoms such as sweating and palpitations are not usually prominent, probably because prolonged hypoglycemia down-regulates counterregulatory responses.[42] Weight gain is not a reliable clinical sign, occurring in only 20% of cases.[43] Many patients fail to recognize that eating prevents attacks.

Diagnosis

The rarity of insulinomas and the nonspecific nature of the symptoms of hypoglycemia can result in erroneous diagnoses—notably neurologic or psychiatric. On the other hand, there are many other causes of hypoglycemia-type symptoms and hypoglycemia (Table 56–2), and a poorly authenticated diagnosis of insulinoma could result in futile surgical exploration and pancreatic surgery. Biochemical hypoglycemia has to be demonstrated: patients with supposed episodes of hypoglycemia and no evidence of organic disease have symptoms that correlate very poorly with the concentration of blood glucose.[44]

The patient's history needs to establish whether symptoms occur mainly during fasting, in which case insulinoma is the most likely pathologic cause. If hypoglycemia occurs 4 to 5 hours after ingestion of food, the cause is more likely to be reactive hypoglycemia due to previous gastric surgery, glucose intolerance/early diabetes mellitus, or of idiopathic origin in some thin subjects. Once fasting hypoglycemia has been established, other causes such as non-islet tumors, endocrine deficiency, cirrhosis, and drugs (e.g., β-adrenergic blocking agents) need to be excluded. Only the demonstration of inappropriately high insulin concentrations in the face of biochemical hypoglycemia can distinguish insulinoma from most other causes of fasting hypoglycemia. Factitious hypoglycemia caused by self-administration of insulin or sulfonylurea drugs needs to be excluded with particular care. A careful history that looks for evidence of psychiatric disease, easy access to hypoglycemic medication, or both, is important in the assessment of such patients, although

Table 56–2. Causes of Hypoglycemia

Hyperinsulinemic/high C peptide
Insulinoma
Islet cell hyperplasia
Nesidioblastosis
Sulfonylurea treatment
Neonatal
  Prematurity
  Children of diabetic mothers
Hyperinsulinemic/low C peptide
Exogenous insulin
Insulin autoimmune syndrome
Hypoinsulinemic
Drugs
  Salicylates
  β-blocking agents
  Quinine
  Disopyramide
  Trimethoprim/sulfamethoxazole
  Alcohol (with preexisting malnutrition)
Tumors (insulin-like activity in serum and plasma)
  Mesenchymal tumors (e.g., retroperitoneal sarcomas)
  Hepatoma
Insulin-receptor antibodies
Metabolic
  Hepatic disease
  Addison's disease
  Hypopituitarism
  Isolated growth-hormone deficiency
  Renal failure
  Starvation
  Galactosemia
  Glycogen storage disease
  Fructose intolerance

such evidence will, of course, not be sufficient in itself. The possibility of MEN1 should be investigated, since patients with MEN1 are more likely to have multiple pancreatic tumors at presentation.

Nesidioblastosis is a rare neonatal condition in which nesidioblasts differentiate from pancreatic duct epithelium and form endocrine cells that are separate from the true islets, giving rise to hyperinsulinism and hypoglycemia.[45] Infants presenting with hyperinsulinism and hypoglycemia are more likely to have nesidioblastosis than insulinoma. The condition rarely occurs in adults,[46] in whom the appearance of nesidioblastosis in a pathologic specimen usually indicates the presence of an insulinoma elsewhere.

Four methods of screening patients for suspected insulinoma may be used:

1. *Overnight fasting blood sample for glucose, insulin, and C-peptide.* The majority of patients with insulinomas have biochemical hypoglycemia (<3.5 mM/L is very unusual in normal subjects and <4.0 mM/L is suggestive in a symptomatic patient). The diagnosis can be made if the fasting plasma glucose concentration is <2.5 mM/L with an insulin level of >5 mU/L, while an insulin level of >3 mU/L is suggestive of an insulinoma.[47] It is important that a sensitive insulin assay be used; assays with a lower limit of detection of 3 to 5 mU/L should be avoided. For a definitive diagnosis, measurements must be made on two occasions. It should be noted that a normal blood glucose value after an overnight fast does not exclude fasting hypoglycemia.

2. *Fasting plasma proinsulin.* This is a useful screening test, since virtually all patients with insulinomas have a raised proinsulin level, even when the fasting glucose level is normal.[48]

3. *Hypoglycemia/C-peptide suppression test.*[49,50] The infusion of insulin (0.05 U/kg per hour) for 2 hours should result in a plasma glucose level of <2.5 mM/L and suppression of C-peptide level by >50% to a value of <150 pM/L. Blood samples are taken at 30-minute intervals, and when the glucose levels becomes <2.5 mM/L, the final sample is taken and glucose is administered. An intravenous cannula should be used to ensure venous access in the unlikely event of a seizure. The degree to which the hypoglycemic symptoms during this test match the usual symptoms is of interest. Normal C-peptide suppression excludes an insulinoma but not other causes of fasting hypoglycemia, which should be sought if clinically indicated.

4. *Admission of the patient for a prolonged supervised fast for up to 72 hours.* In most patients a hypoglycemic episode will occur during the first 24 hours of a fast. The patient should be kept active, and if by 72 hours no symptomatic hypoglycemic episode has occurred, a period of vigorous exercise is undertaken (e.g., 30 minutes of continuous walking up and down flights of stairs). If the combination of a prolonged fast and exercise does not induce clinical hypoglycemia, investigations need be taken no further, as 98% of patients with an insulinoma will have had a symptomatic hypoglycemic episode by 72 hours after their last meal.[43] If the patient does have symptoms of hypoglycemia, blood must be taken immediately for simultaneous determinations of plasma glucose, insulin, and C-peptide levels. Invalidation of the study by well-intentioned nursing or medical staff offering food or administering glucose without first taking blood is an ever-present risk. In normal subjects a blood glucose level of ≤2.2 mM/L will be associated with suppressed serum insulin level of ≤2 mU/L. Thus, if patients have a normal or elevated insulin level in the face of hypoglycemia (preferably on more than one occasion), the biochemical criteria for insulinoma have been satisfied. Appropriate simultaneous concentrations of C-peptide (>300 pM/L) will help exclude the self-administration of insulin as the cause of hypoglycemia. Urine should be screened for sulfonylureas, as self-administration of these gives biochemical indices indistinguishable from those produced by an insulinoma.

Other biochemical tests that have been proposed for use in difficult cases include the administration of tolbutamide, which results in an exaggerated fall in blood glucose level and rise in plasma insulin[51]; and the intravenous administration of calcium, to which the response is also exaggerated.[52] Neither of these tests offers significant improvements in diagnostic accuracy in routine clinical practice.

Tumor Localization

The aims of localization studies are 1) to define the number and location of tumors and 2) to assess whether metastasis has already occurred. High-resolution CT scanning of the abdomen, usually with intravenous contrast, will identify up to 50% of pancreatic tumors and also will permit assessment of possible metastases. However, many insulinomas are too small to be detected by CT scans. Ultrasound examination has a slightly better chance of detecting small tumors. The optimal preoperative localization technique is celiac and superior mesenteric arteriography—looking for the characteristic tumor blush of both primary tumor and hepatic metastases. This technique is highly sensitive and specific in experienced hands, giving positive confirmation of up to 80% of cases. Now that intraoperative ultrasound technology[53] is available, it may be reasonable in centers where this is well established to proceed straight to laparotomy in patients with no unusual features.

Other techniques are required only when specific problems have arisen. Transhepatic portal vein sampling, in which a local gradient in insulin concentration is looked for, has been reported as giving results as good as those from angiography.[54] It may be particularly useful when no tumor has been found at operation and when β-cell hyperplasia or nesidioblastosis is suspected. Iodine 131-labeled antibody to insulin has been used in an attempt to identify insulinomas and their metastases with only limited success.[55]

Treatment

Surgical resection and cure are the aims of treatment in most patients. Medical treatment can be used to control symptoms before surgery or in patients with metastatic disease.

Medical Treatment

Before presenting to the physician, some patients have evolved their own quite effective treatment of eating small and frequent meals. Diazoxide, a thiazide compound that inhibits insulin release, is an effective and useful agent in the medical treatment of insulinoma. Doses of between 150 and 800 mg/day control hyperglycemia in most patients. Adverse effects include fluid retention (a diuretic is usually prescribed in combination with diazoxide), nausea, and vomiting, and hypertrichosis in females. Diazoxide is only effective in about 50% of patients. Calcium antagonists,[56] phenytoin, and propanolol may also be useful in addition to diazoxide.

Octreotide has been used in patients with insulinoma,[57] but it is effective in only approximately 50% of cases and may exacerbate hypoglycemia because of its inhibitory effect on counterregulatory hormone secretion.[58] The probable reason for this lack of efficacy is that only a certain proportion of insulinomas express enough receptors for somatostatin and/or octreotide. This con-trasts with the efficacy of octreotide in nesidioblastosis, in which it has been exceptionally useful in controlling hyperinsulinism and hypoglycemia.[59,60]

Palliative Treatment

Chemotherapy can be effective in the palliative treatment of metastatic insulinoma. Streptozotocin (500 mg/m^2 per day) has been most commonly used in 5-day courses (in combination with fluorouracil (400 mg/m^2 per day) repeated at 2- to 3-month intervals. Hepatic embolization may be used as a means of debulking hepatic metastases if present.

Surgical Treatment

With the exception of those tumors associated with MEN1, the great majority of insulinomas are single and pancreatic, and up to 95% are successfully enucleated at surgery. Therefore, there is a case for "blind" surgery in patients for whom there is biochemical evidence of a tumor but no success in preoperative localization. The tumor or tumors can usually be palpated by an experienced surgeon. Intraoperative ultrasonography[61,62] may be useful both for identifying an insulinoma and for searching for possible multiple tumors. When no tumor is identified, it is not advisable to perform a "blind" distal pancreatectomy, as the tumor is likely to be hidden in the head of pancreas. In some centers the patient may subsequently be referred for localization by transhepatic portal vein cannulation. This can also be done at the time of operation via a splenic vein radicle.[63] An alternative strategy when no tumor is found is to treat medically and to perform additional localization tests at annual intervals or if medical treatment is unsuccessful.

GASTRINOMA

The existence of a substance that promoted production of gastric acid was first postulated in 1905.[64] Fifty-five years later Gregory and Tracy succeeded in extracting material from gastric antral mucosa that stimulated acid secretion.[65] Gregory and colleagues subsequently purified, sequenced, and synthesized a 17-amino-acid peptide showing minimal amino acid substitutions between the peptide in humans and that in other mammals, as well as a 34-amino-acid form of gastrin, called "big" gastrin or G34.[66] The gastric atrium contains the highest concentration of gastrin-producing cells, but the duodenum also contains these cells and is the major source of extra-antral gastrin.[67] The gastrin gene and immunoreactive gastrin are expressed in normal pancreatic islet cells during fetal life but not after birth.[68]

Zollinger and Ellison[69] were the first to hypothesize that a humoral factor was the link between non-β-cell islet tumors of the pancreas and a fulminating ulcer diathesis. It is now known that these tumors contain gastrin[66] and are accompanied by raised concentrations of circulating immunoreactive gastrin (predominantly G34).[70] Sensitive and specific radioimmunoassays for plasma gastrin have become the cornerstone of the diagnosis of this syndrome.

Gastrinomas are the second most commonly diagnosed pancreatic islet cell tumors after insulinoma. Approximately 60% of gastrinomas are malignant at the time of diagnosis.[71] One-third of patients with gastrinoma have MEN1. A minority of gastrinomas occur in the duodenum; approximately one-third of a series of 33 patients with endocrine duodenal tumors had presented with the gastrinoma syndrome, whereas an additional one-third had tumors that stained for gastrin but did not produce the gastrinoma syndrome.[72]

Clinical Features

Except in the terminal stages of malignant disease, the clinical features of the Zollinger-Ellison syndrome are due entirely to the overproduction of gastrin. Patients may present with a relatively short (<2-year) history of peptic ulceration, often multiple and atypical in site and refractory to standard medical or surgical treatment. Complications include perforation, pyloric stenosis, hemorrhage, and gastrojejunocolic fistulas. Diarrhea and malabsorption caused by acid-related inactivation of enzymes and mucosal damage in the upper small bowel may predate ulceration. Effective anti-ulcer drugs and early diagnosis through the routine availability of the gastrin radioimmunoassay have resulted in a decreased incidence of the catastrophic complications of the disease.

Diagnosis

The relatively uncommon patients with gastrinoma need to be differentiated from the mass of patients suffering from peptic ulcers. Suspicion should be heightened by the occurrence of multiple ulcers in unusual sites, diarrhea, complications of peptic ulcer, recurrence after gastric surgery, and a family history of peptic ulcer or endocrine disorders.

The biochemical diagnosis requires a finding of an elevated fasting plasma gastrin level together with a high basal output of gastric acid. A normal fasting plasma gastrin level (e.g., <40 pM/L in the author's laboratory), in one or more samples, effectively excludes the diagnosis in the great majority of cases. Other causes of raised gastrin levels need to be excluded (see Table 56–3). Some of the highest plasma gastrin values seen are attributable to nonmalignant causes such as achlorhydria

Table 56–3. Causes of Hypergastrinemia

With low gastric acid production
Vagotomy
Antisecretory treatment
Hypochlorhydria
Short gut syndrome
With normal/slightly elevated acid production
Renal failure
Hypercalcemia
With elevated acid production
Excluded antrum syndrome
G cell hyperplasia
Zollinger-Ellison syndrome

or impaired gastrin metabolism in chronic renal failure. The presence of elevated concentrations of pancreatic polypeptide; of other gut hormones, such as glucagon; or of nonspecific neuroendocrine tumor products, such as chromogranins, provides valuable additional evidence for the possible presence of a tumor. Demonstration of the presence of circulating gastrin precursors or abnormally processed gastrin may also prove useful in distinguishing between tumors and other causes.[73,74]

A raised plasma gastrin level is significant only in the presence of increased gastric acid secretion. Patients with gastric hypersecretion in association with the gastrinoma syndrome usually secrete >100 mM of acid in a 12-hour overnight collection. In practice a 1-hour basal acid output (BAO) determination is sufficient, and the amount of acid should exceed 10 mM/hour. If the patient has undergone a previous gastric surgical procedure, the diagnosis should be considered when the BAO exceeds 5 mM/hour. Low-normal or diminished acid production in a patient not receiving antacid or antisecretory therapy excludes the diagnosis of gastrinoma. Borderline elevation of gastric acidity may give a false-positive result; a few patients with duodenal ulceration may exhibit gastric acid production of >15 mM/hour. Patients with a duodenal ulcer may be distinguishable from those with gastrinoma by having a more marked response to pentagastrin (patients with gastrinoma are said to have a BAO that is ≥60% of the pentagastrin-stimulated peak output). However, up to 50% of patients with gastrinoma fail to show this pattern, and in our experience a determination of response to pentagastrin stimulation adds little to the diagnostic value of a determination of BAO.

Provocative tests for gastrin release have been advocated in cases in which plasma gastrin elevation is borderline. The best known of these is the secretin test, in which intravenous injection of secretin (2 units/kg) causes a characteristic increase in plasma gastrin level within 10 minutes in patients with gastrinoma that is not seen in normal subjects.[75] However, false-positive results may occur,[76] and the routine use of this test is not justified except in cases in which the diagnosis is still in question after the measurement of plasma gastrin and BAO. A number of other tests, such as the gastrin response to a test meal[77] or to a calcium infusion,[78] have been suggested but have generally not been shown to be of discriminatory value, either in sporadic gastrinomas or in patients with MEN1.[79]

There are other conditions in which gastrin level is elevated in the presence of a high gastric acid output. The condition of G-cell hyperplasia is of unknown origin and is diagnosed histologically from a gastric biopsy specimen. The excluded antrum syndrome occurs after surgery when a portion of antrum is left isolated from the gastric lumen; feedback inhibition of gastrin production by acid is lost, and hypergastrinemia and hyperacidity ensue.

Tumor Localization

Once a firm biochemical diagnosis of the gastrinoma syndrome is made, further investigations are aimed at identifying the site of the primary tumor, the extent of tumor spread, and the possibility of operative cure.

The majority of gastrinomas are situated in the "gastrinoma triangle," which is bounded by the junction of the cystic and common bile ducts superiorly, the junction of the second and third parts of the duodenum inferiorly, and the junction of the neck and body of the pancreas medially. Tumor localization is, however, a difficult problem in many patients with gastrinoma; tumors are often very small (3 to 5 mm) and may be extrapancreatic, e.g., in the duodenum.

Sensitivity is the major problem for all radiologic investigations in patients with clinical evidence of the gastrinoma syndrome, with the sensitivity ranging from 20% with ultrasound to 72% with CT scanning. Once a tumor is located, specificity is >90%, whatever method is used.[80] Nuclear magnetic resonance (NMR) scanning has been reported to be as effective as CT scanning[81] but needs further evaluation.

In the hands of operators experienced at recognizing a tumor blush, selective arterial angiography (Fig. 56–5), in combination with CT scanning, is the most effective preoperative investigation, with a sensitivity of up to 86%.[82] Intra-arterial infusion of secretin is currently under investigation as a means of localizing occult small tumors. Secretin (30 units) is injected during selective arteriography, and blood is taken within 1 minute from hepatic and peripheral veins. Injection of secretin into the region of the gastrinoma leads to a rapid rise in gastrin levels.[83,84] This procedure may prove to be of value in localizing tumors in difficult cases. It is, however, expensive and time-consuming in terms of both radiologic and laboratory procedures, and further evaluation is required before it is accepted into general practice.

Published experience suggests that portal vein sampling may give useful positive information in cases in which a single tumor is present in the pancreas or duodenum or hepatic metastases are present, but it is of less value in other cases.[85]

Thus, a combination of CT scanning—preferably dynamic scanning with contrast—and selective arteriography should be used to locate tumors. Portal vein sampling and intra-arterial secretin testing may be useful in difficult cases. Despite these investigations many tumors remain elusive, in which case hypergastrinemia should be controlled medically and CT scanning should be repeated annually to pick up any small tumor that might become apparent.[86]

Treatment

The aims of treatment are 1) the control of the hypersecretion of gastrin and 2) the removal of the tumor if this will effect a cure or at least alter the natural history of the condition.

Medical Treatment

High-dose blockers of histamine H_2 receptors and, more recently, the Na^+/K^+-ATPase inhibitor omeprazole have revolutionized the management of gastrinoma. Urgent laparotomy for the removal of tumor and/or gastrectomy is now obsolete. The symptoms of gastrinoma can be alleviated and its complications avoided with antisecretory treatment while the location of a resectable tumor is sought.

The aim of medical treatment is to reduce basal acid production to within the normal range. Acid production should be formally monitored, particularly during the initiation of treatment, the aim being to decrease basal

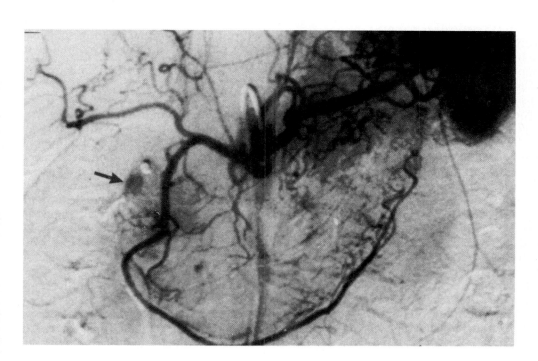

Fig. 56–5. Celiac axis arteriogram demonstrating a small arterial blush (arrow) in a patient suspected of having a gastrinoma. At laparotomy a small duodenal tumor was removed, resulting in the complete resolution of the patient's hypergastrinemia (courtesy of Dr. James Jackson, Royal Postgraduate Medical School).

acid production to a peak of 10 mM/hour. Usually the doses of H_2 blockers required are higher than those used for the treatment of peptic ulcer disease, and periodic increases in dosage are often necessary.[87] A variety of H_2 blockers are available and have been used for patients with gastrinoma. The rate of treatment failure in different series varies, but these differences may reflect inadequate dosage rather than variations in the efficacy of different H_2 blocking drugs.[88,89]

Omeprazole is a substituted benzaminidine that suppresses acid production by inhibiting parietal cell Na^+/K^+-ATPase. Compared with H_2 blockers, omeprazole is a more potent acid suppressant, has a longer duration of action, and is less likely to require increases in dosage once optimal acid suppression is achieved.[90–92] Omeprazole, at a dosage of 80 to 120 mg daily, effectively produces a medical gastrectomy, reducing basal acid output to <5 mM/hour after 2 days of treatment and healing 98% of ulcers within 2 weeks and 100% within 1 month of initiation of therapy. These do not recur if treatment is maintained.[91] Concerns about the advisability of complete suppression of acid output were fueled by the development of gastric carcinoids in rats receiving long-term therapy with omeprazole[93] but have not been borne out in humans to date.

Somatostatin is produced by cells within the gastric antrum, where it may act as paracrine inhibitor of gastrin production. Treatment with octreotide has been shown to suppress gastrin production in patients with gastrinoma.[94] However, treatment with octreotide is no more effective than treatment with H_2 blockers or omeprazole at relieving symptoms and has not been shown to alter the natural history of islet cell tumors or their metastases. Its value in patients with tumors that secrete only gastrin therefore seems limited.

Palliative Treatment

Distant metastases generally involve the liver but may be found further afield. Patients with metastatic disease can lead a normal life while receiving antisecretory treatment; thus, further therapeutic intervention should be considered only if clinical improvement is likely, e.g., if metastatic tumor bulk is causing symptoms as a result of compression or infiltration. The major options for palliation are cytotoxic chemotherapy and hepatic embolization.

Chemotherapeutic regimens have proven less useful in patients with gastrinoma than in those with other hormone syndromes: only 20% of patients with gastrinoma respond to chemotherapy, as compared with 80% of those with the VIPoma syndrome. The most commonly used regimen is a combination of the islet cell toxin streptozotocin and fluorouracil.[29] The main indication for chemotherapy is the failure of other treatment to control the effects of hypergastrinemia or the presence of symptoms caused primarily by tumor bulk.

Hepatic artery embolization is directed at the relief of local symptoms and the reduction of hormone output by liver metastases and may provide effective palliation if all other measures fail.

Surgical Treatment

The major decision to be made is whether to operate to locate and remove the primary tumor. In patients who present with good clinical and biochemical evidence of the gastrinoma syndrome and have no family history suggesting the possibility of MEN1 and in those in whom a pancreatic or duodenal tumor is identified preoperatively, little controversy surrounds the decision to operate. Operation and tumor resection have a good chance of effecting a complete cure[95,96] even when affected lymph nodes are discovered at laparotomy.[97] Operation is rarely justified in patients who are known to have hepatic metastases, although some authors have claimed a beneficial effect of tumor debulking. Total gastrectomy does not prolong survival and is not justified unless all other treatment options have failed.[98]

Problems arise in patients in whom no tumor can be demonstrated preoperatively, particularly when MEN1 is suspected on clinical grounds. The main argument for early operation and a careful search for a tumor by an experienced surgeon (including introperative ultrasound) is that up to one-third of such patients have been found to have resectable pancreatic or extrapancreatic gastrinomas at operation.[99] These include small duodenal tumors that are difficult to detect preoperatively and yet potentially curable if resected. If a tumor cannot be identified, the duodenum should be carefully examined[100]—probably by duodenotomy and possibly by transillumination.[101] Preoperative upper gastrointestinal endoscopy usually fails to reveal these tumors. Blind resection of the tail of pancreas is not justified, since the great majority of pancreatic tumors are in the head of pancreas. Neither should patients be routinely exposed to the morbidity and mortality associated with pancreatoduodenectomy (Whipple's procedure).

Experience has shown that the prognosis for patients whose gastrinomas cannot be located is relatively good. A strong case can be made for not undertaking "blind" exploratory surgery: CT scanning and arteriography may be repeated at intervals while the patient continues to receive antisecretory treatment.

Patients with Suspected MEN1 Syndrome

The presence of the MEN1 syndrome in patients with gastrinoma has important clinical implications. Patients with MEN1 are likely to present with multiple tumors, frequently microscopic and difficult to detect at operation, and may be particularly prone to the development of multiple small gastrinomas in the duodenum.[102] The policy in most centers is to investigate patients with MEN1 syndrome in the same manner as that applied to patients with gastrinoma and to operate when well-defined pancreatic or duodenal tumors are positively identified.[103] When no tumor is found, the justification both for early operation and exploration may be even less than that for sporadic gastrinomas, since multiple and recurrent tumors commonly occur.

In summary, management of the gastrinoma syndrome has been greatly improved by increased clinical awareness, the ready availability of gastrin radioimmunoassay, and effective medical treatment. The optimal surgical management of patients with gastrinoma, particularly those whose tumors cannot be located preoperatively or who may have the MEN1 syndrome, remains controversial.

VIPOMA

Vasoactive intestinal polypeptide (VIP) is a linear, 28-amino-acid peptide with considerable homology with secretin and other members of the secretin family. In 1967 Said and colleagues found a potent vasodilating peptide in aqueous extracts of mammalian lungs and eventually purified VIP from porcine duodenum in 1970.[104] VIP has a widespread distribution in the central and peripheral nervous system but is not found in mucosal endocrine cells of the gastrointestinal tract. The physiologic role of VIP in the intestine appears, therefore, to be as a local neurotransmitter and probable modulator of intestinal ion and water transport, as well as being a splanchnic vasodilator.[105]

Priest and Alexander in 1957[106] and Verner and Morrison in 1958[107] described patients in whom severe watery diarrhea was associated with non-insulin-producing islet cell tumors. The syndrome subsequently was shown to be associated with VIP-producing tumors and circulating VIP,[108] and such tumors were found to comprise 3 to 5% of pancreatic endocrine tumors. Infused VIP simulates the tumor syndrome, causing a secretory diarrhea, hypokalemia, and metabolic acidosis.[109] Thus, VIPoma has superseded the previous designation of Verner-Morrison—that of watery diarrhea hypoglycemia hypochlorhydria (WDHA) or pancreatic cholera syndrome. The majority of patients have pancreatic tumors; the rest have primarily neuroblastomas or ganglioneuromas or, rarely, phaeochromocytomas. Peptide histidine methionine (PHM) is derived from the same precursor as VIP (pre-pro VIP), has similar effects on intestinal secretion, and may contribute to the clinical picture in patients with the VIP-producing tumors,[110,111] 10% of which also secrete the neuropeptide neurotensin.[112]

Pancreatic VIPomas are often large—up to 7 cm in diameter. Immunocytochemical staining shows evidence for VIP and PHM production, which in many cases is seen together with pancreatic polypeptide. Immunocytochemical staining that uses region-specific antibodies to the pre-pro VIP molecule can now be used for histologic diagnosis and has replaced nonspecific stains.

Clinical Features and Diagnosis

The diagnosis of VIPoma is suggested by the presence of intractable watery diarrhea, without steatorrhea, and hypokalemic acidosis caused by the loss of both potassium and bicarbonate into the stool. Hypochlorhydria, which is present in 50% of patients, can be helpful in distinguishing VIPoma syndrome from the secretory diarrhea due to gastrinoma. In severe cases the combination of severe fluid depletion and electrolyte disturbance can be sufficient to cause death. VIP has a glucagon-like effect on hepatic gluconeogenesis, and hyperglycemia

may occur. Hypercalcemia has also been noted and may be due to production of a parathyroid-related peptide by the tumor.[113]

Diagnosis requires the demonstration of unequivocally elevated levels of plasma VIP, preferably with elevated PHM, by radioimmunoassay. VIP is relatively unstable, and samples should be protected with a protease inhibitor, separated, and frozen almost immediately to prevent loss of peptide. Other conditions with diarrhea, such as short bowel syndrome or inflammatory bowel disease, can give rise to mildly elevated VIP concentrations, but these are generally lower than those in patients with VIP-secreting tumors. Patients with watery diarrhea but who show no elevation of VIP in a carefully collected and reliably assayed sample do not have VIPomas[114] and another cause should be sought.

Tumor Localization

The localization of pancreatic VIPomas rarely presents a problem; CT scanning and selective angiography have proved to be the most useful approaches. The possibility of a neuroblastoma or ganglioneuroma needs to be considered, particularly in children.

Treatment

Medical Treatment

Diarrhea due to VIPoma will respond to a number of agents, notably corticosteroids and clonidine. However, octreotide has dramatically improved the medical control of VIPoma symptoms by both reducing tumor VIP output and diminishing VIP-induced chloride secretion by the intestine.[115,116] Resistance to octreotide can occur, however, and an increase in dose is often required, culminating finally in treatment failure.

Palliative Treatment

For patients with inoperable tumors, cytotoxic treatment with streptozotocin and fluorouracil can be extremely effective in reducing VIP secretion and improving symptoms. Hepatic embolization can reduce hormone output by hepatic metastases and may relieve symptoms caused by hepatomegaly.

Surgical Treatment

Resection of the pancreatic tumor is the optimal treatment for VIPoma in the absence of hepatic metastases. Surgery is not indicated in patients with hepatic metastases (about 50% of patients at presentation). In a patient who has severe symptoms and for whom biochemical and clinical evidence of the VIPoma syndrome is present but no tumor can be localized, "blind" laparotomy with or without intraoperative ultrasound is justifiable. This is the case even in the rare patients with MEN1 and VIPoma syndrome in whom the chances of finding and excising the pancreatic tumor appear to be good.[117] If a tumor is not found at laparotomy, the choice between performing a "blind" distal pancreatectomy and leaving the pancreas in situ and relying on medical treatment is difficult and will depend on local experience and prejudices.

GLUCAGONOMA

Glucagon, a 29-amino-acid peptide with an important physiologic role in the control of hepatic carbohydrate metabolism, is produced by α-cells located on the periphery of pancreatic islets. Processing of proglucagon in the pancreatic α-cell yields glucagon as well as some other peptides that have uncertain biologic activity. Elsewhere, notably in the small intestine, processing of preproglucagon may yield the glucagon precursor enteroglucagon or glucagon-like peptides 1 and 2,[118] the physiologic actions of which are under investigation.[119] In patients with glucagon-secreting tumors, abnormally large forms of glucagon, together with glucagon-like peptides, are found in the circulation.[120]

The glucagonoma syndrome is rare, slightly more common in women than in men, and associated in most cases with large (3 to 5 cm), single, pancreatic tumors found predominantly in the body and tail of the pancreas. Up to 60% of tumors have metastasized by the time of presentation, mainly to regional lymph nodes and the liver, although more-remote sites such as bone or the adrenals can be involved. The glucagonoma syndrome is rarely found in association with MEN1.

Clinical Features

Most commonly, patients are between the ages of 40 and 70 years at presentation. The syndrome is distin-

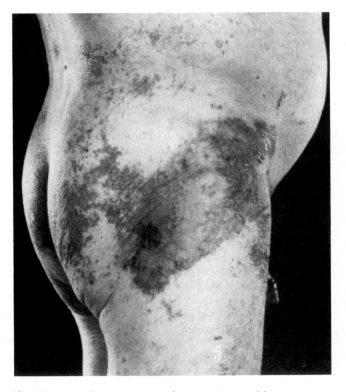

Fig. 56–6. Glucagonoma rash in a 53-year-old man.

Table 56–4. Clinical Features of Glucagonoma

Necrolytic migratory erythema
Reduced amino acids
Glucose intolerance
Recurrent thromboembolism
Anemia
Raised erythrocyte sedimentation rate
Personality changes

guished by its characteristic physical sign, the necrolytic erythematous rash (Fig. 56–6), whose relationship to glucagon-secreting pancreatic tumors was not firmly established until 1974.[121] This rash occurs in 80% of the known cases and may be the major source of disability for the patient. The most common sites are the extremities, intertriginous areas, and periorificial sites. The rash is initially erythematous and scaly, later raised and bullous, and finally crusty and confluent. Healing results in hyperpigmentation and induration. Superinfection can occur. Glossitis, angular cheilitis, nail dystrophy, and hair thinning often coexist with the rash.

The precise cause of the rash is not known. Raised circulating concentrations of plasma glucagon appear to be of central importance: the rash improves dramatically with the decrease in glucagon concentrations following treatment. Nutritional deficiencies may be partly responsible; the rash is strikingly similar to the rash that occurs in other conditions associated with decreased zinc availability (e.g., acrodermatitis enteropathica).[122] Generalized depletion of amino acids to <25% of normal values, which is a characteristic feature of the glucagonoma syndrome, may contribute to the rash and may be useful for diagnostic purposes.[123] The cause of this depletion in amino acids is thought to be an increased demand for amino acids for glucagon-stimulated hepatic gluconeogenesis.[124]

Other specific clinical problems affecting patients with glucagonoma include profound weight loss, anemia, and depression (Table 56–4). Deep venous thrombosis, which is not associated with coagulation disorders, is relatively common and may lead to pulmonary embolism.

Although patients may present with diabetes mellitus, it is usually mild and non-ketotic, despite high circulating levels of glucagon. This suggests that raised glucagon concentrations are not sufficient to cause sustained hyperglycemia.[125]

Diagnosis

The diagnosis of glucagonoma is based on the demonstration of high concentrations of plasma glucagon—usually well above the upper limit of normal (approximately 50 pM/L) and much higher than the levels seen in most benign conditions associated with hyperglucagonemia (Table 56–5). Patients may have been extensively investigated for the cause of their chronic skin rash in association with mild diabetes mellitus and, occasionally, for recurrent thromboemboli. Other plasma gut hormones should be measured, partly to look for increases in other hormones such as pancreatic polypeptide that may

Table 56–5. Causes of Hyperglucagonemia

Renal impairment
Stress
Fasting
Biologically inactive high-molecular-weight hyperglucagonemia
Drugs (danazol/oral contraceptives)
Glucagonoma

suggest the presence of a tumor and partly to exclude the presence of other, clinically significant, hormone syndromes such as VIPoma or gastrinoma. Barium studies may show excessive mucosal-fold thickening and delayed transit, which may be due to the biologic effects of enteroglucagon-like substances secreted by the tumors.[126]

Tumor Localization

Tumor localization is rarely a problem in patients with the glucagonoma syndrome. A combination of ultrasound, CT scanning, and occasionally arteriography is usually sufficient to demonstrate the pancreatic tumor and the presence of hepatic metastases (Fig. 56–7).

Treatment

The aim of medical treatment is a reduction in the elevated plasma concentrations of glucagon, which in most cases will lead to improvement in the skin rash. Octreotide can be extremely effective in achieving this aim.[123,127] Zinc supplementation and amino acid infusions often are used to diminish the rash, although this is probably of little use if glucagon levels remain high.[128] Associated diabetes should be treated. Recurrent thromboembolism should be treated with aspirin or other antiplatelet medication, and formal anticoagulation therapy should be considered.

Surgery is indicated in those patients in whom metastasis has not occurred. In patients with metastatic disease, surgery is unlikely to be of value, although successful resection of the pancreatic primary combined with hepatic transplantation has been reported and may be a promising treatment strategy for the future.[129]

In addition to octreotide, arterial embolization of hepatic metastases[130,131] and cytotoxic treatment with streptozotocin and fluorouracil may be valuable in reducing the hormone output of the tumor. In many patients all of these measures will be necessary as the tumor burden gradually and inexorably increases over a period of 2 to 10 years from diagnosis. Hepatic metastases may switch to the production of other hormones. Production of gastrin may lead to particular difficulties in clinical management, the patient being placed precariously between the risks of thrombosis if left untreated and those of gastrointestinal hemorrhage if anticoagulant therapy is used.[132]

SOMATOSTATINOMAS

Somatostatin is produced by δ-cells, which make up approximately 10% of islet cells. The physiologic role of somatostatin within the islet is not known. Comparison with its actions elsewhere suggest that it may act as a local paracrine modulator of hormone secretion by α- and β-cells, but this requires confirmation. Somatostatin-secreting tumors are rare.

Clinical Features and Diagnosis

Somatostatin-secreting tumors are slow-growing and rarely diagnosed. Like gastrinomas they may arise from the pancreas or the small bowel. They may be incidental findings, up to 50% being asymptomatic. The somatostatinoma syndrome was first recognized in 1979, and 31 cases had been reported by 1987.[133] When symptoms

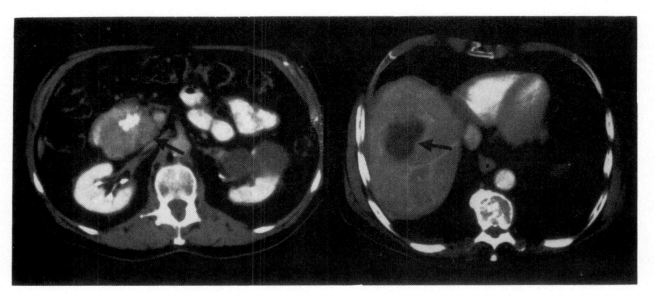

Fig. 56–7. Computed tomographic scans of patient in Figure 56–6 demonstrating a large pancreatic tumor and a necrotic secondary lesion in the liver (arrows).

occur they consist of diarrhea, gallstones, carbohydrate intolerance, and hypochlorhydria, all side effects of exogenous somatostatin administration. The mild and relatively nonspecific nature of symptoms may lead to prolonged delay in diagnosis, by which time the patient may present with end-stage disease resulting from overwhelming metastases.[134] In rare cases, duodenal somatostatinomas may be found in association with neurofibromatosis.[135]

Treatment

The principles of treatment of somatostatinomas are similar to those for any pancreatic endocrine tumor. Patients who present with hepatic metastases will require palliative treatment with hepatic embolization or chemotherapy. Octreotide is not effective.

PANCREATIC POLYPEPTIDE

Pancreatic polypeptide (PP) is a carboxyamidated 36-amino-acid peptide first identified as a contaminant during experiments aimed at the purification of insulin preparations.[136] PP is one of a family of structurally related polypeptides that includes neuropeptide Y and peptide YY, both of which are widely distributed in the central and peripheral nervous system. PP is produced by the PP cell, which forms approximately 10% of islet cells and is situated at the periphery of the islets of Langerhans predominantly in the head of pancreas.

No physiologic role has been established for PP. It is released in response to food, particularly to protein, a response that is blocked by atropine, suggesting that it is controlled by the vagus nerve.[1] Infused PP has only a weak effect on glycogenolysis, as well as on gastric and pancreatic exocrine function, but these effects are unlikely to have physiologic importance.[137] Symptoms of diarrhea have been described in patients with malignant PP-secreting tumors, although the great majority of patients are asymptomatic.[138]

Nearly 100% of pancreatic endocrine tumors contain significant amounts of extractable PP,[139] which has been shown to be localized in secretory granules together with the primary tumor product.[140] Thus, the major potential value of measuring plasma PP is as a nonspecific marker in the diagnosis of neuroendocrine tumors. Discovery of raised plasma concentrations of PP provides useful corroborative evidence for the presence of an endocrine tumor: in a series of 323 patients with islet cell tumors,[141] 45% had raised circulating levels of PP. Compared with patients without tumors who had raised PP levels, patients with tumors had higher PP levels that were not suppressed by atropine.

OTHER PEPTIDES

In keeping with the multipotential nature of islet cell peptide production,[142] there are reports of the secretion of numerous other peptides by pancreatic tumors. These include growth hormone-releasing factor with secondary acromegaly,[143] as well as corticotropin-releasing factor and adrenocorticotropic hormone (ACTH) with associated Cushing syndrome.[144]

SECOND HORMONE SYNDROMES

Multiple hormone production is a common feature of islet cell tumors.[145] In most cases the additional peptides produced by tumor cells are of no clinical relevance. Second and subsequent clinical hormone syndromes may occur, however. In the series at the Hammersmith Hospital, 7% of patients with islet cell tumors developed elevated levels of other hormones; in 50% of these patients the elevated hormone was gastrin.[145] Although a series of patients with gastrinoma followed up for a median duration of 84 months at another center[146] found that the incidence of secondary hormone syndromes was rare (1 in 45 cases), the implication of these findings is that safe clinical practice requires periodic screening for the development of second and subsequent hormone syndromes.

MULTIPLE ENDOCRINE NEOPLASIA TYPE 1

Multiple endocrine neoplasia type 1 (MEN1) is one of a variety of pluriglandular neoplasias; these may be either inherited or sporadic. The coexistence of acromegaly, a pituitary tumor, and enlarged parathyroids has been noted since 1903, and in 1953 Underdahl suggested the presence of a common underlying disorder.[147] Family studies by Wermer[148] and Ballard et al.[149] established that this was inherited in an autosomal dominant fashion. The prevalence of the syndrome has been estimated at 0.25%.[150]

Clinical Features

The predominant clinical manifestation of MEN1 is the co-existence of hyperparathyroidism with pancreatic islet cell tumors and/or anterior pituitary tumors (Fig. 56–8).

The pattern and presentation of disease varies considerably[151] but its severity may run true within individual families, a characteristic that may be useful in planning clinical management.[152,153] In most studies, the syndrome was found to present by the age of 40 years in 80% of the patients.[154]

Pancreatic Disease

Islet cell tumors are found in 40 to 100% of patients with MEN1 and are estimated to cause 80% of deaths of these patients—largely as a consequence of hypergastrinemia.[155] Tumors or their metastases may secrete more than one hormone or may be nonfunctioning, despite immunocytochemical evidence of hormone storage.[156] Different members of the same family may have pancreatic tumors that produce different hormone syndromes, and hepatic metastases may produce hormones different from those produced by the primary tumor. There are no definite histologic markers for malignancy in MEN1 pancreatic tumors: apparent malignancy may be more accurately described as tumor multicentricity, and although up to 30% of pancreatic tumors have been described as malignant, MEN1-associated pancreatic tu-

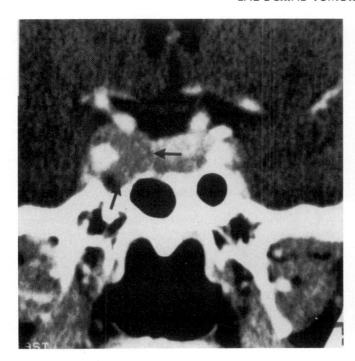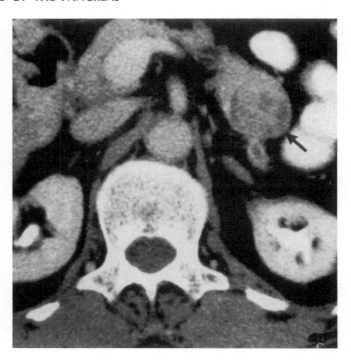

Fig. 56—8. Computed tomographic scans of the pituitary (coronal section; left) and the abdomen (right), demonstrating a right-sided pituitary tumor and a large tumor in the tail of pancreas, respectively (arrows). The patient was a 60-year-old woman with a strong family history of multiple endocrine neoplasia type 1 (MEN1). Hyperparathyroidism had been diagnosed several years previously. The patient had documented hypergastrinemia. The pituitary tumor was "functionless."

mors generally carry a better prognosis than sporadic tumors.[155]

The pancreatic tumor syndromes most commonly associated with MEN1 are gastrinomas and insulinomas. Approximately 66% of pancreatic tumors in MEN1 secrete gastrin, and between 20 and 60% of patients with the gastrinoma syndrome may have MEN1.[157] Insulinomas account for approximately one-third of islet cell tumors in MEN1,[158] some of which also secrete gastrin, but only comprise approximately 6% of all insulinomas. Compared with sporadic tumors, pancreatic tumors in MEN1 are more likely to be multiple and malignant. Hyperplastic changes in the surrounding islet cells have been demonstrated, including nesidioblastosis,[156] suggesting that widespread abnormalities are present in islet cells. The glucagonoma syndrome is rare, although patients may have hyperglucagonemia.[159] Tumors that produce other pancreatic hormones such as VIP have been reported in patients with MEN1 but are very uncommon. Multiple hormone production is frequent, however, including the production of the combination of gastrin and insulin.

The possible presence of MEN1 has an important influence on clinical management of islet cell tumors. In MEN1, gastrinomas are likely to be multicentric, probably more likely to be sited in the duodenum,[160] and less likely to be cured by resection than are sporadic gastrinomas. These considerations have led to a more conservative approach to surgery in patients with MEN1 than in patients with sporadic gastrinomas. In contrast, in patients presenting with insulinoma (approximately 30%

of MEN1 pancreatic tumors), the presence of MEN1 increases the likelihood of malignancy and the prevalence of multicentric pancreatic tumors. Thus, more extensive pancreatic surgery is likely to be required than in sporadic cases, in which insulinomas are more commonly small, single, and benign. Exploration is warranted in patients with MEN1 and glucagonomas or VIPomas even when a tumor cannot be easily located preoperatively.[117]

Nonpancreatic Disease

Hyperparathyroidism, defined as the combination of hypercalcemia and an inappropriately elevated level of circulating parathyroid hormone, is the most common manifestation of MEN1, being present in 90 to 100% of patients at presentation.[151,161] The histologic hallmark of MEN1-associated hyperparathyroidism is the presence of four-gland hyperplasia, although adenomas also may occur. The complications of hyperparathyroidism in patients with MEN1 do not differ from those in patients with sporadic tumors. If surgery is required, the excision of all parathyroid glands that can be identified is necessary. Surgical implantation of parathyroid tissue into the deltoid muscle was a favored option for ensuring continued parathyroid function but has been superseded by lifelong replacement of vitamin D, as it has become apparent that implantation can lead to recurrence of hyperparathyroidism.[162] Hyperparathyroidism and hypercalcemia can cause elevations in plasma gastrin levels, which reverse following parathyroidectomy.[163] However, recent clinical studies suggest that significant hypergastrinemia in such patients is rarely attributable to hyperparathyroidism alone.[164]

Pituitary tumors due to MEN1 account for less than 3% of surgically resected pituitary tumors[164] but have been reported to be present at autopsy in up to 95% of patients with MEN1 and at clinical investigation in 65%. The histologic spectrum ranges from hyperplasia to adenoma to invasive tumors. The hormones most commonly produced by MEN1-associated tumors are prolactin (60%), growth hormone (25%), and ACTH (3%).[166] The complications and treatment of pituitary tumors do not differ from those of sporadic pituitary tumors, although the possibility of ectopic production of releasing factors by pancreatic tumors and subsequent, reversible, pituitary hyperplasia needs to be noted.[166,167]

Other tumors for which there is good epidemiologic evidence for an association with MEN1 are foregut carcinoid tumors[168] and lipomas. Despite case reports, an increased prevalence of thyroid disease and adrenal hyperplasia or adenomas in patients with MEN1 remains unproven.

Genetic Basis of MEN1

MEN1 is inherited in an autosomal dominant fashion with varying degrees of age-related penetrance. Comparison of restriction fragment length polymorphisms (RFLPs) obtained from pancreatic insulinoma DNA with RFLPs from circulating leukocytes has demonstrated a loss of RFLPs from chromosome 11,[169] which is also the chromosome that contains the gene for parathyroid hormone. Studies in both pancreatic[170,171] and parathyroid[172] tumors have shown the recessive loss of genetic tissue from the pericentromeric region of the long arm of chromosome 11 (11q13).

How this chromosomal abnormality in affected tissue is related to hyperplasia and adenoma formation is not clear. One possibility is a two-stage recessional mutation process in subjects who have inherited a deletion on the other gene, whereby somatic mutation leads to loss of the intact gene in the unaffected chromosome. In patients with sporadic MEN1, spontaneous mutations would be required that affect both chromosomes 11 in affected tissues.[173] The precise nature of the events allowing simultaneous or consecutive development of multicentric and multi-organ tumors in affected individuals is unclear. There is evidence for the presence of a circulating "mitogenic" factor in patients with MEN1 that has been shown to stimulate proliferation of bovine parathyroid cells.[174] In addition, there is some evidence that the development of a monoclonal tumor in the parathyroid may follow a period of polyclonal hyperplasia.[175] The near-universal presence of hyperparathyroidism in patients with MEN1 may signify that hyperparathyroidism is a prerequisite for the development of tumors elsewhere. Animal models such as transgenic mice that bear oncogenes resulting in the development of multiple endocrine tumors may be of value in providing the answer.[176]

Screening for MEN1

Screening is necessary for first-degree relatives of patients with probable MEN1. Until a readily accessible genetic marker is available, the major questions concern which test to use and at what age patients and relatives should be tested. Hyperparathyroidism is present by the age of 40 years in nearly 100% of patients with MEN1.[177] Thus, measurements of serum calcium, and where appropriate, determination of parathyroid hormone are the most useful screening tests both in patients presenting with pancreatic tumors and in relatives of patients thought to have MEN1.[160] In screening for pancreatic tumors, both fasting plasma gastrin levels[178] and the response of plasma gastrin levels to a test meal[77] may be of limited value. Measurement of serum prolactin may be of use in screening for pituitary tumors in women.[178] Radiologic studies of the pituitary fossa are unnecessary in the absence of raised pituitary hormone levels. Testing should be continued until the subject is at least 50 years old.

REFERENCES

1. Adrian TE, Bloom Sr, Bryant MG, et al. Distribution and release of human pancreatic polypeptide. Gut 1976; 17:940–4.
2. Hamid QA, Bishop AE, Sikri KL, et al. Immunocytochemical characterization of 10 pancreatic tumours, associated with the glucagonoma syndrome, using antibodies to separate regions of the pro-glucagon molecule and other neuroendocrine markers. Histopathology 1986; 10:119–33.
3. Wilander E. Diagnostic pathology of gastrointestinal and pancreatic neuroendocrine tumours. Acta Oncol 1989; 28:363–9.
4. Bishop AE, Polak JM, Facer P, et al. Neuron specific enolase: a common marker for the endocrine cells and innervation of the gut and pancreas. Gastroenterology 1982; 83:902–15.
5. O'Connor DT, Deftos LJ. Secretion of chromogranin A by peptide-producing endocrine neoplasms. N Engl J Med 1986;314:1145–51.
6. Suzuki H, Christofides ND, Chretien M, et al. Developmental changes in immunoreactive content of novel pituitary protein 7B2 in human pancreas and its identification in pancreatic tumors. Diabetes 1987;36:1276–9.
7. Sekiya K, Ghatei MA, Salahuddin MJ, et al. Production of GAWK (chromogranin-B 420–493)-like immunoreactivity by endocrine tumors and its possible diagnostic value. J Clin Invest 1989;83:1834–42.
8. Tateishi A, Funakoshi A, Jimi A, et al. High plasma pancreastatin-like immunoreactivity in a patient with malignant insulinoma. Gastroenterology 1989;97:1313–8.
9. Bishop AE, Bretherton-Watt D, Hamid QA, et al. The occurrence of pancreastatin in tumours of the diffuse neuroendocrine system. Mol Cell Probes 1988;2:225–35.
10. Erikkson B, Oberg K, Skogseid B. Neuroendocrine pancreatic tumors: clinical findings in a prospective study of 84 patients. Acta Oncol 1989;28:373–7.
11. Howard TJ, Stabile BE, Zinner MJ, et al. Anatomic distribution of pancreatic endocrine tumors. Am J Surg 1990;159:258–64.
12. Boyce GA, Sivak MV Jr. Endoscopic ultrasonography in the diagnosis of pancreatic tumors. Gastrointest Endosc 1990;36(Suppl 2):S28–32.
13. Klotter HJ, Ruckert K, Kummerle F, Rothmund M. The use of intraoperative sonography in endocrine tumors of the pancreas. World J Surg 1987;11:635–41.
14. Bloom SR, Polak JM. Somatostatin localization in tissues. Scand J Gastroenterol Suppl 1986;119:11–21.

15. Patel YC, Wheatley T, Ning C. Multiple forms of immuno-reactive somatostatin: comparison of distribution in neural and nonneural tissues and portal plasma of the rat. Endocrinology 1981;109:1943–9.

16. Reichlin S. Somatostatin. N Engl J Med 1983;309:1495–501.

17. Kvols LK, Buck M, Moertel CG, et al. Treatment of metastatic islet cell carcinoma with a somatostatin analogue (SMS 201–995). Ann Intern Med 1987;107:162–8.

18. Gorden P, Comi RJ, Maton PN, Go VLW. NIH conference. Somatostatin and somatostatin analogue (SMS 201–995) in treatment of hormone-secreting tumors of the pituitary and gastrointestinal tract and non-neoplastic diseases of the gut. Ann Intern Med 1989;110:35–50.

19. Lamberts SW, Pieters GF, Metselaar HJ, et al. Development of resistance to a long-acting somatostatin analogue during treatment of two patients with metastatic endocrine pancreatic tumours. Acta Endocrinol (Copenh) 1988;119:561–6.

20. Wynick D, Anderson JV, Williams SJ, Bloom SR. Resistance of metastatic pancreatic endocrine tumours after long-term treatment with the somatostatin analogue octreotide (SMS 201–995). Clin Endocrinol (Oxf) 1989;30:385–8.

21. Marteau P, Chretien Y, Calmus Y, et al. Pharmacological effect of somatostatin on bile secretion in man. Digestion 1989;42:16–21.

22. Wood SM, Kraenzlin ME, Adrian TE, Bloom SR. Treatment of patients with pancreatic endocrine tumours using a new long-acting somatostatin analogue: symptomatic and peptide responses. Gut 1985;26:438–444.

23. Reubi JC, Hackl WH, Lamberts SWJ. Hormone-producing gastrointestinal tumors contain a high density of somatostatin receptors. J Clin Endocrinol Metabol 1987;65:1127–34.

24. Lamberts SWJ, Bakker WH, Reubi J-C, Krenning EP. Somatostatin-receptor imaging in the localization of endocrine tumors. N Engl J Med 1990;323:1246–9.

25. Krenning EP, Bakker WH, Breeman WAP, et al. Localisation of endocrine-related tumours with radioiodinated analogue of somatostatin. Lancet 1989;1:242–4.

26. Lamberts SWJ, Hofland LJ, van Koetsveld PM, et al. Parallel in vivo and in vitro detection of functional somatostatin receptors in human endocrine pancreatic tumors: consequences with regard to diagnosis, localization and therapy. J Clin Endocrinol Metab 1990;71:566–74.

27. Allison DJ. Therapeutic embolization. Br J Hosp Med 1978;20:707–15.

28. Mendelson DS, Rubinoff SW, Dan SJ, et al. Inadvertent pancreatic embolization as a complication of hepatic carcinoid treatment—computed tomography appearance. Clin Imaging 1989;13:212–4.

29. Ajani JA, Carrasco CH, Charnsangavej C, et al. Islet cell tumors metastatic to the liver: effective palliation by sequential hepatic artery embolization. Ann Intern Med 1988;108:340–4.

30. Moertel CG, Hanley JA, Johnson LA. Streptozocin alone compared streptozocin plus fluorouracil in the treatment of advanced islet cell carcinoma. N Engl J Med 1980;303:1189–94.

31. Hanse R, Helm J, Wilson JF, Wilson S. Nonfunctioning islet cell carcinoma of the pancreas: complete response to continuous 5-fluorouracil infusion. Cancer 1988;62:15–7.

32. Broder LE, Carter SK. Pancreatic islet cell carcinoma. II. Results of therapy with streptozotocin in 52 patients. Ann Intern Med 1973;79:108–18.

33. Altimari AF, Badrinath K, Reisel HJ, Prinz R. DTIC therapy in patients with malignant intra-abdominal neuroendocrine tumors. Surgery 1987;102:1009–17.

34. Eriksson B, Oberg K, Alm G, et al. Treatment of malignant endocrine pancreatic tumours with human leucocyte interferon. Lancet 1986;2:1307–8.

35. Oberg K, Eriksson B. Medical treatment of neuroendocrine gut and pancreatic tumors. Acta Oncol 1989;28:425–31.

36. Sheehan-Dare RA, Simmons AV, Cotterill JA, Janke PG. Hepatic tumors with hyperglucagonemia: response to treatment with human lymphoblastoid interferon. Cancer 1988;62:912–4.

37. Watson RGP, Johnston CF, O'Hare MMT, et al. The frequency of gastrointestinal endocrine tumours in a well-defined population—Northern Ireland 1970–1985. Q J Med 1989;72:647–57.

38. Service FJ. Insulinoma. In: Service FJ, Ed. Hypoglycemic disorders: pathogenesis, diagnosis and treatment. Boston: GK Hall, 1983.

39. Stefanini P, Carboni M, Patrassi N, Basoli A. Beta-islet cell tumors of the pancreas: results of a study on 1,067 cases. Surgery 1974;75:597–609.

40. Service FJ, Nelson RL. Insulinoma. Compr Ther 1980;6(2):70–4.

41. Broder LE, Carter SK. Pancreatic islet cell carcinoma. I. Clinical features of 52 patients. Ann Intern Med 1973;79:101–7.

42. Amiel SA, Sherwin RS, Simonson DC, Tamborlane WV. Effect of intensive insulin therapy on glycemic thresholds for counterregulatory hormone release. Diabetes 1988;37:901–7.

43. Service FJ, Dale AJD, Elveback LR, et al. Insulinoma: clinical and diagnostic features of 60 consecutive cases. Mayo Clin Proc 1976;51:417–29.

44. Snorgaard O, Binder C. Monitoring of blood glucose concentration in subjects with hypoglycaemic symptoms during everyday life. BMJ 1990;300:16–8.

45. Aynsley-Green A, Polak JM, Bloom SR, et al. Nesidioblastosis of the pancreas: definition of the syndrome and the management of the severe neonatal hyperinsulinaemic hypoglycaemia. Arch Dis Child 1981;56:496–508.

46. McHenry C, Newell K, Chejfec G, et al. Adult nesidioblastosis. An unusual cause of fasting hypoglycemia. Am Surg 1989;55:366–9.

47. Turner RC, Harris E. Diagnosis of insulinomas by suppression tests. Lancet 1974;2:188–93.

48. Cohen RM, Given BD, Licinio-Paixao J, et al. Proinsulin radioimmunoassay in the evaluation of insulinomas and familial hyperproinsulinemia. Metabolism 1986;35:1137–46.

49. Gin H, Brottier E, Dupuy B, et al. Use of the glucose clamp technique for confirmation of insulinoma autonomous hyperinsulinism. Arch Intern Med 1987;147:985–7.

50. Ipp E, Sinai Y, Forster B, et al. A glucose reduction challenge in the differential diagnosis of fasting hypoglycemia: a two-center study. J Clin Endocrinol Metab 1990;70:711–7.

51. McMahon MM, O'Brien PC, Service FJ. Diagnostic interpretation of the intravenous tolbutamide test for insulinoma. Mayo Clin Proc 1989;64:1481–8.

52. Brunt LM, Veldhuis JD, Dilley WG, et al. Stimulation of insulin secretion by a rapid intravenous calcium infusion in patients with B-cell neoplasms of the pancreas. J Clin Endocrinol Metab 1986;62:210–6.

53. Gorman B, Cahrboneuau JW, James EM, et al. Benign pancreatic insulinoma: preoperative and intraoperative sonographic localization. AJR Am J Roentgenol 1986;147:929–34.

54. Fajans SS, Vinik AI. Insulin-producing islet cell tumors. Endocrinol Metab Clin North Am 1989;18:45–74.

55. Chapman CE, Fairweather DS, Keeling AA, et al. An evaluation of anti-insulin radioimmunodetection in patients with suspected insulinoma. Clin Endocrinol (Oxf) 1987;26:433–40.

56. Stehouwer CDA, Lems WF, Fischer HRA, et al. Malignant insulinoma: is combined treatment with verapamil and the long-acting somatostatin analogue octreotide (SMS 201-995) more effective than single therapy with either drug? Neth J Med 1989;35:86–94.

57. Glaser B, Rosler A, Halperin Y. Chronic treatment of a benign insulinoma using the long-acting somatostatin analogue SMS 201-995. Isr J Med Sci 1990;26:16–9.

58. Stehouwer CD, Lems WF, Fischer HR, et al. Aggravation of hypoglycemia in insulinoma patients by the long-acting somatostatin analogue octreotide (Sandostatin). Acta Endocrinol (Copenh) 1989;121:34–40.

59. Glaser B, Landau H, Smilovici A, Nesher R. Persistent hyperinsulinaemic hypoglycaemia of infancy, long-term treatment with the somatostatin analogue sandostatin. Clin Endocrinol (Oxf) 1989;31:71–80.

60. Delemarre-van de Waal HA, Veldkamp EJM, Schrander-Stumpel CTRM. Long-term treatment of an infant with nesidioblastosis using a somatostatin analogue [Letter]. N Engl J Med 1987;316:222–3.

61. Galiber AK, Reading CC, Carboneau JW, et al. Localization of pancreatic insulinoma: comparison of pre- and intraoperative US with CT and angiography. Radiology 1988;166:405–8.

62. Norton JA, Cromack DT, Shawker TH, et al. Intraoperative ultrasonographic localization of islet cell tumors: a prospective comparison to palpation. Ann Surg 1988;207:160–8.

63. Turner RC, Lee EG, Morris PJ, et al. Localisation of insulinomas. Lancet 1978;1:515–8.

64. Edkins JS. On the chemical mechanisms of gastric secretion. Proc Roy Soc Lond [Biol] 1905;76:376.

65. Gregory RA, Tracy HJ. The preparation and properties of gastrin. J Physiol (Lond) 1961;156:523–53.

66. Gregory RA, Tracy HJ. Isolation of two "big gastrins" from Zollinger-Ellison tumour tissue. Lancet 1972;2:797–9.

67. Bloom SR, Polak JM. Gut hormone overview. In: Bloom SR, Polak JM. Gut hormones. 1st ed. London: Churchill Livingstone, 1978:3–17.

68. Wang TC, Brand SJ. Islet cell-specific regulatory domain in the gastrin promoter contains adjacent positive and negative DNA elements. J Biol Chem 1990;265:8908–14.

69. Zollinger RM, Ellison EH. Primary peptic ulcerations of the jejunum associated with islet cell tumors of the pancreas. Ann Surg 1955;142:709–28.

70. Yalow RS, Berson SA. Further studies on the nature of immunoreactive gastrin in human plasma. Gastroenterology 1971;60:203–14.

71. Modlin IM, Brennan MF. The diagnosis and management of gastrinoma. Surg Gynecol Obstet 1984;158:97–104.

72. Capella C, Riva C, Rindi G, et al. Endocrine tumors of the duodenum and upper jejunum: a study of 33 cases with clinico-pathological characteristics and hormone content. Hepatogastroenterology 1990;37:247–52.

73. Kothary PC, Fabri PJ, Gower W, et al. Evaluation of NH_2-terminus gastrins in gastrinoma syndrome. J Clin Endocrinol Metab 1986;62:970–4.

74. Bardram L. Progastrin in serum from Zollinger-Ellison patients: an indicator of malignancy? Gastroenterology 1990;98:1420–6.

75. McGuigan JE, Wolfe MM. Secretin injection test in the diagnosis of gastrinoma. Gastroenterology 1980;79:1324–31.

76. Feldman M, Schiller LR, Walsh JH, et al. Positive intravenous secretin test in patients with achlorhydria-related hypergastrinemia. Gastroenterology 1987;93:59–62.

77. Skogseid B, Oberg K, Benson L, et al. A standardized meal stimulation test of the endocrine pancreas for early detection of pancreatic endocrine tumors in multiple endocrine neoplasia type 1 syndrome: five years experience. J Clin Endocrinol Metab 1987;64:1233–40.

78. Frucht H, Howard JM, Slaff JI, et al. Secretin and calcium provocative tests in the Zollinger-Ellison syndrome. A prospective study. Ann Intern Med 1989;111:713–22.

79. Frucht H, Howard JM, Stark HA, et al. Prospective study of the standard meal provocative test in Zollinger-Ellison syndrome. Am J Med 1989;87:528–36.

80. Wolfe MM, Jensen RT. Zollinger-Ellison syndrome: current concepts in diagnosis and management. N Engl J Med 1987;317:1200–9.

81. Tjon A, Tham RT, Jensen RT, Lamers CB, CT and MR imaging of advanced Zollinger-Ellison syndrome. J Comput Assist Tomogr 1989;13:821–8.

82. Maton PN, Miller DL, Doppman JL, et al. Role of selective angiography in the management of patients with Zollinger-Ellison syndrome. Gastroenterology 1987;2:913–8.

83. Imamura M, Takahashi K, Adachi H, et al. Usefulness of selective arterial secretin injection test for localization of gastrinoma in the Zollinger-Ellison syndrome. Ann Surg 1987;205:230–9.

84. Doppman JL, Miller DL, Change R, et al. Gastrinomas: localization by means of selective intraarterial injection of secretin. Radiology 1990;174:25–9.

85. Vinik AI, Moattari AR, Cho K, Thompson N. Transhepatic portal vein catheterization for localization of sporadic and MEN gastrinomas: a ten-year experience. Surgery 1990;107:246–55.

86. Doppman JL, Shawker TH, Miller DL. Localization of islet cell tumors. Gastroenterol Clin North Am 1989;18:793–804.

87. Jensen RT. Basis for failure of cimetidine in patients with Zollinger-Ellison syndrome [Editorial]. Dig Dis Sci 1984;29:363–6.

88. Vinayek R, Howard JM, Maton PN, et al. Famotidine in the therapy of gastric hypersecretory states. Am J Med 1986;81(Suppl 4B):49–59.

89. Jensen RT, Collen MJ, McArthur KE, et al. Comparison of the effectiveness of ranitidine and cimetidine in inhibiting acid secretion in patients with gastric hypersecretory states. Am J Med 1984;77(Suppl 5B):90–105.

90. Lamers CBHW, Lind T, Moberg S, et al. Omeprazole in Zollinger-Ellison syndrome: effects of a single dose and of long-term treatment in patients resistant to histamine H_2-receptor antagonists. N Engl J Med 1984;310:758–61.

91. McArthur KE, Collen MJ, Maton PN, et al. Omeprazole: effective, convenient therapy for Zollinger-Ellison syndrome. Gastroenterology 1985;88:939–44.

92. Brunner G, Creutzfeld W. Omeprazole in the long-term management of patients with acid-related diseases resistant to ranitidine. Scand J Gastroenterol Suppl 1989;166:101–5.

93. Ekman L, Hansson E, Havu N, et al. Toxicological studies on omeprazole. Scand J Gastroenterol Suppl 1985;108:53–69.

94. Mozell E, Woltering EA, O'Dorisio TM, et al. Effect of somatostatin analog on peptide release and tumor growth in the Zollinger-Ellison syndrome. Surg Gynecol Obstet 1990;170:476–84.

95. Delcore R Jr, Hermreck AS, Friesen SR. Selective surgical

management of correctable hypergastrinemia. Surgery 1989;106:1094–102.

96. Wise SR, Johnson J, Sparks J, et al. Gastrinoma: the predictive value of preoperative localization. Surgery 1989;106:1087–93.

97. Howard TJ, Zinner MJ, Stabile BE, Passaro E Jr. Gastrinoma excision for cure. a prospective analysis. Ann Surg 1990;211:14.

98. Fox PS, Hofmann JW, DeCosse JJ, Wilson SD. The influence of total gastrectomy on survival in malignant Zollinger-Ellison tumors. Ann Surg 1974;180:558–66.

99. Norton JA, Doppman JL, Collen MJ, et al. Prospective study of gastrinoma localization and resection in patients with Zollinger-Ellison syndrome. Ann Surg 1986; 204:468–79.

100. Thompson NW, Vinik AI, Eckhauser FE. Microgastrinomas of the duodenum: a cause of failed operations for the Zollinger-Ellison syndrome. Ann Surg 1989;209:396–404.

101. Frucht H, Norton JA, London JF, et al. Detection of duodenal gastrinomas by operative endoscopic transillumination: a prospective study. Gastroenterology 1990; 99:1622–7.

102. Pipeleers-Marichal M, Somers G, Willems G, et al. Gastrinomas in the duodenums of patients with multiple endocrine neoplasia type 1 and the Zollinger-Ellison syndrome. N Engl J Med 1990;322:723–7.

103. Thompson NW, Bondeson A-G, Bondeson L, Vinik A. The surgical treatment of gastrinoma in MEN I syndrome patients. Surgery 1989;106:1081–6.

104. Said SI, Mutt V. Potent peripheral and splanchnic vasodilator peptide from normal gut [Letter]. Nature 1970; 225:862–4.

105. Said SI. Vasoactive intestinal peptide. J Endocrinol Invest 1986;9:191–200.

106. Priest WM, Alexander MK. Islet-cell tumour of the pancreas with peptic ulceration, diarrhoea and hypokalaemia. Lancet 1957;2:1145–7.

107. Verner JV, Morrison AB. Islet cell tumor and a syndrome of refractory, watery diarrhea and hypokalemia. Am J Med 1958;25:374–80.

108. Bloom SR, Polak JM, Pearse AGE. Vasoactive intestinal peptide and watery-diarrhoea syndrome. Lancet 1973; 2:14–6.

109. Kane MG, O'Dorisio TM, Krejs GJ. Production of secretory diarrhea by intravenous infusion of vasoactive intestinal polypeptide. N Engl J Med 1983;309:1482–5.

110. Bloom SR, Christofides ND, Delamarter J, et al. Diarrhoea in vipoma patients associated with cosecretion of a second active peptide (peptide histidine isoleucine) explained by single coding gene. Lancet 1983;2:1163–5.

111. Yiangou Y, Williams SJ, Bishop AE, et al. Peptide-histidine-methionine-immunoreactivity in plasma and tissue from patients with vasoactive intestinal peptide-secreting tumors and watery diarrhea syndrome. J Clin Endocrinol Metab 1987;64:131–9.

112. Blackburn AM, Bryant MG, Adrian TE, Bloom SR. Pancreatic tumors produce neurotensin. J Clin Endocrinol Metab 1981; 52:820–2.

113. Wynick D, Ratcliffe WA, Heath DA, et al. Treatment of a malignant pancreatic endocrine tumour secreting parathyroid hormone related protein. BMJ 1990;300:1314–5.

114. Long RG, Bryant MG, Mitchell SJ, et al. Clinicopathological study of pancreatic and ganglioneuroblastoma tumours secreting vasoactive intestinal polypeptide (vipomas). BMJ 1981;282:1767–71.

115. Wood SM, Kraenzlin ME, Adrian TE, Bloom SR. Treatment of patients with pancreatic endocrine tumours using a new long-acting somatostatin analogue: symptomatic and peptide responses. Gut 1985;26:438–44.

116. Santangelo WC, O'Dorisio TM, Kim JG, et al. VIPoma syndrome: effect of a synthetic somatostatin analogue. Scand J Gastroenterol 1985;103:363–7.

117. Sheppard BC, Norton JA, Doppman JL, et al. Management of islet cell tumors in patients with multiple endocrine neoplasia: a prospective study. Surgery 1989; 106:1108–18.

118. Bell GI, Santerre RF, Mullenbach GT. Hamster preproglucagon contains the sequence of glucagon and two related peptides [Letter]. Nature 1983;302:716–8.

119. Kreymann B, Williams G, Ghatei MA, Bloom SR. Glucagon-like peptide-1 7-36. a physiological incretin in man. Lancet 1987;2:1300–4.

120. Uttenthal LO, Ghiglione M, George SK, et al. Molecular forms of glucagon-like peptide-1 in human pancreas and glucagonomas. J Clin Endocrinol Metabol 1985;61: 472–9.

121. Mallinson N, Bloom SR, Warin AP, et al. A glucagonoma syndrome. Lancet 1974;2:1–5.

122. Miller SJ. Nutritional deficiency and the skin. J Am Acad Dermatol 1989;21:1–30.

123. Boden G. Glucagonomas and insulinomas. Gastroenterol Clin North Am 1989;18:831–45.

124. Boden G, Rezvani I, Owen OE. Effects of glucagon on plasma amino acids. J Clin Invest 1984;73:785–93.

125. Bloom SR, Polak JM. Glucagonoma syndrome. Am J Med 1987;82(Suppl 5B):25–36.

126. Lax E, Leibovici V, Fields SI, Gordon RL. Neglected radiologic signs of the glucagonoma syndrome. Diagn Imaging Clin Med 1986;55:321–6.

127. Rosenbaum A, Flourie B, Chagnon S, et al. Octreotide (SMS 201–995) in the treatment of metastatic glucagonoma: report of one case and review of the literature. Digestion 1989;42:116–20.

128. Roth E, Muhlbacher F, Karner J, et al. Free amino acid levels in muscle and liver of a patient with glucagonoma syndrome. Metabolism 1987;36:7–13.

129. Makowka L, Tzakis AG, Mazzaferro V, et al. Transplantation of the liver for metastatic endocrine tumors of the intestine and pancreas. Surg Gynecol Obstet 1989; 168:107–11.

130. Assaad SN, Carrasco CH, Vassilopouylou-Sellin R, et al. Glucagonoma syndrome: rapid response following arterial embolization of glucagonoma metastatic to the liver. Am J Med 1987;82:533–5.

131. Freimann J, Pazdur R. Hepatic arterial embolization for treatment of glucagonomas: antineoplastic and palliative benefits. Am J Clin Oncol 1990;13:271–5.

132. Wynick D, Williams SJ, Bloom SR. Symptomatic secondary hormone syndromes in patients with established malignant pancreatic endocrine tumors. N Engl J Med 1988; 319:605–7.

133. Harris GJ, Tio F, Cruz AB. Somatostatinoma: a case report and review of the literature. J Surg Oncol 1987;36:8–19.

134. Krejs GJ, Orci L, Conlon JM, et al. Somatostatinoma syndrome: biochemical, morphologic and clinical features. N Engl J Med 1979;301:285–92.

135. Stephens M, Williams GT, Jasani B, Williams ED. Synchronous duodenal neuroendocrine tumors in von Recklinghausen's disease—a case report of co-existing gangliocytic paraganglioma and somatostatin-rich glandular carcinoid. Histopathology 1987;11:1331–40.

136. Kimmel JR, Pollock Hg, Hazelwood RL. Isolation and characterization of chicken insulin. Endocrinology 1968; 83:1323–30.

137. Szecowka J, Tatemoto K, Rajamaki G, Efendic S. Effects of PYY and PP on endocrine pancreas. Acta Physiol Scand 1983;119:123–6.

138. Tomita T, Friesen SR, Kimmel JR, et al. Pancreatic polypeptide-secreting islet-cell tumors: a study of three cases. Am J Pathol 1983;113:134–42.

139. Polak JM, Bloom SR, Adrian TE, et al. Pancreatic polypeptide in insulinomas, gastrinomas, VIPomas and glucagonomas. Lancet 1976;1:328–30.

140. Ooi A, Katsuda S, Nakanishi I, et al. Electron microscopic and immunoelectron microscopic demonstration of pancreatic polypeptide cells in glucagonoma: colocalization of pancreatic peptide and glucagon in single secretory granules. Ultrastruct Pathol 1989;13:15–22.

141. Adrian TE, Uttenthal LO, Williams SJ, Bloom SR. Secretion of pancreatic polypeptide in patients with pancreatic endocrine tumors. N Engl J Med 1986;315:287–91.

142. Philippe J, Powers AC, Jojsov S, et al. Expression of peptide hormone genes in human islet cell tumors. Diabetes 1988;37:1647–51.

143. Thorner MO, Perryman RL, Cronin MJ, et al. Somatotrophin hyperplasia. Successful treatment of acromegaly by removal of a pancreatic islet tumor secreting a growth hormone-releasing factor. J Clin Invest 1982;70:965–77.

144. Lokich J, Bothe A, O'Hara C, Federman D. Metastatic islet cell tumor with ACTH, gastrin and glucagon secretion: clinical and pathologic studies with multiple therapies. Cancer 1987;56:2053–8.

145. Friesen SR. Tumors of the endocrine pancreas. N Engl J Med 1982;306:580–90.

146. Chiang H-CV, O'Dorisio TM, Huang SC, et al. Multiple hormone elevations in Zollinger Ellison syndrome: prospective study of clinical significance and of the development of second symptomatic pancreatic endocrine tumor syndrome. Gastroenterology 1990;99:1565–75.

147. Underdahl LO, Woltner LB, Black BM. Multiple endocrine adenomas: report of 8 cases in which the parathyroids, pituitary, and pancreatic islets were involved. J Clin Endocrinol Metab 1953;13:20–47.

148. Wermer P. Genetic aspects of adenomatosis of endocrine glands. Am J Med 1954;16:363–71.

149. Ballard HS, Frame B, Hartsock RJ. Familial multiple endocrine adenoma-peptic ulcer complex. Medicine (Baltimore) 1964;43:481–516.

150. Lips CJM, Vasen HFA, Lamers CB. Multiple endocrine neoplasia syndromes. Crit Rev Oncol Hematol 1984; 2:117–84.

151. Samaan NA, Ouais S, Ordonez NG, et al. Multiple endocrine syndrome type I. Clinical, laboratory findings, and management in five families. Cancer 1989;64:741–52.

152. Tisell LE, Ahlman H, Jansson S, Grimelius L. Total pancreatectomy in the MEN-1 syndrome. Br J Surg 1988; 75:154–7.

153. Tisell LE, Ahlman H. Treatment of the pancreatic disease of multiple endocrine neoplasia type 1 (MEN 1). Acta Oncol 1989;28:415–7.

154. Shepherd JJ. Latent familial multiple endocrine neoplasia in Tasmania. Med J Aust 1985;142:395–7.

155. Oberg K, Skogseid B, Eriksson B. Multiple endocrine neoplasia type 1 (MEN-1). Clinical, biochemical and genetical investigations. Acta Oncol 1989;28:383–7.

156. Kloppel G, Willemer S, Stamm B, et al. Pancreatic lesions and hormonal profile of pancreatic tumors in multiple endocrine neoplasia type I. An immunocytochemical study of nine patients. Cancer 1986;57:1824–32.

157. Lamers CB, Stadil F, Van Tongeren JH. Prevalence of endocrine abnormalities in patients with the Zollinger-Ellison syndrome and in their families. Am J Med 1978;64:607–12.

158. Rasbach DA, van Heerden JA, Telander RL, et al. Surgical management of hyperinsulinism in the multiple endocrine neoplasia, type 1 syndrome. Arch Surg 1985;120: 584–9.

159. Marx SJ, Spiegel AM, Brown EM, Aurbach GD. Family studies in patients with primary parathyroid hyperplasia. Am J Med 1977;62:698–706.

160. Pipeleers-Marichal M, Somers G, Willems G, et al. Gastrinomas in the duodenums of patients with multiple endocrine neoplasia type 1 and the Zollinger-Ellison syndrome. N Engl J Med 1990;322:723–7.

161. Marx SJ, Vinik AI, Santen RJ, et al. Multiple endocrine neoplasia type I: assessment of laboratory tests to screen for the gene in a large kindred. Medicine (Baltimore) 1986;65:226–41.

162. Mallette LE, Blevins T, Jordan PH, Noon GP. Autogenous parathyroid grafts for generalized primary parathyroid hyperplasia: contrasting outcome in sporadic hyperplasia versus multiple endocrine neoplasia type I. Surgery 1987;101:738–45.

163. Norton JA, Cornelius MJ, Doppman JL, et al. Effect of parathyroidectomy in patients with hyperparathyroidism, Zollinger-Ellison syndrome, and multiple endocrine neoplasia type I: a prospective study. Surgery 1987; 102:958–66.

164. Lamers CBHW, Rotter JI, Jansen JBMJ. Gastrin cell function in familial multiple endocrine neoplasia type I. Gut 1988;29:1358–63.

165. Scheithauer BW, Laws ER Jr, Kovacs K, et al. Pituitary adenomas of the multiple endocrine neoplasia type I syndrome. Semin Diagn Pathol 1987;4:205–11.

166. Maton PN, Gardner JD, Jensen RT. Cushing's syndrome in patients with the Zollinger-Ellison syndrome. N Engl J Med 1986;315:1–5.

167. Ramsay JA, Kovacs K, Asa SL, et al. Reversible sellar enlargement due to growth hormone-releasing hormone production by pancreatic endocrine tumors in an acromegalic patient with multiple endocrine neoplasia type I syndrome. Cancer 1988;62:445–50.

168. Duh Q-Y, Hybarger CP, Geist R, et al. Carcinoids associated with multiple endocrine neoplasia syndromes. Am J Surg 1987;154:142–8.

169. Larsson C, Skogseid B, Oberg K, et al. Multiple endocrine neoplasia type 1 gene maps to chromosome 11 and is lost in insulinoma [Letter]. Nature 1988;332:85–7.

170. Nakamura Y, Larsson C, Julier C, et al. Localization of the genetic defect in multiple endocrine neoplasia type 1 within a small region of chromosome 11. Am J Hum Genet 1989;44:751–5.

171. Bystrom C, Larsson C, Blomberg C, et al. Localization of the MEN1 gene to a small region within chromosome 11q13 by deletion mapping in tumors. Proc Natl Acad Sci USA 1990;87:1968–72.

172. Thakker RV, Bouloux P, Wooding C, et al. Association of parathyroid tumors in multiple endocrine neoplasia type 1 with loss of alleles on chromosome 11. N Engl J Med 1989;321:218–224.

173. Friend SH, Dryja TP, Weinberg RA. Oncogenes and tumor-suppressing genes. N Engl J Med 1988;318: 618–22.

174. Marx SJ, Sakaguchi K, Green J III, et al. Mitogenic activity on parathyroid cells in plasma from members of a large kindred with multiple endocrine neoplasia type 1. J Clin Endocrinol Metab 1988;67:149–53.

175. Friedman E, Skaguchi K, Bale AE, et al. Clonality of

parathyroid tumors in familial multiple endocrine neoplasia type 1. N Engl J Med 1989;321:213−8.

176. Murphy D, Bishop A, Rindi G, et al. Mice transgenic for a vasopressin SV40 hybrid oncogene develop tumors of the endocrine pancreas and the anterior pituitary: a possible model for human multiple endocrine neoplasia type 1. Am J Pathol 1987;129:552−66.

177. Benson L, Ljunghall S, Akerstrom G, Oberg K. Hyperparathyroidism presenting as the first lesion in multiple endocrine neoplasia type 1. Am J Med 1987;82,:731−7.

178. Vasen HFA, Lamers CBH, Lips CJM. Screening for the multiple endocrine neoplasia syndrome type I. A study of 11 kindreds in the Netherlands. Arch Intern Med 1989;149:2717−22.·

Appendix

FINDINGS OF THE DIABETES CONTROL AND COMPLICATIONS TRIAL

JAMES L. ROSENZWEIG,
RICHARD BEASER,
SUSAN CROWELL,
EMMIE FRIEDLANDER,
OM P. GANDA,
BEVERLY HALFORD,
ALAN JACOBSON,
LAWRENCE I. RAND,
CARRIE STEWART,
AND JOSEPH I. WOLFSDORF*

With the discovery of insulin in 1921, patients with insulin-dependent diabetes (IDDM) were saved from the immediate threat of death. However, as patients with IDDM lived longer, they were afflicted with a host of devastating chronic complications, including retinopathy, nephropathy, neuropathy, and an increased risk of atherosclerotic disease. Over the years, debate has continued concerning the role of hyperglycemia in the pathogenesis of the chronic complications of diabetes. The "glucose hypothesis" assumed that glucose itself was the major mediator of most of these complications and that specific treatment of diabetes to reduce chronic hyperglycemia could significantly slow or prevent these complications. This has not been easy to prove convincingly. Several epidemiological studies have shown a relationship between the severity of complications and the degree of glycemic control in patients with diabetes,[1,2] and studies of retinopathy and nephropathy in animal models have supported this hypothesis.[3-5] Nevertheless, to prove this hypothesis, it was essential to demonstrate that a randomized, prospective intervention that lowered average blood glucose to levels near the normal range could slow the onset or progression of the chronic complications of diabetes.

Until recently, the only prospective clinical trials comparing one or more forms of intensive insulin therapy with conventional therapy involved small numbers of patients, almost all of whom had evidence of retinopathy and/or nephropathy at the onset of the trials.[6-9] None of these trials could show an amelioration of retinopathy with intensive therapy. Indeed, to the contrary, with intensive therapy a transient worsening of retinopathy was often seen in the first 6 to 12 months.[6-8] Some of the studies demonstrated that intensive therapy did ameliorate the increase in urinary albumin excretion,[10,11] but this was without any clear effect on the development of overt clinical nephropathy.

The Diabetes Control and Complications Trial (DCCT) was designed to conclusively test the glucose hypothesis

and resolve controversies raised by these earlier studies.[12] The principal study goal was to determine whether intensive insulin therapy, with the aim of lowering blood glucose levels as close as possible to the nondiabetic range, could either prevent or decrease the development of the long-term complications of diabetes. Retinopathy was examined as the main clinical endpoint. Secondary endpoints included nephropathy, neuropathy, macrovascular complications, cognitive function, and quality of life assessment. Two distinct cohorts of patients were recruited for the study—a primary prevention cohort and a secondary intervention cohort (Table A–1). To determine whether intensive therapy could prevent the development or subsequent progression of retinopathy, a group of patients with no preexisting retinopathy as determined by stereoscopic fundus photography, with urinary albumin excretion less than 40 mg/24 hr, and with diabetes duration between 1 to 5 years was recruited as the primary prevention cohort. A secondary intervention cohort was recruited to determine whether intensive therapy could decrease the progression of preexisting retinopathy. These patients had mild to moderate nonproliferative retinopathy as identified on stereoscopic fundus photography, albumin excretion of less than 200 mg/24 hr, and diabetes duration of 1 to 15 years.

Between 1983 and 1989, 1441 patients with IDDM, confirmed by C-peptide deficiency, were recruited for the study in 29 participating clinics in the United States and Canada. Of these subjects, 726 were assigned to the primary prevention cohort and 715 to the secondary intervention cohort. Subjects were randomized to either

Table A–1. Characteristics of DCCT Patient Cohorts

Primary Prevention	Secondary Intervention
13 to 39 years of age	13 to 39 years of age
Diabetes duration 1–5 years	Diabetes duration 1–15 years
No retinopathy	Minimal to moderate retinopathy
Albuminuria <40 mg/24 hr	Albuminuria ≤200 mg/24 hr

*Members of the DCCT Research Group at the Joslin Diabetes Center

a conventional or intensive treatment regimen. In general, subjects with conventional treatment took one or two injections of insulin a day, and treatment goals were to maintain clinical well being and absence of symptoms of hyperglycemia and hypoglycemia. Daily self-testing of blood or urine was performed, but insulin doses were not adjusted daily by the patients to achieve target blood glucose levels. Subjects randomized to the intensive treatment group used treatment regimens designed to maintain blood glucose levels as close as possible to the nondiabetic range, while avoiding severe or recurrent hypoglycemia.

The specific target goals for blood glucose are outlined in Table A-2. Hemoglobin A_{1c} was measured monthly and subjects were encouraged to achieve hemoglobin A_{1c} levels of less than 6.05% (the upper limit of the normal range in the assay used). To achieve these goals, subjects used either multiple daily insulin regimens (MDI) with 3, 4, or more insulin injections per day, or continuous subcutaneous insulin pump therapy (CSII) employing an external insulin infusion device. Blood glucose monitoring was performed at least four times per day, and insulin doses were adjusted by the patient based upon blood glucose levels, meal content, and exercise. Subjects were admitted to the hospital to initiate intensive therapy. They were seen at least monthly in their local clinics, and frequent telephone contact was used to help with blood glucose management. Extensive dietary instruction was used to help improve glycemic control. Study patients could, at their discretion, and on the advice of their physicians, choose between pump therapy and multiple daily injections, and could change between these forms of therapy. Fifty-nine percent of the subjects used pump therapy for at least part of the study, and pump therapy was used for approximately 34% of the total duration of intensive therapy.

The level of glycemic control of both the intensively and the conventionally treated patients was assessed with quarterly hemoglobin A_{1c} measurements. The median hemoglobin A_{1c} level for all subjects at entry into the study was approximately 8.9%, and remained at this level for those subjects randomized to conventional therapy. The median hemoglobin A_{1c} level of experimental patients, however, decreased quickly to about 7.2%,[13] and remained at that level for the full 9-year duration of the study.[14,15] A separation of 1.5 to 2.0% between the two treatment groups was maintained during the entire study. There was no difference in glycemic control between the primary prevention and secondary intervention groups. Adolescent subjects in both treatment groups had hemo-

globin A_{1c} levels that were about 1.0% higher than adult subjects.

Although the duration of the study was 9 years, patients were recruited into the study over a 6-year period. The mean length of participation for the whole patient population was 6.5 years. Adherence by patients to their assigned treatment regimens was high; there were relatively few deviations from assigned therapy. Although 93 of the patients temporarily switched from conventional to intensive therapy either in preparation for or treatment during pregnancy, the results of treatment were evaluated according to the patients' original treatment assignments.

RETINOPATHY RESULTS

Retinopathy was the primary outcome evaluated in the DCCT. All subjects in the study had seven-field stereoscopic fundus photography performed at 6-month intervals, and these were graded at a central reading unit. A scale of retinopathy, adapted from the Early Treatment Diabetic Retinopathy Study, was used with a total of 25 gradations, or steps, ranging from microaneurysms only to severe proliferative retinopathy requiring laser treatment. Clinically meaningful worsening of retinopathy was defined as a change of three steps or greater between measurements. This was felt to be particularly significant if the three-step change was sustained (not reversed) over two consecutive measurement intervals of 6 months' duration. In addition, patients were evaluated annually by ophthalmologists in the individual DCCT centers with direct and indirect ophthalmoscopy and measurement of visual acuity.

The cumulative incidence of sustained three-step changes in retinopathy in the primary prevention group is illustrated in Figure A-1A. Cumulative incidence refers to the accumulated proportion of the patients who underwent an event at least once during the study. As can be seen for the first 3 years of the study, there were very few events. Subsequently, the percentage of patients in the conventionally treated group with sustained three-step changes increased progressively, as compared with the intensively treated patients, and the difference between the groups widened by the end of the study. By then, intensive therapy had reduced sustained three-step progression by 76%. Similarly, intensive therapy reduced the risk of total (sustained and unsustained) three-step changes by 60% in the primary prevention cohort, and the risk of developing at least one microaneurysm was decreased by 27%.

The severity of retinopathy in individual subjects may sometimes improve, and cumulative incidence, which treats events as irreversible, does not take this into account. Point prevalence data shows the actual percentage of patients with three-step changes at specific times in the study. In the primary prevention cohort, point prevalence of three-step changes in the conventional treatment group progressively increased with time to about 60% by the end of the study, whereas in the intensive treatment group, it increased more slowly and appeared to level off at a lower level (Fig. A-2A). It

Table A-2. Clinical Goals of Intensive Insulin Therapy

1. Clinical well-being and absence of symptoms of hyperglycemia or hypoglycemia
2. Blood glucose control as close as possible to nondiabetic levels:
   Pre-meal: 70-120 mg/dl
   Post-meal: <180 mg/dl
   3 AM: >65 mg/dl
3. Hemoglobin A_{1c} <6.05%

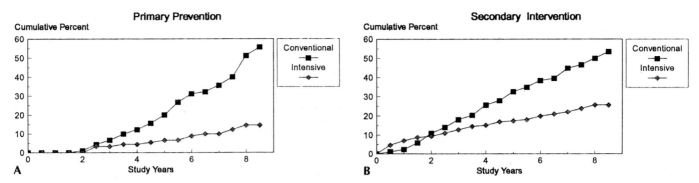

Fig. A–1. The cumulative incidence of sustained three-step retinopathy change in subjects in the DCCT. (A) Primary prevention cohort. (B) Secondary intervention cohort. Data is taken from reference 14 (DCCT Research Group. DCCT Update Symposium. Presented at the 53rd Annual Meeting of the American Diabetes Association, Las Vegas, Nevada, June 13, 1993).

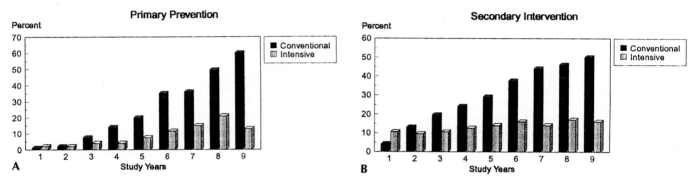

Fig. A–2. Point prevalence of three-step retinopathy change in subjects in the DCCT. (A) Primary prevention cohort. (B) Secondary intervention cohort. Adapted from reference 14 (DCCT Research Group. DCCT Update Symposium. Presented at the 53rd Annual Meeting of the American Diabetes Association, Las Vegas, Nevada, June 13, 1993).

should be noted, however, that only 268 patients participated for the full 9 years of the study. Therefore, the data presented for the last few years of the study represented a relatively small portion of the total patients.

More severe retinopathy outcomes, such as severe nonproliferative or proliferative retinopathy or macular edema, were relatively uncommon in the primary prevention cohort. Since only 15 cases had severe retinopathy, the number was too small for statistical analysis of an effect between treatment groups.

In the secondary intervention cohort, intensive therapy also had a dramatic effect in reducing progression of retinopathy (Fig. A–1B). In this group, the cumulative incidence of sustained three-step changes was transiently increased with intensive therapy during the first 2 years, confirming the findings of previous studies.[6-8] Subsequently, intensive therapy was associated with a decrease in the incidence of retinopathy progression, as compared to conventional therapy, so that by the end of the study, retinopathy was reduced by 54%. A similar pattern was seen with the less stringent definition of total three-step changes, although in this analysis the early transient worsening of retinopathy with intensive therapy had a greater impact on the results and thus the effect of intensive therapy was less beneficial, with a 34% reduction.

In the secondary intervention group, point prevalence of three-step progression of retinopathy is shown in Figure A–2B. The percentage of conventionally treated subjects with clinically significant progression of retinopathy steadily increased during the course of the study, reaching 50% by the last year. In the intensively treated patients, however, the percentage of patients with three-step progression remained relatively constant, between 10% and 15% during the entire duration of the study. The beneficial effect of intensive therapy was maintained in all patient subgroups, and was not affected by patient age, sex, duration of diabetes, or clinic location.

Intensive therapy also had a beneficial effect in ameliorating the more severe retinopathy events (Table A–3). The risk of developing severe nonproliferative retinopathy was decreased by 46%, and more severe retinopathy requiring laser treatment was reduced by 54%. In addition, the incidence of macular edema appeared to be reduced, but the change did not reach statistical significance. As summarized in Table A–3, intensive therapy had a major effect in reducing the risk of almost all retinopathy outcome variables.

NEPHROPATHY

At entry into to the study, subjects in the primary prevention cohort were selected to have 24-hour albumin excretion of less than 40 mg. Subjects in the secondary intervention group, by contrast, could have albumin excretion rates of up to 200 mg/24 hr, but in fact,

Table A–3. Summary of Risk Reduction with Intensive Therapy

Outcome	Risk Reduction
Retinopathy	
Primary Prevention Group	
≥ 1 microaneurysm	27%
≥ Three-step progression	60%
Sustained ≥ three-step progression	76%
Secondary Intervention Group	
≥ Three-step progression	34%
Sustained ≥ three-step progression	54%
Proliferative or severe retinopathy	46%
Requiring laser treatment	54%
Nephropathy (Combined Group)	
Microalbuminuria	35%
Macroalbuminuria	56%
Neuropathy	
Primary Prevention Group	70%
Secondary Intervention Group	56%

Data taken from reference 14 (DCCT Research Group. DCCT Update Symposium. Presented at the 53rd Annual Meeting of the American Diabetes Association, Las Vegas, Nevada, June 13, 1993).

only 10% of these patients actually did have albumin excretion greater than 40 mg/24 hr at baseline. The cumulative incidence of microalbuminuria, as defined by albumin excretion rate of greater than 40 mg/24 hr, was substantially reduced by intensive therapy in both cohorts, individually, and when they were combined (Fig. A–3). During the study, very few of the subjects in the primary cohort developed clinical grade albuminuria (300 mg/24 hr or greater). In the secondary intervention cohort, and when both primary and secondary groups were combined, intensive therapy had a potent effect in decreasing the incidence of clinical proteinuria (Fig. A–3). Only seven patients in the study developed clinical grade proteinuria associated with a serum creatinine of 2

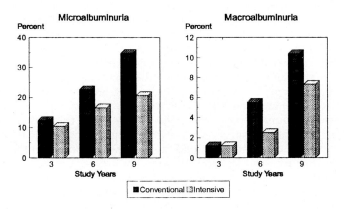

Fig. A–3. Percent of study patients in the DCCT combined cohort who fulfill criteria for albumin excretion at years 3, 6, and 9. The figure on the left represents microalbuminuria (albumin excretion between 40 mg/24 hr and 300 mg/24 hr) and the figure on the right shows macroalbuminuria (excretion of 300 mg/24 hr of greater). Data is adapted from reference 14 (DCCT Research Group. DCCT Update Symposium. Presented at the 53rd Annual Meeting of the American Diabetes Association, Las Vegas, Nevada, June 13, 1993).

mg/dl or greater; five were in the conventional treatment group and two were in the intensive group.

NEUROPATHY

Neuropathy was measured in the DCCT with clinical neurologic examinations and sensory and motor nerve conduction tests at baseline, year 5, and at the end of the study. Cardiovascular autonomic function tests were performed every 2 years; the test battery included measurements of heart rate variation with Valsalva and respiration, and orthostatic testing. The outcome of clinical sensorimotor polyneuropathy was defined in the study as the presence of definite signs and symptoms on clinical examination, associated with abnormal conduction in at least two distinct peripheral nerves or abnormal autonomic function tests.

Intensive treatment substantially lowered the prevalence of confirmed clinical neuropathy in both primary and secondary treatment groups (Fig. A–4). In addition, when each of the individual tests were examined separately, there was a 55% reduction in risk of neuropathy on physical examination alone, a 50% reduction in abnormal nerve conduction, and 43% reduction of abnormal autonomic function. The results shown here were obtained after 5 years, and were confirmed in those patients followed for longer periods of time in the study.

MACROVASCULAR DISEASE

Because the DCCT population consisted of relatively young patients, the incidence of macrovascular events in the study was low. There were a total of 59 cardiovascular and peripheral vascular events, with 21 in subjects receiving intensive treatment and 38 in subjects treated conventionally. This represented a 44% overall reduction in risk with intensive therapy. The reduction in risk for cardiac events alone was 80%, but the results did not achieve statistical significance. Although a beneficial effect of intensive therapy could not be conclusively proved, the trend appeared positive, and it appears that

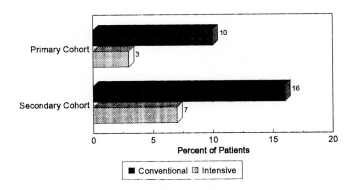

Fig. A–4. The prevalence of clinical neuropathy in the DCCT after 5 years of follow-up. Adapted from reference 14 (DCCT Research Group. DCCT Update Symposium. Presented at the 53rd Annual Meeting of the American Diabetes Association, Las Vegas, Nevada, June 13, 1993).

intensive therapy does not pose any added risk for macrovascular disease.

The risk of developing hypercholesterolemia, defined as LDL-cholesterol greater than 160 mg/dl, was reduced by 35% in the combined cohort. There was no significant difference in the incidence of hypertension or clinical hypertriglyceridemia between the two groups. Further analyses of the stratified data are not yet available.

COGNITIVE FUNCTION AND QUALITY OF LIFE

In order to evaluate whether intensive therapy and the increased frequency of hypoglycemia had any effect upon cognitive function, patients in the DCCT underwent an extensive array of neurobehavioral tests. These included evaluations of memory, dexterity, attention, and verbal fluency. In addition, a quality of life questionnaire was administered at regular intervals to determine whether the increased stresses and demands of intensive therapy had any adverse effects upon quality of daily life. No significant differences between the two treatment groups were seen in either cognitive functioning or quality of life.

ADVERSE EFFECTS OF INTENSIVE THERAPY

The principal adverse effect of intensive therapy in the DCCT was an increased frequency of severe hypoglycemia.[16] Hypoglycemic episodes were classified as severe if they could not be treated by the patient alone, and if their management required the assistance of another person. Intensive therapy increased the risk of severe hypoglycemia three-fold in the combined cohort (Fig. A–5). Those severe episodes of hypoglycemia involving seizure and coma, and those with injury requiring emergency room or hospital treatment were also increased with intensive therapy. Approximately 53% of the episodes of severe hypoglycemia occurred during sleep, and another 35% happened when patients were awake but had no adrenergic warning symptoms. There was no difference on neurobehavioral testing between those subjects who experienced severe hypoglycemia and those who did not.

Although no patient deaths were directly attributable to hypoglycemia, there were traffic accidents, episodes of

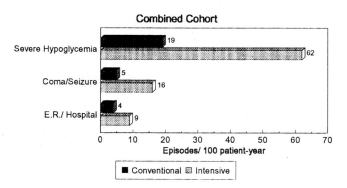

Fig. A–5. The effect of intensive therapy on the incidence of severe hypoglycemia in subjects in the DCCT. Adapted from reference 14 (DCCT Research Group. DCCT Update Symposium. Presented at the 53rd Annual Meeting of the American Diabetes Association, Las Vegas, Nevada, June 13, 1993).

physical injuries, and property damage. The death of one individual not in the DCCT was caused by a motor vehicle accident by a hypoglycemic patient on intensive therapy. The increased risk of hypoglycemia with intensive therapy was not affected by patient age, gender, duration of diabetes, or presence of clinical neuropathy. Those patients on intensive therapy who had the greatest decline in hemoglobin A_{1c} were at the greatest risk for severe hypoglycemia. In addition, those patients who had severe hypoglycemia prior to entry into the study were at increased risk for severe hypoglycemia during the study.

The other adverse effects of intensive therapy were weight gain[17] and catheter infections. Patients in both treatment groups gained weight during the study, but the patients on intensive therapy gained about 10 lbs more than the conventionally treated patients. Excessive weight gain (greater than 120% of ideal body weight) was more common in the intensive treatment group. Patients on insulin pump therapy also developed local infections at catheter sites at a rate of 12 episodes per 100 patient years of pump use. Contrary to previous reports,[18,19] diabetic ketoacidosis was not seen with increased frequency in patients using insulin pumps.

IMPLICATIONS FOR DIABETES TREATMENT

The DCCT has conclusively shown that the use of intensive diabetes therapy results in substantial reductions in the onset and progression of retinopathy, nephropathy, and neuropathy.[14,15] It is possible that intensive therapy may reduce macrovascular disease as well. The study demonstrated that intensive therapy can be safely and practicably implemented in a large patient population, resulting in a significant decline in mean hemoglobin A_{1c} concentration, albeit to levels still higher than normal. Intensive therapy was accepted by these study volunteers without any perceived change in their quality of life.

Nevertheless, intensive therapy has certain risks and disadvantages. Serious hypoglycemia was increased three-fold in the study population, despite the fact that the patients were under close supervision by the research staff responsible for supervising their diabetes care. The weight gain seen with intensive therapy had less clinical importance, but was of concern to many patients. Successful implementation of intensive therapy requires a great amount of motivation and diligence on the part of the patient. Comprehensive care was given by teams of experienced, highly trained nurses, physicians, mental health professionals, and dietitians in a structured environment, with close and frequent patient contact. Successful translation of this approach to the general population of patients with diabetes will require major investments to support education, supplies such as testing equipment and insulin pumps, and training skilled professional staff to deliver and coordinate the required care.

The results of the DCCT show, however, that for most patients with IDDM, the benefits of intensive therapy clearly outweigh its risks. The majority of patients with IDDM should be treated with the aim of lowering blood glucose levels as near to normal as possible, within the boundaries of good clinical judgment and concern for patient safety. Secondary analyses of the DCCT data have shown that there is no specific hemoglobin A_{1c} "cut-off," or level of glycemic control above the normal range that confers full protection from retinopathy. The lower the hemoglobin A_{1c}, the lower the risk of microvascular complications. It is clear that most patients on intensive therapy regimens are unable to achieve the idealized goal of near-normoglycemia. Nevertheless, any decrease in hemoglobin A_{1c} will have a significant impact on retinopathy progression.

Specific subgroups of patients with IDDM would not benefit from intensive therapy and are at an especially high risk of severe hypoglycemia. These include patients with a history of recurrent severe hypoglycemia and hypoglycemia unawareness. Patients with severe irreversible microvascular complications, such end-stage renal disease and/or blindness, are also less likely to benefit from intensive therapy. Hypoglycemia may present added risks to patients with severe coronary artery disease or cerebrovascular disease, and intensive therapy should be used with caution in such patients. It is not clear whether prepubertal children are appropriate candidates for intensive therapy. Variability of patient activity and diet, and the inability of very young children to recognize and independently treat hypoglycemia, would increase the risk of recurrent and severe hypoglycemia, with possible deleterious effects upon central nervous system development. The DCCT did not study children under 13 years of age, and it is not known whether tight glycemic control has the same beneficial effects prior to puberty.

An important question to be answered is how to apply the findings of the DCCT to the treatment of noninsulin-dependent diabetes mellitus (NIDDM). Although patients with NIDDM were not studied in the DCCT, there is no reason to assume that the pathogenesis of microvascular and macrovascular complications is different in the two forms of diabetes. The DCCT tested the "glucose hypothesis," and it is likely that the conclusions from the DCCT also apply to NIDDM. Treatment of diabetes to restore glycemia to near normal levels may be a reasonable goal in these patients. In most NIDDM patients, this can be achieved with diet, weight loss, exercise, oral agents, or simple insulin regimens rather than with insulin pumps or MDI. The weight gain associated with intensive therapy may exacerbate the insulin resistance of NIDDM. Because the risks of hypoglycemia with intensive therapy are particularly high in patients with advanced age and atherosclerosis, it should be used with great caution in this population.

REFERENCES

1. Klein R, Klein B, Moss S, et al. Glycosylated hemoglobin predicts the incidence and progression of diabetic retinopathy. JAMA 1988; 260:2864.

2. Chase H, Jackson M, Hoops S, et al. Glucose control and the renal and retinal complications of insulin-dependent diabetes. JAMA 1989; 261:1189.

3. Cohen A, McGill P, Rossetti R, et al. Glomerulopathy in spontaneously diabetic rat: Impact of glycemic control. Diabetes 1987; 36:944.

4. Engerman R, Bloodworth J, Jr., Nelson S. Relationship of microvascular disease in diabetes to metabolic control. Diabetes 1977; 26:760.

5. Gray B, Watkins E, Jr. Prevention of vascular complications of diabetes by pancreatic islet transplantation. Arch Surg 1976; 111:788.

6. Kroc Collaborative Study Group: Blood glucose control and the evolution of diabetic retinopathy and albuminuria. N Engl J Med 1984; 6:365.

7. Lauritzen T, Frost-Larsen K, Larsen HW, et al. The Sten Study Group: Two-year experience with continuous subcutaneous insulin infusion in relation to retinopathy and neuropathy. Diabetes 1984; 34(suppl 3):74.

8. Brinchmann-Hansen O, Dahl-Jorgensen K, Hanssen K, et al. The response of diabetic retinopathy to 41 months of multiple insulin injections, insulin pumps, and conventional insulin therapy. Arch Ophthalmol 1988; 106:1242.

9. Reichard P, Rosenquist U. Nephropathy is delayed by intensified insulin treatment in patients with insulin-dependent diabetes mellitus and retinopathy. J Int Med 1989; 226:81.

10. Feld-Rasmussen B, Mathiesen E, Deckert T. Effect of two years of strict metabolic control on progression of incipient nephropathy in insulin-dependent diabetes. Lancet 1986; 2:1300.

11. Reichard P, Rosenquist U. Nephropathy is delayed by intensified insulin treatment in patients with insulin-dependent diabetes mellitus and retinopathy. J Int Med 1989; 226:81.

12. DCCT Research Group. The Diabetes Control and Complications Trial (DCCT): Design and Methodological Considerations for the Feasibility Phase. Diabetes 1986; 35:530–545.

13. DCCT Research Group. Diabetes Control and Complications Trial (DCCT): Results of Feasibility Study. Diabetes Care 1987; 10:1–19.

14. DCCT Research Group. DCCT Update Symposium. Presented at the 53rd Annual Meeting of the American Diabetes Association, Las Vegas, Nevada, June 13, 1993.

15. DCCT Research Group. N Engl J Med 1993; in press.

16. DCCT Research Group. Epidemiology of severe hypoglycemia in the Diabetes Control and Complications Trial. Am J Med 1991; 90:450.

17. DCCT Research Group. Weight gain associated with intensive therapy in the Diabetes Control and Complications Trial. Diabetes Care 1988; 567–573.

18. Mecklenburg RS, Benson EA, Benson JW, et al. Acute complications associated with insulin infusion pump therapy: Report of experience with 161 patients. JAMA 1984; 252:3265–3269.

19. Peden NR, Bratten JT, McKendry JB. Diabetic ketoacidosis during long-term treatment with continuous subcutaneous insulin infusion. Diabetes Care 1984; 7:1–5.

INDEX

Note: Page numbers in italics indicate figures; numbers followed by "t" indicate tables. Greek letters preceding index entries have been spelled out and are alphabetized according to the spelled-out version. Entries preceded by other letters or by numerals are alphabetized by the root entry.